DUBOIS' LUPUS ERYTHEMATOSUS

DUBOIS' LUPUS ERYTHEMATOSUS

Fourth Edition

DANIEL J. WALLACE, M.D.

Clinical Chief of Rheumatology
Cedars-Sinai Medical Center, Los Angeles;
Associate Clinical Professor of Medicine
UCLA School of Medicine
Los Angeles, California

BEVRA HANNAHS HAHN, M.D.

Chief of Rheumatology
Professor of Medicine
UCLA School of Medicine
Los Angeles, California

Associate Editors:
FRANCISCO P. QUISMORIO Jr., M.D.
JAMES R. KLINENBERG, M.D.

Lea & Febiger • Philadelphia • London •

Lea & Febiger
Box 3024
200 Chester Field Parkway
Malvern, Pennsylvania   19355-9725
U.S.A.
(610) 251-2230

Executive Editor—R. Kenneth Bussy
Project Editor—Frances M. Klass   •
Production Manager—Samuel A. Rondinelli
Developmental Editor—Tanya Lazar

Library of Congress Cataloging-in-Publication Data

Dubois' lupus erythematosus / [edited by] Daniel J. Wallace, Bevra H.
   Hahn. — 4th ed.
        p.   cm.
      1. Lupus erythematosus.   2. Systemic lupus erythematosus.
   I. Wallace, Daniel J. (Daniel Jeffrey), 1949–   . II. Hahn, Bevra H.
   III. Dubois, Edmund L. Lupus erythematosus.
      [DNLM: 1. Lupus Erythematosus, Discoid.   2. Lupus Erythematosus,
   Systemic.   WR 152 D8152]
   RC924.5.L85L87   1992
   616.7′7—dc20
   DNLM/DLC
   for Library of Congress   92-12529
                                                                      CIP

First Edition, 1966
Second Edition, 1974
Second Revised Edition, 1976
Third Edition, 1987

> Reprints of chapters may be purchased from Lea & Febiger in quantities of 100 or more. Contact Sally
> Grande in the Sales Department.

PRINTED IN THE UNITED STATES OF AMERICA

Print number: 5   4   3

DEDICATION

We dedicate the third edition of this textbook to Dr. Edmund Dubois, whose untimely death has saddened the rheumatology community and his devoted patients.

Edmund Lawrence Dubois was born in Newark, New Jersey, on June 28, 1923, and died in Los Angeles, California, on February 2, 1985. During his short 61 years, he published 175 papers and revolutionized our concepts of diagnosis and treatment of systemic lupus erythematosus. A graduate of The Johns Hopkins School of Medicine in 1946, his postgraduate training included service at Johns Hopkins, University of Utah (under Maxwell Wintrobe), Parkland Hospital in Dallas (under Tinsley Harrison), and finally at the Los Angeles County General Hospital.

While setting up a private practice in Los Angeles in 1950 as an internist, he volunteered his time at the County Hospital. Dr. Paul Starr, then Chairman of the Department of Medicine, asked him to start a clinic consisting of eight patients who had a host of mysterious symptoms and signs. The common thread was that they all had a positive new blood test called an LE prep. Ed Dubois built this assignment into the largest lupus center in the world. At one time, he was following 500 SLE patients each in his private practice and at LAC-USC Medical Center. He was kept busy coordinating drug, clinical, and laboratory studies. His work established protocols that are still utilized for the treatment of central nervous system lupus, autoimmune hemolytic anemia, and other lupus subsets. He was the first to describe avascular necrosis of bone and peptic ulceration from steroid use in lupus. Pioneering work from his clinic firmly established the efficacy of antimalarial drugs in SLE. He helped analyze the NZB/NZW mouse model of lupus in the early 1960s. Twenty-year follow-ups on his series of hundreds of patients have established the natural course of the disease.

Along with these commitments, he found time to travel widely, become an expert photographer and yachtsman, entered into an enduring and happy marriage to Nancy Kully, and helped raise wonderful children (Lindy, Larry, Robby, Jeannie, and granddaughter Maria). His second granddaughter, Emily, was named in his memory.

One of his greatest legacies is this textbook. The first edition in 1966, second edition in 1974, and second revised edition in 1976 sold widely, and it is considered the definitive lupus textbook. Ed Dubois spent much of his last two years working on this 3rd edition, and we feel he would approve of the expansion that characterizes this 4th edition.

Los Angeles, Calif.
1985

Daniel J. Wallace

PREFACE

The fourth edition represents a major expansion of the third edition. The number of chapters has been increased from 24 to 62, including the writings of 39 new contributors. The basic science section (Chapters 2 to 29) has doubled in length and incorporates new sections covering genetics, tolerance, B and T lymphocytes, cytokines, natural killer cells, arachidonic acid metabolites, idiotype networks, and sex hormones. Autoantibody chapters now number 11, as opposed to 3 in the third edition. The basic science section consists of a comprehensive series of state-of-the-art reviews. Chapters 30 to 62 in the clinical section are compendiums that cite nearly every important peer-reviewed publication ever written for the area. This section includes new chapters on pediatric rheumatology, infection, and supportive management. The long, unwieldy 132-page Chapter 18 of the third edition has been replaced with 10 tightly organized chapters that use an organ system approach. Less than 15% of the text of the third edition is used in the fourth.

An effort has been made to make this edition more "user friendly." There are many more summary boxes and tables; algorithms are used for the first time. The alphabetized bibliography, long a unique feature of the Dubois texts, has been complemented with an author and subject index. The number of references cited has increased from 5000 to over 8000.

We wish to acknowledge the support of The American Lupus Society and to commend Ellie Clements for her excellent editing and computer skills. In addition, Dr. Wallace wishes to acknowledge the support of his wife, Janice and his children, Naomi, Phillip, and Sarah. He is also indebted to the late Edmund L. Dubois, under whose tutelage he had the privilege of learning about lupus erythematosus. Dr. Hahn expresses her loving gratitude to her husband, Dr. Theodore J. Hahn, her children Alysanne and April, and the inspiring mentors who originally instructed her about lupus—Drs. Mary Betty Stevens and Lawrence E. Shulman.

Los Angeles, California   DANIEL J. WALLACE, M.D.
Los Angeles, California   BEVRA H. HAHN, M.D.

CONTRIBUTORS

S. Ansar Ahmed, M.D.
Assistant Professor of Immunology
Virginia-Maryland Regional College of Veterinary
  Medicine
Blacksburg, Virginia

Cynthia Aranow, M.D.
Albert Einstein College of Medicine
Bronx, New York

Frank C. Arnett, Jr., M.D.
Professor of Internal Medicine
Director, Division of Rheumatology and Clinical
  Immunogenetics
University of Texas Medical School at Houston
Houston, Texas

Ronald A. Asherson, M.D.
Director of Clinical Research, The Lupus Arthritis
  Research Unit
The Rayne Institute
Honorary Consultant Physician
St. Thomas Hospital
London, United Kingdom, and
Division of Rheumatology
The St. Luke's/Roosevelt Hospital Center
New York, New York

Harry G. Bluestein, M.D.
Professor of Medicine
Director, Division of Rheumatic Diseases
University of California School of Medicine
San Diego, California

Richard Cervera, M.D., Ph.D.
Systemic Autoimmune Diseases Research Unit
Department of Internal Medicine
Hospital Clinic
Barcelona, Spain

Joseph Craft, M.D.
Section of Rheumatology
Department of Internal Medicine
Yale University School of Medicine
New Haven, Connecticut

Betty Diamond, M.D.
Professor, Department of Microbiology and
  Immunology
Albert Einstein College of Medicine
Bronx, New York

Fanny M. Ebling, Ph.D.
Adj. Associate Professor
Department of Medicine
University of California Los Angeles
Los Angeles, California

Woodruff Emlen, M.D.
Associate Professor of Medicine
Department of Medicine, Division of Rheumatology
University of Colorado
Denver, Colorado

Donald I. Feinstein, M.D.
Professor and Chief of Medicine
USC University Hospital, and
Norris Cancer Hospital and Research Institute of the
University of Southern California
Los Angeles, California

Phillip D. Fernsten, Ph.D.
University of North Carolina
Chapel Hill, North Carolina

Robert B. Francis, Jr., M.D.
Associate Professor of Medicine
Director, Coagulation Laboratory
University of Southern California
Los Angeles, California

Marvin J. Fritzler, M.D.
Professor of Medicine
Head, Division of Rheumatology, Clinical Immunology
  & Dermatology
University of Calgary
Calgary, Alberta
Canada

J. Dixon Gray, Ph.D.
Assistant Professor of Research Medicine
University of Southern California Medical School
Los Angeles, California

Bevra H. Hahn, M.D.
Professor of Medicine
Chief of Rheumatology
University of California Los Angeles School of Medicine
Los Angeles, California

John A. Hardin, M.D.
Chairman, Department of Medicine
Medical College of Georgia
Augusta, Georgia

John B. Harley, M.D., Ph.D.
Associate Professor, University of Oklahoma, and
Associate Member, Oklahoma Medical Research
    Foundation, and
Clinical Investigator, Oklahoma City Veterans Affairs
    Medical Center
Oklahoma City, Oklahoma

Evelyn L. Hess, M.D.
McDonald Professor of Medicine
Director, Division of Immunology
Department of Medicine
University of Cincinnati Medical Center
Cincinnati, Ohio

Marc C. Hochberg, M.D., M.P.H.
Professor of Medicine and Epidemiology and Preventive
    Medicine
University of Maryland School of Medicine
Baltimore, Maryland

David A. Horwitz, M.D.
Chief, Rheumatology and Immunology
Professor of Medicine and Microbiology
University of Southern California School of Medicine
Los Angeles, California

Kenneth C. Kalunian, M.D.
Assistant Professor of Medicine
University of California Los Angeles School of Medicine
Los Angeles, California

Rodanthi C. Kitridou, M.D.
Professor of Medicine
University of Southern California School of Medicine,
    and
Directress of Clinical Rheumatology
LAC + USC Medical Center
Los Angeles, California

James Klinenberg, M.D.
Senior Vice President
Academic Affairs
Cedars-Sinai Medical Center, and
Professor of Medicine and Associate Dean
University of California Los Angeles School of Medicine
Los Angeles, California

Dennis M. Klinman, M.D., Ph.D.
Senior Investigator
Division of Virology
CBER/FDA
Bethesda, Maryland

John H. Klippel, M.D.
Clinical Director
National Institute of Arthritis and Musculoskeletal and
    Skin Diseases
Bethesda, Maryland

Thomas J. A. Lehman, M.D.
Associate Professor of Pediatrics
Cornell University Medical Center, and
Chief, Division of Pediatric Rheumatology
The Hospital for Special Surgery
New York, New York

Daniel P. McCauliffe, M.D.
University of Texas Southwestern Medical Center
Dallas, Texas

Allen L. Metzger, M.D.
Associate Clinical Professor of Medicine
University of California Los Angeles, and
Attending Physician, Cedars-Sinai Medical Center
Los Angeles, California

Toshihide Mimura, M.D.
Research Assistant, Professor of Medicine
Division of Rheumatology and Immunology
Thurston Arthritis Center
University of North Carolina at Chapel Hill
Chapel Hill, North Carolina

Gregorio Mintz, M.D.
Professor and Chairman
Department of Rheumatology
Centro Medico Naciional, IMSS
Mexico City, Mexico

Anne Barbara Mongey, M.B., B.Ch., B.A.O., D.C.H.
Instructor in Medicine
Division of Immunology
Department of Medicine
University of Cincinnati Medical Center
Chief, Immunology Section, Veterans Administration
    Hospital
Cincinnati, Ohio

Elahna Paul
Department of Microbiology and Immunology
Albert Einstein School of Medicine
Bronx, New York

Conrad L. Pirani, M.D.
Professor Emeritus of Pathology
Consultant in Pathology and Special Lectures
Columbia University—College of Physicians and
    Surgeons
New York, New York

Victor E. Pollak, M.D.
Emeritus Professor of Medicine
Attending Physician
University of Cincinnnati Hospital
Cincinnati, Ohio

Thomas T. Provost, M.D.
Noxell Professor and Chairman
Department of Dermatology
Johns Hopkins Medical Institutions
Baltimore, Maryland

Francisco P. Quismorio, Jr., M.D.
Professor of Medicine and Pathology
Vice Chief, Division of Rheumatology and Immunology
University of Southern California School of Medicine,
    and
Attending Physician, LAC + USC Medical Center
Los Angeles, California

Morris Reichlin, M.D.
Professor and Chief, Immunology Section
Oklahoma University Health Sciences Center
Head, Arthritis/Immunology Program
Oklahoma Medical Research Foundation
Oklahoma City, Oklahoma

Dwight R. Robinson, M.D.
Professor of Medicine
Harvard Medical School, and
Physician in Arthritis Unit
Department of Medicine
Massachusetts General Hospital
Boston, Massachusetts

Linda J. Rosinsky, B.S.
Founder and President
Lupus Network, Inc.
Bridgeport, Connecticut

Robert L. Rubin, Ph.D.
Associate Member
Department of Molecular and Experimental Medicine
The Scripps Research Institute
La Jolla, California

Jane E. Salmon, M.D.
Associate Professor of Medicine
Cornell University Medical College, and
Associate Attending Physician
The Hospital for Special Surgery and The New York
    Hospital
New York, New York

Peter H. Schur, M.D.
Professor of Medicine
Harvard Medical School
Boston, Massachusetts

Howard S. Shapiro, M.D.
Assistant Clinical Professor Psychiatry and Human
    Behavior
Department of Psychiatry
University of Southern California
Attending Staff
Cedars-Sinai Medical Center
Los Angeles, California

Akira Shirai, M.D.
Division of Virology
Center for Biologics Evaluation and Research
Federal Drug Administration
Bethesda, Maryland

Richard D. Sontheimer, M.D.
Professor of Dermatology and Internal Medicine
Vice-Chairman, Department of Dermatology
University of Texas Southwestern Medical Center
Dallas, Texas

William Stohl, M.D., Ph.D.
Assistant Professor of Medicine
USC School of Medicine, and
LAC + USC Medical Center
Los Angeles, California

Norman Talal, M.D.
Professor of Medicine and Microbiology
Head, Division of Clinical Immunology
Department of Medicine
University of Texas Health Science Center
San Antonio, Texas

John D. Talbott, M.D. (deceased)
Clinical Professor of Medicine
University of Miami School of Medicine
Miami, Florida

Betty P. Tsao, Ph.D.
Assistant Professor of Medicine
Division of Rheumatology
University of California Los Angeles School of Medicine
Los Angeles, California

CONTRIBUTORS

Daniel J. Wallace, M.D.
Clinical Chief of Rheumatology
Associate Clinical Professor of Medicine
University of California School of Medicine
Los Angeles, California

Rosemarie Watson, M.D.
Associate Professor
Department of Dermatology
Johns Hopkins University School of Medicine
Baltimore, Maryland

John B. Winfield, M.D.
Herman & Louise Smith Professor of Medicine
Chief, Division of Rheumatology and Immunology
Director, Hurston Arthritis Research Center
Attending Physician
University of North Carolina Hospitals
Chapel Hill, North Carolina

CONTENTS

Section IV.   AUTOANTIBODIES

Section V.   CUTANEOUS LUPUS

Section VI.   SYSTEMIC LUPUS ERYTHEMATOSUS

PART A.   CLINICAL AND LABORATORY FEATURES

Section VII. MANAGEMENT AND PROGNOSIS

Section VIII.   APPENDIX

Section IX.   BIBLIOGRAPHY

Section I

THE HISTORY OF LUPUS ERYTHEMATOSUS

Chapter 1

HISTORICAL BACKGROUND OF DISCOID AND SYSTEMIC LUPUS ERYTHEMATOSUS

JOHN H. TALBOTT*

The term lupus has been used in descriptions of morbid cutaneous conditions for at least seven centuries. In the distant past, several physicians wrote, or at least have been credited with writing, about lupus—the term being a Latin derivative (*lupus*, wolf) referring to erythematous ulcerations about the face—a disease that eats away, bites, and destroys. Rogerius (c. 1230), Paracelsus (1493 to 1541), Manardi (c. 1500), and Sennert (1611), are included in the historical list.[V88] Hebra and Kaposi, in their comprehensive treatise of lupus vulgaris,[K65] referred to the *herpes esthiomenos* of Hippocrates (460 to 370 B.C.) and *herpes ulcerosus* of Amatus Lusitanus (1510 to 1568) as synonyms for lupus. The noteworthy communications and observations on lupus in the nineteenth century were reported by pupils or followers, not by the original observers. Bateman[B121] presented the observations of Willan, Cazenave those of Biett, and Kaposi those of his father-in-law, Hebra. In one of the first monographs of cutaneous diseases (1813), the companion volume to the first section of a series planned by his teacher Willan, Bateman noted:[B121]

> Of this disease (lupus) I shall not treat at any length; for I can mention no medicine, which has been of any essential service in the cure of it, and it requires the constant assistance of the surgeon in consequence of the spreading ulcerations, in which the original tubercules terminate.
> The term was intended by Dr. Willan to comprise, together with the "*noli me tangere*" (do not touch me) affecting the nose and lips, other slow tubercular affections, especially about the face, commonly ending in ragged ulcerations of the cheeks, forehead, eyelids, and lips, and sometimes occurring in other parts of the body, where they gradually destroy the skin and muscular parts to a considerable depth. Sometimes the disease appears in the cheek circularly, or in the form of a sort of ringworm, destroying the substance, and leaving a deep and deformed cicatrix: and I have seen a similar circular patch of the disease, dilating itself at length to the extent of a handbreadth or more, upon the pectoral muscle.

In 1826, Rayer, in a description of lupus "Fluxus Sebaceus," identified the facial distribution and scaly eruption.[R78] Biett[B301] is credited with a description of lupus, as one of the erythemas, in 1828. In an exhaustive review of historical documents, Jarcho[J55] found no evidence that Biett published this report, but that the reference by Cazenave and Schedel to lupus and Biett concerns an oral communication only.[C168] The term "érythème centrifuge," following Biett, was introduced in the second edition (1833).[C169] In 1851 to 1852, Cazenave changed the term to "lupus érythémateaux" and gave credit to Biett for distinguishing three principal varieties:[C172]

> (1) lupus which destroys the surface, (2) lupus which destroys in depth, and (3) lupus without ulcers but accompanied by hypertrophy of the involved parts.
> We are following this classification with a slight modification which is justified by the necessity to bring into this consideration a disorder of which Biett had a foreboding, and which was designated by him with the term "érythème centrifuge" and which evidently belongs to lupus.
> Lupus erythematosus (érythème centrifuge according to Biett, gnawing dermatosis which destroys the surface) is characterized by red spots which disappear temporarily on digital pressure.
> Lupus erythematosus presents itself in two forms, sufficiently distinct. In one form which seems to pertain more to women, to persons with a fine, white skin, the disease is erythematosus, and its aspect resembles that of urticaria or of the chilblain. The other form is more common in men, and seems to affect the deeper layers of the skin.

In the preceding year, Cazenave discussed the case of a 38-year-old male admitted to the Hôpital Saint-Louis.[C171] A portion of the protocol has been translated by Shelley and Crissey:[S348]

> The eruption with which he is at present affected dates from 1841; it appeared without appreciable cause, and began with red spots, without elevation, without itching, the spots occupying at times the cheeks and at other times the ears, and which disappeared readily under the influence of a soft diet and tisanes. According to the patient, it is especially since he used a strong cantharidos ointment that the disease has extended, and that the redness has spread more and more, and has reached the nose and all those parts of the face which it occupies today.

* Dr. Talbott died in 1990. The editors have updated the text.

In the diagnosis of lupus, Cazenave noted that:[C173]

> A diagnostic error is possible because of the predilection of lupus for the face, a characteristic which it has in common with other forms.
>
> That, which characterizes lupus, in general, is its onset particularly during adolescence, and rarely after: an important characteristic which often should be an aid in diagnosis in order to differentiate the lupus from certain forms which furthermore share with lupus a great similarity of aspect, but which affect in general adults, 25 to 30 years of age.
>
> At the onset lupus erythematosus may be characterized by its urticarial, or erythematous plaques, particularly of erythema pernio or chilblain type. But the persistence of the plaques of lupus, their purplish color, their exclusive location, will be indicative until the time when the skin becomes atrophic and shiny, exfoliation appears and finally scarring.

The first illustration of discoid lupus erythematosus appeared in the third edition of the monograph by Cazenave and Schedel, published in 1838 (Fig. 1–1).[C170] The original color picture, probably prepared from a copper plate, shows a bilateral rash on the cheeks and forehead that does not cross the bridge of the nose in a butterfly distribution.

In 1845, Hebra discussed seborrhea congestiva, which most surely was lupus erythematosus, and used the butterfly simile for the facial lesion. The correct reference was identified by Jarcho[J55] after it had been incorrectly identified for many years.[H236] A generation after Hebra's discussion of lupus, his son-in-law Kaposi (Moriz Kohn) listed a number of terms that had been used to identify or qualify the disorders.[H237]

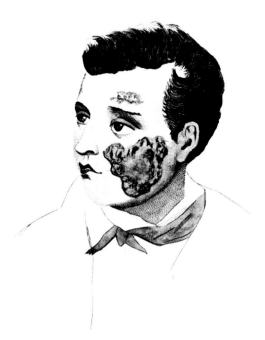

Fig. 1–1. The first illustration of discoid lupus erythematosus. It appeared in an 1838 edition of a monograph by Cazenave and Schedel.[C170]

Hebra, having regard to the fact that all the above-named varieties are neither more nor less than different stages of development of lupus, did not consider them as distinct species, but looked on the affection in all its forms as one disease.

No confusion in our ideas regarding lupus need be caused by the circumstance that, since 1850, a cutaneous affection, thoroughly distinct from Lupus vulgaris, has been included under the designation of Lupus, after the example of Cazenave, with the title of Lupus erythematosus. It is quite sufficient, when we wish to indicate the form described by Willan, to speak of it as Lupus vulgaris, or simply as Lupus.

Kaposi differentiated discoid lupus from the "aggregated form" and, in describing the facial lesion, noted that it resembled a butterfly in shape and that:[H237]

> Lupus Erythematosus may not only extend more deeply locally, and be attended by altogether more severe pathological changes than were known of at that time; but that also various grave and even dangerous constitutional symptoms may be intimately associated with the process in question, and that death may result from conditions which must be considered to arise from the local malady.
>
> More or less fever of an irregularly remittent type is almost constantly associated with acute or subacute eruptions, whether they are accompanied by severe or slight local symptoms... attended by general prostration and disturbed consciousness, resulting in coma or sopor or complicated with pleuropneumonia, and ending in death.
>
> Chlorosis, tuberculosis, and anemia may be considered as complications of lupus erythematosus, inasmuch as they not only exist in combination with it, but also seem to alternate in association with it.

Jonathan Hutchinson was especially interested in lupus, and in the 1870s observed that it was a "somewhat rare disease." In commenting upon the illustrations in Hebra's "Atlas," instead of using the butterfly simile, Hutchinson likened the facial lesions to:[H521]

> Large bat's-wing patches on cheeks and nose... I may here observe also that the special type of lupus erythematosus is determined to some extent by age. The more purely erythematous type occurs in early life almost exclusively, the sebaceous and less vascular types in middle life.

The concept of the pathogenesis of lupus has experienced extensive changes during the past century. Initially, lupus was believed to be a type of cancer. At the beginning of the nineteenth century, Willan listed it under the class "tuberculae" where it remained for more than a century.[V88] In 1880, Hutchinson was on the verge of differentiating tubercular lupus vulgaris from lupus erythematosus, but he failed to pursue the argument to a firm conclusion.[H519,H520,H521]

Anyone who has seen half a dozen examples of common lupus and of lupus erythematosus is able with ease to distinguish the one from the other, and both in turn from scrofula, syphilis and psoriasis; but let him wait awhile and see more, and he will find before long that there are examples of mixed forms of disease which it is impossible to denote correctly without employing hybrid names or qualifying adjectives. The reason of this is, as already stated, that lupus is not in any of its forms specific, it is not produced by any one definite cause, but is a result of various modifications of vital endowment existing in its subject.

I have tried to prove that lupus is mainly a scrofulous malady; that it is influenced by the causes which induce chilblains; and that in some cases it has an alliance with psoriasis. . . . From these data, the rules for treatment, or at any rate for constitutional treatment, are easily evolved.

We just improve the patient's state of nutrition by tonics, good food, bracing air, cod-liver oil, and the judicious use of stimulants.

In a series of three communications published between 1895 and 1903, William Osler discussed the visceral complications of erythema exudativum multiforme.[O107,O108,O109] Not all of these patients suffered from what is now identified as systemic lupus erythematosus (SLE), but he expanded the concept of a systemic disease and mentioned extensive and critical visceral complications.

By exudative erythema is understood a disease of unknown etiology with polymorphic skin lesions—hyperaemia, oedema, and hemorrhage—arthritis occasionally, and a variable number of visceral manifestations, of which the most important are gastrointestinal crises, endocarditis, pericarditis, acute nephritis and hemorrhage from the mucous surface. Recurrence is a special feature of the disease and attacks may come on month after month or even throughout a long period of years. Variability in the skin lesions is the rule, and a case may present in one attack the features of an angioneurotic edema, in a second of a multiforme or nodose erythema, and in a third those of peliosis rheumatica. The attacks may not be characterized by skin manifestations; the visceral symptoms alone may be present, and to the outward view the patient may have no indications whatever of erythema exudativum.

The third communication in Osler's series described arthritis, pneumonia, central nervous system symptoms, delirium, aphasia, and hemiplegia in affected patients. Mild joint symptoms were reported, but the arthritis did not progress to crippling deformity. Although Osler reported no postmortem examinations, he speculated that the symptoms possibly were due to vascular changes in the brain, similar to vascular changes in the skin:[O108] "The essential process is a vascular change with exudate, blood, serum, alone or combined."

At the time that Osler was assembling and reporting his studies from Baltimore, Jadassohn, in Vienna, was engaged in a similar pursuit.[J33a] No longer was there any doubt of the diffuse distribution of affected structures and organs in a patient with SLE. Jadassohn's communication was a typical German review and listed more than 400 references.

Libman and Sacks, in 1923, reported to the Association of American Physicians their findings of four cases of "A Hitherto Undescribed Form of Valvular and Mural Endocarditis."[L269] Although it was assumed that a new disease had been described, Libman-Sacks disease, it was soon recognized that the syndrome was a variant of SLE. Each patient complained of arthralgia. Two showed an erythematous eruption of butterfly distribution on the face, resembling acute lupus erythematosus disseminatus. Pulmonary symptoms were present in each patient. Three complained of pleurisy, and a pericardial friction rub was detected in a similar number, one of whom developed a pericardial effusion. The first patient had been seen in 1911. The endocardial lesion suggested neither acute rheumatic endocarditis nor subacute bacterial endocarditis. Histologically, the heart muscle was free from Aschoff bodies, and the kidney showed no embolic glomerular lesions. Obliteration of the loops of the glomeruli with hyalinization, fibrosis, and adhesions to Bowman's capsule were characteristic of the kidneys in one case. Many of the glomeruli were obliterated.[L269]

In the deeper layers (of the heart valves), there were focal and diffuse cellular infiltrations, chiefly of round cells in three of the cases, and predominantly of polymorphonuclear cells in the remaining one. . . . The valves in several instances showed diffuse fibrous thickening of the type resulting from previous attacks of endocarditis. In the older lesions, there were areas of fibroblastic invasion, hyalinization of the newly-formed connective tissue and extensive vascularization. . . . In one case, many of the blood vessels in the mitral valve showed marked endothelial proliferation of the intima. . . . There were cellular accumulations in the subendothelial tissues and extensive fibrosis in the deeper layers, indicating healing.

These observations were extended by Gross, who reviewed the protocols and pathologic findings in 11 cases and reported in the Libman Festschrift volume in 1932:[G405]

It will be seen that, taken as a whole, this clinical picture is unique even though many phenomena are common to a number of diseases. . . . Occasionally there were seen intermingled with the granular substance several spindle-shaped fairly dense masses, staining moderately deeply with hematoxylin. These will be referred to as "hematoxylin stained bodies.". . . There are frequently seen minute myocardial infarcts due to the "granular plugged vessels" so that all stages in the healing of these minute infarcts are encountered in various parts of the myocardium.

A significant contribution to the understanding of the clinical and pathologic findings of lupus was a communication, also to the Association of American Physicians. At the 1935 meeting, Baehr, Klemperer, and Schifrin[B18] described the "wire-loop" appearance of the glomeruli in 13 of 23 postmortem examinations at Mt. Sinai Hospital in New York, structural changes noted by others previously, but not distinguished from the more common findings in renal disorders and not previously identified specifically with the natural history of SLE.

> The commonest and most characteristic glomerular alteration was a peculiar hyaline thickening of the capillary walls which is striking even in sections stained with hematoxylin eosin. The thickened wall appears rigid, as if made of heavy wire. We have, therefore, called it the "wire-loop lesion.". . . This very characteristic lesion has not been seen by us in any other human disease, except perhaps in eclampsia. It resembles the glomerular and vascular lesions described by Wadsworth in horses which have been immunized by repeated intravenous injections of live bacteria, especially of the pneumococcus-streptococcus group. It is quite different from the hyaline degeneration seen in glomeruli of arteriosclerotic kidneys or of chronic glomerulonephritis.

The vascular lesions, particularly in the kidneys, showed a variety of alterations that included proliferation of the endothelium of the capillaries, arterioles, and venules associated with thrombi and degenerative necrotizing lesions and sometimes hemorrhage into the adjacent tissues. They were considered stages of the same underlying morbid process.

Also from the Mt. Sinai Hospital, Friedberg, Gross, and Wallach reported on four females who, in retrospect, were recognized to have SLE.[F246] The investigations suggested:

> that a condition belonging to the same general type as that described by Baehr and his co-workers, might occur without the striking cutaneous lesions, but with the other associated clinical and pathological features of the disease.

The unusual features included absence of skin lesions, deforming peripheral arthritis (rheumatoid), endothelial proliferation, endothelial degeneration with granular degeneration and swelling, narrowing or obstruction of the lumen by plugs, internal proliferation and necrosis of the vessel wall. In 1940, Gross modified his interpretation and suggested that the two groups of cases previously called acute disseminated lupus erythematosus and atypical verrucous endocarditis, respectively, should be placed into the single category of Libman-Sacks disease.[G406]

Nearly 15 years earlier, Keith and Rowntree had studied the renal function and histologic findings in four cases of SLE and had thought that the functional findings were consistent with a clinical diagnosis of nephrosis and the pathologic findings consistent with chronic glomerular nephritis:[K147]

> The glomeruli showed beginning hyalinization of the capillary loops with marked formation of lobules. There was swelling of the epithelial cells covering the loops and atrophy of the endothelial cells. The loops, in general, were atrophied and the capsular spaces dilated; only an occasional loop was patent, and in some places the loop was practically obliterated. The capsular epithelium contained evidences of swelling and proliferation. No evidences of tuberculosis were found.

The term diffuse collagen disease, especially popular a generation ago, but in recent years largely replaced by diffuse connective tissue disorders, was introduced by Klemperer, Pollack, and Baehr in 1941 to identify the lesion under consideration.[K284]

> These fiber changes have been called fibrinoid degeneration, a term first applied by Neumann. We shall continue the use of this term in its purely descriptive sense. It can also, therefore, be properly applied to the altered ground substance giving the same tinctorial reactions as the altered fibers.
>
> The thick, gelatinous, adherent pericardium owes its arresting gross appearance not alone to proliferative and infiltrative tissue changes but even more to a series of alterations affecting the pre-existing and the newly formed connective tissue. Here the usual sharp contrast between fibers and ground substance is obliterated. In hematoxylin-eosin preparations the fibers, cell cytoplasm and ground substance can be optically isolated under high magnification only by "stopping down" the diaphragm of the substage condenser. In the Mallory trichrome stain the ground substance assumes a pale blue homogeneous appearance, in which the deeper blue collagen fibers stand out quite clearly. The ground substance may be thought to have become "collagenized."

Although some believed that discoid lupus and disseminated lupus had a close relationship, the majority felt that they were two distinct entities. Keil, on the other hand, emphasized what should have been apparent to those who followed patients with discoid lupus for long periods: dissemination in discoid lupus is not a unique consequence:[K144] "Clinical and pathologic data are presented to support the belief that the acute variety of the disease is related to the ordinary fixed atrophic forms." Keil[K143] also rejected, as others had done previously,[M554] the theory that SLE was related to tuberculosis:

> On the basis of the necropsies[K143] which I studied, as well as of those reported in the literature, I must conclude that the occurrence of tuberculosis in cases of lupus erythematosus is coincidental and unrelated. There is no justification, in my opinion, for the assumption that active tuberculosis is present merely because the patient has lupus erythematosus.

The development of SLE following splenectomy in idiopathic thrombocytopenia purpura or the association of thrombocytopenic purpura in fully developed instances of SLE was reported also in the 1930s. Lyon, in 1933, described the clinical course of idiopathic thrombocytopenic purpura with leukopenia in a 12-year-old boy, who subsequently revealed the skin lesions of SLE.[L434] In a general discussion of the treatment of purpura hemorrhagica in 1936, Jones and Tocantins noted:[J107a]

> A thrombopenia is said to be associated with the disease lupus erythematosus. The patient . . . developed a lupus of the face, neck, mouth and less extensively on other parts of the body five months after splenectomy and when her platelet count was normal. Another

patient developed lupus during a chronic thrombopenic state which was known to have existed at least three years. A third patient had lupus and then developed symptoms and signs of purpura haemorrhagica after intravenous gold injections.

Similar in name to idiopathic thrombocytopenic purpura, but quite different clinically, is thrombotic thrombocytopenic purpura. A number of examples of this usually fatal malady, with clinical or histologic evidence of SLE, have been reported since Fordyce, in 1899, observed capillary thrombosis in a patient with SLE. The case described by Fordyce might well have been an example of thrombotic thrombocytopenic purpura in a patient with SLE.[F165a]

> The Capillary Vessels in the middle and deeper regions of the derma are in places partially or completely obliterated; in some of them organizing thrombi are met with. In others, coagulum, red and white blood corpuscles, partially disorganized.

The literature on the association was reviewed by Gitlow and Goldmark in 1939,[G169] in conjunction with the study of two cases, one a combination of thrombotic thrombocytopenic purpura and systemic lupus. More recently, Laszlo, Alvarez, and Feldman[L87] in reporting a similar case, "suggested that thrombotic thrombocytopenic purpura may belong in the category of 'collagen diseases,'" a sentiment expressed by Beigelman in 1951.[B170] A 6-year followup of a patient, with good evidence in support of a diagnosis of each of these conditions, was provided from personal communication with Schwartz, one of the writers in the communication by Siegel and associates.[S412] The clinical and biopsy findings in a 29-year-old black woman with thrombohemolytic thrombocytopenia purpura were presented in a paper published in 1957.[S412] A biopsy of the left gastrocnemius muscle showed findings highly suggestive of thrombohemolytic thrombocytopenic purpura. After a good clinical response to adrenocorticotropic hormone, the spleen was removed. Histologic study of the organ confirmed the biopsy findings. After the operation, however, clinical findings of SLE appeared, substantiated by demonstration of the LE-cell phenomenon. In 1962, the patient remained under treatment with steroids for SLE; meanwhile the LE test remained positive.

The variety and number of diffuse clinical characteristics that have been observed in SLE have given rise to the overworked cliché "diffuse systemic disease." This includes involvement of the heart, lungs, central and peripheral nervous system, gastrointestinal system, splenolymphatic system, and musculoskeletal system. Except in instances noted specifically, clinical and laboratory findings cannot be considered characteristic of SLE. However, clinical and histologic changes in the eye constitute one of the few specific diagnostic criteria. Bergmeister, in 1929, noted white patches along the retinal veins in a patient with lupus, shortly before death from tuberculosis.[B239] The eyes were not studied histologically. In the following decade, fluffy white patches and hemorrhages were reported in the fundus of lupus patients, usually without clinical evidence to support a diagnosis of glomerulonephritis or malignant hypertension. One of the first histologic studies of the globus, by Semon and Wolff, described round-cell infiltration of the choroid, with a partially organized subretinal exudate of inflammatory cells at the site of one of the fluffy white patches observed ophthalmoscopically. Only postmortem changes were noted in the retina.[S272] White, raised lesions were apparent in the fundus. Histologically, there was invasion of the choroid with inflammatory cells. At the site of the lesion was a well-marked subretinal exudate containing inflammatory cells (lymphocytes, a few polymorphonuclears and a few large mononuclears). There were no changes in the retina.

In 1940, Maumenee reported the structural changes in the eye in four cases of SLE and one case of discoid lupus:[M215]

> The yellowish-white to white spots seen with the ophthalmoscope... were found to be typical areas of cytoid bodies in the nerve-fiber layer of the retina.... One or more groups of cytoid bodies were found in every case. The sizes of these lesions varied from a few globular elements that caused no localized elevation of the hyaloid membrane to areas about 1 mm in diameter and almost double the thickness of the nerve-fiber layer. Three of the lesions were noted to be in the proximity of retinal vessels but none touched a vessel. A few red blood cells were found at the edges of two of the lesions, but in no instance were the areas related to large hemorrhages. In two cases very small hemorrhages were seen among the inner fibers of the nerve-fiber layer. Slight papilledema was histologically evident in case 2 and moderate papilledema in case 5. Only in case 2 were any notable changes found in the retinal vessels, in which case there was a slight hyaline degeneration of the intima of the retinal arteries typical of arteriolar sclerosis. No hemorrhages nor exudates were found in the nuclear or plexiform layers of the retina. The ganglion cells appeared to be normal. There was no subretinal exudate in any of the cases. A slight round-cell infiltration of the choroid, "septic choroiditis," was present in all five cases. In case 2 there were serous exudates and hemorrhages in the stroma of the choroid extending about two to three disc diameters out from the optic nerve.... The choroidal vessels in this case exhibited a moderate hyaline degeneration of the intima and a proliferation of the adventitia.

In addition to these characteristic findings in the eye and the wire loop lesion in the kidney, necrosis of lymph nodes, "onion-ring" lesions in the spleen, and hematoxylin-staining bodies in various structures are intimately identified with SLE. Extensive destruction in the lymph nodes of one case of SLE was described by Short in 1907:[S394]

> *Mesenteric glands* show marked evidence of acute inflammatory change.... The lymphoid cells are, to a great extent, replaced by large cells with a considerable amount of protoplasm, the nuclei of which are large and oval, often duplicated, and frequently showing mitotic figures. There are areas of haemorrhage and other areas of complete necrosis.

The onion-ring lesion of the arteries of the spleen was described first by Libman and Sacks without specific comment:[L269]

> The spleen in three was enlarged—In two of these, the malpighian bodies were enlarged, and in one, the enlargement was due not to hyperplasia of the lymphoid elements, but to a peculiar hyaline thickening around the arterioles.

The hematoxylin-staining bodies in heart valves, already observed by Gross,[G406] were reported by Ginzler and Fox in lymph nodes, spleen, and other structures:[G156]

> One section showed areas of endothelial swelling close to the pocket of the tricuspid leaflet, with adherent masses of pink-staining granular material containing mononuclear cells and numerous dark-staining round or oval nuclei, some of which were pyknotic.

In the kidney:

> The endothelial cells showed pronounced swelling and proliferation, completely filling some of the loops and contributing to a distinct increase in cellularity of many of the glomeruli. The cells showed occasional hyaline droplet degeneration, but much more severe and extensive were pinkish-violet-staining granular degeneration and necrosis of these cells, associated with nuclear pyknosis and karyorrhexis.

Three critical laboratory procedures are of great interest in this malady. A false-positive serologic test for syphilis may prove to be a diagnostic clue, and the LE-cell phenomenon most surely is of great diagnostic significance. The antinuclear antibody test and related serologic findings have greatly improved our understanding of the disease.

Two instances of a false-positive Wassermann reaction in patients with lupus were reported shortly after the reaction was described. In each instance, there was no evidence to support a diagnosis of syphilis.[H206,R140] A decade later, Gennerich attributed particular significance to a positive serologic reaction and associated it with the pathogenesis of lupus.[G88a]

> That disintegration of the lymph glands does indeed cause lupus erythematosus, in a way to be discussed later on, is indicated by the presence of a positive serologic reaction. This is true of all those cases where invasion of the organism by lymphocyte ferments becomes overabundant. Positive serologic reaction in these cases of acute lupus erythematosus, which take a particularly vehement development, is the key to the lupus erythematosus etiology.
>
> As early as 1910, I had reason to assume, on the strength of observations made on salvarsan provocation, that a positive serologic reaction is based on disintegration of lymphocytes.

Keil reported false-positive reactions in ten cases of SLE: one showed a paretic-type colloidal gold curve without clinical or other evidence of syphilis.[K146] In a majority of instances, the false-positive serologic reactions, supported by a negative treponema immobilization reaction, are associated with hypergammaglobulinemia. The incidence of false-positive reactions has been observed to be as high as 35% in the acute stage when a battery of serologic tests were applied.[R135] In some of the more interesting examples, a false-positive reaction has been observed months or years before any clinical evidence of SLE appeared.[H183]

The discovery of the LE and the tart cells by Hargraves, Richmond, and Morton, reported in the *Proceedings of the Staff Meetings of the Mayo Clinic* in 1948, was a most important event in the history of lupus.[H129]

> In the last two years we have been observing a phenomenon in our bone marrow preparations which, to our knowledge, has never been described in the literature. Actually there are two phenomena involved and, while their significance is not definitely understood, it seems wise to record a description of the involved cells so that others may contribute their observations on bone marrow to clarify the significance of these findings further. During this period we have shown preparations containing these cells to numerous visiting hematologists as well as presented them to the Hematology Club in Chicago in the Fall of 1946 and 1947, and none have previously observed them. It is important that both cells be described because of the possible confusion that may result if a distinction is not clearly made.
>
> The second cell which we wish to present has been called an "L.E." cell. . . in our laboratory because of its frequent appearance in the bone marrow in cases of acute disseminated lupus erythematosus. This cell undoubtedly represents a process which is going on in such bone marrows and is the end result of one of two things: either phagocytosis of free nuclear material with a resulting round vacuole containing this partially digested and lysed nuclear material or, second, an actual autolysis of one or more lobes of the nucleus. . . of the involved cell so that it presents essentially the same appearance as the one which has phagocytized nuclear material. The "L.E." cell is practically always a mature neutrophilic polymorphonuclear leukocyte in contradistinction to the "tart" cell, which is most often a histiocyte. . . While most of these cells characteristically show a homogeneous, purple-staining mass in the vacuole there are instances in which the chromatin pattern is still visible.
>
> We have not yet found either of these cells in the peripheral blood. It would seem reasonable that the "L.E." cell, being the result of phagocytosis of nuclear material, should be found in circumstances in which there is any active destruction of body tissue.

The discovery of the LE cell gave impetus to the concept that SLE was an autoimmune disease and that the phenomenon, as revealed by findings in the peripheral blood and bone marrow, offered an excellent procedure to pursue this possibility in depth. Rheumatoid arthritis, intimately or casually related to SLE, was one of the first disorders to be studied. A number of reports of LE cells in patients with rheumatoid arthritis have appeared. Kievits, Goslings, Schuit, and Hijmans, in one of the first large series of patients with rheumatoid arthritis, reported an incidence of 16% positive reactors.[K198] The LE cell in this disorder seems indistinguishable morphologically from the cell in SLE. Is the LE cell in rheumatoid arthritis a prophetic phenomenon of the development subsequently of SLE? The LE cell is transmissible to the infant of a mother afflicted with SLE but is not heritable. Bridge and Foley observed the LE phenomenon in the newborn of a mother who suffered from lupus for 30 months.[B488] The blood of the mother gave a positive cell response on several occasions. The LE cells and LE rosettes were observed in the cord blood at delivery and persisted in the child for seven weeks. They were absent four months post-partum. Subsequently the mother died while the child was known to be in apparent good health at the age of nine. Therefore, the LE factor (IgG, which binds DNA-histone) is transmitted to the fetus from maternal blood. When maternal IgG is metabolized, the infant no longer has LE cells. This antibody appears to be harmless to the fetus, in contrast to anti-Ro, which can cause fetal lesions.

The LE-cell phenomenon and a rheumatoid-like arthritis syndrome has been observed as an untoward reaction of potent therapeutic agents. In 1954, Dustan, Taylor, Corcoran, and Page reported the development of an LE-like syndrome following treatment with the antihypertensive drug hydralazine hydrochloride (Apresoline).[D365] LE cells were detected in the plasma or bone marrow; sometimes LE cells were present without associated symptoms.

> Another striking complication of treatment has appeared in some of our patients; this seems to be related to the use of large doses of hydralazine over long periods of time. The syndrome in its less severe form resembles rheumatoid arthritis; in its severer febrile aspect, it stimulates acute systemic lupus erythematosus.... The process usually disappeared spontaneously on withdrawal of therapy with the drug or on reduction in dosage.

The term lupus hepatitis has been introduced into the literature, already burdened with names. Joske and King[J134] reported LE cells in the blood of two patients with chronic hepatitis. At the time of the report, neither patient had developed lupus. It is uncertain whether this was an isolated observation associated with an abnormal antibody-producing mechanism following hepatitis or an early manifestation of SLE. In some patients a past history of hepatitis, with an intervening period of good health, has been noted in their protocols. The association remains as unclear as the association between arthritis and SLE. It is now clear that ANA and LE cells can be a manifestation of chronic hepatitis.

In 1957, Witebsky et al.[W310] discussed autoimmunization in selected cases of chronic thyroiditis. This concept later received support, but not indisputable proof, from the speculation that the phenomenon involved forbidden clones,[B584a] self-reactive cells with immunologic properties capable of overcoming a normal response of the body, which survived rather than perished.

In addition to the Wassermann and LE-cell tests, the third critical laboratory test, which has essentially replaced the LE-cell test, is the detection of ANA by fluorescent staining.[F270]

The discovery by Coons[C380] of immunofluorescence and its subsequent application by Friou[F270] to blood and tissues of SLE patients was another landmark in the evolution of defining lupus as an autoimmune disease. The value of this technique in the intervening years has been firmly established.

The production of LE cells experimentally by Finch, Ross, and Ebaugh[F92] gave credence to the hypothesis that lupus is in some measure an autoimmune response. Heteroimmune antibodies were produced in rabbits against human granulocytic leukemic leukocytes that produced phagocytosis of normal human granulocytes by polymorphonuclear leukocytes. Upon incubation of the cells with antileukocytic serum, LE cells developed. The cells seen are more typically "tart" cells than LE cells. Dameshek[D24] predicated an autoimmune pathogenesis upon the presence of onion-ring lesions in the spleen in selected patients with idiopathic thrombocytopenic purpura, the development of SLE following splenectomy in patients with typical idiopathic thrombocytopenic purpura, the false-positive serologic tests for syphilis, the presence of a positive Coombs' test, and the presence of hemolytic anemia and thrombocytopenic purpura in selected patients.

An experimental model of SLE in the hybrid New Zealand mouse (NZB/NZW), described by Bielschowsky, Helyer, and Howie[B298] in 1958, closely resembles the human disease. Studies of this animal model have yielded increased insight into understanding the human counterpart.

Treatment of SLE was symptomatic and supportive until adrenocorticotropic hormone and the corticosteroids became available. Not long after the introduction of ACTH and cortisone into clinical medicine, in the treatment of arthritis, Thorne and associates[T160] found new agents equally helpful in treatment.

Between 1960 and 1990, 1000 to 2000 articles dealing with lupus appeared annually in peer-reviewed literature. These studies provided a treasure trove of new insights in four major areas: family and genetic studies, cellular immunology, the discovery of new autoantibodies, and improved clinical investigation.

The description of the HLA system was followed by the first assessments of HLA haplotypes in SLE by McDevitt's[G416] and Walford's[W94] groups in 1971. Major breakthroughs eluded investigators until DR2 and DR3 were associated with lupus by Reinertsen et al. in 1978.[R139] Family studies were pioneered by Siegel et al. in 1965.[S417] These landmark works laid the groundwork for the molecular genetic probes and pedigree surveys that followed. It is now clear that SLE has a complex genetic basis, with several predisposing single genes and extended haplotypes.

In the 1970s, lymphocytes were classified as T cells, B cells, and null cells by the presence or absence of surface receptors. Assisted by the development of monoclonal antibodies, use of cell sorters, elucidation of idiotype networks, discovery of cytokines, evolution of theories of tolerance-induction mechanisms, and the availability of immunoblot techniques, our whole approach to cellular and humoral research has been completely transformed. These studies have revealed multiple abnormalities in T and B cell functions which are probably required for disease expression.

New important autoantibodies have permitted us to define previously unrecognized clinical subsets of LE. The false-positive syphilis serologies appreciated among LE patients in the 1940s (see above) was further explored with the description of the circulating lupus anticoagulant by Conley and Hartmann in 1952.[C367a] In 1983, Harris and colleagues identified a group of antibodies to phospholipid in many of these patients.[H152] They were able to correlate its presence with spontaneous abortions, thromboembolic phenomena, and thrombocytopenia. The antiphospholipid syndrome as we now know it is treated differently from active SLE. Tan and Kunkel's 1966 identification of the Sm antigen, followed by Mattioli and Reichlin's discovery of anti-RNP in 1971, as well as the work of Sharp and Holman,[H38,M209,S336,T48] allowed the delineation of a subgroup with mixed connective tissue disease and opened the door to a host of new disease specificities. Although first described by Jones in 1958,[J104] anti-Ro/SSA and anti-La/SSB were ultimately characterized by Alsbaugh and Tan and Mattioli and Reichlin[M211] in 1974. Sjögren's syndrome, neonatal lupus,[L352] and subacute cutaneous lupus subsets[S568] were subsequently defined as associated with these antibody systems.

The first edition of this monograph in 1966 was almost completely the work of one individual, Edmund L. Dubois. It was largely an anecdotal compendium reflecting his immense experience with the disease. Many of his prejudices were well founded, others were not. The primitive quality of clinical studies was gradually improved with the introduction of life table analysis by Merrell and Shulman in 1955,[M359] adoption of provisional American Rheumatism Association criteria for SLE in 1971 (revised in 1982),[C325,T46] the use of multivariate analysis by Fries in a textbook in 1975,[F256] and the evolution of clinical indices for assessing disease activity beginning with the Lupus Activity Criteria Count by Urowitz et al. in 1984.[U37a] Perhaps the most important clinical undertaking was the large, controlled, prospective lupus nephritis trial initiated by the National Institutes of Health in the early 1970s,[S638] which was still yielding useful results in 1991[B64,S652] and changed our perception of cytotoxic therapies. Thus, current therapy of severe, life-threatening disease is more aggressive than it was 15 years ago, with frequent "standard" use of cytotoxic regimens, combination cytotoxics/steroid regimens, intermittent high-dose boluses of intravenous steroids, and experimental protocols that use multiple immunomodulatory techniques, such as apheresis and monoclonal antibodies against T cells. Organized medicine recognized rheumatology as a subspecialty within internal medicine in 1972, which allowed the expansion of fellowship programs and research opportunities.

The 1990s will see the development of cytokine receptor antagonists and monoclonal antibodies against cellular and humoral components that mediate the inflammatory process. Lupus has come a long way over the last 150 years, even though at times it seems that we will need another 150 years to really understand it.

Section II

THE GENETICS, EPIDEMIOLOGY, AND CLASSIFICATION OF LUPUS

Chapter 2

THE GENETIC BASIS OF LUPUS ERYTHEMATOSUS

FRANK C. ARNETT, JR.

Over the last two decades, it has become clear that genetic factors play important roles in the etiopathogenesis of lupus erythematosus. Earlier reports documented that SLE frequently clustered in families and that asymptomatic relatives often had circulating immunologic abnormalities; however, no classical pattern of inheritance was obvious from these studies. In parallel with new knowledge of the genetics of the immune response, associations of SLE with actual genetic markers became apparent. Most notable were increased frequencies of certain human leukocyte antigens (HLAs), encoded from the major histocompatibility complex (MHC), in patients with SLE. Additionally, hereditary deficiencies of early components of the complement system, several of which also mapped to the MHC, were found to increase disease susceptibility. Over the same interval, the clinical heterogeneity of lupus was recognized, and a variety of disease subsets, associated primarily with different autoantibody profiles, were recognized. With recent advances in molecular biology, it is now possible to examine these previous associations at a more basic level. Indeed, the concept is now evolving that lupus is a multigenic composite disease of several overlapping autoimmune responses, each mediated by distinct genetic profiles.

It is the purpose of this chapter to describe the structure and function of those genetic systems currently most relevant to SLE and to review current knowledge of their roles in disease pathogenesis.

MAJOR HISTOCOMPATIBILITY COMPLEX (MHC)
Genetic Organization and Definitions

The MHC or HLA region in humans, is located on the short arm of human chromosome 6 (Fig. 2–1).[C110,D362, G131,H123,K360] At least three functionally distinct regions have been defined, MHC (or HLA) class I, II, and III. MHC class I genes include the HLA-A, B, and C loci, which encode glycoprotein molecules noncovalently bound to β_2-microglobulin, expressed on all nucleated cells. A variety of other class I genes have been found (HLA-E, F, and G), but they are probably pseudogenes which do not encode cell-surface molecules.[K360] The MHC class II region includes the α and β genes (Fig. 2–2) (as well as several DO and DN pseudogenes) for three types of structurally similar $\alpha\beta$ heterodimers, HLA-DR, DQ, and DP molecules[H123] (Fig. 2–3). Class II antigens are expressed on antigen-presenting cells, especially macrophages/monocytes and B lymphocytes, and activated T lymphocytes.[G131] Recently, genes for transporter proteins, which

carry MHC class I molecules to the cell surface, have been mapped within the class II region.[T226] The MHC class III region, lying between the HLA-B and HLA-DR loci, does not contain histocompatibility loci but rather the structural genes for the early complement components C4 (C4a and C4b), C2, and factor B (Bf), as well as steroid hormone 21-hydroxylase (21-OHB), a 21-OHA pseudogene,[A370,C51,C108,C109,O82] tumor necrosis factor (TNF) α and β (lymphotoxin),[S597] heat-shock protein (hsp) 70,[S80] and RD, a gene whose function is unknown.[L212] Five additional genes of unknown function, termed "B-associated transcripts" (BATs), have recently been mapped between the TNF and HLA-B loci and may constitute an MHC "class IV" region.[S596]

The multiple genes of the HLA region are inherited "en bloc" in a Mendelian codominant fashion, and the contribution from each parent is referred to as a "haplotype." Recombinational or crossover events at the time of meiosis occur in approximately 2% of matings. Thus, the haplotype inherited from each parent will carry a linked cluster of relatively unique MHC alleles.

The HLA region, especially class I and II, is the most *polymorphic* genetic system yet recognized in humans.[B375,D362] Multiple alleles which code different antigenic forms (specificities) exist for each locus. The molecular basis for this polymorphism will be discussed later. HLA antigens detected on cell surfaces are designated (WHO nomenclature) by the letters of the locus from which they are coded followed by a number, i.e., HLA-A2, HLA-B8, HLA-Cw1, HLA-DR4, HLA-DQw8, HLA-DPw1, etc. A "w" or international "workshop" assignment is maintained until a specificity is determined to be reasonably homogeneous. HLA alleles, as determined by DNA sequencing, are given a more precise numerical designation prefixed by the exact locus that confers the polymorphism. Examples of class I alleles include HLA-A*0201 (HLA-A2), HLA-B*0801 (HLA-B8), HLA-Cw*0101 (HLA-Cw1), etc. For some alleles, such as HLA-B27, additional subtypes have been found and are designated as HLA-B*2701, *2702, *2703, etc.

HLA class II nomenclature follows similar rules but is somewhat more complex (Table 2–1).[B375] The polymorphism for HLA-DR is conferred only by the beta genes since the DR α gene (DRA1) is invariant. There are several functional DR β genes including DRB1, DRB3, DRB4, and DRB5. HLA-DRB1 is the most polymorphic and determines the majority of conventional DR molecules, i.e., DR1 through DRw18. Many of these DR specificities have

13

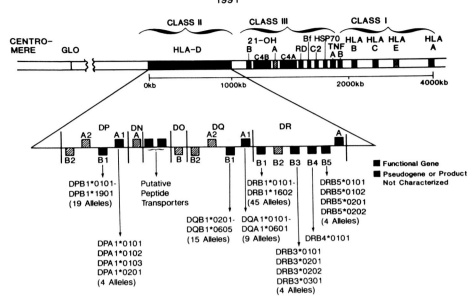

Fig. 2–1. Schematic representation of the human major histocompatibility compatibility complex (MHC) or HLA region located on the short arm of chromosome 6. The multiple genes and their order are shown. The area between HLA-A and HLA-DP spans approximately 3.5×10^6 base pairs of DNA and represents a distance of approximately 2 centimorgans (map or recombinational units).

multiple subtypes, first detected by mixed lymphocyte culture (MLC) techniques (Dw types) and later by DNA sequencing. An example is HLA-DR4 with its serologic specificity (MLC subtype) and specific alleles designated as follows: DR4 (Dw4) = DRB1*0401, DR4 (Dw10) = DRB1*0402, DR4 (Dw13) = DRB1*0403, etc. HLA-DRB2 is a pseudogene. HLA-DRB3 is found only on HLA haplotypes bearing DRB1 alleles for DR3, DR5, and DRw6 (DRw13 and DRw14) and encodes several subtypes of the supertypic specificity HLA-DRw52, while DRB4, which encodes DRw53, is found only on DR4- and DR7-bearing haplotypes. HLA-DRB5 is found only on DR2 (DRw15 and DRw16) haplotypes. Only DRB1 loci exist on HLA-DR1, DRw8, and DRw10 haplotypes.

CLASS II GENE

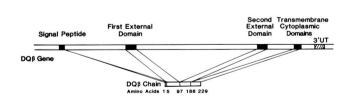

Fig. 2–2. Organization of an MHC class II gene (HLA-DQβ) showing exons (darkened areas) which encode the major structural components of class II molecules. The nucleotides encoding the polymorphic amino acids are located in the first external domain.

Polymorphism for HLA-DQ and DP molecules is conferred by both the α and β chain loci, i.e., DQA1 and DQB1, and DPA1 and DPB1, respectively (Table 2–2). There are fewer DQA1 than DQB1 alleles (DPA1 and DPB1, similarly); therefore, some DQA1 alleles will be associated with several different DQB1 alleles (Fig. 2–4); however, the serologic specificities of DQ molecules are primarily determined by the DQB1 chain.[B375,D362,G360] In addition, it is possible in vivo for a DQA1 chain inherited from one parental haplotype to physically pair on the cell surface with the DQB1 chain inherited from the alternative parental haplotype, thus forming a new "trans-associated hybrid" DQ molecule not present in either parent.[G130,K492] The genetics of the HLA-DQ genes is highly relevant to SLE and will be discussed further later. A number of other class II genes have been mapped, including DQA2, DQB2, DPA2, and DPB2, and others (DO, DN) which are probably pseudogenes.[H123]

Population Differences and Linkage Disequilibrium. HLA antigens (or alleles) occur in differing frequencies in various ethnic populations.[B129,D362,L148,L149] For example, HLA-DR3 (DRw17 or DRB1*0301) is found in approximately 25% of normal American and European Caucasians but is rarely found in Japanese. Another HLA-DR3, designated DR3 (DRw18 or DRB1*0302), differs from DR3 (DRw17) by four conservative amino acid substitutions and occurs exclusively in African blacks.[H510,H511] Because of racial admixture, American blacks may possess either DR3 (DRw17) or DR3 (DRw18). Another example is HLA-DR4, which in Ameri-

CLASS II HLA MOLECULE

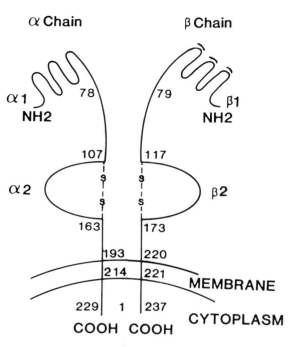

Fig. 2–3. Schematic representation of an MHC class II heterodimer comprised of alpha and beta chains. The amino (NH_2) terminus is the most external domain, while the carboxy (COOH) terminus is intracytoplasmic. There are two external domains on each of the α and β chains, with the most outermost containing the polymorphic amino acid sequences. Figures 2–6 and 2–7 provide three-dimensional schemas of MHC molecules. Reprinted from Arnett, F.C.: The HLA system and cutaneous disease. In Immunologic Diseases of the Skin. Edited by R.E. Jordon. Norwalk, Connecticut, and San Mateo, California, Appleton and Lange, 1991.

cans and Europeans is usually represented by the DR4 (Dw4 or DRB1*0401) or DR4 (Dw14 or DRB1*0404) subtypes, while in Japanese the DR4 (Dw15 or DRB1*0405) subtype is most common, and in Ashkenazi and Israeli Jews the DR4 (Dw10 or DRB1*0402) subtype predominates.[G361] Because of these ethnic and, at times, regional differences in allelic distributions, disease association studies require locally obtained normal controls that are ethnically matched.

Another phenomenon observed in different populations is *linkage disequilibrium*, or the frequent occurrence of certain alleles together on the same HLA haplotype. Given a constant recombination rate (2%) and a long evolutionary time period, it would be anticipated that different alleles from each of the HLA loci would be randomly distributed. That is, no HLA class I, II, or III alleles would occur together any more often than by chance alone, i.e., the product of their respective frequencies in the population. An evolutionary explanation for the occurrence of certain "extended haplotypes" in certain ethnic groups is not yet apparent; however, certain combinations of HLA alleles with their repertoire of immune responses may have afforded a selective advantage, possibly against certain local infections. The major example of an "extended haplotype" in Caucasians of Northern and Western European descent is that of *HLA-A1, B8, Cw7, DR3 (DRw17), DRw52a, DQw2.1*, which also carries a

Table 2-1. HLA-DR Alleles

HLA Alleles	HLA-DR Specificities	HLA-D–associated (T-cell or MLC-defined) Specificities
DRB1*0101	DR1	Dw1
DRB1*0102	DR1	Dw20
DRB1*0103	DR"BR"	Dw"BON"
DRB1*1501	DRw14(2)*	Dw2
DRB1*1502	DRw15(2)	Dw12
DRB1*1601	DRw16(2)	Dw21
DRB1*1602	DRw16(2)	Dw22
DRB1*0301	DRw17(3)	Dw3
DRB1*0302	DRw18(3)	Dw"RSH"
DRB1*0401	DR4	Dw4
DRB1*0402	DR4	Dw10
DRB1*0403	DR4	Dw13
DRB1*0404	DR4	Dw14
DRB1*0405	DR4	Dw15
DRB1*0406	DR4	Dw"KT2"
DRB1*0407	DR4	Dw13
DRB1*0408	DR4	Dw14
DRB1*1101	DRw11(5)	Dw5
DRB1*1102	DRw11(5)	Dw"JVM"
DRB1*1103	DRw11(5)	—
DRB1*1104	DRw11(5)	Dw"FS"
DRB1*1201	DRw12(5)	Dw"DB6"
DRB1*1301	DRw13(w6)	Dw18
DRB1*1302	DRw13(w6)	Dw19
DRB1*1303	DRw13(w6)	Dw"HAG"
DRB1*1401	DRw14(w6)	Dw9
DRB1*1402	DRw14(w6)	Dw16
DRB1*0701	DR7	Dw17
DRB1*0702	DR7	Dw"DB1"
DRB1*0801	DRw8	Dw8.1
DRB1*0802	DRw8	Dw8.2
DRB1*0803	DRw8	Dw8.3
DRB1*0901	DR9	Dw23
DRB1*1001	DRw10	—
DRB3*0101	DRw52a	Dw24
DRB3*0201	DRw52b	Dw25
DRB3*0202	DRw52b	Dw25
DRB3*0301	DRw52c	Dw26
DRB4*0101	DRw53	Dw4, Dw10, Dw13, Dw14, Dw15, Dw17, Dw23
DRB5*0101	DRw15(2)	Dw2
DRB5*0102	DRw15(2)	Dw12
DRB5*0201	DRw16(2)	Dw21
DRB5*0202	DRw16(2)	Dw22

From Bodmer, J.G., Marsh, S.G.E., Parham, P. et al.: Nomenclature for factors of the HLA system, 1989. Human Immunol., 28:326, 1990.[B375]
* Numbers in parentheses represent former HLA-DR designations, i.e., (2) = former DR2, (3) = former DR3, etc.

Table 2–2. HLA-DQA1 and DQB1 Alleles

HLA Alleles	HLA–DQ Specificities	HLA-D–associated (T-cell–defined) Specificities	Previous Equivalents
DQA1*0101	—	Dw1,w9	DQA1.1, 1.9
DQA1*0102	—	Dw2,w21,w19	DQA1.2, 1.9; 1.AZH
DQA1*0103	—	Dw18,w12,w8,Dw"FS"	DQA1.3, 1.18; DRw8-DQw1
DQA1*0201	—	Dw7,w11	DQA2, 3.7
DQA1*0301	—	Dw4,w10,w13,w14,w15,w23	DQA3, 3.1, 3.2; DR9-DQw3
DQA1*0401	—	Dw8,Dw"RSH"	DQA4.2, 3.8
DQA1*0501	—	Dw3,w5,w22	DQA4.1,2; DQA1*0202
DQA1*0601	—	Dw8	DQA4.3; DQA1*0302
DQB1*0501	DQw5(w1)*	Dw1	DQB1.1; DRw1C-DQw1.1, DQB1*0101, DQw1.AZH
DQB1*0501	DQw5(w1)	Dw21	DQB1.2, 1.21; DQB1*0102
DQB1*0503	DQw5(w1)	Dw9	DQB1.3, 1.9; DQB1*0103
DQB1*0601	DQw6(w1)	Dw12,w8	DQB1.4, 1.12; DQB1*0104
DQB1*0602	DQw6(w1)	Dw2	DQB1.5, 1.2; DQB1*0105
DQB1*0603	DQw6(w1)	Dw18,Dw"FS"	DQB1.6, 1.18; DQB1*0106
DQB1*0604	DQw6(w1)	Dw19	DQB1.7, 1.19; DQB1*0107
DQB1*0201	DQw2	Dw3,w7	DQB2
DQB1*0301	DQw7(w3)	Dw4,w5,w8,w13	DQB3.1
DQB1*0302	DQw8(w3)	Dw4,w10,w13,w14	DQB3.2
DQB1*0303	DQw9(w3)	Dw23,w11	DQB3.3
DQB1*0401	DQw4	Dw15	DQB4.1, Wa
DQB1*0402	DQw4	DW8,Dw"RSH"	DQB4.2, Wa

From Bodmer, J.G., Marsh, S.G.E., Parham, P. et al.: Nomenclature for factors of the HLA system, 1989. Human Immunol., 28:326, 1990.[B375]
* Numbers and letters in parentheses represent previous HLA-DQ designations, i.e., (w1) = former DQw1, (w3) = former DQw3, etc.

deletion of the *C4A, 21-OHA* genes in the class III region.[A370,C111] Other examples of linkage disequilibrium are numerous and include the *HLA-B18, DR3, DRw52b, DQw2.1* haplotype in Southern Europeans, *HLA-B7, DR2, DQw6* in Northern Europeans, and *HLA-B42, DR3 (DRw18), DRw52a, DQw4* in African blacks.[A123,A370,B129, D362,H510,H511] The two haplotypes primarily associated with SLE in Americans and Western Europeans are shown in Figure 2–5. Linkage disequilibrium is particularly strong between HLA-DR and DQ genes[G360] (Fig. 2–4), while HLA-DP alleles show little if any association with

the other HLA loci because of a proposed high frequency of recombination between the HLA-DQ and DP loci.[K329]

Disease associations have been confounded by linkage disequilibrium. For example, the *HLA-B8, DR3* haplotype has been associated with many autoimmune diseases, including lupus.[S204,T165] Localization of the precise disease-conferring locus from among these multiple linked alleles

HLA-DQ, DR HAPLOTYPES

Fig. 2–4. Several representative haplotypes of HLA-DQA1 and DQB1 alleles are shown. The WHO allelic designations are given under each allele (darkened areas). To the left are the DQ specificities resulting from these DQA1 and DQB1 alleles, while to the right the usual DR alleles, which are in linkage disequilibrium with these DQ combinations, are shown.

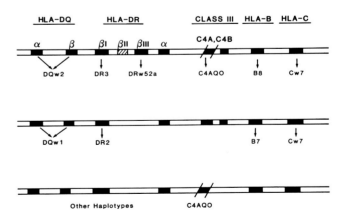

HLA HAPLOTYPES ASSOCIATED WITH SLE

Fig. 2–5. The major HLA haplotypes associated with SLE in American and Western European Caucasians are shown. There are multiple alleles in linkage disequilibrium on the HLA-B8, DR3 haplotype, including a gene deletion of C4A in the class III region. The HLA-DR2 haplotype does not possess a C4A null allele. Other haplotypes possessing C4A null genes, as well as other MHC class I and II alleles are also found in SLE patients.

is nearly impossible in Caucasian populations. Studies in other ethnic groups, where these alleles are not tightly held together, is one means of determining the primary disease-associated allele.

Determination of HLA Alleles

Tissue typing for HLA-A, B, and C antigens has conventionally been performed on peripheral blood lymphocytes in a microcytotoxicity assay utilizing a panel of anti-HLA sera obtained from multiparous women or multiply transfused donors. HLA-DR and DQ typing is similar, but only B lymphocytes are typed using antisera from which HLA-A, B, or C antibodies have been removed. Monoclonal reagents are becoming increasingly available for both class I and II typing. Mixed lymphocyte cultures (MLCs) have been used to detect HLA-DR subtypes (Dw), and primed lymphocyte typing was originally necessary to define HLA-DP alleles.[A123,B129,D362]

With the recent cloning and sequencing of most of the HLA alleles, more accurate methods are now available for typing at the DNA level, especially for HLA class II alleles.[D362] These techniques are being applied more widely and include the use of restriction fragment length polymorphisms (RFLPs) and/or small allele- or sequence-specific oligonucleotide probes hybridized to polymerase chain reaction (PCR) amplified DNA.

HLA Class II Structure-Function Relationships

The MHC contributions to SLE appear to come primarily from HLA class II and class III alleles. Therefore, the structure and function of MHC class II alleles will be given emphasis here. It should be clear, however, that only certain HLA class I alleles (A2, Aw68, and B27) have had their three-dimensional structure defined by crystallography at the time of this writing[B323,B324] (Fig. 2–6). The precise structure of class II molecules has yet to be defined, and the proposed model for class II structure is only inferred from that of class I[B521] (Fig. 2–7).

The MHC class II molecule is a heterodimer composed of non-covalently bound α and β chains[B521] (Figs. 2–3 and 2–7). The molecule's outermost or first domains form a "cleft" or "groove" with a "floor" of β-pleated sheets surrounded on each side by α helices. This cleft is believed to hold an antigenic peptide of 10 to 12 amino acids in length which is presented to the T-cell antigen receptor on CD4-positive helper T lymphocytes (Fig. 2–8). Amino acids forming the "floor" bind the peptide being presented, while those of the α helices could bind either portions of the peptide or the T-cell receptor.

The polymorphic amino acid sequences that determine each of the multiple class II alleles (Tables 2–3 and 2–4 show those for DQα and DQβ alleles) are found in this outermost domain of the class II molecule and confer fine

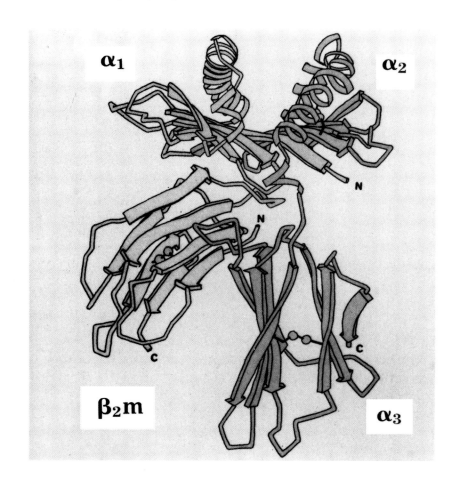

Fig. 2–6. Three-dimensional structure of the MHC class I molecule, HLA-A2. The nonpolymorphic α3 region and β2-microglobulin (β2m) function as an anchoring platform on the cell surface on top of which rest the polymorphic α1 and α2 domains. Note that α1 and α2 form an antigen-binding "groove" or "cleft" with a floor of β-pleated sheets surrounded by α helical walls. From Bjorkman, P.J., Saper, M.A., Samraoui, B. et al.: Nature (London). 329:506, 1987. With permission.[B323]

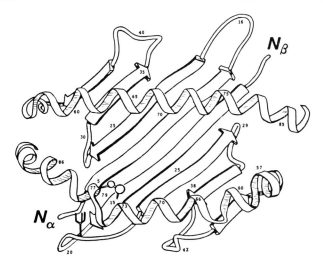

Fig. 2–7. Hypothetical model of the antigen-binding "groove" or "cleft" of an MHC class II molecule. Numbers indicate amino acid positions. Note that polymorphic amino acids constituting the first (positions 9 to 13) and second (positions 25 to 38) hypervariable regions map to the floor of the groove where they could contact and bind peptide, while those of the third (positions 57 to 86) hypervariable region are found along the α helices, where they could bind either the peptide or the T-cell antigen receptor (TCR). From Brown, J.H., Jardetzky, T., Saper, M.A. et al.: Nature (London), *332*:845, 1988. With permission.[B521]

conformational differences in the antigen-binding cleft.[G359] These polymorphisms are found primarily in three major hypervariable or diversity regions, the first including amino acids 9 to 13; the second, amino acids 25 to 38; and the third, amino acids 57 to 86. The first and second hypervariable regions map to the floor of the cleft, and the third to the α helices of the proposed model for class II structure (Fig. 2–7). These hypervariable regions, which contain the polymorphic sequences dictating different HLA antigens, (alleles) constitute the molecular basis for HLA associations with autoimmune diseases.[G359,T168] Within the *trimolecular complex* of MHC molecule, antigenic peptide, and T-cell receptor (Fig. 2–8), there appears to be a failure to discriminate self from nonself peptides. A variety of autoimmune responses thus ensue. HLA and disease associations are now centered on the molecular fine structure of disease-conferring HLA alleles and how these polymorphisms might predispose to abnormal immune responses.

HLA and Disease Associations

A variety of HLA and disease associations have been defined.[T165] In most instances, the diseases in question are believed to be immunologic in origin. Associations are based on a particular HLA antigen (allele) being statistically significantly increased in an ethnically and clinically homogeneous group of patients with a disease as compared to an ethnically matched group of normal individuals from the same locale.[T165] A probability (p) value is generated for any alleles that appear to be increased or decreased in the disease group compared to the controls.

Because there are so many HLA antigens being compared between the disease and control groups, there is a high likelihood that at least one HLA type will be increased based on chance alone (type I statistical error). Therefore, it has become conventional that a p value be corrected by multiplying it by the number of comparisons. Once an association has been so established, if it is confirmed in another different study, a correction of the p value is not necessary.

An additional calculation is also traditionally made,

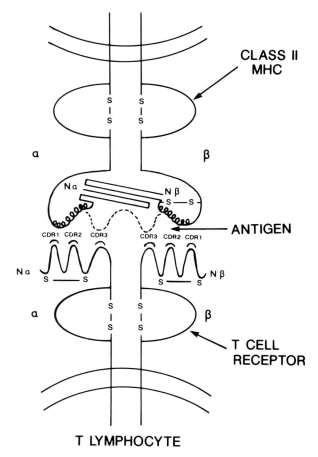

Fig. 2–8. Schematic representation of the trimolecular HLA class II antigen T-cell receptor complex. Processed antigen (indicated by the curved dotted line) is presented by the HLA class II αβ heterodimer (top) to the T-cell receptor αβ heterodimer (bottom). The first two complementarity-determining regions (CDR1 and CDR2, indicated by the double loop) interact with the α helix of the HLA class II heterodimer containing the third hypervariable amino acid segment of the outermost (first) domains and forming the wall of the antigen-presentation cleft. The putative contact points for antigen include CDR3 on the T-cell receptor and, in the floor of the antigen-presentation cleft of the HLA class II heterodimer (in β-pleated configuration), the first and second hypervariable amino acid segments of the outermost domains. Reprinted from Reveille, J.R., and Arnett, F.C.: Immunogenetics of systemic autoimmune diseases. *In* Systemic Autoimmunity. Edited by M. Reichlin and P. Bigazzi. New York, Marcel Dekker (In press).

Table 2–3. HLA-DQ α First Domain Amino Acid Sequences

	20	30	40	50	60	70	80	
DR1, 10, 14; DQw5; DQA1*0101	CGVNLYQFYG	PSGQYTHEFD	GDEEFYVDLE	RKETAWRWPE	FSKFGGFDPQ	GALRNMAVAK	HNLNIMIKRY	NSTAATN
DR4; DQw7, 8; DQA1*0301	Y	S	S	V Q L L	RR RR	F T I L	V	S
DR9; DQw9; DQA1*0301	Y	S	S	V QL L	RR RR	F T I L	V	S
DR7; DQw2.2; DQA1*0201	Y	S	F	V KL L	HR LR*	F T I L	L	S
DR2, 13; DQw6; DQA1*0102			Q					
DR5, 13; DQw6; DQw6; DQA1*0103		F	Q	K				
DR3 (DRw17); DQw2.1, DQA1*0501	Y	S	Q	G V CL V	LRQ R*	F T I L	SL	S
DR5 (DRw11), DRw14; DQw7; DQA1*0501	Y	S	Q	G V CL V	LRQ R*	F T I L	SL	S
DRw8, DR3 (DRw18); DQw4; DQA1*0401	Y	S	Q	G V CL V	LRQ R*	F T I T	L	S
DRw8; DQw4; DQA1*0601	Y	S	F Q	G V CL V	LRQ R*	F T I T	L	S

One-letter code abbreviations for amino acids: F = Phe, L = Leu, S = Ser, Y = Tyr, C = Cys, P = Pro, H = His, Q = Gln, R = Arg, I = Ile, M = Met, T = Thr, N = Asn, K = Lys, V = Val, A = Ala, D = Asp, E = Glu, G = Gly, and W = Trp.

namely *relative risk*.[T165] This is usually calculated as an *odds ratio* and quantifies the likelihood of disease in persons who possess a risk factor (HLA antigen) as compared to persons without it. A relative risk of 1 implies no association. The strength of an HLA association is directly related to the height of the relative risk.

HLA alleles may show positive or negative correlations with a disease. A positive association implies that an allele predisposes to the disease, while a negative correlation suggests that the HLA allele may be "protective," especially if it has a "dominant" effect and is not found in affected individuals in heterozygous combination with a putative disease-promoting allele. HLA alleles whose frequencies are not significantly disturbed and/or do not appear to be protective are considered "neutral" in promoting disease.

MHC associations have recently been examined at the molecular level in several autoimmune diseases and may provide guidance to studies in SLE.[G359,G361,T168] Predisposition to rheumatoid arthritis in different ethnic groups has been associated with similar amino acid sequences in the third hypervariable region shared by several HLA-DRB1 alleles, including DR4 (Dw4, Dw14, and Dw15 sequences only), DR1, DRw10, and DRw6 (Dw16). Thus, a "shared epitope" among several different HLA alleles may promote disease, but the specific alleles carrying the "epitope" may be different among affected individuals in different ethnic groups.[G359,G361] Pemphigus vulgaris shows an association with two entirely different amino acid sequences, one in HLA-DR4 (Dw10) and another in a rare DQβ allele.[T168] Protection from acquiring type I diabetes mellitus appears to be conferred by an aspartic acid in

Table 2–4. DQ β First Domain Amino Acid Sequences

	10	20	30	40	50	60	70	80	90	
DR1, 10; DQw5; DQB1*0501	RDSPEDFVYQ	FKGLCYFTNG	TERVRGVTRH	IYNREEYVRF	DSDVGVYRAV	TPQGRPVAEY	WNSQKEVLEG	ARASVDRVCR	HNYEVAYRGI	LQRR
DR2, 8; DQw6; DQB1*0601	P	L AM	Y Y	D		D	DI	R T EL T	F	
DR2, DQw5; GQB1*0502					S					
DRw14; DQw5; DQB1*0503					D					
DR4, 5, 14; DQw7; DQB1*0301		AM	Y Y	A	E	L P D		R T EL T	QLEL	TT
DR4; DQw4; DQB1*0401	F	M	LG Y	A		LLD	DI	E D T	QLEL	TT
DRw8, 18; DQw4; DQB1*0402	F	M	G Y	A		LLD	DI	E D T	QLEL	TT
DR3; DQw2; DQB1*0201		M	L S S	I	EF	LLLA		R T EL T	G	
DR2; DQw6; DQB1*0602	F	M	L Y	A		D	DI	R K A	QLEL	TT
DRw13; DQw6; DQB1*0603			L	A		D		T EL T	F	
DRw13; DQw6; DQB1*0604		M	L	A				T EL T		
DR4; DQw8; DQB1*0302		M	L Y	A		LPA		R T EL T	QLEL	TT
DR7, 9; DQw9; DQB1*0303		M	L Y	A		LPD		R T EL T	QLEL	TT

One-letter code abbreviations for amino acids: F = Phe, L = Leu, S = Ser, Y = Tyr, C = Cys, P = Pro, H = His, Q = Gln, R = Arg, I = Ile, M = Met, T = Thr, N = Asn, K = Lys, V = Val, A = Ala, D = Asp, E = Glu, G = Gly, and W = Trp.

position 57 of the DQβ chain, while alleles having neutral amino acids in position 57 confer susceptibility.[T168] Thus, it is now critical that HLA and disease associations be examined at the molecular level and in different ethnic groups.

THE T-CELL ANTIGEN RECEPTOR (TCR)

The genetics of another set of molecules involved in T-cell recognition, the T-cell antigen receptors (TCRs), also may be relevant to autoimmune diseases. TCRs have heterodimeric structures similar to MHC class I and II molecules, as well as immunoglobulins and β$_2$-microglobulin, and are classified within what has been termed the immune "supergene" family.[D59,D87,F72,H503,M188,R64] The most common TCR, present on over 95% of T cells, is the αβTCR. The αβTCR heterodimer, when expressed on CD4-positive T helper cells, recognizes antigen presented by MHC class II molecules (Fig. 2–8), but when expressed on CD8-positive cytotoxic T cells, recognizes antigens in the context of MHC class I molecules. A second type of T-cell receptor, the γδTCR, is present on a subset of CD4- and CD8-negative T lymphocytes, and has been shown to recognize self and myobacterial stress or heat-shock proteins.[V28] Although originally believed not to be MHC restricted, recent evidence suggests that interaction with MHC molecules does occur for at least some immune responses.[D87,R64]

The human genes for the TCR are not linked to the MHC on chromosome 6. The TCRα gene resides on human chromosome 14 and overlaps the gene for TCRδ, while TCRβ and γ map to human chromosome 7.[D87] Like immunoglobulin genes, the TCR genes are divided into arrays of interchangeable coding sequences scattered over large segments of DNA (Fig. 2–9). Each of these genes is composed of constant (C), junctional (J), and variable (V) regions, and TCRβ and δ also possess diversity (D) regions. Within T cells, translated TCR V, D, and J segments are rearranged and then fused together to form a V-coding domain adjacent to a particular C region, which is then expressed on the cell surface as αβ or γδ heterodimers (Fig. 2–8). These rearrangements in T cells

T CELL RECEPTOR BETA CHAIN

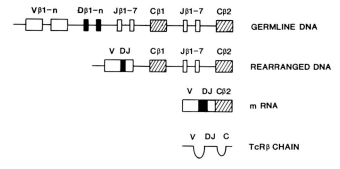

Fig. 2–9. Schematic representation of the transcription, translation, and rearrangement of a T-cell receptor β chain gene.

are very similar to those of immunoglobulin genes in B lymphocytes.

Although the MHC and TCR genes are not genetically linked, it is theoretically possible that combinations of certain MHC and TCR haplotypes, which conferred a selective advantage, could have co-evolved. If this were the case, individuals with certain MHC alleles should show associations with certain germline TCR haplotypes. One study in normal Caucasians homozygous for HLA-DR2, DR3, or DR4 demonstrated no such correlations with TCR haplotypes.[C212] Nonetheless, distinct MHC and TCR, especially V region, associations may still exist, and future disease studies should control for this possibility.

MHC ASSOCIATIONS WITH SLE

HLA Class I and II Alleles

Knowledge of HLA associations with SLE has paralleled that of the MHC itself. The first reports[G416,W94] in 1971 and shortly thereafter[G242,N94,S620] described increased frequencies of certain HLA class I specificities, at a time when only two allelic series, later to be designated HLA-A and B, were detectable by serologic HLA typing. Multiple weak associations with various specificities were reported. HLA-B8 was found most consistently[G242,G416,W94] but was later found to reflect only linkage disequilibrium with the class II alleles HLA-DR3 and DQw2. Mixed lymphocyte culture (MLC) was first used to determine alleles of the HLA-D region; however, attempts to type SLE patients were unsuccessful because of poor viability of lymphocytes.[S622] When products of HLA-D were discovered on B lymphocytes (B-cell alloantigens, Ia antigens, D-related or DR antigens), serologic HLA-DR typing became possible.

Reinertsen et al.[R137] first determined HLA-DR specificities in Caucasians with SLE and found HLA-DR2 and HLA-DR3 each significantly increased in frequency. In addition, another B-cell alloantigen, detected by alloantiserum Ia-715, was also increased. This specificity soon thereafter was designated MBI (MTI) but was later shown to represent an HLA-DQ molecule, DQw1, which was in linkage disequilibrium with HLA-DR2 and DRw6. Another serum, Ia-172, was reactive in the majority of SLE patients, and this specificity was later designated MT2 and thereafter HLA-DRw52, an allelic series from the DRB3 locus in linkage disequilibrium with HLA-DR3, DR5, DRw6, and DRw8 haplotypes.

Gibofsky et al.[G121] found that 75% of 24 whites with SLE had either HLA-DR2 or DR3, or both, and Stasny[S622] and Schur et al.[S205] noted these same antigens to be slightly increased in their patients. Other studies by Scherak et al.[S123,S124] and Celada et al.,[C177] however, found only HLA-DR3 to be significantly associated with SLE, and Gladman et al.[G175] noted an excess of HLA-DR2.

Ahearn et al.[A66] and Alvarellos et al.[A169] could show significant correlations with HLA-DR2 and DRw52 but not HLA-DR3 in 87 SLE patients. Several studies of whites have found no significant HLA-DR associations with SLE.[B118,B184] When all of these studies are viewed together, the consensus is that HLA-DR2 and DR3 are increased in Caucasian SLE patients of Western European descent. More recent studies using molecular genetic methods to define HLA class II alleles in SLE patients have confirmed previous reports which used serologic HLA typing. Dunckley et al.[D355] reported HLA-DR3, but not HLA-DR2, defined by restriction fragment length polymorphisms (RFLPs), to be increased in white Australians with SLE. Using similar techniques, So et al. found both HLA-DR2 and DR3 alleles to be increased in an English lupus population.[S530] Neither of these studies determined HLA-DQ or DP alleles. Reveille et al.[R169] used RFLPs to define HLA-DR, DQ, and DP alleles in 60 Caucasians from Alabama; HLA-DR3 (DRw17) and DQw2.1, which are in linkage disequilibrium, were the only MHC class II alleles increased in this patient population. Reinharz et al.,[R141] using oligonucleotide probes, found only HLA-DR3 increased in Swiss patients, and in a surprising observation found no HLA-DR2/DR3, DR2/DR7, or DQB1*0602/*0201 heterozygotes in their patients. Others have not found this to be the case and, in fact, these haplotypic combinations provide the strongest association with the anti-Ro and La autoantibody responses in SLE and Sjögren's syndrome (to be discussed later).

Studies of HLA associations with diseases across ethnic and racial groups are important in removing the confounding effects of linkage disequilibrium and helping to localize the actual disease-conferring alleles.[G359, G361,S204,T168] This approach has been helpful in other autoimmune diseases such as rheumatoid arthritis, type I diabetes mellitus, and pemphigus vulgaris. Unlike these other disorders, which result from one or a limited number of abnormal autoimmune responses, SLE is a composite of multiple autoimmune phenomena. Thus, HLA studies of this heterogeneous disease in peoples of non–Western European origin have yielded only limited information.

Alarif et al.[A118] reported HLA-DR3 increased in 57% of 31 blacks with SLE, compared to 27% in local black controls in Washington, D.C. Kachru et al.[K4] studied 37 Chicago blacks and found HLA-DR3 in 62% (control frequency 18%). Gladman et al.[G175] noted an excess of HLA-DR2 in Toronto blacks, which was not statistically significant. Wilson et al.[W276] reported HLA-DR7 increased (50%) in 28 Louisiana blacks compared to a local normal frequency of 17%. Hochberg et al.[H347] found no disturbances of HLA class II antigen frequencies in 37 Baltimore blacks, and utilizing RFLPs Reveille et al.[R176] reported no associations in 63 Alabama blacks. A similar negative study has been reported in blacks from the French West Indies.[M547] No studies have yet been reported from Africa.

The Japanese population has a negligible frequency of HLA-DR3, yet SLE is not uncommon. Kameda et al.[K44] examined 55 patients with SLE for HLA-A and B specificities and found none to be increased. HLA-DR typing in 45 Japanese SLE patients and 36 controls revealed HLA-DR2 in 51 and 25%, respectively.[K44] This difference was not statistically significant; however, if these frequencies were to be maintained in a larger series, statistical significance would be attained. Hashimoto et al.[H188] and Kawai et al.[K127] also reported an increased frequency of HLA-DR2. On the other hand, Hirose et al.[H327] reported an increased

frequency of HLA-DR2/DR4 heterozygotes in Japanese SLE patients of young disease onset. Nishikai and Sekiguchi[N103] found a significant excess of HLA-DQw3 in 88% of 32 Japanese SLE patients compared to 48% in normals.

Among 75 Chinese SLE patients, HLA-B17 was associated with severe and HLA-B13 with mild SLE; however, HLA-DR antigens were not tested.[C202] More recently, Hawkins et al.[H215] studied 100 Chinese patients and found HLA-DR2 to be significantly increased (62 versus 38% in controls).

Olsen et al.[O74] have recently determined HLA-DR, DQ, and DP alleles in 31 Greek patients with SLE and 27 Greek controls. HLA-DR2 occurred in 61% of SLE patients and 37% of controls (p = NS). In these patients, an unusual DR2 (DRw15), DQw5 (DQB1*0502 or DQB1.AZH) haplotype was found which is uncommon in Americans and other Europeans. In 32 Mexican-Americans from Texas with SLE, Reveille et al.[R175] found no HLA-DR, DQ, or DP associations with disease by DNA typing. It must be emphasized that in all of the ethnic groups studied thus far (Western Europeans, American Caucasians, American blacks, Mexican-Americans, Greeks, Japanese, and Chinese), associations with C4A null alleles in the MHC class III region have been found.[A298] In fact, C4 null alleles correlate far stronger with SLE itself across racial lines than any other MHC factor, and this is discussed in Chapter 13. The MHC class II associations correlate more strongly with autoantibody subsets of SLE rather than with the disease itself (to be discussed).

Attempts to find particular clinical manifestations of SLE that might assort more strongly with HLA genes have been largely unrewarding. The cutaneous lupus subsets are the exception and will be subsequently discussed. Ahearn et al.[A66] detected no HLA specificities that correlated with lupus-related sicca complex, nephritis, cerebritis, or vasculitis in 70 patients. Schur et al.[S205] reported that lupus arthritis might be associated with HLA-DQw1 and a low frequency of HLA-DR5, and pericarditis with HLA-Aw32 in a series of 63 patients. Kawai et al.[K127] have reported increased frequencies of HLA-B7 and Bw61 in Japanese patients with central nervous system involvement.

Recently, Fronek et al.[F289] studied 44 SLE patients with and 25 without nephritis for HLA-DR and DQ alleles using RFLPs and DNA sequencing of selected alleles. HLA-DR2 was significantly increased in those with (59%) versus those without renal disease (36%). HLA-DR3 was not increased in this SLE series, and HLA-DR4 was significantly reduced in frequency. Certain HLA-DQβ alleles, the DQw65 and DQw6 subtypes of DQw1, were found to show the strongest associations with lupus nephritis when compared to normal controls (but not when compared to lupus patients without nephritis). One particular DQw5 type (DQw1.AZH or DQB1*0502), occurring in 25% of nephritis patients, was significantly increased as compared to the nonrenal patients (6%). HLA-DQw1 itself (including the DQw5 and DQw6 subtypes), which is in linkage disequilibrium with HLA-DR1, 2, and w6, was even more strongly associated with lupus nephritis. The authors postulated that shared amino acids in the first or third hypervariable regions of the DQβ chain of certain DQw1-associated alleles might promote lupus nephritis. Unfortunately, this study relied on historical rather than local, ethnically matched controls. Others have not found DQw5 or DQw6 to be associated with nephritis.[R141,R169] Moreover, the DQw1.AZH (DQB1*0502) allele is very rare in other American SLE studies (5 of 254 SLE patients studied in Houston and Alabama), but it is very common among Greeks with and without SLE and among Ashkenazi Jews.[F289,O74]

Age of onset appears to discriminate different genetic subsets of SLE. Bell and colleagues[B187] reported that HLA-B8 and HLA-DR3 were significantly increased in white women with SLE whose disease onset was over the age of 35 (mean 48 years). HLA-DR3 was not significantly increased in younger-onset (mean 22 years) females compared to sex-matched controls. Moreover, 14 males showed increased frequencies for HLA-B8 and DR3 compared to normal males.

Hochberg et al.[H347] have confirmed and extended these data in 113 white patients with SLE whose ages at diagnosis were correlated with HLA status. The frequency of HLA-DR2 was 48% in the youngest disease-onset quartile (<22 years) and 23% in the oldest (>44 years). The local control frequency for HLA-DR2 was 24%. Similarly, HLA-DQw1 (which is in linkage disequilibrium with DR2) occurred in 76% of the younger-onset group, 55% of the older group, and 55% of controls. Altered frequencies of HLA-DR2 were more impressive when the youngest-onset quartile (48% positive) was compared to patients diagnosed over age 50 (16% positive). The prevalence of HLA-DQw1 was also decreased (42%) in those over age 50. Its frequency in younger-onset patients (24%) did not differ from controls (25%). Thus, while Bell et al.[B187] noted a bimodality in age of onset and Hochberg et al.[H347] a unimodal distribution, both showed a segregation of HLA-DR3 into those with older onset, and Hochberg et al.[H347] revealed an association of HLA-DR2 and DQw1 with younger disease onset.

MHC CLASS II ASSOCIATIONS WITH AUTOANTIBODIES IN SLE

Because SLE is characterized by a myriad of autoantibodies, the concept of serologic subsets has been evolving recently. Indeed, many clinical features of disease appear to correlate with certain autoantibodies, and in some cases the autoantibody is believed to participate directly in the pathogenesis of the clinical manifestation. Moreover, since HLA molecules participate in T-cell–dependent antigen-specific immune responses, stronger correlations have been found between HLA alleles and certain autoantibodies (Table 2–5).

Anti–Double-Stranded (ds) DNA Antibodies

Anti-dsDNA antibodies are found in 40 to 60% of SLE patients, are highly specific for SLE, and correlate with glomerulonephritis. Anti-dsDNA–DNA immune complexes have been found in the glomerular lesions.

Griffing et al.[G376] first reported a strong correlation of HLA-DR3 with antibodies to dsDNA detected by a millipore filter assay. Ahearn et al.[A66] and Alvarellos et al.[A169] reported that high levels of anti-dsDNA detected by Farr and *Crithidia luciliae* assays were associated with HLA-DR2, and possibly DQw1, in their series of patients. Schur et al.[S205] noted HLA-DR7 to be increased in anti-DNA positives.

In a recent study of 126 SLE patients, whose MHC class II alleles were determined by DNA oligotyping, Khanduja et al.[K190] reported the strongest correlations between anti-dsDNA antibodies and certain HLA-DQβ alleles. HLA-DQB1*0201 (linked to DR3 and DR7), DQB1*0602 (linked to DR2 and DRw6), and DQB1*0302 (linked to some HLA-DR4 haplotypes) occurred in 96% of patients having high levels of anti-dsDNA antibodies. None of these HLA-DQ alleles were specifically associated with nephritis, although anti-dsDNA itself was significantly correlated with renal involvement. There was a trend suggesting that HLA-DQB1*0201 (linked to DR3 and DR7) was more frequent in patients with anti-dsDNA who do not develop renal disease. The HLA-DQB1 allele *0502 (AZH), as well as other DQw6 alleles (DQB1*0501 and *0503) reported by Fronek et al.[F289] to be increased in lupus nephritis patients, were infrequently found in the series reported by Khanduja et al.[K190] On the other hand, Olsen et al.[O74] recently found an increased frequency of HLA-DQB1*0502 (AZH) in Greek SLE patients with anti-dsDNA, and this allele has a high background frequency in this population.

The three HLA-DQβ alleles (*0201, *0602, and *0302) associated with anti-dsDNA antibodies by Kunduja et

Table 2–5. Associations of MHC Class II Alleles and Outer Domain Amino Acids with Specific Autoantibodies in Systemic Lupus Erythematosus

Autoantibodies	Previous Associations with MHC Specificities	Currently Associated MHC Alleles (Specificities)	Proposed Critical Amino Acid Residues Within MHC Molecules
Anti-dsDNA	DR3, DR2	DQB1*0201, *0602, and *0302	DQβ *methionine* 14 and *leucine* 26
Anti-Sm	None	DQw6 (DQB1*0602 and/or DQA1*0102)	Unknown
Anti-nRNP (U1-RNP)	DR4	DQw5, DQw8	Unknown
Antiphospholipid	DR4, DR7	DQw7 (DQB1*0301), DQw8 (*0302), DQw9 (*0303), and DQw6 (*0602)	DQβ positions 71–77
Anti-EBA (type 7 procollagen)	DR2	DR2	Unknown
Anti-Ro (SSA) and anti-La (SSB)	DR3, DR2, DQw1/DQw2	DQA1*0501, *0101–*0104, *0402 DQB1*0201, *0601, 0604, and *0302	DQα1 *glutamine* 34 DQβ1 *leucine* 26

al.[K190] share in common a *methionine* in position 14 and a *leucine* in position 26 of the DQβ outermost domain, which might represent the critical residues for this autoimmune response; however, HLA-DQB1*0502 (AZH) found in Greeks does not share this same molecular motif.

Anti-Sm and nRNP Antibodies

Autoantibodies to the small nuclear ribonucleoproteins (snRNPs) involved in splicing of mRNA occur frequently in SLE patients, especially blacks.[A297] Anti-Sm antibodies are directed against U1, U2, U4, U5, and U6 snRNPs and are highly specific for SLE. Anti-nRNP (U1-RNP) often accompanies anti-Sm in lupus patients, but frequently is found in SLE patients without anti-Sm, as well as in mixed connective tissue disease (MCTD), scleroderma, and polymyositis. In some SLE series, these autoantibodies, especially anti-nRNP (U1-RNP), have been correlated with complicating Raynaud's phenomenon, myositis, and/or myocarditis.

Previous HLA associations with anti-Sm and nRNP based on serologic HLA typing have been few and weak. Schur et al.[S205] reported a correlation of anti-Sm with HLA-DR7. Bell and Maddison,[B184] and Ahearn et al.[A66] found no HLA correlations with anti-Sm or nRNP, and Hamilton et al.[H187] noted only a negative correlation with HLA-DQw1/DQw2 heterozygosity. Smolen et al.[S520] found an increased frequency of HLA-DR4 in white SLE patients with anti-Sm or anti-nRNP, and Nishikai and Sekiguchi[N103] reported an excess of HLA-DQw33 (now DQw7, 8, or 9) in Japanese patients with anti-nRNP. Hoffman et al.[H363] have recently found HLA-DR4 to be associated with an anti−70 kD protein of U1-RNP reported to be more common to MCTD than to SLE patients.[P162]

Olsen et al.[O73] using RFLPs and oligotyping of American whites and blacks have recently found a correlation of anti-Sm (with or without anti-nRNP) with HLA-DR2. More striking, however, was the correlation with a subtype of HLA-DQw6 (DQA1*0102 and DQB1*0602), which is in linkage disequilibrium with some HLA-DR2 and DRw6 haplotypes. In contrast, there was a significantly decreased frequency of this HLA-DQw6 subtype in SLE patients having anti-nRNP without anti-Sm. Anti-nRNP in the absence of anti-Sm appeared to show increased frequencies of HLA-DQw5, DQw8, and DQw7; however, these studies are still in progress.

Antiphospholipid Antibodies

Antiphospholipid antibodies (APAs), as determined by anticardiolipin assays or detection as a circulating lupus anticoagulant, are being appreciated increasingly as playing a role in certain manifestations of SLE. APAs have been associated with a tendency for spontaneous intravascular thrombotic events, thrombocytopenia, Libman-Sacks endocarditis, livedo reticularis, recurrent miscarriages and fetal wastage. These same clinical features may occur in association with APAs in individuals without SLE, necessitating the recent introduction of the diagnostic term, primary antiphospholipid antibody syndrome.

Studies of HLA antigens in patients with APAs are few. Savi et al.[S98] reported an increased frequency of HLA-DR7

in Italian patients with anticardiolipin antibodies, and McHugh et al.[M290] found HLA-DR4 to be increased in English patients. Both of these studies utilized serologic HLA typing, and HLA-DQ frequencies were not reported. A potentially unifying HLA allele common to the findings of both of these studies could be the HLA-DRB4 allele, DRw53, which is represented on both DR4 and DR7 haplotypes, and a recent preliminary report by Goldstein et al.[G273] using RFLPs in Canadian patients supported this possibility by finding an increased frequency of HLA-DRw53. In another recent study using RFLPs, Arnett et al.[A299] found HLA-DR5, DQw7 haplotypes, which do not carry DRw53, to be significantly increased in American patients with the lupus anticoagulant. Patients with SLE, other connective tissue diseases, and primary APA syndrome were included, and the HLA specificity showing the strongest association was HLA-DQw7, specifically the HLA-DQB1*0301 allele occurring in 70% of patients with the lupus anticoagulant. Among the HLA-DQw7−negative patients, all possessed HLA-DQw8, DQw9, and/or DQw6. All of these HLA-DQβ alleles share the same amino acid sequence in positions 71 to 77 of the HLA-DQβ third hypervariable region, and this may represent the major "epitope" promoting this autoimmune response. In a more recent study of Mexican-American patients with SLE and anticardiolipin antibodies, HLA-DQw7 and/or DQw8 were again associated with APA.[M227]

Anti-EBA or Type 7 Procollagen

The autoimmune bullous skin disease, epidermolysis bullosa acquisita (EBA), has recently been shown to result from autoantibodies to epidermal type 7 procollagen. Rarely, patients with SLE develop bullous skin lesions and the same autoantibody appears to be present. Gammon et al.[G26] have studied HLA antigens in white and black patients with autoantibodies to type 7 procollagen. HLA-DR2 is strongly associated with this autoantibody in both patients with primary EBA and those with bullous lupus.

Anti-Ro (SSA) and La (SSB) Antibodies

Anti-Ro and anti-La are linked autoantibody responses which occur frequently in both SLE and Sjögren's syndrome. Anti-La rarely if ever occurs in the absence of anti-Ro, and is present more often in Sjögren's syndrome than in SLE.

Bell and Maddison[B184] first reported a high frequency of HLA-DR3 (and HLA-B8) in white anti-Ro−positive SLE patients, which was not significantly increased in their SLE patient group as a whole. Ahearn et al.[A66] and Alvarellos et al.[A169] confirmed the association of HLA-DR3 with the Ro antibody response in white SLE patients, but also demonstrated an increased frequency of HLA-DQw2 (then MB2) linked to DR3, as well as an increased frequency of HLA-DR2 in HLA-DR3−negative patients. The presence of the co-occurrence of HLA-DR2 and DR3 was even more strongly correlated with anti-Ro. The presence of anti-Ro, but not the HLA antigens, was also statistically significantly correlated with the sicca-complex, hyperglobulinemia, and the presence of rheumatoid factor in these SLE patients.

Catoggio et al.[C158] first demonstrated that anti-Ro, usually accompanied by anti-La, was more common in elderly SLE patients. Hochberg et al.[H347] showed that anti-Ro without anti-La and HLA-DR2 both occurred in SLE patients with young age of disease onset, while anti-Ro with anti-La and HLA-DR3 were present in patients with older ages of onset. The association of HLA-DR3 with anti-Ro in SLE was further confirmed in other Caucasians of Western European descent by Smolen et al.[S520]

In Louisiana blacks with SLE, Wilson et al.[W276] found HLA-DR7 in 13 of 17 (76%) with anti-Ro but in only 1 of 11 patients without this antibody. Hochberg et al.[H347] found no increased HLA specificities, including DR3, DR2, and DR7 in Baltimore blacks with SLE and anti-Ro. Nishikai and Sekiguchi[N103] could correlate no HLA-DR or DQ antigens with anti-Ro in Japanese patients, a population in which HLA-DR3 is only rarely found.

Sjögren's syndrome frequently complicates the course of SLE, and primary Sjögren's syndrome shares many overlapping clinical and serologic features with SLE. Moreover, anti-Ro and La autoantibodies occur in both disorders and appear to demonstrate the same HLA associations. Reveille and Arnett recently have reviewed the genetics of Sjögren's syndrome.[R170]

Primary Sjögren's syndrome was first demonstrated to have significantly elevated frequencies of HLA-B8 and Dw3 (determined by MHC).[C265,F325,M117] Subsequently, Moutsopoulos et al.[M637] demonstrated a stronger association of HLA-DR3 with primary Sjögren's syndrome. Even more impressive, however, was the demonstration of HLA-DRw52 (MT2), defined by antisera Ia-172 and Ia-350, in 100% of 22 such patients. In addition, while HLA-DR3 was not increased in 11 rheumatoids with secondary sicca, the DRw52 (MT2) specificity was found in significant excess. (82%)

Wilson et al.[W273] examined 102 patients with Sjögren's syndrome: 55 with primary disease, 20 with rheumatoid arthritis and sicca, 20 with SLE and sicca, and 7 with PSS and/or myositis and sicca. HLA-DR3 was increased in blacks (80%) and whites (50%) with primary Sjögren's syndrome but was not elevated in patients with secondary sicca. On the other hand, HLA-DRw52 (MT2) occurred in 87% of those with primary Sjögren's syndrome, and was also significantly increased in the secondary sicca complex occurring in rheumatoid arthritis (80%), SLE (90%), and PSS-myositis (86%) compared to normal frequencies of 46% in whites and 65% in blacks. HLA-DRw52 (MT2) was also significantly increased in white patients with rheumatoid arthritis and SLE who had secondary sicca compared to their counterparts without sicca complaints.

In Sjögren's syndrome, anti-Ro has been found to correlate strongly with vasculitis, hematologic cytopenias, and, like in SLE, rheumatoid factor and hyperglobulinemia.[A133,W273] When Wilson et al.[W273] examined the relationships of HLA antigens to Ro and La antibodies, they found that anti-Ro was, as in SLE, strongly associated with HLA-DR2 and DR3. In fact, 96% of anti-Ro positives with primary Sjögren's syndrome had HLA-DR2, DR3, or both, as well as 80% of those with secondary sicca. Thus, while HLA-DRw52 (MT2) was the strongest HLA correlate with the disease (primary and secondary sicca), the DR2 and DR3 specificities were more closely allied to the Ro antibody response. La antibody was strongly associated only with HLA-DR3.

Harley et al.[H134] examined 86 of these same sera using a sensitive ELISA assay to detect Ro and La antibodies. Both antibodies were found in the sera of over 95% of these Sjögren's syndrome patients. Titers of Ro and La antibodies closely paralleled each other, as well as levels of rheumatoid factor, IgG, and IgA. Patients having the highest levels of anti-Ro and La had a significant excess of HLA-DR3 compared to their counterparts with lower antibody levels. Harley et al.[H137] later examined frequencies of the newly serologically defined HLA-DQ alleles in the same anti-Ro and La-positive patients with primary Sjögren's syndrome. A striking association was found between heterozygosity for HLA-DQw1/DQw2 and the highest Ro and La autoantibody levels. Since DQα and DQβ chains are both polymorphic, it was hypothesized that trans-associated "hybrid" DQαβ molecules[G130] might account for this quantitative effect. Using the same ELISA, Hamilton et al.[H87] examined anti-Ro and La levels in SLE patients in relation to HLA-DR and DQ. HLA-DQw1/DQw2 heterozygosity again appeared to exert a quantitative effect on Ro and La autoantibody levels in SLE patients. Moreover, HLA-DR2 was significantly associated with anti-Ro without anti-La, and HLA-DR3 correlated with anti-Ro with anti-La. Levels of Ro antibodies were higher in the HLA-DR3– rather than the HLA-DR2–associated groups.

Utilizing RFLPs to define HLA-DR and DQ alleles in both white and black Americans with SLE or Sjögren's syndrome having Ro and La antibodies, Arnett et al.[A292] demonstrated that the Caucasian *HLA-DR3 (DRw17), DQw2.1* haplotype was associated with these autoantibodies in both races. The African haplotype, *HLA-DR3 (DRw18), DQw4*, was not increased in the black patients. Thus, since HLA-DR3 (DRw17) and DR3 (DRw18) have very similar structures, differing by only four conservative amino acid substitutions,[H510;H511] HLA-DQ alleles, specifically HLA-DQw2.1 rather than HLA-DR3 appeared to be the most relevant MHC class II specificity predisposing to this autoimmune response. Moreover, in many American black patients with this autoantibody response, racial admixture appeared to play a role since they possessed the Caucasian *DR3 (DRw17), DQw2.1* haplotype. In addition, approximately 25% of anti-Ro and La positives were heterozygotes for HLA-DQw6 (a subtype of DQw1) and DQw2.1 (a subtype of DQw2) as compared to only 2 to 5% of anti-Ro–negative SLE/Sjögren's syndrome patients and normal race-matched controls. Fujisaku et al.[F300] subsequently reported the simultaneous occurrence of a DQα RFLP associated with DQw1 and a DQβ RFLP associated with DQw2 in their anti-Ro–positive SLE patients.

Reveille et al.[R174] subsequently defined all HLA-DR, DQ, and DP alleles in white and black patients with anti-Ro antibodies using sequence-specific oligonucleotide probes. HLA-DR3 (DRw17), DQw2.1, and heterozygosity for DQw6/DQw2.1 remained the strongest associations in both races. Among patients who were positive for the autoantibodies but were DQw2.1 negative, HLA-DQw6 emerged as the next most strongly associated specificity. In the remaining Ro antibody positives, the DQB1*0302 allele (linked to some DR4 haplotypes) and the DQA1*0401 allele [linked to some DRw8 and DR3 (DRw18) haplotypes], especially in blacks, were found in the remainder. Moreover, as can be seen in Figure 2–4, the DQB1 allele (*0201) of DQw2.1 is represented on DR7, DQw2.2 haplotypes, and the DQA1 allele of DQw2.1 (*0501) is present on DR5 and some DR4 haplotypes bearing DQw7. Thus, the net effect of heterozygosity for DR5 (or DR4) and DR7 haplotypes could be the transassociation of these DQ alleles to produce the DQw2.1 specificity (see Fig. 2–4). No other DR or DP alleles were significantly increased in either race with these autoantibodies. Thus, the Ro and La antibody responses appear restricted to a limited number of HLA-DQA1 and HLA-DQB1 alleles represented on DR2 and DR3, as well as a variety of other class II haplotypes. (See Tables 2–3 and 2–4.) A gene dosage effect of these alleles was also apparent, with most anti-Ro and La-positive patients having three or four of the relevant DQ alleles and none with less than two. A recent study by Kwok et al.[K492] suggests that α chains of DQw1 (DQw5 and DQw6) cannot pair on the cell surface with β chains of DQw2 (2.1 and 2.2) or DQw3 (DQw7, 8, and 9), while those of DQw2 and DQw3 can. Thus, hybrid DQ molecules is a less likely explanation than gene dosage for the association of HLA-DQw6/DQw2.1 heterozygosity demonstrated for the Ro and La autoimmune responses. The DQB1*0201 (DQw2.1) allele represented on DR3 (DRw17) and DR7 haplotypes appears to be most important to the anti-La response, while the DQA1 of DQw2.1, DQw6, and DQw8 alleles may be more important to anti-Ro alone.

At the molecular level, all of the DQα alleles associated with anti-Ro possess in common a *glutamine* in position 34, and all of the DQβ alleles share a *leucine* in position 26 of the outermost domains (Tables 2–3 and 2–4). These amino acids appear critical to autoreactivity to Ro and La, and both would be predicted to map to the floor of the proposed model for MHC class II molecules (Fig. 2–10). This location would be relevant to binding the putative peptides which initiate and/or perpetuate these autoimmune responses. Finally, only one animal model of SLE (and Sjögren's syndrome), the MRL lpr/lpr mouse, has been found to spontaneously produce autoantibodies to Ro and La. The H-2 I-A alleles of this mouse, which are equivalent to HLA-DQ in humans, have recently been sequenced, and the I-A α chain possesses a *glutamine* in position 34 and the I-A β chain a *leucine* in position 26, similar to humans.

HLA IN OTHER CLINICAL/SEROLOGIC SUBSETS OF LUPUS

Several lupus-like syndromes characterized clinically by a distinctive cutaneous eruption and serologically by the Ro and La antibodies have been described. Applications of HLA studies have helped to confirm their homogeneity. These disorders provide additional clues supporting the likelihood that the MHC exerts its effect on certain autoantibody responses that, in turn, produce or accompany factors leading to clinical manifestations characteristic of lupus erythematosus.

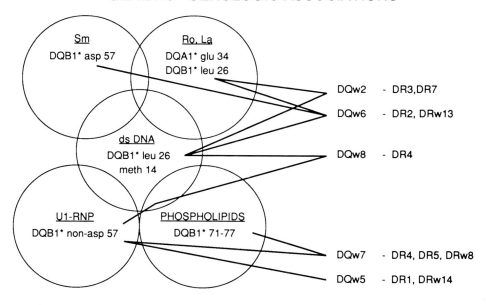

SYSTEMIC LUPUS ERYTHEMATOSUS
GENETIC - SEROLOGIC ASSOCIATIONS

Fig. 2–10. Schematic representation of current HLA associations with autoantibody subsets of SLE. HLA-DR and their linked HLA-DQ alleles are shown outside the autoantibody circles. The currently hypothesized amino acid residues within HLA-DQ molecules which show the strongest associations with specific autoantibodies are shown within the circles.

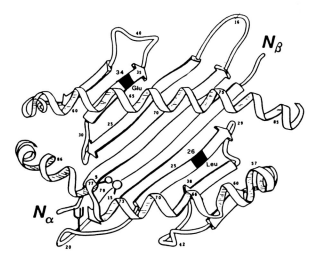

Fig. 2–11. Schematic representation of the proposed structure of the antigen-binding groove or cleft of an MHC class II molecule. The presence of *glutamine* in position 34 of the α chain and *leucine* in position 26 of the β chain appear to be the critical residues for the Ro (SSA) and La (SSB) autoantibody responses [Reveille et al[R174]]. In addition, the *leucine* in position 26 also is associated with anti-dsDNA antibodies [Khanduja et al[K190]]. Adapted from Brown, J.H., Jardetzky, T., Saper, M.A. et al.: Nature (London), *332*:845, 1988. With permission.[B521]

Subacute Cutaneous Lupus Erythematosus (SCLE)

Sontheimer et al.[S568] described a clinically distinct, non-scarring variety of cutaneous LE, which they termed SCLE. The disorder was further characterized by a paucity of systemic manifestations and the frequent absence of antinuclear and anti-DNA antibodies. It is possible that SCLE encompasses the same nosologic group termed "ANA-negative lupus" by Maddison et al.[M48] The skin manifestations of SCLE include large annular, often photosensitive and widespread, lesions and/or a papulosquamous eruption that may be confused with psoriasis.

Sontheimer et al.[S567] separated patients with these two types of skin lesions into two subgroups and studied their HLA phenotypes. HLA-B8 was significantly increased in the 11 patients composing the annular subgroup (81%), but HLA-DR3 was universally found (100%). The papulosquamous subgroup also showed a significant excess of HLA-DR3 (60%). The overall relative risk for HLA-DR3 in SCLE was 10.8, which climbed to 67 in the annular subgroup. The investigators carefully scrutinized patients for Sjögren's syndrome using a questionnaire, ophthalmologic evaluation, and minor salivary gland biopsies. None of their patients had overt or subclinical sicca. Ro antibodies were found in 15 of 24 (63%) SCLE patients, and La antibodies in 6 (25%).[S566] The annular subgroup was more likely to demonstrate anti-Ro (73%) than the papulosquamous subgroup (54%), and HLA-DR3 occurred in all 8 patients having both the annular lesions and anti-Ro antibodies. Thus, anti-Ro and HLA-DR3 are intimately linked in this cutaneous subset of lupus erythematosus. While molecular studies have not yet been reported, in SCLE patients it is likely that the Ro and La autoantibodies

will be found to be associated with the HLA-DQA1 and DQB1 alleles discussed earlier (Table 2–5). (See Chapter 31.)

The Lupus-like Syndrome of Homozygous C2 Deficiency

A cutaneous syndrome with annular lesions similar to those in SCLE is often seen in patients homozygous for deficiency of the second component of complement (C2).[A54] Systemic features are infrequent, and antinuclear antibodies and anti-DNA are usually absent. Provost et al.[P308] determined autoantibodies in the sera of 20 patients with homozygous C2 deficiency. Anti-Ro (but not anti-La) occurred in 9 of 12 (70%) of those with lupus-like diseases. The C2 deficient gene is located on an HLA-*A25, B18, DR2, DQw6* bearing haplotype. Interestingly, in this setting the anti-Ro response is associated with HLA-DR2 by virtue of its linkage disequilibrium with the C2 null allele. Whether HLA-DR2 or DQw6 is playing any role, however, is not known. (See Chapter 13.)

Neonatal Lupus Erythematosus (NLE)

In 1954, McCuistion and Schoch[M254] described an infant girl (originally misprinted as boy) with lupus dermatitis which regressed by age 5 months. The child's mother was asymptomatic before and during pregnancy but developed fatal SLE 11 months postpartum. In 1945, Plant and Steven[P219] described a newborn with congenital complete heart block whose mother was thought to have only coincidental SLE. Multiple reports of neonatal discoid-like lesions and/or congenital heart block appeared in the 1950s, 1960s, and 1970s, along with the demonstration that the LE-cell phenomenon, antinuclear antibodies, and biologic false-positive tests for syphilis could be transplacentally passed from mother to infant.[B151,B248,B488,B584,E6, E119,F218,H372] Hull et al.[H494,J9,M360,M405,N44,N84] showed convincingly that congenital heart block with conduction system fibrosis was associated with maternal lupus erythematosus. The nearly universal presence of Ro antibody in NLE suggests that it may play a pathogenic role in producing the skin and cardiac lesions. The cutaneous lesions of NLE are strikingly similar to the annular subgroup of SCLE[S566] and the lupus-like syndrome of homozygous C2 deficiency.[P308]

Lockshin et al.[L352] performed HLA typing in the family of a child with neonatal rash and heart block whose mother had mild SLE. Both mother and child carried Ro and La antibodies. The mother was HLA-B8 and DR3 positive, but the child did not inherit this maternal haplotype. Lee et al.[L132] studied six NLE families, in which five of the anti-Ro–positive mothers were clinically asymptomatic. Five mothers were positive for HLA-DR3 and HLA-DQw2 (MB2). Compared to an ethnically matched normal control group, HLA-DR3 was significantly associated with anti-Ro–positive mothers having an affected NLE infant (relative risk = 32). On the other hand, the NLE infants did not inherit this maternal HLA-DR3–bearing haplotype any more often than expected by chance. In fact, only one of seven infants was DR3 positive. Thus, it appears that the MHC influences autoantibody production in the mother but is not a prerequisite for expression of NLE in the infant.

Watson et al.[W103] studied HLA antigens in 11 NLE families, contrasting them with those in 10 anti-Ro antibody-positive mothers and infants who did not demonstrate the NLE syndrome. Again, mothers with anti-Ro having infants with NLE had significantly elevated frequencies of the HLA-A1, B8, DR3, DQw2 haplotypes (91%). The infants with NLE again appeared to inherit HLA types randomly. In sharp contrast, anti-Ro–positive mothers of clinically normal infants had significantly increased frequencies of HLA-DR2 (70%) and DQw1 (90%). Arnaiz-Villena et al.[A290] recently presented some additional anti-Ro–positive mothers having children with congenital complete heart block. The HLA-B8, DR3 haplotype bearing deleted *C4A,21-OHA* genes rather than the HLA-B18, DR3 haplotype not having a deleted C4 null allele occurred more frequently in anti-Ro–positive, DR3-positive mothers of children with heart block than in anti-Ro–positive, DR3-positive mothers having normal infants. The data suggested that the C4A null allele might further predispose to the cardiac complication; however, the numbers of patients studied was small.

Harley et al.[H135] determined anti-Ro antibody levels using EIA and HLA antigens in a mother and her pair of dizygous twins in which only one twin developed complete heart block. Anti-Ro levels were significantly lower in the affected twin, suggesting antibody consumption, but both twins were HLA identical (HLA-DR3 positive). Anti-La antibodies were negative in all members of this family. This author has studied a family in which only one pair of proven monozygotic twins developed congenital heart block. The mother had Sjögren's syndrome with anti-Ro and La antibodies. A third child born later developed neonatal lupus rash without heart block. All were HLA-DR3 positive (Arnett FC: Unpublished observations). Thus, there appear to be immunogenetic differences between Ro antibody-positive mothers who produce infants with NLE and those having normal infants.

Recently, using immunoblotting, Buyon et al.[B601] have demonstrated that mothers of infants with congenital heart block almost invariably have autoantibodies to the 48 kD La protein and/or the 52 kD Ro protein. Moreover, the HLA-DR3 haplotype is almost invariably present in the mothers. This suggests a major genetic role for HLA-DQB1*0201, as previously discussed. (See Chapter 52.)

HLA in Drug-Induced Lupus

Drug-induced lupus syndromes provide the opportunity to contrast contributing genetic factors with those in idiopathic SLE. Unfortunately, there are few studies of HLA profiles in patients with drug-induced lupus. Batchelor et al.[B118] studied HLA and acetylator phenotypes in 26 patients with hydralazine-induced lupus. Twenty-five (96%) were slow acetylators. HLA-DR4 was significantly increased in hydralazine-induced lupus (73%) compared to 33% in normal controls, while HLA-DR3 was decreased (none positive). Female sex, present in 81% of this series, was also important in predisposing to hydralazine-induced lupus.

HLA studies in other drug-induced lupus syndromes are few. Chalmers et al.[C191] reported six patients with seropositive, erosive rheumatoid arthritis who developed penicillamine-induced lupus. The drug-induced syndrome more closely resembled idiopathic SLE than does hydralazine-induced disease. HLA-B15 was present in five and HLA-DR4 in three of five tested. It should be noted, however, that DR4 is associated with rheumatoid arthritis itself[S621] and HLA-B15 (Bw62) is often in linkage disequilibrium with DR4. None of these patients had HLA-DR2 or DR3 haplotypes.

Grosse-Wilde et al.[G409] have reported an association of HLA-DR4 with a pseudolupus syndrome induced by phenopyrazone-containing drugs used to treat venous disorders. (See Chapter 45.)

T-CELL RECEPTOR GENES IN SLE

Since MHC class II molecules present antigenic peptides to the T-cell antigen receptor (TCR) on CD4-positive helper T lymphocytes, it is possible that TCR polymorphisms may also contribute to disease susceptibility and/or autoantibody production. Such a contribution from the TCR, when absent, might explain SLE patients who, despite possessing the relevant MHC alleles, do not produce particular autoantibodies.

Knowledge of TCR gene polymorphisms is still in its early stages, unlike that of the MHC. Nonetheless, several studies of TCR genes, primarily determined at the germline DNA level using RFLPs, have been conducted in SLE patients. The first suggestion that TCR genes might be important in lupus came from the discovery of a large deletion in the TCRβ chain gene of New Zealand White (NZW) mice, phenotypically normal animals, which when mated to New Zealand Black (NZB) mice, results in the NZB/NZW F1 hybrid murine model of SLE.[N122] Later studies, however, demonstrated no significant effect of the TCRβ deletion upon autoimmunity in NZB/NZW hybrids, but, instead, reaffirmed the importance of MHC (H-2) genes.[K395] Fronek et al.[F288] found no deletion in the human TCRβ chain gene in SLE and no association of a diallelic TCRβ constant region polymorphism definable by the restriction endonuclease *Bgl* II. Goldstein et al.[G271] also found a normal distribution of this same RFLP pattern in SLE patients; however, SLE patients having HLA-DR3 appeared to show an increased frequency of the larger 9.8 kb *Bgl* II fragment.

Dunckley et al.[D356] studied a variety of TCRα, β, and γ RFLPs in conjunction with MHC class II RFLPs and found no association with SLE overall or with specific MHC class II alleles in these patients. On the other hand, Tebib et al.[T92] examined TCRα RFLPs in American Caucasians and Mexicans with SLE. A TCRα *Pst*I 1.3/3.0 kb constant region RFLP was significantly increased in the American but not the Mexican SLE patients. The RFLP did not correlate with any autoantibody or HLA specificities.

More recently, Frank et al.[F210] reported that the combination of the *Bgl* II TCRβ (Cβ1) 9.8 RFLP and a *Kpn* I TCRβ (Cβ2) 1.75 kb RFLP was significantly increased in SLE patients with anti-Ro antibodies (76%) compared to those without anti-Ro (41%). The combination of TCRβ

RFLPs did not differ between SLE patients as a whole and normal controls, suggesting that the association was only with anti-Ro production. Moreover, the TCRβ RFLP combination occurred significantly more frequently in patients with anti-Ro without anti-La, especially those possessing HLA-DQw1. This study suggests that both MHC and TCR polymorphisms are important in certain autoantibody subsets of SLE, and future studies, especially applying TCR probes of the variable regions, should be pursued. One family study reported thus far has shown no linkage of TCRα, β or γ genes to SLE in multiplex families.[W338]

MHC CLASS III GENES ASSOCIATED WITH SLE

Complement Deficiencies

While MHC class II and perhaps TCR alleles appear to influence the expression of SLE via specific autoantibody responses, it now appears certain that hereditary deficiencies of complement components, especially C4, are additional and independent risk factors for disease susceptibility. The C4A and C4B genes map within the MHC class III region,[C109] and hereditary deficiency of C4A (C4A null alleles or C4A*QO) has been associated with SLE in American and European Caucasians,[B116,F85,G269,H455,K166,K347] and American blacks,[H455,O75,W275] Japanese,[T175,Y8] Southern Chinese,[D354,H215] and Mexicans.[A108,G335,K457,R175] In Caucasians, C4A*QO is most often the result of a large deletion of the C4A and 21-OHA genes on the HLA-B8, DR3 haplotype;[C111,G269,K166] however, in other ethnic groups, C4A null alleles resulting from several molecular mechanisms are associated with SLE and occur on other HLA haplotypes.[K457,O75,Y8] Thus, the strength of the HLA-B8, DR3 association with SLE in Caucasians may relate to the fact that it possesses at least two of the genetic loci (HLA-DQw2 and C4A) relevant to disease predisposition. The relationships among C4, other complement genes, and SLE are discussed further in Chapter 13.

Tumor Necrosis Factor (TNF)

Polymorphism of the TNFα gene, which is located in the MHC class III region,[S597] has recently been demonstrated by both restriction enzyme mapping and functional quantitative assays. Fugger et al.[F296] examined NcoI RFLPs in four autoimmune diseases. A 5.5 kb RFLP was found to be increased in SLE and Sjögren's syndrome patients, while a 10.5 kb fragment was decreased. The 5.5 kb RFLP was found to be in linkage disequilibrium with HLA-B8, a haplotype (B8, DR3) that is known to be increased in both SLE and Sjögren's syndrome.

Of considerable interest are recent studies by Jacob et al.,[J15,J16] who have determined TNFα polymorphisms and serum levels in both murine and human lupus. Low TNFα levels (along with an associated RFLP) were found in NZB × NZW) F1 mice.[J16] This genetic trait was contributed by the NZW parent. Most strikingly, the onset of lupus nephritis was significantly delayed in F1 mice by the replacement of TNFα.[J16] Similar experiments in the nonobese diabetic (NOD) mouse demonstrated that insulinitis and clinical diabetes could be blocked by treatment with TNFα.[J14] Low inducible levels of TNFα were also found in human lupus patients with nephritis, and this genetic trait in both SLE and normal subjects was associated with HLA-DR2, DQw1 haplotypes.[J15] Higher inducible TNF levels were found in SLE patients and normal subjects with HLA-DR3 and DR4 haplotypes.[O75] The NcoI RFLPs described earlier[F296] did not correlate with the quantitative levels of TNFα. These data suggest that genetic differences in TNFα genes, along with those already described for HLA class II and C4, may also contribute to autoimmune diseases, especially SLE.

Heart-Shock Protein (HSP) 70

HSP 70 is one of a family of highly conserved stress proteins that recently have been suspected of playing a role in autoimmunity.[V28,W283] The theoretical mechanisms are beyond the scope of this chapter but have been recently reviewed.[W283] Indeed, autoantibodies to HSP 70 and other stress proteins have been reported in SLE,[M464,M466] however, additional studies of the HSP 70 genes in SLE patients are needed. (See Chapter 26.)

HLA-B–Associated Transcripts (BATs)

The five BAT genes, although mapped to the MHC and possibly constituting a "class IV region," remain ill-defined as to structure and function. Fugger et al.[F297] have recently studied RFLP of BAT1 and BAT2 genes in five autoimmune diseases, including SLE and Sjögren's syndrome. No gross gene deletions or duplications were found. The BAT2 Rsa I 2.17 kb RFLP was more frequently found in SLE, Sjögren's syndrome, and primary biliary cirrhosis; however, it appeared to be in linkage disequilibrium with HLA-B8. Thus, further studies of BAT genes may be warranted, especially when they have been better defined.

OTHER NON-MHC–LINKED GENES AND SLE

Immunoglobulin Genes

Studies of immunoglobulin heavy chain (Gm) and light chain (Km) genes have shown a variety of associations with SLE. Gm maps to human chromosome 14 and Km to chromosome 2; both show moderate polymorphism. Increased susceptibility to SLE has been reported in individuals heterozygous for Gm markers compared to homozygotes. Whittingham et al.[W216] found an association of the Gm (1,2,3;5,21) phenotype in white Australians with SLE, Schur et al.,[S206] Gm (1,3,17;5,13,21) in white Boston SLE patients, and Stenszky et al.,[S662] Gm (3;5,13) in Hungarians with SLE. In other ethnic groups, Gm (1,2;21) was found to be increased in Japanese patients,[N26] and Gm (1,17;5,6,13) in South Carolina blacks.[F42] These differences may relate to the heterogeneity of Gm phenotypes among different ethnic groups, as well as a failure to relate specific immunoglobulin genotypes to specific autoantibody responses.

Reveille et al.[R177] examined the segregation of Gm haplotypes in six large kindreds with Sjögren's syndrome, two of which had SLE members, and found no haplotypes cosegregating with disease or autoantibodies. This lack of Gm haplotype sharing may be similar to that observed for HLA (to be discussed). Nonetheless, these early studies suggest a role for immunoglobulin genes in predisposing to SLE. Moreover, Gm allotype associations have been reported in other autoimmune diseases, including myasthenia gravis,[N25] autoimmune thyroid disease,[F20] Graves' disease,[F19] chronic active hepatitis,[W215] and multiple sclerosis.[P24]

Whittingham et al.[W211] first reported the association of a particular Km phenotype, Km (1), with anti-La antibodies. Genth et al.[G89] reported that both HLA-DR4 and Gm (1,3;5,21) were associated with anti–U1-nRNP. More recently, Hoffman et al.[H364] studied Gm and Km phenotypes in white patients with SLE, MCTD, and scleroderma. The Km (1) phenotype was significantly increased in the SLE patients (69%) as compared to normal white controls (12%), but was not increased in the MCTD or scleroderma patients. Anti-dsDNA antibodies were significantly correlated with Km (1). Gm (1,3,17;5,21) was also increased in SLE and MCTD patients, similar to the study by Schur et al.[S206] Black et al.[B326] previously reported a significant increase in the Gm (1,17,21;3,5,11) phenotype in MCTD patients. Grosse-Wilde et al.[G409] noted an association of both Gm (1;21) and HLA-DR4 with the pseudolupus syndrome induced by phenopyrazone-containing drugs used to treat venous disorders.

The sharing of cross-reactive idiotypes by anti-DNA antibodies in unrelated SLE patients, in SLE families, and in murine lupus strains has been demonstrated,[E51,H74,J35, S380,S383,S544,Z45] suggesting a possible role for immunoglobulin variable genes. High serum levels of one particular anti-DNA idiotype, IdGN2, has been demonstrated in SLE patients with nephritis in contrast to those without renal involvement.[K41,T233] Moreover this pathogenic antibody can be found in the glomerular lesions of SLE patients. No correlation of IdGN2 has been found with HLA class II alleles.[H34] Using molecular methods to examine immunoglobulin variable (V) genes, Olee et al.[O63] have found a homozygous deletion of the human Humhv 3005 gene that is likely to encode heavy chains of rheumatoid factor to be present in approximately 20% of rheumatoid and SLE patients but in only 2% of normal controls.

Estrogen Metabolism

Female sex has been long known to predispose to SLE and other autoimmune diseases.[M177] Studies in murine models and humans have demonstrated important effects of both androgenic and estrogenic hormones.[J145,L19,L21, R361,S695]

Lahita et al.[L18,L19,L21] showed that estrone is preferentially hydroxylated at the C-16 position in males and females with SLE as well as their first-degree relatives. This defect results in the accumulation of 16 hydroxylated metabolites with high estrogenic activity.[F119,L16,L26] Whether this is a genetic or acquired defect remains unknown. (See Chapter 16.)

Acetylator Phenotypes

The slow acetylation of certain aromatic amines and hydrazones has clearly been shown to predispose to hydralazine- and procainamide-induced lupus syndromes.[P148,W348] Fast and slow acetylation is a genetic trait, but its location within the human genome is still unknown. Multiple studies to determine whether the slow acetylator phenotype is associated with idiopathic SLE have been largely negative.[F135,M599] Reidenberg[R126] reviewed and totaled results from the literature and concluded that slow acetylators were significantly overrepresented in the SLE population. Normal matched local controls, however, were not always available from these reports. Reidenberg thus reached his conclusion based on population control frequencies derived from nonlocal sources. This remains a major potential flaw, and the issue has not been satisfactorily settled. (See Chapter 45.)

Genes Associated with Chronic Granulomatous Disease (CGD)

Discoid lupus without ANAs or other autoantibodies has been recorded frequently in patients, as well as their mothers, with CGD.[M119] CGD results from impaired killing of microorganisms by polymorphonuclear leukocytes because of an inability to generate toxic derivatives of oxygen. The basic defect is probably deficient NADPH oxidase activation. The disease occurs in both X-linked and autosomal forms, both of which have been associated with discoid lupus. Manzi et al.[M119] described a boy with X-linked CGD and SLE, including nephritis, associated with a positive ANA and anti-dsDNA antibodies, and reviewed all the previous literature. The reasons underlying this leukocyte defect and predisposition to lupus are unknown.

STUDIES OF FAMILIES WITH LUPUS ERYTHEMATOSUS

Familial SLE

The familial occurrence of SLE has been increasingly recognized over the last three decades. This section reviews those reports and family studies that provide important clues to heritable factors.

Prevalence

In the early 1960s, Siegel et al.[S417] studied the relatives of 66 hospitalized cases of SLE, along with those of 50 patients with rheumatoid arthritis and 91 normal controls. Among approximately 155 relatives in each group, there was no evidence of an increased familial prevalence of SLE. In 1963, however, Dubois[D323] noted that 2% of his 520 index cases of SLE had family members, usually parents or sibs, with the same disorder. By 1974 the prevalence had risen to 5% in this same group.[D323] Estes and Christian[E147] noted 7 (4%) of their 150 cases of SLE to have a similarly affected first-degree relative. In a review of the literature in 1964, Vasey[V48] found 81 cases of familial SLE in 36 families and summarized 27 reports of familial discoid LE. In addition, he found one positive LE-cell test and three positive ANA tests in a study of 79 asymptomatic relatives of 16 patients with SLE.[V49]

There was also early evidence for the familial occurrence of discoid lupus. As early as 1903, Sequeira[S283] described two families in which two sisters in each had discoid lupus erythematosus. In one of these families, one child had intermittent albuminuria and both "suffered from blueness of the extremities and during the winter months from chilblains." In Dubois' series of 520 cases, discoid LE occurred in only three families.[D323] Klemperer et al.[K284] mentioned a family in which the mother had discoid LE and the daughter had autopsy-proven SLE. Becket and Lewis[B160] reported a family in which the daughter, age 32, had discoid lupus and the mother, age 61, had proven SLE. Blaney[B337] collected 15 such reported kinships.

Buckman et al.[B552] systematically sought family histories of lupus in 340 patients with SLE and documented a familial prevalence of 12%. Among these 41 familial cases, 5 had 2 and 36 had 1 affected family member each. Ten (30%) of the 33 male probands and 31 (10%) of the 307 female probands had other affected relatives (p < .05). Discoid lupus was verified in 9 families, 4 of whom had 2 or more members with SLE. More recently, Pistiner et al.[P216] have resurveyed the 570 SLE patients in this private practice. Lupus was found in 18% of all relatives and in 10% of first-degree relatives (3% males and 7% females). Twenty-seven percent of all relatives and 15% of first-degree relatives had other autoimmune diseases, most commonly rheumatoid arthritis and Hashimoto's thyroiditis. LEANON, a lupus support group, circulated a questionnaire among patients diagnosed as having various forms of lupus to determine whether family members were afflicted. Eighty of 561 (14.2%) replied affirmatively, and in 53 (9.9%) SLE existed in first-degree relatives.[H493]

Hochberg et al.[H343,H351] performed a case-control study of 77 SLE patients and 77 age-, race-, and sex-matched normal associate controls. Eight SLE probands (10%) had 1 or more first-degree relatives with SLE as compared to only 1 such relative (1%) among controls (p = .034; relative risk = 8). Nine of the 541 (1.7%) first-degree relatives of lupus probands also had SLE compared to only 1 of 540 (0.2%) relatives of normal controls (p = .02; RR = 9).

More recently, Lawrence et al.[L102] performed a survey of SLE and discoid LE among first-degree relatives of lupus patients as well as those of normal probands. Ten of 335 (3%) relatives of SLE patients were found to have SLE as compared to only 7 of 2512 (0.3%) relatives of healthy individuals (p = 1 × 10⁻⁸; RR = 11). Among the SLE relatives, only 0.6% had discoid lupus, a nonsignificant difference from control relatives (0.5%). On the other hand, discoid LE was significantly increased (3.5%) among the 255 first-degree relatives of discoid LE probands compared to control relatives (0.5%) (p = 1 × 10⁻⁶; RR = 7). Among 61 spouses of SLE and 56 spouses of discoid LE probands, none were found to have lupus, either systemic or discoid. Thus, the studies of both Hochberg et al.[H343,H351] and Lawrence et al.[L102] have formally proven that *familial aggregation* exists for SLE and for discoid LE. The genetic epidemiology of SLE was recently reviewed by Hochberg.[H343] (See Chapter 4.)

Familial Relationships

In 1976, Arnett and Shulman[A301] reviewed the literature and found 7 pairs of identical twins with SLE,[B365,B541,D89,J100,J132,L275,W6] 1 pair of nonidentical twins,[L190] 15 sib-

Table 2–6. Familial Cases of Systemic Lupus Erythematosus

Family Relationships	Buckman et al. No. Individuals	Arnett and Shulman No. Individuals
Sister/sister	12	20
Brother/sister	16	10
Female identical twins	2	16
Male identical twins	2	2
Brother/brother	2	6
Father/daughter	6	10
Mother/daughter	20	30
Mother/son	2	2
Aunt/niece	6	0
Cousin/cousin	4	0
Niece/two aunts	3	0
Sister/sister/mother	3	0
Brother/sister/niece	3	0
Aunt/two nieces	3	0
Son/mother/aunt	3	0
Father/son	0	2
Three sisters	0	9
Four sisters	0	4
Mother/daughter/son	0	3
Total	87	114
Male involvement	19 (22%)	22 (19%)

Modified and reprinted with permission. Buckman, K.J., Moore, S.K., Ebbin, A.J. et al.: Familial systemic erythematosus. Arch. Intern. Med. 138:1674, 1978. Copyright 1978, American Medical Association.[B552]

ships,[B351,B538,D323,L79,L190,L376,M144,P148,R161,T163,W251] and 10 parent-offspring combinations[A31,B28,B538,D323,G180,G375,M144,P208] reported to date. They added 1 set of monozygotic twins, 3 sib pairs, and 5 parent-offspring combinations, including a father and son. The intrafamilial relationships among these cases and those of Buckman et al.[B552] are shown in Table 2–6. Females predominate with mother-daughter and sister-sister pairs being most common. Nonetheless, there may be an excess of males (20%) as compared to series of SLE patients where a female:male ratio of 10:1 is usually found.[D323]

Lahita et al.[L23] reported four families containing fathers and sons with SLE. Clinical disease in males did not appear to differ from that in females, and several daughters also had SLE, other autoimmune diseases, or seroreactivity. Male karyotypes were normal, and no obvious endocrinopathy was found. The writers drew analogies to lupus-like disease in the B × SB murine strain where males are most susceptible.[D233,E64,M667]

Analysis of the occurrence of SLE by birth order in families showed a random distribution.[S416] This is suggestive of a genetic role and tends to exclude host and environmental factors that vary with time, such as parental age, previous pregnancies, maternal disorders, use of new drugs, and other environmental influences during the reproductive period.

Analyses of Familial Cases

Arnett and Shulman[A301] compared the frequencies of 23 clinical and laboratory manifestations in 51 familial cases of SLE (24 families) to those in 51 nonfamilial SLE patients matched for age, race, sex, and disease duration.

No significant differences were found, suggesting to the authors that familial SLE was probably the same disorder as sporadic SLE. On the other hand, when each familial case was compared to his or her affected relative for these same 23 clinicolaboratory attributes, striking concordance for disease expression was found between identical twin pairs and between parent and offspring. No such concordance was found for sib pairs. These findings supported genetic influences on the expression of SLE, especially in twins and parent-offspring who are more obliged to share genetic traits than sibs. Subsequently, this author has observed that affected sibs with SLE show striking concordance for both disease and autoantibody profiles when they share the same two HLA haplotypes. (Arnett FC: Unpublished observations.)

Intervals between ages and actual times of disease onset were also examined.[A301] Disease began in identical twin pairs within an average of 2 years. In nontwin sibs, while the average difference in actual dates of onset was only 3 years, the average interval time between ages of onset was 9 years. Average time and age between disease onset for parents and offspring were 8 years and 20 years, respectively. Kaplan[K59] performed a similar controlled analysis in affected twins and sibs and showed an average 4-year interval between dates of onset and a longer period (6 years) between ages at onset. Thus, these findings are suggestive of environmental effects on disease onset, especially in sibs.

Twins and SLE

Studies of twins have provided important information concerning genetic versus nongenetic factors in the pathogenesis of SLE. Concordance for disease in monozygotic twins and discordance in dizygotic twins provide strong evidence for genetic influences, since both types of twins usually share the same environment. On the other hand, the lack of 100% concordance in monozygotic twins implies the requirement for nongermline factors, either environmental triggers or somatic mutations, such as in immunoglobulin or T-cell receptor genes. Ideally, concordance in monozygotic pairs separated at birth and raised separately would provide the strongest genetic evidence. Only one such instance has been reported by Karoleva et al.[K74] and Ermakova et al.,[E132] who described a pair of identical twins separated at 16 months of age and raised in different foster homes. Both twins developed SLE at age 14 with strikingly similar disease features and courses. Many instances of monozygotic twins discordant for SLE have been reported.[A293,B539,H428] The majority of monozygotic twins described in the literature have been concordant for SLE, while the few dizygotic pairs have usually been discordant.[A301,B347, B365, B368, B539, B541, D89, D328, E132, F121, H395,J100,J132,K74,K349,K358,L79,L190,L275,M389,P159,R172,S29,S183, W6,Y44]

Block et al.[B347] provided an excellent review of all 17 previously reported twin pairs and added 12 additional well-studied sets. Zygosity was proven in 7 monozygous and 3 dizygous pairs. Four of the 7 (57%) monozygotic twins were concordant for SLE, fulfilling preliminary ARA criteria,[C325] while 3 dizygous pairs were discordant for

clinical SLE. Concordance for ANA was 71% and for hyperglobulinemia 87% in the identical twin pairs. One clinically normal dizygotic twin had LE cells, ANAs, and a biologic false-positive test for syphilis. When literature reports were combined with the series of Block et al.[B347] and only proven monozygotic twins with definite SLE considered, concordance rates of 69% for LE cells and/or ANAs and 92% for hyperglobulinemia were found. Although the study of Block et al.[B347] was not a systematic ascertainment of all possible twins from a defined population base, the writers estimated that they had found 7 to 9 of the expected 17 monozygotic twins with SLE from the metropolitan New York area.

Deapen et al.[D103] surveyed a twin registry and found 138 twin pairs where one or both had self-reported SLE. Only 23% of 66 monozygotic twins (14% males and 24% females) were concordant for SLE. Among 44 dizygotic twins, 9% were concordant (0% males and 11% females). It must be emphasized that zygosity was not formally proven in these twins, and the full study has not been published beyond an abstract.

In another report, Block et al.[B346] examined immunologic function in nine twin pairs, emphasizing three discordant monozygotic sets. They attempted to find a genetic marker for SLE that might be differentially expressed in the affected twin. Lymphocyte proliferative responses to three mitogens were generally lower in affected twins as compared to discordant healthy twins. Although a somewhat lessened lymphocyte response was suggested in the healthy twins, this was not a consistent finding when compared to normal controls. Similarly, sera from affected and healthy twin pairs added to each other's lymphocyte cultures did not consistently affect mitogenic response. Electron microscopic surveillance of lymphoid cells for tubuloreticular structures revealed them in 9 of 11 affected twins but also in 1 of 3 healthy identical twins and in a healthy but seroreactive nonidentical twin. Lymphocytotoxic antibodies were found (with one exception) only in sera from affected twins. Mixed lymphocyte cultures of twins' cells with allogeneic and with each other's lymphocytes gave the expected responses, namely stimulation and nonstimulation, respectively. Thus, the writers concluded that depression of cell-mediated immunity related most strongly to clinical disease activity, while anti-lymphocyte antibodies and lymphocyte tubuloreticular structures were associated with serologic phenomena in affected and clinically normal twins.

The autologous mixed lymphocyte response (AMLR) was assessed by Sakane et al.[S29] in two sets of monozygotic twins. The first pair was discordant for SLE but the affected twin had inactive disease, while the second pair was concordant, one having active and the other inactive lupus. Utilizing mixing experiments, the writers concluded that patients with active SLE had a defect in the ability of non-T cells to stimulate as well as a diminished capability in both T γ and T non-γ cells to respond in this in vitro system. Inactive lupus patients were defective only in the responsiveness of their T γ cells.

Schroeder et al.[S183] investigated a pair of clinically discordant prepubertal monozygotic male twins. The affected twin had arthritis, rash, lymphadenopathy, hepatosplenomegaly, nephritis, pancytopenia, high-titer antinuclear antibodies (1/2560), anti-DNA antibodies (1/640), and hypocomplementemia. The asymptomatic twin was serologically active with antinuclear antibodies (1/160) and anti-DNA antibodies (1/10) but normal C3 and C4 levels. Both had HLA-DR2 and DR3. Testosterone, gonadotropin, and estrogen levels were normally low in both. Unfractionated mononuclear cells from the twin with SLE demonstrated a marked increase in spontaneous immunoglobulin synthesis (IgG, IgA, and IgM), which paradoxically declined with pokeweed mitogen stimulation. The healthy twin's cells showed a similar pattern, which was less marked. Coculture experiments were indicative of enhanced suppressor T-cell activity, rather than the usually reported decrease in suppressor cell function. Moreover, in contradistinction to previous studies, the affected twin's T cells showed a brisk proliferative response in the autologous MLR to his own, to his brother's, and to allogeneic stimulator cells. The normal twin had a more subdued autologous MLR, and both twins' sera suppressed the MLR of a normal control by 30 to 65%.

The occurrence of discoid lupus in identical twins has been reported on at least three occasions, and Okun et al.[O51] described a set of identical twins, one of whom had SLE and the other discoid LE.

The reported twin kindreds are representative of other reports that demonstrate the familial occurrence of a variety of autoimmune disorders and serologic reactions in relatives of patients with SLE. Cases of juvenile-onset diabetes mellitus,[D89] multiple sclerosis,[H395] scleroderma with discoid lupus,[D328] myasthenia gravis,[M389] and dermatomyositis[F121] have each been recorded in the identical twin of a patient with SLE. Such observations in twins strongly suggest underlying genetic factors common to all of these disorders of altered immunoregulation.

SLE, Other Autoimmune Diseases, and Serologic Abnormalities in Families

Although familial SLE is not uncommon, more striking is the frequency with which other autoimmune diseases and/or serologic abnormalities occur in relatives of patients with lupus.

Ansell and Lawrence[A257] were not impressed by a sizable increase in the familial prevalence of SLE and rheumatoid arthritis in their family study of 46 male and 81 female relatives of 46 cases of classic SLE. A slight increase occurred in the frequency of positive antinuclear antibody tests in female relatives of the probands with classic SLE, but this was not so marked as in other studies. Holborow and Johnson[H376] restudied the sera of this group of patients using a more sensitive antinuclear antibody technique. They observed a 4% prevalence of positive antinuclear antibody tests in 125 relatives, compared with an 0.8% frequency in the control group.

Bywaters[B613] studied 81 relatives of 24 probands with SLE and found no additional cases; there were, however, four relatives with rheumatoid arthritis and three with discoid LE. Four relatives had sera positive for antinuclear antibodies compared with none in 10 spouses and 91 controls. This is far less than that observed by Pollak et al.[P242]

who found antinuclear antibody in nearly 50% of relatives. Pollak[P237] subsequently studied a larger group of cases, using his original buccal mucosal cell method and the sensitive technique described by Holborow et al.[H377] The results of both methods in his laboratory were similar. Antinuclear antibodies were observed in 91.5% of patients with SLE, 24% of patients with rheumatoid arthritis and other connective tissue diseases, and 17% of those with chronic liver disease or infectious hepatitis. Antinuclear antibodies were found in SLE relatives in 25 of 43 families studied, occurring in 33% of 142 first-degree and 21% of 47 second-degree relatives. The conflicting results of the two laboratories performing these serologic studies are partially due to differing interpretations of a weakly positive fluorescent reaction, which Pollak[P237] considered significant while Holborow et al.[H376] did not.

Larsson and Leonhardt,[L79] in a classic study of two families with SLE, showed a high frequency of hypergammaglobulinemia in these kinships. The prevalence of hyperglobulinemia decreased as the familial relationships weakened, i.e., sibs to nephews and nieces to first cousins and to normal controls. Eight of 10 sibs (80%) had elevation of the γ-globulin, 15 of 38 (39%) nephews and nieces, 9 of 24 (38%) first cousins, 3 of 28 (11%) second cousins, and 5 of 47 (11%) controls. In a detailed monograph on familial studies in SLE, Leonhardt[L191] personally examined 225 first-degree relatives of 57 probands and confirmed his earlier findings of a statistically significantly higher frequency of hypergammaglobulinemia than in normal controls. In addition, the latex-particle test for rheumatoid factor was positive in 13.5% of the probands, 2.7% of the female relatives, and in none of the controls. Fluorescent antinuclear antibodies were observed in 88.9% of the probands, 7.8% of the male relatives, 20.0% of the female relatives, and 2.5% of the female controls. Only 1 of 225 relatives had a false-positive serologic test for syphilis. In addition, Leonhardt[L191] noted a higher incidence of cold sensitivity, sunlight sensitivity, and drug reactions in the relatives than in the control population. These findings suggested a "constitutional diathesis" for the development of SLE.

In an investigation of 59 first-degree relatives of 17 patients with SLE, Rodnan et al.[R261] found seven instances in 6 families of additional major rheumatic disease, two with SLE, four with rheumatoid arthritis, and one with discoid lupus. Hypergammaglobulinemia was found in 20% of the relatives and moderate elevation of the γ-globulin was noted in another 14%. Four individuals had a positive latex-fixation reaction, two of whom had polyarthritis, the other two being asymptomatic. Three false-positive reactions for syphilis were found. In all, there were 17 subjects from 11 families with one or more major clinical or serologic abnormalities.

Morteo et al.[M614] studied 44 relatives of 19 patients with SLE and found that 11% had evidence for connective tissue disease, 36% had positive tests for rheumatoid factor, 11% biologic false-positive tests for syphilis, 18% hypergammaglobulinemia, and 14% antinuclear antibodies. Thirty-nine of these 44 relatives were asymptomatic. The 46 matched control cases showed negligible abnormalities other than a 9% frequency of rheumatoid factor.

Holman and Deicher[H388] investigated 57 relatives of 18 families with SLE and found that 11 (19%) had hypergammaglobulinemia. Individuals in 5 of the families had symptoms, serologic reactions, and x-ray evidence of rheumatoid arthritis.

Clinical thyroid disease was present in 11 (15%) of 72 SLE probands studied by Larsen and Godal[L73] and was four times more frequent in relatives of SLE probands with thyroid disease (27.5%) than in relatives of SLE probands without thyroid disease (7%)—a statistically significant difference. Thyroid disease itself also aggregated in families of patients who had only thyroid disease.

Rheumatoid arthritis may be more frequent in SLE families. Among Dubois' 520 SLE patients, 5.5% had a family history of rheumatoid arthritis.[D323] Siegel et al.[S417] did not find an excess of rheumatoid arthritis (1.3%) among 155 relatives of 66 cases of SLE. Leonhardt[L191] found an 8.2% prevalence of polyarthritis in 225 first-degree relatives of 57 cases of SLE.

Scleroderma and SLE have been described in one pair of twins,[D328] as well as in two mothers and daughters.[H18,T260] Flores et al.[F131] described eight families in which one member had progressive systemic sclerosis (PSS) and another SLE. The scleroderma-SLE combinations included three father-daughters, a pair of sisters, a grandfather-granddaughter, an aunt-niece, and two first cousin pairs. Affected relatives showed no striking concordance for specific clinical features, including Raynaud's phenomenon, except for nearly identical digital calcinosis in two sisters. Antinuclear antibodies, especially to Sm and/or nRNP, were frequently present or absent in the same related pairs. Seven of the eight PSS/SLE pairs did not live in the same household at the onsets of their respective diseases, and three never shared a common environment. HLA haplotypes were shared by five of six pairs studied.

Antinucleic acid and lymphocytotoxic antibodies were determined in SLE probands and their family members by DeHoratius et al.[D125] Among 26 families there were 27 patients with SLE and 124 relatives (94 had close household contact with the proband and 30 did not). Twenty household contacts were related to the proband only by marriage (nonconsanguineous). Control sera from 76 normal individuals in 16 non-SLE families were studied concurrently. Antibodies to nDNA were found in 68% of the SLE probands, 5% of the total family members, 6% of the household contacts, and 1% of control family members. On the other hand, anti-RNA antibodies (single-stranded or antipoly A, and double-stranded or antipoly A:poly U) were found in 16% of family members, 21% of close household contacts, and 82% of the probands with SLE. All of these frequencies were significantly elevated when compared to the 5% prevalence of RNA antibodies in control families.

Similarly, lymphocytotoxic antibodies were elevated in 57% of 124 SLE family members, 68% of the close household contacts, 23% of nonhousehold contacts, 50% of the nonconsanguineous relatives, 82% of SLE probands, and only 4% of control family members. Lymphocytotoxic antibodies correlated strongly with anti-RNA antibodies in the SLE patients and in their relatives but were associated with anti-DNA antibodies only in lupus probands. When household contact and consanguinity were considered, anti-RNA antibodies were significantly increased (27%) in consanguineous as compared to nonconsanguineous (0%) household contacts. Lymphocytotoxic antibodies were increased in both groups as compared to controls but were significantly more frequent in consanguineous contacts. Moreover, lymphocytotoxic antibodies were significantly increased (73%) in consanguineous household contacts as compared to consanguineous nonhousehold contacts (23%). Lymphocytotoxic antibodies may be more common in relatives of patients with childhood rather than adult-onset lupus.[L169]

In a similar study of Russian families, Folomeeva et al.[F144] confirmed the findings of DeHoratius et al.[D125] Of most interest, however, was the detection of lymphocyte antibodies in nine normal controls, four of whom also had polynucleotide antibodies. These controls were all nurses or physicians having close hospital contact with SLE patients.

Over the last two decades, a variety of antinuclear and anticytoplasmic autoantibody specificities found in SLE have been characterized. These include anti-Ro (SSA), La (SSB), Sm, nRNP, antiphospholipid and antiribosomal P, to name the most common. Family studies of these autoantibodies, especially in relation to HLA markers are providing additional insights into the genetic basis of autoimmune diseases.

Reveille et al.[R171,R172] and Arnett et al.[A300] determined autoantibody frequencies in 181 relatives and 34 spouses in 19 SLE kindreds. Using passive immunodiffusion, antibodies to Ro and nRNP were each found only in 1 (0.6%) relative and in none of the spouses, although 26% of the relatives and 9% of spouses had positive antinuclear antibodies, anti—single-stranded (ss)DNA, and/or a biologic false-positive test for syphilis. None had anti-Sm or anti-La.

Lehman et al.[L171] similarly studied autoantibodies in 33 relatives of adult SLE patients and compared their frequencies to those in 94 relatives of children with lupus. Except for antilymphocyte antibodies, which were found significantly more frequently in relatives of children than adults with SLE, there were no significant differences in the frequencies of other autoantibodies between relatives of children and adult SLE patients. Among the total 127 first-degree relatives, anti-Ro occurred in 5 (0.4%), anti-La in none, anti-Sm in 1 (0.08%), and anti-nRNP in 3 (0.2%).

With the development of highly sensitive and specific quantitative enzyme immunoassays (EIAs) for anti-Ro, La and the Sm/nRNP complex, Arnett et al.[A296] determined frequencies for these autoantibodies in relatives of SLE and Sjögren's syndrome patients from two cohorts (Table 2-7). Anti-Ro was detected in 21 to 27% of first-degree relatives of SLE/Sjögren's patients, 11% of second-degree relatives, 11% of spouses, 6% of normal controls. No differences in the frequencies of anti-Ro were found between relatives of probands who were anti-Ro positive and those who were anti-Ro negative. Anti-La was present in 6% of first-degree and 2% of second-degree relatives, and anti-Sm/nRNP occurred in 7 to 13% of these relatives.

Utilizing the same EIA, Lehman et al.[L176] studied serum from 71 children with SLE and 188 of their first-degree

Table 2–7. Frequencies of Autoantibodies in Relatives of Probands with Systemic Lupus Erythematosus (SLE) or Sjögren's Syndrome (SS)

	Anti-Ro Positive	Anti-La Positive	Anti-Sm/RNP Positive
Houston Study			
First-degree relatives of anti-Ro–positive SLE or SS probands	10/48 (21%)*	3/48 (6%)	2/30 (7%)
Second-degree relatives of anti-Ro–positive probands	6/56 (11%)+	1/56 (2%)	0/33
Spouses	1/9 (11%)	0/9	0/6
Unrelated healthy controls	2/67 (3%)	0/67	0/67
Oklahoma City Study			
First-degree relatives of anti-Ro–positive SLE probands	9/33 (27%)‡	ND	4/33 (12%)
First-degree relatives of anti-Ro–negative SLE probands	13/45 (29%)§	ND	6/45 (13%)
First-degree relatives of 10 normal families	3/50 (6%)	ND	1/50 (2%)

*p = .003 compared to unrelated healthy controls.
+p = .09 compared to unrelated healthy controls.
‡p = .009 compared to relatives in healthy families.
§p = .003 compared to relatives in healthy families.
From Arnett, F.C., Hamilton, R.G., Reveille, J.D. et al.: Genetic Studies of Ro (SS-A) and La (SS-B) autoantibodies in families with systemic lupus erythematosus and primary Sjögren's syndrome. Arthritis Rheum., 32:413, 1989.[A296]

relatives. Anti-Ro antibodies as well as their levels were significantly increased in the mothers of male children with SLE (63%) and the mothers of children with SLE onset before age 10 (39%), as compared to mothers of female children (14%) and mothers of children with the onset of SLE after 10 (13%). No relationships between age and sex were found for anti-La or Sm/nRNP. The authors speculated that maternal antibodies to Ro might initiate anti-idiotypic antibodies in the fetus or neonate with subsequent amplification by the idiotype–anti-idiotype network. Previous studies reviewed[L176] have shown that fetal exposure to maternal antigen and neonatal antibody administration both profoundly affect subsequent immune response. It is also likely that the child's MHC genes are also important, since anti-Ro is so strongly associated with specific MHC class II determinants.

An interesting family supporting this possibility was reported by Reichlin et al.[R116] An asymptomatic woman gave birth to a male child with congenital heart block, and 26 years later developed SLE and Sjögren's syndrome with anti-Ro and La antibodies. The son was found to be anti-Ro positive at age 33 but had no disease features. Both mother and son, as well as a healthy anti-Ro–negative daughter, all possessed HLA-DR3. In addition, two previously reported infants with neonatal lupus have subsequently been reported to have developed SLE;[F186,J10] however, it was not reported whether they possessed anti-Ro antibodies or not.

Circulating immune complexes measured by a Clq binding assay were investigated in 85 relatives of 18 SLE patients and in 37 family members of nine families whose index member was known to have no connective tissue disease.[E82] A positive Clq binding test was found in 22 (26%) lupus relatives and in only 2 (5%) healthy family members, a significant difference. Furthermore, levels of immune complexes were similar in SLE relatives and probands. Significantly higher levels occurred in relatives with close household contact than in those not exposed; however, this latter group also had higher immune complex levels than controls. Thus both genetic and environmental effects appeared to be operative. Lehman et al.[L169] also found Clq binding complexes in 8% of 92 relatives of children with SLE.

Familial Abnormalities of Lymphocyte Function

While a variety of circulating serologic abnormalities may be found in family members of patients with SLE, abnormalities of lymphocyte function also have been demonstrated. Miller and Schwartz[M425] studied suppressor T-cell function in vitro (concanavalin A–induced suppression) in 15 SLE patients, 50 of their healthy first-degree relatives, and 41 normal controls. Impaired suppressor function was found in 11 SLE patients (73%) regardless of clinical disease activity and in 13 (26%) relatives, 12 of whom were women. Moreover, 8 of 10 mothers of SLE patients had abnormal suppression and/or antinuclear antibodies. Abnormal suppression was not consistently found in relatives with antinuclear antibodies, and there was no apparent relationship to lymphocytotoxic antibodies. Moreover, lymphocyte abnormalities occurred in relatives having no household contact with the proband. Thus, the authors concluded that these functional lymphocyte defects might be genetically determined. Unfortunately, HLA and other genetic markers were not tested to determine whether they cosegregated with this proposed "trait."

Jabs et al.[J2] found no correlations of similar lymphocyte defects with HLA haplotypes or alleles in a large Sjögren's syndrome kindred in which there were also relatives with SLE. Spencer-Green et al.[S587] also found evidence for suppressor defects in asymptomatic relatives of lupus patients.

More recently, Sakane et al.[S28] have used a PHA-induced interleukin-2 (IL-2) activity assay and a spontaneous plaque-forming cell assay to evaluate T- and B-lymphocyte function in 34 clinically healthy family members of six SLE probands. Impaired IL-2 activity was found in 15 of 29 consanguineous relatives, and there was no relationship with whether they were household or nonhousehold contacts. B cell abnormalities were found in 22 of 29 consanguineous relatives but also in 4 of 5 nonconsanguineous household relatives. No HLA studies were performed. The authors concluded that the data supported a genetic basis for impaired IL-2 activity in these families.

Genetic Analyses in Familial SLE

The multiple reports and striking prevalence of familial SLE, as well as studies in mono- and dizygotic twins, have suggested an important role for genetic factors in disease predisposition. Patterns of inheritance have been difficult to discern in the families studied; however, a dominant model has appeared more likely than a recessive one because of the demonstration of parent-offspring transmission. In fact, multigenic inheritance has been suggested most strongly because of the low penetrance of the disease in families, as well as nonlinkage to HLA alleles which are known to be associated with disease predisposition. Based on the twin studies of Block et al.,[B347] Winchester has proposed that at least four genes are required to produce SLE.[W277,W279] Genetic studies in murine lupus models also suggest that both MHC and non-MHC linked genes are necessary for disease expression.[S369,S647] The multiple varieties of autoimmune disorders that appear in lupus families, as well as healthy relatives with autoantibodies and other immunologic abnormalities, also must be taken into account. Having observed such families, Pirofsky[P206] suggested in 1968 that an immunoregulatory defect might be common to a multitude of autoimmune disorders rather than specific defects for each disease. Only recently has it become possible to apply studies of genetic markers, such as HLA, to such families and to perform the formal genetic analyses so long lacking in large kindreds.

Cleland et al.[C296] examined HLA-A and B antigens in 103 members of four kindreds containing multiple members with SLE. HLA-B8 was found in three families, including 8 of 9 members with SLE. An HLA-A11, Bw35 haplotype occurred in affected members of the fourth family. Antinuclear antibodies were found in greater than 50% of both consanguineous and nonconsanguineous relatives. Linkage of SLE to HLA was explored using Morton's lod scoring method; however, the data were inconclusive.

Reinertsen et al.[R138] studied HLA-A, B, and DR antigens in seven families containing two or more members with SLE. In six families, persons with SLE were homozygous for HLA-DR2 or had two haplotypes bearing HLA-DQw1 (defined by serum Ia-715), or had at least two of three previously identified risk factors, i.e., HLA-DR2, DR3, or DQw1. The authors postulated a role for the coinheritance of several HLA-D region genes in the development of SLE.

Schur and Carpenter[S203] determined HLA haplotypes in 44 SLE families, 9 of which had more than one affected member. Haplotype sharing between members of the same family with SLE and between SLE relatives and healthy antinuclear antibody seroreactors was no greater than expected by chance. One HLA-A, B haplotype was shared by both parents of an SLE patient in 7 of 35 (20%) families. This was significantly greater than the expected rate in local (3.1%) and International Histocompatibility Testing Workshops controls (5%). Only 1 of 19 offspring was homozygous for the shared parental haplotypes instead of the expected 4.75, a difference that was statistically significant. Four of 7 SLE offspring had one of the shared HLA types. The authors concluded that a lethal recessive HLA-linked gene was operative in some SLE families and that heterozygosity for this trait might lead to SLE. Haplotype sharing by parents of SLE patients has not been noted in the families studied by this writer.[A300]

Reveille et al.[R172] examined HLA and complement component profiles in eight families containing 22 members with SLE. Among the 40 relatives, 18% had other autoimmune diseases, 13% high-titer antinuclear antibodies, 28% antibodies to ssDNA, and 2.5% a biologic false-positive test for syphilis. The more specific autoantibodies (anti-dsDNA, anti-Ro, anti-La, anti-Sm, and anti-nRNP) occurred only in members with SLE. HLA-DR2 and DR3 each occurred in 36% of relatives affected with SLE, and heterozygous C2 deficiency was found in one family but occurred in only 1 of the 3 affected members with SLE. HLA haplotype sharing between affected sibs was no greater than expected by chance alone. Thus, genetic factors additional to HLA and C2 deficiency were proposed.

Reveille et al.[R171] then studied C4 null alleles and HLA haplotypes in another eight multiplex SLE families, one of which contained an SLE proband with total C4 deficiency. A high background of C4A null alleles, usually associated with HLA-B8, DR3 haplotypes, was found in these families occurring in 60% of members affected with SLE, 50% of healthy relatives, 24% of spouses, and 19% of normal controls. Specific HLA haplotypes again were not shared by relatives with SLE or those with other autoimmune diseases or circulating autoantibodies. On the other hand, HLA-DR2 and/or DR3 phenotypes, regardless of haplotype, were found in 100% of the relatives with SLE and were significantly increased in SLE as compared to relatives with other autoimmune diseases (79%), asymptomatic relatives with autoantibodies (70%), all asymptomatic relatives (64%), spouses (53%), and normal controls (48%).

Jones et al.[J114] performed a similar analysis of C4 null genes in a large kindred having two sisters with SLE. The two affected sibs shared C4 null alleles, as did four healthy sibs. Eight of 11 members of the sibship had serum autoantibodies (anti-DNA, nRNP, Ro, and/or La) compared to 3 of 13 relatives in the parental generation. The authors concluded that separate loci controlled C4 deficiency and autoantibody production in this family.

Lippman et al.[L324] applied segregation analysis and linkage studies to two large kindreds with multiple members affected by autoimmune diseases. The proband in one had autoimmune hemolytic anemia, and in the other ITP. Seventy relatives and 23 spouses were studied and compared for the frequencies of autoantibodies. Statistically significant differences between relatives and spouses were found for immune-mediated disorders (21 versus 0%), high-titer antinuclear antibodies (≥1/80; 18 versus 0%) and antibodies to ssDNA (18 versus 0%). Although elevations of immunoglobulins occurred more often in relatives (34%) than in spouses (13%), the difference was not statistically significant. Segregation analysis, which viewed high-titer antinuclear antibodies and/or anti-ssDNA as a single trait marking autoimmunity, yielded data most consistent with a Mendelian dominant model having a gene frequency of 0.06 with 91% penetrance. The odds ratio for this dominant prototype versus a recessive one was 500:1. Linkage analysis of the proposed "autoimmune" trait to HLA yielded odds greater than 100:1 against linkage at a recombination fraction of 0.20. When the "trait" was redefined as any immune-mediated disorder, high-titer ANA, anti-ssDNA, a positive direct Coombs' test and/or a biologic false-positive test for syphilis, the trends again supported dominant segregation with a gene frequency of 0.21 with 81% penetrance. A similar analysis of the first eight SLE families described by Reveille et al.[R172] also suggested a dominant model which was not linked to HLA.

These investigators have attempted to confirm the presence of this dominant, non–HLA-linked "autoimmune gene" in 18 new families with SLE, Sjögren's syndrome, or other autoimmune diseases.[A295,A300,B291,R171] The "trait" was defined as any autoimmune disease, high-titer antinuclear antibodies (>1/80), anti-ssDNA and/or a biologic false-positive. Segregation analysis of 50 matings again supported the likelihood of a Mendelian dominant gene that is not linked to HLA, the immunoglobulin heavy chain region (Gm), or the κ chain region (κm). A suggestion of linkage to the MNS blood group on chromosome 4 was suggested. The gene frequency appeared to be approximately 0.10 with penetrance of 92% in females and 40% in males. This proposed "autoimmunity gene" requires definitive mapping and/or elucidation of function before its existence can be confirmed. In addition, these studies showed a profound effect of female sex upon autoimmune phenomena in these families. Moreover, males with SLE were more likely than females to produce offspring with autoimmune diseases, presumably because males require a larger number of the relevant genes to express disease since they lack the effect from estrogens.

The SLE families included in these analyses have previously been reviewed by this author.[A300] Among these 11 new SLE families and the 8 reported by Reveille et al.,[R172] there was an impressive array of other autoimmune diseases in the SLE probands (14%) and their relatives (13%), as well as a myriad of autoantibodies (Table 2–8). HLA haplotypes were inconsistently shared by affected SLE members, relatives with other autoimmune disorders, and seroreactive healthy relatives. In fact, an analysis of HLA haplotype distributions in sib pairs with SLE showed no significant deviation of haplotype sharing from that expected in normals.[A300] On the other hand, HLA-DR2 (and to a lesser degree HLA-DR3) tended to cluster into family members with SLE regardless of HLA haplotype. In the Sjögren's kindreds reported by Reveille et al.,[R177] HLA-DR3 was significantly increased in those relatives with primary sicca syndrome compared to other family members, again unrelated to HLA haplotype sharing.

Table 2–8. Other Immune-mediated Disorders in SLE Patients and Their Relatives in 19 Kindreds

Disorder	SLE (N = 43)	Relatives (N = 208)
Hypothyroidism	5	10
Cutaneous lupus	NA	5
Rheumatoid arthritis	0	3
Scleroderma (PSS)	1	0
ITP	NA	3
Sjögren's syndrome (1°)	NA	1
IDDM	0	2
Hyperthyroidism	0	1
Ulcerative colitis	0	1
Multiple sclerosis	0	1
Total	6 (14%)	27 (13%)

ITP = immune thrombocytopenic purpura, 1° = primary, NA = not applicable, and IDDM = insulin-dependent diabetes mellitus. Reprinted with permission. Arnett, F.C., Reveille, J.D., Wilson, R.W. et al.: Systemic lupus erythematosus: Current state of the genetic hypothesis. Semin. Arthritis Rheum., *14*:24, 1984.[A300]

Table 2–9. Summary

1. SLE is a multigenic disease.
2. HLA – linked and non–HLA-linked genes are involved.
3. Certain extended HLA haplotypes are associated with disease susceptibility but these differ among ethnic groups.
4. A null allele for C4A is the HLA-linked (class III) gene most consistently associated with susceptibility to SLE in different ethnic groups; however, it is not absolutely necessary for disease.
5. HLA class II genes (DR and DQ) are more strongly associated with ability to produce certain autoantibodies than with clinical disease features. These antibodies include anti-dsDNA, anti-Ro/SSA and La/SSB, anti-Sm, anti-RNP, and antiphospholipids.
6. The strongest links between HLA genes and individual autoantibodies are usually found in HLA-DQα and/or DQβ chain alleles and may ultimately be found to correlate with single or short amino acid sequences in immunoreactive regions of these molecules.
7. T-cell receptor genes, whose products interact with HLA molecules, and immunoglobulin genes may also contribute to genetic susceptibility.
8. Relatives of SLE patients have an increased incidence of SLE and other autoimmune diseases, as well as certain autoantibodies including ANA and antilymphocyte antibodies.
9. Family studies show no formal genetic linkage between disease and the HLA complex; however, disease and autoantibody profiles show the same HLA associations in unrelated individuals. Therefore, non–HLA-linked genes are probably quite important. Males appear to need more of these susceptibility genes than females to develop disease.

SUMMARY

Autoimmune diseases are probably multigenic in origin (Table 2–9). If a non-HLA "autoimmunity gene"[B291] is common to many or all, it appears that HLA acts as a modifier of how it is expressed. HLA-DR2 and/or DQw1 haplotypes appear to promote a syndrome recognized as SLE of younger onset and often characterized by a heightened response to single- and double-stranded DNA, as well as anti-Ro antibodies without accompanying anti-La. HLA-DR3, DQW2.1 haplotypes are associated with an older age of onset for SLE with a higher frequency of anti-Ro and La antibodies. HLA-DR3 and DR2 haplotypes are also closely allied with Ro and La antibodies in SCLE, the neonatal lupus syndrome, and in Sjögren's syndrome. It now appears likely that the HLA-DQ alleles in linkage disequilibrium with HLA-DR2, DR3, and other DR alleles are primarily involved in mediating these antibodies. In fact, for each of the autoantibody subsets of SLE studied thus far, different HLA-DQ alleles, or, more often, different shared sequences within DQ alleles, appear to show the primary associations (Table 2–5). HLA-DR and DP alleles do not appear to be directly involved. If these autoantibodies are directly pathogenic in producing the various lesions of SLE, their mediation by the MHC may better explain HLA and disease associations. TCR genes are also potential contributors to these autoantibody responses, but one study thus far has shown no linkage of TCRα, β, and γ genes to SLE in multiplex families.[W338] Additional genes, including C4 and other complement deficiency states, tumor necrosis factor, immunoglobulin, and the proposed "autoimmunity gene" also appear to be additional genetic factors predisposing to SLE.

Chapter 3

THE POTENTIAL ROLE OF ENVIRONMENTAL AGENTS IN SYSTEMIC LUPUS ERYTHEMATOSUS AND ASSOCIATED DISORDERS

Anne-Barbara Mongey
Evelyn V. Hess

The pathogenesis of systemic lupus erythematosus (SLE) is believed to be mediated via the immune system as suggested by the presence of immunologic abnormalities such as polyclonal B-cell activation, production of antinuclear and other autoantibodies, and impairment of T-cell regulation. Genetic influences play an important role as exemplified by the higher incidence of lupus among blacks, Polynesians, and the Sioux nation.[H172,K93,M620,S286] HLA associations especially to DR3 and deficiencies of C2 and C4 also suggest a genetic linkage.[F85,H455] However, factors other than genetic must play a role in the development of SLE as indicated by the incomplete penetrance of SLE observed in families and identical twins. Discordance has also been observed in the prevalence of SLE in the same ethnic groups living in different parts of the world. One study reported an increased prevalence of SLE among Chinese living in Beijing,[N19] but a study of SLE patients in the San Francisco area did not find an increased prevalence among the Chinese population living there.[F74] These observations suggest that environmental factors must play an important role, possibly acting as the trigger for disease induction in susceptible individuals. Many drugs have been implicated in the pathogenesis of a lupus-like syndrome. The first report was in 1945 and sulfadiazine was the implicated drug.[H362] Hydralazine in 1953[M603] and procainamide in 1962 followed.[L9] Some of these, such as procainamide and hydralazine, have been shown to be definitely associated with the development of a lupus-like syndrome in some patients—which is reversible upon discontinuation of the drug—while others, such as estrogens, are believed to occasionally exacerbate or even trigger idiopathic systemic lupus erythematosus. Many of the drugs provoke the development of autoimmune phenomena, such as autoantibody production, without being associated with the development of the clinical syndrome. For example, up to 90% of patients receiving procainamide will develop a positive antinuclear antibody (ANA) within a year of starting therapy, but only about 30% of these patients are likely to develop the lupus-like syndrome.[W140] Many of the drugs that have been proposed as incriminating agents lack definite proof of association. At present, there are six drugs—procainamide, hydralazine, isoniazid, methyldopa, quinidine,

and chlorpromazine—which have been demonstrated in prospective studies to have a definite association with the development of a lupus-like syndrome. Of interest, drug-related lupus does not share the same gender bias since it is found as commonly in men as in women. It also tends to affect an older population. This could of course reflect the higher prevalence of diseases for which these drugs are being prescribed among the elderly male population. Patients receiving these drugs have many of the immunologic features associated with SLE such as autoantibody formation and immune cellular abnormalities. Chapter 45 deals with the topic of drug-related lupus in detail. Observations dating back to 1969 implicated certain metals and chemicals present in food and the environment with the development of a lupus-like syndrome. As early as 1969, infectious agents have been proposed as possible factors. Sex hormone metabolism may also play a role since SLE is most frequently seen in young women. The recent finding of hyperprolactinemia in SLE provides further support to this relationship.[J53] This chapter will review the potential for environmental agents to trigger the onset and possibly exacerbations of SLE (see Table 3–1).

CHEMICAL FACTORS

See Table 3–2 for summary.

Chemical Agents

Aromatic Amines and Hydrazines

Many of the drugs implicated in drug-related lupus (DRL), such as procainamide and hydralazine, are aromatic amines or hydrazines. These drugs are metabolized by means of the acetylation pathway; studies show that DRL and autoantibody formation are more likely to occur in patients who are genetically slow acetylators,[P134] suggesting that the free amine or hydrazine moiety is the inciting agent. Both naturally occurring hydrazines and aromatic amines are potential inciting agents in the development of lupus. Hydrazine and its derivatives are present in a variety of compounds used in agriculture and industry. They have numerous commercial applications as intermediates in the synthesis of products such as plastics, anticorrosives, rubber products, herbicides, pesticides, photographic supplies, preservatives, textiles, dyes, and

37

Table 3–1. Agents with a Potential Role as Triggers of SLE and Associated Disorders

Chemical Factors	Dietary Factors	Radiation	Infectious Agents
Chemical agents	Amino acids	UV light	Viruses
Metals	Fats and caloric intake		Bacteria and their products
Toxins			

pharmaceuticals. Hydrazine itself occurs naturally in tobacco, tobacco smoke, mushrooms, and a penicillium. Reidenberg et al.[R128] reported the development of a lupus-like syndrome due to occupational exposure to hydrazine. The patient was a 25-year-old laboratory technician who used hydrazine sulphate intermittently in her work doing enzymatic determinations of lactate, maleate, and β-hydroxybutyrate. She developed recurrent episodes of arthralgias, photosensitive rash, fever, and a positive ANA. Avoidance of contact with hydrazine resulted in remission of symptoms. Subsequently the patient had recurrences of the symptoms when reexposed to hydrazine, its derivatives, or following ingestion of a tartrazine-containing medication. Of interest, the patient was a slow acetylator. Her twin sister, who had not been exposed to hydrazine, had no evidence of lupus although she did have antibodies to native DNA. She did not develop any features of lupus when subsequently exposed to hydrazine.

Aromatic amines are present in the diet as reduction products of azo food dyes by the intestinal bacteria. Tartrazine or FD&C yellow No. 5 is an azo dye present in thousands of foods and drugs. It is an aniline and *p*-sulfophenylhydrazine derivative, which has been reported to cause asthma, urticaria, angioedema, rhinorrhea, allergic vascular purpura and peripheral eosinophilia, and to have phototoxic potential. Pereyo has described the development of a lupus-like syndrome characterized by photosensitivity, arthralgias, and myalgias following ingestion of tartrazine in a patient who previously had drug-related lupus secondary to procainamide.[P114] Subsequently he reported exacerbations of cutaneous involvement in five patients with SLE after they ingested medicines containing

Table 3–2. Chemical Factors Associated with Development of Autoimmune Disease

Factors	Disease
Hydrazines	Lupus-like syndrome*
Tartrazine	Lupus-like syndrome*
Hair dyes	Lupus-like syndrome*
Silica	Scleroderma*
Polyvinyl chloride	Scleroderma
Hydrocarbon solvents	Goodpasture's syndrome
Mercury	Glomerulopathy*
Gold	Glomerulopathy*
Cadmium	Glomerulopathy*
Rapeseed oil	Toxic oil syndrome*
Colchicine	Myopathy
Eosin	Photosensitive rash
Paraffin/silicone	"Adjuvant disease"*

* Positive ANA reported.

tartrazine.[P116] Another patient developed a lupus-like syndrome consisting of arthralgias, myalgias, malaise, photosensitivity, and a positive ANA after an oral challenge with tartrazine.[P116]

Aromatic amines are also present in permanent hair coloring solutions and can be absorbed through the scalp.[R125] Paraphenylenediamine, which is used commercially as a dyeing compound for hair, has been shown to reproduce features of connective tissue disease in experimental animals. Geschickter et al.[G104] found that following repeated daily brushings of N,N^1-dimethyl-*p*-phenylenediamine to the shaved skins of rats, various focal lesions of the collagen vascular diseases were reproduced histologically. These included Aschoff-like bodies in the heart, rheumatoid nodules, capillary platelet thrombi, glomeruli "wire looping," and focal fibrinoid necrosis. Scleroderma-like lesions were seen in the skin of those animals receiving high doses or those that had been receiving treatment for a very prolonged period.

In a case-control study of environmental factors, Hochberg et al. found an increase in the prior use of hair dyes among 74 patients with systemic lupus erythematosus.[H353] However this difference was not statistically significant. Six years later, Freni-Titulaer et al., in another case-control study, reported a positive association between the use of hair care products with the development of connective tissue diseases.[F235] The study included 23 patients with SLE, 10 patients with scleroderma, 2 with polymyositis, and 9 with undifferentiated connective tissue disease. For each patient, two control subjects of the same age (± 2 years), race, sex, and telephone prefix were selected from lists of possible controls prepared from household telephone surveys. Environmental factors were only considered if the exposure occurred in the 5-year period prior to the onset of the disease for patients or in the equivalent period for the controls. In the crude analyses, exposures to hair dyes, hair permanent solutions, and hair spray all showed statistically significant associations. Using multivariate analyses only the association with hair dyes remained statistically significant. An association of exposure to hair care products with the development of connective tissue disease was found for each of the individual diseases studied and the association with hair dyes was significant for each of these individual groups. The authors postulated that the aromatic amines present in hair dyes may trigger the development of a connective tissue disease by means of absorption through the scalp. The authors concluded by suggesting that family members of patients with connective tissue disorders should be advised to refrain from using hair dyes. There is no information on the effects of these hair care products on the course of connective tissue diseases.

Occupational Exposure–Related Factors

In addition to the aromatic amines and hydrazines, other chemicals and toxins to which people are exposed as part of their occupation have also been implicated in the development of connective tissue–like diseases. Reports have suggested an association between the development of scleroderma and exposure to silica dust. Erasmus[E125] reported the occurrence of 17 cases of scleroderma among underground gold miners in South Africa, which had a predominance of pulmonary features. Chest x rays revealed evidence of pulmonary fibrosis comparable with scleroderma in greater than 50% of patients. Other reports of scleroderma in association with exposure to silicosis have appeared. In reviewing their experience of more than 150 scleroderma patients, Rodnan et al.[R260] found that 43% of their 60 male patients had worked in coal mines or in other occupations marked by prolonged and heavy exposure to silica dust. These patients had pulmonary manifestations more frequently than the other scleroderma patients. Otherwise, the mode of onset, severity, and course of the disease did not differ significantly from the "nonexposed" patients. Similar to the previous study, silicosis was noted on chest x rays in about one third of these patients.

Sclerodermatous-like skin lesions have been found in workers involved in the industrial process of polymerization of polyvinyl chloride (a solid plastic material) from vinyl chloride (a gas). The plastics industry uses polymerized vinyl chloride to manufacture plastics. A small percentage (3% or less) of the workers involved in the polymerization process have been reported to develop occupational acro-osteolysis, which is characterized by Raynaud's-like phenomenon involving the hands, sclerodermatous-like changes involving the skin of the hands and forearms, and osteolytic and sclerotic lesions of the bones, especially the extremities and sacroiliac joints, and in some cases synovial thickening of the small joints of the hands.[D245,M139] Raynaud's phenomenon appears to be the first sign of this syndrome, occurring in one or both hands. Following this, diffuse swelling of the fingers may occur resulting in difficulty with finger flexion. Some patients may be asymptomatic initially, and diagnosis is based on roentgenographic evidence of bony lytic lesions in the hands. Cutaneous involvement is characterized by diffuse, waxy thickening of the skin of the digits and hands, most noticeable over the flexor and extensor tendons. Unlike scleroderma, the skin appendages continue to function and there is an absence of polygonal telangiectasia in the area of active disease. Cutaneous changes may also be seen in the feet but without concomitant Raynaud's phenomenon. The bony lytic lesions are most commonly seen in the distal phalanges of the hands, styloid processes of the ulna and radius and sacroiliac joints, commencing with marginal and/or cortical defects, which may progress to cause transverse defects or fractures and complete resorption of the tufts and shafts of one or more distal phalanges. Extensive erosive and sclerotic changes may occur in the sacroiliac joints. Antinuclear antibodies and rheumatoid factors were negative and immunoglobulins normal. Duration of exposure prior to onset of the disease is variable. The syndrome appears to occur only in workers involved in the manual cleaning of the polyvinyl chloride reactor vessels and not those working with vinyl chloride, the finished polymer polyvinyl chloride, its copolymers, or in the processing of the polymer into its finished plastic products. This suggests that the etiologic agent(s) may be one or more of the incomplete products of polymerization. Patients with vinyl chloride–induced

scleroderma have been reported to have an elevated frequency of HLA-DR5 and an increased linkage disequilibrium between HLA-B8 and HLA-DR3, which is seen in idiopathic scleroderma patients.[B327] This would suggest a genetic influence. No treatment exists except for removal from exposure to the chemical, which is thought to prevent further progression of the skin disease, but has no effect on the further progression of bone lesions.

Exposure to hydrocarbon solvents has been associated with the development of Goodpasture's syndrome. Beirne et al.[B172] reported a history of extensive occupational exposure to various industrial solvents in six of eight patients with antiglomerular basement membrane antibody-mediated glomerulonephritis whom they interviewed. These solvents included paint solvents and sprays, jet propulsion fuel, degreasing solvents, and hair sprays. Exposure duration was a minimum of 1 year in five cases and was generally to a vapor or fine mist form of the solvent in question. Three of four patients tested had antibodies to glomerular basement membrane in the serum. Klavis et al.,[K271] who described a patient with Goodpasture's syndrome who became ill after a single massive exposure to a gasoline-based paint spray, also reported the development of pulmonary hemorrhage and glomerular damage in rats who were chronically exposed to gasoline vapors. It has been suggested that chronic or massive exposure to these chemicals may result in chemical interaction with possible injury to the lung and glomerular basement membranes, which leads to the formation of autoantibodies directed against these membranes in certain susceptible individuals. In a study of rabbits,[Y17] it was found that intratracheal instillation of minute amounts of gasoline resulted in the binding of antibasement membrane antibodies to the alveolar basement membrane. This would suggest that the chemical facilitates the binding of the antibody to the tissue antigen rather than producing an autoimmune response itself.

Cocaine

In vitro and in vivo studies have demonstrated modulation of the immune response by cocaine.[W110] Increased levels of and significant stimulation of NK cell activity was noted in humans after administration of a single dose of cocaine. Cocaine use has been found to reverse the depression of E-rosette formation noted in heroin addicts, presumably by neutralizing the negative effects of heroin. In vivo studies of the effects of cocaine in mice have demonstrated an increase in T-cell and a decrease in B-cell proliferation. Delayed hypersensitivity responsiveness was also increased. Of interest, in vitro studies of mice demonstrated a decrease in T-lymphocyte proliferation. Thus, there is evidence demonstrating an effect of cocaine on the immune response, but the significance of this in vivo has yet to be determined. Cocaine abuse has resulted in the development of clinical features and syndromes that simulate connective tissue diseases such as SLE, vasculitis, and polymyositis.[L273] Examples include optic neuropathy, transverse myelitis, pulmonary granulomatosis, glomerulopathy, and myopathy. Zamora-Quezada et al.[Z6] reported the development of a necrotizing disease affecting the skin and muscle of a 20-year-old woman soon after free-basing cocaine. Some of the features were suggestive of dermatomyositis, and they responded rapidly to high-dose steroids. However, skin and muscle biopsies did not show vasculitis. Three other people who had inhaled cocaine with the patient also became ill. Neurologic complications of cocaine abuse have become increasing recognized, and have included transient ischemic attacks, cerebral hemorrhage and infarcts, anterior spinal artery and lateral medullary syndromes and seizures.[M512] No identifiable pattern with regard to the duration or frequency of cocaine abuse, the preparation, route of administration, or amount of cocaine used has been found. Thrombocytopenia, believed to be immune mediated, has been reported in association with cocaine abuse by intranasal and intravenous routes.[O99] It is as yet unclear whether cocaine produces its effects through direct toxicity, repeated vascular injury, repeated antigenic stimulation, modulation of the immune system, or a combination of all of these. There are some preliminary data on the effects of other recreational drugs.

Metals

Chronic exposure to a variety of chemicals and in particular certain metals has been reported to induce kidney disease in both animals and humans through the formation of immune complexes, which may contain autoantigens and/or autoantibodies, or the production of autoantibodies to renal antigens.[D296,H166]

Mercuric chloride has been demonstrated to induce the development of several types of immune complex—mediated glomerulopathies, such as membranous and mesangial glomerulonephropathy, in susceptible strains of rats. In some cases there was concomitant production of antinuclear antibodies directed against a nuclear nonhistone chromatic protein.[W120] Antibodies to self-antigens, such as ssDNA, laminin, collagen II, and IV and to nonself antigens, such as trinitrophenyl and sheep red blood cells, have been described in the Brown-Norway (BN) rats.[G262] Antilaminin autoantibodies were found to make up the major part of the antiglomerular basement membrane antibodies in the glomerular deposits.[G422] High titers of antinucleolar antibodies, composed of all IgG subclasses, developed in SJL/N and B10.S (H-2^s) mice following mercury administration.[H496,R168] Some mice also had antinuclear antibodies of the IgM class. The staining pattern of both the IgM and IgG antibodies was described as "clumpy nucleolar."[H496] The antinucleolar antibodies induced by treatment with mercuric chloride were found to be directed against a U3-RNP—associated protein believed to be fibrillarin and are very similar to the antibodies found in some patients with scleroderma.[R168] IgM and IgG antibodies to histones were also found in some mice.[H496] It appears that different strains vary in their susceptibility to induce antibody formation and clinical disease. Studies of various strains of mice by Goter Robinson et al.[G312] demonstrated variation in antibody responses to mercuric chloride administration between the strains. Susceptibility appeared to be determined by the H-2^s haplotype. Further work suggested that the I region of the H-2 complex

was the major genetic factor controlling the immune response that resulted in production of antigen-specific antibodies, suggesting a genetic influence. Antinuclear antibodies of the IgG class directed against nucleolar antigen(s) were induced in Swiss ICR mice by the parenteral administration of mercuric chloride.[G311] However, unlike the BN rat, while some renal changes did occur none of the mice developed true glomerulopathy. This may be due to a difference in antigen specificity between the two animal models or to inadequate immune complex formation due to antibody excess. Other strains of mice did develop immune deposits and glomerulonephritis following treatment with mercuric chloride, suggesting a genetic influence. Lindqvist et al. reported the presence of immunoglobulin and complement deposits at the level of the glomerular basement membrane in patients with nephrotic syndrome who had been exposed to mercury through the use of skin-lightening creams containing the chemical.[L304] It is unclear as to the mechanism(s) by which mercury produces its autoimmune effects. The metal has not been found in the immune complexes, and there is no evidence implicating it as the antigen responsible for the formation of these complexes. Mercury has been shown to affect the functions of some of the immune cells—in particular the macrophages, polymorphonuclear leukocytes, and T lymphocytes. In an experimental rat model of mercury-induced immune complex glomerulopathy associated with antinuclear antibody formation and vasculitis, the metal was found to impair T-cell reactivity to mitogenic stimulation and to decrease suppressor T-cell function.[W120] Neonatal thymectomy resulted in acceleration of antinuclear antibody activity as has been described in the spontaneous autoimmune disease in NZB and MRL mice. It also resulted in acceleration of immune aggregate formation and development of glomerular lesions, suggesting a T-cell—mediated effect.

Chronic administration *of gold* may lead to the development of a glomerulopathy and antibody formation. The predominant lesion is membranous glomerulonephritis. Diffuse granular deposits of IgG, IgM, and complement have been found in the glomerular lesions in humans. Particulate matter consistent with gold has been observed in the renal tubules, interstitium, and glomerular tufts. Silverberg et al.[S439] reported the presence of gold deposits in the proximal tubules of four cases of gold-induced nephrotic syndrome and of one patient who had a renal biopsy while receiving gold but who did not have proteinuria. The deposits were more marked in the three patients who had received the largest doses of gold. These three patients (including the patient without proteinuria) also had gold deposits in the interstitium, glomerular tufts, and distal tubules in contrast to the other two patients. The patient who had not developed proteinuria had gold deposits that were similar in location and extent to those found in patients receiving similar amounts of gold who had developed the nephrotic syndrome. The lack of correlation between the dose of gold and proteinuria/nephrotic syndrome would argue against a direct toxic effect and in favor of a hypersensitivity mechanism. Gold also has an effect on neutrophil, monocyte, and lymphocyte function. Of interest, the risk of gold-induced proteinuria is increased 32 times in patients who possess HLA-DR2 and DR3, suggesting a genetic predisposition.[W346] Immune response genes may also play a role in the development of autoimmune diseases induced by other agents. Administration of gold has resulted in the development of immune complex—mediated nephropathy in a large proportion of treated animals, and it has been associated with the production of antibodies to renal epithelial antigens, granular immune deposits consisting of these antibodies and their antigens, and thickening of capillary walls and mesangial cellularity. Antinuclear and antinucleolar antibodies have been induced in some strains of mice and antilaminin antibodies in BN rats following administration of parenteral gold.[G312,S189] Increased mesangial deposits of IgG were reported in C57BL/6 mice.[S189]

Long term oral exposure to *cadmium* has been reported to induce a membranous glomerulonephropathy in rats, which is thought to be mediated by immune complexes.[J133] The nephropathy demonstrates similar morphologic, immune-histochemical, and ultrastructural characteristics to those seen in membranous glomerulonephritis in humans. Granular irregular dense deposits of IgG were found in most glomeruli. In addition, tubular lesions resembling those seen in mercuric chloride—induced nephropathy were also noted. Like mercury and gold, cadmium has also been reported to induce the formation of antinuclear antibodies in mice.[O33] Results suggest that this may be the result of either direct or indirect polyclonal activation of B cells. Others have reported the development of follicular hyperplasia of lymphoid tissue and marked proliferation of B cells in rats receiving high doses of cadmium, which resulted in antibody formation.[P276] Miners and alkaline battery workers are exposed to cadmium in the course of their occupation.

Toxic Oil Syndrome

In 1981, Tabuenca reported the appearance of a new multisystem syndrome in Spain which appeared to be related to the ingestion of rapeseed oil that had been denatured with aniline and contained acetanilide.[T3] This adulterated oil had been sold fraudulently as pure olive oil. Approximately 20,000 people were affected with the syndrome, and over 350 people died as a result of it.[A155] It took 6 weeks to discover the association between the syndrome and ingestion of this adulterated oil. Following removal of the oil from the market, there was a sharp drop in the incidence of new cases. Initially it appeared that both sexes and all ages were affected, but subsequently it was found that there was a marked predominance of females among those with the more severe and chronic disease. Patients initially presented with fever, generalized malaise, headache, cough, dyspnea, exanthems, pruritus, and myalgias.[A155,T799] A diffuse interstitial alveolar pattern was characteristically seen on chest x ray and was associated with hypoxia and peripheral eosinophilia. Other less common features included anorexia, nausea, vomiting, abdominal pain, irritability, facial edema, clouding of consciousness, lymphadenopathy, purpura, thrombocytopenia, and liver abnormalities. With remission of the respiratory and nonspecific initial symptoms, patients developed intense myalgias, severe muscle weakness and atrophy, joint contractures, dysphagia, scleroderma-like cutaneous lesions, alopecia, Raynaud's phenomenon, peripheral neuropathy, sicca syndrome, pulmonary arterial hypertension, and occasionally thromboembolism. The muscle weakness chiefly affected the distal muscles in the upper limbs and proximal muscles in the lower limbs and was associated with atrophy in the majority of cases. Muscle enzymes were generally within normal limits, and electromyography was either normal or showed a mixed pattern of fibrillations at rest. Some patients required mechanical ventilation because of respiratory failure secondary to neuromuscular involvement. Nerve conduction studies demonstrated abnormalities compatible with a predominantly distal axonal motor and sensory polyneuropathy. The sclerodermatous-like cutaneous lesions did not appear until about the third or fourth month. The lesions were preceded by the development of subcutaneous pitting edema affecting predominantly the ankles, legs, forearms, hands, and face. Subsequently the skin became hardened, swollen, indurated, and developed a shiny, wax-like appearance. These changes occurred most commonly in the legs and forearms beginning both proximally and distally, and were found 10 times more commonly in women. The extent of the changes varied from a localized form of scleroderma to diffuse involvement. The majority of these patients also developed flexion contractures—especially of fingers, elbows, knees, ankles, hips, and shoulders—which resulted in restricted joint mobility. Many also had sicca syndrome and/or dysphagia. Oesophageal manometry showed a reduction in primary waves and an increase in tertiary waves. Other concomitant findings were Raynaud's phenomenon and pulmonary hypertension. The skin changes reached this maximal extent 5 to 10 months after onset; following this, atrophy and hyperpigmentation of the skin occurred. Late in the course of the disease, livedo reticularis, carpal tunnel syndrome, and digital tuft changes were seen.

Histologic studies demonstrated vascular lesions, which were found in all organs and at all phases of development of the syndrome. Features of these lesions included 1) swelling and necrosis of endothelial cells followed by proliferation of these cells, which resulted in partial or total obliteration of the lumen of the affected arterioles, capillaries, and veins; 2) predominant lymphocyte and histiocyte infiltration of perivascular tissue of the media or of the intima of vessels, which in the case of the last one was subsequently associated with fibroblastic proliferation of the subintimal; 3) obliterative fibrosis of the intima, which was found in the late phases of the disease. Skin biopsies revealed lymphocytic vasculitis of the small vessels of the dermis and diffuse lymphohistiocytic infiltration of the dermis and fascia initially. Subsequently deposits of fibrillar mucin and eosinophilic fibrosis were found even in patients without evidence of scleroderma. Atrophy of dermal appendages such as sweat glands and hair follicles occurred. The fibrosis extended into the subcutaneous fat tissue in some patients. Many patients had antinuclear antibodies but were negative for rheumatoid factor, anti-DNA, and anti-ENA antibodies including anti-Sm and anti-SSB anti-SS-B antibodies. While the majority of patients have positive ANAs during the early phase of the disease, generally titers subsequently dropped and became negative in most cases. Thus, this so-called toxic oil syndrome has many features of connective tissue diseases and provides evidence for a supporting role for the induction of collagen-vascular diseases by an environmental toxin to which large populations were exposed. The toxic oil syndrome has many similarities to the eosinophilia-myalgia syndrome (EMS) associated with tryptophan ingestion, which is discussed later in this chapter.

Other Chemicals and Toxins

Colchicine, a medication that is derived from a plant source, the autumn crocus, has been reported to cause neuromuscular toxicity.[K459] The myopathy that has been observed is similar to that seen in patients with polymyositis. Patients with colchicine-induced myopathy typically have marked proximal weakness affecting both upper and lower limbs, although distal involvement has also been noted. The weakness is generally associated with a subacute onset and may be severe. Serum creatinine kinase levels are elevated at presentation and fall following discontinuation of the drug in parallel with recovery of muscle strength. Electromyography of proximal muscles of some of these patients demonstrated prominent fibrillations, positive sharp waves, and brief, polyphasic small-amplitude motor unit potentials, which are the typical findings in polymyositis and other necrotizing myopathies. Muscle biopsies reveal a distinct lysosomal vacuolar myopathy but without evidence of myonecrosis. A mild axonal polyneuropathy was seen in association with the myopathy. The myopathy itself generally resolved within 4 weeks of discontinuing the colchicine, but the neuropathy persisted for a longer period of time. Of interest, the patients that developed this neuromuscular toxicity had evidence of renal impairment, which suggests that the toxicity may be the result of elevated plasma colchicine levels. All four patients had been taking colchicine 0.6 mg twice daily for at least 2 years. This provides further evidence of the way in which an environmental agent, in this case plant material, may induce a collagen-vascular–like disease such as polymyositis.

Eosin, which is contained in lipstick and is used in the laboratory for tissue staining, has been reported to cause photosensitivity rashes and contact dermatitis.[B591] It is known to have the ability to bind strongly to body tissue in vitro, and it has been suggested that if the same happened in vivo, through the application of lipstick, it might act as an immunologic trigger for systemic lupus erythematosus. Certainly photosensitivity is one of the recognized features of lupus, and the presence of eosin in lipstick might suggest an explanation for the female predominance seen in lupus if it is indeed a trigger.

Autoimmune diseases have been reported to occur after injection or implantation of *paraffin* or *silicone.*[K18,S289] Miyoshi et al. first described the development of autoimmune phenomena in humans after inframammary injections of paraffin, which he termed "human adjuvant disease."[M506] Characteristics of the disease were the development of features of autoimmune diseases, such as hypergammaglobulinemia, autoantibody formation, including ANA, and granuloma formation, approximately 2 years after injection of foreign substances, such as silicone or related substances, with improvement following removal of these substances. Subsequently, in a review of seven cases of the disease following injections of paraffin/silicone for augmentation mammoplasty, Yoshida also included arthralgias, arthritis, adenopathy, elevated erythrocyte sedimentation rate, and positive rheumatoid factor among the manifestations of the disease.[Y51] Of interest, not all the patients showed clinical improvement following removal of the injected materials. In 1984, Kumagai et al.[K455] reported an association between the injection of either paraffin or silicone and the development of autoimmune diseases in 46 patients. Of these, 24 patients had evidence of a definite connective tissue disease, which included systemic lupus erythematosus, mixed connective tissue disease, rheumatoid arthritis, Sjögren's syndrome, Hashimoto's thyroiditis, and in many cases, scleroderma. The other 22 patients had manifestations suggestive but not diagnostic of collagen-vascular disease. Overall at least 75 reports have appeared of patients developing autoimmune diseases up to 25 years after injection augmentation mammoplasty including augmentation mammoplasty following gel-filled and saline-filled silicone implants. The exact mechanism by which human adjuvant disease is produced remains unknown, but hypotheses have included 1) the release of silica from the hardened silicone or conversion of silicone to silica, and 2) the formation of an antigenic complex with silicone microparticles acting as hapten-like substances. As previously described in this chapter, exposure to silica has been associated with the development of autoimmune diseases. Since only a few patients develop human adjuvant disease following augmentation mammoplasty, other factors, such as genetic susceptibility, may also play a pathogenic role.

DIETARY FACTORS

See Table 3–3 for summary.

Amino Acids

A systemic lupus erythematosus–like syndrome has been described in adult female cynomolgus macaques (monkeys) fed semipurified diets containing 40% (oven-dried) alfalfa sprouts or 45% ground alfalfa seeds.[B92,M92]

Table 3–3. Dietary Factors and Their Possible Role in Autoimmune Disease

Factors	Possible Role
L-Canavanine (alfalfa seeds and sprouts)	Induction of a lupus-like syndrome
L-Tryptophan	Induction of eosinophilic-myalgia syndrome
High caloric diet	Acceleration of renal disease in autoimmune mice
Polyunsaturated fatty acids	Reduction of lupus activity in mice

Features of this syndrome included the development of antinuclear antibodies, elevated anti-dsDNA binding, LE cells in peripheral smears, variable degrees of hypocomplementemia, antiglobulin-positive anemia, alopecia, dermatitis, nephrotic syndrome, and evidence of systemic illness such as anorexia and lethargy. Antinuclear antibodies were present in high titers and were associated with rim, homogeneous, and occasionally speckled patterns of staining. Serum binding to dsDNA using a modified Farr method rose as high as 96.1% in one monkey and was associated with a predominantly rim pattern (with a titre of 1:1920). Decreases in both C3 and C4 were observed. Positive indirect and direct antiglobulin tests were noted in association with anemia. Skin biopsy of one animal revealed a prominent dense band of fine granules deposited along the dermal-epidermal junction, which stained with conjugated antisera to human IgG, IgA, and C3. Renal biopsy of the same animal revealed a diffuse glomerulonephritis, which was characterized by mesangial cell enlargement and hyperplasia and coarse granular deposits of IgG and C3 within the mesangium and along segments of glomerular capillary walls. Withdrawal of alfalfa seeds from the diet resulted in normalization of hematologic parameters and negative antiglobulin tests in two animals, with recurrence of lupus-like disease following a second challenge of alfalfa seeds. Addition of L-canavanine, a nonprotein amino acid that occurs in relatively large amounts in alfalfa seeds and sprouts, to the diet of three monkeys that had previously developed this lupus-like syndrome following ingestion of alfalfa sprouts or seeds, resulted in reactivation of the syndrome.[M92] Not all the monkeys exposed to alfalfa seeds or sprouts in their diet developed this syndrome, suggesting that L-canavanine has the ability to induce a SLE-like syndrome in genetically susceptible primates. The development of antinuclear antibodies and pancytopenia was reported in one human following prolonged ingestion of alfalfa seeds.[M91] Reactivation of systemic lupus erythematosus was observed in two patients with clinically and serologically quiescent diseases following ingestion of alfalfa tablets.[R238] Lupus-like symptoms developed in four previously well individuals, two men and two women, while taking 12 to 24 alfalfa tablets per day.[P289] Symptoms developed between 3 weeks and 7 months after taking the tablets and consisted of arthralgias, myalgias, rash, with positive antinuclear antibodies (titers of 1:20 to 1:320, homogeneous staining pattern) and double-stranded DNA antibodies (20%) in one patient. Patients became asymptomatic after discontinuing the tablets and antinuclear antibodies disappeared in two patients. These data suggest that alfalfa or one of its constituents, such as L-canavanine, may play a role in the induction or reactivation of SLE in humans.

The mechanism by which L-canavanine might exert its effects on the immune system and hence induce a lupus-like syndrome remains unclear. Since L-canavanine is a competitive analogue of L-arginine, an essential amino acid, it has been suggested that it may interfere with protein synthesis or enzymatic reactions involving L-arginine. In vitro studies by Alcocer-Varela et al. revealed dose-related effects of L-canavanine on normal human peripheral blood mononuclear cells, which included diminution of the mitogenic response to both phytohemagglutinin and concanavalin A, but not to pokeweed mitogen, and abrogation of concanavalin A–induced suppressor cell functions, which resulted in increased IgG and DNA binding activity by cells.[A127] Other studies have reported a predominant effect on B cells in autoimmune mice. L-Canavanine was found to stimulate intracytoplasmic immunoglobulin synthesis, autoantibody production including double-stranded DNA antibodies, and antibody-mediated glomerular damage in both normal and autoimmune mice. L-Canavanine has also been noted to increase intracytoplasmic immunoglobulin synthesis by lymphocytes from some normal human subjects and patients taking alfalfa tablets, suggesting a B-cell effect. In contrast to Alcocer-Varela et al., Prete did not find any significant difference in mitogen responses with any dose of L-canavanine between normal individuals and patients taking alfalfa tablets.[P289] Prete also studied lymphocyte responses in the previously described four patients who developed a lupus-like syndrome while ingesting 12 to 24 alfalfa tablets per day. The patients were studied while symptomatic and taking the alfalfa tablets: no significant difference was observed between the mitogen responses of the four patients and the control subjects. It may be that L-canavanine has multiple effects on the immune system, and that the manner in which individual immunoregulatory cells respond may be subject to other factors such as genetic influence.

Tryptophan and Eosinophilia-Myalgia Syndrome

In late 1989, an apparently new clinical entity, which became known as the eosinophilia-myalgia syndrome (EMS) was described by the Centers for Disease Control. Case-control studies demonstrated an association between the syndrome and use of L-tryptophan–containing products.[A237,E30] Similar to the Spanish toxic oil syndrome, the eosinophilic-myalgia syndrome reached epidemic proportions early on; following nationwide withdrawal of L-tryptophan–containing products, there was a dramatic decrease in the number of new cases. Over 1500 cases have been reported, and at least 26 patients have died.[H287]

The syndrome appears to have a subacute onset with symptoms developing over several weeks.[K199] The clinical features, severity of the disease, and duration of L-tryptophan exposure before illness are variable. Patients typically present with fatigue and myalgia, which is often severe enough to be incapacitating. The onset of myalgia is generally acute and rapid (1 to 5 days) with no preceding precipitating event. There may be associated arthralgia and/or marked cutaneous hyperesthesia. The arthralgias, which are generally symmetrical and polyarticular, affect the elbow, knee, and shoulder joints predominantly and are not associated with any joint swelling or morning stiffness. Many patients have respiratory symptoms characterized by dyspnea and a nonproductive cough, which are usually mild and self-limited. Some patients present with edema of the lower extremities, and less commonly, of the hands and forearms. There may be a variety of cutaneous lesions—maculopapular, vesicular, urticarial, or blotchy erythema—that generally resolve spontaneously within a few weeks of onset but may progress to a chronic stage. Other less common symptoms include fatigue, lassitude, recurrent fevers, diarrhea, and mild to moderately severe proximal muscle weakness which is independent of loss of function due to severe myalgia.

Chest roentgenogram may show diffuse interstitial infiltrates or may be normal. Abnormal pulmonary function testing has been observed in patients with and without respiratory symptoms—a reduction in carbon monoxide–diffusing capacity and evidence of a restrictive ventilatory defect are most commonly seen. There may be evidence of an inflammatory pulmonary parenchymal process. Modest transient elevation of hepatic transaminases and other enzymes may occur. Muscle enzymes may also be elevated, although in one review of 17 patients[V44] it was found that while the majority of patients had elevations of the skeletal muscle isoenzymes of lactic dehydrogenase and aldolase, none had elevations of creatine kinase. In another study, creatine kinase levels were normal in 14 of 20 patients.[M163] Electromyographic studies have revealed evidence of acute denervation or myopathic pattern. Muscle biopsies typically reveal perivascular inflammatory infiltrates consisting of mostly mononuclear cells in the perimysium and fascia and less frequently the endomysium. Peripheral blood eosinophilia, often with absolute eosinophil counts greater than 2000 cells/mm³, is invariably seen and may be associated with a modest leukocytosis. Erythrocyte sedimentation rates may be normal or mildly elevated. Positive antinuclear antibodies, most frequently with a speckled staining pattern, may be seen. Antibodies to double-stranded DNA and other nuclear and cytoplasmic antigens are negative as is rheumatoid factor. Antibodies to histones and their subfractions have been found in some patients with a dominance of IgM responses (personal observations).

Following the initial acute phase, a chronic phase may develop in a large number of patients which is characterized by a predominance of cutaneous, neurologic, or pulmonary involvement. Cutaneous involvement, which may resemble scleroderma or diffuse fasciitis, is frequently prominent. Progressive induration of the skin developing in the distal part of the lower extremities initially, and ascending gradually, is followed by involvement of the distal part of the upper extremities and occasionally the trunk. Sparing of the digits has been noted. Involvement may be severe enough to result in joint contractures especially of elbows and wrists. Skin biopsy typically reveals thickening of the fascia, inflammatory cell infiltration of the deep layers of the dermis, the interlobular septa of the adipose tissue, and the fascia. Progressive cutaneous fibrosis may develop. Some patients subsequently have had slow regression of their skin disease.

Neurologic involvement may occur and is characterized by a sensory neuropathy, with evidence of both axonal and demyelinating abnormalities. A number of patients have been reported to develop a progressive and potentially fatal ascending polyneuropathy.[K199]

Chronic pulmonary involvement consisting of interstitial lung disease, obstructive lung disease, pleural effusions, hypoventilation secondary to neuromuscular dysfunction and pulmonary hypertension have been noted in some patients.

The course and progress of the disease is variable. In some patients there is a rapid resolution following discontinuation of L-tryptophan, while in others there is progression of the disease with evolution into a chronic form.

The etiopathogenesis of this syndrome has yet to be elucidated. Case-control studies have found a strong association between the ingestion of L-tryptophan and development of the syndrome, but it is unclear whether it is L-tryptophan itself or a contaminant or impurity that is the etiologic factor. L-tryptophan is present in the average protein diet in the Western world in amounts equal to or greater than that found in the preparations ingested by some affected patients, and has been used commonly in tablet form in the United States over the last decade without the widespread occurrence of the syndrome until 2 years ago. This would argue against the amino acid itself being the inciting factor. It is more likely that, similar to the Spanish toxic oil syndrome, a contaminant is at fault. A recent study found an association between retail lots of L-tryptophan used by 29 patients who developed the syndrome and a reduction in the quantity of powdered carbon used in the purification step.[B193] This would suggest that possible incomplete purification processing of the tryptophan may have resulted in the presence of a contaminant, shown by an absorbance peak on HPLC, in the tryptophan product. This has yet to be confirmed. This postulated contaminant might either incite an inflammatory response or might be autosensitizing in a susceptible host either by direct means or through hapten formation. The same could be postulated for an abnormal metabolite of L-tryptophan. Alternatively, there may be inherited or acquired abnormalities in L-tryptophan metabolism in certain individuals, which might result in the formation and/or accumulation of pathogenic metabolites upon exposure to large amounts of L-tryptophan.

There is evidence to implicate eosinophils in the pathogenesis of the syndrome. Eosinophils are sources of toxic granule-associated proteins that may activate other cells. Elevated levels of these proteins were found in the sera and urine of patients with the syndrome compared with controls.[M163] In situ hybridization studies of affected skin revealed increased expression of Type 1 collagen gene in fibroblasts localized in the fascia, subcutaneous adipose tissue, and deeper layers of the dermis.[V46] This may lead to dermal and fascial fibrosis, as is seen in the patients, giving rise to the sclerodermatous-like skin changes seen in this syndrome.

Other Amino Acids

Restrictions of some amino acids in the diet have been reported to modify the severity of autoimmune disease in mice. Dubois et al.[D337] reported that feeding of low-phenylalanine or low-tyrosine diets prevented the development of renal diseases and prolonged survival of autoimmune-prone (NZB × NZW) F1 (B/W) mice.

Fats

Environmental agents present in the diet may play an important role in the modulation of disease activity. Many factors, such as reduction in dietary fat, caloric intake, and saturated fatty acids, have been shown to modify the severity of murine lupus. The autoimmune disease seen in NZB mice was reported to occur significantly later and be less severe in those mice fed low-fat diets.[F67] In addition, lower titers of autoantibodies and increased cellular cytotoxicity after tumor immunization were noted.[F66]

Studies of the hybrid autoimmunity prone (NZB × NZW) F1 (B/W) mice revealed that restriction of caloric intake initiated from the time of weaning was associated with a significant prolongation of life and alteration of lymphoid cell immune function.[F62,F63] These mice generally die of renal disease; however, caloric restriction to 10 kcal/day more than doubled the life span of the mice on the low-calorie diet. Histopathologic study performed when the mice were 10 months old revealed advanced renal disease with extensive glomerular sclerosis, wire loop lesions, and cellular proliferation in the group receiving the high-calorie diet, whereas those receiving the low-calorie diet had little glomerular proliferation and virtually no wire loops or evidence of glomerulosclerosis. Immunofluorescent studies showed extensive deposits of γ globulin and complement in the glomerular capillaries of mice fed high-calorie diets, while minimal capillary deposits were seen in those on low-calorie diets.[F63] Antibody titers to native DNA were significantly lower in the 10-month-old mice on the low-calorie diet compared with those receiving the high-calorie diet.

Restriction of caloric and fat intake was found to inhibit the development of vasculitis and glomerulonephritis in B/W mice, while high intake of saturated fat in the diet enhanced the development of these lesions.[F62] Diets enriched with the polyunsaturated fatty acid, eicosapentaenoic acid, has been shown to delay the onset of proteinuria and rise of both anti-ssDNA and dsDNA antibody titers, inhibit the development of glomerular disease, and prolong life survival of female NZB × NZW/F1 mice.[P296] Kelley et al.[K151] showed that a diet using fish oil as the exclusive source of lipid suppressed autoimmunity and retarded the development of immune-mediated glomerulonephritis in MRL-lpr mice. The effects of diet on murine lupus are discussed further in Chapter 17.

The effects of caloric restriction and changes in fatty acid consumption on disease severity in humans has been less well defined. There have been only a few studies and these have tended to have had variable results. Thorner et al.[T162] reported the results of an open study in which 17 patients with systemic lupus erythematosus were treated with a diet reduced in polyunsaturated fats and enriched in saturated fat, for 1 year. The patients followed a diet in which the ratio of polyunsaturated to saturated fatty acids was reduced from an average of 0.3 to 0.1. Their total energy intake was not changed. After the 12-month diet, the fatty acid percentage content of linoleic acid was significantly reduced. Serum and low density lipoprotein cholesterol were increased significantly ($p < .05$) but remained within normal limits. High density lipoprotein 2 cholesterol increased, ($p < .05$) and high density lipoprotein 3 decreased. There was a significant reduction in the number of patients with active disease and in prednisolone consumption, suggesting a beneficial effect; however,

the numbers are too small to draw any definite conclusions and a placebo effect cannot be ruled out. More recently, Walton et al.[W62] conducted a prospective, double blind, crossover study to assess the effects of a low-fat, high marine oil (eicosapentaenoic acid was used) diet on the course of the disease in 27 patients with active SLE. Patients were given 20 g daily of eicosapentaenoic acid or 20 g of olive oil in matching capsules which were added to a standardized isoenergetic low-fat diet. Seventeen patients completed the full 34-week study. Fourteen had either "ideal" or "useful" improvement in their disease while receiving eicosapentaenoic acid compared with only 4 of those receiving placebo. Thirteen patients had no change or deterioration in their disease while receiving placebo, compared with only 3 of those receiving eicosapentaenoic acid. A significant difference ($p < .01$) in outcome was found when the "ideal" and "useful" categories were combined and compared with the "static" and "worse" groups, suggesting a beneficial effect from the marine oil–supplemented diet. However two other studies in which patients were supplemented for 6 months with 10 to 20 capsules (dose not given) of eicosapentaenoic acid daily failed to demonstrate any benefit.[K420] Clinical improvement has been reported in rheumatoid arthritis patients receiving a 12-week dietary supplement of eicosapentaenoic acid.[K414]

There have been some suggestions that rheumatoid arthritis and other inflammatory arthropathies may be associated with environmental agents. Of interest is one case report that demonstrated an association between symptomatic exacerbations of inflammatory arthritis and ingestion of milk in a patient with an 11-year history of rheumatoid arthritis,[P33] suggesting that milk or one of its constituents has the ability to trigger flares. (See Chapter 14.)

RADIATION

Exposure to sunlight is a well-established environmental factor in the induction and exacerbation of both cutaneous and systemic lupus erythematosus. An increase in mortality and acceleration of autoimmunity has been reported in B × SB mice exposed to ultraviolet (UV) light.[A256] This agent may be involved in the pathogenesis of lupus. Cutaneous lesions tend to occur in the sun-exposed areas of lupus patients and are often associated with exposure to UV light. Artificial UV radiation has also been implicated with reports of exacerbations of systemic lupus erythematosus in patients who visit tanning parlors.[S672] Experimental reproduction of cutaneous lesions, clinically and histologically consistent with lupus erythematosus, by exposure to ultraviolet radiation, has been reported in both animals and humans.[L164,W42] In one study of 128 lupus patients exposure to UV light induced cutaneous lesions, consistent with lupus, in 64% of patients with subacute cutaneous lupus erythematosus, 42% of patients with discoid lupus erythematosus, and 25% of those with systemic lupus erythematosus.[L164] It was found that both UV-A and B radiation could produce these lesions, although the action spectrum of the induced lesions was more common within the UV-B range. Ultraviolet A radiation has been demonstrated to induce the formation of antinuclear antibodies in mice[B547] and to increase the susceptibility to induction of DNA damage in murine lupus.[G222] Ultraviolet irradiation of DNA can phototransform the molecule and render it immunogenic (UV-DNA). Natali and Tan[N42] were able to induce specific skin lesions of lupus in mice by first immunizing them with UV-DNA to induce high titers of antibody and then irradiating them with UV light. Immunofluorescence studies showed fixation of mouse Ig and complement in the dermal-epidermal areas and in the nuclei of peridermal cells in areas of irradiated skin similar to that seen in SLE. Furukawa et al.[F320] demonstrated augmentation of extranuclear antigen expression on keratinocyte cell surfaces following UV light irradiation. This augmentation was dose dependent, UV-B light dependent, glycosylation dependent, and cell cycle independent, and involved expression of SSA/Ro, SSB/La and U1-RNP antigens. Ultraviolet A light appeared to have no effect. This group also demonstrated binding of antibodies to SSA/Ro, SSB/La, and U1-RNP to human keratinocytes that had been irradiated with UV light. Antibodies to both SSA/Ro and SSB/La have been associated with the development of cutaneous lupus, and it may be that binding of these antibodies to keratinocytes in the skin may provide the immunologic trigger for the development of cutaneous lupus. Thus, evidence exists that implicates both UV-A and B irradiation in the pathogenesis of lupus. Of interest, however, is the report of a controlled study by McGrath et al.,[M285] who found that long term exposure to low dose UV-A light prolonged the survival of NZB/NZW mice. The mice were treated with 3.5 joules/cm^2/day of UV-A light, which had a peak wavelength of 355, for 5 days each week. Those mice who had UV-A irradiation combined with depilation had a significantly augmented in vitro cellular immunologic function and decreased levels of antibodies to DNA compared with the group that received neither treatment. These results suggest a possible beneficial effect of UV-A light on lupus through immune modulation. The apparent discrepancy between these and results of other studies may reflect the administration of smaller doses of UV-A light. Higher doses of UV-A light are required to induce photobiologic reactions compared with UV-B light, and the dose used may have been insufficient to produce effects. Others[L164] have used doses of 100 joule/cm^2/day of UV-A light in order to reproduce cutaneous lesions in lupus patients. The apparent beneficial effects on survival and immune modulation is less easily explained. McGrath et al. suggested that it might result from enhancement of cell-mediated immunity by UV-A light. Of interest is the finding that combining the use of a depilatory agent with the UV-A irradiation augmented the immune response. Photosensitivity to fluorescent light has been reported in a patient with systemic lupus erythematosus. The patient developed a severe skin rash and with avoidance of exposure to fluorescent lighting, the lesions resolved and did not recur.[M160]

Photochemotherapy with longwave UV light and oral 8-methoxypsoralen (PUVA) has been associated with the development of connective tissue diseases, such as lupus and sclerodermatous-like syndromes, in some patients with psoriasis. It is yet unclear whether a causal relationship exists or whether these apparent associations merely represent chance occurrences. In one report of a psoriatic patient, who while receiving PUVA treatment, developed pancytopenia, antibodies to double-stranded DNA and to SSA/Ro, hypocomplementemia, and cutaneous lesions that were clinically and histopathologically consistent with subacute cutaneous lupus erythematosus, there was complete resolution of cutaneous lesions and improvement of the hematologic abnormalities following discontinuation of PUVA therapy, suggesting a temporal association.[D284] A number of studies have suggested an association between PUVA therapy and the development of antinuclear antibodies; however, others have disputed this. Eyanson et al.[E174] reported the development of SLE in a 23-year-old woman with psoriasis during PUVA treatment. The SLE was characterized by an erythematous rash, alopecia, nephritis, seizures, coma, high-titer antinuclear antibodies, and hypocomplementemia; of interest, antibodies to DNA were not detected. Bjellerup et al.[B322] reported the occurrence of antinuclear antibodies in 7 of 34 (21%) patients with severe psoriasis receiving PUVA therapy, compared with a 6% frequency of antinuclear antibodies in 50 patients prior to PUVA treatment. ANA titers were low and antibodies to dsDNA were not detected. Kubba et al.[K440] reported the incidence of antinuclear antibodies in a sequential study of 99 patients who received PUVA therapy. Thirty-one patients developed a positive ANA during the study. The majority had low titers and homogeneous staining patterns. Antibodies to DNA and ENA were negative. None of the patients developed systemic disease. However, Stern et al.,[S673] as part of a prospective study of 1023 patients who were treated with PUVA, failed to detect a significant incidence of positive ANAs in these patients over a 2-year period. Levin et al.[L216] did not find any association between antinuclear antibodies and PUVA treatment in their 2-year study of 22 patients. Thus, at present the relationship remains equivocal. (See Chapters 29 to 32.)

INFECTIOUS AGENTS

See Table 3–4 for summary.

Viruses

Viruses have been proposed as possible trigger factors for the induction of connective tissue diseases, in particular, systemic lupus erythematosus. This concept was supported by reports of virus-like intracellular inclusions in glomerular endothelial cytoplasm and virus-like extracellular particles in electron-dense deposits within the glomerular membranes in patients with lupus.[F239,G340,G442]

Table 3–4. Infectious Agents

Viruses	Bacteria
Myxoviruses	Streptotococcal cell walls
Reoviruses	Freund's adjuvant
Measles	Bacterial lipopolysaccharide
Rubella	
Parainfluenza	
Mumps	
Epstein-Barr	
Type C oncornaviruses	
Type C retroviruses	

These inclusions, termed lupus inclusions, are tubuloreticular structures that bear a resemblance to the filamentous forms of myxoviruses and reoviruses. In addition to renal tissue, they have also been described in vascular walls and circulating leukocytes of lupus patients and have been associated with disease activity. While these particles have been observed most frequently in SLE patients, they have also been seen in patients with idiopathic membranous nephropathy, infectious mononucleosis, neoplasia, and AIDS suggesting that they are not specific for SLE. Rich et al.[R192] found that α-interferon endogenous to SLE patients had the ability to induce lupus inclusions in the human B lymphoblastoid cell line, Daudi, and suggested that the same might occur in the circulating leukocytes in SLE patients in vivo. They also demonstrated an association between the ability of SLE serum to induce lupus inclusions and disease activity. Persistent, high, endogenous levels of α-interferon have been reported in SLE and AIDS patients, and it may be that the occurrence of these lupus inclusions may be a nonspecific marker of elevated levels of α-interferon and thus a manifestation of disease activity rather than evidence of viral disease.

Other evidence supporting a viral etiology comes from reports of significant elevations of antibody titers to a number of viruses in lupus patients. Raised antibody titers to measles, rubella, parainfluenza types 1, 2, and 3, reovirus type 2, mumps, and Epstein-Barr virus have all been reported;[H384,P178,R351] however, no specific virus has yet been implicated. The raised antibody titers seen may represent nonspecific activation of B lymphocytes in lupus patients. Of interest was the lack of correlation between virus antibody titers and IgG levels with disease activity.

Type C oncornaviruses have been implicated in the pathogenesis of glomerulonephritis in NZB mice.[L232,M348] Immunochemical studies have reported evidence of type C RNA virus expression in human tissues from SLE patients.[M349,P26] However, further studies using electron microscopy, tissue culture, DNA-DNA hybridization, and reverse transcriptase assays have failed to provide confirmatory evidence of type C virus infection.[H299]

A number of studies have investigated a possible role for type C retroviruses in the pathogenesis of lupus with conflicting results. Recently Krieg et al.[K421] reported an association between murine lupus and expression of an endogenous retroviral transcript which, in the case of NZB mice, was expressed from day one of life, suggesting that it is not due to disease expression, but is in fact a primary manifestation of lupus. However, a causal relationship has yet to be demonstrated. Talal et al.[T30] reported the presence of antibodies to the p24 gag protein of HIV-1 in 22 of 61 patients with systemic lupus erythematosus using Western blotting. Twenty (91%) of these patients also expressed an immunodominant idiotype (Id 4B4), which had been previously demonstrated on a human anti-Sm monoclonal antibody called 4B4. Sm antigen partially inhibited antibody binding of p24 gag, which suggests cross-reactivity between the two antigens. Serum antibodies to HIV-1 proteins have also been described in patients with primary Sjögren's syndrome. Talal et al.[T28] reported moderate to strong reactivity to p24 gag protein, but not to gp41 or gp120 (env), in 14 of 47 (30%) patients with primary Sjögren's syndrome and only 1 of 120

controls. No difference with regard to immunoglobulin concentrations or clinical features was noted between those patients with and without the antibody. It is of interest that in humans HIV/AIDS infection, SLE is extraordinarily rare and antinuclear antibodies infrequent.[S542] In animal studies, transgenic mice containing the HTLV-I *tax* gene have been shown to develop an exocrinopathy involving the salivary and lacrimal glands, which histologically resembles Sjögren's syndrome—which further supports an etiologic association.[G350] Human T-cell lymphotropic virus type I (HTLV-I), the etiologic agent of adult T-cell leukemia, has been associated with a number of immune and connective tissue diseases. Danao and colleagues have recently shown that some of the descriptions of antibodies to HTLV-I in SLE most likely represent artifactual reaction with cellular components in the antigenic extract.[D31] Possible relationships to the retroviruses are worth pursuing, especially because of the recent finding of the detection of HTLV-I proviral DNA and its gene expression in synovial cells in a special type of inflammatory arthritis.[K256]

Several studies have looked for a possible association between Epstein-Barr virus (EBV) and Sjögren's syndrome with variable results. Fox et al.,[F185] using immunochemical techniques, detected the EBV early antigen in the salivary glands 8 of 14 patients with Sjögren's syndrome but not in controls. Saito et al.[S26] reported increased levels of EBV-DNA in salivary gland biopsies and peripheral blood mononuclear cells in 6 of 33 patients with Sjögren's syndrome using the polymerase chain reaction; EBV-DNA was only detected in 3 of 50 controls. Most recently, using in situ hybridization, Mariette et al.[M131] detected EBV-DNA in epithelial cells of labial salivary biopsies from 4 of 8 (50%) patients with primary Sjögren's syndrome, none of 6 with secondary Sjögren's syndrome, and 3 of 39 (8%) of controls. The same authors, using a polymerase chain reaction technique, detected EBV-DNA in labial salivary gland specimens from 6 of 7 (86%) patients with primary Sjögren's syndrome, 3 of 5 (60%) of those with secondary Sjögren's syndrome, and 7 of 24 (29%) of controls. Schuurman et al.[S209] detected EBV-DNA in sublabial salivary gland biopsies of 4 of 8 patients with primary Sjögren's syndrome, 2 of 5 patients with secondary Sjögren's syndrome using hybridohistochemical techniques; however, they failed to detect the presence of EBV-encoded proteins (nuclear antigen, early antigen R membrane antigen, or viral capsid antigen) in any of the tissue by immunohistochemical means. This is in contrast to the report by Fox et al.[F185] of the presence of EBV early antigen D in epithelium of the sublabial salivary gland of about 50% of their patients with Sjögren's syndrome. Venables et al.[V64] using the in situ hydrization method, detected EBV-DNA in salivary gland biopsies of 2 of 12 patients with primary Sjögren's syndrome, 1 of 3 with secondary Sjögren's syndrome, and 5 of 7 controls. All of the biopsies containing EBV-DNA and four additional biopsies were positive for early diffuse antigen (EA-D). Other EBV-specific antigens, such as the restricted component of early antigen (EAR) viral capsid antigen and Epstein-Barr nuclear antigen, were not detected although membrane antigens were detected in 2 primary Sjögren's syndrome patients with EA-D. This group[V63] subsequently reported normal levels of antibodies to the EB virus measured by ELISA, in sera of 20 patients with Sjögren's syndrome. A significant increase in the germline heavy chain idiotype G6 was found in patients with both Sjögren's syndrome and infectious mononucleosis, suggesting activation of similar B-cell subsets, although this has yet to be proven. The apparent discrepancies in the results of these studies may result from differences in the control groups and the relatively small numbers of both patients and control subjects included in these studies. Certainly there appears to be evidence of an increased EBV load in the salivary glands of patients with primary Sjögren's syndrome. But, in view of the fact that EB virus is found in the tissues of many apparently healthy individuals, it is extremely unlikely that it is the sole cause of Sjögren's syndrome, although it may be one of many possible cofactors. However, there is as yet insufficient evidence to definitively implicate this virus in the etiopathogenesis of Sjögren's syndrome, and its presence may simply be a manifestation of the generalized B-cell activation associated with this disease.

A role for a viral agent in the pathogenesis of SLE has also been proposed by Plotz, suggesting that the autoantibodies found in lupus patients are anti-idiotype antibodies to antiviral antibodies.[P224] However this mechanism would not explain the polyclonal B-cell activation seen in SLE.

Bacteria

Chronic polyarthritis has been induced in animals by injecting cell walls from certain bacteria, such as streptococci and Freund's complete adjuvant, which consists of a dispersion of dried heat-killed tubercle bacilli in mineral oil, with or without an emulsifying agent.[K345,P86] The polyarthritis resembles human rheumatoid arthritis. In addition to the articular features, nodular skin lesions, weight loss, malaise, uveitis, iritis, dermatitis, urethritis, and alopecia may also be present. Although the exact pathogenetic mechanism remains unknown, a delayed hypersensitivity to constituents of the bacterial cell wall is most likely responsible; whether a similar event is responsible for the induction of rheumatoid arthritis in humans remains unclear.

It has been suggested that bacterial products may play a role in the pathogenesis of lupus nephritis. Cavallo and Granholm[C165] noted an enhancement of polyclonal B-cell activation, elevation of anti-DNA antibodies, and development of a diffuse proliferative glomerulonephritis in the NZB/W mice who received bacterial lipopolysaccharide. The potential significance of this in relation to human disease has yet to be determined.

A large body of circumstantial evidence exists therefore to strengthen the clinical observations that infections may be associated with the onset and flare-ups of SLE.

MECHANISMS

While SLE is believed to be immunologically mediated, the exact etiopathogenic mechanisms remain unknown. A strong genetic influence is believed to exist as suggested by reported associations with MHC antigens. It is likely

Table 3–5. Mechanisms by Which Environmental Agents Might Induce Immune Dysregulation

1. Nonspecific polyclonal B cell activation
2. Direct cellular toxicity
3. Molecular mimicry
4. Modulation of the immune response

that SLE develops as a result of a genetically controlled immune response following exposure to certain "trigger" factor(s), most likely environmental agent(s), in a susceptible, genetically primed individual. These agents may produce their effects in a variety of ways:

1. The agent, such as a virus, which normally elicits an antigen-specific immune response, may in certain individuals induce polyclonal B-cell activation resulting in autoantibody production.
2. Agents may mediate their effects by means of direct cellular toxicity. Examples of this would be damage to DNA and alteration of nuclear antigen(s) by agents such as UV light or toxins. This could result in increasing the generally poor immunogenicity of DNA and other nuclear material, thus inducing autoantibody production. There may also be direct toxic effects directed towards cells of the immune system, especially lymphocytes, such as seen in patients with HIV virus or following ingestion of toxin.
3. Another possible mechanism involves molecular mimicry where cross-reactivity may occur as a result of structural similarities between the agent(s) and cellular constituent(s) or through sharing of molecular epitopes by the agent, such as a microbe and the host. Examples include the similarity between hydralazine, a drug associated with the development of a lupus-like syndrome, and adenosine; and the sharing of epitopes between the heart and the streptococcus.
4. There may be modulation of the immune response by many environmental agents, which results in amelioration or acceleration of the disease. Examples include the modulation of lupus activity by changes in dietary factors such as polyunsaturated fats. It has been suggested that the effects of fatty acids may be mediated through alterations in the composition of cellular membranes, especially lymphocytes (see Table 3–5).

SUMMARY

Despite intensive research, the etiology and pathogenesis of systemic lupus erythematosus and other connective tissue diseases remain to be elucidated. Evidence of autoimmunity and immune dysregulation has been demonstrated but not the actual inciting agents that are most likely ubiquitous in the environment. Many environmental agents have the ability to induce autoimmune disease in both humans and animals but probably require certain conditions, such as genetic predisposition, in order to do so. It may be that more than one agent has the potential to trigger a disease like SLE.

Chapter 4

THE EPIDEMIOLOGY OF SYSTEMIC LUPUS ERYTHEMATOSUS*

MARC C. HOCHBERG

Epidemiology can be defined as the study of the frequency and distribution of disease and the determinants (factors) associated with disease occurrence and outcome of disease in populations. Epidemiologists design and conduct four major types of studies to evaluate chronic disease: 1) descriptive studies to estimate incidence and prevalence of and mortality from disease in relation to characteristics of person, place, and time; 2) observational studies, either retrospective or prospective in design, to derive inferences about etiologic factors associated with the occurrence of disease; 3) observational cohort studies to determine the course and prognosis of a disease; and 4) experimental studies to evaluate preventive or therapeutic measures.

Epidemiologic studies of systemic lupus erythematosus (SLE) have focused on the following areas: 1) development and validation of criteria for disease classification; 2) estimation of morbidity and mortality rates in different populations at different times; 3) determination of etiologic factors, both host and environmental; 4) estimation of prognosis and survivorship of patients with SLE; and 5) evaluation of treatments for SLE in randomized controlled trials. This chapter will review major findings in the epidemiology of SLE in some of the above areas: disease classification, morbidity and mortality rates, etiologic factors, and prognosis and survivorship. The reader is referred to Chapters 2 and 3 for a detailed discussion of the mechanisms underlying the association of genetic and environmental factors, respectively, with SLE.

CLASSIFICATION CRITERIA

As noted in previous reviews of the epidemiology of SLE, a proper case definition for the disease is required for both the conduct and interpretation of epidemiologic studies.[F78,H346,M174,N110] In 1971, the American Rheumatism Association published preliminary criteria for the classification of SLE.[C325] Presently, the 1982 revised criteria for the classification of SLE (Table 4-1) are used for case definition; the authors of that report noted that the criteria "should be used mainly for the purpose of classifying patients in reports relating to clinical, serologic, cellular, or pathogenetic studies of SLE."[T46] The original 1982 data set has been reanalyzed by Edworthy and colleagues, using the method of recursive partitioning to generate two classification trees, in an effort to "identify simpler and more explicit rules to classify patients with [SLE]."[E40] The resultant simple classification tree requires knowledge of only two variables, immunologic disorder and malar rash; a more complex tree requires knowledge of six variables including serum complement levels, an item not included within the 1982 revised criteria. Based on the criteria data set (Table 4-1), the sensitivity, specificity, and accuracy of the 1982 revised criteria and the simple classification tree were 96 and 92%, respectively. Perez-Gutthann and colleagues studied the sensitivity of the 1982 revised criteria and both classification trees in 198 patients with SLE.[P124] The 1982 revised criteria were significantly more sensitive than the simple classification tree, correctly identifying 184 (93%) compared to 168 (85%) cases, respectively (p = .016); the full classification tree correctly identified 186 (94%) cases. Of interest, the simple classification tree had a significantly lower sensitivity among black than Caucasian patients, correctly identifying 92 (80%) of 113 and 76 (92%) of 84 cases, respectively (p = .038). This finding is attributed to a lower frequency of malar rash among black compared to Caucasian SLE patients.[H347,P156] Thus, these data support the use of the 1982 revised criteria for purposes of classifying patients with SLE for basic or clinical epidemiologic studies.

None of these methods for classifying patients with SLE was designed, however, for diagnostic purposes. In addition, both lack the sensitivity for recognizing milder cases of SLE. Although this is a virtue for purposes of analytic epidemiologic studies of etiologic features, so to assure homogeneity of the case population, it may alternatively be a limitation in descriptive studies of morbidity and observational studies of prognosis, since subjects with a multisystem disease consistent with SLE will not be included if they fail to fulfill the criteria. Several authors have introduced potentially confusing terminology such as suspected SLE,[M391] incomplete lupus,[G357] or "latent lupus"[G29] to describe groups of patients with one or more symptoms or signs of SLE who fail to fulfill the 1982 revised criteria. This author prefers the term "unclassified connective tissue disease" for such patients. (See Chapter 5.)

PREVALENCE AND INCIDENCE

The overall prevalence of SLE in the continental United States has been reported to range between 14.6 and 50.8 cases per 100,000 persons; the individual studies vary over time and place and used different methods of case

* Adapted with permission from Hochberg, M.C.: Systemic lupus erythematosus. Rheum Dis Clin N.A., 16:617, 1990.

Table 4–1. 1982 Revised Criteria for Systemic Lupus Erythematosus*

	Sensitivity	Specificity	Accuracy
1. Malar rash	57	96	76
2. Discoid rash	18	99	57
3. Photosensitivity	43	96	68
4. Oral ulcers	27	96	60
5. Nonerosive arthritis	86	37	63
6. Pleuritis or pericarditis	56	86	70
7. Renal disorder	51	94	71
8. Seizures or psychosis	20	98	57
9. Hematologic disorder	59	89	73
10. Immunologic disorder	85	93	88
11. Positive antinuclear antibody	99	49	77
≥4 of above criteria items	96	96	96
Simple classification tree	92	92	92
Full classification tree	97	95	96

* For definitions of individual criterion items, see Tan et al.[T46]
Data from Tan, E.M., Cohen, A.S., Fries, J.F. et al.: The 1982 revised criteria for the classification of systemic lupus erythematosus. Arthritis Rheum. 25:1271, 1982. Edworthy, S.M., Zatarain, E., McShane, D.J. et al.: Analysis of the 1982 ARA lupus criteria data set by recursive merit of individual criteria. J. Rheumatol. 15:1493, 1988.[E40]

Table 4–3. Prevalence of SLE: Selected International Studies

Authors	Country	Date	No. Cases	Rate*
Meddings and Grennan[M322]	New Zealand	1980	16	15
Nived et al.[N111]	Sweden	1982	61	39
Helve[H257]	Finland	1978	1323	28
Hochberg[H341]	England	1982	20	12†
Nakae et al.[N21]	Japan	1984	NS	21

* Rate per 100,000 box sexes combined.
† Females only, as no cases identified among males.
NS = Not stated.

ascertainment.[F74,K473,M391,S416] The studies conducted in San Francisco and Rochester, Minn., utilized both inpatient and outpatient records for case identification and published criteria for case validation; the major differences were the sampling frame, members of Kaiser Foundation Health Plan, and residents of Rochester, respectively, and the racial composition of the populations, 81 and 99% Caucasian, respectively. The sex- and race-specific prevalence estimates for Caucasian males and Caucasian females, however, are comparable as 95% confidence intervals for these ratios overlap; estimates for the overall prevalence in Caucasians were 44 and 40/100,000 respectively (Table 4–2). The most current estimate in American blacks is that from the San Francisco study, but it is based on only 19 cases, 16 in black females. Thus, the confidence intervals are wide, limiting the reliability of the estimate.

Applying the rates obtained from the San Francisco

study to the 1985 U.S. population, the National Arthritis Data Workgroup estimated that 131,000 cases of SLE were present in the United States; 7,000 Caucasian males, 7,000 black males, 43,000 black females, and 74,000 Caucasian females.[L105] The Workgroup acknowledged that these figures were likely to be underestimates; specifically, the number of cases with suspected SLE was not estimated. Data from Rochester suggest that the prevalence of suspected SLE is comparable to that of definite SLE: 64 versus 54/100,000 in Caucasian females and 33 versus 40/100,000 overall, respectively.[M391] In addition, the National Arthritis Data Workgroup did not include estimates for Hispanics and Orientals; both of these groups have been reported to have higher prevalence compared with Caucasians (vide infra).

International studies to estimate the prevalence of SLE have been conducted in Sweden,[L191,N111] Finland,[H257] Iceland,[T99] New Zealand,[H172,M322] Malaysia,[F209] England and Wales,[H341] China,[N19,N20] and Japan[N21] (Table 4–3). Of studies conducted in countries with predominantly Caucasian populations, there is variability in prevalence estimates from a low of 12.5/100,000 females in England[H341] to 39/100,000 both sexes combined in Sweden.[N111] Variability may be due to different methods of case ascertainment, including use of general practice diagnostic registries,[H341] hospital discharge records,[H257,M322,N21] outpatient clinic records or combinations thereof.[N111] In comparing studies using similar methodology for case identification and validation, the prevalence of SLE is almost identical.[M391,N111] However, true geographic differences in prevalence of SLE among Caucasians cannot be excluded.

Table 4–2. Prevalence of Systemic Lupus Erythematosus by Sex/Race Group in the United States*

Authors	Location	Date	WM	WF	BM	BF	Overall
Siegel and Lee[S416]	New York, N.Y.	July 1965	3	17	3	56	14.6
Fessel[F74]	San Francisco, Calif.	July 1973	7	71	53	283	50.8
Michet et al.[M391]	Rochester, Minn.	Jan. 1980	19	54	ND	ND	40.0

* Rates per 100,000 persons.
ND = No data.
Abbreviations: WM = white males, WF = white females, BM = black males, BF = black females.
Modified from Lawrence, R.C., Martins, L., Kelsey, J.L. et al.: Estimates of prevalence of selected arthritis and musculoskeletal diseases in the United States. J. Rheumatol., 16:427, 1989.[L105]

Table 4–4. Incidence of Systemic Lupus Erythematosus by Sex/Race Group in the United States*

Authors	Location	Date	WM	WF	BM	BF	Overall
Siegel and Lee[S416]	New York, N.Y.	1956–1965	0.3	2.5	1.1	8.1	2.0
Fessel[F74]	San Francisco, Calif.	1965–1973	ND	ND	ND	ND	7.6
Michet et al.[M391]	Rochester, Minn.	1950–1979	0.9	2.5	ND	ND	1.8
		1970–1979	0.8	3.4	ND	ND	2.2
Hochberg[H340]	Baltimore, Md.	1970–1977	0.4	3.9	2.5	11.4	4.6

* Incidence rates per 100,000 persons per year.
ND = No data.
Abbreviations: WM = white males, WF = white females, BM = black males, BF = black females.

The average annual incidence of SLE in the continental United States has been estimated in several studies; incidence rates vary from 1.8 to 7.6 cases per 100,000 persons per year[F74,H340,K473,M391,S416] (Table 4–4). As noted previously, several reasons may help to explain differences between studies. Of particular interest are the differences in incidence reported by Kurland and colleagues[K473] and Michet and colleagues[M391] for the same population utilizing the identical medical record retrieval system; Michet attributed these differences to changes in diagnostic classification. Nonetheless, a temporal trend in incidence among white females can be inferred from the Rochester data; rates increased by a factor of 2.5 from 1950 to 1954 to 1975 to 1979.[M391] The higher rates reported by Fessel from the Kaiser Permanente Health Maintenance Organization in San Francisco,[F74] when compared to those reported in Baltimore,[H340] may in part be attributed to the different methods of case ascertainment: community-based outpatient medical records system and hospital discharge records, respectively.

Recent studies from Iceland[T99] and Sweden[N111] reported similar incidence rates for the years 1971 to 1975 and 1981 to 1982, respectively. In the Swedish study, Nived and colleagues used a system for case identification that employed review of not only the inpatient and outpatient computerized registers, but also the outpatient clinic files. These authors identified 15 cases of SLE for an incidence of 4.8 cases per 100,000 per year.

Effects of Age, Sex, and Race on Morbidity Rates

Among Caucasian females, age-specific incidence rates have been estimated in four studies and showed maximum rates per 100,000 per year of 3.8 in the 15- to 44-year age group,[S416] 6.3 in the 25- to 44-year age group,[M391] 7.0 in the 35- to 54-year age group,[H340] and 15.9 in the 45- to 64-year age group.[N111] Median age at diagnosis for Caucasian females in the first three studies was 39, 39, and 42 years, respectively. Age-specific incidence rates in Caucasian males are difficult to interpret because of small numbers of cases in these studies, but peak rates of 4.5 and 0.9/100,000/year in the age group 65 and above have been reported in the New York City[S416] and Rochester studies,[M391] respectively. Furthermore, that SLE develops later in Caucasian males than Caucasian females was also noted in the Baltimore population study.[H340]

Age-specific incidence rates in black females were greatest in the 15- to 44-year age group in New York City[S416] and the 25- to 34-year age group in Baltimore, exceeding 20/100,000/year;[H340] age-specific rates in black males can only be reliably estimated from the Baltimore study and reached a peak in the 45- to 64-year age group of 5/100,000 per year.

Age-specific prevalence rates for females in the United States are best estimated by the data of Fessel: approximately 1 and 4/1,000 for Caucasian and black females, aged 15 to 64 years, respectively.[F74] Comparable prevalence rates for Caucasian females in southern Sweden of 99/100,000 were noted by Nived and colleagues as of December 31, 1982.[N111]

Clinical studies have consistently demonstrated a female predominance approaching 90% of SLE cases. This excess is especially noteworthy during the 15- to 64-year age group wherein ratios of age- and sex-specific incidence rates show a six- to tenfold female excess in Caucasians and blacks. No such excess was noted in the age groups 14 and below and 65 and above in New York City,[S416] Rochester,[M391] or Sweden.[N111] A fourfold excess incidence rate in females age 65 and above was found among Baltimore Caucasians but not blacks.[H340] These age-related differences in the ratio of sex-specific incidence rates have been felt to be related to hormonal changes occurring during puberty and the childbearing years (vide infra).

A greater incidence and prevalence of SLE has consistently been found among American blacks compared with American Caucasians.[F74,H340,S416] Studies in both New York City[S416] and San Francisco[F74] found three- to fourfold greater prevalence in females aged 15 to 64 (Table 4–2), and a study in Baltimore found a threefold greater age-adjusted average annual incidence rate[H340] (Table 4–4). In this latter study, the age distribution of incident cases differed significantly with a younger mean age in black females of 35.5 years compared with 41.7 years in Caucasian females, and a corresponding earlier peak incidence rate in the 25- to 34-year age group compared with the 35- to 54-year age group, respectively. A mean age at diagnosis of 31 years with a peak age of diagnosis in the 21- to 30-year age group was found in 93 Jamaican black SLE patients; no comparison with Jamaican Caucasians was available.[W274]

The reasons for the excess morbidity from SLE in American blacks are unknown but may be related to differences in exposure to environmental factors rather than differences in genetic predisposition.[H345] A possible role for natural selection in explaining the difference between blacks and Caucasians has also been suggested.[P233]

Conflicting data exist regarding excess prevalence of SLE among Orientals as compared to Caucasians.[C152,C250,H172,M620,N19,N20,N21,S286] Serdula and Rhoads identified 107 cases of SLE hospitalized in civilian hospitals on Oahu from 1970 through 1975; the estimated age-adjusted prevalence was 5.8/100,000 in Caucasians compared to 17.0/100,000 among Orientals.[S286] These data have been updated through 1980 with more recent age-adjusted prevalence estimates of 10.3 and 22.4/100,000 in Caucasians and Orientals, respectively[C152] (Table 4–5). Prevalence of SLE in Auckland, New Zealand, was estimated in 1980 based on 96 Caucasian and 34 Polynesian hospital-discharged cases of SLE; age-adjusted rates were 14.6 and 50.6/100,000 in Caucasians and Polynesians, respectively.[H172]

Casting doubt on real differences between Orientals, specifically Chinese, and Caucasians are the findings of Fessel[F74] and Nai-Zheng.[N19,N20] In the San Francisco study, the prevalence of SLE was not apparently increased among Chinese compared with Caucasians.[F74] Data from China, based on population surveys, suggest a prevalence of SLE between 40 to 70/100,000.[N20] Finally, a survey in Taiwan identified only one case of SLE among 1,836 residents and no cases among 2,000 female students.[C250] Thus, population-based data in three countries fail to support an excess prevalence of SLE among Chinese. Prevalence data from Japan also fail to support the observations in Hawaii of excess prevalence in Japanese.[N21]

An excess incidence and prevalence of SLE among North American Indians compared with Caucasians was suggested by two studies.[A349,M620] However, this excess was isolated to only 3 of 75 American Indian tribes,[M620] and a single Pacific Northwest Indian population, the Nootka.[A349] These isolated observations could represent chance findings; on the other hand, inbreeding and/or environmental factors may explain this clustering. Further studies of Native American Indian populations could identify additional clusters with excess morbidity from SLE in an effort to test hypotheses regarding risk factors for SLE.

Table 4–5. Prevalence per 100,000 of Systemic Lupus Erythematosus in the State of Hawaii by Ethnic Group

Group	Year 1975	Year 1980
Caucasians	5.8*	10.3*
Chinese	24.1	33.5
Filipinos	19.9	44.0
Japanese	18.2	27.5
Total Oriental	17.0*	25.8*

* Total Oriental and Caucasian rates significantly different with p < .01. Data for 1975 from Catalano, M.A. and Hoffmeier, M.: Frequency of systemic lupus erythematosus (SLE) among the ethnic groups of Hawaii. Arthritis Rheum. 32(Suppl 4):S30, 1989.[C152] Data for 1980 from Serdula, M.K., and Rhoads, G.G.: Frequency of systemic lupus erythematosus in different ethnic groups in Hawaii. Arthritis Rheum., 22:328, 1979.[S286]

Table 4–6. Mortality from Systemic Lupus Erythematosus by Sex/Race Group in the United States*

Authors	Years	WM	WF	BM	BF
Cobb[C313]	1959–1961	1.1	4.0	1.8	10.6
Siegel and Lee[S416]	1956–1965	1.6	6.6	4.4	20.0
Kaslow and Masi[K93]	1972–1976	1.5	5.2	2.2	14.8
Gordon et al.[G298]	1972–1976	1.2	4.5	1.9	13.1
Lopez-Acuna et al.†[G298]	1968–1978	1.8	6.0	3.0	17.6

* Rates per million persons per year.
† Includes deaths attributed to both discoid and systemic lupus. Abbreviations: WM = white males, WF = white females, BM = black males, BF = black females.

MORTALITY DATA

Mortality attributed to SLE in the continental United States has been estimated from community-based[S416] as well as national data[C313,G298,K93,L378] (Table 4–6). The most recent data analysis was performed by Lopez-Acuna and colleagues, who identified all deaths attributed to both discoid and systemic lupus erythematosus from National Center for Health Statistics (NCHS) data tapes for the period 1968 to 1978.[L378] A total of 11,156 deaths were identified; 2,568 (23.0%) attributed to discoid lupus and 8,588 (77.0%) to SLE. There were no differences in the distribution of deaths from discoid LE and SLE by sex/race group, region, or year; therefore, the authors combined results for their analysis. There were a total of 6,452 deaths in Caucasian females, 2,573 in black females, 1,760 in Caucasian males, and 371 in black males with average annual age-adjusted mortality rates of 6.0, 17.6, 1.8, and 3.0 per million persons per year, respectively (Table 4–6). Age-specific average annual mortality rates showed a unimodal distribution for all sex/race groups with maximum rates occurring in the 45- to 54-year age group in blacks and 65- to 74-year age group in Caucasians (Fig. 4–1).

Kaslow analyzed a subset of these mortality records and examined deaths attributed to SLE alone from 1968 through 1976 in 12 states that have 88% of the U.S. residents of Asian descent.[K92] Mortality rates were threefold greater among blacks and twofold greater among Asians as compared with Caucasians: 8.4, 6.8, and 2.8 per million person-years, respectively. The age- and sex-adjusted mortality rates for Chinese, Japanese, and Filipinos were 7.5, 6.8 and 5.1 per million persons-years, respectively. Age- and sex-adjusted, race-specific mortality rates for the state of Hawaii were greater among Filipinos and the combined Asian group than for the U.S. mainland population, confirming previous observations.[S286] It is unclear whether the differences in mortality rates between Orientals and Caucasians mirror true differences in incidence rates as is seen with American blacks (vide supra).

Siegel and Lee noted greater mortality and morbidity from SLE among Puerto Ricans in New York City compared with Caucasians.[S416] Lopez-Acuna and colleagues analyzed mortality from SLE in Puerto Rico from 1970 through 1977 as well as a subset of the NCHS data set for five southwestern states: Arizona, California, Colorado,

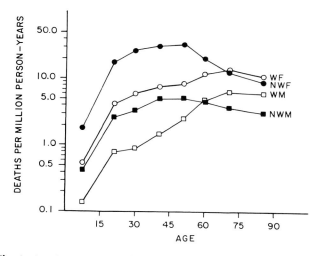

Fig. 4–1. Average annual age-specific mortality rates attributed to lupus erythematosus by sex/race group in the United States, 1968 to 1978. (White males □, white females ○, black males ■, black females ●).

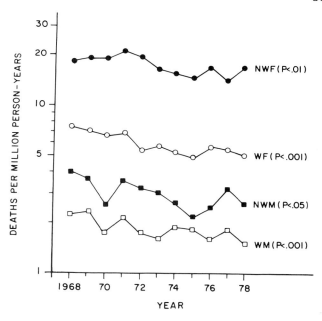

Fig. 4–2. Trends in age-adjusted annual mortality rates from lupus erythematosus by sex/race group in the United States between 1968 and 1978. (White males □, white females ○, black males ■, black females ●).

New Mexico, and Texas.[L377] A total of 92 deaths from SLE occurred in Puerto Rico; the average annual age-adjusted mortality rates of 7.5 and 2.0 deaths per million person-years in females and males, respectively, were not significantly different from those noted among U.S. Caucasians over this time period. A correlation between the proportion of Spanish-heritage population and county-specific mortality rates from SLE was noted for females but not males in the five states; the implications of this finding may reflect both ethnic/racial and socioeconomic factors. Mortality studies from Latin American countries have not been reported.

Nationwide mortality data from SLE have been reported from Finland[H257] and England and Wales;[H342] average annual mortality rates were 4.7 and 2.5 per million person-years, respectively. Patterns of age-specific mortality rates in both countries were similar to those in U.S. Caucasians; the fourfold greater age-adjusted mortality among English females compared to males is similar to that seen in the United States.

Temporal trends in mortality rates have been examined in both the United States[G298,H378] and England and Wales.[H342] In the United States there was a significant decline in age-adjusted annual mortality rates between 1968 and 1978 for all sex/race groups[L378] (Fig. 4–2). A significant temporal decline in age-adjusted annual mortality rates from SLE was also observed among females in England and Wales from 1974 to 1983 but not among males, probably because of small numbers of deaths.[H342] The decline in mortality rates observed in these developed countries is probably because of improved survival in patients with SLE as reflected by 1) a temporal increase in mean age at death from SLE in the United States between 1968 and 1978[L378] (Fig. 4–3), and 2) 10-year cumulative survival rates approaching or exceeding 90% in some studies[R360] (vide infra). (See Chapter 62.)

ETIOLOGIC FACTORS

Epidemiologic studies of etiologic factors in SLE have focused on three broad areas: 1) endocrine-metabolic factors, 2) environmental factors, and 3) genetic factors.

Endocrine-Metabolic Factors

The strongest risk factor for the development of SLE is female gender. In a review of five series of juvenile-onset SLE and seven series of adult-onset SLE totaling 317 and 1177 cases, respectively, Masi and Kaslow showed that the sex ratio at age of onset or diagnosis rises with puberty from 2:1 to approximately 6:1, peaks in young adulthood at 8:1, and then declines with the female menopause in the sixth decade (Table 4–7).[M177] The authors felt these data indicated that study of sex-related factors offered a clue to pathogenesis of SLE. Studies in the NZB/W F_1 hy-

Table 4–7. Female-to-Male Sex Ratio at Age of Onset or Diagnosis in Systemic Lupus Erythematosus

Age of Onset	No. Female	No. Male	F:M Ratio
0–9	39	19	2.0
10–19	220	39	5.6
20–29	369	49	7.5
30–39	298	37	8.0
40–49	183	35	5.2
50–59	98	25	3.9
60 +	58	25	2.3
Total	1265	229	5.5

Modified from Masi, A.T., and Kaslow, R.A.: Sex effects in systemic lupus erythematosus: A clue to pathogenesis. Arthritis Rheum., *21*:480, 1978.[M177]

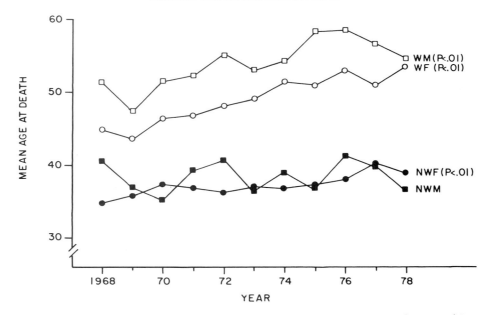

Fig. 4–3. Trends in mean age at death from lupus erythematosus by sex/race group in the United States between 1968 and 1978. (White males □, white females ○, black males ■, black females ●).

brid mouse, a murine model of SLE, support a role for female hormones in the modulation of autoantibody production and development of renal disease and death.[R365] Indeed, Lahita and colleagues[L16,L18,L19,L20,L21,L26] as well as others[J145,M432] have reported abnormalities in the metabolism of estrogens and androgens in both males and females with SLE.

Two case-control studies have been performed to investigate the role of clinically recognizable endocrine factors in the etiology of SLE.[G388,H353] Grimes and colleagues studied 109 newly hospital-diagnosed cases and an equal number of controls discharged from Emory University Hospital between 1973 and 1982; cases differed significantly in age distribution and race distribution from controls.[G388] The investigators found no association of age at menarche, parity, history of infertility, fetal wastage, or oral contraceptive usage with SLE. Hysterectomy appeared to be protective with a crude odds ratio of 0.55; however, after adjustment for age, the odds ratio was 0.73 with 95% confidence intervals of 0.4 and 1.5. Simultaneous adjustment by age and race was not performed. A history of endometriosis was more common in women with SLE, but the odds ratio did not significantly differ from unity.

Hochberg and Kaslow interviewed 74 women with SLE and an equal number of age-, race-, and neighborhood-matched unrelated associate controls to determine menstrual, sexual, and reproductive histories prior to diagnosis.[H353] Cases had a mean age of 30 years, 51 (70%) were Caucasian, 61% were married, and 78% were high school graduates. There were no significant differences between cases and controls in age at menarche, age at first intercourse, and proportion with irregular menses, history of infertility, or usage of oral contraceptives. History of pregnancy ending in miscarriage was associated with SLE

(Table 4–8), as was the condition of being pregnant on one or more occasions without having a live birth—i.e., being a habitual aborter (Table 4–9). The possible mechanisms explaining these observed associations have been reviewed by others,[M473,P48,R32] and are discussed further in Chapters 16, 24, 33, 50, and 51.

Environmental Factors

Historically, SLE has been considered to probably have a viral etiology;[P193,P177] however, despite several decades of investigations, no firm documentation of a definite viral etiology has been identified. Some studies have focused on human retroviruses, especially human T-lymphotropic virus, type I (HTLV-I); however, the majority of studies have failed to demonstrate an association between antibodies to HTLV-I and SLE.[B435,K354,M269,M668] Nonetheless,

Table 4–8. Pregnancy Outcome in Cases of Systemic Lupus Erythematosus and Age-, Race-, and Neighborhood-Matched Controls*

Pregnancy Outcome	Cases (N = 46)	Controls (N = 45)
Miscarriage	39	21
Live birth	75	108
Total pregnancies	114	129
No. pregnancies per subject (mean ± 1 SE)	2.5 ± 0.3	2.9 ± 0.3

* Odds ratio for the association of miscarriage with SLE = 2.7 (95% confidence interval: 1.4, 5.2).
Data from Hochberg, M.C., and Kaslow, R.A.: Risk factors for the development of systemic lupus erythematosus. Clin. Res., 32:732A, 1983.[H353]

Table 4–9. Proportion of Cases with Systemic Lupus Erythematosus and Age-, Race-, and Neighborhood-Matched Controls Not Having a Living Offspring Prior to Diagnosis*

No. Living Offspring	Cases (N = 46)	Controls (N = 45)
0	7	0
≥1	39	45

* Estimated odds ratio = 17.3 (p = .006).
Data from Hochberg, M.D., Kaslow, R.A.: Risk factors for the development of systemic lupus erythematosus. Clin Res., *31*:732A, 1983.[H353]

investigations employing molecular biologic techniques to identify viral proteins including reverse transcriptase continue.

The presence of a transmissible agent, presumed viral, was hypothesized to explain the co-occurrence of human and canine SLE in the same household.[B141] An epidemiologic study comparing households owning dogs with lupus to households owning healthy dogs, matched on veterinarian, failed to find any excess cases of SLE or asymptomatic, seropositive subjects with anti-DNA antibodies among household contacts of index dogs.[R136] Similarly, in the study of Hochberg and Kaslow (vide supra), there was no association of either dog or cat ownership with SLE.[H353]

The most likely noninfectious environmental factors to have an etiologic role in SLE are chemicals. The syndrome of drug-induced lupus, most commonly reported with hydralazine, procainamide, and isoniazid,[H289,S541,S724] provides a model to study the possible effects of other chemicals, especially aromatic amines.[R126] In a recent case-control study of 44 subjects with connective tissue disease, including 23 with SLE and a further 9 with unclassified connective tissue disease, and 88 age-, sex-, race-matched controls, Freni-Titulaer and colleagues determined exposure to occupational and environmental factors including medications associated with drug-induced lupus and chemicals with structural similarities to these medications.[F235] Results of matched univariate analyses demonstrated significant associations between use of hair dyes, use of hair permanent solutions, and use of hair spray with connective tissue disease; in the multivariate analysis, the association of use of hair dyes with connective tissue disease remained significant with an odds ratio of 7.1 (95% confidence interval: 1.9, 26.9). Some hair dyes contain aromatic amines, which are absorbed through the scalp and then metabolized through acetylation. Reidenberg hypothesized that slow acetylation was a risk factor for SLE as an explanation for the occurrence of drug-induced lupus and the possible association of exposure to aromatic amines with SLE;[R126] however, a recent study failed to confirm an independent association of slow acetylation with SLE.[B19] Further studies are needed to confirm whether use of hair dye is a risk factor for SLE and to investigate the mechanism for the association should it exist.

Finally, although dietary factors have not been explored in epidemiologic studies, alfalfa sprouts have been re-

ported to induce an SLE-like syndrome in adult female macaques[M80] and cause disease exacerbation in a single patient with SLE.[R238] The active component of alfalfa sprouts is the nonessential amino acid L-canavanine, which exerts an immunomodulatory effect in vitro.[A127] The role of nutritional factors in immunology, in both normal and disease states in animals and humans, is the subject of active investigation.[V11] As chemical exposures and dietary factors are potentially modifiable risk factors, future epidemiologic studies should investigate their possible association with SLE.

A detailed review of possible environmental triggers and the proposed mechanisms underlying the association of these agents with SLE can be found in Chapter 3.

Genetic Factors

The application of genetic epidemiology to SLE has generated strong evidence of a hereditary predisposition to this disorder; these data have been reviewed by this author elsewhere.[H343,H344]

Familial aggregation of SLE has been demonstrated in two studies.[H352,L102] Hochberg and colleagues studied the occurrence of SLE among first-degree relatives of 77 patients with SLE, and age-, sex-, and race-matched controls without a history of rheumatic disease.[H352] Eight (10.4%) of the SLE probands had 1 or more first-degree relatives with SLE compared to only 1 (1.3%) of the controls: relative risk (rr) = 8, p = .03. SLE occurred in 9 (1.67%) of 541 first-degree relatives of SLE probands but in only 1 (0.18%) of 540 first-degree relatives of controls: rr = 9, p = .01. Of the 9 affected first-degree relatives of SLE probands, 7 were female and 2 male, while the only affected control first-degree relative was female; thus, the prevalence of SLE in female first-degree relatives was 2.64% versus 0.40%: rr = 6.8, p = .04.

Lawrence and colleagues studied 41 consecutive patients with SLE, identified from hospital registers, who had 147 available first-degree relatives, aged 15 and above, of whom 128 were fully evaluated with examinations and serologic studies.[L102] Control relatives were selected from family surveys of probands with osteoarthritis, psoriasis, and colitis. Definite SLE was found in 5 (3.9%) of first-degree relatives of SLE probands compared with only 1 (0.8%) of 128 matched first-degree relatives of controls: p = .001.

Twin studies have demonstrated a greater concordance rate among monozygotic than dizygotic twin pairs providing further support for a genetic contribution to the mechanism of familial aggregation of SLE.[B347,D103] Block and colleagues studied 12 twin pairs, and reviewed data on 17 additional published pairs.[B347] Concordance of clinical SLE occurred in 4 (57%) of the 7 monozygotic pairs and none of the 3 dizygous pairs. Of the 12 monozygotic pairs in the literature, concordance for SLE was documented in 7 (58%); thus, concordance for SLE was present in 11 (58%) of 19 total monozygous pairs. The authors interpreted these results as strong evidence for a genetic contribution to SLE; however, they also acknowledged a role for nongenetic factors in the expression of the illness. Another study, based on self-reported diagnoses in per-

Chapter 5

DEFINITION, CLASSIFICATION, AND ACTIVITY INDICES

KENNETH C. KALUNIAN

DEFINITION OF SYSTEMIC LUPUS ERYTHEMATOSUS

Systemic lupus erythematosus is a multisystem disease caused by tissue damage resulting from antibody and complement-fixing immune complex deposition. There is a wide spectrum of clinical presentations characterized by remissions and exacerbations. The pathogenic immune responses probably result from environmental triggers acting in the setting of certain susceptibility genes. Ultraviolet light and certain drugs are the only known environmental triggers to date.

SLE CLASSIFICATION CRITERIA

In 1971, the American Rheumatism Association published preliminary criteria for the classification of SLE. The criteria were developed for the purposes of clinical trials and population studies rather than for diagnostic purposes.[C325] The criteria were based on information from 52 rheumatologists in clinics and hospitals in the United States and Canada; each physician provided 74 items of data on five patients in each of the following categories: unequivocal SLE, probable SLE, classic RA, and medical patients with nonrheumatic diseases.[C325] Based on computer analysis of the data, 14 manifestations were selected. The committee proposed that a person can be said to have SLE if any four or more of these manifestations are present, serially or simultaneous, during any period of observation:

1. Facial erythema (butterfly rash). Diffuse erythema, flat or raised, over the malar eminence(s) and/or bridge of the nose; may be unilateral.
2. Discoid lupus. Erythematous-raised patches with adherent keratotic scaling and follicular plugging; atrophic scarring may occur in older lesions; may be present anywhere on the body.
3. Raynaud's phenomenon. Requires a two-phase color reaction, by patient's history or physician's observation.
4. Alopecia. Rapid loss of large amount of the scalp hair, by patient's history or physician's observation.
5. Photosensitivity. Unusual skin reaction from exposure to sunlight, by patient's history, or physician's observation.
6. Oral or nasopharyngeal ulceration.
7. Arthritis without deformity. One or more peripheral joints involved with any of the following in the absence of deformity: a) pain on motion, b) tenderness, c) effusion or periarticular soft tissue swelling. (Peripheral joints include feet, ankles, knees, hips, shoulders, elbows, wrists, metacarpophalangeal, proximal interphalangeal, and terminal interphalangeal and temporomandibular joints.)
8. LE cells. Two or more classical LE cells seen on one or more occasions or one cell seen on two or more occasions, using an accepted published method.
9. Chronic false-positive STS. Known to be present for at least 6 months and confirmed by TPI or Reiter's tests.
10. Profuse proteinuria. Greater than 3.5 g/day.
11. Urinary cellular casts. May be red cell, hemoglobin, granular, tubular, or mixed.
12. One or both of the following: a) pleuritis, good history of pleuritic pain; or rub heard by a physician; or x-ray evidence of both pleural thickening and fluid, b) pericarditis, documented by EKG or rub.
13. One or both of the following: a) psychosis, b) convulsions, by patient's history or physician's observation in the absence of uremia and offending drugs.
14. One or more of the following: a) hemolytic anemia, b) leukopenia, WBC less than $4000/mm^2$ on two or more occasions, c) thrombocytopenia, platelet count less than $100,000 \ mm^3$.

These criteria were selected because of their high sensitivity and specificity; the committee noted a 90% sensitivity and 99% specificity against rheumatoid arthritis and 98% specificity against a miscellany of nonrheumatic diseases.[C325] In a retrospective pilot study of 500 male veterans with scleroderma, only 10 patients satisfied the SLE criteria at the time of diagnosis.[C325]

These criteria were subsequently tested in other centers; sensitivities varied between 57.2 to 98%.[C324,D91, F264,G126,L294] The studies with the lowest sensitivities involved patients seen either initially or at only one particular point in time;[F264,L274] these investigators noted that a higher proportion of their patients eventually demonstrated four or more criteria with time. Lom-Orta et al.[L368] studied 31 patients who were thought to have SLE who did not fulfill the ARA criteria; 21 of them fulfilled criteria within a few years.

Numerous suggestions were made for the improvement of the classification criteria, including the inclusion of antinuclear antibodies and other autoantibodies[C61,L261,W141] and the use of a weighted scoring system in which certain criteria were given more weight than others.[T53] An ARA subcommittee was created to evaluate these considerations; their study led to the publication of revised criteria in 1982 as shown in Table 5–1.[T46] Thirty potential criteria were studied including numerous serologic tests and histologic descriptions of skin and kidney as well as each of the original 1971 criteria. These 30 variables were compared in SLE patients and matched controls. Eighteen investigators representing major clinics contributed patient report forms; the forms indicated the presence or absence of each variable at the time of examination or at any time in the past. Abnormalities that could be attributed to comorbid conditions or concurrent medications were not reported.[F259] Each investigator was instructed to report data on 10 consecutive patients and the next age, race and sex-matched patient with a nontraumatic, nondegenerative connective tissue disease seen at that clinic. This generated data from 177 SLE patients and 162 control patients from 18 institutions. Cluster and other multivariate analysis techniques were utilized in studying the variables; numerous potential criteria sets were analyzed. The final revised criteria consists of 11 criteria compared to 14 in the preliminary criteria; 5 of the criteria are composites of one or more abnormalities. As in the preliminary data, patients must fulfill 4 or more of the criteria; no single criterion is absolutely essential. The new criteria in many cases provided improved clarity and reduced ambiguity in definition of terms. A weighting system was not utilized in order to maintain simplicity and easy applicability.

Skin and kidney biopsies were not used in the final criteria set because they were infrequently obtained. Raynaud's phenomenon and alopecia were eliminated because their combined sensitivity/specificity scores were low. Renal criteria were consolidated. In the preliminary criteria set, cellular casts and proteinuria were separate criteria; in the revised criteria set, there is only a single renal criterion. This single criterion is satisfied if a patient has cellular casts and/or proteinuria. In addition, the revised criteria reduced the amount of proteinuria needed for fulfillment from >3.5 g/day in the preliminary criteria to >0.5 g/day (or >3+ if quantitation is not performed).

Antinuclear antibodies, anti-DNA, and anti-Sm antibodies were included and the importance of false-positive serology for syphilis and LE-cell preparations were downgraded. Antinuclear antibodies were felt to be the most important addition to the criteria set as they were positive at some point during the course of the disease in 176 of the 177 patients. Despite their nonspecificity (they were present in 51% of the controls studied), the subcommittee felt their almost universal positivity made them a required criterion.

Using the patient data base on which the revised criteria were based, the revised criteria were 96% sensitive and specific compared with 78% and 87%, respectively, for the 1971 criteria.[T46] The subcommittee further tested the revised criteria against an ARA data base of 590 patients with SLE, scleroderma, or dermatomyositis/polymyositis. Using the revised criteria against this data base population, sensitivity in SLE patients was 83% and specificity against the combined scleroderma and dermatomyositis/polymyositis patients was 89%; utilizing the preliminary criteria,

Table 5–1. The 1982 Revised Criteria for Classification of SLE*

Criterion	Definition
1. Malar rash	Fixed malar erythema, flat or raised.
2. Discoid rash	Erythematous raised patches with keratotic scaling and follicular plugging; atrophic scarring may occur in older lesions
3. Photosensitivity	Skin rash as an unusual reaction to sunlight, by patient history or physician observation
4. Oral ulcers	Oral or nasopharyngeal ulcers, usually painless, observed by physician
5. Arthritis	Nonerosive arthritis involving two or more peripheral joints, characterized by tenderness, swelling, or effusion
6. Serositis	a. Pleuritis (convincing history of pleuritic pain or rub heard by physician or evidence of pleural effusion) OR b. Pericarditis (documented by ECG or rub or evidence of pericardial effusion)
7. Renal disorder	a. Persistent proteinuria >0.5 g/day or >3+ OR b. Cellular casts of any type
8. Neurologic disorder	a. Seizures (in the absence of other causes) OR b. Psychosis (in the absence of other causes)
9. Hematologic disorder	a. Hemolytic anemia OR b. Leukopenia (<4000/mm³ on two or more occasions) OR c. Lymphopenia (<1500/mm³ on two or more occasions) OR d. Thrombocytopenia (<100,000/mm³ in the absence of offending drugs)
10. Immunologic disorder	a. Positive LE-cell preparation OR b. Anti-dsDNA OR c. Anti-Sm OR d. BFP (false-positive serologic test for syphilis positive for at least 6 months with negative TPI or FTA)
11. Antinuclear antibody	An abnormal titer of ANA by immunofluorescence or an equivalent assay at any time and in the absence of drugs known to be associated with "drug-induced lupus syndrome"

* For the purpose of identifying patients in clinical studies, a person shall be said to have SLE if any 4 or more of the 11 criteria are present, serially or simultaneously, during any interval or observation.

From Tan, E.M., Cohen, A.S., Fries, J.F. et al.: The 1982 revised criteria for the classification of SLE. Arthritis Rheum., 25:1271, 1982.[T46] the sensitivity for SLE was only 78% and specificity was only 87%.[F259]

In a subsequent comparison of the relative sensitivities of the 1971 and 1982 criteria, Levin et al.[L217] studied 156 SLE patients at the University of Connecticut (a participating center in devising the revised criteria); 88% met the preliminary criteria, whereas 83% met the revised criteria when arthritis was strictly defined (nonerosive arthritis), and 91% met the revised criteria when arthritis was more liberally defined (nondeforming arthritis). These differences were not statistically significant. Their analysis also noted that of the three serologic tests added in the revised criteria (ANA, anti-Sm, and anti-DNA antibodies), the ANA accounted for the increased sensitivity of the revised criteria. Levin et al.[L217] noted that both the preliminary and revised criteria were inappropriate for diagnostic purposes in that over 50% of their patients fulfilled neither set of criteria when tested at the time of diagnosis. These patients subsequently fulfilled both sets of criteria at the same rate (77.5% fulfilled preliminary criteria and 78.5% fulfilled revised criteria 5 years after diagnosis; 84.5% and 83.0% for preliminary and revised criteria, respectively, at 7 years).

Passas et al.[P62a] compared the specificity of the preliminary and revised criteria in 207 University of Connecticut patients with non-SLE rheumatic diseases important in the differential diagnosis of SLE. The specificity was 98% for the preliminary criteria and 99% for the revised criteria.

The preliminary and revised criteria were tested on 285 Japanese SLE patients and 272 control patients with non-SLE connective tissue diseases;[Y45] the preliminary criteria had a sensitivity of 78% and a specificity of 98% compared to a sensitivity of 89% and specificity of 96% for the revised criteria. Davis and Stein[D94] applied the preliminary and revised criteria to 18 of the 31 Zimbabwean SLE patients reported up to 1989; they noted a sensitivity of 83% for the preliminary criteria and 94% for the revised criteria. When serologic criteria were excluded, the sensitivity of the revised criteria was only 78%. They concluded that in many areas of Zimbabwe where serologic tests are not readily available, the preliminary criteria may be more valuable than the revised criteria in the classification of SLE patients as the preliminary criteria set relies more on clinical rather than serologic variables. An Iranian study[D58] noted an improvement in sensitivity with the revised criteria (90% compared to 81% for the preliminary criteria) in a study of 135 SLE patients in Tehran. They noted that this improvement was attributed to the inclusion of antinuclear antibodies, anti-DNA antibodies, and the decrease in the level of proteinuria needed to fulfill the renal criterion.

The patient data set on which the revised criteria were based were reanalyzed by Edworthy and colleagues using recursive partitioning methodology to develop a classification tree; the intent was to provide a simpler means of classifying SLE patients.[E40] This approach has been recommended by the ARA for classifying knee osteoarthritis,[A166] and the 1987 revised ARA criteria for classifying rheumatoid arthritis are presented in both traditional and a classification tree format[A294] as are the 1990 American College of Rheumatology criteria for classifying the various vasculitides.[F261]

Edworthy and colleagues[E40] developed two classification trees (Fig. 5–1). The simple tree requires knowledge of only two variables: immunologic disorder and malar rash. If a patient has an immunologic disorder (defined as the presence of LE cells, a false-positive VDRL, anti-DNA antibodies, or anti-Sm antibodies), then the patient meets classification criteria; if the patient does not fulfill the immunologic criterion but has a malar rash, then the patient is classified as SLE. A more complex classification tree was also derived that requires the knowledge of six variables, including antinuclear antibodies, anti-DNA antibodies, malar rash, discoid rash, pleurisy, and hypocomplementemia; all of these variables were included in the revised criteria set except hypocomplementemia. When applied to the patient data sets used in the development of the 1982 revised criteria, the sensitivity and specificity of the simple classification tree were both 92%. Using the complex tree, they noted 97% sensitivity, 95% specificity, and 96% accuracy. Antibodies to DNA were found to be the best overall discriminator.[E40] Davatchi and colleagues[D57] studied the sensitivity of the 1982 revised criteria and the complex classification tree in 135 SLE patients at the Tehran University hospitals. The 1982 revised criteria were significantly more sensitive than the classification tree, correctly identifying 90% compared to 73% of patients, respectively. With a modified version of the complex tree using the same six variables, the investigators were able to increase the sensitivity to 91%. The specificities of both the revised criteria and both classification trees were 96%. Perez-Gutthann and colleagues[P124] studied the sensitivities of the revised criteria and both the simple and the original complex trees in 198 SLE patients; they also found the revised criteria to be more sensitive than the simple classification tree with 93% sensitivity for the revised criteria as compared to 85% for the simple tree (p = .016). The complex classification tree had a sensitivity of 94%, which did not significantly differ from the sensitivity of the revised criteria. The findings of the Perez-Gutthann and the Davatchi groups support the use of the 1982 revised criteria for purposes of classifying SLE patients for investigative studies.

None of the methods for classifying SLE patients were intended to be used for diagnostic purposes. The findings of Levin et al.[L217] underscore the problems associated with the use of classification criteria for diagnostic purposes. Over 50% of their SLE patients did not fulfill criteria at one particular point in time; all eventually did but it required 9 to 20 years in some cases. The sensitivity of these classification criteria for milder cases of SLE is not known. Jonsson et al.[J121] in their study of Swedish SLE patients noted that the number of criteria of the 1982 revised set fulfilled by their patients was similar to or higher than other reported series despite overall mild disease; however, no strict measure of disease activity was applied and no comparisons of disease activity in other populations were made.

SLE ACTIVITY INDICES

Defining the degree of disease activity is essential in quantitating changes in patients, standardizing differences

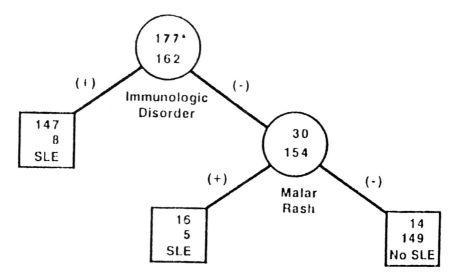

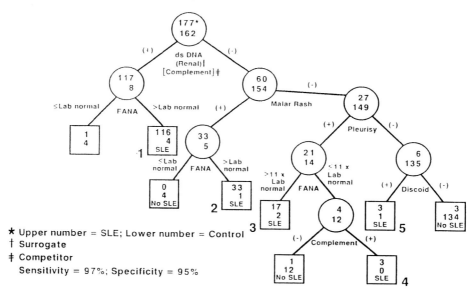

Fig. 5–1. Classification trees for systemic lupus erythematosus.

between patients, and evaluating clinical responses to therapy, especially in therapeutic trials. Although over 60 systems to assess disease activity in SLE exist, agreement on a definition for SLE activity has not been reached.[1,263] The ACR created a committee on disease activity in SLE, which met in 1989 to define the concept of activity, to outline conceptual and measurement differences between currently available disease activity indices, and to develop a new simple ACR Disease Activity Index; these goals have not yet been met.

Most studies of the usefulness of the various available indices have focused on four indices: the British Isles Lupus Assessment Group scale (BILAG), the Systemic Lupus Erythematosus Disease Activity Index (SLEDAI), the Systemic Lupus Activity Measure (SLAM), and the Uni-

versity of California, San Francisco/Johns Hopkins University Lupus Activity Index (LAI).

The BILAG system, developed by clinical investigators from four centers in the United Kingdom and one in the Republic of Ireland, rates the activity of SLE in eight organ systems.[5796] Scoring in each organ system is based on the principle of intention to treat using the following ratings: A = disease that requires urgent disease-modifying therapy; B = disease that demands close attention and perhaps modification of minor therapy (addition of such medications as low-dose corticosteroids or hydroxychloroquine) with maintenance of but not institution of new major modalities (including medications such as high-dose corticosteroids or cytotoxic agents); C = static or inactive disease requiring no therapy or only symptomatic therapy (including pain medications and nonsteroidal anti-inflammatory agents); and D = absence of symptoms or laboratory abnormalities. Ratings are made based on the patient's clinical condition within the last month prior to evaluation. For purposes of statistical comparison with other numerically based indices, the following weights have been given to the four categories: A = 9, B = 4, C = 1, D = 0.[K39] Possible scores with this system vary from a minimum of 0 to a maximum of 72.

SLEDAI was developed at the University of Toronto. Several clinicians rated the importance of 37 variables in defining SLE activity.[B396,C359] Using the highest-ranking 24 variables, 39 fictitious patients were created and 14 rheumatologists ordered the patients in terms of amount of disease activity. The implied weights of each variable in contributing to the judgment of activity in the group of fictitious patients were derived from multiple regression analysis. The resultant index utilizes the best variables identified by this analysis. Real patients were then used to compare the instrument with the physician's global assessment of activity and significant correlations were seen. The index is a one-page form with 24 items. Definitions of the items are provided on the form. Items that are present are noted, and scoring is calculated by summing the predetermined weights for the items that are present. Items that are life threatening have higher weights. Possible scores using this instrument vary from 0 to 105. Manifestations must be present in the month preceding evaluation.

SLAM, developed at Brigham and Women's Hospital,[L262] lists 33 clinical and laboratory manifestations of SLE, and each manifestation is assessed as either active or inactive. Graded estimates of activity are based on severity of increasing disability, organ destruction, need to follow the patient more closely, or need to consider major treatment change. Possible scores with this instrument vary from 0 to 86. Manifestations must be present in the month prior to evaluation.

The LAI[P152] is a five-part scale. Part one is the physician's global disease activity assessment on a 0- to 3-point visual analog scale (VAS); part two is an assessment of four symptoms (fatigue, rash, arthritis, serositis), each on a 0- to 3-point VAS; part three scores the activity of four organ systems (neurologic, renal, pulmonary, and hematologic), each on a 0- to 3-point VAS; part four involves medication, i.e., prednisone (1 point for 0 to 15 mg/day, 2 points for 16 to 39 mg/day, 3 points ≥40 mg/day) and cytotoxic agents (3 points for use of cyclophosphamide, chlorambucil, azathioprine, or methotrexate); part five scores for three laboratory parameters: proteinuria (0 points for negative or trace, 1 point for 1+, 2 points for 2 to 3+, and 3 points for 4+ on urine dipstick), anti-DNA (0 to 3 points assigned according to range used in local laboratory), and C3, C4, or CH50 (0 to 3 points assigned according to range used in local laboratory). The LAI summary score is the arithmetic mean of a) the part one score, b) the mean of the four values in part two, c) the maximum of the four values in part three, d) the mean of the two values in part four, and e) the mean of the three laboratory values. Possible LAI scores range from 0 to 3. Scores reflect

manifestations, laboratory abnormalities, and medications during the 2-week period prior to scoring.

In a study that did not include the LAI, Liang and colleagues[L262] studied six indices for their reliability and validity in assessing disease activity in SLE patients at one center. Twenty-five patients, who were selected to represent a spectrum of disease activity, were independently evaluated by two physicians on two occasions approximately 1 month apart. Validity of the six instruments was demonstrated by significant correlations of scores among the different indices (r = 0.81 to 0.97). BILAG, SLEDAI, and SLAM demonstrated the best intervisit and inter-rater reliability.

An international group sponsored by the North Atlantic Treaty Organization (NATO) is involved in the ongoing study of the operational validity, reliability, and sensitivity to change of several indices when used by physicians at different centers; this group chose to limit their studies to BILAG, SLEDAI, and SLAM because of the prior work of Liang and colleagues noted above,[L262] which did not study LAI.

The NATO group initially studied the validity of the three indices when used by physicians from eight different centers to assess the same patients; the indices were tested using data on patients from chart review.[K39] The indices were compared to the clinician's judgment of disease activity using a visual analog scale (VAS). The three indices correlated significantly with each other and with the VAS (p < .05 for all correlation coefficients). However, the activity scores for the same patients using different indices varied widely among two of the eight physician scorers. This suggested that the indices are complex and require familiarity for effective use, and that the considerable intra- and interobserver variation may make the indices difficult to correlate in multicenter comparison studies of SLE patient groups or treatment protocols in which different investigators use different indices to assess activity. The group suggested that uniform use of one or two of the indices might improve the ability to compare results of studies from different centers.

The NATO group next studied the same three indices for their reproducibility and validity in the assessment of patients in an actual clinical setting.[G172] Seven patients representing a spectrum of disease activity and disease manifestations were each examined by four of seven physicians from seven different centers; physicians from the center where the study patients received their care were excluded. Each observer completed the three indices and a VAS of disease activity on each of the examined patients. The indices all significantly correlated with each other, and there was no significant interobserver variation with any of the indices. All three indices detected differences among patients. This study suggested that physicians from different countries and health care systems can evaluate patients reproducibly, regardless of the instruments used and the disease activity of the patients, without significant interobserver variation. Differences in the findings of the two NATO studies may be attributable to the methodologies used; the problems with inter- and intraobserver variations seen in the first study may have been due to difficulties associated with chart abstraction of clinical information, and these problems may not exist when the indices are used in an actual clinical setting. The NATO group is currently studying the sensitivities of the three indices to change by having the same seven physicians use the three indices to assess disease activity on the same seven patients examined 20 months after the initial study.

Petri and colleagues[P152] have demonstrated that LAI and SLEDAI are sensitive to change. As part of an ongoing prospective study, the physicians's global assessment of disease activity, LAI and SLEDAI have been completed at least quarterly on 185 SLE patients followed by rheumatologists at Johns Hopkins Hospital. Using a definition of disease flare as a change of ≥ 1.0 in the physician's global assessment of disease activity (measured on a 0 to 3 scale) from the previous visit or from a visit within the prior 93 days, mean SLEDAI scores increased by 3.0, and mean LAI scores (modified to omit the physician's global assessment) increased by 0.26 at times of flare; these increases in SLEDAI and LAI scores were found to be significant increases. These findings suggest that both SLEDAI and LAI can detect changes in activity with time, and they may be useful in following changes in disease activity in the clinic setting.

It appears that the four most commonly used activity indices have clinical utility when they are used in the assessment of actual patients. The indices are reliable, valid, and correlate with each other; SLEDAI and LAI are sensitive to change, and tests of the sensitivity to change of SLAM and BILAG are pending. Index preference among clinicians will depend on familiarity and ease of usage; it is the aim of the ACR Committee on Disease Activity in SLE to develop an index that is simple, while maintaining the reliability, validity, and sensitivity to change of the existing indices.

A future goal of both clinical investigators of the NATO group and the investigators involved in the development of LAI is to develop a damage index of SLE; the goal is to provide clinicians with a single index that is valid, reliable, sensitive to change, and simple. Like activity indices, a damage index can be used to compare patient groups and measure outcome in treatment protocals.

Section III

IMMUNOLOGICAL ABNORMALITIES IN SYSTEMIC LUPUS ERYTHEMATOSUS

Chapter 6

AN OVERVIEW OF THE PATHOGENESIS OF SYSTEMIC LUPUS ERYTHEMATOSUS

BEVRA H. HAHN

Systemic lupus erythematosus (SLE) probably results from multiple events, which begin as interactions between susceptibility genes and environmental stimuli.[H22,S640,T191a] These interactions result in abnormal immune responses that produce autoantibodies and immune complexes, with pathogenic subsets of both causing tissue damage. In healthy individuals, abnormal immune responses of this type (consisting of hyperactive T-cell help and hyperactive B-cell synthesis of immunoglobulins) are down-regulated, and potentially harmful immune complexes are eliminated. During periods of disease flare in patients with SLE, these suppressive control mechanisms are defective. These abnormalities are illustrated in Figure 6–1.

The relative contribution of susceptibility genes and of environmental triggers is unknown. It is possible that a sizable "dose" of either susceptibility genes or a potent environmental stimulus can by itself cause SLE. Perhaps an individual who inherits multiple predisposing genes does not require an environmental trigger to develop disease. Similarly, some potent infectious agent or environmental toxin may be capable of causing SLE in any individual, with the disease manifestations being influenced by the genetic background. This process would resemble the ability of hydralazine or procainamide to induce lupus-like syndromes in Caucasians. However, to date no single gene, gene combination, or environmental agent has been shown to be the sole cause of idiopathic SLE.

The multiple abnormalities required for development of SLE are listed in Table 6–1, and in more detail in Table 6–2. Each is considered in depth in one or more chapters of this book (as indicated in Table 6–2). Extensive references are provided in those chapters; only recent overview discussions of pathogenesis are listed as references at the end of this chapter. Each abnormality that contributes to SLE will be discussed briefly in the following paragraphs.

Table 6–1. Factors Required for Development of SLE

1. Susceptible genetic background
2. Available "correct" environment factors
3. Abnormalities of B lymphocytes
4. Abnormalities of T lymphocytes
5. Abnormalities of immunoglobulin repertoire
6. Defective down-regulation of immune response

SUSCEPTIBLE GENETIC BACKGROUND

As discussed in Chapter 2, several different single genes are known to increase the relative risk for SLE. The strongest correlations are between individual HLA class II and the ability to make certain autoantibodies, such as anti-Ro (SSA), anti-DNA, and antiphospholipid. The autoantibody profile in each individual patient plays a role in the clinical manifestations of SLE (e.g., high-titer IgG anti-DNA correlates with nephritis, antiphospholipid antibodies with hypercoagulability). Therefore, if HLA class II genes shape autoantibody repertoires, they also shape clinical subsets of disease. Single amino acids and amino acid sequences, found most frequently in DQ β chains, may be common to the class II haplotypes specifically associated with certain autoantibodies.

The C4AQO gene is the single gene most frequently associated with SLE in different populations (some Caucasian, some black, and some Asian groups). However, to date C4AQO has not been associated with specific autoantibodies or clinical subsets, and many susceptible haplotypes have normal complotypes. At least two extended haplotypes are associated with SLE, e.g., A1.B8. DR3.DQw1.C4AQO, which occurs mainly in Caucasians with a Northern European background and tends to be associated with late-onset disease and antibodies to Ro/SSA.

Genes outside the HLA loci, and on chromosomes other than chromosome 6, may also confer increased risk for SLE. These include several genes or gene deletions that relate to the structure of immunoglobulins, and possibly genes that encode T-cell receptors.

The influence of sex hormones, discussed in Chapter 16, may be at least partly genetic. The propensity for SLE to develop in women of child-bearing ages may reflect the influence of sex hormones on expression of certain genes. In addition, mature females of certain animal species and strains make higher quantities of antibodies in response to antigenic stimulation than do males. The abnormal metabolism of testosterone and estradiol, which occurs in patients with SLE, is probably under genetic control, and may in itself influence immune responses that favor sustained production of pathogenic autoantibodies.

AVAILABLE "CORRECT" ENVIRONMENTAL FACTORS

The nature of environmental stimuli for induction of SLE, discussed in Chapter 3, is the least well understood

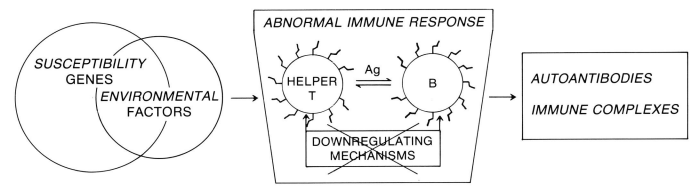

Fig. 6–1. An overview of the pathogenesis of SLE. Interactions between susceptibility genes and environmental factors lead to abnormal immune responses. Those responses consist of hyperactive T-cell help for hyperactive B cells, with both polyclonal activation and specific antigenic stimulation of both types of cell. Down-regulating mechanisms that shut off such hyperactive responses in normal individuals are impaired in patients with SLE. The result of the abnormal immune response is production of autoantibodies, some of which form immune complexes. Pathogenic subsets of the autoantibodies and the immune complexes deposit in or on tissues and initiate the damage that is characteristic of SLE.

aspect of disease pathogenesis. Investigations for infectious agents as a primary cause of SLE have been largely fruitless, although there is current interest in retroviruses. Ultraviolet light (especially UVB) clearly flares disease in some individuals, but it is not clear that this stimulus can initiate disease. Exposure to ultraviolet light increases the antigenicity of DNA, stimulates keratinocytes to express Ro antigen on their surfaces, and induces the release of numerous cytokines from skin cells. The lupus-like syndromes caused by certain drugs, discussed in Chapter 45, differ clinically and genetically from idiopathic SLE and usually disappear when the offending drug is withdrawn. Environmental "toxins" such as aromatic amines may be important.

Femaleness is clearly permissive for development of SLE. Sex hormone status can influence the magnitude of immune responses and can modify immune tolerance. However, sex hormones alone are probably not the sole predisposing factor for SLE. Boys and men develop the disease, their clinical manifestations are similar to those in women, and their prognosis may be somewhat worse.

The environment, external and internal, must present antigens to the immune system in order to drive the abnormal responses characteristic of SLE. It is likely that there are some true self-antigens in SLE. Autologous cells provide DNA/histone (at least in nucleosome form), U1-RNP, and other RNA/protein particles that individuals predisposed to SLE can recognize. These antigens are probably released from cells undergoing apoptosis (programmed cell death) and/or disruption. It is possible that external viruses alter endogeneous DNA and/or RNA to render them antigenic, but there is little evidence to support this hypothesis. Endogenous retroviruses may be important; one retroviral protein is expressed in thymuses of mice predisposed to lupus but not in healthy strains. Bacterial DNA can induce anti-DNA responses directly, and could theoretically induce that autoantibody. In contrast, mammalian DNA is a poor antigen. Ultraviolet light exposure alters the chemical structure of DNA in a man-

ner that increases its antigenicity; it also stimulates keratinocytes to present Ro/SSA antigen on their surfaces, where antibody can access it. Finally, some external antigens may mimic self. For example, some anti-RNP recognize p30 gag antigens of type C retroviruses. An immune response against the virus would then cross-react with U1-RNP self-antigen. it is also possible that the antigen(s) that initiate SLE are external, whereas the antigen(s) that perpetuate the disease are self—provided by activated cells with increased MHC class II (and other) antigens on their surfaces, and by increased quantities of intracellular self-antigens released during cell death.

Ethnic and socioeconomic factors also play a role in SLE, as discussed in Chapter 4. Generally, the disease is more prevalent and more severe in many non-Caucasian populations, compared to North American Caucasians. Overall, patients with low educational levels and low incomes tend to have more severe disease and higher mortality rates. The relative importance of genetics and of socioeconomic/environmental factors in these different populations has not been clarified.

Abnormalities of B Lymphocytes.

B cells of patients (and mice) with SLE are hyperactive, and spontaneously secrete abnormally large quantities of polyclonal immunoglobulin (Ig). Some of the hyperactivity probably results from enhanced responses to cytokines released from T cells, such as IL-5. B cells from individuals with SLE also secrete increased quantities of B-cell growth factors, thus favoring their own expansion. In addition, B cells with surface Ig that binds self-antigens with high avidity are selected for clonal expansion, escaping normal mechanisms of tolerance. Those cells then secrete the autoantibodies characteristic of the disease.

In some strains of mice that develop lupus, there are inherited stem cell abnormalities that lead to activated B and T lymphocytes at early ages. However, abnormal microenvironments in which immature forms of these cells develop also play a role in hyperactivation.

Table 6–2. Details of Abnormalities Contributing to the Pathogenesis of SLE

Abnormalities	Chapter(s) with Discussion
1. Susceptible Genetic Background	
HLA class II and/or III genes	2
Additional, non–HLA-linked genes	2
Genes that influence sex hormone status	16
2. Available "Correct" Environmental Factors	
Antigens, exogenous and self	3, 17, 19–29
Ultraviolet light	3, 17
Female sex	4, 16, 17
Socioeconomic class	4
Ethnicity	2, 4
3. Abnormalities of B lymphocytes	7, 8, 17
Hyperactivation	
Ability to recognize certain self-antigens	
Ability to make autoantibodies containing lupus-specific and pathogenic subsets	
Autoreactive clones escape tolerance	
4. Abnormalities of T lymphocytes	7, 9, 17
Hyperactivation of helper function	
Ability to recognize certain self-antigens	
Skewing of multiple subsets of different phenotypes toward help for autoantibody responses	
Autoreactive clones escape tolerance	
5. Abnormalities of Immunoglobulin Repertoire	11, 15, 18, 19–29
Skewing of repertoire toward subsets that bind certain self-antigens with high-avidity and/or form pathogenic immune complexes	
Skewing of repertoire toward IgG	
Skewing of repertoire toward complement-fixing isotypes of Ig	
Somatic mutations and/or N additions that increase binding of self-antigens with high avidity	
Production of subsets with charges that favor binding to membranes/tissues of opposite charge	
6. Defective Down-regulation of Immune Responses	
Abnormal MPS function	11, 12
Abnormal T-cell suppressive mechanisms	9, 17
Abnormal NK cell function	10
Abnormal immune tolerance	7
Abnormal idiotypic networks	15

In addition to nonspecific hyperactivation, B cells from individuals with SLE respond to specific antigenic stimulation. Thus, the general hyperactivation of B cells sets the stage for brisk responses to selected antigens. Reactivity to antigenic stimuli is probably not global, but is restricted to certain self-antigens such as RNA/protein particles. At least some of the antigen-specific response is controlled genetically. The antibody responses are quantitatively high; certain autoantibody subsets may also be qualitatively different so that they are pathogenic. B-cell clones that make these undesirable autoantibodies are probably positively selected for expansion—possibly by helper T cells.

The features of B-cell functions characteristic of human and murine SLE are reviewed in Chapters 7, 8, and 17.

ABNORMALITIES OF T LYMPHOCYTES

As with the B-lymphocyte repertoire, T cells are hyperactivated in patients with SLE and in some murine lupus strains. Whether the hyperactivation is encoded in stem cells or results from environmental stimuli is unknown. Cells expressing surface T-cell receptors (TCRs) with high avidity for self-antigens escape the deleting and anergizing mechanisms of immune tolerance.

Are the T cells that up-regulate autoantibodies clonal? Most investigations of TCR restriction in human SLE have been negative, but there is preliminary evidence for restriction in the TCR repertoire in one clinical subset of patients.

Part of the T-cell abnormality in SLE patients is quantitative. Individuals with active disease have lymphopenia, which correlates with titers of antilymphocyte antibodies. CD8+ cells and CD4+ CD45R+ suppressor-inducers are particularly affected. Therefore, there is a relative decrease in cells with suppressor phenotypes compared to cells with helper phenotypes.

T-cell help is critical for development of full-blown disease. In murine lupus, the elimination or inactivation of helper T-cell repertoires is effective in preventing or suppressing disease in virtually every strain in which it has been tested. Interestingly, T cells of several different surface phenotypes can provide help for B-cell synthesis of autoantibodies—not only the classic CD4+ CD8− helper T cells, but also CD4− CD8+ and CD4− CD8− T cells. Further, cells with either αβ or γδ TCRs can belong to these helper phenotypes in individuals with SLE. Therefore, the T-cell repertoire is heavily skewed toward help.

An interesting paradox occurs, in that T-cell help is excessive in individuals with SLE, and yet some T-cell functions are abnormal. Clearly, some antibodies to lymphocytes react with surface molecules on T lymphocytes and impair cell responses to various stimuli (see Chap. 26). Indeed, some of the antibodies correlate with lymphocytopenia, and lymphocytopenia itself may be important in defective T-cell regulatory circuits. Release of IL-2 and surface appearance of IL-2R is abnormally low in some populations of lupus T cells after exposure to some (but not all) activating signals. This may reflect intrinsic, autoantibody-independent abnormalities in cell activation circuits. There is evidence for hypomethylation of DNA and for abnormal synthesis of intracellular second messengers in SLE lymphocytes, including protein kinase C, cyclic AMP, and protein kinase A.

Cytotoxic T cells may participate directly in development of tissue lesions (in SLE patients with polymyositis or Ro-mediated dermatitis, for example). However, T cells that normally suppress hyperactive B- and T-cell circuits either do not develop normally from their precursor cells, or are ineffective.

T-cell abnormalities characteristic of SLE are reviewed in Chapter 9.

ABNORMALITIES OF IMMUNOGLOBULIN REPERTOIRE

Multiple studies of nucleotide and amino acid sequences of variable (V) regions of the heavy (H) and light

(L) chains of autoantibodies from patients and mice with SLE are available. Ig structure is reviewed in Chapter 18. Interpretation of these data suggests that most autoantibodies are encoded by normal germline DNA with no unique elements that are restricted to individuals with autoimmune diseases. Similarly, there is nothing unique about the choice of individual V_H or V_L genes that distinguishes autoantibodies from normal antibodies to exogenous antigens. However, it is likely that nucleotide (N) additions at junctional areas in the V regions (especially in humans), and single and multiple somatic mutations of nucleotides in assembled molecules (in humans and mice), promote the development of high-avidity autoantibodies. Some autoantibodies, especially IgM, are encoded directly from germline DNA with no mutations; others, especially IgG, are highly mutated or altered by N additions. It is suspected that pathogenic subsets of autoantibodies are of the latter type, but this has not been definitely established.

Whatever the mechanisms of autoantibody assembly, certain subsets are more likely than others to bind to tissues and promote antibody-mediated damage. Factors that play a role in pathogenicity include epitope specificity, high avidity for the epitope, and ability to fix complement. Charge is probably important: cationic antibodies or immune complexes can fix to anionic regions in membranes independent of epitope specificity.

Finally, the ability of antibodies to form high-avidity immune complexes with their antigens is critical to some manifestations of SLE, such as vasculitis and some forms of glomerulonephritis. The size, charge, and complement-fixing capabilities of the complexes determine whether they are cleared, or fix to tissues and initiate damage. Immune complexes are discussed in Chapter 11 and their clearance in Chapter 12.

DEFECTIVE DOWN-REGULATION OF IMMUNE RESPONSES

Immune complexes (ICs) are transported via fixation to complement receptors (primarily CR1 on erythrocytes) and cleared by cells of the mononuclear phagocytic system (MPS). Individuals with SLE have defects in both mechanisms. CR1-mediated binding is impaired because of low numbers of available receptors, secondary to stripping of receptors by large quantities of complexes, and in some cases to inherited low receptor numbers. The ability of the MPS to clear particulate ICs is impaired in SLE patients with active disease, and in those with nephritis. Healthy individuals with DR2 and DR3 haplotypes have reduced capacity for Fc-mediated IC clearance compared to healthy individuals of other genetic backgrounds. Similarly, SLE patients cannot process soluble ICs normally: there is reduced binding to CR1 on erythrocytes and defective clearance by the MPS. These abnormalities clearly favor persistence of ICs and deposition in tissues.

In individuals with SLE, T lymphocytes (usually CD8 +) with suppressive capabilities for autoantibody-synthesizing B cells are defective or absent. This could result from

lymphocytopenia, from inactivating antibodies on cell surfaces, from inadequate maturation of precursor CD8 + suppressors (which require signals from CD4 + cells to mature), and/or from abnormal intracellular messages following cell activation. Whatever the mechanism, CD8 + cells deliver help rather than suppression.

Large granular lymphocytes (LGLs), also known as natural killer (NK) cells, normally participate in regulating antibody production. These cells mediate both antibody-dependent and antibody-independent cytotoxicity. They can both enhance and suppress B-cell synthesis of Ig; suppression may depend on interaction with T cells. In SLE patients, especially those with active disease, numbers of and cytotoxic effects of LGLs are decreased. This might result from immune complexes modulating CD16 expression on NK cell surfaces, from anti-NK antibodies in SLE sera, from intrinsic cell activation defects, or from absence of the CD8 + T cells required to mediate suppression of B cells. In any event, as in the T-cell population, the LGLs may be skewed toward B-cell help rather than suppression. The defects in LGL cells associated with SLE are discussed in Chapter 10.

The abnormalities of B- and T-cell function in SLE, specifically the ability to react with high avidity to self, indicate that normal immune tolerance mechanisms have failed. Most T and B cells expressing surface receptors with high avidity for self are either deleted or anergized. Deletion is a more efficient mechanism of tolerance, since anergized B cells can be activated by appropriate signals to secrete antibodies to self. The abnormalities that cause tolerance to fail are not clearly understood. It is possible that production of IgG anti-self bypasses deletion, since surface IgG expression is quantitatively less than IgM expression. In addition, the presence of polyclonal T- and B-cell activation in SLE may continually oppose anergy. Tolerance mechanisms are discussed in Chapters 7 and 9.

Another control mechanism that fails in individuals with lupus is idiotypic regulation, discussed in Chapter 15. Individual antibodies and T cells express idiotypes (Ids) which are immunogenic and induce anti-idiotypic antibodies and T cells. A network based on Ids arises and participates in regulation of B- and T-cell function. Certain public Ids, shared by multiple different antibody molecules, can dominate autoantibody populations; some of those Ids are enriched in pathogenic subsets. Presumably, healthy individuals, who can make the same Ids as SLE patients, down-regulate high quantities of antibodies expressing those public Ids and patients with SLE do not. Certain populations of anti-Ids contain the internal image of the inciting antigen, and can themselves act as antigen. These anti-Ids could therefore up-regulate the Id-positive antibody responses.

In general, the defective down-regulating mechanisms discussed in this section are more easily demonstrated in patients with active disease than in those whose disease is controlled. Therefore, the defects may be secondary rather than primary phenomena. Clearly, all of them contribute to disease.

Chapter 7

TOLERANCE ABNORMALITIES IN SYSTEMIC LUPUS ERYTHEMATOSUS

AKIRA SHIRAI AND DENNIS M. KLINMAN

Considerable progress has been made in delineating the immunologic defects and pathologic mechanisms associated with the development of systemic lupus erythematosus (SLE). Nevertheless, the etiology of this disease remains obscure. Different lines of study indicate that autoimmunity can be induced and/or perpetuated by a variety of genetic and environmental factors.[A225,S511,S643,T130] Common to each of these processes is a loss of tolerance for self resulting in the abnormal production of pathogenic autoantibodies.[A225,P196]

An active immune response is elicited when the immune system encounters foreign antigen. In contrast, the immune system is tolerized following exposure to self.[O129] Considerable effort has been directed toward elucidating the mechanism(s) responsible for developing and maintaining self tolerance and determining how it is lost in autoimmune states.

Early studies provided evidence that murine lupus was associated with one or more generalized abnormalities in the induction of experimental tolerance to foreign antigens.[H98,L84,S614] Other pioneering work suggested that antigen-specific suppressor T cells were involved in this process.[A313,C454,D267,G99,G348] More recently, researchers have established that T-cell tolerance develops in the thymus through a process of positive[K252,S299] and negative selection[A6,B329,K68,K251,P333] and is maintained in part through a peripheral mechanism of anergy.

Recent advances in molecular immunology have contributed enormously to our understanding of immune recognition and the processes by which self tolerance is acquired and maintained. Such work includes the analysis of transgenic mice whose expression of neoautoantigens and generation of lymphocytes reactive with those antigens is under experimental control.[F73] Additional studies involving murine models of organ-specific autoimmune disease—e.g., experimental allergic encephalomyelitis (EAE) as a model for multiple sclerosis and nonobese diabetic mice (NOD) as a model for insulin-dependent diabetes mellitus (IDDM)—have further improved our understanding of how tolerance to specific autoantigens is lost in autoimmune states.[S479] To better understand the tolerance abnormalities in SLE, we will describe recent advances in these related areas and consider the etiologic significance of self-nonself discrimination in the disease process.

DEFECTS IN EXPERIMENTAL TOLERANCE INDUCTION

An immunologic abnormality common to many strains of lupus-prone mice is an inherent resistance to experimentally induced tolerance.[H98,L84,S614,S641] Historically, NZB and B/W F_1 mice were observed to manifest a defect in experimental tolerance induction.[S613,S614,S615,S645] Those studies involved challenging animals with heterologous serum proteins. Results showed that a tolerance defect was detectable before the onset of clinical disease, suggesting it might represent a primary immune disorder.[L84]

The cell type(s) responsible for the diminution of experimental tolerance was a matter of contention. Experiments in which recipient mice were irradiated and reconstituted with different populations of immunologically relevant cells implicated NZB T cells or pre-T cells in the abnormal development of tolerance to bovine gamma globulin (BGG).[L83,L84,T81] T-cell abnormalities were also associated with tolerance defects in B/W F_1 mice.[S613,S645] However, when an in vitro system was used to study tolerance induction, B cells from NZB and B/W F_1 mice were found to be intrinsically abnormal.[G254,G255] In vivo studies using a DNP-carrier system also found intrinsic abnormalities in B-cell tolerance induction among NZB (but not B/W F_1) mice.[M249]

These conflicting results are partly attributable to differences in the tolerization protocol being used (e.g., the nature of the tolerizing antigen, the method by which the antigen was prepared, and the density of epitopes expressed by the tolerogen). An additional variable in studies of experimental tolerance concerned the route by which the antigen was administered, a variable that influences whether an agent acts as immunogen or tolerogen. For example, intraperitoneal, intravenous, and oral administration of certain antigens favors the induction of tolerance, whereas intracutaneous and intramuscular administration favors the induction of immunity.

Unfortunately, it is uncertain to what degree abnormalities in the induction of experimental tolerance correlate with the development of SLE.[I69] In several animal models, these two processes were found to be independent. For example, (NZW × BXSB)F_1 female and B6-*lpr/lpr* mice showed no tolerance defect to HGG but did develop an

Table 7–1. Possible Sources of Tolerance Defects in Systemic Lupus Erythematosus

I. Abnormalities in T-cell deletion/anergy
  A. Abnormalities in the intrathymic selection/deletion of self reactive T cells
  B. Abnormalities in the development of peripheral T-cell anergy
  C. Defects in suppressor T-cell function
  D. Increased activation of T helper cells, leading to the overproduction of B-cell–activating factors
II. Abnormalities in the development of B-cell tolerance
  A. Increased B-cell responsiveness to (or production of) immunostimulatory signals
  B. Decreased B-cell responsiveness to (or production of) tolerogenic signals
  C. Selective expansion of an atypical subset of self reactive B cells, such as those expressing the Ly-1/CD5 membrane markers
III. Other immune abnormalities
  A. Differences in the quality or quantity of self antigen
  B. Exposure to environmental antigens that cross-react with self
  C. Abnormalities in MHC-restricted presentation of self antigen (within or outside the thymus)

SLE-like syndrome.[169] By comparison, (NZB × B10.D2)F_1, (NZB × NFS)F_1, and SJL/J mice expressed abnormalities in the induction of experimental tolerance but did not develop SLE.[F301,169,M249]

MECHANISMS OF T-CELL TOLERANCE

At least three mechanisms have been proposed to explain how T-cell tolerance might be established and maintained: clonal deletion, direct clonal inactivation (anergy), and indirect clonal inactivation through the intervention of regulatory cells.[A313,C454,K68,K69,K251,M4,N139,S299,W128] T cells (Table 7–1) recognize "nonself" antigens primarily in the context of "self" MHC molecules.[B323,B324,B521,S215,Z32] This MHC-restricted recognition is "learned" in the thymus by a process whereby T cells which bind to self MHC with moderate affinity are positively selected while T cells binding with very high affinity to self MHC or self MHC plus self antigen (i.e., autoreactive clones) are negatively selected.[B329]

Numerous studies have shown that potentially self reactive T cells are clonally deleted in the thymus, and that this is the main mechanism used by normal animals to prevent autoreactive T cells from reaching the periphery.[K68] However, clonal deletion is not 100% efficient and could not explain how T cells specific for self antigens not expressed in the thymus were rendered tolerant. A second mechanism—clonal anergy—has been implicated in the inactivation of autoreactive lymphocytes that reach the periphery.[B485,B579,J67,M566] Although less well understood, this mechanism induces unresponsiveness among autoreactive T cells that have escaped deletion in the thymus. Whereas considerable evidence supporting these two mechanisms has been obtained, a third hypothesis suggesting that suppressor cells are responsible for directly inhibiting the activation of autoreactive clones[A313,B117,C454,D267,G99,G348,L433] has received much less experimental support.

THE ROLE OF THE T-CELL RECEPTOR IN TOLERANCE

The heterodimeric T-cell receptor (TCR) is generated when noncontiguous germline gene elements (V, D, J) are recombined to form a continuous variable region gene.[D86,D87,K432,W270] Evidence suggests that certain TCRs play a significant role in the pathogenesis of selected autoimmune diseases.[A25,K363,K458] For example, one of the TCR gene families (VB6) is associated with the development of type II collagen-induced arthritis in mice,[B72] and the VB8.2 TCR gene family plays a dominant role in EAE.[A24,U26] In the latter model, elimination of T cells expressing disease-associated TCRs reduces susceptibility to EAE.[A24,O131,U26] Such restriction is not absolute, however, in that T cells capable of eliciting EAE may be present that express alternative TCRs. Moreover, some murine strains susceptible to this disease do not show TCR restriction.

The role of particular TCRs in the pathogenesis of systemic lupus erythematosus is less clear. A striking abnormality in NZW T-cell receptor β chain genes has been detected, but does not seem to be involved in the disease process.[K392,N122,Y28] MRL-*lpr/lpr* mice express skewed TCR repertoires,[G435,M633,S467] and the V β gene repertoires of other autoimmune strains become skewed with age.[S468] It is as yet uncertain, however, whether these changes play a meaningful role in the development of autoimmune disease.

Restriction fragment length polymorphism (RFLP) analyses have been used to search for associations between particular genes and disease states. RFLP studies of the human TCR repertoire successfully documented an association between an RFLP pattern and several autoimmune diseases—IDDM,[H411,M443] Graves' disease,[D147] hypothyroidism,[W121] multiple sclerosis,[B136,O45] myasthenia gravis,[O45,S503] membranous nephropathy,[D148] and rheumatoid arthritis.[G35] RFLP analyses have not identified an association between TCR β chain genes and the development of SLE,[D356,F288,W333] although one recent study reported a significant correlation between expression of a specific RFLP band derived from the TCR α chain and the presence of lupus in a subset of Caucasians.[T92] Continued research will be needed to verify these observations and to identify the TCR(s) that might contribute to the development of SLE.

CLONAL T-CELL DELETION IN SLE

The possibility that autoimmunity arises from a defect in the intrathymic deletion of self reactive T cells has been investigated.[S468,T134] Experiments indicate that thymic deletion of self reactive T cells occurs normally in autoimmune mice.[K393,K394,S468] This result is based upon analysis of specific VB families that encode TCR reactive with Mls (mouse mammary tumor virus–encoded) superantigens.[D380,F216,J42,M148,W342] In normal animals, T cells expressing such TCRs are specifically deleted in the thymus. Similarly, autoimmune-prone (NZB × NZW)F_1, (NZB × SWR)F_1, and *lpr* animals appropriately delete their Mls-reactive T cells intrathymically.[K393,K394] These results indicate that there is no global defect in superantigen-induced clonal deletion of T cells in lupus-prone mice. One exception to this conclusion may have been uncovered in studies of SNF_1 mice, where T-cell clones that supported the production of pathogenic IgG anti-DNA antibodies were found to express "forbidden" TCRs reactive against Mls autoantigens.[A33] Thus, the escape of self reactive T cells may contribute to the development of autoimmune disease in some forms of lupus.

THE INFLUENCE OF T CELLS ON B-CELL TOLERANCE

Many investigators believe that T lymphocytes represent the principal cell type responsible for establishing and maintaining self tolerance.[N141,S418] They view B-cell tolerance as a secondary event, reflecting an absence of T-cell help rather than clonal anergy/deletion. Supporting this model is evidence that pathogenic autoantibodies express many of the characteristics commonly associated with T-cell–dependent responses: they tend to be of the IgG heavy chain class,[P37,S687] bind to self antigens with high affinity,[D51,E16] and be encoded by Ig variable region genes that have undergone somatic mutation.[B168,E17,M537,S375,S376,S377,V31]

T cells could contribute to a loss of B-cell tolerance in either an antigen-dependent or antigen-independent manner. In organ-specific autoimmune diseases, T cells have been shown to moderate an autoantigen-specific loss of tolerance.[A25,K363,K458] This may also occur in SLE—T cells capable of specifically augmenting the production of anti-DNA antibodies have been isolated in both murine and human lupus.[A33,A215,D51,R17,S373] T cells could also interfere with the clonal deletion of autoreactive B cells by producing polyclonal activating factors. This mechanism has been implicated in the autoantibody production associated with graft-versus-host disease (GVH) and the early stages of murine lupus.[D242,P319,R308,V35,V76]

The role of T-cell–derived factors in determining whether B cells are stimulated or tolerized was codified by Bretcher and Cohn.[B485] They hypothesized that a B cell would be rendered unresponsive after encountering antigen unless T-cell helper signals were also provided. Numerous experiments support this hypothesis and have clarified the conditions that predispose to the development of B-cell anergy. These include the maturation stage of the lymphocyte, its affinity for antigen, and the valency of binding between antigen and the B cell's sIg receptor.[L32,N140]

FACTORS INFLUENCING THE DEVELOPMENT OF B-CELL TOLERANCE

Although T cells contribute to the development and maintenance of B-cell tolerance, evidence suggests that autoreactive B cells may be stimulated under conditions where T cells have been rendered tolerant.[A38] In autoimmune animals in particular, the induction of B-cell tolerance may be intrinsically abnormal. Thus, B cells from autoimmune mice transferred to nonautoimmune recipients continue to secrete autoantibodies under conditions where normal B cells would not.[K301] In a recent series of experiments, B cells from MRL/lpr and congenic MRL-±/± mice were mixed and transferred to lpr or ±/± recipients. On the basis of Ig allotype differences, it was shown that the lpr-derived B cells were activated to produce autoantibodies under conditions where the ±/± lymphocytes remained quiescent.[S533] These findings strongly suggest that B cells from autoimmune mice may be intrinsically abnormal and are either hyperresponsive to activating signals or hyporesponsive to tolerogenic signals.[K293,L35,M634,S533,U17]

Recent studies involving transgenic mice have furthered our understanding of B-cell tolerance.[G291] In one study, a transgene encoding the production of high-affinity antibody against the protein hen egg lysozyme (HEL) was introduced into mice.[G292] A majority of the B cells from these transgenic mice could produce anti-HEL antibodies. These animals were then mated to mice that constitutively synthesized the HEL protein (again due to the introduction of a transgene). The double transgenic offspring of this mating had HEL-reactive B cells in their peripheral circulation, but these cells were functionally silent and expressed an abnormal IgM^{lo}, IgD^{hi} surface phenotype.

In a separate series of experiments, HEL–anti-HEL double transgenic mice were created in which the production of HEL was experimentally regulated.[G293] In the absence of HEL production, large numbers of mature B cells in the peripheral circulation secreted anti-HEL antibodies. When HEL production was turned on, these mature B cells were rendered tolerant (rather than being stimulated). The induction of tolerance required that the surface Ig receptor on the HEL-specific B cells be occupied by HEL above a critical concentration threshold.[G293] A similar mechanism might account for the tolerization of autoreactive B cells that arise during normal antigen-driven immune responses.

Results from a number of other experiments involving transgenic mice lead to the following series of conclusions. 1) Contact with self-antigen can lead to clonal deletion[N65] or a state of anergy in B cells.[G292] 2) Anergy is more easily induced in immature than mature B cells.[G293,K304,K305] 3) This differential sensitivity to tolerance induction reflects differences in the threshold of antigen occupancy required to down-regulate the sIg receptors on immature versus mature B cells.[G293] 4) Tolerant B cells express a distinctive sIg phenotype—IgM^{lo}, IgD^{hi} [G292,G293] 5) T cells are rendered tolerant at a much lower antigen concentration than that required to induce B-cell tolerance.[A38]

These findings have implications both for the production of "natural" autoantibodies by normal animals and the production of pathogenic autoantibodies by autoimmune animals. The finding that natural autoantibodies are present in the serum of virtually all individuals has led some to conclude that B cells are not tolerant of self antigens. Yet these natural autoantibodies are generally IgMs of low affinity, unlike pathogenic autoantibodies, which tend to be high-affinity IgGs.[D51,E16,H49,W286] Our understanding of B-cell tolerance suggests that the low-affinity clones might fall below the threshold needed to down-regulate receptor expression (or moderate tissue damage). A surprising high proportion (up to 30%) of the B cells in the peripheral circulation of normal animals reportedly express the IgM[low], IgD[hi] phenotype associated with anergy.[H209] It is interesting to speculate that such cells may actually be anergic, and that they were tolerized following contact with self antigen.

Our understanding of tolerance induction in vivo, while dramatically improved, remains incomplete. It appears that B cells may be rendered tolerant either through clonal deletion or clonal anergy, with the choice of mechanism apparently dependent upon 1) the maturation stage of the B cell, 2) its affinity for (auto)antigen, 3) the concentration of (auto)antigen, and 4) the presence or absence of helper/suppressor signals from T lymphocytes and other immunocompetent cells.

DEFECTIVE CLONAL DELETION OF B CELLS IN SLE

SLE is characterized by an increase in the level of pathogenic autoantibodies present in the circulation. Whether defective B-cell tolerance/anergy contributes to the production of lymphocytes capable of producing pathogenic autoantibodies is an issue of considerable interest. Age-associated changes occur in the B-cell repertoires expressed by autoimmune animals. In young (2- to 10-week-old) lupus-prone mice, the absolute number of B cells actively secreting Ig is significantly increased over that of age-matched controls.[M103,M634,T130] However, the specificity of the antibodies produced by these activated cells is qualitatively similar to that of normal mice.[K303] These findings suggest that B cells are being nonspecifically activated in young autoimmune animals but that autoreactive B cells are not escaping tolerization/anergy.

By comparison, older autoimmune animals express repertoires skewed toward the overproduction of specific autoantibodies.[K294,K296] Such repertoire skewing is not detected in young autoimmune mice or normal adult mice.[K303] To examine whether repertoire skewing reflects an age-associated decrease in the susceptibility of B cells to tolerization, a comparison was made between the frequency of anti-ssDNA precursors in the bone marrow (representing immature B cells) versus the spleen.[C420] Whereas normal adult DBA/2 mice had significantly fewer anti-DNA–secreting cells in the spleen than in the bone marrow, autoimmune NZB mice showed no reduction in the frequency of anti-ssDNA precursors in the spleen. Similar results were obtained in studies of autoimmune NZB/W F$_1$ mice.[R66,T249]

Direct evidence of a defect in B-cell tolerance induction in autoimmune mice was found in studies of transgenic mice. A transgene encoding a pathogenic IgM anti-DNA antibody was introduced into normal Balb/c and autoimmune MRL-*lpr/lpr* mice.[E131] In the normal animals, B cells expressing the transgene were blocked in their ability to differentiate into antibody-secreting cells.[E131] When the same transgene was introduced into lupus-prone mice, the DNA-specific B cells were activated to secrete antibodies.[E131] These findings provide definitive evidence that DNA-reactive clones that are tolerized in normal animals can escape this process in lupus-prone mice. Recent studies involving the introduction of a transgene encoding an IgG anti-DNA antibody indicate that tolerance in normal animals requires the expression of sIg (and perhaps sIgM).[T234a]

POSSIBLE ROLE OF THE MAJOR HISTOCOMPATIBILITY COMPLEX IN THE BREAKDOWN OF SELF TOLERANCE

Susceptibility to many autoimmune diseases is associated with the expression of specific class II MHC genes.[T165] This association reflects the critical importance of the trimolecular complex of TCR, MHC molecule, and antigen in the generation of immune responses. Two mechanisms have been proposed to account for the influence of specific MHC molecules in the development of autoimmunity.[M513] First, a specific MHC allele might be uniquely configured to bind to and present self antigen in an immunogenic form. Individuals expressing such an allele would thereby be predisposed to mount a cellular or humoral immune responses to a particular self antigen. Alternatively, specific MHC alleles might influence the intrathymic selection of T cells. In that case, lymphocytes reactive with particular self antigens might be rescued rather than clonally deleted when they arise in the thymus.

A striking association has been found between the expression of the HLA-DQB gene and development of IDDM in mice and humans.[T169] Analysis of the amino acid sequence expressed by these HLA molecules shows that an aspartic acid at position 57 provides resistance to diabetes, while the presence of other amino acids at this site accounts for disease susceptibility.[T169] This observation was confirmed in experiments involving the introduction of a transgene-bearing aspartic acid at position 57 into IDDM-prone mice.[L418,M505,S489] The transgene prevented the development of disease.

The possibility that MHC-encoded genes contribute to the development of SLE has received limited experimental support. In one study, a 90% association was found between the expression of an MHC-linked gene and the development of lupus in (NZB × F$_1$) backcross mice.[K393] However no specific MHC gene was identified in that work. In humans, DR3 (and possibly DR2) were found to be significantly associated with SLE.[A300,D355,D356,F300,S205] This apparent association between MHC genes and lupus does not necessarily implicate MHC molecules in the disease process however, since disease susceptibility genes might exist in linkage disequilibrium with the MHC.

TARGET ANTIGEN IN TOLERANCE BREAKDOWN

A critical issue in SLE is whether autoantibody production results from autoantigen-specific immune stimulation. The target antigens of many autoantibodies have been defined. These include intranuclear determinants such as DNA, histone, Ro, La and Sm, cytoplasmic antigens such as myosin, actin and thyroglobulin, and membrane-bound proteins, such as those on erythrocytes and WBCs. Yet it has been difficult to determine whether these autoantigens are responsible for the production of their corresponding autoantibodies.

Autoantibody-secreting B cells have many characteristics that suggest they are being stimulated in an antigen-dependent manner. They can 1) produce high-affinity antibodies,[E16] 2) undergo isotype switching from IgM to IgG,[D51,P37,S687] and 3) be overexpressed in the B-cell repertoire.[E59,E67,S218] Moreover, sequence analysis of the Ig variable region genes from these autoreactive B cells indicates that somatic mutations have accumulated in a nonrandom fashion, consistent with a process of antigen-driven affinity maturation.[B168,M537,R38,R66,S375,V31]

Although considerable effort has been expended in trying to document intrinsic differences in either the quantity or quality of autoantigen present in lupus patients, such work has met with little success. For example, DNA from lupus patients is no more immunogenic than DNA from normal controls. There is some evidence that particular autoantigens may be present at higher than normal concentrations in the serum of animals with active lupus,[C361] but this may be the simple result of tissue injury induced during periods of active lupus.

It is therefore unclear whether pathogenic autoantibodies are induced by the autoantigens to which they bind. Whereas IgG anti-DNA antibodies are characteristic of active lupus, attempts to induce anti-DNA antibodies by immunizing normal mice with native DNA have generally been unsuccessful.[S218,S705] Conventional immunization protocols have similarly been unable to induce autoantibodies with binding characteristics of those from lupus patients.[E65,R400,S391] This has led some to hypothesize that autoantibody production results from the stimulation of cross-reactive B cells by foreign (rather than self) antigens. Alternatively, autoantibody production might arise from a generalized process of polyclonal B-cell activation resulting from the overproduction of immunostimulatory factors (or increased responsiveness of autoreactive B cells to normal levels of such factors).

While the precise mechanism involved in the stimulation of autoreactive B cells is unclear, the pathologic changes induced by their autoantibody products are well known. In particular, IgG anti-DNA antibodies (especially those of high affinity and pI) have been implicated in the development of glomerulonephritis in both humans and mice with lupus.[D51,E16,P37] Several attempts have been made to treat systemic autoimmune disease by suppressing the production of these autoantibodies. In the context of this chapter's analysis of self tolerance, one of these approaches deserves special attention.

Researchers have attempted to induce and maintain tolerance to DNA by repeatedly treating autoimmune-prone animals with a tolerogenic form of that molecule. Early work showed that DNA or oligonucleotides, alone or cross-linked to a variety of tolerogenic carriers (including lysine, glutamic acid, and gamma globulin), could induce a state of unresponsiveness in mice that were subsequently challenged with nucleotides presented in an immunogenic form (coupled to KLH or BSA).[E142,T63] Cell transfer experiments indicated that both T cells and bone marrow—derived cells were actively tolerized by this procedure.[T63]

Longterm high-dose administration of DNA (especially when coupled to IgG) was then shown to maintain a state of tolerance in NZB/W mice. This resulted in a diminution in IgG anti-DNA production by treated animals, a prolongation in their survival, and a diminution in renal pathology.[P52] Of interest, the beneficial effects of these treatments persisted for several months after the cessation of tolerogen administration.[B417] Cells from patients with SLE have also been exposed to tolerogenic IgG-DNA complexes in vitro. Results suggest that such treatment reduces polyclonal anti-DNA production by over one-half and virtually eliminates antigen-driven anti-DNA production.[B415] It remains uncertain, however, whether high-affinity anti-DNA—producing cells that have already been stimulated in vivo can be inhibited by such therapy.

SUMMARY

The loss of tolerance to self antigens, manifest by the production of autoantibodies reactive with DNA and other cellular constituents, plays an important role in the pathogenesis of SLE. Despite considerable investigation, the processes and cells responsible for this loss of self tolerance remain uncertain.

Tolerance can be established and maintained in a variety of ways, including intrathymic T-cell deletion and peripheral anergy. Since the immune system is highly interactive, a defect in one cell type can result in an even greater (and clinically more relevant) abnormality in other cells. We have argued that lupus represents the culmination of a two-stage process that is initiated by abnormal polyclonal B-cell activation and perpetuated by (auto) antigen-specific immune stimulation.[S644] This model explains a large number of the divergent findings associated with tolerance defects in lupus. On the one hand, there is ample evidence that a generalized breakdown in tolerance mechanism(s) is present in humans and mice with lupus. On the other hand, active disease is frequently accompanied by a dramatic increase in the activity of a small subset of autoreactive lymphocytes.

Adding to this confusion are differences in the pathogenicity of various lymphocyte subsets. B cells which produce polyreactive IgM autoantibodies are present in normal individuals. Although the number of such cells is significantly increased in patients with autoimmune disease, their presence may have no pathologic consequence. Indeed, their antibody product might be of such low affinity that it falls below the threshold needed to induce tolerance following exposure to self antigen. The activation of these low-affinity lymphocytes could result from the excess production of B-cell—stimulating factors in the autoimmune animal and thus be unrelated to a tolerance defect. Whether high-affinity autoreactive clones arise from the hypermutation of these low-affinity self reactive B cells is uncertain.[K296] It is also unclear whether polyclonal activation interferes with B-cell tolerance, although polyclonal activating factors create an environment that favors B-cell stimulation over suppression.[H97]

Unlike the situation with polyreactive lymphocytes, the number of B cells producing high-affinity IgG autoantibodies is negligible in normal animals.[K299] The strict regulation of such clones suggests that their activation is detrimental, a finding confirmed by studies in which B cells producing IgG autoantibodies were down-regulated following transfer to normal recipients.[K302] The excess production of IgG autoantibodies in human and murine lupus necessarily implies a breakdown in self tolerance.

Whether this breakdown is at the level of the helper T cell, the antigen-presenting cell, or the B cell itself has been a matter of contention for many years. The answer may vary as a function of the nature, severity, and duration of disease. Other important parameters involved in self-nonself discrimination include the specificity of the T-cell receptor, the antigen-binding and antigen-presenting properties of MHC-encoded molecules, and the nature and concentration of autoantigen. Each of these factors has been shown to play a role in the development of organ-specific autoimmune diseases. Unfortunately, definitive evidence linking these factors to the development of systemic autoimmunity has not yet been obtained. Continued study of these issues using recently developed transgenic technology should significantly further our understanding of tolerance abnormalities in SLE.

Chapter 8

B-CELL ABNORMALITIES CHARACTERISTIC OF SYSTEMIC LUPUS ERYTHEMATOSUS

DENNIS M. KLINMAN

Early immunologists believed that autoreactive B cells were immediately deleted from the immune repertoire to prevent the development of a "horror autotoxicus." It is now known that lymphocytes capable of secreting autoantibodies are present and functional in normal individuals but that their activation is strictly regulated. Two types of evidence support this conclusion: 1) low but detectable levels of autoantibody are present in the serum of healthy individuals,[D209,G423] and 2) B cells removed from their normal in vivo regulatory environment secrete large amounts of autoantibody when cultured in vitro or when transferred into animals with diminished immunoregulatory capacity.[F106,K301,K302,S100]

Systemic lupus erythematosus in humans and animals is characterized by the increased activation of B cells secreting Ig reactive with a variety of self antigens, including cell membrane molecules, cytoplasmic proteins, and nuclear determinants.[T133,Z62] Two divergent models have been proposed to account for the stimulation of autoreactive lymphocytes in patients with SLE. The first holds that self reactive B cells are intrinsically abnormal, being either hyper-responsive to normal activation signals or unresponsive to tolerogenic signals.[S644] The second model holds that autoreactive B cells are similar to those of conventional antigenic specificity and that their stimulation is caused by abnormalities in the immune environment.

Analyzing the causes of B-cell activation in humans is complicated. Individual patients have widely divergent genetic backgrounds and have been exposed to dissimilar environmental/self antigens. It is also difficult to identify and study patients during the initial stages of disease when autoantibody production is initiated but clinically recognizable abnormalities have not yet arisen. To circumvent these problems, murine models of SLE have been developed in which every member of a strain reproducibly develops systemic autoimmunity. This chapter will rely heavily on studies of murine lupus to examine the causes of B-cell activation in SLE and to investigate the nature and properties of autoreactive B cells.

B-CELL HYPERACTIVATION IN SYSTEMIC LUPUS ERYTHEMATOSUS

Patients with SLE commonly have increased numbers of Ig-secreting B cells present in their peripheral blood when compared to normal controls.[B330,G155,I44,K300, K452,S33] These lymphocytes produce antibodies reactive

with a wide variety of self antigens, including cell membrane molecules, cytoplasmic proteins, and nuclear determinants (most notably DNA).[T133,Z62] The autoantibodies produced are responsible, in whole or part, for moderating the tissue damage that is characteristic of lupus (including hemolytic anemia, glomerulonephritis, and vasculitis) and for inducing abnormalities in other elements of the immune system (i.e., antibodies that interfere with T-cell function).[H30,P37]

Patients with SLE have increased numbers of B cells at all stages of maturation.[B330,B557,K452,S635] The rate of B-cell proliferation, activation, and Ig secretion is also profoundly increased in many patients with SLE.[B330,B557,G155, K452,T54] For example, the frequency of Ig-secreting B cells in patients with very active disease is elevated up to 50-fold over normal. Individuals with inactive lupus have an average of one- to threefold more lymphocytes secreting Ig in their peripheral blood than normals (Fig. 8–1). Studies of lupus-prone mice suggest that B-cell abnormalities are present at birth or within the first few weeks of life. Increased B-cell activation may therefore represent a primary immune abnormality.[K299,M103,M634] Longitudinal studies of twins and family members of SLE patients support the view that B-cell abnormalities precede the onset of clinically detectable autoimmunity.[D124,F25]

Lymphocytes in the peripheral circulation of patients with active lupus spontaneously secrete IgG, IgA, and to a lesser extent IgM when cultured in vitro.[B330,G155] In the absence of further stimulation, IgG production ceases after 24 hours. The frequency of Ig-secreting cells has been used as a measure of disease activity. At least one study suggests that the number of Ig-secreting B cells more accurately reflects disease activity than more classic serologic markers such as C3 level or anti-DNA concentration.[B159,F53] The association between serum Ig levels and disease status is less impressive, perhaps because the concentration of Ig in serum reflects a balance between Ig catabolism and production, both of which are increased in lupus patients.[Q18] For this reason, the number of cells secreting Ig more accurately reflects disease activity and correlates more closely with the development of proliferative lupus nephritis than does serum Ig concentration.[B66,F53]

Despite increased numbers of Ig-secreting cells in their peripheral blood and elevated levels of serum Ig, some patients with SLE have impaired primary antibody re-

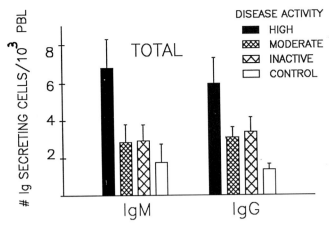

Fig. 8–1. An ELISA spot assay was used to quantitate the number of IgM- and IgG-secreting B cells present in the peripheral blood of lupus patients versus sex- and age-matched normal controls. Results represent the mean ± standard deviation of results from a minimum of 15 patients per group. Note that patients with the most active disease have the greatest number of Ig-secreting cells (p < .01). Klinman, D. M., Shirai, A., Ishigatsubo, Y. et al.: Quantitation of IgG and IgM secreting B cells in the peripheral blood of patients with systemic lupus erythematosus. Arthritis Rheum (In press).

sponses to standard immunizations in vivo and to challenge with polyclonal B-cell activators in vitro.[B127,B372, K33,L226,W238] This paradoxic reduction in B-cell responsiveness may reflect changes in the immunoregulatory milieu of such patients—including an increase in suppression,[C70] exhaustion of B-cell growth factors,[B372,N95] and/or refractoriness of stimulated B cells to further activation.[S644] In this context, studies of patients treated with gamma globulin indicate that high circulating Ig levels can lead to immunosuppression and blunted responses to exogenous antigens.[L230,W207]

POSSIBLE CAUSES OF B-CELL HYPERACTIVATION

Three general mechanisms have been proposed to account for the B-cell hyperactivation characteristic of SLE (Table 8–1). 1) A unique subset of B cells predisposed toward the production of autoantibodies might be abnormally expanded in animals with systemic autoimmunity.[H220] 2) Self reactive B cells might be triggered by autoantigen, or by an antigen cross-reactive with self, to proliferate and secrete Ig. Such stimulation may be due to a loss of self tolerance arising from decreased suppressor T-cell function or increased T-cell help.[C70,T31,T81] 3) A generalized process of B-cell hyperactivation (caused by polyclonal B-cell stimulators in the immune environment) could lead to the increased production of antibodies reactive with all antigens, including those against self.[171,K303,P318,T133]

It is presently unclear which (if any) of these three mechanisms is primarily responsible for autoantibody production in human SLE. Due to the diverse laboratory and clinical manifestations of lupus, it is possible that distinct processes are responsible for autoantibody produc-

tion among different subsets of patients or in the same patient over time.[S521,S639] Indeed, there is evidence that the mechanism that initiates B-cell activation in murine lupus differs from that responsible for the perpetuation of autoantibody production late in disease.[K296,K298]

B-CELL SUBSETS

The antigenic specificity of a B lymphocyte is determined by the light and heavy chain variable region genes used to encode its antibody product. The mouse and human genome encode several thousand variable region genes that can associate independently to produce millions of different antibody molecules. Additional repertoire diversification occurs when the Ig genes of activated B cells undergo somatic hypermutation. Since both Ig variable region gene selection and somatic mutation are random events, lymphocytes capable of producing autoantibodies could potentially arise from all lineages of B cells.

A particularly interesting subset of lymphocytes expressing the Ly-1/CD5 surface marker (Ly-1 in mice, CD5 in humans) has been described. B cells with this surface marker reportedly manifest a number of unusual properties. They are described as being long-lived, self-reconstituting, and predisposed to constituently synthesize IgM antibodies of low affinity and high cross-reactivity.[H125,H220,S410] The Ly-1 surface marker is present on 1 to 2% of splenic B cells and up to 30% of peritoneal B lymphocytes in normal adult mice.[H219] CD5⁺ B cells constitute approximately 20% of the B cells in normal human peripheral blood.[H126] Cells with this surface phe-

Table 8–1. Possible Causes of Increased B-cell Activation in SLE

I. Expansion of a unique subset of B cells
  A. Ly-1⁺ B cells in mice
    1. Long-lived and self-reconstituting
    2. Produce cross-reactive IgM autoantibodies
    3. Present at increased frequency in some autoimmune strains
  B. CD5⁺ B cells in humans
    1. Produce both cross-reactive and monospecific autoantibodies
    2. Implicated in the production of autoantibodies in RA and perhaps SLE
II. Intrinsic B-cell abnormalities
  A. Increased susceptibility to (or production of) growth factors
  B. Decreased susceptibility to inhibitory factors
III. Microenvironmental growth factors
IV. Autoantigen-driven immune stimulation
  A. A limited repertoire of autoantibodies is specifically overproduced in advanced lupus
  B. These autoantibodies have undergone isotype switching and affinity maturation
  C. Molecular genetic analyses indicate
    1. Possible skewing of the IgVh gene repertoire used in the production of autoantibodies.
    2. The ratio of replacement/silent nucleotide mutations in the autoantibody-combining site indicates selection of high-affinity clones
V. Polyclonal activation
  A. Young lupus-prone mice have increased numbers of B cells secreting Ig but do not selectively overproduce autoantibodies
  B. Patients with lupus produce autoantibodies against different and sometimes multiple autoantigens
  C. Polyclonal activators can break B-cell tolerance

notype are even more common in newborns, where they may be responsible for producing much of the natural (i.e., presumably uninduced) autoantibody found in the serum of young animals.[H125]

Several pieces of evidence implicate Ly-1+ B cells in the development of SLE. Increased numbers of these cells are present in autoimmune NZB and motheaten mice where they have been shown to produce anti-DNA and antierythrocyte autoantibodies.[H221,S410] Similarly, autoantibody production in patients with active RA and SLE has been attributed (at least in part) to CD5+ B cells.[C125,C126, H126,S773] Supporting the view that Ly-1 B cells are autoreactive is evidence that monoclonal antibodies derived from such cells commonly bind to self antigens.[V3]

Despite these findings, the association between Ly-1/ CD5 B cells and lupus remains uncertain. There is no increase in the number of Ly-1+ B cells present in most strains of autoimmune mice, and mice experimentally induced to express large numbers of Ly-1 B cells do not develop autoimmune disease.[H270,W317] Moreover, a direct comparison between Ly-1+ and Ly-1− splenic lymphocytes revealed that these two populations contributed equally to the production of autoantibodies in normal adult mice.[K297] It now appears that the primary role of Ly-1 B cells might be to produce highly cross-reactive antibodies early in life (when young animals have only a limited number of lymphocytes to provide protection against the universe of environmental pathogens)[C125] and to respond to T-independent antigens. The contribution of the antibodies produced by such cells toward the development of clinically relevant autoimmune disease remains to be established.

INTRINSIC B-CELL ABNORMALITIES

Other abnormalities have been detected among B cells from autoimmune mice. For example, B cells arise from the bone marrow of NZB mice at an extremely rapid rate and proliferate more rapidly than normal in vivo and in vitro.[R66,Y54] Lymphocytes from MRL/*lpr* mice also proliferate rapidly, and have a growth advantage over normal lymphocytes when transferred into irradiated recipients.[P126] Significantly, other *lpr* cells of myeloid lineage (such as erythrocytes) do not demonstrate this growth advantage.

INFLUENCE OF THE INTERNAL MICROENVIRONMENT ON B-CELL ACTIVATION

While these in vivo studies suggest that autoreactive B cells may be intrinsically abnormal, other evidence indicates that the environment in which autoreactive lymphocytes mature is responsible for their unusual properties. In a series of cell transfer experiments, purified B cells from normal mice were placed into autoimmune-prone recipients, and vice versa (Fig. 8–2). Normal B cells in the autoimmune environment secreted large amounts of autoantibody over a 4-week period (Fig. 8–2).[K299,K302] Conversely, B cells from autoimmune mice transferred into normal recipients produced very little autoantibody.[K301] B cells from young autoimmune mice (<2 weeks of age) did not effectively transfer autoantibody

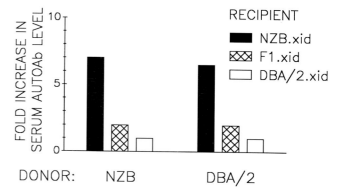

Fig. 8–2. B cells from autoimmune NZB and normal DBA/2 mice were transferred into animals with impaired autoantibody production (from the presence of the X-linked immunodeficiency gene). When placed in autoimmune-prone NZB.*xid* recipients, B cells from either donor proliferated rapidly and secreted large amounts of serum autoantibody. The rate of proliferation and autoantibody production by the transferred B cells was significantly reduced in (NZB.*xid* × DBA/2.*xid*)F₁ and nonautoimmune DBA/2.*xid* recipients. Thus, recipient environment rather than B-cell origin exercised the major influence over autoantibody production. Klinman, D. M., and Steinberg, A. D.: Similar in vivo expansion of B cells from normal DBA/2 and autoimmune NZB mice in xid recipients. J Immunol, 139:2284, 1987.

production into any recipient.[K302] However when bone marrow from normal DBA/2 and autoimmune NZB mice were cotransferred into irradiated F₁ recipients, B cells from the autoimmune strain demonstrated a proliferative advantage over those from the normals.[R66] These findings suggest that B cells or stem cells from autoimmune animals might be intrinsically hyper-responsive to stimulatory signals and that such signals are increased in an autoimmune-prone environment. While the nature of the internal factor(s) influencing B-cell development remains obscure, evidence suggests that it is genetically predetermined and may be linked to the MHC.[G113,G155]

ANTIGEN-SPECIFIC B-CELL ACTIVATION

A variety of mechanisms could potentially be responsible for the autoantibody production characteristic of SLE. In graft-versus-host disease, B-cell activation results when alloreactive T cells are induced to secrete an excess of immunostimulatory factors.[A262,B532,R280] Autoantibody production can also result when the normal B-cell repertoire is polyclonally activated, for example by infectious agents or specific lymphokines.[H97] Yet autoantigen-specific immune stimulation has historically been considered the primary force driving the production of autoantibodies in human and murine lupus.

Several lines of evidence support the view that (auto)antigen plays an important role in SLE. 1) The expressed B-cell repertoires of patients and mice with active lupus are frequently skewed toward the overproduction of specific autoantibodies.[E59,E67,G113,S218] Such skewing may be predictive of disease progression[B402,F53,H138,S33, S521,S639,W91] and can be experimentally reproduced by stimulating normal animals with antigen. 2) Autoantibody-secreting B cells from lupus-prone mice undergo affinity maturation, isotype switching, and idiotype selection over time. These changes are conventionally associated with antigen-driven immune responses.[D51,E15,K41, P37,S687] 3) A restricted portion of the IgVh gene repertoire may be utilized in the production of autoantibodies (although there are conflicting data on this point).[C420,D174,M135] 4) The ratio of replacement to silent nucleotides in the hypervariable domains of IgG anti-DNA and IgG anti-RF autoantibodies is consistent with a process of random somatic mutation followed by antigen-driven selection.[M135,M537,R38,S376,S377,V31,V78] 5) Organ-specific autoimmune diseases are induced when self antigen is presented to the immune system in an immunogenic rather than tolerogenic form.[T167]

Despite these findings, it has been difficult to demonstrate that specific self antigens are required to initiate and/or perpetuate autoantibody production. Individual lupus patients express B-cell repertoires reactive against widely divergent autoantigens. Some develop high levels of anti-DNA antibodies, others manifest increased anti-myosin or anticardiolipin production, while still others develop a generalized hypergammaglobulinemia without apparent antigenic bias.[K339,M228,P196] A similar pattern has been described in autoimmune mice. In the MRL-*lpr/lpr* strain for example, one-third of adults express repertoires skewed against the autoantigen Sm, one-sixth against DNA, and the remainder against a variety of other foreign and self antigens.[E60,E63,K296] Despite these differences in autoantibody specificity, the natural history of disease and longevity of all these animals is indistinguishable. It is also noteworthy that when normal and autoimmune-prone mice are experimentally immunized with self antigens, the fine specificity (and frequently the concentration) of autoantibodies they produce differs dramatically from those produced spontaneously by animals with active lupus.[E65,R400,S391]

POLYCLONAL B-CELL ACTIVATION

Increased numbers of B cells producing antibodies against nonself as well as self antigens are frequently present in patients and mice with active lupus.[B557,I44,K300,K303] This finding suggests that some form of antigen-independent polyclonal B-cell stimulation is present in SLE. Additional studies indicate that this generalized process of B-cell activation precedes the more selective stimulation of autoantibody-secreting cells.[K294,K296,K298,K303] In MRL/*lpr* mice, for example, the number of B cells producing antibodies reactive with TNP, ovalbumin, sheep red blood cells, and other nonself antigens is significantly elevated by 3 weeks of age, whereas the preferential production of anti-Sm and anti-DNA antibodies does not appear until 3 to 4 months of age (Fig. 8–3).[K296] It is also noteworthy that a B-cell repertoire similar to that expressed by young lupus-prone mice can be induced in normal mice by treatment with polyclonal immune activators such as lipopolysaccharide.

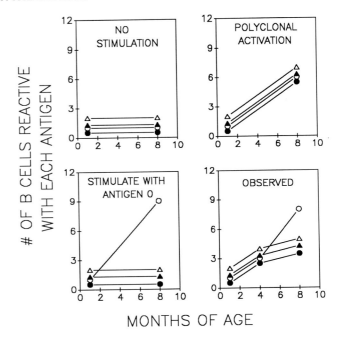

Fig. 8–3. Each panel shows an idealized representation of the number of B cells reactive with four different antigens (△, ○, ▲, ●) in mice of increasing age. The B-cell repertoire of normal unmanipulated mice (*upper left*) is relatively constant over time. In the presence of a polyclonal B-cell activator (*upper right*), B cells of all specificities are induced to proliferate. In the presence of a specific antigenic stimulus (*lower left*), only B cells reactive with that antigen (○) increase in number. The experimentally observed B-cell repertoire of autoimmune mice is shown in the lower right panel. The autoimmune repertoire seems to reflect polyclonal B-cell activation at early time points but specific autoantigenic stimulation once disease becomes established. Klinman, D. M.: Current Advances in Murine Lupus. Cur Op Immunol, *1*:740, 1989.

To determine the contribution of polyclonal activation to the pathogenesis of murine lupus (NZB × NZB/W)F$_2$ mice were studied. Approximately one-half of these animals develop fatal lupus glomerulonephritis by 6 months of age, while the other half live for greater than 1 year. The degree of polyclonal B-cell activation present in young F$_2$ mice was significantly correlated with the early onset lupus nephritis ($R^2 = .78$).[K294] In contrast, young mice with increased anti-DNA antibody production were not statistically more likely to develop rapidly progressive SLE. Among (NZB × NZB/W)F$_2$ mice that survived until 1 year of age, IgG anti-DNA levels did correlate with the severity of renal disease ($R^2 = .89$).[K294] These findings support the view that antigen-independent polyclonal B-cell activation is an important manifestation of early lupus, whereas the preferential expansion of autoantibody-secreting clones dominates during the latter stages of disease.

There is additional evidence suggesting that polyclonal activators could stimulate the B-cell activation found in early lupus. At high concentrations, such activators induce Ig production in the absence of T-cell help.[H97] At lower concentrations, polyclonal activators facilitate antigen-

Table 8–2. Cytokines that Affect Murine B-cell Maturation, Proliferation, and/or Secretion

Cytokine	Effect
IL-1	Costimulant of B-cell proliferation and maturation (especially when used with IL-2)
IL-2	Implicated in the stimulation of B-cell proliferation and differentiation to Ig-producing cell
IL-4	Costimulant for proliferation; promotes isotype switching (to IgG1 and IgE); induces expression of IA
IL-5	Promotes proliferation and maturation to Ig production in vitro of germinal center and Ly-1 B cells
IL-6	Stimulates terminal differentiation to Ig-producing cell
IL-7	Growth factor for pre-B cells
IL-10	Induces IA expression; may enhance the proliferation of Ly-1 B cells
γ-Interferon	Promotes isotype switching (to IgG2a). Inhibits B-cell proliferation and maturation to Ig production
TNFα	May stimulate Ig production by human B cells
TGFβ	Markedly inhibits B-cell proliferation; induces isotype switch (to IgA).

driven B-cell responses.[A181] Evidence suggests that autoreactive B cells (which are normally quiescent or rendered tolerant due to a lack of T-cell help) can be triggered by polyclonal activators to secrete large amounts of autoantibody.[H97,I70] There is also evidence that normal mice treated with polyclonal activating factors develop symptoms of autoimmune disease, especially when challenged with common environmental pathogens.[L46] Thus, polyclonal activators might act by 1) creating an environment conducive to the expansion of autoreactive clones[K296] and/or 2) contributing to the generation of autoreactive memory cells, which are subsequently stimulated by autoantigen.[J93]

Several questions concerning the importance of polyclonal activators in autoimmune disease remain. Although elevated levels of polyclonal activating factors have been detected in humans with autoimmune disease and in lupus-prone mice,[H317,J147,P319] the nature and source of the putative activating factors have not been established. Evidence suggests that T cells may be responsible for excess lymphokine production, although other cells of the immune system (or even enteric bacteria) can produce factors that cause polyclonal B-cell activation. Also unclear is the number of activating factors involved. Recent studies suggest that different cytokines are responsible for moderating B-cell proliferation, differentiation, and isotype switching (Table 8–2).[C421,S527]

B CELLS PRODUCING PATHOGENIC VERSUS NATURAL AUTOANTIBODIES

Not all autoreactive B cells contribute equally to the development of autoimmune disease. In general, the pathogenicity of an antibody reflects its affinity,[D51,E16] charge,[D51] heavy chain class (IgM, IgG, IgA, etc.),[H5] idiotype,[E15,H5] and antigenic specificity.[E60] B cells that secrete low-affinity IgM autoantibodies (such as those that predominate in normal individuals) are relatively inefficient

at inducing tissue destruction. By comparison, B cells that produce high-affinity IgG antibodies (particularly those that are cationically charged or form immune complexes) are effective moderators of tissue injury.[D51,E16] When charged immune complexes lodge in the kidney or vascular endothelium, they fix complement and induce a strong inflammatory response.[H5,P37]

In studies of lupus-prone mice including MRL/*lpr*, BXSB, C3H/*gld*, and NZB/W, a strong temporal association has been observed between the appearance of B cells producing IgG autoantibodies and the development of glomerulonephritis.[D51,H30,K296,K298,S18] Several groups have demonstrated that IgG anti-DNA antibodies of high pH are present in the nephritic kidneys of autoimmune mice, and that the transfer of antibodies with these properties into susceptible animals accelerates disease development.[D51,H30] IgG anti-DNA antibodies bearing particular idiotypes (e.g., the dominant GN1 and GN2 idiotypes)[H30] have also been implicated in the disease process.

The appearance of specific autoantibodies, however, does not always herald an acceleration of disease. For example, the presence or absence of anti-Sm or antihistone antibodies in MRL/*lpr* and NZB/W mice, respectively, does not seem to affect disease progression or mortality.[E60,E63] Similarly, disease is not prevented (but may be delayed) when the production of IgG anti-DNA antibodies bearing specific idiotypes is blocked (e.g., by anti-idiotypic therapy). These observations suggest that certain autoantibody responses may play a role in disease progression, while others reflect (but do not actively contribute to) the disease process. In the latter case, the interaction of environmental stimuli with self MHC products may be responsible for determining which autoantibodies are produced.

CROSS-REACTIVITY OF AUTOREACTIVE B CELLS

Antibodies produced by some B cells are highly cross-reactive; i.e., they bind to a variety of apparently unrelated antigens.[M190,M228,S708] Frequently this binding is of low affinity since cross-reactivity tends to decrease as affinity increases.[K295,M540,S500] In some studies, 10 to 50% of the hybridomas produced from the fusion of normal B cells were found to cross-react against a panel of 6 to 10 self antigens.[F232,U20] This observation led investigators to suggest that cross-reactivity was an inherent characteristic of self reactive B cells.

To examine this issue more carefully, the cross-reactivity of lymphocytes from normal DBA/2 and autoimmune NZB mice was compared. B cells from these strains were cloned and tested under identical conditions for binding to a large panel of self and nonself antigens. Results showed that B cells from these two strains were equally cross-reactive, and that B cells producing autoantibodies were no more cross-reactive than those secreting antibodies of conventional antigenic specificity[K295] (Fig. 8–4).

To further examine the nature of autoreactive B cells, several groups have analyzed the Ig variable region genes utilized by lymphocytes producing conventional antibodies versus autoantibodies. Results from this work are somewhat contradictory. One group has documented ex-

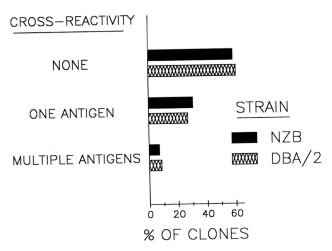

Fig. 8–4. B-cell clones from autoimmune NZB and normal DBA/2 mice were analyzed for the production of cross-reactive antibodies using the splenic fragment assay system. Klinman, D. M., Banks, S., Hartman, A. et al.: Natural murine autoantibodies and conventional antibodies exhibit similar degrees of antigenic cross-reactivity. J Clin Invest, 82:652, 1988. Individual B-cell clones from these strains were equally cross-reactive. Moreover, autoantibodies were found to be no more cross-reactive than antibodies of conventional antigenic specificity. Klinman, D. M.: B cells and autoimmune disease. ISI Atlas of Science: Immunology, 1:185, 1988.

treme bias in V_H gene utilization among B cells producing antirheumatoid factor and anti-DNA antibodies in MRL/ lpr mice,[S376,S377] while other investigators found that anti-DNA–secreting B cells utilize a random sampling of the V_H and J_H gene pool.[D174,P31,T214] Similarly, V_H gene utiliza- tion by B cells from autoimmune NZB, MRL/lpr, and motheaten mice was not found to differ from that of nor- mal Balb/C mice.[K100,P11] It is reasonable to conclude that autoimmune mice can selectively expand a small popula- tion of B cells late in the disease process. Analysis of such individuals would reveal a biased utilization of germline Ig genes. However this bias would not be present during the early stages of SLE, and does not appear to be a funda- mental characteristic of the autoimmune repertoire.

SUMMARY

There is clear-cut evidence of B-cell hyperactivation in humans and mice with lupus. During periods of active disease, a limited number of B-cell clones are stimulated preferentially to secrete pathogenic IgG autoantibodies. The antigenic specificity, isotype, idiotype, and Ig gene mutations manifest by these lymphocytes indicate they are activated in an (auto)antigen-specific manner.

Prior to the stimulus provided by (auto)antigen, B cells in lupus-prone mice are exposed to polyclonal activating factors. These factors are capable of interfering with toler- ance induction and accelerating the rate of B-cell matura- tion/activation. Indeed, B cells exposed to polyclonal acti- vating factors have a diminished need for T-cell help and can be stimulated by suboptimal (tolerogenic?) concen- trations of autoantigen.

We postulate that an individual's genetic makeup, expo- sure to polyclonal activating factors, and interactions with environmental and/or self antigens all contribute to the development of autoimmune disease. The production of autoantibodies is seen to primarily arise from abnormal immune stimulation rather than from an intrinsic defect of autoreactive B cells.

Chapter 9

T LYMPHOCYTES, CYTOKINES, AND IMMUNE REGULATION IN SYSTEMIC LUPUS ERYTHEMATOSUS

DAVID A. HORWITZ AND WILLIAM STOHL

SLE is a systemic disease characterized by generalized autoimmunity. Unlike other autoimmune diseases such as insulin-dependent diabetes mellitus or myasthenia gravis, which are organ specific, SLE is characterized by autoantibodies against nuclear, cytoplasmic, or cell surface molecules that transcend organ-specific boundaries. It is the inflammatory responses triggered by local formation and/or deposition of antigen-antibody immune complexes that are responsible for the clinical manifestation of vasculitis and multiorgan system disease.[G184]

For the past 20 years SLE had been considered to be primarily a B-cell disease as reflected by hyperactivity of the humoral component of the immune response and concomitant T-cell hypoactivity.[B330,S647a,T25,T130] It has become increasingly evident, however, that this belief is erroneous and that most, if not all, autoimmune diseases are, in fact, T cell dependent. In murine models of SLE, depletion of CD4+ T cells blocks disease onset[W320] and athymic mice do not develop SLE.[M404,S384] As a consequence, concepts concerning antigen recognition by T cells have had to be revised. Formerly, self-recognition was considered to be pathologic, and self-reactive T cells were believed to be normally eliminated during ontogeny. Indeed, it is now appreciated that the mechanisms that enable T cells to recognize and respond to foreign and self-antigens are similar. Self-reactivity by T cells is not only physiologic, but is indispensable to the generation of normal immune responses. Due to the obligatory autoreactive property of T cells, some T cells capable of triggering autoimmune disease may escape thymic deletion and mature and migrate to peripheral lymphoid tissues.[B580]

With the realization that every individual harbors T cells with the potential to induce autoimmune disease, it is not surprising that previous efforts to identify the specific inherent T-cell defect in SLE predisposing to autoimmunity have been unsuccessful. What actually appears to be abnormal in SLE is the breakdown of self-tolerance. Contrary to old dogma, B cells with the potential to make autoantibodies are not normally deleted during ontogeny.[G291] IgM autoantibodies with anti-DNA or anti-IgG (rheumatoid factor) specificities may arise through nonspecific (T-cell–independent) stimulation of B cells.[B557,G155] Because they are of the IgM class, these autoantibodies generally are not pathogenic. Class switching to pathogenic IgG autoantibodies requires T-cell help. In SLE, normally quiescent T cells become activated through what appear to be antigen-driven processes.[B320,G113,M601] The end result is that these activated T cells can now supply the necessary help to the autoreactive B cells to produce pathogenic IgG anti-DNA autoantibodies.[M601,T19] As indicated below, many discrete and seemingly disparate T-cell abnormalities may lead to this same common end result. Moreover, ineffective attempts by the immune system to down-regulate the ongoing autoimmunity may lead to a variety of secondary T-cell abnormalities.

Before reviewing specific T-cell abnormalities in SLE, present concepts of cellular immunity in normals will be summarized to provide the reader with the background needed for understanding the immunopathogenesis of this disorder. Topics considered will include thymic and post-thymic mechanisms of T-cell development, mechanisms of tolerance induction and maintenance, and the principles involved in T-cell activation and development of effector functions.

One important caveat must be offered at the outset. Present concepts of immune dysregulation in SLE have been largely derived from studies of murine models of SLE. Two great advantages of murine models are that 1) in vivo studies can be undertaken, and 2) the lymphoid organs where autoimmunity is generated and sustained can be studied directly. In contrast, most of the information concerning human SLE is derived from the study of blood lymphocytes *ex vivo*. The functional properties of lymphocytes circulating in blood may not precisely reflect lymphocyte function in lymphoid organs, and in vivo studies may, therefore, not precisely reflect the immune status in vivo. Certain cytokines, for example, may have opposite regulatory effects when added to lymphocytes in tissue culture than when administered to the experimental animal.[C47] Confusing the picture further is the heterogeneity of SLE syndromes and differences in patient populations studied by individual investigators. Nonetheless, in vitro studies of blood lymphocytes in human SLE have, in general, complemented in vitro and in vivo studies in murine lupus and have shed considerable light on the immune dysfunctions underlying SLE.

GENERAL PROPERTIES OF T CELLS

T cells are thymus-derived lymphocytes that participate in a variety of cell-mediated reactions. The principal T-

Table 9–1. Human Peripherial Blood T Lymphocyte Populations*

Population	Normal Values	TCR Chains	Comment
All	65–80%	Mostly αβ, few γδ	
CD4+	40–55%	αβ, very rare γδ	Recognize peptide antigens complexed to self-MHC class II structures; in SLE, can provide help for DNA antibody production.
CD8+	15–30%	αβ, few γδ	Recognize peptide antigens complexed to self-MHC class I structures; in SLE, can provide help for ANA production with CD4+.
CD4−CD8−	<10%		Provide MHC nonrestricted antigen recognition.
		1/3 αβ	In SLE, cells within this subset can provide specific help for anti-DNA antibody production.
		2/3 γδ	In healthy subjects, these cells can be potent suppressors of antibody production, whereas in SLE, cells within this subset can provide specific help for anti-DNA antibody production.

* All T cells express CD3 and CD2 structures on their cell surface. TCR = T-cell receptor.

cell populations are listed in Table 9–1. Unlike B cells, T cells are unable to bind antigen directly, but rather recognize antigen in conjunction with self–class I or class II molecules of the major histocompatibility complex (MHC). The T-cell antigen receptor (TCR) is expressed on the surface of T cells as the CD3/TCR complex. This complex consists of a two-chain heterodimer antigen-binding unit (either α and β chains or γ and δ chains), which is noncovalently complexed to the signal-transducing CD3 structure. CD4+ lymphocytes recognize antigen in combination with self–class II (HLA-DR, DP, DQ) MHC gene products (Table 9–1). Typically, phagocytic cells ingest, e.g., bacteria, and, after antigen-processing, small peptides are expressed on the cell surface complexed to MHC class II for presentation to CD4+ cells. Monocytes, dendritic cells, and other HLA-DR+ antigen-presenting cells interact with CD4+ cells in this manner.

CD8+ T cells differ from CD4+ cells in that they recognize peptide fragments bound to class I (HLA-A, B, C) MHC molecules. In this way CD8+ cells can eliminate cells infected by intracellular organisms. Viral proteins synthesized by infected cells are degraded by proteases, and these peptides are complexed to MHC class I molecules where they are translocated to the cell surface for recognition by CD8+ cells.

CD4+ cells were originally called inducer or helper cells, and CD8+ cells were called cytotoxic or suppressor cells.[M578] Although CD4+ and CD8+ cells usually perform these respective functions, the principal difference between these two T-cell subsets is, as discussed above, the way they recognize antigen. Under certain conditions, CD4+ cells can function as suppressor or killer cells, and CD8+ cells can provide help for B lymphocytes.[K83,T12] In addition, some T cells have the capacity to recognize antigen receptors on lymphocytes. The peptide fragments of the antigen receptor recognized are called idiotypes, and idiotype-specific helper T cells have been identified. Anti-idiotypic self-recognition is important in immune regulation as discussed elsewhere in this volume.

MECHANISMS INVOLVED IN TOLERANCE INDUCTION AND MAINTENANCE

Clonal Deletion

During ontogeny, pluripotent stem cells migrate to the thymus and become thymocytes, potentially capable of differentiating into mature T cells. However, only a small percentage of thymocytes actually survive intrathymic development and achieve full maturation into an immunocompetent T cell. This is the result of two processes called positive and negative selection. Positive selection refers to those events through which only those T cells that recognize self-MHC class II or class I molecules are allowed to survive.[B329] These T cells recognizing self-MHC class II or class I molecules become CD4+ or CD8+ cells, respectively. Through a sequence of events called negative selection, these T cells then migrate to the thymic medulla where those T cells that bind strongly to self-peptide MHC complexes presented by stromal cells are eliminated.[B329] In this manner, only T cells capable of recognizing self-MHC molecules reach the periphery, but those T cells with exceptionally avid autoreactivity (potential autoaggressive T cells) are physically deleted from the T-cell repertoire (Table 9–2).

Clonal Anergy

Since thymic stromal cells lack many important tissue-specific autoantigens, clonal deletion of potential autoag-

Table 9–2. Mechanisms Involved in Tolerance Induction and Maintenance

Mechanism	Site	Comment
Clonal deletion	Thymus	Not all potentially autoaggressive T cells are deleted from the repertoire.
Clonal anergy	Thymus and periphery	T cells that recognize self-peptides (signal 1) without the required costimulatory signal (signal 2) become nonresponsive. Clonal anergy, however, is reversible.
T suppressor cells	Periphery	Although there is unequivocal evidence of antigen-specific suppression, the cellular mechanisms involved are poorly understood.

gressive T cells in the thymus is incomplete. Studies with transgenic mice have revealed that some potential autoaggressive T cells do physically exist, but are rendered anergic (immunologically nonresponsive).[B580] T cells require at least two signals to proliferate or develop effector function. In addition to specific antigen (signal 1), some costimulatory signal (signal 2), such as interleukin-1 (IL-1), is also needed. If T cells bind antigen but do not receive a proper costimulatory signal, not only will they fail to proliferate or develop effector function, but they will undergo a series of events that prevents them from becoming activated by antigen at some subsequent time.[S216] This is called *clonal anergy* and is probably the principal mechanism accounting for immunologic nonresponsiveness after birth.

Since anergic cells may not be physically deleted, the possibility remains that anergy could be reversed. Indeed, recent studies with experimental animals have revealed that T-cell anergy can be reversed by IL-2.[N133] Thus, IL-2 produced by T cells stimulated by foreign antigens could convert local bystander anergic potential autoaggressive T cells to competent autoaggressive T cells capable of promoting an autoimmune response.

T Suppressor Cells

A third mechanism through which potential autoaggressive T cells could be kept in check is through a separate population of cells with functional suppressor activity. Suppressor T cells have the capacity to inhibit antibody synthesis by B cells or suppress responses by effector T cells. CD8+ cells have been considered to be the principal source of suppressor cells, but CD4+ coexpressing Leu 8 can develop this function as well.[K52]

At present, the existence of antigen-specific T suppressor cells is controversial because putative T suppressor clones do not demonstrate rearrangement of genes that encode the T-cell antigen receptor. Regardless of whether true antigen-specific suppressor T cells exist, or whether functional suppression is predicated through more conventional mechanisms such as auto–anti-idiotypic responses, there is persuasive evidence that one or more T-cell subsets in the adult have a surveillance function and suppress autoimmunity. In murine models, passive transfer of T cells from nonautoimmune strains to genetically identical athymic adult animals induces autoimmunity[M300] because the recipients lack the necessary suppressor cells to down-regulate autoaggressive donor T cells. Second, in the induction of arthritis by the passive transfer of auto-immune T-cell clones, the recipients must be first irradiated or pretreated with cyclophosphamide to eliminate T cells that block autoimmunity.[T80]

Post-Thymic T-Cell Maturation

T-cell functional properties were formerly believed to be fully programmed in the thymus. It is now evident, however, that T-cell maturation is not complete when a T cell leaves the thymus but requires exposure to antigen in the periphery to complete the maturation process. Neonatal CD4+ peripheral T cells have low avidity for antigen, and upon stimulation they produce interleukin-2 but

few other cytokines.[E42] These T cells are considered to be "virgin" or "naive." After antigenic stimulation, avidity for antigen increases, presumably as a result of up-regulation of adhesion molecules, which promote contact with antigen-presenting cells. Such CD4+ cells can respond well to soluble antigens and support B-cell differentiation and are now called "memory" cells.[A83,B279,B610,C299] These memory T cells can produce γ-interferon, interleukin-4, and other cytokines.[E42] Corresponding memory CD8+ cells are also generated which are the precursors of antigen-specific killer cells.[M356,Y21]

Naive and memory T cells can phenotypically be identified by reciprocal expression of CD45 isoforms on their cell surfaces. (CD45 is a membrane tyrosine phosphatase that has a vital role in signal transduction). All leukocytes express CD45 isoforms which vary in the size of the component external to the cell surface. Naive T cells display the high-molecular-weight CD45RA isoform, and memory T cells express the low-molecular-weight CD45RO isoform.[A83,B279,B610,C299] Some T cells express both the CD45RA and RO isoforms. These cells may reflect a recently activated T cell undergoing conversion from the naive to the memory state, or possibly CD45RO+ cells reverting to the naive phenotype.

CD29 has also been used to identify memory T cells. The CD29 molecule is the β chain common to the very late antigen (VLA) family which appears on the T-cell surface after activation. CD29+ T cells overlap substantially, but not completely, with the CD45RO isoform expressed by memory T cells.[B279]

This distinction between naive and memory T cells is especially important in the development of autoimmunity because T cells capable of recognizing self-peptides are presumably in the immature, naive state. As discussed above, through clonal anergy or T-cell suppression, these cells will not have been permitted to proliferate and mature into memory cells. Once autoreactive T cells are able to reach the memory stage, autoimmunity would be easy to sustain because of the relative ease of their activation by antigen.

PHYSIOLOGIC T-CELL REGULATION OF ANTIBODY PRODUCTION

Generation of antibodies in response to most antigens is T cell dependent. The T-cell contribution to antibody synthesis can be subdivided into antigen presentation to CD4+ T cells; T-cell activation; and cell to cell interactions among activated T cells, B cells, and other cells resulting in the production of cytokines, which modulates B-cell differentiation. Antigen presentation to CD4+ cells was discussed above.

Early Activation Events

Binding of ligand to T-cell surface CD3/TCR triggers a sequence of events leading to phospholipase C activation with hydrolysis of phosphatidylinositol-1, 4-bisphosphate (PIP_2) to diacylglycerol (DAG) and inositol 1,4,5-triphosphate (1,4,5-IP_3).[S689] DAG is the physiologic activator of protein kinase C (PKC);[N105] 1,4,5-IP_3 promotes calcium mobilization from internal stores[U5] and, in T cells, may promote calcium influx across the plasma membrane as well.[K466] In addition to the role of PIP$_2$ hydrolysis in generating intracellular DAG, a major portion of intracellular DAG generation (leading to PKC activation) may also arise via hydrolysis of phosphatidylcholine.[B374,R322]

Changes in intracellular free calcium concentration play a key role in T-cell activation. Elevations in intracellular free calcium levels through mobilization of intracellular stores may not generate the same functional consequences to the cell as elevations of intracellular free calcium through influx of extracellular calcium.[G83] Influx of exogenous calcium is critical, since depletion of extracellular calcium with chelating agents or pharmacologic blockade of calcium channels profoundly inhibits lymphocyte activation,[G82,W161] and calcium chelators added even 4 to 6 hours after stimulation may affect gene expression and production of vital lymphokines such as IL-2.[G264]

Other early activation-associated biochemical events include activation of PKC and generation of cyclic AMP (cAMP). Activation of PKC is absolutely essential for IL-2 production,[T230] and inhibition of PKC activity correlates well with inhibition of T-cell proliferation.[N57] Conversely, increased intracellular levels of cAMP correlate with inhibition of IL-2 production by and proliferation of T cells, presumably by activating protein kinase A (PKA).[A365]

Cell to Cell Interactions

As indicated above, T cells do not recognize isolated antigen. Rather, they recognize antigen only in the context of self-MHC molecules expressed on the surface of the antigen-presenting cell. In addition to the binding of antigen to CD3/TCR, T cells require a costimulatory signal(s) for proliferation and differentiation supplied by antigen-presenting cells and other interacting cells.[S216] Cytokines such as interleukin-1 (IL-1) and IL-6 are important costimulatory factors for T cells, but other signals generated by direct cell to cell interactions may be equally important. For example, CD28 is a cell surface structure expressed by CD4+ cells and most CD8+ cells which can transduce activation signals.[H109] An identified ligand (binding site) for CD28 is the BB1/B7 structure which is expressed on B cells, especially those committed to produce IgG.[D28] Perturbation of CD28 by BB1/B7 can result in enhanced IL-2 production by T cells, thereby leading to enhanced IgG production by B cells.[G149]

An increasing number of cell surface antigens called adhesion molecules have been described that promote contact between T cells and B cells. In some cases adhesion molecules may have signal transducing properties.[O130] These molecules can profoundly affect avidity of T cell/B cell interactions that, in turn, can profoundly affect antibody production. Examples of such adhesion molecules include lymphocyte function antigen 3 (LFA-3 or CD58), which binds to the signal transducing CD2 molecule, and intracellular adhesion molecule (ICAM-1 or CD54), which binds to another T-cell surface structure called LFA-1 (or CD11a). Cell to cell interactions via adhesion molecules increase the binding capacity of T cells to antigen-presenting cells and supply costimulatory signals needed for T-cell activation.

In addition to the positive effects that may ensue from certain T cell/B cell interactions, activated T cells may be down-regulated by CD8+ T cells through incompletely understood mechanisms. Of importance, CD8+ cells require help from CD4+ cells to become suppressor cells.[M577] In the absence of appropriate help from CD4+ cells, CD8+ T cells actually become helper cells instead.[K83] The ramifications of CD8+ T cells as helper cells in SLE are discussed below.

The Role of Cytokines

Cytokines are hormone-like factors produced and secreted by various cell types during the course of an immune response. They generally act at short distances to affect the function of the cells that produce them (i.e., autocrine effects) and the function of other cells in the immediate vicinity (i.e., paracrine effects). They exert their effects by binding to specific cell surface receptors expressed by target cells. Since many different cell types express receptors for a given cytokine, any given cytokine can have pleiotropic effects. Depending on whether individual cytokines are predominantly secreted by lymphocytes or macrophages, they are classified as lymphokines or monokines, respectively.

Table 9–3 indicates the principal source of the growing number of cytokines. Lymphokines such as Interleukin-2 (IL-2), IL-4, IL-5, and IL-10 are produced by predominantly by T cells. Gamma interferon (γIFN) is predominantly produced by both T cells and natural killer (NK) cells and the latter also produce αIFN. IL-1, IL-6, and tumor necrosis factor α (TNFα) are produced predomi-

Table 9–3. The Principal Cytokines Regulating Antibody Production

Source	Cytokine	Effects on Human B Cells
T cells		
Naive and memory	IL-2	Growth and maturation
Memory	IL-4	Supports B cell differentiation; inhibits early B cell activation blocks CD5 expression
	IL-5	Minimal effects on human B cells
	IL-6	Synergistic effects with IL-2 and other cytokines
	IL-10	Blocks antigen presentation to T cells
	γIFN	Inhibits growth, stimulates maturation
B cells		
	IL-1	Cofactor for growth and maturation
	IL-6	Produced by EBV-transformed B cells
	αIFN	Produced by virus-infected B cells
Natural killer cells		
	γIFN	Inhibits growth, stimulates maturation
	αIFN	Inhibits growth, stimulates maturation
	TNFα	Cofactor for maturation
Nonlymphoid cells		
	TGFβ	Inhibits growth and maturation
	IL-1, IL-6 IL-10, TNFα αIFN	Same as above

nantly by mononuclear phagocytes[D222] and by certain other cells as well. Transforming growth factor β (TGFβ) is also produced predominantly by nonlymphoid cells, but can be synthesized by T cells.[R235]

The functional properties of T cells are largely determined by the cytokines they produce. For example, murine CD4+ T cells can be divided into two subsets, TH1 and TH2. TH1 cells, the mediators of delayed hypersensitivity, produce IL-2 and γIFN. TH2 cells, the helper cells for antibody production, produce IL-4, IL-5, IL-6, and IL-10.[F68] Although human T cells can not be categorized as TH1 or TH2 cells on the basis of the cytokines they produce, nonetheless, the function of human T-cell clones also appears to depend upon their cytokine profiles. γIFN up-regulates the response of CD4+ and CD8+ T cells to antigen by enhancing the expression of MHC class II and class I structures on antigen-presenting cells and can induce epithelial cells and fibroblasts cells to express MHC class (HLA-DR) structures on their cell surface, thereby becoming potential antigen-presenting cells for CD4+ cells.[G91] Of importance, γIFN can inhibit helper cytokines for antibody production and IL-4 and IL-10 can inhibit delayed hypersensitivity. TGFβ has diverse effects on T-cell proliferation and helper activity.[L130,T4]

Cytokines can also up-regulate or down-regulate B-cell function. IL-1 and IL-2 enhance the growth and differentiation of B cells in addition to their effects on T cells.[D222] IL-4 is an important B-cell growth factor in mice, but may not be as important in humans. This cytokine up-regulates IgG4 and IgE production, but inhibits production of other Ig isotypes,[C18] perhaps through its inhibitory effects on monocytes.[B158,S610] Moreover, IL-4 appears to facilitate tolerance induction,[P277] an effect that can be abrogated by anti–IL-4 antibody.[S208] IL-6 serves as an important growth factor for activated B cells in the late phase of B-cell differentiation.[V36] γIFN inhibits B-cell proliferation, but enhances B-cell differentiation. TGFβ generally down-regulates B-cell function.[K142,W8]

The biologic effect of a given cytokine is complex because its action will depend upon the composition and/or the maturation state of other cells in the immediate vicinity. For example, γIFN produced by a CD4+ T helper cell may facilitate B-cell differentiation. However, if T suppressor cells are in the vicinity, γIFN may induce these cells to inhibit B-cell differentiation.

A given cytokine may up-regulate the production of other cytokines. IL-2 induces the production of IL-1α, IL-1β, IL-5, IL-6, γIFN, TNFα, TNFβ, and granulocyte-macrophage colony-stimulating factor (GM-CSF).[H288,K90] IL-1, IL-6, and TNFα have cascade effects upon each other in that TNFα stimulates IL1-production, and IL-1 stimulates IL-6 production.[D222] Conversely, certain cytokines inhibit the production of others. For example, γIFN and transforming growth factor β (TNFβ) inhibit IL-1 production.[D222] Certain cytokines act synergistically with one another. IL-1 and IL-6, or IL-2 and IL-6 have potent synergistic effects on T cells and B-cell function.[H399,R159,S359] An important feedback regulatory circuit in the inflammatory response involves IL-1 via IL-6 in stimulating the release of glucocorticoid hormones which in turn down-regulate cytokine production.[B119]

IMMUNOREGULATORY ABNORMALITIES IN SLE

Antigen Recognition by T Cells

As discussed above, T-cell recognition of and response to foreign and self-antigens is determined by class I and II MHC gene products of the host. T-cell cytokine production and subsequent helper activity is, therefore, influenced by expression of MHC alleles on antigen-presenting cells. For example, expression of HLA-DR3 is associated with decreased production of IL-1 and IL-2,[H193] expression of HLA-DR2 and DQw1 gene products correlates with elevated anti–double-stranded (ds)DNA autoantibody titers, decreased production of TNFα in vitro, and lupus nephritis,[J15] and expression of HLA-DR3 and DQw2 correlates with detectable anti-Ro/SSA and anti-La/SSB antibodies.[A136,A292]

Since the recognition processes of T cells for self- and foreign antigens are similar, one must consider whether antigen-presenting cells in SLE may aberrantly process self-antigens or whether there may be an increase in T cells capable of responding to self-peptides. Regarding the former possibility, abnormalities of SLE monocytes have been described. Depletion of monocytes decreased anti-DNA antibody production in vitro, and adding the SLE monocytes back into cultures increased production of this autoantibody.[S85] Regarding the latter possibility, there is no evidence to date of oligoclonal expansion of T cells in human SLE as manifested by restricted usage of T-cell antigen receptor variable region genes.[P272,W338] Although restriction fragment length polymorphism studies have revealed an association between one framework gene encoding the constant region of the T-cell receptor α region and SLE,[T92] the significance of this observation is not yet clear.

Defects in tolerance induction have been reported in murine SLE,[L84] but analogous studies are difficult, if not impossible, to perform in humans. It is possible to down-regulate autoantibody production in SLE by adding DNA complexed with human gamma globulin.[B415] These workers have suggested that the principle of carrier-determined tolerance could be applied as a specific therapy for SLE.[B415]

Percentage and Absolute Numbers of T-Cell Subsets

Decreased numbers of T cells, B cells, and natural killer (NK) cells is a common manifestation of active SLE.[A5,G199,H435,M373,M569,R227,R228] Most patients with active SLE have total lymphocyte counts less than 1000 cells/mm³. Because of the relative decrease of lymphocytes in SLE in comparison with monocytes, the percentage of CD3+ T cells is often decreased in mononuclear cells prepared by Ficoll/Hypaque density centrifugation. The apparent percentage of T cells may be further decreased by the presence of immature granulocytes which sediment with mononuclear cells in patients with active disease.

Within the context of T-cell lymphopenia, certain T-cell subsets may be affected more than others in SLE. Early reports indicated a relative decrease in CD8+ cells in SLE.[M581,T239] One group indicated that patients with sicca syndrome, central nervous system disease, lung disease, and muscle disease exhibit increased CD4:CD8 ratios.[S519] Other studies have indicated that the relative percentage of CD8+ cells is normal or increased, and that CD4+ cells are often decreased in active SLE.[B40,M295,S519] In such cases the decrease in CD4+ cells results in an abnormally low CD4:CD8 ratio, a finding frequently observed in patients with severe lupus nephritis.[F167,S519] Corticosteroid therapy preferentially decreases CD4+ cells and thus decreases the CD4:CD8 ratio.[B40] Decreased CD4+ cells correlate with antilymphocyte antibodies (ALAs) specifically reactive against this T-cell subset,[M580,Y5,Y7] and a strong relationship exists between high titers of ALAs, lymphopenia, and disease activity.[B598,D126,G199,M372,O84, S642,W288,W292]

In addition to alterations in the number or percentages of CD4+ cells, we reported an association between SLE and expression of a genetically determined variant of the CD4+ molecule.[S699,S700] This association was most dramatic in Jamaican black individuals. Whether expression of this variant CD4 molecule truly predisposes certain individuals to develop SLE or simply acts as a marker for some other SLE predisposing factor remains unknown at this time.

Naive and Memory T Lymphocyte Subsets

CD4+ T cells with the naive phenotype (CD45RA+) were reported to be decreased in SLE.[M584,R84,S93] Since serum from SLE patients contain autoantibodies against CD45RA, it was suggested that this subset, which has suppressor-inducer activity, was deleted.[M453,T56] However, as stated above, it was later determined that following activation, T cells lose the CD45RA marker and become memory cells. Surprisingly, therefore, another group reported decreased percentages of cells with a more mature phenotype (CD29+), and this finding correlated with increased production of anti-DNA antibodies in patients with active SLE.[G306] In our laboratory, we confirmed decreased expression of CD45RA by CD4+ cells and also noted decreased expression of CD45RA by CD8+ cells in these patients. In some patients with lupus nephritis, there was an increased percentage of CD4+ and CD8+ cells that expressed both CD45RA and RO. Neither patients with inactive SLE nor controls with tuberculosis or with non-SLE nephritis exhibited increased percentages of CD45RA+ RO+ cells.[H431] Increased numbers of CD45RA+ RO+ cells could possibly reflect a partial transition of naive cells to memory cells or a reversion of memory cells to naive cells as described in rats.[S580] Whichever explanation is correct, patients with increased CD45RA+ RO+ cells had decreased numbers of CD45RA− RO+ memory cells. The failure of T cells from these patients to become fully developed memory cells may be important because antigen-specific suppressor-inducer cells are memory cells.[D27]

CD4− CD8− (Double-Negative) T Cells in SLE

In addition to CD4+ and CD8+ T cells, there are small numbers of T cells that express neither CD4 nor CD8. These have been called CD3+ double-negative (DN) cells [B205] and consist of two principal subsets. Two-thirds of these cells express T-cell receptors (TCRs) comprised of γ and δ chains and one-third bear α and β TCR chains.[B474,L63] Since CD3+ DN cells may develop outside the thymus,[B188] clones of such T cells with autoreactivity may escape thymic deletion. Both αβ CD3+ DN cells and γδ CD3+ DN cells can provide help for anti-DNA antibody production,[R17] and αβ CD3+ DN cells are increased in patients with active SLE.[S373] In contrast to increased numbers of αβ CD3+ DN cells in SLE, there is a preliminary report of decreased numbers of γδ T cells in SLE.[L417] This may have profound ramifications for regulation of autoantibody production, since after a brief exposure to IL-2, γδ CD3+ DN cells in healthy subjects may develop potent suppressor activity.[R223]

Early Activation Events in SLE

Despite the obvious importance of intracellular second messengers to T-cell function in SLE, relatively little is known regarding their levels, their generation, or their regulation in SLE. Impaired calcium responses to mitogenic lectins and anti-CD3 monoclonal antibody (MAb) in T-cell−enriched populations in SLE have been reported,[S422] and PKC activity in response to phorbol ester may be somewhat lower in SLE T cells than in normal T cells.[T5] Generation of intracellular cAMP levels in response to multiple different stimuli is impaired in SLE PBMC and T-cell−enriched populations,[M90,P174] and PKA activity has been suggested to be abnormal in T cells from active SLE patients when compared to T cells from either normal donors or patients with rheumatoid arthritis or Sjögren's syndrome.[H195]

Activated T Cells in SLE

Blood lymphocytes isolated from subjects with active SLE exhibit signs of previous in vivo activation as documented by increased expression of MHC class II molecules, increased IL-2 receptor (IL-2R) expression, the release of soluble IL-2R into the serum, and ongoing IL-2 synthesis (Table 9−4). Activated, but not resting, T cells express HLA-DR on their cell surfaces, and as much as 20% of T cells from subjects with active SLE are HLA-DR positive. Some workers have reported increased CD4+ DR+ cells;[R83] others, an increase in CD8+ DR+ cells;[T251] and we and others, an increase in both CD4+ DR+ and CD8+ DR+ cells.[I16,L312] Surface expression of HLA-DP is also increased in SLE[H329] as is the early activation antigen TLiSA1.[T1] In addition, patients with active

Table 9−4. Evidence of T-cell Activation *in vivo* in Subjects with Active SLE

1. Increased cell surface expression in unstimulated T cells of MHC class II (HLA-DR, DP) structures, and, to a lesser extent, interleukin-2 receptor expression and TLiSA1
2. Increased expression of proliferating cell nuclear antigen in unstimulated T cells
3. Increased levels of mRNA transcripts for interleukin-2 in unstimulated T cells
4. Increased serum levels of interleukin-2, soluble interleukin-2 receptors, and γ-interferon

SLE have increased expression of proliferating cell nuclear antigen (cyclin),[M664] a finding consistent with the observation of increased numbers of spontaneously proliferating lymphocytes in SLE.[H437]

Studies using radiolabeled IL-2 have revealed significantly increased levels of cell surface IL-2R in patients with active disease compared with inactive disease.[W223] Other studies using anti–IL-2 monoclonal antibodies that recognize the p55 component of IL-2R have indicated that the increase in IL-2R expression is more modest than the increase in HLA-DR+ cells in patients with active SLE.[L312,V101] This is probably because IL-2 receptors tend to disappear from the cell surface after chronic stimulation of lymphocytes.

Serum-soluble IL-2R levels are also increased in SLE[C52,M108,S271,T109,W323] and this correlates with disease activity.[C52,T109] In addition, using the polymerase chain reaction to document cytokine gene expression, we have detected increased IL-2 mRNA synthesis by CD4+ T cells in patients with active SLE (see below). Others have reported that serum levels of IL-2 are increased in these patients.[H468]

Cytokine Production and Responsiveness in SLE

For the following discussion it is important to distinguish the properties of freshly isolated SLE mononuclear cells from the properties of cells stimulated in vitro. The former presumably reflects the activities of mononuclear cells in vivo, whereas observed defects of in vitro–stimulated cells may be explained by the refractory nature of in vivo–activated cells to further stimulation (Table 9–5).

T-Cell–Derived Cytokines

T-cell–derived cytokines include IL-2, IL-4, and γIFN.

INTERLEUKIN-2

CD4+ lymphocytes are the principal producers of IL-2. CD8+ cells are generally poor producers of IL-2 in response to antigens or mitogens, but do generate substantial amounts of this cytokine when phorbol esters are added to the cell cultures.[L412,M375] CD3+ DN cells also produce IL-2 in response to mitogenic stimulation, but to a lesser extent than CD4+ cells.[B205]

Table 9–5. Cytokine Production in Patients with Active SLE

Cytokine	Serum Level	Spontaneous Release	After Stimulation of PBMCs In Vitro
T cell derived			
Interleukin-2	Increased	Low	Decreased
γ-Interferon	Increased	Low	Decreased
Non-T cell derived			
Interleukin-1	Not known	Increased	Decreased
Tumor necrosis factor α	Normal or increased	Normal or slightly increased	Decreased
Interleukin-6	Increased	Increased	Not known

IL-2 activity in culture supernatants of mitogen-stimulated PBMC is decreased in SLE.[A126,H329,H467,L311,M503,M662,M663,S422,W89] This decrease reflects decreased production and is not simply because of increased passive absorption by activated mononuclear cells.[H467] Decreased IL-2 activity may correlate with disease activity,[W223] but not all investigators have been able to confirm this observation.[L311,V101] Relatives of SLE patients also exhibit decreased levels of in vitro–induced IL-2 levels.[S28] This abnormality in family members, however, disappeared when antibodies to the α chain of the IL-2R (CD25) were added to the cultures.[R222] This defect, therefore, can most simply be explained by increased absorption of IL-2 rather than decreased production.

Decreased IL-2 production in vitro may be explained by decreased numbers of IL-2 producer cells, dysfunctional IL-2 producer cells, or factors external to the IL-2 producer cell. Although CD4+ cells are frequently decreased in number in active SLE (see above), decreased IL-2 production in patients with normal percentages of CD4+ cells has been documented.[L311]

There is now general agreement that decreased IL-2 production is not due to some intrinsic defect in the IL-2 producer cell. Rather impaired IL-2 production appears to be a result of factors external to the IL-2–producing cell. Three nonmutually exclusive mechanisms may be operative. Removal of radiosensitive CD8+ cells normalizes IL-2 production in SLE,[L312] and the suppressor cells were identified as CD8+ DR+ T cells or CD8+ CD16+ NK cells.[L315,L316] A partially characterized suppressor factor produced by CD8+ cells can substitute for intact cells.[L313] Thus, non–IL-2–producing cells in SLE can inhibit IL-2 production. These cells might reflect a normal feedback regulatory mechanism to down-regulate IL-2 produced by stimulated autoreactive T cells (see below).

A second mechanism to explain decreased IL-2 production in SLE deals with the increased numbers of activated T cells in SLE (see above). Recently activated T cells are refractory to further stimulation. Indeed, resting SLE PBMCs for 2 or 3 days before stimulating these cells with phytohemagglutinin (PHA) plus phorbol ester normalized IL-2 production.[H467] Others reported the decreased IL-2 production correlated with increased surface expression of the MHC class II marker, HLA-DP. After culturing SLE lymphocytes, decreased numbers of HLA-DP+ cells correlated with increased IL-2 production.[H329] By contrast, two other groups have also reported that the addition of phorbol esters to PHA could correct the IL-2 defect in SLE.[M662,S422] Phorbol esters directly activate protein kinase C and apparently bypass the refractoriness of activated SLE T cells.

A third mechanism involves serum factors. Antibodies in SLE serum have been described that inhibit IL-2 production by normal cells.[M500] Conversely, the levels of IL-2 inhibiting activity normally present in human serum is decreased in SLE.[F305,K442]

Although freshly isolated T cells from SLE patients produce only small amounts of IL-2 without stimulation, there is increasing evidence that activated T cells are producing this cytokine in vivo. First, increased levels of IL-2 in the serum of SLE patients has been reported.[H468]

Although this could be explained by decreased IL-2 clearance in SLE, the more likely explanation is that more IL-2 is being produced in SLE than in normals. Increased production by SLE PBMCs cultured at low cell densities has been documented.[W87] In addition, IL-2 mRNA transcripts can be detected in unstimulated PBMCs only from patients with SLE, but not from healthy controls or patients with tuberculosis.[W68] Although the presence of IL-2 mRNA does not prove IL-2 protein synthesis, it certainly supports the notion of increased IL-2 production in SLE. Additional indirect evidence that unstimulated SLE PBMCs do produce increased amounts of IL-2 is that anti–IL-2 antibodies markedly decreases spontaneous Ig production by SLE B cells.[L317]

RESPONSIVENESS TO IL-2

The lymphocyte response to IL-2 is decreased in SLE.[A126,I43,J79] This is because of decreased expression of IL-2 receptors following mitogenic stimulation. IL-2R is comprised of a p55 α chain (CD25) and a p70–75 β chain. Lymphocytes may express each of these components separately or together as a high-avidity IL-2R. Although freshly isolated T cells from patients with active SLE may have increased expression of the α chain, the β chain is not increased.[T58] Moreover, in response to mitogenic stimulation there is less up-regulation of both α chain and the β chain,[I43,S17,T58] predominantly in CD4+ cells.[M663,T10] This abnormality may also reflect a regulatory defect. The precursor frequencies of IL-2–responsive cells increased after "resting" them for 24 hours before mitogenic stimulation.[W89] Of interest, although T cells are hyporesponsive, B cells in SLE show increased responsiveness to IL-2 because of increased expression of the IL-2 receptor β chain.[H468]

INTERLEUKIN-4

In contrast to the substantial body of information regarding IL-2 in SLE, there is little information available concerning IL-4. In contrast to increased IL-2 mRNA transcripts in SLE PBMCs, IL-4 mRNA transcripts are decreased.[W68] This putative decrease in IL-4 production in SLE is of interest in that IL-4 has been reported to decrease CD5 expression by B cells, and increased numbers of this autoantibody-forming B-cell subset are present in SLE.[F224]

INTERFERONS

Although, like IL-2, isolated PBMCs from normals produce only minimal amounts of IFN, there is evidence of increased αIFN production in SLE. Serum levels of an acid-labile αIFN are increased in SLE,[P282] and the levels correlate with activity of disease.[K49,K205,M183,V113,Y39] The acid lability of αIFN in SLE is caused by a serum factor rather than reflecting an unusual IFN. Serum levels of γIFN are also increased in SLE, but do not correlate with clinical activity.

Production of γIFN by mitogen-stimulated PBMCs in vitro is usually decreased in SLE.[S710,T244,T247] Decreased in vitro production of γIFN correlates well with decreased natural killer activity.[T244] Also like the IL-2 abnormality described above, the addition of phorbol ester to the cultures reversed the defect.[S405,S710] Anti-IFN antibodies have also been described in the serum of SLE patients.[S404]

The effects of IFN on lymphocytes depend upon their state of activation or maturation. Although γIFN inhibits T- and B-cell proliferation in healthy subjects,[B333] inhibition of B-cell proliferation is not observed in SLE.[F312] Both γIFN and IL-2 augment B-cell maturation,[K250] and these cytokines enhance spontaneous IgG production by purified B cells from SLE patients.[G225] Interestingly, the addition of γIFN to unseparated PBMCs decreases both polyclonal IgG and anti-DNA antibody production in SLE,[B462] suggesting that the net effects of this cytokine also depend on the regulatory cells that are cultured with B cells.

At present, there is no information concerning the activities of IL-5 and IL-10 in subjects with SLE.

Cytokines Principally Produced by Non-T cells

Although T cells can produce IL-1, TNFα, IL-6, and TGFβ, these cytokines are produced predominantly by non-T cells.

INTERLEUKIN-1

Increased spontaneous release of IL-1 from SLE monocytes has been reported by several groups[A263,H328,J41,T57] with one exception.[S423] In one study, increased release of IL-1α and β correlated with serum antibodies to ribonucleoprotein.[A263] Adherent cells release factors such as IL-1 and IL-6, which support anti-DNA antibody synthesis in SLE. Although these factors do not usually have a direct stimulatory effect, they greatly enhance the ability of T cells to provide help to B cells in autoantibody production.

In addition to monocytes as a rich source of IL-1, SLE B cells also produce IL-1 and IL-6 and are reported to sustain B-cell activity in an autocrine fashion.[T57,T59,P96] It should be noted that there is controversy whether sustained antibody production by SLE B cells can occur without T-cell help. Others have reported that T-cell help is essential.[C334,L317,M601,T19]

In contrast to increased spontaneous release of IL-1, there is general agreement that the ability of monocytes or adherent cells to produce detectable IL-1 after stimulation is decreased.[A128,M681,S423,T16,W202] In our laboratory, we found that decreased in vitro IL-1 production in SLE could be reversed by indomethacin, a finding suggesting that prostaglandins might be responsible for decreased IL-1 production. Increased prostaglandin production by monocytes has, indeed, been reported in SLE.[M138,T16] Decreased IL-1 activity in vitro can be explained by either defective synthesis, or IL-1 receptor antagonists. Of note is that monocytes stimulated by immune complexes produce an IL-1 receptor antagonist,[A284] so SLE monocytes, having been exposed in vivo to circulating immune complexes, may be primed for production of IL-1 receptor antagonist.

TUMOR NECROSIS FACTOR α.

Serum levels of TNFα in SLE are normal or increased.[M217] Spontaneous in vitro release of TNFα by SLE

PBMCs is also normal or slightly increased.[M78,M216] In contrast, production of TNFα in vitro by stimulated PBMCs is decreased.[J15,M78,M681] In response to mitogenic stimulation, SLE patients with MHC class II antigens HLA-DR2 and DQw1 produce low levels of TNFα, a phenotype associated with lupus nephritis.[J15] Taken together, TNFα production in vivo and following stimulation of PBMCs in vitro appears to mirror that of IL-1.

INTERLEUKIN-6

Spontaneous in vitro release of IL-6 is increased in SLE, and neutralizing anti–IL-6 antibodies decrease spontaneous Ig production.[K269,L314] Nevertheless, no correlation between in vitro levels of IL-6 and Ig production could be demonstrated,[H184] and, in a retrospective study, IL-6 levels and exacerbations of disease did not correlate.[S780] Moreover, IL-6 stimulates the liver to produce the acute-phase–reactant C-reactive protein, but this protein is not usually increased in active SLE. Although serum levels of IL-6 are elevated in SLE,[L314] high serum IL-6 concentrations are found in a wide variety of conditions such as bacterial infections, burns, and alcoholic cirrhosis.[K429] For these reasons, IL-6 may be an important cofactor in sustaining B-cell hyperactivity, but likely is not a primary factor.

Studies with IL-6 have provided evidence of a B-cell abnormality is SLE. Although low-density (resting) B cells from healthy subjects did not respond to this cytokine, low-density B cells from active SLE patients directly differentiated into Ig-secreting cells without an additional costimulatory signal.[K258] Whether SLE B cells have been primed in vivo for IL-6 responsiveness, or are inherently more responsive to IL-6, remains to be clarified.

TRANSFORMING GROWTH FACTOR β

In one preliminary report, the addition of anti-TGFβ antibodies to SLE PBMCs resulted in increased spontaneous Ig synthesis.[D142] Since TGFβ can have marked inhibitory effects on T- and B-cell function, forthcoming information regarding levels of this cytokine in SLE will be of great interest.

CYTOKINES AND CLINICAL DISEASE

There are several examples where specific cytokines may play a causal role in SLE or SLE-like disease. Administration of γIFN to a patient with presumed rheumatoid arthritis has induced an exacerbation of SLE.[M8] Administration of αIFN to patients with hematologic malignancies has also led to the appearance of autoantibodies and even clinical SLE.[R270,S141] Moreover, αIFN has also been implicated as a pathogenetic factor in lupus central nervous system (CNS) disease, in that a strong correlation has been reported between αIFN levels in the cerebrospinal fluid (CSF) and lupus CNS disease.[S367] Although IL-6 can also be detected in the CSF, levels of this cytokine did not correlate with CNS disease.[H324] Finally, IL-1 and TNF have been implicated in the pathogenesis of lupus nephritis. Increased IL-1β and TNF gene expression have been detected in the kidneys of mice with lupus nephritis. Unstim-

ulated isolated glomeruli from mice with autoimmune lupus nephritis, but not control glomeruli, released TNF.[B422]

T Lymphocyte Functional Responses

In the early 1970s workers from several laboratories reported that patients with active SLE respond poorly to intradermal injected skin test antigens.[H26,H428,P70] This observation was followed by numerous reports of abnormal defects in the T-cell proliferative responses to mitogens,[H433,L357,M138,R313,U39] to soluble antigens,[G315] and to MHC class II antigens on both allogeneic[K454,S754,T238] and autologous antigen-presenting cells.[K468,S29,S30,T10] Generation of antigen-specific cytolytic T cells was also found to be decreased.[A112,C213] These observations could be explained by regulatory defects or an inherent T-cell defect in SLE. In support of an inherent defect, impaired capping of membrane CD3, CD4, and CD8 following incubation with the corresponding monoclonal antibodies was, in fact, noted in T cells from patients with SLE.[K45] This lead to the identification of a defect in cAMP metabolism of CD4 + cells in SLE,[M90] and this defect has been documented in patients with inactive as well as active disease.[K46] Regulatory abnormalities have also been described, as summarized in Table 9–6.

The Proliferative Response to Mitogens

Most investigators have reported decreased proliferative responses of SLE blood leukocytes or mononuclear cells in vitro to mitogenic lectins (phytohemagglutinin [PHA], concanavalin A [Con A], and pokeweed mitogen [PWM])[B180,H85,H433,L357,M77,M138,P69,P70,R313,S754,U39]

Table 9–6. T Lymphocyte Functional Activities In Vitro

Function	Activity
Proliferation	
Mitogenic lectins	Decreased or normal
Anti-CD3	Decreased or normal*
Anti-CD2	Decreased
Soluble antigens	Decreased
Allogeneic mixed lymphocyte reaction	Decreased
Autologous mixed lymphocyte reaction	Markedly decreased
Response to interleukin-2	Decreased or normal
Helper cell activity	
Nonspecific	Decreased or normal
Antigen specific	Decreased
Suppressor cell activity	
Con A induced	Decreased or normal
Antigen specific	Decreased
Spontaneous inhibitors of IL-2 production	Increased
Cytotoxic cell activity	
In response to allogeneic or xenogeneic antigens	Decreased
In response to hapten-modified antigens	Increased
In response to anti-CD3	Decreased
In response to IL-2	Decreased

* When isolated T cells are used instead of PBMCs, the response to αCD3 is normal or increased.

Table 9–7. Initiation of Systemic Lupus Erythematosus

1. Inciting factor(s) ↓	• Infectious agents or other environmental trigger factors
2. Genetic Predisposition ↓	• Major histocompatibility complex class II susceptibility alleles (for autoantibodies) • Deletion of genes encoding serum complement components and/or protective autoantibodies • Female sex hormones
4. Defective immune response ↓	• Failure to eliminate inciting agent (virus or bacteria) • Chronic inflammation with T-cell dysfunction and polyclonal B-cell activation
4. Breakdown of tolerance (nonresponsiveness) ↓	• Reversal of clonal anergy and activation of self-reactive autoaggressive T cells because of defective suppressor cell activity
5. Pathogenic autoantibodies and immune complexes	• Onset of clinical disease

(Table 9–7). The significance of these observations is unclear, however, because most, but not all,[U39] observers have been unable to correlate decreased mitogenic activity with clinical activity. Moreover, several groups have reported normal responsiveness to mitogens.[G258,L50,S281,T241]

The discrepant results could be attributed to differences in patient populations studied, differing cell preparation procedures, and culture conditions. Regarding the last possibility, several factors that may explain decreased mitogenic reactivity include suboptimal concentrations of mitogen,[H433,M77,U39] inhibitory monocytes,[M138] hypergammaglobulinemia,[B180] and inhibitory antibody and nonantibody serum factors.[H430,H432,H434] Along these lines, studies conducted in our laboratory revealed that impaired mitogenesis in SLE was most easily demonstrated when comparing cells from patients and controls cultured in a standard lot of human AB serum and in the presence of suboptimal doses of mitogens. Decreased responses were observed, especially in those patients who were anergic to skin test antigens. Although depressed mitogenic reactivity did not correlate with clinical activity, the degree of serum suppression was positively correlated with disease activity, and the principal serum inhibitor was found in the IgG fraction.[H430]

In addition to studies with mitogenic lectins, the proliferative responses to mitogenic anti-CD3 and anti-CD2 monoclonal antibodies have been examined. Although proliferation of unfractionated PBMCs to anti-CD3 MAbs may be depressed in SLE,[K52,T194] isolated T cells exhibit normal to increased responsiveness in SLE.[S660,S698] The observed impaired proliferative responses of SLE PBMCs to anti-CD3 MAbs, therefore, appear to be a result of an abnormality in accessory (non-T) cells rather than a T-cell defect.

To date, there is only one reported study of T-cell proliferation in response to anti-CD2 MAbs in SLE that documented decreased responsiveness.[F178] It remains to be determined whether this impaired response is because of

a T-cell defect, or as the case for anti-CD3 MAbs, is from an abnormality in accessory cells. In our laboratory, the response of PBMC to anti-CD2 is decreased or normal.

The Proliferative Response to Soluble and Cell Surface Antigens

There is general agreement that lymphocyte proliferation in response to soluble antigens is decreased in patients with active SLE.[G315,O16,P70] The one report of normal responsiveness to recall antigens also noted intact delayed hypersensitivity.[G258] The SLE patients described in this latter study were possibly less active than were patients of the other studies documenting poor responses to soluble antigens.

The reasons why the T-cell proliferative response in SLE to soluble antigens is decreased to a greater extent than is the response to mitogens are not well understood. Since memory T cells are the lymphocytes that respond to soluble antigens, it is possible that this proliferative defect can be attributed to decreased numbers or defective function of this T-cell subset. As stated above, some SLE patients have decreased percentages of CD45RA − RO + memory cells.[H431]

T-cell responsiveness to both allogeneic and autologous lymphocytes is decreased in SLE.[K454,K463,S754,T10,T238,W180] In the autologous mixed lymphocyte reaction (AMLR), CD4 + T lymphocytes recognize self-MHC class II major histocompatibility antigens on non-T cells. They respond by secreting IL-2, which promotes the proliferation of IL-2R + T cells. Considerable precaution must be taken in setting up the AMLR because foreign antigens contained in fetal calf serum (used as culture growth factors) can also stimulate T cells to proliferate. However, with care, the AMLR can reflect a physiologic response that results in induction of B-cell differentiation and the activation of T suppressor cells.[K467] Impaired AMLR in SLE may be caused by the inability of SLE T cells to produce adequate amounts of IL-2.[T10] In addition, naive (CD45RA +) CD4 + T cells, which proliferate in response to self-antigens, are decreased in SLE.[M584,R84,S93]

T Helper Cell Activity in SLE

T helper cell activity induced by pokeweed mitogen is decreased[G155,T52] or normal[F25,N95] in SLE. T helper cell activity induced by specific antigens is decreased in SLE. Unlike normal lymphocytes, SLE cells immunized in vitro with trinitrophenyl polyacrylamide beads were unable to generate antigen-specific antibody-forming cells. SLE B cells responded when cocultured with normal T cells, but SLE T cells were unable to provide help for normal B cells.[D140] The ability of SLE T cells to support B-cell colony formation is also defective in SLE.[K452] Again, the failure of SLE T cells to respond normally to mitogens or antigens may be explained by the fact that in vivo–activated T cells respond poorly to subsequent in vitro stimulation. Alternatively, suppressor cells generated by chronic antigenic stimulation in vivo may inhibit T-cell activation in vitro.

Freshly isolated T cells from SLE peripheral blood will sustain polyclonal (including autoantibody) production by B cells. Studies from our laboratory revealed that CD4+ DR+ cells and, surprisingly, CD8+ DR+ T cells supported polyclonal IgG synthesis. Moreover, in the concentrations added, CD4+ cells by themselves were unable to sustain anti-DNA antibody production. The addition of CD8+ cells or NK cells to CD4+ cells was necessary to support autoantibody production.[L317] (In normals, CD8+ cells and NK cells down-regulate antibody synthesis.) Thus, these observations point to dysregulation of both CD8+ cells and NK cells in SLE.

T Suppressor Cell Activity

During the 1970s assays to measure T suppressor activity were developed[B483,S395] and numerous investigators reported a defect in SLE.[T240] Here "suppressor" activity was generated in vitro by culturing mononuclear cells with concanavalin A, and the effects of these activated cells on other lymphocytes was determined. However, the relevance of this information to the regulation of antibody production in SLE has been seriously questioned.

As stated above, defective suppression of antibody production may be explained by dysregulation of CD4+ cells and/or CD8+ cells. Abnormalities involving one or the other of these T-cell subsets were described by one group. These workers reported that high concentrations of CD4+ cells suppressed antibody synthesis in normals, but not in SLE patients with decreased percentages of CD4+ cells. This suggested a defect of suppressor-inducer cells or CD4+ Leu 8+ suppressor cells in these SLE patients. In addition, these workers described a separate abnormality involving CD8+ cells in SLE patients with normal percentages of CD4+ cells,[M295] suggesting that multiple suppressor abnormalities exist in SLE.

It is clear that CD8+ cells from patients with active SLE are often unable to down-regulate polyclonal Ig synthesis[L317,M295] and autoantibody production.[L280,L317,T19] Several factors probably account for the inability of CD8+ cells to down-regulate antibody production. The vast majority of CD8+ cells are naive cells that, without sufficient stimulation, may provide help for B cells.[T12] Naive CD8+ cells require cytokines such as IL-2 or γIFN to develop this suppressor function, and the majority of CD4+ T cells in patients with active SLE may be defective in producing these cytokines. In addition, CD8+ cell differentiation to suppressor-effector cells require interaction with other cells via cell surface adhesion molecules. Defective expression of crucial adhesion molecules by CD8+ T cells in SLE could contribute to the inability of these cells to develop normal suppressor function.

DNA-induced antibody synthesis has been analyzed in a pair of identical twins discordant for SLE in which only B cells from the SLE co-twin could produce anti-DNA antibodies. Addition of SLE co-twin's T cells to her B cells promoted anti-DNA antibody production induced by calf thymus DNA. On the other hand, T cells from the nonaffected co-twin did not promote anti-DNA antibody synthesis unless CD8+ cells were depleted. This finding suggested that the healthy co-twin did have anti-DNA–specific T helper cells, but they were kept nonfunctional by CD8+ suppressor cells.[T19] Whether all normal

individuals harbor T cells capable of helping an anti-DNA antibody response, or whether only those individuals with a "SLE genetic constitution" harbor such T cells remains uncertain.

A T suppressor cell defect in first-degree relatives of SLE patients has been documented that correlates with increased levels of 16/6, a cross-reactive idiotype of monoclonal anti-DNA antibodies.[S114] This observation reinforces the notion of genetic predisposition to SLE.

T-Cell Cytotoxic Activity

Numerous abnormalities pertaining to cytolytic activity have been described in SLE.[C213,F285,H368,K114,S406,S442,T245,W88] Most of these reported abnormalities in cytolytic function lie within the non–T-cell population, including impaired NK activity[H368,K114,S406,S442,T245] and impaired lymphokine-activated killer activity.[F285] Nevertheless, abnormalities in T-cell–dependent or T-cell–mediated cytolytic activity in SLE have also been described, including abnormal PWM-induced cytotoxicity,[W88] impaired generation of cytotoxic T cells against allogeneic or xenogeneic targets,[C213,T245] and impaired anti-CD3–induced cytotoxicity.[S698]

This latter report may be especially important in that anti-CD3 MAbs, which activate all T cells, could lead to *normal* T-cell proliferation in SLE despite *abnormal* T-cell–mediated cytolytic activity. This may have important ramifications for SLE pathogenesis. In a murine graft-versus-host (GVH) model, inoculation of F_1 recipient mice with T cells from parent A resulted in an immunosuppressive GVH reaction with no clinical autoimmune features, whereas inoculation of recipient F_1 mice with T cells from parent B resulted in an immunostimulatory GVH with clinical features resembling SLE. Further analysis revealed that the number of anti-F_1 cytotoxic T lymphocyte precursor cells (CTLp) was markedly lower in the SLE-like GVH reaction than in the non–SLE-like GVH reaction, and elimination of CD8+ T cells (presumably containing the relevant CTLp) derived from parent A prior to inoculation of the F_1 recipients also resulted in a SLE-like response.[V75] Thus, based on this murine GVH model, the absence of an adequate *polyclonal* T-cell–mediated cytolytic response may be an important contributing factor to the development of SLE.

SLE patients, never having received foreign tissues, obviously do not experience GVH reactions per se. Nevertheless, polyclonal T-cell activation leading to autoreactivity and help for autoantibody production could arise following exposure to environmental infectious agents. A compelling argument has been offered for the role of microbial superantigens (which, like anti-CD3 MAbs, activate T cells via surface CD3/TCRs) in the triggering of polyclonal T-cell autoreactivity, which, under the proper setting, could result in SLE.[F253] Moreover, as has been documented for the human immunodeficiency virus (HIV)[M3] but likely also the case for other viruses, T cells—following their infection with certain viruses and their incorporation of the viral genomes—can become potent unrestricted helpers for Ig production. In either of these two scenarios, T cells would become activated through *antigen-independent* processes (i.e., in the absence of specific antigenic peptides in the context of self-MHC molecules), for which *antigen-independent* activation of T cells by anti-CD3 MAbs may be an excellent model. Thus, the observed in vitro defect in anti-CD3—induced polyclonal T-cell—mediated cytolytic activity may reflect similar in vivo defects in generating polyclonal T-cell—mediated cytolytic activity, resulting in dysregulated polyclonal T-cell helper activity and predisposing to the development of SLE.

Serum Inhibitors of T-Cell Function

SLE sera inhibit lymphocyte proliferation in response to mitogenic lectins,[B180,H430,H432] soluble antigens[Y7] and allogeneic[S659,W180,W244] and autologous MHC antigens.[H37,O49,S27,S664,S754] These sera also block the generation of cytotoxic T cells,[C213] and interfere with antigen presentation by macrophages.[B528] Much of this inhibitory capacity can be ascribed to IgM and IgG antibodies, which react with various lymphocyte cell surface molecules. SLE antilymphocyte antibodies (ALAs) react with activated lymphocytes more strongly than resting lymphocytes.[C334,L335,Y7] IgG ALAs inhibit suppressor cell generation and activity.[O49,S15] In addition, IgG ALAs inhibit mitogen and MLR-induced proliferation [H430,H432,L335,O49,S15, W180,W244] and preferentially inhibit the T-cell response to soluble antigens.[Y7]

Although initially reported to react with only T suppressor cells,[M575,S32] ALAs react with both CD4+ and CD8+ cells[M580,Y6] and actually appear to preferentially react with CD4+ cells.[Y5] Such autoantibodies may result in altered CD4:CD8 ratios, leading to altered immune function. In addition, IgM autoantibodies reactive with the membrane tyrosine phosphatase CD45 molecule have been described in SLE.[M453,T56] These antibodies preferentially react with the high-molecular-weight CD45RA isoform expressed on naive T cells.[B279] Such autoantibodies may interfere with T-cell signal transduction. Autoantibodies against the MHC class I—associated β_2-microglobulin[M371] and MHC class II molecules[O49] have also been described. Such autoantibodies could inhibit T-cell function by blocking cell to cell interactions.

THE ROLE OF T CELLS IN PATHOGENESIS AND PERPETUATION

The defects of T-cell function described above presumably contribute to the pathogenesis and perpetuation of SLE. Current views are summarized in this section.

The Development of Autoreactive Memory T Cells

To understand the pathogenesis of SLE, two fundamental issues must be clarified: 1) the mechanisms responsible for the breakdown of immunologic tolerance; and 2) the factors responsible for numerous autoantibodies to nuclear, cytoplasmic, and cell surface antigens (i.e., generalized autoimmunity). As stated above, T cells with the potential to respond to self-peptides exist in peripheral lymphoid tissue but are normally rendered anergic or tolerant. In subjects who develop SLE, a breakdown of tolerance to certain self-peptides leads to generalized autoimmunity.

The nuclear antigens recognized by SLE cells are beginning to be characterized. Even though anti—double-stranded DNA antibodies are characteristic of SLE, it is unlikely that self-DNA is the triggering antigen. Mammalian DNA is poorly immunogenic, and T cells recognize only peptide antigens, not oligonucleotides. Bacterial DNA, however, can induce anti-dsDNA antibodies in nonimmune mice,[G133] and DNA-protein complexes can trigger pathogenic anti-DNA antibodies in SLE. DNA bound to histone or complexed to other proteins, in fact, is a common target of autoantibodies in SLE.[J20,J22] Anti-DNA antibodies similar to those detected in human SLE have been raised in nonautoimmune mice immunized with a human DNA-protein complex present in high levels in the circulation of SLE patients,[R205] and certain nucleoprotein fractions isolated from immunoblots can also stimulate SLE T cells.[P171]

It has been proposed that autoimmunity actually is an immune deficiency disorder [S644] in that the failure of the immune system to neutralize an antigenic challenge lays the foundation for the development of an autoimmune disease (Table 9—7). If the antigen is an infectious organism, persistence of this agent will result in continuous immune stimulation.

In favor of this hypothesis is the observation that individuals with genetic deficiencies of early serum complement components have an increased susceptibility to SLE.[S196,S538] In addition to their role in autoimmune disease, certain autoantibodies may have a protective role in host defense.[C326] The genes encoding many IgM anti-IgG antibodies are transcribed directly from germline and are highly conserved in phylogeny. Mature B cells expressing these receptors are concentrated in the mantle area of lymphoid tissue. Carson and colleagues have proposed that the role of B cells with surface IgM anti-IgG may be to capture immune complexes bearing infectious agents, thus serving as antigen-presenting cells for T cells.[C115] Deletion of these germline genes may, therefore, have profound effects on T-cell responses to foreign antigens. A homozygous deletion of one such autoantibody-associated IgG light chain variable gene has been reported in SLE.[O63] This group suggested that the absence of these antigen-presenting B cells may impair the ability of the host to eliminate infectious agents and predispose to autoimmunity.

Persisting infectious organisms induce a chronic inflammatory reaction setting up conditions suitable for a breakdown of self-tolerance and the induction of autoimmunity for three reasons. First, the adjuvant-like effects of the organisms persisting in the inflammatory exudate would stimulate the lymphocytes and macrophages present to secrete cytokines, including IL-2, which can convert anergic T cells to immunocompetent lymphocytes capable of proliferation and differentiation. Some of these anergic T cells are likely to be autoreactive and capable of recognizing self—nucleoprotein peptides. Second, in the inflammatory exudate, dead cells will be phagocytosed by macrophages, and peptides from degraded nuclear structures will be complexed to self-MHC class II molecules for presentation to T cells. Under such circumstances, therefore, autoreactive T cells not only recognize self-peptides and receive one activation signal, but simultaneously receive appropriate costimulatory signals provided by other activated immune cells in the inflammatory exudate. Third, the chronic inflammatory response, at least in SLE, alters the function of T suppressor cells. Activated CD8+ T cells (CD8+ DR+ T cells) in peripheral blood down-regulate IL-2 production rather than inhibit antibody production.[L315,L316,W288] If this is also the case in lymphoid tissues, then CD8+ T cells might be unable to inhibit deleterious antiself immune responses.

Thus, conditions permitting the transformation of anergic T cells to competent T cells in the absence of functional suppressor mechanisms would allow naive autoreactive T cells to undergo clonal expansion and become memory T cells. In fact, T cells which provide specific help for anti-DNA antibody production in SLE display the memory phenotype.[S373] Since memory cells have a low threshold for activation, subsequent exposure to nucleoprotein antigens along with the appropriate costimulatory factors can precipitate the onset of autoimmune disease.

Other mechanisms besides chronic inflammation can reverse anergy. As stated above, certain retroviruses may have this capacity.[M3] Some drug-induced lupus syndromes may be triggered by the conversion of anergic autoreactive T cells to immunocompetent ones through a mechanism involving DNA methylation. Inhibitors of DNA methylation induce gene expression, and it has been reported that drugs such as procainamide and hydralazine induce self-reactivity in cloned T-cell lines by this mechanism.[C388,R196]

Generalized Autoimmunity in SLE

Studies of experimental animals that develop chronic graft-versus-host disease (GVHD) following bone marrow transplantation have provided important clues regarding mechanisms underlying generalized autoimmunity. Mice undergoing chronic GVHD develop lupus-like disease.[G192,G193] In this model, donor CD4+ T cells recognize and respond to foreign MHC class II determinants expressed by the recipient's B cells. The activated CD4+ cells provide the help needed for the recipient's B cells to become antibody-forming cells. In this manner, self-reactive B cells are activated to become antibody-forming cells in the presence of self-antigen (Table 9–8).

Table 9–8. Generalized Autoimmunity in SLE

1. IgG autoantibodies which are directed against self-antigen structures that can cross-link B-cell Ig receptors.
2. These self-antigens include cell surface molecules, such as CD4 or CD5; intracellular molecules with a repetitive structure, such as DNA; and highly charged molecules with a repetitive structure, such as the phospholipid target of the lupus anticoagulant.
3. In normals, binding of these self-antigens to B-cell receptors induces nonresponsiveness.
4. In SLE, activated CD4+ T cells bind to self-reactive B cells and provide the costimulatory signals that trigger autoantibody formation.
5. Microbial superantigens are likely agents that bring CD4+ T cells and B cells into close contact and induce T-cell activation.
6. In the absence of functional suppressor cells, autoantibodies will be produced.

Features of the molecules that induce autoantibodies in SLE are their highly charged nature, such as RNA, DNA, or histones, or their highly repetitive nature such as cell surface carbohydrates. These antigens can cross-link the Ig receptors on those B cells which recognize these molecules. Such cross-linking by antigen would result in nonresponsiveness under normal conditions, since an appropriate T-cell–derived costimulatory signal needed for activation would be absent. In GVHD, however, activated donor CD4+ cells can provide this second signal. These conditions, therefore, permit the development of expanded clones of memory B cells capable of making specific autoantibodies. As stated above, once memory cells have been generated, the opportunity for further autoantibody production is substantially increased.

Unlike GVHD, there is no evidence of increased responsiveness of CD4+ T cells to self–HLA-DR molecules in human SLE. In fact, the converse is the case. The autologous mixed lymphocyte reaction is decreased in SLE. There are other mechanisms, however, that permit CD4+ T cells to activate B cells. Certain bacteria such as staphylococci, streptococci, and mycoplasmas bear structures called superantigens that simultaneously bind to specific structures on the variable (V) region of the T-cell receptor β chain and bind to the class II MHC molecules of antigen-presenting B cells. These structures, therefore, can bring CD4+ cells into close contact with B cells. Such bridging of T cells and B cells by microbial superantigens can induce polyclonal IgM and IgG formation. Moreover, specific autoantibodies may be produced if there is also concurrent cross-linking of the B-cell receptor by autoantigen.[F253] The superantigen hypothesis, in fact, can now be tested. Since techniques have been developed to quantitate the usage of TCR V region genes, one may find selective changes in profile of Vβ gene products antigen receptors expressed by T cells.

T Cells and Perpetuation of SLE

Once SLE is induced, it must be sustained by one or more clones of autoreactive memory T cells that can respond to self-peptides derived from nuclear structures (Table 9–9). As indicated above, such autoreactive T-cell clones are normally down-regulated through suppressor mechanisms, but such mechanisms are dysfunctional in active SLE.[H436,T19] Activated CD4+ and CD8+ cells detected in the peripheral blood of patients with active SLE are likely the products of an autoimmune response to nuclear autoantigens. As stated above, both CD4+ DR+ and CD8+ DR+ support B-cell activity in SLE. A simplified

Table 9–9. Perpetuation of SLE

1. Immune responses by clonally expanded T and B memory cells are directed against self-antigens for which tolerance has been broken.
2. Because of T-cell dysfunction, CD8+ T cells (and NK cells) can provide help for B cells instead of down-regulating antibody production.
3. Other down-regulating circuits are defective (MPS* function, idiotype networks, etc.).

* MPS indicates mononuclear phagocyte system.

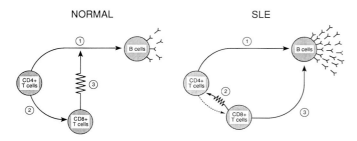

NORMAL   SLE

Fig. 9–1. Regulation of antibody production in normals and subjects with SLE. In healthy individuals, antigen-stimulated CD4 + lymphocytes provide help for antibody production (*1*) and also provide help for CD8 + cells (*2*) to down-regulate the antibody response (*3*). In subjects with active SLE, CD4 + T cells become abnormal for reasons summarized in the text and are unable to provide help for CD8 + cells. In the absence of the proper inductive influence of CD4 + cells, CD8 + cells become helper cells for B cells and, paradoxically, down-regulate CD4 + cells. This pathologic circuit sustains B-cell activity. Unbroken arrows indicate helper activity. Arrows with zigzags indicate suppressor activity.

model of the pathologic immune circuit in SLE is shown in Figure 9–1. CD8 + cells (and NK cells not shown) may support B-cell function as a consequence of inadequate help provided by CD4 + cells.

One would predict that interruption of this pathologic circuit and restoration of normal immune function would correlate with disease remission. Remissions with reconstitution of T-cell function have been observed in patients treated with oral cyclophosphamide. In these patients, clinical improvement, disappearance of anti-DNA antibodies, normalization of complement, and disappearance of the sequelae of chronic inflammation were followed by normalization of T-cell proliferation in SLE.[H429] A case was described in which clinical remission correlated with normalization of IL-2 production, serum IL-2 receptor levels, and increase in CD8 + DR + memory cells.[D53] This last finding could reflect the emergence of CD8 + cells with intact effector functions and suggests that CD4 + cells have reappeared with the ability to provide help needed for normal maturation of CD8 + T cells. Although a considerable effort remains to clarify mechanisms involved in normal and pathologic immune regulation, an effective strategy in treating patients with SLE should be to disrupt pathologic immune circuits and allow normal homeostatic mechanisms to become re-established. Novel approaches to accomplish this goal are in development.[S384]

Chapter 10

NATURAL KILLER CELLS AND SYSTEMIC LUPUS ERYTHEMATOSUS

J. DIXON GRAY AND DAVID A. HORWITZ

Natural killer (NK) cells have the ability to lyse particular tumor target cells in the absence of any activating stimulus[J103,T13,W192] and can kill certain cells infected by intracellular organisms.[B314] In addition to their cytotoxic properties, NK cells can enhance or suppress antibody production.[A12,K488,V118] The purpose of this chapter is to consider whether NK cells play a role in regulating B-cell hyperactivity characteristic of SLE. After the features of NK cells are described, their cytotoxic activities and regulatory effects in SLE will be reviewed. Finally, current views to explain why NK cells contribute to suppression of antibody production in healthy subjects, but have the opposite effect in SLE, will be discussed.

FEATURES OF NK CELLS

It is now evident that NK cells comprise a separate lymphocyte population clearly distinct from T cells and B cells. NK cells were originally identified by their ability to lyse a certain panel of tumor target cells in short-term cytotoxicity assays.[J103,T13,W192] Because activated T cells also have cytotoxic activity and NK cells and T cells share certain common surface markers (such as CD2),[G374,Z13] it was initially suspected that NK cells represented a subpopulation of T cells. However, unlike T cells, they lack specific receptors capable of recognizing peptide antigens.[L58]

The monoclonal antibodies to CD11b, CD16, and CD56 react predominantly with NK cells.[H272,K132,L60,P140] CD11b is a receptor for the complement component C3bi called the complement type 3 receptor or CR3.[R324] This molecule is also a member of the integrin or LeuCAM family of adhesion molecules and is expressed on approximately 15 to 20% of peripheral blood lymphocytes.[D366,P64] CD16 is a low-affinity receptor for IgG termed type III Fc receptor (FcRs) and is expressed on approximately 10 to 15% of peripheral blood lymphocytes.[R73] CD56 is a neural cell adhesion molecule (NCAM) and is expressed on approximately 15 to 20% of peripheral blood lymphocytes.[L62] All CD16+ lymphocytes are CD11b+ and CD56+, that is, CD16+ lymphocytes are a subpopulation of CD11b+ and CD56+ lymphocytes.[B39,L60] Both CD11b and CD56 identify virtually identical lymphocyte populations.[W177]

There is a small percentage of CD11b+ or CD56+ lymphocytes that co-express the T-cell marker, CD3.[G341,L60] However, the most highly cytolytic population is CD3−.[G341,L60] It is the CD11b+CD3− or CD56+CD3− lymphocytes that are NK cells, and these cells represent a distinct, third population of lymphocytes in addition to T and B lymphocytes.[L61]

Another important feature that distinguishes NK cells from T and B cells is their ability to respond directly to interleukin-2 and γ-interferon.[D255,T219] Resting T and B cells generally require a first signal to be able to respond to these cytokines. Surface markers that characterize NK cells are reviewed in Table 10–1.

NUMBERS OF NK CELLS IN SLE

Both the percentage and absolute numbers of NK cells are generally decreased in patients with active SLE. The percentages of CD16+ cells are decreased [A113,F26,G342,S738] and the percentages of CD3−CD11b+ lymphocytes are also decreased.[B39] In patients with inactive SLE, values for NK cells are usually normal.

CYTOTOXIC ACTIVITY IN SLE

In comparison to normal donors, SLE patients are found to have decreased NK cytotoxic activity; the decrease tends to be more pronounced in more active patients.[G313,H368,K114,O106,R289,S442] Several explanations have been proposed to explain this abnormality, and these explanations are not necessarily mutually exclusive. Decreased NK activity may be explained by decreased percentages of NK cells. As stated above, CD16+ cells are often decreased in active SLE.[A113,F26,G342,S738] This finding, however, may reflect modulation of CD16 from the cell surface by immune complexes rather than decreased numbers of this subset. Fc receptors on the cell surface are modulated following exposure to immune complexes, and this results in a loss of cytotoxic activity.[H368,P138,S442] In support of modulation of CD16, rather than a decrease in the number of NK cells, is the finding that the numbers of lymphocytes binding NK-sensitive target are comparable between normal donors and SLE patients.[K114] Cytotoxic activity, nonetheless, was decreased; a finding suggesting a defect in the actual lytic event in SLE.[K114] Therefore, NK cells in patients with active SLE may be defective in their capacity to lyse target cells.

Alternatively, "serum factors" can also account for decreased cytotoxic activity in SLE. One such serum factor is immune complexes which are elevated in patients with

Table 10–1. Characteristics of NK Cells

Definition	Natural Killer (NK) cells are a population of lymphocytes distinct from T and B cells which spontaneously lyse tumor target cells.	
Phenotype	CD3 –	Lack T-cell receptors (TCR/CD3 complex)
	CD2 +	50% of NK cells express receptors for sheep red blood cells
	CD11b+	Type 3 complement receptors
	CD16+	Type 3 Fc receptors for IgG
	CD56+	Neural cell adhesion molecule
Normal values	10–15% of blood lymphocytes	Decreased in active SLE
Cytotoxicity	Endogenous	Decreased in active SLE
	IL-2 stimulated	Normal or decreased in active SLE
	IFN stimulated	Decreased in active SLE
	Antibody-dependent cellular cytotoxicity (ADCC)	Decreased in active SLE

active disease.[S200] Immune complexes, when added to normal donor peripheral blood mononuclear cells (PBMC), suppress or decrease NK cytotoxic activity.[H368,P138,S442] However, most of the studies with SLE PBMC implied, rather than actually demonstrated, that it was immune complexes in the serum that decreased NK cytotoxic activity.

Antilymphocyte antibodies in SLE serum have also been considered to decrease NK activity. Several groups have reported that incubation with SLE patients' serum followed by treatment with complement greatly decreased NK cytotoxic activity.[G313,O106,R289] The inability of serum alone to decrease the NK activity suggested that immune complexes were not involved. Whether or not the antilymphocyte antibodies are specific for NK cells is unknown. One study demonstrated that SLE patients' serum plus complement did kill a substantial number of NK cells.[R289] In this study preincubation of the serum with T lymphocytes removed the cytotoxic activity suggesting that the antibodies were not NK cell specific. However, another study described the presence of autoantibodies specific for CD16.[S481] As stated elsewhere in this volume, there are antilymphocyte antibodies in SLE that react with a variety of cell surface structures, some of which may have the potential to react with NK cells specifically or prevent mediation of full functional activity.

As the majority of NK cells express FcRs, these cells are also capable of mediating *antibody-dependent cellular cytotoxicity* (ADCC). This activity is also decreased in SLE,[D200,F54,S120,S153] a finding that would be expected because of decreased expression of CD16 by NK cells in SLE.

SLE sera can contain IgG antilymphocyte antibodies capable of sensitizing cells for ADCC. There is one report demonstrating that active SLE patients sera can induce ADCC activity against peripheral blood lymphocytes.[K453] This finding provides a mechanism that could explain, at least in part, the observed lymphopenia in SLE.

Certain cytokines such as interleukin-2 (IL-2) or interferon can augment NK cytotoxic activity.[B534,D255,P176,S776,T218,T219] One group reported that NK cell activity can be restored to normal levels by IL-2, whereas interferon is more variable and usually less effective.[T245] Another group, however, was unable to correct the defect with either IL-2 or γIFN.[S406] Although the ability of SLE PBMC to produce IL-2 in vitro in response to mitogenic stimulation is impaired in SLE,[A126,L311] whether, indeed, there is a relationship between IL-2 production and NK cytotoxic activity is not known.

NK cells have the ability to kill almost all tumor target cells after a brief culture with IL-2.[G391,P175,R307] This is called *lymphokine-activated killer cell* (LAK) activity. Only two studies on the generation of LAK cell activity in SLE patients have been reported, and these are contradictory with one describing decreased LAK cell generation and the other finding normal levels.[F285,J79] Clearly, there is simply a paucity of data to make any conclusions regarding the status of LAK cell generation in SLE.

NK CELL SUPPRESSOR ACTIVITY

Early studies on B-cell regulation by NK cells demonstrated that NK cells could suppress antibody production. By far the majority of these studies measured the effect of NK cells on antibody production in pokeweed mitogen (PWM) cultures, although similar results were obtained when Epstein-Barr virus (EBV) transformed B cells were used as a source of antibody-producing cells.[A12,A276,B489,K488,T164] A further reduction in the amount of antibody produced resulted if the NK cells were pretreated with α-interferon or IL-2.[A12,K488] Some studies reported that suppressive activity was augmented by stimulating the NK cells with immune complexes.[T164] As NK cells express one class of receptor for the Fc portion of Ig (FcR III), it was suggested that stimulation through this receptor could induce suppressor activity. This would have been an attractive possibility with respect to SLE since elevated levels of immune complexes are associated with this disease. However, not all investigators have found that immune complexes stimulate or enhance suppressor activity.[A12,A276] Moreover, this mechanism is clearly absent or impaired in SLE since a major problem in this disease is the lack of antibody suppression.

The finding that α-interferon and IL-2 enhance suppressive activity as well as cytotoxic activity suggested that a possible mechanism of suppression was cytolysis. However, the majority of studies conclude that this is not a likely mechanism. In cultures where purified NK cells were added to purified B cells in the presence of T-cell–derived supernatants, no suppression of antibody was found.[A276] In fact, the addition of NK cells enhanced antibody production in these cultures. Suppression only became evident when T cells were included in the cultures. This finding suggested that suppression of antibody production by NK cells is mediated indirectly by T cells, and one group has demonstrated that the NK cells induce or augment T suppressor cell activity.[K113]

While the mechanism by which NK cells regulate T suppressor activity is unknown, one potentially important cytokine is γ-interferon. In a detailed study of the induction of suppressor cell activity in PWM cultures, Elmasry et al. reported that the sequential exposure of CD8+ lymphocytes to prostaglandin E_2 and γ-interferon was required to generate suppressor T cells.[E89] The finding that NK cells are a potent source of γ-interferon suggests a possible role of this cytokine in the regulation of suppressor cell activity by NK cells.

NK CELL HELPER ACTIVITY

The first report that NK cells may stimulate rather than suppress the activity of B cells was that of Vyakarnam et al.[V118] These authors demonstrated that NK cell clones, when added to a B-cell–enriched population, induced the production of antibodies. Subsequently, Kimata et al. reported that freshly isolated human peripheral blood NK cells could enhance the production of antibody by various B lymphoblastoid cell lines.[K207] Moreover, as mentioned above, in studies trying to determine the mechanism of suppression, it was found that in the absence of T cells, NK cells enhanced, rather than suppressed, antibody production.[A276,K113]

Studies of patients receiving bone marrow transplants have also suggested that NK cells can support antibody production in vivo.[B475] Recipients of T-cell–depleted allogeneic bone marrow can synthesize high titers of antibody. While they have few detectable T cells, these patients do have normal levels of NK cells that appear to be activated and can induce autologous B cells to produce antibody in vitro. That B-cell hyperactivity in SLE may similarly be supported, at least in part, by NK cells is indicated by the studies from this laboratory where full restoration of antibody production by purified B cells required the presence NK cells as well as T cells.[L317] Thus, the regulatory effects of NK cells in SLE are not related to the cytotoxic activities. Consistent with this are the studies of Procopio et al., which demonstrated that NK clones could mediate helper activity in the absence of cytotoxic activity.[P303]

Several investigators have described B-cell factors in the supernatants of NK cells or their clones.[B155,K208,P303,V118] These factors include supernatants that support B-cell growth and/or support B-cell differentiation. Of the supernatants that support B-cell differentiation, two have been characterized, at least to some degree. Becker et al. using NK clones and B cells activated by stimulation with Staphylococcus aureus Cowan (SAC) and IL-2 reported that neutralizing antibodies to tumor necrosis factor alpha

(TNFα) inhibited the enhancement of antibody production.[B155] Moreover, activated, but not resting, B cells stimulated TNFα production from the NK clones. Also using SAC- and IL-2–stimulated B cells, Jelinek and Lipsky reported that TNFα could augment antibody production.[J63] The TNFα enhancement was found to be late acting and effective only after initial B-cell activation. Kimata et al. also described a late-acting B-cell differentiation factor produced by purified NK cells. Although the factor was not identified, TNFα did not have activity in their system.[K208]

SUMMARY

The ability of NK cells to either suppress or support antibody production at first seems paradoxical. However, virtually all the studies on B-cell regulation are consistent with the following mode of action. In the absence of T cells, any regulatory effect of NK cells on B cells is one of help, whether it is support of B-cell growth and/or differentiation. In the presence of functional CD8+ T cells, however, NK cells enhance the suppressive effects of these T cells. Thus, direct helper effect of NK cells is to enhance antibody production while the suppressive effect is indirect.

In determining the lymphocyte population(s) supporting antibody production in SLE, we have found T-cell–depleted lymphocytes still produce antibody, although purified B cells did not. Moreover, the addition of SLE NK cells to B cells enhanced antibody production.[L317] These observations suggest that NK cells are involved in sustaining antibody production in SLE. In Chapter 9, studies from our laboratory demonstrating that CD8+ cells in patients with active SLE are dysfunctional and act as helper cells rather than suppressor cells are summarized.[L317] Thus, it is not surprising that NK cells enhance rather than suppress antibody production in SLE.

The effects of NK on B cells are reviewed in Table 10–2.

Table 10–2. Regulatory Properties of NK Cells on Antibody Production

Direct	NK cells can directly help B cells differentiate into antibody-forming cells. This direct effect is probably important in sustaining B-cell hyperactivity in SLE.
Indirect	NK cells can enhance the suppressor activity of CD8+ T cells resulting in down-regulation of antibody production. Because of dysregulation of CD8+ cells in SLE patients with active disease, the suppressive effect of NK cells is decreased or absent.

Chapter 11

IMMUNE COMPLEXES IN SYSTEMIC LUPUS ERYTHEMATOSUS

WOODRUFF EMLEN

Systemic lupus erythematosus (SLE) is considered the prototype of human diseases that are mediated by immune complexes (ICs).[C317] Notwithstanding the many abnormalities of the immune system that have been described in SLE, the final common pathway of many of these abnormalities is the production of autoantibodies and the tissue deposition of ICs. Once in tissues, ICs initiate inflammation through activation of the complement cascade and cellular chemotaxis, resulting in tissue damage and ultimately in disease manifestations. Clinical manifestations of SLE felt primarily to be due to tissue deposition of ICs include glomerulonephritis, arthritis, dermatitis, serositis, vasculitis, and possibly cerebritis. The formation of ICs is the normal part of the immune response, however, and occurs in all individuals as a mechanism to remove foreign antigens.[D137,J46] It is the deposition of excess ICs in target tissues, such as the kidney, skin, and joints, which leads to disease in SLE. This chapter will briefly review what is known of the normal physiology of ICs, review the evidence for the role of ICs in causing SLE disease manifestations, discuss mechanisms for the tissue deposition of excess ICs in SLE, and review the data on the clinical usefulness of measurement of ICs in SLE patients.

PHYSIOLOGY OF IMMUNE COMPLEX FORMATION AND CLEARANCE

Immune complexes form when an antibody binds noncovalently to its cognate antigen. In the normal immune response, when a organism is exposed to a foreign antigen, antibodies are produced that bind to antigen, leading to the formation of ICs. IC formation results in the clustering of multiple immunoglobulin (Ig) molecules around the antigen; by bringing the Fc portions of many Ig molecules into close proximity, the IC acquires new biologic properties, including the ability to fix complement and to interact with cellular and complement Fc receptors.[M95,M97] IC interaction with these receptors facilitates IC clearance by mediating binding to the fixed tissue macrophages of the mononuclear phagocyte system (MPS) (Fig. 11–1).[A285,L100,M95,M98,M99] Binding of ICs to erythrocyte complement receptors acts to keep circulating ICs in the intravascular space until they can be cleared by the MPS[C390,H233] (discussed below and in Chap. 12). Under normal conditions, ICs are cleared rapidly, antigen is eliminated, and the immune response abates. However, a number of factors such as excess production of ICs, or blockade of the MPS, may result in incomplete clearance of ICs, resulting in spillover of ICs into tissues other than the

MPS.[H2,K210,M95,M100] Alternatively, some antibodies may bind or cross-react with tissue antigens, resulting in *in situ* IC formation.[C415] Once in these tissues, the ability of ICs to fix complement and interact with cellular receptors can result in initiation of inflammation and tissue damage (Fig. 11–1). Thus, although the formation of an IC is part of the normal immune response and is designed to facilitate antigen removal, perturbation of this system can result in the deposition of ICs in tissues other than the MPS, leading to tissue inflammation and "immune complex disease."

A number of factors govern the physical characteristics of ICs and hence their biologic properties (Table 11–1). These include the nature of the antibody in the complex, the nature of the antigen, and the nature of the antigen-antibody interaction. These factors in turn govern the ability of ICs to fix complement, the efficiency with which they are cleared by the MPS, and the propensity they have to deposit in tissues other than the MPS. The antibody response to different antigens in different individuals may differ quantitatively and qualitatively. IC formed with IgG or IgM antibody can activate complement by the classical pathway; IgA-containing complexes can activate complement by the alternative pathway, but IgD and IgE cannot activate complement.[B419] Furthermore, the IgG1, IgG2, and IgG3 subclasses of IgG fix complement better than IgG4. The nature of the antibody response can therefore significantly affect the ability of ICs to elicit tissue inflammation. In SLE, antibodies to double-stranded DNA (dsDNA), which are felt to play an important role in the pathogenesis of lupus nephritis, show a subclass restriction to IgG1, IgG2, and IgG3 and are efficient complement activators.[R398,W304] The quantity of antibody produced to a given antigen will control the amount of IC produced, as well as affect the molar antigen to antibody ratio (see below). The strength with which an antibody binds to antigen (avidity) can affect the nature of the IC formed; in general, low-avidity antibodies are more likely to form small ICs. Finally, the net charge of the antibody (or antigen) in an IC can alter the *in vivo* properties of an IC by influencing binding of the IC to specific tissues. For example, ICs containing cationized (positively charged) antibody or antigen bind to the renal glomerulus to a much greater degree than ICs containing uncharged (neutral) antibodies.[G70,G71,G72]

The antigen contained within an IC can also markedly affect the properties of that IC. The valence of an antigen is defined as the number of antibody binding sites per

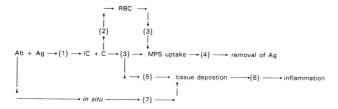

Fig. 11–1. Formation and Clearance of IC. The combination of antigen and antibody results in the formation of ICs {1}, some of which are capable of fixing complement (C). C-containing ICs are carried in the circulation bound to erythrocytes {2} and are cleared from the circulation or from the erythrocyte surface by the phagocytic cells of the MPS {3}. Under normal conditions, this results in efficient removal of antigen {4}. However, if MPS clearance of ICs is incomplete, ICs may deposit in other tissues {5}, resulting in inflammation {6}. Alternatively, antibody may directly bind or cross-react with tissue antigens, resulting in *in situ* IC formation {7}.

molecule. Small antigens with low valence form small ICs, whereas large, complex antigens can bind multiple antibodies, resulting in the formation of large ICs containing multiple antigens and antibodies. The lattice of an IC is defined as the number of antigen and antibody molecules in a given IC. ICs with a high degree of lattice (large-latticed complexes) are more efficient at fixing complement, are cleared from the circulation rapidly via binding to cellular receptors, and are potent initiators of inflammation. Small (low-lattice) ICs may persist in the circulation, but are relatively poor inducers of inflammation.[J77,M95,M97] Antigens may also alter the properties of ICs independent of their combination with antibody. Certain antigens such as DNA may be specific ligands for their own receptors, such that clearance of ICs containing these antigens may be mediated not only by FcRs, but also by antigen receptors.[E98,E102] Antigen in an IC may also preferentially bind to a specific tissue either on the basis of charge or direct tissue tropism, thereby directing the deposition of ICs containing these antigens.

Finally, the molar ratio of antigen to antibody in an IC plays a major role in determining the lattice of ICs. At molar equivalence, the chances for cross-linking antigen and antibody are maximized, resulting in the formation of large-latticed precipitates. At moderate degrees of antigen excess, soluble ICs are formed that are still relatively large latticed, and are therefore active in complement activa-

Table 11–1. Factors Influencing Characteristics of ICs

A. Antibody
  1. Quantity
  2. Class, subclass (valence, complement fixation)
  3. Avidity
  4. Charge
B. Antigen
  1. Availability
  2. Valence, size
  3. Tissue tropism/charge
C. Antigen-antibody interaction
  1. Molar ratio

Table 11–2. Biologic Properties of ICs

A. Complement activation
  1. Covalent binding to C3b
  2. Chemotaxis (C5a)
  3. Anaphylaxis (C3a, C5a)
  4. Cytotoxicity (C5–9)
B. Binding to cell receptors
  1. Phagocytic cells (CR, FcR)
  2. Lymphocytes (CR, FcR)
  3. Erythrocytes (CR)

tion and binding to cellular receptors. At extreme antigen or antibody excess, small ICs with low inflammatory potential are formed. Experimental models of serum sickness suggest that ICs formed at moderate antigen excess may be most important for eliciting tissue inflammation.

Once an IC forms, it acquires biologic properties distinct from the properties of isolated antigen or antibody that comprise the IC. These properties, which occur as a result of clustering of Fc regions of the Ig molecule within the IC, include activation of complement and stable binding (via multivalent receptor-ligand interactions) to cell receptors for Fc and complement (Table 11–2). While these characteristics serve to facilitate IC clearance, they also lead to the initiation of inflammation.[B153,C317,M270] Complement activation leads to generation of anaphylatoxins C5a and C3a and can lead to direct and indirect cell lysis by activation of the terminal complement components (C5–C9).[H494] By virtue of ICs binding to C3b and clustering of Fc, ICs bind to neutrophils and monocytes, resulting in the release of lysosomal enzymes.[S166] Interaction with the Fc receptors on platelets results in the release of vasoactive amines and activation of the clotting and kinin cascades.[B153] Interaction of ICs with basophils and mast cells can result in degranulation with the release of heparin and histamine.[B153] If ICs are present in tissues, the release of these factors, which is normally designed to facilitate IC removal and destruction, can result in inflammation and damage to the tissue itself.

The diversity of factors that determine the characteristics and biologic properties of ICs results in the potential for tremendous IC variability. This variability influences the efficiency with which ICs are cleared, the tendency of ICs to deposit in specific tissues, and the ability of ICs to be detected in IC assays employed clinically (see section below). One can speculate that this diversity of ICs may contribute in part to the diverse spectrum of disease seen in different SLE patients and in the same patient at different times in the disease course.

SLE AS AN IMMUNE COMPLEX DISEASE

This first description of IC disease in humans was made by Von Pirquet in 1911 while studying the illness that followed the injection of diphtheria antitoxin in children.[V112] He postulated that the observed illness was because of the immune response of the host in which a serum factor (antibody) reacted with the injected antigens and caused tissue damage. Nearly 50 years later, Dixon and colleagues established an experimental model

Table 11–3. Evidence that SLE is an IC Disease

A. Similarity of clinical/pathologic features to serum sickness
B. Evidence of complement activation
　　1. Anticomplementary activity of SLE sera
　　2. Hypocomplementemia during disease
　　3. Presence of C3 and factor B split products in lupus sera
C. Demonstration of IC in tissues
　　1. IgG and C3 in glomeruli and skin by IF
　　2. Elution of IgG, anti-DNA from kidneys
　　3. Similarity of lesions to experimental IC disease
D. Animal model of disease
E. Demonstration of ICs in circulation

of serum sickness and demonstrated that the symptoms of serum sickness—including glomerulonephritis, arthritis, and vasculitis—were caused by the tissue deposition of circulating ICs.[D232,D234] The similarity of the clinical manifestations of serum sickness and human SLE raised the possibility that these two conditions might be caused by a common mechanism. Over the past 30 years, a significant amount of evidence has accumulated to suggest that much of the tissue inflammation and damage seen in human SLE is mediated by the tissue deposition of ICs (Table 11–3).

In experimental serum sickness, a fall in serum complement level occurs at the time at which ICs form in circulation and inflammatory lesions develop in tissues.[D232,D234] In SLE, the first correlation between disease activity and hypocomplementemia was noted by Vaughn and colleagues in 1951.[V50] Since then multiple studies have confirmed that in many patients, increased disease activity, particularly glomerulonephritis, is associated with a fall in serum complement.[K350,L341,S782] In addition, it has long been noted that serum from SLE patients has the ability to activate complement *in vitro*, an observation that has been interpreted as indirect evidence for the presence of ICs in SLE sera. However, measurement of the level of serum complement does not always provide an accurate picture of complement activation since the serum complement level represents the steady-state balance between complement synthesis and consumption. More sensitive methods to detect complement activation are to directly measure catabolism of complement components or to measure the production of breakdown products of C3 or factor B that are generated during complement activation. A number of studies have shown hypercatabolism of C3 and C4[C209] and increased serum levels of C3a, C5a, and Bb in SLE patients.[B192,K176,N53] Further, the level of these complement breakdown products correlates with disease activity. Thus, there is ample evidence that there are factors (presumably ICs) that are present in SLE sera that are capable of activating complement, and that in general, complement activation parallels disease activity.

Convincing evidence that tissue lesions in SLE are caused by the deposition of ICs comes from the demonstration of IC components in affected tissues. Deposits of immunoglobulin and complement have been found in glomeruli and at the dermal-epidermal junction of the skin in patients with SLE.[A221,C317,D232,K341] The granular pattern of Ig and complement deposition seen along the glomerular basement membrane (GBM) is similar to that observed in experimental models of serum sickness and glomerulonephritis, and suggests the deposition of circulating ICs in these areas. Electron microscopy of the glomeruli of patients with SLE has shown electron-dense deposits in the subendothelial and/or subepithelial spaces, consistent with the appearance of tissue ICs seen in experimental models.[G97] Experiments have also been performed to elute IC components from the glomeruli of lupus patients. Early studies showed that antibodies to nuclear antigens, in particular antibodies to dsDNA and ssDNA, were concentrated in renal eluates relative to serum.[K425] This suggests that these antibodies are selectively concentrated in the kidneys and may play a direct role in the inflammatory response. More recently, staining of glomeruli with antibodies directed against the idiotypes of specific DNA antibodies has indicated that renal deposits are enriched in certain anti-DNA idiotypes, which are felt to play an important role in the pathogenesis of disease.[K41] Evidence for the presence of antibodies to other antigens including antibodies to RNA, nuclear proteins, and some retroviral proteins has also been presented,[O114,S487] but the role of ICs containing these antigens is presently unclear. Although the antigen-antibody composition of tissue-bound ICs remains uncertain in SLE, there is a large amount of experimental evidence that suggests that components of ICs and their activation products (immunoglobulin, complement) are present in affected tissues in a pattern identical to that seen in experimental models of serum sickness and glomerulonephritis.

Murine models of SLE, originally described in the 1960s, have provided additional experimental support for the concept that SLE is an IC disease. A number of inbred mouse strains (NZB/NZW, MRL-lpr/lpr, BXSB) develop an illness with striking similarities to SLE clinically, pathologically, and serologically[A225,D235,T133] (see Chap. 17). Immunofluorescence studies of the tissues of these animals have shown deposits of immunoglobulin and complement in a granular pattern identical to that seen in human SLE. Studies have documented circulating ICs in these animals which increase as disease progresses.[N22] In addition, recent experiments have suggested that inhibition of anti-DNA antibody synthesis by the administration of anti-idiotypic antibodies transiently decreases glomerulonephritis and proteinuria.[H29] The similarity between murine disease and human SLE, and the additional evidence that murine SLE is mediated by ICs further strengthens the argument that human SLE is an IC-mediated disease. Finally, numerous studies have demonstrated the presence of increased levels of IC in the circulation of patients with active SLE (see below).

FACTORS PREDISPOSING TO THE TISSUE DEPOSITION OF IMMUNE COMPLEXES IN SLE

During the course of an immune response in normal individuals, ICs are formed and rapidly cleared by the MPS, thereby resulting in efficient clearance of exogenous antigen. If, however, ICs are present chronically or recurrently in the circulation, gradual accumulation of ICs in target tissues occurs, eventually triggering an inflammatory response. A number of factors influence the level of

Table 11–4. Factors Favoring Tissue Localization of ICs in SLE

A. Excess IC formation
   1. Increased Ab synthesis
   2. Increased Ag availability
B. Decreased IC clearance/catabolism
   1. Decreased MPS clearance (FcR and CR)
   2. Decreased IC solubilization (complement)
   3. Decreased erythrocyte CR1
C. Tissue tropism of ICs
D. Tissue localization of Ag and Ab (*in situ* IC formation)
   1. Tissue tropism
   2. Direct reactivity or cross-reactivity of Ab

ICs in the circulation and their propensity to localize in tissues outside the MPS (Table 11–4). As is evident from Figure 11–1, either excess production of ICs or decreased removal of ICs could result in increased levels of circulating ICs. In addition, the tendency for an IC to bind to a specific tissue other than the MPS may favor tissue IC deposition. A number of studies have demonstrated that the charge of an IC can directly influence renal IC deposition.[G19,G70,G71,G72] Moreover, a specific antigen or antibody may also bind directly to tissues (tissue tropism), resulting in *in situ* formation of ICs. Finally, local hemodynamic factors such as increased blood flow and increased vascular permeability secondary to inflammatory mediators may favor tissue localization of ICs. There is evidence to suggest that all of these factors may be operative in SLE and contribute to formation of tissue ICs. In any given patient, however, only one or a few of these factors may contribute to disease. Thus, even though the final common pathway of tissue damage in SLE is tissue deposition of ICs, the mechanisms by which tissue IC formation occurs in highly variable. This may be yet another factor that contributes to the wide variability in the spectrum of clinical disease observed in SLE.

EXCESS IMMUNE COMPLEX FORMATION

The hallmark of SLE is B-cell hyperactivity, the production of multiple antibodies, and hypergammaglobulinemia. While it has been suggested that the B-cell activation in SLE is the result of polyclonal B-cell activation, there is increasing evidence to suggest that antibodies produced in SLE are directed to a relatively limited number of self antigens.[B63,S374,T43] B-cell hyperactivity results in the continuous production of high levels of antibodies to these antigens. Antibodies to many autoantigens have recently been described in normal individuals, and have been termed "natural autoantibodies."[C7,P212] However, in SLE these natural autoantibodies appear to be modified by the processes of somatic mutation and T-cell help, resulting in the production of high-avidity IgG autoantibodies with an increased capacity for initiating tissue inflammation. By virtue of producing these antibodies, the immune system is poised to produce ICs with high phlogistic potential whenever antigen is released into the circulation.

A large number of antigens have been implicated in the formation of pathogenic ICs in SLE. These include nuclear antigens such as DNA, histones, and a variety of nuclear enzymes, cell surface antigens, and antigens to retroviral proteins.[O114,O115,T133] Despite a voluminous literature on the subject, it is not yet clear which antigen-antibody systems are dominant in eliciting tissue damage in SLE. It is likely that multiple antigen-antibody systems are involved, and that the predominant ICs involved in tissue injury may vary from individual to individual and at different times within the same individual. A characteristic common to many of the antigens is that they are autoantigens, and are therefore potentially present in large amounts. An exogenous antigen is removed by the formation of ICs, thereby resulting in abrogation of the immune response. However, autoantigens can never be completely eradicated, leading to ongoing immunologic stimulation and the potential for chronic formation of ICs. The most frequently implicated and most well-studied antigen-antibody system in SLE is DNA–anti-DNA. Antibodies to dsDNA are seen almost exclusively in SLE, and increased levels of these antibodies correlate with clinical disease activity in most studies.[A48,B535,L341,S782] Detailed analysis of the levels of DNA antibodies present in the circulation over time was conducted by Swaak et al., who demonstrated that just prior to a clinical flare, the level of DNA antibodies decreased.[S782] They proposed that the decrease in antibody level was the result of release of antigen, binding of free antibody to the antigen, and the formation of ICs.

The nature and behavior of DNA in the circulation has been studied over the past 15 years. Studies in experimental animals have shown that DNA is rapidly and efficiently cleared from the circulation.[E100,F173] In SLE patients, however, low levels of circulating DNA have been demonstrated,[D79,F175,M248,R48,S655a] and some studies suggest that levels of DNA increase with increased disease activity.[F174,M582] Analysis of the circulating DNA has indicated that it is of host origin, and may be present as histone-DNA complexes resembling nucleosomes.[L258,R48,R420,S655a] Protein binding of DNA may protect DNA from circulating endonucleases and prevent rapid clearance. Indeed, in SLE patients, binding of IgG antibodies to DNA protects small fragments of DNA from nuclease digestion, resulting in the persistence of small DNA–anti-DNA ICs in the circulation.[E97,E98] Release of DNA into the circulation has been associated with cytolysis occurring after hemodialysis,[S656] surgical trauma,[D79] and after LPS injection or UV exposure in experimental animals.[F173,F174,I66] It is of interest that a number of these factors have also been implicated in triggering clinical flares of disease activity. Thus, in the case of the DNA–anti-DNA IC system, increased levels of antibody are present in the circulation, and antigen may be periodically released into the circulation resulting in the formation of ICs and tissue damage. Analogous mechanisms may be operating with other antigen-antibody systems, although the nature of these systems remains unclear at the present time.

DECREASED IC CLEARANCE/CATABOLISM

The steady-state level of circulating ICs is a function of the rate of IC production and the efficiency of IC removal. Removal of circulating ICs is performed primarily by the

MPS of the liver and spleen, mediated by binding of ICs to tissue-fixed Fc receptors (FcRs) and complement receptors (CRs). In addition, complement can inhibit tissue deposition of ICs and facilitate IC clearance by mediating solubilization of ICs and binding of ICs to CRs on erythrocytes. Erythrocyte-bound ICs are transported to fixed tissue macrophages,[A199,C390,D73,I59,K212,N63,S136,W111] where they are bound by FcRs and CRs, phagocytosed, and degraded.[K176,L100,M95] Abnormalities, either genetic or acquired, have been described for almost all of these IC clearance pathways in SLE.

These abnormalities include reduced numbers of CR1 receptors on erythrocytes (the reduction is largely acquired but may also be inherited), hypocomplementemia (acquired or inherited), which impairs both solubilization and opsonization of ICs,[C464,N2,N153,S139] saturation of CR1 and FcRs by pre-existing ICs,[I12,M97,M100] and abnormal function of several of the isoforms of FcR on various cells, resulting in impaired phagocytosis of ICs.[S53] Multiple studies have shown that SLE patients have reduced clearance of Ig-coated particles and of soluble immune complexes.[F213,F214,G4,K219,L344,L345,S51,S54,S136] The resultant increase in IC levels in the circulation probably enhances their deposition in glomeruli and other tissues. The FcR- and CR-mediated binding and degradation of ICs are discussed in detail in Chapter 12.

In addition to the role of CRs in IC phagocytosis, several additional functions of complement in the clearance of circulating ICs have received increasing interest in the past 10 years. Incorporation of complement into ICs can prevent the formation of immune precipitates, and solubilize immune precipitates that have already formed.[C464,N2] Since very large, precipitable ICs appear to have the greatest phlogistic potential, solubilization of ICs or prevention of the formation of large lattice complexes may act to decrease the inflammatory potential of these complexes. This mechanism may also act in situ to inhibit the formation of large lattice immune aggregates in tissues. The relevance of this action of complement to SLE becomes evident when one considers that SLE is associated with complement deficiencies—both acquired and genetic (see Chap. 13). Serum from SLE patients has a decreased ability to inhibit immune precipitation because of acquired hypocomplementemia,[N153,S139] and serum from patients with hereditary deficiencies of the early complement components are unable to inhibit immune precipitation.[S139] Thus, complement deficiency may contribute to the initiation or exacerbation of disease in SLE patients by compromising the ability of the host to inhibit the formation of large, phlogistic immune aggregates, as well as by decreasing clearance of circulating ICs via the MPS complement receptors.

The IC binding capacity of erythrocyte CR1 is also compromised in SLE. IC binding capacity is proportional to the CR1 number on the erythrocyte, which in turn is controlled by a genetic polymorphism.[H393,W268] While there is no evidence that a genetically low CR1 number contributes to the pathogenesis of SLE,[M525,T93] the erythrocytes of SLE patients exhibit decreased CR1 number, primarily on an acquired basis. The decrease in erythrocyte CR1 number parallels disease activity,[R326,W51] and transfusion of erythrocytes bearing high CR1 number into SLE patients with active disease resulted in a rapid loss of CR1 from the transfused red cells.[W48] The mechanism of CR1 loss in SLE is not known, but the decreased CR1 number results in decreased IC-carrying capacity,[M54] and one would therefore predict decreased buffering capacity and decreased efficiency of MPS IC clearance. Evidence for a role of erythrocyte CR1 in the clearance of circulating ICs in humans comes from several studies. Clearance of soluble heat-aggregated IgG in humans is associated with rapid initial binding of these model ICs to red cells followed by MPS clearance.[D73,H70,L344,S136] In SLE patients with low erythrocyte CR1 number, rather than binding to red cells, ICs appear to distribute to the extravascular space immediately after infusion.[H70,S137] These observations support the concept that binding of ICs to erythrocytes functions to maintain ICs in the intravascular space to prevent their binding to vessel walls or extravasation into the extravascular space. In addition, other studies have demonstrated that the administration of erythrocytes bearing high CR1 numbers to patients with high levels of circulating ICs results in decreased IC levels.[I13] These data support in vitro studies that suggest that binding of ICs to erythrocyte CR1 facilitates clearance of ICs by the MPS.[E99]

Thus, complement plays a role in the clearance and processing of ICs in at least three ways: facilitation of FcR-mediated phagocytosis of ICs, inhibition of immune precipitation, and mediation of binding of ICs to erythrocyte CR1. In SLE, hereditary complement deficiencies, acquired hypocomplementemia, and decreased erythrocyte CR1 number may all contribute to compromise of IC clearance. As with other abnormalities in SLE, the contribution of each of these factors to clinical disease may vary from patient to patient and from time to time within the same patient.

IN SITU IMMUNE COMPLEX FORMATION

Experimental models of glomerulonephritis, in which circulating ICs deposit in tissues, cannot account for all of the types of glomerulonephritis seen in SLE. In particular, membranous glomerulonephritis, characterized by large numbers of subepithelial deposits, is not associated with increased levels of circulating ICs.[O85] Furthermore, intravenous administration of preformed ICs to experimental animals results primarily in mesangial and subendothelial localization of ICs rather than subepithelial localization of ICs.[C415,M95,M97,M100] Work by Couser and others in the 1970s, using the isolated perfused kidney in the rat, demonstrated that sequential perfusion of antigen and antibody into the kidney could result in the formation of subepithelial ICs.[C413,C414,C417] The formation of ICs directly in the tissues has been termed in situ IC formation, and likely plays a role in some forms of lupus nephritis, and may also contribute to other manifestations of SLE.

At least two different mechanisms have been demonstrated that can lead to the formation of ICs in situ in SLE: 1) sequential binding of antigen and antibody to tissue, occurring as a result of tissue binding (tissue tropism) of one of the ligands; and 2) direct reactivity or cross-reactivity of antibody to tissue antigens (Table 11–4). Tissue tropism refers to the preferential binding of circulating antigen (or antibody) to a specific tissue, followed by a binding of the appropriate antibody (or antigen) to the fixed ligand. If a tissue binds one component of an IC, it can serve to concentrate ligand, thereby facilitating binding of the other IC component and enhancing IC formation. Binding of antigen or antibody to tissues may be on the basis of charge or through specific ligand binding interactions. In the isolated perfused rat kidney, concanavalin A (Con A) binds to the GBM when perfused into the kidney.[O36] Subsequent perfusion with antibodies to Con A resulted in antibody binding to the GBM-bound Con A and elicited glomerulonephritis. Other studies have shown that cationized (positively charged) antigen or antibody infused into the kidneys binds to the negatively charged GBM, and if this is followed by perfusion of the appropriate ligand, in situ subepithelial IC formation occurs.[A59,B122,B414] Thus, positively charged antigens or antibodies may bind to the negatively charged GBM, and thereby provide a target for the appropriate circulating ligand, resulting in the in situ formation of ICs. The presence of positively charged ligands within a circulating IC can also facilitate deposition of ICs in the skin[J130] or the GBM.[G70,G71]

In animal models of SLE, several studies have demonstrated that DNA can bind directly to the GBM,[C89,H418,I67] and there is some evidence that circulating DNA antibodies can bind to the tissue-fixed DNA.[D33,I67] Since DNA is negatively charged, it is unlikely that charge-charge interactions are the basis for the binding of the DNA to the GBM. Whether DNA binds to the GBM via some other interaction or potentially binds to tissue-fixed DNA antibodies remains unclear. However, studies have demonstrated that DNA antibodies eluted from the kidneys of mice with SLE demonstrate an increased isoelectric point (positive charge) relative to DNA antibodies obtained from the sera of the same mice.[H21] These studies suggest that the positive charge of certain DNA antibody subsets may favor localization of these antibodies in the kidneys and contribute to their pathogenicity. Whether these antibodies are binding directly to the GBM (see below) or binding to tissue-fixed DNA is not clear.

In addition to the sequential binding of antigen and antibody to tissues as a result of tissue tropism, in situ IC formation can occur by direct binding of autoantibodies to intrinsic tissue antigens. This is a well-recognized mechanism for tissue-specific autoimmune diseases such as myasthenia gravis, pemphigus, and autoimmune thyroiditis. Furthermore, this mechanism of tissue damage has long been recognized as accounting for some of the disease manifestations of lupus such as thrombocytopenia, lymphopenia, and hemolytic anemia in which binding of antibodies to cell surface antigens results in accelerated cell clearance. However, data suggest that similar mechanisms may play a role in other organ lesions, such as glomerulonephritis, which were previously thought to occur only as a result of deposition of circulating ICs. The experimental model for this form of glomerulonephritis is Heymann nephritis, in which antibodies to proximal tubular epithelial cell antigen are perfused into the kidney with

the resultant formation of subepithelial IC deposits and glomerulonephritis.[C413] Studies searching for antibodies to similar intrinsic renal antigens in human glomerulonephritis and in SLE have been unsuccessful. However, data on the antigenic cross-reactivity of some antibodies in lupus patients have raised the possibility that circulating antibodies, in particular anti-DNA, may bind directly to the kidney as a result of antibody cross-reactivity with intrinsic renal antigens.[E49] Monoclonal antibodies to DNA have been shown to be broadly cross-reactive with a variety of non-DNA antigens including other nucleotides, some proteins, and negatively charged molecules such as heparan sulfate.[A230,C113,F2,L10] This latter observation led to experiments suggesting that DNA antibodies bound directly to the heparan sulfate present in the renal GBM.[F2,N29] Other investigators have also argued that cross-reactive DNA antibodies may be more pathogenic in eliciting renal disease, presumably as a result of their ability to bind directly to renal antigens.[E49,P30] Recently, Raz and colleagues perfused monoclonal DNA antibodies or sera from SLE patients containing anti-DNA into rat kidneys and demonstrated renal deposition of immunoglobulin and complement and induction of proteinuria.[R80] Although this mechanism for IC formation remains intriguing, other studies have argued that pathogenic DNA antibodies are poorly cross-reactive, and that the behavior of DNA antibodies demonstrated using monoclonal antibodies is not relevant to the DNA antibodies which are pathogenic in SLE.[B496,E24,E101] Direct binding of antibodies to tissue antigens has been more convincingly demonstrated with other antigen-antibody systems in lupus. For example, antibodies to SSA (Ro), which are associated clinically with cutaneous lupus and neonatal heart block, have been shown to bind directly to skin[L135] and to fetal cardiac conduction system tissue,[B602] directly accounting for the clinical manifestations observed.

In summary, formation of ICs in situ can occur by several mechanisms, and may play an important role in certain aspects of SLE, in particular thrombocytopenia, lymphopenia, hemolytic anemia, and possibly membranous glomerulonephritis. Since SLE is a disease characterized by the production of antibodies to autoantigens, in situ IC formation can account for the presence of active disease in the absence of circulating ICs. This is an important factor when considering the value of measuring levels of circulating ICs to predict disease flares. The pattern of disease activity observed clinically as well as the level of measurable circulating ICs will depend upon the degree to which disease is initiated by tissue deposition of circulating ICs compared with in situ formation of ICs.

CLINICAL MEASUREMENT OF CIRCULATING IMMUNE COMPLEXES IN SLE

With increasing evidence supporting the concept that SLE was an IC disease, the 1970s and early 1980s saw an explosion of techniques designed to measure circulating ICs in SLE. It was hoped that the measurement of circulating ICs would allow clinicians to more closely follow disease activity and predict disease outcome. Currently, greater than 40 assays for circulating ICs have been developed and have been applied to SLE as well as to many other potential IC diseases. Ideally, if the antigen within an IC is known, it should be possible to isolate the ICs and directly measure the amount of antigen and specific antibody present. Such methodology has been applied to detect circulating ICs in hepatitis B infection, where hepatitis B surface antigen-containing ICs can be demonstrated.[G428,122] However, in SLE, the nature of the antigen in the circulating IC is not known, with the possible exception of DNA–anti-DNA. Therefore, the detection of ICs must rely on the antigen-nonspecific properties of the IC. When an immunoglobulin molecule binds to and aggregates around an antigen, the physical and biologic properties of the IC change. It is these changes, which occur when immunoglobulin molecules aggregate, that allow one to distinguish an IC from monomeric immunoglobulin. Some of the most frequently used antigen-nonspecific methods to detect circulating ICs are listed in Table 11–5.

Each of these different methods relies on a slightly different property of the IC for detection.[118,119,M270,T127,T132] Considering the extremely large degree of variability in IC structure and characteristics, it should not be surprising that IC assays are not always in agreement with each other on the presence or absence of ICs in any given sample. In addition to the large amount of IC variability that is possible *in vivo*, problems with standardization of IC assays have arisen since no universally applicable "standard" IC is available. Arbitrarily, heat-aggregated IgG has been used as a standard, but different preparations of aggregated IgG can vary significantly. This has created additional problems in comparing one assay to another and comparing the same assay between different laboratories. Finally, since the nonantigen-specific IC assays depend upon the aggregation of immunoglobulins, factors that lead to nonspecific aggregation of immunoglobulin will cause false-positive results. Factors known to increase immunoglobulin aggregation include freezing/thawing of samples and high concentrations of immunoglobulin, as may be seen in SLE. Despite these limitations, a large amount of data on the clinical applicability of these assays in SLE have been amassed. This section will briefly discuss the major methods used to measure ICs in biologic fluids, and review the usefulness of these assays in SLE.

Table 11–5. Methods for Detecting Immune Complexes

A. Physical properties
  1. Size
  2. Solubility
    a. PEG
    b. Cold
B. Biologic properties
  1. Properties due to aggregation of Fc
    a. Complement fixation
    b. C1q binding
    c. RF binding
    d. Platelet aggregation
  2. Properties due to incorporation of C3 into the IC
    a. Raji cell binding
  b. Conglutinin binding
    c. Binding to anti-C3 antibodies

One of the first demonstrations of ICs in SLE was based on the precipitability of some ICs in the cold to form cryoprecipitates.[C255] A number of studies have since confirmed that a small percentage of patients with SLE have cryoglobulinemia.[A48,M318,W287] However, cryoprecipitation is a property of only a small fraction of ICs, and is therefore an insensitive assay for the detection of circulating ICs. Also, this assay is not specific, since other proteins can also precipitate in the cold. The differential solubility of aggregated compared to monomeric immunoglobulin in 3.5 to 4.0% polyethylene glycol (PEG) has also been used to measure ICs.[118,H270,T127] Increased amounts of PEG-precipitated Ig have been reported to be positive in up to 60 to 70% of SLE patients.[D208] However, some other serum proteins are also precipitated with PEG, and high concentrations of serum IgG resulting in aggregation can also give false-positive results.

When ICs form, the biologic properties of the immunoglobulin molecule are altered by virtue of bringing the Fc portions of multiple immunoglobulin molecules into close proximity. Aggregation of Fc facilitates binding of immunoglobulin to C1q, and activates the complement cascade both by the classical and potentially by the alternative pathway. Complement fixation tests measure consumption (activation) of a standard amount of complement that is added to the patient's serum. However, serum complement activity must be first inactivated by heating, a process that itself can aggregate IgG, potentially resulting in a false-positive test. Alternatively, binding of ICs to purified C1q can be directly measured. In the C1q binding assay (C1q-BA) labeled C1q is added to serum, followed by the precipitation of IC-bound C1q with PEG.[N154,X1] Binding of C1q to other proteins as well as to DNA will also yield positive results. In the solid-phase C1q assay (C1q-SP), C1q is adsorbed to the wall of tubes. ICs in sera bind to the adsorbed C1q, nonbound proteins are removed by washing, and ICs are detected by probing with labeled anti-immunoglobulin.[G4,H217] The solid-phase C1q assay has been reported to be positive in 40 to 60% of SLE patients, whereas the C1q binding assay has shown a considerably higher frequency of positive results.

In addition to having the potential to bind C1q and activate complement *in vitro*, ICs may also activate complement *in vivo*, resulting in the covalent binding of C3b and/or C3b breakdown products to the ICs. A number of assays utilize this property of ICs to allow their detection. Raji cells are lymphoblastoid B cells derived from patients with Burkitt's lymphoma, which have a high number of receptors for the C3b cleavage product C3d (CR2). Consequently, these cells will bind ICs in the biologic fluids that have incorporated C3d. Once bound, the bound complexes can be detected by probing with labeled antibodies to immunoglobulins. This test is easy to perform and has yielded evidence of increased levels of circulating ICs in a high percentage of SLE patients.[T136] However, enthusiasm for the assay has decreased since the demonstration that antilymphocyte antibodies, and some antinuclear antibodies may interact directly with Raji cells resulting in false-positive tests.[A199,H426] Conglutinin is a bovine protein that has a strong affinity for C3bi, a cleavage product of C3b. ICs can be detected by binding to conglutinin, followed by probing with labeled antibodies to Ig.[E66] Similar assays have been established employing antibodies to specific C3 components as a method to capture complement-containing ICs.[S487,X1]

Aggregation of immunoglobulins also increases the avidity of IgG binding to rheumatoid factor, thus providing the basis for RF binding assays.[G4,M270] These assays vary significantly depending upon the source of RF used for the assay and appear to be relatively insensitive for detecting ICs in SLE sera. The ability of aggregated IgG to bind to platelet Fc receptors and trigger platelet aggregation has also been used as a measurement of circulating IC activity.[P110] However, antiplatelet antibodies, which may be found in SLE, can also result in platelet aggregation and give a false-positive test.

Direct comparison of these different assays has been undertaken in a number of studies, the most complete of which was performed by the WHO in 1978.[L37] This study compared 18 IC assays performed in a number of laboratories on standardized samples. With the exception of the Raji assay, bioassays that required viable intact cells or platelets were less reproducible than assays using more stable reagents. There was a significant amount of variability in the sensitivity of the different assays. In a subsequent study by McDougal et al. 5 IC assays were compared.[M268] All assays were shown to detect large ICs better than small ICs. Not surprisingly, this was most marked in assays that required complement activation. In direct comparisons, a large range of correlations between assays was found, with assay methods based on similar principles correlating more closely than those based on different principles.[L37,M268,M270,T127]

From the above discussion, it should be evident that the application of various IC assays to patients with SLE will give variable results depending upon the status of the patient and the type of IC assay used. Numerous studies have shown that IC levels are increased in 20 to 100% of patients with SLE. In general, the Raji cell assay is the most sensitive, and the rheumatoid factor binding assay the least sensitive. Studies examining the correlation between clinical disease activity and levels of circulating ICs have yielded conflicting results. Early studies suggested that there was a good correlation between active disease and elevated levels of circulating ICs.[A20,B91,C12,L341] However, subsequent studies, although demonstrating increased levels of circulating ICs in SLE patients, failed to show a correlation between disease activity and IC levels.[C60,D92,]

[H517,I20] Lloyd and Schur studied 27 patients serially, and although they showed a correlation between circulating IC levels as measured by C1q binding assay and renal disease, they concluded that the measurement of serum C4 and CH50 were more predictive of disease flares than measurement of IC levels.[L341] The picture is further clouded by the demonstration that some SLE patients have antibodies to C1q present in their sera, and that these antibodies can alter the results of C1q binding assays.[U41] A recent study has argued that the level of antibodies to C1q correlates with renal disease,[S419] raising the question of whether previous correlations between renal disease and circulating ICs as measured by the C1q binding assay may have been caused by the presence of these antibodies rather than caused by ICs.

Thus, there is considerable disagreement as to whether circulating IC levels correlate with or are predictive of disease activity. Several issues should be raised when considering this question. First, the definition of disease activity in SLE patients was fraught with difficulty in the past, making comparisons of different studies difficult. Second, these studies have used different IC assays, and since different assays detect different subpopulations of ICs, it is to be expected that the studies would have varied degrees of correlation between IC levels and disease activity. Finally, IC-mediated organ damage in SLE is mediated by tissue ICs. One cannot assume that the level and type of ICs present in the circulation is representative of the pathogenic ICs that deposit in tissues. As is evident from previous discussions in this chapter, ICs may form in tissues not only by the deposition of circulating ICs, but also *in situ*. ICs formed in this way would be treated undetected by assays to measure circulating ICs.

In summary, increased levels of circulating ICs have been well documented in SLE using a variety of different techniques for measuring ICs. These data support the concept that many of the manifestations of SLE are mediated by ICs. However, no single assay gives an adequate picture of disease, since different IC assays detect different subpopulations of ICs. Although a rough correlation exists between the level of circulating ICs and SLE disease activity, the correlation is not strong enough to justify basing clinical or therapeutic decisions on the results of these assays. The measurement of IC levels in SLE will continue to be of only limited value until we have a better understanding of the specific antigen-antibody systems involved in eliciting disease, and can specifically measure those pathogenic complexes.

Chapter 12

ABNORMALITIES IN IMMUNE COMPLEX CLEARANCE AND Fc RECEPTOR FUNCTION*

JANE E. SALMON

Systemic lupus erythematosus (SLE), the prototype human disease mediated by immune complexes, is characterized by circulating antigen-antibody complexes which may be removed by the mononuclear phagocyte system or deposited in tissues. The fate of circulating immune complexes depends upon the lattice of the immune complexes (number of antigens and antibody molecules in a given complex), the nature of the antigen and antibodies composing the immune complexes (see Chap. 11), and the status of the mononuclear phagocyte system. The efficiency of mononuclear phagocyte system immune complex clearance depends upon the function of the Fcγ receptors, receptors recognizing the Fc region of immunoglobulin, and the complement receptors. In SLE inadequate clearance results in tissue immune complex deposition, detected by immunofluorescence and electron microscopy, which initiates release of inflammatory mediators and influx of inflammatory cells. If sustained, this leads to tissue damage with resultant clinically apparent disease, such as glomerulonephritis. Through *in vivo* and *in vitro* studies with SLE patients, it is clear that there is both Fcγ receptor (FcγR)-dependent and complement-dependent mononuclear phagocyte dysfunction in SLE, which have inherited and acquired components. The purpose of this chapter is to review the role of the mononuclear phagocyte system in immune complex clearance, describe the abnormalities in the mononuclear phagocyte function in SLE, and discuss mononuclear phagocyte system Fcγ receptor dysfunction as a mechanism for abnormal immune complex clearance in SLE.

THE ROLE OF THE MONONUCLEAR PHAGOCYTE SYSTEM IN THE CLEARANCE OF IMMUNE COMPLEXES

Historical Perspective

Early studies of blood clearance of bacteria in mice, rabbits, and guinea pigs demonstrated that the mononuclear phagocyte system (previously known as the reticuloendothelial system) performed this function for opsonized particles. Infused bacteria were phagocytized by hepatic and splenic phagocytes.[B202] The rate of clearance of bacteria from the blood and the site of clearance de-

pended upon the level of antibodies to the bacteria in the serum of the animal. Rapidly cleared, well-opsonized bacteria were principally phagocytosed in the liver, while the more slowly cleared, less efficiently internalized bacteria (presumably less opsonized) were removed by splenic phagocytes. These observations are remarkable for their similarity to the models of immune complex clearance in animals and humans that are described below.

The role of the mononuclear phagocyte system in the clearance of soluble immune complexes infused into the circulation has been defined in several experimental animal models. In mice and rabbits, a major portion of infused immune complexes made with rabbit antibodies is taken up by the liver, indicating that the mononuclear phagocyte system serves an important role as a site for complex removal.[A285,M99] This system may be saturated with increasing amounts of infused immune complexes, resulting in glomerular deposition of immune complexes.[H2] These early studies suggested that modulation of mononuclear phagocyte system function regulates the localization of immune complexes.

Several lines of evidence support this model and demonstrate that defective mononuclear phagocyte system clearance of immune complexes may be important in the development of immune complex diseases, especially glomerulonephritis. Increased glomerular deposition of immune complexes is found when rates of clearance of infused immune complexes are decreased by blockade of the mononuclear phagocyte system with colloidal carbon,[F160] by cortisone treatment,[H1] and by reduction and alkylation of antibodies.[H3,H4] In mouse strains with intrinsically lower clearance rates, there is a high degree of immune complex glomerular deposition.[F161] In contrast, decreased deposition of immune complexes in the kidney is found when mononuclear phagocyte system clearance is enhanced by pretreatment with C. parvum[B88] or zymosan.[R11]

Animal models of endogenous immune complex deposition support the relationship between depressed mononuclear phagocyte system clearance and the genesis of glomerulonephritis. In chronic serum sickness there is decreased clearance of aggregated albumin[W256] and aggregated human IgG.[W79] Decreased clearance of heat-aggregated IgG in murine nephritis (associated with lymphocytic choriomeningitis virus infection)[H369] and

*I thank Dr. Robert P. Kimberly and Dr. Jeffrey C. Edberg for thoughtful discussions and for their review of this manuscript.

of polyvinyl pyrrolidine in NZB/W mice[M570] has been observed, although some studies of endogenous immune complex–mediated disease have not found mononuclear phagocyte system dysfunction. Studies of Heyman nephritis[O95] and NZB/W nephritis[F89] have concluded that mononuclear phagocyte system function is either normal or supranormal. These results, however, are not in conflict; rather they highlight the importance of the mononuclear phagocyte system probe, the site of clearance, and the timing of the study in relationship to the genesis of disease (see below). In addition, properties of clearance may vary with endogenous versus exogenous administration of immune complexes and with acute versus chronic disease models. Sequential studies during the development of rodent malaria have clearly demonstrated the importance of the test particle and the timing of the test clearance relative to the disease state in determining the experimental result.[P38] In this model, decreased mononuclear phagocyte system clearance function is seen only when the animal is at risk for immune complex–mediated complications of malaria.

The principle derived from these animal models of immune complex disease, whether from infused immune complexes or endogenous disease, is that immune complex deposition is influenced by mononuclear phagocyte system clearance efficiency. Specifically, impairment of mononuclear phagocyte system clearance function is associated with tissue deposition of immune complexes and glomerulonephritis.

MECHANISMS OF IMMUNE COMPLEX CLEARANCE

Antigen and antibodies in the circulation may rapidly form immune complexes, but the immunochemical properties of these circulating immune complexes determine their ultimate fate. Specifically, their potential to interact with FcγRs, to fix complement, and to react with complement receptors influences their rate of clearance. An immune complex without complement will be cleared primarily by FcγRs on fixed tissue macrophages. An immune complex opsonized with sufficient complement may bind to the receptor for C3b on circulating erythrocytes and subsequently be removed by FcγRs and complement receptors. Thus, two classes of receptors, the FcγRs on phagocytes and the complement receptors on both erythrocytes and phagocytes, participate in the clearance of immune complexes (Fig. 12–1).

Complement Mechanisms: Immune Adherence and Erythrocyte CR1 System

Complement component 3 and the receptor for C3b on erythrocytes are important in processing and transporting large immune complexes.[H231] Incorporation of complement components, in particular C3b, modifies the solubility of large immune complexes[S135,S139] and mediates the binding of immune complexes to human and other primate erythrocytes. Though the liver and the spleen are the major sites of immune complex uptake, erythrocytes in primates[C390,H231] (and platelets in rodents)[M113,T87] are important in clearing/processing immune complexes from the circulation. It has long been known that large complement-opsonized immune complexes bind to human erythrocytes.[N62,N63,P92] This reaction, termed immune adherence, has recently been shown to participate in the handling of nascent circulating immune complexes in primates.[E20] Human erythrocytes express complement receptor type 1 (CR1), which permits binding of complement-fixing immune complexes.[P92] CR1 on erythrocytes can be conceptualized as having three main functions, which are not mutually exclusive: buffering, transporting, and processing (Fig. 12–1). The role as immune complex buffer has been suggested because erythrocyte-bound immune complexes are unavailable for tissue deposition, whereas nonbound complexes can deposit in the tissues. The bound immune complexes are transported to the liver or spleen where fixed tissue phagocyte FcγRs and complement receptors strip the immune complexes from the erythrocytes, which then return to the circulation to continue this process, thus performing transporting function. Finally, CR1 promotes degradation of captured C3b on immune complexes, thereby modifying their subsequent handling.

The human CR1, the complement receptor for C3b/C4b and to a lesser degree iC3b, is a single-chain intrinsic membrane glycoprotein expressed on several different cells, including erythrocytes, granulocytes, monocytes and macrophages (see Chap. 13). There are four codomi-

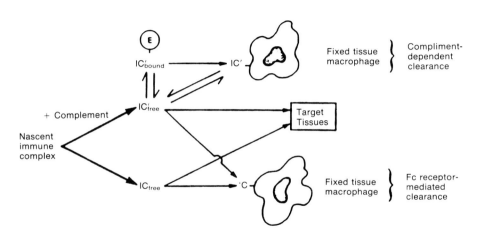

Fig. 12–1. Framework for immune complex handling. Nascent immune complexes (IC) that fix complement efficiently are rapidly bound by erythrocytes (E). IC containing complement may cycle between E-bound and unbound; they are usually rapidly taken up in the liver. Unbound complexes may also deposit in the tissues. With impaired complement-dependent uptake, they may also be taken up by Fc receptor–dependent mechanisms. IC that do not bind complement are either taken up by Fc receptor–dependent mechanisms or deposited in tissues.[K210] From Kimberly, R.P.: Immune complexes in rheumatic diseases. Rheum. Dis. Clinics of North America, *13*:583, 1987.

nantly expressed alleles of CR1 with molecular weights of 220,000, 250,000, 190,000 and 280,000 daltons.[D373,D376,D377,F36,F38,H379,R324,W339] This structural polymorphism reflects differences in the number of long homologous repeat units comprising the receptors.[K287] Inherited and acquired differences in numeric expression of CR1 on erythrocytes have also been described and associated with SLE.[W53,W264,W265,W267,W268] Two alleles with codominant expression determine erythrocyte CR1 number in healthy individuals.[W267,M525] Though the CR1 number expressed on erythrocytes is low compared to that on leukocytes, because there are far more erythrocytes than leukocytes in the circulation, approximately 90% of total circulating CR1 is on erythrocytes.[H233,S138,S413]

The binding of immune complexes to CR1 occurs rapidly *in vivo* and represents multivalent binding between multiple C3b molecules on the complex and clusters of CR1 on erythrocytes.[C230,C399,E20,E21,E27,H419,N182,P2,P4] *In vivo* studies have demonstrated that immune complexes preferentially bind to circulating erythrocytes that express multiple CR1 clusters and that the capacity of each erythrocyte for binding correlates with the density of cell surface CR1.[C399] Since CR1 on erythrocytes tends to cluster more than that on resting neutrophils, the majority of immune complexes bound to circulating cells are bound to erythrocytes.[B313,C390,C398,D73,E20,H233,K212,P3,S136,S137,S138,W111,W112] A reduction in the number of functional CR1 limits the capacity of erythrocytes to transport and buffer immune complexes. *In vivo* studies have demonstrated that repeated administration of antigens in immunized humans and primates with immune complex formation results in a decrease in erythrocyte CR1 levels.[D73,H234] Studies with primates have suggested that circulating immune complexes not bound to erythrocytes are more easily trapped in the microvasculature and can be recovered in the lungs and kidneys.[W111,W112] Together these findings have obvious implications for immune complex–mediated diseases.

The efficiency of immune complex binding to erythrocytes via CR1 is related to the nature of the immune complex, particularly the ability to activate complement and capture C3b, the spatial organization of the captured C3b, and the final size of the complex.[E21,E26] Several models have been used to analyze the characteristics of immune complexes interacting with the erythrocyte CR1 system, including DNA–human anti-DNA, BSA–anti-BSA, tetanus toxoid/human antitetanus toxoid, and hepatitis B surface antigen/human antihepatitis B surface antigen.[C390,E20,M55,P4,S136,W111] In each system large immune complexes bind to erythrocytes better than small immune complexes.[E20,S140] The antigen and antibody also influence this reaction, because the capacity to fix complement varies with antibody class and certain antigens alone may capture C3b.[L218] Erythrocyte CR1 immune complex binding is avid but reversible, and the rate of dissociation also varies according the particular immune complex, which dictates the nature of C3b capture.[E27,H417,M331]

The erythrocyte CR1 system may have a second physiologic function, i.e., it provides a processing mechanism for immune complexes.[M326] In addition to being a carrier for opsonized immune complexes, CR1 has a potent inhibi-

tory function in the complement cascade that may enhance clearance. It participates in the inactivation of C3b and may thereby alter the size of complexes, affecting their subsequent handling. Specifically, CR1 is a cofactor for factor I in the cleavage of C3b to iC3b and then to C3dg.[M324,M326,M327,M329,M331,M332,R323] Thus, binding of immune complexes containing C3b to erythrocyte CR1 facilitates proteolytic cleavage of the C3b to iC3b and C3dg, which do not bind to CR1. This reaction is the basis for the degradation of complement on immune complexes with their subsequent release from the receptor,[D77] and its rate varies with the physicochemical properties of individual complexes.[H417,M331,M332] If the immune complex can again activate complement and bind C3b, it can rebind to CR1.[M328,M329] Although repeated cycles of binding and release are likely, these immune complexes are not constantly bound to erythrocytes and are thereby available for either deposition or (enhanced) removal by the mononuclear phagocyte system. The fraction of immune complexes in whole blood that is erythrocyte bound depends on several dynamic processes: complement fixation and C3b capture, erythrocyte binding, and C3b degradation and immune complex release.

Fcγ Receptor Mechanisms

Immune complexes are removed from the circulation by the mononuclear phagocyte system of the liver and spleen through engagement of FcγRs and complement receptors. The interaction of immune complexes with the phagocyte involves a qualitatively different process than that with erythrocytes.[K212] The relative contribution of each receptor system depends upon the immunochemical properties of the complex. The liver, which is much larger than the spleen, is the principal site of uptake of immune complexes.[C390,H438,L344,W112] However, immune complexes that escape clearance by hepatic macrophages (which may be smaller and of lower valence) are taken up by the spleen.[H438] The role of FcγRs in immune complex clearance of both soluble and particulate immune complexes is shown by studies wherein blockade of FcγRs by infusion of aggregated IgG into the portal venous system [H233] or infusion of antibodies against FcγRs[K212] suppresses uptake of these immune complexes (Fig. 12–2). To support the pivotal role of FcγRs in handling certain immune complexes, studies of complement depletion show no effect on the efficiency of uptake of immune complexes by the liver or spleen and actually show an acceleration in the rate of removal of complexes from the circulation, presumably due to "trapping" in the microvasculature.[W111]

FcγRs appear to play a key role in the transfer and retention of immune complexes by mononuclear phagocytes. Studies of DNA–anti-DNA complexes bound to radiolabeled erythrocytes and injected into chimpanzees show that while immune complexes are removed by the mononuclear phagocyte system, the erythrocytes are not sequestered but are stripped of immune complexes and promptly recirculate.[C390] Though the mechanism of the stripping of complexes is not well defined, the involve-

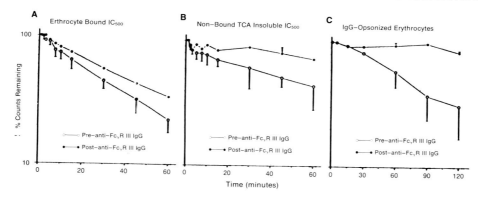

Fig. 12–2. Effect of anti-FcγRIII MAb on the handling of soluble IC. The effects of anti-FcγRIII MAb infusions on the handling of several different radiolabeled model IC probes in chimpanzees are presented with the data expressed as the percentage counts remaining relative to the counts infused. *A,* Following intravenous infusion of soluble radiolabeled IC, clearance of E-bound IC was measured and found to be slowed by treatment with anti-FcγRIII MAb IgG. *B,* After intravenous infusion of soluble IC, clearance of non–E-bound IC was more slowed by anti-FcγRIII MAb IgG. *C,* Clearance of IgG-opsonized E was most markedly slowed by anti-FcγRIII infusions.[K212] From Kimberly, R.P., Edberg, J.C., Merriam, L.T. et al.: In vivo handling of soluble complement fixing Ab/dsDNA in immune complexes in chimpanzees. J. Clin. Invest., *84*:962, 1989. Copyright 1989, The American Society for Clinical Investigation, with permission.

ment of complement proteases has been implicated.[M330,R326] In this model of immune complex clearance, infusion of erythrocyte-bound DNA–anti-DNA complexes after treatment with anti-FcγR monoclonal antibody results in a significant amount of nonerythrocyte-bound circulating immune complexes documenting the participation of FcγRs in the retention of immune complexes by phagocytes (Fig. 12–2B).[K212] In addition to stripping erythrocyte-bound complexes, FcγRs as well as CR3/CR4 are responsible for the clearance of those complexes unable to bind to erythrocyte CR1 because of inadequate C3b capture or degradation of C3b. This interpretation is supported by experiments in primates treated with anti-FcγR monoclonal antibodies showing impaired clearance of infused immune complexes, which was most pronounced in the fraction of complexes that did not bind to erythrocytes.[K212] It has been shown that immune adherence is not a prerequisite for efficient handling of immune complexes by the mononuclear phagocyte system,[E21,E25,W112] but immune complexes that do not fix complement or fix complement poorly cannot be cleared if FcγR function is impaired (Fig. 12–1).

ABNORMAL IMMUNE COMPLEX CLEARANCE IN SLE

Human Models of Immune Complex Clearance

The probes that have been used to assess the efficiency of immune complex clearance in humans are 1) autologous erythrocytes sensitized with IgG antibodies directed against the D antigen of the Rh system, 2) preformed immune complexes or aggregated IgG, and 3) antigen infused into passively immunized subjects. As expected, since each of these probes has distinct immunochemical properties, they interact differently with the complement and FcγR systems. Thus, the results of *in vivo* studies comparing immune clearance in SLE patients and healthy individuals vary depending upon the model probe.

Analysis of Clearance of IgG-Sensitized Autologous Erythrocytes

The technique introduced by Frank et al. to measure mononuclear phagocyte system function employs autologous ^{51}Cr-radiolabeled erythrocytes sensitized with IgG anti-(Rh)D antibodies injected into study subjects, and clearance or removal of these cells from the circulation is determined by serial bleeding.[F213,F214,F215] External surface counting of sensitized radiolabeled erythrocytes shows initial rapid sequestration in the liver, followed by splenic accumulation of most of the injected cells.[M529] Semilogarithmic plot of the mean data for clearance of sensitized cells in normal controls is curvilinear, with a rapid initial loss of radiolabeled cells followed by a slower sustained loss of radioactivity (Fig. 12–3).[K218,M363,S175]

Though originally conceptualized as a measure of FcγR capacity, kinetic analysis of *in vivo* clearance studies and *in vitro* studies with IgG anti-(Rh)D-coated erythrocytes suggest that complement also plays a role in clearance of this probe. Further support for this is provided by studies of C4-deficient patients who show delayed clearance relative to normals.[F215] A proposed model to describe the series of steps in handling of IgG anti-(Rh)D-sensitized erythrocytes is as follows. Circulating cells initially sequestered by a complement-dependent process are either deactivated and released back into the circulation or are phagocytosed. Released cells are sequestered and phagocytosed by an FcγR-mediated process. Circulating cells may also be directly sequestered and phagocytosed by FcγRs.[K218,M363,M365]

The role of complement in the clearance of anti-(Rh)D-sensitized erythrocytes is a function of the level of antibody sensitization.[H483,M366] Erythrocytes prepared with a low density of surface anti-(Rh)D are cleared primarily by splenic FcγRs, while at higher density sensitization hepatic complement receptor-mediated clearance

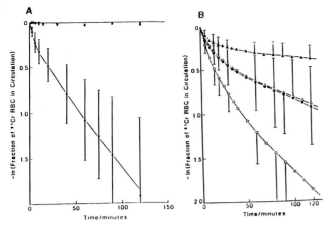

Fig. 12–3. *A*, Survival of ⁵¹Cr-labeled autologous erythrocytes (±SD) in normal controls. Unsensitized erythrocytes in six normal controls (*upper curve*); Anti-Rh(D)–sensitized erythrocytes in 49 normal controls (*lower curve*). *B*, Survival of ⁵¹Cr-labeled autologous anti-Rh(D)-sensitized erythrocytes in 32 SLE patients: comparison between disease active subgroups. (0---0 inactive/nonrenal [n = 5], ●---● active/nonrenal [n = 7], △---△ active/nonrenal [n = 12], ▲---▲ active/renal [n = 8]).[K218] From Kimberly, R.P., Maryhew, N.L., and Runquist, O.A.: Mononuclear phagocyte function in SLE I. Bipartite Fcs and complement-dependent dysfunction. J. Immunol., *137*:91, 1986.

becomes increasingly important. This observation is highlighted in studies of splenectomized patients, showing that clearance of erythrocytes sensitized with low levels of anti-(Rh)D antibody is more markedly prolonged than that of more densely opsonized erythrocytes, which fix complement and may be cleared by hepatic C3b receptors.[H438] Since density of opsonization determines the relative contribution of FcγRs and complement mechanisms in clearance, the results of *in vivo* clearance studies in SLE patients must be interpreted in the context of the level of sensitization of the probe.

In Vivo Studies of IgG-Sensitized Autologous Erythrocytes in SLE

Abnormal mononuclear phagocyte system function in SLE patients has been demonstrated in several studies performed with IgG anti-(Rh)D[F213,K219,H80,P55,V24] sensitized erythrocytes. Clearance half-times for radiolabeled autologous IgG-sensitized erythrocytes were prolonged in SLE patients compared to normals and were longer in patients with renal disease than in those without renal disease (Figs. 12–3 and 12–4). In these studies, the prolongation of clearance half-time of erythrocytes (low-density sensitization) was attributed to impaired splenic FcγR function.[F213] At this low sensitization level, hepatic complement-mediated clearance is negligible, and the rate of clearance indeed reflects the efficiency and capacity of FcγRs. The abnormality in clearance is receptor specific, because clearance of heat-damaged erythrocytes and aggregated albumin was not prolonged in these SLE patients.[E80,F213] In a contrasting study, clearance of more heavily sensitized erythrocytes in SLE patients was similar

to that of normal controls.[K3] At this higher level of sensitization, clearance half-times are primarily a measure of hepatic complement receptor function rather than splenic FcγR function.[M366] Because complement-dependent clearance is often normal in SLE patients without renal involvement (see below), the overall clearance of heavy opsonized erythrocytes may be normal despite marked FcγR dysfunction.

When clinical activity in SLE patients was assessed, there was a significant but independent association between impaired FcγR clearance and level of both renal and nonrenal disease activity.[P55] Increased activity along either parameter was associated with more impaired clearance. As shown on Figure 12–4, patients with active renal and nonrenal disease are most likely to have the highest degree of clearance dysfunction. Longitudinal studies in SLE patients showed that mononuclear phagocyte system function changed concordantly with changes in clinical status, indicating that clearance dysfunction is dynamic and closely related to disease activity.[H80,K219]

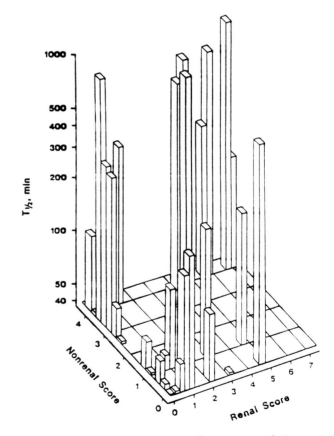

Fig. 12–4. Relationship of clinical activity and Fc receptor–mediated mononuclear phagocyte system dysfunction. Clinical activity was assessed in terms of both renal and nonrenal manifestations. Longer (taller) clearance half-time values represent greater degrees of dysfunction. Patients with active renal and nonrenal disease showed the greatest degree of Fc-mediated clearance impairment.[K222] From Kimberly, R.P., Salmon, J.E., Edberg, J.C. et al.: The Role of Fcγ receptors in mononuclear phagocyte system function. Clin. Exp. Rheum., 7:S-3:S105, 1989.

Semilogarithmic plots of the mean data for clearance in SLE patients, grouped according to disease activity and presence or absence of renal involvement, show differences in slope and duration of initial rapid loss of radiolabeled cells from the circulation (predominantly complement-dependent clearance) and in the slope of the slow sustained clearance reaction (predominantly FcγR-mediated clearance) (Fig. 12–3B). Rate constants governing the FcγR- and complement-dependent steps of the clearance process were derived from kinetic analysis of these curvilinear clearance data. Rate constants were evaluated for four steps: complement-dependent sequestration, C3b deactivation and release, complement-mediated phagocytosis, and FcγR-mediated sequestration and phagocytosis. Such analysis of the studies of SLE patients grouped by disease activity revealed both FcγR- and complement-dependent dysfunction.[K218] Impaired FcγR function was evident in all SLE patients except those with neither renal involvement nor any other manifestation of activity. Complement-mediated phagocytic dysfunction was seen only in patients with renal disease. These data suggest that altered complement-mediated phagocytosis in combination with abnormal FcγR-mediated phagocytosis by fixed tissue macrophages contribute to the pathogenesis of lupus nephritis.

In hypocomplementemic SLE patients, examination of clearance rate constants revealed a good correlation between disease activity and FcγR-mediated clearance function.[M365] With decreased complement levels there may be deficient complement opsonization of complexes, impaired binding and processing by erythrocytes, and reduced clearance by hepatic complement receptors. Such circulating immune complexes with little or no complement must be cleared by FcγRs. While rapid hepatic complement-dependent clearance appears to be the first line of defense against immune complex deposition, when this mechanism fails FcγR-mediated clearance becomes pivotal. In disease processes associated with hypocomplementemia, tissue immune complex deposition and increased disease activity occurs when there is a concomitant defect in FcγR clearance. Similar to human SLE, studies in four murine models of lupus demonstrated an early progressive defect in FcγR-mediated clearance of IgG-sensitized erythrocytes, whereas efficiency of complement-mediated clearance varied among the murine strains.[M367] The consistent finding of impaired FcγR-specific clearance in patients with active SLE emphasizes the potential importance of the mechanism for immune complex disease.

Given the role of immune complex deposition in the pathogenesis of SLE, circulating immune complex levels in patients were measured by a series of different assay systems (C1q binding, staphylococcal protein A binding assay, Raji cell assay) at the time of *in vivo* erythrocyte clearance in many studies. There was a relationship between levels of immune complexes and FcγR dysfunction in some, but not all groups of SLE patients.[F213,M365,H80] The lack of direct correlation between mononuclear phagocyte system function and immune complex level in all studies is not surprising given the complexity of im-

mune complex handling and the range of variables determining net complex levels.[K219,P55]

Although partly acquired and related to disease activity, the FcγR mononuclear phagocyte dysfunction may also have a genetic component. Normal individuals with an HLA haplotype containing either DR2 or DR3, which are some gene products found with increased frequency in SLE populations, (see Chap. 2), are more likely to have an abnormally prolonged FcγR-mediated clearance of IgG-sensitized erythrocytes than their normal counterparts without these haplotypes[K213,L101] (Fig. 12–5). The ability

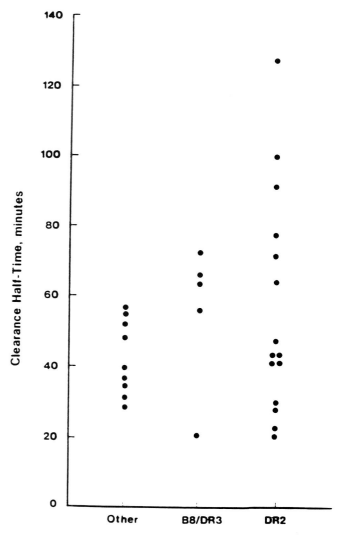

Fig. 12–5. Mononuclear phagocyte system clearance half-times in disease-free individuals by immunogenetic subgroups. HLA-B8/DR3 individuals (p = .027) and DR2-positive individuals (p = .037) each contain more individuals than expected with abnormally long clearance times compared to upper 95% confidence limit of the control group ("other," non-DR2, DR3).[K213] From Kimberly, R.P., Gibofsky, A., Salmon, J.E. et al.: Impaired Fc-mediated mononuclear phagocyte system clearance in HLA-DR2 and MT1-positive healthy adults. J. Exp. Med., *157*:1698, 1983. Copyright 1983, the Rockefeller University Press.

to detect these differences may depend upon the study probe.[V24] While the magnitude of the FcγR dysfunction is substantially larger in SLE patients and has a large dynamic component associated with disease activity,[F213,K219,P55] individuals with an immunogenetically determined decrease in FcγR function might be more susceptible to the secondary FcγR abnormalities associated with SLE. Thus, basal immunogenetically determined mononuclear phagocyte clearance in normal individuals may contribute to the predisposition and pathogenesis of SLE.

Analysis of Clearance of Infused Soluble Immune Complexes

As another measure of mononuclear phagocyte system function, the clearance of preformed large, soluble complement-fixing immune complexes has been studied in humans. Radiolabeled tetanus toxoid/antitetanus toxoid, hepatitis B surface antigen-antibody, or aggregated human IgG are infused and sequential blood samples are obtained and analyzed for whole blood and erythrocyte-bound radioactivity to monitor clearance.[H70,M55,S136] Clearance of these preformed immune complexes (free or erythrocyte bound) from the circulation of humans has been shown to involve activation of complement with capture of C3b, binding to erythrocyte CR1 receptors, uptake by complement and FcγR tissue mononuclear phagocytes as described above (see Complement Mechanisms). The site of clearance is predominantly the liver.[L345] Factors that cause the erythrocyte transport system to fail, such as hypocomplementemia or CR1 deficiency, are associated with an initial more rapid disappearance of immune complexes presumably caused by trapping in capillary beds outside the mononuclear phagocyte system. For example, clearance of injected hepatitis B surface antigen-antibody complexes in patients with essential mixed cryoglobulinemia is accelerated compared to normal subjects, presumably due to immune complex deposition in tissues outside the liver and spleen as a result of impaired immune adherence. The basis for defective erythrocyte transport and buffering of complexes in these patients appear to be a result of complement depletion and monoclonal rheumatoid factor inhibition of immune complex opsonization and binding.[M55]

Because the relevance of these large preformed complexes (>40S) to human SLE is not entirely clear, studies of clearance of smaller (19S) complexes formed *in vivo* have been performed. Patients with ovarian cancer were infused with murine antitumor antibodies followed by human antimurine IgG.[D73] In this model, complexes were cleared rapidly by the liver, though the role of erythrocyte CR1 was unclear. *In vivo* immune complex formation was associated with systemic complement activation, reduction in erythrocyte CR1, and increased erythrocyte C3 and C4 (similar to the findings in SLE—see below), which could predispose to less efficient handling of further complexes. Given the different kinds of information obtained from each of these *in vivo* probes, examination of multiple models of immune complex clearance is necessary to define the mechanisms of immune complex deposition in SLE.

In Vivo Studies of Infused Soluble Immune Complexes in SLE

In vivo studies of infused soluble immune complexes complement the sensitized erythrocyte model of clearance and demonstrate multifactorial mononuclear phagocyte dysfunction. Abnormalities in erythrocyte CR1 system, the early buffer for circulating immune complexes are described in patients with SLE. For the purposes of these models, it is important to recognize that SLE patients tend to have an acquired decreased numeric expression of CR1 on erythrocytes, which correlates with disease activity,[R326,W51] and may be a consequence of repeated immune complex/erythrocyte CR1 interactions.[D73,H234] There is also evidence for an inherited deficiency of CR1 in some SLE patients.[M502,W265,W268] Diminished CR1 resulting in impaired immune adherence is one of the mechanisms of abnormal clearance of infused soluble complexes in SLE. For example, SLE patients infused with radiolabeled aggregated human IgG show decreased binding of the probe to erythrocytes and a more rapid initial distribution phase compared to that in normal controls.[H70,L344] Similarly, complement-mediated binding of tetanus toxoid/antitetanus toxoid immune complexes to erythrocytes was decreased in SLE, and this correlated with erythrocyte CR1 number.[S136] With these model immune complexes a rapid first phase of elimination was noted in patients with low complement, low CR1, and low immune adherence, which was ascribed to inappropriate tissue deposition of complexes.[S137]

The second, slower elimination phase of infused aggregated IgG is also abnormal in SLE, presumably because of impaired splenic uptake as well as generalized mononuclear phagocyte dysfunction. Whereas studies in normals show preferential hepatic uptake of aggregated IgG, and splenectomized normals show hepatic compensation for splenic loss with normal elimination half-times, SLE patients have both minimal splenic uptake and prolonged clearance half-times.[H70,H71,L344] Abnormalities in both splenic and hepatic clearance function allow for spillover of complexes beyond the mononuclear phagocyte system in SLE.

Blockade of FcγRs by elevated levels of IgG interferes with this key mechanism of elimination of soluble circulating immune complexes.[K165,K221] The observation that serum concentrations of IgG are an important factor predicting the rate of aggregated IgG clearance in SLE[H70] emphasizes the importance of FcγR mechanisms in this model and supports the conclusions derived from the sensitized erythrocyte model of immune complex clearance. Specifically, FcγR-mediated clearance efficiency is crucial in SLE because of the defects in complement-dependent function.

ABNORMALITIES IN Fcγ RECEPTORS IN SLE

FcγR saturation by circulating immune complexes with decreased receptor availability was initially proposed as a potential mechanism for defective FcγR-mediated clearance.[F213,F214,P55] Support for this hypothesis was derived from *in vitro* induction of loss of surface FcγRs in monocytes by culture with immune complexes[M347,M393,R3] and

FcγRs by immune complex, there are both heterotypic and homotypic receptor clusters resulting in intracellular interactions between the signals generated by each receptor family. Indeed, there is evidence that engagement of the different classes of receptors leads to quantitatively and perhaps qualitatively distinct cell functions in relation to engagement of either receptor alone.[E22] In monocytes, FcγRI and FcγRII cooperate in triggering activation, presumably by heterotypic clustering.[K374] In neutrophils FcγRIIIB acts synergistically with FcγRII to mediate phagocytosis.[C436,E22,S46] Interactions between FcγRs and other leukocyte receptors modulate FcγR-initiated functions. For example, engagement of complement receptor type 3 enhances FcγR-mediated phagocytosis by monocytes.[G332] In the interaction of immune complexes with leukocytes, effector function capacity is a consequence of cooperation among FcγR families and between FcγRs and other receptors, all of which may be simultaneously engaged.

The FcγR system has sufficient overlap of function that major genetic abnormalities have been described without clinical sequelae. Four members of a family were identified lacking FcγRI on their monocytes.[C186] In spite of this, these individuals were free of clinical disease, circulating immune complexes, or increased susceptibility to infection. Similarly, patients with paroxysmal nocturnal hemoglobinuria who have decreased surface FcγRIIIB because of defective expression of glycosyl-phosphatidylinositol–anchored molecules,[E23,H490,S270] as well as other individuals lacking FcγRIIIB because of abnormalities in the FcγRIIIB gene, have no evidence of immune complex disease.[H489] Although one patient with SLE was found to lack FcγRIIIB, its role in the pathogenesis of her illness is unclear since FcγRIIIA expression on mononuclear phagocytes was unaffected.[C281] These experiments of nature clearly demonstrate the redundancy of the FcγR system. Simultaneous abnormalities in FcγRs and other receptor mechanisms, such as the complement system, however, appear to predispose to immune complex disease and argue for therapy directed at enhancing FcγR clearance function.

STRATEGIES FOR MODULATING FcγR-MEDIATED IMMUNE COMPLEX CLEARANCE

The emerging picture of extensive structural delivery of human FcγRs, the importance of FcγRs in immune complex clearance, and the evidence for FcγR dysfunction in SLE presents the opportunity for novel treatment strategies. Though our present understanding of FcγR structural forms in relation to their function is insufficient to outline a specific therapeutic approach, potential directions are evident. A variety of cytokines can regulate total receptor expression,[H371,V21] modulate relative isoform predominance,[H491,W139] and modulate receptor function.[E126] For example, in vivo and in vitro studies have shown that γ-interferon up-regulates FcγRI expression[G438,G439,H491,P139] and TGFβ up-regulates FcγRIIIA on monocytes,[A149,W168] while IL-4 down-regulates expression of all three classes of FcγRs.[T90] In contrast, IL-6 and γ-interferon enhance antibody-dependent cytotoxicity triggered by FcγRI and FcγRII, respectively, without altering receptor expression.[E126,F17]

Cytokines can also interact with endogenous or pharmacologic agents to alter net FcγR function.[G166,S51] Steroid hormones have major effects on FcγR expression and function, estrogens augment and progesterones inhibit,[F249,R220,S177] but steroid effects may vary with the level of activation of the mononuclear system.[H409,W83] For example, glucocorticoids enhance the γ-interferon–induced augmentation of monocyte FcγR function, whereas alone they are inhibitory for normal donors.[A351,A353,C422,F266,G166,H463,S181,W83] Interestingly, for monocytes from SLE patients, which may be primed in vivo with γ-interferon,[H409,P282,P283] glucocorticoids enhance function. Patients with active SLE treated with high-dose intravenous pulse methylprednisolone have improved clearance of IgG-sensitized autologous erythrocytes, enhanced monocyte FcγR expression and phagocytosis, and decreased levels of circulating immune complexes.[S51] These data raise the possibility that pharmacologic therapies can act synergistically with endogenous cytokines to achieve the desired outcome. With such a range of receptor modulating agents, successful therapeutic intervention will be feasible and form the basis for further advances in the treatment of SLE.

Chapter 13

COMPLEMENT AND SYSTEMIC LUPUS ERYTHEMATOSUS

PETER H. SCHUR*

Considerable evidence shows that much of the pathology in patients with systemic lupus erythematosus (SLE) can be attributed to immune complexes. These immune complexes either may form in the circulation and later deposit in tissues or form in situ. Immune complexes do not appear to cause tissue inflammation directly but rather through activation of the complement system. This causes release of various mediators, promotes cell interaction, and ultimately results in inflammation. Evaluation of the complement system (which can serve as an indirect measure of the presence of immune complexes) often correlates with clinical aspects of SLE. Monitoring blood levels of complement may be useful in adjusting therapy for the patient.

THE COMPLEMENT SYSTEM

The complement system consists of a group of at least 28 plasma proteins that interact sequentially to both facilitate clearance of immune complexes but also effect systems of inflammation.[C383,F37,F39,F211,M652,M653,O9,R406,S138,S194] Some of these activities occur on cell surfaces, some on the surface of immune complexes, and others in various body fluids.

The complement system (see Fig. 13–1) consists of three pathways: the classic pathway and the alternative (or properdin) pathway; these two pathways enter into the terminal (or membrane) attack pathway. The classic complement pathway involves complement components C1, C4, and C2. Human immune complexes containing IgM and/or the IgG subclasses IgG1, IgG2, or IgG3 will bind the C1q portion of C1. Such binding leads to the sequential activation of C1r, C1s, cleavage of C2 and C4 into C2a, C2b, C4a, C4c, C4d and the eventual cleavage of C3 by C3 convertase (i.e., the complex C4b2a) into C3a and C3b. There are natural controls or modulators of activation of this system such as C1 inhibitor (C1INH), C4b binding protein (C4bp), and factor I (C3b inactivator (C3bINA), KAF).

Cleavage of C3 can also come about through an alternative pathway, the properdin system. This phylogenetically older system can be activated by some immunoglobulins, including aggregated IgA and possibly IgE, as well as polysaccharides, including bacterial endotoxin. The pathway involves a number of proteins including properdin, factor B, factor D, and C3, that interact to create another C3 convertase (C3bBb), which cleaves C3. Interaction of both of these pathways leads to cleavage of the third component into C3a and C3b—and by various enzymes into even smaller fragments: C3c, C3d, C3dg, C4dk, C3e, and C3g (some of which may still have biologic properties). The larger fragment, C3b, can interact further with components of the properdin system, causing a positive feedback cycle, resulting in further activation and cleavage of C3.

The terminal pathway also begins at C3. Activation of C3 via C3b results in sequential cleavage or activation of C5, C6, C7, C8, and C9. An inactivator of C3b (C3bINA) (factor I) in concert with β IH (factor H) can block the hemolytic potential of C3b by cleaving it into two inactive fragments: C3d, which remains bound to the antigen-antibody complex, and C3c, which is released into the fluid. Properdin (P) and C3 nephritic factor (C3NEF) stabilize C3 convertases, and thus facilitate the progression of the system. Deposition of the multimolecular complex consisting of C5 through C9 on a cell membrane leads to the formation of cell membrane defects that cause increased permeability and release of intracellular contents, such as hemoglobin. Release of hemoglobin thus provides a means for assaying the overall function of the complement system.

Many cells have receptors for complement components or fragments including C1q, C3a, C3b, C3d, C3bi, C3e, H, and C5a.[F39,O9,S138] Receptor CR1 reacts with C3b, iC3b, and C4b; CR2 reacts with iC3b, C3dg, and C3d; CR3 reacts with iC3b; C3a receptor reacts with C3a and C4a; there are individual receptors for C1q, C3e, factor H, and C5a. Receptors are found on erythrocytes, polymorphonuclear leukocytes, monocytes, lymphocytes, mast cells, and glomerular podocytes. The receptors appear to have a role in clearing immune complexes, enhancing phagocytosis, augmenting antibody-dependent cellular cytotoxicity (ADCC), chemotaxis, leukocyte respiratory bursts, secretion, and B-cell proliferation.

IMMUNOBIOLOGIC ASPECTS OF THE COMPLEMENT SYSTEM[C383,F37,F39,F211,M652,M653,O9,R406,S138,S194]

A number of biologic functions have been ascribed to various complement components. C1, C4, and C2 are involved in viral neutralization. The interaction of C1, C4, and C2 produces a peptide that increases local vascular permeability. The cleavage products C3a and C5a have anaphylatoxic properties and release histamine from mast

* The author thanks Dr. A. Kumar for his critical evaluation and comments and Ms. J. Davis for her excellent secretarial assistance.

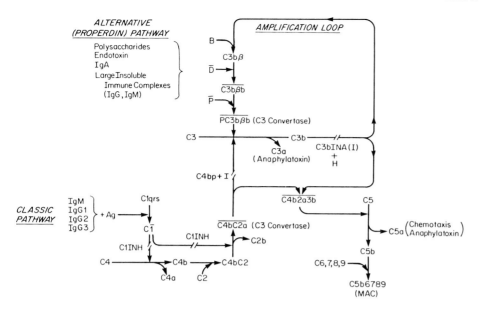

Fig. 13-1. The complement cascade.

cells. In addition C5a is also chemotactic for monocytes and polymorphonuclear leukocytes. Both C3a and C5a have been implicated in the regulation of the humoral immune response.

The presence of C3b on antigen-antibody complexes helps bind these to specific receptors on erythrocytes, B lymphocytes, monocytes, or polymorphonuclear leukocytes, and promotes clearance and subsequent phagocytosis of these complement complexes—with release of lysosomal enzymes. Immune complexes coated with C3b may bind to platelets, causing release of vasoactive amines, resulting in inflammatory reactions. These biologic activities of C3b can be blocked by C3bINA.

MEASUREMENT OF COMPLEMENT[R406,S194]

The complement system can be assessed by measurement of total hemolytic complement activity (CH50), immunochemical or hemolytic measurement of individual components, measurements of complement breakdown products, and determination of complement metabolism.

The total hemolytic complement level (CH50) represents the sum of all components of the system. By adding diluted serum to antibody-sensitized sheep erythrocytes, and quantitating the amount of released hemoglobin, one can measure this level in units which represents the reciprocal of that dilution of serum that causes 50% of cells to lyse (i.e., CH50). A CH100 represents that dilution of serum that lyses 100% of sensitized cells; this measurement is not nearly as accurate as a CH50, which reflects actual hemolysis in a more linear fashion than does a CH100.

Separate complement components are generally measured by immunochemical means: radial immunodiffusion, electroimmunodiffusion, or nephelometry. However, such determinations yield no information about the functional biologic integrity or hemolytic potential of the components being measured. Such functional tests are rarely employed because of their difficulty in routine clinical assays.

When measuring CH50 or components, it is important to remember that some components are thermolabile. Serum stored at room temperature, even for a few days, is adequate for immunochemical measurement of individual components as proteins (as, for instance, by immunodiffusion). However, it is essential to store samples as soon as possible at −70° C when measurement of the hemolytic levels of individual components is desired. The CH50 will remain relatively stable for a few hours at room temperature or overnight at −20° C; however, samples are best stored at −70° C as soon as possible. Heating for 30 minutes at 56° C is also known to inactivate complement components and decrease/abolish CH50 activity.

The above assays give but a glimpse of the dynamic state of the complement system. Serial values may be helpful in assessing this dynamic state: falling values suggest more catabolism (e.g., via immune complex fixation) than synthesis, while rising levels suggest that less catabolism is taking place. Measurement of split, or activation, products of individual components is a way of assessing the catabolic state of the complement system, without necessarily doing serial measurements. The split or conversion products are generally measured by ELISA using monoclonal antisera.[A305,S263]

Complement metabolism is a better way of assessing the dynamic state (i.e., synthesis and catabolism) of individual complement components.[R407] However, these studies are rarely performed because of the great difficulty in isolating hemolytically and biologically active purified components and in maintaining their activity after radiolabeling. The liver is the primary source of synthesis of complement components.[C353]

COMPLEMENT ABNORMALITIES

Understanding the role of complement in disease requires analysis of the whole system, i.e., CH50 levels and levels of individual components. For instance, a depressed CH50 level could be the result of inherited depletion of a single component and/or acquired depletion of multiple components through immune and nonimmune processes. Further, static measurements of serum CH50 levels or of individual complement components should be confirmed whenever possible by serial studies to estimate the metabolism of these proteins. Since most disorders of the complement system affect either the classic or the alternative pathway, I recommend for routine serum analysis a serum hemolytic CH50 and immunochemical analysis of C1q, C4, C3, and factor B proteins. Late or terminal components are rarely affected unless C3 is affected as well; measurement of C5 protein has been useful in this regard. Generally, a decrease in CH50 activity corresponds well with a decrease in C1q, C4, C2, and C3 component levels and vice versa. When, on the other hand, CH50 levels do not correlate with the levels of these components, one should consider abnormalities of one of the other components, or serum-handling problems.

INHERITED DEFECTS OF COMPLEMENT[A54,A350,C50, C354,G182,H334,M306,R65,R219,R327,R405,S194,S198]

Four types of inherited complement abnormalities are most readily recognized: homozygous deficiency, heterozygous deficiency, dysfunctional proteins, and allotypy (i.e., electrophoretically defined alleles). Certain allotypes are also expressed as null genes (i.e., the "gene" is present but the protein is not) resulting in either hetero- or homozygous deficiency. Molecular biologic techniques including restriction fragment length polymorphism (RFLP) have revealed more heterogeneity and abnormalities among complement genes than were recognized by immunochemical techniques.

Persons who are homozygous deficient in a complement component generally show virtually no CH50 activity and are missing one component (assessed hemolytically or immunochemically); the levels of all other components are normal. Those who are heterozygous deficient in a component—in particular C1, C4, C2, or C3—have approximately half the normal levels of that component and approximately half the normal CH50 levels; levels of all other components are normal[S194] (Table 13–1). The inherited nature of the defect needs to be confirmed by family studies demonstrating either homozygous and/or heterozygous defects in other family members. Inheritance of most complement abnormalities and deficiencies is autosomal dominant. In most of the studies performed in Caucasian populations, the frequency of complement deficiencies is approximately the same among males and females. However, C3 deficiency is found mostly in females[R327] and factor B deficiency is found in males.[R327] Many of the cases of recurrent neisserial infection in patients with terminal complement deficiencies have occurred in blacks.[R327]

The frequency of complement deficiencies in the general population is probably low. In an attempt to determine this frequency, 10,000 English blood bank donors were screened for CH50 levels. Only one person was found to have a deficiency of a complement component C2.[S723] In a study of 146,000 Japanese blood bank donors, 16 late-acting deficiencies were found: 2 cases of C5, 4 cases of C6, 6 cases of C7, and 4 cases of C8 deficiency—without any deficiencies of early complement components. Twelve individuals were asymptomatic.[114] These observations suggest that complement deficiencies may differ by race and also that disease associations with early complement component deficiencies do not represent ascertainment bias. One can estimate the frequency of homozygous deficiency in a population by determining the frequency of the (more common) heterozygous deficiency.

To determine whether there is possible association between a particular complement deficiency and some clinical entity, it is important to determine whether the association is a real phenomenon or is a result of an ascertainment bias. This becomes relevant when one recognizes that physicians tend to order complement levels primarily in patients with immune, rheumatic, renal, and infectious disorders. It is also important to remember that deficiency of a particular component may not be associated with any disease. The first case of homozygous complement deficiency (C2) was described in an immunologist who donated his blood to a colleague for a (complement-fixing) experiment that did not work![S443] Nevertheless, about two-thirds of individuals with homozygous deficiency of the classic pathway suffer from immune/rheumatic disorders such as SLE, glomerulonephri-

Table 13–1. Complement Profiles in Hereditary and Acquired Deficiencies in SLE

Condition	CH$_{50}$*	C1q†	C4†	C2†	C3†	Factor B†
Normal	150–250	35–56	26–83	1.6–3.9	91–198	19–39
Homozygous C2 deficiency	0	35–56	26–83	0	91–198	19–39
Heterozygous C2 deficiency	100–150	35–56	26–83	1–1.5	91–198	19–39
Homozygous C4 deficiency	0	35–56	0	1.6–3.9	91–198	19–39
Heterozygous C4 deficiency	100–150	35–56	10–25	1.6–3.9	91–198	19–39
SLE						
Arthritis	100–150	18–34	10–25	1.6–3.9	91–150	19–39
Vasculitis	50–100	5–25	5–15	1–1.5	80–120	19–39
Glomerulonephritis	25–125	10–30	5–20	1–1.5	70–75	12–18
Nephrotic syndrome‡	100–150	18–34	26–83	1.6–3.9	91–198	19–39

* μ/ml.
† mg/dl.
‡ Any nephrotic syndrome.

Table 13–2. Complement Component Deficiencies

Component	Clinical Associations*
Classical pathway	
C1q	SLE, GN
C1r	SLE, GN, infection
C1r and C1s	Infection, SLE
C4	SLE, infection, GN
C2	SLE, infection, various immune disorders, normality
Alternative pathway	
C3	Infection, GN
P	Infection
D	Infection
Effector (terminal) pathway	
C5	Infection (Neisseria)
C6	Infection (Neisseria)
C7	Infection (Neisseria), GN
C8	Infection (Neisseria), normality, xeroderma
C9	Normality, infection (Neisseria)
Control proteins	
C1 INH	Hereditary angioedema, SLE
I	Infection
H	Normality, hemolytic uremic syndrome
Complement receptors	
CR1	SLE

* Only the more common associations are given.
SLE = systemic lupus erythematosus, GN = glomerulonephritis.
This table is based on references R-65, G182 and H334.

tis, anaphylactic purpura/vasculitis, and related disorders (see Table 13–2).[A54,A350,C50,C354,G182,H334,M306,R65,R219,R327,R405,S194,S198] The strongest associations are between systemic lupus erythematosus and C2 and C4 deficiency. Terminal component deficiencies are significantly associated with recurrent pyogenic infection, particularly that caused by Neisseria[R327] (see Table 13-2). However, infections are also noted among individuals with classic component deficiencies, and immune/rheumatic diseases are found in individuals with terminal component deficiencies. It is not clear whether these associations are greater than would be expected by chance alone.

C1

At least 14 pedigrees of C1 (i.e., C1q, C1r, or C1s subunit) deficiencies have been described.[R327] The clinical profile of many of these families reveals lupus erythematosus or a lupus-like disease, glomerulonephritis, and skin lesions. Many of the children have had infections, and many of the siblings died young of either infections or lupus-like diseases. Heterozygotes within families are difficult to identify.

C4

Less than 1 in 10,000 Caucasians (in Boston) are homozygous C4 deficient.[M126] Homozygous C4 deficiency has been recognized in at least eight families.[R327] Lupus (or lupus-like) erythematosus disease is found in most of them. The analysis of C4 is more complicated as it consists of two isotypic forms, C4A and C4B. At least 13 C4A alleles

and 16 C4B alleles as well as a null allele at each locus are presently known.[M213] Null alleles are ascertained both by electrophoresis (allotyping) and family studies to confirm the null state—a necessary test to prove that the apparent C4A or C4B null state is not acquired, as may happen in SLE due to immune complex binding and activation. Further, there is no good relationship between C4A or C4B null states and serum C4 levels—and most SLE patients have low C4 levels.[S194] C4A null is probably the most common inherited complement deficiency occurring in varying frequency in different populations (e.g., Japan 0.067, blacks 0.071–0.221, England 0.284, France 0.132, Germany 0.087).[B129,B130] The frequency of homozygous C4A deficiency in normal Caucasians (in Boston) is 3% and for C4B is 2%.[M126] An increased frequency (50 to 80%) of C4A (protein) null alleles has been noted in patients with SLE in studies of predominately Anglo-Sazon populations,[D98,F85,H455,K166] blacks,[H455,O95,W275] Chinese and Japanese,[D354,H215] and Swedes,[S748] but not in our study in Boston,[S204] nor in French,[G320] French Canadians,[G272] or in (other) Japanese.[Y8] However, when our Boston SLE patients were categorized into two groups based on their European ancestry (English/Irish versus other) there was an increased frequency of C4AQ0, HLA-DR3, and the complotype SC01 in SLE patients of English/Irish descent as compared to ethnically matched controls.[S204] The increase in C4AQ0 (and DR3) could be accounted for by their being part of the extended haplotype [HLA-B8;SC01;DR3].[S204] Most of the (other) early observations of increased C4AQ0 were indeed in SLE patients of English/Irish descent in whom an association with DR3 was also noted. Other studies of SLE patients have reported an increase of the C4A protein null allele without an increase in DR3. Most of these studies have not confirmed the inheritance of the C4A null state by family studies.

RFLP analysis of individuals with C4A null allele (C4AQ0/C4AQ0Q0) and DR3 using the restriction enzyme HindIII and a 5' C4 cDNA probe has revealed loss of a 15 kb restriction fragment and the appearance of a 8.5 kb fragment.[G269,K166,K457] However, in non-DR3 individuals, C4A gene deletion failed to account for the C4A protein deficiency.[K457] Further analysis of the C4d region of the C4A gene by polymerase chain reaction (PCR) and RFLP using the N1a IV enzyme revealed that homoexpression of C4B at both loci was also not responsible for C4A deficiency in non-DR3 individuals.[K457]

Patients with genetic deficiency of C4 tend to have antibodies to Ro.[M381] There is an increased frequency of the C4A null allele in patients with hydralazine-induced SLE.[S595]

In summary, the role of C4AQ0 is not entirely clear. C4AQ0 undoubtedly contributes to the pathogenesis of SLE. Some ethnic groups express it as part of an extended haplotype and thereby are at increased risk for developing SLE. However, C4AQ0 is not a necessary risk factor for lupus in all ethnic groups.

C2

Deficiency of complement component C2 is the second most common genetic complement deficiency in Caucasians; 1% of individuals are heterozygous deficient, and approximately 1 in 10,000 have homozygous deficiency.[G183,S723] Homozygous C2 deficiency has been recognized in over 60 families, while heterozygous deficiency is found in many more.[G183,R327] It is inherited as an autosomal dominant. Well over 50% of the homozygous C2-deficient individuals have SLE, or lupus-like disease.[A54] Most homozygous C2-deficient SLE patients have mild disease with mostly skin and joint manifestations; renal disease is uncommon.[A54] One patient developed severe lupus nephritis after a transfusion, which suggests that the lack of C2 prevented immune complex–mediated glomerulonephritis.[R242] Many patients had either absent or low-titer antinuclear antibodies (ANAs); this often made it difficult to diagnose lupus.[G183] The frequency of C2 heterozygous deficiency (which is relatively easy to establish) was increased among SLE patients and juvenile rheumatoid arthritis (JRA) patients but not RA patients —6%, 3%, and 1% respectively; the frequency is 1% in normals.[G183] Clinically there was no difference between SLE patients with or without heterozygous C2 deficiency, except for the aforementioned tendency toward low ANA titers[G183] and a high frequency of antibodies to Ro.[M381,W275] Infections do not appear to be a major problem for most C2-deficient families.[A54]

C2 deficiency is found in strong linkage disequilibrium with HLA-A10, B18, DR2, C4A4, C4B2, BFS.[A371] C2 deficiency had been shown not to be caused by a major gene deletion, insertion, or rearrangement but was believed to be from a specific and selective pretranslational regulatory defect in C2 gene expression, leading to lack of detectable C2 mRNA and a lack of protein.[C343] However, more recently C2 deficiency has been shown to be caused by a splicing defect resulting from a 28 bp genomic deletion, leading to excision of a 134 bp exon and predicted premature termination of the C2 translation product.[J89]

C3–9

SLE has occasionally been noted in association with C3, C5, C6, C7, C8, and C9 deficiency;[K126,R327,T94] however, these deficiencies are usually associated with infections.[R327] SLE has occasionally also been noted in individuals with C1INH deficiency associated with hereditary angioedema.[R327]

CR1

Deficiency of the erythrocyte receptor for C3b (CR1) has also been described in patients with SLE. Whether this deficiency is acquired, inherited, or both, in patients with SLE, and normals, has become an area of some controversy. Utilizing functional studies and later immunoassays, investigators in Japan concluded that erythrocyte CR1 deficiency is inherited in patients with SLE.[M467,M502] Subsequently, using immunoassays, investigators in New York City demonstrated low levels in patients with SLE that correlated with disease activity.[15]

In our own studies, we have demonstrated, using both polyclonal and monoclonal antisera to the C3b receptor, that a significant number of relatives of probands (of both

patients and normals) had reduced levels of CR1 and that three phenotypes could be identified, having high, intermediate, and low levels of CR1.[W268] Family studies indicated that the levels were inherited in an autosomal codominant manner. These observations were confirmed when the original population were restudied 3 years later, and the population group expanded.[W267] Further, to help confirm the genetic influence on erythrocyte CR1 levels, a probe for CR1 was developed and used to assess genomic DNA from normals and SLE patients and their relatives. A restriction fragment length polymorphism was identified utilizing HindIII, whereby a 7.4 kb fragment correlated with high erythrocyte CR1 levels and a 6.9 kb fragment was associated with low erythrocyte CR1 levels.[15] In addition, the mean numbers of Yz-1 sites/erythrocyte for patients and relatives who were homozygous (p < .02) and heterozygous (p < .05) for the 7.4 kb allele were significantly lower than those for normal persons matched for the HindIII RFLP, suggesting the existence of additional hereditable factors that decrease CR1 expression.[W267]

In a study of normals and SLE patients in Great Britain, utilizing a monoclonal anti-CR1, patients had low erythrocyte CR1 levels.[W53] In family studies of normals, relatives often had low levels, suggesting that erythrocyte CR1 levels were inherited in normals; however, this inheritance was not demonstrable in SLE families.[W53] In a study of patients from Great Britain and North Carolina, there were no significant differences between erythrocyte CR1 levels in SLE relatives and normals.[R325] A 7.4/6.9 RFLP pattern, using a CR1 probe similar to the Boston one, was strongly correlated with erythrocyte CR1 levels in normals, patients, and relatives in patients from Great Britain,[M525] much as in the Boston study. In another study of SLE patients in Greece, utilizing the same reagents as used in the Boston study, no significant differences between SLE relatives and normals were observed, suggesting that the Greek population was similar to the Great Britain/ North Carolina study in respect to their CR1 genetics.[J137,W263] Studies from Australia, using adherence hemagglutination showed low erythrocyte CR1 levels that correlated with anti-DNA levels and complement activation and varied with time, thus presumably reflecting clinical activity; no family studies were performed.[U13] In another study from Great Britain, using monoclonal antibodies, of 56 normals and 26 SLE patients, it was concluded that low erythrocyte CR1 levels were inherited in normals and acquired in SLE.[H393] Normal erythrocytes transfused into SLE patients lost 60% of CR1 within 5 days.[W48] In a study of normals and hypertensive patients who developed hydralazine-induced SLE, low erythrocyte CR1 levels were noted in some relatives. However, in the patients, low CR1 levels were inversely correlated with circulating immune complex levels and were thought to be acquired defects.[M485]

How to reconcile these differences of acquired versus inherited abnormalities of erythrocyte CR1 levels in SLE patients is not clear.[W263,W264] However, ethnic analysis of our Boston SLE patients suggests that while the C4A null SLE patients tend to have an Anglo-Saxon heritage, the erythrocyte CR1 deficient patients have mostly a non–Anglo-Saxon heritage.[S201] However, in more recent studies of Mexicans with lupus, there was no association of RFLP (associated with low erythrocyte CR1) and SLE,[T93] further substantiating the hypothesis that genetic associations with SLE usually have an ethnic basis. In summary, both inherited (probably ethnically defined) and acquired factors contribute to low erythrocyte CR1 levels in SLE.[R326]

CR1, CR2

CR1 and CR2 deficiencies on SLE B lymphocytes and CR1 deficiencies on SLE neutrophils have also been noted;[W266,Y52] some of these deficiencies may be familial.[W266] Low levels of lymphocyte CR3 have been observed in active SLE.[G342]

POSSIBLE MECHANISMS OF INHERITED COMPLEMENT DEFICIENCY DISEASE ASSOCIATIONS

What is the role of these inherited complement component deficiencies in predisposing to disease? The association of deficiency of either C3, C5, C6, C7, C8, C3b inactivator with repeated infections is easiest to understand in light of the importance of these complement components in chemotaxis and phagocytosis. The nature of the association between the inherited complement component deficiencies, particularly the early components and SLE, is not as clear, however. These early components, including C4 and C2, do play a role in immune complex solubilization (especially C4A), the clearance of immune complexes, the generation of immunoregulatory factors, and viral neutralization.[F37,F39,F212,M220,M264,M365] Porter speculated that relatively inefficient particular C4 alleles in individuals may predispose to SLE[P267] and Briggs et al.[B491] observed that C4A null SLE patients tended to have low C4d levels. However, while C4 null individuals have deficient C4-dependent function, they have normal C3 convertase activity, which suggests a normal ability to activate C3 and all the biologic functions associated with that.[W169] The association of immune disease with heterozygous C2 and C4 deficiency, where there is adequate complement to participate in the usual complement-dependent reactions, suggests that the complement deficiency represents primarily a genetic rather than a biologic marker, and that the association between complement deficiency and SLE is due to some other factor(s).

The genes for C4 and C2 (and factor B) are on the short arm of the sixth chromosome between HLA-B and HLA-DR. The linkage of C4 and C2 null genes with HLA-DR3 and DR2, respectively, provides a clue to another possible inter-relationship. There is now increasing evidence that immune response genes may be closely linked to those of HLA.[B201] Further, a number of studies have shown that there is an increased frequency of either HLA-DR3 and DR2 (or both) in patients with SLE.[S205,A66] Therefore, the HLA-linked complement deficiencies may also be linked to immune response genes that may express themselves as immunologically mediated disease. In a sense, C2 and C4 may be only a marker gene for a subset of patients with SLE. On the other hand, C4A deficiency may also not be associated with HLA-DR3 or other HLA. In these instances, the C4A deficiency may indeed contribute to SLE directly.

SLE is also associated with deficiencies of other complement components (C1, C5, C6, C7, C8, C9, C1INH).[A54,D98,G182,H334,K126,M306,R65,R219,R327,S194,S198,T94] However, the frequency of association is so low that ascertainment bias, or chance, probably accounts for it.

The mechanism whereby deficiency of C3b receptors (CR1) on erythrocytes predisposes to SLE is not clear, but the fact that these proteins are important in immune complex clearance mechanisms provides a rationale for their association.[W264] These receptors promote immune complex clearance by binding immune complexes with the red blood cell surface and bringing them to the reticuloendothelial system where the immune complexes are stripped from the erythrocyte.[C390] The erythrocytes of SLE patients bind immune complexes of DNA–anti-DNA less well than in normals, probably because of the low number of CR1 receptors.[H419,T86] Thus the low number of C3b receptors may result in increased levels of pathogenic immune complexes in the circulation of SLE patients.

In addition to genetic reasons, acquired C2, C4, and C3b receptor deficiencies may themselves magnify clinical expression of disease. In summary, complement deficiency, such as C4A, C2, and CR1 can contribute to predisposition directly and also by their linkage to immune response (sixth chromosomal) genes.

ACQUIRED SERUM COMPLEMENT ABNORMALITIES

Vaughan et al.[V50] were among the first to show that serum complement levels are decreased in patients with SLE. Subsequently, many studies have demonstrated the association of CH50 C1q, C4, C2, and C3 levels with clinical activity,[L341,S784] although some studies have not observed this association.[A20,C12,C38,V6] SLE patients with renal disease tend to have lower mean levels of CH50, C1q, C4, and C3 than those without renal disease.[L341,S784]

Patients with active SLE who are pregnant tend to have somewhat decreased levels of CH50, C3, and C4,[B603,L353] whereas patients with pre-eclampsia (but not LE) have normal levels.[B603] Patients with primary habitual abortion and high serum levels of anticardiolipin antibodies had low (presumably acquired) C4 levels.[U19]

The complement component profile in patients with active lupus nephritis differs somewhat from that seen in other forms of glomerulonephritis. In SLE there are usually marked depressions of C1q and C4 and less substantial depressions of C3. While there may be early depressions of C1q and C4 in patients with acute poststreptococcal glomerulonephritis, this disease, as well as chronic membranoproliferative glomerulonephritis, is characterized by marked depressions of C3.[L243]

In one study,[L341] we observed the lowest mean levels of CH50, C1q, C4, and C3 in patients who had both active nephritis and active extrarenal manifestations. Of those patients with active renal disease (with or without active extrarenal manifestations) 87% had low CH50 levels, 80% had low C1q and C4 levels, and 68% had low C3 levels. By contrast, of those with only active extrarenal manifestations, 50% had low CH50 and C1q levels, 62% had low C4 levels, and 37% had low C3 levels. Associations have been noted between low levels of individual components and various facets of SLE (Table 13–3). Low factor B levels were found to be one of the best (complement) indicators of active nephritis. Patients with active vasculitis and/or cryoglobulinemia have especially low C1q and C4 levels. A normal C3 level suggests the absence of active renal disease. These studies demonstrate the qualitative and quantitative differences in the complement system of SLE patients depending on the presence of either active nephritis and/or active extrarenal disease. Patients with both renal and extrarenal manifestations tend to have the lowest levels. Patients with extrarenal manifestations alone have the most minor abnormalities. Some patients (10%) may have minor depressions of complement components without apparent clinical activity—this is especially true for C4.

Serial measurements of complement parameters have demonstrated that complement levels often increase coincidentally with clinical improvement and decreased with exacerbation.[L341] We have noted low C4 levels prior to exacerbation in 25% of patients who developed extrarenal manifestations, 67% of patients who developed active nephritis alone, and virtually all patients who developed active nephritis and active extrarenal manifestations. The most significant fall in C4, CH50, and C1q occurred early in exacerbation, whereas C3 continued to decline during the height of clinical illness. We and others have also observed exacerbations associated, or even preceded by falls in CH50 levels and/or rises in anti-dsDNA antibody levels.[S207] Normal C3 and anti-DNA levels are usually associated with inactive disease and carry a good prognosis.[L341]

We and others have also observed an inverse relationship between C1q binding immune complex levels and CH50, C1q, C4, and C3 levels.[L341] Patients with low complement levels, low titers of anti-DNA antibodies, and low levels of immune complexes may not have active disease.[L341] Immunologic tests have been used as a guide to therapy for SLE patients. Lange et al.[L48] administered steroid therapy to 15 lupus nephritis patients based on the degree of hypocomplementemia and hypergammaglobulinemia. They observed normalization of gamma globulin, anti-DNA levels, and CH50 by 21 months.[L48] Appel et al.,[A265] in a prospective study of 25 patients, guided immunosuppressive therapy by changes in CH50 and antibody to double-stranded DNA. The 5-year followup suggested that normalization of complement resulted in a trend toward stabilization of renal histology, creatinine clearance, and serum creatinine at a lower final mean dose of prednisone.[J56]

In summary, we[L341] have concluded that an isolated value of any one serologic parameter may assist in diagnosis but is not of any great therapeutic consequence. Clinical exacerbations may be predicted by serial monitoring of either C4, CH50, C1q binding assay, C3, or anti-DNA antibodies, ranked in that order of usefulness (Table 13-4).[L341] We feel that different serologic profiles exist for different types of clinical exacerbation. Combinations of serologic tests appear to be more useful in predicting exacerbations and in guiding therapy—a view shared by others.[M608,S784] In our hands, CH50, C4, C3, and C1q binding assay appeared to be the most helpful.

OTHER STUDIES ON SLE SERUM

As noted above, static measurements and even serial measurement of complement may not accurately reflect the metabolism of complement in the individual with SLE. Metabolic studies are the key, but are infrequently done because of the difficulty in isolating biologically active complement components. In the few studies performed, SLE patients with active disease generally had increased catabolism and increased synthesis of C3 and C4 even though serum levels were normal or decreased.[A156,C353,S491,T253] Several patients had low synthetic rates of certain complement components.[A156] Another approach to evaluation of the complement system in patients with SLE is quantitation of complement breakdown products, which reflect activation of the complement system. Generally the presence of these breakdown products correlated with the presence of active disease, often more so than decreased levels of the intact component. These have included studies of plasma factor Ba;[K19] plasma C4d and C3d;[K177,S275,S745] plasma iC3b neoantigen, especially with nephritis;[N53] serum terminal complement complex C5b–9,[F11,G60,H20,S67] especially in cases of nephritis;[H420] and C3a and C5a.[B192]

Atkinson et al.[A352] described two SLE patients with low CH50 levels, low levels of complement components measured by hemolytic assay, but normal levels of complement components measured as proteins (antigenically).

Table 13–4. Ability of Immune Tests to Predict Clinical Exacerbations in SLE

CH50	C3	Anti-DNA	Immune Complexes	Clinical Evidence
↓↓	↓	↑↑	Slight ↑	None necessarily
↓↓	↓↓	↑↑↑	↑↑↑	Active nephritis
↓	↓ (but normal)	↑↑↑	Slight ↑	Active extrarenal
↓↓↓	↓↓↓	↑	↑↑↑	Active nephritis and extrarenal

Table 13-3. Associations with Low Serum Levels of Complement Components

C1q	C4	C3	Factor B
Azotemia	Anti-NP*	Anti-DNA	Azotemia
Casts	Casts	Casts	Casts
High ANA		Leukopenia	Pyuria
			Hematuria
			Anemia

Other Associations	
C1q	C4
Cryoglobulins	Arthritis
Vasculitis	Rashes
Immune complexes	Nephritis

* Anti-NP = antibodies to nucleoprotein.

Plasma had normal complement levels as did serum incubated at 37° C. These sera could be shown to activate complement in vitro at 5° C. These observations re-emphasize that not all patients with low complement have active SLE; some may have genetic deficiencies, while others have complement activation in vitro but not in vivo.

Patients with drug-induced LE-like syndromes generally have normal complement levels.[B349] However, hydralazine and isoniazid (drugs implicated in drug-induced LE) inhibit the binding of C4 to an in vitro activating system,[S447] and patients with hydralazine-induced lupus tend to have (inherited) low erythrocyte CR1 levels, thereby, perhaps, reducing their ability to efficiently clear immune complexes.[M485] One can speculate that this has a genetic basis, recognizing that drug-induced LE is often associated with DR4 and that certain C4 alleles are associated with DR4. Thus complement may be directly or indirectly involved in this entity. A minority of SLE patients with isolated hemolytic anemia and/or idiopathic thrombocytopenic purpura may have mildly depressed CH50 levels.

Complement levels tend to be inversely related to cryoglobulin concentration.[G322,S623] These mixed cryoglobulins, which are considered to be cold-precipitable immune complexes, may consist of IgG, IgM, Clq, C4, and/or C3.[S192,S623] Some cryoglobulins fix complement in vitro resulting in falsely low hemolytic (e.g., CH50) but not antigen (viz. C3, C4 protein) measurements.

Although Davis and Bollet[D83] observed an inverse correlation between low complement levels and the presence of rheumatoid factors in patients with lupus nephritis; others, including ourselves, have not been able to confirm this observation.

Antibodies to complement components have been observed, including in patients with SLE. Antibodies to C1q may cause false-positive (C1q binding) assays for immune complexes.[A259,U49] Anticardiolipin antibodies correlated inversely with low levels of erythrocyte CR1 levels[H90] and directly with low levels of C4[H225] and activation of complement.[N123] (See Chapter 48.)

COMPLEMENT IN THE CSF OF SLE PATIENTS

Complement levels have been measured in the cerebrospinal fluid (CSF) of SLE patients. Because of the low protein levels in this fluid, it is impossible to do CH50 levels. However, individual components have been measured. Petz et al.[P167] noted that CSF hemolytic C4 levels were low in patients with SLE and central nervous system (CNS) involvement, while normal levels were found in those SLE patients without CNS involvement. The authors commented on the rapid (7.5%/day) decay of C4 in spinal fluids from normals even when stored at −50° C and thus reported on samples stored for 7 days or less. Hadler et al.[H13] found normal levels of CSF hemolytic C4 in both normal individuals and SLE patients with and without CNS involvement. However, when serial C4 levels were determined on patients who went from active CNS involve-

ment into remission, it was apparent that C4 levels went from a low normal value to either normal or high normal levels, suggesting that serial C4 levels might be of value in evaluating patients with definite or questionable CNS involvement in SLE. Hadler's study suggests that these assays must be done within a few hours after spinal tap, as hemolytic activity was nearly all lost within 24 hours after routine storage of CSF from SLE patients with CNS involvement, while C4 in other CSF specimens decayed less rapidly. Hadler also concluded that serum C4 values were not helpful in evaluating his four SLE patients with active CNS involvement. More recently, activated terminal complement component C5b−9 has been found in the CSF of patients with SLE with active CNS disease.[S67]

In summary, there is complement activation in the CSF of SLE patients; however, practical methods to measure these phenomena are not currently available. (See Chapter 38.)

COMPLEMENT IN TISSUES IN SLE

Further evidence for the participation of complement in SLE has been the detection of complement components in inflamed tissue particularly in the same locations as immunoglobulins and antigens. Complement components detected in renal lesions include C1q, C1s, C4, C2, C3, C5, C6, C9, properdin, and factor B.[C317,K338,L243,R345,S193,V72] However, C4 and factor B were seen infrequently, despite the fact that serum levels of these components were often low in patients with nephritis. There was no apparent difference in the components deposited in those with predominantly membranous or proliferative nephritis.[V72]

Similar complement components have been found at the dermal-epidermal junction of patients with skin lesions.[G141,P314,R345,S193,T47] The presence of C4 is highly suggestive of SLE.

SUMMARY

SLE is characterized by a host of immune abnormalities. It is not clear to date which of these are primary and which are secondary. The observation of a number of genetic defects suggests that they are primary. Multiple genetic defects may then lead to abnormal immune responses to common pathogens, antigens, or even autoantigens. As a result of this abnormal immune response, immune complexes form with resultant complement fixation and activation. These immune complexes interacting with cells and complement initiate an inflammatory response. One can also speculate that this inflammatory response represents a normal response to an abnormal event, or is also abnormal in the SLE patient. The ultimate result is tissue inflammation and often damage.

While at present our therapy is aimed at controlling these secondary inflammatory phenomena mediated by immune complexes and complement, ultimately therapy may be more successful after the primary defects are corrected.

Chapter 14

EICOSANOIDS; PROSTAGLANDINS, LEUKOTRIENES, AND RELATED LIPID MEDIATORS*

DWIGHT R. ROBINSON

The eicosanoids are a class of mediators that are derived from enzymatic reactions of polyunsaturated fatty acids (PUFAs) with molecular oxygen. Although each compound has its own characteristics, there are some general properties that apply to all eicosanoids.[C247,N49,S63] These compounds are ubiquitous and are produced by all mammalian tissues, and each type of cell produces certain eicosanoids. In general, the eicosanoids are not preformed and stored in cells. Rather, upon stimulation cells initiate the biosynthesis and secretion of these compounds. The eicosanoids are autocrine or paracrine agonists, acting at or near their sites of origin. They are often potent agents and only accumulate in low concentrations in body fluids. They are generally labile, either because of chemical instability, or because of enzyme-catalyzed metabolism in the blood or tissues. These properties lead to some difficulties in eicosanoid measurements. The most meaningful measurements would involve eicosanoid concentrations at local sites of action, which may be inaccessible. Eicosanoid measurements require highly specific and sensitive assays, which may not always be available. As an alternative to direct measurements, it may be necessary to measure a metabolite of a given eicosanoid in the blood or urine, but these measurements may not reflect correctly the quantities of an eicosanoid at its site of action.

Because of their potency and the nature of their actions, the levels of eicosanoids must be closely regulated in tissues.[M153] Their synthesis must be rapid when called for, and their metabolism to inactive products must occur when their actions are no longer desired. The substrates for the synthesis of eicosanoids, the PUFAs, are present in large quantities in tissues, but only small proportions of the available substrate are usually utilized for eicosanoid synthesis at any given time. The major substrate for eicosanoids, arachidonic acid (AA) is abundant in tissues, predominantly in ester linkage in cell phospholipids. It has been generally accepted that activation of eicosanoid synthesis requires the induction of arachidonic acid release from phospholipids, since the levels of nonesterified arachidonic acid in resting cells is low, and it is insufficient to provide sufficient substrate for the production of the quantities of eicosanoids that many cells are capable of producing when certain stimuli are present. Eicosanoids

are only produced from the free, nonesterified forms of AA. The release of AA and other PUFAs is catalyzed by phospholipases of two major types, phospholipase A_2 and phospholipase C. Phospholipase A_2 hydrolyzes fatty acids from the $sn2$, or middle carbon of the glycerol moiety of phospholipids to yield the free or nonesterified fatty acids and lysophospholipids (Fig. 14-1). Phospholipase C hydrolyzes phospholipids at the $sn3$ carbon of glycerol to yield phosphorylated bases and diacylglycerol. A particularly important group of phospholipases C are the enzymes that act on phosphatidylinositol (PI) phosphates to produce the second messengers, diacylglycerol and inositol phosphates. The action of the C phospholipases do not result in the release of free fatty acid directly, but the subsequent action of lipases on diacylglycerol breaks that compound down into free fatty acids and glycerol. Phospholipases are activated by a large number of cell stimuli, such as hormones and other agonists.[G148] The C phospholipases acting on PI phosphates are activated by agonists interacting with receptors linked to specific G proteins, gp, and to C phospholipases. Other phospholipases, such as the A2 phospholipases, are activated by agonists that induce the influx of calcium ion.

BIOSYNTHESIS OF EICOSANOIDS

The eicosanoids are synthesized through the cyclo-oxygenase and several lipoxygenase pathways.[L247,N49,S63] These reactions are initiated by abstraction of hydrogen from a PUFA, usually arachidonic acid, followed by the addition of oxygen and rearrangements of the structure of the original fatty acid.[K447,S290] The best-known products are produced according to the biosynthetic pathways outlined in Figures 14-2, 14-3, and 14-4). The cyclo-oxygenases are ubiquitous in tissues and carry out the initial reactions on the pathways of synthesis of prostaglandins (PGs) and thromboxanes.[N49] This enzyme adds two molecules of molecular oxygen to AA to produce PGG_2, an unstable endoperoxide intermediate. In the cyclo-oxygenase reaction, a five-membered ring is formed that is characteristic of the prostaglandins. The PGG_2 is converted to PGH_2 in a peroxidase reaction, which is also catalyzed by the same cyclo-oxygenase molecule that catalyzes the formation of PGG_2. This second endoperoxide, PGH_2, is then converted to PGs and thromboxane by either isomerase or synthase enzymes, which differ in different cells. For example, the major cyclo-oxygenase

* Supported by grants from the NIH (AR 03564, AI 28465) and the Davis Family Foundation.

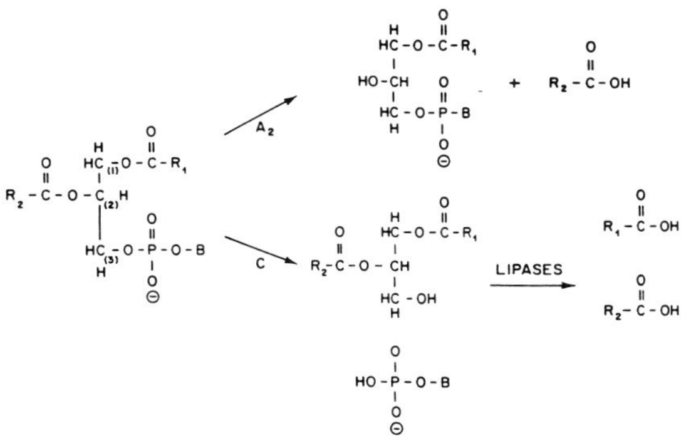

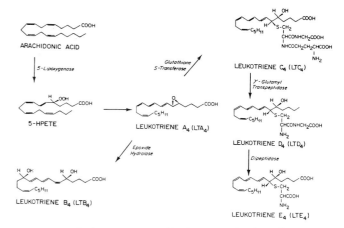

Fig. 14–1. The actions of phospholipase A_2 and phospholipace C on phospholipids. Either pathway can result in the release of arachidonic acid from the *sn2*, or middle carbon atom of the glycerol moiety of phospholipids. From Robinson, D.R., and Zvaifler, N.J. (eds.): Rheumatic disease clinics of North America. Vol. 13. *In* Pathogenesis of chronic inflammatory arthritis. New York, W.B. Saunders, 1987. With permission.

Fig. 14–3. The biosynthesis of leukotrienes by the 5-lipoxygenase pathway. From Robinson, D.R., and Zvaifler, N.J. (eds.): Rheumatic disease clinics of North America. Vol. 13. *In* Pathogenesis of chronic inflammatory arthritis. New York, W.B. Saunders, 1987. With permission.

product of blood platelets is thromboxane A_2, which is produced by thromboxane synthase in platelets acting on PGH_2. In vascular tissues, the major cyclo-oxygenase product is prostacyclin, or PGI_2, produced by the enzyme, prostacyclin synthase. Thus the nature of the cyclo-oxygenase produced in tissues depends on the cellular composition of that tissue and its enzyme complement. The lifetime of the cyclo-oxygenase products under physiologic conditions is generally transient. Some of the products are chemically unstable, such as thromboxane A_2 and PGI_2, which break down rapidly under physiologic conditions into thromboxane B_2 and 6-keto-$PGF_{1\alpha}$, respectively. Other products are chemically stable but are converted by enzymes in tissues to inactive metabolites, of which there may be large numbers. Urinary metabolites have often been useful as an estimate of eicosanoid pro-

duction, although usually any single metabolite represents a small proportion of the original eicosanoid produced.[L331] Nonetheless, the quantities of a metabolite may reflect the overall production of a given metabolite in the body, assuming that changes that are taken to reflect changes in the production of an eicosanoid take place in the absence of any changes in the metabolism of the eicosanoid.

The products of the cyclo-oxygenase pathway differ greatly in their biologic properties.[N49,R251] Some cyclo-oxygenase products have effects on the vasculature, which may contribute to inflammation (Table 14–1). The vasodilator PGs, primarily PGE_2 and PGI_2, not only increase blood flow to the microvasculature, but they may

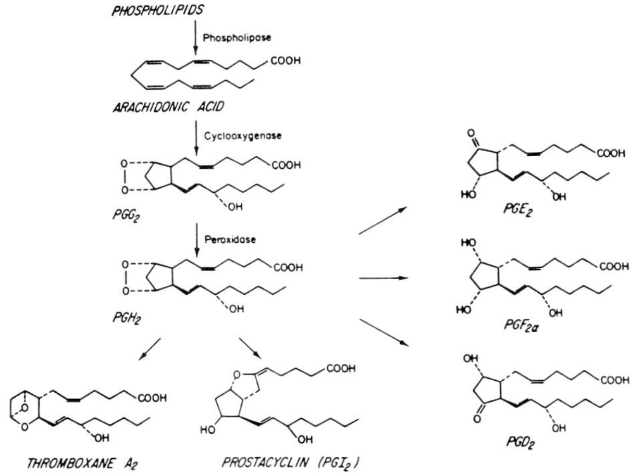

Fig. 14–2. The biosynthesis of prostaglandins and thromboxane A_2 through the cyclo-oxygenase pathway. From Robinson, D.R., and Zvaifler, N.J. (eds.): Rheumatic disease clinics of North America. Vol. 13. *In* Pathogenesis of chronic inflammatory arthritis. New York, W.B. Saunders, 1987. With permission.

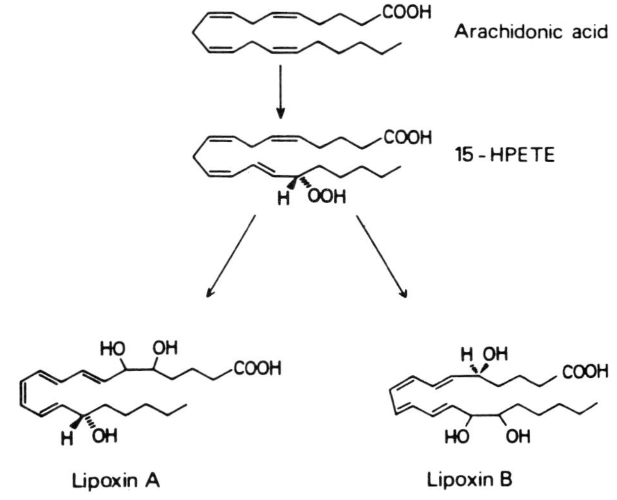

Fig. 14–4. The biosynthesis of lipoxins. From Robinson, D.R., and Zvaifler, N.J. (eds.): Rheumatic disease clinics of North America. Vol. 13. *In* Pathogenesis of chronic inflammatory arthritis. New York, W.B. Saunders, 1987. With permission.

Table 14–1. Some Functions of Eicosanoids Related to Inflammatory Reactions

PGE_2, PGI_2	Vasodilation
	Act synergistically with other mediators, including bradykinin, histamine, $C5_a$, and LTB_4 to increase vascular permeability
	Bronchodilation
	Inhibition of platelet aggregation
	Stimulation of osteoclastic bone resorption
PGD_2	Vasodilation
	Increased vascular permeability
	Bronchoconstriction
	Stimulation of random migration of neutrophils and eosinophils
LTC_4, LTD_4, LTE_4	Vasoconstriction, bronchoconstriction
	Production of wheal and flare reaction in skin
	Augment bronchial mucous secretion
LTB_4	Chemotaxis and chemokinesis of neutrophils, eosinophils, and monocytes
	Promotion of leukocyte adhesiveness and adherence to endothelium
	Promotion of secretion of reactive oxygen species and hydrolytic enzymes by neutrophils

From Robinson, D.R., and Zvaifler, N.J. (eds.): Rheumatic disease clinics of North America. Vol. 13. In Pathogenesis of chronic inflammatory arthritis. New York, W.B. Saunders, 1987. With permission.

act synergistically with other mediators to enhance microvascular permeability, perhaps through vasodilation. These PGs sensitize nocioeptors to painful stimuli, and they produce fever through stimulation of thermoregulatory centers in the midbrain. Therefore PGE_2 and PGI_2 can duplicate the cardinal signs of inflammation, but evidence also indicates that they may have anti-inflammatory effects as well. These PGs may inhibit the production of other inflammatory products from leukocytes.[R62] The increased microvascular permeability induced by certain experimental immediate hypersensitivity reactions appears to be mediated by histamine and sulfidopeptide leukotrienes. The release of these mediators from tissue mast cells is inhibited by PGE_2, and the increased microvascular permeability following antigen challenge in sensitized animals is augmented by inhibition of PGE_2 synthesis by the nonsteroidal anti-inflammatory drugs. Similarly, systemic anaphylaxis induced by antigen challenge in vivo is aggravated by cyclo-oxygenase inhibitors, and the latter result in marked enhancement of the production of sulfidopeptide leukotrienes in tissue fluids.[L150,R250] Thus PGE_2 and PGI_2 may enhance inflammatory reactions through vasodilation, but these mediators also have the potential to modulate or inhibit inflammation by inhibiting the secretion of other inflammatory mediators produced by leukocytes. The basis for the aggravation of allergic reactions by cyclo-oxygenase inhibitors in aspirin-hypersensitive individuals may reside in the removal of the inhibition of mediator release by prostaglandins. While the latter hypothesis may account for this infrequent effect of the NSAID, clearly these drugs are anti-inflammatory under most conditions. As is discussed below, it seems likely that cyclo-oxygenase inhibition also has anti-inflammatory effects through removal of the vasodilator actions of the prostaglandins, but this conclusion remains a hypothesis

rather than an established fact. Other studies have shown that administration of the E prostaglandins to experimental animals can suppress inflammation. While these findings point out that the E prostaglandins may have pharmacologic effects that are anti-inflammatory, issues of dose, distribution, and other considerations make it difficult to extrapolate these effects to the effects of these prostaglandins when they are produced endogenously.

The prostaglandins may also modify immune reactions.[G296,R251] The mitogen-induced proliferation of T cells is inhibited by PGE_2, and the proliferation and maturation of B cells is also inhibited by PGE_2, in association with elevations of the levels of cyclic $3',5'$-AMP that are induced by PGE_2 in cells.[M73,M454,R46,S453] The inhibition of T-cell mitogenesis produced by PGE_2 was shown to be secondary to elevations in the levels of $3',5'$-cyclic AMP, which inhibits the production of the cytokine, interleukin-2 by T cells.[M73] These in vitro observations suggest that the production of PGE_2, and probably other prostaglandins that stimulate $3',5'$-cyclic AMP should have immunosuppressive effects. Thus, cyclo-oxygenase inhibitors should be capable of enhancing or activating immune responses. Such immune stimulation has not been obvious in clinical settings. In fact, the use of therapeutic doses of NSAIDs has been associated with suppression of serum levels of rheumatoid factor in patients with rheumatoid arthritis, although the mechanism of this suppression is unknown.[C187,C460] Thus, although lymphocyte activation is inhibited by prostaglandins in vitro, the inhibition of prostaglandin synthesis that is associated with the clinical use of NSAIDs does not seem to activate the immune system in any obvious way. Further investigation is needed to reconcile this apparent discrepancy.

Finally, PGE_2 and PGI_2 stimulate osteoclastic bone resorption. Since the rheumatoid synovial pannus produces large quantities of PGE_2, the development of erosions in juxta-articular bone may be mediated in part by this mechanism.[R251] Several cytokines, such as interleukin-1, stimulate prostaglandin production as well as stimulate osteoclastic bone resorption in bone cultures. At least some of the cytokine-stimulated bone resorption may be mediated by the PGE_2 resulting from IL-1 stimulation, but evidence also exists that some cytokines may also stimulate bone resorption by prostaglandin-independent mechanisms.

LIPOXYGENASE PRODUCTS

The lipoxygenases are named for the position of the AA molecule into which they introduce molecular oxygen to produce lipid hydroperoxides. Three major lipoxygenases are present in mammalian tissues, the 5-, 12-, and 15-lipoxygenases.[S63,S290] The major leukotrienes (LTs) are products of the 5-lipoxygenase pathway following the formation of 5-hydroperoxyeicosatetraenoic acid (Fig. 14–3). The same enzyme molecule converts this initial product into an epoxide, the first leukotriene, LTA_4. The LTA_4 is an intermediate compound that may react with additional enzymes to form several important LTs. In one reaction, LTA_4 is converted to LTB_4 by LTA_4 hydrolase. The second pathway from LTA_4 is its conversion to LTC_4 through addition of glutathione to the 6-carbon position of AA by the

Table 14–2.   Role of AA-Derived Lipids in SLE

Eicosanoid Alterations in SLE
1. Patients with nephritis
   Elevated urinary PGE$_2$
   Elevated urinary thromboxane B$_2$
   Reduced urinary levels of 6-keto-PGF$_{1\alpha}$ (metabolite of PGI$_2$)
   Treatment with NSAIDs/salicylates inhibits production of PGE$_2$, PGI$_2$ and thromboxane A$_2$ and reduces creatinine clearance.
2. Mice with lupus nephritis
   Nephritis is associated with increased production of LTB$_4$, LTC$_4$, and LTD$_4$ by renal cells.
   Administration of LT antagonist improves renal function.
Dietary Modifications that Influence SLE
1. Mice with lupus
   Addition of n-3 marine lipids to diets reduces severity of nephritis. γ-Linolenic acid (evening primrose oil) supplementation prolongs life in MRL/lpr mice.
2. Patients with lupus
   High doses of fish oil supplement may reduce disease activity in some settings.

enzyme glutathione-S-transferase. The product, LTC$_4$, is converted to two other compounds, LTD$_4$ and LTE$_4$, by the sequential removal of γ-glutamyl and glycine residues. The three compounds, LTC$_4$, LTD$_4$, and LTE$_4$, are called the sulfidopeptide leukotrienes, compounds that account for the activity previously known as slow-reacting substance of anaphylaxis, an important mediator of immediate hypersensitivity reactions.

Products of the 5-lipoxygenase pathway are important mediators of inflammation.[L247,S63,S290] One of these compounds, LTB$_4$, is a strong chemoattractant for leukocytes, and it also promotes the adherence of leukocytes to endothelial cells, which is a necessary preliminary step prior to migration of leukocytes into extravascular sites of inflammation. Conversely, the sulfidopeptide derivatives, LTC$_4$, LTD$_4$, and LTE$_4$, contract smooth muscle in several tissues. These LTs have similar actions, but they vary in potency in some cases. They cause vasoconstriction, but they increase microvascular permeability. They are thought to be important mediators of bronchial asthma since they also cause bronchoconstriction and they increase the flow of bronchial mucus. The sulfidopeptide LTs may affect several organs; for example, they stimulate mesangial cells contraction and they exert negative inotropic and arrhythmogenic actions on the heart.

Several other lipoxygenase products are known that have biologic activity.[L247,S63,S290] Among them are products that arise from the combined activity of more than one lipoxygenase, such as the 5- and the 15-lipoxygenases, the lipoxins (Fig. 14–4). The lipoxins A$_4$ and B$_4$ are vasodilators, and they have modest chemotactic activity. They inhibit the cytotoxic activity of natural killer cells. As an intracellular mediator, lipoxin A$_4$ may activate protein kinase C with a potency comparable to diacylglycerol. It has been also postulated that the lipoxins may have counterregulatory properties toward the LTs. As an example, lipoxin A$_4$ inhibits the chemotactic responses of neutrophils to both a chemotactic peptide and LTB$_4$. The precursor of lipoxin A$_4$, 15-hydroxyeicosatetraenoic acid, has anti-inflammatory activity in psoriasis lesions, and in experimental carrageenan-induced arthritis.[S290]

Finally, AA may be oxidized by several microsomal cytochrome P$_{450}$ mono-oxygenase enzymes to form a large number of compounds, many of which are biologically active (Fig. 14–5). Three classes of products formed are 1) epoxyeicosatraenoic acids, which may each react with epoxide hydrolases to form vicinal diols of eicosatraenoic acid; 2) hydroxyteraenoic and ketotrienoic acids; and 3) the 19- and 20-hydroxy derivatives of arachidonic acid. Several of these compounds have biologic activities including vasodilatation, vasoconstriction, angiogenesis, Na$^+$-K$^+$-ATPase stimulation, activation of immediate early response genes, stimulation of peptide hormone release, mobilization of microsomal calcium, and inhibition of platelet aggregation. Since a mono-oxygenase reaction could take place at each double bond in AA, each leading to several products, a complex array of products is potentially available from these reactions, and the biologic significance of these compounds is not yet well understood. Some of these products can participate in inflammatory reactions, and several are known to be produced by the kidney and to have effects on renal cell function.

MODIFICATION OF EICOSANOID SYNTHESIS

Eicosanoid synthesis must be highly regulated. Since there are large quantities of AA in cell membranes, exces-

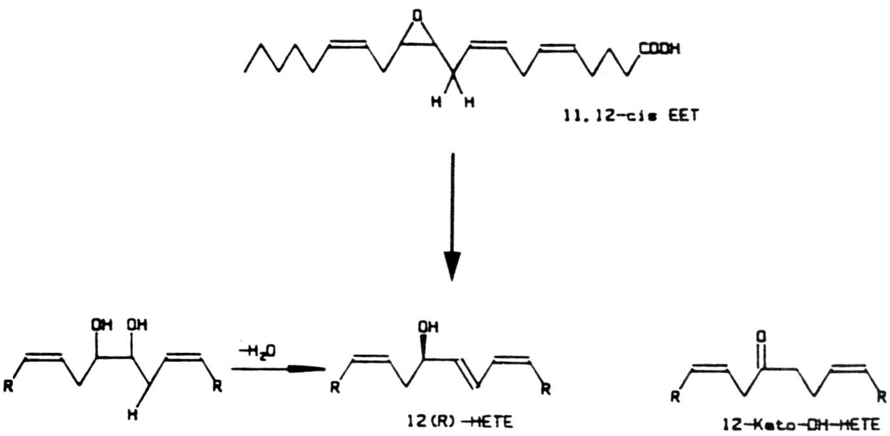

Fig. 14–5. Epoxyeicosatraenoic acid and some of its derivatives formed by a cytochrome P$_{450}$–dependent reaction of arachidonic acid.[M670] Adapted from Murphy, R.C., Fakk, J.R., Lumin, S. et al.: 12(R)-Hydroxy eicosatrienoic acid: A vasodilator cytochrome P-450-dependent arachidonate metabolite from the bovine corneal epithelium. J. Biol. Chem., 263:17197, 1988.

sive production of eicosanoids could damage cell membranes by removal of PUFAs, and excessive quantities of eicosanoids could lead to drastic tissue reactions.[M153] A wide variety of physical and chemical stimuli lead to the synthesis of eicosanoids. Some of these stimuli are receptor-mediated, highly specific events and others are more general. Receptor activation in some cases may activate phospholipases and release AA for eicosanoid synthesis. Other stimuli may induce the synthesis of the enzyme cyclo-oxygenase, which may enhance the capacity of the cell to produce cyclo-oxygenase products.[R81] The best-known pharmacologic manipulations of eicosanoid synthesis are the use of nonsteroidal anti-inflammatory drugs (NSAIDs) and glucocorticoids, both of which inhibit prostaglandin synthesis. Another manipulation that alters eicosanoid synthesis is to change the intake of PUFAs in the diet, which can in turn change the composition of the PUFAs in tissues. We will consider these approaches to manipulating eicosanoid synthesis at this point.

The NSAIDs, including aspirin and related drugs, have the common property of inhibiting PG synthesis by inhibiting the enzyme cyclo-oxygenase. Inhibition of cyclo-oxygenase by these drugs was first described by Vane and coworkers, who subsequently postulated that the major pharmacologic effects of these drugs could be accounted for by their ability to inhibit PG (and thromboxane) synthesis.[F70] Several lines of evidence have continued to support this hypothesis since it was proposed over two decades ago. Some of the evidence in favor of the Vane hypothesis may be summarized as follows.[F70,R251] Many of these drugs, although they differ in chemical structure and pharmacologic potency, have similar clinical indications and effects, such as their use in the treatment of patients with rheumatoid arthritis. Extensive correlations have shown that the relative anti-inflammatory potency of different NSAIDs parallels their potency as inhibitors of PG synthesis in vitro. For example, indomethacin, a potent cyclo-oxygenase inhibitor, is used in lower doses than aspirin, a weak cyclo-oxygenase inhibitor, in the treatment of rheumatoid arthritis. Yet both indomethacin and aspirin can achieve similar therapeutic efficacy in rheumatoid arthritis when used in appropriate doses. Both drugs can also effectively inhibit PG synthesis, but much higher concentrations of aspirin than indomethacin are required to achieve a comparable degree of inhibition. Correlations between anti-inflammatory effects and PG synthesis inhibition by some NSAIDs have a high degree of specificity. For example, the d-stereoisomer of naproxen is active both as an anti-inflammatory agent and as a cyclo-oxygenase inhibitor, whereas the l-isomer is relatively inactive in both respects. These and similar correlations demonstrate that subtle changes in structure result in dramatic and parallel changes as both anti-inflammatory agents and a cyclo-oxygenase inhibitors. Another important observation is that for several NSAIDs the peak concentrations of free, non–protein-bound drug that are achieved under clinical circumstances are in the range of the concentrations that inhibit PG synthesis in vitro. Therefore, it is reasonable to conclude that the NSAIDs as used clinically are capable of inhibiting PG synthesis in vivo, in inflammatory exudates. Thus, the hypothesis that the NSAIDs

exert their therapeutic effects through inhibition of PG synthesis is reasonable and well supported, and alternative mechanisms that have been proposed lack this degree of support. It has been suggested that nonacetylated salicylate is an exception to the Vane hypothesis, since salicylate has comparable anti-inflammatory efficacy to aspirin but lacks inhibitory effects on cyclo-oxygenase. Actually, studies of an experimental model of inflammation, carageenan-impregnated sponges in rats have shown that aspirin and nonacetylated salicylate have similar abilities to inhibit the inflammatory response in this model system, and the anti-inflammatory effects of both drugs is paralleled by similar reductions in the levels of PGE_2 in these tissue exudates.[H300] It has also been shown that salicylate and aspirin are comparable inhibitors of PG synthesis in humans, based on measurements of a urinary PGE metabolite.[H175] Thus, salicylates need not be considered exceptional to other NSAIDs. Nonacetylated salicylate is comparable to aspirin both as a cyclo-oxygenase inhibitor in vivo, and as an anti-inflammatory agent, both experimentally and in the treatment of rheumatoid arthritis. It might be pointed out the high potency of aspirin as an inhibitor of thromboxane synthesis in platelets is specific for those elements. Studies have shown that platelet cyclo-oxygenase is irreversibly acetylated by aspirin in the mesenteric circulation, as a presystemic compartment.[P89a] The inability of platelets to synthesize new enzyme results in permanent loss of cyclo-oxygenase activity for the lifetime of the platelet.

Several other mechanisms have been proposed to account for the actions of NSAIDs, but none of these mechanisms have been presented with compelling support.[A17,B511] The secretion of mediators and enzymes by activated neutrophils can be inhibited by various NSAIDs in vitro. However, these changes do not correlate with anti-inflammatory effects, and the inhibitions are seen at concentrations of non–protein-bound drug, which are higher than levels that are achieved in vivo.[A17] Thus, there is no persuasive evidence that inhibition of secretion of these neutrophil products contributes significantly to the pharmacologic effects of NSAIDs.

It is also well accepted that many of the toxic side effects of the NSAID can also be accounted for by PG inhibition. For example, inhibition of gastric PG synthesis can account for the upper gastrointestinal toxicity of these drugs by reducing the cytoprotective actions of PGE_2 on the gastric mucosa. These cytoprotective effects of PGE_2 can be attributed to several actions of this compound on the mucosa,[S267] including inhibiting acid secretion by the parietal cells, augmenting the protective phospholipid and mucous layers on the mucosal surface, increasing the secretion of bicarbonae, and enhancing gastric mucosal blood flow through vasodilation. One practical application of these findings was the development of orally ingested PGE derivatives for the prophylaxis and treatment of gastric mucosal injury induced by NSAIDs.[G331]

Renal toxicity may also may be mediated by inhibition of renal PG synthesis.[C305] Although deleterious effects on renal function are not generally seen in individuals with normal cardiovascular and renal function, patients in whom the circulating blood volume has been reduced by various pathologic states may suffer deterioration of renal function when treated with NSAIDs. Renal synthesis of the vasodilator PGs are important for maintaining adequate renal blood flow under conditions where effective renal blood flow is reduced. These states include the nephrotic syndrome, cirrhosis of the liver with ascites, and congestive heart failure with diuretic therapy. Under these conditions, PG inhibition may precipitate or aggravate renal failure. Early studies pointed out that patients with systemic lupus with some degree of renal involvement had evidence of elevated PGE production by the kidney, and that aspirin treatment decreased glomerular function in association with reduction in the levels of urinary PGE (see below).

A final example that we shall consider is the inhibition of platelet function by NSAIDs. As noted above, this is especially prominent in the case of aspirin because of the irreversible inhibition of platelet cyclo-oxygenase by acetylation. Other cells are able to compensate for this inhibition for two major reasons. First, nucleated cells are generally capable of synthesizing new cyclo-oxygenase. Second, the levels of aspirin in the bloodstream are transient since plasma esterases rapidly hydrolyze aspirin to salicylate following absorption. Because of this platelets in the mesenteric circulation are exposed to higher levels of aspirin than many peripheral tissues.[P89a] Thus, doses of aspirin in the range of 30 mg/day was shown to completely and irreversibly inhibit platelet cyclo-oxygenase, with no significant effect on the synthesis of PGI_2, which is produced by sources other than platelets.[P67] In spite of nearly complete inhibition of platelet cyclo-oxygenase by aspirin, platelet function is only mildly impaired, and becomes of clinical significance only if other coagulation defects, such as anticoagulant therapy, are simultaneously present. The combined use of NSAIDs and anticoagulants probably increases the risks of massive upper gastrointestinal bleeding, but definitive evidence to define this risk is lacking.

GLUCOCORTICOIDS

The most potent anti-inflammatory drugs, the glucocorticoids, also inhibit the production of both cyclo-oxygenase and 5-lipoxygenase products. This has been attributed to the formation of intracellular proteins termed lipocortins, which are augmented by glucocorticoids.[C272,D70] The lipocortins inhibit phospholipases and therefore would be expected to inhibit the formation of eicosanoids on this basis. Studies have also demonstrated that the glucocorticoids inhibit the stimulated synthesis of the enzyme cyclo-oxygenase by interleukin-1.[F293] An additional effect that would be expected to reduce eicosanoid synthesis is the ability of glucocorticoids to inhibit the synthesis of cytokines, including interleukin-1 and tumor necrosis factor α, both of which strongly stimulate PG synthesis.[K175,L410] Thus, glucocorticoids may inhibit eicosanoid synthesis through several possible mechanisms. The ability of these agents to inhibit LT production[L247] as well as PG synthesis may account in part for their greater potency than NSAIDs, but mechanisms other than inhibition of eicosanoid synthesis probably contribute to the anti-inflammatory actions of glucocorticoids.

EICOSANOID ALTERATIONS IN SLE

As noted above, patients with SLE with active renal disease were found to have elevated levels of urinary PGE, presumably reflecting enhanced synthesis of PGE_2 by the kidney, compared to normal individuals. In addition, treatment with aspirin caused deterioration of renal function and sodium retention, and these changes were interpreted to be secondary to inhibition of renal PG synthesis.[K214] Subsequent studies by others have demonstrated that SLE patients with nephritis had elevated urinary levels of thromboxane B_2, the inactive metabolite of the potent vasoconstrictor thromboxane A_2, and elevated levels of urinary PGE_2, consistent with the previous studies by others.[P68] Conversely, urinary levels of 6-keto-$PGF_{1\alpha}$, the stable metabolite of the vasodilator PGI_2, or prostacyclin, were reduced in these SLE patients. The cyclo-oxygenase inhibitor, ibuprofen, was associated with reduced excretion of these three metabolites, as well as reduction in glomerular filtration rates. Apparently, the inhibition in production of renal PGI_2 and PGE_2 by ibuprofen outweighed the potentially deleterious effects of the vasoconstrictor and mesangial cell contracting agent, thromboxane A_2, since the net result of inhibition of all three of these cyclo-oxygenase products was associated with deterioration of renal function, as reflected in reduced creatinine clearance rates.[P68] Thus, patients with lupus nephritis frequently respond to NSAIDs with deterioration of renal function, and thus these drugs must be used with caution, if at all, in this setting. Individuals with mild renal impairment of other causes often tolerate NSAIDs well, but the possible aggravation of renal insufficiency must be monitored for in all patients with any degree of renal impairment, even if their cardiovascular status is normal. Patients with contracted circulating blood volume and high renin states must receive NSAIDs with extreme caution, even if their renal function tests are normal.

Evidence from studies in murine lupus indicate that LTs may contribute to the pathogenesis of renal disease in this animal model.[S602] The spontaneous renal disease in MRL-1pr/lpr mice was accompanied by enhancement of ionophore-stimulated production of LTB_4 and the sulfidopeptide LTs, LTC_4 and LTD_4, in vitro. Administration of a specific sulfidopeptide antagonist to mice with renal dysfunction resulted in improvement in renal function. Other studies demonstrated that administration of a thromboxane A_2 antagonist had little effect on renal dysfunction in this animal model, and therefore the beneficial effect of sulfidopeptide LT blockade is not likely to be secondary to an indirect effect on thromboxane production. Likewise, chronic administration of a cyclo-oxygenase inhibitor had no significant effect on the development of the glomeulonephritis in MRL-1pr/lpr mice.[K153] Therefore, cyclo-oxygenase inhibitors may be deleterious to patients with lupus renal disease, as discussed above, but studies with murine lupus suggest that LT blockade could be useful for improving renal function in human SLE. (See Chapter 41.)

DIETARY LIPID MODIFICATION IN SLE

The PUFAs are necessary constituents of cell membranes for the maintenance of normal health. These fatty

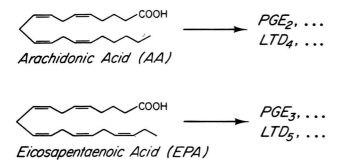

Fig. 14–6. Arachidonic acid and eicosapentaenoic acid are important members of the n-6 and n-3 fatty acids, respectively. Alternatively, these fatty acids may be referred to as omega-6 and omega-3, since the double bond in each molecule nearest the methyl terminal carbon atom is 3 and 6 carbon atoms from the terminal carbon atom. From Robinson, D.R., and Zvaifler, N.J. (eds.): Rheumatic disease clinics of North America. Vol. 13. *In* Pathogenesis of chronic inflammatory arthritis. New York, W.B. Saunders, 1987. With permission.

acids are primarily members of two classes, either n-3 or n-6, determined by the location of the double bond that is nearest to the terminal carbon atom of the molecule (Fig. 14–6). These PUFAs are referred to as essential fatty acids, since they are required for normal health. They must be obtained in the diet, since mammalian tissues cannot insert double bonds into the n-3 or the n-6 positions of fatty acids, whereas plants are capable of producing these compounds.[L112] It is notable that the fatty acid composition of tissue lipids is dependent upon the dietary intake. Terrestrial food sources in Western diets are generally plentiful in n-6 PUFAs, whereas marine sources, as well as certain plants and grains, are enriched in n-3 fatty acids. These fatty acids are sufficiently abundant that dietary essential fatty acid deficiency is rare, but under certain extreme or experimental conditions, essential fatty acid deficiency may result in a disease state consisting of skin rashes, growth retardation, reproductive failure, and other manifestations.[Z25] Under these conditions, the n-3 and n-6 PUFAs are depleted from tissue fats, and are replaced at least in part with n-9 PUFAs. With diets containing PUFAs, the quantities of n-3 and n-6 fatty acids in tissues may be altered depending upon the relative quantities of these classes of fatty acids in the diets. There has been considerable interest in recent years in the possibility that the composition of dietary PUFAs may influence susceptibility to various diseases.[L112,S459] Epidemiologic studies of Greenland Eskimos called attention to this possibility when it was recognized that although these individuals ingested a high-fat diet, comparable to the fat content of the diets in Western industrialized societies, they were found to have a much lower prevalence of cardiovascular disease compared to individuals ingesting Western diets.[K432,L112] The most obvious difference between the diets of Western and Eskimo societies was the high content of n-3 fatty acids in the Eskimo diet, which was derived from cold water marine sources. Since these early

observations a large number of epidemiologic and experimental observations have established that diet-induced changes in the ratios of n-3 to n-6 fatty acids in tissue lipids have important consequences for cell function and disease susceptibility.[L112,S459] The enrichment of tissues in n-3 fatty acids usually is accompanied by reductions in the contents of AA and other n-6 PUFAs, and this change may be associated with reductions in the capacities of cells to produce the eicosanoids that are derived from AA. In addition, the n-3 fatty acids, especially the AA analoge eicosapentaenoic acid, may be converted into eicosanoids that are analoges of those eicosanoids derived from AA. Since the n-3 eicosanoids frequently differ in their functions from their n-6 eicosanoid analoges, these changes in the nature of the eicosanoids produced as a consequence of increasing the n-3 fatty acid content of tissues may contribute to the differences in cell function and disease states that are induced by diets enriched in n-3 fatty acids. In addition, other changes in cell membranes apart from changes in eicosanoids may also contribute to the observed functional changes.[H65,L112,L183,L147]

In addition to the beneficial effects on cardiovascular diseases, the n-3 fatty acid diets lead to anti-inflammatory effects in several experimental disease states, and in a small number of clinical trials. Such effects were suggested by observations of the health statistics of Greenland Eskimos. These data revealed a reduced frequency of psoriasis and allergic diseases, compared to Danish controls.[K431] Studies of murine lupus then demonstrated that dietary marine lipids markedly reduced the severity of the autoimmune glomerulonephritis in several murine lupus strains.[R248] The anti-inflammatory effects of marine lipid diets were not observed in all disease models, however, in that the severity of type II collagen-induced arthritis in rats was not modified by a marine lipid diet. In fact, the incidence of the arthritis was increased in the fish oil fed rats.[P297] Subsequently however, other investigators reported that type II collagen-induced arthritis in female mice was alleviated by dietary fish oil.[L198] It was also shown that a fish oil diet suppressed the elevation of the amyloid P component during the acute-phase response.[G281a]

These studies in experimental inflammatory and autoimmune disease suggest that dietary alterations of PUFAs could modify the course of SLE and perhaps other autoimmune diseases. Several controlled trials of the treatment of patients with rheumatoid arthritis with dietary fish oil supplements have demonstrated modest clinical anti-inflammatory effects.[C297,K415,K416,V19] Thus far, these benefits were associated with the ingestion of modest quantities, up to approximately 6 g/day of n-3 fatty acids, in the form of refined fish oil triglycerides or ethyl ester preparations. Several studies of peripheral blood leukocytes from human volunteers or from patients with rheumatoid arthritis have demonstrated that these dietary preparations are capable of reducing the production of inflammatory mediators ex vivo.[L147,S589] The production of LTB$_4$ by neutrophils and monocytes after stimulation with a calcium ionophore is significantly reduced from cells from individuals ingesting fish oil preparations compared to controls. Although some LTB_5, a product derived from eicosapentaenoic acid, was produced by cells taken from the fish oil–treated individuals, the quantities were small, and other studies have shown that LTB_5 is much less biologically active than LTB_4. This reduction in the capacity of inflammatory cells to produce LTB_4 by dietary n-3 fatty acids would be expected to exert an anti-inflammatory effect. Additional cellular effects that might be anti-inflammatory include reduction of monocyte production of platelet-activating factor, reduced neutrophil adherence to endothelial cells, and reduced neutrophil chemotactic responsiveness, all of which were seen with cells from fish oil–treated individuals.[L147,S589]

There has been little study of the effects of n-3 fatty acids on patients with SLE. This is unfortunate in view of the dramatic degree of effectiveness of n-3 fatty acids on the glomerulonephritis of murine lupus. An initial pilot study of SLE patients for 1 year revealed no significant clinical benefits, but active renal disease was infrequent in these patients.[M557] Another study involved 12 patients with SLE and nephritis ingesting up to 18 g of a fish oil preparation for periods of 5 weeks.[C288] Changes in serum lipids were seen that were considered to be antiatherogenic, and decreased platelet aggregation was induced, consistent with many previous studies on individuals without SLE. No significant changes in anti-DNA antibodies, immune complex levels, or albuminuria were observed, and clinical symptoms were not described in this study. These authors suggested that antiatherogenic effects could be useful, but that the chronic nature of the proteinuria and the brief duration of the fish oil treatment both could have precluded the induction of other beneficial results. Finally, in a report of a 34-week placebo (olive oil) controlled trial of 20 g of a fish oil supplement daily in SLE patients, significant improvement in clinical symptoms were reported based on individual patient assessments, although no objective data were reported.[W62] This study suggests that the ingestion of fish oil supplements may be beneficial in patients with SLE, but the effects of this intervention on nephritis and other serious organ system involvement has not yet been adequately investigated. (See Chapters 3 and 55.)

OTHER POLYUNSATURATED FATTY ACIDS

Another alteration in dietary PUFAs that has been investigated is the supplementation of the diet with oils containing γ-linolenic acid, 18:3 n-6 (GLA). This fatty acid is formed from the desaturation of linoleic acid and is present in various plant oils, although usually in lower abundance than linoleic acid. The GLA is then elongated to dihomogammalinolenic acid (DGLA), which is in turn desaturated to AA.[Z58] The DGLA is an analog of AA containing 20 carbon atoms but lacking a double bond in the 5,6 position. Reactions of DGLA with cyclo-oxygenase forms the one series PGs, e.g., PGE_1, which contains only one double bond, and has properties that differ in some respects from PGE_2. Ingestion of oils enriched in GLA elevate the levels of GLA in tissues as well as the GLA metabo-

lites, DGLA and AA. These changes, with their accompanying increases in eicosanoids derived from DGLA, especially PGE_1, are postulated to modify cell functions and many disease states, with beneficial results. Anti-inflammatory effects of GLA supplements have been reported on carrageenan-induced footpad edema, and in urate-induced inflammation in the rat subcutaneous air pouch.[Z58] Perhaps the best-established therapeutic benefit of the GLA-enriched oils is the effect of evening primrose oil, a GLA-enriched oil, on atopic eczema.[M612] In addition, a controlled trial of an evening primrose oil dietary supplement in rheumatoid arthritis patients appeared to produce modest anti-inflammatory effects.[B175] Some of these and other preliminary reports of therapeutic effects of GLA oils are promising, but more definitive studies are needed to establish the role of this intervention in inflammatory and other diseases. Studies in lupus patients have not yet been reported, but evening primrose oil was reported to prolong the lifespan of MRL/1pr mice.[G210]

INHIBITION OF LIPOXYGENASE PRODUCTS

A great deal of effort has been directed toward the development of agents that specifically inhibit lipoxygenase products, and studies have begun to appear describing the clinical investigation of some of these compounds. Although glucocorticoids have been reported to inhibit the production of both prostaglandins and leukotrienes, these hormones have a broad range of activities that may contribute to their undesirable side effects, and it seems likely that specific inhibitors of leukotrienes and certain other lipoxygenase products may have anti-inflammatory effects with fewer undesirable actions. The agents of most interest have been specific inhibitors of 5-lipoxygenases and leukotriene antagonists. The 5-lipoxygenase inhibitor A-64077 reduced symptoms of nasal congestion in allergic rhinitis,[K318] and the same drug ameliorated the asthmatic response to inhaled cold, dry air.[150] In another study, the LTD_4 receptor antagonist MK-571 reduced exercise-induced bronchoconstriction.[M101] These results indicate both that the LTs have a significant role in human allergic diseases, and that drugs that inhibit these mediators may be useful therapeutic agents.

SUMMARY

A large body of evidence now supports an important role for the eicosanoids in inflammatory rheumatic diseases, and in a variety of other disease states. Eicosanoids with important functions in these diseases include products of the cyclo-oxygenase and lipoxygenase pathways, including the prostaglandins, thromboxanes, and leukotrienes. Many of these compounds act on the vascular phases of inflammation, inducing vasodilation and increased vascular permeability, but others are vasoconstrictors, and alter inflammatory cell function, and a variety of other important cell functions in tissues. Modification of production of eicosanoids results from the use of a number of anti-inflammatory drugs, including non-steroidal anti-inflammatory drugs, glucocorticoids, and inhibitors and antagonists of the leukotrienes. The modification of eicosanoid pathways by these drugs is likely to account for at least some of the therapeutic and toxic actions of these compounds, and further development of lipoxygenase inhibitors promises to yield some useful therapeutic agents. The production of eicosanoids also may be modified by changes in the polyunsaturated fatty acid composition of phospholipids in cells induced by changes in dietary lipids. These dietary alterations, such as the substitution of marine lipids for most terrestrial lipid sources, may alter cell functions and disease susceptibility through mechanisms that involve changes in eicosanoid production as well as other not yet well-defined mechanisms.

Chapter 15

IDIOTYPES AND IDIOTYPE NETWORKS

BEVRA H. HAHN AND FANNY M. EBLING

HISTORY

In 1963, Oudin and Michel[O124] proposed the concept of idiotypes (Ids) and anti-idiotypes (anti-Ids) when describing rabbit antibodies inducing antibodies against themselves. In the same year, Kunkel et al.[K464] described Ids on human antibodies. In 1974, Jerne[J72] suggested the idea that Ids and anti-Ids participate in self-regulatory immune networks. Since then, many investigators have established the importance of Ids in immune regulation, and in experimental manipulation of cell function and immune responses.

DEFINITIONS

Terms used in defining idiotypes and idiotypic networks are listed in Table 15–1. Idiotopes are antigenic regions located in the variable regions of immunoglobulin (Ig) molecules or T-cell antigen receptors (TCRs). Single Ig molecules can express several different idiotopes; the series of idiotopes is referred to as the idiotype for that molecule. Since the exact structural basis of most idiotopes is unknown, the term idiotype is widely used to describe the entire antigenic region on Igs or TCRs. An antibody produced in response to antigen expresses Id and is called Ab1 to define its place in the Id immune network.

Idiotypes are divided into two general classes—private and public. Private Ids are expressed on Igs or TCRs that expand from a single parent clone. Therefore, private Ids define antibodies or T cells that are clonal and specific for a single stimulating antigen. In contrast, public Ids (also called cross-reactive Ids) are expressed on Igs and TCRs deriving from different parental cells. Therefore, Igs and TCRs displaying public Ids bind several different antigens and are likely to appear in many different individuals of the same species. Further, public Ids may be found on antibodies in individuals of different species. For example, public Ids on anti-DNA antibodies derived from certain mouse strains are found on anti-DNA and other Igs in humans.[E15,E53]

Since idiotypes are antigenic, they stimulate production of anti-idiotypic antibodies (anti-Ids), which are referred to as Ab2. Ab2 molecules are divided into at least two subtypes, depending upon whether they mimic Ag.[J74] $Ab2_\alpha$ binds Ab1 but otherwise shares no properties of the initial stimulating Ag. $Ab2_\beta$ binds Ab1 and also behaves in other ways like Ag. They can stimulate production of more Ab1 and can bind to receptors that ordinarily bind Ag. This property was first noted in insulin systems;[S250] some Ab2 against anti-insulin Ab1 could bind the insulin receptor on cell surfaces and actually trigger glucose metabolism by those cells. $Ab2_\beta$ anti-Ids are also called internal image anti-Ids, after a suggestion of Nisonoff and Lamoyi,[N106] implying that they share structural similarities with Ag. Some authors refer to them as "epibodies" or "homobodies."

Since Ab2 molecules express Ids, they stimulate production of anti–anti-Ids (Ab3).

Within the variable region of each Ab1 is a region that binds the epitope of the stimulating antigen. The region on Ab1 that binds Ab2 is called a paratope. If the paratope- and epitope-binding regions of the Ab1 molecule overlap or are located close to each other, binding of either (by epitope of Ag or paratope of Ab2) may inhibit binding of the opposite molecule.

IDIOTYPE NETWORKS

Idiotype networks are complex. Two features are particularly important. First, members of the network regulate each other, thus serving to control immune responses. Second, the network links immune responses to self with immune responses to the external environment.

Antigen-Antibody Id Networks

There are at least two major concepts of Id networks. The most widely held view, suggested originally by Jerne[J72] and later expanded him and others,[J73,J74,K170,N106,R258,S250,U25] is illustrated in Figure 15–1. This concept is based on information suggesting that convex epitopes on Ags are bound by concave regions in the antigen-binding groove of Ig molecules, as suggested by x-ray crystallographic studies of an Ag-Ab complex.[A185] Similarly, convex regions on Ab1 molecules are bound by concave regions in the binding groove of Ab2; the same process permits binding of Ab3 to Ab2.

This Id network regulates itself in at least two ways, as shown in Figure 15–1. First, as discussed above, some Ab2 molecules behave like Ag; they stimulate Ab1 production, bind Ag receptors, and can probably trigger cell activation under certain conditions. As illustrated in the figure, these $Ab2_\beta$ internal image anti-Ids have sequences or conformations highly similar to those on Ag. This property of anti-Id serving as surrogate Ag has been used to isolate and characterize receptors[S250] and to stimulate production of neutralizing Ab1—thus using Ab2 as a vaccine.[N106,K170]

Table 15–1. Definitions

1. *Idiotope.* A region on the variable portion of an immunoglobulin molecule or T-cell antigen receptor that is antigenic. When present on an antibody molecule, the antibody may be referred to as Ab1.
2. *Idiotype.* A series of idiotopes on the same molecule.
3. *Private idiotype.* An Id expressed only on the products of a single B- or T-cell clone. Antibodies and T cells bearing private Ids will be specific for only one antigen (Ag).
4. *Public idiotype.* An Id expressed on different B- and T-cell clones which interrelates them. Antibodies and T cells bearing public Ids are in sum able to recognize multiple different Ags. These are also referred to as cross-reactive Ids or shared Ids.
5. *Anti-idiotype.* An antibody directed against the idiotope on immunoglobulin, B-cell surface, or T-cell antigen receptor. This antibody may be referred to as Ab2.
6. *Anti-Id type 1.* Also called Ab2$_\alpha$, this Ab2 binds to Ab1 but does not otherwise behave like antigen (Ag).
7. *Anti-Id type 2.* Also called Ab2$_\beta$; also called homobody, internal image anti-Id, or epibody. This Ab2 binds Ab1 and behaves in additional ways like Ag. For example, it can bind to receptors for Ag and by so doing can trigger cell activation.
8. *Anti–Anti-Id.* An antibody against Ab2. It may also be referred to as Ab3. Some Ab3 molecules share structural similarities to and behave like Ab1; for example, they may bind the Ag to which the original Ab1 is directed.
9. *Epitope.* The region of an antigen bound by Ab1.
10. *Paratope.* The region of an antibody or T-cell receptor bound by anti-Id.
11. *Connectivity.* The property of one Id network influencing the development of another. For example, the Ids on mature immune responses develop in sequence to different Ids expressed on Ig in fetal mice.
12. *Parallel sets.* A network of Ab1-Ab2-Ab3 that is interactive.
13. *Network antigen.* An Ab2 that can react either with Ag or with Ab1 and therefore can regulate the entire Ag-Ab1-Ab2-Ab3 Id network.

Second, some Ab3 molecules have properties of Ab1, in that they can bind the original Ag. An elegant demonstration of the entire network, from Ag to Ab3, has been reported in a study using the O-specific polysaccharide side chain of Pseudomonas aeruginosa as Ag to raise Ab1 and Ab3 in mice; both Ab1 and Ab3 were opsonizing, protective antibodies that prevented lethal infection.[S178] Structural mimicry between Ag and Ab2 has been reported in the GAT system;[M222] an amino acid motif in GAT was present in Ab2 and recognized by Ab3.

Although experimental results in many Id–anti-Id systems fit the Jerne hypothesis, numerous exceptions have occurred. For example, some Ab2 molecules can serve as surrogate Ags even though their binding to Ab1 is not Ag inhibitable, suggesting that they are not internal image anti-Ids. Such observations have led to another hypothesis of Ag-Id–anti-Id interactions, reviewed by Kohler and colleagues.[K348] This hypothesis suggests that interactions between Ag, Ab1, Ab2, etc., can occur via side chains/conformations outside the Ag-binding groove of Ig. Such side chains can serve variably as Ag or as Ab. For example, Ab2 might have a side loop on the variable region of the molecule that is similar to one on Ag and on Ab1. Whether Ab2 binds Ab1 or Ag will depend primarily on the relative avidity for each reaction. Ab3 might share a side chain with Ab1 by which it could bind Ag. None of these interactions depend upon the ability of Ag or sequences on Ig molecules to fit into the Ag-binding groove.

Both hypotheses regarding Id interactions may be correct, and they may occur simultaneously. Further, three-dimensional shapes of Ag, Ab1, Ab2, etc., may change as interactions occur, exposing new sequences/conformations to the immune system for extension of the network.

T Cells in Idiotypic Networks

The preceding discussion addressed Ag induction of circulating Ab1, Ab2, and Ab3. Naturally, B lymphocytes secreting the Abs express the same Ids on their surface Ig. In addition, T lymphocytes are involved in Id–anti-Id networks. Several experiments have shown that Ab2 can bind to and in some cases activate T cells.[B311,E46] Figure 15–2 illustrates the mechanisms by which B and helper T cells interact to activate each other and to up-regulate production of Igs bearing certain Ids. Current concepts of T-cell activation require interaction between antigenic peptides presented by the MHC to the TCR of T cells. In general, helper T cells (TH) recognize Ag presented by MHC class II; cytotoxic T cells (Tcyt) recognize Ab presented by MHC class I. B lymphoma cells can internalize their surface Ig, process it, and present immunoglobulin-derived, *idio*peptides to TCRs.[W162] Activation of a TH cell by this method is shown in Figure 15–2. In addition to the presentation of idiopeptides, B cells may be able to activate T cells via intact surface Ig. In the antiphosphocholine (PC) antibody response of BALB/c mice, Ab1 molecules bear a dominant Id called T15. Helper T (L3T4+) cells can bind intact T15+ Ig, but not isolated heavy (H) or light (L) chains, and can detect different conformational idiotopes.[D358,C182] The same principle applies to Ab2: dendritic cells (which presumably cannot process Ig) can present Ab2 to helper T cells.[F208] Ig can probably stimulate both B and T cells; in the reovirus system, a B-cell epitope has been defined in the CDR2 region of the Ig light chain, and a T-cell epitope in the CDR2 of the heavy chain.[B531,W247]

Activation of Id-recognizing TH cells is probably necessary for full-scale production of Id-bearing antibodies, as shown in Figure 15–2. Activation of TH cells releases B-cell growth and differentiation lymphokines, which in combination with cell-cell contact results in B-cell production of Ab1, Ab2, etc.[W342]

TCRs can serve as immunogens for developing the Ab1/Ab2/Ab3 network, as well as a regulatory T network, as shown in Figure 15–2. For example, immunization of B10.D2 mice with an anti-Id made against the Id on the TCR of a TH clone specific for Sendai virus was effective in producing virus-specific 1) neutralizing antibody, 2) delayed-type hypersensitivity, 3) cytotoxic T cells, and 4) protection against infection.[E135]

Id-recognizing TH cells may be distinct individual cells, or the recognition of Id may be a property of cells that can also recognize Ag epitopes. In several murine antibody systems, including anti-PC and anti–(T,G)A-L, there is collaboration between TH cells that recognize the Ag and the Id or anti-Id. However, TH cells that bind to Ab1 or Ab2 and specifically enrich Id+ antibodies have been detected.[D358,K125]

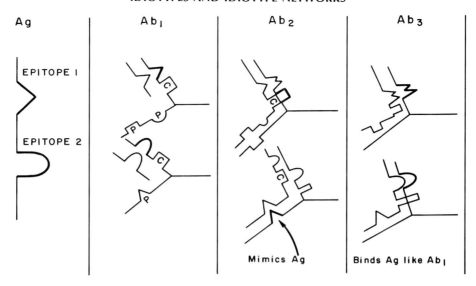

Fig. 15–1. The antibody idiotype network. In the first panel, an antigen (Ag) with two epitopes is shown. In the second panel, two antibodies (Ab1) against the antigen are shown: the top Ab1 recognizes epitope 1 and the bottom Ab1 recognizes epitope 2. Each Ab1 has a idiotope specific to that clone—a private Id (p). Both Ab1 contain an identical sequence or conformational idiotope, designated as a cross-reactive (C) or public Id. Thus, the private Ids identify distinct clonal Ab specific for one Ag, and the public Ids identify related families of Ab that derive from different clones and can recognize different epitopes. In the third panel, two anti-idiotypic antibodies (Ab2) have been induced by Ab1. The upper Ab2 is an α type; it binds Ab1 but does not mimic Ag. The lower Ab2 is a β type; it contains a sequence that mimics an epitope on the original Ag and can behave like Ag (bind receptors for Ag, stimulate Ab1, etc.) It is called Ab$_B$ or internal image anti-Id, or an epibody. In the fourth panel, two antibodies (Ab3) induced by Ab2 are shown. The upper Ab3 binds only Ab2. The lower Ab3 has a sequence or conformation that mimics a sequence/conformation in Ab1; it can bind Ag. Some, but not all, members of the network have the capacity to regulate other members. From Hahn, B.H.: Idiotype and antiidiotype antibodies. *In* Autoimmunity and Molecular Biology. Edited by E. Brahn. Boston, Little, Brown & Co. In press. With permission of the publisher.

T-cell participation in Id networks is not confined to cells with helper function. Manipulation of the Id network can produce T cells that participate in delayed-type hypersensitivity, suppress Ab1 responses, kill cells expressing surface Ag or Ab2, and suppress proliferation of cells expressing the target Ids on their TCRs.[B117,D250,D251, E135,K125]

THE STRUCTURAL BASIS OF IDIOTYPES

Definition of exact amino acid sequences on H or L chains of Ig molecules which define idiotopes has been possible in only a few systems. Anti-Ids react exclusively with H or L chains of some monoclonal antibodies, indicating that sequences/conformations confined to those chains confer idiotypy. Examples of public Ids located on H chain include 1) antidextran Abs in BALB/c mice[C302] (two amino acids and/or carbohydrates in the CDR2 of the H chain), 2) anti-*p*-azoarsonate antibodies[M335,C74,S512] (amino acids in the D region), 3) antigalactan antibodies in mice[R410] (sequences in the D region of the H chain), and 4) macroglobulins with blood group I and i specificities.[237] Ids associated with L chains have been described on 1) inulin-binding myeloma proteins,[L277] 2) antibodies to streptococcal group A carbohydrate,[N16] and 3) the 8.12 Id on some human anti-DNA antibodies.[L338] Interestingly, some anti-Ids react with both V_H and V_L:

such reactivity has been described for antithyroglobulin antibodies[Z9] and a monoclonal cold agglutinin.[K330]

It is clear that Ids can be separated from Ag specificity in some antibodies. Amino acid substitutions at two to three locations in the CDR2 of the H chain of BALB/c anti-a($1 \rightarrow 6$) dextran MAbs abolished expression of the public idiotope without changing Ag binding.[S427]

However, the structural basis of most Ig and T-cell Ids has eluded definition. Many anti-Ids apparently recognize conformations, since both V_H and V_L are required for their expression. Since public Ids are found on Abs with different specificities, in different individuals of the same species, in unrelated individuals, and even across species, it is assumed that they are products of highly conserved germline genes. Such public Ids can be assembled from different V_H and V_L gene families.[P31,V79] Therefore, it is likely that different genes code for similar or identical amino acid sequences in idiotopes, or that several different noncontiguous sequences, especially when presented in the context of two Ig chains, assume conformations that are recognized by anti-Id Ig or anti-Id T cells. By analysis of hydrophilic side groups unique to certain Ig molecules, Kieber-Emmons et al.[K194,K195] have postulated that five regions on V_H and six on V_L can participate in Id structure. These are called IDRs, for idiotype-determining regions. Using that model, and applying sequence data from eight different MAbs expressing the A48 Id of anti-

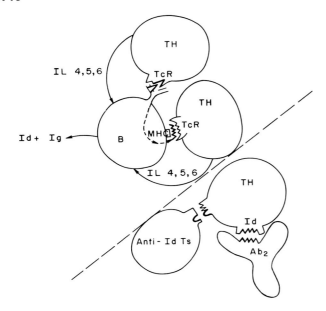

Fig. 15–2. The T/B-Cell idiotypic network. In the top panel, T helper cells that augment autoantibody production are shown. They are idiotypic TH cells. The upper TH cell has a TCR that recognizes an Id on the surface immunoglubulin (Ig) of an Id+ B cell. The lower TH cell has a TCR that recognizes an idiopeptide processed by the B cell from its surface Ig and presented by a MHC class II molecule. Both Id TH cells secrete B-cell stimulatory factors (IL-4, 5, and 6) that up-regulate production of the Id+ antibody. In the lower panel, the Id TH cell recognizes the idiotope on an Ab2 in one region of its TCR; another region of TCR has induced an anti-Id suppressor T cell (Ts), which can suppress the Id TH cell. Thus, both B and T cells participate in cellular and humoral regulatory networks governed by idiotypes. From Hahn, B.H. Idiotype and antiidiotype antibodies. In Autoimmunity and Molecular Biology. Edited by E. Brahn. Boston, Little, Brown & Co. With permission of the publisher. (In press.)

fructan antibodies in BALB/c mice, Victor-Kobrin and colleagues[V79] found one subset of Id+ MAbs with identical amino acid replacements in hydrophilic residues in three of the IDRs of L chain. They confirmed earlier information that Id expression is also influenced by a lysine or asparagine at position 73 in the H chain. However, some Id+ MAbs did not follow these rules, so that some regions that confer idiotypic specificity in this system are not completely defined.

IDIOTYPIC REGULATORY CIRCUITS

Some Ids are regulatory, in that they can be suppressed or up-regulated by other members of the circuit, and can in turn regulate the other members. Early information regarding regulation suggested that anti-Ids served to suppress expression of their complementary Ids on antibodies to specific antigens.[P80,W129] On the other hand, some anti-Ids can up-regulate target Ids, even to extent of activating silent B-cell clones that normally do not express their Id-bearing Ig. For example, BALB/c mice usually do not express the A48Id on their antifructosan Abs. However, administration of any of the following can force expression of that Id: 1) A48Id at birth, 2) polyclonal or

monoclonal anti-Ids at birth, or 3) KLH-linked polyclonal anti-Id in adults.[V79] In some systems, certain Ids or anti-Ids are either enhancers or suppressors of Id expression, whereas other Id-bearing MAbs do not regulate the circuit.

In many experiments with Ids and anti-Ids, the dose and timing of administration are critical to the results. In general, administration of small quantities of Ids or anti-Ids up-regulates Id expression, whereas administration of large quantities suppresses Id expression. For example, as shown in Figure 15–3, immunization of young NZB/NZW F_1 (BW) mice with small quantities (200 ng) of anti-IdX (a public Id on anti-DNA in BW mice) in Freund's adjuvant resulted in accelerated appearance of two autoantibodies—IdX+ anti-DNA and IdX+ antihistone.[H24] In contrast, as shown in Figure 15–4, repeated administration of large doses of anti-IdX (100 μg every 2 weeks) to adult BW mice suppressed IdX+ Ig, anti-DNA, and the lupus-like nephritis associated with anti-DNA in this mouse strain.[H29,H32] Thus, the same MAb anti-Id could be used to either enhance or suppress the Id-bearing Ig.

Id-recognizing T cells can also be used to alter immune responses. For example, infusion of T cells that have been sensitized to Ids of CD4+ T cells that recognize alloanti-

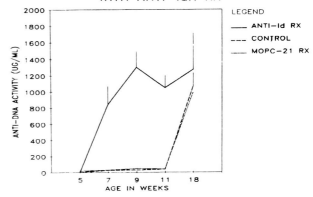

Fig. 15–3. Up-regulation of Id+ antibodies to DNA by administration of anti-idiotypic antibodies in NZB/NZW F_1 mice. This is an example of an up-regulating Id network. Small doses (200 ng) of a monoclonal anti-IdX (made by immunization with an IdX+ antibody to DNA) were injected into young BW mice, and the appearance of anti-DNA in their sera was compared to littermates injected with the carrier or with an Id-negative monoclonal antibody (MOPC-21). Injections were made at 4 weeks of age. Anti-Id–treated mice developed high titers of antibody to DNA by 7 weeks of age. In the control groups anti-DNA appeared at 11 weeks (when the mice ordinarily begin to develop antibody); 95% of the anti-DNA in the anti-Id–treated mice expressed IdX. The same mice also made IdX+ antihistone antibodies at an earlier age than the controls. Thus, the anti-Id activated an Id+ autoantibody network that resulted in production of different autoantibodies expressing the same cross-reactive, public Id. From Hahn, B.H.: Idiotype and antiidiotype antibodies. In Autoimmunity and Molecular Biology. Edited by E. Brahn. Boston, Little, Brown & Co. With permission of the publisher. (In Press.) (The experiments were performed by Karen Dunn, M.D.)

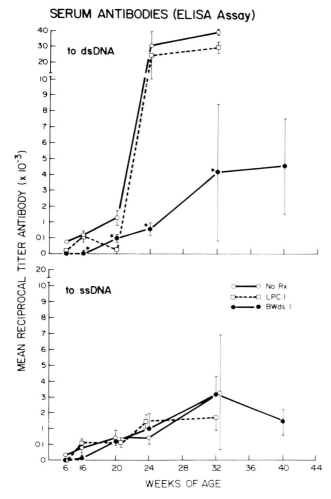

SERUM ANTIBODIES (ELISA Assay)

Fig. 15–4. Down-regulation of autoantibody responses by anti-idiotypic antibodies. The idiotypic system is being studied in these experiments and the experiments shown in Figure 15–3. In this case, high doses of monoclonal IdX (200 μg weekly), which induce anti-IdX, were given repeatedly to NZB/NZW F₁ females beginning at 20 weeks of age. Antibodies to dsDNA (*upper panel*) were significantly suppressed in IdX-treated mice (*solid line, closed circles*) compared to two control groups (*open symbols*). This is an example of an anti-Id induced by Id down-regulating an autoantibody. From Hahn, B.H., and Ebling, F.M.: J. Clin. Invest. *71*:1728, 1983. With permission of the publisher.

gens results in suppression of the ability of TH cells to proliferate to those Ags, and prolongs allograft survival.[B117]

Although regulatory properties of public Ids can be used to alter in vivo immune responses, in some systems, the Id network escapes from such regulation.[H129,H132,L236] One mechanism of escape is somatic mutation of the Id so that it is no longer recognized by anti-Id.[L236] Since mutation of Ig molecules is common in B cells, whereas it is yet to be demonstrated in the TCR of T cells, this escape mechanism probably applies only to Ids on Ig. In NZB/NZW mice treated with anti-Ids, escape of Id + antibodies from suppression occurs without evidence of mu-

tation of the Ig; this might represent a change in Id-directed T-cell help.

ROLE OF IDIOTYPES IN MATURATION OF THE IMMUNE RESPONSE

In adults, the normal B-cell repertoire is probably dependent on establishment of essential idiotypic networks during fetal life. Studies of B-cell hybridomas obtained from fetal and 1- to 2-week-old normal BALB/c mice have defined early antibody responses in the pre-immune and early immune states.[H392,V3] Two properties are clear: 1) many early Ig molecules bind to self antigens, including V regions of Ig, and 2) this pre-immune network is highly connected via idiotypy. In general, antibodies produced during the first week of gestation bear Ids that are not positively selected later: responses to similar Ag in the neonate or 1- to 3-week-old mouse carry different Ids, and those Ids are positively selected for expansion, even in adult life. This idiotype switch is probably independent of environmental stimuli. In fetal Ab responses to dextran or phosphocholine (the first Ag from E. cloacae and the second from the pneumococcus) the entire network of Ag, Ab1, Ab2, and Ab3 can be found. Further, a single Ab2 can react with Ab1 from different B cells, i.e., with both anti-PC and antidextran Ab1. Such Ab2 molecules are regulatory;[V3] they can either suppress the fetal Id + Ig or enhance the more mature public Ids characteristic of 2- to 3-week-old mice, depending on the MAb Ab2 and the timing of administration. The interplay of the different Ab2 molecules in suppressing or enhancing fetal or mature Ids has been called connectivity. It suggests that the original Ab1 responses in the fetus express determinants that activate the Id network and are critical for determining the idiotypic profiles of the adult immune response. Kearney has referred to the early multispecific B cell as a superorganizer, influencing many generations of B cells that follow. This early network can be influenced by administration of Id + Abs that do not bind the initiating Ag, so the network is at least partly independent of Ag and can operate via recognition of Id alone. Any interference with the newborn network (by administration of Ag, Ab1, Ab2, or Ab3) results in impairment of normal antibody responses in adult life.

USE OF IDIOTYPIC NETWORKS TO PREVENT INFECTIOUS DISEASES

There has been great interest in using the Id network to raise protective B- and T-cell responses to infectious agents.[E135,F207,G67,K169,K170,K171,K172,M310,M351,N106,N138,R88,R266,S11,S178,S634,T125,V42,V43,W195] There are at least three situations in which this approach has advantages over standard immunizations with attenuated, killed, or carrier-linked infectious agents. First, some organisms are so highly infectious that a batch that is not adequately killed or attenuated can produce disease. This is of special concern for organisms with a high mutation rate that allow new virulent forms to emerge that escape immune surveillance, such as HIV. Second, patients who are immunosuppressed are not only poor responders to standard attenuated vaccines (e.g., vaccinia), but may be subject to infection by them. Third, neonates and infants are unable to make good immune response to T-independent antigens, such as polysaccharides in cell walls of enteric bacteria. For example, infants with cystic fibrosis are predisposed to Pseudomonas superinfection. Finally, anti-Id vaccines would be useful in infectious diseases for which there are currently no effective immunizations, such as rabies, certain gram-negative bacteria, meningococcus, HIV, etc.

The use of Id networks to protect against infectious disease relies mainly on immunizations with Ab2 (anti-Ids), raised against Ab1 or against T cells. Ab2 molecules are chosen that bear the internal image of the Ag, or induce Ab1, Ab3, and/or cytotoxic T cells that are Ag specific. These concepts are discussed above. For bacterial infections, opsonizing antibody responses are probably adequate to prevent infection; for viral infections, both neutralizing antibodies and cytotoxic T cells are desirable. Id or anti-Id vaccines effectively protect animal models from infection with trypanosomes, some viruses (hepatitis B, reovirus encephalitis, Sendai, Venezuelan equine encephalitis virus) and certain bacteria (pneumococcus, E. coli, capsular polysaccharide of Neisseria meningitidis C, O-polysaccharide of Pseudomonas aeruginosa).[E135,F207, G67,K172,M310,N138,R88,R266,S11,S178,S634,T125,V43,W195] Some Id –anti-Id vaccines activate only Id-based antibody circuits, others only T cells, and still others the entire antibody/ T-cell Id network.[E135,N138,G67]

The idiotype approach to vaccination may prove to be useful; however, in one series of experiments, immunization with Ab2 *increased* susceptibility of mice to infection with herpes simplex.[K169] Such a result is predictable, based upon the Id regulatory circuits discussed above.

To date, no direct attempts to induce immunity in humans with anti-Id have been published. Ab2 molecules raised in an antirabies system have been shown to activate human CD4 + T cells,[J42] and the antihepatitis B Ab1 molecules of humans react with Ab2 made in mice.[K171] The closest work to human use is the demonstration that Ab2 in a hepatitis B mouse system could induce protective immunization in chimpanzees—a species that is susceptible to clinical hepatitis B.[K171] Therefore, anti-idiotype vaccines remain an interesting but unproven approach to prevention of infectious diseases in humans.[M351]

IDIOTYPES ON MONOCLONAL PARAPROTEINS AND MALIGNANT CELLS

Monoclonal paraproteins and malignant cells both possess idiotypes. They are described below.

Idiotypes on Paraproteins

The initial studies defining Ids in humans were performed on monoclonal paraproteins. Rheumatoid factor (RF) activity is common among paraproteins from unrelated individuals. Further, many RF+ paraproteins express one of a few public Ids, suggesting that genes capable of encoding them are frequent in unrelated humans. Germline information that codes for those Ids has been identified.[A227,B225,C116,C223,C225,G280,K462,K465] An Id designated Wa by Kunkel and colleagues is present on 60% of

IgM-RF cryoglobulins; a second Id designated Po is expressed on an additional 10%.[K462] A common Id on human IgM paraproteins was designated 17.109 by Carson and colleagues.[C116] Both Wa + and 17.109 + RF use restricted V_H, V_L, and J segments.[C116,C223,C225,G280,K465,N72] One human germline V_κ gene encodes the 17.109 Id; that gene is designated V_κRF or V_κ325 or humkv325.[C223,C116] Most monoclonal RFs utilizing V_κRF also use an H chain derived from the V_H1 germline gene region designated hv1263 or 783 V_H.[C225,N72] Most are synthesized by CD5 + B cells. The V_κ and V_H rearranged genes encoding these RFs vary from germline by 2 to 11 amino acids. Therefore, it is possible that closely related but different V gene families are used. In summary, human paraproteins with RF activity are oligoclonal and use highly restricted germline gene material from both V_H and V_κ regions.

One would predict from such data that the mono- or oligoclonal RF products of lymphoproliferative malignancies would display idiotypic restriction, and that is the case. The majority express the public Ids 17.109, PSL2, or PSL3.[C116] About 20% of neoplastic CD5 + B cells from patients with chronic lymphocytic leukemia express κ chains on their surfaces derived from the V_κRF gene.[K245]

In contrast to the situation with monoclonal RFs, the anti–gamma globulins that appear during infections or in autoimmune diseases are polyclonal. The V_κRF and V_H1 genes are usually found on a minority of those RFs.

Idiotypes on Tumors

Analysis and therapy of tumor cells can be approached using Id–anti-Id strategies. First, any malignant cell that expresses an Ig or TCR molecule on its surface should be able to elicit anti-Id responses. Second, since some Ab2 molecules either contain internal image of antigens or can recognize other sequences/conformations neighboring the Ag-binding site, some tumor-associated surface antigens (TAAs) might also react with anti-Ids. The approach of using surface Ags of various types to raise anti-Ids, and then using selected Ab2 molecules to identify malignant cells, predict tumor spread, and treat disease, has been tried by many laboratories. Tumors analyzed in this manner include human B-cell lymphomas and leukemias, murine B-cell lymphomas, human T-cell leukemias, and human and murine mammary virus-associated tumors.[B228,B287,B524,B525,C48,C49,C71,M337,R77,S522,S685]

The largest body of work has been done in B-cell leukemias and lymphomas, both in humans and in mice.[B524,B525,C48,C49,C71,M337,R77,S685] Patients with various types of B-cell lymphomas have been treated with anti-Ids.[B525] In initial studies, an anti-Id specific for each patient's tumor cells (obtained from biopsy specimens) was made. Of 15 patients treated repeatedly with one to three different anti-Ids, two entered longterm remissions (>6 years), and 7 others showed partial remissions lasting 1 to 12 months. Later studies combined anti-Ids with lymphokines such as α-interferon, with a higher rate of partial responses.[B524] Another investigator[S685] has suggested a strategy for defining public, rather than private, idiotopes on human lymphomas, which would make the production of therapeutic reagents more practical. Vaccination with idiotypes, H or L chains of Id + Ig, or a peptide derived from that Ig, has been successful in suppressing lymphoma growth in mice.[C48] Mice immunized with Id coupled to KLH and administered in adjuvant had 90% survival 50 days after transfer of lymphoma cells, compared to 50% survival in mice immunized with Id-KLH alone, and 0% in mice immunized with an irrelevant Id vaccine. Even after tumors were established in the mice, immunization with Id-KLH in adjuvant, especially if followed by cyclophosphamide, prolonged survival.[C49] Another group [R77] has been successful in prolonging life of lymphoma-bearing mice immunized with a selected anti-Id that caused production of Id-specific antibodies, delayed hypersensitivity, and cytotoxic T lymphocytes. As in the preparation of antiviral vaccines, manipulation of the Id network should ideally result in both B- and T-cell responses to the target cell.

In addition to activating Id networks for therapy, anti-Ids may be used to identify tumor cells in the circulation or in tissue biopsies. In some systems, high serum levels of the tumor-associated Id correlate with large tumor burden and poor prognosis.[B525]

One of the problems with using anti-Ids as therapy is escape of tumor from regulation by the anti-Id being administered. Such escape could result from 1) somatic mutation of V_H or V_L, or both, which may be driven by the Id vaccines or anti-Ids, or by cytotoxic/radiation therapies; 2) heterogeneity of the initial B-cell tumor with Id-negative subpopulations selected for survival; and 3) ability of surviving cells to use different germline rearrangements to assemble the Ig on their surfaces. There is evidence that all of these processes occur.[B242,B525,C114,L237,R404] In spite of these problems, some tumors remain remarkably stable with regard to expression of Id as various therapies are introduced, and those may be most susceptible to the therapeutic strategies outlined.

An additional problem with administration of monoclonal mouse reagents to humans as therapeutic agents is the development of antimouse antibodies, which can block the efficacy of the MAb. A minority of lymphoma patients have developed antimouse responses, probably because they are immunosuppressed by therapy and by their disease. However, several investigators have developed chimeric antibodies containing the $F(ab')_2$ or Fv of the mouse MAb (to provide Ag specificity), combined with the Fc portion of a human antibody. Such preparations have been less immunogenic than mouse MAbs.[S686]

IDIOTYPES AND TRANSPLANTATION IMMUNOLOGY

Rejection of allogeneic transplants is initiated when CD4 + helper T cells recognize foreign HLA class II antigens and are activated. Activation is followed by release of cytokines, which ultimately leads to B-cell production of antialloantibodies that can lead to tissue damage via antibody-dependent cellular cytotoxicity (ADCC), and generation of cytotoxic T cells that directly damage the allograft. It is interesting that major actions of glucocorticoids and cyclosporine include blockade of early activation stages of the CD4 + cell.[K419] It is therefore appealing

to theorize that anti-Id Igs or anti-Id T cells, which inhibit initial recognition of alloantigens by TCRs on CD4 + cells, might prevent graft rejection.

One strategy used MHC class I and II molecules (from mice) as Ids to induce Ab2. A few such Ab2 molecules recognized MHC molecules, including one designated 14-4-4, which recognizes the Ia.7 specificity, which is present in all mice that express I-E.[S10] In vivo treatment with Ab2 resulted in production of Id in all recipients, and Id could bind the relevant MHC antigen. No cellular immune responses occurred; therefore skin graft rejection was not altered. In contrast, a different anti-Id MAb made against a murine Ab2 against MHC antigen was highly effective in prolonging skin graft survival,[H112] whereas other Ab2 molecules in that same system were ineffective.

More recent Id network manipulations have centered on the T cell as target. In rats, long-surviving renal allografts are associated with splenic T cells capable of transferring alloantigen-specific nonresponsiveness to naive rats.[B117] One group[M519] has grown human CD8 + T cell lines and clones that proliferate specifically to autologous CD4 + cells obtained from in vitro mixed leukocyte reactions (MLRs). Those CD8 + cells do not respond to the alloantigens, but they inhibit the CD4 + cells from proliferating in response to the alloantigen. This effect occurs in the absence of cytotoxicity. Presumably the CD8 + cells are anti-Id T suppressors. Similar CD8 + cells have been implicated in protection of LEW rats from EAE induced by MBP-specific CD4 + cells.[S763] Presumably, anti-Id (also called anticlonotypic) T cells recognize an idiopeptide derived from the TCR (not from alloantigens), which is presented in the context of MHC class I.[B117]

To date, there are no published studies of use of such anti-Id T-cell reagents in humans to prevent allotransplant rejection. Success would depend in part upon restricted clonality of the CD4 + T-cell targets, or similarities in TCR peptides from different clones, and some universality in the ability of multiple MHCs to present those peptides.

IDIOTYPES, AUTOIMMUNITY, AND SYSTEMIC LUPUS ERYTHEMATOSUS

The Role of Idiotypes in Autoimmunity

There are several mechanisms by which idiotype networks may be important in autoimmune diseases such as SLE. First, many autoantibodies are characterized by public as well as private Ids. A partial list of autoantibodies containing subsets expressing public Ids is presented in Table 15–2. Second, the Id on any Ab1 that arises may induce internal image Ab2 (Ab2$_\beta$, epibodies, homobodies). These internal image anti-Ids can then behave as antigens, thus inducing other Ab1 molecules that react with multiple self antigens. For example, rabbits immunized with human polyclonal anti-DNA or with monoclonal anti-DNA derived from MRL/1pr mice developed autoantibodies that reacted with DNA, cardiolipin, SmRNP, and glomerular extract. All these reactivities were contained in the rabbit anti-Id against the immunizing Ig.[P328] Certain Id + monoclonal anti-DNAs (16/6 for example) when used as an immunogen can induce multiple autoantibodies and nephritis in susceptible strains of normal

Table 15–2.   Public Idiotypes on Human Autoantibodies

Autoantibody	Ids	References
Anti-DNA	GN2, GN1, X, 16/6, 32/15, PR4, 3I, 8.12, H130, A52, TOF, DNA3, O-81, NE1, 3E10	C9,D34,D49,D63,D66,E15, E17,E51,E53,H24,H133, I35,I40,K41,L338,M34, M675,R57,S380,S383, S544,W106,W151,Z45
Rheumatoid factor	Wa, Po, 17.109, PR4, PSL2, PSL3, RQ, H3	A227,B225,C116,C223,C225, G280,K462,K465,N22
Antithyroglobulin	62	Z8,Z10
Anticardiolipin	H3	S769
Antiacetylcholine receptor	See references	L156,S764,Z66
Anti-MBP	See references	L271,O131
Anticollagen	See references	A288,N13
Anti-Sm	Y2, 4B4	D34,P214,T-30

mice.[M353,M354] Only mice that develop anti-Id responses to the immunogen develop SLE-like disease. Third, Id networks are probably defective in patients with active SLE. Anti-Ids are detected during disease remission but not during disease activity.[A5] This is probably another example of an immunoregulatory abnormality that contributes to SLE. Restoration of Id circuitry to normal might abrogate the disease. Anti-Ids have been effective in suppressing autoantibody production by human B cells in vitro[A5] and murine B cells in vivo.[H29] Mechanisms by which Ids might participate in the pathogenesis of SLE are reviewed in Table 15–3.

Idiotypes in Systemic Lupus Erythematosus (SLE)

Since SLE is considered the prototype systemic autoimmune disease, the Id–anti-Id profiles of its most characteristic autoantibody, anti-DNA, have been studied by many investigators.[D49,E17,H30,I35,I40,K41,M136,R59,S380,S383,S544,T233,Z45] Although most normal individuals, human and murine, can make anti-DNA, and anti-DNA is part of polyreactive neonatal antibodies, most individuals with SLE have a different anti-DNA repertoire. In general, anti-DNA in healthy individuals is composed largely of IgM with low affinity for single-stranded DNA (ssDNA). In contrast, anti-DNA in mice or humans with active SLE is largely IgG with high affinity for both ssDNA and double-stranded DNA

Table 15–3.   Mechanisms by Which Idiotypic Networks Participate in the Pathogenesis of SLE

1. Many autoantibodies express public idiotypes. These Ids may be targets of up-regulation, thus keeping the levels of the autoantibodies high.
2. Some public Ids on Ab1 induce anti-Ids (Ab2) that bear internal image of Ags. Those Ab2 molecules in turn induce Ab1 molecules that react with multiple self antigens. Thus, Id + anti-DNA can induce Id + anti-Sm, Id + anticardiolipin, etc.
3. Certain public Ids are markers of autoantibodies enriched in pathogenic subsets.
4. Idiotypic regulation is skewed toward up-regulation of undesirable autoantibodies during periods of disease activity. Restoration of normal Id circuitry might abrogate disease.

(dsDNA). In fact, anti-dsDNAs are relatively specific for SLE.

There is substantial evidence that autoantibodies in SLE arise both from polyclonal hyper-reactivity of helper T and B cells, and from specific antigenic stimulation.[E17] It is thought that some structure on dsDNA and/or the proteins (histones) that often accompany it, may be specifically immunogenic in individuals genetically predisposed to this disease. This is probably true both for the human disease and for at least most of the murine lupus models that have been studied.

Several laboratories have defined public Ids on anti-DNA originating either in human or murine systems (see Table 15–4). Many such Ids, especially those occurring near the epitope-binding regions of the Ig molecule, occur both in murine and human SLE. Further, they are found in humans with virtually all known connective tissue diseases (most frequently in Sjögren's syndrome), in first-degree relatives, and in small proportions of healthy individuals.[D49,I40,S380] The presence of the same Id in unrelated individuals, in addition to the presence of the same Ids in mice and humans,[E18,E51,I40,W109] suggests that at least some of these Ids are derived from highly conserved germline genes with minimal mutations. Another characteristic of the lupus Ids is that none are confined to anti-DNA; in fact, in healthy individuals the Id may be found, but rarely on anti-DNA. The 16/6 lupus anti-DNA Id has been found on antibodies to cardiolipin, platelets, cytoskeleton, lymphocytes, brain gangliosides, and mycobacteria.[S380] With a few exceptions, such as 16/6, serum levels of the lupus Ids do not correlate well with disease activity, nor do they accurately predict clinical characteristics of a patient.

Sequencing of several Id-bearing anti-DNAs from humans and mice have shown that some are derived from germline with minimal mutation, whereas others have undergone somatic mutation (see Chaps. 18 and 20). These two populations could represent those arising from polyclonal activation and those responding to specific antigenic stimulation. Not all anti-DNAs are pathogens; only certain subsets can induce disease directly, especially immune glomerulonephritis.[E17,T233] There is substantial evidence that certain Ids are enriched in pathogenic autoantibody subsets. For example, we found that IdGN2 dominates the Ig in glomeruli of renal biopsies from almost all patients with proliferative histologic forms of lupus nephritis.[K41] IdGN2 accounts for 28 to 50% of the anti-DNA deposited in glomeruli of patients with DPGN.[K41] Other investigators have searched for Id + Ig in tissue lesions of mice or humans with active SLE. Ids 16/6, 32/15, 3I, GN2, and V-88 have been found in glomerular Ig deposits and/or at the dermal-epidermal junction in patients with the rash of SLE[K41,S380,W109] (see Table 15–4). It is likely that each of these Ids is enriched in pathogenic antibody subsets. This is also true in animal models of SLE. In NZB × Swiss Webster F₁ mice, lupus nephritis is associated with glomerular deposition of IgG anti-DNA which is highly enriched in a family of Ids designated IdLN.[G75] In nephritic NZB/NZW mice, 50% of the glomerular Ig contains IdGN2 and IdGN1 + antibodies. In addition, administration of some (but not all) IdGN2 +

Table 15—4. Public Idiotypes in Patients with Systemic Lupus Erythematosus

Id	Source	Found in Tissue Lesions of SLE Patients	Location of Id	Special Characteristics	Percent of SLE Patients with Ids in Serum	Percent of Normals with Ids in Serum	References
GNs	Glomerular eluate, NZB/NZW mice	+ +(G)	H chain	Dominant Id on glomeruli of patients with DPGN	67	13	H30,140, K41
X	MAb anti-dsDNA, NZB/NZW mouse	0	?	Dominant Id on serum IgG of nephritic NZB/NZW mice; anti-Id suppresses disease in mice	42	21	H30,140,K41
16/6	MAb anti-DNA, SLE patient	+ +(G, S)	H chain germline DNA	Immunization of normal mice may cause SLE-like disease	30	7	S383,I35, S380,I40, C224, M353, M354
0—81	MAb anti-ssDNA, SLE patient	+ +(G)	?	Found in NZB/NZW mice	72* (with GN) 19 (without GN)	0	H116,M675
NE-1	MAb anti-dsDNA, SLE patient	+ +(G)	?	Found in NZB/NZW mice; αIds to 0—81 plus NE-1 suppress disease in mice	33* (with GN) 6 (without GN)	0	H116,M675
3I	Polyclonal anti-DNA, SLE patient serum	+	κ chain	3I+ anti-DNA enriched in cationic IgG	50	7	D63,140,S544
F4	Polyclonal anti-DNA, SLE patient sera	?	H chain	Expressed only by IgG, enriched in cationic IgG	35	?	D63,D64,D66
KIM4.6.3	MAb IgM anti-ssDNA, normal human tonsil	?	L chain	Id derived from normal human is found in SLE	17 (90)* (12)	7 (24)* (7)	C9,140
134	MAb anti-DNA, SLE patient	?	?		42	0	I40,R57
AM	Polyclonal anti-DNA serum, SLE patient	?	Conformational		25	13	H133,140
BEG-2	MAb anti-DNA, human fetal liver	?	L chain	Fetal antibody persists in human SLE	8	7	I40,W106
8EY	MAb anti-DNA, patient with leprosy	?	?	Id from patient with infection occurs in SLE	25	0	I40,M34
3E10 (DNA spld)	MAb anti-dsDNA, spleen of MRL/lpr mouse	?	Conformational	Anti-Id suppresses SLE in MRL/lpr mice; may be specific for anti-DNA	75* (with GN) 25* (without GN)	2*	W151
A52	MAb anti-DNA, NZB/NZW mouse	?	Conformational	Id from NZB/NZW mouse found in human SLE	>50*	?	E51
Y2	MAb anti-Sm MRL/lpr mouse	?	?	Id from MRL/lpr mouse found in human SLE	41*	6*	D34,P214
4B4	MAb anti-Sm, human	?	?	Cross-reacts with Sm and p24 gag protein of HIV-1	52*	?	T30

* Prevalence in human populations studied by authors, but not by multinational group.
Abbreviations: G = glomerulus, S = skin.

monoclonal IgG2 anti-DNA to normal BALB/c mice produces Id+ Ig deposits in their glomeruli and clinical nephritis.[T233] In contrast, monoclonal IgG2 anti-DNA bearing another public Id, IdX, do not induce nephritis in normal mice.

As with ids on antibodies to external Ag, the structural basis of Ids on autoantibodies is known for only a few MAbs. It is clear that the assembly of autoantibodies does not require any special genetic information. They can be constructed from ordinary germline DNA, with or without somatic mutation; they can be assembled from different V_H and V_L gene families (although there may be some bias toward utilization of certain families); they can resemble antibodies to external Ag.[B397,C8,D173,G426,K344,M540,P31, S375,T214,T215,T233] Expression of public Ids can depend on amino acid sequences on the H or L chains, or both, or may be conformational.[C224,L338] Finally, the structural characteristics of an antibody that make it pathogenic, perhaps related in part to Id expression, are yet to be defined.

Manipulation of Clinical Disease in Mouse Models of SLE by Altering the Idiotypic Network

Idiotype networks have been manipulated by several investigators, by administering Ids or anti-Ids, in attempts to alter disease in the NZB/NZW and MRL/lpr mouse models of SLE. Successful experiments in which nephritis was delayed were performed in our laboratories. IdGN2, commonly found on glomerular Ig in human lupus DPGN and in nephritic NZB/NZW mice, was down-regulated in NZB/NZW mice by administration of a closely related anti-Id (see Fig. 15–5). Serum levels of IdGN2 were initially

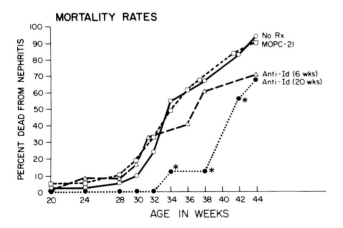

Fig. 15–5. Suppression of clinical nephritis in NZB/NZW mice by administration of anti-idiotypic antibody. In these experiments, NZB/NZW F1 females were treated once every 2 weeks with injections of a monoclonal anti-IdX or an Id-negative monoclonal antibody (MOPC-21). Some littermates were untreated. Mice treated with anti-IdX (*dotted line with solid circles*) lived about 10 weeks longer than other groups. Their production of anti-dsDNA and IdX+ IgG was suppressed during that period, but escaped from control. The appearance of IgG anti-DNA in serum was followed within a few weeks by lethal nephritis. Thus, anti-Id therapy was successful, but only as long as the Id network was sensitive to it. From Hahn, B.H., and Ebling, F.M.: J. Immunol., *132*:2110, 1987. With permission of the publisher.

suppressed, but escaped from control, and mice died of nephritis with deposits of IdGN2+ and IdGN1+ Ig in their glomeruli. Their lives were prolonged a mean of 10 weeks compared to controls treated with an irrelevant murine MAb.[E15] There was no evidence for emergence of mutated or unrecognized Ids in the mice with escape nephritis. It may be that the ability of certain Ids to escape from suppression is a feature that partially explains their enrichment in pathogenic antibody subsets.

Although much work has focused on attempts to suppress expression of pathogenic Ids in murine lupus, recent experiments with the 16/6 Id–anti-Id system have shown that lupus can be induced in normal mice by manipulating this Id network.[B539,M353,M354] Immunization of some normal mice (BALB/c, C3H.SW, AKR, and SJL—but not C57B/6 or C3H/He) with Ids or anti-Ids resulted in development of circulating Ids and anti-Ids, multiple autoantibodies (including anti-DNA, anti-Sm, and anticardiolipin), leukopenia, and nephritis. The susceptibility of strains to induction of disease did not seem to correlate with MHC or Ig allotype genes, but did correlate with ability to make immune responses within the Id network. That is, susceptible strains immunized with Id or anti-Id responded by producing high-titer anti-Id or Id, respectively; resistant strains did not. The different susceptibilities could be accounted for by varying abilities of Id–anti-Id immunization to form pathogenic immune complexes, to activate suppressor T-cell circuits, or to activate extraordinary T-cell help. Clearly, activation of certain Id networks can induce pathogenic reactivity to self.

Idiotypes in other Autoimmune Disorders

Antibodies to thyroglobulin (anti-TG) may play a role in autoimmune thyroiditis; many such Ab1 molecules express public Ids. Zanetti and colleagues have shown that a mature anti-TG obtained in mice after immunization can bear the same Id as a natural Ab1 in unstimulated neonates. Further, both MAbs used unmutated germline genes in their V_H regions.[S54] The public Id62 on murine anti-TG is regulatory and can be used as an immunogen to induce T cells that suppress formation of Ab1; Ab2 can induce the appearance of Ab1 in naive mice or rats.[Z8,Z10]

Antibodies to the acetylcholine receptor of muscle probably cause the autoimmune disease myasthenia gravis in humans and in experimental murine models.[Z66] Several public Ids have been found on anti-AcR, and on non-AcR Ab1 molecules in patients with myasthenia; some are regulatory.[L156,L157,S769] One study[L157] identified Ab2 at the onset or before onset of disease, followed by the appearance of Ab1 (Id) as clinical symptoms appeared or worsened.

In experimental allergic encephalomyelitis (EAE), neurologic disease resulting in weakness, paralysis, and death in susceptible murine and rat strains is probably caused exclusively by T cells, although antibodies are produced. Anti-Id Ig or anti-Id T cells made by immunization with effector T cells can both prevent disease induced by Ag (myelin basic protein, MBP) in certain strains.[L271,O131]

Antibodies to Sm antigen (anti-Sm) are relatively specific for SLE in patients; they are also found in MRL/lpr mice. Like anti-DNA, some populations express public Ids.[D34,P214] A public Id (Y2) defined on a murine MAb anti-Sm was found in 41% of SLE patients, 27% of their relatives, and 6% of normals. In mice, Y2 is found on both anti-Sm and non-anti-Sm in MRL/lpr mice, as well as in sera of some normal mouse strains. These observations are similar to those for anti-DNA. One group has reported that a public Id, 4B4, on a monoclonal human anti-Sm is found in sera of SLE patients who also have antibodies to the p24 gag protein of HIV-1.[T30] This brings to mind the possibility that anti-4B4 (anti-Id) may have induced Ab1 molecules that react with a wide variety of self and nonself antigens.

Antibodies to type II collagen (anti-CII) are produced by mice and rats susceptible to collagen-induced arthritis, which is considered by some experts to be a model for human rheumatoid arthritis. There is evidence that these antibodies can be important in inducing and perpetuating disease, but it is also clear that some T cells can induce joint destruction independent of the antibody response. Twenty to 25% of anti-CII in DBA/1 mice immunized with bovine CII bear a public Id. That Id can be regulated by Ag, but Ab1 molecules that express it are apparently not involved in disease induction, since their suppression does not alter disease.[N13] In contrast, administration of a different anti-Id to rats at the time of immunization with CII suppressed anti-CII and disease; however, the AB2 was not effective if given 7 days after immunization.[A288] Interestingly, the effective anti-Id protocol was not associated with suppression of DTH to CII, so the anti-Id may have had a greater effect on Ab2 formation than on the cellular component of the disease.

In human rheumatoid arthritis (RA) several public Ids have been described. See page 142 for a discussion of the idiotypic characteristics of paraprotein rheumatoid factors (RFs). Patients with RA usually have polyclonal RFs, with only a small proportion expressing the public Ids characteristic of monoclonal RFs. The polyclonal RF repertoire contains both private and public Ids. Ids defined in other autoantibody systems, such as PR4 on anti-DNA and the H3 Id on anticardiolipin, are increased in patients with RA.[S769,Y58] Some public Ids predominate in the sera of patients with RF-positive disease; others can be found in similar proportions of patients with seropositive or seronegative RA, and in hidden RF (contained in immune complexes and not detected as free populations).[B400,H95,I9,M562,R414,S769,Y58] No public Ids have been defined that are disease specific (as for the other human diseases discussed), and no studies have been conducted attempting to alter human disease by administration of Ids, anti-Ids, or idiopeptides.

Clinical Utility of Idiotypes—Anti-idiotypes in SLE

The extensive information about Ids and their roles in autoantibodies, immune networks, and SLE reviewed in this chapter has provided increased understanding of immune regulation and the dysregulation characteristic of SLE. It was hoped that measuring certain Ids or anti-Ids in patient sera would provide valuable clinical data regarding predisposition of patients to nephritis or other clinical disease manifestations. Further, serum levels of selected Ids or anti-Ids might be used to detect early disease flares.[A5,E18,I40] Unfortunately, none of these hopes have yet been realized. The ultimate utility of this information would be to devise new therapies or preventive strategies. However, idiotypic manipulation in animal models of SLE has been disappointing in that longterm disease suppression has not been achieved. This might be due to participation of multiple different Id—anti-Id networks in the disease, resistance of pathogen-enriched Ids to suppression, or inadequately designed interventions. The use of internal image anti-Ids, or peptides derived from them, as vaccines to induce active immune responses that might prevent formation of pathogenic autoantibodies is still being studied, and may yet prove to be a useful clinical intervention.

Chapter 16

IMPORTANCE OF SEX HORMONES IN SYSTEMIC LUPUS ERYTHEMATOSUS

S. ANSAR AHMED AND NORMAN TALAL*

HISTORICAL PERSPECTIVES

The immune system is influenced by several non-lymphoid systems (e.g., endocrine and nervous). The immune system, in turn, influences the endocrine and nervous systems. The first clue that the lymphoid system is regulated by endocrine factors (gonadal hormones) dates back approximately to the turn of the century when Calzolari in 1898[C32] and subsequently Hammar in 1906[H188] noticed that gonadectomy of animals resulted in augmented thymic growth (size and weight). This seminal finding did not generate enthusiasm during the next several decades as the thymus at that time was regarded as an organ of no biologic function (perhaps similar to the appendix). During this period, because the thymus was only of academic interest (primarily to anatomists), the work on this crucial lymphoid organ (particularly the effect of hormones) proceeded at a slow pace. In 1940, Chiodi indirectly confirmed Calzolari/Hammar's work when he observed that administration of gonadal hormones to animals resulted in thymic atrophy.[C240] These findings have now been confirmed in numerous laboratories and illustrate the bidirectional relationship of the immune system with the gonadal hormones.

The second clue to support interactions of sex hormones with the immune system comes from the observations of both basic scientists and clinicians who noted that males as a group, overall, responded less well to a variety of antigens compared to females. Male laboratory animals succumbed to a variety of infectious diseases earlier or with greater severity than their female cohorts. Clinicians observed that men more than women were susceptible to a variety of infections. Nevertheless, the concept of sex hormone regulation of the immune system escaped scientific scrutiny as, at that time, interactions of the immune system with a discrete endocrine system was not yet appreciated. Indeed these observations were made during a period when the field of immunology was in its infancy. In subsequent years the concepts of immunology were rapidly expanding and posed fundamental challenges. This includes the concept of autoimmunity, which suggested that the immune system is not always a protector of the body. Not surprisingly, clinicians noted that women were more susceptible to autoimmune diseases than age-matched men, presumably because of vigorous response to self-antigens. These sex-related differences in autoimmune disease were also noticed and recorded in anecdotal context in certain animal models of autoimmune diseases. Despite compelling evidence to suggest the involvement of sex steroids in autoimmune disease, there were no definitive studies directed at addressing this issue. A report by the National Advisory Committee on the future of arthritis research, sponsored by the Arthritis Foundation in 1972, urged that an explanation *"be sought for the remarkable female to male ratio in systemic lupus."*

The availability of genetically determined laboratory animal models of human disease such as NZB and (NZB × NZW)F_1 or B/W mice, which spontaneously develop autoimmunity, launched intensive research in the field of immune dysregulation. Animal models provide an excellent system to study the role of sex factors in the induction, progression, and treatment of autoimmune diseases. Definitive studies documenting the regulation of murine lupus by sex steroids were reported in B/W mice, a classic animal model of systemic lupus erythematosus (SLE).[R364,R365,S646] These findings rejuvenated interest in the field of hormonal regulation of the autoimmune response and further solidified a new emerging subbranch of immunology, immunoendocrinology (neuroimmunoendocrinology). The influence of sex hormones on a variety of experimental autoimmune diseases has since been reported.[A246,A247,A249,A250]

We believe interactions of sex hormones with the immune system are of biomedical importance because of the following reasons. First, sex hormones regulate the initiation and course of autoimmune diseases such as SLE. As sex hormones modulate the immune system, it is likely that they also affect the course of certain oncopathologic and allergic processes. Second, sex hormones are natural immunomodulators, which are present in varied but defined concentrations throughout life and thus are likely to contribute to altered immune status relative to age. These agents may be employed as tools to dissect complex immunoregulatory pathways. Third, modified sex hormone analogs with desired levels of immunosuppression, with diminished or absent endocrinologic effects and antagonists, may be viable options in designing therapeutic strategies for autoimmune diseases.

* We acknowledge the support of the General Medical Research Service of the Veterans Administration and BSRG grants.

SEXUAL DIMORPHISM IN IMMUNE RESPONSES AND SUSCEPTIBILITY TO AUTOIMMUNE DISEASE: SEX HORMONE BASIS

Physiologic gender differences in immunocapabilities have been noted not only in vertebrates such as birds and mammals[A246,A247,A249,A250,G411] but also in invertebrates.[R186] In general, females of various species have better immunocapabilities (particularly antibody-mediated immunity) than their male counterparts[E48,T122] For example, females have higher immunoglobulin levels (IgM and IgG)[B115,B599,R187] and stronger antibody responses to a wide range of foreign antigens than age-matched males. Further, females resist a variety of infections more successfully than males presumably because of their ability to mount effective immune responses. There is also evidence that females reject allografts more rapidly,[A204,G330] have reduced incidence of certain tumors,[G407,M343] demonstrate greater cytotoxicity against certain viruses,[H471] and are relatively resistant to the induction of immune tolerance.[D324] It is tempting to postulate that greater longevity of females compared to males[V91] may be attributed, in part, to their better immunocapability.

Human Data

The greater immune responsiveness of the female gender group is also reflected in their increased susceptibility to most autoimmune disease. Women during their reproductive years are some 9 to 13 times more susceptible to the development of SLE than men.[D324,L15,S669] The female to male susceptibility ratio (F:M) falls during prepubertal and postmenopausal stages, which in itself strongly suggests the regulation of the disease by sex steroid hormones. Women are also more susceptible to other rheumatic autoimmune syndromes such as Sjögren's syndrome (F:M = 9:1) and rheumatoid arthritis (F:M = 2–4:1). Women are also more susceptible to the development of autoimmune thyroiditis, a relatively common organ-specific autoimmune disease.[D264] Preferential susceptibility of women to other organ-specific autoimmune diseases such as myasthenia gravis, idiopathic adrenal insufficiency (autoimmune adrenal disease), autoimmune diabetes mellitus (insulin dependent), and scleroderma[A246,A247,A249] has also been noticed. The F:M ratio in these diseases is 2–5:1.

There is strong evidence to implicate the involvement of sex steroid hormones in the pathogenesis of autoimmune diseases in humans. For example, episodes of flares in lupus have been reported in pregnant and postpartum patients (a period during which major sex hormone change occurs).[M657] Pregnancy also modulates the course of many autoimmune diseases including rheumatoid arthritis[H260,O37] Graves' disease, idiopathic thrombocytopenic purpura,[L384] polymyositis,[G433] and autoimmune thyroiditis.[A184] Menses also alters the degree of severity of lupus.[R299] Exogenous estrogens, such as in oral contraceptives, modify the course of the disease.[C205,J141] Interestingly, estrogen-containing contraceptives when taken orally by apparently normal women have been linked to the development of rheumatic symptoms or LE cells, a feature of lupus. The presence of autoimmune diseases (e.g., SLE,

myasthenia gravis) in patients with Klinefelter's syndrome, a genetically determined disease in males (XXY) characterized by sex hormone abnormalities, small testes, and gynecomastia, adds support to the involvement of sex hormones.[M389,S669] However, the effects of pregnancy on SLE are variable.[M657] Further, reduction of estrogen to androgen ratio in female SLE patients by the administration of cyproterone acetate reduces the episodes of exacerbations,[J143] thus supporting the role of sex hormones in SLE. Moreover, in a study of monozygotic twins with Klinefelter's syndrome, it was observed that one twin developed SLE while the other had symptomatic myasthenia gravis, thus suggesting sex hormone involvement in autoimmune diseases.[M389] Estrogen enhances binding of specific anti-Ro and La autoantibodies to cultured human keratinocytes, a finding that has led to the suggestion that estrogen may be an in vivo trigger factor for immunologic damage in cutaneous and neonatal lupus.[F321]

SLE patients, as well as those with Klinefelter's syndrome, have abnormal metabolism of estrogen to yield an excess production of 16-α-hydroxyesterone and estrol metabolites.[L15,L19] These metabolites are thought to induce a chronic hyperestrogenic state. Of relevance to lupus, which tends to exhibit familial susceptibility, there is an increased level of 16-α-hydroxylation in first-degree relatives.[L15] Increased serum levels of prolactin, a reproductive polypeptide pituitary hormone, have also been reported in SLE patients.[L95] It is not known whether hyperprolactinemia is the consequence of estrogen stimulation of prolactin. Abnormal metabolism of androgens in SLE patients has also been documented.[J145,L21] Male SLE patients have been reported to have lower basal levels of testosterone[L95,M33] and reduced dehydroepiandrosterone and dehydroepiandrosterone sulfate.[L25] Similarly, the above two hormones are decreased in female SLE patients; levels of these hormones correlate with the activity of the disease.[J145,L15,L21] It is not clear whether abnormal metabolism of androgens in SLE patients would culminate in the formation of estrogenic compounds.

The possible involvement of sex hormones in other autoimmune diseases has been provided by the following observations. First, male rheumatoid arthritis patients (like SLE patients) have decreased concentrations of serum testosterone and dehydroepiandrosterone.[C462] Replacement with testosterone in male RA patients brought about clinical improvement as noted by reduction in numbers of affected joints and levels of IgM rheumatoid factor, and increase in numbers of CD8+ cells.[C463] Further, postmenopausal RA patients have significantly diminished levels of testosterone, dehydroepiandrosterone sulfate, and esterone when compared to normal postmenopausal women.[S56] Second, there is an inverse relationship between levels of testosterone in the serum with the development of antinuclear and anti–smooth muscle autoantibodies in patients with alcohol-induced cirrhosis. Third, some male Graves' disease patients have an imbalance of androgens and estrogens.[C245]

Together these data suggest that an abnormal level of estrogen, coupled with diminished levels of androgens

Table 16–1. Evidence to Support the Involvement of Sex Hormones in Human SLE

1. SLE occurs 9 to 13 times more frequently in women (in reproductive years) than men.
2. The ratio female to male susceptibility to SLE falls in prepubertal and postmenopausal women.
3. Pregnancy, estrogen-containing oral contraceptives, and menses may modify the course of SLE.
4. SLE patients have abnormal metabolism of androgen and estrogen.
5. Klinefelter's syndrome patients who have depleted androgen levels are also susceptible to SLE.

with immunosuppressive effects, may regulate the onset or course of human autoimmune diseases (Table 16–1).

Animal Data

Analogous to the clinical situation, autoimmune diseases occur or exacerbate preferentially in female animals in the majority of experimental animal models (Table 16–2). In particular, female B/W mice have an accelerated expression of lupus and Sjögren's syndrome–like disease compared with their male counterparts.[R363,R365,S646] Female B/W mice have increased autoantibodies (e.g. anti-DNA) and die several months earlier (at least by 5 months) than males. Histopathologically, deposition of immune complexes in the glomeruli is more diffuse and of brighter fluorescent intensity in females than male B/W mice. The accelerated glomerulonephritis in females is often associated with proliferation of renal capsular cells and fibrinoid necrotic changes.

A similar sex-related expression of SLE and RA-like syndromes that occurs spontaneously has been noted in other murine models including (NZB × SJL/J)F₁, PN, (NZB × DBA/2)F₁ and to a lesser extent MRL/n and MRL/1pr. For example, at 1 year of age, lupus nephritis in (NZB × SJL/J)F₁ mice characterized by immunoglobulin deposits in the renal glomeruli and proteinuria is clearly evident in about 80 to 90% of females compared to 10 to 20% in males.[D352] These female, but not male, mice demonstrate thymic abnormalities including the presence of plasma cells and B cells. MRL/1pr mice that develop an aggressive disease do not show dramatic sex differences, although a similar trend is evident. The mean survival time of MRL/1pr females is 143 days while that in males is 154 days. MRL/n mice that have delayed onset of autoimmune syndromes have a mean longevity period of 476 days in fe-

Table 16–2. Evidence to Support the Role of Sex Hormones in the Pathogenesis of Murine SLE

1. Female B/W mice have an accelerated development of lupus syndrome and die prematurely compared to male B/W littermates.
2. Sex differences in autoantibody synthesis have been noted in several murine strains prone to develop lupus. Female mice develop autoantibodies to nuclear antigens earlier than males.
3. Depletion of male hormone levels by orchiectomy or an increase of female hormone (estrogen) levels in B/W mice accelerates lupus.
4. Administration of a variety of androgens delays the onset of the disease. Delayed androgen therapy of B/W mice also prolongs life.

males as compared to 546 days in males of this strain.[T131] Further, sex differences in autoantibody production have been noted in another "1pr" strain of mice, C57BL/6-1pr/1pr. Females of this strain develop higher levels of anti-DNA, rheumatoid factor, and anti-gp70 than males.[W84] However, no sex differences have been demonstrated in AKR-1pr/1pr or C3H-1pr/1pr mice.[W84] These results suggest that sex hormones do not play an equal role in all lupus-prone mice. This may reflect differences in the characteristics of the disease among various types of 1pr mice. Further, unlike human SLE and most of its animal models, the lupus-like disease in BXSB mice is accelerated in males compared to females.[M667] This is thought to be because of a Y chromosome–linked gene which is not regulated by sex hormones. However, in crosses between BXSB and nonautoimmune CBA/J mice, the female F₁ offspring has comparatively more severe disease.[S641] Thus, it has been suggested that the effect of the Y chromosome of BXSB mice is evident only when other appropriate background genes are present.[S641]

Definitive evidence attesting to the role of sex hormones in the pathogenesis of autoimmune disease has been provided by the animal models of autoimmune diseases where sex hormone manipulation could be performed. The best-studied animal model in this regard is B/W mice. More than a decade ago, we showed that subjecting B/W mice to orchidectomy or estrogen treatment[R365] accelerates the course of lupus. Conversely, the course of the disease was significantly delayed in highly susceptible female B/W mice (or orchiectomized males) by prolonged exposure to 5-α-dihydrotestosterone (DHT). Importantly, the beneficial effects of DHT are evident even in mice with established autoimmune disease.[R364] Various types of androgens have been shown to be of therapeutic or prophylactic value in murine lupus. Dehydroisoandrosterone (DHA) administered orally to B/W mice reduced anti-DNA antibody levels and prolonged survival period[L406] but did not prevent hypergammaglobulinemia or affect macrophage functions.[M191] The precise mechanism of action underlying the beneficial effect of DHA is not readily apparent, but it is unlikely that it involves macrophage arachidonate metabolism. Conversion of DHA to other beneficial steroids appears to be an attractive possibility.[M191] Others have shown that 19-nortestosterone (nandrolone, decanoate), an anabolic steroid with minimal virilizing effects, when administered to B/W mice prolongs survival, improves renal function, and reduces anti-DNA autoantibodies.[V67]

The beneficial value of androgens has been documented in other murine models of lupus, including NZB × SJL/J, NZB × CBA, NZB × C3H, NZB × DBA/2 and even in MRL/1pr mice.[R69,R70,S649] Treatment of MRL/1pr mice with DHT brought about improvement in levels of autoantibodies, renal function, and survival rate but did not improve the clearance of erythrocytes sensitized with IgG.[S338,S648] However, DHT treatment of MRL/n (MRL/+/+) mice improved immune clearance. These studies indicate that the beneficial effect of DHT therapy in MRL/1pr mice is not a result of improved clearance of immune complexes. The potential role of sex hormones has also been demonstrated in an alternative murine model of SLE induced by the injection of human anti-DNA (16/6 idiotype +) antibody.[B340] Estrogen- but not testosterone-treated mice had an earlier expression of the disease characterized by an elevated level of autoantibodies to nuclear components.

Sex Hormone Therapy in SLE and Related Autoimmune Diseases

Preliminary and unconfirmed studies in the 1950s suggested that testosterone esters may be useful in SLE and Sjögren's syndrome in women with SLE.[F287] Testosterone undecanoate had beneficial effects in patients with Klinefelter's syndrome who also manifested SLE or Sjögren's syndrome.[B321] Testosterone therapy normalized CD4:CD8 ratios and reduced titers of rheumatoid factor and antinuclear antibodies. However, even if testosterone is highly effective, it cannot be employed because of confounding virilizing effects. Alternatively, nandrolone decanoate (19-nortestosterone) with minimum virilizing effects did have promising desired effects in women (but not men) with SLE[L25] and rheumatoid arthritis.[P200] Danazol, an attenuated male sex hormone, which is effective in some cases of idiopathic thrombocytopenia[A74,A75] had varied effects in SLE patients.[M615] Danazol has been reported to have beneficial effects in women with SLE-like disease in conjunction with hereditary angioedema.[Y57] Interestingly, administration of danazol (100 mg/kg) to autoimmune-prone MRL/1pr mice significantly increased longevity and reduced proteinuria and serum amyloid protein (an acute-phase reactant)[C372] only in female, but not in male, mice. These studies are reminiscent of clinical findings of disparate effects of danazol on hereditary angioedema relative to gender. While the danazol was highly effective in female patients, it exacerbated the disease in male patients.[F241,F240] In a case study, a female patient with SLE and autoimmune hemolytic anemia, who previously failed to respond to aggressive therapy (corticosteroids, immunosuppressive drugs, and splenectomy) derived significant benefit from danazol.[C197] The underlying mechanisms for the preferential gender effect are not clear. Perhaps danazol requires the collaboration of female hormones for optimal effects. Alternatively, male sex hormones may interfere with the action of danazol. Perhaps danazol activates different immunoregulatory pathways or transduces different types of signals in males and females. It is likely that danazol alters the subsets of T helper cells or synthesis of cytokines and response to these cytokines.

Danazol had beneficial effects on patients with autoimmune hemolytic anemia.[A72] Twelve of 15 patients responded well to danazol therapy. Interestingly 2 out of 3 patients from these groups who also manifested SLE responded well to danazol but not prednisone. The above clinical studies thus suggest that danazol therapy may be an option in formulating a therapeutic regimen. Although mechanisms underlying the therapeutic effects of danazol on autoimmune hemolytic anemia are not readily apparent, a few suggested mechanisms include refractoriness of erythrocyte membranes to osmolysis, interference (negative signaling) via Fc receptors on monocytes,[S174] or nor-

malization of helper to cytotoxic/suppressor cell ratios.[M683] In order to conclusively evaluate the potential beneficial effects of danazol in SLE, a larger study is required that takes gender influence into account. The beneficial effect of danazol cannot be generalized as it had no therapeutic value in murine lupus[R363] and was unable to dampen the lymphocytic infiltrations in salivary/lacrimal glands that spontaneously develop in MRL/1pr mice (Sullivan, personal communication).

Sex Hormones and Non-SLE Autoimmune Diseases

Preferential female susceptibility to autoimmune arthritis induced in LEW/N rats by the injection of peptidoglycan polysaccharide derived from streptococci (group A) has been observed.[A148] Male rats can be rendered susceptible to the induction of polyarthritis by estrogen treatment or by orchidectomy. Importantly, estrogen also rendered refractory strain F-334/N susceptible to the development of autoimmune arthritis following injections of peptidoglycan polysaccharide. Genetic studies discounted the role of X chromosomes and indirectly supported the role of sex hormones in the pathogenesis of autoimmune arthritis. Further, in another model of arthritis is was shown that female, rather than male F_1 hybrids of good responder DA (RT1^{avi}) and poor responder BN (RT1^n) strains of rats are highly susceptible to collagen-induced arthritis.[G384] Female susceptibility to arthritis in a nonhuman primate model (cynomolgus monkeys) induced by injections of chick type II collagen has also been reported.[T117] In this study 100% of female monkeys (10 of 10) developed severe arthritis, while 1 out of 5 male monkeys (1 of 5) developed mild and transient arthritis. Further, female rhesus (Macaca mulatta) monkeys are susceptible to the development of arthritis and manifest high levels of antibodies to bovine type II collagen.[Y46] Male monkeys, conversely, are refractory to the induction of arthritis and demonstrate low levels of autoantibodies. Taken together, these studies suggest a sex hormone influence on the pathogenesis of the disease.

In contrast to the clinical situation and other animal models male DBA/1 (H-2^q) but not female, mice are susceptible to the induction of type II collagen arthritis.[L76] Interestingly, kinetic studies demonstrated that both sexes develop early histopathologic lesions with detection of autoantibodies by 2 weeks post-immunization.[B387] This suggests that the disease is down-regulated in the female environment while it progresses in males. Oophorectomy renders the mice susceptible while estrogen administration reduces the incidence.[J49,L76] Even physiologic doses of estrogen delay the onset or reduce the severity of arthritis. Delayed-type hypersensitivity to collagen was decreased, while immunoglobulin-secreting cells were increased in estrogen-treated mice. Delayed estrogen treatment had minimal effects on autoantibodies to collagen. Estrogen could have down-regulated T-cell functions, which may have significantly contributed to the amelioration of the disease. It is noteworthy that the potential role of other autoantibodies in the disease process cannot be fully discounted.[J49]

Earlier studies showed that estrone administration (at

relatively high doses) inhibited the development of adjuvant arthritis induced by the administration of heat-killed mycobacteria pHLEI in paraffin oil.[T171] Interestingly, pregnancy may at times ameliorate rheumatoid arthritis. Overall, these observations demonstrate the inherent complexity of sex hormone effects on the pathogenesis of autoimmune disorders.

B/W mice, in addition to SLE, also develop Sjögren's syndrome–like glandular lesions characterized by mononuclear cellular infiltration of salivary glands.[K180,S167] Androgen (nandrolone decanoate) effectively suppresses the expression of the disease and is of therapeutic benefit.[154,S167] Several other steroids such as ethylestrenol (progestational anabolic steroid with minimal virilizing effects), tibolone (org OD14: with less potent androgenic, progestational effects with no androgenic or little estrogenic effects) also diminish the incidence of salivary glandular autoimmune lesions as well as lupus in B/W mice.[V67,V68]

MRL/1pr mice also spontaneously develop Sjögren's syndrome–like lesions in addition to lupus and massive lymphadenopathy. Testosterone treatment of MRL/1pr mice after the onset of the disease impressively reduced the lymphocytic infiltrations in the lacrimal tissue.[A286] Analysis of lymphocytes in the lacrimal gland of testosterone-treated MRL/1pr mice revealed that the total number of pan T cells, CD4, CD8, class II, immature T and immunoglobulin-positive B cells were reduced.[S92] The beneficial effects of testosterone were also evident by a two- to threefold increase in glandular weight concomitant with a significant reduction in acinar density/field. Importantly, the output of IgA into the tears was increased following testosterone therapy, which reflects the gradual rebuilding of lacrimal tissue. The therapeutic effect of testosterone was mimicked by nortestosterone and but not by danazol, estradiol, or dexamethasone, suggesting selective effects of certain types of androgenic compounds (Sullivan, personal communications).

Early studies have shown that normal female rats subjected to early thymectomy and irradiation were at least four to six times more susceptible to the development of autoimmune thyroiditis than age-matched males.[A245,P101] Female Tx-X rats had higher levels of autoantibodies to thyroglobulin and a greater degree of autoimmune thyroid lesions than males. The higher incidence of thyroiditis in female Tx-X rats is not a result of intrinsic localized defects of thyroids as confirmed by thyroid transplantation studies (Ahmed and Penhale, unpublished observations). Rather it is a result of the effects of sex hormones.[A245,A253] Testosterone not only prevented the expression of thyroiditis but also significantly ameliorated established thyroid lesions.[A245,A253]

Sex hormone effects have also been demonstrated in other models of thyroiditis.[G68,O41,P102] The expression of spontaneous autoimmune thyroiditis in obese strain chickens can be prevented by testosterone treatment.[C345] Testosterone appears to act on bursal epithelial cells and quite likely on other tissues.[F22] Others have reported that female obese strain (OS) chickens develop persistent levels of autoantibodies to thyroglobulin.[G69] Administration of testosterone to OS chickens suppresses the develop-

Table 16–3. Sex Hormones Modulate Other (non-SLE) Experimental Autoimmune Diseases

1. Females are more susceptible to the induction of arthritis in the rat and subhuman primate experimental models.
2. Androgens (and other related steroids) ameliorate the spontaneous expression of Sjögren's syndrome in B/W and MRL/lpr mice.
3. Male thymectomized and irradiated (Tx-X) rats develop a lower incidence of thyroiditis and autoantibodies to thyroglobulin and have a reduced degree of severity index (mononuclear cellular infiltration) than age-matched female Tx-X rats. Manipulation of androgen levels in Tx-X rats alters the susceptibility to spontaneous induction of thyroiditis.
4. Sex hormone effects have also been noted in the murine model and chicken (OS strain) models of thyroiditis.

ment of autoimmune thyroiditis.[F22,G330] Both testosterone and estrogen, at relatively high does, suppressed autoimmune thyroiditis induced in guinea pigs by the administration of thyroid extract in adjuvant.[K66]

Estrogen-containing oral contraceptives can prevent the induction of experimental autoimmune encephalitis.[A291] Manipulation of testosterone levels (by orchidectomy or testosterone administration) of mice modulates autoantibodies to acetylcholine receptors induced by parenteral administration of acetylcholine receptors in Freund's complete adjuvant.[T152]

The foregoing studies clearly demonstrate that sex hormones have a profound effect on the expression of not only lupus but also on several rheumatic and nonrheumatic autoimmune disorders (Table 16–3).

Mechanisms of Sex Hormone Action

While the relationship between sex hormones and the immune system is becoming clear, the mechanisms by which they act are relatively obscure. It has been hypothesized, often supported by experimental evidence, that sex hormones could modulate the immune system via several different target sites.[A248,A249,G411] Sex hormones could act directly on lymphoid organs such as thymus and bursa or could act indirectly by acting initially on several non-lymphoid organs that affect the functioning of the immune system. Sex hormones may act on 1) the central nervous system to release immunoregulatory peptides or compounds, 2) the macrophage-monocyte system to regulate their function and elaboration of monokines, and 3) other endocrine glands to release immunomodulatory hormones. Although the mechanisms by which sex hormones regulate the immune system are not well known, it is, however, clear that they do not act by a simple pathway. Thus, sex hormones can affect the final outcome of immune responses through acting on different sites.

Sex Steroid Receptors

Data from endocrinologic studies performed on classic reproductive tissues revealed that sex hormones act on target cells through interaction with specific intracellular receptors to form a steroid-receptor complex. This steroid-receptor complex acquires increased binding affinity for nuclear acceptor sites (steroid-responsive elements) and triggers events that modulate the transcription of specific genes.[Y15] These hormones can be viewed as agents that "activate" the receptor proteins to become DNA regulatory molecules. Specific sex steroid–binding proteins have been reported in the thymus of normal rats, mice, and guinea pigs, and in the spleens of mice by biochemical and autoradiographic techniques.[S90,S744] Radiolabeled estrogen sex steroid receptors localized to the supporting connective tissues of the baboon spleen but not to the red pulp or lymphocytes. In yet other studies, these estrogen-binding receptor proteins were demonstrated in human mononuclear cells, splenic lymphocytes, and thymocytes.[D36] Further, nuclear uptake and retention of ³H-estrogen has been reported in lymphocytes and thymocytes of germinal centers and in the connective tissue capsules of the guinea pig lymph nodes.[S744] These receptors have been detected in human thymomas and leukemic cells.[R140] Further, by employing a modified binding assay, estrogen receptors were found predominantly in CD8 (suppressor/cytotoxic) rather than CD4 (helper/inducer) human lymphocytes.[C328,S694] However, in most cases the binding of sex steroid receptors was low.

Unlike the reproductive tissues, sex hormone receptors have not been unequivocally demonstrated in lymphocytes, despite the known effects of sex hormones on these cells. In general, it has been difficult to demonstrate sex hormone receptors (measured by ligand binding techniques) in lymphocytes, perhaps because of low capacity (i.e., number). Additionally, only a selected population may possess these receptors, as differential sensitivity to sex hormones among lymphocytes is apparent.[A243,N150,S233] Therefore, the use of whole lymphocytes may mask the expression of receptors in a small yet significant population of lymphocyte subsets. In our laboratory, we have been unable to convincingly demonstrate the presence of sex steroid receptors in highly purified murine lymphocytes (Chen, Ahmed, Sheridan, Talal, unpublished observations). Further, it is not known whether sex hormone receptors in the immune system differ from those in classic endocrinologic tissues. More importantly, it is hoped that future studies will unambiguously resolve the presence of sex hormone receptors in the cells of the immune system.

That sex hormones act on lymphoid cells is also suggested by studies that show that nonsteroidal antiestrogens (domiphen) inhibit the proliferation of neoplastic lymphoid cell lines (EL4 [lymphoma] and Raji [derived from Burkitt's lymphoma]) and normal splenic lymphocytes.[H373] Estrogen receptors have been reported in patients with acute lymphoid leukemia and acute myeloid leukemia.[L67] A second type of estrogen receptor, type II estrogen binding sites, has been demonstrated in human lymphoblastoid cell line (IM9).[S103] These type II estrogen binding sites presumably have lower-affinity/higher-binding capacity for estrogen compared to classic estrogen receptors.[C278] It is believed that pharmacologic doses of estrogen may act on these binding sites to induce growth-inhibitory effects. It is not known, although conceivable, whether type II estrogen binding sites exist in normal lymphoid cells. It is interesting that estrogen receptors are relatively difficult to detect in normal lymphoid cells

compared to that in neoplastic lymphoid cells (vide supra).

MRL/1pr mice may have malfunctioning estrogen receptors in the uterus, which may be caused by local levels of polyamines. MRL/1pr mice have higher levels of uterine polyamines than BALB/c mice, which is inversely related to DNA-binding activity of estrogen receptors.[T152] Treatment of mice with difluoromethylornithase, which irreversibly reduces the level of polyamines, restores the DNA-binding activity of estrogen receptors. It is not known whether there are malfunctioning sex hormone receptors in the cells of the immune system of these mice.

Thymus and T-cell–Mediated Immunity

Even within the immune system, sex hormones act on several lymphoid organs. However, the thymus appears to be a primary lymphoid target through which sex hormones may mediate their effects throughout the system (Table 16–4). Historic findings in this field have shown that thymus gland size varies with sex hormone status. Depletion of sex hormone levels by gonadectomy (e.g., orchiectomy) induces thymic hyperplasia, while excessive supplementation (e.g., sex hormone injections) induces thymic atrophy.[A243,C32,C150,D352,G411,S533] Further, the maximal size of the thymus gland is attained prior to puberty followed by gradual diminution in size during postpubertal life and shrinking to a remnant with advanced age.

Interestingly, the thymic hyperplasia induced by orchiectomy is caused by an equal expansion of thymocyte subsets in normal, but not in autoimmune, mice[D352] suggesting differential effects of sex hormones in health and disease. Orchiectomy of autoimmune-prone (NZB × SJL/J)F₁ mice led to differential expansion of Thy-1.2^dull, CD5+, and immature PNA dull thymocytes, which suggests that T-cell development in an autoimmune environment may be skewed by sex hormones.[D352] It is still not clear whether or not thymocytes themselves are targets of sex hormones. A likely target site for sex hormones is thymic stromal cells (epithelial or macrophages). Sex hormones could act on these stromal cells (which are sex hormone receptor positive) to regulate the synthesis of monokines and other factors that nurture developing thymocytes.[H57] Serum from estrogen-treated mice with an intact thymus, but not from estrogen-treated mice with thymus ablated, had inhibitory effects when added to lymphocyte cultures stimulated with T-cell mitogens,[G411,S695] suggesting thymic involvement in sex hormone action. Sex hormones could affect the production of IL-6 or IL-7 from thymic stromal cells. An additional mechanism by

Table 16–4. Sex Hormone–induced Alterations of the Cells of the Immune System

1. Sex hormones induce thymic atrophy and alter thymic subsets.
2. Sex hormones (at pharmacologic doses) reduce T-cell–mediated immune functons.
3. Estrogens increase autoantibody production.
4. Estrogens increase macrophage functions.
5. Estrogens inhibit NK cell functions.

which sex hormones could regulate thymic function is by inducing the release of neuropeptides, which can act on the thymus.

Sex hormones alter thymic subsets.[A243,K129,N150,S233,W146] Estrogen reduces CD8+ murine thymocytes as demonstrated by single color flow cytometry.[A243,N150] By dual color flow cytometry it appears that CD4+8+ thymocytes are depleted following exposure to excessive estrogen.[S233] Androgens maintain CD8+ thymocytes.[B533,T29] It is likely that sex hormone effects on the thymus eventually influence the T-cell immunocompetence. Interestingly, prepubertal boys (with incomplete descent of testes) whose androgen, but not estrogen, levels are elevated to physiologic concentrations by the administration of human chorionic gonadotropin have decreased CD4:CD8 ratios in peripheral blood.[D357] This alteration of lymphocyte subsets disappeared after puberty suggesting complex effects of other hormones.

Administration of testosterone to mice of certain H-2 haplotype reduced the ability of lymphocytes to proliferate to T-cell mitogens.[A251] In this context it is interesting that genes of the H-2 complex not only regulate immune functions but also several nonimmune functions such as testosterone levels, sex hormone–binding globulins, expression of uterine estrogen receptors, and H-Y antigens.[A248] Thus, it is not surprising that one MHC supratype in humans, involving the C4AQO allele, is associated with depleted testosterone levels and increased manifestations of autoimmune diseases.[D98] In several systems, various steroids (particularly at high doses) have been found to inhibit the proliferation of T lymphocytes in response to T-cell mitogens.[A246,S411,S488,W361] Our preliminary results have shown that T cells derived from testosterone- or estrogen-treated mice had reduced ornithine decarboxylase (ODC) enzyme activity, an early enzyme in polyamine synthesis, when stimulated with the T-cell mitogen concanavalin A (Con A), when compared with similarly treated T cells from control mice (5-α- dihydrotestosterone 28.89, pM/h/10^6 T cells; estrogen 14.4 pM/hr/10^6 T cells; control 92.76 pM/hr/10^6 T cells). (Ansar Ahmed, Talal and Fischbach, unpublished observations). A similar trend was noticed in sex hormone–treated C57BL/6-1pr mice, albeit the ODC values in general after Con A stimulation were low in these SLE-prone mice. Estrogenic sex hormones (at pharmacologic doses) also depress IL-2 levels, presumably produced by CD4+ T cells.[P334] Androgens can maintain IL-2 levels. Autoimmune mice have decreased IL-2 production by T cells, which can be normalized by androgen treatment.[T29] Further, in vitro studies using human peripheral blood have shown that estrogens act on suppressor T cells.[P1]

The age of an individual when exposed to sex hormones could have a major effect on the outcome of immune responses. Neonatal administration of estrogen-induced profound thymic atrophy, depletion of Thy-1.2+ cells,[K26] reduced ability to respond to delayed-type hypersensitivity (DTH) and inability to generate cytotoxic CD8+ T cells against mammary tumor virus–infected cells.[B331,K29,W113] Prenatal exposure of mice to diethylstilbestrol, a synthetic estrogen agonist, also reduced DTH.[L425] We have found that prenatal exposure of C57BL/ 6J mice to estrogens induced earlier expression of Sjögren's syndrome–like lesions.[A241]

Sex hormones can also affect the immune system of animals deprived of their thymus suggesting extrathymic sites of action. For example, testosterone not only inhibited the spontaneous expression of autoimmune diseases in thymectomized and irradiated (Tx-X) rats but also had therapeutic effects.[A245,A253]

Antibody-Mediated Immunity

Sex hormones also regulate the expression of antibody and autoantibody levels, suggesting their effects on B-cell functions.[K28,K439,M411] Female normal mice (C3H, C57BL/ 6J) produce greater numbers of cells producing autoantibodies to erythrocytes than do males.[A242,E134] These autoantibody producing cells are present in large numbers in the peritoneal cavity of female mice.[A242,D55,E134] Accessory cells (macrophage or other cell types) were found to be necessary for autoantibody production by B cells suggesting a positive signal(s) (cell contact or secretion of cytokines) delivered from accessory cells to B cells.[E134]

Estrogen regulates the synthesis of serum and uterine immunoglobulin.[B115,B599,S744] In general, estrogen enhances while male hormones inhibit or have no effect on autoantibody levels.[A247,A299,B487] Estrogen has been shown to increase a variety of autoantibodies in autoimmune mice as well as to increase autoantibodies to erythrocytes (presumably phosphatidylcholine) in nonautoimmune mice.[A247] Estrogen administration per se had little effect on numbers of immunoglobulin-bearing B cells. We found that B cells derived from estrogen-treated mice had increased lipopolysaccharide- (LPS-) induced ODC activity when compared to sham-treated mice (sham, 16.7 pM/ hr/10^6 cells; estrogen, 76.1 pM/hr/10^6 cells) (Ansar Ahmed, Talal and Fischbach, unpublished observations). It is still not clear whether sex hormones affect autoantibody production by acting directly on B cells or indirectly by affecting T cells, macrophages, and other cell types. Also not known are the effects of hormones on B-cell activation, proliferation, or differentiation.

Phagocytic and Natural Killer Cells

Phagocytic cells are also targets of sex hormone action.[B410,L426,M59] Estrogens are potent activators of certain functions of macrophages.[V71] Estrogen also enhances clearance of immunoglobulin G–coated erythrocytes[F249] and stimulates the reticuloendothelial cells.[D102] Estrogen is also believed to stimulate suppressor macrophages, which in turn may suppress T-cell functions. Estrogen stimulates the synthesis of IL-1 as well as increased expression of class II (Ia) molecules on macrophages.[F133] It is not clear whether estrogen alters the class II antigenic expression on lymphocytes (unpublished observations). The Ia induction by estrogen may be mediated by effects on γ-interferon (γINF) or IL-4. Female hormones such as estrogen, progesterone, and prolactin have been shown to increase Ia on mammary gland epithelium.[K268] Ectopic expression of class II antigens on target organs such as thyroid epithelial cells[B424] may be indirectly mediated by estrogen through the modulation of γINF. Lymphocytes from female mice produce greater quantities of γINF than those from males.[M276] Studies from our laboratory have not conclusively shown that estrogen regulates γINF. (Ahmed, Talal, Baron, unpublished results). Studies, however, have shown that estrogen is thought to regulate the γINF promotor.[S83] The importance of ectopic Ia expression in the induction of autoimmunity has been suggested in the experimental model of autoimmune thyroiditis. Culturing of normal thyroid lobes with INF induced Ia expression on thyroid tissue. Transplantation of these thyroids, but not control thyroids, to syngenic recipients induced thyroid autoreactive destruction.[F286]

The local production of cytokines, particularly those involved in inflammation, may be of importance in regulating the expression of an autoimmune lesion. These cytokines could be produced by nonlymphoid cells (e.g., thyroid or salivary gland epithelial cells) or by infiltrates of mononuclear cells. In this context, IL-6 and IL-1 are produced by thyroid epithelial cells of Hashimoto's thyroiditis.[Z24] Also, IL-6, but not IL-1, has been found in joint exudates of rheumatoid arthritis patients.[B285] The IL-6 of multiple isoforms appears to be produced by synovial lining cells. Monocytes, but not lymphocytes, produce IL-6 only when stimulated with LPS. This suggests that bacterial infection or possibly unknown stimuli may induce activation of monocytes. IL-1 may be produced by synovial lining or other types of infiltrating cells and could be rapidly consumed. Sex hormones such as estrogen may alter the synthesis of these cytokines or response to these cytokines in a manner that affects the outcome of autoimmune diseases. In a related context, it was shown that estrogens inhibited the secretion of IL-6 by endometrial stromal cells exposed to inflammation-associated cytokines.[T2] This may relate to the reported beneficial effects of administration of relatively high levels of estrogen in rodent model of thyroiditis and arthritis.[A252,K66,L76]

Natural killer (NK) cells are regarded as "primitive" innate immune defense against viral-infected or tumor cells.[H271] NK cells possess nonclonally distributed effector recognition mechanisms. These cells require no prior sensitization, lack specific immunologic memory, and can kill aberrant cells in a non–MHC-restricted fashion.[H27] The wider biologic importance of NK cells is now becoming apparent. The NK cells 1) kill certain virus-infected cells[B560] and tumor cells; 2) destroy cells that lack class I antigen and contribute to the cytotoxic effector repertoire; 3) directly lyse certain bacterial cells;[G44] 4) may regulate hemopoiesis (through the recognition of gene products mapping between H-2S and H-2D), and [R156] 5) possess Fc receptors and therefore can bind to antibody-coated target cells.[G44] NK cells are non-T and non-B cells. However, there is some evidence to suggest a phenotypic relationship with T cells. For example, NK cells possess a ζ chain, an invariant polypeptide found on most hemopoietic cells including T cells (associated with the T-cell receptor).[A210,J43] Further, NK cells, like T cells, express the CD2 surface marker, which is involved in the alternate pathway of T-cell activation. These observations have led to the suggestion that cytotoxic T cells may have evolved from NK cells.

Natural killer (NK) cells are also important targets of sex hormones.[K27,K29] The precise role of NK cells in autoimmune disease is not readily apparent. One possibility is that they may down-regulate B-cell functions.[A21] Autoimmune-prone MRL/1pr mice have decreased splenic NK cell activity.[L259] Defective NK cell functions in autoimmune mice may represent a facet of generalized immunoregulatory dysfunction. There is a negative correlation between NK cell function and increased B-cell functions. Estrogens have been shown to reduce NK cell functions in both normal as well as autoimmune-prone mice.[A242,S238] The precise mechanism by which estrogens down-regulate NK cell functions is not clear. Several possibilities have been suggested. For example, estrogens 1) may alter T-cell lymphokines (e.g., IL-2 or γINF), which affect NK cell activity, 2) may affect suppressor cells regulating NK cell activity, although this possibility remains unproven, 3) may alter NK cell development and 4) may alter the response of NK cells to cytokines.

Hypothalamus-Pituitary-Thymus-Gonadal Axis

It is now recognized that the immune (thymus), central nervous (hypothalamus-pituitary), and endocrine (gonadal) systems influence each other in a bidirectional fashion.[B334,S578] Space limitations prohibit extensive review of this subject. Some evidence includes observations that the brain and the pituitary can influence the immune system by sending signals via innervation of lymphoid organs or by the release of various neuroendocrine peptides.[B334] Studies in rats have shown that testosterone-induced stimulation of IgA synthesis in the eye can be abrogated by hypophysectomy, which supports the existence of a hypophysis-gonadal immune axis.[S760] It is relevant that stress is considered one of the contributing factors in autoimmune diseases such as SLE. Stress may induce the release of various immunoregulatory neuropeptides that can modify autoimmune responses. Similar mechanisms mediated by sex hormones possibly may be operative in nonstress situations.

The sex steroid hormone binding at σ receptors (exclusive of sex hormone receptors) in the nervous and lymphoid systems consolidates the relationship of endocrine, nervous, and the immune systems.[S751] Sex steroid hormones could affect the immune system by binding to σ receptors in the lymphoid tissue or indirectly by binding to σ receptors in the brain. The binding of PCP, a behavior-altering drug, to σ receptors in lymphoid tissue may be responsible for the reported immunosuppressive effects of PCP.[K191] Sex steroid hormone–induced mental alterations could indirectly affect the functioning of the immune system.

Estrogen induces the synthesis of prolactin, a hypothalamic hormone known to have a profound immunomodulatory effect. Prolactin has been shown to up-regulate IL-2 receptors on rat splenic lymphocytes without affecting the synthesis of IL-2,[M643] suggesting that response to IL-2 may be altered. This effect of prolactin is highly dependent upon estrogen status (i.e., seen only in ovariectomized and diestrus animals).

Other Factors

Autoimmune diseases, particularly arthritis, have been linked to mycobacterial infections.[R290] Studies have shown that a 67 kD protein of mycobacteria cross-reacts with autoantigens (e.g., lactoferrin).[E137] Rheumatoid arthritis patients have raised levels of antimycobacterial antibodies.[T248] Synovial T cells (likely δ)[G66] derived from synovial membranes of RA patients respond impressively to the 65 kD mycobacterial heat-shock proteins.[R163] The involvement of microbial agents in autoimmune diseases such as SLE is not proven but cannot be fully discounted. Future studies (molecular, genetic, and biochemical) may answer this question. The regulation of the normal immune system by sex hormones may affect infectious agents as well as autoantigens. Thus, it is conceivable that the normal immune response directed against infectious agents, which can be regulated by sex hormones, also affects biochemically related autoantigenic epitopes.

SUMMARY

Clinical studies on SLE provide compelling evidence to support the involvement of sex hormones in the modulation of the disease process. Unequivocal evidence for the regulation of lupus by sex hormones comes from appropriate animal models of SLE. In general, estrogens enhance, while male hormones retard, the expression of murine lupus. Detailed studies in several laboratories have established that mechanisms by which sex hormones regulate the immune system are highly complex. Sex hormones could conceivably act on multiple target sites (including nonlymphoid tissues) to alter the functioning of the immune system. Diverse types of cells of the immune system appear to be affected by sex hormones. It is hoped that studies on hormonal regulation of lupus will provide valuable insights into the immunologic mechanisms involved in the disease process.

Data from both clinical and experimental studies urge careful consideration for the development of a clinical hormone program as an adjunct therapy. Likely candidates in this regard may be modified androgens, with or without estrogen antagonists. For example, it may be possible to appropriately alter (chemically) male hormones to eliminate virilizing but to retain the desired level of immunosuppressive effects. It must be, however, emphasized that even if the above-mentioned sex hormone therapy becomes successful in SLE, it still remains a nonspecific approach like most forms of therapy for autoimmune diseases. Hopefully, with rapid advances of biomedical research it may become possible to develop immunotherapeutic strategies to selectively "switch off" or delete only those clones of lymphocytes involved in pathogenic autoreactivity, sparing normal reactive lymphocytes.

Chapter 17

ANIMAL MODELS OF SYSTEMIC LUPUS ERYTHEMATOSUS

BEVRA H. HAHN

Since the derivation of the autoimmune NZB/Bl mouse in 1959,[B298] there has been great interest in New Zealand and newer mouse models of SLE-like disease. Studies in these animals have shown that genetic factors govern development of autoimmunity; however, multiple genes are involved, and they are probably influenced by environmental and hormonal factors. Many different immunologic abnormalities have been reported, each of which plays a role in disease. Each model differs from the others in genetic, immunologic, and clinical manifestations of autoimmunity. Information from studies of these animals has contributed to understanding human disease. Further, studies of efficacy of therapeutic interventions in murine SLE have formed the basis of similar interventions in human disease. Spontaneous SLE also occurs in dogs, and drug- or diet-induced SLE has been reported in cats and monkeys. Investigations are most extensive in mice, so most of this chapter is devoted to murine SLE.

In the paragraphs that follow, the five most widely studied murine models of SLE are described. These include NZB/Bl, NZB/NZW F_1, NZB/SWR F_1, MRL/lpr, and BXSB. See Table 17–1 for an overview of abnormalities in those strains.

CLINICAL DISEASE, HISTOLOGIC ABNORMALITIES, AND AUTOANTIBODIES IN MURINE SLE

Numerous murine models of SLE have been studied. This section reviews the principal characteristics of the most important models.

NZB/Bl (NZB) Mice

The New Zealand Bielchowsky Black (NZB/Bl) mouse was bred by Bielschowsky, who was mating mice by coat color to derive cancer-susceptible strains. In 1959, she reported that NZB mice died early from autoimmune hemolytic anemia.[B298] Shortly thereafter[H258,H259] her colleagues described a hybrid between NZB and the unrelated strains—including the New Zealand White (NZW)—characterized by early death in females from nephritis associated with LE cells, thus providing the first animal models of SLE.

The characteristics of NZB mice are shown in Tables 17–1 and 17–2, and are discussed in several review articles.[A225,S641,T133,Y53] NZB mice are characterized by hyperactive B cells, present in fetal life, that produce primarily IgM antibodies to thymocytes, erythrocytes, single-stranded DNA (ssDNA), and the gp70 glycoprotein of murine leukemia virus.[A225,D121,D122,M617,M168,S641,T133,Y53] In comparison to normal mice, there are increased numbers of IgM-secreting cells, and increased synthesis of IgM by individual B cells; these two characteristics are controlled by different genes.[A225,M103,M634,S641,T78,T133, T135,Y53] NZB mice also have dramatic involution of thymic tissue; thymic epithelium is atrophied and immunologically defective by 1 month of age. The combination of B-cell hyperactivity and thymic loss probably results in abnormal shaping of adult T- and B-cell repertoires.[S641,T133,Y53]

The first antibody to appear in serum is NTA (natural thymocytotoxic antibody),[M410,S370] by 3 months of age 100% of mice have this antibody. NTAs are cytotoxic for all thymocytes, for 50 to 60% of thoracic duct and peripheral blood lymphocytes (both CD4+ and CD8+ populations), for 50% of lymph node cells, 33% of spleen cells, and 5% of bone marrow cells, which is similar to the reactivity of anti–Thy-1 sera that recognize all T cells. The antigens recognized by NTA are varied; some NTAs react with cell surface molecules on B lymphocytes, granulocytes, and bone marrow myeloid cells; some react with a 55 kDa molecule on most T cells. Other reactivities reported include an 88 kDa glycoprotein thought to be a T-cell differentiation antigen, and surface molecules of 33 kDa and 30 kDa size.[B466,B467,L180,O26,Y53]

The primary clinical problem in NZB mice is hemolytic anemia, which is fatal in the majority between 15 and 18 months of age.[A225,B298,Y53] There is mild disease acceleration in females, with death about 1 month earlier than in males. Antibodies to erythrocytes cause the hemolysis[M364] and can be directed against the erythrocyte surface antigen designated X, or can recognize cryptic antigens. The exact structure of the RBC-derived antigens has not been determined.[D120,D122,H374,L302] Anti-RBCs appear in the serum by 3 months of age and are found in 100% of mice by 12 to 15 months. Clinical hemolysis begins 1 to 5 months after the antibodies appear. Severe anemia occurs in 87% of virgin females, 56% of breeder females, and 77% of males.[H460] The expected sequelae of hemolysis occur; i.e., erythrocyte sequestration and extramedullary hematopoiesis in liver and spleen, splenomegaly, hepatomegaly, and deposits of hemosiderin in multiple tissues.

Clinical nephritis may be observed in some NZB mice, but it is mild in comparison to the nephritis of other lupus murine models, probably because the IgM anti-ssDNA that dominates the NZB response does not contain many nephritogenic subsets of anti-DNA, in contrast to the IgG

Table 17–1. Major Characteristics of Murine Strains Developing SLE

Strain:	NZB/Bl	NZB/NZW F₁ (BW)	NZB/SWR F₁ (SNF₁)	MRL-lpr/lpr (MRL/l)	BXSB
Coat color	Black	Brown	Brown	White	Brown
H-2 locus	d/d	d/z	d/q	k/k	b/b
Mls-1 locus	a	a/b	a/a	b	b
Age for 50% mortality (months)	16	8.5	6	6	5
Sex dominance	Sl F	F	F	Sl F	M
Cause of death	Hemolytic anemic	GN	GN	GN	GN
Autoantibodies	NTA	IgG anti-DNA	IgG anti-DNA	CIC	IgG anti-DNA
	Anti-RBC			Anti-DNA	
	Anti-gp70			RF	
				Anti-Sm	

Abbreviations: F = female; M = male; GN = glomerulonephritis; CIC = circulating immune complexes; RF = rheumatoid factors.

anti-dsDNA that arise in the other strains. However, histologic changes of glomerulonephritis, nephrotic syndrome, and renal insufficiency occur in some mice late in their life span, especially in virgin females.[B297,H298]

Dramatic histologic changes occur in the thymus, with

Table 17–2. Characteristics of NZB/Bl Mice

A. Clinical
  1. Females live a mean of 431 days, males 467 days.
  2. Death is usually caused by autoimmune hemolytic anemia.
  3. Fifty percent mortality by 15 to 17 months of age.
B. Histologic
  1. Glomerulonephritis with Ig and C3 deposits.
  2. Marked thymic atrophy.
  3. Mild lymphoid hyperplasia.
C. Autoantibodies
  1. IgM natural antithymocyte (NTA).
  2. IgM and IgG antierythrocyte.
  3. IgM anti-ssDNA.
  4. Anti-gp70.
  5. ANAs by late life.
  6. Modest elevations of circulating immune complexes.
D. Immune abnormalities
  1. B cells are unusually mature, hyperactivated, and secreting Ig spontaneously from very early age (in fetus and in newborn mice). This abnormality is required for autoimmune disease in the NZB and hybrids mated with NZB mice.
  2. Numbers of CD5 + (ly-1 +) B cells in spleen and peritoneum are increased.
  3. B cells resist tolerance to T-independent antigens.
  4. Older mice develop aneuploidy in CD5 + B cells.
  5. Thymic epithelium is atrophic by 1 month of age. This is a striking abnormality in the NZB mouse.
  6. Antithymocyte antibodies react with immature T cells and may inactivate/delete precursors of suppressor T populations.
  7. T cells are required for maximal autoantibody formation.
  8. A unique form of retroviral gp70 antigen is secreted and found in serum in high quantities.
  9. Clearance of immune complexes by Fc-mediated mechanisms is defective.
E. Genetics
  1. Multiple dominant, codominant, and recessive genes participate in the immune abnormalities.
  2. One set of genes controls the constellation of polyclonal B-cell activation, expression of gp70, and antithymocyte antibodies. Another set of genes controls B-cell tolerance defects, antibodies to gp70, anti-ssDNA, and anti-RBCs. The gene sets segregate independently. Neither of these sets is dependent on H-2.
  3. Two separate genes control the increase in CD5 + B cells.
  4. The Igh allotype is linked to ability to make high quantities of IgM anti-ssDNA.

epithelial cell degeneration, accumulation of TdT + large immature T cells in the subcapsular region of the cortex, cortical atrophy, and increased lymphoid and plasma cell infiltrates in the medulla.[A225,D193,G102,H396,M410,W217] These changes are evident at 1 month of age, before detectable NTAs arise. NZB thymic epithelial cells are functionally defective compared to cells from normal mice, with low expression of surface Ia molecules, low secretion of IL-1, high secretion of PGE_2 and PGE_3, and diminished ability to educate nonthymic cells to express Thy-1.[G102,M461,M462,M463,W217]

Antibodies against cerebellar cells have been reported,[H118] and some monoclonal NTAs react with Purkinje cells of the cerebellum.[O26] Histologic changes in the cortex of the brain similar to those seen in dyslexic humans have been described.[S356]

Other abnormalities highly characteristic of NZB mice are the appearance of aneuploidy in B cells as the mice age, and the high frequency of CD5 + (also designated Ly-1 +) B cells, which produce many of the IgM autoantibodies. Hyperdiploid CD5 + B cells with additional chromosomes 10, 15, 17 and X are common.[R67] CD5 + B cells are increased in numbers in spleen and in peritoneum;[H219,H221,W317] these cells can make IgM autoantibodies to RBCs, thymocytes, and ssDNA.[H219,H220,H221] (CD5 − B cells make antibodies to self and to nonself and are likely to be the source for IgG autoantibodies.[C366,M104] Lymphoid malignancies are more common in NZB than in other murine lupus strains, varying in different colonies between 1 and 20%.[D159,H396,M410] Most of the mice demonstrate hyperplasia of lymphoid follicles in multiple organs, including salivary glands.

The incidence of antinuclear antibodies (ANAs) in NZB mice is variable. ANAs are not regularly present in high titers as they are in other lupus-prone strains, but about 80% of mice are positive by 9 months of age.[A225]

In summary, NZB mice are characterized by a fatal hemolytic anemia induced by antierythrocyte antibodies. Other autoantibodies in their repertoire include predominantly IgM NTA, anti-ssDNA, and anti-gp70. Their dominant immunologic abnormalities are hyperactivated B cells from fetal life onward, early degeneration of thymic epithelium, and increased numbers of CD5 + B cells that develop aneuploidy with age. These manifestations are controlled by multiple different genes, as discussed later.

Sex differences are not marked; disease is slightly accelerated in females.

NZB/NZW F₁ Mice (BW)

The F₁ hybrid cross between NZB and New Zealand White (NZW) mice is considered by many to be the murine model most closely resembling human SLE. The disease is more severe and earlier in females; high titers of IgG anti-dsDNA, ANA, and LE cells occur in virtually all females; death results from immune glomerulonephritis.[A225,B585,D332,H298,S641,T133,Y53] (see Table 17–3).

Both NZB and NZW parents contribute genetically to the immune abnormalities that cause disease.[H326,K320,K395,M172,S132,Y28,Y49,Y53] The NZW parent has a slightly

Table 17–3. Characteristics of NZB/NZW F₁ Mice

A. Clinical
  1. Females live a mean of 280 days, males 439 days.
  2. Death is usually caused by immune glomerulonephritis.
  3. Fifty percent mortality by 8 months in female, 15 months in male.
B. Histologic
  1. Glomerulonephritis with proliferative changes in mesangial and endothelial cells of glomeruli, capillary basement membrane thickening, and chronic obliterative changes.
  2. Glomerular immune deposits of IgG (predominantly IgG2a) and C3; similar deposits in tubular basement membrane and interstitium.
  3. Thymic cortical atrophy by 6 months of age.
  4. Myocardial infarcts with hyaline thickening of small arteries.
  5. Mild lymph node hyperplasia and splenomegaly.
C. Autoantibodies
  1. IgG anti-dsDNA (also binds ssDNA), enriched in IgG2a and 2b.
  2. ANA and LE cells in all.
  3. Antithymocyte in most females, some males.
  4. Renal eluates contain IgG anti-dsDNA concentrated 25 to 30 times greater than in serum.
  5. Modest elevations of circulating immune complexes; these include gp70–anti-gp70.
  6. Low serum complement levels by 6 months of age in females.
D. Immune abnormalities:
  1. Polyclonal B-cell activation.
  2. B cells are resistant to tolerance fo some antigens.
  3. Strict dependence on T-cell help for formation of pathogenic IgG anti-DNA. CD4+CD8− and CD4−CD8− cells can provide help.
  4. IgG repertoire becomes restricted with age to certain public idiotypes; there may be some restriction of B-cell clonality in the IgG anti-DNA response.
  5. Thymic epithelial atrophy by 6 months of age; medullary hyperplasia; effect of thymectomy on disease varies.
  6. Clearance of immune complexes by Fc-mediated and complement-mediated mechanisms is defective.
  7. Disease and autoantibody production is sensitive to sex hormone influences.
E. Genetics
  1. The expression of high-titer IgG anti-dsDNA requires heterozygosity at MHC, namely H-2$^{d/z}$.
  2. Additional complementary non–H-2–linked genes are required from both NZB and NZW parents to permit full expression of the IgG anti-DNA response.
  3. Renal disease, linked to high-titer IgG anti-DNA, depends upon at least 2 dominant genes (at least 1 on chromosome 17) from NZB parents and 2 from NZW (at least 1 of which is also on chromosome 17 and linked to MHC).
  4. The large deletion in the β chain of the TCR of the NZW parent probably does not predispose to disease.
  5. Nephritis may depend on the I-E^z β chain from the NZW parent.

shortened life span, and develops intermittent autoantibodies. Some NZW mice develop clinical nephritis late in life.[H39,K153a] A large portion of the β chain of the T-cell receptor is deleted in NZW mice.[K395,N122,Y28] Genetic backcross studies showed lupus-like disease segregating with the abnormal TCRs in the hands of one group,[Y28] but not in extensive backcross studies performed by another group.[B3,K393,K395] The B-cell hyperactivity characteristic of the NZB is inherited by the BW, with abnormally high secretion of Ig detectable by 1 month of age.[S641,T135] However, the T-cell dependence of the response is more striking than in the NZB parent, and is probably responsible for the isotype shift from IgM anti-DNA to IgG anti-DNA that precedes clinical disease.[P137,S687] The large quantities of IgG antibodies that bind both dsDNA and ssDNA, and are widely designated anti-dsDNA, are striking and can be abrogated by removal of CD4+ (L3T4+) T cells.[W319,W320] The IgG antibodies to dsDNA clearly contain subsets that cause nephritis: transfer of certain monoclonal BW IgG2a anti-dsDNA antibodies to normal BALB/c mice induces nephritis in the recipients.[T233] Characteristics of pathogenic subsets of anti-DNA are discussed in detail in Chapter 20. The B-cell repertoire that expresses anti-DNA may be somewhat restricted. Public idiotypes expressed on total serum IgG become increasingly restricted as the mice age.[H310] Some investigators have noted that many monoclonal anti-DNAs from individual BW mice are similar enough in structure to have derived from a small number of B-cell clones;[M135] other investigators have found little evidence of such restriction.[P31]

Anti-DNAs are the most important autoantibodies made by BW mice that contribute to nephritis.[E17] However, ANAs are detectable in most females by 2 to 3 months of age and include antibodies that bind dsDNA, ssDNA, dsRNA, tRNA, polynucleotides, histones and nucleic acid-protein complexes (including chromatin and DNA/histone).[B53,B486,F110,M410,M659] IgM anti-DNAs arise in females between 3 and 5 months of age; by 5 to 7 months IgG anti-DNAs appear.[A225,E17,P37,S687] The IgG2a and 2b subclasses are most frequent, a fact of great importance because these subclasses fix complement well. The IgM to IgG switch, and the dominance of IgG2a and 2b thereafter, occur in BW females responding not only to DNA but also to other thymic-independent and dependent antigens.[P42] Shortly after the switch to IgG, IgG and complement deposit in the mesangia of BW glomeruli, spreading later to capillary loops and interstitial tubular regions.[A225] Proteinuria appears between 5 and 7 months; azotemia followed by death occurs at 6 to 12 months of age. Approximately half of the females are dead by 8 months and 90% at 12 months.[A225,B585,T133] The antibodies eluted from glomeruli are composed predominantly of IgG anti-DNA; 50% of the total IgG is anti-DNA according to some reports;[D235,L36] in our colonies anti-DNA accounts for as much as 85% of the total glomerular IgG.[E16] IgG2a is the dominant isotype in glomerular deposits. Other antigens and antibodies have been reported in glomerular eluates, including gp70[G20,M172,T133] and anti-RNA polymerase.[S675] The high serum levels of IgG anti-DNA occur about the same time as hypocomplementemia, and levels of circulating immune complexes are elevated.[A225] Histologic changes in kidneys include chronic obliterative changes in glomeruli, mesangial and peripheral proliferative changes, capillary membrane thickening, glomerular sclerosis, tubular atrophy, interstitial inflammation and vasculopathy (primarily degenerative, occasionally inflammatory)[A225,H460] (see Fig. 17–1).

Antibodies to erythrocytes occur in 35 to 78% of BW females, but they rarely develop hemolytic anemia.[T133] About 50% develop NTAs by 6 months of age. Since genes governing NTA, anti-DNA, and antierythrocyte antibodies segregate separately,[D50,M172,M435,R68,S641,Y53] New Zealand mouse strains have been bred that have high-titer NTAs but no autoimmune disease. However, NTAs may serve as an accelerator of the disease process that occurs in mice with IgG anti-DNA, since NTAs may alter T-cell function.

The lymphoproliferative features of NZB mice occur in BW hybrids, which exhibit mild lymphadenopathy and splenomegaly.[A225,T133] Lymphoid neoplasia is far less common than in NZB mice. Some investigators have reported a relatively high incidence of thymoma, from 1 to 5%,[T31] but that has been rare in the author's colonies, unless mice are treated with immunosuppressive interventions.[H35] The degeneration of thymic epithelial cells characteristic of NZB mice occurs in BW mice, but at 6 months of age in contrast to 1 month of age in the NZB parent.[Y53]

Extrarenal lesions occur in BW mice, including lymphocytic infiltration of salivary glands, mild inflammation around bile ducts in the liver, pancarditis, vasculitis (less common than in MRL/lpr and BXSB mice), myocardial infarcts, and deposits of DNA and anti-DNA in the dermoepidermal junction of skin and in the choroid plexus.[A225]

The "femaleness" of spontaneous BW disease has been studied extensively. Most BW males develop ANAs, including antibodies to DNA, but they are predominantly IgM. The IgM to IgG switch occurs relatively late in life, usually after 12 months. Histologic evidence of nephritis can be found in males, and most die of slowly progressive chronic nephritis by 15 to 20 months of age.[A225,H460,M410]

The BW mouse is particularly sensitive to the effect of sex hormones on disease. In general, androgens are protective and suppress the expression of autoantibodies and disease; estrogens are permissive. Male BW mice (and other hybrids of NZB) do not fully express genes controlling autoantibody production unless they are castrated.[S641] Males castrated and/or treated with estrogens assume a female pattern—early IgM to IgG switch of anti-DNA antibodies and early, fatal nephritis.[R362] Females treated with castration and androgens, or with antiestrogens, have prolonged survival with suppression of IgG anti-DNA and nephritis.[D370,R364,R365,S646] In old females, androgens can suppress disease without altering the elevated levels of IgG anti-DNA.[R364] The effects of sex hor-

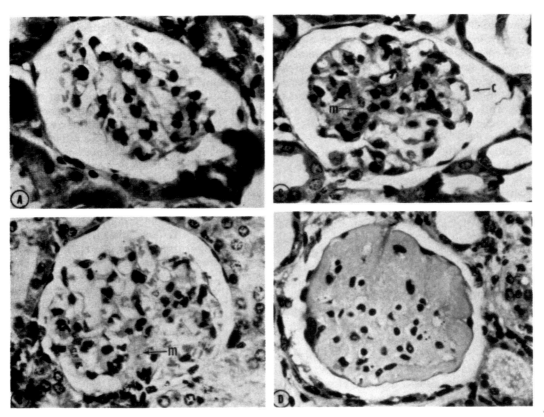

Fig. 17–1. Glomerulonephritis in New Zealand Mice. *A*, Normal mouse glomerulus. *B*, Mesangial proliferation and thickening (m). *C*, Proliferative glomerulonephritis with thickened glomerular capillaries (c). *D*, End state glomerulopathy; the glomerulus is obliterated. Each of these samples is from sections of kidneys from NZW mice.

mones on immune responses are complex and poorly understood. Sex hormones alter function of the reticulo-endothelial system and of lymphocytes, and regulate the expression of certain genes.

In summary, BW mice develop fatal glomerulonephritis, mediated primarily by IgG antibodies to dsDNA, which is earlier and more severe in females and can be modulated by sex hormones. Multiple genes inherited from both NZB and NZW parents, some of which are linked to MHC, are required for development of high-titer IgG anti-dsDNA and clinical nephritis. Abnormalities in both T- and B-cell compartments are required for the disease to be fully manifest.

NZB × SWR F₁ (SNF₁) Mice

The SNF₁ mouse is a model of lupus nephritis produced by mating NZB with the normal SWR mouse;[D47,D48,E7,G73,G74,G75,O42] it does not matter which parent is female and which is male. In contrast to NZW mice, SWR mice are completely healthy, with normal life spans, low levels of serum gp70, and no evidence of autoimmune disease.[D47,D48] Their B cells can produce Igs bearing the same public Ids that dominate serum Igs in MRL/lpr mice.[R59]

SNF₁ mice are similar to BW mice. Females are dead by 10 to 12 months of age (50% mortality at 6 months) from an immune glomerulonephritis that is mediated primarily by IgG2b antibodies to dsDNA.[E7,G74] The model has been of particular interest because of the oligoclonality of the IgG anti-DNA deposited in glomeruli.[G73,G75] Activated B cells of NZB mice make anti-DNAs that are predominantly IgM, bind ss rather than dsDNA, and are anionic in charge.[G74] In contrast, B cells of SNF₁ mice make predomi-

Table 17–4. Characteristics of NZB × SWR F₁ (SNF₁) Mice

A. Clinical
   1. Mean survival in females is 297 days; mean survival in males is 531 days.
   2. Females die from immune glomerulonephritis between 5 and 13 months of age.
B. Histologic
   1. Glomerulonephritis with proliferative and obliterative lesions.
C. Autoantibodies
   1. IgG anti-dsDNA is made by all females.
   2. Anti-dsDNA is dominated by IgG2b cationic populations with restricted idiotypes.
   3. ANAs in all females.
D. Immune Abnormalities
   1. B cells are hyperactivated.
   2. The development of nephritis depends upon presence of T-cell help for production of IgG anti-DNA.
   3. Cationic IgG anti-dsDNA may use allotype of either NZB or healthy SWR parent.
   4. Anti-dsDNA deposited in glomeruli cluster into two main groups defined by their idiotypes.
   5. CD4+CD8− and CD4−CD8− T cells can provide help for synthesis of cationic IgG anti-dsDNA.
E. Genetics
   1. Heterozygosity at H-2 is required, namely H-2^{d/q}.
   2. Nephritis is also influenced by genes linked to the TCR β and MHC I-A β chain of the SWR parent.

---

nantly IgG2b anti-dsDNA that is cationic.[G74,G75] Cationic charge is probably important in initiating nephritis, since cationic antibodies (or antigens or immune complexes) can bind to polyanions in glomerular basement membrane.[E17,G70] IgG in glomerular eluates from BW mice is also enriched in cationic subpopulations,[E16] and it is those populations that bind directly to glomeruli when infused into old BW mice.[D33] (One group of investigators failed to find cationic IgG in glomerular eluates of BW mice, although they were present in MRL/lpr and BXSB mice.[Y50]

The presumed pathogens, IgG2b cationic anti-dsDNA, are also restricted in idiotype expression. The IgG in glomeruli of SNF₁ mice can be grouped into two families of Ids.[G73,G75] The first, Id564, is composed entirely of cationic IgG and most bear the Igh allotype of the SWR parent. The second Id cluster, Id512, contains Ig of anionic, neutral, and cationic charge; the allotypes expressed are both SWR and NZB derived. Id564 is unique to SNF₁ mice and is not found in either parent. Again, this Id restriction is similar to that reported by our group in BW mice, where only two public Ids (IdGN1 and IdGN2) dominate the glomerular Ig deposits.[H30]

Sequence data show that the expression of Id564 depends upon the V_H region of the Ig molecule; Id564+ monoclonal antibodies are closely related structurally and probably derive from a germline gene that is unique to the SNF₁ mouse.[O42]

The expression of disease in SNF₁ mice requires T-cell participation, as in most (possibly all) of the mouse models discussed in this chapter. B cells from SNF₁ spleens (or BW spleens) secrete IgG anti-dsDNA (including cationic subsets) only when stimulated by T cells in culture.[A215,D51] Those T cells may bear the classical CD4+CD8− phenotype of helper T cells, or they may be CD4−CD8−. The CD4+CD8− cells bear the αβ TCR, but the CD4−CD8− cells bear γΔ.[D51] This contrasts with the MRL/lpr mouse, in which the unusual, hyperproliferating T cell is CD4−CD8− but αβ positive.[S466,T134]

As in the BW mouse, genes contributed from both parents are necessary for disease in the SNF₁.[E7] Some genes are clearly linked to H-2. However, one study suggests that nephritis is also influenced by the TCR β chain (which contains a large deletion similar to the NZW), as well as the I-A β chain of the SWR parent.[G117]

In summary, the SNF₁ mouse is another example of female-dominant, T-cell–dependent lupus nephritis in a hybrid mouse with an NZB background. The nature of the antibodies that deposit in glomeruli has been particularly well studied and is somewhat oligoclonal, thus providing important information about the characteristics and genetic control of pathogenic subsets of autoantibodies.

MRL/Mp-lpr/lpr Mice (MRL/lpr)

The MRL/lpr strain and the congenic MRL (+/+), also called MRL/n, were developed by Murphy and Roths in 1976.[M665] They are derived from LG/J mice crossed with AKR/J, C3HDi, and C57Bl/6. The lpr (lymphoproliferation) trait occurred as a spontaneous mutation in a single autosomal recessive gene; it causes massive lymphoproliferation in virtually any recipient. By the twelfth generation of inbreeding, the MRL/lpr was derived and was characterized by marked lymphadenopathy and splenomegaly, large quantities of antibodies to DNA, and lethal immune nephritis. MRL/+ + mice, lacking the lpr gene, share over 95% of the genetic material of MRL/lpr.[T133] MRL/+ + mice are abnormal and develop late-life lupus. They make anti-DNA, anti-Sm, and rheumatoid factors, but serum levels are lower than those of MRL/lpr mice. Male and female MRL/+ + are similarly affected; most develop clinical nephritis with advancing age and are dead by 24 months.[A225,M665,T133]

In MRL/lpr mice, the quantities of antibodies provided by the MRL/+ + background are greatly amplified, probably by the T-cell help delivered by the cells expanded by lymphoproliferation.[M610] The dominant cells that pack lymph nodes and spleen bear the surface phenotype

Table 17–5. Characteristics of MRL/lpr Mice

A. Clinical
 1. Massive lymphadenopathy.
 2. Early death in males and females (50% mortality at 6 months).
 3. Congenic strain MRL/+ + lacks lpr, 50% mortality at 17 months.
 4. Deaths are usually due to immune glomerulonephritis.
 5. About one-half develop acute necrotizing polyarteritis.
 6. In some colonies, about 25% develop destructive polyarthritis.
B. Histologic
 1. Subacute proliferation of mesangial and endothelial cells, occasional glomerular crescents, basement membrane thickening. Deposits of Ig and C3 in glomeruli, especially in capillary walls.
 2. Acute polyarteritis of coronary and renal arteries.
 3. Proliferative synovitis, pannus formation, and destruction of articular cartilage.
 4. Thymic atrophy.
 5. Massive hyperplasia of all lymphoid organs, sometimes with hemorrhage and cystic necrosis.
C. Autoantibodies
 1. Monoclonal paraproteins in about 40%.
 2. Most marked elevations of serum IgG, IgM, and immune complexes of all the murine models of SLE.
 3. ANAs at highest levels of all murine SLE models.
 4. IgG and IgM anti-dsDNA and anti-ssDNA.
 5. Anti-Sm in 10% of females, 35% of males.
 6. IgM and IgG rheumatoid factors in 65%; some IgG-IgG complexes.
 7. gp70–anti-gp70 complexes.
 8. Hypocomplementemia.
D. Immune Abnormalities
 1. Lymphoid hyperplasia is primarily due to expansion of an unusual CD2+, weak CD4+ or CD4−, CD8−, B220+, αβ+ T cells.
 2. Appearance of these T cells and of early disease is strictly thymus dependent.
 3. High numbers of hyperactivated B cells appear just before onset of clinical disease.
 4. Defective Fc-mediated phagocytosis and clearance of immune complexes.
E. Genetics
 1. Accelerated disease is produced by a single autosomal recessive gene, lpr. Mice homozygous for this gene develop lymphoproliferation on most backgrounds, but clinical autoimmune disease appears primarily in backgrounds that are permissive, such as MRL/+ + and NZB.
 2. The congenic MRL/+ + has a B-cell repertoire that makes anti-DNA, anti-Sm, and rheumatoid factors. These autoantibodies are probably controlled by multiple genes, as in the NZB.
E. Genetics
 1. An autosomal recessive gene, lpr, controls the lymphoproliferation in MRL/lpr mice.

CD3+, CD4− (or weakly +), CD8−, and B220+. They bear αβ T-cell receptors and are therefore part of the T-cell lineage.[M610,S466,T134]

Both male and female MRL/lpr mice develop high serum levels of immunoglobulins, monoclonal paraproteins, ANAs, and immune complexes (the highest of all murine lupus strains).[A225,T133] They make IgM and IgG anti-ss and anti-dsDNA and die from immune nephritis at a young age (90% dead by 9 months of age). Other antibodies in their repertoire include IgG2a antichromatin, anti-RBCs, antithyroglobulin, antilymphocyte, anti-Sm antiribosomal P, and anti-RNA polymerase I.[B486,E77,F110,S532,S676] The following features are found in MRL/lpr and never or rarely in NZB mice and their hybrids: 1) massive lymphoproliferation, 2) destructive inflammatory polyarthritis, 3) rheumatoid factors, 4) severe necrotizing arteritis, and 5) anti-Sm.[A225,T133,T134]

In females, anti-DNAs are detectable in the circulation by 6 to 8 weeks of age, proteinuria begins at 1 to 3 months, and death associated with azotemia occurs at 3 to 6 months.[A225,T133] Males lag behind females by approximately 1 month. IgG2a antibodies to DNA deposit in glomeruli. The IgG and anti-DNA repertoire is dominated by a public idiotype, H130.[R59] These features are reminiscent of the nephritis of BW and SNF₁ mice. Histology of the kidneys shows proliferation of mesangial and endothelial cells in glomeruli, occasional crescent formation, and basement membrane thickening.[A225] IgG, C3, and anti-DNA are deposited in glomeruli; the presence of gp70 is variable and less constant than in NZB and related strains.[A228] Antibodies to RNA polymerase I may also contribute to nephritis.[S676] Renal failure is the primary cause of death.

Lymphoproliferation is the hallmark of MRL/lpr mice. In both males and females, lymphadenopathy begins by 3 months of age.[A225,T133] Nodes can reach one hundred times normal size, and may develop hemorrhage and necrosis (see Fig. 17–2). Lymphoid malignancies are rare. Normal mouse strains upon which the lpr gene is engrafted yield homozygotes that have lymphoproliferation; most develop anti-DNA, and varying proportions develop nephritis (not as universal or severe as in MRL/lpr mice).[164,T133] Therefore, the lpr gene confers characteristics on T cells that increase their proliferation[K104,M610] and probably provide help for B cells that make autoantibodies. In fact, T-cell help for syngeneic B cells is more marked in MRL/lpr than in NZB or BXSB mice.[T133] The most prominent cell found in the large nodes is unusual in that it bears both T- and B-cell surface markers (CD3+, B220+).[M610,S446,T134] Since the cells express the T-cell αβ receptor, they are T cells. Expression of CD4 is absent or weak; CD8 is not expressed. There may be some clonal restriction among these cells; the genes used to assemble their TCRs are diverse,[S467] but the autoreactive Vβ 8.2 and 8.3 are over-represented, being found in 60%.[S467] CD4 and CD8 surface molecules may be lost late in thymic maturation. Highly autoreactive T cells should be deleted early from the thymic repertoire. There is evidence that this early deletion process is normal in MRL/lpr mice,[K391,M633] suggesting that escape of relatively mature, late-stage cells from the thymic selection process is pro-

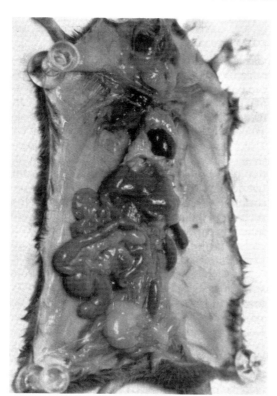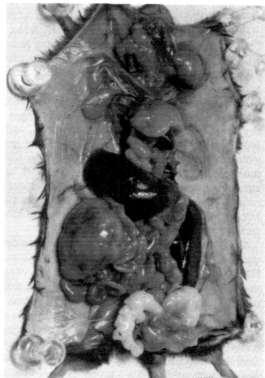

Fig. 17–2. Massive lymphoproliferation induced by the lpr gene. On the left is a mouse with a normal lymphoid system; on the right is a mouse with massive enlargement of cervical, auxiliary, and mesenteric lymph nodes, liver, and spleen. The picture on the left would be typical of an MRL/n mouse; the picture on the right would be typical of an MRL/lpr mouse. The mice pictured are C57Bl/lpr mice fed restricted calories (left) or a normal diet (right). (Provided by Dr. Normal Talal through the courtesy of Drs. Gabriel Fernandez and Robert Good from the Texas Health Sciences Center, San Antonio, and the Oklahoma Medical Research Foundation.)

vided by the lpr gene.[S469] The ability of MRL/lpr T cells to cap, proliferate, express IL-2 surface receptors, and secrete IL-2 after antigenic or mitogenic stimulation is impaired.[A165,D76] Some work suggests this may be due to deficient signaling via the phophoinositide pathway.[S163]

Classic CD4 + CD8 − T cells also play a role in the disease, and probably provide functional T-cell help to lpr B cells.[C335,F111,S392] Treatment with anti-CD4 decreases IgG anti-DNA, lymphadenopathy, and splenomegaly,[S75] so these cells also proliferate in response to the lpr gene.

Polyarthritis occurs in MRL/lpr mice in some but not all colonies. The prevalence varies between 15 and 25% in susceptible colonies.[A225,H99,O117,T133] Clinically, the mice develop swelling in the hind feet and lower legs. Histology[O117] shows, by 14 weeks of age, synovial cell proliferation with early subchondral bone destruction and marginal erosions. Cartilage is intact in this early lesion, and the synovial stroma is devoid of inflammatory cells. By 19 weeks of age, there is destruction of cartilage and subchondral bone associated with proliferating synovial lining cells and pannus formation. Mild inflammation occurs in synovial stroma but is remote from areas of cartilage damage. Focal arteriolitis can occur. By 25 weeks of age, the inflammatory response in synovium is more marked, but proliferating synovial lining cells continue to

be present; joint destruction has progressed to development of periarticular fibrous scar tissue and new bone formation. The animals have rheumatoid factors and antibodies to collagen type II.[A225,O117,T133] There is a correlation between the presence of IgM rheumatoid factor and arthritis.[H99] The rheumatoid factors in MRL/lpr mice differ from those in MRL/ + + and C57Bl6-lpr/lpr in that they are more likely to bind IgG2a than other IgG isotypes.[A61] All these features raise the possibility that MRL/lpr mice are a model of spontaneous, genetically controlled arthritis similar to human rheumatoid arthritis. However, since mice in some colonies do not develop the arthropathy, even though they have rheumatoid factors, it seems likely that additional environmental factors are required to trigger disease. It is particularly fascinating that the initial destructive lesions are formed by proliferating synovium without inflammatory cells.

Antibodies to Sm antigen occur only in the MRL/lpr and MRL/ + + models of SLE.[A225,T133] They are found in approximately 25% of animals. The reasons some MRL/lpr mice express anti-Sm and others do not is not clear; there are no demonstrable genetic or environmental factors that account for the differences.[E61] There may be a role for antibody specificities; the D epitope of Sm may contain helper epitopes that permit antibody expression;

the B epitope may contain suppressor epitopes.[E65] Antigen specificity for components of the polypeptide-snRNP complex are similar to the specificities of human anti-Sm. The anti-Sm response is dominated by public idiotypes (e.g., Y2), which can be found on human anti-Sm and on other human and murine autoantibodies.[D34,P214] The ability to make anti-Sm does not correlate with clinical nephritis.

Acute necrotizing arteritis, primarily of coronary and renal arteries, is found in over half of MRL/lpr males and females.[A225,T133] Many have myocardial infarctions, but these seem more related histologically to small vessel vasculopathy than to inflammation of medium-sized arteries. The degenerative vascular disease consists of PAS-positive, eosinophilic deposits in the intima and media of small vessels, without inflammation. Ig, C3, and occasionally gp70 can be found in the walls of medium and small arteries, venules, and arterioles. Thymic cortical atrophy is severe, and medullary hyperplasia common, as in NZB and BW mice.[A225]

An additional interesting abnormality in MRL/lpr and MRL/++ mice is the development of band keratopathy and of posterior uveitis in as many as one-third of mice.[H365]

The immunologic abnormality in MRL/lpr mice is complex. There is excessive T-cell help.[C335,S392,T133] The anti-Sm response is strictly T-cell dependent; both it and the anti-dsDNA response are dominated by the IgG2a isotype.[S392] In contrast, the antichromatin response is not T-cell dependent,[F111] suggesting that abnormalities in B-cell repertoire are also necessary for full expression of autoantibody repertoires and disease. B-cell hyperactivation occurs, but later and less dramatically than in mice of other lupus strains. Recent studies in chimeric mice show that the lpr B cell is necessary for autoantibody production in the absence of MRL background;[S532] in MRL/lpr mice the contribution of the MRL background apparently provides B cells with appropriate antibody repertoires to cause autoimmunity.

The disease is more thymus dependent than in other strains. Thymectomy of newborn MRL/lpr mice prevents development of lymphoproliferation and autoimmune disease;[S498,S641,S648,T133] MRL/lpr thymus engrafted into MRL/++ mice causes lymphoproliferation and early death from autoimmune nephritis.[T133]

Abnormal cell functions extend to populations other than lymphocytes.[G370] Neutrophils from MRL/lpr mice (but not MRL/++) have a marked defect in FcR-mediated phagocytosis, which develops at the time of onset of autoimmune disease; this may be due to elevated levels of TGFβ in the serum. Their ability to access areas of inflammation may also be impaired.

The genetics of MRL/lpr disease are fairly well understood. Backcross studies have shown (as in NZB and NZB hybrid mice) that the ability to secrete large quantities of Ig, and the ability to make several different autoantibodies, segregate independently of each other.[T134,K393,E61] Therefore, several independent genes are involved in creating B-cell repertoires. The T-cell defect, on the other hand, may be conferred entirely by a single gene, lpr, which is inherited as an autosomal recessive.[M610,M665,S498,S641]

In summary, MRL/lpr mice are particularly interesting as a model of the accelerating factor for autoimmunity that can be provided by a single gene added to a susceptible host. The lymphoproliferation associated with the autosomal recessive lpr gene results in excessive T-cell help. This help engrafted on a B-cell repertoire that can make pathogenic autoantibodies results in accelerated autoimmunity and early death from lupus-like nephritis, probably mediated by IgG2a antibodies to DNA. Some MRL/lpr mice develop destructive polyarthritis, often associated with IgM rheumatoid factors. MRL mice are the only strains that make anti-Sm.

BXSB/MpJ (BXSB) Mice

Like the MRL/lpr mouse, the BXSB strain was developed by Murphy and Roths.[M666,M667] BXSB is a recombinant inbred (RI) strain; RI mice are derived by brother-sister matings within each generation, usually extending 12 to 20 generations. RI are used to produce strains with high frequencies of homozygosity at many loci in order to see expression of recessive genes. The initial mating was between a C57Bl/6 female and an SB/Le male (BXSB).

The unique features of BXSB mice are that their disease is much worse in the male than the female, and the disease-accelerating gene responsible for that difference is located on the Y chromosome. The gene is called Yaa for Y chromosome autoimmunity accelerator. The female BXSB gets late-life lupus; therefore additional genes contribute to disease, as in all the other lupus models studied to date.

BXSB mice make an autoantibody repertoire that includes IgG antibodies to ssDNA and dsDNA, antichromatin, ANAs, and antibodies directed against brain cells.[A225,H366,M71,T133] In addition, a small proportion make antierythrocytes, NTAs, monoclonal paraproteins, and gp70–anti-gp70 immune complexes.[A225,T133] By an early age (3 months) they have elevated levels of circulating immune complexes and hypocomplementemia.[A225] They are the only lupus mouse strain that has serum levels of C4 that diminish as clinical disease appears.[G52]

Death is caused by immune glomerulonephritis.[A225,M71,S641,T133] Histologically, the disease is more exudative than in other mouse models. That is, there are neutrophils invading glomeruli along with IgG and C3 deposition, proliferative changes in mesangia and endothelial cells, and basement membrane thickening.[A225] The progression from nephritis to death is rapid, with 50% of males dead by 5 months of age.[A225,M71,T133] In fact, of the most widely studied SLE mouse models, the BXSB has the most fulminant disease.

Lymphoproliferation occurs in BXSB mice; it is more marked than in BW but less dramatic than in MRL/lpr.[A225,T133] In contrast to MRL/lpr mice, the hyperplastic nodes contain predominantly B cells,[S641,T133] and for some time it was thought that the B-cell defects are the primary abnormality in BXSB mice. As in the other models, B cells are hyperactivated, higher portions are mature (expressing IgD and IgM on their surfaces), and secretion of IgG and IgM is increased.[S641,T133] The B cells are resistant to tolerance with human gamma globulin;

Table 17-6. Characteristics of BXSB Mice

A. Clinical
   1. Males die early of lupus (50% mortality at 5 months; 90% at 8 months).
   2. Females have late onset lupus (50% mortality at 15 months; 90% at 24 months).
   3. Major cause of death is immune glomerulonephritis.
B. Histologic
   1. Males show severe acute to subacute glomerulonephritis with proliferation and exudation of neutrophils into glomeruli.
   2. In males, IgG and C3 deposit in mesangium and glomerular capillary walls by 3 months of age; deposits in tubular basement membranes and interstitium also.
   3. Lymph node hyperplasia (10 to 20 times normal size) in males.
   4. Myocardial infarcts in 25%, without arteritis.
   5. Thymic cortical atrophy with medullary hyperplasia. Thymic epithelial cells contain crystalline inclusions.
C. Autoantibodies
   1. All males develop ANAs and IgG anti-dsDNa and anti-ssDNA.
   2. Less than half of males develop monoclonal paraproteins, anti-erythrocyte antibodies, gp70–anti-gp70, thymocytotoxic antibodies.
   3. Hypocomplementemia in males by 3 months of age; low C4 levels.
   4. Elevated levels of circulating immune complexes.
D. Immune Abnormalities
   1. B cell is the most frequent cell in hyperplastic lymph nodes.
   2. B-cell hyperactivation and advanced maturity.
   3. B cells are resistant to tolerance with some antigens.
   4. Male bone marrow transferred to female BXSB mice produces accelerated disease: female marrow confers late lupus when transferred to males. Mature male B cells do not accelerate disease; abnormality is contained in marrow stem cells.
   5. Monocytosis occurs.
   6. Elimination of CD4 + T cells diminishes anti-DNA, monocytosis, nephritis, and mortality.
   7. Disease is not influenced substantially by thymectomy.
   8. Disease is not influenced substantially by sex hormone therapies and/or castration.
   9. Defective Fc-mediated immune complex clearance.
E. Genetics
   1. A single gene that accelerates disease, Yaa, is present on the Y chromosome.
   2. Additional genes that behave as X-linked recessives confer susceptibility to disease. They may account for late-life SLE in females.

the resistance is a property of the B cell itself and does not reflect abnormalities in antigen-presenting cells or in T cells.[G55] However, it is now clear that T cells play a necessary role in disease[D353,V18] removal of CD4 + T cells with an appropriate monoclonal antibody suppresses autoantibody formation and disease.[W314] Thymectomy has accelerated disease in some hands and has not altered it in others;[S508,T135] the effects are not as consistent and dramatic as the protection from disease conferred by thymectomy in MRL/lpr mice.[S498,S641,S648,T133]

An additional feature of BXSB mice is monocytosis. Further, the monocytes/macrophages are abnormal; they make unusually large quantities of procoagulants, which might contribute to the rapid damage of glomeruli that characterizes lupus in this strain.[C342]

Thymic cortical atrophy occurs in BXSB mice as it does in all the other lupus strains.[A225] Crystalline structures have been described in thymic epithelial cells of BXSB males; they are thought to represent abnormal storage of thymic hormones.[D44]

There is good evidence that a stem cell abnormality is crucial to the development of disease in BXSB mice,[S234,T133] since bone male BXSB bone marrow can transfer disease, and normal marrow grafted into male BXSB mice can prevent disease.[H130,I6,S234,T133] This is reviewed in more detail in the Pathogenesis section of this chapter. This stem cell defect, or other factors, must also influence T cells. They provide help for autoantibody formation, even though as mice age they develop the typical T-cell defects of SLE mice (abnormally low proliferative responses to antigens/mitogens, reduced production of IL-2, etc.). The elimination of CD4 + T cells suppresses autoantibodies, monocytosis, and nephritis.[W314]

The genetics of BXSB lupus are complex, as in the other models. There is an inherent tendency to autoimmune disease in BXSB mice of both sexes; that tendency is dramatically accelerated by the introduction of Yaa—a gene on the Y chromosome. This accounts for the earlier, more severe disease in males. Manipulations such as castration and androgen therapy do not dramatically alter outcome.[E62,S641,T133] The Yaa gene alone is probably not sufficient to permit development of autoimmunity: C57Bl/J mice mated with male BXSB do not develop autoantibodies or disease. In contrast, male BXSB mated with (NZW × C57Bl/6) F_1 hybrids produce males with anti-DNA, gp70–anti-gp70 immune complexes and early death from nephritis.[164] Therefore, genes contributed from the NZW background seem essential for the Yaa gene to exert its accelerating effect. Susceptibility to autoimmunity is transmitted as an autosomal dominant trait in some F_1 hybrids derived from BXSB,[E62,E64,M666] and in others susceptibility behaves as if it were controlled by autosomal recessive genes.[T133]

In summary, BXSB mice are unique in that lupus nephritis is more severe and earlier in males than in females; this is from the accelerating effect of a single gene, Yaa, which is located on the Y chromosome. Expression of disease acceleration is not influenced by sex hormones. Evidence for a stem cell defect that makes B cells autoimmune is strong; whether that same stem cell defect accounts for abnormalities in T-cell and monocyte/macrophage functions is unclear.

Other Models of Murine SLE

Chronic Graft-versus-Host Disease (GVH)

GVH is produced in mice by injecting lymphocytes from a parent into an F_1 hybrid differing at one MHC locus from that parent. Acute GVH is runting disease with failure to thrive, diarrhea, wasting, and early death. If injections are made after the recipient F_1 has reached at least 6 weeks of age, and if certain H-2 genes are represented in the parent and F_1, chronic GVH results. Chronic GVH resembles SLE.[G193,G195,K227,P264,R279,V29] Several IgG autoantibodies are made, including anti-dsDNA, anti-ssDNA, and antihistone.[P264,V29] In some combinations, fatal lupus-like nephritis mediated by the IgG anti-DNA occurs.

CD4 + effector cells provided by the donor are required for induction of chronic GVH,[M601,R279,V29] they must be activated by appropriate MHC class II gene products on the surface of recipient cells.[G193,G195,K227,P264]

Table 17–7. Pathogenesis of Autoimmunity in Murine Models of SLE

Immune Abnormality	Mouse Strains	Genetic Basis of Abnormalities
1. Individual B-cell hypersecretion of Ig	NZB NZB/NZW F_1 Female NZB/SWR F_1 Female BXSB Male (MRL/lpr)	Two or more unlinked genes, both semidominant and recessive. Increased IsM production linked to NTA, increased gp70, increased CD5+ B cells. Increased IgG2a synthesis linked to anti-dsDNA and nephritis.
2. Increased numbers of B cells secreting Ig	Same as 1	Two or more unlinked genes, unlinked to genes in 1, both semidominant and recessive.

3. Production of autoantibodies (initially polyclonal, later Ag specific)
  Natural thymocytotoxic (NTA)
  Antierythrocyte
  Anti-DNA (anti-ssDNA)
    (anti-dsDNA)
  Antihistone
  Antichromatin
  Antibrain cells
  Anti-RNA polymerase I
  gp70–anti-gp70
 	
  Anti-Sm
  Rheumatoid factors
  Switch from IgM to IgG
	
	All, especially NZB
	All except SNF_1
	All, especially BW, SN, MRL/l
	All except NZB
	All
	All
	All
	BW, MRL/l
	All except SNF_1, especially NZB, NZB/NZW F_1
	MRL only
	MRL only
	All except NZB
		NTA: NZB contributes 1 or more dominant genes, correlates with anti-dsDNA but not anti-ssDNA in NZB hybrids.
		Antierythrocyte: Multiple genes required: segregates with anti-ssDNA, anti-gp70, and defects in tolerance.
		Anti-DNA, anti-ssDNA: Multiple genes, segregates somewhat differently from anti-dsDNA.
		anti-dsDNA: Requires MHC-linked genes, including some linked to MHC class II. Probable linkage to I-A and or I-E gene products (equivalent to human DR and DQ HLA class II). Controlled by at least 2 genes from NZB, NZW, and SWR parents in NZB hybrids—at least 1 linked to chromosome 17 from each parent. Linked to nephritis in all strains, but IgG anti-dsDNAs are neither absolutely necessary or sufficient for development of severe GN.
		IgM to IgG switch: Depends on T cells. Probably controlled by MHC-linked genes.

4. Fatal immune glomerulonephritis	All except NZB	Fatal nephritis: linked to anti-dsDNA, IgM to IgG switch, anti-gp70 in some strains. Linked to H-2 in NZB and in BW and SNF_1. Requires $H-2^{d/z}$, $H-2^{d/q}$, $H-2^{bm12}$ in NZB backgrounds. Autoantibody production and glomerulonephritis are accelerated on many backgrounds by lpr or Yaa genes. lpr causes lymphoproliferation and is an autosomal recessive. Yaa is an autoimmunity accelerating gene in the Y chromosome of BXSB mice. Neither gene is sufficient by itself to cause autoimmunity.

The most effective combination that results in fatal nephritis is H-2^d donor lymphocytes into an H-2^b recipient.[G195,P279] Most recipient H-2^k haplotypes are resistant. The development of clinical nephritis and the development of autoantibodies can be separated. Many parental hybrid combinations result in ability of the recipient to make high-titer IgG anti-DNA, but class II genes I-A and I-E (probably equivalent to human HLA class II DR and DQ) must contain the b haplotype for severe nephritis to result.[P264] Animals without nephritis confine renal deposits of IgG to mesangial regions of glomeruli; animals with nephritis have IgG deposits along capillary loops.[P264] Whether the differences in I-A/I-E are correlated with differences in antibody subsets or in ability of glomerular cells to react to them is unknown.

This model provides perhaps the best example of lupus nephritis resulting from interactions between helper T cells and antigen-presenting cells with certain MHC-determined genetic characteristics.

Palmerston North Mice (PN)

PN mice are descendants of albino mice purchased from a pet shop in 1948 and raised at the Palmerston North Hospital in New Zealand. Inbreeding was started in 1964, with animals selected for ANA positivity. Autoantibodies and nephritis were characterized by Walker in 1978.[W15] Fifty percent survivals are 11 months for females and 15 months for males. The mice develop two main lesions—necrotizing vasculitis of small and medium arteries, and proliferative glomerulonephritis with fibrinoid necrosis, crescent formation, and glomerular deposits of IgG and C3. Arteritis occurs in spleen, thymus, kidneys, ovaries, and lungs, with sparing of the aorta. Lymph nodes are hyperplastic in some mice, and malignant lymphoma

Table 17–7. Pathogenesis of Autoimmunity in Murine Models of SLE—*(Continued)*

Immune Abnormality	Mouse Strains	Genetic Basis of Abnormalities
5. Stem cell abnormalities	BXSB, possibly all	Stem cell abnormalities: Linked to Yaa.
6. Thymic cortical atrophy	All, especially NZB	For other features on list on left, genetics are not known.
7. Lymphoproliferation	MRL/lpr > BSXB > NZB > BW, SNF₁	For other features on list on left, genetics are not known.
8. Excessive T-cell help	All, especially BW, MRL	For other features on list on left, genetics are not known.
9. Defective T-cell activation	All	For other features on list on left, genetics are not known.
10. Expansion of an unusual T cell (CD3+, CD4−, CD8−, B220+, αβ)	MRL/lpr, C57/lpr, all lpr-bearing mice	Expansion of an unusual cell: Linked to lpr and to Yaa.
11. Defective clearance of immune complexes	All	For other features on list on left, genetics are not known.
12. Defective neutrophil phagocytosis	MRL/lpr	For other features on list on left, genetics are not known.
13. Monocytosis/macrophage abnormalities	MRL/lpr, BXSB	For other features on list on left, genetics are not known.
14. Sex hormones have major role in enhancing autoantibody expression and clinical nephritis.	NZB/NZW F₁	For other features on list on left, genetics are not known.

In all strains:

Two or more unlinked genes, both semidominant and recessive, are required for full immunologic and clinical manifestations of SLE.

Genetic requirements for individual autoantibodies and/or clinical manifestations in mice with NZ background are as follows:

Natural thymocytotoxic antibodies (NTA): NZB contributes 1 or more dominant genes, correlates with anti-dsDNA but not anti-ssDNA in NZB hybrids.

Anti-erythrocyte: Multiple genes required: segregates with anti-ssDNA anti-gp70 and defects in tolerance.

Anti-DNA: anti-ssDNA: Multiple genes, segregates somewhat differently from anti-dsDNA.

anti-dsDNA: Requires MHC-linked genes, including some linked to MHC Class II. Probable linkage to I-A and or I-E gene products (equivalent to human DR and DQ HLA Class II). Controlled by at least 2 genes from NZB, NZW and SWR parents in NZB hybrids— at least 1 linked to Chromosome 17 from each parent. Linked to nephritis in all strains, but IgG anti-dsDNA are neither absolutely necessary or sufficient for development of severe GN.

IgM to IgG Switch: Depends on T cells. Probably controlled by MHC-linked genes.

Fatal Nephritis: Linked to anti-dsDNA, IgM to IgG switch, anti-gp70 in some strains. Linked to H-2 in NZB and in BW and SNF1. Requires H-2$^{d/z}$, H-2$^{d/q}$, H-2^{bm12} in NZB backgrounds.

Genetic Requirements in Mice with backgrounds other than NZ: AUTOANTIBODY PRODUCTION AND GLOMERULONEPHRITIS ARE ACCELERATED ON MANY BACKGROUNDS BY lpr OR Yaa GENES. lpr causes lymphoproliferation and is an autosomal recessive. Yaa is an autoimmunity accelerating gene in the Y chromosome of BXSB mice. NEITHER GENE IS SUFFICIENT BY ITSELF TO CAUSE AUTOIMMUNITY.

Stem Cell Abnormalities: LInked to Yaa.

Expansion of an unusual lymphocyte: Linked to lpr and to Yaa.

occurs. Thymic cortical atrophy occurs late (about 11 months) in males at 20 months.

Anti-DNA and ANAs may be present at birth in some PN mice, and increase with age until most animals are positive. The anti-DNA response is predominantly IgM. LE cells have been reported. As the mice age, the proliferative responses of their T cells tends to diminish, as in other lupus strains.[W16] The most remarkable finding in PN mice is the appearance of autoantibodies and Ig deposition in glomeruli in the first few weeks after birth.

PATHOGENESIS OF MURINE LUPUS—GENETICS AND IMMUNE ABNORMALITIES

Murine lupus is a genetically determined disease.[A225, B3, C90,C233, D47,D48, D50,E7, E61,G74,G75,G101,G117,G195,H326, I64, K104,K227, K320,K395, K396,L36, M172,M355, M435,M610,M665,M666, M667,O34,P264,R68,S132,S641,T78,T79,T133, T134,V29, Y28,Y48,Y49,Y53]

In all strains, more than 90% of animals at risk develop a similar profile of autoantibodies and clinical manifestations of disease. (The only major exception occurs in MRL/lpr mice,[A225,E61,H49,I64,K104,O117,S392,T133,T134] with the incidence of arthritis varying between colonies in different environments, and anti-Sm appearing in only 25%

of animals.) There is evidence that environmental factors that add to the antigen, antibody, immune complex load can accelerate disease, but in general those contributions are minor.[C166,T133] Sex hormones also play a role—more important in some strains than others.[D370,R362,R364,R365]

In these primarily genetic diseases, multiple genes are required for full-blown disease to develop.[T134] No single gene, even lpr or Yaa, is sufficient to cause severe, uniformly fatal autoimmune diseases. Attempts to identify exact genes that control the multiple abnormalities that lead to autoimmune disease have been partially successful. In the next paragraphs, the immune abnormalities that characterize mice with lupus, and the proposed genetic basis for those abnormalities will be discussed. They are summarized in Table 17–7.

Methods for Performing Genetic Studies in Mice

Genetic studies in autoimmune and other mice may be performed in several ways. Mice with an abnormality that is under genetic control can be mated with healthy mice; if 50% of the hybrids have the abnormality, a single autosomal dominant gene may be responsible. Such studies are limited by the presence of multiple genetic differences in the two parental strains; one must assume that none of those differences affect disease or autoantibody formation, and that is unlikely to be true. Additional backcrosses with one of the parents allow analysis of the contribution of that parent. Examples include the F_1-Fn generations of NZB/SWR mice backcrossed to SWR mice.[E7] This technique maximizes the ability to define the contributions from the SWR parent to the disease of NZB/SWR F_1 mice. Recombinant inbred (RI) mice are made by 12 to 20 generations of brother-sister matings. This maximizes the expression of autosomal recessive genes. Congenic mice are made by mating mice for selected traits. For example, NZB mice are mated with CBA/N mice bearing the *xid* recessive gene that deletes CD5+ B cells.[T79] Matings within each generation are selected for expression of NZB Ig allotypes and of *xid*. This breeds out non-*xid* CBA/N genes. After several generations, NZB.*xid* mice should differ genetically from NZB mice only at the *xid* locus. Recombinant inbred lines and congenic mice are informative in analyzing the contribution of single genes to autoimmunity. The information regarding the genetics of the immune abnormalities discussed in the following paragraphs is based on multiple studies using backcross, RI, and/or congenic mice.

Abnormalities of Hematopoietic Stem Cells

Stem cells that evolve into B lymphocytes are clearly abnormal in BXSB and NZB mice, and they may be abnormal in all the lupus strains.[A225,D121,E7,E64,H310,K296,M617, M618,S234,S532,Y53,Y54] B cells in all are hyperactivated, with higher numbers of cells secreting Ig and each cell secreting higher quantities of Ig than is normal.[A225,K296,M634, T133,Y53] This "defect" appears earliest in the NZB and has been noted in B cells from fetal liver.[M634] In BXSB mice it is identifiable a few weeks after birth.[E64,M667,S234] The importance of stem cells is shown by the fact that transfer of bone marrow cells (but not spleen cells) from male, Yaa-bearing BXSB mice to females accelerates the female autoimmune disorders.[E64] Female bone marrow protects males from early lupus-like disease.[E64] Male BXSB mice can also be protected by bone marrow transplants from normal mice made tolerant to BXSB cells and depleted of T cells that mediate graft-versus-host disease.[H130,16] Therefore, BXSB stem cells play a major role in early autoimmune disease. The data are less clear for NZB mice;[Y53] there is some evidence that the microenvironment in which stem cells develop influences their ability to be hyperactivated.[K299,K302] The nature of the stem cell defect(s) is not known. One could postulate that a single abnormality leads to abnormal function (generally toward hyperactivation) of B and helper T cells, as well as monocytes/macrophages (abnormalities of which are most notable in MRL/lpr and BXSB mice). The B-cell abnormalities observed in murine lupus include autoantibody synthesis, abnormalities of B-cell tolerance, and restricted clonality.

B-Cell Abnormalities

Hyperactivation and Increased Ig Synthesis

As mentioned in the preceding paragraph, B cells in all SLE mouse models are hyperactivated, with increased surface IgD and IgM expression, increased synthesis of Ig per cell, and increased numbers of cells secreting Ig.[K296,M103,M410,M634,S532,S641,T128,T133,Y53] In NZB mice and their hybrids, the population of CD5+ (Ly-1+) B cells is increased.[H219,H221,R67,Y53] That may be relevant because CD5+ B cells make autoantibodies, chiefly of the IgM class. The ability of each B cell to secrete high quantities of IgM is controlled by at least two genes from the NZB mouse; it is linked to the ability to make NTA, gp70 antigen, and to increases in CD5+ B cells.[B585,D50,M435,R68,Y53] The increased numbers of cells synthesizing IgM is inherited independently of the genes controlling Ig secretion per cell, and requires at least two genes from NZB mice. None of these genes is linked to MHC.[M435,R68,Y53] Neither abnormality is linked to clinical nephritis.[M172,M435,R68,S641,Y53] However, the ability to secrete increased quantities of IgG2a, in contrast to IgM, is linked to the ability to make IgG2 anti-dsDNA and to nephritis; these manifestations are linked to H-2.[A225,B3,E7, G101,H326,K320,K395,K396,M172,O34,S641,T133,T134,Y48,Y49,Y53]

B cells may also appear hyperactivated in lupus-prone mice because they hyper-respond to B-cell growth factors, released primarily from helper T cells but also from the B cells themselves. For example, spleen cells from young BW mice make more Ig in response to supernatants of TH-2 type T-cell clones, or to recombinant Il-5.[H283,H284] However, hyper-reactivity to IL-5 is not a feature of B cells from BXSB or MRL/lpr mice.[U17]

Autoantibody Production

The major consequence of B-cell abnormalities is synthesis of autoantibodies in high quantities, some of which contain pathogenic subsets that cause disease. Many of the autoantibodies made by mice with SLE are inherited independently of other autoantibodies; some are linked. The ability to make IgG anti-dsDNA and to develop nephritis are linked to each other, to NTA and to H-2.[A225,B3, E7, G101,H326,K320,K395,K396,M71,M172,O34,S641,T133,T134, Y49,Y53]

Mice with an NZB background must inherit the H-2 haplotype H-$2^{d/z}$ or H-$2^{d/q}$ to develop severe nephritis.[B3,E7,H326, K395,K396,Y49] These are the haplotypes of BW and SNF_1 mice. Therefore, contributions from all parents (NZB, which is H-$2^{d/d}$; NZW, which is H-$2^{z/z}$; SWR, which is H-$2^{q/q}$) are required. In fact, in SNF_1 mice, some of the putatively most nephritogenic subsets of cationic IgG2b anti-dsDNA are made from Ig genes contributed by the normal SWR parent; others use the Ig allotype of the NZB.[G73,G74,G75] There may be further linkage of anti-dsDNA and nephritis to the MHC class II molecules I-A and I-E,[C233,G117,S132] which are equivalent to HLA-DR and DQ in humans. The I-E^z molecule of NZW mice is different from a normal I-E^u molecule by one amino acid at position 72 in its β chain.[S132] An NZB recombinant, NZB^{bm12}, differs from NZB by expressing an I-A molecule that has a similar change at position 72 in its β chain, probably derived from the I-E chain by gene conversion. Normally, NZB mice do not develop IgG anti-dsDNA and few develop severe nephritis; in contrast, NZB^{bm12} mice develop both.[C233] These data imply that amino acids at the 72 position in the I-E or I-A β chain play an important role in susceptibility to autoimmunity. However, extensive studies using NZB/NZW F_1 mice backcrossed with NZB mice showed that correlations between nephritis, H-$2^{d/z}$, I-A$^{d/z}$, and I-E$^{d/z}$ are incomplete; nephritis occurs in a small proportion of H-$2^{d/d}$ mice.[B3]

Genetic contributions of MHC class II genes were sought because products of those genes on surfaces of antigen-presenting cells present peptides to the T-cell receptors (TCRs) on surfaces of helper T cells to activate T-cell help. Since nephritis in all murine lupus models depends on T-cell help,[A215,C335,D51,D353,G193,G195,K227, M601,P264,R279,S75,S469,S648,V29,W314,W319,W320,Y53] it is tempting to postulate that certain genetically controlled structures within TCRs predispose to murine lupus. NZW and SWR mice have large deletions in the β chains of their TCRs.[G117,K395,N122,T134,Y28] In BW mice, one study showed a positive correlation between inheritance of the deletion and development of anti-dsDNA and nephritis;[Y28] another large series showed no correlation.[K395] In SNF$_1$ mice, anti-dsDNA and nephritis do not segregate with the TCR deletion,[G117] so that most evidence suggests that the TCR deletion is not important to disease.

The only other autoantibody that correlates with severe nephritis is anti-gp70, usually complexed with the murine leukemia virus antigen gp70.[A225,A228,D47,D48,D50,G20,M172, M435,R68,S641,T133,Y53] It seems to worsen nephritis in NZB mouse backgrounds, but not in MRL backgrounds.[A224,A228,G201,S641,T133,Y53] It is linked to ability to make IgG anti-ssDNA in NZ mice. The ability to make anti-ssDNA is weakly linked with anti-dsDNA, but probably requires at least some differences in genetic background. It segregates with ability to make antierythrocyte antibodies and with defects in tolerance, and is controlled by multiple genes.[H326,K320,K395,M172,Y49,Y53]

Abnormalities of B-Cell Tolerance

B-cell tolerance is abnormal in mice with SLE-like disease. As NZB, BW, SNF$_1$, and MRL/lpr mice age, their ability to develop tolerance to some T-independent antigens, such as human gamma globulin, diminishes.[B506,G55, G253,S641] Our group was able to tolerize newborn BW mice to sonicated ssDNA presented on a tolerogenic carrier molecule, which prevented formation of anti-dsDNA and development of nephritis. However, once the mice were more than 2 weeks old, tolerance was difficult to achieve.[P52,T63] Most investigators have attributed these abnormalities of tolerance to primary B-cell defects. However, a recent study in MRL/lpr mice suggested that T-cell populations were able to abrogate tolerance induced directly in B cells.[M434] The tolerance defects are not universal for all antigens. See Chapter 7 for a detailed discussion of abnormalities of tolerance in SLE.

Restricted Clonality in B Cells

A final consideration regarding B cells is the possibility that certain clones that make pathogenic autoantibodies are selected for expansion. Normally, a few days after specific antigenic stimulation, clonal selection of B cells begins.[T65] Responder B cells express surface Ig with increasing avidity for the antigen, antigen binds tightly to their

surfaces; those cells are activated and preferentially expanded. There is evidence in NZB, BW, SNF$_1$, MRL/lpr, and BXSB strains that young mice have polyclonal activation of B cells.[B422,E7,E64,K296,M617,M618,M634,O34,S532,S641, S644,S757,T78,T79,T133,T135,W317,Y53,Y54] As they age, the polyclonal antibody response is increasingly replaced by antigen-driven B cells, thus establishing the autoantibody pattern characteristic of each strain.[E59,E65,K296,K298,M135,P42, P179,S376,S644] It is logical then to expect that only certain clones are expanded. There has been interest in the possibility that CD5 + (Ly-1 +) B cells are the source of autoantibodies in murine lupus.[C366,H219,H220,H221,M104,R67, W317,Y53] NZB and BW mice bearing the *xid* gene, which deletes Ly-1 + B cells and eliminates IgM synthesis, have substantially less autoantibody formation and nephritis than non-*xid* NZB and BW mice.[O34,T78,T79] However, approximately 20% of old NZB.*xid* and BW.*xid* mice develop autoantibodies and some die of nephritis.[O34] Other studies show that Ly-1 − B cells can make autoantibodies in mice.[C366,K297] Therefore, although Ly-1 + B cells may be important in making some of the autoantibody repertoire, they are not the exclusive source of pathogenic subsets.

Other evidence for restricted B-cell clonality includes the limited numbers of public idiotypes that dominate autoantibodies in most of the murine lupus strains.[H30,G73, G75,O42,R59] Some of these Ids are probably conformational; in general they do not define selected Ig V_H genes. A few studies analyzing anti-DNA repertoires in individual MRL/lpr or BW mice have concluded that frequent usage of highly similar V_H, D, J_H and light chain V regions by the majority of B cells demonstrates the clonality of the B-cell response.[M135,S376] In contrast, studies from our laboratory showed usage of multiple different V region genes in both heavy and light chains of antibodies from individual BW mice.[P31] The author is unconvinced that pathogenic autoantibody responses are restricted to a few B-cell clones. However, we agree with many other investigators who have shown preferential use of certain gene families in murine autoantibody construction.[E17,P31,T134] (See Chap. 8 for a more extensive discussion of the role of B cells in SLE.)

Abnormalities in T Cells

All the mouse strains that develop SLE-like disease develop abnormalities of T-cell function that are required for full expression of their syndromes. The importance of the abnormality varies somewhat; autoantibody production and nephritis are virtually abrogated by removal of CD4 + T cells in BW and MRL/lpr mice.[S75,W319,W320] Even in the NZB and BXSB strains with their remarkable B-cell/stem cell abnormalities, T-cell help can be demonstrated and definitely permits full expression of disease.[D51,D353,W314] T cells are required for the development of lupus nephritis in mice with chronic GVH disease.[G193,R279,V29]

Increased T-Cell Help

Switch of autoantibody isotype from IgM to IgG is essential for the development of nephritis in BW, SNF$_1$,

BXSB and MRL/lpr mice.[A215,C335,D51,D353,F117,M71,P37,P42,S75,S262,S697,T134] This switch is dependent on T-cell help, and occurs in all lupus-prone strains as they age, with the exception of NZB mice. We have shown that T cells isolated from spleens of nephritic BW mice greatly augment the production of IgG anti-dsDNA and anti-ssDNA by B cells from BW mice.[A215] CD4+ T cell clones and lines obtained from spleens of nephritic mice, either BW or SNF$_1$, help syngeneic B cells produce autoantibodies.[D51,S262] In fact, B cells obtained from old BW, SNF$_1$, or MRL/++ mice cannot synthesize IgG anti-dsDNA (including the cationic subsets) unless syngeneic old T cells are present.[A215,D51,S262] The phenotype of helper T cells includes at least two populations—the classic CD3+CD4+CD8− helper cell, and double-negative T cells (CD3+CD4−CD8−). The first population expresses the αβ T-cell receptor; the second expresses γΔ.[D51] These differ from the CD3+ CD4− CD8− B220+ αβ T cells that dominate MRL/lpr repertoires. T cells from young, non-nephritic mice cannot provide help to old B cells.[A215,D51,S262] Young B cells cannot produce IgG anti-dsDNA (they can make IgM and IgG anti-ssDNA), even when stimulated with old T cells or mitogens. Therefore, both T and B cells develop the ability to make pathogenic autoantibody repertoires as they age. Note that this excessive help is demonstrable at a time when T cells show impaired ability to proliferate and secrete IL-2 in response to mitogenic, allogenic, or antigenic stimuli.[A165,C40,C90,D76,K103,M463,N18,S163,V18,W16] Thus, the ability to provide help and the ability to proliferate are probably dissociated in these pathogenic T helper cells.

Strong evidence for the requirement for L3T4+ (CD4+ in humans) cells to develop full autoimmune syndromes has been provided by studies in which they are eliminated or inactivated by administration of anti-L3T4 monoclonal antibodies to lupus-prone mice.[S75,W314,W319,W320] Deletion or inactivation of these cells prevents autoantibody formation and disease in young BW mice,[C122,W319] and suppresses established disease in significant proportions of old BW mice.[W320] Treatment of pre-morbid young MRL/lpr mice lessens subsequent lymphoproliferation (but does not abolish it totally), prevents IgG (but not IgM) deposition in glomeruli, prevents diffuse proliferative glomerulonephritis, reduces the incidence of vasculitis, prolongs life, and reduces the levels of IgG anti-dsDNA and IgG anti-Sm.[S75] In BXSB mice, anti-CD4 therapy reduces anti-DNA, nephritis, monocytosis, and mortality.[W314]

A final piece of evidence supporting the necessity for T-cell help in murine lupus has been studied in nude mice of susceptible strains. BW nu/nu mice cannot make IgG anti-ssDNA; they do not develop nephritis. Their BW nu/+ littermates, in which T cells are not depleted, develop lupus in the same manner as unmanipulated BW mice.[G101,M404]

Additional Abnormalities in T Cells, Including Expansion of Abnormal Subsets by lpr Gene

The major effect of the lpr gene is to expand T-cell populations.[I64,K104,M355,M610,M665,S498] Chief among these is a T cell with an unusual surface phenotype CD3+, CD4−, CD8−, B220+, αβTCR. The presence of the TCR indicates this is a T cell, regardless of the expression of the B-cell marker, B220. There is no evidence that these cells, which are heterogeneous,[K20] participate in the acceleration of autoimmunity that characterizes the MRL/lpr compared to the congenic MRL/++. Many T-cell populations are expanded in mice bearing the lpr gene;[C166,S467] analysis of TCRs of lymph node cells has shown clonal diversity.[S467] CD4+CD8− classic helper T cells are expanded,[C335,S75,S392] and these probably play a more direct role in disease, as discussed in the preceding paragraph. The lpr gene is an autosomal recessive;[M610,M665,S641,T133] mice heterozygous for the lpr gene also have lymphoproliferation and autoantibodies, albeit milder than in homozygous mice.[M665] The Yaa autoimmunity accelerating gene, which is transmitted on the Y chromosome and characterizes BXSB mice, causes lymphoproliferation, primarily of B cells.[M355,M667,S641,T133,Y53]

As mice predisposed to lupus age, numerous abnormalities of T-cell populations appear, in addition to the excessive T-cell help discussed in the previous section. These abnormalities include 1) markedly reduced proliferation in response to T-cell mitogens, allogeneic cells, soluble antigens and IL-2;[A165,C40,K103,M463,N18,U18,W16] 2) reduced production of IL-2 after stimulation;[A165,K103,N18,V18] and 3) reduced numbers of surface IL-2 receptors after stimulation. These abnormalities occur in BW females, MRL/lpr and MRL/++ males and females, and in BXSB males. They are absent or less striking in NZB and BXSB females. The defective proliferative responses cannot be restored in vitro by incubation with IL-2.[A165]

The ability to assemble intracellular RNA message for IL-2 is probably normal in lupus mice.[U16] Con A stimulation of spleen cells induced RNA message and protein for IL-2, IL-4, and γIFN in old MRL/lpr and male BXSB mice, although levels of IL-2 were low in MRL/lpr.[B553] The high production of γIFN and IL-4 could cause increased expression of Ia molecules on cell surfaces (with increased antigen presentation), and increased maturation of activated B cells, respectively. Expression of oncogenes associated with cell activation is normal to high in autoimmune mice.[M631] Lymph nodes of lpr/lpr mice have greatly elevated levels of *myb* expression, probably associated with the expansion of the unusual T-cell population, since it is not elevated in nodes of other lupus mice. Mice with expanded B-cell populations (NZB, BXSB) have increased expression of *myc, bas,* and *abl* oncogenes. Whether the differences in oncogene expression are related to abnormal function, or primarily to activation of T- or B-cell subsets that occur in different frequencies in different strains, is unknown. Administration of cyclosporin A, an inhibitor of IL-2 production, to MRL/lpr mice restores the ability of T cells to proliferate in concanavalin A and reduces lymphoproliferation.[B232,M632] Therefore, early in life, IL-2 may be required for the lpr gene to expand the populations of lymphocytes that cannot proliferate and release IL-2. Administration of cyclosporin did not diminish production of antibodies to DNA. In one report, nephritis was not prevented;[B232] in another it was significantly diminished.[M632]

The etiology of the abnormalities of T-cell proliferation and IL-2 release is not clear. They have been attributed to production of anti–IL-2 or other antilymphocyte antibodies by B cells (B-cell hyperactivation precedes T-cell abnormalities), but most data suggest that contribution is minor.[A165] There may be suppressor or helper factors that are abnormal, secreted by lymphoid and nonlymphoid cells that populate lymphoid organs as disease evolves.[C40,M62,N18] For example, T-cell clones from BW mice are more likely to secrete B-cell growth factors (IL-4, 5, and 6) than T-cell growth factors (IL-2), thus favoring B-cell activation rather than development of suppressor T cells. The expanded T cells in MRL/lpr lymph nodes are enriched in memory T cells (determined by the surface marker CD44), which make high quantities of γIFN and, in association with CD4, high levels of IL-4.[B553] T cells from NZB mice secrete a factor that enhances IgA synthesis by NZB B cells.[M560]

Most appealing to the author is recent evidence suggesting that activation mechanisms that result in proliferation are abnormal.[D76,K20,K103,S163] T lymphocytes from lpr/lpr mice bind phytohemagglutinin (mitogen) normally, express TCR-CD3 surface complex (required for cell activation), translocate protein kinase C from cytosol to intracellular particles normally, but do not hydrolyze phosphoinositide.[S163] This could be due to defective function of the TCR-CD3 complex, GTP-binding proteins, or phosphoinositide phosphodiesterase. Yet, in spite of these defects, T-cell help is increased. This could be explained by the cells capable of giving help and of proliferating becoming a minor population of lymphocytes as the disease progresses, or by the possibility that the cells that cannot proliferate can still give help.

In spite of these T-cell defects, levels of soluble IL-2 receptor are elevated in the sera of old lpr/lpr, BXSB, and BW mice with clinical autoimmune disease.[B44] The IL-2R may be released from activated B cells, with a contribution from the T-cell populations that do not display these defects.

Role of the Thymus and Defects in Thymic Tolerance of T Cells

Early degeneration of thymic cortical epithelium occurs in all murine lupus strains, being most dramatic in NZB mice.[A225,D44,D193,G101,G102,H259,K21,S641,T133,Y53] The importance of this phenomenon to disease is not clear. Increased numbers of immature prothymocytes bearing the TdT surface marker are found in thymic cortex of NZB and BW mice.[W217] Thymic epithelium from NZB mice incubated with early T cells does not produce normal maturation signals.[G102,M461,M465] However, since most of the abnormalities in T-cell function and morphology appear after at least several weeks of age in mice with SLE, the influence of thymic tissue in fetal and neonatal life may not be critical. The influence of thymectomy on disease is variable. In MRL/lpr mice, thymectomy clearly prevents development of lymphoproliferation, autoantibodies, and disease.[A225,S641,S648] Therefore, the influence of the thymus may be critical in that model. In NZ background and BXSB mice, influence of thymectomy or thymus trans-

plants has varied in different reports, the majority of which suggest that removal of the thymus permits disease to accelerate.[S508,S645] On the other hand, nude BW mice do not develop lupus (although they have B-cell hyperactivation) unless they are reconstituted with thymus cells, indicating that thymus is essential for the eventual emergence of T-cell help required for development of nephritogenic autoantibodies.[M404]

Several groups have studied T-cell tolerance at the thymic level, and it appears to be normal in lupus-prone mice. In normal mice, the thymus deletes T cells with high avidity for self antigens. Certain TCRs are over-represented in the self antigen–binding repertoire. These include, in various mouse strains, TCR Vβ 3, 6, 8.1, 11, and 17a. The TCRs on cells from lymph nodes and spleens are depleted of the appropriate self reactive Vβ families in MRL/+ +, MRL/lpr, NZB, BXSB, BW, and SNF$_1$ mice.[K391,K393,K394, M633,S466] These data imply that self reactive T cells are selectively expanded in the periphery, after release from thymus, and that thymus can perform normal negative selection of highly autoreactive cells.

Role of Monocytes/Macrophages and Neutrophils in Murine Lupus

Monocytosis is a feature of the full-blown autoimmune syndrome in BXSB and MRL/lpr mice.[M665,M666,M667] It may result from T-cell stimuli, since it is abrogated by administration of anti-CD4.[W314] However, monocytes/macrophages probably play important roles in disease. The glomeruli of MRL/lpr are infiltrated with monocytes/macrophages.[B423] Expression of IL-1 and thromboxane (which is induced by IL-1), and of TNF, are greatly increased in glomeruli of MRL/lpr mice.[B422,B423,K153] Monocytes/macrophages from BXSB mice also release increased quantities of procoagulants.[C342] The combined effects of these cytokines would obviously contribute to glomerular damage and accelerate disease. Kupffer cells from livers of MRL/lpr mice also secrete high levels of TNF.[M62]

Neutrophils from MRL/lpr mice, but not from MRL/+ +, have reduced Fc receptor–mediated phagocytosis, which is acquired with advancing age. This effect may be mediated by high levels of TGFβ released by MRL/lpr T cells.[G370] Another consequence of this abnormality is reduced ability to migrate to sites of inflammation.

Defects in Clearance of Immune Complexes

As in humans with SLE, the clearance of circulating immune complexes, and of cells coated with antibodies, may be abnormal in murine lupus. The Fc-mediated clearance of radiolabeled, Ig-sensitized RBCs is delayed in NZB, BW, MRL/lpr, and BXSB mice by the time they reach 6 months of age. Complement receptor–mediated clearance was delayed in MRL/lpr mice but not in the other strains.[F83,M367] Clearance of heat-aggregated IgG is reduced in old MRL/lpr, but not old MRL/+ +, BXSB, or BW mice.[M71,M655]

The Role of Environmental Factors

The microenvironment is important in some strains, especially with relation to sex hormones. In all murine lupus strains (except BXSB), disease is earlier in females than males.[A225] In NZB and MRL/lpr mice, the difference in disease onset is only 1 to 2 months. In BW and SNF$_1$ mice, the difference is several months, and the female predominance in these two strains is striking. Disease in BW mice can be dramatically altered by sex hormone manipulation; estrogens accelerating disease and androgens delaying it.[D370,R362,R364,R365,S646]

With regard to exogenous stimuli, there is evidence that infections can accelerate murine lupus.[L36,T133] This probably results from formation of additional immune complexes that can add to the Ig deposits in glomeruli and blood vessels. Polyclonal activation by in vivo administration of lipopolysaccharide (similar to the effects of endotoxin) can also accelerate disease in MRL/lpr mice.[C166] However, these effects are probably minor. Lupus in mice is almost entirely a genetic disease.

In summary, multiple abnormalities are required for a mouse to develop lupus-like disease. These include disturbances in the function of hematopoietic stem cells, B lymphocytes, T lymphocytes, and phagocytic cells. The abnormalities are determined primarily by genetic influences; most require multiple genes provided by both parents of a susceptible strain. Two accelerating genes, lpr and Yaa, are not sufficient to cause disease unless engrafted onto a host that is genetically susceptible to autoimmunity. The most important results of the abnormalities are production of pathogenic subsets of autoantibodies and immune complexes, which depend upon both abnormal B-cell repertoires and unopposed T-cell help. Environmental factors may accentuate these abnormalities, but are of minor importance.

THERAPEUTIC INTERVENTIONS IN MURINE LUPUS

A major advantage of each of the mouse models of SLE is their availability for studies of therapeutic interventions. These interventions will be considered as studies of immunosuppressive drugs, immunosuppressive antibodies and other strategies, nutritional interventions, sex hormone therapies, gene manipulations, and miscellaneous interventions. All are summarized in Table 17–8. All successful interventions are most effective when introduced prior to development of full-blown clinical lupus. The most interesting ones are also effective in mice with established disease, especially those who have advanced to proteinuria.

Immunosuppressive Drugs

Drugs that are standard in the management of SLE in patients have been studied in murine models of lupus. These include glucocorticoids, azathioprine, and cyclophosphamide. Glucocorticoids suppress hemolysis and prolong life in NZB mice.[C140] In BW mice, and murine chronic GVH, they suppress IgG anti-dsDNA, proteinuria, glomerular Ig deposits and nephritis, with resultant prolonged survival.[A271,C137,G85,H25] They are effective even in animals with established nephritis, although better when introduced before clinical disease appears.

Azathioprine as a single agent does not prolong survival in NZB, BW, or chronic GVH mice; in combination with

glucocorticoids and/or cyclophosphamide it is more effective than any single drug alone.[C138,G85,H25]

As a single drug intervention, cyclophosphamide is superior to glucocorticoids or azathioprine in suppressing nephritis and IgG autoantibodies, and prolonging life in NZB, BW, and chronic GVH mice.[A271,A281,C139,G85,H25,H424,R432] It is equally effective if given daily or intermittently[H125] (see Fig. 17–3). Administration of cyclophosphamide in any regimen is associated with substantial increases in malignancies; in some colonies azathioprine also has this effect.[C138,H35,W14] Any combination therapy that includes cyclophosphamide suppresses lupus nephritis effectively.[G85,W2]

A recently developed cytotoxic drug, 15-deoxyspergualin suppresses immune complex formation, anti-DNA, nephritis, and lymphoproliferation in MRL/lpr and male BXSB mice.[I55,M72] It has been administered primarily to mice before onset of florid disease.

The effects of cyclosporin A (Cy-A) in MRL/lpr, BXSB, and NZB mice have been studied. Cy-A is highly effective in suppressing lymphoproliferation; the unusual CD2+ CD4− CD8− B220+ lymphocytes associated with the lpr gene do not expand when IL-2 is inhibited by Cy-A.[B232,M632] Cy-A in high doses can suppress synthesis of anti-DNA in vitro.[P210] However, B-cell hyperactivation with production of high levels of Ig, circulating immune complexes, rheumatoid factors, and anti-DNA was not suppressed when the drug was given in vivo.[B232,B237,H69,M632] The effects on nephritis were variable: one group reported no suppression of nephritis and no improvement in survival in either MRL/lpr or BXSB mice,[B232] whereas two groups reported reduction of nephritis and prolonged survival.[B237,M632] Apparently, renal damage can be suppressed without diminishing B-cell activation and autoantibody synthesis, suggesting that autoantibodies alone may be necessary but not sufficient for the development of lethal lupus nephritis. Since many T cells that are found in spleen and lymph nodes at the time of clinical disease do not release IL-2 or display many IL-2 receptors on their surfaces, it is interesting the Cy-A is effective at all in MRL/lpr and BXSB mice. These findings suggest either that early in the evolution of autoimmunity IL-2 responsive cells are present, or that in established disease they represent a small subset of T cells that are essential to organ damage. A compound that also suppresses IL-2, FK506, was given to young MRL/lpr mice; it prevented lymphoproliferation and nephritis, and also reduced titers of anti-dsDNA.[Y14]

Immunosuppressive Antibodies and Total Nodal Irradiation

One of the most interesting recent advances in therapy of murine lupus has been the demonstration of the efficacy of monoclonal antibodies that either deplete or inactivate L3T4+ T cells (CD4+ in humans). Administration of these antibodies prolongs survival, suppresses IgG anti-dsDNA and other autoantibodies, and suppresses nephritis and lymphoproliferation in BW, MRL/lpr, and BXSB mice.[S75,W314,W316,W319] Anti-L3T4 therapy is efficacious when given before clinical disease appears, and is also effective after nephritis is established.[W320] The mono-

Table 17–8. Therapeutic Interventions in Murine Lupus

Intervention	Strains Studied	Effects
Immunosuppressive Drugs		
1. Glucocorticoids	NZB, BW, MRL/lpr, BXSB, chronic GVH	Prolong survival
		Suppress GN
		Suppress AutoAb
		Suppress T abnormalities
2. Cyclophosphamide	Same as 1	Same as 1
3. Azathioprine	BW, chronic GVH	Not effective as single drug; effective in combination
4. Combinations 1–3	BW	More effective than 1 drug alone
5. 15-Deoxyspergualin	MRL/lpr, BXSB	Suppresses B activity
		Suppresses lymphoproliferation
		Suppresses CIC, anti-DNA
		Suppresses GN
6. Cyclosporin A	MRL/lpr, BXSB BW	Suppresses lymphoproliferation
		No suppression of anti-DNA, CIC*
		Suppresses GN, arthritis*
		Prolongs survival*
7. FK506	MRL/lpr	Prolongs survival
		Suppresses lymphoproliferation
		Suppresses anti-DNA
		Suppresses nephritis
Immunosuppressive Antibodies and Other Strategies		
1. Anti-L3T4	BW, MRL/lpr, BXSB	Prolongs survival in pre-dz and post-dz mice
		Depletes or inactivates L3T4 +, suppresses accumulation of CD8 +, B and monocytes in lymphoid organs and kidneys
		Suppresses anti-DNA
		Suppresses GN
2. Anti-idiotypes	BW, MRL/lpr	Prolong survival*
		Suppress anti-DNA*
		Suppress GN*
3. Anti-Ia	BW	Anti-IAᶻ prolongs survival
		Suppresses anti-DNA
		Suppresses GN
		Anti-IAᵈ less effective
5. Anti–Ly-2	BW	No effect on survival, autoAbs, nephritis. Depletes Ly-2 + T cells
6. Total nodal irradiation	BW	Prolongs survival
		No suppression of anti-DNA
		Suppresses GN
		Reduction of T-cell help for months, suppression for weeks
Nutritional Interventions		
1. Calorie reduction	NZB, BW, MRL/lpr, BXSB	Prolongs survival
		Suppresses lymphoproliferation
		Suppresses CIC
		Suppresses nephritis
2. Fat-restricted diet	BW	Same as 1
3. Omega-3 fatty acid–BW, MRL/lpr enriched diets (includes fish oil, eicosopentanoic acid)	BW, MRL/lpr	Prolong survival
		Suppress lymphoproliferation
		Suppress anti-DNA, CIC
		Suppress nephritis
		Suppress vasculitis
4. Omega-9 and 6 fatty acid–enriched diets	BW, MRL/lpr	Reduce survival
		Enhance oncogene expression
		Enhance lymphoproliferation
5. Casein-free diet	BW	Prolongs survival
		Suppresses anti-DNA
		Suppresses nephritis
6. Alfalfa sprouts/ʟ-canavanine-enriched diet	NZB, BW	Decrease survival
		Increase IgG anti-DNA
		Increase IgG synthesis
Sex Hormone Therapies		
1. Estrogens, castration	BW, MRL/lpr, BXSB	Accelerate male dz
		Increase IgG anti-DNA
		Increase nephritis
		Decrease survival
		Dramatic in BW, modest effects in MRL/lpr, no effect in BXSB males

(continued)

Table 17–8. Therapeutic Interventions in Murine Lupus—(*Continued*)

Intervention	Strains Studied	Effects
2. Androgens plus castration or antiestrogens	BW, MRL/lpr	Suppress female dz Prolong survival Delay IgG anti-DNA Delay nephritis Dramatic in BW, modest effects in MRL/lpr females
Gene Therapies		
1. Introduction of *xid* NZB, BW gene	NZB, BW	Deletes Ly-1 + B cells Decreases IgM synthesis Suppresses AutoAbs Prolongs survival Suppresses nephritis, hemolysis
2. Introduction of nu/nu genes	BW	Deletes T cells Prolongs survival Decreases IgG anti-DNA Suppresses nephritis Decreases lymphoproliferation
3. Administration of α TNF	BW	Prolongs survival Inhibits T and NK function No suppresson of anti-DNA Delays nephritis
Miscellaneous Interventions		
1. Prostaglandin E	BW	Prolongs survival Suppresses nephritis
2. UVA light exposure	BW	Prolongs survival Reduces lymphoproliferation Suppresses anti-DNA

clonal antibody used is a rat antimouse L3T4; it has the advantage of inducing tolerance to itself in the recipient by preventing antibody responses that require T-cell help.[S75,W314,W319] In earlier studies using antibodies against lymphocytes or thymocytes or Thy-1 + cells (CD2 + in humans), results were often obscured by the development of inactivating antibodies, and of serum sickness nephritis caused by the immune response to the antilymphocyte globulin.[D160,D161,H36,W318] In the setting of tolerance to anti-L3T4, the effect of removing T-cell help

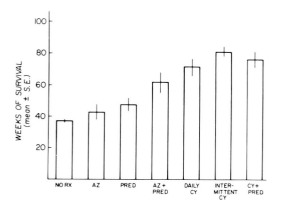

Fig. 17–3. Survival in NZB/NZW F$_1$ female mice treated from six weeks of age with daily oral doses of azathioprine (Az), prednisolone (Pred), cyclophosphamide (Cy), or combination therapies. Bars indicate mean weeks of survival; vertical lines are one SEM. Survival was significantly better in Pred vs no R$_x$, Az and Pred vs Az, Pred, or no R$_x$, and best in all groups receiving Cy, whether daily or intermittent. (See reference H25 for details.)

can be clearly seen. The rat anti-L3T4 monoclonal antibody is cytotoxic to helper T cells and deletes them from the repertoire. The F(ab')$_2$ fragment of the monoclonal antibody is not cytotoxic, since it cannot fix complement, but it inactivates L3T4 + T cells and is as effective as the whole antibody molecule in preventing the development of anti-DNA and nephritis in BW mice.[C123] In addition to the predictable effects of anti-L3T4 on diminishing T-cell help and autoantibody formation, non-L3T4 + cells that infiltrate renal and lymphoid tissue as lupus evolves are also influenced. Ly-2 + (human CD8 +) T cells and B220 + B cells, as well as L3T4 + T cells, are all diminished.[C123,W316] This could be interpreted as indicating a central role for L3T4 + T cells in the evolution of activated Ly-2 + and B cells, or as evidence that anti-L3T4 recognizes additional cell surface markers, or both. In any case, these studies have shown that L3T4 + T cells are critical to the development of lupus-like lymphoproliferation and nephritis, as well as to production of pathogenic autoantibodies, in most if not all of the murine models of SLE.

In contrast to the efficacy of anti-L3T4, administration of anti–Ly-2 to tolerized BW mice depleted Ly-2 + cells but did not influence autoantibody titers, nephritis, or survival.[W315]

Another method of interfering with B- and/or T-cell repertoires that participate in disease has been the administration of anti-idiotypic antibodies. See Chapter 15 for a discussion of idiotypic networks and their manipulation. Manipulation of the idiotypic network by administration of idiotype (Id) or anti-idiotype (anti-Id) can have profound effects on the immune system, and those effects can result in either up-regulation or down-regulation of autoantibodies. Administration of carefully chosen Ids or anti-Ids in proper doses at the correct time can suppress Id+ anti-dsDNA and delay the onset of nephritis in BW mice.[E15,H28,H29,S84,S87] Similar suppression of anti-DNA by injection of anti-Ids has been reported in MRL/lpr mice.[M65] Treatment with anti-Ids conjugated to cytotoxic compounds such as neocarzinostatin is also effective in suppressing autoantibodies and nephritis in BW mice, particularly if multiple anti-Ids are included in the regimen.[S84,S87] Anti-Ids can also suppress in vitro synthesis of autoantibodies by human B cells.[S86] There are limitations to Id–anti-Id therapies. Some anti-Ids up-regulate autoantibodies.[T98] Variations in dose and time of administration to lupus mice can profoundly influence whether immune responses are enhanced or suppressed. Some anti-Ids do not affect antibody synthesis.[M589] Beneficial responses can be short-lived, abrogated either by escape of pathogen-enriched Ids from suppression or by the emergence of pathogenic autoantibodies bearing different Ids.[E15,H29] Finally, pathogenic autoantibodies can express different Ids, so that suppression of multiple public (and possibly some private) Ids may be required for prolonged efficacy of these interventions.

One group has published a study of the efficacy of antibodies to Ia in murine lupus.[A37] NZB/NZW F₁ mice express I-A and I-E MHC class II molecules with two alleles, d and z. Administration of antibodies directed against I-A^z suppressed production of anti-DNA and development of nephritis in BW mice. Anti-I-A^d was somewhat immunosuppressive, but less effective than anti–I-A^z. These data add to the evidence that the class II molecules derived from the NZW parent may play a major role in permitting formation of IgG anti-dsDNA and clinical nephritis, as suggested by many genetic studies reviewed earlier in this chapter.

Another antibody that has been used to treat murine SLE is anti–MEL-14.[M630] This antibody blocks the homing of lymphocytes to lymph nodes. Administration to MRL/lpr mice suppressed adenopathy (but increased splenomegaly); it did not alter autoantibody production.

Total nodal irradiation has been studied in murine as well as human SLE. Irradiation of BW or MRL/lpr mice, even after clinical disease is established, results in prolonged survival and markedly diminished nephritis, associated with decreased serum levels of anti-DNA.[K390,K397,M621,S490,T129] In MRL/lpr mice, lymphoproliferation is reduced.[M621] Both suppressing and enhancing cell circuits are suppressed for a few weeks after therapy is stopped, but helper circuits return to supernormal, with increased antibody production and proliferation to antigens and mitogens. However, the mice are protected from recurrent high levels of ANA production, and from disease for several months after this help appears, in spite of the fact that suppressive circuits cannot be demonstrated.[K390] In one study comparing total node irradiation to cyclophosphamide therapy in BW mice, irradiation was superior in prolonging life because the incidence of malignant tumors was lower.[W2]

Nutritional Interventions

Dietary factors have a major influence on murine lupus. Calorie reduction alone, to about 40% of the usual laboratory mouse dietary intake, significantly prolongs survival and suppresses lymphoproliferation, autoantibody production, and nephritis in NZB, BW, MRL/lpr, and BXSB mice.[F64,H509,J88] (see Fig. 17–2). The important restriction appears to be in dietary fat, rather than in protein.[A138,F64,G209,H509,M605,Y27] Diets rich in unsaturated fats, and in omega-3 fatty acids such as fish oil, menhaden oil, and eicosapentanoic acid, are associated with improved survival and markedly less lymphoproliferation, autoantibody production, nephritis, and vasculitis in BW and MRL/lpr mice.[A138,F64,G209,J88,M605,P295,R249,W98,W194,Y27] In contrast, diets enriched in unsaturated fats and in omega-9 and omega-6 fatty acids are associated with reduced survival, enhanced oncogene expression, and severe lymphoproliferation.[A138,F64,G209,J88,M605,W98,W194,Y27]

The most likely explanation for the profound effects of diet in murine lupus relate to the conversion of dietary fats to various arachidonic acid metabolites (prostaglandins and leukotrienes). Presumably the omega-3 fatty acids are precursors of molecules that are less inflammatory and/or immunostimulatory than the products of omega-9 and omega-6 fatty acids. A detailed discussion of arachidonic acid metabolites and their potential roles in SLE can be found in Chapter 14. The administration of prostaglandins to BW mice influences their SLE. Repeated injections of PGE₁ suppress nephritis and prolong survival.[Z59,Z60] Whether this clinical benefit relates to the ability of PGE₁ to suppress the accumulation of immature prothymocytes (TdT+ cells) in the thymus and bone marrow of NZB and BW mice is unknown.[W217] However, PGF_{a2}, which does not alter SLE in BW mice, also does not prevent the expansion of TdT+ cells.[W217]

Dietary factors unrelated to lipids also influence murine lupus. BW mice raised on a casein-free diet have diminished anti-DNA and nephritis and improved survival.[C99] The mechanism of this effect is not known. Alfalfa seeds fed to cynomolgus macaque monkeys were associated with the development of autoimmune hemolytic anemia and ANA;[M80] when the seeds were autoclaved before administration the disease did not occur.[M81] Several investigators have attributed this phenomenon to the presence of L-canavanine, a nonprotein amino acid, in alfalfa. L-Canavanine is immunostimulatory and increases proliferation of lymphocytes to mitogens and antigens.[A127,M80,P292] The importance of this finding in human SLE is unknown.

Sex Hormone Therapies

The influence of sex hormones on murine lupus is highly variable depending upon the strain. This was discussed previously in this chapter in the section on pathogenesis. Briefly, hybrid mice derived from NZ backgrounds, especially BW mice, are exquisitely sensitive to the effects of sex hormones. Females are protected from severe early-life lupus by castration plus androgenic hormone, or by antiestrogens.[D370,M189,R362,R364,R365] Males develop early-life severe SLE, rather than their usual late-onset disease, if castrated and treated with estrogenic hormones.[D370,R362,R364,R365,S646] Whether this relates to modification of immune responses by sex hormone receptors in immune cells, or modification of gene expression, is unclear. In contrast, male BXSB mice develop rapid-onset early-life lupus whether or not they are castrated or receive sex hormones.[E62] MRL/lpr mice are intermediate between BW and BXSB; that is, estrogenic hormones tend to worsen and androgenic hormones to suppress disease manifestations, but the effects are less dramatic than in BW mice.[S648]

Gene Therapies

As discussed under pathogenesis, several genetic manipulations influence murine lupus. The introduction of the *xid* gene into NZB or BW backgrounds results in inability to synthesize normal levels of IgM, and near-deletion of Ly1 + B cells. In that setting, NZB.*xid* and BW.*xid* mice do not develop their characteristic early-life severe lupus.[T78,T79,Y53] They are not disease free: a few animals develop autoantibodies and nephritis late in life.[O34,Y55] These studies support evidence for a stem cell defect in NZ mice that leads to B-cell abnormalities, for the potential role of the Ly-1 + B cell in disease, and for the influence of autoimmune microenvironments, since normal pre-B cells transferred into the NZB.*xid* animal develop hyperactivation as though they were NZB B cells.[K302]

BW mice have also been bred with nude mice to produce BW.nu/nu offspring. Nu/nu homozygotes are athymic and develop T-cell repertoires that are small in number and uneducated in the thymus. BW-nu/nu mice, without T-cell help, have prolonged survival associated with decreased levels of IgG anti-DNA and with little development of nephritis or lymphoproliferation.[G101,M404] However, like BW.*xid*, the animals are not completely disease free and develop some autoantibodies. These data together suggest that both B- and T-cell abnormalities underlie SLE in this strain—and probably in all the others as well.

Another approach to gene therapy has been to provide the recombinant product of a defective gene. BW mice produce abnormally low quantities of TNFα—a defect that correlated with an unusual restriction fragment length polymorphism in the TNFα gene.[J16] Initial studies reported that administration of normal recombinant TNFα delayed development of nephritis.[J16] The ability of the recombinant molecule to suppress established nephritis somewhat and prolong survival in BW mice was shown, but the benefit was lost after a few months.[G301] Another study reported that low doses of TNFα could accelerate nephritis.[B473] Treatment of normal mice with TNFα reduced the ability of monocytes to support lymphocyte proliferative responses to mitogens, and inhibited T-cell cytotoxicity and NK cell activity.[G302] Such effects, if they occur in autoimmune mice, could confer substantial protection from organ damage.

Miscellaneous Interventions

Several additional strategies that affect murine lupus should be noted. Exposure of BW mice to UVA light, especially if mice are shaved to maximize the exposure, was

associated with prolonged survival, reduced lymphoproliferation, and suppression of anti-DNA antibodies.[M285] There is some interest currently in this strategy for treatment of human lupus. In contrast, exposure of BXSB mice to UV light that included UVA and UVB, and was reproduced with UVB alone, exacerbated disease.[A256]

Disease in MRL/lpr mice has been successfully suppressed by administration of cholera toxin[F15] and of a PAF (platelet-activating receptor) antagonist.[B45] The value of these strategies, and other strategies not mentioned here, will depend upon whether the findings can be confirmed and whether the role of these compounds in altering disease can be elucidated.

LUPUS IN ANIMALS OTHER THAN MICE

Spontaneous lupus-like disease has been reported in dogs, cats, rats, rabbits, guinea pigs, pigs, monkeys, hamsters, and Aleutian minks.[A85,H67,S307] The largest body of literature addresses SLE in dogs. In that animal, the disease can be sporadic or familial.[L251,L252,M546,T97] There is a colony of dogs created by breeding a male and female German shepherd, each of which had SLE. As healthy sires were introduced to mate with F_1 and F_2 generations, the disease prevalence declined.[M546,T87] There is a genetic association with MHC, as in mice and in humans. The DLA-A7 MHC class I gene confers a relative risk of approximately 12 for SLE, whether found in sporadic or familial disease; DLA-A1 and B5 are negatively correlated with disease.[T87] Dogs can develop clinical manifestations similar to those in humans, including membranous and proliferative forms of glomerulonephritis.[C180,C401,H64,M546] Bullous, discoid, and systemic type skin lesions can occur. The autoantibodies described in canine lupus include ANA, anti-dsDNA, antihistone, anti-Ro/SSA, anti-Sm, and antilymphocyte.[B494,C401] The H130 idiotype characteristic of MRL/lpr mice has been found on anti-DNA in dogs.[Z47] Apheresis has been a fairly successful therapeutic strategy in canine lupus.

Because of concern that SLE may be transmitted by viruses, studies have been done to determine whether SLE in humans is more common among owners of dogs with SLE. A study of 83 members of 23 households with 19 dogs that had high-titer ANAs showed no excess in the number of cases of human SLE.[R136]

SLE in cats is usually a spontaneous disease. However, there has been interest in a series of experiments in which administration of propylthiouracil to cats induces autoantibodies and autoimmune hemolytic anemia.[A356]

SLE in monkeys can be induced by feeding macaques alfalfa seeds, probably because of the immunostimulatory properties of the L-canavanine nonprotein amino acid contained in the seeds.[A127,M80,M81,P292]

Attempts have been made to induce SLE in animals by transferring plasma from patients with SLE. Histologic evidence of glomerulonephritis was produced by repeated infusions of human plasma containing LE factors into healthy dogs in one set of experiments[C303] but not in another.[B204] Similar experiments were unsuccessful in guinea pigs.[B204]

Efforts to induce lupus-like disease in various animals

by administering lupus-inducing drugs have been largely unsuccessful. Hydralazine or procainamide have been given to dogs, guinea pigs, swine, and rats with little evidence of autoimmune responses.[D333]

Finally, dogs have been studied for evidence of vertical transmission of infectious agents that cause SLE. In breeding studies performed by Lewis and colleagues,[L251] the incidence of positive LE-cell tests in inbred backcrosses and outcross matings was not consistent with any conventional mechanisms of inheritance. The investigators concluded that the results could be explained by vertical transmission of an infectious agent in a genetically susceptible individual. Cell-free filtrates of tissues from seropositive dogs were injected into newborn mice.[L250] These mice developed ANAs and, in some cases, lymphomas. Passage of cells or filtrates from the tumors to normal newborn puppies resulted in ANA production or positive LE-cell tests. C type RNA viruses were identified in the tumors. In cats, autoimmunity is highly associated with the feline leukemia virus.[H67] It may be that autoimmune disease similar to human SLE is more closely linked to viral infections in dogs and cats than in humans.

Section IV

AUTOANTIBODIES

Chapter 18

THE STRUCTURE AND DERIVATION OF ANTIBODIES AND AUTOANTIBODIES

CYNTHIA ARANOW
ELAHNA PAUL
BETTY DIAMOND

The normal humoral immune response protects an organism from environmental pathogens. Antibodies neutralize microbial agents and facilitate phagocytosis of foreign antigens. To be effective, the antibody repertoire must recognize a large spectrum of antigenic specificities. Not only must the immune system generate a panel of high-affinity antibodies to the seemingly limitless world of foreign antigens, but it must do so without generating high-affinity antibodies to self.

The production of high-affinity autoantibodies, antibodies that bind to self determinants, is a prominent feature of systemic lupus erythematosus (SLE).[T42] Some autoantibodies in SLE are markers for disease (anti-Sm, ANA, anti-DNA) or disease manifestations (anti-Ro), while some are thought to play a role in pathogenesis and tissue damage.[G115,K36,K335,T44,W286]

In recent years there has been extensive investigation of autoantibodies in SLE. These studies address a number of specific questions:

1. Is the autoantibody response polyclonal or oligoclonal?
2. Do polymorphisms of immunoglobulin variable region genes contribute to disease susceptibility?
3. Can the same immunoglobulin variable region genes encode both autoantibodies and protective antibodies? Can B cells producing autoantibodies be clonally related to B cells producing protective antibodies?
4. Do autoantibodies result from polyclonal activation or do they represent an antigen-selected response? If antigen selection occurs, is the initiating antigen a self antigen or a foreign, perhaps microbial, antigen?
5. What B-cell lineage(s) produce autoantibodies?
6. What defects in immune regulation permit the expression of pathogenic autoantibodies?

This chapter discusses some of the recent advances in our understanding of autoreactivity, and the relationship of autoantibodies to the normal immune response.

THE ANTIBODY MOLECULE

Antibodies are protein molecules produced by B lymphocytes. They are composed of two heavy (H) chains and two light (L) chains that associate to form a molecule with two functional regions: an antigen-binding region and a constant region that determines the effector functions of the molecule (Figure 18–1).[S592] Each heavy chain and each light chain is composed of a variable region and a constant region. The heavy chain constant region defines the isotype of an antibody molecule (IgM, IgD, IgG, IgA, or IgE). IgM is the first isotype produced by a B cell, and IgM antibodies are characteristic of the primary immune response. Since the μ constant region can activate complement, IgM antibodies can mediate lysis of cells expressing target antigens. Under appropriate conditions, B cells producing IgM can switch to the production of different isotypes (discussed below). IgG is the predominant isotype of the secondary immune response. In addition to activating complement, IgG antibodies can promote Fc receptor-mediated phagocytosis and can cross the placenta, thereby transferring passive immunity to the fetus and neonate. IgA is the only isotype that can migrate across epithelial cells and enter secretions. IgA is, therefore, the primary isotype found in saliva and intestinal secretions. Antibodies of the IgE isotype can trigger mast cells. These antibodies are important in the immune response to extracellular parasites. There are also two light chain isotypes, κ and λ. Light chain isotypes are not known to mediate antibody function.

The second functional domain of an antibody, the antigen-binding region, is specific to each antibody molecule. Every antibody has two such domains, each composed of the variable regions of one heavy and one light chain (Figure 18–1). A variable region is divided into complementarity-determining regions (CDRs), also called hypervariable regions and framework (FW) regions. The CDRs contain amino acids that are contact residues for antigen binding and are, therefore, the most variable portion of the antibody molecule.[K1,P235] The FW regions maintain the spatial orientation of the antigen-binding pocket by determining the folding of the polypeptide chain. These regions are less polymorphic than the CDRs and probably contribute little to antigenic specificity. Several years ago Kunkel and Oudin made antibodies called anti-idiotypes, against the variable region of antibody molecules.[C73,O123, O124] The epitopes in the variable region that are recognized by these anti-idiotypes are called idiotopes. Idi-

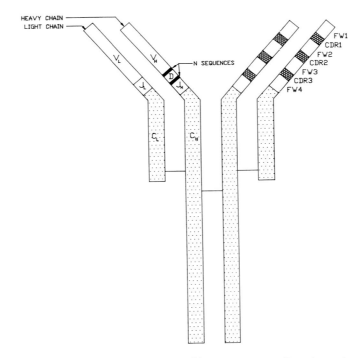

Fig. 18–1. A prototypic antibody molecule. V = variable region, D = diversity region, J = joining region, C = constant region, FW = Framework region, CDR = complementary-determining region.

otopes are markers of the antigen-binding region; some are in the antigen-binding site itself, while others are determinants in FW regions. Private idiotypes are unique to a given antibody; cross-reactive idiotypes are shared among antibodies of different antigenic specificities and among antibodies present in different individuals. Presumably, antibodies that share the same idiotype have a high degree of structural homology within their variable regions and are encoded by similar or related immunoglobulin variable region genes.[M12,S131] Idiotypic determinants are thought to be important in the regulation of the immune response as they are recognized by both T and B cells.[B426,J72,R19,U24]

ANTIBODY GENES

The assembly of an antibody molecule begins with the rearrangement of three heavy chain gene segments, the variable (V), diversity (D), and joining (J) segments.[E3, K478,S34] In humans, V, D, and J gene segments are grouped in three gene clusters that are tandemly arrayed on chromosome 14 (Figure 18–2).[B29,K334,W59] Heavy chain V region genes are classified into families whose members share 80% homology by DNA sequence. Six human chain variable region families have been identified to date.[B249,P60,W59] Homology between family members oc-

curs primarily in the FW regions, while CDRs can vary considerably.

Each V, D, and J gene segment is flanked by a heptamer/nonamer consensus sequence that is crucial for rearrangement of the gene segment. The assembly of the complete heavy chain gene begins with the joining of a D segment from the D cluster to a J segment in the J cluster downstream, deleting the intervening DNA. In a similar manner, a V gene segment is next rearranged to the DJ unit to form a complete VDJ variable region.[H406,T182] During rearrangement, nontemplate-derived nucleotides (N sequences) may be inserted at the VD or DJ junctions of the heavy chain by the enzyme terminal deoxytransferase (Figure 18–1).[D176,L42] Such N sequences are fairly common in antibodies of the adult immunoglobulin repertoire, but are less frequent early in ontogeny.[F43] The rearranged heavy chain VDJ segment encodes the three CDRs and the four FW regions of the immunoglobulin heavy chain: the heavy chain V region gene encodes two FWs and two CDRs, the D region encodes the third CDR, and the J segment encodes the fourth FW region (Figure 18–1).

Every B cell produces a single heavy chain and a single light chain. While all somatic cells are endowed with two of each chromosome, only one rearranged heavy chain

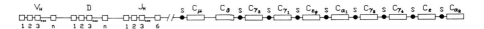

Fig. 18–2. The heavy chain immunoglobulin gene locus on chromosome 14. V = variable gene locus, D = diversity gene locus, J = joining gene locus, C = constant region, S = switch region.

gene and one rearranged light chain gene is expressed by a normal B cell. This phenomenon is known as allelic exclusion. A productive rearrangement on one chromosome presumably inhibits additional rearrangements on the alternate chromosome. However, rearrangements are sometimes unproductive because of frameshifts that can occur during DNA rearrangement or through the use of aberrant V gene segments called pseudogenes. If rearrangement on the first chromosome is unproductive and cannot lead to the formation of a functional polypeptide chain, then the immunoglobulin genes on the second chromosome can rearrange.

Initially the rearranged VDJ segment is transcribed with a μ constant region gene to encode an IgM heavy chain. During the secondary immune response, the VDJ unit can undergo a second kind of gene rearrangement to associate with a different constant region gene downstream of Cμ (Figure 18–2).[G400,M197,S365] Switch sequences located 5' to each constant region gene mediate heavy chain class switching.[D88]

After the generation of an intact heavy chain, the light chain gene segments rearrange.[S257] The light chain variable region is composed of two gene segments, V and J. Genes for the variable and joining region of the light chain are located at two genetic loci: κ chain genes are on chromosome 2 and λ chain genes are on chromosome 22. There are, to date, four identified κ variable region gene families[J35,K315,K316,M339] and seven λ variable region gene families.[C259] V and J elements of the light chain loci also rearrange by recombination at heptamer/nonamer consensus sites. Rarely N sequences can be inserted at the VJ junction of the light chain genes.[H251] The light chain V gene segment encodes the first three FWs and CDR1 and CDR2. The VJ junction encodes CDR3. The fourth FW is encoded by the J segment (Figure 18–1). Genes of the κ locus are the first light chain genes to rearrange. If κ gene rearrangements are nonproductive on both chromosomes, then the V and J segments of the λ locus rearrange to produce an intact light chain.[H246,K385]

GENERATION OF ANTIBODY DIVERSITY

The immune system has a variety of mechanisms to produce antibodies with a large spectrum of antigenic specificities. Antibodies of the primary immune response are assembled in B cells before exposure to antigen. Diversity of the primary immune response results from 1) the assembly of different gene segments into intact heavy and light chain genes, 2) junctional diversity of the heavy and light chains produced by N sequences insertion and/or by imprecise joining of gene segments, and 3) the random pairing of heavy and light chains (Table 18–1).

B cells are amplified and triggered to secrete IgM upon initial exposure to antigen. These IgM antibodies of the primary immune response are generally polyreactive and display low affinity to a multitude of antigens, even antigens without obvious structural homology. Upon re-exposure to antigen and T-cell factors, B cells produce antibodies with greater specificity and with increased affinity for antigen.[B234,M111] This process of affinity maturation is achieved by somatic mutation, an additional mechanism

Table 18–1. Mechanisms of Antibody Diversity

Primary Immune Response
1. Combinatorial diversity of V, D, and J gene segments for heavy chain variable region, and V and J gene segments for light chain variable region
2. Junctional diversity of rearranged heavy and light chain variable regions
3. Random association of heavy and light chains

Secondary Immune Response
1. Somatic point mutation
2. Gene conversion
3. Gene replacement

for diversifying germline immunoglobulin genes (Table 18–2 and Figure 18–3).[F234,K333,M82] Somatically mutated antibodies of the secondary immune response have usually undergone heavy chain class switching, predominantly to IgG. Class switching and somatic mutation occur during a similar time in B-cell development and are both thought to require the interaction of B cells with activated T cells, although they can occur independently of each other.[C431,G78,L430,S420]

Mechanisms of somatic mutation in the secondary immune response include somatic point mutation, gene conversion, and gene replacement.[C290,C291,R180] Somatic point mutations are single nucleotide substitutions that can occur randomly throughout the heavy and light chain variable region genes. The ramifications of such nucleotide substitutions are discussed below in greater detail. Gene conversion is the incorporation of a discrete portion of one gene (or pseudogene) into an already rearranged gene.[C291,D213,K321,K413,R181,S130] Gene replacement is the replacement of the V segment in a rearranged heavy chain VDJ or light chain VJ with a different upstream V region gene.[K276,R164] It is thought that most somatic mutation in the mouse is a consequence of somatic point mutation,[C290,G380,K203,S7] while in chickens, gene conversion is clearly the dominant mechanism.[R180,R181,T155] There is insufficient information to know which process dominates in humans. Point mutations are believed to occur randomly in both FW and CDR regions. Only those nucleotide substitutions that encode amino acid substitutions can affect an antibody's affinity for antigen. Genealogies or lineages of B cells with serial mutations in their immunoglobulin gene sequences demonstrate how point mutations lead to antibodies with altered affinity for antigen (Figure 18–3).[F234,G380,K332,S7] B cells producing antibodies with decreased affinity will be rare in vivo, as they are not amplified further in the immune response, while B

Table 18–2. Distinguishing Features of Autoantibodies

Natural Autoantibodies	Pathogenic Autoantibodies
IgM	IgG
Polyreactive	Monospecific
Low affinity	High affinity
Germline encoded	Somatically mutated
3' V genes	Interspersed V genes
CD5 + B-cell lineage	CD5 − B-cell population

FIRST GENERATION B CELL

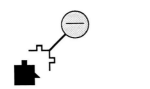

SOMATICALLY MUTATED PROGENY

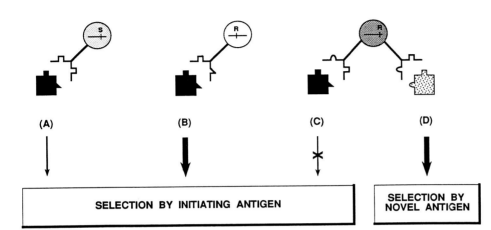

(A)   **(B)**   **(C)**   **(D)**

SELECTION BY INITIATING ANTIGEN

SELECTION BY NOVEL ANTIGEN

Fig. 18–3. B-cell genealogy. The progenitor B cell depicted at the top of the figure expresses an antibody that is encoded by germline immunoglobulin genes and that has low affinity for antigen. When antigen and T-cell factors trigger B-cell proliferation, class switching and somatic mutation, numerous B-cell progeny are possible. Three examples are schematized here. *A,* A B cell with a silent (S) point mutation. This nucleotide substitution does not encode a new amino acid, therefore the antibody molecule is unaffected and affinity for antigen does not change. *B,* A B cell whose point mutation encodes an amino acid replacement (R) leading to increased affinity for antigen. This mutated antibody exemplifies affinity maturation. *C,* A B cell with a replacement mutation that alters antigenic specificity. This antibody can no longer bind to the initial triggering antigen. As shown in *D,* however, the same antibody can acquire specificity for a novel antigen.

cells producing antibodies of higher affinity will continue to be amplified. Mutated antibodies can acquire novel antigenic specificities. In one in vitro system, a somatic point mutation changed a protective antipneumococcal antibody into an antibody with reduced binding to pneumococcal polysaccharide but with a newly acquired affinity for double-stranded DNA.[D197]

It is possible to follow the footprint of antigen selection by calculating the ratio of replacement mutations (R) to silent mutations (S) (i.e., point mutations that lead to alterations in amino acid sequence versus point mutations that alter codons without altering the amino acid sequence). If mutations occur randomly or as a result of polyclonal activation, one would predict an R/S ratio of approximately 3:1.[S377] If, however, B cells are acted upon by selective forces, one sees an increased R/S ratio, with amino acid substitutions that lead to greater affinity for antigen. Additionally, if mutation is random, then the R/S ratio should be uniform throughout the variable region, whereas, with antigenic selection, CDRs have higher R/S ratios than framework regions. Thus, molecular analysis provides insight into the forces that drive a given antibody response.

B-CELL LINEAGES

Recent studies suggest that there may be more than one B-cell lineage involved in the production of antibody molecules. B cells expressing CD5 on their surface constitute a population that undergoes limited heavy chain class switching and little, if any, somatic mutation. A large percentage of the B cells in the peritoneal cavity are CD5+ cells, but only a small percentage of B cells in secondary lymphoid organs express the CD5 marker.[H218,K244] CD5+ B cells predominantly express 3' heavy chain V region genes, genes used early in the ontogeny of a B-cell repertoire.[H308,J70,K335,S182] While much controversy exists over the physiologic function of this B-cell population, it seems that CD5+ B cells are responsible for production of "natural" autoantibodies[H218] (see below).

Other studies have recently suggested that the B-cell lineage activated in a primary antibody response may differ from the lineage producing the somatically mutated antibodies of the secondary immune response.[L320] This remains an area of active investigation.

NATURAL AUTOANTIBODIES

It has become apparent that autoreactive antibodies are part of a normal B-cell repertoire.[A367,D209] They are not unique to SLE nor to any autoimmune disease. Transformed B cells and hybridomas derived from normal individuals produce antibodies in vitro that bind to self determinants.[C7,S259] B cells producing "natural" autoantibodies can also be found in vivo in healthy individuals; however, estimates of autoantibody titers in normal serum are variable.[G423] There is no evidence that natural autoantibodies are pathogenic, and their physiologic significance remains unknown.

Natural autoantibodies resemble the antibodies of a primary immune response. They are IgM and display low affinity to self antigens. Further, they are polyreactive, binding to a wide variety of both autoantigens and foreign antigens that often have no apparent structural homology.[A230,B182,S259,T120] Sequence analysis shows that they are encoded by germline genes,[B7,D63,H339,M110,S77] frequently using a heavy chain V region gene from the 3' end of the immunoglobulin gene locus. It appears that the CD5+ population of B cells is responsible for production of natural autoantibodies.

PATHOGENIC AUTOANTIBODIES

The autoantibodies of SLE differ from natural autoantibodies (Table 8–2). SLE autoantibodies tend to be IgG antibodies that possess high affinity for antigen. While they are not necessarily monospecific, they cross-react with structurally homologous molecules.[A222,V9] Anti-DNA antibodies, for example, also bind other phosphate-rich antigens such as cardiolipin and phospholipid.[J21,L10,R59] The pathogenicity of these autoantibodies is inferred from their association with pathologic findings in SLE and from their presence in affected tissue. Antiphospholipid antibodies are associated with fetal wastage and with vascular compromise. Anti-Ro antibodies are associated with the development of neonatal SLE and may cause cardiac conduction abnormalities during fetal development. Anti-DNA antibodies, believed to contribute to glomerulonephritis and serositis, can be eluted from kidneys of lupus patients and can also be found in affected skin and pericardium.

To a great extent the structural basis for pathogenicity remains unknown: clearly not all SLE autoantibodies are pathogenic. Presumably, the fine specificity of the antibody as well as its affinity for antigen are critical parameters of pathogenicity. The heavy chain isotype also helps determine an antibody's potential for pathogenicity. In murine lupus the switch from serum IgM anti-DNA activity to IgG anti-DNA activity heralds the onset of renal disease.[P37,S687] Similarly, human IgG antibodies present in the immune complex deposits in SLE kidneys appear to trigger mesangial cell proliferation and subsequent tissue damage to a greater extent than IgM antibodies, perhaps because mesangial cells have Fc receptors for IgG. The role of isotype in SLE anticardiolipin antibodies is intriguing.[G38,G115] Several groups have noted that IgG antiphospholipid antibodies correlate better with clinical thrombosis than other isotypes (see Chap. 24); one investigator has associated IgA antiphospholipid antibodies with fetal loss.[K42] Thus, heavy chain class switching may be critical to the pathogenicity of lupus antibodies and distinguish them, in large part, from natural autoantibodies.

DERIVATION OF SLE AUTOANTIBODIES

Despite the apparent differences between natural autoantibodies and pathogenic autoantibodies, there are indications that the two populations may be clonally related. Idiotypic analyses of natural anti-DNA antibodies from normal individuals and anti-DNA antibodies in SLE demonstrate that cross-reactive idiotypes are present in both populations.[H74,I37] While CD5+ B cells, the population responsible for the production of natural autoantibodies, are less likely than conventional B cells to undergo heavy chain class switching and somatic mutation, these processes have been reported in CD5+ B cells, and, in SLE, might occur in this cell population even more frequently. While some investigators have speculated that natural autoantibodies are the precursors to pathogenic autoantibodies,[D174,N28] there are data suggesting that the two classes of autoantibodies arise from distinct B-cell populations, and that the SLE autoantibodies arise by somatic mutation of genes that encode protective antibodies.[D62,D65,D197,M135,M137,O42,S374,S375,S376,S377,S378]

GENETIC AND MOLECULAR ANALYSIS OF ANTI-DNA ANTIBODIES

Genetic analyses of anti-DNA antibodies in human and murine lupus have provided important information regarding the production of autoantibodies. There is no evidence that a distinctive set of disease-associated autoreactive V region genes, present only in individuals with a familial susceptibility to autoimmunity, is used to encode the autoantibodies of autoimmune disease. Analysis of restriction fragment length polymorphisms (RFLPs), a powerful tool to identify similarities and differences among particular genes in a population, has revealed no distinct polymorphisms that associate with SLE.[S78,S574,W233,Z46] Although such results cannot prove that autoimmune immunoglobulin genes do not exist, they suggest that there is no dramatic change in the number of V region gene segments and no easily identifiable allelic differences that distinguish the immunoglobulin genes of autoimmune patients from those of normal individuals. Moreover, it is clear that the immunoglobulin genes present in a nonautoimmune animal are capable of forming pathogenic autoantibodies. The offspring of a nonautoimmune SWR mouse and an NZB mouse, characterized by the spontaneous production of autoantibodies, produce autoantibodies. A large percentage of the anti-DNA antibodies deposited in the kidneys of (NZB × SWR) F_1 mice are encoded by genes from the nonautoimmune SWR parent.[G74]

In addition to the genetic studies suggesting that there are no disease-associated alleles, or at least no particular immunoglobulin V region genes absolutely required for the production of autoantibodies, both idiotypic and molecular studies show that the V region genes used to produce autoantibodies can also be used in a protective antibody response.[G344,N28,S388] Autoantibodies bear cross-reactive idiotypes that are also present on antibodies made in response to foreign antigens, and V region genes used to encode autoantibodies also encode antibodies to foreign antigen.[K344,M34,M536,N30] In fact, in the literature there are several examples of autoantibodies that also bind foreign antigens, demonstrating that the same V region gene segments can be used in both protective and potentially pathogenic responses.[C113,K2,Q7]

Although there is no evidence that specific genes encode only autoantibodies, there are data to suggest that autoantibodies are, nevertheless, encoded by a restricted number of immunoglobulin V region genes.[A279,R59,S76,T214] In murine lupus, extensive analyses of anti-DNA producing B cells show that only 15 to 20 heavy chain

V region genes encode most anti-DNA antibodies.[E52,Y34] While molecular studies of human antibodies are more limited, idiotypic analyses also suggest restricted V gene usage. Cross-reactive idiotypes are present in many individuals with SLE and represent a substantial proportion of the relevant autoantibodies.[H74,I37,P72,W246] It should be emphasized that this restricted V region gene usage does not appear to be skewed toward 3' V region genes or particular gene families.

While the V region genes used for anti-DNA antibodies appear unremarkable, there have been a few reports of unusual D regions. In some anti-DNA antibodies, D region gene segments are read in an uncommon reading frame.[E52,S375] Additionally, the D regions of some autoantibodies are produced by the fusion of two D region gene segments.[D63,M336,N88] Whether or not D-D fusion and the reading of D regions in unusual frames are more common in autoantibodies is not known.

AUTOANTIBODY REGULATION

It appears that the autoantibodies present in SLE do not exist in an unstimulated B-cell repertoire. Rather, autoantibodies in SLE seem to reflect the process of somatic mutation, and are apparently made by B cells following exposure to antigen and T cells. For some autoantibodies it is clear that mutation of the germline sequences is crucial in generating antigenic specificity.[V30] These antibodies have a high R/S ratio, primarily in their CDRs. However, there are also lupus autoantibodies that have a high R/S ratio in FW regions.[B169] As these FW mutations are unlikely to alter antigenic specificity, it is tempting to speculate that they may instead facilitate escape from a putative regulatory mechanism.

There are several hypotheses regarding the nature of the eliciting antigen(s) in SLE (Table 18–3), but much evidence points to a role for microbial antigens. For example, lupus prone strains of mice carrying a mutant *xid* gene, which impairs production of the antipolysaccharide antibodies required for antibacterial immunity, develop much lower titers of anti-DNA antibody and decreased renal disease.[S654] Similarly, lupus-prone mice raised in a germfree environment also produce reduced titers of anti-DNA antibodies and show delayed onset of autoimmune manifestations.[U22]

Some autoantibodies cross-react with foreign antigens. Although numerous examples of such molecular mimicry have been noted, it is not possible to determine whether such observations have etiologic significance in autoimmunity. Further, patients with Klebsiella infections and individuals vaccinated with pneumococcal polysaccharide develop antibacterial antibodies expressing anti-DNA cross-reactive idiotypes.[E92,G344] Anti-DNA antibodies may arise by somatic mutation of antimicrobial antibodies. This process would lead to antibodies with altered antigenic specificity without a change in idiotypic reactivity. Alternatively, an idiotypic network activated by a microbial antigen might stimulate cells to secrete antibodies bearing the cross-reactive idiotype but with no specificity for the eliciting antigen.[J72]

It is possible that the anti-idiotype itself might be an autoantibody.[B29,P328] For example, the Ku antigen is a DNA binding protein.[M451] Studies of anti-DNA and anti-Ku antibodies suggest that the anti-Ku antibodies are anti-idiotypic to anti-DNA antibodies.[R104] Significantly, experiments have shown that mice immunized with an anti-DNA antibody and mice immunized with an anti-idiotypic antibody to an anti-DNA antibody each develop autoantibodies.[M353,M354] These findings strongly suggest that the idiotypic network may contribute to the production of autoantibodies.

Finally, it remains true that autoantibodies need not arise inadvertently in a response to exogenous antigen; it is certainly possible that autoantigens themselves elicit autoantibody responses.[T113] The study of autoantigens suggests that autoantibodies are directed to highly conserved regions of the antigens and that, in general, the same epitopes are recognized by autoantibodies from genetically different individuals. Since the known autoantigens in SLE are nonpolymorphic, it appears that all individuals have immunoglobulin V region genes capable of producing pathogenic autoantibodies, and because foreign antigens hypothesized to be important in eliciting autoantibody production are essentially ubiquitous, it is important to ask why all individuals do not continually generate high-affinity autoantibodies.

CONCLUSIONS

Studies on the origins of pathogenic autoantibodies in autoimmune disease have demonstrated several salient points. It is clear that a restricted subset of variable region genes encodes antibodies with high affinities for a given autoantigen, and that these genes are used repeatedly in unrelated patients with SLE. It is also clear that these V region genes do not encode pathogenic autoantibodies exclusively, as they are also expressed in healthy individuals. At least some of these V region genes also encode antibodies against environmental pathogens, presumably participating in protective as well as pathogenic humoral responses. It is likely that somatic mutation of such V region genes is an important mechanism for the production of pathogenic autoantibodies; even a single amino acid substitution can change an antibacterial antibody into an antibody that binds DNA. Molecular genetic analyses further implicate antigen selection, but such an approach cannot identify the agent(s) that triggers disease.

Is there an unusual autoantigen specific to SLE patients, or is there a foreign antigen capable of breaking tolerance and inducing disease in genetically susceptible individuals? Further, what is the nature of the genetic predisposition to autoimmune disease? If "normal" genes can encode pathogenic autoantibodies, then a normal immune system must encompass regulatory mechanisms that sup-

Table 18–3. Triggers of Autoantibody Production

1. Environmental antigens
   Antigenic cross-reactivity
   Idiotypic cross-reactivity
2. Idiotypic network (anti-id = autoantibody)
3. Autoantigen

press expression of pathogenic autoreactivity. Perhaps there are subtle changes in B-cell differentiation in SLE, leading to a prolonged period of somatic mutation or to a diminished sensitivity to negative regulatory signals.[B510] Alternatively, SLE may be a disease with no intrinsic B-cell defect, but with an abnormality in the regulatory mechanisms that maintain peripheral B-cell tolerance. Mice transgenic for monoclonal autoantibodies will be useful in unraveling the networks that regulate autoantibody expression. To date, the studies of lupus autoantibodies favor a model predicting that genetic defects in SLE are of a permissive nature: abnormal regulation of antigen-driven responses or a breakdown in peripheral tolerance yield the pathogenic antibodies of autoimmune disease.

Chapter 19

ANTINUCLEAR ANTIBODIES: An Overview

MORRIS REICHLIN
JOHN B. HARLEY

The serology of systemic lupus erythematosus (SLE) originated with the discovery of the LE-cell phenomenon by Hargraves in 1948.[H129] The LE phenomenon was the first serologic marker utilized in the clinical diagnosis of SLE and, while rarely performed today, launched studies that have produced a powerful array of diagnostic tools that are still in evolution. The LE phenomenon as a diagnostic tool has been largely replaced by the antinuclear antibody (ANA) test, which in the first applications employed indirect immunofluorescence (IFA) on cryostat sections of animal tissues, usually rodent liver or kidney.[F279,H377,H390] Several other concurrent developments have occurred that have both refined the applications and illustrated the limitations of the ANA test.

From the beginning it was recognized that different patterns of immunofluorescence were produced by the sera of patients with SLE as well as other connective tissue diseases.[B150] These patterns reflected the heterogeneity of autoantibodies directed to discrete nuclear antigens. The history of the serology of SLE has been the resolution of this heterogeneity and the identification of the various nuclear targets of the autoimmune response. It was also recognized that some SLE sera also bound to the cellular cytoplasm and these have been termed anticytoplasmic antibodies (ACAs). The subsequent utilization of human tissue culture cells as substrates proved to be not only a more sensitive method for the detection of ANAs and ACAs but also capable of easier pattern recognition because of the larger size of the individual cells and the more discrete fluorescence displayed by subcellular organelles. Finally, an IFA test has been developed for the specific detection of antibodies to native or double-stranded (ds) DNA, which is still the most specific serologic marker for SLE.

This chapter will review present concepts of the use and interpretation of ANA testing in the clinical diagnosis of SLE. The current status of our understanding of the strengths and limitations of ANA determination, pattern recognition, the significance of variation in ANA titer, the specificity and sensitivity of positive tests, the recognition of false-positive and false-negative tests, the choice of substrate, and a view of the future of ANA testing will be explored. Where relevant to the diagnosis of SLE, ANA patterns and specificities characteristic of other systemic rheumatic diseases will also be described.

ANA TESTS IN THE DIAGNOSIS OF SLE

The first step in the interpretation of an ANA test is the recognition of what is "background" among normals. This varies with the substrates used, which includes rodent tissues, typically liver or kidney or monolayers of human cell lines. Tissue culture lines have a higher background with sera from normal populations. With rodent tissue substrates, 5 to 10% of normals will have a positive test at the screening dilution of 1/20 but only about 1% will have a positive test at 1/100. With tissue culture cells, 10 to 15% of normals will have a positive test at the screening dilution of 1/40 but only about 1% will have a positive test at 1/320. A positive ANA test without a systemic rheumatic disease is not rare and may reflect aging, unrecognized chronic infection, chronic liver disease, or ingestion of certain drugs (e.g., procainamide hydrochloride [Pronestyl], hydralazine, isoniazid, chlorpromazine), among the more common causes.

As illustrated in Table 19–1, all the systemic rheumatic diseases have positive ANA tests, although they occur most frequently and have the highest titers in SLE patients. Thus, the proper use of the tests requires that clinical findings suggestive of SLE be present when the tests are ordered. To put this in its most absurd light, a positive ANA test does not mean a patient with typical rheumatoid arthritis has SLE nor that a patient with only nonspecific clinical findings and a positive ANA test any rheumatic disease.

A working algorithm utilizes the association of characteristic findings of SLE (as the ARA criteria) and positive ANA tests. If patients have three of the revised preliminary criteria of the American Rheumatism Association (ARA), a positive ANA test adds evidence for and supports the clinical diagnosis.[T46] If patients have four or more of the revised preliminary ARA criteria (excluding a positive ANA), a positive ANA confirms and reinforces the evidence for SLE, but is unnecessary for the clinical diagnosis.

Patients with two or less ARA criteria and a positive ANA may or may not have SLE and clinical followup usually results in a diagnosis with the accumulation of more clinical findings within a year or two. Typical clinical situations include patients with only polyarthritis or a pleural effusion or a Coombs' positive hemolytic anemia, in association with a positive ANA. The differential diagnosis is still broad in such patients, and a diagnosis in the absence of other clinical or more specific serologic findings is untenable.

ANTIBODIES TO NATIVE DNA

Antibodies to native or double-stranded (ds) DNA are in a class by themselves in terms of diagnostic power, and

Table 19–1. Positive ANA Tests

	Frequency of Positive Tests Rodent Epithelial Tissues	Hep-2 Cells
SLE	90–95%	98%
PSS	50–70%	95%
RA	30–50%	50–75%
Primary Sjögren's syndrome	50%	75%
Polymyositis	30%	90%
JRA	25%	ND
Chronic active hepatitis	50%	ND
Infectious mononucleosis	5–20%	ND
Lepromatous leprosy	5–20%	ND
Vasculitis	5–20%	ND
Subacute bacterial endocarditis	5–20%	ND

ND = No data.

in many patients such antibodies fluctuate with disease activity. High titers of these antibodies rarely occur in patients who are asymptomatic or in diseases other than SLE. In family studies we have conducted, anti-nDNA antibodies measured in the Crithidia luciliae assay are unique in not occurring in asymptomatic first-degree relatives; they only occur in SLE patients. Positive ANA tests occurred in 25% of such relatives (Reichlin, M., and Harley, J.B. unpublished data). This frequency of positive ANA tests is significantly higher than in random normals. Thus, determination of a strongly positive anti-nDNA test has the greatest diagnostic power of any available serologic test, and one is rarely, if ever, faced with evaluating the meaning of a positive test associated with few or no clinical findings of SLE.

One must be certain, however, that the test for anti-dsDNA measures only antibodies to dsDNA and the test DNA is free of single-stranded regions. Antibodies to single-stranded (ss) DNA occur in a broad spectrum of rheumatic diseases and are not specific for SLE. The most reliable tests for anti-dsDNA are those involving circular double-stranded DNA as in the Crithidia assay or radioimmunoassay with PM-2 DNA or alternatively S_1 nuclease treatment of mammalian DNA just prior to the performance of the assay to remove single-stranded regions. One current good method for the determination of antibodies to dsDNA is IFA using the Crithidia luciliae organism as substrate.[T46] There are some technical problems with the reading of the Crithidia test. Identification of the kinetoplast is the key to proper interpretation of a positive test. Technicians must be carefully instructed about the distinction between the kinetoplast, the nucleus, and the polar body. Counterstaining with ethidium bromide facilitates identification in the training stages. Fluorescence of the polar body is common and has no clinical meaning. Fluorescence of the nucleus alone occurs with some sera and may even occur in the absence of a positive ANA on standard substrates. This finding has no known clinical significance. There are rare sera that intensely stain the kinetoplast and yet the activity is not due to anti-dsDNA. One suspects this when the standard ANA test on the same serum is negative. One can prove this fluorescence is not a result of anti-DNA by the failure of an excess of native DNA added to the serum to inhibit the binding of antibody

and thus the fluorescence. Fluorescence due to anti-dsDNA is easily blocked by added native DNA. Such positive tests must reflect antibodies to some antigen other than dsDNA and are of unknown significance. With these limitations in mind, the Crithidia test is a convenient way to measure anti-dsDNA, can be made semiquantitative by the use of titer determination, and utilizes the same equipment as that employed in the standard ANA test. An alternative method, also in wide use, is the ELISA assay in which double-stranded DNA is fixed to the wells of microtiter plates, and test sera are added. Presence of IgG or IgM binding the DNA is detected with enzyme labeled anti-human Ig reagins.

Anti-DNA antibodies are discussed in detail in Chapter 20.

DRUG-INDUCED ANAs

Drug-induced ANAs represent an important area in which determination of the specificity of the ANA is helpful in establishing the diagnosis. It has long been known that the pattern of fluorescence seen in drug-induced ANAs with the common inducing agents (e.g., hydralazine, Pronestyl, isoniazid) is homogeneous. Early studies showed that the reactive antigen is histone dependent. Acid extraction of nuclei from tissue sections abolishes fluorescence, and addition of purified histone restores the antigenic activity of acid-extracted nuclei.[F280] Chromatin efficiently absorbed out antibody activity and purified histones can react directly with sera from drug-induced lupus sera.[R392]

While antihistone antibody-specific ELISA tests are available, the presence of a homogeneous pattern ANA after patients have been treated with one of the common drugs that induce ANAs is highly suggestive of a drug-induced ANA. Resolution of SLE symptoms upon discontinuation of the drug in association with a decline in ANA titer is diagnostic of drug-induced SLE. In our experience, however, the decline in ANA titer may be slow, and in some patients low ANA titers of homogeneous pattern may linger for years in the absence of clinical symptoms. The presence of antibodies to histone does not distinguish patients with drug-induced LE from those with spontaneous SLE, since the antibodies are frequent in both groups.[B263,G165,H121,K423,R392]

Complexity is the major serologic difference between drug-induced and idiopathic SLE. The response in drug-induced disease is highly restricted with antibody to histone-dependent antigens and ssDNA being the major and usually the only antibodies measurable. The presence of any of the common highly characteristic autoantibodies seen in idiopathic SLE such as those directed to dsDNA, U_1-RNP, Sm, Ro/SSA, La/SSB, or ribosomal P proteins provides strong evidence for the diagnosis of idiopathic SLE and against the diagnosis of drug-induced disease.

PATTERNS OF IMMUNOFLUORESCENCE

Different patterns of nuclear immunofluorescence were first noted by Beck in 1961,[B150] and in the ensuing 30 years this variability in staining patterns has been determined to reflect the heterogeneity of the autoantibodies present in rheumatic disease sera. This pattern variability

Table 19–2. Patterns of Immunofluorescence in SLE

Pattern	Related Antigen Specificities
Nuclear	
Homogeneous	Chromatin, histone, deoxyribonucleoprotein
Peripheral or rim	DNA, lamins
Speckled	U1-RNP, Sm, Ro/SSA, La/SSB, Ku
Cytoplasmic	
Homogeneous or finely granular with or without nucleolar staining	Ribosomal P protein

is obvious in SLE sera, and Table 19–2 lists the common patterns that have been appreciated. It is well known to clinical serologists that single sera can show multiple patterns depending on dilution. These SLE sera frequently show homogeneous and/or peripheral patterns at low dilution and a speckled pattern at higher dilution. This reflects the relative concentrations of the autoantibodies responsible for these patterns. Antibodies to the RNA protein antigens such as U$_1$-RNP, Sm, Ro/SSA, and La/SSB, which are associated with speckled patterns, have much higher autoantibody concentrations[M49] than do chromatin[T198] and DNA, which are responsible for the homogeneous and peripheral or rim patterns, respectively.

While present in the great majority of SLE sera, antibodies to chromatin are also present in the other systemic rheumatic diseases to variable extents. These antichromatin antibodies produce the homogeneous nuclear fluorescence that is especially common in patients with classic rheumatoid arthritis with high titers of rheumatoid factor (RF). In many cases, these autoantibodies have

been shown to have a surprisingly dual specificity, binding both nucleosomes and the classical RF epitope, the Fc fragment of IgG.[A56,A80,H105,H107]

The peripheral pattern of IFA is highly correlated with SLE and can be due to either anti-dsDNA,[C127] antilamins,[G425,R103] or both.[S280] Rarely, a peripheral pattern can be seen unrelated to either anti-dsDNA or antilamins and has been shown to be caused by antibody to the molecular pore complex.[D9] Clinical significance of such autoantibodies is unknown, but molecular studies have revealed its presence in a single case of polymyositis[D9] and in several cases of primary biliary cirrhosis.[C412,L86]

Speckled patterns of ANAs are common in SLE but are not diagnostically specific and can be seen in progressive systemic sclerosis (PSS), particularly and to lesser extents in all the systemic rheumatic diseases. In PSS sera, nuclear speckled patterns that are related to the centromere complex are easily identified morphologically and exhibit the presence of antigen in the chromosomes of mitotic cells.[M593] Other PSS sera have nuclear speckled patterns, many of which are caused by autoantibodies to the Scl-70 antigen now known to be caused by the nuclear enzyme topoisomerase I.[D283,G427,M214,S354] (These patterns of fluorescence are illustrated—see in Figure 19–1).

About 10% of SLE sera have autoantibodies that display a characteristic finely granular fluorescence in the cytoplasm of all cells. In tissue culture cells there is frequently an accompanying nucleolar fluorescence. These autoantibodies are directed to the ribosomal P proteins[E79] and are of clinical interest since they occur in a subset of SLE patients enriched for neuropsychiatric disease.[B402,S152] In all these instances, the IFA patterns become meaningful in the presence of clinical data but rigorous demonstration of the particular specificity responsible for the pat-

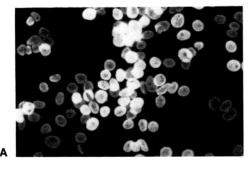

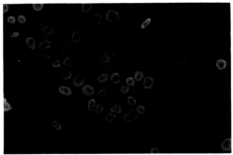

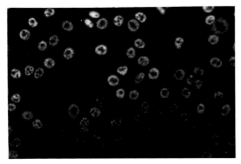

Fig. 19–1. Patterns of nuclear fluorescence seen on Hep-2 cells. *A*, Homogeneous. *B*, Peripheral or rim. *C*, Speckled. All three patterns are common in patients with SLE.

tern requires the appropriate antigen-specific serologic test. This finely granular cytoplasmic fluorescence seen with antiribosomal antibody is also seen with autoantibodies to molecular components of the translation apparatus as seen in polymyositis with or without interstitial lung disease. These patterns are seen in Figure 19–2A. Antigenic targets whose cognate autoantibody produces such IFA patterns include Jo-1 (histidyl-tRNA synthetase)[R115,T69] PL-7 (threonyl-tRNA synthetase),[M185] PL-12 (alanyl-tRNA synthetase),[B570] KJ antigen,[T68] and signal recognition particle.[T70] None of these autoantibodies has yet been recognized in SLE sera, but the clinical picture as well as molecular definition of the particular specificity establish the clinical significance of finely granular cytoplasmic fluorescence.

Precipitating antibodies to Ku were first described in scleroderma-polymyositis overlap in Japanese patients[M446] and are rare in Caucasians with scleroderma-polymyositis overlap syndromes. The antigenic target is a dimer, composed of 86 kD and 70 kD proteins, which binds internucleosomal segments of DNA.[M450,R102,Y32] Although precipitating anti-Ku is rare in both SLE and scleroderma, sensitive ELISA and/or Western blotting methods detect antibodies in sizable numbers of SLE[F206,R102,Y31] and scleroderma sera.[R102,Y31] The human proteins are the preferred antigenic targets, and this species specificity is strong evidence for the immune response being antigen driven. These autoantibodies are associated with a nuclear speckled pattern of fluorescence.

Finally, a rare but characteristic nuclear staining pattern seen in about 2 to 5% of SLE sera is caused by antibodies to proliferating cell nuclear antigen (PCNA).[M493] This pat-

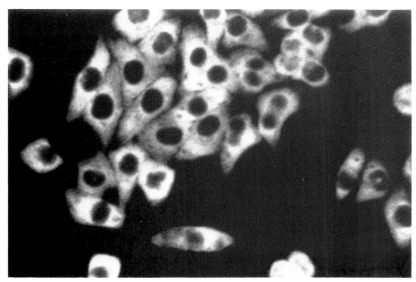

A

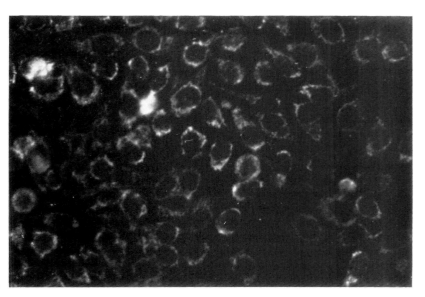

B

Fig. 19–2. *A*, The finely granular pattern of cytoplasmic fluorescence. *B*, In contrast, the reticular lacy cytoplasmic staining characteristic of antibody to mitochondria is shown. This pattern is typical of primary biliary cirrhosis. The substrate in both panels is Hep-2 cells. (See also Figure 19–5*A*.)

Table 19–3. Patterns of Immunofluorescence That Rarely Occur in SLE

Pattern	Clinical Association	Related Antigen specificities
Nuclear		
Centromere	CREST variant of PSS	Centromere-related proteins 17, 80, and 140 kD proteins
Pseudocentromere	Undifferentiated connective tissue syndromes	Same appearance as centromere but chromosome negative
Nuclear dots	Primary biliary cirrhosis	95 kD nuclear protein not associated with chromosomes: lesser number of dots than in centromere or pseudocentromere
Nucleolar	Scleroderma	RNA polymerase I Fibrillarin NOR-90
	Scleroderma polymyositis overlap	PM-Scl
Cytoplasmic		
Filamentous, reticular	Primary biliary cirrhosis	Mitochondrial lipoamide dehydrogenase

tern is caused by autoantibody to the nuclear protein cyclin and is seen only in interstitial cells in rodent substrates and recognized by the variable staining of nuclei in tissue culture cells, the so-called harlequin pattern.[P284] The variable staining is caused by the varying concentration of cyclin present in the different stages of the cell cycle. Because of the low frequency of positive tests for anti-PCNA, it is difficult to establish its disease specificity, but it clearly occurs in SLE sera.

IMMUNOFLUORESCENT PATTERNS RARELY SEEN WITH SLE SERA

In Table 19–3 are listed a number of IFA patterns that are rarely seen in SLE sera. Their usefulness in the clinical diagnosis is that their presence makes the diagnosis of SLE unlikely. In early disease with limited clinical findings,

these patterns lead the clinician away from SLE and toward the diagnosis suggested by the IFA pattern.

Thus, the centromere (see Fig. 19–4) and nucleolar (Fig. 19–3) patterns are highly suggestive of PSS and are seen only rarely in SLE patients. In the two lupus patients that the authors have seen that have antibody to centromere, neither has the CREST syndrome but one has subacute cutaneous lupus erythematosus (SCLE), polyarthritis, and Raynaud's phenomenon, while the other has primary Sjögren's syndrome, SCLE, and a mother who has CREST syndrome with high titers of anticentromere antibody. Similarly, only two of our SLE patients have antibodies to nucleoli as the dominant ANA pattern. Several antigenic targets in the nucleolus have been characterized at the molecular level, and these are listed in Table 19–3 and seen in Figure 19–3.[R112] In general, such autoantibody

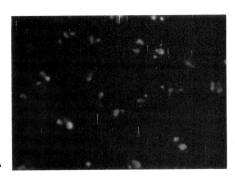

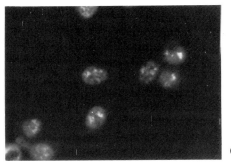

A

B

C

Fig. 19–3. Three different nucleolar patterns are illustrated on Hep-2 cells. A, Shaggy nucleolar staining typical of anti-fibrillarin. B, Speckled nucleolar staining characteristic of antibodies to RNA polymerase I. C, Homogeneous nucleolar staining accompanied invariably by nucleoplasmic staining as seen with antibodies to Pm-Scl. Patterns in A and B are most frequently seen in scleroderma. The pattern in C occurs in patients with polymyositis-scleroderma overlaps.

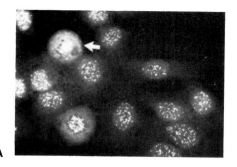

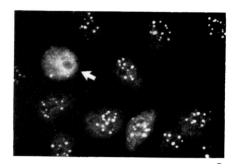

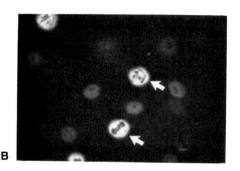

A

B

C

Fig. 19–4. *A,* Anticentromere antibodies produce a discrete speckled pattern of immunofluorescence on both interphase and metaphase (arrow) cells. They are most commonly seen in CREST syndrome. *B,* The NSp1 "pseudocentromere" antibody produces a speckled pattern of immunofluorescence, but the number of speckles is fewer than anticentromere and there is no staining of metaphase chromatin (arrow). *C,* The NSpII antibody is characterized by large speckles on metaphase chromatin (arrows) and a fine speckled pattern in interphase cells. Antibodies in *B* and *C* are not associated with defined rheumatic diseases. The substrate was Hep-2 cells. From Fritzler, M.J., Valencia, D.W., and McCarty, G.A.: Speckled pattern antinuclear antibodies resembling anticentromere antibodies. Arthritis Rheum., *27*:92, 1984. With permission.[F282]

specificities direct the clinician's attention to other diagnoses. Autoantibodies that are designated antipseudocentromere are directed to an as yet unidentified nuclear target, are rarely present in SLE sera, but are thus far not associated with any systemic rheumatic disease. Morphologically, the large speckles characteristic of the pseudocentromere (NSP-1) pattern are indistinguishable from the centromere pattern, but in NSP-1 the chromosomes of mitotic cells do not contain the antigen that makes the distinction certain.[F282] These centromere and pseudocentromere patterns are illustrated in Figure 19–4.

One described pattern, designated nuclear dots, is recognized by a small number (10 or less) of large uniform staining bodies that are not associated with the chromosomes in mitotic cells.[E158,S802] Representative staining patterns are seen in Figure 19–5. The antigenic target has been identified as a 95 kD protein, and these autoantibod-

ies have thus far been described only in patients with primary biliary cirrhosis. Finally, a characteristic pattern of cytoplasmic fluorescence in a reticular network is easily identified in HEp-2 cells, which has been shown to be highly associated with autoantibodies to mitochondria (Figure 19–5*A;* see also Figure 19–2*B*). High titers of these antimitochondrial antibodies are also seen in primary biliary cirrhosis.

ANA-NEGATIVE SLE

With the advent of the use of tissue culture cells for the determination of ANA, the occurrence of patients with clinical SLE and a negative ANA test is unusual but still occurs.[F76,G171] When rodent epithelial cells were used as the principal substrate for IFA, a negative ANA test occurred in about 5% of SLE patients' sera, and these patients had a characteristic clinical picture. This ANA negativity was not caused by therapy or disease inactivity, but was related to the fact that the major immune response of such LE patients was to the antigens poorly represented in rodent tissues. These two antigens were the RNA protein antigen Ro/SSA and ssDNA.[M48] The Ro/SSA protein is present in mouse tissues but is evolutionarily divergent from the human Ro/SSA protein as evidenced by the appropriate immunochemical studies.[R121,R122] Thus, mouse and rat Ro/SSA react poorly with human anti-Ro/SSA and in standard immunofluorescence tests are undetectable. In immunofluorescence, it is presumed that the DNA in the resting chromosomes of interphase nuclei is in its characteristic double-stranded helical conformation so that autoantibodies specific for ssDNA would not react.

Thus, it is part of the biology of this subset of lupus that leads to the fact that the ANA test is negative on rodent substrates. Widespread use of human tissue culture cells

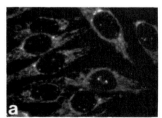

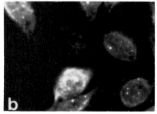

a b

Fig. 19–5. Indirect immunofluorescence on Hep-2 cells with two representative sera displaying the nuclear dot pattern. *A,* The serum shown produces mitochondrial staining in addition to staining of nuclear dots. *B,* The serum shown produces a weak homogeneous pattern plus a nuclear dot pattern. Nuclear dots are most commonly seen in patients with primary biliary cirrhosis.

has led to a lower prevalence of ANA-negative SLE since 70% of such sera that have a negative ANA on rodent tissues are strongly positive on the human tissue culture cells, reflecting the adequate structure and concentration of the Ro/SSA antigen in the nuclei of such cells. Thus, the ANA test is negative in only about 2% of SLE sera when human tissue culture cells are used and the patients have active untreated disease.

Finally, it should be noted that some SLE patients develop a negative ANA when their disease remits, either spontaneously or after immunosuppression. Disappearance of a positive ANA test only occurs in about 10 to 20% of cases, but is especially prevalent in SLE patients who experience renal failure in which at least a third to a half become ANA negative. Experienced clinicians are familiar with the phenomenon that SLE patients who experience clinical remission usually maintain high ANA titers, and that this is not an indication for therapy. Except for anti-dsDNA, the titer of most of the other autoantibody specificities do not correlate with disease activity.

THE FUTURE OF ANA TESTING AND THE CHOICE OF SUBSTRATE

Because of the widespread availability and the diagnostic power of the ANA test when coupled with the clinical data, it is likely that ANA determination as a screening test will be useful for many years to come. The major direction of ANA research will likely remain the development of simple inexpensive quantitative tests for the measurement of individual autoantibody specificities. A decision for ANA determination is the choice of substrate. In Table 19–4 are listed the known autoantibody specificities detected by rodent substrates compared to human tissue culture lines. The advantages of the tissue culture cells are manifold. 1) As they are of human origin they detect autoantibodies that have species specificity. 2) Pattern recognition is easier, and some patterns (e.g., centromere) are not present on rodent organ section substrates. 3) The presence of mitotic cells enables the observer to distinguish chromosome-associated from non–chromosome-associated antigenic targets. The only recognized disadvantage of the tissue culture lines is a somewhat higher sensitivity for determining ANAs, so that the false-

Table 19–4. Autoantibody Specificities Detected by Mouse Kidney and Hep-2 Substrates

	MK	Hep-2
ANA % positive in active		
untreated SLE	90–95%	98–99%
Normal Sera	5% + 1/20	10–15% + 1/40
DNA histone	+	+
U1-RNP	+	+
Sm	+	+
La/SSB	+	+
Ro/SSA	−	+
PCNA	−	+
Ribosomes	+	+
Ku	−	+

positive rate is higher. This latter problem is mitigated by the fact that positive ANA tests without clinical findings should be treated by clinicians with reserve and patience since they are common. Low-titer ANAs with no symptoms infrequently are the harbingers of future disease. Even should clinical investigation develop the knowledge that would enable them to differentiate positive ANA tests that are predictive of future disease from those that are not, this knowledge will have little impact on clinical practice until safe interventions become available that could prevent disease expression.

On balance, then, when faced with the decision as to which substrate should be used for ANA determination, the tissue culture cells are the clear choice.

CONCLUSIONS

Determination of antinuclear antibodies (ANAs) is an integral part of the diagnosis of SLE and is also an important tool in the diagnosis of other systemic rheumatic diseases. The presence of a positive ANA test confirms the diagnosis of SLE in the presence of appropriate clinical findings. The evolution of ANA testing has featured the use of human tissue culture cells and the recognition of diagnostically useful immunofluorescent patterns. Associated with these developments has been the molecular definition of the antigenic targets.

Chapter 20

ANTIBODIES TO DNA

BEVRA H. HAHN
BETTY P. TSAO

Antibodies to DNA (anti-DNA) are the classic autoantibodies that characterize SLE. High-avidity IgG antibodies to double-stranded DNA play a major role in inducing some of the disease manifestations of SLE (especially nephritis), are specific for the disease, and are good markers of disease activity.

HISTORICAL CONSIDERATIONS

The LE-cell phenomenon identified the first autoantibody recognized in patients with SLE;[H129] LE cells result from the action on nuclei of antibodies to DNA-protein complexes; the major antigen recognized is a histone DNA complex.[H377] The altered nuclei are then ingested by phagocytic cells.

The first reports of anti-DNA in sera of lupus patients appeared in 1957—discovered in four different laboratories almost simultaneously.[C181,M397,R234,S265] The clinical importance of circulating anti-DNA was soon recognized. Certain subsets were found to be specific for SLE and correlated with disease activity and nephritis.[R354,S207] Evidence mounted that anti-DNA cause some of the tissue lesions characteristic of SLE, especially lupus nephritis. Anti-DNA was eluted from tissue lesions (glomeruli, skin, choroid plexus) of patients and mice with SLE.[A225,L35,T41,W286] In mouse models of SLE, disease was prevented by blocking immune responses to DNA and accelerated by increasing those responses.[B416,L35,P521]

The development of monoclonal antibody technology permitted expanded studies of DNA antibodies[H31] and has provided new information regarding the characteristics of different antibody subsets, the presence of anti-DNA in unstimulated immune repertoires of healthy individuals, and the features of individual antibodies that contribute to their pathogenicity. The central role of these antibodies in the disease process in some patients seems clear.

CHARACTERISTICS OF SUBSETS OF ANTIBODIES TO DNA

There are many different individual antibodies to DNA. They differ in isotype, complement-fixing capabilities, avidity for DNA, antigenic specificities, charge, and idiotypes[E17] (see Table 20–1). Healthy individuals, both human and mouse, make antibodies to DNA as part of their normal, resulting immune repertoires.[C10,F106,H203,H338,P213a,R391,S218,S509,S630] These natural autoantibodies are largely IgM class and react primarily with single-stranded DNA (ssDNA). They have low avidity for DNA, and are polyreactive. In fact, monoclonal antibodies to DNA have been shown to react with multiple polynucleotides, Sm antigen, cytoskeletal proteins, histones, laminin, phospholipids, the Fc of IgG, cell surface structures (on platelets, lymphocytes, and Raji cells), proteoglycans such as heparan sulfate, myelin, gangliosides, bacterial polysaccharides, and proteins.[A222, B496, C113, F1, F2, F223, J20, J22, J23, K357, L10, P211, P213, R61, R80 R401,S3,S218, S385] Most of these "natural" autoantibodies are probably derived directly from rearranged germline DNA with little somatic mutation. However, activation of the resting B-cell repertoire in mice and in humans yields not only IgM low-avidity anti-ssDNA, but also some IgM and IgG subsets that bind dsDNA.[C10,F106,H338,P213a,R391,S509,S630] Therefore, the ability of human and murine B cells to make antibodies to DNA is not "forbidden," but is normal. In fact, IgM and IgG antibodies to ssDNA can be found in many healthy individuals, and in many disease states other than SLE that are associated with B-cell activation, such as infections, chronic inflammatory states, and aging.[V30]

CHARACTERISTICS OF PATHOGENIC ANTIBODY SUBSETS

Some individuals with SLE probably make increased quantities of anti-DNA and synthesize subsets of anti-DNA that differ from those of the normal repertoire. Several investigators have shown that antibodies associated with active disease and with nephritis are IgG, complement fixing, and have high avidity for dsDNA.[A225,E16,K41, R354,S562] Such antibodies usually bind both dsDNA and ssDNA; only a small proportion bind dsDNA alone. These antibodies also lack the wide, low-avidity polyreactivity of the IgM anti-DNA in the resting repertoire. It is likely that many of the IgG high-avidity anti-dsDNAs have undergone numerous somatic mutations.[B169,D63,G426,S374,S375] A high number of somatic mutations suggest that specific antigens are driving B-cell maturation and secretion. The nature of those antigens is unknown.

Antigenic Specificities

The antigens with which a particular antibody to DNA react are probably important in determining pathogenicity. For example, when rodent or human kidneys are perfused in vivo or incubated in vitro with antibodies to DNA,

Table 20–1. Different Subsets of Antibodies to DNA

Probable Nonpathogens The Normal Repertoire	Probable Pathogens The SLE Repertoire
IgM	Complement-fixing Ig Isotype
IgG non–complement fixing	(IgG1 in humans, IgG2a and
Low avidity for ssDNA	IgG2b in mice, some IgM)
Wide cross-reactivity (low	High avidity for dsDNA and
avidity) to	ssDNA
Polynucleotides	Ability to bind directly to
Sm/RNP	glomeruli
Cytoskeleton	Cationic charge
Histones	High-avidity binding to
Fc of IgG	DNA
Laminin	DNA/histone
Proteoglycans	Laminin
Phospholipids	Heparan sulfate
Cell surfaces	Phospholipids
Myelin	DNA receptors
Gangliosides	Ability to form immune
Bacteria	complexes of correct size and
Polysaccharides	charge to avoid clearance and
Phospholipids	fix to GBM
Proteins	Enrichment in certain idiotypes
	IdGN2
	16/6
	32/15
	3I
	O-81

some antibodies fix to glomeruli and others do not.[D33,J20, R80,S3] Some monoclonal antibody (MAb) anti-dsDNAs inoculated into normal mice cause clinical nephritis; others do not.[T233] Differences between pathogens and nonpathogens include 1) polyreactivity in pathogens (with DNA, RNA, Sm/RNP, gp70, phospholipids, and proteoglycans;[P30] 2) ability of pathogens to bind directly to components of glomerular basement membrane such as laminin or heparan sulfate;[F2,R80,S3] and 3) ability of pathogens to bind DNA planted in glomerular structures.[D33] We have shown that antibodies to dsDNA that bind positively charged histone can then bind negatively charged heparan sulfate; the MAb-DNA-histone complexes bind to glomerular basement membranes in vitro, and cause clinical nephritis when injected into normal mice.[O29]

Charge

Charge may also be important. There are many regions of the glomerular basement membrane that are polyanionic. Therefore, antigens, antibodies, or immune complexes with cationic charges can bind to GBM via charge.[D33,E16,B70,G75,M96] If a cationic anti-DNA is trapped by this mechanism, and DNA is available, then an immune complex forms in the GBM, complement is activated, and damage occurs. One group has reported that one antibody with a cationic charge in an immune complex is sufficient to permit trapping in the GBM.[G70] Several investigators have noted an enrichment of cationic anti-DNA populations in IgG of glomerular eluates from mice with lupus nephritis;[E16,D33,G75] other groups disagree.[P30,Y50] A study of Japanese patients with lupus nephritis showed that cationic clonotypes of anti-DNA (pI 7.0 to 8.5) were found

in glomeruli but not in circulating immune complexes.[M675]

Idiotypes

Finally, the idiotypic characteristics of anti-DNA may also contribute to pathogenicity.[D63,E17,G75,H30,I35,K41, M353,M354,M675,S380,S544,W151] Idiotypes are antigenic sequences in the V regions of antibodies; they induce B- and T-cell anti-idiotypic responses that are important in regulating antibody production. Idiotypes and idiotypic networks are reviewed in Chapter 15. As discussed there, public idiotypes that characterize many antibodies to DNA have been identified in murine and human lupus. Certain idiotypes have been found in tissue lesions (IdGN2, 16/6, 32/15, 3I, 0-81) of patients with lupus.[D63,I35,K41,M675,S380] One human public idiotype or anti-idiotype (the 16/6 system), when injected into certain strains of normal mice, can activate an Id–anti-Id network. This results in production of multiple Id-positive antibodies (including anti-DNA), and the mice develop nephritis.[M353,M354] Therefore, pathogenic anti-DNA subsets are enriched in certain idiotypic markers, and those idiotypes can be targets of regulation that permit abnormal up-regulation of pathogenic subsets of anti-DNA.

STRUCTURE AND ORIGIN OF ANTIBODIES TO DNA

The structures of many monoclonal (MAb) human and murine antibodies to DNA have been studied[B169,B397,C8, C224,D63,D174,E52,G426,K343,K344,S374,S375,T215,T233,V30] (see Table 20–2). As reviewed in Chapter 18, the heavy (H) chains of immunoglobulins (Igs) are encoded by rearrangements of variable (V_H) region gene segments with diversity (D) and joining (J_H) segments that combine with constant (C_H) regions for the Ig isotype. Light (L) chains are formed by rearrangements of V_L and J_L with C_κ or C_λ. Joining of the H and L chains forms an intact Ig molecule. Diversity in antibody binding is generated by 1) variations in the information contained in germline DNA in different individuals; 2) different rearrangements of V, D, and J segments for H, and V and J for L chains; 3) addition of nucleic acids at the junctions (N additions) between variable and constant regions in H or L chains; and 4) somatic mutations of single nucleic acids in rearranged H and L chains. In general, antigen-driven antibody responses undergo increasing numbers of somatic mutations with each cell di-

Table 20–2. Structure of Antibodies to DNA

Genes Encoding Immunoglobulin
1. Germline DNA—no unique information.
2. Rearrangement of germline:
   No unique rearrangements.
   Many different V_H, D, J_H, V_L and J_L can be used.
   Enriched in V_H J558 in mice, V_H3 in humans.
3. Somatic mutations—can be none, a few, or many.

Amino Acid Sequences in Heavy and Light Chains
1. CDR of H and L chains are enriched in Arg, Asp, and Tyr.
2. Ser-Tyr found frequently in CDR1 of V_H.
3. Tyr-Tyr-Gly-Gly-Ser-Tyr found frequently in CDR3 of V_H.

bose-phosphate backbone alone, or particular conformations in dsDNA.[M659,S218,S709] Multiple different conformations occur; dsDNA may form twisted supercoiled closed circular molecules, relaxed circular forms, left-handed Z-DNA segments, and cruciform structures. These polymorphisms are associated with different base pair sequences, and with the physicochemical characteristics of the environment. It is not known which of these reactivities is associated with the most pathogenic antibodies.

When dsDNA is denatured, compact single chains are formed, which can present bases, nucleotide sequences, backbone, short regions of base-paired secondary structures, and short helices. Anti-ssDNA can therefore react with bases, nucleosides, nucleotides, oligonucleotides, and ribose-phosphate backbone.[M659,S218] Antibodies to ssDNA react predominantly with individual bases, and even better with polynucleotides containing multiples of that base. The largest proportions of anti-ssDNA in sera react with guanosine and thymidine, but others recognize polyA, polyC, polyI, Z-DNA, ssRNA, RNA-DNA hybrids, and poly(ADP)ribose.

Antibodies to DNA induced by immunization with bases, nucleosides, or oligonucleotides are usually highly specific for the immunogen. In contrast, spontaneous antibodies to DNA that arise in individuals with SLE are usually polyspecific and react with multiple oligonucleotides and several forms of DNA. This wide reactivity could result from similar epitopes shared by multiple different molecules (probably conformational) or a single antibody-combining site having multiple contact regions for unrelated epitopes. An example of shared epitopes would be the cross-reactivity of many MAbs for DNA and cardiolipin. There are shared phosphodiester groups in the ribose-phosphate backbone of DNA and in phospholipids.

Is DNA Altered to Become Antigenic?

Does self DNA become antigenic, and if so, how (see Table 20–3)? Abnormalities in DNA have been suggested in patients with SLE. It has been hypothesized that DNA is altered structurally to become more antigenic. Unaltered mammalian DNA does not induce high-titer anti-DNA when inoculated into normal animals as an immunogen. In contrast, bacterial DNA can induce good antibody responses in mice.[G133] I have mentioned in an earlier section that some anti-DNAs cross-react with Klebsiella polysaccharides,[S218] with Escherichia coli β-galactosidase,[P211] and with phospholipids of streptococci and staphylococci.[C113] Further, the structure of many MAb anti-DNA

Table 20–3. Possible Antigens Inducing Anti-DNA

Altered self DNA
DNA-histone (nucleosomes)
Bacterial
    DNA
    Polysaccharides
    Phospholipids
Molecules that share epitopes with phosphate-ribose backbone (phospholipids)
Other molecules, antibodies to which cross-react with conformations in DNA

molecules is similar to that of antibacterial antibodies.[G426,K343,K344] Therefore, it is possible that ordinary bacteria are the antigens that induce anti-DNA responses in humans. In fact, immunization of normal mice with bacterial phospholipids/polysaccharides incudes antibodies to DNA.[166] It is also possible that integration of viral nucleic acids into the human genome results in antigenic self DNA. Finally, DNA-histone complexes, abundantly present in nucleosomes, may be the true antigen.[H120,R420] Negatively charged DNA noncovalently linked to positively charged proteins such as histone is a good antigen.[L35] DNA found in the circulation of patients with SLE consists of small populations (100 to 150 base pairs), and units of 200 base pairs and their multiples.[R420,S71] The 200 bp and multiples are usually present in nucleosomes. Cell apoptosis releases DNA of this size; cell necrosis does not. Therefore in SLE, cell apoptosis may be induced by immunologic abnormalities, and the nucleosomes released from those cells provide the antigenic stimulus that results in somatically mutated high-affinity IgG anti-DNA antibodies.

DNA may be different in individuals with SLE from DNA in normals. The quantities of DNA released by cultured lymphocytes from humans and mice with SLE are significantly greater than quantities released by normal cells.[G223,P23,S711] The circulating DNA in SLE patients is richer in guanosine and cytosine than DNA from healthy controls.[S71] Such a change could increase the ability to form Z-DNA.

Degradation of DNA

The degradation of DNA may be slower than normal in individuals with lupus. The ability of nucleases to digest DNA may be impaired in patients with SLE. DNA is probably cleared in two phases, based on studies in normal mice.[E100] In the first phase, large pieces of DNA (more than 15 base pairs) rapidly bind to various organs (primarily the liver for ssDNA, other soft tissues for dsDNA). In the second phase, DNA is degraded in the circulation and in tissue by nucleases. ssDNA is cleared more rapidly than dsDNA—20 minutes compared to 40 minutes. The second, digestion phase of clearance is similar for both. Several conditions may prolong the half-life of DNA. Hepatic uptake of DNA is saturable with excess DNA or excess immune complexes, which results in a prolonged half-life. If DNA is present in small size, organ binding is impaired. In patients with active disease, excess quantities of circulating DNA and of small immune complexes have been detected. Therefore, clearance of antigenic DNA is probably impaired.[E100]

Another factor that allows DNA to persist in patients with SLE is its existence as protected fragments.[E97] Small DNA fragments, 30 to 40 base pairs, are bound by the two arms of IgG anti-DNA and are thus protected both from organ binding and from the action of nucleases.

DNA may serve as a target antigen, beyond its participation in immune complexes. There is a DNA receptor on a number of cells, including glomeruli.[B217,J20] DNA bound into that receptor might well be a target of pathogenic anti-DNA. There is some evidence that DNA molecules can be trapped in collagen or other structures in glomeruli.[H408,167]

In summary, DNA, DNA-histone complex, or small immune complexes containing protected fragments of DNA may persist for abnormally long periods in individuals with SLE for a variety of reasons. Such a situation could result in prolonged antigenic stimulation, and in availability of DNA to bind to target tissues or to circulating anti-DNA, thus perpetuating the disease process.

DNA–anti-DNA Immune Complexes

Immune complexes containing DNA have been found in the circulation of a small proportion of patients with active SLE.[B535,F173] For other immune complexes, small soluble complexes in slight antigen excess that can fix complement are the most pathogenic. For DNA, complexes in slight antibody excess may be most stable and therefore most pathogenic.[L186,T88] The complexes should be bound by Fc and CR1 receptors and cleared by the mononuclear phagocyte system. However, during periods of active SLE, clearance of immune complexes is defective. The abnormalities are complex (see Chap. 12) and include a combination of high quantities of complexes, decreased numbers of receptors, saturation of receptors that are present, and defective phagocytosis of the complexes fixed to receptors.[F213] Genetic abnormalities in quantities of CR1 receptors have been suggested,[W268] but the low numbers on cells of SLE patients probably reflect stripping of occupied receptors.[A350] No structural defects in CR1 or in Fc receptors have yet been found in patients with SLE. As discussed in the preceding paragraph, immune complexes containing cationic antigen or antibody, or protected DNA fragments that cannot be bound by cells that clear DNA, are probably important pathogens. These features stabilize the complex and permit its persistence.

METHODS OF MEASURING ANTIBODIES TO DNA

Several techniques are available to measure antibodies to DNA in serum or plasma[E101,S381,S499] (see Table 20–4). The ones chosen by service or research laboratories are critical, because some detect primarily high-avidity subsets of anti-DNA that are enriched in pathogens, and others detect both low- and high-avidity anti-DNA. The following tests measure primarily high-avidity antibodies: precipitation, complement fixation, and the Farr assay. The second group of tests detects both high- and low-avidity antibodies; ELISA, Crithidia luciliae, hemagglutination, and radioimmunoassays with precipitation of DNA-containing immune complexes by polyethylene glycol

(the PEG assay). In general, the first group is less sensitive than the second (being positive in 50 to 60% of SLE patients), but correlates better with disease flares and with high risk for glomerulonephritis. The second group is more sensitive, being positive in 70 to 85% of patients with SLE; however, they correlate less well with disease activity and manifestations. These differences account for much of the discrepancy in the literature regarding the clinical utility of anti-DNA testing.

The tests most commonly used in service laboratories are Farr, ELISA, and Crithidia luciliae.[S381] In the Farr assay, radiolabeled DNA is added to diluted serum or plasma, and Ig is precipitated by ammonium sulfate. Radioactivity in the precipitate indicates binding of DNA by anti-DNA; unbound DNA is not precipitated by the ammonium sulfate. DNA can be purified to contain primarily dsDNA, although a few ss nicks develop during the assay. Both IgG and IgM high-avidity precipitating antibodies are captured in this assay, which is probably the best of the widely available tests to detect primarily high-avidity antibodies to DNA.

In the ELISA assay, DNA is bound to wells in plastic microtiter plates. In general, ssDNA sticks directly to the wells. The adherence of dsDNA is variable, and many laboratories coat the wells with negatively charged molecules such as protamine sulfate, poly-L-lysine, or methylated BSA before dsDNA is added to ensure uniform entrapment of the antigen. Then, diluted patient plasma or sera are incubated with DNA in the wells. After several hours, the wells are washed and bound Ig is incubated with enzyme-labeled antihuman Ig, IgG, or IgM. The binding of the second antibody is detected by a color change following addition of a substrate upon which the enzyme acts, the color being read in a spectrophotometer. This assay allows measurement of low-avidity and high-avidity antibodies and detection of IgG, IgM, and total populations of anti-DNA. The substrate fixed to the wells can be highly purified dsDNA (which can be from mammalian or bacterial sources); a few ss nicks develop during the incubations. Commercial substrates often contain significant quantities of ssDNA as well as dsDNA. Therefore, low quantities of anti-DNA detected in this assay may be primarily directed against ssDNA. Clinical correlations are best if confined to interpretation of high titers of anti-DNA detected in this manner.

The Crithidia luciliae test takes advantage of the presence of a kinetoplast containing circular dsDNA in this flagellate. Test sera or plasma are incubated with the or-

Table 20–4. Methods of Measuring Antibodies to DNA

Test	Sensitive	Specific	Correlates with Disease Activity and Nephritis	Availability
Precipitation	+	+ + +	+ + +	Highly limited
Hemagglutination	+ +	+	+	Highly limited
Complement fixation	+ +	+ + +	+ + +	Limited
Farr assay	+ +	+ + +	+ + +	Limited
PEG assay	+ +	+ +	+	Limited
Crithidia luciliae immunofluorescence	+ +	+ + +	+	Good
ELISA assay	+ + +	+ +	+	Good

ganisms on a glass slide. After washing, fluoresceinated antihuman Ig, IgG or IgM are added. After appropriate incubation, Ig bound to the DNA structure is detected by examining the glass slide for fluorescence using an ultraviolet microscope. Although even this circular DNA structure can contain one or two ss nicks, this assay is the most specific for anti-dsDNA. Therefore, positive tests are highly specific for SLE. However, in our laboratories the sensitivity is not as good as the ELISA assay. The Crithidia assay can be modified to detect complement-fixing antibody subsets. However, both low- and high-avidity anti-dsDNA are measured. Titers of anti-DNA measured by this method have little correlation with clinical disease activity.

In summary, several different assays for anti-dsDNA are available commercially; each has advantages and disadvantages. No standardized test is used uniformly in all service laboratories. The ideal anti-DNA assay would detect primarily IgG high-avidity complement-fixing anti-dsDNA; however, none of the assays available in most service laboratories do so. Therefore, the physician should determine which assay is used in the laboratory to which the specimens are sent, and understand the specificity, sensitivity, and clinical correlations of that method. With methods that detect most populations of anti-dsDNA (and some anti-ssDNA), weakly positive tests can be obtained in patients with chronic liver disease, rheumatoid arthritis, nonlupus connective tissue diseases, drug-induced lupus, infections, and aging.

CLINICAL USE OF ANTIBODIES TO DNA

Detection of antibodies to dsDNA is often useful in diagnosis and management of patients with SLE (see Table 20–5). Their interpretation is limited by lack of a standardized assay to measure them, inability to equate results of assays with the most pathogenic subsets of anti-DNA, and the fact that antibodies other than anti-DNA participate in the tissue lesions of SLE. *Antibodies to ssDNA should not be measured, since they have no specificity for the disease.* There is considerable controversy in the literature regarding the clinical utility of anti-DNA testing. Earlier work employed techniques that detected high-avidity antibodies; good correlations with disease activity were demonstrated.[E101,G103,R354,S207,S381] More recent papers show weaker correlations, partly because more sensi-

tive assays that detect more subpopulations of anti-dsDNA, such as the ELISA assay, were used.[136]

In studies comparing the clinical utility of different tests in management of patients with SLE, sensitive tests indicating complement activation (especially those that measure activated components directly, such as C3a, C5a, or C3d) correlate better with disease flares than do high titers of anti-DNA.[A265,H414,M609] One prospective study showed that normalization of serum complement levels is more strongly correlated with good longterm outcomes in renal function than is normalization of serum anti-DNA.[A265] Clearly, there are patients who have active SLE and deteriorating organ function in whom antibodies to dsDNA are never detectable. This could result from removal of anti-DNA from the circulation when it is fixed to tissue, or other antigen-antibody systems being responsible for the glomerular damage. Conversely, there are patients with sustained high serum levels of anti-dsDNA who do well over long periods.[G29,G179] Nevertheless, in most patients, increasing quantities of anti-dsDNA in the serum are likely to herald a flare of disease, and patients with high anti-DNA titers are at increased risk for lupus nephritis.[W76]

In summary, measurement of anti-dsDNA in sera has two useful clinical applications (Table 20–5). First, high titers of these antibodies have >90% specificty for SLE; they are therefore useful in making the diagnosis. Second, rising levels should alert the clinician to the possibility of an imminent disease flare, and high levels (especially associated with low levels of serum complement) suggest increased risk for lupus nephritis. I recommend that in each SLE patient, the physician establish whether the pattern of serum anti-DNA titers correlates with clinical manifestations and disease activity. If such correlations are present, serial measurements of anti-DNA are useful. (See Chapter 48.)

FUTURE DIRECTIONS

Since antibodies to DNA are important in disease pathogenesis in some individuals with SLE, further characterization of the pathogenic antibody subsets, their function and their structure, can be anticipated. This should provide new insights into how antibodies cause disease. Equally exciting are the studies of why pathogenic antibody subsets are up-regulated in patients with SLE, and the genetic basis of that abnormal regulation. Understanding such interactions should lead to novel therapeutic interventions that specifically suppress undesirable autoantibodies while leaving normal components of immune responses intact.

Clinically, standardized tests for anti-dsDNA would represent an important advance, and would allow us to compare data between different series of patients and settle the issue of the clinical utility of measuring these antibodies. There is continual search for a different assay that will identify disease flares and risk for organ damage more accurately than measurement of anti-dsDNA. Finally, there are experts who argue that assessment of clinical characteristics is a better measure of clinical activity and effects of therapies than any currently available laboratory measurement of autoantibodies, complement, or products of inflammation.[L262]

Table 20–5. Clinical Utility of Measuring Anti-DNA

High Titers of Anti-dsDNA
1. Have >90% specificity for SLE
2. Often indicate clinically active disease and increased risk for nephritis

Low Titers of Anti-dsDNA
1. Can be detecting anti-ssDNA
2. Can be found in
    Drug-induced lupus
    Rheumatoid arthritis
    Sjögren's syndrome
    Other CTD
    Chronic infections
    Chronic liver disease
    Aging

Chapter 21

HISTONE ANTIBODIES

MARVIN J. FRITZLER

In 1884, Albrecht Kossel isolated a basic, peptone-like component from a water and ether lysate of goose erythrocyte nuclei.[D246] This proteinaceous material was called histone. Ten years later, Leon Lilienfeld described the extraction of calf thymocyte histones and suggested that histone was a highly basic protein as evidenced by its solubility in acidic water. In 1908, the International Nomenclature Body listed histones as a class of proteins along with albumins and other proteins. In the following half century, histones received little interest until 1950, when Stedman and Stedman compared the histone from a wide variety of species and suggested that it was not a homogeneous protein.[S628] The following year, state-of-the-art paper chromatography was used to distinguish two classes of histones, the arginine-rich main histones and the lysine-rich subsidiary histones.[S629] These findings sparked an increase in histone research, eventually leading to the publication of the first primary structure of calf thymus histone 4 (H4, originally designated F2A1) in 1968[D130] and pea embryo H4 in 1969.[D129]

The renewed interest in the biochemistry and cell biology of histones in the 1950s and 1960s coincided with the description and popularization of the LE-cell phenomenon and the LE-cell test in SLE. Eventually, it became apparent that the LE cell formed in vivo,[H129] and the LE-cell phenomenon demonstrated in vitro,[H82,H387,M396] was dependent on the presence of histone and was mediated by histone antibodies.[F272,R234] In the next 30 years, these observations were followed by a proliferation of observations on histones as targets of the immune response in SLE, drug-induced lupus (DIL) and other diseases (Table 21–1).

HISTONES

The histones are by far the best understood of the structural proteins in the eucaryotic nucleus.[B596,C195,N76,V110,W204] They occur in such abundance that it is traditional to classify them into two classes: the histones and the nonhistone chromosomal proteins (NHCPs). The NHCPs, such as high-mobility-group proteins, low-mobility-group proteins, chromosome scaffold proteins, centromere proteins, ubiquitin and protein A24, are present in quantities of approximately 100 to 1000 molecules per nucleus.[D379,G294,W224] By dramatic contrast, the mass of each histone is 60 million molecules per cell and is about equal to the cellular DNA content.[C195] However, attention to histones as autoantigens postdated

extensive studies of DNA and other nonhistone autoantigens such as Sm and U1RNP.

On the basis of their primary structure, the five types of histones can be divided into three main groups. Two of the three groups, referred to as the core or nucleosomal histones, are the slightly lysine-rich histones H2A and H2B and the arginine-rich histones H3 and H4. The core histones are responsible for coiling the DNA into higher-order structures known as nucleosomes (Fig. 21–1). The third and least conserved group is the lysine-rich histones H1 and H1 variants. The amino acid sequences of all classes of histones from a variety of plant and animal tissues have been determined.[141,S447]

The high proportion of positively charged amino acids of these relatively small proteins helps them bind tightly to DNA. Since histones only rarely dissociate from DNA, they are believed to play a key role in control of gene expression and cell division.

Higher-Order Chromatin Structure

The Nucleosome

If the DNA in a single nucleus were stretched out, it would span the nucleus thousands of times. Histones play a key role in packaging, in an orderly way, the entire genome into a single nucleus. However, the role of packaging DNA is complex because not all DNA is folded in the same way. The manner in which portions of the DNA are folded in specific cells appears to influence gene activation.

The basic repeating structural subunit of eukaryotic chromatin is known as the nucleosome. The nucleosome, which has the appearance of beads on a string in the electron microscope, consists of approximately 166 to 240 base pairs (depending on the source) of DNA helix wound around an octameric complex of two molecules each of histones H2A, H2B, H3, and H4 (Figure 21–1).[B596,K378] The path that DNA takes around the nucleosome core reduces its length by fortyfold.[B596,K377,M281] A tetrameric complex of two molecules each of H3 and H4 comprise the interior of the nucleosomal core particle (Figure 21–1), and a dimer of H2A-H2B sits on each face of the nucleosome. Histone H1 occupies a position on the top of the nucleosome and serves to bind the incoming and outgoing strands of helical DNA (Figure 21–2).

The Chromatosome, Core Particles, and Octameric Complex

Brief digestion of chromatin with micrococcal nuclease cleaves the linker DNA between nucleosomes producing

Table 21–1. Human Diseases Associated with Histone Autoantibodies

Disease	Frequency (%)	References
Rheumatic Diseases		
SLE	24–95	B263,E118,F55,F107,F280, G165,G218,G394, H121,R392 A81,K346,K371,M647,S159a B594,G279
DIL-procainamide	67–100	C427,E118,F280,G218,G413, P262,P265,R394,T193
DIL-hydralazine	50–100	C427,H336,P262
DIA	22–81	E118,K267,R394,R403,T193
RA	0–80	A80,B594,C403,F278,K267 C331,C402,M680,S159b
RA plus vasculitis	75	B263
Felty's syndrome	79	C53,C331
JRA	42–75	M83,M539,0113,P77,T256
UCTD*	90	M524
Immune Disease		
Monoclonal gammopathy	14	S158
Neoplastic Disease	79	K267
Hepatic Diseases		
PBC	50–60	K368,P106
Cirrhosis	0–50	K368,P106

* Patients selected for a certain speckled staining pattern on cryopreserved rodent sections referred to as variable large speckled.
Abbreviations: DIL = drug-induced lupus, DIA = drug-induced autoimmunity, RA = rheumatoid arthritis, JRA = juvenile rheumatoid arthritis, PBC = primary biliary cirrhosis, UCTD = undifferentiated connective tissue disease.

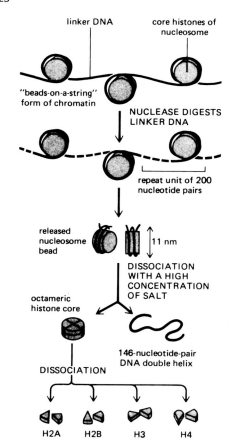

Fig. 21–1. The schematic structure of the nucleosome. The nucleosome consists of two full turns of DNA wound around a core of histones, plus adjacent linker DNA. The nucleosome bead can be released from chromatin by digestion of the linker DNA with micrococcal nuclease. In each nucleosome bead, approximately 146 nucleotide pairs of DNA remain wound around an octameric histone core. The histone core is composed of two each of histones H2A, H2B, H3, and H4.[C195] From Chambon, P., Elgin, S., Felsenfeld, G. et al.: The cell nucleus. In Molecular Biology of the Cell. 2nd Ed. Edited by B. Alberts, D. Bray, J. Lewis et al. New York, Garland Publishers Co., 1989. With permission.

the chromatosome (Figure 21–1).[B131,B596,M281M282] Thus, the chromatosome consists of a molecule of H1, the core histones, and approximately 166 base pairs of DNA.[S462] Additional digestion of the nucleosome releases H1 and approximately 20 base pairs of DNA, resulting in a structure referred to as the core particle. The core particle is made up of approximately 146 base pairs of DNA and an octamer containing two molecules of H2A, H2B, H3, and H4.[M474] Several models of nucleosome core particles have been based on neutron scattering, neutron diffraction, raman spectroscopy, x-ray crystallograpy, and image reconstruction from electron micrographs.[B132,B581,G211,H222,M282,P43,R200,S462,U1,U2]

When nucleosome core particles are suspended in 2 M NaC1 at neutral pH, the DNA is dissociated, leaving an octameric complex that contains two molecules of the core histones H2A, H2B, H3, and H4 (Figure 21–1). In solutions of low ionic strength, or non-neutral pH, the octamer dissociates further to form a tetramer of H3-H4 and two dimers of H2A-H2B.[U2] Evidence has indicated that this dissociation may not be as straightforward as once thought.[Y1]

Nonhistone Chromosomal Proteins (NHCPs)

The mechanisms responsible for the dynamic process of chromatin condensation and decondensation are not entirely understood. While the interactions between DNA and histone result in approximately a 40-fold shortening of the DNA, there is a further 250-fold shortening that

must be accounted for. This additional compaction is thought to be caused in large part by NHCPs that bind to chromatin at every 60 to 100 kb and anchor the loops of chromatin to their periphery.[E4] Some of these proteins have been identified as scaffold protein 1 (170 kD) and scaffold protein 2 (135 kD).[L240] Other proteins involved in chromatin condensation are the centromeric proteins CENP-B (80 kD), CENP-C (140 kD), and LMG160.[C377,E5,W224] Although many proteins play a role in chromatin condensation, the exact mechanisms leading to the initiation and termination of this dynamic process have yet to be determined.[G404,M514,W76] Even less information is available on the mechanisms leading to chromosome decondensation. One protein involved in this process is nucleolin.[L65] This protein, which has a highly acidic domain, displaces H1 from chromatin presumably by

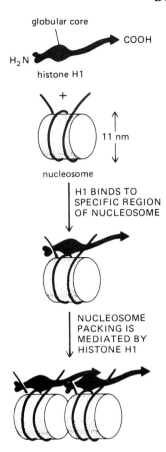

Fig. 21–2. The structure and function of H1. H1 helps pack adjacent nucleosomes together. The globular core of H1 binds to each nucleosome near the site where the DNA helix enters and leaves the octameric complex. When H1 is removed, an extra 20 DNA nucleotide pairs are exposed and can be removed by micrococcal nuclease digestion.[C195] From Chambon, P., Elgin, S., Felsenfeld, G. et al.: The cell nucleus. *In* Molecular Biology of the Cell. 2nd Ed. Edited by B. Alberts, D. Bray, J. Lewis et al. New York, Garland Publishers Co., 1989. With permission.

competing for H1 binding to DNA. Of interest, nucleolin is a recently described autoantigen that reacts with SLE and other rheumatic disease antibodies.[M465]

Conclusions

The nucleosome is composed of subunits including two H2A-H2B dimers that surround an H3-H4 tetramer. This complex of histones is surrounded by a third subunit comprised of approximately two turns of double-stranded DNA. The structure of the nucleosome is locked by a molecule of H1 that is able to associate with other H1 molecules on adjacent molecules, forming a compact chromatin mass referred to as the chromatosome. The variable length of DNA between adjacent nucleosomes is referred to as linker DNA. Further compaction of the polynucleosome and compaction of the chromatin results in the familiar higher-ordered structures known as chromosomes.

Histone H1 and Variants

Histone H1, the most variable of the histones, has an approximate molecular weight of 21.5 kD (Figure 21–3), and has been found in all cells with the exception of yeasts. H1 is a family of outer or linker histones (Figure 21–2) that consist of H1, H1⁰, H5, and other variants. The number of H1 variants can vary from tissue to tissue and species to species.[C274,O25,S337,T89] However, three major domains can be distinguished within the primary structure of all H1 variants: an amino terminal region that is highly basic, variable, and rich in alanine and proline; a central globular domain that is hydrophobic and nonvariable; a carboxyterminal region that is highly basic and variable.

The function of H1 is to stabilize the formation of two complete turns of DNA around the histone octamer, which in turn is essential for the formation of higher-order structures.[A144,T143] (Figure 21–2). Peptides from the globular and carboxy terminal domains of H1 have been shown to be just as effective in inducing higher-order structures as the intact protein.[A144] Since the globular domain of H1 alone cannot induce chromatin folding, the carboxy terminal domain of the molecule is believed to play a primary role in DNA packaging.[K378,M282] The evidence suggests that the globular domain serves to locate H1 in the nucleosome at the point where the DNA-strands leave the chromatosome and that the carboxy terminal domain is necessary for the stabilization of the fold.[S588] Vertebrate species have from four to six different H1 subtypes that are derived from a set of primary amino acid sequence variants.[C274,S337,T89] The functional significance of having multiple subtypes is not fully understood, although it is speculated that they are responsible for the different transcriptional potentials of eucaryotic cells.[C347,R50,S309] The function of H1 can be better understood when examined in the context of its variants, H1⁰ and H5. H1⁰ is a mammalian protein present mainly in quiescent, nonreplicating cells. There appears to be a direct correlation between the presence of H1⁰ and the termination of cell division.[B438,P128]

H5 is an extreme variant of H1 and is present only in transcriptionally inactive cells of some species.[A52,R417] Although H5 was at one time thought to be present in mammals,[L268] it is most commonly associated with the nucleated erythrocytes of birds, reptiles, amphibians, and fish. H5 confers high stability and transcriptional inactivity to chromatin. Immunocytochemical studies have been used to identify interactions of H5 with structural and functional components of chromatin.[C273,T140,Z43] H5 demonstrates limited sequence homology with an H1 subfraction from bovine thymus, but extensive homology with the globular domain and the terminal portion of the carboxy terminus of H1⁰.[C344,N48] Therefore, observations of polyclonal and monoclonal antibodies directed against H5[M352b,M538,Y36] could be explained on the basis of their cross-reactivity with H1⁰.

Although H5 and H1⁰ share sequence identity, it appears that not all reactivity with H5 can be accounted for on the basis of cross-reactivity with H1⁰. In studies of SLE, DIL, and JRA sera where H5 reactivity was demonstrated,

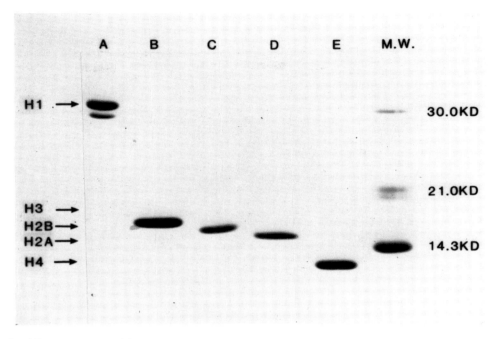

Fig. 21–3. Histones extracted from calf thymus nuclei can be fractionated into the 5 main groups as illustrated in this photograph of an SDS gel. Lane A: H1 (Mr = 33 kD) often represented as doublet; Lane B: H3 (Mr = 18 kD); Lane C: H2B (Mr = 17 kD); Lane D: H2A (Mr = 15.5 kD); Lane E: H4 (Mr = 13 kD); M.W. = molecular weight markers. One of the reasons why the relative mobility (Mr) of the histones differs in SDS-PAGE from the actual molecular weights (see text) is that the basic amino acids, especially in H1, bind to SDS used in the electrophoresis, thereby retarding their mobility through the polyacrylamide gel.

no reactivity with H1[0] was observed.[P76,P77] Subsequent studies have suggested that the reactivity of SLE and DIL sera with H5 is likely directed against conformational epitopes.[P75] Therefore, in diseases like SLE where conformational epitopes are the target of the autoantibody response, comparison of sequences from closely related or widely divergent proteins may provide little meaningful information to explain cross-reactive antibodies.

Core Histones: H2A, H2B, H3, H4

The slightly lysine-rich histones H2A and H2B have two domains, which include an amino terminus made up of predominantly basic residues and a carboxy terminus that is rich in hydrophobic residues. Histones H2A and H2B have molecular weights of approximately 14 and 13.8 kD, respectively (Figure 21–3), and are considered to be the most variable of the core histones.[C195]

The arginine-rich histones H3 and H4 are the most highly conserved histones and, like H2A and H2B, they contain two domains, a basic amino terminal region and a hydrophobic carboxy terminal region.[S588] Histones H3 and H4 have molecular weights of approximately 15.4 and 11.3 kD, respectively (Figure 21–3), and they interact with each other to form a H3-H4 tetramer (Figure 21–1).[W359]

Like all eucaryotic gene messages, histone messenger RNAs are translated in the cytoplasm. After transport of newly synthesized histones across the nuclear membrane, they are combined with older histones into an octameric

nucleosome.[S755,Y23] For example, newly synthesized histones H3 and H4 deposit as a tetramer and will associate only with old histones H2A and H2B.[J13] Similarly, newly synthesized histones H2A and H2B will only deposit as a dimer associated with old histones H2A, H2B, H3, and H4.[J11,J12] During formation of the octamer, the core histones are deposited onto the DNA.[A274]

The role of core histones in stabilization of the nucleosome and folding of chromatin is not clearly understood. One method employed to analyze this role uses selective trypsinization [A358,S515] and radiolabeling.[H303] Trypsinization studies have shown that after removal of the histone tails (generally the amino terminal regions of the core histones), the stability of the nucleosome core particle was not affected.[A358] However, studies of the thermal stability of nucleosomes indicate that the amino terminal tails play a significant structural role.[H303] Evidence suggests that thermal stability can be attributed to the binding of the amino terminal tails of H2B and H3 and the carboxy terminal tail of H2A to linker DNA.[H303,L306]

Postsynthetic Modification of Histones

Postsynthetic modifications of histones are important because they may be crucial in our understanding of the autoimmune responses directed against these proteins. For example, it is possible that the induction of postsynthetic modification of histones is triggered by drugs or other environmental agents implicated in the pathogenesis of SLE.

As described above, all four of the core histones have randomly coiled, unstructured amino terminal tails and globular structured carboxy terminal domains. The tails of the histones are of particular interest because they include most of the sites that undergo post-translational modifications. Post-translational modification of histones includes methylation, acetylation, phosphorylation, and ADP ribosylation.[D237,W359]

Acetylation

Acetylation occurs at specific lysine residues located in the amino terminal half of the core histones. Acetylation of lysine residues neutralizes the positive charge of histones. This suggests that acetylation modulates the interaction of histone amino termini with the negatively charged DNA backbone, although acetylation alone does not change the structure or stability of nucleosomes.[A359,M283] Increased acetylation of histones is correlated with transcriptional activity.[L295,P169,R207] Antibodies specific for acetylated histones have also been used to study acetylation in transcriptionally active chromatin.[H230,L295,P169,T274]

Methylation

Methylation is a relatively stable modification and has been reported in all the histones.[F290,W359] The sites of methylation are only known for H3 and H4.[H404] Methylation occurs after DNA synthesis in the late S or G_2 phase and after assembly into chromatin, suggesting that it is not essential in the assembly of chromatin. On the other hand, methylation has been suggested to be important in chromatin condensation, other mitotic events,[H404] and activation of gene transcription.[D181]

Phosphorylation

Unlike most other modifications, phosphorylation of histidine, lysine, serine, and threonine residues occurs in all of the histones.[W359] Amino acids subject to phosphorylation include histidine, lysine, serine, and threonine.[W359] Phosphorylation, which reduces the net positive charge of the N-terminal region of the core histones, and the N- and C-termini of H1, is thought to alter histone-DNA interaction.[D237,F23] It is still not known whether the loosening of DNA-histone interaction after histone phosphorylation is sufficient to account for enhanced template activity in DNA.[F23] In addition to its role in affecting histone interaction with DNA, the phosphorylation of histone appears to alter DNA primase activity.[T9]

Poly(ADP)ribosylation

Poly(ADP)ribosylation is another important post-translational modification of histones.[L303] The covalent addition of an ADP-ribose moiety of NAD to proteins is catalyzed by poly(ADP)ribose polymerase.[B429] The major acceptor proteins for poly(ADP)ribose are H1 and H2B, although ribosylation of H2A and H3 have also been reported. Modification by poly(ADP)ribosylation has been postulated to play a role in DNA replication, DNA repair, DNA amplification, and cell differentiation. Correlation of the rate and extent of poly(ADP)ribosylation with DNA repair activity and relaxation of chromatin structure has been experimentally confirmed.[G1,G2,H492,L31] An increase in the activity of poly(ADP)ribose synthetase has been correlated with the appearance of DNA strand breaks produced by nucleases and other agents.[B429] This is interesting in light of observations that drugs associated with DIL induce extensive DNA strand breakage. In addition, ADP ribosylation, which essentially adds a ribose-phosphate moiety to acceptor proteins, may increase the immunogenicity of histones. Evidence for this is based on the observation that free histones are weakly immunogenic, but when they are coupled to ribose nucleic acids (i.e., tRNA) are highly immunogenic.[M352a,M649]

Ubiquitination

Ubiquitin, a protein of 76 amino acids found in all cells, has been shown to be bound to lysine 119 of H2A and lysine 120 of H2B.[N86] The major arrangement of ubiquitin in the polyubiquitinated histone H2A appears to be a chain of at least four ubiquitin molecules bound to the ϵ-amino group of lysine 119.[N87] Since ubiquitination in the cytoplasm is involved in controlled proteolysis, it is thought that ubiquitinated histones are involved in the same process.[H285] Ubiquitinated histones may also play a role in maintaining the structure of transcriptionally active chromatin.[N86] The observation that antibodies to ubiquitin are found in some SLE sera[M646,M648] provides supporting evidence for the concept that the nucleosome is an important immunogen in SLE.

Conclusions

The histones are small proteins with a large content of positively charged amino acids lysine and arginine. The core histones H2A, H2B, H3, and H4 are responsible for folding DNA into structures known as nucleosomes, whereas H1 is believed to induce higher-order structures in chromatin. The histones may be divided into three groups based on their amino acid content. H1 is lysine rich and has the most interspecies amino acid sequence variability. H2A and H2B are slightly lysine rich and moderately conserved throughout evolution. H3 and H4 are arginine rich and are the most highly conserved of the histones.

HISTONE AUTOANTIBODIES

In order to appreciate the growing data on the clinical and pathologic significance of histone autoantibodies, an understanding of the techniques and methods used to demonstrate them is important. In most clinical laboratories, an indirect immunofluorescence (IIF) assay is used as a screening test to identify antinuclear antibodies.[F276,F281] Most histone autoantibodies are detected by this screening test and are commonly correlated with a homogeneous or diffuse staining pattern (Fig. 21–4). The clinician should appreciate two exceptions to this generalization. First, the homogeneous or diffuse pattern is seen with other autoantibodies, notably those directed against dsDNA.[F276,F281] Second, sera that have antibodies to only H1, H3, H4, or hidden determinants on native

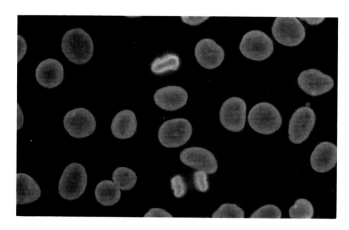

Fig. 21–4. Indirect immunofluorescence of autoantibodies from a patient with DIL produces a homogeneous pattern of nuclear staining on human epithelial cells. Note that the staining is particularly intense over chromosomes of a dividing cell and the cytoplasm displays no detectable staining.

or fixed histones (cryptotopes) may show only weak or negative ANAs.[C162,M524,P77,P265] Therefore, the identification of histone antibodies must rely on more specific assays.

The seminal studies of Kunkel, Holman, and Deicher[H389,K463,R234] used a complement depletion assay to identify free histones as autoantigens. Many of the studies that followed continued to rely on unfractionated histones. Reactivity of SLE antibodies with unfractionated DNP was demonstrated with a double immunodiffusion technique by Tan[T39] and a complement fixation assay by Rothfield and Stollar.[R354] These early investigations suggested that histone antibody titers in SLE fluctuated in concert with disease activity, were predominantly reactive with H1, but that they occurred infrequently and were of low titer.[K463,S703,S704] One explanation of these conclusions was that histones themselves demonstrated procomplementary activity.[H248]

The insensitive features of the complement fixation assays used in early studies of histone autoantibodies led to a general disinterest in histone antibodies until Tan and his colleagues modified an IIF assay to demonstrate histone antibodies.[T49] This assay, which used cryopreserved sections of rodent kidney as substrate, employed dilute acid to extract histones and other proteins from the nuclei. Purified histones could then be reconstituted onto the retained nuclear DNA by incubating the acid-extracted substrate in solubilized histones. Conventional indirect immunofluorescence was then used to demonstrate histone reactivity. For example, sera containing antihistone antibodies demonstrated positive staining on untreated and reconstituted sections but not on acid-extracted sections. By comparison, sera that contained antibodies to double-stranded DNA (dsDNA) were positive on the untreated, the acid-extracted, and the reconstituted sections. This assay was used to demonstrate that high titers of histone antibodies are found in SLE[F278,F280] and procainamide-induced lupus.[F280,M403] It later became clear that this assay had limitations since it detected pri-

marily antibodies to H2A, H2B, and H2A-H2B complexes. Sera containing antibodies to H1, H3, or H4 are relatively nonreactive with reconstituted histone substrates because these proteins are not adequately reconstituted under the experimental conditions of this assay.[C427,H336,P262,P265]

In the decade that followed the introduction of the extraction-reconstitution assay, solid-phase assays became the predominant method for demonstrating histone antibodies. The most popular assays include ELISA[A81,R282,R392] and solid-phase radioimmunoassays (SPRIAs).[K463,R393] These assays were relatively easy to establish because purified histone, histone complexes, and chromatin components were easily adsorbed to the polystyrene. Fluorochrome-, enzyme-, or radioisotope-conjugated, class-specific antibodies were then used to provide a quantitative and qualitative analysis of antihistone reactivity. The studies using ELISA and SPRIA were followed by Western blotting (immunoblotting) of histones that were separated by polyacrylamide gel electrophoresis (Figure 21–3).[G218,R403,T42] This technique has required substantial refinement because of the highly cationic nature of histones and their propensity to bind a variety of anionic proteins.[D348,M352a,S151,S752,W4] In addition, it is not clear if all epitopes are available for binding after the proteins are blotted since higher-order structures may be altered after the heating and sodium dodecyl sulfate treatment used to prepare proteins for electrophoresis.[B273,S715] However, some evidence has suggested that secondary structures are restored when histones and other proteins are transferred to the nitrocellulose paper used in the immunoblotting experiments.[G100,T195,T196]

Despite these advances in histone antibody assays, certain technical problems remain. The discrepancies reported in the frequency and titers of histone antibodies within disease groups are likely related to a number of factors. First, the selection of sera for studies, diagnostic criteria, ethnic or regional variation, and therapeutic agents provide an important source for intraobserver variation. As described above, the protocols employed to detect histone antibodies are primary among these factors.

Another significant variable is the use of different secondary antibodies as detecting reagents. Some studies have used polyvalent antisera, others have used immunoglobulin class-specific reagents, whereas others have used protein A. The potential discordant results with protein A are important because it binds primarily to IgG1, IgG2, and IgG4, but only weakly with IgG3 and IgM.

The quality and purity of the histone used in the assays is of importance. Contamination of histones with DNA and other NHCPs is common but can only be controlled by scrupulous attention to characterization of the antigen.

Other technical concerns include the effect of histone denaturation on antigenicity, the solubility of histones and nucleohistones in biologic fluids, and the susceptibility of purified histones to degradation by serum proteases during the performance of assays.[W4] Differences in the procedures to determine the cutoff between normal and pathologic sera are likely another variable that accounts for intralaboratory variation. Last, most studies have used histones prepared from calf thymus, chicken erythrocytes, and other animal sources. Ideally, human histones should be used for studies of true histone autoantibodies.

Despite all these concerns and variables, there is remarkably good agreement on the frequency of histone antibodies in systemic rheumatic diseases. As with many other areas in clinical medicine, attempts to standardize these variables through interinstitutional collaboration and discussion will be important in the future.

Histones and the LE Cell

The relationship between antibodies to histones and SLE is of interest because most evidence suggests that histone autoantibodies, and histones themselves, are responsible for the LE-cell phenomenon.[H106,H387,R154,T38] A central role for histones was suggested when Holman and Kunkel,[K390] and then Holborow and Weir,[H375] demonstrated abrogation of the LE-cell phenomenon after histones were replaced by protamine. In addition, the LE-cell factor and certain antinuclear antibodies (ANAs) were absorbed by DNase-digested deoxyribonucleoprotein (DNP).[A79,H387] These early studies implied that DNP antibodies were directed against DNA-histone complexes and this reactivity was responsible for the LE-cell phenomenon. Additional evidence for the accuracy of these observations was provided by studies of Hannestad and his colleagues,[H106,R154] who demonstrated that histones were responsible for the LE-cell phenomenon. These observations have been substantiated by clinical observations because LE cells and histone antibodies have been associated with other diseases such as drug-induced lupus (DIL) (see Chap. 28) and rheumatoid arthritis.[A80,C331,M680]

Histone Autoantibodies in SLE

Histone antibodies have been found in 24 to 95% of patients with SLE. SLE patients have antibodies directed against all classes of histones, but particularly H1 and H2B.[B263,C402,G218,H121,H336,K371] In some studies H1[H336,S159a] or H2B[M646] did not show predominant reactivity, whereas H3 did.[B263,S159a,S159b] As is discussed earlier in this chapter, the reasons for these interobserver differences are numerous.

Studies on the correlation of clinical features and disease activity with histone antibody titers or class reactivity have been inconsistent. When SLE patients who only have histone antibodies were compared to those who have other ANAs, it was found that the former have a higher frequency of joint disease and a lower incidence of renal disease, central nervous system disease, alopecia, anemia, and hypocomplementemia.[F278] The correlation of histone antibodies with skin and/or joint involvement has been reported by others.[A81,K371] In other studies, histone antibody activity was correlated with renal disease activity[K346] and neuropsychiatric manifestations of SLE.[F107] Studies attempting to correlate histone antibodies with specific clinical symptoms have not shown any clear-cut associations.[B263,E118,F278,K423] A high correlation of histone antibodies with disease activity has been suggested in some studies[G165,K267,K371,M646,R354] but not in others.[G279] The studies of Muller et al.[M646] observed a corre-

lation of disease activity with antibodies to the core histones but not with H1 or ubiquitin antibodies. In contrast to one study,[F278] SLE patients in the other studies were not selected on the basis of monospecific antihistone antibody activity.

Histone Autoantibodies in Drug-Induced Lupus (DIL) and Drug-Induced Autoimmunity (DIA)

Histone antibodies have been reported in 67 to 100% of DIL patients. The drugs most commonly implicated in DIL include procainamide, hydralazine, quinidine, and isoniazid, although a variety of other drugs have been implicated as well (see Chap. 45). DIL is characterized by the presence of antibodies to single-stranded DNA and histones.[T43] This profile is distinguished from that observed in SLE because antibodies to double-stranded DNA, Sm, U1-RNP, Ro/SSA, La/SSB antigens, and others characteristic of the autoimmune state are typically absent in DIL. Serologically, it is not difficult to differentiate DIL from SLE except in the rare situation when SLE patients possess only antibodies to single-stranded DNA and histones.

Patients treated with procainamide eventually develop antihistone antibodies, but symptomatic disease occurs in only 10 to 20% of procainamide-treated patients.[T193] Thus, the majority of antihistone antibodies are apparently benign, and examination of their class and fine specificity revealed that antihistone antibodies in asymptomatic patients are predominantly IgM and display broad reactivity with all the individual histones.[H336,R393,R394] In contrast, patients with symptomatic procainamide-induced lupus develop a unique type of IgG antihistone antibody which, rather than reacting predominantly with individual histones, displays pronounced reactivity with the histone complex H2A-H2B (Table 21–2).[B583,P265,R393] Antibodies to this complex have a high (>90%) sensitivity and specificity for symptomatic procainamide-induced lupus compared to asymptomatic patients[T193] and an even higher specificity when a H2A-H2B/DNA complex is used as the antigen.[B583] The antibodies to these complexes are remarkable because they do not appear to be a feature of the immune response in SLE or hydralazine-induced lupus,[R395,T193] although they are found in other DIL syndromes.[B583]

Hydralazine-induced lupus has been characterized by

Table 21–2. Reactivity of Histone Classes with Autoantibodies from Patients with Systemic Rheumatic Diseases*

Disease	H2A-H2B/DNA	H1	H2B	H2A	H3	H4
SLE	ND	5	4	2	1	1
PIL	25	5	4	2	1	1
HIL	ND	1	3	2	5	5
JRA	—	5	2	1	—	—

* Units of reactivity are based on the least reaction assigned an arbitrary unit of 1. Data compiled and extracted from references [A81,B263,C402, C427,G165,H336,K371,M83,M539,M646,O113,P77,P262,P265,R392,R394,T193,T256].

Abbreviations: JRA = juvenile rheumatoid arthritis, HIL = hydralazine-induced lupus. ND = none detected, PIL = procainamide-induced lupus.

the presence of antibodies to H2B, H3, H1 and H2A,[C427] H3 and H4 but not H2b,[P262] H1 and H5,[P75] or the absence of any particular pattern of histone reactivity at all.[H336]

A comparison of the reactivity of SLE and DIL sera with different histone fractions is shown in Table 21–2. To facilitate an understanding of the data, the histone classes and histone complexes have been assigned an arbitrary activity unit that corresponds to their reactivity with sera from different disease groups. An arbitrary unit of 1 is assigned to a reaction intensity that is clearly above background in ELISA or other solid-phase assays. Using this approach, it can be appreciated that the reactivity of procainamide-induced sera with the H2A-H2B/DNA complex, as reported by Rubin, his colleagues, and others,[B583,P262, R394,T193] is five- to tenfold greater than reactivity observed with fractionated histones. In addition, this reaction is not seen in asymptomatic patients with drug-induced autoimmunity (DIA).[R394,T193]

Histone Autoantibodies in Other Diseases

Histone antibodies have been reported in a wide range of diseases (Table 21–1).[M651,R403,T43,T44] Studies by Tan and his colleagues[M524] used sera from certain patients with an undifferentiated connective tissue disease produced a staining pattern on cryopreserved liver sections referred to as variable large speckles. The autoantibody producing this staining pattern was correlated with H3 antibodies.

The frequency of histone antibodies reported in rheumatoid arthritis (RA) has been reported to be as high as 80%. One of the first studies by Aitcheson et al.[A80] reported that 14% of unselected RA patients and 24% of RA patients with a positive ANA had histone antibodies as demonstrated by the extraction-reconstitution assay. Other studies have reported similar frequencies in unselected RA patients (Table 21–1) but higher frequencies in ANA-positive RA.[C331,M680] Unlike patients with SLE and DIL, the titer of histone antibodies tends to be low.

Campion et al.[C53] reported histone antibodies in the sera of 20 of 32 (68%) patients with Felty's syndrome (FS). The frequency of antihistone antibodies in FS in this study was compared to 12% in RA and 54% in SLE. The histone antibodies in this syndrome appear to be directed against conformational histone determinants since reactivity was lost when the histones were denatured in detergent. The high frequency of histone antibodies in Felty's syndrome is of interest because they commonly have high levels of rheumatoid factor, an autoantibody believed to cross-react with histones,[A80,F205,P61] especially H3.[M164]

Goshen et al.[G308] reported histone antibodies in 17% of patients with IgA nephropathy, 11% with mesangiocapillary glomerulonephritis, and 20% with membranoproliferative glomerulonephritis. Since the study populations were small, the incidence of histone antibodies in these diseases did not reach statistical significance even though the normal control population had no histone antibodies at all.

In a study of 249 patients with monoclonal gammopathies, Schoenfeld et al.[S159] found 34 (13.6%) were positive for histone antibodies. When monoclonal antibodies were purified from 12 sera, all but 1 demonstrated antihistone activity. However, the observation that the majority of these antibodies also demonstrated anti-DNA activity, as measured by the Crithidia luciliae assay, brings into question the specificity of the assay used to detect the histone antibodies.

Antibodies to chymotrypsin-treated H2B have been reported in a 29-year-old male with vasculitis.[C162] Similarity, 75% of RA patients with vasculitis have histone antibodies.[B263] These reports are of interest because vasculitis has been associated with the presence of myeloperoxidase antibodies and, like histones, myeloperoxidase is a highly basic protein (pH > 11). This raises the possibility that myeloperoxidase antibodies cross-react with histone and vice versa. Evidence supporting this notion is based on the observations that antibodies to neutrophil myeloperoxidase, one of the antigens in the neutrophil cytoplasm recognized by antineutrophil antibodies (ANCAs),[R24,V25] have been reported in patients on hydralazine,[N35] a syndrome characterized by histone antibodies.

A search for histone antibodies in JRA has led to various conclusions.[L323] In early studies, when the acid extraction–histone reconstitution technique[F280] was used, JRA sera were found to bind histones infrequently.[H223,S95] A subsequent study using immunoblotting techniques showed that six of nine JRA sera with a homogeneous ANA-staining pattern bound to histones. Further, the majority of these sera reacted with the amino terminus of histone H2B.[B537] Another study, using immunoblot techniques on nuclear extracts of Hep-2 cells, demonstrated that the predominant reactivity of JRA sera was with a 33 kD doublet thought to be H1.[M83] Weaker reactivity to lower-molecular-weight bands was attributed to antibodies binding the core histones. A study using ELISA for detection of antibodies to only the core histones reported the overall frequency of antibodies to histones in JRA was 44%, and 62% of the sera bound to the amino terminus of H3. An interesting observation in this study was that not all sera that bound the 1 to 21 residues of H3 demonstrated reactivity to the intact histones.

The studies of histone antibodies in juvenile rheumatoid arthritis (JRA) are of interest because of their potential to aid in the subclassification of this disease. Histone antibodies have been reported in 67 to 93% of JRA patients with uveitis[M83,M539,O113,P77] compared to 33% of patients without uveitis.[O113] However, either a weak or no association with uveitis was observed in other studies.[M83,T256] When other clinical subsets were compared, histone antibodies tended to be more common in the pauci- or polyarticular subset than in the systemic onset (Still's disease) subset.[M83,P77]

Studies of histone antibodies in other diseases include primary biliary cirrhosis,[K368,P106] other chronic liver disease,[K368,P106] and patients with neoplastic disease selected on the basis of a positive ANA.[K267] A report suggests that scleroderma patients with anticentromere antibodies who have concomitant histone antibodies have a more severe form of the disease and a poor clinical outcome.[M162] Anti-H2A reactivity has been reported in patients with secondary Sjögren's syndrome. Considering the similarities between a number of systemic rheumatic diseases and the considerable clinical overlap, it is surprising that histone antibodies have not been generally reported in primary Sjögren's syndrome, progressive systemic sclerosis, mixed connective tissue disease, or polymyositis.

Conclusions

Numerous studies have conclusively shown that antibodies to all classes of mammalian histones, H1, H2A, H2B, H3, and H4 are predominantly, but not exclusively, present in SLE and DIL (Table 21–1). Studies of the clinical correlates of histone antibodies suggest several conclusions. First, antihistone antibodies are not a specific marker for a single disease. The determination of histone reactivity, especially IgG antibodies to H2A-H2B/DNA complexes, can be used to differentiate procainamide-induced lupus from DIA and idiopathic SLE. Second, the presence of histone antibodies is likely not correlated with disease activity. Third, disease activity may correlate with the levels of histone antibodies. Multicenter collaborative studies, using standardized measures of SLE disease activity and of antihistone antibodies, are required to provide a clearer understanding of all these parameters.

ARE HISTONE AUTOANTIBODIES PATHOGENIC?

In the past two decades, considerable attention has focused on the pathogenesis of SLE. One of the primary mechanisms of tissue inflammation and injury has implicated the deposition of immune complexes and activation of a wide range of mediators, including complement, in target organs (see Chaps. 11 and 13). Anti-DNA antibodies have received most of the attention since they were identified in eluates of human and animal organs affected by lupus. Evidence has suggested a key role for histones and antihistone antibodies in the pathogenesis of SLE. The attention to histones was inevitable because they are most likely bound to circulating DNA and are present in DNA–anti-DNA complexes.[R419] Circumstantial evidence is provided by the observation that histone antibodies are commonly associated with antibodies to dsDNA.[C402,K346,K423] Some reports support a phlogistic role for antihistone-histone complexes because they are able to bind glomerular basement membranes[B496,S151,T118] and cell surfaces.[J22,R151] Recent studies have also shown that histones are chemotactic for polymorphonuclear leukocytes.[N151] The pathogenic potential of histone antibodies has also been implied by studies demonstrating a correlation of rising histone antibody titers with SLE disease activity,[G165] with decreasing antihistone levels after therapy,[F107] and with vasculitis in rheumatoid arthritis.[B263] Evidence against a pathogenic role for histone antibodies comes from studies of drug-induced autoimmunity (see Chap. 45) where the presence of histone antibodies is not necessarily accompanied by evidence of disease activity, and none of the patients with high titers of antihistone monoclonal gammopathies[S158] developed symptoms of lupus.

Histone Determinants and Epitopes

An investigation of the histone epitopes reactive with SLE and DIL autoantibodies has been undertaken by a number of investigators. There is general agreement that SLE and DIL antibodies bind to all classes of intact histone with H1 being the most reactive and H4 being the least reactive.[G218,H121] The epitope mapping studies have used peptides derived from the enzymatic and chemical cleavage of core histones. By using this approach, it can be concluded that most DIL and SLE sera bind to determinants in the amino termini but not to those in the central hydrophobic or carboxy termini (Figure 21–5).[G218,P262,T145] More specifically, the reactive epitope of H2B lies within peptides 1 to 20.[B384,H121,P262,T145] Although similar analyses have provided a less clear picture of H2A epitopes, the bulk of the evidence suggests that they are present in peptides 1 to 11 and 119 to 129. When viewed in the context of intact chromatin, the epitopes on H2A and H2B are in relatively exposed areas of the nucleosome. Epitopes on H3 were mapped to amino terminal residues 1 to 26 and the carboxy terminal 6 amino acids, whereas residues 1 to 29 of H4 were the most reactive.[C427,G218,M647,P262,T145,T256] Last, the epitopes on H1 and H5 are localized in the carboxy terminal residues 123 to 220.[C403,G219,H121,P76] One report demonstrated significant reactivity with H1 amino terminal peptides.[K371] One conclusion from many of these studies is that the histone epitopes reacting with DIL sera are no less restricted than those reacting with SLE sera.

The results summarized here are a simplification of a large body of data where discrepancies do exist. As with the assays for histone antibodies themselves, the reactivity with histone epitopes is fraught with similar limitations and interobserver variability. The significance and limitations of epitope mapping studies in relation to the etiology and pathogenesis of SLE is discussed later in this chapter.

HISTONE ANTIBODY GENES

Antihistone antibodies can be found in all the major immunoglobulin classes, but there is little agreement as to the predominant isotype. A clearer understanding of the origin and induction of histone autoantibodies may come from studies that identify the sequences of their V region genes. Earlier studies have indicated that some DNA antibodies, a common serologic feature of SLE arise from unmutated germline genes whereas others contain multiple somatic mutations[S374] (see Chaps. 18 and 20).

Two reports of the nucleotide sequences of murine antihistone monoclonal antibodies demonstrated that these antibodies were not clonally related and diverse V, D, and J genes were represented.[K344a,M535] Of interest, seven of the eight antibodies had V_H segments encoded by genes from the J558 family. This is a remarkable finding, since J558 represents approximately 50% of the V_H gene repertoire, and it is commonly used among autoantibodies of various specificities.[K343,K362,M540]

The isoelectric points of two IgG histone antibodies ranged from 6.0 to 7.0.[M535] The second complementarity-determining region (CDR) of the V_H gene of MRA12 (the most acidic and the strongest histone-reactive antibody) included only two positively charged, but five negatively charged, amino acid residues. This feature is unusual since the CDR of most V_HJ558 genes is not comprised predomi-

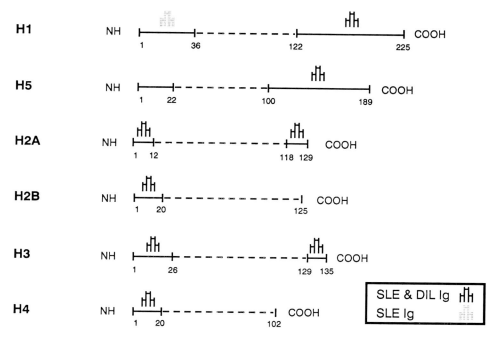

Fig. 21—5. Histone domains bound by systemic lupus erythematosus and drug-induced lupus antibodies.

nantly of acidic residues. A simplistic view of the role of these negatively charged residues is that they are responsible for binding to the basic region of histones. However, since the monoclonal MRA12 bound specifically to H1 and not other histones, it is likely that factors other than charge-charge interactions are important for antibody specificity and binding.

A theme that arises from the early studies of the V genes of histone antibodies bears remarkable resemblance to the current knowledge of anti-DNA antibodies. For example, the anionic isoelectric points of the histone antibodies that react with H1 parallels observations that anionic antigens such as DNA elicit cationic anti-DNA antibodies.[D66,H27,M40] Last, the sequence of the CDR of the heavy chain of the histone monoclonal antibody MRA12 differed from an IgG1 antinitrophenyl antibody by only six amino acid residues.[K344a] This observation is reminiscent of the report of a base substitution in the CDR of the antiphosphorylcholine antibody that resulted in DNA antibody-binding activity.[D65,D197] It is interesting to speculate that antinitrophenyl antibodies, which might arise by immunization with drugs or other agents, cross-react with histones.

INDUCTION OF HISTONE AUTOANTIBODIES

The mechanisms that underlie the induction of histone antibodies are not clearly understood. Even when an inciting agent, such as procainamide or hydralazine, is identified, the events that lead to induction of histone antibodies are not clear. The immunogenicity of histones is somewhat remarkable considering that they are highly conserved among species.

A number of theories have been espoused to account

for the origin of histone antibodies. At the outset, it should be appreciated that none of these theories are independent and features of each may result in the production of histone antibodies. The first theory is that environmental agents, drugs, or chemicals bind to endogenous macromolecules and alter their physical basic properties causing them to become antigenic. In this model the drug may act as a hapten or a carrier. The second theory is that autoantibody production is a result of a process referred to as molecular mimicry. The third is that autoantibody responses are generated and driven by true autoantigens. And fourth, autoantibody production is primarily the outcome of an aberration in the control of the immune network and cellular dysregulation.

Altered Antigen

This hypothesis suggests that drugs or other environmental agents bind to nucleoprotein and then cause some portion of the macromolecule to become immunogenic or form an antibody recognition site.[S706] Hydralazine and procainamide covalently bind to DNA and alter its viscosity, optical rotation, and melting point.[E71,T40] Other studies demonstrate that hydralazine interacts with and alters pyrimidine bases.[D345] In the case of DIL, this theory has limitations. If the drug functioned as a carrier, it might be expected to bind to other macromolecules and result in a variety of autoantibodies. In addition, drugs such as hydralazine and procainamide are small molecules, whereas carriers are typically large molecules. Attempts to induce antinuclear antibodies by immunizing animals with procainamide bound to protein were unsuccessful. Although immunization with a procainamide-deoxyribonucleoprotein (DNP) complex did produce antibodies to procainamide and DNP, the stability of this complex in vivo was not demonstrated.[G228]

Molecular Mimicry

Molecular mimicry can be defined as the products from dissimilar genes that share structural similarity or immune identity.[D378,O56] For example, linear or conformational epitopes on macromolecules from different organisms, (i.e., human and viral proteins), or from different cellular compartments (i.e., nucleus, cytoplasm, and cell surface) that bear striking similarity can be said to demonstrate molecular mimicry. The macromolecules might be nucleic acids, proteins, glycoproteins, lipoproteins, or phospholipids. Similarities between proteins have been described on the basis of immunologic reactions at the humoral or cellular level or by identifying similar amino acid sequences of antigens that are stored in computer data banks. The rapid expansion of gene sequence data banks is providing a constantly changing and growing resource to study molecular mimicry and the possible role of viruses and other microorganisms in the etiology of systemic rheumatic diseases.

Molecular mimicry as a mechanism of inducing autoimmunity has been proposed by a number of authors.[O56,O57,O58,Z69] In the case of DIL, the structure of certain drugs is similar to that of the purine bases, suggesting crossreactivity in the induction of antibodies to DNA. Immunization of rabbits with a hydralazine human serum albumin complex resulted in high levels of antihydralazine antibodies, that were cross-reactive with denatured and native DNA, suggesting the presence of common antigenic determinants.[Y26] However, these studies did not block antibody binding by preincubating sera with the drug. Evidence against this theory was provided by prospective studies of patients on hydralazine which did not show development of antihydralazine antibodies.[L333]

In the past, viruses and other microorganisms have been the favorite topic of research aimed at identifying the cause of autoimmune disease through the mechanism of molecular mimicry.[W108] Indeed, histones and histone-like proteins are found in yeast[S471] and on bacterial chromosomes.[P164] One of the mechanisms by which viruses or other microorganisms may induce or perpetuate autoantibody production is through viral persistence. Careful searches for offending viruses in a number of autoimmune diseases, including SLE, have proven unrewarding. The concept of molecular mimicry, however, does not depend solely on viral persistence, although it does not exclude it either. Various pathways leading to autoimmunity after viral infection have been proposed.[D378,O56] One of these is the hit-and-run concept. In this model, a virus initiates the autoimmune event but is rapidly cleared or enters a cryptic state by the time the disease is clinically manifest. The disease is then perpetuated through the autoimmune assault on normal tissues with the release of antigen, the production of additional autoantibodies, and so on. In some cases of viral persistence, the virus might periodically re-express antigens that again become the target of the immune response, thus initiating flares or relapses.

Despite the preoccupation with viruses as etiologic agents, it is not necessary to restrict one's view to the viral or bacterial pathogenesis of autoimmunity. The probability that molecular mimicry operates at a higher evolutionary level (i.e., between humans and other mammalian species or between macromolecules in different cellular compartments) is as likely as the notion that it operates between widely evolved organisms, such as viruses and humans.[F279]

Other studies of histone autoantigens provide evidence to support the concept of intracellular molecular mimicry. The conventional view of histones is that they are restricted to the nucleus. As discussed earlier, histones are synthesized in the cytoplasm and then transported to the nucleus where they are assembled into nucleosomes. The stores of cytoplasmic histones are not large, and histone antibodies are not commonly associated with cytoplasmic staining by immunofluorescence (see Fig. 21–4). However, it is reasonable to anticipate that DNA in other cytoplasmic structures, such as mitochondria and centrioles, have histone-like proteins bound to them. In addition, there is evidence that certain nuclear and cytoplasmic structures share sequence similarity and antigenic reactivity with histones. The 17 kD centromeric protein CENP-A, which reacts with scleroderma sera,[T43] has been shown to be a histone-like molecule having significant sequence identity with H3.[P19] A H1-like molecule has been identified in the nuclear membrane. Human monoclonal histone antibodies, which react with cytoplasmic microfilaments[M414] and antibodies to myeloperoxidase, a highly basic cytoplasmic protein, are seen in high frequency in the sera of hydralazine-induced lupus.[N35] Further, there is growing evidence that the cell surface of lymphocytes and other cells bears DNA and histones.[B214,B215,J22,M186,R151,R155] Some evidence suggests that this nucleosome-like material is derived from nuclei via the process of programmed cell death known as apoptosis.[B185,B186,W363] Other evidence suggests that the material is not nuclear in origin.[R151] These features of histone antigens support the concept of intracellular molecular mimicry.[F279] Similar features are illustrated by a number of other autoantigens including DNA, Ro/SSA, Th, and others.[F279]

The observations in DIL are germaine to the topic of molecular mimicry. Like the events in the viral etiology hypothesis, the inciting agent need not be present for the persistent or continued production of autoantibodies. This parallels the concept of the hit-and-run virus theory, which has become a theme of molecular mimicry.[D378,O56] In this setting the virus or drug is considered to be responsible for breaking tolerance to self antigens with the only remaining fingerprint being an antibody that binds to an epitope bearing identity or similarity to the infecting agent. The fact that a drug is related to the induction of autoantibodies against a self protein such as histone suggests, among other theories, that on exposure to drugs changes occur to the protein that renders it immunogenic. In support of this concept, is the observation that hydralazine alters the physical and physicochemical properties (e.g., decreased sensitivity to protease and nuclease digestion) of chromatin.[T40,Z1] It is possible that similar drug-induced alterations of antigens might expose epitopes not present on the native protein or nucleic acid. Thus, unlike the notion that microorganisms themselves bear the cross-reacting epitopes, alteration of endogenous macromolecules may occur during drug treatment or exposure to certain environmental agents such as viruses.

One approach to a study of molecular mimicry is to study the epitopes on specific antigens.[W235] The determinants on H5, a nonmammalian variant of histone H1 that reacts with antibodies from SLE sera, demonstrated that the determinants are primarily located in the carboxy terminus.[G220,T145] When computer analysis of the complete H5 sequence in the Protein Identification Research Databank was performed, high degrees of similarity with a variety of mammalian proteins were observed.[H222] As expected, the greatest similarity was with H1° and other histone variants. However, a scan for sequence identity to only the C-terminus of chicken H5 demonstrated that goose H5 has a 27.2% similarity, but scores for all other histones and proteins were less than 10%. Only three regions of similarity to other H1 sequences were noted. Of these sequences, amino acids 148 to 155 (SPKKAKKP), 183 to 189 (RKSPKKK), and 167 to 172 (KAKKVK) were identical. All three of these regions are similar only to nonmammalian (chicken, goose, sea urchin, and annelid) H1 variants. This analysis did not support the concept that histones share epitopes with viral or bacterial peptides. Even if sequence identity was found with viral or bacterial peptides, the significance of that finding would be limited because sequence similarities between widely divergent species occur more commonly than once thought.[O30]

In another study the epitopes on H5 were synthesized in an attempt to determine if reactive epitopes were shared by other proteins.[P75] To accomplish this, the synthesis of H5 hexamers was undertaken and reactivity with overlapping peptides determined. After the reactive H5 epitopes were identified, sequence similarities with other proteins were investigated to determine the existence of cross-reactivity or mimicry. These studies showed that the linear epitopes in H5 were in the globular domain. This is in contradistinction to immunoblotting data that had mapped the immunodominant determinants of H5 to the carboxy terminus.[P76] No significant sequence similarity between H5 epitopes and other nonmammalian or nonhistone proteins was identified. This study also suggested that evidence for molecular mimicry may be difficult to obtain since many of the epitopes on histone appear to be conformational rather than linear.

The epitopes on other nuclear antigens and most other autoantigens studied to date are primarily linear or continuous. This does not imply that conformational epitopes are unlikely targets of autoimmune responses but rather that they are somewhat more difficult to study. Like the evidence for histone antibodies, there is growing evidence that conformational epitopes might be as important, or more important, as autoantigen recognition structures than are linear conformations.[L98,M421,R107,S221]

Autoantigen-Driven Responses

The preceding discussion has provided evidence suggesting the potential of molecular mimicry as an integral event in the development of histone antibodies. There is equally compelling evidence that the autoantibody response is initiated and driven by autoantigens.[H120,P75,W235] The evidence in favor of this conclusion is fourfold. First, many ANA responses are highly specific and restricted to specific disease. Second, certain diseases are characterized by unique ANA profiles. For example, SLE is characterized by a wide diversity of autoantibody responses, whereas drug-induced lupus is characterized by a relative homogeneity of antibodies. Third, even when certain diseases, such as SLE or scleroderma, appear to be associated with a wide range of autoantibody responses, careful analysis of the antigens shows that the diverse antibodies are either directed to physically associated or functionally related macromolecules. For example, the antigens involved in SLE (histones, DNA, RNP, ribosomes) are related to gene expression. Fourth, purified or cloned nuclear antigens have multiple epitopes on a single molecule. For example, SLE autoantibodies recognize epitopes on both the carboxy and amino terminus of H1,[G219] PCNA,[O17] and La/SSB.[B465] Adding more weight to these observations is the demonstration that autoantibodies from DIL patients bind to determinants on different histone molecules, a response indistinguishable from that of idiopathic SLE.[G220] Evidence at the cellular level supports these observations in that different proteolytic fragments of autoantigen are capable of inducing lymphoproliferative responses.[T43] These and other observations indicate that the autoantibody response is polyclonal, and it is also directed against more than one determinant. These observations provide a challenge for the proponents of molecular mimicry, especially if widely divergent interspecies antigens (i.e., virus versus human) are thought to be targets of autoantibodies. It would be difficult to envision a process of interspecies molecular mimicry being exercised several times in one disease,[T43,W235] much less in one individual. The obvious caveat held by the proponent of molecular mimicry is the hit-and-run concept, which suggests that determinants on the infecting agent shared by an endogenous macromolecule are sufficient to break tolerance.[F125,F230]

Another important observation is that naturally occurring human autoantibodies recognize different epitopes or domains than do monoclonal antibodies or immunization-induced antibodies. This is especially true when purified antigens (proteins, nucleic acids) rather than native macromolecules (nucleosomes, ribsosomes) are used as immunogens. For example, human autoantibodies to proliferating cell nuclear antigen (PCNA/cyclin) recognize different epitopes than do murine monoclonal antibodies or polyclonal antibodies to the amino terminal peptide of the protein.[T36] Only the human autoantibody directed against PCNA/cyclin inhibits the auxiliary protein-dependent DNA polymerase δ function.[T36] Similar observations have been made with antibodies directed against histidyl-tRNA synthetase,[G294] threonyl-tRNA synthetase,[D32] and La/SSB.[T43] These observations suggest that the induction of autoantibodies is different from the classic immunization.[R400]

The strong reactivity of DIL and SLE sera with the H2A-H2B/DNA complex, H1, and H2B compared with other histones suggests that nucleosomes, rather than free histones, act as immunogens in SLE or DIL. In the intact nucleosome, H1, H2A, and H2B occupy particularly exposed external positions. In studies where the exposure of histones in native chromatin was measured by the adsorption of antibodies specific for individual histone by chromatin, it was shown that H1 and H2B were more available to interact with homologous antibody than H3 or H4. Typically, free histones are weakly immunogenic, but when they are coupled to a nucleic acid they are highly immunogenic.[E54,M649] Immunization of rabbits with avian erythrocyte nucleosomes resulted in the production of antihistone antibodies represented by the strongest response to H5, and followed in intensity by H2B, H2A, H3, and H4.[E54] These observations are similar to the hierarchical binding activity of SLE, JRA, and DIL antibodies reported by Gohill et al.[G218] and Pauls et al.[P77] Whether the nucleosome itself or its digestion products were responsible for the antihistone antibodies is unclear.

The suggestion that the nucleosome is the immunogen in SLE and PIL is also supported by mapping the antigenic domains of histones. The domains have been localized to the extreme amino terminal segments of H2B and H4, and the amino and/or carboxy terminal ends of histone H3 and H2A.[C427,G218] These domains are exposed on the nucleosomal structure, which would provide an appropriately exposed epitope to the immune system.

Epitopes on a number of autoantigens that react with systemic rheumatic disease antibodies, including histone, Ro/SSA,[M421] Ku,[R107] and histidyl-tRNA synthetase[M421] have been identified. Although linear epitopes in some of these antigens have been suggested, it appears that the immunodominant epitopes are conformational structures. These conclusions are based on observations that there is a disparity between antibody binding to proteins in intact macromolecules, purified proteins, and peptide fragments when compared to binding to small synthetic peptides.[P75] These observations also suggested that endogenous proteins are responsible for driving the autoimmune response. On the other hand, peptides in autoantigens such as Ro/SSA have been identified that bear striking resemblance to viral protein sequences.[S221] These observations have been taken to support the concept of molecular mimicry.[L98]

With the argument supporting the autoantigen-driven hypothesis aside, it is important to point out some difficulties with the autoantigen-driven concept and some possible resolutions. As pointed out above, the autoantibody response in SLE and some other autoimmune diseases appears to be directed against functionally or physiologically related cellular processes. Earlier reference was made to observations that histone or histone-like proteins are located in multiple cellular compartments, including the cell surface of certain cells. Histone or histone-like proteins almost certainly are bound to DNA in these sites.[B186] Although these observations are conceptually difficult for proponents of the autoantigen-driven autoantibody response, it does provide some cause for reappraisal of both the autoantigen-driven and the molecular mimicry concepts. For one thing, these observations provide an alternative to the concept that the autoantigen

is nuclear in origin, although through the mechanism of apoptosis[B185,M240,W362,W363] or necrotic cell death, there is ample means by which intracellular antigens are exposed to the immune system. The observation that some, and perhaps all, nuclear antigens are represented widely throughout intercellular and intracellular compartments gives support to the concept that molecular mimicry may operate at an intracellular rather than an interspecies level.[F279] An attractive part of this concept is that it may give more insight into the pathogenic role of autoantibodies, especially if nuclear proteins are represented or mimicked as cell surface or cytoplasmic structures with similar physiologic and functional properties. This concept raises the possibility that the pathophysiology of SLE includes the recognition of cell surface proteins by antibodies, thus leading to an inflammatory response.

Immune Dysregulation

The last hypothesis suggests that inducers of autoimmunity have a direct effect on the cells involved in immunoregulation. The function of the cell may be altered, thereby altering lymphocyte subpopulations through the mechanisms of cytotoxicity. This theory has credibility in light of the observation that normal individuals and the relatives of patients with autoimmune disease have circulating autoantibodies,[D32,D129] and that in autoimmune animal models the primary defect lies in the bone marrow stem cells.[F278]

Of interest, BK virus, a human polyomavirus containing dsDNA and host cell histones, has been shown to terminate tolerance to dsDNA and histone antigens.[F230] The reactivity of antibodies in this rabbit model were primarily directed to virus structural proteins, dsDNA and ssDNA, H1 and H3. Although the autoantibody response was transient, it reappeared after a second boost in one of the rabbits. These studies suggest that the anti-DNA and antihistone antibodies that are induced in this model are not a result of nonspecific polyclonal B-cell activation. Further, this model provides a convenient merging of the molecular mimicry and immune dysregulation theories.

In another animal model of viral-related histone antibody induction, rabbits infected with the rinderpest virus also developed anti-DNA and histone antibodies.[110] The histone responses were directed predominantly to H2A-H2B/DNA or H2B/DNA complexes in some rabbits. Since the appearance of histone-reactive antibodies appeared in only some rabbits, the investigators suggested that the genetic background was likely an important factor in the induction of the autoantibody response.

In the past decade, much interest has focused on the human immunodeficiency virus and its alteration of the immune system. Impetus for the study of histone antibodies in these patients may come from observations that a chimpanzee persistently infected with HIV-1 developed H2B antibodies that correlated with the appearance of thrombocytopenia, CD4+ lymphopenia, and hypocomplementemia.[F310]

Although the evidence for viral induction of SLE is not clear, more clear-cut evidence has implicated a number of drugs, most notably procainamide and hydralazine. Patients treated with procainamide for longer than 6 months demonstrate impairment of B-cell function.[Y60] Other studies demonstrated enhanced T helper cell function in procainamide-treated patients with positive antinuclear antibody profiles.[M424] Increases in spontaneous IgG synthesis in patients with active PIL have also been reported.[F168] Procainamide and hydralazine have been shown to induce self reactivity in antigen-specific CD4 + cell lines.[C388] On the other hand N-acetyl procainamide, a drug that is not associated with DIL, was less effective at inducing T-cell autoreactivity.[R195] Although these studies provide evidence of immune cellular abnormalities in drug-induced lupus, the results are inconsistent. For a thorough discussion of this subject, refer to Chapter 45.

Chapter 22

ANTI-snRNP ANTIBODIES

JOE CRAFT*
JOHN HARDIN*

Autoantibodies to the U1 RNP and Sm antigens are dominant features of the autoimmune responses that occur in some patients with systemic lupus erythematosus (SLE). These antibodies have attracted considerable attention because of their usefulness as diagnostic markers, their value as molecular probes for the study of gene expression, and the possibility that they hold clues to the basic etiologic mechanisms for the connective tissue diseases. The present chapter will review how our understanding of these autoimmune responses developed, summarize our present knowledge of the structure and function of the U series of *small nuclear ribonucleoproteins* (UsnRNPs), and cover clinical uses of anti–U1 RNP and anti-Sm antibodies. In addition, we will discuss some of the present ideas that address the genesis of these autoantibodies. In the preparation of this chapter, the authors have relied heavily upon a review of antibodies to snRNPs.[C422a]

DISCOVERY OF AUTOANTIBODIES TO U SERIES snRNPs

Antibodies to the Sm antigen, named after a prototype serum, were first identified by Tan and Kunkel in 1966 using immunodiffusion.[T48] The specificity known as nRNP (nuclear RNP; originally called anti-Mo after the prototype serum) was identified in sera of patients with SLE by Mattioli and Reichlin in 1971.[M209] The term RNP stems from the early observation that its antigenic activity could be destroyed by treatment with ribonuclease and trypsin,[M209] thus it was a ribonucleoprotein or "RNAprotein" antigen,[R119] whereas the Sm antigen was resistant to such treatment.[T48] During the same period, Sharp and colleagues described a group of patients with a syndrome characterized by features of SLE, inflammatory muscle disease, and scleroderma, which they called mixed connective tissue disease (MCTD).[S333] The sera of these patients contained antibodies to extractable nuclear antigens (ENA) as measured by passive hemagglutination. Subsequent studies showed that ENA contained both the Sm and nRNP antigens,[N132,R118,S335,S336] and that the patients described by Sharp and co-workers were reacting with the latter component.[S336]

It is important to note that the original discovery of these specificities was based on the application of the technique of immunodiffusion, and the present clinical associations are based on studies conducted with this methodology. It is of interest that the careful early studies of Reichlin and colleagues, while based on this relatively insensitive technique, revealed that the nRNP and Sm antigens were physically associated.[M210] The molecular nature of these antigens began to become clear in 1979 when Lerner and Steitz demonstrated that both the Sm and nRNP antigens were located on the U1-snRNP (thus the modification of the term anti-nRNP to anti–U1-RNP antibodies), a complex of a small nuclear RNA, the U1-RNA, and associated polypeptides that carry the antigenic determinants.[L196] In addition to being a principal target of the autoimmune response in SLE, this particle, along with a series of closely related U snRNP particles, also plays a key role in splicing of premessenger RNA.[L195,L414,S657,S658]

STRUCTURE AND PROTEIN COMPONENTS OF THE Sm snRNPs

The U snRNPs are all intranuclear and are comprised of a small RNA (small nuclear RNA, or snRNA) and at least several polypeptides[L413] (Table 22–1). The RNA components were initially called U snRNAs because the most abundant of them had a high *uridine* content. These RNAs are still grouped together, since with the exception of the U6-snRNA, they have a unique, 5′ terminal trimethylguanosine cap.[R92] At least 13 U snRNAs (U1-U13) have been found in mammalian cells, and several others have been tentatively identified;[M553] the majority of these snRNAs have been shown to exist within snRNP particles (complexes of RNA and proteins). Two of these snRNAs, U4 and U6, exist in the same duplex particle, commonly referred to as the U4/U6 snRNP. Three of the U snRNPs, the abundant U3 snRNP and the less abundant U8 and U13 snRNPs, are found in the nucleolus.[B112,L327,T284]

The most abundant U-snRNPs, the U1, U2, U4/U6, and U5 particles, share a number of polypeptides that associate into a common structure and are referred to as the Sm core proteins[H315,L196,L413] (Table 22–1). This name reflects their recognition by anti-Sm antibodies. The intranucleolar U3, U8, and U13 snRNPs do not contain these core proteins. In human cells, the Sm core group consists

* Supported in part by grants from the NIH (AR 40072 and AI 26853) and the Connecticut Chapters of the Arthritis Foundation and the Lupus Foundation.

Table 22–1. Polypeptide Components of the Abundant Sm snRNPs in Human Cells

Particle	Protein Components	Antibody Reactivity
U1 snRNPs	*70K, A, C,* B′/B, D, E–G*	Anti-Sm, anti-U1 RNP†
U2 snRNPs	*A′, B″,* B′/B, D, E–G*	Anti-Sm, anti-U2 RNP‡
U5 snRNPs	*8 proteins,*§ B′/B, D, E–G*	Anti-Sm, anti-U5 RNP§
U4/U6 snRNPs	*150 kD,*¶ B′/B, D, E–G*	Anti-Sm, anti-U4/U6 RNP¶

* The B′/B and D–G proteins are common to all Sm snRNPs.[H315,L196,L413] Each of the abundant snRNPs listed here also contains unique proteins that are italicized. Anti-Sm antibodies principally bind the B′/B and D proteins, although they sometimes bind the E protein.[P161] Occasional sera also bind F and G.[R167] The B′ protein is a tissue-specific variant of B and is not found in nonhuman species,[C423,F275,G377,H315,L196,S148,Z20] for example, the proteins common to all Sm snRNPs in mouse cells are B, D, and E–G. Another protein similar to B, the N polypeptide has been identified, and is found on Sm snRNPs in neural tissues in at least humans and rodents.[M223,M224,S148,S149] Two additional D proteins, D2 and D3, also have been identified, and are bound by anti-Sm antibodies.[A191,B495,L179]

† Anti-U1 RNP antibodies bind the 70K, A, and/or C proteins of the U1 snRNP.[P161]

‡ Anti-U2 RNP antibodies bind the A′ and B″ proteins of the U2 snRNP.[C425,H8, M452]

§ The U5 snRNP contains 8 unique proteins, and anti-U5 antibodies bind at least 4 of them, including polypeptides of 100, 102, and a doublet of 200 kD.[B9,B10] The exact frequency of anti-U5 snRNP antibodies is unknown at present, but these antibodies are likely to be quite unusual.[B10]

¶ The U4/U5-snRNP apparently contains 1 unique antigenic protein bound by anti-U4/U6 autoantibodies. The molecular weight of this polypeptide was reported as 150 kD in one instance,[O39] and 120 kD in another.[M449] Only 2 patients have been identified with anti–U4/U6 RNP antibodies and the clinical significance of this specificity is unclear.[M449,O39]. From Craft, J.: Antibodies to snRNPs in SLE. Rheum. Dis. Clinics N. Amer., 18: 311–336, 1992.[C422a]

of the B′/B (29 and 28 kilodaltons [kD], D [16 kD], E [12 kD], F [11 kD], and G [9 kD]) polypeptides. Thus, by polyacrylamide gel electrophoresis, the B′ protein is the largest of the Sm group, and G is the smallest. Of note, the B′ polypeptide is not found in nonhuman species,[C423,F275,G377,H315,L196,S148,Z20] and its expression is tissue specific in human cells, where it is absent in brain.[M224,S148] In the latter tissue, the Sm snRNPs contain a polypeptide referred to as N[M223,M224,S149] which has close homology with B′ and B but which is encoded by a separate gene.[S148] The tissue-specific variations of these common Sm proteins may reflect the differential splicing needs of cells.

The array of Sm snRNP polypeptides appears to be more complex than was originally apparent. For example, Lührmann and his colleagues have identified two additional D polypeptides, of 16.5 and 18 kD, and have shown that they are components of the abundant Sm snRNPs.[B495,L179] Zieve and co-workers have also described a variant of D, called D′2. Although the nomenclature is somewhat confusing, the original 16 kD D polypeptide identified in 1979 by Lerner and Steitz[L196] is now referred to simply as D, or D1, and the more recently discovered larger D proteins as D2 and D3.[L179] There is also some evidence that there may be another as yet unnamed Sm core protein that has approximately the same molecular mass as G.[L179]

The common polypeptides of Sm snRNPs are highly conserved evolutionarily, as would be expected because of the crucial role these particles play in splicing premessenger RNA. For example, the B and D polypeptides are found in a variety of eukaryotic species, including humans,[H315,M204] rodents,[H315,L196] *Xenopus,*[F275,Z20] and *Drosophila.*[C423] When sought, these proteins also are found in all tissues and cell lines from these species.[C423,F275,G377,H315,L196,M223,M224,S148,Z20] Proteins of similar size to the B and D polypeptides, and immunologi-

cally reactive with anti-Sm antibodies, are also found in plants.[P14] In addition, human anti-Sm antibodies immunoprecipitate U snRNAs from cells of species as diverse as humans to *Drosophila* to yeasts,[T178,W356] indicating that the epitopes bound by these antibodies, which are constituted by proteins bound to the RNAs, are conserved in all eukaryotes.

The Sm core of polypeptides binds to their U RNAs at a conserved single-stranded nucleotide stretch consisting of purineAu$_{>3–6}$Gpurine, a sequence referred to as the Sm binding site[L267,M202,M203,R92] (Fig. 22–1). It is uncertain whether the Sm core proteins bind this nucleotide motif directly, since the B, N, D, and E proteins lack an amino acid sequence[M224,O32,R276,S611,V14] called an RNA recognition motif (RRM)[Q5] (or RNP consensus-sequence)[B71] that is found in certain proteins that bind RNA directly.[K141] The core protein F may play a role in direct RNA binding,[W349] however, its amino acid sequence is not yet known. Like the proteins that bind it, the Sm binding site is highly conserved evolutionarily; for example, this RNA sequence is found in organisms as diverse as humans and yeast (*S. cerevisiae*),[R206] as well as in certain viral RNAs.[L141]

In addition to the common core proteins, individual Sm snRNPs also contain unique polypeptides[L413] (Table 22–1 and Fig. 22–1). For example, the U1 snRNP contains polypeptides known as 70K, A, and C.[H315,K235,K236] The U2 snRNP contains polypeptides A′ and B″, so-named because they were identified after the A and B′/B proteins and because they migrate closely to these polypeptides on polyacrylamide gels.[K235,K236,M452] The U4/U6 snRNPs contain at least one unique protein, reported to be of either 150 or 120 kD in molecular weight.[M449,O39] The U5 snRNPs, when found in large 20S particles, also contain eight unique proteins.[B9,B10] Like the Sm core polypeptides, the snRNP specific proteins also appear to be highly

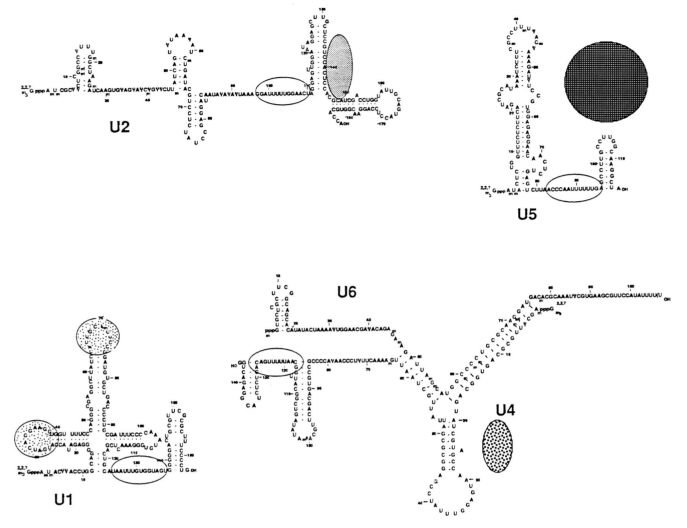

Fig. 22–1. Schematic of the abundant U1, U2, U5, and U4/U6 snRNPs. All contain a common Sm core group of proteins (in human cells, B', B, D1–D3, and E–G) represented by the open circles. These core proteins bind to a conserved single-strand RNA region purineAU$_{>3-6}$Gpurine. Additionally, each snRNP shown has unique proteins represented by the shaded areas. The U1 snRNP contains the 70K and A proteins that bind to the first and second stem loops of the U1 RNA, respectively;[L427,Q6] the binding site of the U1 snRNP protein C is not precisely known and thus it is not shown. The A' and B'' proteins together are associated with a 3' stem loop of the U2 RNA. The binding site of the unique proteins of the U4/U6 and U5 snRNPs are not known at present. (See text and Table 22–1 for details). Modified from Lee, S.I.: Four novel U RNAs are encoded by a herpes virus. Ph.D. thesis, Yale University, 1990.

conserved. For example, an A protein homologue is found in plants,[P14] and a protein that corresponds to the 70 K protein is found in yeast (*S. cerevisiae*).[S516]

As shown in Figure 22–1, the 70K and A proteins of the U1 snRNP bind directly to the first and second stem loops of the U1 RNA, respectively.[L427,L429,Q5,Q6,S127,S765] Both of these polypeptides contain the RNA-recognition motif mentioned above. This motif is also found in the B'' protein, which binds directly to the U2 RNA. This interaction is enhanced by binding of B'' by the A' protein, likely via a repetitive leucine motif found in A.[B226,B377,F238,S126,S128] The binding site of the C protein to the U1 RNA is not known, but it appears to require other snRNP proteins for association with the U1 particle.[N58]

The primary structure of the majority of the proteins of the U1 snRNP, including the 70K,[Q7,S601,T126] A,[S431] and C[S432,Y13] proteins, and the B'/B,[O32,V14] N,[M223,M224,S149] D,[R276] and E[S611] polypeptides common to all Sm snRNPs, has now been determined; the unique proteins of the U2 snRNP, A'[S433] and B'',[H10] have also been cloned. Features of interest of these proteins are shown in Table 22–2 (reviewed in [L415,V41]).

FUNCTION OF THE U snRNPs

The U1, U2, U5, and U4/U6 snRNPs are the most abundant (amounts range from 2×10^5 copies/mammalian

Table 22–2. Structural Characteristics of the Polypeptide Components of Sm snRNPs

Proteins	Proteins Notable Structural Features*
U1-snRNP–Specific Proteins	
70K	Contains RNA binding domain (RNA-recognition motif) involved in U1 RNA binding; also contains mixed-charge amino acid clusters, including one at COOH end responsible for aberrant migration by SDS-PAGE of this 52 kD protein at 70 kD[A2,S601,T126]
A	Contains RNA-recognition motif involved in U1 RNA binding[S431]
C	Lacks RNA-recognition motif; binding to U1 RNA likely requires the presence of other proteins; true molecular weight is ~17 kD, thus it also migrates aberrantly by SDS-PAGE[S432,Y13]
U2-snRNP–Specific Proteins	
A'	Leucine-rich region involved in protein-protein interaction with the B" polypeptide[F238,S433]
B"	Homology with A protein of U1 snRNP, with which it shares a common autoimmune epitope; contains RNA-recognition motif involved in U2-RNA binding[H110]
Common Sm Proteins	
B'/B	Arises from same gene by alternative splicing of common RNA transcript,[C258,O32,V14,V15] contains repetitive proline-rich motif in COOH end around which common B-cell epitope resides,[E78,R278] also has proline-rich epitope that is cross-reactive with the A and C proteins of the U1 snRNP[H9]
N	Neuron specific; high degree of homology with B'/B[M223,M224,R277,S149]
D	Lacks primary sequence homology with B'/B,[R276] despite the fact that these proteins share a cross-reactive B-cell epitope commonly recognized by anti-Sm sera
E	Lacks the above-noted RNA-recognition motif,[S611] also lacking in the other Sm proteins

* See text for details and for references relative to RNA binding of the U1 and U2 snRNP specific proteins; also see Figure 22-2.
From Craft, J.: Antibodies to snRNPs in SLE. Rheum. Dis. Clinics N. Amer., 18:311–336, 1992.

cell for U5 and U4/U6, to 1×10^6 copies/cell for the U1 snRNSP[R92]) and play a central role in the splicing of premRNA.[L414,S657,S658] Genes of higher organisms contain regions, called introns, that are noncoding and that separate the coding regions, or exons. Although the noncoding regions are transcribed wholesale along with the coding regions into premessenger RNA, the introns must be removed for effective translation of the messenger RNA into protein. The process of intron removal is called splicing, and is mediated in the nucleus by the abundant Sm snRNPs prior to export of the mature messenger RNA to the cytoplasm for translation into proteins on ribosomes.[D46,L414,S657,S658,W358]

The less abundant U7 snRNP (2.5×10^4 copies/cell) participates in the processing of 3' ends of histone mRNAs.[M638] The function of the even less abundant U11 and U12 snRNPs (10^3 to 10^4 copies/cell) is unknown at present.[M553] The nucleolar U3-snRNP is involved in ribosomal RNA processing;[K95] presumably the closely related U8 and U13 particles have a similar function. The U9- and U10-RNAs are likely components of Sm snRNPs, but they have not been further characterized.[R93]

INTRACELLULAR ASSEMBLY OF Sm snRNP PARTICLES

The Sm snRNPs are assembled in the cytoplasm.[A190a,W97] Work by Zieve, Mattaj, Lührmann, Keene and their colleagues, as well as others, have shed valuable insights into this assembly pathway. Formation of these particles begins with transcription of the appropriate U small RNAs in the nucleus, a step mediated through RNA polymerase II with the exception that the U6 RNA is synthesized by RNA polymerase III. RNA polymerase II is the enzyme complex that also transcribes messenger RNA, while RNA polymerase III transcribes tRNAs, 5S ribosomal RNAs, and other small RNAs including the RoRNAs. The U RNAs are transported to the cytoplasm where they interact with snRNP polypeptides in an ordered assembly process. The Sm core proteins self-associate in cytoplasmic pools. Binding of the resulting complex to the U snRNAs is associated with conversion of the 5'-guanosine residue of the latter molecules from a monomethyl to a trimethyl form (referred to as a trimethyl guanosine cap). Both of these steps are required for entry of the assemblies of the snRNPs into the nucleus. Additional individual proteins such as 70K, A, and/or C of the U1 particle either enter the nucleus independently prior to binding their respective snRNAs or are incorporated into the snRNP while the new complex remains in the cytoplasm. This highly programmed assembly pathway ensures that partially assembled snRNP complexes will not interact with pre-mRNA.[N97]

ANTIGENIC POLYPEPTIDES OF THE U snRNPs

Dominant autoimmune reactions in patients with SLE are often directed against the abundant snRNPs. The anti-Sm response involves production of antibodies that immunoprecipitate the U1, U2, U4/U6 and U5 snRNPs through interactions with some combination of the B', B, N, D1–D3, and E polypeptides which are shared among these particles.[L196,M223,P161] In contrast, anti-U1 snRNP antibodies bind the 70K, A, and/or C proteins of the U1-snRNP,[P161] while anti–U2-RNA antibodies recognize the A' and B" polypeptides of the U2 particle[C425,H8,M452] (Table 22–1). Similarly, autoantibodies bind the proteins specific to the U4/U6- and U5-snRNPs,[B10,M449,O39,O40] but these latter specificities appear to be rare. Thus, as discussed below, these latter antibodies immunoprecipitate individual snRNPs because they recognize unique proteins of each respective snRNP. In contrast, the nucleolar U3, U8, and U13 snRNPs lack the common Sm proteins, but share the polypeptide fibrillarin, and are immunoprecipitable with antibodies that bind this polypeptide.[T284]

DETECTION OF ANTI-SM AND ANTI-U1 RNP ANTIBODIES

Anti-Sm and anti-U1 RNP antibodies stain the nucleus of cells in a fine speckled pattern, with sparing of nucleoli, when examined in indirect immunofluorescence (Fig. 22–2). This staining pattern reflects the location of the Sm snRNPs in the nucleoplasm. Certain anti-Sm and anti-U1 RNP sera also appear to stain the nucleus with brighter intensity in more discrete, larger speckles on the background of diffuse speckling (J. Craft, unpublished observation), possibly reflecting the observation that the major components of the splicing machinery appear to exist, perhaps as storage pools, in discrete foci within the nucleus.[C91,F294,G12] Similarly, sera specific for the U2, U5, and U4/U6 snRNPs also produce an identical speckled staining pattern[M449,O39,O40] consistent with the role these particles play in pre-mRNA splicing.

Presently, most laboratories rely on the technique of immunodiffusion for the routine detection of anti-Sm and anti-U1 RNP antibodies. The sensitivity of immunodiffusion can be enhanced with the technique of counterimmunoelectrophoresis.[R114] This method is of particular use in the detection of anti-Sm and anti-U1 RNP antibodies. It is important to recall that the currently accepted clinical associations of these antibodies with various diseases are largely based on data developed with immunodiffusion.[R114] In immunodiffusion, a prototype anti-Sm or anti-U1 RNP serum is placed into a well cut into agarose. The soluble fraction of a tissue extract (such as rabbit or calf thymus or spleen) prepared by sonication in a saline buffer is placed in an adjacent well. During a 24- to 48-hour incubation period, diffusion brings the antibodies together with their respective antigens (so-called extractable nuclear antigen[s] or ENA) and as they bind, a lattice structure develops that appears as a visible precipitin band. Antibodies in a particular serum can be identified through comparison with a serum of known specificity. In other words, if the two sera are binding the same antigen, the precipitin lines will fuse to form a line of identity;

otherwise, they will spur across one another. When anti-U1 RNP antibodies are compared with anti-Sm antibodies, a line of partial identity is often observed (*i.e.*, the Sm line spurs over the U1 RNP line, but the latter fuses with the Sm line). This pattern occurs when some soluble particles contain both antigens (bound by anti-Sm and anti-U1 RNP sera), and others contain Sm determinants alone (bound by anti-Sm sera).

More recently, ELISA assays for detection of anti-Sm and anti-U1 RNP antibodies have been developed. In these assays a highly pure antigen is allowed to adhere to the surface of wells in a plastic tray. Dilute patient serum is then added, and antibodies that bind the antigen on the plastic surface can be detected by the use of a second, antihuman antibody tagged with an enzyme that catalyzes a color change in an indicator substrate. Originally, these assays depended upon biochemically or affinity-purified antigen, which is often difficult to prepare. The recombinant forms of the snRNP polypeptides that are now available may soon alleviate this difficulty.

ELISA methods have the advantages of speed (results are available within hours rather than 1 to 2 days required for immunodiffusion) and sensitivity (approximating that of radioimmunoassays). They are also easier and safer to perform than most radioimmunoassays. Their major limitations are the requirement for a completely pure antigen to serve as substrate and a relatively high rate of false-positive results, compared to immunodiffusion.

IMMUNOPRECIPITATION AND IMMUNOBLOT ASSAYS FOR THE DETECTION OF ANTIBODIES TO THE Sm snRNPs

Antibodies that bind polypeptides present on an individual snRNP can be used to specifically remove, or immunoprecipitate, that particle from solution and thus ascertain its function. A practical application of such an experiment was the use of lupus patient sera to inhibit pre-mRNA splicing by the selective removal of U1- or U2-snRNPs from splicing extracts. Such experiments helped to determine the role of the individual snRNPs in the splicing pathway.

The protein components of the Sm snRNPs were also initially demonstrated using immunoprecipitation assays.[H315,L196,P161] Immunodiffusion data had previously shown that the Sm and RNP determinants were physically associated, but were different antigens.[M209,M210] These observations were explained by the finding from immunoprecipitation experiments that both these determinants were located on the U1 snRNP. In these experiments, both anti-Sm and anti-U1 RNP antibodies were used to immunoprecipitate radiolabeled snRNPs. In such experiments, commonly used in research laboratories, cells are labeled *in vivo* with ^{35}S-methionine, which places a radioactive tag in all cellular proteins. The radiolabeled cell extracts are then mixed with human sera containing anti-Sm or anti-U1 RNP antibodies (or sera of other specificities) bound to a particulate carrier such as protein A-sepharose.[C424] After binding of the antibody to its antigenic target, the antibody-antigen complex can be immunoprecipitated via the particulate carrier. Immunoprecipitated

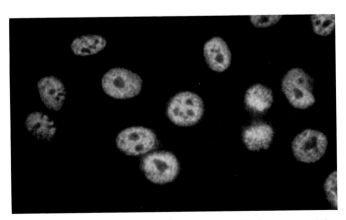

Fig. 22–2. Indirect immunofluorescence of a human anti-Sm serum diluted 1:40; note the fine speckled staining. Anti-U1 snRNP and U2 snRNP sera would produce an identical pattern of immunofluorescence. From Craft, J.: Antibodies to snRNPs in SLE. Rheum. Dis. Clinics N. Amer., 18:311–336, 1992. With permission.

antigens, bearing the ^{35}S-methionine tag can then be detected by polyacrylamide gel electrophoresis and autoradiography. An example of such an experiment is shown in Figure 22–3. Immunoprecipitates formed with an anti-U1 RNP serum and with anti-Sm serum are shown in lanes 2 and 3, respectively. Both immunoprecipitate from solution all the components of the U1 snRNP, since their antigenic targets (B′, B, D, and E for anti-Sm antibodies and the 70K, A, and C proteins for anti-U1 RNP antibodies; Table 22–1) are associated via their common RNA backbone (Fig. 22–1). The 70K protein and the D2 and D3 proteins are not visualized under the conditions of this experiment. The N protein is also absent in these non-neural cells.

Cells also can be labeled *in vivo* with ^{32}P to tag RNAs with radioactivity.[C424] In a fashion similar to that described for immunoprecipitation of ^{35}S-methionine–labeled proteins, autoantibodies can then be used to immunoprecipitate selective RNAs via their associated antigenic proteins. Recall that autoantibodies are usually directed toward the protein components of the snRNP complex, rather than the RNA itself. After immunoprecipitation, bound RNA(s) can be visualized by gel fractionation followed by exposure of the gel to X-ray film. Since anti-U1 RNP antibodies only bind the 70K, A, and C proteins which are unique to the U1 snRNP (Table 22–1 and Fig. 22–1), the U1 RNA component is visualized on the gel when these antibodies are used to form immunoprecipitates (Fig. 22–4, lane 3). Note that this serum also immunoprecipitates the U2 RNA via low titers of antibodies directed toward the antigenic A′ and B″ proteins of the U2 snRNP (Table 22–1 and Fig. 22–1). An immunoprecipitate formed with a serum containing high titers of anti-U2 snRNP antibodies is also shown (Fig. 22–4, lane 5); this anti–U2-snRNP serum also contains anti-U1 RNP antibodies in low titer, so the U1 RNA is also seen in immunoprecipitates formed with this serum. In contrast, anti-Sm antibodies immunoprecipitate all the Sm snRNAs via epitopes that are found on the common B′/B, D (D1–D3), and E proteins (Fig. 22–4, lane 4). The amount of each of the Sm snRNAs (U1, U2, U4, U5, and U6) in the immunoprecipitate at least partly reflects their relative abundance within the nucleus, as discussed above under the characterization and function of Sm snRNPs.

Radioimmunoprecipitation assays can be used as a sensitive means to screen sera for the presence of anti-Sm and anti-U1 RNP antibodies, as well as for other antibodies directed against ribonucleoproteins, such as anti-Ro, anti-La, or anti–Jo-1. Immunoprecipitation assays are extremely sensitive and specific, since the radiolabeled antigen can be detected in minute quantity and visualized directly. A major disadvantage of immunoprecipitation assays is that they typically require use of radioactivity. Although this latter problem can now be circumvented through the use of sensitive staining procedures to identify immunoprecipitates in gels, these assays are somewhat laborious compared to ELISA or immunodiffusion, and thus their usage is usually limited to research laboratories.

Immunoblots can also be used for detection of anti-Sm and anti-U1 RNP antibodies.[P161] Cell nuclei, a source of

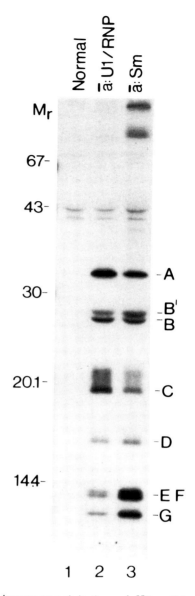

Fig. 22–3. Immunoprecipitation of ^{35}S-methionine–labeled HeLa cell extracts with human antisera. Cells were labeled *in vivo* with ^{35}S-methionine, followed by sonication and centrifugation to remove particulate debris. Sera from patients with SLE were mixed with protein A-sepharose beads, allowing the IgG fraction of sera to specifically bind to the beads. IgG-coated sepharose beads were then incubated with radiolabeled cell extracts. Bound proteins were then fractionated by gel fractionation, and detected by autoradiography. Lane 1 shows an immunoprecipitate formed with a normal control serum, whereas lanes 2 and 3 show immunoprecipitates formed with anti-U1 RNP and anti-Sm sera, respectively. Although these sera bind different polypeptide components of the U1 snRNP, they both immunoprecipitate all the proteins of this particle via their link on the U1 RNA backbone. The 70K protein is not labeled under the conditions used here, and is therefore not seen in the immunoprecipitates. Similarly, the D2 and D3 proteins are not visualized under the gel conditions used. From Craft, J.: Antibodies to snRNPs in SLE. Rheum. Dis. Clinics N. Amer., 18:311–336, 1992. With permission.

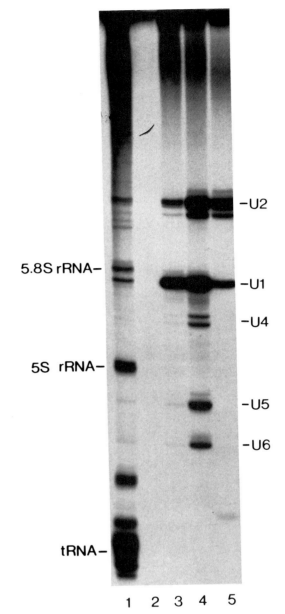

Fig. 22–4. Immunoprecipitation of ^{32}P-labeled HeLa cell extracts with human antisera. Cells were labeled *in vivo* with ^{32}P, followed by sonication and centrifugation to remove particulate debris. Sera from patients with SLE were mixed with protein A-sepharose beads, allowing the IgG fraction of sera to specifically bind to the beads. IgG-coated sepharose beads were then incubated with radiolabeled cell extracts; snRNP particles bound by the IgG via antigenic polypeptides were then extracted to remove protein, and the radiolabeled RNAs recovered, followed by gel fractionation, and autoradiography. Shown in lane 1 are total radiolabeled RNAs present in the soluble cell extract, including the abundant Sm/snRNAs. Lane 2 shows the immunoprecipitate formed with a normal control serum. Lanes 3–5 show immunoprecipitates formed with an anti-U1 RNP serum, an anti-Sm serum, and an anti–U2-RNP serum, respectively. Note that the anti-U1 serum primarily immunoprecipitates the U1-RNA since this specificity binds the 70K, A, and/or C polypeptides unique to the U1-snRNP. In contrast the anti-U2 snRNP serum, via antibodies that target the A' and B'' proteins (see text), only immu-

Table 22–3. Association of Diseases and Antibodies to the Sm snRNPs

Antibody	Disease or Clinical Syndrome
Anti-Sm	SLE*
Anti–U1-RNP	SLE,* MCTD†
Anti-70K‡	MCTD, SLE (paucity of nephritis)
Anti-A‡	Unclear
Anti-C‡	Unclear
Anti–U2-RNP	MCTD, SLE, or scleroderma with myositis

* In SLE, anti-Sm antibodies frequently occur with anti-U1 RNP; the latter antibodies may occur alone.
† In MCTD, anti-U1 RNP antibodies are found alone and typically in high titer.
‡ The anti-U1 RNP response is comprised of three separate antibody populations: anti-70K, anti-A, and anti-C.
From Craft, J.: Antibodies to snRNPs in SLE. Rheum. Dis. Clinics, 1991. (In press.)^{C422a}

snRNPs, can be fractionated on polyacrylamide gels, followed by transfer to nitrocellulose and probing with diluted patient sera. Bound antibodies can be detected with a second antibody coupled to an enzyme that produces a color when its substrate is added, or via a second antibody that can be detected with a ^{125}I tag. A major advantage of immunoblots is their specificity, since the antigenic protein targets of these antibodies can be visualized directly. Additionally, in comparison to immunoprecipitation assays, immunoblots can provide information about which polypeptide carries the specific epitope that is being recognized, since the antigens are probed with antisera after electrophoretic separation, whereas immunoprecipitation assays reveal only the total protein or RNA composition of the bound antigen.^{P161} For example, antibodies specific for the B or D proteins on the U1 snRNP will immunoprecipitate all the polypeptide components of this particle, via their association on an U1 snRNA backbone (e.g., refer to Figs. 22–1 and 22–3). However, in general, immunoblots are not any more sensitive than ELISA assays, and their performance is more laborious. Like immunoprecipitation assays, immunoblots for the detection of anti-Sm and anti-U1 RNP antibodies are typically limited to the research lab.

CLINICAL ASSOCIATION OF ANTI-Sm ANTIBODIES

Anti-Sm antibodies are an important diagnostic marker for SLE^{N149} (Table 22–3). When sera are examined in immunodiffusion, these antibodies are found in approximately 25% of all patients with lupus, and their presence has been included as part of the revised ARA (American College of Rheumatology) criteria for the diagnosis of this disorder.^{T46} In comparison to immunodiffusion,

noprecipitates the U2 snRNA; this serum also contains a low titer of anti-U1 RNP antibodies. Finally, the anti-Sm serum immunoprecipitates all the abundant Sm/snRNPs via the Sm core proteins common to all the Sm/snRNAs. From Craft, J.: Antibodies to snRNPs in SLE. Rheum. Dis. Clinics, N. Amer., 18: 311–336, 1992. With permission.

ELISA assays increase detection of these antibodies[A297,F84,H402,R105] by about 10%[F84,H402] to twofold[R105] without sacrificing their specificity as a disease marker for SLE.[F84,H402] Anti-Sm antibodies are more common in peoples of African and Asian descent, in comparison to those of European origin,[A297,F84] and in the American SLE population, occur about twice as often in the former versus the latter group.[A297] Overall, the incidence of these antibodies ranges from approximately 10 to 20% of Caucasian patients with SLE, compared to the 30 to 40%, or more, of Asian and black patients, respectively.[A22,A297,F84,H402] Although anti-Sm antibody titers may fluctuate over time,[B82,F115,T14] it is unusual for them to completely disappear when measured by sensitive immunoprecipitation assays.[F115] However, they may become undetectable by standard immunodiffusion tests.[B82]

Several clinical studies have sought to correlate anti-Sm antibodies with disease activity and individual disease parameters. Early studies using immunodiffusion assays suggested that patients with these antibodies may have milder renal disease and less CNS involvement than patients with anti-DNA antibodies.[W305] Other studies have found that rising anti-Sm titers are predictive of disease flares or more active disease.[B380] However, in a subsequent study based on ELISA, these antibodies did not correlate with particular disease manifestations.[F84] A large study involving over 100 Japanese patients found that when detected by ELISA, anti-Sm antibodies correlated with a low frequency of progression to end-stage renal disease (and thus milder renal disease), despite a high prevalence of late-onset proteinuria, and despite a poorer prognosis overall than patients without anti-Sm.[H402] This finding was supported by an evaluation of a group of American patients, which suggested that these antibodies, when detected by ELISA, were associated with renal disease, the progression of which was not defined.[T14]

The sum total of current evidence indicates that the presence of anti-Sm antibodies is a helpful adjunct in making the diagnosis of SLE. While their role in predicting or following the course of the illness is much less clearly defined, in certain populations, these antibodies may identify a group of patients with a propensity to develop certain disease manifestations.

CLINICAL ASSOCIATION OF ANTI-U1 RNP ANTIBODIES

Anti-U1 RNP antibodies are found in about 30 to 40% of patients with SLE whose sera are tested in immunodiffusion[A297,B380,N149,S22] (Table 22–3). These antibodies may occur alone but are often present in conjunction with other specificities. They are almost always demonstrable in patients who have anti-Sm antibodies; conversely, the latter specificity rarely occurs without anti-U1 RNP antibodies.[M210,P161,R105] This pattern suggests that when the U1 snRNP particle acts as an autoimmunogen, initial responses are induced against U1 RNP determinants and are propagated, particularly in SLE patients, to include Sm determinants. Thus, an ability to expand autoimmune responses to a wide array of epitopes on the U1 snRNP appears to characterize SLE.

The major clinical association of anti-U1 RNP antibodies is with mixed connective tissue disease where they typically occur in high titers and are not associated with other specificities[R105,S334,S336] (Table 22–3). Indeed, this illness is defined by the presence of these antibodies. Anti-U1 RNP antibodies may also occur in a small fraction of patients with Sjögren's syndrome, rheumatoid arthritis, scleroderma, and polymyositis.[N149,R105,S334] Like anti-Sm, anti–U1-RNP antibodies are more common in SLE patients of African descent than those of European descent.[A297]

The three unique proteins of the U1 snRNP, 70K, A, and C, do not share known cross-reactive epitopes,[H8] and are recognized by at least three separate antibody populations (referred to as anti-70K, anti-A, and anti-C), which may occur together or singly in a given patient.[R161] In other words, all three antibodies contribute to the anti-U1 RNP response. ELISAs that detect antibodies to individual 70K, A, and C proteins have now been established, and they demonstrate these antibodies in a small percentage of patients whose sera are negative in immunodiffusion.[S22]

Antibodies to the 70K protein, which are detectable in immunoblots, occur in 75 to 95% of patients with MCTD who are preselected because they have the anti-U1 RNP specificity as determined by immunodiffusion or by counterimmunoelectrophoresis[A123,H7,P162] (Table 22–3). These antibodies may be less frequent in comparable groups of SLE patients where immunoblot-detectable anti-70K antibodies appear to occur in as few as one-fifth to as many as one-half of individuals.[H7,P162,R123] However, ELISA assays, based upon either gel-purified 70K polypeptides, or recombinant 70K fusion proteins expressed in *E. coli*, reveal that up to 85% of patients with SLE, with anti-U1 RNP antibodies detectable by immunodiffusion, will have anti-70K antibodies.[S22,T14] Among patients not preselected for the anti-U1 RNP specificity, anti-70K antibodies are found in around 12% of patients with SLE[E44] and occasional patients with rheumatoid arthritis, polymyositis, and scleroderma.[S22] When patients with MCTD and SLE are grouped together, anti-70K antibodies appear to correlate with myositis, esophageal hypomotility, Raynaud's phenomenon, lack of nephritis, and the HLA-DR4 phenotype.[H363,R123,T14] Longitudinal studies have indicated that anti-70K antibody titers vary over time, but it is uncertain whether these levels reflect underlying disease activity.[D172,H452,P162,S22,T14] There is no experimental evidence that the antibodies themselves are involved in tissue injury. Thus, anti-70K antibodies occur in both MCTD and SLE, they may be markers for the former diagnosis when present in high titer, and they may correlate with overlap features in patients otherwise thought to have SLE.

Antibodies to the A polypeptide are also quite common in patients who have anti-U1 RNP antibodies. Among patient populations selected for the presence of anti-U1 RNP, anti-A and anti-70K antibodies occur with approximately the same overall frequency, when measured by immunoblots.[P161] However, among patients selected because they have SLE, anti-A antibodies appear to be twice as common as anti-70K antibodies,[E44,P162] appearing in approximately 23% of such patients overall,[E44] or in approximately 75% of lupus patients who have anti-U1 RNP antibodies by immunodiffusion.[T14] Presently, it is unclear whether anti-A antibodies are associated with specific disease manifestations.[T14] Like antibodies to the 70K polypeptide, those against A also vary over time, and these changes in titer do not necessarily reflect disease activity.[D172,T14]

Antibodies to the C polypeptide occur in almost the same frequency as anti-70K and anti-A antibodies in patients with either MCTD or SLE who are preselected for the anti-U1 RNP specificity.[P161] Clinical associations of these antibodies have not been recognized as yet.

In summary, it appears that antibodies to all of the three unique proteins of the U1-snRNP contribute to the anti-U1 RNP response as measured by immunodiffusion, or by other assays that do not detect antibodies to the specific proteins. The contributions of the anti-70K and anti-A response to the overall anti-U1 RNP response may vary depending upon disease, MCTD versus SLE, as well as perhaps upon manifestations of SLE.

CLINICAL ASSOCIATION OF ANTI-U2 RNP ANTIBODIES

Anti-U2 RNP antibodies were first described by Mimori and colleagues in a patient with scleroderma-polymyositis overlap syndrome.[M452] Habets and co-workers subsequently identified four patients whose sera contained these antibodies, although they did not find a specific disease association.[H8] However, later studies found that these antibodies were associated with overlap syndromes,[C425,P162,R106] occurring in about 15% of patients with MCTD[C425,P162] and approximately the same frequency in patients with SLE or scleroderma plus myositis[C425] (Table 22–3). Like anti-U1 RNP or anti-Sm, these antibodies produce a speckled immunofluorescence pattern;[C425,H8,M452] however, they can be distinguished in immunodiffusion, where they give partial identity with control anti-Sm sera.[M452] In the latter assay, they have lines of nonidentity with control anti-U1 RNP sera, unless they contain these latter antibodies in addition to anti-U2 RNP. The best available methods to confirm the presence of anti-U2 RNP antibodies are immunoprecipitation or immunoblotting.

GENESIS OF THE ANTI-U1 RNP AND ANTI-Sm RESPONSES

As we have conceptualized,[C422a] the accumulating information about the spectrum of antibodies to the Sm snRNPs and their relationship to the architecture of these particles make it possible to speculate about the underlying mechanisms that account for the production of these autoimmune responses. Several indirect lines of evidence support the idea that anti-Sm and anti-U1 RNP responses

arise as a result of antigen drive by the U1 snRNP.[E58,H120] In other words, it seems quite possible that these responses are engendered by T-cell–dependent B-cell activation, a process initiated by presentation of these antigens by class II MHC molecules.

The support for this scenario includes the following data and rationale. Anti-Sm and anti-U1 RNP antibodies often occur in high titer, may represent the majority of detectable autoantibodies present in a patient, are responsible for a significant proportion of the total serum immunoglobulin,[M49] and are polyclonal;[E63] all these features are similar to immune responses seen after immunization of animals with exogenous antigens. Additionally, anti-Sm antibodies virtually always occur in linkage with anti-U1 RNP antibodies, and individual antibodies to the 70K, A, and C polypeptides likewise occur in linkage;[C426] these linked responses suggest that the U1 RNP particle initiates their production.[H120] Such focused responses are not compatible with autoantibodies that result from polyclonal B-cell activation;[C426,H120] rather, the pattern of antibodies to the U1 snRNP can most easily be reconciled by postulating that the antigen *per se* determines which B-cell clones are activated. This concept is supported by the finding that U1 snRNPs as immunogens in mice elicit antibodies that target the same epitopes as those bound by anti-Sm and anti-U1 RNP antibodies in patients with SLE.[R166] In addition, *in vitro* anti-Sm responses can be augmented when immune cells are exposed to Sm antigen,[S391] and other autoantibody responses in humans with SLE appear to arise independent of polyclonal B-cell activation.[R108]

The T-cell dependence of the anti-U1 RNP and anti-Sm response is also supported by several observations. First, both types of antibodies are restricted to the IgG1 heavy chain isotype, suggesting that these responses are T-cell dependent and likely antigen dependent.[E63] Additionally, B cells from patients with anti-U1 RNP antibodies produce these antibodies *in vitro*, a response that is enhanced by coculture with patient T cells and adherent cells.[O31] O'Brien, Harrison, and colleagues have isolated human T cells that are specific for the 70K protein of the U1 RNP, and have identified an immunodominant epitope at the carboxyl end of this protein.[O4]

Although all these lines of evidence are suggestive that the anti-Sm and anti-U1 RNP responses are secondary to response to self-U1 snRNP particles, it should be emphasized that direct evidence for this scenario is not currently available. To support this view, evidence that shows processing by antigen-presenting cells and presentation of peptides derived from self-U1 snRNP proteins (extracellular U1 snRNPs via cell death, or fully or partially assembled intracellular U1 snRNPs via targeting of their constituent polypeptides to class II MHC molecules as they assemble within cells) is necessary.

Chapter 23

ANTIBODIES TO RO/SSA AND LA/SSB

JOHN B. HARLEY
MORRIS REICHLIN*

Anti-Ro (or SSA) and anti-La (or SSB) are important autoantibodies in systemic lupus erythematosus. They are respectively found in just less than half and nearly a fifth of these patients in concentrations sufficient for precipitin formation. These autoantibodies are also closely allied with particular clinical findings. They are such an intrinsic component of disease expression that one is led to the conclusion that an understanding of the immune response to these and other autoantigens would reveal the mechanism of the autoimmune dysregulation of lupus, if not also the etiology of the disease.

A precipitin, likely to have been Ro or La, was first described over 30 years ago in a patient with Sjögren's syndrome.[J104] This observation was expanded upon by Anderson and colleagues, who defined both antigens, which they called SjT and SjD.[A205,A206] In addition, they observed a "lupus" precipitin that in retrospect is likely to have been an anti-nRNP or anti-Sm specificity. Unfortunately, these observations lay fallow until the anti-Ro and anti-La specificities were independently described by M. Reichlin and colleagues.[C277,M211] The Ro and La specificities have been under continuous investigation since. They have also been described as Sjögren's syndrome A (SSA) and Sjögren's syndrome B (SSB) antigens.[A162,A163] An Ouchterlony immunodiffusion showing an example of the anti-Ro and anti-La responses is represented in Figure 23–1. Beyond this the most fundamental contribution has been the marriage of autoimmune serology with molecular biologic approaches for the analysis of these antigens.[L196]

The clinical relevance of anti-Ro has been particularly well established. The data are less compelling for anti-La, though clearly, this autoantibody is also important. The associations of clinical findings with anti-Ro and anti-La, as presented in Table 23–1, do not in themselves constitute a direct evidence for an immunopathogenic role in any aspect of the disease. Nevertheless, at the very least these associations are important as aids for diagnosis and prognosis.

Photosensitive skin rash as an association with anti-Ro was first appreciated by Maddison[M47] and has been confirmed in a more comprehensive evaluation of this manifestation of lupus. Lee and colleagues have established that anti-Ro is specifically deposited in human skin and, therefore, likely to be directly involved in injury to the skin.[L135,L139]

Chest radiographs with changes of interstitial pneumonitis have been shown to be associated with anti-Ro.[H242] There is no evidence directly implicating anti-Ro in pulmonary disease of lupus, though the association of anti-Ro with pulmonary disease has been previously appreciated.[S521]

Idiopathic thrombocytopenic purpura is well known to present before lupus can be diagnosed in some patients. These patients tend to have anti-Ro precipitins.[A29,A207,M590] Both anti-Ro and a positive antinuclear antibody test may be present at presentation with immune thrombocytopenia and precede fulfilling the diagnostic criteria for lupus by as much as 14 years.[A29] How long before presentation with immune thrombocytopenic purpura these patients develop anti-Ro is not known.

Indeed, the temporal relationship of the appearance of anti-Ro or anti-La to the clinical presentation with lupus or Sjögren's syndrome is not known. Anti-Ro or anti-La appear after the diagnosis in the rare patient. In addition, most mothers of infants with congenital heart block or neonatal lupus dermatitis who have anti-Ro or anti-La have never had clinical manifestations of any of the disorders associated with these autoantibodies.[S230,W103] Many mothers, however, develop lupus in the years following the birth of the affected infant.[M255] This leads one to suspect that anti-Ro and anti-La autoantibodies may arise before the clinical illness appears. Perhaps in many cases these autoantibodies are present for years before patients become ill.

In addition to thrombocytopenia, other hematologic cytopenias have been associated with anti-Ro. In lupus patients who in any way satisfy the hematologic criterion for classification of systemic lupus erythematosus,[T46] but particularly those with lymphopenia, tend to have anti-Ro.[H138] In Sjögren's syndrome, thrombocytopenia, anemia, and lymphopenia are associated with anti-Ro.[A133] In rheumatoid arthritis, though anti-Ro is uncommon (about 5% of patients[B262]), this autoantibody is associated with leukopenia.[B386]

There are data supporting a role for anti-Ro in nephritis. In a series of anti-Ro precipitin-positive patients, only those who had anti-Ro without an anti-La precipitin developed renal disease.[W91] Acid-eluted immunoglobulin from the renal tissue of two anti-Ro precipitin-positive patients

* We are grateful to our many colleagues who have contributed to the work discussed herein. Our efforts are supported by the NIH (AR39577, AI14717, AI21568, AI31584, AR32214, AR31133) and the U.S. Department of Veterans Affairs.

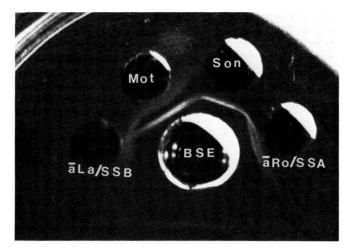

Fig. 23–1. Anti-Ro and anti-La precipitins. The mother (Mot) has both anti-Ro and anti-La autoantibodies while the affected son (Son) has only a faint anti-Ro precipitin. Precipitins from reference anti-La (aLa/SSB) and anti-Ro (aRo/SSA) sera are also presented against a bovine spleen extract (BSE). The anti-La precipitin is light and diffused in this example. Pedigree described in Reichlin, M., Friday, K., and Harley, J.B.: Complete congenital heart block followed by the development of antibodies to Ro/SSA in adult life: Serological clinical and HLA studies in an informative family. Am. J. Med., *84:*339, 1988.

Table 23–1. Associations with Anti-Ro and Anti-La Autoantibodies in Systemic Lupus Erythematosus and Related Disorders*

Specificity	Clinical or Genetic Association
Anti-Ro (or anti-SSA)	Photosensitive skin rash (lupus)
	Interstitial pneumonitis (lupus)
	Thrombocytopenia (lupus, Sjögren's syndrome)
	Lymphopenia (lupus, Sjögren's syndrome)
	Nephritis (lupus)
	C2 complement deficiency (lupus)
	HLA-DQ1/2
	T-cell receptor β gene (lupus)
	Vasculitis (Sjögren's syndrome)
	Thrombocytopenic purpura (Sjögren's syndrome, subacute cutaneous lupus)
	Primary biliary cirrhosis
Anti-La (or SSB)	Absence of nephritis (lupus)
	HLA-B8, DR3 (lupus)
	HLA-DQ1/2 (Sjögren's syndrome)
Anti-Ro and anti-La	Rheumatoid factor (lupus, Sjögren's syndrome)
	Sjögren's syndrome
	Subacute cutaneous lupus erythematosus
	Neonatal lupus dermatitis
	Complete congenital heart block

* Associations are presented for systemic lupus erythematosus (lupus) unless the data are derived from patients with another diagnosis such as Sjögren's syndrome.

contained anti-Ro that had been concentrated in the antibody deposited in the kidney.[M50] This is prima facie evidence to support a direct role for anti-Ro in the nephritis of some patients. Anti-Ro deposited in the tissue either as an immune complex or by virtue of binding to a specific antigen has the potential to be phlogistic and mediate the inflammatory response that follows antibody binding.

Over the past decade a compelling association has been demonstrated between congenital complete heart block and both anti-Ro and anti-La precipitating autoantibodies.[F204,K173,S230] The anti-Ro IgG clearly originates with the mother, who is likely to be asymptomatic for an autoimmune rheumatic disorder. In a few cases normal conduction has been demonstrated before the third trimester.[B604,T227] Heart block often appears late in the second trimester or early in the third trimester, coincident with the active transport of maternal IgG across the placenta. Complete congenital heart block is found in about 1 of every 20,000 births.[M388]

In the largest series of congenital heart block cases, anti-Ro and/or anti-La has been found in 83%.[S230] Survey studies estimate that an anti-Ro precipitin is present in 1% of pregnant women.[C30,T85] An expectant mother with an anti-Ro precipitin has an increased risk of bearing a child with congenital heart block, but even so this risk remains small.

The mechanism of heart block is unclear. Cardiac conduction tissue binds anti-Ro more avidly than other cardiac cell types.[D155] Data from a set of fraternal twins discordant for heart block have shown depletion of anti-Ro

in the serum of the affected twin consistent with the possibility that anti-Ro is specifically being deposited in cardiac tissue.[H135] This observation strongly suggests that critical contributions are made toward the generation of heart block by the fetus in a way that varies from patient to patient. One theory of pathogenesis holds that the basic process is a nonspecific endomyocarditis, which involves the atrioventricular node by extension at a time when the node is in an anatomically vulnerable position.[H135] If true, then many additional fetuses may have the endomyocarditis while only a fraction of these involve the atrioventricular node and develop heart block.

There are at least three ways that congenital heart block is relevant to lupus. First, pregnant female lupus patients with anti-Ro, by virtue of having this autoantibody, have a 1 in 20 risk of having a child with congenital complete heart block.[R34] Second, the mothers of children with heart block are at increased risk of developing a systemic autoimmune rheumatic disorder even if they are asymptomatic when the child is born.[M255] Indeed, we have seen a patient whose lupus developed 26 years after delivery of an infant with congenital heart block and coincided with her retiring from Ohio to bask in the sunshine of Florida.[R116] Third, a study of adult lupus patients has revealed an increased prevalence of conduction abnormalities among anti-Ro precipitin-positive patients.[L362]

Infants of mothers with anti-Ro may also develop neonatal dermatitis. This rash most often appears after birth. Areas of sun exposure predominate, but are not exclusively involved. Skin lesions are often similar to those found in subacute cutaneous lupus with arcuate erythematous macules or papulosquamous lesions. Occasionally they may leave hypopigmented skin, but generally the lesions resolve without sequela. In infants all of the lesions that appear usually develop and resolve together. As the maternal IgG, which in these patients nearly always contains anti-Ro, is cleared from the infant's circulation the likelihood of developing the rash diminishes. Maternal IgG is almost undetectable in the infant by 6 months of age, and the onset of neonatal lupus dermatitis is unheard of at this stage. It is important to note that a few cases of neonatal dermatitis have been reported associated with an anti-nRNP precipitin in the absence of an anti-Ro precipitin.[P315]

The diagnosis of subacute cutaneous lupus erythematosus is established on the basis of a characteristic erythematous macular, arcuate, or papulosquamous skin rash (Figure 23-2) along with consistent histology. About 75% of patients with subacute cutaneous lupus have anti-Ro precipitins.[S566] These patients may or may not satisfy the classification criteria for systemic lupus.[T46] The rash of subacute lupus erythematosus is not ordinarily accentuated by sun exposure, and many patients will have lesions in areas of their skin protected from skin exposure. The lesions are erythematous and may or may not be raised. In some patients the lesions have central clearing. Lesions at all the different stages of maturity may be present simultaneously. Some of these patients develop petechia or purpura, particularly of the lower extremities, which on biopsy often reveals small vessel vasculitis. Those with vasculitis seem to be a subgroup with greater hypergammaglobulinemia and more likely to have Sjögren's syndrome than the remaining patients.

Of the disorders associated with anti-Ro and anti-La perhaps none is more intriguing than Sjögren's syndrome. Depending upon the assay performed and the population selected from 40 to over 95% of these patients have anti-Ro and 15 to over 85% have anti-La.[H134] The finding of dry eyes and dry mouth associated with a lymphocytic infiltrate of the salivary or lacrimal glands is not uncommon in a number of autoimmune rheumatic disorders including systemic lupus erythematosus, rheumatoid arthritis, progressive systemic sclerosis, primary biliary cirrhosis, and autoimmune myositis. Hence, Sjögren's syndrome is a feature shared by a minor proportion of the patients with each of these disorders, which suggests that these diseases must also have fundamental aspects in common.

Primary Sjögren's syndrome is considered to be present when the diagnostic criteria for Sjögren's syndrome are satisfied [M114] in the absence of another rheumatic disease with autoimmune features. Since the etiology and pathogenesis of all of these diseases are unknown, and since there is great latitude in applying the diagnostic standards, the relative composition of patient groups used by different investigators is likely to vary greatly between institutions. This situation does not seem to have been helped by the current criteria for the classification of rheumatoid arthritis,[A294] which are more broadly inclusive than the previous criteria.[R296]

There are a number of patients whose predominant disease process over time is Sjögren's syndrome who then develop features consistent with systemic lupus erythematosus.[A136,P312,P313] As a group they are highly enriched for HLA-DR3 and commonly have both anti-Ro and anti-

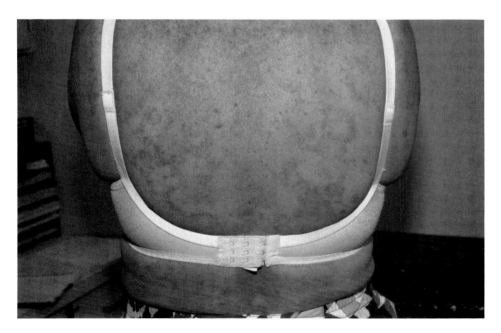

Fig. 23-2. The rash of subacute cutaneous lupus erythematosus showing erythematous macules and papulosquamous lesions. The typical arcuate lesions can be appreciated on this middle-aged woman's back at presentation.

La. The usefulness of the distinction between primary and secondary Sjögren's syndrome is lost in this situation. Indeed, these are commonly referred to as having lupus-Sjögren's overlap disease. The important point is that these and other patients with lupus or Sjögren's syndrome form a continuous spectrum of disease expression, from classic Sjögren's syndrome through the overlap with shared features to a more ordinarily recognizable lupus process. The failure of existing nosology to straightforwardly separate patients demonstrates the inadequacy of present diagnostic practices and the need to understand etiology and pathogenesis.

Systemic lupus erythematosus is also associated with hereditary deficiencies of the early components of the classic complement cascade.[A55,M381] Patients with component C2 deficiency tend to have an anti-Ro precipitin, but not an anti-La precipitin. Anti-Ro may be more common in homozygous C2-deficient patients than ordinarily found in the remainder of lupus patients.[P308] Lupus patients with complement component deficiencies also tend to have a mild form of lupus with cutaneous manifestations, but with neither anti–double-stranded DNA autoantibody nor nephritis. Patients with lupus and the other early complement component deficiencies also have anti-Ro without an anti-La precipitin, but this has not been evaluated in a sample large enough to be conclusive.[M381]

Anti-Ro and anti-La are clearly related to autoimmune rheumatic disease expression. In only a few situations has strong evidence been obtained for its phlogistic potential. In individual tissues anti-Ro has been shown to be concentrated in the parotid gland and kidney.[M50,P107] Affinity-enriched anti-Ro has been shown to deposit specifically in human skin transplanted onto nude and scid mice.[L135,L139]

Immunogenetic associations with individual autoantibodies have led to model building in an effort to understand the possible molecular events in the context of what has been learned of the immune response. The first relationship appreciated has been the association of anti-Ro with HLA-DR3.[B184,M44] Subsequently it has been appreciated that anti-Ro is also related to HLA-DR2 in both lupus and Sjögren's syndrome.[A66,A169] These multiple associations have been reconciled in two ways. First, a gene interaction effect has been defined between HLA-DQw1 and HLA-DQw2 such that lupus or Sjögren's syndrome patients who have both of these alleles tend to have anti-Ro. This has been extended in lupus to show that particular subsets of the DQA1 and DQB2 genes mediate this effect, which therefore is consistent with a gene complementation mechanism. This result leads to the prediction that in some patients the capacity to form a particular DQ molecule is important to their having anti-Ro. For them the predicted MHC class II surface molecule is composed of a DQ α peptide encoded from one parental chromosome and a DQ β peptide encoded from the other parental chromosome, resulting in a molecule composed of an α chain from DQw1 and a β chain from DQw2.

Reveille and colleagues have taken a more inclusive approach and have tried to define the common structural sequences related to anti-Ro relative to a control population.[R174] They have also mapped the most powerful associations to the DQ locus and found that nearly all the patients with an anti-Ro response also had a glutamine at amino acid 34 of at least one of their DQ α chains and a leucine at amino acid 26 of at least one of their DQ β chains.

The HLA associations with the anti-La response are a little different. In primary Sjögren's syndrome anti-La is related to HLA-B8, DR3, and DR2,[H134,W214,W273] much as for anti-Ro. Indeed, the association of anti-La with the HLA-DQw1/w2 heterozygous state was as powerful as it was for anti-Ro.[H137] In lupus, however, the strongest association is with the B8, DR3 haplotype.[H138] The basis for this discrepancy is not known.

Humoral autoimmunity is revealed by the presence of autoantibodies. It is much more difficult to be confident that human diseases with lymphocytic infiltrates but without autoantibodies are also autoimmune, though work in animal models has provided convincing and overwhelming evidence that this mechanism of disease pathogenesis is a practical possibility. Here the prevailing suspicion is that T lymphocytes are mediating autoimmunity without stimulating B lymphocytes to differentiate and produce autoantibodies. T lymphocytes appear to determine not only whether a cellular as opposed to an antibody response results from immunogen exposure, but in many circumstances whether tolerance is maintained or broken. For these and other reasons most investigators suspect that T lymphocytes have an obligate role in the immunoregulatory decision to synthesize autoantibody against protein autoantigens. Defining this role in human lupus has been difficult, as it has been in other inflammatory, possibly autoimmune, disorders of unknown etiology. For example, in lupus there is no evidence to suspect linkage of lupus with T-lymphocyte receptor genes in multiplex families.[W338]

On the other hand, just as the histocompatibility associations are different for risk of disease than they are for the production of individual autoantibodies, there may be analogous differences at the level of the T-cell receptor. Recent work has shown that alleles of the T-cell receptor β chain gene are related to the presence of anti-Ro in lupus.[F210] Interestingly, the association is most significant for those patients who have an anti-Ro precipitin without an anti-La precipitin and does not exist for those who have both anti-Ro and anti-La precipitins. Preliminary analysis is consistent with synergy between the T-cell receptor association and the HLA-DQ alleles associated with anti-Ro.[H136] Other work with the 70 kD U1 ribonucleoprotein has shown that lymphocytes proliferate after exposure to this peptide when it is presented as a fusion protein, and that a region from the carboxyl terminus is more stimulatory than other regions of the molecule.[O4]

In aggregate these data are consistent with a model of the generation of lupus autoantibodies, in general, and of anti-Ro, in particular, which requires the participation of HLA-DQ and T-cell receptor alleles along with the autoantigen to form a trimolecular complex (Figure 23–3). Human Ro is suspected to be directly involved since Ro from other species is less antigenic with human autoantibodies.[R121] From these data the conclusion is compelling

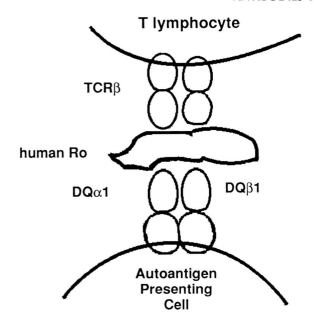

T lymphocyte

TCRβ

human Ro

DQα1   DQβ1

**Autoantigen
Presenting
Cell**

Fig. 23–3. The trimolecular complex model for autoantigen presentation of the human Ro autoantigen based upon associations of anti-Ro with alleles at HLA-DQ and the β peptide of the T-lymphocyte receptor.

that the anti-Ro autoimmune response is Ro autoantigen-driven in lupus. Similar conclusions have been reached using other experimental strategies for the anti-Sm and anti-DNA responses in lupus.[E63,P212] Accordingly, autoantigen-driven autoimmune responses appear to be the general rule in lupus.

Some of the genetic risk factors have been defined for the generation of individual autoantibodies. Associations with clinical manifestations are also known. The question remains to be determined, however, how the clinical features, immunogenetics, and autoantibodies are interrelated in lupus, though one would suspect that relationships should flow from the genetic features to the autoantibodies and from the autoantibodies to disease manifestations. This concept of the disease predicts, for example, that HLA alleles are generally related to clinical manifestations through the autoantibodies, and that the relationships of autoantibodies with HLA alleles and of autoantibodies with clinical manifestations will be stronger than HLA alleles with clinical manifestations.

This hypothesis was confirmed in a group of 40 lupus patients in which the anti-La, anti-Ro, anti-Sm, anti-nRNP, anti–single-stranded DNA, and anti–double-stranded DNA were measured.[H138] Primary relationships were found between HLA-DQw1/w2 and anti-Ro, between HLA-B8, DR3, and anti-La, between anti-Ro and lymphopenia, and between anti-La and the absence of nephritis. No statistically relevant relationships were present between any of the HLA antigens determined and any of the criteria for the classification of lupus. Logistic regression analysis established that the presence of lymphopenia was best explained by considering the combined contributions of anti-Ro and anti–single-stranded DNA.[H138]

The relationship of anti-La to the absence of nephritis was analyzed by an analogous approach. The literature inconsistently shows an association of anti–double-stranded DNA with nephritis, though there is convincing evidence that some anti–double-stranded DNA antibodies are deposited in the kidney.[E15,H34,K340,K341,W286] On the other hand, both anti-La and anti-nRNP have been associated with a decreased incidence of nephritis in lupus.[R119,R123,W91] In this group of 40 lupus patients, there was no simple association between anti–double-stranded DNA and nephritis.[H138] Logistic regression analysis, however, produces an interesting result (Table 23–2). The association of anti-La with the absence of nephritis is powerful. However, once this effect is incorporated into the logistic model, then anti–double-stranded DNA makes an important contribution. Here anti-La and anti–double-stranded DNA have opposing effects, which is demonstrated in the resulting logistic equation presented in the legend to Figure 23–4. These data support a mechanism of disease expression in which the clinical manifestations are the result of complicated interactions of various kinds of autoantibodies. The autoantibodies, in turn, are strongly influenced by the particular HLA and T-cell receptor alleles present.

In clinical practice, Ouchterlony double immunodiffusions is the traditional method of determining whether anti-Ro or anti-La are present (Figure 23–1). Most of the data relating these serologies to clinical manifestations have been developed using this technique or the closely related procedure of counterimmunoelectrophoresis. Double immunodiffusion is specific and sufficiently sensitive for nearly all clinical applications. Unfortunately, the procedure requires 2 days to complete, and its performance requires specialized training. Not infrequently, an anti-Ro precipitin is missed because poor quality reagents have been used or because an inexperienced person is performing the test.

These difficulties and inefficiencies have provided an incentive for the development and marketing of alternative methodologies. Immunoprecipitation, immunoblotting, and solid-phase enzyme-linked immunosorbent as-

Table 23–2. Logistic Regression Model of Renal Disease in 40 Patients with Lupus*

Step	Term	Improvement		Goodness of Fit		Coefficient	Standard Error
		X^2	P	X^2	P		
1	Anti-La	8.7	0.003	33	0.50	−1.22	0.52
2	Anti-dsDNA	6.9	0.008	26	0.79	2.75	1.19

* Anti-La is presented as the $\log_{10}$ of the enzyme-linked immunosorbent assay units of the La solid-phase binding activity (range 2 to 7.03). Anti–double-stranded DNA (dsDNA) is a dichotomous variable (1 = present and 0 = never detected). The standard error of the mean of the coefficient is given.
From Harley, J.B., Sestak, A.S., Willis, L.G. et al.: A model for disease heterogeneity in systemic lupus erythematosus. Relationships between histocompatibility antigens, autoantibodies, and lymphopenia or renal disease. Arthritis Rheum., 32:826, 1989. With permission.[H138]

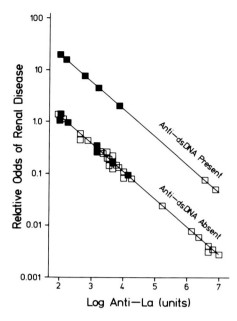

Fig. 23–4. Relative odds of lupus nephritis in 40 lupus patients as calculated from the anti-La and anti–double-stranded DNA (dsDNA). Anti-La titer is expressed as the $\log_{10}$ of the relative binding in a solid-phase assay using purified bovine La. The presence or absence of anti-dsDNA is indicated. The presence (*closed squares*) or absence (*opened squares*) of renal disease is indicated. The relative odds of renal disease are calculated from the logistic regression model presented in Table 23–2 (n = 40): ln (relative odds of renal disease) = − 1.22 (anti-La) + 2.75 (anti-dsDNA) + 2.67. From Harley, J.B., Sestak, A.S., Willis, L.G. et al.: A model for disease heterogeneity in systemic lupus erythematosus. Relationships between histocompatibility antigens, autoantibodies and lymphopenia or renal disease. Arthritis Rheum., *32*:826, 1989. With permission.

says (ELISAs) are available in research laboratories. Of these only the anti-Ro and anti-La ELISAs have been marketed to clinicians and clinical laboratories. These assays appear to provide as much as a ten- to hundredfold increase in sensitivity over double immunodiffusion. There is greater potential for interfering binding in ELISA, and the specificity of these assays is reduced relative to double immunodiffusion. The increased sensitivity means that half or more of lupus patients and, perhaps, over three-quarters of Sjögren's syndrome patients clearly have anti-Ro, instead of the 30 to 40% with lupus and more than 40% with Sjögren's syndrome who have precipitating antibodies in double immunodiffusion. Anti-La precipitins are less prevalent, being found in 10 to 20% of lupus and 15 to 30% of Sjögren's syndrome patients. The anti-La ELISAs may identify twice as many patients as having this autoantibody.

The importance of identifying patients who have anti-Ro or anti-La by an ELISA is problematic for those who do not form precipitins. A significant proportion of normals may fall into this category. This level of anti-Ro does not, at present, assist in formulating diagnosis or prognosis. The ready availability and relative ease of performing these solid-phase assays dictates their increasing use.

Nevertheless, whatever assay the clinician chooses, he should fully understand the meaning of the results obtained and the limitations that are important to impose upon his interpretation.

At present there is no clinical situation where monitoring the level of anti-Ro or anti-La is warranted. Mildly affected patients have been known or inferred to have had anti-Ro or anti-La precipitins for decades. It is rare to observe the appearance or disappearance of an anti-Ro or anti-La precipitin after disease onset unless the patient has had aggressive cytotoxic therapy, longterm corticosteroids at high doses, heavy proteinuria or renal failure. It is clear that the levels of anti-Ro and anti-La vary over time by as much as ten- to twentyfold during the disease course, but the relevance of this to disease expression is not known.

Important progress has also been made in defining molecular properties of the Ro and La antigens. All four of the human Ro-associated RNAs, known as hY RNAs, have been sequenced (Fig. 23–5). Each of these is a product of RNA polymerase III and is from 84 to 112 bases in length. The hY RNAs have a triphosphate 5′ terminus and a polyuridine 3′ terminus.[K107,W326] Two highly conserved regions of 24 bases paired with one another are found in each hY RNA sequence.[O3] Part of this conserved region is thought to bind to the Ro protein by virtue of its being protected from RNAse digestion.[W326] From two to four Y RNAs have been isolated from other species,[M86] leading to the impression that there is substantial heterogeneity in Y RNAs between species.

The peptide with a molecular weight of about 60 kD is thought to be the major peptide in the Ro RNA-protein particle.[Y10] Two sequences of this species have been obtained that are essentially identical except for a small region of sequence divergence at the amino terminus of the predicted protein.[B198,D185] The 60 kD Ro peptide has a putative ribonuclear protein binding domain and a zinc finger. Itoh and colleagues have presented evidence for two antigenically related forms of 60 kD Ro.[157]

Three other peptides have been related to anti-Ro autoantibodies. A 52 kD peptide has been identified from lymphocytes by immunoblot,[B197] and its cDNA has been cloned and sequenced.[C200,156] Though affinity-isolated anti–52 kD autoantibodies immunoprecipitate the hY RNAs, it is probably premature to conclude that the hY RNAs are directly bound by this peptide.

In erythrocytes 60 kD and 54 kD peptides are variably identified in immunoblot by different anti-Ro containing sera.[R7] The 54 kD erythrocyte Ro peptide appears to be antigenically related to 52 kD lymphocyte Ro.[157] Interestingly, only hY1 and hY4 RNAs are immunoprecipitated from erythrocytes where they are slightly smaller than in other cell types. This difference is probably because of the shorter polyuridine 3′ end on the Y RNAs found in erythrocytes. The Y RNAs in human platelets have been demonstrated to be restricted to hY3 and hY4.[158]

Finally, a 46 kD protein has been identified and sequenced using patient sera that contain anti-Ro activity. This sequence appears to be the human form of calreticulin, a calcium binding protein.[M229]

Ro particles have been studied without exposure to

A
```
                    10              30              50
hY1    GGCUGGUCCGAAGGUAGUGAGUUAUCUCAAUUGAUUGUUCACAGUCAGUUACAGAUCGAA
hY3         GU C   GUG U A.   C A   A   AC          UU..
hY4      T  T     T  T  T G ..TTAT .GAACTTATTA   TT.   TGT   ... T
hY5      A  U     GU U   G ..U A........   A......    ... UU


                    70              90             110
hY1    CUCCUUGUUCUACUCUUUCCCCCCUUCUCACUACUGCACUUGACUAGUCUUU
hY3    .. U  .....U C  .U AC C   G  U          C
hY4    AG..TT GTAT AA...      ..... TG TAA TTT   TG CTT
hY5    A..  ...... ..       ..ACA  CG G...      CU GC
```

B

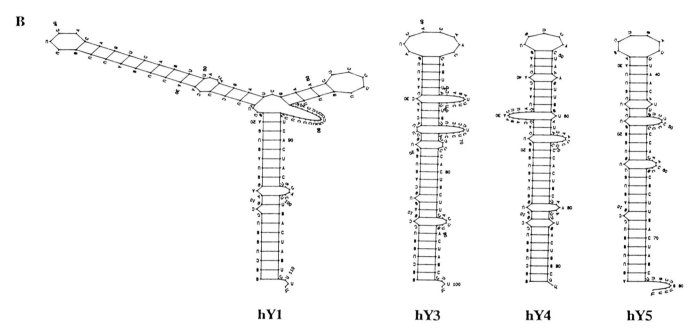

hY1   hY3   hY4   hY5

Fig. 23–5. hY RNAs. *A*, Shows sequence comparison of the four hY RNAs. The complete sequence of hY1 is presented and the changes found in hY3, hY4, and hY5 are indicated. Periods indicate gaps in the sequence arranged to maximize sequence alignment. *B*, Shows proposed secondary structure of the hY RNAs. From O'Brien, C.A., and Harley, J.B.: A subset of Y RNAs are associated with erythrocyte Ro ribonucleoproteins. EMBO J., 9:3683, 1990. With permission.

denaturing conditions to allow an evaluation of in vivo Ro particle composition. In gel filtration these particles range from 230 to 350 kD, thus supporting the position that there may be more than one peptide in a Ro particle.[B385] At least one of these isolated Ro particles also contains the La peptide, thereby providing a structural basis for their association with one another.

The La peptide contains 408 amino acids and has a predicted molecular weight of 46.7 kD.[C193,C194,C201] La also has an 80 amino acid conserved element referred to as the RNA recognition motif.[Q5] The carboxyl end of the protein is methionine free and phosphorylated while the amino end is methionine rich.[C199] The La peptide appears to bind any RNA with a polyuridine 3' end.[M184,S663] In addition to the Y RNAs, these include the precursors of 7S, 5S, U6, and transfer RNAs. The RNAs bound are gener-

ally the immature transcription products of RNA polymerase III except for U1-RNA, which is an RNA polymerase II product that binds La.[M511] Some virus-encoded RNAs also bind La from adenovirus, Epstein-Barr virus, and vesicular stomatitis virus.[K470,R292]

While there is evidence for multiple roles for La in the molecular economy of the cell, none has yet been delineated for Ro. La may function as a shuttle protein to carry RNA transcripts from the nucleus to the cytoplasm.[B12,B14] Others have obtained evidence that La is a termination factor for RNA polymerase III.[G316,G317] La has been shown to melt an RNA-DNA hybrid in a reaction that requires ATP hydrolysis.[B15]

With more detailed structural information available, attention has turned to the fine specificity of anti-Ro and anti-La autoantibodies. By expressing fragments of the recombinant La cDNA clone, a number of groups have shown that there are multiple epitopes on the La peptide distributed throughout the primary structure.[C193,K352,R63,S21,S750]

The 60 kD Ro peptide also appears to have multiple linear epitopes.[S221] Unexpectedly these tend to occur in regions of Ro that share short sequence homology with the nucleocapsid protein of vesicular stomatitis virus. Whether this or some other possible precursor antigenic exposure is important in the immune dysregulation that leads to Ro or La humoral autoimmunity will be an important question for the 1990s.

Chapter 24

ANTICARDIOLIPIN ANTIBODIES, CHRONIC BIOLOGIC FALSE-POSITIVE TESTS FOR SYPHILIS AND OTHER ANTIPHOSPHOLIPID ANTIBODIES

RONALD A. ASHERSON
RICARD CERVERA

The study of the anticardiolipin antibodies, (aCLs) the antibodies detected in the chronic biologic false-positive serologic tests for syphilis (BFP-STS) and autoantibodies directed against other phospholipids (aPLs), such as phosphatidylserine, phosphatidylinositol, or phosphatidic acid, has received much attention over the last few years not only because of their relatively high prevalence in patients with SLE, but also, particularly with aCLs, because of their strong association with recurrent episodes of venous and arterial thrombosis, spontaneous fetal losses, and thrombocytopenia.[L392,S57] The antibodies responsible for the lupus anticoagulant (LA) phenomenon, whose detection is also associated with thrombotic complications, comprise closely related aPLs, and they are reviewed in depth in another chapter.

ANTICARDIOLIPIN ANTIBODIES

Of the various aPLs, the aCLs have received more attention because of their easy detection by means of sensitive, reproducible, and reliable tests.

Historical Considerations

In the early 1980s, studies carried out at London's Hammersmith Hospital in search of simple reproducible tests to study more closely patients with SLE presenting with thrombosis, abortions, and cerebral disease[H474] led to the development of solid-phase immunoassays to detect aCLs.[G114,H152,L364]

Subsequently, a close relationship between these antibodies and the presence of LA was demonstrated.[T221] Most of these aCL- and LA-positive patients also demonstrated antibodies against other negatively charged phospholipids, namely phosphatidylserine or phosphatidic acid.[L379] Additionally, some of these patients were shown to have transient or, more commonly, chronic BFP-STS[C183,K356] because, in fact, these tests also detected the presence of antibodies against cardiolipin in the cardiolipin-phosphatidylcholine-cholesterol antigen used in that assay.

The high correlation between the IgG isotype of aCLs and clinical thrombosis was first documented in 1986,[H150] and this observation was confirmed in subsequent stud-

ies.[A100,C183,F151,F170] A minority of patients, however, demonstrated high levels of the IgM isotype, which was also accompanied by thrombotic complications. In addition, the frequency of fetal losses[D175,H150,L350,L354,W49] and thrombocytopenia (usually moderate)[C183,D138,D139,H147,H150] was increased in this group of patients.

These findings led in 1986 to the recognition of the so-called anticardiolipin syndrome,[H476] later termed the antiphospholipid syndrome, (APS)[H149] which included those patients with thrombosis, recurrent abortions, and/or thrombocytopenia, who had aCLs and/or LA.

This syndrome was seen mostly in patients with SLE, but it soon became clear that other patients not suffering from defined SLE might exhibit features of APS. Many of these had some clinical or serologic features of SLE but failed to fulfill four of the 1982 revised criteria for the classification of SLE. These patients were considered to suffer from a lupus-like illness or "probable" SLE.[A334] Other patients with aPLs and thrombosis or recurrent abortions did not have any of the typical clinical or serologic features of SLE or any other defined connective tissue disease. These patients were subsequently defined as having "primary" APS.[A115,A316,A336,F155,M31]

Frequency

The prevalence of aCLs in SLE varies between 20 and 50%.[A100,C183,C439,H150,L392,S57] This wide range of variation may be because of difference in the sensitivity of laboratory assays, in the cut-off positive level, or may reflect the effects of patient selection, e.g., ethnic and racial differences as well as treatment. Additionally, age also influences the prevalence of aCLs in SLE. Font et al.[F156] have described a higher prevalence of aPLs (including aCLs and LA) in SLE patients over 50 years old (62.5%) as compared with a younger group (38.7%). However, most SLE patients with aCL do not have aPL-related symptoms. Approximately one-third of SLE patients with these antibodies may have a history of, or will develop, clinical manifestations of APS. Patients with persistently moderate to high titers of aCLS of the IgG isotype seem to be at higher risk.[C183,H150,I46], although occasionally IgM or IgA isotypes only may be seen.

The presence of aCLs is not limited to SLE or lupus-

Table 24–1. Diseases in Which aPLs Have Been Found

Autoimmune diseases
  Systemic lupus erythematosus
  Rheumatoid arthritis
  Scleroderma
  Dermatomyositis-polymyositis
  Mixed connective tissue disease
  Sjögren's syndrome
  Temporal arteritis/polymyalgia rheumatica
  Takayasu's arteritis
  Behçet's disease
  Autoimmune hemolytic anemia
  Idiopathic thrombocytopenic purpura
  Diabetes mellitus
  Hashimoto's thyroiditis
  Myasthenia gravia
Drug-induced lupus (D.I.L.)
  Chlorpromazine
  Procainamide
  Hydralazine
  Quinidine
  Phenytoin
  Sulphonamides
Infectious diseases
  Bacterial (tuberculosis, leprosy, syphilis, Lyme disease, infective endocarditis, Klebsiella infections)
  Protozoal (Pneumocystis carinii, plasmodium)
  Viral (AIDS, mononucleosis, hepatitis, rubella, parvovirus)
Hematologic diseases
  Thrombotic thrombocytopenic purpura
  Sickle cell disease
  Polycythemia vera
  Myelofibrosis
  Monoclonal gammopathies
  von Willebrand's disease
Malignant diseases
  Hairy cell leukemia
  Malignant lymphoma
  Waldenström's macroglobulinemia
  Epithelial malignancies (lung, maxilla, prostate, esophagus, colon, cervix)
  Hypernephroma
  Thymoma
Other conditions
  Renal failure undergoing dialysis
  Degos' disease

like disease. They have been reported in other connective tissue disorders, as well as in drug-induced, malignant, and infectious diseases (Table 24–1).[F151,F170,Z14] The majority of these patients however have low positive titers, often transient and mainly the IgM isotype. Therefore, the aCLs are usually of little clinical relevance in these patients.

Positive aCL titers have also been found in 10 to 30% of women with idiopathic repeated spontaneous abortion.[B42,B87] They have also been detected in 19% of patients with venous or arterial thrombosis attending a routine anticoagulation clinic who do not suffer from SLE or any other well-delineated autoimmune disorder.[E169] In addition, it has been estimated that approximately 9,000 young people in the United States per year suffer from an ischemic cerebral episode associated with aPLs (500,000 new strokes per year with 4% occurring in people under the age of 50 and nearly 45% of these associated with aPLs). As many as 1,260 will go on to develop recurrent

strokes despite conventional therapy.[A240a] Interestingly, aCLs may be detected in cerebrospinal fluid, but studies to date have not demonstrated a relationship with cerebral thrombotic events.

Elevations of serum aCLs may also occur in up to 7.5% of normal populations. Harris et al. recently found a prevalence of only 1.7% (IgGaCL) and 4.3% (Ig MaCL) when testing 1,449 pregnant women. The results were low (<2 SD) in all positives.[H161a] In all studies the antibodies usually exhibit low avidity for cardiolipin and the titers are low. The frequency rises with increase in age.[F87,K42,M109] Salivary IgA aCLs have also been detected in normal populations.[C228]

Finally, the presence of aCLs has also been demonstrated in experimental mouse models of SLE.[R59] Smith et al.[S510] found that the MRL-lpr/lpr mouse had significantly elevated levels of aCLs when compared to normal mice. These authors also observed histologic evidence of central nervous system thromboses, perivascular infiltrates of the choroid plexus, and thrombocytopenia in their experimental mouse model. Gharavi et al.[G116] reported increased fetal loss in mice with aCL elevations.

Methods of Detection

A solid-phase radioimmunoassay (RIA) for the detection of aCLs was first described in 1983.[H152] Subsequently, the enzyme-linked immunosorbent assay (ELISAs) were developed.[G115,L364] Essentially, these assays involve coating plastic plates with pure cardiolipin dissolved in ethanol, blocking nonspecific binding by incubation with fetal calf or adult bovine serum, and then incubating with diluted patient test sera. Finally, antibody bound to the phospholipid is identified using ^{125}I-labeled or enzyme-labeled antihuman antibody.

The aCL assays, compared to the LA tests, are more sensitive, have less observer error, and can be performed using stored sera. However, three main problems arise: 1) the presence of nonspecific binding of antibodies, especially of the IgM isotype, to the plastic wells; 2) the influence of temperature on aCL binding; and 3) the reporting of results.

In order to exclude false-positive aCL results caused by nonspecific binding of other antibodies (e.g., rheumatoid factor) to the wells, several technical considerations are important. The use of 10% fetal calf serum or 10% adult bovine serum in phosphate-buffered saline (PBS) rather than Tween as buffers, high (1/50, 1/100) rather than low (1/10, 1/25) test sera dilutions, and short (1 to 2 hour) incubation times will reduce nonspecific binding.[H146]. In addition, the assay was modified by inclusion of measurement of binding to the wells without coated cardiolipin. The value for the samples from the wells without cardiolipin was considered as nonspecific binding. The calculated value from wells with cardiolipin is referred to as total binding. The specific binding is calculated after correction by the subtraction of the nonspecific binding from the total binding.

Additionally, it has become evident that binding of aCLs to cardiolipin is temperature dependent. Heat treatment of serum and plasma before testing consistently induces

Table 24–2. Semiquantitative Manner of Reporting aCL Results

	IgG aCLs	IgM aCLs
High positive	>80 GPL	>50 MPL
Medium positive	15–80 GPL	6–50 MPL
Low positive	5–15 GPL	3.5–6 MPL
Negative	<5 GPL	<3.5 MPL

an increase of aCL binding and can give false-positive results in the ELISA even in normal populations.[H201] This phenomenon is dependent on the duration and degree of heating, optimum levels being reached at 3 hours at 56°C. The heating effect is more pronounced for IgG aCL than for IgM aCLs. This finding suggests that the presence of a serum or plasma heat-sensitive component may prevent aCL binding in ELISA. High temperature inactivates this component and allows the binding of aCLs to cardiolipin.

On the other hand, when sera incubations in the second step of the ELISA are performed at 4 to 22°C, both IgG and IgM aCLs are easily detectable in positive patients. In contrast, when the incubations are done at 37 to 45°C, IgG aCL binding markedly decreases, but IgM aCL binding does not. Although the reason for this change of binding may relate to some change in the configuration of the antigen or the antibody, a satisfactory explanation is not yet available.[L355]

In summary, it is now possible to recommend the following conditions for performing accurate ELISA assays for aCLs: 1) do not heat test sera; 2) after incubating cardiolipin in plastic wells, block nonspecific binding with 10% fetal calf serum or 10% adult bovine serum in PBS; 3) add test sera to the wells at dilution of 1/50 to 1/100; 4) incubate the mixture for 1 to 2 hours at around 22°C (room temperature); and 5) measure immunoglobulin bound to cardiolipin with ^{125}I- or enzyme-labeled antihuman IgG and IgM.

Finally, a number of systems of reporting the results of the aCL assays have been described. These include binding index units, standard deviations, etc. In order to standardize the assay and to ensure both an easy and reliable way of reporting results, 30 laboratories from seven countries held an International Workshop in 1986.[H157] They recommend the use of GPL and MPL units, where 1 GPL unit was taken as the binding activity of 1 μg/ml of affinity-purified IgG aCL and 1 MPL unit, the binding activity of 1 μg/ml of affinity-purified IgM aCL.

However, a relatively wide variation of results still occurs for a single sample, both on interassays and between different laboratories performing the test. In an attempt to achieve better concordance of results, a semiquantitative manner of reporting results was recommended by the Second Standardization Workshop conducted in 1988. It was then suggested that sample results should be reported as high, medium, or low positive (Table 24–2).[H160]

Characteristics

It has become evident that aCLs are a heterogeneous group of autoantibodies with different characteristics.[H154]

As only a minority of patients with aCLs develop thrombotic complications, possible explanations for the differences between "innocent" and pathogenic antibodies may be attributed to isotypic diversity as well as to differences in binding specificities, avidities, idiotypes, and associated genetic and environmental factors. Although no definitive correlations between these aCL characteristics and clinical features have been clearly demonstrated, some of these may be considered in more detail.

Isotype

Various investigators have shown that aCLs in SLE are predominantly of the IgG—mainly IgG2 and IgG4—and the IgM isotypes.[A100,C183,F151,G115,L392,S57] The development of thrombosis, fetal loss, and thrombocytopenia is mainly related to the presence of the IgG isotype. On the other hand, some authors have found an association between the IgM isotype and the development of hemolytic anemia and neutropenia.[A91,C183,D138,D139] In certain diseases, such as Sjögren's syndrome, there may be a predominance of the IgA isotype. This latter isotype has also been correlated with severe forms of the Guillain-Barré syndrome[F194] and with recurrent abortions.[K42]

Quantity

High levels of IgG aCLs are the most predictive and specific markers for thrombosis, recurrent fetal loss, and thrombocytopenia.[C183,H150] However, serial measurements show fluctuations in aCL levels. Two aspects related to this fact have received special attention. First, some patients demonstrate persistently positive levels of IgG aCLs, while other patients show elevated levels only during active phases of SLE, which regress with treatment.[146,O125] Still others exhibit wide fluctuations in titer independent of disease activity and of therapy. Those with persistently positive levels seem to be more predisposed to develop the above-mentioned complications. Second, some aCL-positive patients show a drop in level immediately prior to the time when the thrombotic complication occurs, suggesting possible aCL "consumption" by the thrombotic event.[A100] This interesting finding must be taken into careful consideration because if the aCL level is only measured during or immediately following a thrombotic event, some aCL-positive patients might be misconstrued as negative.

Binding Specificity

Most aCLs bind to cardiolipin and also to other negatively charged phospholipids, such as phosphatidic acid, phosphatidylserine, or phosphatidylinositol, and a minority even bind to neutral phospholipids, such as phosphatidylethanolamine. This cross-reactivity may be because of similarities in structure, charge, or configuration. However, the exact site of binding of aCLs is unknown. Although it was thought that the phosphodiester groups were the sites bound by these antibodies, removal of the glyceride portion of the molecule also results in loss of antigenicity. This suggests that the glyceride moiety is essential for antibody binding, probably helping the orien-

Substituted Group

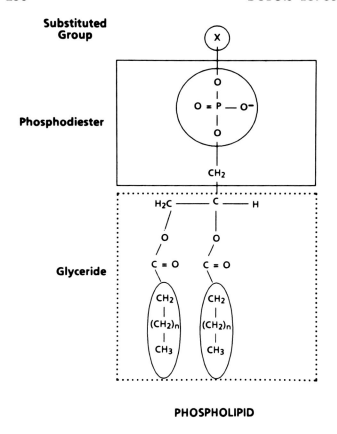

Phosphodiester

Glyceride

PHOSPHOLIPID

Fig. 24–1. Diagrammatic representation of a phospholipid molecule. Access of antibody to the phosphodiester group may depend on the charge of the substituent X. If X is positively charged (e.g., choline, ethanolamine), there may be charge-charge interaction between X and the negatively charged phosphodiester group. The latter interaction will block access to the phosphodiester group by aPLs. If X has no charge (serine, inositol) or is a hydrogen (phosphatidic acid), the phosphodiester group is available for binding.

tation of the phosphodiester group into a configuration best bound by aCLs (Fig. 24–1). In addition, studies with monoclonal aCLs have shown considerable conformational specificity, with the ability to distinguish between phospholipids in lamellar and hexagonal forms.[H146]

Avidity

Some investigators have reported positive titers of aCLs in patients with high levels of anti-DNA antibodies. In these cases, inhibition studies with pure cardiolipin and DNA disclosed a partial cross-reactivity between these two groups of antibodies.[H158] Therefore, it has been suggested that some aCLs with low avidity for cardiolipin may also react with DNA and vice versa. However, it has been confirmed that monoclonal aCLs with high avidity for cardiolipin have no reactivity against DNA. In addition, some low-avidity aCLs may also react with other antigens (mitochondria, endothelial cells, etc.) and exhibit a partial cross-reactivity with type M5 antimitochondrial antibod-

ies,[M358] antiendothelial cell antibodies,[C185a,V90] or IgM rheumatoid factor.[A60]

Idiotype

Some interesting considerations have come from the work of Krause et al.[K412] These authors have examined the presence of two idiotypes of aCLs—the so-called 1.10 and H3—in four groups of subjects: patients with SLE, with primary APS, with monoclonal gammopathies, and a healthy population. Patients with SLE and primary APS carry aCLs that are thought to participate in the pathogenesis of the disease, while patients with monoclonal gammopathies represent a population that produces aCLs, but usually does not develop any aCL-related complications. The idiotype 1.10 is a mouse monoclonal antibody generated following immunization of mice with polyclonal aCLs derived from a patient with active SLE. It was detected more frequently among patients with primary APS and SLE than in patients with monoclonal gammopathies. The idiotype H3 is another mouse monoclonal antibody that was generated following immunization of mice with a human monoclonal aCL called H3. Conversely, this was mainly detected in patients with monoclonal gammopathies. These findings indicate that idiotypic diversity exists among aCLs derived from different sources, and some of these may be more pathogenic than others.

Genetic Factors

An increased prevalence of raised aCL levels has been found in the first-degree relatives of SLE and primary APS patients compared with normal subjects.[F155] Conflicting reports have been published on the association between aCLs and HLA antigens. Savi et al.[S98] found an increased prevalence of HLA-DR7 in northern Italian SLE patients with aCLs. McHugh and Maddison[M290] described an association with DR4 in patients from Great Britain. In another study from Australia,[M313] the prevalence of DR3 and DRw52 was found to be reduced, whereas DR4 and DRw53 were increased in nonlupus aCL-positive patients undergoing coronary artery bypass graft surgery. A trend for a negative association between aCLs and both DR2 and DR3 was also found by Sebastiani et al.[S246] in Italian SLE patients, while Galleazzi et al.[G10] demonstrated that aCLs were positively associated with DPB14 and negatively associated with DPB13. Arnett et al.[A299] have determined the HLA-DR and DQ alleles by restriction fragment length polymorphisms in SLE patients with and without aPLs. The HLA-DQw7 (DQB1*0301) allele, linked to HLA-DR5 and DR4 haplotypes, was significantly increased compared to race-matched normal controls. Moreover, its frequency was significantly higher in SLE patients with aPLs as compared with patients without aPLs but with other autoantibodies. The discrepancies in some of these results might be purely methodologic, perhaps depending on the regional frequency of the various HLA alleles, or patient samples from different regions may differ in part in their genetic composition. Genes encoding a human monoclonal aCL have been sequenced,[S452] opening new avenues in the study of genetics of aCLs.

Environmental Factors

It has been postulated that aPLs may arise in response to foreign antigens. Not only is cardiolipin an effective immunogen in experimental animals,[L10] but raised levels of aCLs are frequently found in a number of infections, e.g., spirochetal, such as Lyme disease,[M30] and in certain conditions caused by "envelope" viruses. Only on rare occasions do these patients present thrombotic complications. Unpublished data from our laboratory support the concept that lipids present on the outer coating of these viruses lead to elevations of aCLs as well as to antibodies directed against glycolipids. (Asherson RA. Personal communication, 1992.)[A314a]

CHRONIC BIOLOGIC FALSE-POSITIVE SEROLOGIC TESTS FOR SYPHILIS

BFP-STS are frequently found in patients with SLE. Conversely, it is well established that some patients with chronic BFP-STS will eventually develop a connective tissue disease, most commonly SLE. As these tests detect the presence of antibodies against cardiolipin mixed with phosphatidylcholine and cholesterol, their study shares some similarities with that of aPLs detected by a solid-phase assay.

Historical Considerations

In 1906, Wassermann discovered "reagin," an antibody that reacted with an antigen located in alcohol extracts of liver from a fetus with congenital syphilis. Over the succeeding 3 to 4 decades, it was apparent that other tissues were also a good source of this antigen, especially beef cardiac muscle. In 1941, Pangborn[P28] showed that the antigen was a phospholipid which was named cardiolipin. The subsequent use of pure cardiolipin with phosphatidylcholine and cholesterol enabled the development of several precipitation and complement-fixation techniques to detect reagin.

Keil's 1940 classic paper[K146] was the first to demonstrate BFP-STS in SLE in 10 patients. Subsequently, during World War II several people were identified with positive tests, but without clinical evidence of syphilis.[M559] In 1948, the development by Nelson and Mayer[N64] of a specific test for the detection of Treponema pallidum, the treponemal immobilization (TPI) test, allowed better identification of these false-positive reactors. It was apparent that the BFP-STS may occur transiently, usually as a result of an acute infection (Table 24–3), or might last

Table 24–3. Acute Infections in Which BFP-STS May Occur Transiently

Bacterial	Plasmodial
Leprosy	Malaria
Chancroid	Rickettsial
Scarlatina	Typhus
Tuberculosis	Protozoal
Pneumonia	Trypanosomiasis
Endocarditis	Viral
Spirochetal	Vaccinia
Relapsing fever	Lymphogranuloma venereum
Rat-bite fever	Infectious hepatitis
Leptospirosis	Measles
	Rubella

for greater than 6 months (chronic BFP-STS reactors). In 1955, Moore and Lutz[M558] showed that patients in the latter category had a high incidence of autoimmune disorders, especially SLE.

Frequency

BFP-STS in SLE Patients

The prevalence of BFP-STS in SLE patients varies between 11 and 29%, as assessed in the largest series.[D340,E147] This range of variation may be explained by 1) the sensitivity of the test performed; 2) the number of different tests done on each serum sample; 3) the stage of the disease (BFP-STS may disappear with treatment or remission); 4) the frequency of the tests during the course of the disease; and 5) the accuracy of the exclusion of syphilis by more specific tests.

Interestingly, BFP-STS may also be observed in drug-induced SLE although this is unusual.[A194] The prevalence of BFP-STS in discoid lupus is also low. Rowell[R376] reported a prevalence of 5% in patients with discoid lupus, as compared to 22% in patients with SLE. In addition, the frequency of BFP-STS in other rheumatic conditions, such as rheumatoid arthritis, Sjögren's syndrome, or ankylosing spondylitis seems to be extremely low.

The presence of BFP-STS has also been demonstrated in certain experimental mouse models of SLE. Norins et al.[N128] reported positive tests in 3% mice of the NZB strain but not in mice of the A/J strain. However, in the (A/J × NZB) F_1 hybrid, the prevalence was 15%.

SLE in BFP-STS Reactors

The prevalence of SLE among BFP reactors varies between 5 and 19% in the largest series.[C160,M558] A smaller percentage of BFP reactors develop other autoimmune disorders, such as rheumatoid arthritis.[C160]

Methods of Detection

The Wassermann test for the diagnosis of syphilis employed the complement-fixation technique to detect the reaction between a lipid-tissue antigen and an antibody (reagin) in syphilitic serum. When first introduced, the test utilized extracts of human syphilitic organs as antigen. Subsequently, it was found that suitable antigen could be prepared from normal organs of humans and other mammals. The Wassermann reaction was modified, refined, and simplified by the use of flocculation techniques and the development of new serologic tests. Designed to give maximal sensitivity and specificity for the clinical diagnosis of syphilis, each test, for the most part, bears the name of the developer; e.g., Eagle, Hinton, Kahn, Kline, Kolmer, and Mazzini.

Related tests have replaced those listed above. The standard in use today is the Veneral Disease Research Laboratory (VDRL) test, an easily quantitated slide flocculation procedure. Others frequently used include the rapid plasma reagin (RPR), circle card agglutination screen, and unheated serum reagin (USR). All are simple, inexpensive, and well standardized.

Characteristics

The exact relationship between aPLs responsible for positive STS and those for LA and/or aCL tests is not clearly determined. Antibodies from patients with both SLE or related disorders and with syphilis bind to cardiolipin in solid-phase immunoassays, but only aPLs from patients with autoimmune disorders are associated with thrombosis and recurrent fetal losses. In addition, the VDRL titer correlates with aPL levels in sera from syphilis patients, but not from those with autoimmunity.[L365] Finally, LA activity is uncommon in patients with syphilis. The reasons for these discrepancies probably relate not only to the different composition of the antigens used in these tests but also to the great heterogeneity of aPLs associated with autoimmune diseases and syphilis.

Although the aPLs present in syphilis patients do not bind phosphatidylcholine or cholesterol, inclusion of these auxiliary lipids in the VDRL antigen increases the binding to cardiolipin. In contrast, aPLs in patients with autoimmune disorders bind cardiolipin less well when cardiolipin is mixed with phosphatidylcholine and cholesterol.[H159] Hence, mixing cardiolipin with these auxiliary lipids to form the VDRL antigen somehow alters the conformation of cardiolipin to enable more avid binding by syphilis sera and less avid binding by autoimmune sera.

On the other hand, while aPLs in patients with autoimmune disorders mainly bind cardiolipin and other negatively charged phospholipids, which are essential cellular components involved in a variety of cellular functions,[H159] binding to neutral phospholipids is largely restricted to sera from patients with syphilis[L365] (Table 24–4).

Taking all these studies together strongly suggests that

Table 24–4. Different Characteristics of aPLs in Patients with Syphilis and with Autoimmune Disorders

	Syphilis	Autoimmune Disorders
Binding to cardiolipin when mixed with phosphatidylcholine and cholesterol	↑	↓
Binding to negatively charged phospholipids	↓	↑
Binding to neutral phospholipids	↑	↓

the primary structure of the phospholipid as well as the configuration and charge are important for the binding of aPLs, probably both in the solid-phase assays and in vivo.

OTHER ANTIPHOSPHOLIPID ANTIBODIES

Although aCLs are the best-studied aPLs, antibodies directed against other negatively charged and neutral phospholipids may also be detected in patients with SLE and a thrombotic tendency.[S626,T221] Some of the best studied include antibodies to phosphatidylserine, phosphatidylinositol, phosphatidic acid, thromboplastin, phosphatidylcholine, phosphatidylethanolamine, and sphingomyelin. These phospholipids share some similarities in structure with cardiolipin (Fig. 24–2). Moreover, the presence of these aPLs, although variable, is usually associated with the presence of aCLs. Weidmann et al.[W125a] confirmed the strong relationship of these other aPLs with aCLs, with the exception of antibodies directed against phosphatidylethanolamine. Reports of patients with thrombotic complications demonstrating other aPLs in the absence of aCLs are unusual.[S626]

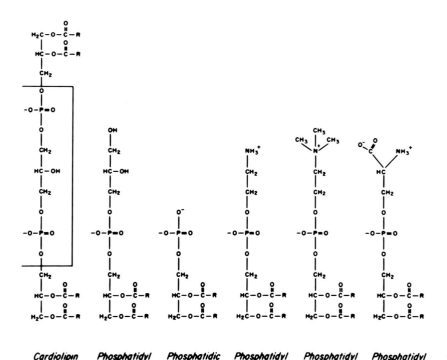

Cardiolipin	*Phosphatidyl Glycerol*	*Phosphatidic Acid*	*Phosphatidyl Ethanolamine*	*Phosphatidyl Choline*	*Phosphatidyl Serine*

Fig. 24–2. Diagrammatic representation of several phospholipid molecules.

Methods of Detection

Detection of these antibodies may also be performed by means of ELISA using either the pure phospholipid or a mixture of phospholipids (diluted in chloroform) as antigens. López-Soto et al.[L379] found that the detection of antibodies against bovine thromboplastin (mixture of phospholipids) is more closely related to the detection of LA activity than that of aCLs or other aPLs. However, detection of these other aPLs generally provides little additional information and few laboratories perform these tests routinely.

MECHANISMS OF ACTION

The exact mechanism by which aPLs cause the antiphospholipid syndrome is still unknown. In fact, whether these antibodies are the main cause of the clinical manifestations related to the antiphospholipid syndrome, or epiphenomena accompanying more basic underlying immunologic disturbances, is still unclear.

Since phospholipids are essential constituents of cell membranes and also play an integral part in the major hemostatic pathways, most of the efforts to elucidate the mechanisms of thrombosis in patients with aPLs have been based on the effects of these antibodies on endothelial cell and platelet functions. In addition, the requirement for a serum cofactor in order to enhance the binding of aPLs to phospholipids has been demonstrated. However, it has become evident that there may be more than one mechanism causing thrombosis in patients with aPLs, and that these mechanisms may vary from patient to patient[K184] (Fig. 24–3).

Effects of aPLs on Endothelial Cells

Endothelial cells are strategically positioned to play an important role in the regulation of vascular homeostasis. They have been considered as possible targets for immune-mediated attacks because they are constantly in contact with circulating immune effectors. Carreras and Vermylen[C105] postulated that aPLs may bind to endothelial cells and thereby reduce the release of prostacyclin, which is a potent vasodilator and inhibitor of platelet aggregation. Other authors, however, could not confirm this hypothesis.[H198,R437] It has subsequently been proposed that aPLs may interfere with the function of several endothelial cell proteins that play an important role in the procoagulant or fibrinolytic pathways. These include thrombomodulin, protein C and S, tissue plasminogen activator and its inhibitor, von Willebrand factor, and the placental anticoagulant protein.[B611,C87,C360,K187,R415,S57]

Vismara et al.[V90] demonstrated that affinity-purified aCLs from SLE sera bind living human endothelial cells, and that the binding does not occur nonspecifically via the Fc receptors since blocking of Fc receptors with rabbit IgG did not affect the endothelial cell reactivity.

Additional support for this hypothesis comes from a study of antiendothelial cell antibodies. These are a group of autoantibodies directed against antigens located in the cytoplasmic membrane of endothelial cells. Their physiologic and clinical importance relates to the fact that they have been detected in a variety of immunologic disorders that have in common the presence of vascular lesions. Vismara et al.[V90] found in a group of SLE patients having both aCLs and antiendothelial cell antibodies that cardiolipin liposomes inhibited not only aCL activity but also, partially, antiendothelial cell antibody activity. Studies by the groups from Hospital Clínic in Barcelona and St. Thomas' Hospital in London[C185a] have detected a high prevalence of antiendothelial cell antibodies not only in patients with SLE but also in patients with primary APS. However, these antibodies were not found in patients with thrombosis without aPLs. In contrast to this, Rosenbaum et al.[R302] found no relationship between antiendo-

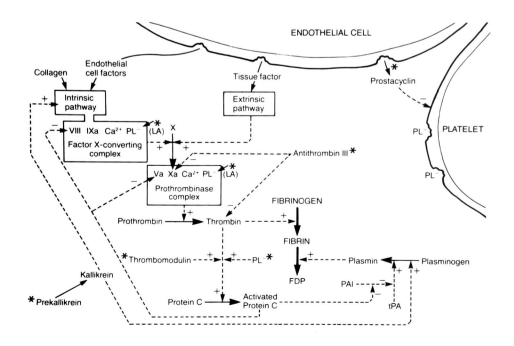

Fig. 24–3. Highly simplified diagram illustrating possible sites of interaction (X) of antiphospholipid antibodies in the clotting process. (PAI = plasminogen activator inhibitor, tPA = tissue plasminogen activator, FDP = fibrin degradation products, PL = anionic phospholipids, LA = lupus anticoagulant, __+__ > indicates promotion and __−__ > inhibition of a pathway [→]). From Mackworth-Young, C.: Antiphospholipid antibodies: More than just a disease marker? Immunol. Today, 11:60, 1990.

thelial cell antibodies and aPLs or thrombosis in patients with SLE, scleroderma, and rheumatoid arthritis. Therefore, although aPLs and antiendothelial cell antibodies seem to be two different families of antibodies, some aPLs may be part of the antiendothelial cell antibody family in certain patients with SLE or primary APS. On the other hand, the role of endothelial cell adhesion molecules in the genesis of platelet aggregation in patients with APS remains to be elucidated.

Effects of aPLs on Platelets

Another hypothesis is that aPLs may bind to platelets causing activation and thrombosis,[H147] or simply increase destruction in the reticuloendothelial system.[H153] Pierangeli et al.[P183] have demonstrated binding of affinity-purified IgG aCLs to intact platelet membranes by electron microscopy using gold-labeled protein A probes. Other studies have also demonstrated binding of murine monoclonal aPLs to both resting and activated platelets.[K353,R58,R334]

However, other authors have reported that aPLs can only bind to activated or partially destroyed platelets. Mikhail et al.[M407] demonstrated binding of affinity-purified aCLs to activated but not resting platelets. Khamashta et al.[K187] showed that aCLs may be absorbed by, and subsequently eluted from, freeze-thawed but not intact platelets. These authors also showed that aCLs bind to phospholipids located in the inner leaflet of the platelet membrane only. This indicates that this type of damage to the platelets may shift negatively charged phospholipids to the outer leaflet, and is necessary for aCLs to react with the platelets. Haga et al.,[H17] by flow-cytometric studies, confirmed that there was no significant specific binding of IgG aCLs to resting or to activated platelets, while significant binding was observed to freeze-thawed platelets.

The effect of aPLs on in vitro platelet aggregation has also been studied. Frampton et al.[F191] reported that purified aPLs enhanced production of thromboxane—a pro-aggregating factor—by activated, but not unstimulated, platelets. Escolar et al.[E138] also showed that the presence of aPLs in SLE plasma promotes platelet aggregation under flow conditions. However, others[H17] found no increased platelet aggregation responses to ADP by turbidometric techniques in vitro.

These conflicting reports emphasize the methodologic problems involved in studying binding of immunoglobulins to platelets in general. Additionally, they may reflect the heterogeneity of aPLs used. Interestingly, Rote et al.[R334] demonstrated that monoclonal IgM antiphosphatidylserine but not aCLs reacted slightly with resting, but significantly more with thrombin-activated platelets.

The Role of a Cofactor on the Effect of aPLs

It has been demonstrated that aPLs require the presence of a serum cofactor in vitro in order to bind to phospholipids. Galli et al.[G15] found that, in comparison with nonspecific IgG, there was no net binding of affinity-purified aCLs to cardiolipin-coated ELISA plates or cardiolipin-containing liposomes unless plasma or a protein purified from plasma was present.

Working in another laboratory, McNeil et al.[M15] also noted that when aCLs containing fractions derived from ion-exchange chromatography of plasma were applied to phosphatidylserine or cardiolipin affinity columns, there was no binding of the antibody, despite the fact that when plasma containing these antibodies was applied to these columns, aCLs could be purified. This also suggested that there was a cofactor present in plasma or serum which was required for aCLs to bind to the affinity columns. Addition of normal (aCL-negative) plasma or serum to the ion-exchange fractions resulted in aCLs binding to the columns, supporting this hypothesis. Subsequently, both groups were able to purify the cofactor to homogeneity and identify it as β_2-glycoprotein I, also known as apolipoprotein H.

There is thus strong evidence that aPLs from patients with autoimmune disorders are directed against a complex antigen of which β_2-glycoprotein I is an essential component. Affinity-purified aPLs from these patients fail to bind to cardiolipin coated on ELISA wells unless exogenous β_2-glycoprotein I is added. In contrast, aPL fractions from patients with infections, including syphilis, bind directly to the phospholipids in the absence of β_2-glycoprotein I.[M314]

This glycoprotein is well known to inhibit the intrinsic pathway of coagulation, to act as an antiprothrombinase in vitro, to bind to activated protein C, to interact with heparin and to inhibit ADP-dependent platelet aggregation. This raises the possibility that β_2-glycoprotein I may bind to platelets and this could be a cellular epitope for aPL binding, thus predisposing to thrombotic events. Alternatively, since β_2-glycoprotein I demonstrates homology with a number of complement receptors and some cell surface adhesion molecules, the possibility of cross-reactions with these structures represents an attractive hypothesis.[M314]

CLINICAL SIGNIFICANCE

Vascular occlusive manifestations, spontaneous fetal losses, and thrombocytopenia are the main complications associated with the presence of aPL.[A323] In fact, these are relatively frequent events in the course of SLE and their prevalence, clinical characteristics, treatment, and prognosis are reviewed in other sections of this book. Several specific considerations relating to their association with aPLs require special attention.

Occlusive Vascular Manifestations

The majority of clinical manifestations described as being associated with aPLs may be explained by the coexistence of vascular occlusions or thrombosis, either of veins, arteries, or endocardium.

It was originally thought that large vessels seemed to be mainly affected in patients with these antibodies. Deep vein thrombosis (occasionally superficial thrombophlebitis) particularly affecting the veins of the lower limbs were the commonest venous occlusions seen.[C183,H150] Strokes, often preceded by transient ischemic attacks, were the most frequent arterial events encountered in these patients.[A334,A339,B493,C410,F86,L221,L223]

Table 24–5. Main Occlusive Vascular Manifestations Associated with aPLs

Vessel Involved	Clinical Manifestations
Veins	
Limbs	Thrombophlebitis
Liver	
Large vessels	Budd-Chiari syndrome
Small vessels	Hepatomegaly, enzyme elevations
Adrenal glands	Addison's disease, hypoadrenalism
Lungs	Pulmonary embolism, thromboembolic pulmonary hypertension
Skin	Livedo reticularis, skin nodules, superficial macules resembling vasculitis, chronic leg ulcers
Eyes	Retinal vein thrombosis
Arteries	
Limbs	Ischemia, gangrene
Brain	
Large vessels	Stroke, transient ischemic attacks, Sneddon's syndrome*
Small vessels	Acute ischemic encephalopathy, multi-infarct dementia
Heart	
Large vessels	Myocardial infarction
Small vessels	
Acute	Circulatory collapse, cardiac arrest
Chronic	Cardiomyopathy, arrhythmia, bradycardia
Kidney	
Large vessels	Renal artery thrombosis
Small vessels	Renal thrombotic microangiopathy
Liver	Hepatic infarction
Aorta	
Arch vessels	Aortic arch syndrome
Abdominal	Claudication
Skin	Digital gangrene
Eyes	Retinal artery and arteriolar thrombosis
Endocardium	
Valves	
Acute	Vegetations, pseudoinfective endocarditis
Chronic	Valve dysfunction (regurgitation, stenosis), cerebral embolism
Chambers	Thrombus, pseudotumour, cerebral embolism

* Sneddon's syndrome is the association of cerebrovascular accident, hypertension, and livedo reticularis.

However, it soon became evident that not only may a large variety of both veins and arteries be affected but that small vessels might also be involved. Therefore, many diverse clinical manifestations due to vascular occlusions in the liver,[A130,A335,G365,M565,N23,P125] adrenal glands,[A157,A183,A329,A330,C79,I15,L229,R42,Y35] lungs,[A208,E74,J61] heart,[A322,A333,A338,A343,B520,C183,C185b,G24,K185,L205,M669,N98,S527a] kidney,[F192a,K54,K229,L114,O116] skin[A130,A338b,M292,Q7a,W142] eyes,[J102] etc., may now be associated with the presence of aPLs (Table 24–5). Other conditions, where no definitive histopathologic or radiologic evidence of vascular occlusions has as yet been confirmed, are less strongly associated[A321,A326,A332,F194,I96,N5,R190,Z38b] (Table 24–6). The evolving concepts of APS have recently been reviewed in detail.[A318a]

Spontaneous Fetal Losses

Recurrent fetal losses occur in patients with the APS whether in association with defined SLE, lupus-like disease

Table 24–6. Other Manifestations Possibly Associated with aPLs

Neurologic
  Chorea
  Transverse myelitis
  Guillain-Barré syndrome
  Psychosis
Bone
  Avascular necrosis
Pulmonary
  Nonthromboembolic pulmonary hypertension
Hepatic
  Nodular regenerative hyperplasia
Hematologic
  Thrombocytopenia
  Hemolytic anemia
  Evans's syndrome*
  Neutropenia

* Evans's syndrome is the association of autoimmune thrombocytopenic purpura and hemolytic anemia.

(probable SLE), or in the context of primary APS. They can occur in any trimester of pregnancy, although they are commoner in the second and third trimester.

There are a number of mechanisms that have been proposed in order to explain how these fetal losses occur. The most accepted implies that fetal losses are associated with thrombosis of the placental vessels and subsequent infarction resulting in placental insufficiency, fetal growth retardation, and ultimately fetal loss.[L350,L354,W49] Not all placentas examined, however, have shown areas of thrombosis or infarction and other mechanisms may be operative in these patients. See Chapters 50–52.

Thrombocytopenia

Several authors[C183,D138,D139,H147,H150] have demonstrated a strong association between thrombocytopenia and the presence of aPLs, mainly IgG aCLs, in patients with SLE. It is usually mild (70,000 to 120,000 platelets/mm^3), benign, and does not require any active intervention. In addition, aPLs have also been detected in patients with idiopathic thrombocytopenic purpura (ITP).[F151,H153] These may represent a separate and distinct subset of ITP patients prone to develop full-blown APS with thrombotic events or SLE in the future.[C182a] See Chapter 43.

The Antiphospholipid Syndrome

This term was introduced as a means of categorizing and studying those patients with vascular occlusive manifestations, recurrent fetal losses, and/or thrombocytopenia associated with raised levels of aPLs.[H149,H476] The diagnosis of APS should be based both on clinical and serologic criteria (Table 24–7).

This condition may superficially resemble other thrombotic conditions such as thrombotic thrombocytopenic purpura (TTP), disseminated intravascular coagulation (DIC), cryoglobulinemia and other hypercoagulable states, or Raynaud's phenomenon with digital infarcts secondary to vascular pathology occurring particularly in pa-

Table 24–7. Criteria for Classification of the Antiphospholipid Syndrome (APS)*

Clinical	Laboratory
Venous thrombosis	IgG aCLs (moderate/high levels)
Arterial thrombosis	IgM aCLs (moderate/high levels)
Recurrent fetal loss	Positive LA test
Thrombocytopenia	

* Patients with the syndrome should have at least one clinical plus one laboratory finding during their disease. The aPL test must be positive on at least two occasions more than 3 months apart.

tients with "overlap" syndromes. The presence of extensive purpura, fluctuating neurologic signs and hemolytic anemia may assist in the differentiation of TTP. The diagnosis of DIC depends to a large extent on the presence of elevated fibrin split products as well as thrombocytopenia. DIC is rarely associated with aPLs, although several patients with SLE have developed this complication[A315] and occult pulmonary embolism, common in patients with APS, may be the only manifestation of DIC.[M678a] The presence of cryoglobulins or the deficiency of protein C or S or antithrombin III will lead to the diagnosis of specific hypercoagulable states. Finally, the diagnosis of Raynaud's phenomenon with digital infarcts will be made more in the setting of the typical clinical pattern of an overlap syndrome than on laboratory findings.

The Primary Antiphospholipid Syndrome

Since 1988, several series have been documented detailing the major clinical and serologic characteristics of this syndrome.[A115,A316,A336,F155,M31] Essentially, these patients present features of any patient with APS, e.g., thrombosis (venous and/or arterial) and/or recurrent fetal losses, but without SLE or any other well-defined disease. A followup longer than 5 years is now considered necessary in order to rule out SLE and the other autoimmune disorders.

Some of these patients may, however, have a few clinical manifestations resembling SLE or other connective tissue disorders. The clear separation of this group of patients and those with SLE and lupus-like disease is important. They may also demonstrate valve lesions (affecting mitral valves particularly) but not as frequently as in APS patients associated with SLE.[B473a,C185b] Patients with primary APS essentially do not have any of the flares (fever, arthralgias, myalgias), polyserositis, immune complex type nephritis, or noncerebrovascular neurologic disease seen in patients with SLE and lupus-like disease. They do not usually have other features closely associated with SLE such as Raynaud's phenomenon, alopecia, mouth ulcers, or butterfly rashes, but they may demonstrate vasculitic skin rashes. Serologically, the antinuclear antibody level may be negative or low positive. Antibodies to dsDNA, estimated by the Crithidia or Farr assays, are usually negative. However, in some patients, presumably in those more closely related to SLE, low-affinity anti-dsDNA antibodies may be demonstrable by ELISA. Antibodies to ENA are absent. Other immunologic disturbances such as

rheumatoid factor, cryoglobulinemia, or immune complexes may also be present. A number of patients may demonstrate a low C4 level. In these cases, further studies are awaited in order to determine whether the low complement levels are because of complement activation or to a null allele at the C4a or C4b locus. A family history of SLE or other autoimmune disease may be elicitable.

The value of aPL determination in a variety of thrombotic conditions has been the realization that:

1. Patients previously identified as suffering from so-called idiopathic vascular occlusions are now classifiable as suffering from primary APS—thus, some patients with Sneddon's syndrome, Budd-Chiari syndrome, pregnancy-related or postpartum renal failure, and Addison's disease/hypoadrenalism are now clearly identifiable as belonging to this category.
2. A percentage of patients suffering from these conditions now have a basic identifiable coagulopathy that may require specific treatment.

The "Catastrophic" Antiphospholipid Syndrome

A minority of patients with aPLs may develop an acute and catastrophic APS characterized by widespread vascular occlusions involving multiple organs. Ten such patients are documented and reviewed in the literature.[A315] These patients have in common the following:

1. Clinical evidence of multiple organ involvement (three or more): severe renal dysfunction often accompanied by accelerated or malignant hypertension; central nervous system symptomatology often heralded by behavior disturbances, but ending in disturbances of consciousness such as stupor and evidence of focal vascular disturbances, e.g., hemiparesis; respiratory difficulties such as the clinical and radiologic picture of adult respiratory distress syndrome; skin manifestations such as livedo reticularis, acrocyanosis, or ischemic ulcerations and gangrene; or other organ failure from multiple fibrin thrombi occluding small vessels, e.g., myocardial arteriolar thromboses, adrenal vessel occlusion, hepatic infarction and, rarely, ischemic bowel ulceration.
2. Histopathologic evidence of multiple large and small vessel occlusion.
3. Serologic confirmation of the presence of aPLs, usually in high titer. Other features of APS, such as thrombocytopenia, are also frequent. If the patient has SLE, activity of the disease is usually mild or absent, with low levels of antibodies to dsDNA.

Pediatric Antiphospholipid Syndromes

Unlike the study of adults with APS, there are comparatively few reports on the frequency of aPL-associated conditions in the pediatric literature.

Shergy et al.[S352] have reported that up to 50% of children with SLE have aPLs and that the clinical manifestations are similar to those encountered in adults, particularly recurrent deep vein thrombosis, strokes, chorea, renal artery thrombosis, or hypoadrenalism. These may be seen in infants as young as 9 months of age[R256a] ranging through childhood to adolescence.[K148a,P95a]

Additionally, there have been several reports of aortic thrombosis in neonates caused by maternal transfer of IgG aCLs.[F88a,S352a]

Management

An approach to the management of patients with aPLs, who essentially present with features common to other hypercoagulable states, could be to proceed as in patients with known risk factors for the development of vascular occlusions, such as excessive smoking, hypertension, or hypercholesterolemia. This implies, first, attempting to eliminate the aPLs, and, second, the appropriate use of antiaggregant, anticoagulant, and fibrinolytic drugs, following indications previously established for prophylaxis and therapy of occlusive venous and arterial disease. Several specific comments are necessary.

Elimination of aPLs

Although energetic immunosuppression, e.g., with pulse cyclophosphamide, plasmapheresis, or gamma globulin infusions is sometimes effective in reducing elevated antibody levels, there is usually a rapid rebound to pretreatment levels shortly after discontinuation of the therapy. In addition, only about one-third of patients with aPLs will develop thrombotic manifestations, and there is no evidence based on adequate clinical trials that the administration of steroids or immunosuppression will prevent these thrombotic events. Finally, it is still unclear whether the aPLs themselves are pathogenetic or occur as epiphenomena related to more basic underlying disturbances. Therefore, prophylaxis and therapy should not primarily be directed at reducing these antibody levels, and the use of immunotherapy is generally not indicated, unless required for the treatment of the underlying condition, e.g., SLE.

Removal of Additional Risk Factors

Energetic attempts must be made to avoid or to treat any associated risk factors—e.g., antihypertensives, cholesterol-lowering agents, treatment of active nephritis, avoidance of smoking or sedentarism, etc. Care should be also taken with the administration of oral contraceptives in patients with aPLs. There is some evidence that their administration may result in complications such as vascular occlusions or chorea.[A325]

Prophylaxis to Prevent Occlusive Vascular Complications in Patients Who Have Not Experienced Thrombosis

Prophylaxis of arterial thrombosis in the general population is controversial, as it is in patients with aPLs. In some trials within the general population and in patients with arteriosclerotic or hypertensive vascular disease,[A260] the longterm use of aspirin has proven useful in the prevention of arterial occlusions, mainly of coronary vessels. Comparison between these groups of patients with overt

vascular disease and those with aPLs may be invalid. However, there may be a case for the prophylactic treatment of individuals with high levels of IgG aCLs or persistent LA activity using antiaggregants such as aspirin, especially in those with added risk factors. Hydroxychloroquine has also been shown to have an antiaggregant effect and its use may be considered.

On the other hand, prophylaxis of venous thrombosis is required for patients undergoing surgical procedures or who require a long stay in bed. In the general population, the use of low-dose subcutaneous heparin (10,000 to 15,000 units/day) is recommended in those circumstances. However, patients with aPLs may show some resistance to these doses, as in other hypercoagulable states, and these doses may be insufficient for the prevention of recurrent thrombosis. It is therefore suggested that higher doses of subcutaneous heparin (25,000 units/day) or the use of intravenous heparin (40,000 units/day) be administered to these patients.

Treatment of Occlusive Vascular Complications

In the general population, indications for antiaggregant, anticoagulant, or fibrinolytic agents, for the treatment of arterial and venous thrombosis depend on the localization of the occlusion and its clinical characteristics. Experience in the treatment of patients with aPLs and vascular complications is short and based mainly on retrospective studies. Until prospective and controlled studies become available, the same procedures as apply to the general population should be followed. However, four special considerations must be emphasized in case of anticoagulation for patients with venous or arterial thrombosis:

1. Because of the tendency to recurrence, patients require anticoagulation on a longterm basis, and probably for life.
2. Warfarin resistance has been encountered in several of these patients, who may require up to 20 mg/day of warfarin in order to achieve an international normalization ratio (INR) within a therapeutic range—the INR in patients with aPLs should be kept at a level of 3 to 4 rather than at 2 to 2.5.
3. In the case of using heparin, anticoagulation should be controlled by the recalcification test (Howell test) and not by the activated partial thromboplastin test (APTT) because of the interference of the LA with the latter. The principle of the recalcification test depends on the addition of calcium chloride to platelet-rich plasma, which will initiate the coagulation process. The time taken for a "soft" clot to form is compared with normal standards from patients without heparin (5 to 7 minutes). Ideally, heparinized patients will take 10 to 15 minutes for clot formation. This is not an exact test but, in fact, is the only possible method of monitoring patients with prolonged APTT because of LA.
4. Because of the common finding of fluctuating levels of the anticoagulation control tests, frequent and regular visits to anticoagulation clinics must be recommended, as well as instruction of patients and

medical personnel as to the dangers of noncompliance.

Treatment of Catastrophic APS

This depends on early recognition of the syndrome and the early administration of effective anticoagulation, plasmapheresis, and perhaps, pulse steroids and immunosuppression. The use of streptokinase or other fibrinolytic agents in these resistant hypercoagulable patients may have to be considered. Concomitant hypertension and renal failure also need effective treatment.[A315]

Prevention of Fetal Losses

The presence of aPLs in pregnant women in the absence of a previous history of fetal loss is not an indication for treatment. In those with previous spontaneous fetal losses or miscarriages, several therapeutic approaches have been proposed, including subcutaneous heparin,[L401,R322d] steroids,[O92,P285] azathioprine,[B456] etc., but no controlled studies have as yet been performed.[W49] However, low-dose (30 to 80 mg/day) aspirin administered from the beginning of pregnancy has proven useful and safe in an acceptable number of women with aPLs, and we concur with this view, as our experience thus far has mirrored that of others.[B42,E70] Because of the risk of hemorrhagic complications in both the newborn and the mother, aspirin should be ideally discontinued at least 48 to 72 hours prior to delivery. Some authorities advocate the use of moderate doses of prednisone (15 to 20 mg/day) in the face of a rising titer of aCLs. In addition, close monitoring of pregnancy with Doppler technique, in order to detect placental vascular insufficiency, and early delivery by Caesarean section with the first signs of fetal distress are mandatory. If the patient is receiving warfarin because of previous thrombotic manifestations, this must be changed to subcutaneous heparin, at least in the first trimester, since warfarin is teratogenic.

Treatment of Thrombocytopenia

Thrombocytopenia associated with aPLs is usually mild and does not require intervention. However, in a minority of cases it can be severe and refractory to prednisone therapy. Low-dose aspirin has proved useful in some cases,[A116,D182a,I63a] but its administration may not be without risk, especially in patients with less than 20,000 platelets/mm^3. In our experience, immunosuppressive therapy, i.e., with azathioprine, has been effective. Intravenous gamma globulin or danazol therapy can also be considered. In contrast, splenectomy should be considered with caution in patients with aPLs, because of the increased thromboembolic risk related to postsplenectomy thrombocytosis.[E171].

Summary 1.   Anticardiolipin Antibodies

1. Anticardiolipin antibodies (aCLs) are highly prevalent in SLE, being demonstrated in 20 to 50% of patients. However, they are not specific for SLE but may also be found in other connective tissue diseases, as well as in drug-induced lupus, and in malignant and infectious diseases.

2. The enzyme-linked immunosorbent assay (ELISA) is the most sensitive technique to detect aCLs. It is recommended that sample results should be reported as high-, medium-, or low-positive because of the correlation between the quantities of aCLs and the clinical manifestations.

3. Immunologically, aCLs are a heterogeneous group of autoantibodies with different characteristics. As only a minority of patients with aCLs develop complications, some possible explanations for the differences between innocent and pathogenic antibodies may be attributed to isotypic diversity as well as to differences in the quantities, binding specificity, avidity, idiotype, and associated genetic and environmental factors.

Summary 2.   The Chronic Biologic False-positive Serologic Tests for Syphilis

1. As the standard tests for syphilis detect the presence of antibodies against cardiolipin mixed with phosphatidylcholine and cholesterol, their properties share some similarities with those of the antiphospholipid antibodies (aPLs) detected by a solid-phase assay.

2. Chronic biologic false-positive standard tests for syphilis (BFP-STS) are found in 11 to 29% of cases of SLE.

3. Between 5 and 19% of BFP-STS reactors develop SLE. A smaller percentage develop other autoimmune disorders.

4. The exact relationship between aPLs responsible for positive STS and those for lupus anticoagulant and/or anticardiolipin antibody tests is not clearly determined. Antibodies from both patients with SLE and with syphilis bind to cardiolipin in solid-phase immunoassays, but only aPLs from patients with SLE are associated with thrombosis and recurrent fetal losses.

Summary 3.   Mechanisms of Action of the Antiphospholipid Antibodies

1. It is not known whether antiphospholipid antibodies (aPLs) are directly involved in the pathogenesis of the thrombotic events related to their presence or epiphenomena accompanying more basic underlying immunologic disturbances.

2. Since phospholipids are essential constituents of cell membranes and play an integral part in the hemostatic pathways, most of the efforts to elucidate the mechanisms of thrombosis in patients with aPLs have been based on the effects of these antibodies on endothelial cell and platelet function as well as on the fibrinolytic system.

3. The requirement for a serum cofactor in order to produce the effect of aPLs has been demonstrated. However, at this time it has become evident that there may be more than one mechanism causing thrombosis in patients with aPLs.

Summary 4.   Clinical Significance of the Antiphospholipid Antibodies

1. Vascular occlusive manifestations, spontaneous fetal losses, and thrombocytopenia are the main clinical complications associated with the presence of aPLs.

2. The term antiphospholipid syndrome (APS) was introduced as a means of categorizing and studying those patients with vascular occlusive manifestations, recurrent fetal losses, and/or thrombocytopenia associated with raised levels of aPLs.

3. This syndrome was seen mostly in patients with SLE or lupus-like illness, but other patients not suffering from SLE might exhibit features of APS. These patients are considered to suffer from primary APS. A followup longer than 2 years is now considered mandatory in order to rule out SLE and the other autoimmune disorders.

4. A minority of patients with aPLs may develop an acute catastrophic coagulation syndrome, which is characterized by vascular occlusions involving multiple organs.

Summary 5. Management of Patients with the Antiphospholipid Syndrome

1. Prophylaxis and therapy of the antiphospholipid syndrome (APS) should not primarily be directed at reducing the antiphospholipid antibody (aPL) levels. The use of immunotherapy is generally not indicated, unless required for the treatment of the underlying condition, e.g., SLE.
2. There may be a case for prophylaxis of thrombosis in individuals with high levels of aPLs of the IgG isotype, or persistent lupus anticoagulant activity, with antiaggregants, especially in those with added risk factors.
3. Treatment of patients with aPLs and vascular complications follows the same indications as in the general population. However, because of the tendency to recurrence, patients undergoing anticoagulation will require this on a longterm basis—probably for life—and, usually, higher doses of oral anticoagulants are necessary.
4. Low-dose (30 to 80 mg/day) aspirin administered from the beginning of pregnancy has proved useful and safe in an acceptable number of women with aPLs. Close monitoring of pregnancy with Doppler technique, in order to detect placental vascular insufficiency, and early delivery with the first signs of fetal distress are mandatory. If the patient is receiving warfarin because of previous thrombotic complications, this should be changed to subcutaneous heparin.

Chapter 25

THE LUPUS ANTICOAGULANT AND ANTICARDIOLIPIN ANTIBODIES

DONALD I. FEINSTEIN
ROBERT B. FRANCIS

GENERAL CONSIDERATIONS

The so-called lupus anticoagulant is an antibody (IgG or IgM or both) that prolongs phospholipid-dependent coagulation tests by binding to epitopes on the phospholipid portion of prothrombinase (a complex of factor Xa, factor Va, phospholipid, and calcium.)[F47,F48,S324] It was given this name in 1972 because clear proof of its site of action was lacking and because the anticoagulant had been recognized initially in patients with SLE. Although this name has persisted, it is clearly a misnomer, since it is now known that the lupus anticoagulant is more frequently encountered in patients without lupus[F47,F48,S324] and is associated with thrombosis rather than abnormal bleeding.[F47,F48,S324] Immunoglobulins reacting with other hemostatic factors such as von Willebrand factor,[S456] factor VIII,[R231] factor IX,[F47] factor XI,[F47] and inhibitors of fibrin polymerization[F47] have also been described in patients with SLE, but they are rare compared to the lupus anticoagulant.

The patients with the lupus anticoagulant who do not have established SLE fall into several different categories:

1. Patients with lupus-like chronic autoimmune disorders but without findings that fit the criteria for the diagnosis of SLE.[B379,C15,S146]
2. Patients presenting with a venous or arterial thrombotic event for which no underlying cause may be apparent.[B261,G53,G203,H173,L234,M105,M641,P250]
3. Patients receiving certain drugs, of which procainamide[B19,D95] (a well-known cause of drug-induced SLE) and phenothiazine[Z14] are most important. A high prevalence of the lupus anticoagulant and of a positive antinuclear antibody test has been reported in psychotic patients receiving longterm chlorpromazine therapy.[Z14] Other drugs that may induce the lupus anticoagulant on occasion include hydralazine and quinidine.
4. Children with a recent acute viral infection[B149,B500] in whom the anticoagulant is usually transient.
5. Patients with human immunodeficiency virus infection.[B352,C66,C323]
6. Women with recurrent fetal wastage.[B379,B456,C419,D175,D194,F103,H148,H150,L350,L401,N100]
7. Patients seeking medical attention for a variety of disorders in whom the anticoagulant is discovered

as an incidental finding. A high percentage of patients fall into this category. Frequently such patients are discovered because of a prolonged PTT performed as a routine preoperative evaluation of hemostasis.

The prevalence of the lupus anticoagulant in patients with SLE in which the PTT test was used for its detection is approximately 10%.[B379,R109,G170] However, a higher prevalence of approximately 50% is found when a modified PTT test with a reduced concentration of exogenous phospholipid is used to detect the anticoagulant.[B379] Moreover, when the kaolin clotting time—a test with increased sensitivity for detecting low-titer lupus anticoagulants because it contains no added exogenous phospholipid (i.e., low antigen concentration)—is utilized, evidence of inhibitor activity can be demonstrated in the plasma of the majority (>50%) of randomly selected patients with SLE.[E170,N392] Interestingly, this percentage approximates the 42 to 44% incidence of the frequency of anticardiolipin antibodies in patients with systemic lupus erythematosus.[L392]

PROPERTIES AND MECHANISM OF ACTION

There is unequivocal evidence that the lupus anticoagulant is an immunoglobulin. In some patients, e.g., those in which it arises secondary to longterm chlorpromazine therapy, it is IgM;[Z214] in other patients it is IgG;[F47,S324] and in still other patients it may be both IgG and IgM.[F47,S324] Although IgA anticardiolipin antibodies have been well described, IgA anticoagulant activity has never been studied.

A large body of indirect evidence supports the conclusion that the immunoglobulins responsible for the lupus anticoagulant effect react in in vitro assay systems against procoagulant phospholipids. This evidence may be summarized as follows:

1. Reducing the phospholipid component of clotting mixtures disproportionately potentiates the anticoagulant's effect. Thus, the most sensitive tests for detecting the inhibitor contain only limited amounts of procoagulant phospholipid: the recalcification time of platelet-free plasma;[M129] the kaolin clotting time of platelet-poor plasma;[E167,E168,E170] and the

prothrombin time performed with dilute tissue factor, the so-called tissue thromboplastin inhibition (TTI) test.[S146,E168]

2. Increasing procoagulant phospholipid in clotting mixtures diminishes the effect of the anticoagulant. Many years ago it was reported that adding an exogenous source of procoagulant phospholipid corrected the abnormal prothrombin consumption test of blood containing the lupus inhibitor.[B442] Adding liposomes containing phosphatidylserine[K159] rabbit brain phospholipid,[R323b] or freeze-thawed platelets,[H454,T220] markedly shortens the prolonged PTT time of plasma containing the lupus anticoagulant.

3. Patients with the lupus anticoagulant also have evidence of plasma immunoglobulin reacting with the nonprocoagulant phospholipid, cardiolipin. This was first recognized as a high prevalence of an associated chronic biologic false-positive test for syphilis,[F47,L90,M129,S324] a test in which cardiolipin is the antigen. With the use of a sensitive quantitative radioimmunoassay for anticardiolipin antibodies, it has become clear that most patients with the lupus anticoagulant have raised levels of anticardiolipin antibodies in their plasma.[H152]

Thiagarajan, Shapiro, and De Marco[T139] have provided direct evidence that a lupus anticoagulant can react with phospholipid in studies of a patient with macroglobulinemia and a monoclonal IgM that behaved like a lupus anticoagulant. The purified immunoglobulin gave precipitin lines in a double immunodiffusion system with phosphatidylserine, phosphatidylinositol, and phosphatidic acid and inhibited calcium-dependent binding of prothrombin and factor X to phospholipid vesicles. In their review of the lupus anticoagulant,[S324] Shapiro and Thiagarajan also refer to further studies in which plasma from 17 patients with the lupus anticoagulant had precipitin activity against anionic phospholipids on analysis by double diffusion, whereas plasma from none of 22 control patients with SLE, but without the lupus anticoagulant, exhibited such activity. In addition, Yamamoto et al.[Y16] have shown that immobilized anionic phospholipids will deplete plasma of lupus anticoagulant activity.

Phospholipid participates in coagulation at several known steps: as a component of the prothrombin activator complex, as a cofactor with factor VIIIa for factor IXa in the intrinsic activation of factor X, as a cofactor with protein S for activated protein C's proteolytic inactivation of factor Va and factor VIIIa, and as a cofactor for activation of factor VII by factor Xa or factor IXa.[M182,R6] It is possible, therefore, that the lupus anticoagulant impedes each of these reactions of blood coagulation. The exact biochemical mechanism whereby the lupus anticoagulant inhibits the prothrombin activator is not completely understood. However, it does appear that the anticoagulant is able to inhibit the binding of both factor X and prothrombin to the negatively charged phospholipid surface.[L392,P100,T139] Thus, inhibition of prothrombinase is caused by both deficient formation of the prothrombinase complex and poor substrate binding. Whether the lupus anticoagulant can interfere with the procoagulant activity of activated platelets continues to be debatable.[G16] However, some studies strongly suggest that the anticoagulant is capable of affecting platelet-dependent prothrombinase activity, particularly when platelets are present in reduced numbers.[G16]

POTENTIATION OF THE LUPUS ANTICOAGULANT BY A COFACTOR

Loeliger[L361] first showed that normal plasma contains a cofactor potentiating the activity of the lupus anticoagulant. The finding that a prolonged PTT or kaolin clotting time of a patient's plasma lengthens further when normal plasma is added to it represents the presence of the cofactor in coagulation assays. Several groups have shown that this plasma cofactor is also required for anticardiolipin antibodies to bind cardiolipin.[B280,B281,G15,M198,M315] This cofactor has been characterized as β_2-glycoprotein I,[G15,M198,M315] and in anticardiolipin or antiphospholipid assays, it appears that the antibody is directed against either a complex consisting of β_2-glycoprotein I bound to anionic phospholipid or a cryptic epitope formed during the interaction of β_2-glycoprotein I with phospholipid. The antibody, however, does not appear to bind β_2-glycoprotein I independent of the presence of phospholipid. The physiologic function of β_2-glycoprotein I is uncertain, but it is known to bind to lipoproteins, anionic phospholipids, platelets, heparin, DNA, and mitochondria.[M315] Because this protein is associated with lipoproteins of various classes, it has been designated apolipoprotein H. Interestingly, β_2-glycoprotein I has been found to inhibit the intrinsic coagulation pathway and to bind platelets and inhibit ADP-mediated platelet aggregation.[M315]

MECHANISM OF HYPOPROTHROMBINEMIA IN THE HYPOPROTHROMBINEMIA–LUPUS ANTICOAGULANT SYNDROME

A small subset of patients with the lupus anticoagulant will also have a specific deficiency of plasma prothrombin (factor II). It was known for many years that the plasma of such patients does not contain anticoagulant material capable of neutralizing the coagulant activity of prothrombin added in vitro.[F47,R43] It was also shown that plasma prothrombin antigen is decreased to the same extent as prothrombin activity,[F47,F139,L289,N43] i.e., that the reduced activity reflects a reduced concentration of the prothrombin molecule. However, a reason for this remained obscure until Bajaj and colleagues[B32] demonstrated that the plasma from patients with the hypoprothrombinemia–lupus anticoagulant syndrome contained antibodies that bind prothrombin without neutralizing its in vitro coagulant activity. The data of Bajaj and colleagues have been confirmed, and in addition, altered mobility of prothrombin antigen on crossed immunoelectrophoresis indicative of the presence of plasma prothrombin antigen-antibody complexes has been demonstrated in other patients with the lupus anticoagulant in whom plasma activity was not substantially decreased.[E33] In these latter patients, prothrombin synthesis presumably keeps pace with the clearance of prothrombin antigen-antibody complexes, and the plasma prothrombin level remains within the normal range. In all patients studied to date with the acquired hypoprothrombinemia–lupus anticoagulant syndrome, the prothrombin antibodies have all reacted with epitopes on the carboxy terminal segment of the prothrombin molecule.[B32] Fleck and coworkers[F128] have provided suggestive evidence that the antibodies responsible for the lupus anticoagulant phenomenon exhibit polyreactivity for epitopes on both prothrombin and anionic phospholipids. However, other data suggest that these antibodies are different antibodies and can be separated from each other.[B31]

LABORATORY DIAGNOSIS

The pattern of screening coagulation laboratory test results usually found in patients with the lupus anticoagulant may be summarized as follows:

1. Activated partial thromboplastin time (APTT).
   a. Prolonged.
   b. Prolonged when the patient's plasma is mixed with equal parts of normal plasma. Sometimes the clotting time of the mixture may be longer than that of the patient's plasma alone (cofactor effect).
   c. Incubation of a mixture of the patient's plasma and normal plasma does not lengthen the clotting time further.
2. Quick prothrombin time.
   a. Minimally to moderately prolonged (0.5 to 3 seconds) but occasionally normal when carried out with standard full-strength tissue factor.
   b. Prolonged more than normal plasma when diluted tissue factor is used as in the tissue thromboplastin (TTI) test.[S146]
3. Thrombin time: normal.

Why the APTT test is more sensitive to the effects of the lupus anticoagulant than the prothrombin time test has not been specifically studied. It may reflect differences in lipid concentration and/or lipid composition between phospholipids in APTT reagents and phospholipids in tissue factor reagents, or it may result from inhibition of the phospholipid that markedly accelerates the intrinsic factor X activating complex (factor VIIIa, factor IXa, phospholipid, Ca^{2+}). It should also be noted that the sensitivity of the APTT for detecting the lupus anticoagulant varies with the commercial reagent used for the test.[M102,M520,S674] This probably reflects, at least in part, variation in the phospholipid composition of different APTT reagents.[S674]

It is extremely important to prevent platelet activation in plasma samples, since procoagulant phospholipid, either in the patient's plasma or the normal plasma used for mixing studies, may neutralize weak lupus anticoagulant activity.[E172,E173] Thus, it is recommended that test plasma and normal plasma be initially centrifuged at 5,000 to 15,000 g for 10 to 15 minutes and/or filtered through 0.22 μm screens to remove platelets prior to freezing.[E173]

CONFIRMATION OF THE DIAGNOSIS

The screening test pattern of the lupus anticoagulant is often indistinguishable from that of an anticoagulant directed against any one of the several clotting factors that influence the APTT but not the prothrombin time test result. Therefore, further tests are needed to confirm that the prolonged APTT time of a mixture of patient's plasma and normal plasma results from the lupus anticoagulant.

Tests based upon the observation that excess phospholipid substantially shortens the prolonged APTT of lupus anticoagulant plasma have been advocated as a means to differentiate the lupus anticoagulant from other inhibitors. The excess phospholipid has been added either as freeze-thawed platelets,[T220] as liposomes containing phosphatidylserine,[K159] or as rabbit brain phospholipid.[R322b] The latter test, in which the capacity of a fourfold increase in phospholipid concentration is used to normalize an abnormal standard APTT is particularly promising, since it can be easily done in most clinical laboratories. Sensitivity of this test was superior to that of the tissue thromboplastin inhibition test (97 versus 58%). False-positive results were frequently encountered with heparinized patients. No positive results were obtained from patients with other clotting factor inhibitors, congenital factor deficiencies, hepatic insufficiency, or with patients receiving warfarin therapy.

Another diagnostic approach to confirm the diagnosis is to perform several of the specific one-stage clotting factor assays based upon the APTT technique (e.g., factors VIII, IX, and XI). The following pattern of results is frequently found:

1. Low values not for a single factor, as would be obtained if the screening test pattern resulted from an anticoagulant against a specific clotting factor, but low values for several clotting factors. These are artifactually decreased values, reflecting the ability of the lupus anticoagulant in the test sample to impair the reactivity of the phospholipid reagent common to each assay system.
2. Increasing values for each clotting factor with increasing dilution of the test plasma in the assay system. This reflects a decreased carryover of the lupus anticoagulant into the assay system with a higher dilution of the patient's plasma. Occasionally, however, the lupus anticoagulant may be in such high titer that low values are obtained in specific assay systems. This may be seen at the highest dilution of a test plasma that is technically feasible to use in the assay systems. Then, special techniques, in which mixtures of decreasing concentrations of patient's plasma in normal plasma are assayed immediately and, after incubation, may be needed to rule out an anticoagulant directed against a specific clotting factor.

Prothrombin time tests using dilute tissue thromboplastin have also been used to confirm the presence of the lupus anticoagulant.[S146,T138] The dilute Russel's viper venom time test, in particular, appears to be a simple, sensitive, and relatively specific assay for the detection of the lupus anticoagulant.[T138] In contrast, the tissue thromboplastin inhibition test appears to be less sensitive and specific.[E167,E168,L200,R320,R322b]

An enzyme-linked immunoadsorbent assay, using partial thromboplastin derived from human brain as the antigen, was developed for detection of the lupus anticoagulant.[B455] This assay circumvents some of the disadvantages of coagulation assays and is highly sensitive and specific.

DETECTION OF LOW-TITER LUPUS ANTICOAGULANTS

It should be emphasized that the PTT may be normal in patients with a low-titer and/or low-avidity lupus anticoagulant. Since the recognition of a lupus anticoagulant may be important in the management of patients, with or without SLE, who experience unusual thrombotic events or thrombotic events at a younger age than expected, one should not accept a normal APTT test as ruling out a low-titer inhibitor in such patients. This requires also demonstrating a normal clotting time in a more sensitive system containing limited amounts of phospholipid and by demonstrating the absence of anticardiolipin antibodies (described below) in the patient's plasma. The most sensitive assay for detecting the presence of the lupus anticoagulant is the kaolin clotting time mixture test as described by Exner et al.,[E170] and the dilute phospholipid APTT described by Alving et al.[A173] Moreover, both assays are also useful in identifying patients with the lupus anticoagulant who are anticoagulated with warfarin.[A173,M279] In direct comparisons with the thromboplastin inhibition test, the dilute Russel's viper venom test, and APTT with and without high concentrations of phospholipid, the assay described by Exner is most sensitive in detecting low titers of the lupus anticoagulant.[L200]

In summary, the following are recommended criteria for detecting a lupus anticoagulant[T138]:

1. It is important that platelets and platelet debris be removed from both the patient's plasma and the normal plasma used for mixing studies before any testing is carried out.
2. If sensitivity is important, then a screening test with high sensitivity such as the kaolin clotting time should be used.
3. The clotting time of a mixture of test and normal plasma should be significantly longer than that of the normal plasma mixed with various nonlupus anticoagulant plasma.
4. In order to increase specificity, there should be a relative correction of the defect by the addition of lysed washed platelets or phospholipid liposomes containing phosphatidylserine or hexagonal-phase phospholipids.

RECOGNITION OF THE HYPOPROTHROMBINEMIA–LUPUS ANTICOAGULANT SYNDROME

Although minimal to moderate prolongation of the prothrombin time, up to about 3 seconds beyond a control

value, can be accounted for by the lupus anticoagulant, the finding of a substantially prolonged prothrombin time, e.g., in the 18 to 20 second range with a control value in the 11 to 12 second range, represents presumptive evidence of an associated specific prothrombin deficiency. Unlike the specific clotting factors assayed in modified APTT test systems, the specific clotting factors affecting the prothrombin time test—prothrombin itself, factor VII, factor X, and factor V—are assayed in clotting systems that are affected only by rare, high-titer lupus anticoagulants. Therefore, the finding of a low value in a specific prothrombin assay may be taken as convincing evidence of an associated prothrombin deficiency. If, however, further evidence is desired one may demonstrate three additional findings: 1) a mixture of equal parts of patient's plasma and normal plasma gives the expected value calculated from the mean of the levels in individual plasma, 2) prothrombin activity and prothrombin antigen measured by electroimmunoassay are concordantly decreased, or 3) prothrombin has abnormal mobility on crossed immunoelectrophoresis.[F128]

RELATIONSHIP OF THE LUPUS ANTICOAGULANT TO OTHER ANTIPHOSPHOLIPID ANTIBODIES

Relationship of the Lupus Anticoagulant to Anticardiolipin Antibodies

As noted previously, the lupus anticoagulant and anticardiolipin antibodies are both antiphospholipid antibodies that are frequently associated with thrombosis, fetal wastage, or thrombocytopenia with or without autoimmune disorders. Some investigators[A334,H148,H155] have renamed this clinical entity the antiphospholipid syndrome. In contrast to the antiphospholipid syndrome, the "primary" antiphospholipid syndrome is defined as venous and/or arterial thrombotic disease or recurrent fetal wastage associated with elevated levels of antiphospholipid antibodies in the absence of any definite autoimmune disease.[A334] These patients do not demonstrate any other clinical or serologic evidence of autoimmune disease except for occasional low-titer (<1:160) antinuclear antibodies.

There are considerable data to suggest that anticardiolipin antibodies and lupus anticoagulants are related groups of antibodies. Both bind negatively charged phospholipids,[A334,H155,T139] and antibodies purified with cardiolipin liposomes demonstrate lupus anticoagulant activity.[H158,P100] In addition, the majority of patients who test positive for the lupus anticoagulant have elevated levels of anticardiolipin antibodies. However, although there is significant correlation between the two, many patients have been reported who test positive for lupus anticoagulant activity, but do not have elevated levels of anticardiolipin or other antiphospholipid antibodies and vice versa.[A174,D169,L347,M311,R322a,T221] Moreover, some data suggest that anticardiolipin antibodies and lupus anticoagulants comprise separate antibody subgroups that can be isolated from one another in vitro and possess different phospholipid binding characteristics.[K42]

In addition, since it has been reported that anticardiolipin antibody levels can fluctuate significantly,[K42] it is im-

synthesis (see below). There is a single report of reduced antithrombin III activity in a subject with APA-associated thrombosis.[C397] Since an increased incidence of venous thrombosis,[R306] and perhaps arterial thrombosis as well,[C348,S9,U10] has been reported in some subjects with inherited deficiencies of antithrombin III, protein C, and protein S, it is possible that impaired activity of natural anticoagulant pathways may contribute to thrombosis in subjects with antiphospholipid antibodies. However, as with impaired prostacyclin release, a close correlation between abnormalities of natural anticoagulant mechanisms and thrombosis in subjects with antiphospholipid antibodies has not been clearly demonstrated. It would be useful to investigate whether indices of in vivo coagulation activation, which are known to be abnormally increased in subjects with inherited deficiencies of antithrombin III and protein C,[B123] are also abnormally increased in subjects with antiphospholipid antibodies with or without thrombosis. Such studies have been hampered by the fact that most subjects with antiphospholipid antibody-associated thrombosis receive long-term anticoagulant therapy, which is known to suppress indices of abnormal coagulation activation in subjects with hypercoagulable conditions.[B123]

It has been proposed that impaired fibrinolysis contributes to thrombosis in subjects with antiphospholipid antibodies.[A233,T231] However, one of these studies investigated subjects with active SLE,[A233] which is independently associated with impaired fibrinolysis.[G181] Other studies of subjects with antiphospholipid antibody-associated thrombosis without SLE have failed to document either impaired fibrinolysis in vivo,[F201] or any effect of plasma containing antiphospholipid antibodies on in vitro endothelial secretion of either tissue-type plasminogen activator (tPA) or its rapid inhibitor (type 1 plasminogen activator inhibitor, or PAI-1).[F202]

Antibodies against endothelial cells have been reported in some subjects with antiphospholipid antibody-associated thrombosis.[C337,H199] These could conceivably cause thrombosis by directly damaging endothelial cells, by impairing endothelial, antiplatelet, and/or anticoagulant activities (see below), or by causing procoagulant changes in endothelial function such as expression of tissue factor.[T62] In addition to prostacyclin, thrombomodulin, protein S, tPA, and PAI-1, vascular endothelial cells express or secrete many other hemostasis-related substances that modulate platelet activity (thromboxane A2, platelet-activating factor, endothelin, endothelial-derived relaxing factor, von Willebrand factor, fibronectin, and thrombospondin); stimulate coagulation (tissue factor and receptors for procoagulant clotting factors); and inhibit coagulation (heparin-like substances and the extrinsic pathway inhibitor).[B565,V27,W82] None of these have yet been studied either in vivo or in vitro in subjects with antiphospholipid antibody-associated thrombosis.

The possibility that antiphospholipid antibodies might cross-react with serine-phosphorylated proteins (see above) has potentially interesting implications for the pathogenesis of antiphospholipid antibody-associated thrombosis. The association between antiphospholipid antibodies and antiplatelet and antiendothelial antibodies, for example, could represent binding of antiphospholipid antibodies to phosphoproteins on the platelet or endothelial membrane, rather than to anionic phospholipids, which are normally sequestered in the inner or cytoplasmic leaflet of the red cell, platelet, and presumably endothelial cell membranes (see below), and therefore theoretically not available to bind antiphospholipid antibodies. Also, several important hemostasis-related proteins, including fibrinogen and the extrinsic pathway inhibitor, are serine phosphorylated,[B348,G167] and thus could represent potential targets of antiphospholipid antibodies. These possibilities are of course speculative at present.

Antiphospholipid Antibodies as a Secondary Consequence of Thrombosis

Thrombosis is associated with increased in vivo activity of procoagulant pathways, which involves binding of native and activated procoagulant clotting factors to anionic phospholipids exposed in fragments of membrane derived from activated platelets (so-called platelet procoagulant activity or platelet factor 3.[Z65] Perhaps it is more than coincidental that antiphospholipid antibodies are specifically directed against these same procoagulant anionic phospholipids, which are normally not exposed in the outer membrane leaflet of unactivated platelets and other blood cells, but rather are actively sequestered in the inner or cytoplasmic leaflet.[O87] Conceivably, antiphospholipid antibodies in some subjects with thrombosis arise as an immune response to increased exposure of normally hidden procoagulant anionic phospholipids. Some support for this hypothesis is provided by the transient occurrence of antibodies to other products of coagulation activation such as thrombin in postsurgical subjects,[F125a,S730,S731] and by the occurrence of antiphospholipid antibodies in subjects with sickle cell anemia[F199] who have abnormal exposure of anionic phospholipids in the external leaflet of the red blood cell membrane as a result of sickling.[C242] It is also conceivable that antiphospholipid antibodies that originally arise as a secondary consequence of thrombosis may then induce abnormalities of hemostasis (see above). These possibilities are unproven at present, however.

Antiphospholipid Antibodies as Markers of Other Causative Factors of Thrombosis

If antiphospholipid antibodies can arise as an immune reaction to increased coagulation activation and thrombosis (see below), then they would presumably be more frequent in subjects with underlying hypercoagulable states. This could explain the reported associations between antiphospholipid antibodies and reduced antithrombin III and free protein S.[C397,W60] An intriguing but speculative possibility is that both antiphospholipid antibodies and thrombosis might arise as a result of an underlying inherited or acquired defect in the molecular mechanisms that normally sequester procoagulant anionic phospholipids in the cytoplasmic membrane leaflet of platelets, red cells, and presumably vascular endothelial cells.[C358,M394] Abnormal exteriorization of procoagulant anionic phospholipids in cells exposed to flowing blood could give rise to both abnormal coagulation activation and thrombosis, and to antiphospholipid antibodies. This sequence of events may in fact occur in sickle cell anemia.[C242,F199,F200] Another purely speculative possibility is that antiphospholipid antibodies might arise in response to thrombogenic functional alterations of hemostasis-related plasma, platelet, or endothelial proteins induced by abnormal serine phosphorylation.

The recent finding that anticardiolipin antibodies are directed against an antigen, that in some as yet undefined way, includes β_2-glycoprotein I[B280,B281,G15,M198,M315] suggests that possibly the antihemostatic effect is caused by inhibition of β_2-glycoprotein I function. Since the latter protein appears to inhibit the intrinsic pathway of blood coagulation and ADP-dependent platelet aggregation, it is possible that this inhibition leads to a prethrombotic state.[M315]

TREATMENT OF PATIENTS WITH THE LUPUS ANTICOAGULANT

The lupus anticoagulant usually persists in the untreated adult patient. However, it frequently disappears spontaneously when it occurs in children who develop the anticoagulant after a viral infection.

When the anticoagulant is found in patients with underlying autoimmune disease, treatment of the underlying disease with immunosuppressive therapy frequently results in reduction or disappearance of inhibitor activity.[F47,L90,M321,M383,S146,S324] When the anticoagulant is found in association with evidence of severe prothrombin deficiency or severe thrombocytopenia, ($<$20,000/μl) treatment with adrenal corticosteroids to correct the prothrombin deficiency or thrombocytopenia is indicated. However, when the lupus anticoagulant is discovered as an isolated finding and not associated with thrombosis, then treatment is not indicated.

Therapy of patients with thrombosis associated with the lupus anticoagulant and/or anticardiolipin antibodies should be guided by the fact that recurrence is common. Therefore, it is recommended that patients with venous thrombosis receive longterm anticoagulation (probably for life) with oral anticoagulants. Because of the efficacy of warfarin therapy in preventing recurrence of venous thrombosis, and because these patients may require therapy for life, the use of corticosteroids and other immunosuppressive agents to suppress antibody production is not recommended. In contrast to venous thrombosis, the treatment for arterial thrombosis is unknown. There are few reports of the efficacy of antithrombotic treatment in these patients. However, it is reasonable and rational to at

least give the patient low-dose aspirin (80 mg) daily or every other day. The efficacy of oral anticoagulant therapy in patients with the lupus anticoagulant is as questionable as its use in arterial thrombosis not associated with the lupus anticoagulant.

A pregnant patient with or without SLE with the lupus anticoagulant and/or elevated levels of anticardiolipin antibodies associated with a history or recurrent fetal wastage probably should be treated. However, the exact regimen to be used is not clear. Lubbe and coworkers[L403] first described successful pregnancy outcomes in patients with the lupus anticoagulant and fetal wastage who were treated with prednisone (40 to 60 mg/day) and low-dose aspirin (approximately 80 mg). Subsequently, the same regimen led to successful pregnancy outcomes in 10 of 16 pregnancies in 12 patients, some of whom had lupus.[L404] Other investigators, utilizing a similar regimen in patients without lupus also reported a decrease in fetal wastage.[B456] However, longterm high-dose corticosteroids during pregnancy is associated with significant side effects including severe pre-eclampsia, infections, gestational diabetes, cushingoid features, and osteoporosis.

Wallenburg and Rotmans[W44] used low-dose aspirin (60 to 80 mg) plus dipyridamole (75 mg tid) in 37 patients with obstetric histories similar to those with antiphospholipid antibodies, with a 92% success rate. Unfortunately, these patients were not systematically examined for the presence of antiphospholipid antibodies. Similarly, Elder et al.[E70] reported similar success using low-dose aspirin alone in 42 patients of whom 16 had SLE (13 with antiphospholipid antibodies).

However, a report by Lockshin et al.[L351] cast significant doubt regarding the efficacy of aspirin with or without corticosteroids in high-risk patients with high-titer anticardiolipin antibodies. In 11 pregnant patients receiving corticosteroids and low-dose aspirin, there were 9 fetal losses, whereas in 10 pregnancies receiving aspirin alone or no therapy there were 5 fetal losses.

Rosove et al.[R322c] reported 14 of 15 successful pregnancy outcomes in 14 patients with recurrent fetal wastage (5 with lupus) utilizing adjusted full-dose heparin therapy throughout pregnancy. None of the patients were treated with aspirin, and only two patients received a short course of corticosteroids for concomitant autoimmune disease.

Thus, different therapeutic regimens in uncontrolled trials have resulted in what appears to be a significant decrease in fetal wastage. However, it is probably necessary to do a careful randomized prospective trial in such patients to determine the optimum therapeutic regimen.[F49]

Chapter 26

ANTILYMPHOCYTE AUTOANTIBODIES

JOHN B. WINFIELD
TOSHIHIDE MIMURA
PHILIP D. FERNSTEN*

Most patients with SLE develop antilymphocyte autoantibodies** at some point in their illness. As a group, they probably represent a type of natural autoantibody that exhibits a disease-related increase in titer. Contrary to popular misconception, such autoantibodies are not necessarily of low avidity and, therefore, biologically irrelevant. Indeed, the multivalency of IgM autoantibodies, together with the local density of reactive antigens on the cell surface, confers a capacity for a variety of immunoregulatory and nonspecific physiologic roles in the immune system and in autoimmune disease.[A368] There are several major types of antilymphocyte autoantibodies with distinct specificities for different lymphocyte and monocyte populations, but the exact degree of heterogeneity is unknown. Best studied are cold-reactive IgM lymphocytotoxic autoantibodies, which vary in titer with disease activity status in the same fashion as anti-dsDNA autoantibodies.[B598,W292] This association with disease flares and lymphopenia (Figure 26–1) forms one line of evidence for a role of IgM lymphocytotoxic autoantibodies in T-cell depletion and the myriad functional abnormalities of T cells, B cells, and monocytes in SLE (Table 26–1), although other factors undoubtedly contribute as well, e.g., suppressor cells selective for CD3+, CD4+ helper cells, decreased levels of IL-2 inhibitors, soluble IL-2 receptors, etc.[A132,K430,T237,W197] Consistent with this thesis is the capacity of antilymphocyte autoantibodies in SLE serum to alter the function of normal peripheral blood lymphocytes and monocytes in vitro in ways closely paralleling those of freshly isolated lymphocytes and monocytes from patients with SLE. Mechanisms underlying such functional effects while poorly understood, may include those listed in Table 26–2: elimination of cells by complement-mediated lysis, antibody-dependent cell-mediated cytotoxicity (ADCC) and/or opsonization; alteration of lymphocyte migration patterns; modulation of surface determinants; surface receptor blockade; interaction with soluble products of activated cells; and up-regulation or down-regulation by cross-linking cell surface receptors.

Thus, while clearly not the cause of SLE, autoantibodies to lymphocyte and monocyte surface determinants may constitute one of the pathogenetically significant extrinsic elements that alters cellular immune function in this disorder. Of special interest in this regard is the discovery of IgM autoantibodies in SLE that are directed against different isoforms of CD45,[M453] the major protein tyrosine phosphatase on the surface of hemopoietic cells.[C275,H504,S25] CD45, known for years as leukocyte-common antigen,[T148] has been implicated in the regulation of lymphocyte functional activity, including cytotoxicity, proliferation, and differentiation via interaction of its variable extracellular domains with as yet undefined ligands and through its phosphatase action on intracellular tyrosine kinases and other substances.[B251,K270,L119,M171,M491] Whereas previous studies of the effects of antilymphocyte antibodies on lymphocyte function in SLE have been descriptive and phenomenologic, the identification of different isoforms of CD45 as specific antilymphocyte autoantibody targets should permit a more precise understanding of the mechanisms by which such autoantibodies influence lymphocyte behavior.

IS THERE AN INTRINSIC CELLULAR DEFECT IN SLE?

Cellular immune abnormalities are generally most apparent in patients with active SLE and return to or toward normal during disease remission. This fundamental observation argues against an underlying intrinsic cellular defect(s) in this disorder. Although seemingly intrinsic abnormalities in capping and cell surface receptor regeneration[K45] and in suppressor function[S27] have been reported, participation of in vivo humoral effects which carry over in vitro, such as autoantibody-mediated surface receptor modulation, have not been formally excluded. Similarly, it has been suggested that reduction in the production of and/or response to IL-2 reflects intrinsic abnormalities of SLE T cells,[A126,L311,L312,M663] but against this are demonstrations that the pathways responsible for this critical proliferation mechanism are intact when SLE T cells are given the proper stimulus,[S405] when suppressor elements are removed,[L312] or when SLE peripheral blood mononuclear cells are given several days of rest before

* Experimental work from the authors' laboratory was supported in part by National Institutes of Health grants R01 AM30863, T32 AR7416, and P60 AR30701, and a Biomedical Research Center grant from the Arthritis Foundation.

** A more precise terminology is "autoantibodies to surface molecules of lymphocytes and other nucleated mononuclear cells in the blood." The term "antilymphocyte autoantibodies" reflects the historical antecedents of this system, and is retained for convenience.

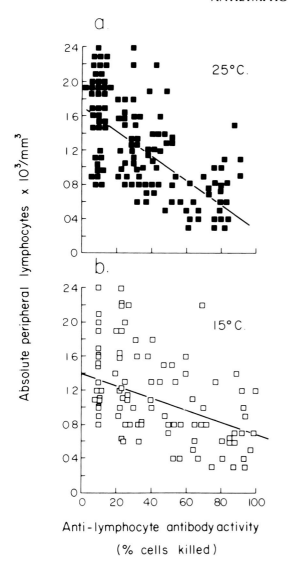

Fig. 26-1. Inverse linear correlation between serum cytotoxicity and peripheral lymphocyte counts in SLE. *A,* Shows data obtained with undiluted sera assayed at 25° C against peripheral blood mononuclear cells ($r = 0.6667$). *B,* Shows data obtained with serum diluted 1:4 in 15° C assays ($r = 0.4664$). From Winfield, J.B., Winchester, R.J., and Kunkel, H.G.: Association of cold-reactive anti-lymphocyte antibodies with lymphopenia in systemic lupus erythematosus. Arthritis Rheum., *18*:587, 1975.

Table 26-1. Cellular Immune Defects in SLE

T lymphopenia, especially CD4+, CD45RA+ cells*
Increased numbers of CD4−, CD8−, CD3+, TCRαβ cells
Impaired T-cell proliferation to mitogens, antigens, and other stimuli*
Spontaneously activated T cells*
Impaired response to and/or production of IL-2 in vitro*
Increased IL-2 production in vivo
Decreased production of cytotoxic T cells*
Decreased nonspecific T-cell suppressor phenomena*
Impaired autologous mixed leukocyte reaction*
Defective T helper function
Excessive monocyte suppression (in vivo preactivated monocytes)
Defective monocyte production of IL-1*
Impaired monocyte metabolism and phagocytosis*
Impaired antigen presentation by monocytes (decreased expression of DR antigens)*
Decreased NK and LAK cell activity*
Decreased ADCC*
Spontaneous B-cell Ig secretion*

* Antilymphocyte or antimonocyte autoantibody effect demonstrated experimentally or inferred through correlation.

based on their immunoglobulin class. IgM autoantibodies are the major type detected in conventional two-stage complement-dependent cytotoxicity assays performed at 15° C, and react broadly with autologous lymphocytes and with lymphocytes from unrelated donors.[M490,T116,W293] Originally described as naturally occurring cold lymphocytotoxins in patients with viral infections to emphasize their distinct properties with respect to warm-reactive IgG alloantibodies to HLA antigens developing as a consequence of pregnancy or multiple transfusions,[T115] it is now recognized that such autoantibodies are produced almost universally in disorders of persistent immune system stimulation. Although IgM antilymphocyte autoantibodies bind maximally at 4° C, complement-dependent cytotoxic activity is optimal at 15° C, which represents a compromise between the lower and higher temperatures required for autoantibody binding and complement-mediated cell lysis, respectively.[W293] This cold reactivity has been exploited for isolation and purification of antilymphocyte autoantibodies by elution from cells at warm temperatures,[W288] and is useful in the operational discrimination of this class from IgG alloantibodies and relatively more warm-reactive, noncytotoxic IgG autoantibodies. Carryover of cold-reactive IgM autoantibody bound to cells during lymphocyte isolation procedures performed at temperatures less than 37° C can

stimulation.[H329,H467] Conversely, defects in production of and/or response to IL-2 can be reproduced in normal cells by extrinsic factors in SLE serum. For example, IgG fractions from SLE sera inhibit T-cell IL-2 production by binding to adherent cells, thereby reducing their production of IL-1.[M500] It is possible that autoantibodies to IL-2 receptors[H394,K8] can inhibit the IL-2 response by acting directly on T cells as well.

GENERAL CHARACTERISTICS OF ANTILYMPHOCYTE AUTOANTIBODIES

A convenient paradigm for describing the special properties of antilymphocyte autoantibodies in SLE is

Table 26-2. Mechanisms by Which Antilymphocyte Autoantibodies Could Alter Cell Function

Elimination of cells
  Complement-mediated lysis
  ADCC
  Opsonization with phagocytosis or altered migration
Modulation of surface determinants
  Shedding
  Interiorization
Surface receptor blockade
Up-regulation or down-regulation by cross-linking a receptor
Interaction with soluble products of activated cells

lead to artifacts in enumerating B cells as surface IgM + cells,[W280] and may influence in vitro assays of lymphocyte function.

IgG antilymphocyte autoantibodies exhibit certain unusual antigenic specificities, e.g., HLA class II antigens,[O47] IL-2 receptors,[K8,S72] soluble products of activated T cells,[L335] and have the potential to kill target cells in vivo by ADCC.[K453,M66] IgG antilymphocyte autoantibodies do not lyse lymphocytes in the presence of complement.[P6,W293] Immunofluorescence assays for detection and characterization of IgG antilymphocyte autoantibodies require special approaches to avoid artifactual Fcγ or complement receptor binding, e.g., use of F(ab')$_2$ antiimmunoglobulin reagents [W278] and/or isolation of 7S monomeric IgG from serum or plasma using acid pH buffers to dissociate immune complexes.[W242]

CELL TYPE SPECIFICITY OF ANTILYMPHOCYTE AUTOANTIBODIES

Autoantibodies in SLE react with essentially all types of blood cells, including resting and activated T cells, B cells, and monocytes.

Autoantibodies to T Cells and T-Cell Subsets

Early studies emphasized a relative specificity of lymphocytotoxic autoantibodies in SLE for T cells, especially thymocytes.[L283,P6,S624,T144,W179,W180,W242] The existence of autoantibodies to discrete T-cell subsets was suggested initially by the demonstration that T cells in a discrete layer of discontinuous Ficoll gradient-fractionated peripheral lymphocytes were reduced in patients with antilymphocyte autoantibodies in their serum directed to this fraction.[G198,G199] Autoantibodies to this lymphocyte fraction inhibited concanavalin A (Con A)–induced T-cell suppression of the allogeneic mixed leukocyte reaction.[T283] This observation, together with discoveries that 1) IgG anti–T-cell autoantibodies in SLE serum inhibited the allogeneic MLR,[W179,W180,W244] and 2) autoantibodies to Tγ cells (Fcγ receptor positive) prevented the generation of Con A–stimulated nonspecific T-cell suppressor activity,[K355,O46,O50,S31,S32] were among the first to emphasize the potential contribution of antilymphocyte autoantibodies to immune system dysfunction in this disorder. This possibility was further underscored by the discovery that a T-cell subset staining brightly with IgM from patient serum was markedly depleted in active SLE.[S642]

The application of monoclonal antibody technology to characterization of T-cell subsets and their function during the 1980s enabled substantial clarification of the nature of autoantibodies to T cells and their potential significance. Early work suggested that anti–T-cell autoantibodies in SLE were more reactive with CD8 + (cytotoxic/suppressor) cells than with CD4 + (helper/inducer) cells, a finding consistent with the idea that autoantibody-mediated CD8 + cell depletion was responsible for reduced T-cell suppressor function.[M576,M579,S27] However, when highly purified peripheral CD4 + and CD8 + T cells and CD4 + and CD8 + T cell clones are used as targets in complement-dependent cytotoxicity assays, overall cytotoxicity by SLE sera for these two subsets is

similar, indicating that reactivity of T cells to classic cold-reactive antilymphocyte autoantibodies is determined primarily by the presence of antigen(s) that are shared by CD4 + and CD8 + subsets.[Y5] Superimposed on this major antigen-antibody system common to both subsets is a slight, but consistent, preferential reactivity with CD4 + T cells,[Y5] especially CD4 + T cells expressing high levels of CD45RA (2H4, suppressor/inducer phenotype).[M578,T20] IgM autoantibodies to CD4 +, CD45RA + T cells are associated with relative depletion of this subset in the circulation of patients with active disease [T56,W291] and with a reduced capacity for suppressor/inducer function in the regulation of PWM-driven B-cell Ig secretion in vivo.[M584,T22,T56] Such data promise to clarify some of the immunoregulatory abnormalities in SLE, but additional complexity is suggested by the observation that most SLE sera, while more cytotoxic for CD4 + T cells at cold temperatures, kill CD8 + T cells preferentially when assays are performed at higher temperatures.[P84]

Autoantibodies to Activated T Cells

Because activated T cells exhibit a higher density of most surface membrane antigens than do resting cells, and also develop neoantigens, such cells may become the special targets of autoantibodies. This was demonstrated first by experiments showing increased binding of SLE serum IgG to phytohaemagglutinin (PHA)- or PWM-stimulated lymphocytes as detected in ^{125}I-labeled protein A radioimmunoassays.[W242] Such autoantibodies preferentially react with activated lymphocytes at physiologic temperatures[L335] and suppress mitogen and soluble antigen-induced T-cell activation and proliferation.[Y7] SLE sera also contain IgG autoantibodies with the capacity to develop reverse hemolytic plaques in mitogen-activated T-lymphocyte preparations, indicating reactivity with products released by activated T cells.[L335] The elimination of the ability of SLE sera to develop plaques after absorption with viable T-cell blasts, but not with resting cells, suggests that these autoantibodies are directed toward activation neoantigen(s) shed from the surface membrane, such as IL-2 receptors.[F243,S72] Other molecules may be involved as well, but their exact nature has not been defined.[M468]

Autoantibodies to B Cells

SLE sera frequently contain cold-reactive IgM cytotoxic autoantibodies to B cells from a variety of sources, including peripheral blood, tonsils, lymph nodes, chronic lymphocytic leukemia, and lymphoblastoid cell lines.[M371,O136,T116] Anti–B-cell autoantibodies are at least partially distinct from autoantibodies to T cells, as demonstrated in differential absorption experiments using B- and T-cell lines. This type of IgM anti–B-cell autoantibody develops in many immunologic diseases other than SLE, and in normal individuals.[O136,P45,T11] IgG autoantibodies to B cells also have been described,[A199,P6,T18,W242] and may play a role in B-cell activation.[T18] At least some of the IgG binding to B cells undoubtedly represents IgG/Fcγ receptor interactions rather than true antibody, however.

Autoantibodies to Other Cells

Relatively less emphasis has been directed toward monocyte-specific autoantibodies and autoantibodies cross-reactive with monocytes and lymphocytes[A283,S371] and NK cells.[R289] Autoantibodies to determinants shared by brain tissue or neuronal cell lines and lymphocytes have been described as well.[B354,B360,W260]

NATURE OF TARGET ANTIGENS

Elucidation of the nature of antilymphocyte autoantibody target antigens should eventually evolve into a fuller understanding of the functional significance of this system in the pathogenesis of SLE.

Autoantibodies to CD45

That CD45 might be a target of IgM antilymphocyte antibodies was suggested initially by studies using the monoclonal antibody anti-2H4 (anti-CD45RA), which showed 1) that patients with active SLE had significantly decreased percentages of circulating T cells bearing the CD4+, 2H4+ phenotype,[M584] and 2) that antilymphocyte antibodies from these patients reacted preferentially with the CD4+, 2H4+ subset.[T56] In blotting experiments utilizing T-cell glycoproteins isolated by lectin chromatography techniques, approximately one-third of SLE sera were found to contain IgM antibodies to different isoforms of the CD45 molecular complex.[M453] At least some of the autoreactive epitopes appeared to be distinct from the CD45RA epitope(s) (expressed on p220 and p205 isoforms) and the CD45RO epitope(s) (expressed on the p180 isoform), recognized by monoclonal antibodies anti-2H4 and UCHL-1, respectively (see below). Thus, of nine SLE sera studied in detail, four reacted with p220 and p205, but the others reacted with p205 alone (one serum), p220 alone (two sera), p205, p190, and p180 (one serum), and p220, p205, and p190 (one serum). This dominant specificity of SLE autoantibodies for the p220 and p205 isoforms suggests that they may recognize the CD45RA epitope encoded, at least in part, by exon 4. However, it should be pointed out that there are two p205 isoforms expressed by human cells (exon 4+, 5+, 6− and 4−, 5+, 6+) and the reactivity of SLE anti-CD45 autoantibodies may be more complex. The isoform specificities of SLE autoantibodies suggests that they could mimic certain ligands and stimulate or inhibit phosphatase activity, a hypothesis consistent with our earlier data showing that SLE antilymphocyte autoantibodies inhibit early phase activation events in the T-cell proliferative response to tetanus toxoid.[Y7] Alternatively, such autoantibodies could sterically hinder ligand binding or influence the association of CD45 with other lymphocyte surface molecules.

CD45 Structure and Function

CD45 is a transmembrane protein expressed at high levels ($>10^6$ molecules per cell) in all hemopoietic cells except erythrocytes.[T148,T183] The extracellular portion of CD45 consists of three subdomains: a variable, highly O-glycosylated region and two cysteine-rich subdomains.[S14]

Its highly conserved intracytoplasmic segment consists of two internally homologous tyrosine phosphatase domains. CD45 is encoded by a single gene, which generates five different isoforms by alternative splicing of exons 4, 5, and 6 (also called exons A, B, and C).[S14,S729,T149] These isoforms have molecular weights of 180 kDa (4−, 5−, 6−), 190 kDa (4−, 5+, 6−), 205 kDa (4−, 5+, 6+), 205 kDa (4+, 5+ 6−), and 220 kDa (4+, 5+, 6+). The variable splicing of exons 4 to 6 alters the number of potential N- and O-glycosylation sites, and qualitative differences in the glycosylation patterns of the higher-molecular-weight isoforms have been demonstrated.[B526,C238,E166,M586] The polymorphism of the O-glycosylated domain may allow specific associations with other cell surface receptors to regulate transmembrane signaling.[L121] Thus, the arrangement of the molecule suggests that the cytoplasmic enzymatic activity is under the control of extracellular ligand binding structures with discrete ligands for the different CD45 isoforms.[T184]

Monoclonal antibodies against restricted epitopes (CD45R) have been used to subdivide T cells into functionally distinct subsets that express either the higher-molecular-weight p220 and p205 isoforms that bear the CD45RA epitope(s) encoded by exon 4, or its junction, or the p180 isoform that bears the CD45RO (or CD45R−) epitope encoded by the junction of exons 3 and 7.[T148] For example, CD4+, CD45RA+ cells are active in IL-2−related activities and graft-versus-host reactions, whereas CD45RO+ cells respond to recall antigens and provide help for antibody production.[A308,B427,B428,M357,M578,S591] It was initially postulated that these subsets represented maturation stages of naive and memory T cells, but data in the rat suggest that either subset can generate cells of the opposite phenotype and that phenotype corresponds to the function of the cells, not their parentage.[B189]

While no ligands for CD45 have yet been identified, CD45 appears to play a central role in proximal signal transduction in T cells and other lymphocytes. One view is that CD45 regulates cell activation via selective action on several intracellular substrates, possibly including phosphatidylinositol-specific phospholipase C (PI-PLC).[L120] Biochemical observations also suggest that CD45 may activate at least two members of the *src* family of tyrosine kinases, *lck* and *fyn*, which are noncovalently associated with CD4 (or CD8) and the TCR, respectively.[G13,K270] In a speculative model for the action of CD45 in T-cell signaling via the TCR, it has been proposed[K270] that engagement of the TCR with antigen bound to MHC molecules facilitates interaction of the *fyn*/TCR complex and the CD4(8)/*lck* with CD45, which activates the *fyn* and *lck* tyrosine kinases by dephosphorylating a tyrosine residue at their carboxy terminals. These kinases rapidly phosphorylate tyrosine residues on several intracellular substrates, including PI-PLC and the ζ chain, a TCR/CD3 complex subunit whose cytoplasmic tail appears to be essential for antigen-stimulated signaling.[129] Breakdown of PI leads to the generation of diacylglycerol (activates protein kinase C, a serine/threonine kinase) and inositol phosphates (e.g., IP_3, which mobilizes $[Ca^{2+}]_i$) in the ensuing cascade of T-cell activation. CD45 also may act in analogous fashion in CD2-mediated T-cell activation,[M199,M376,S170,S171,S172] in surface immunoglobulin-mediated signal transduction in B cells,[L47,Y18] in FcγRIII (CD16)-mediated signaling in NK cells,[V96] and in IL-2/IL-2R) signaling.[H416,T273]

CD45 is absolutely required for soluble antigen-induced T-cell proliferation[P198] and is centrally involved in the function of cells of the immune system generally. CD45 may play a role in autoimmunity as well, as suggested by differences in the carbohydrate composition of CD45 on double-negative T cells in lpr mice[Y22] and by the capacity of anti-CD45 MAbs to reduce IgG production, renal histopathology, and mortality when administered to male BXSB autoimmune mice.[Y3] Depending on the nature of the activation signals, the experimental conditions of the assays, and the state of lymphocyte activation, different anti-CD45 MAbs profoundly influence cell function. Examples include inhibition or augmentation of T-[B251,K197,L119,M171,S171,T21] and B-[A161,G415,H322,L423,M491,P171] cell activation and proliferation to various stimuli; inhibition of NK activity;[G127] and inhibition of T-cell–mediated cytotoxicity.[L158,L159] In some cases, such actions of anti-CD45 MAbs have been related to their specificity for glycoproteins,[B251,G127,L159,P330,P331a,P332] which constitute a heterogeneous molecular complex with epitopes that are selectively expressed by different cell types and at different stages of maturation. This raises the question that the apparent heterogeneity of SLE antilymphocyte autoantibodies for different cell types and their diverse functional effects both might reflect specificities for different forms of CD45.

Other Antilymphocyte Autoantibody Specificities

Other antilymphocyte autoantibody specificities that have been reported in SLE include the IL-2 receptor;[K8,S72] β$_2$-microglobulin;[M371,O83,R178,Y6] HLA class I heavy chains;[M371,P209] a DR framework epitope;[O47] IgD, which functions as an antigen receptor on B cells;[P257] and determinants on plasma membrane molecules that cross-react with histones and DNA.[J20,L10,R151,R152, R153] Cold agglutinins with Ii specificity represent a type of IgM antilymphocyte autoantibody since Ii antigens are expressed on lymphocytes, but contribute relatively little to the lymphocytotoxic activity of SLE sera as detected in conventional assays performed at cold temperatures.[T144,W293] Although vigorously pursued, neither viral antigens nor antiviral antibodies have been convincingly implicated as part of the antilymphocyte autoantibody system.

In immunoblotting experiments using T-cell glycoproteins eluted from solid-phase wheat germ agglutinin columns as substrate, a 46 kD molecule (gp46) has been identified that, together with isoforms of CD45, accounts for a major proportion of the IgM antilymphocyte autoantibody activity in SLE sera.[M453a] Thus, IgM autoantibodies to gp46 were detected in 15 of 24 unselected patient sera and were strongly correlated with the presence of IgM antilymphocyte autoantibodies reactive with both E6-1 cells and peripheral blood mononuclear cells, as determined in independent indirect immunofluorescence and complement-dependent microcytotoxicity assays. Inter-estingly, gp 46 was not expressed by the primitive T-cell line, HSB-2, which lacks most of the differentiation antigens of mature peripheral T cells. The identify of gp46 remains to be determined.

CONTRIBUTION OF ANTILYMPHOCYTE AUTOANTIBODIES TO ABNORMAL CELLULAR FUNCTION

T-Cell Depletion

IgG autoantibodies can sensitize target cells for ADCC[K453,M66] and lyse activated T cells in the presence of complement,[L335] but there is no evidence that either mechanism obtains in vivo. IgM autoantibodies are responsible for most of the complement-dependent cytotoxic activity against resting and activated lymphocytes in vitro and are highly correlated with lymphopenia, despite their relatively low thermal amplitude of binding. Certain evidence suggests that IgM autoantibodies to CD4 +, CD45RA + T cells may be causally related to depletion of this subset in patients with active SLE and with a reduced capacity for suppressor/inducer function in the regulation of PWM-drive B-cell Ig secretion in vitro.[M583,M584,T22,T56,W291,W292,Y5] CD45RA obviously is a potential autoantibody target in this regard, but this has not been shown directly. Although the relationship between antilymphocyte autoantibodies and a proportional and absolute reduction in CD4 + cells is well established,[W291] it is unclear whether the decrease in CD4 +, CD45RA + T cells in active SLE is a consequence of depletion of this subset, a shift to CD45RO + cells, or both mechanisms.

Modulation of Lymphocyte Surface Antigens

Antilymphocyte autoantibodies modulate membrane determinants by promoting shedding from the cell surface[V932] or interiorization.[L375,W290] Shedding of surface antigens in association with antilymphocyte autoantibodies in SLE was first demonstrated by the recovery of allogeneic mixed leukocyte reaction (MLR) responsiveness by T cells exposed to MLR-blocking autoantibodies after short-term culture.[W179] In subsequent studies antilymphocyte autoantibodies were shown to be specifically enriched in purified cryoprecipitates from patients with SLE and chronic lymphocytic leukemia,[D100,W294] suggesting the existence of circulating complexes of shed surface antigen and autoantibody. In a detailed analysis of the modulation by IgM autoantibodies wherein preincubation of T cells with SLE serum at 37° C reduced their reactivity with IgM antilymphocyte autoantibodies at cold temperatures, loss of autoantibody target antigen from the cell surface was found to be rapid, but transient.[W290] A nadir is reached after approximately 120 minutes of 37° C preincubation, followed by essentially complete re-expression of the target antigen several hours later. Modulation is inhibited by sodium azide, but not by colchicine and cytochalasin D, suggesting that integrity of the cytoskeleton is not essential for this process. While speculative at present, it is possible that autoantibody-mediated alteration of surface membrane determinants occurs in vivo in SLE, as has been demonstrated experimentally in other systems.

Functional Autoantibody-Receptor Interactions

There are several potential consequences of autoantibody-receptor interaction in addition to receptor blockade or receptor modulation. Cross-linking of receptors may stimulate cellular function, as has been documented with antibodies to the thyroid-stimulating hormone receptor,[M94] the insulin receptor,[H168] CD3,[V42] and different isoforms of CD45.[T172] F(ab')$_2$ fragments of IgG from SLE serum have been shown to enhance immunoglobulin synthesis in vitro through direct effects on B cells[T18] and to induce secretion of γIFN by normal mononuclear cells.[R23] Alternatively, antilymphocyte autoantibody binding to a given receptor might deliver an "off" signal, or interfere with receptors involved in essential processes upon which cell activation or proliferation are dependent, e.g., the transferrin receptor, which enables iron uptake.[T283]

Are Antilymphocyte Autoantibodies Responsible for Cellular Immune Abnormalities in SLE?

As discussed at the beginning of this chapter, there is no solid evidence for an underlying intrinsic defect in SLE lymphocytes and monocytes. But whether any of the above mechanisms by which antilymphocyte autoantibodies could alter cellular function *in vivo* actually occurs also is speculative, since essentially all of the data in this regard derive from experiments in which SLE serum or plasma is combined with peripheral blood mononuclear cells in short-term culture in vitro. In general, the abnormal immunologic function observed in this type of experiment parallels that seen with SLE patient cells cultured in the absence of added antilymphocyte autoantibody. Examples include reduced T-cell proliferation to a variety of stimuli;[H432,H470,O49,W180,W244,Y7] reduced T suppressor activity;[O46,S15,S31,S32,T283] inhibition of NK activity[G313,K84] and ADCC;[D199,S120] inhibition of antigen presentation and other macrophage functions;[B528,M500,M676,S371] inhibition of generation of alloreactive cytotoxic T cells;[H470] and enhancement of B-cell immunoglobulin secretion.[T18] On the other hand, the IL-2 defect in SLE may be largely an in vitro phenomenon; in vivo there is IL-2 hyperproduction and increased IL-2 responsiveness.[K430] It is entirely possible that antilymphocyte autoantibodies arise as a consequence of a physiologic attempt by the immune system to restore homeostasis in the face of aggressive autoimmune stimulation.

ANTILYMPHOCYTE AUTOANTIBODIES IN OTHER DISEASES

Truly disease-specific antilymphocyte autoantibodies in SLE have not been identified, and at least several of the major types commonly occur in a wide variety of immunologic, neoplastic, or infectious diseases, and in normal subjects following immunization.[D123] In this respect, antilymphocyte autoantibodies are analogous to rheumatoid factors and cold agglutinins. For example, reports have described antilymphocyte autoantibodies in diseases as diverse as rheumatoid arthritis,[V89] aplastic anemia,[C97] the vasculitides,[P322] leprosy,[P275,R49] autoimmune and alcohol-induced hepatic injury,[D263,L85] and viral infections (*e.g.*, infectious mononucleosis),[M475,M628,Q8,T210] acute parvovirus infection,[S547] and HIV infection. Autoantibodies to lymphocytes in HIV-infected individuals and patients with AIDS have attracted considerable interest because of their possible contribution to clinical and immunologic pathophysiology.[C457,D37,D38,D274,K317,O135,P275,R288,S261,S445,S518,W231] A systematic analysis of the similarities and differences between antilymphocyte autoantibodies in SLE and those in other conditions has not been performed.

ORIGIN OF ANTILYMPHOCYTE AUTOANTIBODIES

The basis by which autoantibodies to lymphocytes arise is unknown. Possible mechanisms include molecular mimicry between self antigens and cross-reactive molecules of infecting microorganisms[B27,F299,O55,O57] and the creation of autoimmunogenic sites on cell surface receptors during receptor-ligand interactions.[S261] For example, gp120 may induce a conformational change in the C-terminal domain of CD4 molecules during HIV attachment, thereby leading to the development of anti-CD4 autoantibodies in HIV-infected individuals.[S261] Molecular mimicry may obtain in the development of antilymphocyte autoantibodies in infectious mononucleosis, where it has been shown that affinity-purified anticardiolipin antibodies react with activated lymphocytes.[M475] Also of interest in this regard is a report that 6 of 214 monoclonal antibodies raised against eight common viruses reacted with human T cells; all 6 were IgM monoclonals directed to various constituents (matrix, phosphoprotein, nucleocapsid D) of measles virus.[B27] Usage of immunoglobulin V region genes in the SLE antilymphocyte autoantibody system has not been studied in sufficient detail for firm conclusions to be drawn.[L192,L431,S389]

CONCLUSIONS

Patients with SLE frequently develop IgM and IgG autoantibodies to molecules on the surface of lymphocytes and monocytes. Best studied are cold-reactive antilymphocyte autoantibodies of the IgM class, which may deplete circulating T cells, modulate target antigens, and, in vitro, have profound effects on cellular immune function. Both of the major IgM and IgG classes occur in highest titer during phases of active disease, and their presence correlates closely with essentially the entire spectrum of SLE immune system functional abnormalities that are characteristic of lymphocytes and monocytes from patients with SLE when cultured in vitro. Of special interest in this regard are IgM autoantibodies to different isoforms of CD45, a plasma membrane—associated protein tyrosine phosphatase that delineates functionally discrete T-cell subsets and regulates proximal events in cell signaling. It is still unclear, however, whether antilymphocyte autoantibodies cause abnormal immunoregulation in SLE, or reflect an abortive attempt to restore immunoregulatory homeostasis.

Chapter 27

ANTIBODIES TO NEURONS

HARRY G. BLUESTEIN

Interest in neuron-reactive antibodies in systemic lupus erythematosus derives from studies of the pathogenesis of its wide variety of neuropsychiatric manifestations. Beginning with the landmark study of Johnson and Richardson,[J96] neuropathologic investigations have consistently shown that immune complex–mediated small vessel inflammation, the hallmark of lupus-induced tissue injury in the kidney and other organs, is not the usual mechanism for tissue damage within the central nervous system. Despite the commonly used term lupus cerebritis, autopsy studies have shown remarkably little inflammation, particularly in those patients with the most characteristic lupus CNS manifestations of organic mental syndromes, psychoses, and seizures. In considering alternative pathologic mechanisms to vasculitis, autoantibodies to neurons are a logical candidate. The role of some cell-reactive antibodies as mediators of autoimmune manifestations has long been recognized in SLE where autoantibodies to red cells, platelets, and lymphocytes are responsible for hemolytic anemia, thrombocytopenia, and lymphocytopenia, respectively. Studies over the past 20 years have also documented and characterized neuron-reactive antibodies in SLE, identified the specific molecules with which some of them react, and demonstrated the close association between some of those reactivities and the major lupus CNS manifestations. The reader is referred to Chapters 38 and 39 for a review of the clinical features of lupus and the nervous system.

ANTIBRAIN REACTIVITIES

The earliest studies documenting the presence of brain-reactive antibodies in SLE sera used an immunofluorescent technique on brain tissue[D204,Q17] to reveal an association between lupus neurologic involvement and antineuronal activities. The antibodies detected with those techniques reacted with intracellular antigens and, where tested, lacked specificity for brain. Absorptions with stomach, liver, and kidney removed the antineuronal reactivity. Those early studies did not generate much enthusiasm for the idea that brain-reactive antibodies participated in the pathogenesis of CNS lupus, in part because of the lack of brain specificity and in part because the antibodies were directed at intracellular antigens which were not likely to be accessible to the antibodies in vivo.

The concept of a pathogenic role for neuron-reactive antibodies was revived by studies documenting a high degree of cross-reactivity between cell membrane–reactive lymphocytotoxic antibodies in SLE sera and human brain tissue.[B360,B482] Bluestein and Zvaifler showed that homogenates of human brain tissue effectively deplete lymphocytotoxic activity from the sera. There was a high degree of brain specificity for the absorptive capacity with comparable volumes of homogenized liver and red blood cells having little effect. In addition, the titer of the lymphocytotoxic antibodies was significantly higher in serum samples from lupus patients with neuropsychiatric manifestations than in those without.[B360] The demonstration by Bresnihan et al. that the extent of cross-reactivity between lymphocytotoxic antibodies and brain was significantly greater in sera from lupus patients with CNS involvement gave additional support to the pathogenic potential of those antibodies.[B482]

ANTINEURONAL MEMBRANE REACTIVITIES

The potential involvement of neuron-reactive antibodies in the pathogenesis of neuropsychiatric lupus requires that those antibodies react with intact living cells. A variety of detection systems including complement-dependent cytotoxicity, immunofluorescence, and radioligand binding have been used to detect antibodies reactive with cultured human neuroblastoma cells.[A366,B354,B359,H453,W260] Several different cell lines have been used, but the SK-N-SH line has proven to be the most sensitive for detecting neuron-reactive antibodies in lupus. Cells from that line have retained differentiated features of normal neurons including the action potential sodium ionophore characteristic of electrically excitable membranes, and the presence of normal neuronal differentiation antigens in their cell membranes. In a complement-dependent neurocytotoxicity assay using those cells as the target, neuron-reactive antibodies were found in 75% of the sera from an unselected population of lupus patients.[B354] Some of the antibodies cross-react with membrane molecules on lymphocytes, and some are specific for nervous system–derived cells. A series of absorption experiments with different glial and neuroblastoma cell lines[B355] reveal a number of different antineuronal specificities, most of which react with antigens expressed on at least some of the glial and neuronal lines. The neurocytotoxic antibodies do not cross-react with molecules on erythrocytes or platelets.

While documenting a variety of neuron-reactive antibody specificities in SLE sera, neurocytotoxic antibody assays did not show a relationship between those antibodies and clinically apparent CNS involvement. However, subsequent studies using the same cell lines in an immunofluorescence detection system did reveal an association between IgG neuron-reactive antibodies and diffuse CNS manifestations of lupus.[W260] The IgM antineuronal activity detected by immunofluorescence, like the neurocytotoxicity assay (which also detects predominantly IgM antibody), did not correlate with the clinical manifestations. Other antibody-binding assays show that neuron-reactive antibodies are present in many sera from lupus patients without active CNS disease, but the amount of neuron-reactive antibody is often higher during flares of neuropsychiatric manifestations.[A366,D42,H100,H453] These studies have made it clear that the presence of neuron-reactive antibodies in the serum by itself is not enough to induce CNS disease.

A hypothesis that links neuron-reactive antibodies to the pathogenesis of neurologic disorders must demonstrate the presence of those antibodies within the nervous system. The desire to pursue that hypothesis led to the development of a sensitive radioimmunoassay for detecting antineuronal activity in cerebrospinal fluid.[B359] Using the SK-N-SH neuroblastoma cells as target, neuron-reactive antibody of the IgG class is present in much higher concentration and is much more likely to occur in the CSF from patients with active CNS disease than it is in CSF from lupus patients who are free of neuropsychiatric manifestations. CSF antineuronal activity is detected in approximately 75% of samples from all patients diagnosed with a neuropsychiatric manifestation of lupus, as compared with less than 10% of lupus patients without clinically apparent neuropsychiatric problems. Those false-positive samples have low levels of neuron-reactive antibody, and the frequency of their occurrence is similar to the 5% positive rate detected in several hundred control CSF samples from patients with a wide variety of non-lupus neurologic disorders. Thus, there is a high degree of specificity for lupus-related CNS involvement. Neuron-reactive antibody of the IgM class is also elevated in SLE CSF, but it does not discriminate well between those with and without neuropsychiatric manifestations.

The sensitivity of the CSF IgG neuron-reactive antibody radioimmunoassay is greatest for the detection of the most common diffuse neuropsychiatric manifestations of lupus, including organic mental syndromes with or without psychosis and generalized seizures. Approximately 90% of patients with one or more of those features have IgG antineuronal activity, and samples from those patients have the highest titers of the antibody.[B359] In contrast, antineuronal activity is elevated in less than half of the patients presenting with the focal neurologic features such as stroke, cranial neuropathy, or transverse myelitis (Table 27–1). There is limited longitudinal data regarding CSF neuron-reactive antibody levels during the course of lupus activity. In one published study involving 8 patients whose spinal fluid was obtained during the acute phase of the illness and again 3 to 4 weeks later after aggressive immunotherapy, there was a dramatic fall in the CSF antibody levels in the post-therapy specimens.[Z22] Our own experience (data unpublished) in a similar number of cases confirms a fall in antineuronal activity in parallel with clinical improvement, but sustained elevation of antibody levels in patients with persistent organic brain dysfunction despite aggressive therapy.

Taken as a group, these studies documenting fluctua-

Table 27–1. Prevalence of Antibodies Relevant to Nervous System Involvement in SLE

Antibody	Source	Type of NP SLE	Prevalence*
Antineuronal (membrane)	CSF	Diffuse	90%
		Focal	40%
		None	<10%
Antiribosomal P	Serum	Psychosis/depression	80%–90%
		Other	10%
		None	15%
Antineurofilament	Serum	Diffuse	60%
		Focal	17%
		None	20%

* Antineuronal (membrane) and antiribosomal P data are based on a large number of samples with results confirmed by at least two independent laboratories.
Antineurofilament data are based on a small number of samples (<25) from one research group.

tions in serum levels of neuron-reactive antibodies, in concert with alterations in clinical expression of CNS lupus, together with the strong correlation of the presence of those antibodies within the nervous system with diffuse neuropsychiatric manifestations, suggest that they are playing a pathogenic role. The origin of the antibodies remains undefined. The antigens stimulating the production of neuron-reactive antibodies may be present on the neurons themselves, but a number of observations suggest that it is more likely that they are induced by antigens outside the nervous system which share epitopes with neuronal molecules. We have reviewed much of the data, documenting cross-reactivity between neuron-reactive antibodies and blood cells, particularly lymphocytes and fetal erythrocytes.[B354,B360,B482,B483] Another report documents that a subset of neuron-reactive antibodies cross-reacts with epitopes on mycobacterial antigens.[A366] Antigens capable of inducing neuron-reactive antibodies have also been identified in SLE cryoglobulins.[B357] Antibodies reactive with lymphocyte and neuronal membrane antigens are generated in rabbits immunized with the SLE cryoprecipitates. The pattern of reactivity of the anticryoglobulin sera against a panel of neuronal and glial cell lines is similar to the pattern of reactivity exhibited in the sera from patients with SLE. Thus, there are a number of potential antigens accessible to the immune system that have the potential to induce antineuronal antibodies.

ANTINEURONAL INTRACYTOPLASMIC REACTIVITIES

An interest in lupus antibodies that react with intracellular neuronal antigens has been rekindled by several studies over the past several years. Of particular importance has been analysis of antibodies to ribosomal P proteins.[B402,G276] Interest in this area was stimulated by the demonstration of antibodies to saline soluble cellular antigens in the CSF of lupus patients. Analysis of the fine specificities of some of those antibodies revealed antiribosomal P protein reactivity in specimens specifically from lupus patients with psychosis.[G276] The lupus sera was shown to react with a carboxyl terminal peptide on the 60S ribosomal subunit phosphoproteins P0, P1, and P2.[E79,E81] Synthesized peptides reproducing the C-terminal end amino acid sequence have been used as the antigenic substrate in an ELISA assay for confirmatory tests of the association of anti-P protein antibodies and lupus psychosis.[B402,S152] In one such study, 90% of 20 sera from patients with psychosis secondary to SLE had elevated anti-P levels compared with 3 of 20 sera from patients with other central nervous system manifestations, and none of 8 sera from lupus patients with transient nonpsychotic behavioral abnormalities related to lupus.[B402] In another study of a much larger number of patients[S152] anti-P levels were elevated in 19% of 269 patients with SLE, and among them, those with CNS dysfunction were approximately twice as likely to have elevated levels of anti-P antibodies (29% of 82 patients with versus 14% of 187 patients without neuropsychiatric manifestations). There was a stronger correlation with lupus psychosis, but the frequency of positives (45%) was not as dramatic as reported in the earlier study. Even more striking in this study is the association of antiribosomal P activity with severe depression (88% of 8 patients). These investigations did not find an accumulation of anti-P antibody within the nervous system. In the limited number of cases with active CNS disease for which serum and CSF samples were matched, anti-P activity was much lower in CSF than in serum even when calculated as a function of the IgG concentration in the samples.[S152] This contrasts with other studies describing the association of antiribosomal P and lupus psychosis where the concentration of that antibody activity was enriched in spinal fluid in relationship to the IgG concentration.[B402,S590]

Analysis of fluctuations of antiribosomal P antibody activity during the course of lupus suggests a correlation between the anti-P antibody levels and activity of psychiatric disease. Anti-P levels generally increased before and during the active phase of either psychosis or depression, but did not change appreciably with exacerbations of other manifestations of SLE or during bouts of systemic infection.[B402,S152] A prospective study of antiribosomal P protein levels in two family members with recurrent lupus psychosis has documented a rise and then rapid fall in the antibody levels just prior to the onset of recurrent psychosis, with the result that the antibody levels were normal by the time the patients presented for care.[D168] That rapid decline in antibody levels may account for some of the lack of sensitivity of the anti-P protein assay for the detection of lupus psychosis.

Neurofilaments are another group of intracytoplasmic molecules of neurons that serve as targets of lupus antibodies.[B179,K472,N27] Antineurofilament activity was looked for because of the earlier studies documenting antibodies against unidentified cytoplasmic antigens of neurons in SLE patients with neurologic manifestations, and because in certain chronic neurologic diseases there are alterations of the neurofilament architecture with the resultant production of circulating antibodies against neurofilaments.[B26,C207,K325,N27] Using purified neurofilament polypeptides as target in an ELISA assay, IgG antineurofilament antibodies were identified in the sera of approximately 20% of SLE patients as compared to 6% of patients with rheumatoid arthritis and none of 40 blood donors.[K472] In

that first small study, one-third of the patients with the antibody had a neurologic complication. In subsequent studies, using an immunoblotting assay, a correlation of antineurofilament antibody with diffuse neuropsychiatric disease was documented.[B179,R233] In a study of 19 patients with lupus neuropsychiatric disease, sera from 8 of them had elevated levels of antineurofilament antibodies, but that antibody was especially associated with the diffuse CNS manifestations. Of the 11 lupus patients who fit in that category, sera from 7 of them (65%) had high antibody levels compared to only 1 of the 8 patients with focal neurologic disease. Thus, antibodies to the intracytoplasmic neurofilament antigens share with antibodies to ribosomal P protein, as well as antibodies to as yet undefined neuronal membrane antigens, an association with the diffuse neuropsychiatric manifestations of SLE.

ROLE IN PATHOGENESIS

Antibodies to a variety of molecules on or within neurons occur in patients with systemic lupus erythematosus, and their presence in the circulation and/or the spinal fluid correlates with clinically active neuropsychiatric disturbance. As a group, these antibodies are of great interest both for their potential to provide insights into the pathogenesis of CNS dysfunction in SLE and also as potential diagnostic tests to help resolve difficult diagnostic dilemmas.

In considering the pathogenesis of neuropsychiatric dysfunction in SLE, it is useful to divide the clinical manifestations into focal and diffuse categories. Both the pathology and diagnostic findings are generally straightforward in those patients with focal involvement. Vasculopathy of small- and medium-sized muscular arteries either by immune complex–mediated vasculitis or thrombosis related to antiphospholipid antibodies have caused cerebrovascular accidents, transverse myelitis, cranial neuropathies, and mononeuritis multiplex.[A47,E85, J96,K149] It is with the diffuse neuropsychiatric manifestations, organic mental dysfunction, encephalopathy, psychosis, or other severe psychiatric disturbance and nonfocal seizures that the difficulties in defining the pathogenesis and making the diagnosis persist.

How is one to explain the sometimes dramatically rapid reversal of organic mental dysfunction and bizarre behavior? Pathologic studies of patients who have died with neuropsychiatric dysfunction have been more remarkable for what they do not show, than for the pathologic changes revealed.[E85,J96] As already mentioned, true vasculitis of small vessels, the hallmark of lupus pathology in other organ systems, is generally missing. There are widely scattered microinfarcts and a noninflammatory vasculopathy characterized by intimal proliferation and perivascular gliosis, but this bland vasculopathy generally does not correlate with the clinical findings, and it may be present in patients who did not demonstrate neuropsychiatric involvement. Reactivity with neurons by antibodies that may gain entry into the nervous system through an alteration in the blood-brain barrier (perhaps because of the damage visualized as bland vasculopathy) provides an attractive potential mechanism for producing the reversible diffuse CNS manifestations. The antibodies are present within the nervous system in correlation with those clinical features. A direct effect of lupus neuron-reactive antibodies on neuronal function has not yet been documented. Experiments in animals, however, have documented that antibodies to CNS antigens can induce pathologic changes in the nervous system and alterations in behavior that are quite similar to those that characterize lupus CNS involvement. When injected into spinal fluid of normal rabbits, antibodies to brain produce foci of cerebral edema accompanied by motor discoordination and epileptic seizures.[S455] Similarly, antibody to synaptosomal plasma membranes caused significant memory impairment while intracerebral injection of antibodies to brain gangliosides generated seizures in rats.[K81,K328] Thus, there is a reasonable basis for implicating antibodies reactive with molecules on neuronal membranes in the pathogenesis of neuropsychiatric dysfunction.

A pathogenic role for antibodies directed at intracytoplasmic molecules in neurons is less plausible. True, intracellular injection of antibodies to these molecules can have profound effects; for example, microinjection of anti-ribosomal P antibodies into cultured human fibroblasts inhibits protein synthesis,[K328] and injection of antibodies to neurofilament proteins into a single blastomere of a two-cell stage Xenopus embryo results in unilateral retardation of peripheral nerve development in the resultant tadpoles as well as an abnormal accumulation of intermediate filament proteins only in neuronal cell bodies derived from the injected blastomeres.[C207] In vivo, however, the intact membrane of the living cells prevents interaction between the antibody and its target intracellular antigen, unless, of course, the antigen itself or another molecule expressing cross-reactive epitopes is also present on the cell surface. Knowledge of the sequence of the antigenic C-terminal polypeptide of ribosomal P protein permitted a computerized search for other molecules on the neuronal surface with a similar structure,[S152] and no known candidates were identified. However, more direct approaches have provided some evidence that neuronal membranes bear molecules that are reactive both with antiribosomal P and antineurofilament antibodies. In a preliminary study, affinity-purified antibody to ribosomal P protein bound specifically to the surface of live cultured neuroblastoma cells.[K71] Similarly, a monoclonal antibody to the high-molecular-weight neurofilament protein isolated from the serum of a patient with an IgA monoclonal gammopathy cross-reacted with a 65 kD protein expressed on the membrane of neuroblastoma cells.[S13]

The membrane-bound molecules reactive with the antiribosomal P and antineurofilament antibodies have not yet been fully characterized, but preliminary evidence suggests that they are not identical to, but share epitopes with, the intracytoplasmic molecules. Whether the surface molecules are different or the same as the intracytoplasmic molecules, their presence on the surface provides a target for the binding of antiribosomal P and antineu-

rofilament antibodies to neurons. If these antibodies are internalized, they have the potential to disrupt cellular function through their interaction with their intracytoplasmic targets. While there is yet no documentation that those antibodies can be internalized, there is evidence that other IgG and IgM antibodies reactive with molecules on the neuronal surface can be internalized and transported in a retrograde fashion from the axon to the cell body.[F3] Thus, either through cell surface interactions directly, or after internalization through reaction with their intracellular antigens, it is plausible that the antiribosomal P protein or antineurofilament antibodies could participate in the pathogenesis of neuropsychiatric lupus.

Independent of their role in the pathogenesis of CNS lupus, the neuron-reactive antibodies play an important role in diagnosis. The assay of membrane-reactive IgG antineuronal antibody in the spinal fluid is the most sensitive and specific test for the diagnosis of the diffuse neuropsychiatric manifestations.[B359,Z22] Antibodies to ribosomal P proteins have a narrower specificity for severe psychiatric disturbances. In a comparison of those two tests in a small number of patients, the antiribosomal P assay was abnormal in three of six patients with psychosis and in four of nine patients with any diffuse CNS manifestation, while the antineuronal antibody assay was present in five of six patients with psychosis and eight of nine patients with all diffuse manifestations.[S590] There were no patients in that study with severe depression where the antiribosomal P assay is very sensitive.[S152] The antineuronal binding assay in CSF has generally not been abnormal in patients whose only neuropsychiatric manifestation is depression. Thus, the antiribosomal P protein assay may be most useful for implicating lupus as the cause of that psychiatric problem. These antineuronal antibody assays are becoming more widely available in commercial laboratories. Their appropriate role in the diagnosis of neuropsychiatric lupus will evolve as experience with them increases.

SUMMARY

In conclusion, a strong association of antineuronal antibodies, with the clinically apparent neuropsychiatric manifestations of SLE; the occasionally documented rise in antineuronal activity just prior to the onset of lupus CNS disease; and the absence of those antibodies in similar kinds of neuropsychiatric dysfunction associated with other disorders provides strong circumstantial evidence in support of the hypothesis that neuron-reactive antibodies participate in the pathogenesis of neuropsychiatric dysfunction. Identification of the specific membrane molecules that are the target of the pathogenic antibodies, and the mechanisms by which antibody interaction with those molecules deter neurologic function, will be needed for the development of more effective strategies for the treatment and prevention of these problems.

Chapter 28

OTHER SEROLOGIC ABNORMALITIES IN SLE

FRANCISCO P. QUISMORIO, Jr.

ANTIERYTHROCYTE ANTIBODIES

Antibodies to red blood cells (RBCs) are detected by the antiglobulin (Coombs') test, of which there are two variations. The direct Coombs' test measures the presence of antibodies bound to the surface of circulating RBCs. The antiglobulin reagent, usually rabbit antibody to human gamma globulin, is added to a saline suspension of washed erythrocytes of the patient and if the erythrocytes are coated with antibodies, cell agglutination ensues. The indirect Coombs' test measures for free anti-RBC antibody in the serum of the patient. Test serum is incubated with suspension of a mixture of washed normal group O red cells that express most of the known RBC antigens. Thereafter, the cells are allowed to react with antihuman gamma globulin, and cell agglutination indicates the presence of free anti-RBC antibodies in the patient's serum.

Anti-whole human gamma globulin is usually employed as the antiglobulin reagent, but monospecific antisera to human IgG and other IgG classes, IgG subclasses, C3, and C4 are also being used. In certain situations, immune complexes unrelated to RBC antigens may bind to erythrocytes giving rise to a positive direct Coombs' test. The limited sensitivity of the antiglobulin test has led to the development of other methods with improved sensitivity such as the ELISA and radioassay[H111,L182,Y4]; however, in most clinical laboratories, the Coombs' test remains the standard test for anti-RBC antibodies.

Characteristics of Anti-RBC Antibodies in SLE

Autoantibodies to RBCs are classified into two major types according to their thermal requirements:[H111] warm antibodies react optimally with surface membrane antigens at 37°C,[L182] and cold-type autoantibodies react more avidly with RBC antigens at 0 to −5°C than at higher temperatures.[A374,S173]

Autoantibodies to RBC in SLE as well as in idiopathic autoimmune hemolytic anemia (AIHA) are warm antibodies. Warm antibodies belong most commonly to the IgG class.[C206] All four subclasses of IgG are represented, although IgG1 is the predominant IgG subclass while IgG2 and IgG3 are found less frequently. Warm anti-RBC antibodies belonging to IgG4 subclass are uncommon. Cold-reacting antibodies to RBCs are mostly IgM antibodies and rarely of IgG class. A few cases of SLE patients with hemolytic anemia associated with cold agglutinins have been reported.[D305,V81] The agglutinin titers in some of the patients are relatively low.[V81]

Warm antibodies bound to the surface of RBCs in vivo can be eluted and examined for biologic properties. In vitro, warm antibodies do not fix complement when allowed to react with normal allogeneic erythrocytes; however, often these antibodies are detected bound in vivo to autologous RBCs together with complement components.[A374,W350] In vitro, warm antibodies do not cause red cell agglutination, cell lysis, or alteration of red blood cell membranes.[A374] In patients with idiopathic AIHA, the warm antibodies react with antigenic determinants of the Rh complex.[D4,V115] The specificity of warm antibodies in SLE is not completely known; however, it has been noted that warm antibodies eluted from erythrocytes containing both IgG and complement on their surface (including that from SLE patients) react with Rh null cells.[L112] This observation suggests that the specificity is directed against determinant(s) unrelated to the Rh complex.[B559,C270]

Prevalence of Anti-RBC Antibodies in SLE

Mongan et al. examined the frequency of a positive direct Coombs' test in patients with various types of systemic rheumatic diseases.[M542] Five of 103 (5%) of RA and 15 of 23 (65%) SLE patients had a positive test. None of 6 systemic sclerosis patients and 2 with polyarteritis nodosa were positive. Two of 3 cases of thrombotic thrombocytopenic purpura and only 1 of 103 subjects with nonrheumatic conditions were positive. Worlledge[W350] found positive antiglobulin tests in 16 of 35 (44%) SLE patients. Among normal blood donors, the frequency of a positive Coombs' test was estimated to be 1 in 14,000.[G307]

Despite the high frequency of positive direct antiglobulin tests among SLE and RA patients, Mongan et al.[M542] found no clinical evidence of active hemolysis. This observation illustrates the frequent dissociation between abnormal serologic findings and occurrence of tissue injury. A positive direct Coombs' test in the absence of hemolysis should be regarded as one of the multiple serologic abnormalities frequently seen in SLE.

Pattern of Reaction With Antiglobulin Serum

With the use of antisera of different specificities, three patterns of reactivity are commonly identified in the direct Coombs' test: type I: IgG, IgM, IgA, either singly or in combination are present on the RBC surface; type II: both immunoglobulin and complement components are bound on the RBC surface; type III: RBCs are coated with complement components (C3, C4) alone. Type I is the pattern most commonly found in patients with idiopathic AIHA, while types II and III are patterns generally associated with SLE.[E176,R329,W350]

Of 180 patients with warm-type AIHA, Worlledge[W351] found 83 (46%) patients had IgG coating alone on their RBCs, 64 (36%) had both IgG and complement, and 33 (18%) had complement coating alone. Of the 17 SLE patients included in her series, none had bound IgG alone, 12 patients showed bound IgG and complement, and the remaining 5 subjects had complement reactivity alone. Chaplin and Avioli[C206] suggested that a diagnosis of SLE is unlikely in a patient with immune hemolytic anemia if complement components are not detectable on the RBC surface.

Among SLE patients with a positive direct Coombs' test but without evidence of overt hemolysis, 12 of 13 showed complement reactivity alone, 3 patients had both IgG and complement, and none showed IgG alone. Of 103 RA patients tested, 5 had a positive direct Coombs' test and all showed complement reactivity alone.[M542] The pattern of red cell autosensitization in RA was confirmed by Gilliland and Turner,[G147] who found 12 of 75 consecutive RA patients tested reacted with anti-C' antiserum exclusively.

Two independent investigations established that RBCs coated with complement components alone as determined by the standard direct Coombs' test contain IgG antibody as well, suggesting that complement deposition was in fact antibody mediated. Gilliland and associates[G146] devised a sensitive complement-fixing antibody consumption test, based on the principle of the antiglobulin test, which detected as few as 20 IgG molecules on the red cell surface. On the other hand, MacKenzie and Creevy[M25] detected IgG antibody on the surface of complement-coated RBCs, when the standard Coombs' test was performed at 4 but not at 37°C. The IgG antibody was not eluted from RBCs at 37°C; however, it apparently underwent a thermal-dependent conformational change so that agglutination with the Coombs' antiglobulin reagent did not occur. SLE patients with combined warm reacting IsG and cold reacting IgM anti-RBC antibodies have been reported (see Chap. 43).[S400,S537]

Pathophysiology of Immune Hemolytic Anemia

The pathogenesis of red blood cell damage by anti-RBC autoantibodies has been extensively investigated.[F215,H309,R330] Erythrocytes sensitized with warm-reactive IgG antibodies are cleared from the circulation by macrophages in the splenic sinusoids. Macrophages express surface receptors for Fc portion of the IgG molecule and C3b fragment of complement. The macrophage Fc receptors bind erythrocytes with bound IgG anti-RBC antibody, causing membrane damage, spherocytosis, and phagocytosis of some RBCs. Microspherocytes have a shortened life span because of their increased rigidity and increased osmotic fragility. As the amount of surface-bound antibody increases, splenic trapping becomes more efficient, and red cell survival shortens significantly. When the density of bound IgG antibody is substantial, complement activation occurs. RBCs coated with IgG and complement are cleared by two distinct macrophage receptors, C3b and Fc receptors, causing an accelerated

Table 28–1. Antierythrocyte Antibodies in SLE

1. A positive direct Coombs' test in the absence of active hemolysis is a frequent serologic finding in SLE.
2. The direct Coombs' test frequently shows reactivity with complement alone or with immunoglobulin plus complement.
3. Antierythrocyte antibodies in SLE are IgG antibodies, warm type, and react with non–Rh-related antigens on red cell surface.
4. These antibodies can be associated with significant hemolysis in some patients.

clearance of RBCs from the circulation resulting in extravascular hemolysis. Sequestration of sensitized RBCs by hepatic macrophages with complement but no Fc receptors may also occur at this stage.

The IgG subclass of the anti-RBC antibody is an important determinant in RBC destruction because splenic macrophages have IgG Fc receptors for IgG1 and IgG3 subclasses. The macrophage FcR avidity for IgG3 is greater than for IgG2 antibodies. RBCs with critical quantities of IgG1 and or IgG3 antibodies on their surface are destroyed. It has been calculated that RBCs coated with IgG1 antibody alone or with additional IgG2 and IgG4 antibodies require at least 2000 molecules per RBC to initiate phagocytosis or rosette formation with monocytes in vitro. In contrast, as low as 230 molecules of IgG3 anti-RBC antibodies per cell are required for binding to monocytes.[Z53] Moreover, the clearance of RBCs sensitized with IgG antibody and complement is accelerated, and IgG1 and IgG3 antibodies fix complement efficiently, while IgG2 antibodies are less efficient and IgG4 antibodies do not activate complement.

Erythrocytes coated with IgM anti-RBC antibody, as in the case of cold hemagglutinin disease, are cleared by a mechanisms dependent on complement activation. IgM-coated RBCs bind to C3b receptors of macrophages and are cleared rapidly in the liver.[S175,S176] When the amount of IgM antibody on the RBC surface is high, complement activation is rapid and extensive so that the terminal components of complement become activated, resulting in intravascular hemolysis.

PLATELET ANTIBODIES

A special relationship exists between SLE and chronic immune thrombocytopenic purpura (ITP), both of which primarily afflict young females. Some patients with thrombocytopenic purpura labeled as idiopathic at the onset later develop classic SLE,[B46,K75] suggesting that ITP may be an early manifestation of the disease. Further, a thrombocytopenic purpura, indistinguishable from chronic ITP, may develop along the course of SLE.

Thrombocytopenia in SLE, as in chronic ITP, is caused by increased peripheral destruction of platelets brought about by autoimmune mechanisms. Platelet survival studies in SLE with ^{51}Cr-labeled platelets have demonstrated shortened life span.[C333]

In 1951, Harrington and co-workers[H144] transfused normal human volunteers with plasma from patients with chronic ITP and noted a significant and prompt drop in the platelet counts. Autologous plasma from chronic ITP subjects, obtained during disease exacerbations and stored, produced thrombocytopenia when reinfused to the same patients during periods of disease remission.[S401] The humoral antibody nature of the antiplatelet factor in this disorder has been established. Shulman and associates[S401] showed that the factor was a 7S gamma globulin, reactive to autologous as well as to allogeneic platelets, and it produced in vivo effects quantitatively and qualitatively similar to those exhibited by known antiplatelet antibodies. These findings indicated that the platelet-depressing factor in the plasma is an antiplatelet antibody.

Similar plasma transfusion experiments have not been performed in SLE patients with thrombocytopenia. However, Nathan and Snapper[N44] reported an analogous situation in a premature infant born of a mother with SLE who at the time of delivery had thrombocytopenia. At birth the infant had low platelet counts that persisted up to 3 weeks of age. Both mother and infant had platelet agglutinins and positive LE-cell tests. It was suggested that transplacental transfer of both platelet antibody and antinuclear antibody had occurred from the mother to the baby.

Tests for Antiplatelet Antibodies in SLE

Although the transfusion experiments provided strong argument for the autoimmune nature of chronic ITP, some investigators remained unconvinced because reliable in vitro tests for the detection of antiplatelet antibodies are not available. Over the years, many in vitro tests have been introduced, indicating that a test of reasonable specificity, reproducibility, and sensitivity is yet to become widely accepted. Of the many in vitro tests for antiplatelet antibodies, few have been employed in SLE: platelet agglutination,[H143,W137] direct antiglobulin consumption test,[D56,V20] dextran agglutination test,[H103] platelet factor 3 method,[K79] and indirect immunofluorescence method.[P218,V106]

Karpatkin and Siskind[K78] introduced the platelet factor 3 "immunoinjury" technique to detect antiplatelet antibodies in SLE and chronic ITP. The method is based on the property of antiplatelet antibodies to damage normal platelets releasing factor 3. In turn, this factor is made available to the coagulation cascade, and its effect is measured as a shortening of the clotting time. The gamma globulin fraction of serum isolated by ammonium sulfate precipitation rather than whole serum was tested for antiplatelet antibodies. With this sensitive method, they found platelet antibodies in 65% of patients with chronic ITP (of whom 96% were thrombocytopenic at the time of testing). The antiplatelet antibody was removed with prior incubation of the serum with rabbit antihuman IgG or absorption with normal human platelets. Further, the antiplatelet activity can be eluted from normal platelets after prior incubation with positive but not with a negative serum.[K79] Karpatkin suggested that SLE patients who test positive for antiplatelet antibodies but have normal platelet counts represent a subset of patients with a compensated thrombocytolytic state, in which an increased turnover of platelets is compensated by increased platelet production.[K80] On the other hand, Kutti and co-workers[K486] showed that the abnormal values of platelet factor 3 assay in nonthrombopenic SLE patients correlated with

the amount of circulating immune complexes, suggesting that the assay measured not only antiplatelet antibodies but also immune complexes that presumably bind to surface Fc receptors.

The direct antiglobulin consumption test detects the presence of gamma globulin fixed onto the surface of platelets. Used extensively by early workers, this test appears to be sensitive, but it is technically complex and may yield false-positive results.[M398] Van de Wiel et al.[V20] found that 13 of 23 chronic ITP patients and all 6 SLE patients with thrombocytopenia were positive by this test. Dausett and co-workers[D56] reported that 46 of 93 chronic ITP subjects and 23 of 24 SLE patients were positive.

Platelet-Bound IgG in SLE

In 1975, Dixon and co-workers[D238] introduced a quantitative method of measuring the IgG bound on the surface of platelets that is based on the inhibition of complement lysis. All 17 patients with chronic ITP showed elevated platelet-associated IgG when compared to that of the healthy controls. Moreover, an inverse relationship between platelet count and the concentration of platelet-associated IgG was observed before and during drug therapy. These observations were soon confirmed by several investigators using other methods of measuring platelet-bound IgG.[K160,K161]

Platelet-associated IgG has been shown to be increased in practically all SLE patients with thrombocytopenia.[F8,H241,K162,M656] Kelton and co-workers[K162] reported an inverse correlation between platelet count and platelet-associated IgG in 10 thrombocytopenic SLE patients. Mulshine et al.[M656] confirmed this inverse relationship, and further observed that SLE patients with normal platelet counts had platelet-associated IgG even lower than that seen in normal controls. Conversely, Bonacossa and associates[B398] found elevated platelet-bound IgG in SLE patients with normal platelet counts. Subjects with high amounts of platelet-associated IgG had significantly higher anti-DNA antibodies than those with normal or slightly elevated platelet-bound IgG. However, they found no correlation between disease activity and platelet-bound IgG.

The IgG antiplatelet antibodies in the sera of chronic ITP patients appear to be restricted to the IgG3 subclass,[K77] whereas in SLE sera, all the four IgG subclasses are represented.[D240] Conversely, all four IgG subclasses are bound in vivo to platelets of patients with chronic ITP, suggesting that the circulating antiplatelet IgG and platelet-associated IgG may represent different populations of platelet antibodies.[H523,R331]

The nature of the platelet-associated IgG is not completely known. It may represent IgG antibody bound to platelet-specific surface antigens (autoantigens), IgG antibody bound to HLA or blood group antigens or to exogenous antigens absorbed on the surface of platelets, IgG nonspecifically fixed to damaged platelets, or circulating immune complexes attached to platelet surface Fc receptors.[K70,K160]

McMillan and co-workers[M309] showed that IgG platelet antibodies synthesized by splenic lymphocyte cultures of patients with chronic ITP bind to platelets through their Fab terminus, indicative of a specific antibody reaction. Moreover, eluates from platelets of the same patients contained IgG that bound to normal allogeneic platelets.[M309] Kelton and associates[K163] reported that the increased amounts of platelet-associated IgG in malaria were partly caused by binding of IgG-specific antibody to malarial antigens absorbed on the surface of platelets. Thrombocytopenic purpura in HIV-infected patients is associated with increased platelet-associated IgG. Walsh and associates[W55] presented evidence to show that the platelet-associated IgG in these patients is not due to bound antiplatelet antibodies, but to deposition of complement and immune complexes on the surface of platelets.

The nature of platelet-associated IgG in SLE has not been fully studied, but may in part represent bound immune complexes.[K160] This is supported by the observation that the antiplatelet antibody found in SLE sera fixes complement, unlike that found in the sera of patients with chronic ITP, which is non-complement fixing.[D240] Moreover, preformed complexes of DNA–anti-DNA antibodies bind to the surface of platelets.[C289] Puram et al.[P335] noted a positive relationship between platelet counts in SLE with immune complex–like material in serum measured by polyethylene glycol (PEG) precipitation but not with platelet-associated IgG. On the other hand, no correlation was evident between the level of circulating immune complexes measured by C1q binding[M656] or Raji cell assay[B398] and the amount of platelet-bound IgG in SLE, indicating that platelet-bound IgG was not entirely caused by antigen-antibody complexes.

Elevated levels of platelet-associated IgG are not necessarily diagnostic of chronic ITP or thrombocytopenia as a result of SLE. High values can be seen in patients with thrombocytopenia considered to be nonimmune in origin[K160] as well as in some patients with normal platelet counts.[B398] Conversely, a diagnosis of ITP is unlikely in a thrombocytopenic patient if the platelet-associated IgG is low or normal.

Specificity of Antiplatelet Antibodies in SLE

To date, a limited number of studies have examined the antigenic specificity of autoantibodies to platelets in SLE.[B230,H459,K58] Multiple platelet antigens including surface membrane and cytoplasmic proteins have been identified, implying heterogeneity of these antibodies in SLE.

Howe and Lynch[H459] examined the binding specificities of circulating antiplatelet antibodies in SLE by Western blotting. All SLE patients studied who were thrombocytopenic and with increased amounts of platelet-bound IgG had serum antibodies that reacted with platelet protein fractions with molecular weights of 120 and 80 kDa. SLE patients with normal platelet counts but with elevated platelet-associated IgG were also positive for serum antiplatelet antibodies. Absorption of sera with whole platelets or platelet lysates removed the antibody activity. The binding pattern was found to be relatively specific for SLE and was not seen in healthy controls. Sera from patients with chronic ITP reacted with multiple platelet fractions with no consistent pattern unlike that seen in SLE, suggest-

ing that the specificities of platelet antibodies in the two conditions are different. Using a similar methodology, Kaplan et al.[K58] confirmed the presence of serum antibodies to platelets in 3 of 10 thrombocytopenic SLE patients. The antigens involved were cytoplasmic proteins from normal platelets with molecular weights of 108 and 66 kDa, respectively.

In chronic ITP, target antigens of circulating as well as platelet-bound IgG have also been identified by immunoblotting and by using monoclonal antibodies. Antigenic epitopes on the GPIIb-IIa complex have been the most frequently observed, while GP1b and GPV antigens have occasionally been reported.[W345] These glycoproteins belong to a complex of membrane proteins on the surface of platelets that function as receptors for fibrinogen, fibronectin, and other proteins and are important in hemostasis. Berchtold et al.[B230] examined the specificity of antiplatelet antibodies in patients with disease-related immune thrombocytopenia including SLE, other connective tissue diseases, and lymphomas. Autoantibodies against platelet GPIIb-IIIa complex were found in two SLE patients and one patient each with MCTD and Sjögren's syndrome, showing that the specificity of the antiplatelet antibodies in some patients with systemic rheumatic diseases is similar to that seen in chronic ITP.

Antiphospholipid Antibodies and Antiplatelet Antibodies

The presence of antiphospholipid antibodies including anticardiolipin (ACA) and lupus anticoagulant in SLE is strongly associated with thrombocytopenia. For this reason, it has been hypothesized that ACA may cross-react with platelet phospholipids, resulting in inactivation and/or subsequent sequestration in the reticuloendothelial system. Rupin and associates[R423] examined the significance of specific platelet antibodies and ACA in SLE patients with thrombocytopenia. Although half of their patients with low platelet counts tested positive for ACA, the thrombocytopenia correlated better with the presence of serum IgG antibody to an 80 kDa platelet antigen. Moreover, absorption of the serum with platelets removed the ACA activity in only half of the sera with antiplatelet antibodies. Jouhikainen et al.[J136] examined 71 consecutive SLE patients for platelet antibodies by immunoblotting. The most common antibody found reacted with a 65 kDa platelet antigen and its presence was significantly associated with lupus anticoagulant, a history of thrombocytopenia, and thrombosis, especially arterial occlusions. Out and co-workers[O126] observed that IgG eluted from platelets of SLE patients had antibody activity against negatively charged phospholipids. Nevertheless, there was no evidence of in vivo activation of platelets, and platelet aggregation was not impaired. Thus, in vivo binding of antiphospholipid antibodies to platelets does not necessarily result in thrombocytopenia.

The above data indicate a heterogeneity of platelet antibodies in SLE, some of which cross-react with cardiolipin phospholipids and others react with specific platelet glycoproteins, as well as other membrane and cytoplasmic antigens. Further studies to characterize the antigens and

Table 28–2. Platelet Antibodies in SLE

1. In vitro tests for platelet antibodies such as agglutination, direct anti-globulin consumption test, platelet factor 3 method, and immuno-fluorescence are frequently positive in thrombocytopenic SLE patients. These tests are of limited clinical application because of technical deficiencies.
2. Tests that measure platelet-associated IgG are widely used and show elevated values in practically all SLE patients with thrombocytopenia and in some patients with normal platelet counts.
3. The nature of platelet-associated IgG is not completely known but may represent antiplatelet antibodies and bound immune complexes.

to clarify the relative importance of the different antibodies in the pathogenesis of the thrombocytopenia are needed.

ANTINEUTROPHIL ANTIBODIES

The frequent occurrence of leukopenia in SLE, possibly mediated by immunologic processes similar to that described in autoimmune hemolytic anemia or autoimmune thrombocytopenia, led to investigations on the presence of antileukocyte antibodies. Various conventional serologic methods such as agglutination, complement fixation, antiglobulin consumption test, and cytotoxicity have been utilized for this purpose.[Q18] Early studies employed whole leukocyte preparations rather than purified fractions (e.g., lymphocyte subsets) as substrate. Differences in their specificity and sensitivity make it difficult to compare results of the various tests. Further, the presence of isoantibodies against leukocytes, which may be a consequence of multiple pregnancies and/or blood transfusions, must be differentiated from genuine leukocyte antibodies in interpreting the results.

Technical improvements in fractionation of peripheral blood leukocytes led to the development of new procedures to detect antibodies to lymphocytes. In 1970, Mittal and co-workers employed the lymphocyte microcytotoxicity test developed for histocompatibility testing for the detection of cytotoxic antibodies to lymphocytes in SLE.[M490] They found a high prevalence of specific lymphocytotoxic antibodies in SLE, and this observation soon became confirmed independently by other workers[N94,S625,T116] (see Chap. 26). In contrast, techniques to detect specific immune reactions to granulocytes have been slow to develop and more importantly more difficult to standardize.[L363]

Tests for antineutrophil antibodies fall into two major types: immunochemical and functional.[L363] The former detects immunoglobulins bound to the surface of the patient's neutrophils (direct) or free antibodies in the serum (indirect test) using normal allogeneic neutrophils as substrate. In interpreting the results of these tests, immune complexes binding via Fc and complement receptors on leukocytes should be excluded from binding of specific antineutrophil antibodies. The latter type measures in vitro sequelae of granulocyte antibodies such as lysis of sensitized cells, phagocytosis, etc.

Both IgM- and IgG-specific antineutrophil autoantibodies have been found in SLE. Drew and Terasaki[D289] de-

scribed cytotoxic granulocyte-specific antibodies in 53% of 57 SLE patients using a panel of 70 granulocytes from random normal persons. The antibodies were of IgM class, complement fixing, exhibited optimum activity at 4°C and were present in 10% of healthy nonimmunized individuals. The clinical significance of these antibodies in SLE was not examined. Starkebaum et al.[S647] studied the mechanism of neutropenia in an SLE patient and found increased amounts of IgG bound on the surface of PMNs. The patient's serum caused opsonization of normal neutrophils for ingestion by other neutrophils. Fractionation of the serum showed that both immune complexes and monomeric IgG antineutrophil bound to PMNs, however only the latter cause opsonization of neutrophils. The F(ab')$_2$ fragment of the IgG reacted to the PMNs, confirming the true antibody activity.[S616] Although IgG neutrophil-binding activity of serum was found to be common in SLE, there was no association between the level and neutropenia.[S616] Two independent groups of investigators confirmed the absence of correlation between neutrophil count in SLE and the titer of PMN-binding IgG in the serum.[H14,R435] In contrast, there is some correlation between antilymphocyte antibody titers and lymphopenia (see Chap. 26). However, the ability of SLE sera to opsonize normal PMNs to be phagocytosed by monocytes,[H14] as well as the capacity of serum antineutrophil antibodies to fix C3 on allogeneic normal PMNs, were both found to be inversely correlated with neutrophil count in SLE.

The specificity of antineutrophil antibodies in SLE was examined by Sipos et al.[S481] by Western immunoblots. The antibodies reacted with two membrane antigens with molecular weights of 50 to 60 and 30 kDa, respectively. Moreover, the antineutrophil antibodies inhibited the binding of mouse monoclonal antibodies to CD15 (granulocyte antigen) and CD16 (FcR) to normal neutrophils. Whether the antigens seen in the immunoblots are identical to CD15 or CD16 or not remains to be clarified.

The lack of correlation between titer of antineutrophil antibodies and neutrophil count suggests that factors other than antineutrophil antibodies are important in the pathogenesis of neutropenia in SLE. Antibody-coated PMNs may remain longer in the circulation because of the defective reticuloendothelial function in SLE. The role of antibody avidity, specificity, as well as density of membrane antigens may be important. A study of neutrophil kinetics is needed to determine whether peripheral destruction of neutrophils in SLE is compensated by increased production, such that the net result is a normal peripheral neutrophil count.

Autoantibodies directed against cytoplasmic antigen(s) of human neutrophils and monocytes (ANCAs) are associated with Wegener's granulomatosis.[N116] These antibodies are detected by indirect immunofluorescent test using ethanol-fixed normal neutrophils as substrate. Two fluorescent patterns are seen, a cytoplasmic (C-ANCA) and perinuclear or nuclear (P-ANCA). C-ANCAs are detected in the majority of patients with Wegener's granulomatosis and react with proteinase 3 although other antigens are also involved. P-ANCAs are found in patients with idiopathic necrotizing crescentic glomerulonephritis and polyarteritis nodosa and react predominantly with mye-

Table 28–3. Antineutrophil Antibodies in SLE

1. Circulating antineutrophil antibodies are prevalent in SLE; however, the antibody titer does not correlate with neutrophil count.
2. Ability of SLE sera to opsonize as well as to fix C3 on normal allogeneic PMNs is inversely correlated with the neutrophil count.
3. Most antineutrophil antibodies are directed to surface antigens on PMNs. However, some react with cytoplasm of PMNs; P-ANCAs may be found, but not C-ANCAs.

loperoxidase, a lysosomal enzyme, although other antigens such as elastase are probably involved.[J68] Antinuclear antibodies may interfere with the interpretation of the immunofluorescent test for P-ANCAs.

None of 96 SLE patients studied by Nassberger et al.[N36] by immunofluorescent test had C-ANCAs, while 93% had ANAs. Antimyeloperoxidase antibodies were found in 21% of the patients by a specific ELISA test. The serum titers were generally low, and the presence of the antibody did not correlate with any particular disease feature. Both antibodies to elastase and to myeloperoxidase were found to be prevalent in hydralazine-induced LE.[N36] Thus, the presence of C-ANCAs suggests a systemic vasculitic disease other than SLE. P-ANCAs, however, can be found in patients with SLE.

RHEUMATOID FACTORS

Rheumatoid factors (RFs) comprise a heterogenous group of antibodies reactive with antigenic determinants on the Fc portion of human or animal IgG. Although RFs belonging to the IgM class are the most commonly measured isotype by clinical tests, RFs belonging to the IgA, IgG, IgD, and IgE classes have been identified.[H96,W241] RFs can react with autologous and isologous as well as homologous IgG.

Serum RFs are measured by a variety of serologic methods including agglutination, ELISA, radioimmunoassay, and nephelometry. Agglutination tests such as the latex fixation test, preferentially measure IgM RFs reactive with human IgG. The sheep cell agglutination test measures IgM RFs using rabbit IgG as an antigen. Clinical laboratories prefer nephelometry over the latex fixation test because the former is automated and less labor intensive.

Prevalence of RFs in SLE

The prevalence of RFs in large series of SLE patients measured by the latex fixation test varies from 20 to 60% (mean = 33%). Singer[S464] reviewed several earlier reports and found that 20.5% of SLE patients tested were positive. Estes and Christian[E147] found a positive latex fixation test in 21% of their 150 SLE patients. The serum antibody titer was relatively low, and unlike RA (in which the titer persists), the majority of their patients did not have a sustained titer. Lee et al.[L140] reported positive RFs in 36.7% of 110 SLE patients. In 31.2% of their patients, the titer was equal to or greater than 1:160, and in 28.8% the serum titer was greater than 1:320. On the other hand, Feinglass et al.[F46] described a higher frequency of RFs among their patients. Sixty-one percent of their 122

SLE patients had a positive latex fixation test. In agreement with other studies, the RF titers were modest with a titer of 1:80 seen in half of the patients. Further, the serum titer fluctuated intermittently in patients in whom serial determinations were performed.

The sheep agglutination test (SCAT) for RFs is less sensitive than the latex fixation test, but a positive SCAT is considered to be more characteristic of RA.[W241] None of 25 SLE patients studied by Cathcart et al.[C155] had a positive SCAT, and only 3 SLE patients had borderline titers of less than 1:32.

RFs belonging to isotypes other than IgM are not commonly seen in SLE. If present, they tend to have lower serum titers than those observed in RA patients. IgG RFs, which are implicated in the pathogenesis of synovitis and extra-articular lesions of RA such as vasculitis, are generally absent in SLE.[P258,W181] IgE RFs that are also associated with the extra-articular manifestations of RA are not seen in SLE.[H128,Z54] Dunne and associates[D359] found elevated levels of IgA RFs in sera of patients with RA, Sjögren's syndrome, and SLE. The serum level of IgA RFs in SLE was lower than that seen in RA.

Potential Significance of RFs in SLE

In vitro experiments, as well as studies in experimental animal models, point to a dual effect of RFs on immune-mediated tissue injury.

On one hand, RFs have been shown to exert protective effects by competing with complement for binding to immune complexes.[D82,Z63] RFs binding to antigen-antibody complexes may result in more efficient removal from the circulation by the reticuloendothelial system.[P53,V37] Bolton et al.[B394] showed that RFs blocked 1) the attachment of C3 to aggregated IgG and 2) formation of C3b capable of reacting with C3b receptors of glomeruli in vitro. This phenomenon can potentially shield the glomerulus from the deposition of pathogenic immune complexes.

Conversely, others have found RFs to enhance immune-mediated tissue injury in different experimental animal models.[F132] Floyd and Tessar[F132] showed that the administration of IgM RFs aggravated cutaneous Arthus reaction in animals. RFs and immune complexes injected into the mesenteric arteries of rats induced thrombosis and hemorrhage.[B126] In a series of experiments, Ford and co-workers[F162,F164,F165] showed that RFs bind in situ to immune complexes bound to renal glomeruli in experimental glomerulonephritis. They postulated that bound RFs subsequently act as an immunosorbent, trapping circulating antigen-antibody complexes that may be unrelated to the initial renal insult and, by fixing complement, contribute to the chronicity of the renal disease. Birchmore et al.[B309] noted that RFs enhanced the binding of anti-DNA-DNA immune complexes to C3b receptors on red blood cells in vitro by fixing complement by way of its own Fc region. Their finding suggested that RFs may potentiate renal injury in SLE.

Miyazaki et al.[M504] found IgM, IgA, and IgG RFs in the serum of five patients with diffuse lupus nephritis but not in two patients with membranous lupus nephritis. More importantly they observed the binding of fluorescein-labeled normal human IgG and Fc fragment but not $F(ab')_2$ fragment to the renal glomeruli in diffuse lupus glomerulonephritis. No binding was observed in membranous lupus nephritis or in IgA nephropathy. They interpreted this to mean the presence of RF activity in the glomerular deposits which bind the labeled IgG, suggesting that RFs may be important in the development of diffuse lupus nephritis. This study confirms earlier observations by Agnello et al.,[A58] who showed glomerular deposits of IgM RFs in lupus nephritis by reacting fluorescein-labeled aggregated human IgG and anti-idiotypic antibody to RFs with renal biopsy specimens.

Clinical Correlates of RFs in SLE

Which of the many and varied biologic effects of RFs in vitro or in experimental models are important in the pathogenesis of lesions in SLE remain to be seen. Nevertheless, several investigators have examined clinical correlates of RFs in SLE. In 1966, Davis and Bollet[D83] noted that nephritis was less prevalent in a group of SLE patients who were RF positive by the latex fixation test. They suggested that RFs exerted a protective role in vivo in SLE and other immune complex deposition diseases. A retrospective analysis of their patients confirmed their initial observation, and in addition they found that SLE patients who are rheumatoid factor negative and cryoglobulin positive are likely to develop renal disease, whereas those who are rheumatoid factor positive and cryoglobulin negative were unlikely to do so.[H458] Hill and associates[H305] found that SLE patients with nephritis who were RF positive (latex fixation test) had milder morphologic renal lesions compared to RF-negative SLE patients with nephritis. This protective effect of RFs on lupus nephritis was likewise observed in a study using the sheep cell agglutination test for measuring RFs.[H249] Corke[C385a] found that proteinuria was less frequent in RF-positive SLE patients than in RF-negative patients. Mustakallio et al.[M679] described a negative correlation between RFs and anemia, skin disease, and the LE-cell test. Moreover, the RF-positive SLE patients tended to have a more benign and chronic clinical course. In the foregoing studies, the tests used for detecting RFs preferentially measured IgM RFs. Tarkowski and Westberg[T72] used an enzyme immunoassay to measure the different isotypes of RFs in SLE and found that the presence and serum level of IgG RFs, IgA RFs, and IgM RFs correlated significantly with the absence of renal disease.

Other investigators, however, have failed to confirm a protective role of RFs in SLE nephritis or in other organ involvement. Kantor et al.[K55] measured RFs in 51 consecutive SLE patients and found that the frequency as well as the antibody titer of RFs in those with nephritis did not differ from those without clinical renal disease. Baldwin and associates[B50] confirmed these observations and found that the presence of RFs was not associated with histologic type of nephritis. Estes and Christian[E147] reported that the frequency of renal disease as well as the 5-year survival rate of RF-positive SLE patients did not differ from that of the general SLE population. Two other studies using the sheep cell agglutination test for RFs[P199] and radioimmuno-

assay for IgM, IgA, and IgG RF isotypes[S701] failed to find a protective effect of RFs from developing nephritis (see also Chaps. 53 and 54).

Certain observations not only refute the protective role of RFs but in fact point to the participation of RFs in the pathogenesis of tissue lesions in SLE. Cryoglobulins, which represent a subset of circulating immune complexes in SLE, often contain RF activity. Agnello and associates[A58] identified RFs in glomerular immune deposits in SLE patients with nephritis, hypocomplementemia, and cryoglobulinemia. Deposition of antiglobulins (including RFs) in the renal glomeruli was observed in lupus nephritis and in other types of glomerulonephritis, and their presence appeared to be associated with a relatively severe renal injury.[R332,R333] We found that immune deposits in the walls of pulmonary arteries in SLE patients with pulmonary hypertension were eluted when incubated with aggregated human IgG suggesting the presence of RFs in the vascular immune deposits.[Q21]

In addition to renal disease, a correlation between RFs and other clinical features of SLE has been examined. Moutsopoulos et al.[M636] described a high frequency of RFs in SLE patients with histologic evidence of sicca syndrome on lip biopsy. The prevalence of RFs in 35 SLE patients positive for anti-Ro/SSA antibody (63%) was significantly higher than in 77 SLE patients negative for anti-Ro/SSA antibody (7%). Zizic et al.[Z36] reported a high frequency of RFs among SLE patients presenting with acute abdomen secondary to vasculitis and/or serositis. We found a high prevalence of RFs in SLE patients presenting with pulmonary hypertension.[Q21] Conversely, Feinglass et al.[F46] observed no correlation between RFs and neuropsychiatric involvement in SLE. SLE patients with a persistently positive latex fixation test for RFs tended to have less severe clinical manifestations of the disease, were less likely to have received high-dose steroids or cytotoxic drugs for treatment, and were less likely to have had an episode of herpes zoster, than SLE patients who had persistently negative or inconsistently positive tests for RFs.[F52]

The discrepancy in the results of the various investigations on the relationship between RFs and lupus nephritis or SLE in general is probably caused by several factors. Differences in the methods used measure RFs, selection of patients, ascertainment of activity of the renal disease, and the retrospective design of most of the studies are some of the factors. The titer of the RFs may fluctuate or even disappear along the course of the illness, thus timing of the test will affect the result of the study. Moreover, it is now well recognized that RFs are heterogenous with respect to the immunoglobulin class, reactivity with IgG of different species, complement-fixing property, avidity, and other characteristics. Conceivably, varying types of RFs may differ on their effects on renal disease and other tissue lesions. Our own observations, showing that IgM RFs specific for rabbit IgG correlates positively with arthritis and negatively with other clinical manifestations, suggest a dual effect of RF.[S70]

RFs Cross-Reactive with Nuclear Antigens

In 1963, McCormick and Day[M246] observed that exhaustive absorption of certain sera containing both RF and

Table 28–4. Rheumatoid Factors in SLE

1. The latex fixation test for IgM rheumatoid factors is positive in 33% of SLE patients. Serum titers are generally lower than those seen in RA patients, tend to fluctuate, and may become negative.
2. RFs have been identified in serum cryoglobulins and glomerular deposits of some SLE patients.
3. The hypothesis that renal disease tends to be less frequent and less severe in RF-positive than in RF-negative SLE patients has not been consistently confirmed by other investigators and remains controversial.
4. IgM RFs cross-reactive with nuclear antigens including single-stranded DNA and histone are found in SLE, RA, and in other rheumatic conditions.

ANA activities with aggregated gamma globulin removed the RF activity and was accompanied by a substantial loss of ANA titer. They suspected that the phenomenon was due to the presence of IgG ANAs associated with the IgM RFs as an immune complex. Subsequently, Hannestad[H104,H105] established that was not caused by complexed IgG ANAs, but rather to the dual reactivity of certain polyclonal IgM RFs with both IgG and nuclear antigens. Other investigators confirmed these findings[J94] and showed that isolated IgM RFs reacted with DNA-histone complex,[A56,A80] with histones,[H337] and/or with non-histone nuclear polypeptides.[M178] Cross-reactive IgM RFs have been found most frequently in RA patients and in some cases of overlap syndromes and mixed connective tissue disease.[A56] Kinoshita et al.[K241] found IgM RFs cross-reactive with single-stranded DNA to be prevalent in a variety of rheumatic diseases including SLE; however, the serum titer was highest among RA patients with extra-articular features. Johnson[J94] suggested that the cross-reactive IgM RFs are of limited immunopathogenic significance because such antibodies are non-complement fixing and react optimally at pH 8 or 9 and fail to bind at pH 6.5.

CRYOGLOBULINS IN SLE

It has long been recognized that serum specimens from certain groups of patients develop a precipitate spontaneously when allowed to incubate in a test tube at low temperatures. Lerner and co-workers[L194] described this phenomenon in patients with leukemia, pneumonia, bacterial endocarditis, and other diagnoses. Having identified gamma globulin as the serum protein fraction that reversibly precipitates at 5°C, the term cryoglobulin was introduced to refer to the cold-insoluble precipitates.

Frequency of Cryoglobulins in SLE

Barr and co-workers[B101] examined sera from patients with various diagnoses as well as normal subjects for cryoprecipitation. Sera from 8 of 121 patients, but none from 57 healthy controls had significant amounts of cryoglobulins. Half of the six SLE patients in this early series had cryoglobulins. Christian and associates[C255] reported the presence of cryoglobulins in 10 of 12 SLE patients, with protein concentrations ranging from 7 to 38 mg/dl. In a larger series, Stastny and Ziff[S623] studied 137 sera from 31 SLE patients. Thirty-seven sera from 11 patients had cryoglobulins. Lee and Rivero[L145] observed cryoglobulinemia in 9 of 57 SLE sera, while Barnett et al.[B97] found cryoglobulins in 16 of 18 unselected SLE sera.

Components of Cryoglobulins

Immunochemical analysis of the cryoprecipitate[B513] have revealed three major types of cryoglobulins. 1) Type I cryoglobulins consist of a single monoclonal immunoglobulin: IgG, IgM, IgA, or Bence Jones protein. Type I cryoglobulins are associated with lymphoproliferative disorders. 2) Type II cryoglobulins are mixed cryoglobulins with one of the components a monoclonal Ig. Monoclonal IgM with polyclonal IgG is the most common combination, and frequently the monoclonal component has anti-immunoglobulin (rheumatoid factor) activity. Type II cryoglobulins are found in patients with lymphoproliferative diseases and autoimmune disorders. 3) Type III cryoglobulins are mixed cryoglobulins with polyclonal components. This type is the most common and is associated with infections and autoimmune disorders such as SLE, RA, systemic sclerosis, and Sjögren's syndrome. Types II and III may contain rheumatoid factor, other autoantibodies and complement components, C1q, C3, and C4.

Hanauer and Christian[H94] analyzed isolated serum cryoprecipitates from six SLE subjects and observed that these consisted largely of IgG, IgM, and C1q. When the washed cryoglobulins were used as immunogens in rabbits, the resulting antiserum reacted with IgG, IgM, C1q, and α_2-macroglobulin. Some of the antisera reacted also with C4, C3, and IgA.

Barnett et al.[B96] found IgG and IgM in all 156 SLE cryoprecipitates studied. Eleven contained IgA and C3. Stastny and Ziff[S642] reported that IgM was not a prominent component in SLE cryoprecipitates, but the complex consisted mainly of IgG and C1q. Although IgG was the predominant immunoglobulin, relatively more IgM than IgG was concentrated when compared with the corresponding Ig levels.[E128]

The formation of cryoprecipitates in SLE sera was shown to require the presence of C1q.[C255] Prior incubation of SLE serum at 56°C for 30 minutes to inactivate complement resulted in the loss of cryoprecipitability but was restored when either fresh human serum or purified C1q was added to the test serum.

Fibronectin, a normal plasma protein and a major cell surface membrane protein of fibroblasts, has been shown to be a component of cryoglobulins from patients with connective tissue diseases and other illnesses[A193,B145,W341] Plasma fibronectin can bind to other molecules such as collagen, fibrin, and heparin and the binding may result in the formation of a precipitate at low temperatures. Kono and co-workers[K370] showed that fibronectin is capable of binding to C1q, including C1q fixed to immune complexes. Because fibronectin and C1q frequently coprecipitate in SLE cryoglobulins, this reaction and/or binding of fibronectin to other serum proteins may be important in the formation of cryoglobulins.

Clinical Correlates of Cryoglobulinemia in SLE

Cryoglobulinemia is associated with clinical disease activity. Eight of 11 patients with cryoglobulins reported by

Stastny and Ziff[S438] had active nephritis, and the remaining three had evidence of extrarenal involvement. Nine of the 12 patients with cryoglobulins studied by Christian et al.[C255] had active nephritis. Cryoglobulinemia in SLE has also been associated with reduced serum levels of C3 and C1q.[W282] Cryoglobulins and rheumatoid factor have independent and opposite association with lupus myelitis.[H458]

Cryoglobulins as Circulating Immune Complexes

The association between cryoglobulinemia and disease activity and hypocomplementemia in SLE led to investigations on the potential pathogenicity of the cryoprecipitates. Mixed cryoglobulins are considered to represent circulating immune complexes for several reasons. In certain conditions such as essential mixed cryoglobulinemia, the property of cryoprecipitability does not reside on either moiety of the cryoglobulin but requires the combination of the separated components.[L385] Complement components are required for cryoprecipitability and, further, isolated cryoglobulins have the property of activating the complement system.[M650,R338] Cryoglobulins isolated from the sera of patients with lupus nephritis activate the complement system in vitro either through the classic or alternative pathway.[A49] Despite similarities in immunoglobulin content, SLE cryoglobulins differ from RA cryoglobulins in their complement-binding property. Whereas SLE cryoglobulins frequently bind C1q in vitro, isolated RA cryoglobulins do not.[E128] The difference may reflect varying properties of antigen-antibody systems involved in the cryoglobulin formation in the two conditions.

Antibody Activity of SLE Cryoglobulins

The deposition of antinuclear antibodies and their corresponding antigens in target organs is implicated in the pathogenesis of organ injury in SLE. Cryoprecipitates in SLE patients during periods of disease activity may represent circulating immune complexes of ANAs and nuclear antigens. Lee and Rivero[L145] found no ANA activity in the cryoprecipitates of nine SLE sera that contained high titers of ANAs. Stastny and Ziff[S623] reported ANA IgG component in two out of three SLE cryoglobulins tested; however, they failed to find a preferential concentration of ANAs in the cryoglobulins. Conversely, Winfield and associates[W287] found that SLE cryoglobulins were highly enriched with antibodies to ssDNA and dsDNA and less frequently with antiribonucleoprotein antibodies, relative to the concentration of these autoantibodies in the corresponding sera. Ehrhart et al.[E128] confirmed these findings and reported that 95% of isolated SLE cryoglobulins studied contained antibodies to dsDNA.

Hanauer and Christian[H94] found anti-IgG antibody (rheumatoid factor) in SLE cryoglobulins. This finding has been confirmed by several investigators.[A58,M318,W294,Z64] In addition, rheumatoid factor activity was found to be preferentially enriched in the cryoprecipitates when compared to the antibody activity of the matching serum specimen.[W294] Similarly, cold-reactive IgM antilymphocyte antibodies are found to be selectively concentrated in SLE cryoglobulins.[W294] Lymphocytotoxic activity of SLE cry-

oglobulins did not correlate with clinical severity of the disease, serum complement level, or with the serum titer of anti-DNA antibody.[Z64]

Specific Antigens in SLE Cryoglobulins

To identify specific antigens that may be complexed with corresponding antibody in the cryoprecipitate, experimental animals were immunized with cryoprecipitates isolated from SLE patients.[W294] After absorption with pooled normal human serum, anti-SLE cryoglobulin antisera did not recognize any "unique" antigens except for two antisera that contained antibody activity against intrinsic determinants in IgM molecules. Using a similar approach, Klippel and associates[K309] detected reactivity of anti-SLE cryoglobulin antiserum against lymphocytes, suggesting that lymphocyte membrane antigens, or antigens that cross-react with cell surface determinants, were present in SLE cryoprecipitates. McPhaul and Montgomery[M319] found that anti-SLE cryoglobulin antisera reacted not only against nuclear antigens, but also to reticulin and idiotypic determinants of immunoglobulin deposits in the renal glomeruli. These observations indicate the multiplicity of antigen-antibody systems involved in the formation of cryoglobulins in SLE.

Lee and Rivero[L145] reported the presence of DNA in SLE cryoprecipitates in only one of nine specimens, using ultraviolet light absorption, diphenylamine reaction, and immunoprecipitation. Employing specific antiserum to ssDNA, Barnett et al.[B97] identified DNA in 2 of 16 SLE cryoprecipitates. The DNA was demonstrable only with prior heating of the specimen, presumably to denature the DNA. In contrast, Davis and associates[D84] identified DNA in most SLE cryoglobulins tested, but only after digestion of the precipitate with pronase, suggesting the DNA was bound to anti-DNA antibodies and thus inaccessible to biochemical or immunologic detection. The major portion of the DNA—anti-DNA antibody system in cryoglobulin from patients with lupus nephritis consisted predominantly of low-molecular-weight complexes.[R241]

The presence of DNA in cryoprecipitates is not specific for SLE. DNA has also been identified in cryoglobulins isolated from patients with bacterial endocarditis, Sjögren's syndrome, and non-SLE glomerulonephritis.[B34,B363] Free DNA has been demonstrated in sera of normal individuals,[B34] patients receiving high doses of corticosteroids for a variety of medical conditions, and in patients undergoing cardiac surgery.[D79,H480] Not only was DNA found in non-SLE cryoglobulins, but Roberts and Lewis[R239,R240] identified anti-DNA activity in cryoglobulins isolated from patients with nonlupus glomerulonephritis, bacterial infections, and essential cryoglobulinemia. IgG anti-DNA antibody was demonstrable in cryoglobulins after preincubation of the precipitate in acid buffer or after digestion with deoxyribonuclease, suggesting that anti-DNA antibody in the cryoglobulin was bound to antigen.

Pathogenetic Significance of Cryoglobulins

In addition to complement activation, mixed cryoglobulins possess other biologic properties that suggest a po-

Table 28–5. Cryoglobulins in SLE

1. Serum cryoglobulins in SLE are usually on type III (mixed polyclonal) consisting of immunoglobulins, complement components, and fibronectin.
2. Elevated levels of serum cryoglobulins are associated with hypocomplementemia and clinical disease activity, especially active nephritis.
3. Cryoglobulins represent cold-precipitable circulating immune complexes. Antinuclear antibodies (including anti-DNA), antilymphocyte antibodies, RFs as well as DNA and lymphocyte antigens have been identified in SLE cryoglobulins.

tential pathogenic role. Intradermal injection of redissolved cryoglobulins in unsensitized animals caused localized skin edema, erythema, and hemorrhage within 24 hours, and the intravenous administration caused either anaphylaxis or a glomerulitis.[M296] Whitsed and Penny[W210] described the development of a cutaneous vasculitis following the intradermal injection of autologous cryoglobulin into clinically normal skin of a patient with mixed cryoglobulinemia. The deposition of cryoglobulin in target organs in vivo is supported by the demonstration of a distinctive crystalline fibrillar structure in renal glomeruli, identical to that found in the serum cryoglobulins of the same patient with essential mixed cryoglobulinemia. Using an anti-idiotypic antibody, Agnello et al.[A58] demonstrated the deposition of IgM rheumatoid factor moiety of cryoglobulin in the renal glomeruli of a patient with SLE nephritis.

Cryoglobulins may contribute to the susceptibility of SLE patients to bacterial infections. Nivend and associates[N109] found that the impairment of opsonization of Staphylococcus aureus by SLE serum was associated with cryoglobulinemia. When the cryoglobulin fraction of the immune complexes was removed from SLE serum, normal opsonic capacity was observed. Moreover, reduction of opsonic property was transferred with SLE cryoglobulins to normal serum. The binding of cryoglobulins to protein A of Staphylococcus probably blocked contact between surface receptors of phagocytic cells and opsonized organisms, resulting in defective phagocytosis and killing.

THE LE CELL

In February 1946, Dr. Malcolm M. Hargraves, a hematologist at the Mayo Clinic, examined a bone marrow aspirate from a boy with an obscure medical problem. Part of his report read:[H128]

> The outstanding thing in this bone marrow is the phagocytic reticuloendothelial cells which contain a blue-staining material which we have not previously observed. Some cells are markedly filled with this material gathered together in round vacuoles or droplets. An occasional cell has been ruptured, with the material in discrete globules scattered out among the other cells. This material stains from a light blue to a very dark, almost indigo blue. There is an occasional reticuloendothelial cell that has other phagocytized material as well as that noted above, but most of the reticuloendothelial cells involved seem to be specifically concerned with this material and do not show other phagocytic activities.

Upon learning that the patient probably had SLE, Dr. Hargraves went on to examine bone marrow specimens from two other patients with definite SLE in the next 4 days. He observed that the "striking feature is the marked phagocytic activity of neutrophils containing a muddy purple homogenous material. Some of the cells are so filled with the material that the nucleus is crowded to the periphery."

This is the initial description of the LE cell and 2 years later, Hargraves et al.[H129] reported their experience in 25 SLE patients and noted the frequent appearance of the LE cell in acute cases. The inclusion body of the LE cells, as well as the extracellular material stained with Feulgen stain, showed that both contained DNA and were presumed to be nuclear in origin. Hargraves postulated that the phagocytosis of the material resulted in the formation of LE cells.

The LE-cell phenomenon occurs in vitro during the incubation of peripheral blood or bone marrow aspirate. It is completed in two distinct stages (see Fig. 1), with the initial phase involving the immunologic reaction of the LE-cell factor present in the serum of the patient with the nuclear material of damaged or traumatized leukocytes. Trauma allows the nuclear penetration of the LE-cell factor. The reaction leads to nuclear swelling accompanied by the disintegration of the normal chromatin pattern and basophilia. The altered nucleus then detaches itself from the cytoplasm and appears as a free extracellular LE body. In the second stage, the LE body is engulfed by a neutrophil (occasionally a monocyte) in the presence of complement. The cytoplasm remains outside and is not taken up by the phagocyte.[R247] When stained with Wright's stain, the globular inclusion body appears as a homogenous, pale blue to deep purplish material, pushing the nucleus of the phagocyte to one side of the cell (see Fig. 2).

In 1951, Lee et al.[L144] observed a striking morphologic resemblance of the LE-cell inclusion body to the hematoxylin bodies found in the tissues of SLE patients at autopsy. The latter, described earlier by Klemperer and associates,[K283] consist of altered nuclear material containing DNA in a depolymerized state. The LE-cell inclusion body and the tissue-bound hematoxylin body were found to have diminished affinity for methyl green, a dye that binds stoichiometrically with DNA. Studies by Godman and Deitch[G212] have established that the diminished affinity was not a result of DNA polymerization, but a result of interference by proteins that were bound to the DNA moiety of the inclusion body.

LE-Cell Factor

Haserick et al.[H182] fractionated SLE plasma by electrophoresis and identified the serum factor that participated in the LE-cell phenomenon as gamma globulin, implying it to be an antibody. Other investigators, using ultracentrifugation and chromatography separation methods, confirmed the LE factor to be a serum 7S gamma globulin,[F12,G288] while the 19S was inactive. Subsequent studies established that IgG but not IgM antibody to deoxyribonucleoprotein induces LE-cell formation in vitro.[G246]

A METHOD OF FORMATION OF LE CELLS

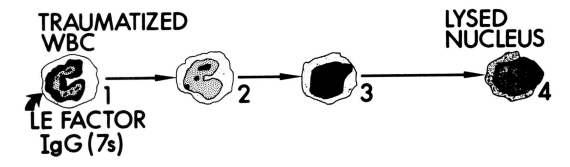

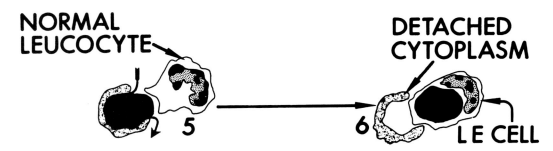

Fig. 28–1. Scheme of the LE cell formation.

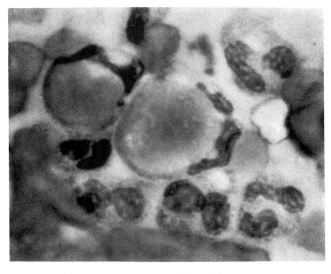

Fig. 28–2. Two typical LE cells (× 1700).

LE-Cell Antigen

In 1954, Miescher and Fauconnet[M398] noted that the capacity of SLE serum to induce LE cells in vitro diminished when the serum was preabsorbed with nuclei isolated from human leukocytes. This observation and the information that the LE-cell factor is a gamma globulin led to definitive investigations that established the antinuclear antibody activity of the LE-cell factor. The application of the fluorescent antibody technique by Friou et al.[F273] contributed significantly in understanding the nature of the LE-cell factor and other antinuclear antibodies.

In a series of elegant studies, Holman et al.[H387,H389,H390] firmly established that the LE-cell factor is an antibody to deoxyribonucleoprotein of cell nuclei, requiring both DNA and histone for the reaction. In their experiments, purified nucleoprotein was used to absorb the LE-cell factor from SLE serum to form an immune complex. By stepwise elution, it was shown that the complete removal of the LE-cell factor from the complex required a two-step procedure. Digestion of the complex with deoxyribonuclease led to the release of gamma globulin, a large amount of DNA, and histone. However, the isolated gamma globulin did not have the property of inducing an LE cell, although it reacted with DNA and cell nuclei. A second elution step employing the incubation of the DNase digest with 2N NaCl at 37°C or in saline at 56°C liberated more gamma globulin, which had a strong LE-cell activity. The released gamma globulin was shown to be reactive with nucleoprotein but not with DNA. Selective removal of either DNA or histone from the nucleoprotein resulted in the loss of the ability to absorb the LE-cell factor. Reconstitution of the two components, DNA and histone, resulted in partial recovery of the activity. Nucleoprotein fully saturated with LE-cell factor from the serum of one patient lost its property to absorb the LE-cell factor of a second patient.

Role of Complement in LE-Cell Formation

In 1959, Aisenberg[A79] reported that the incubation of SLE serum at 56°C for 30 minutes diminished its capacity to induce LE-cell formation in an indirect LE-cell test. Instead of classical LE cells, the preparation showed homogenous, globular, purplish extracellular material. Addition of fresh human serum to isolated cell nuclei complexed with LE-cell factor caused formation of LE cells in the presence of viable phagocytes. This observation suggested that a heat-labile factor in normal serum is required for completion of the LE cell. It remained for Golden and McDuffie[G246,M274] in 1967 to establish the importance of complement in the LE-cell phenomenon. Frozen and thawed human leukocytes were incubated with gamma globulin fraction of SLE serum containing antideoxyribonucleoprotein antibody. Viable leukocytes were then added to the system to complete the second or phagocytic stage of the LE-cell phenomenon. Typical LE cells formed even after thorough washing of the phagocytes and the leukocyte nuclei with saline. They assumed that small amounts of complement remained adherent to the viable phagocytes. Nevertheless, when antiserum to human C3 was added to the system, there was inhibition of LE-cell formation. Addition of excess fresh human serum abrogated the inhibitory effect of anti-C3 antiserum. Thus, it is evident that complement is required for the second stage of the LE-cell phenomenon and the amount required is probably relatively small.

Extracellular Nuclear Material

Extracellular basophilic aggregates of amorphous or ovoid shape are sometimes seen in LE-cell preparations. This extracellular material (ECM), sometimes referred to as a hematoxylin body, may occur alone or accompanied by typical LE cells. It has been assumed that ECMs represent products of the initial stage of the LE-cell phenomenon (complex of the LE-cell factor and nucleoprotein) left unphagocytosed.

Arterberry et al.[A306] found hematoxylin bodies without typical LE cells in 358 subjects out of 3000 patients with various diagnoses who had an LE-cell test done. Three morphologic types were identified: homogenous round hematoxylin body, a lacy type, and an amorphous variety. The homogenous round body was the most common, found in 259 patients. Forty-five percent of the patients in

this group had definite SLE, and another 46% had rheumatoid arthritis or some disease variant.

By block titration of serum, Golden and McDuffie[G246] have shown that the number of LE cells produced by lupus serum decreased as the number of ECMs increased, while keeping the amount of complement and the number of viable phagocytes constant in the indirect LE-cell test. IgG and IgM antideoxyribonucleoprotein antibodies were purified, and both antibody preparations produced ECMs. In contrast, only the IgG antibody had the property to induce the classic LE cell. McDuffie et al.[M274] suggest that the inability to induce typical LE cells may be related to the lack of complement-fixing property of IgM antideoxyribonucleoprotein antibody.

In Vivo Occurrence of LE Cells

The LE-cell factor and most other antinuclear antibodies are not capable of penetrating intact and viable cells to react with their corresponding antigens in the nuclei. Lachman[L5] observed no morphologic changes in actively dividing HeLa cells when grown in tissue culture medium containing lupus serum. Rapp[R44] showed that antinuclear antibodies reacted with the nuclei of air-dried but not viable HeLa cells. Direct smears of peripheral blood of SLE patients showed absence of in vivo binding of immunoglobulin with the nuclei of leukocytes.[Z67] However, in vivo LE cells have occasionally been described in direct smears of pericardial fluid,[S237] pleural fluid,[P25] joint fluid,[H498] ascitic fluid,[M374] and cerebrospinal fluid[N137] of lupus patients. LE cells may form in areas of local inflammation as within the pleural cavity, probably as a result of the presence of leukocytes that are subtly altered or damaged to allow nuclear penetration by the IgG antideoxyribonucleoprotein antibody to form LE bodies. These damaged leukocytes may appear active and viable by morphologic criteria.[D372] Phagocytosis of the LE bodies by polymorphonuclear leukocytes or by macrophages will complete the reaction to form classic and sometimes atypical LE cells.[F58]

Clinical Significance of the LE Cell

The LE-cell test has been largely abandoned as a routine clinical test and supplanted by the fluorescent test for antinuclear antibodies. The LE-cell test is labor intensive, and it requires a skilled technician to interpret the cytology. Atypical LE cells are not infrequently seen in clot preparations, and some observers may report this as a positive test, while others will not unless classic LE cells are also present. Among the many modifications that were developed to increase the yield and/or to improve the cytology, the heparinized rotary glass bead method, the 2-hour clot test, and the combined rotated and washed clot technique were the major procedures used for several years.

The frequency of a positive LE-cell test in SLE varies with the method used, the frequency of performing the test, and the duration of time the patient is studied. At some time during the course of the illness, the rotary glass bead LE-cell test was positive in 75.7% of 520 SLE patients studied by Dubois.[D340] With combined rotary glass bead and washed clot methods, LE cells were found in approximately 90% of the patients.

Despite the high frequency in SLE, it is now well recognized that a positive LE-cell test is not entirely specific for the disease. Positive LE-cell tests have been reported in 5 to 10% of adult rheumatoid arthritis patients and in a smaller percentage of patients with systemic sclerosis, polymyositis, polyarteritis nodosa, and mixed connective tissue disease.[T268,Q18,Q23,D323] LE cells have been described in drug reactions secondary to penicillin,[B86,B250,L144,M552,P74,W56] tetracycline,[D254] chlorpromazine,[Q14] anticonvulsants,[D323] hydralazine,[D323] and procainamide[D319] (see Chap. 45 on drug-induced LE). LE cells have been found in a case of intermittent hydrarthrosis with positive ANAs,[S256] in lupoid hepatitis,[M11,R182,S550] in two cases of lymphoma with no autopsy evidence of SLE,[H461] and DiGuglielmo's disease (acute erythroleukemia).[F99]

Positive LE-Cell Test with Negative ANAs

There have been occasional reports of cases in which the LE-cell test is positive despite a negative fluorescent test for ANAs.[F99] Koller et al.[K359] found 20 cases among a large group of patients tested for LE cells. Five met the criteria for SLE, seven had rheumatoid arthritis, and three had drug reactions. Wallace and Metzger[W36] described two patients with biopsy-proven cutaneous mild SLE with major organ involvement who had positive LE-cell and negative ANA tests using both rat liver and Hep-2 cells.

The explanation for this discrepancy in most of the

Table 28–6. The LE Cell: Summary

1. The LE cell is induced in vitro by an IgG antibody to deoxyribonucleoprotein (LE-cell factor).
2. The LE-cell factor reacts with the nuclear material of traumatized white blood cell to form a hematoxylin body. Phagocytosis of the hematoxylin body by a viable phagocyte in the presence of complement leads to the formation of classic LE cells.
3. In vivo LE cells may be seen in pleural, pericardial, synovial, ascitic, blister fluid, and cerebrospinal fluid of SLE patients.
4. The LE-cell test is positive in 90% of all SLE patients at some time during the disease course. A positive LE-cell test may be seen in other conditions including rheumatoid arthritis, scleroderma, mixed connective tissue disease, lupoid hepatitis, and drug-induced LE.

cases studied is not entirely clear.[F99] Nevertheless, when the clinical picture of the patient is compatible or highly suspicious of SLE, and the standard FANA is negative (after using multiple substrates), an LE-cell test should be ordered to corroborate the diagnosis. In addition, other tests that may be of value in this situation include the lupus band test on nonlesional skin and serologic tests for anti-Ro/SSA antibody.

See Table 28–6 for a summary of the LE cells. (Since positive LE cell tests are rare in patients without rheumatic disease, its presence in a patient with a low titer positive ANA may be confirmatory of lupus, and it is still one of the ARA criteria for SLE. The reader is referred to pages 211–226 of the Third Edition of this textbook for a detailed description of LE cell methodologies.)

Section V

CUTANEOUS LUPUS

Chapter 29

PATHOGENESIS OF CUTANEOUS MANIFESTATIONS OF LUPUS ERYTHEMATOSUS

THOMAS T. PROVOST AND ROSEMARIE WATSON

This chapter reviews the data germane to the pathogenesis of various cutaneous features of lupus erythematosus. Direct immunofluorescent studies, monoclonal antibodies to perform phenotypic analysis of the inflammatory infiltrates, and autoantibody studies have provided a good deal of data relevant to the pathogenesis of cutaneous lupus lesions. In addition, a murine model for cutaneous lupus has been developed.

Cutaneous manifestations in lupus erythematosus are common; second only to arthritis and arthralgias in frequency of occurrence. In the past, it has been estimated that as many as 20% of SLE patients demonstrate prominent cutaneous manifestations as the initial presentation of their disease.[D321] Further, in the past it had been estimated that as many as 60 to 70% of SLE patients will demonstrate cutaneous features during the course of their disease. Undoubtedly, with the long-term use of steroids and/or hydroxychloroquine, the frequencies and severity of the various cutaneous manifestations have been markedly altered.[C56]

CLINICAL FEATURES

The cutaneous manifestations are varied. They range from severe scarring lesions on the face to purpuric lesions on the lower extremities. Some of these lesions are specific for lupus erythematosus; others are not. The specific lesions include the discoid, subacute cutaneous, hypertrophic, and lupus profundus lesions. The nonspecific lesions include purpuric, nodular (panniculitis), bullous, urticaria-like, livedo reticularis, mucous membrane ulceration, and, rarely, dystrophic calcification lesions.

The specific lupus lesions occur predominantly on sun-exposed areas. Discoid lupus lesions appear to be closely related to the other specific lupus lesions except those of subacute cutaneous lupus erythematosus. For example, discoid lesions can be found on the scalp producing a scarring alopecia and on the malar eminence producing classic butterfly lesions (involvement of malar eminences, the wings of the butterfly; involvement of the nose, the body of the butterfly). Discoid lesions may also be associated with extension of the inflammatory infiltrate deep into the dermis and subcutaneous tissue (lupus profundus). In addition, some discoid lupus lesions may display prominent hypertrophic verrucous features characterized by thick tenacious scale formation (hypertrophic lupus erythematosus).[U12]

It must be emphasized that discoid lupus lesions (coin-shaped, scarring lesions with adherent scale and telangiectasia) are found in both SLE patients and lupus patients without systemic disease (cutaneous lupus erythematosus) (Fig. 29–1). For example, in Dubois' 520 cases of SLE, 10% demonstrated discoid lesions.[D340] Hochberg et al., in a study of 150 SLE patients, described a 15% frequency of discoid lesions.[H347] The term discoid, which denotes a morphologic feature, has unfortunately been employed incorrectly to distinguish systemic from cutaneous lupus.

The annular polycyclic or psoriasiform photosensitive lupus lesions are clinically distinct from discoid lupus lesions (Fig. 29–1). They are generally, but not always, seen in anti-Ro/SSA–antibody-positive females with or without mild systemic features (i.e., arthralgias and/or arthritis) and are termed subacute cutaneous lupus erythematosus (SCLE).[S568,W104] These lesions, unlike the discoid lesions, are generally nonscarring, lack follicular plugging, an adherent scale, and telangiectasia. These lesions, like the discoid lupus lesions, may present as a photosensitive dermatitis in a butterfly distribution on the face.

It is important to emphasize that acute-onset lupus dermatitis in the malar region generally occurs in association with systemic disease. Acute inflammatory lupus dermatitis in the malar region can also occur in subacute cutaneous lupus patients. Pathologically, these acute-onset lupus lesions demonstrate the interface dermatitis (liquefaction degeneration) common to both discoid and subacute cutaneous lesions. The history and physical examination, plus the serologic studies, and not the morphology and distribution of the lesions, establishes with certainty the systemic nature of the lupus process.

PATHOLOGY

Histopathologically, evidence exists to support the hypothesis that at least two different pathophysiologic mechanisms may be operative in the genesis of the discoid and subacute cutaneous lupus lesions. Studies by the late James Gilliam's group, in which they "blinded" the dermatopathologist, indicated that approximately 80% of the time it was possible to distinguish discoid from subacute cutaneous lupus lesions.[B76] In contradistinction to the discoid lesions, subacute cutaneous lupus lesions displayed a more diffuse inflammatory infiltrate with prominent vacuolar degeneration of the epidermal basal cell layer (Table

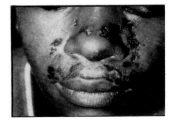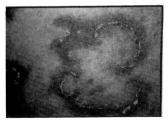

Fig. 29–1. Photomicrograph of severe scarring discoid lupus lesions over face and nose (*left panel*). Nonscarring annular polycyclic lesion of subacute cutaneous lupus erythematosus occurring on upper back (*right panel*).

29–1). Although one cannot absolutely, histopathologically, distinguish between discoid and subacute cutaneous lesions of lupus, there are sufficient pathologic differences, and these differences, together with the distinctive clinical presentations (Fig. 29–1), strongly support the hypothesis that discoid and subacute cutaneous lesions probably are the result of different pathophysiologic mechanisms.

Phenotypic analysis of the inflammatory infiltrate in specific lupus lesions has demonstrated that T cells are the dominant inflammatory cell.[A226,K331,S797] The infiltrate also contains macrophages, but B cells are unusual. The T cells possess HLA-encoded cell surface macromolecules indicating they are activated. One study has demonstrated a slight preponderance of CD8 versus CD4 T cells, but other studies state the reverse. These studies have been performed on discoid and anti-Ro/SSA–positive subacute cutaneous lupus lesions, and the results are comparable.

Table 29–1. Comparison of Clinical, Pathologic and Serologic Features of Discoid and Subacute Cutaneous Lupus Erythematosus

Feature	SCLE	DLE
Morphology	Annular and Psoriasiform	Coin Shaped
Photosensitivity	4 +	2 +
Scarring	±	3–4 +
Follicular plugging	±	3–4 +
Scale formation	+ (Psoriasiform variant)	2–3 +
Telangiectasia	±	3 +
Systemic features	50% (Minor features of SLE)	~10%
Liquefaction degeneration at dermal-epidermal junction	3–4 +	1–2
Inflammatory infiltrate	Diffuse, mild	Prominent superficial and deep
Antibody associations	70% Anti-Ro/SSA	~20–25% ssDNA (IgM isotype)[K451]
Immunopathologic mechanism	(?) Antibody-dependent cellular cytotoxicity	(?) T-cell cytotoxicity

In discussing the pathogenesis of specific lupus lesions, it is also necessary to consider four additional areas of investigation. These are 1) the role of ultraviolet light exposure, 2) the role of deposits of immunoglobulin and complement along the dermal-epidermal junction (lupus band test), 3) the murine model (MRL-lpr/lpr) for the cutaneous lupus lesion, and 4) the experiment of nature—the neonatal lupus syndrome.

ROLE OF ULTRAVIOLET LIGHT

It has been estimated in the past that, clinically, photosensitivity occurs in approximately 20 to 40% of lupus erythematosus patients.[D321] Other studies indicate that as many as 70% of SLE patients are photosensitive.[W365] As noted above, the majority of lupus-specific lesions occur on light-exposed areas. Some patients, especially anti-Ro/SSA–antibody-positive lupus patients are exquisitely sensitive to ultraviolet light. Many give a history of burning through window glass indicating that low-energy long-wave ultraviolet light (UVA >320 nm) is capable of activating their disease. Studies of ours and Rothfield's groups indicate that as many as 90% of anti-Ro/SSA–antibody-positive dermatologic and rheumatologic lupus patients are photosensitive.[M48,M532]

Initial experimental studies by Freeman et al. and Cripps and Rankin demonstrated that monochromatic light was capable of inducing cutaneous lupus lesions in lupus patients.[C434,F226] These lesions, which occurred several weeks after ultraviolet light exposure, demonstrated the classic pathologic features of the lupus lesions. Studies by Lehmann et al. have indicated that ultraviolet light (UVB, sunburn spectrum) as well as UVA (long-wave ultraviolet light) are capable of inducing lupus lesions in approximately 40% of cutaneous lupus and approximately 60% of subacute cutaneous lupus erythematosus patients.[L178] Unfortunately, serologic data were not presented in this paper, but one can safely draw the conclusion that a significant percentage, perhaps 50 to 60% of all lupus patients (both systemic and cutaneous), are photosensitive and that ultraviolet light, both in the sunburn as well as longwave ultraviolet spectrum, is capable of inducing lupus lesions.

At the present time, evidence accumulated by several laboratories indicates that the role of ultraviolet light in the induction of the lupus lesions probably involves the generation of autoantigens by keratinocytes to which the lupus patients are sensitized. For example, in a series of studies, Natali and Tan demonstrated, in mice sensitized with methylated bovine serum albumin coupled to ultraviolet light–denatured DNA (UV-DNA), that following UV epidermal irradiation, denatured DNA (thymidine dimer) was generated in the mouse epidermal nuclei.[N42] This denatured DNA was subsequently removed from the nucleus, presumably by endonucleases (e.g., Uvr ABC endonuclease) and the denatured DNA extruded from the keratinocytes. This denatured DNA diffused back across the basement membrane zone and there, in the region of the dermal-epidermal junction reacted with anti–UV-DNA antibodies producing the deposition of immunoglobulin and complement at the dermal-epidermal junction (lupus band test). There is also some evidence to indicate that native DNA and denatured DNA have a special affinity to bind collagen along the dermal-epidermal junction.[167]

These in vivo studies are important because they provide data regarding the possible etiology of the dermal-epidermal junction immunoglobulin and complement deposits found in cutaneous lupus lesions. These animal experiments also provide evidence to support the clinical observation of the potential deleterious effect of ultraviolet light exposure in inducing flares in systemic lupus erythematosus patients. For example, NZB/NZW mice exposed to ultraviolet light demonstrate fluctuations in anti-ssDNA antibody titers following ultraviolet light exposure.[N40] This presumably reflects immune complex formation. Also, studies demonstrate that the intravenous injection of ultraviolet light–denatured DNA into sensitized rabbits produces glomerulonephritis.[S790] Thus, theoretically, UV exposure of skin of an anti-DNA–antibody-positive SLE patient could conceivably result in denatured DNA being extruded from keratinocytes and gaining entry into the systemic circulation producing circulating DNA–anti-DNA antibody immune complexes.

Studies by the Colorado group have also evaluated the role of ultraviolet light in the generation of ribonuclear protein particles (Ro/SSA, La/SSB, U1-RNP) in keratinocytes.[L154] These studies have demonstrated that keratinocytes in tissue culture exposed to nonlethal doses of ultraviolet light are capable of synthesizing de novo various ribonuclear protein particles including Ro/SSA and U1-RNP. Time-lapsed experiments demonstrate that these particles initially detected in the cytoplasm and the nucleus are translocated to the plasma membrane, where conceivably they can be exposed either to specific antibodies or specific T cells.

In vivo studies by Lee et al. at the University of Colorado have provided evidence to corroborate the presence of Ro/SSA particles on human keratinocytes.[L139] She and her colleagues have demonstrated that human skin transplanted onto nude mice demonstrate by immunofluorescent technology speckled deposits of Ro/SSA antigen on the surface of basal cells in the human, but not mouse, epidermis. The experimental protocol involved intraperitoneally injecting nude mice with human anti-Ro/SSA antibodies. The anti-Ro/SSA antibody is directed at human epitopes and shows little or no cross-reactivity with mouse Ro/SSA macromolecules.[P309,R129] Thus, only the human skin organ transplant demonstrated the speckled immunofluorescent pattern over the basal cell portion of the epidermis. Further, absorption of the human anti-Ro/SSA antibody with purified Ro/SSA antigen prior to intraperitoneal injection of the mice abolished the staining on the epidermis of the skin explant.

The data as recounted above strongly imply that the role of ultraviolet light in lupus erythematosus involves the induction of autoantigen formation either by denaturing DNA or by inducing de novo synthesis of various RNP macromolecules.

Additional studies examining acute and chronic ultraviolet light exposure on autoimmune (MRL-lpr/lpr, [NZB × NZW]F₁, BXSB, and nonautoimmune mice demonstrated a heterogeneous effect.[A256,M285] Acute and chronic ultra-

violet light resulted in significant mortality amongst BXSB but not MRL-lpr/lpr or (NZB × NZW)F₁ mice. The increased mortality in the BXSB mice was associated with an accelerated autoimmune process characterized by an increase in anti-ssDNA antibodies and glomerulonephritis. The deleterious effects of ultraviolet light reside in the UVB (280 to 320 nm) spectrum.

McGrath et al. have presented intriguing data suggesting that UVA (320 to 400 nm) has a beneficial effect on survival of (NZB/NZW)F₁ mice.[M285] This increased survivability was associated with significantly decreased levels of anti-DNA antibodies. These data have stimulated speculation that UVA may have a therapeutic role in the treatment of systemic lupus erythematosus. However, caution should be stressed because clinically many anti-Ro/SSA–positive lupus patients can be activated by UVA window glass–filtered ultraviolet light (i.e., >320 nm in wavelength).

LUPUS BAND TEST

As noted above, immunoglobulin and complement deposits are detected along the dermal-epidermal junction in as many as 90% of cutaneous lupus lesions on light-exposed areas of the body.[B589] This initial observation caused a number of investigators to explore the possible role of these deposits in the pathogenesis of cutaneous lupus lesions. Further studies indicated that the lupus lesions in non light-exposed areas displayed only an approximate 50% frequency of immunoglobulin and complement deposition at the dermal-epidermal junction. It was also noted that only approximately 30% of subacute cutaneous lupus erythematosus lesions are positive for these dermal-epidermal junction deposits.[S568]

In addition to these studies on lupus lesions, other studies examining the presence of immunoglobulin and complement along the dermal-epidermal junction, in noninvolved skin, have demonstrated that systemic lupus erythematosus patients frequently display various classes of immunoglobulins, early and late complement components, as well as components of the alternative complement pathway at the dermal-epidermal junction.[P314] Approximately 60 to 70% of SLE patients possess these immunoglobulin and complement components in noninvolved skin, and these deposits are associated with the presence of native as well as complement-fixing single-stranded DNA antibodies.[G141,P307] Further studies indicated that the frequency of immunoglobulin and complement deposits in noninvolved, non light-exposed areas of the body (e.g., buttocks) of SLE patients was markedly less than in noninvolved, light-exposed areas.[A69]

The antigenic nature of the lupus band test was initially investigated by Tan and Kunkel, who employed enzymatic digest studies. These studies demonstrated that the immunoglobulin and complement deposits at the dermal-epidermal junction in lupus patients could be destroyed by DNaase treatment.[T47] In addition, other studies have demonstrated that the lupus band test is dynamic; the appearance and disappearance of the immunoglobulin and complement deposits correlating with the presence and then the absence of anti-DNA antibodies.[A69] These studies, together with the ultraviolet light data, generated by Natali and Tan, provide a substantial amount of evidence to suggest that DNA is at least a major antigenic component of the lupus band test. Further, these studies indicate a direct relationship between the frequency of the positive lupus band test and ultraviolet light exposure.

Despite the presence of immunoglobulin and complement deposits along the basement membrane zone of non-involved skin of anti-DNA—positive SLE patients, there is no direct evidence to indicate that these immunoglobulin and complement deposits are associated with inflammation. In fact, serial sectioning of the biopsy specimens from a positive lupus band test area demonstrated that these deposits frequently occurred in the total absence of inflammatory cells.[S169] These studies have led to the proposal that the classic scarring discoid cutaneous lupus lesion is a result of a T-cell and not an antibody-mediated immune response.[G139,P306]

Other studies, however, suggest caution in discounting a role for these immunoglobulin and complement deposits at the dermal-epidermal junction in the pathogenesis of the lupus lesions. Biesecker et al., employing direct immunofluorescence studies to detect the neoantigen of the complement membrane attack complex (C5b—C9), have demonstrated the presence of this complement membrane attack complex in lupus skin lesions, whereas a positive lupus band test occurring in normal-appearing skin failed to demonstrate the presence of the complement membrane attack complex.[B300] It is also conceivable that inhibitors of the complement sequence (e.g., factor I and factor H) may prevent the total activation of the complement sequence and thus blunt, or prevent, the development of an inflammatory infiltrate around these deposits.[C93]

The sum total of all these data thus far gathered indicates a lack of a direct role of immunoglobulin and complement deposits at the dermal-epidermal junction in the pathogenesis of the lupus lesions.

THE MRL-LPR/LPR MOUSE MODEL OF CUTANEOUS LUPUS

Japanese investigators have developed a good deal of information strongly suggesting that MRL-lpr/lpr mice develop cutaneous lesions that pathologically demonstrate features similar to human cutaneous lupus lesions. These animals frequently develop alopecia and scab formation over the dorsal surface of the upper back. Pathology studies have demonstrated acanthosis, liquefication, degeneration of the basal cell layer, and the deposition of immunoglobulin beneath the basal lamina of the skin.[H420a] Like human lupus erythematosus lesions, the inflammatory infiltrate is composed predominantly of T cells. Further, this cellular infiltrate is dynamic with L3T4+ (CD4: helper/inducer) cells predominating in early lesions, while in older lesions the percentage of Lyt-2+ (CD8:suppressor/cytotoxic) cells is increased and the L3T4:Lyt-2 ratio decreased.[K48]

THE NEONATAL LUPUS SYNDROME

The neonatal lupus syndrome provides the best evidence for a direct pathologic role of an autoantibody in the genesis of the cutaneous lupus lesions, although the exact pathophysiologic mechanism involving the autoantibodies is unknown. The neonatal lupus syndrome is an uncommon syndrome characterized by the development of cutaneous lupus lesions or isolated heart block in an infant born of an anti-La/SSB— and/or anti-Ro/SSA—or an anti—U1-RNP— (nRNP) antibody-positive mother.[F204,K173,P315,S230] These cutaneous lesions are similar, if not identical, to those seen in subacute cutaneous lupus erythematosus.[S568,W104]

Data supporting a pathologic role of these autoantibodies in the pathogenesis of the neonatal lupus lesions can be summarized as follows:

1. A variety of immunologic techniques including direct immunofluorescence, counterimmunoelectrophoresis, gel double diffusion, and immunoblot studies have demonstrated the presence of Ro/SSA macromolecules in epidermal cells.[D156,L136] Further, as noted above, perturbation of normal keratinocytes with sublethal doses of ultraviolet light induces the de novo synthesis of various RNP particles, including Ro/SSA and U1-RNP macromolecules.[L154] These macromolecules, with time, are translocated from their cytoplasmic and nuclear origins to the plasma membrane of the keratinocytes where, as noted above, they are theoretically exposed to specific antibodies and T cells.

2. Neonatal lupus lesions generally disappear within the first 6 months of life.[W103] This time corresponds to the disappearance of the maternal anti-Ro/SSA, anti-La/SSB, and anti—U1-RNP antibodies from the infant's serum.

3. The overwhelming majority of patients with neonatal lupus have been demonstrated to be born of mothers who possess anti-Ro/SSA antibodies. Approximately 60% of these mothers also demonstrate the presence of anti-La/SSB antibodies.[S230,W103] Thus far, we are aware that four neonatal lupus mothers have demonstrated only anti—U1-RNP antibodies.[P315] No other antibodies (e.g., native DNA, single-stranded DNA, or Sm) have been detected in mothers of neonatal lupus infants.

4. Additional evidence indicating a pathologic role of anti-Ro/SSA and anti—U1-RNP antibodies in the pathogenesis of the neonatal syndrome has been obtained from specific antibody depletion studies. For example, in one study comparing the quantity of anti-Ro/SSA antibody from the serum of an infected infant with isolated congenital heart block with that of his normal fraternal twin sibling and mother, it was determined that there was an accelerated consumption (depletion) of the anti-Ro/SSA antibody in the affected infant with the congenital heart block, compared to his fraternal twin sibling and mother.[H135] This accelerated consumption (depletion) of the maternally derived IgG anti-Ro/SSA antibody in the infant could not be explained by the normal catabolism of the maternally derived antibody.

A similar study has been performed in a neonatal lupus infant with cutaneous lesions and his U1-RNP–positive mother.[P315] The study, as depicted in Fig. 29–2, demonstrated a 450-fold depletion of the anti–U1-RNP antibody in the infant serum, as compared to the mother's. The normal rate of catabolism of the maternal IgG by the infant, as determined by testing the quantity of tetanus toxoid in the infant's and mother's serum, showed an approximate fifteenfold difference.

In view of the experiments recounted above, indicating the presence of Ro/SSA as well as U1-RNP macromolecules on the cell surface of keratinocytes, it is attractive to hypothesize that the specific depletion of the anti-Ro/SSA and anti–U1-RNP antibodies in these two studies of neonatal lupus are the result of these antibodies binding to cell surface Ro/SSA and U1-RNP macromolecules. The exact mechanisms of this immunologic reaction are unknown at the present time, although there appears to be a good deal of circumstantial evidence supporting the role of antibody-dependent cellular cytotoxicity. For example, studies by Norris' group have demonstrated that both anti-Ro/SSA and anti–U1-RNP autoantibodies can participate in antibody-dependent cellular cytotoxicity reactions, and further, other studies have demonstrated that T cells are excellent effector cells of antibody-dependent cellular cytotoxicity.[N130,W9]

Based upon these studies, and the fact that anti-Ro/SSA–antibody-positive subacute cutaneous lupus erythematosus lesions contain predominantly T cells in the inflammatory infiltrate, it has been postulated that the antibody derived from the mother passes across the placenta, and there in the infant induces an inflammatory process in the skin in which infant-derived T cells act as effector cells. The inflammatory infiltrate that results produces the characteristic cutaneous lesions that we recognize as subacute cutaneous lupus erythematosus.

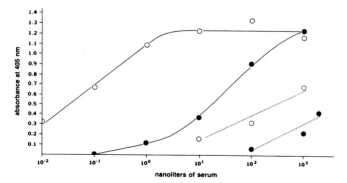

Fig. 29–2. Measurement of antibody concentrations by enzyme-linked immunosorbent assay. Optical density readings (relative absorbance at 405 nm) of anti–U1-RNP (nRNP) (———) and antitetanus toxoid antibodies (– – – –) are plotted on the vertical axis in relation to nanoliters of serum from neonatal lupus infant (●) and his mother (○) on the horizontal axis (see text). Provost, T.T., Watson, R.M., Gammon, R. et al.: Neonatal lupus erythematosus associated with U1RNP (nRNP) antibodies. N. Engl. J. Med., *316*:1135, 1987. With permission.[P315]

Table 29–2. Possible Immunopathologic Mechanisms in Nonspecific Cutaneous Features of SLE

Lesion	Mechanism
Mucosal ulcer	(?) DLE lesion on mucous membrane with ulceration
Bullous lesions	At least 3 potential mechanisms (see text)
Lupus panniculitis	Poorly defined clinically (see text)

Vasculitic lesions
  Microinfarcts
  Periungual telangiectasis
  Osler's nodes
  Janeway's spots
  Palpable and nonpalpable purpuric lesions
  Urticaria-like lesions, nodular lesions ([?] same as febrile relapsing nodular nonsuppurative panniculitis, Weber-Christian disease)
	May all represent manifestations of immune complex disease
	
	(?) Role of antiendothelial cell surface antibodies

Livedo reticularis	Result of vasculitis or anti-cardiolipin Ab—exact mechanism unknown

MUCOUS MEMBRANE ULCERATION

Mucous membrane ulcerations may occur in as many as 25% of systemic lupus erythematosus patients[U31] (Table 29–2). Pathologic examination of these lesions have been performed infrequently, and these studies suggest that the lesions are similar to cutaneous lupus lesions.[J123]

ALOPECIA

There are three forms of alopecia that are frequently detected in patients with lupus erythematosus. One of these forms of alopecia is a scarring alopecia, resulting from the inflammatory destructive infiltrate of discoid lupus lesions. The other two forms of alopecia are transient and nonscarring. These include diffuse hair loss over the entire scalp, as well as a "lupus-hair" phenomenon in which the patients develop a form of alopecia characterized by short, thin strands of hair that easily fracture most prominently at the margins of the scalp, giving the appearance of short, unruly hair.

The diffuse hair loss, in all probability, represents a telogen effluvium. This is a normal shedding process that can be induced by a variety of different stimuli, including the catabolic effect of a chronic or an acute illness. Such a metabolic insult causes the normal growing (anagen) hair to evolve into a resting hair (telogen). This process occurs over a 3-month period and is characterized by the eventual shedding of the resting hair and the emergence of a new growing (anagen) hair in the hair follicle.

The lupus-hair abnormality probably is the result of a similar process. In this case, however, the metabolic insult is not sufficient to induce the growing hair to go through the transition to the resting hair stage, but instead, alters the normal hair growth so that an abnormal weakened hair is produced. It should be noted that diffuse hair loss and the lupus-hair formation are seen in patients who have had, or are recovering from, a severe flare of their systemic lupus disease.

BULLOUS LUPUS ERYTHEMATOSUS

Bullous lesions are unusual cutaneous features in lupus erythematosus. They are generally characterized by small, tense, subepidermal bullae. There are three types of blisters that have been described in lupus patients. On unusual occasions, the severe liquefaction degeneration at the dermal-epidermal junction of cutaneous lupus lesions in anti-Ro/SSA—positive patients results in the formation of blisters.

The second form of blister formation was described by Hall et al. and subsequently by other investigators.[C44,H58,P108] They detected subepidermal blister formation responsive to diaminodiphenylsulfone therapy in four SLE patients. Biopsies demonstrated papillary microabscess formation composed of neutrophils and neutrophil fragments. There was also marked edema and subepidermal vesicle formation. In addition, two of the four patients demonstrated leukocytoclastic vasculitis of the superficial dermal blood vessels. Direct immunofluorescence examination of normal-appearing, non light-exposed skin, as well as perilesional skin, demonstrated heavy granular and linear deposition of various immunoglobulins and C3 at the dermal-epidermal junction. It is conceivable that this form of blister formation in systemic lupus erythematosus patients represents the cutaneous manifestations of a low-grade vasculitic process involving superficial blood vessels in the papillary portion of the dermis.

The third form of blister formation detected in lupus erythematosus has been reported by Gammon et al.[G27] These investigators have reported a subepidermal blistering disease process associated with the presence of an antibody directed against type VII collagen. This antibody appears identical in specificity to the autoantibody found in patients with epidermolysis bullosa acquisita. The antibody appears to react with epitopes on the globular (noncollagenous portion) of the type VII collagen molecule. Blister formation associated with this autoantibody may or may not occur in the presence of an inflammatory response. These data suggest that the antibody, by binding to the type VII collagen may, in the absence of complement activation, interfere with the normal integrity of the type VII collagen resulting in a blister formation.

LUPUS PANNICULITIS

Unfortunately, this is a confusing term that probably encompasses several entities.[T263] For example, inflammatory lesions of lupus panniculitis occur with or without an overlying discoid lupus lesion. In this chapter, we have referred to those lupus panniculitis lesions associated with an overlying discoid lesion as lupus profundus.

Those lupus panniculitis lesions not associated with overlying discoid lupus lesions can present a varied histopathologic picture, some of which may result from a vasculitis.[S64,T263] Other lesions appear to have a distinct histopathologic picture in which a lymphocytic panniculitis

dominates. On occasions, dystrophic calcification may be prominent. Unfortunately, there are no data to suggest an etiopathologic mechanism.

CUTANEOUS MANIFESTATIONS OF VASCULITIS

The cutaneous manifestations of vasculitis include small micro-infarcts at the tips of the fingers, erythematosus urticaria-like nodules at tips of fingers (Osler's nodes), capillary telangiectasia in the periungual region of the nails with or without micro-infarction, erythematous macular palmar lesions (Janeway's spots), livedo and purpuric lesions, most commonly on the lower extremities. In addition, urticaria-like lesions of vasculitis have been detected in patients with systemic lupus erythematosus. These urticaria-like lesions generally demonstrate a leukocytoclastic angiitis, but on uncommon occasions a mononuclear vasculopathy is seen.[O70,P317] In one study, 10 of 143 nontreated SLE patients were found to have urticaria-like vasculitic lesions as their initial cutaneous manifestation.[O70] Direct immunofluorescence examination of these lesions commonly demonstrates the deposition of immunoglobulin and complement in the blood vessels of the upper portion of the papillary and reticular dermis. These findings are consistent with immune complex—mediated leukocytoclastic angiitis as the underlying pathophysiology. Another provocative potential mechanism may be the presence of complement-fixing antiendothelial antibodies (reactive against endothelial cell surface molecules), which could give immunofluorescent findings that mimic immune complex formation.[C271]

LIVEDO RETICULARIS

Livedo reticularis is a term denoting a lacelike, generally violaceous erythematosus vascular pattern most prominent on the lower extremities. Ulceration may or may not be associated. This vascular pattern is seen in a variety of conditions associated with vascular disease, including vasculitis, such as polyarteritis nodosa and the antiphospholipid (cardiolipin) syndrome. Livedo reticularis can also be seen in normal individuals. However, the concomitant presence of ulceration generally indicates a pathologic process. The antiphospholipid syndrome can be seen in association with SLE or exist as a primary syndrome.[A100,A336] The exact cause of the peculiar lacy pattern is unknown.

SUMMARY

In this brief space, we have attempted to present the clinical, pathologic, and immunologic data suggesting the existence of two distinct pathophysiologic mechanisms in the genesis of specific lupus lesions (cell-mediated [discoid] and antibody-dependent cellular cytotoxicity [subacute cutaneous lupus lesions]). Our present-day knowledge suggests immune complexes do not play a primary role in the pathogenesis of either discoid or subacute cutaneous lupus lesions. There are, however, data suggesting that some of the nonspecific cutaneous lesions in lupus erythematosus are mediated by immune complex formation as well as autoantibodies.

Chapter 30

CLINICAL MANIFESTATIONS OF CUTANEOUS LUPUS ERYTHEMATOSUS

RICHARD D. SONTHEIMER

DEFINITION

For the purpose of this discussion, the term lupus erythematosus (LE) will be used to refer to the fundamental underlying autoimmune disease process that is expressed variably as a disease continuum (or spectrum). The clinical expression of this disease continuum can be subdivided into two global forms: cutaneous disease (cutaneous LE) and extracutaneous disease (systemic LE or SLE).

In the past the term discoid LE (DLE) was often used in a generic sense to designate that subgroup of LE patients whose disease is expressed predominantly in the skin. The use of DLE in this sense can create confusion since the same term has also classically been used to designate one of several clinically distinctive forms of cutaneous LE. Thus, in the following discussion the term DLE will be used in the latter, more restricted, sense to refer only to a clinical form of chronic cutaneous LE.

The term SLE has also been used in the past to generically designate all patients suffering from any combination of the systemic manifestations of LE. The term SLE will be used here in the same sense; however, it must be remembered that the large majority of SLE patients will express some form of cutaneous LE during their course, including at times DLE lesions.

It is also important to remember that LE patients can develop dermatologic disorders that are not the direct result of LE activity in the skin. Some such skin disorders can at times simulate the clinical appearance of different varieties of cutaneous LE. Thus, not all skin lesions in LE patients are necessarily forms of cutaneous LE. Corticosteroid-induced acne vulgaris and acne rosacea are examples of dermatologic conditions that are often the result of the treatment of LE rather than the LE autoimmune process itself.

HISTORICAL CONSIDERATIONS

In his scholarly review of the history of LE, Talbott[T33] reminds us that this clinical disorder was originally recognized by its visible cutaneous manifestations long before its systemic manifestations were known to exist. He points out that Cazenave in 1851 is generally given credit for having first used the term lupus érythèmateaux in referring to Biett's earlier description of what appears to have been discoid LE skin lesions.[C172] The term lupus érythè-mateaux helped to further distinguish this entity as a cutaneous malady that was distinct from cutaneous tuberculosis (lupus vulgaris) with which it had been earlier confused. Twenty years later, Kaposi further expanded Hebra's earlier description of what we now recognize as the systemic manifestations of LE and again employed the butterfly simile first used by Hebra to describe the facial skin lesions of LE.[H237] Subsequently, Hutchinson[H520,H521] and later Osler at the turn of the century[O107,O108,O109] further emphasized the multisystem nature of this disorder and the variability from patient to patient with which its cutaneous and systemic manifestations are expressed.

The early part of the twentieth century was dominated by clinical and pathologic descriptions of the various systemic manifestations of LE such as endocarditis, nephritis, and serositis. Freiberg initially presented the somewhat heretical idea in 1936 that the systemic manifestations of LE could occur in the absence of any type of skin disease.[F248] Since that time, the protean cutaneous manifestations of this disorder that had captured the imagination of the earliest students of LE have taken a backseat to the clinical and laboratory manifestations of the systemic involvement that occur in LE patients. This, coupled with the ceding of the autoimmune connective tissue diseases by the dermatologic community to the newly evolving subspecialty of rheumatology, led to a stepchild-like status for the cutaneous manifestations of LE that has existed in the modern era. Rheumatologists should receive more formal training in rheumatic disease dermatology to extend their descriptive prowess beyond the term "rash" when describing and categorizing the cutaneous manifestations of LE. In addition, dermatologists need to make their special knowledge and experience relating to cutaneous LE more available to those who serve as primary-care physicians for LE patients.

Brocq in 1925 initially described a widespread, non-scarring, photosensitive form of cutaneous LE as symmetrical erythema centrifugum[K196] that Gilliam later referred to as subacute cutaneous LE (SCLE), the bridging form of LE-specific skin disease in his revised classification of cutaneous LE.[G140]

In 1934, O'Leary at the Mayo Clinic introduced the term disseminated DLE as part of his new classification of LE that encompassed both its cutaneous and systemic manifestations.[O59] Unfortunately, O'Leary used the term disseminated in this classification scheme somewhat ambiguously to refer to both a widespread distribution of LE skin lesions as well as to indicate the transition from disease limited to skin to the systemic illness that we now recognize as SLE. Thus, several forms of widespread LE-specific skin disease (i.e., generalized DLE and SCLE) were thereafter often lumped together under the designation disseminated DLE or subacute disseminated LE, thereby obscuring the clinical and laboratory correlates of each of these clinically distinctive types of cutaneous LE. As a result, when the large LE population studies were later presented in which the clinical features of LE patients were correlated with the newly identified autoimmune serologic manifestations of the disease, such as the LE cell[H129] and the ANA reaction,[F270] the distinction between patients with generalized DLE and SCLE was often blurred.

Edmund Dubois[D318] was one of the first to apply the "spectrum" analogy to LE, emphasizing that this illness represented a disease continuum extending from localized DLE at the more benign pole to fully expressed SLE at the more severely affected pole. His earlier work with Tuffanelli[D340] emphasized the fact that various transition forms commonly occurred within this spectrum, including the appearance of SLE in patients who had initially presented with DLE lesions alone as well as the development of DLE lesions in patients with pre-existing SLE. These issues are dealt with more extensively by Dubois's student, Daniel J. Wallace, in Chapter 32.

James N. Gilliam later extended the spectrum analogy focusing especially upon the relationships that exist between the various cutaneous and systemic manifestations of LE.[P324] He also stressed the value of the various forms of cutaneous LE as markers for subsetting LE (the exercise of identifying more homogeneous subgroups of LE patients based upon the sharing of common clinical, pathologic, and laboratory features) that had become popular by the 1970s.[G144] Aided by Sontheimer and Thomas in the late 1970s, his description of the rather homogeneous LE subset marked by the presence of SCLE skin lesions[S568] served to highlight the overall value of this approach. The concept of SCLE was originally introduced by Gilliam as a component of a new classification of cutaneous LE that emphasized the histopathologic differences that can exist between different types of LE skin lesions.[G140,G144] Gilliam's earlier work with the dermatopathologist, Alvin Cox, at Stanford, greatly influenced his thinking in this area.

CLASSIFICATION

In most large population studies, the skin is the second only to the synovium as the organ most frequently affected by LE, and skin disease is the second most common way that LE initially presents itself clinically.[D341] In addition, the skin is one of the LE target organs that is most variably affected by this disease process (Table 30–1). Since the various skin manifestations of LE can be intimately linked to different patterns of systemic disease expression, an appreciation of the various cutaneous manifestations of LE is necessary for the fullest understanding of this heterogeneous disease process.

Table 30–1 lists the various clinically distinctive types

Table 30–1. The Gilliam Classification of Cutaneous LE

I. Histopathologically Specific (LE-Specific) Lesions
  A. Acute Cutaneous LE
    1. Localized
    2. Generalized
    3. Classic bullous LE
  B. Subacute Cutaneous LE
    1. Annular
    2. Papulosquamous
    3. Morbilliform or pityriasiform
  C. Chronic Cutaneous LE
    1. Classic DLE
      a. Localized
      b. Generalized
    2. Hypertrophic (verrucous) DLE
    3. Lupus panniculitis (profundus)
    4. Mucosal LE
      a. Oral
      b. Nasal
      c. Conjunctival
      d. Anogenital
    5. DLE-lichen planus overlap
    6. Lupus tumidus
    7. Chilblains LE
II. Histopathologically Nonspecific (LE-Nonspecific) Lesions
  A. Cutaneous vascular disease
    1. Vasculitis
      a. Leukocytoclastic
        (1) Palpable purpura
        (2) Urticarial vasculitis
      b. Periarteritis nodosa-like
    2. Vasculopathy
      a. Dego's disease-like
      b. Atrophy blanche-like
    3. Periungual telangiectasia
    4. Livedo reticularis
    5. Thrombophlebitis
    6. Raynaud's phenomenon
    7. Erythromelalgia
  B. Alopecia (nonscarring)
    1. "Lupus hair"
    2. Telogen effluvium
    3. Alopecia aerata
  C. Sclerodactly
  D. Rheumatoid nodules
  E. Calcinosis cutis
  F. LE-nonspecific bullous lesions
    1. Epidermolysis bullosa acquisita
    2. Dermatitis herpetiformis-like bullous LE
    3. Pemphigus erythematosus
    4. Bullous pemphigoid
    5. Porphyria cutanea tarda
  G. Urticaria
  H. Papulo-nodular mucinosis
  I. Cutis laxa/anetoderma
  J. Acanthosis nigricans (type B insulin resistance)
  K. Erythema multiforme
  L. Leg ulcers
  M. Lichen planus

of skin lesions that occur in LE patients. The dermatologic entities listed in Table 30–1 are ordered along the guidelines first proposed by Gilliam in 1977.[G140] His new classification scheme subdivided cutaneous LE into two broad categories—those that are histopathologically specific for LE (LE specific) and those that are not histopathologically specific for LE (LE nonspecific). The LE-specific skin lesions all share a similar lichenoid pattern of histopathologic changes that is seen to occur only as the result of LE-

Table 30–2. Comparative Histopathologic Features of the Three Major Types of LE-Specific Skin Disease

	ACLE	SCLE	CCLE (DLE)
Epidermal Changes			
Hyperkeratosis	+	+ +	+ + +
Atrophy	−	+ +	+
Liquefactive degeneration of basal cells	+	+ +	+ +
Basement membrane thickening	−	+	+ + +
Dermal Changes			
Lichenoid pattern of mononuclear cell infiltrate	+	+ +	+ + +
Perivascular mononuclear cell infiltrate			
Superficial dermis	+	+ +	+ + +
Deep dermis	−	−	+ +
Periappendageal inflammation	−	+	+ + +
Melanophages	+	+ +	+ + +
Subpapillary edema	+	+	+
Mucin accumulation	+	+	+ +
Subcutaneous Fat Changes			
Perivascular mononuclear cell infiltrate	−	−	+

Abbreviations: ACLE = acute cutaneous LE, SCLE = subacute cutaneous LE, CCLE (DLE) = chronic cutaneous LE (discoid LE).
− absent, + minimal, + + moderate, + + + prominent.
Based on data from Bangert, J.L., Freeman, R.G., Sontheimer, R.D. et al.: Comparative histopathology of subacute cutaneous lupus erythematosus and discoid lupus erythematosus. Arch. Dermatol., *120*:332, 1984.

induced inflammation in the skin[B76] (Table 30–2). Thus, a simple skin biopsy of such lesions can confirm a diagnosis of LE. The one exception is dermatomyositis, whose cutaneous manifestations can share many of the histopathologic features of LE-specific skin lesions. The experienced clinician, however, will usually not have difficulty in distinguishing cutaneous dermatomyositis from LE-specific skin lesions based upon their clinical differences alone.

The LE-nonspecific skin lesions also occur as the result of LE; however they have histopathologic patterns that can be seen in disorders other than LE. For example, the distinctive histopathologic pattern of leukocytoclastic vasculitis that is expressed clinically as palpable purpura or urticarial vasculitis skin lesions is a form of LE-nonspecific skin disease, since such lesions occur as a result of circulating immune complexes that are produced as a manifestation of SLE disease activity. However, leukocytoclastic vasculitic skin lesions can also occur as the result of other immune complex–related clinical disorders not related to LE such as drug hypersensitivity, essential mixed cryoglobulinemia, and Schönlein-Henoch purpura. The focus of the following discussion will be upon the LE-specific skin lesions. The LE-nonspecific skin lesions are addressed in Chapter 37.

As with any arbitrary subdivision of a disease continuum such as LE, overlapping features can be expected to occur in individual patients. Patients who have predominately SCLE lesions but who also develop scarring DLE or acute cutaneous LE lesions at some point in their course are examples of such an overlap. In most cutaneous LE patients, however, one type of LE-specific skin involve-

ment will predominate. Thus, either chronic, subacute, or acute cutaneous LE will usually dominate the clinical picture. Since these cutaneous manifestations correlate with distinct serologic, immunogenetic, and clinical features, it is reasonable to use the classification system discussed above that emphasizes the differences in the clinical expression of the cutaneous LE process for diagnostic, management, and prognostic purposes when dealing with individual patients.

LE-SPECIFIC SKIN DISEASE

Differences in clinical appearance and duration of clinical activity allow LE-specific skin lesions to be subdivided into three major types: acute cutaneous LE, subacute cutaneous LE, and chronic cutaneous LE. These diagnostic entities are not dependent on laboratory confirmation or the presence or absence of systemic disease activity.

An overview of the relationships that exist between the three major types of LE-specific skin disease and the systemic manifestations of SLE are illustrated in Figure 30–1.

Acute Cutaneous LE

For several reasons, acute cutaneous LE is the least well characterized type of LE-specific skin disease in modern immunologic terms. This form of LE skin disease almost always occurs in patients who are acutely ill with active systemic LE, and as such are not often managed by derma-

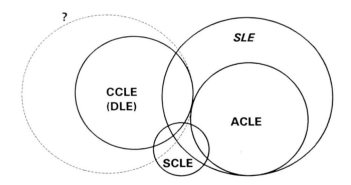

Fig. 30–1. Relationship between the three major types of LE-specific skin disease and SLE. Acute cutaneous LE (ACLE) (the butterfly shaped malar erythema reaction) occurs in 50 to 60% of patients with systemic LE (SLE). Approximately 25% of SLE patients will develop classic scarring discoid LE lesions (DLE), the major clinical variety of chronic cutaneous LE (CCLE), sometimes during their course. Only 10% of patients who present with DLE lesions ever go on to develop SLE later. The circle composed of the dashed line alludes to the fact that there are no population-based data concerning the true prevalence of chronic cutaneous LE (DLE) existing as an isolated clinical finding. Since such patients are often managed by dermatologists alone, it is possible that CCLE (DLE) patients could represent a larger percentage of the total population of LE patients than has been previously recognized. Subacute cutaneous LE (SCLE) occurs in approximately 10% of SLE patients; however, only 50% of patients with SCLE ever develop 4 or more of the American College of Rheumatology classification criteria for SLE. Approximately 15% of SCLE patients will develop CCLE (DLE) during their course, and another 15% will ultimately develop ACLE.

Table 30–3. Disorders Other Than LE That Can Cause a Red Face

Clinical Disorder	Distinguishing Feature(s)
Butterfly Shaped Malar Erythema	
Dermatologic Disorders	
Acne rosacea (including corticosteroid-induced rosacea)	Presence of pustules
Seborrheic dermatitis	Nasolabial fold and eyebrow involvement, histopathology
Photoallergic contact dermatitis	History of contactant exposure, photo patch test results, histopathology
Dermatophyte infection	Positive potassium hydroxide examination, histopathology
Pemphigus erythematosus	Immunopathology, histopathology
Polymorphous light eruption	Histopathology
Systemic Disorders that Involve the Skin	
Dermatomyositis	Violaceous periorbital erythema, Gottron's papules, pruritus
Exaggerated vasomotor flushing reactions (carcinoid syndrome, pheochromocytoma)	Associated symptoms, histopathology
Cushing's syndrome	Body habitus, striae, hypertension
Superior vena cava obstruction	Evidence of collateral venous engorgement, histopathology
Persistent Red Plaques	
Polymorphous light eruption	Histopathology
Sarcoidosis	Histopathology
Granuloma faciale	Histopathology
Pseudolymphoma of Spiegler and Fendt	Histopathology
Benign lymphocytic infiltration of Jessner and Kanof	Histopathology
Lymphocytoma cutis	Histopathology
Lymphoma cutis	Histopathology
Angiolymphoid hyperplasia with eosinophilia	Histopathology

ences of the face. Involvement extending over the bridge of the nose (but sparing the nasolabial folds) completes the body of the classic butterfly. Similar changes can also be seen in the skin of the V-area of the neck. Less commonly, acute cutaneous LE begins as small, discrete macular and/or papular lesions that later become confluent and hyperkeratotic.[M291]

Acute cutaneous LE is commonly precipitated by sun exposure and typically lasts for several hours to several days thereafter, but occasionally is more persistent. The activity of acute cutaneous LE often waxes and wanes in parallel with systemic LE disease activity. Postinflammatory hyperpigmentation and hypopigmentation, which can occur in any racial background, is most prominent in LE patients with darkly pigmented skin. Atrophic dermal scarring does not develop in acute cutaneous LE lesions. Facial swelling may be severe in acute cutaneous LE, sometimes simulating the facial skin changes that are characteristic of dermatomyositis. Some patients with localized acute cutaneous LE will on occasion also have SCLE lesions elsewhere on their body concurrently; however, the simultaneous occurrence of ACLE and active DLE rarely occurs.

Acute cutaneous LE can occasionally present as a more widespread morbilliform or exanthematous eruption (generalized acute cutaneous LE). This presentation may be confused with a drug hypersensitivity reaction, erythema multiforme, or even toxic epidermal necrolysis.

Histopathology and Immunopathology

The histologic picture in acute cutaneous LE is generally less impressive than that seen in SCLE and DLE lesions. A careful examination, however, usually reveals enough evidence of specific epidermal change so that a diagnosis of cutaneous LE can be made (Table 30–2). The dermal cellular infiltrate is usually relatively sparse. The most prominent changes are edema of the upper dermis and

tologists. In such a setting, the cutaneous involvement usually receives much less of the attending physician's attention than do the more life-threatening systemic manifestations of the disease process. In addition, many physicians are reluctant to biopsy the face of a young female for any reason. However, all those who manage systemic LE patients must be aware that the appearance of the "classical butterfly rash" can be simulated by several other benign dermatologic conditions (Table 30–3) and often a simple skin biopsy is the only way to clearly distinguish these disorders.

Clinical Features

Acute cutaneous LE lesions occurs at some time in 30 to 60% of SLE patients.[T264,W100] Localized acute cutaneous LE (the classic butterfly malar rash) is the most common variety of acute cutaneous LE (Fig. 30–2). Most typically, these lesions are characterized by confluent erythema and edema that is focused over the malar emin-

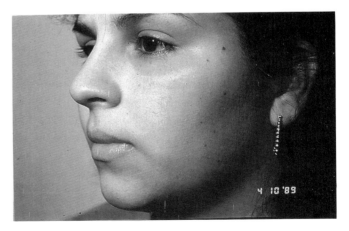

Fig. 30–2. Acute cutaneous LE. The skin overlying the left malar area exhibits confluent, edematous erythema (similar changes were also present on the right side of the patient's face). In this patient, cutaneous involvement does not extend over the bridge of the nose to form a classic butterfly, as it does in many other cases.

focal liquefactive degeneration of the epidermal basal cell layer. In the most severe forms of acute cutaneous LE, epidermal necrosis may occur, producing a histopathologic pattern resembling toxic epidermal necrolysis, a life-threatening pattern of blistering skin disease that most often is triggered by a drug hypersensitivity reaction.

There are few published data concerning direct immunofluorescence findings in acute cutaneous LE biopsy specimens. In one study, five of five (100%) skin biopsies from acute cutaneous LE (i.e., diffuse erythema) lesions were reported to be lesional lupus band test (LBT) positive;[P229] however, another author suggests anecdotally that acute cutaneous LE lesions are usually LBT negative.[W100] The truth probably lies somewhere in between.

Laboratory Findings

The laboratory abnormalities in patients with acute cutaneous LE generally reflect the presence of active systemic disease—high titers/levels of antinuclear and anti-DNA antibodies, low serum complement levels, anemia, leukopenia, hypergammaglobulinemia, elevated erythrocyte sedimentation rate, proteinuria, hematuria, pyuria, and cylindruria.

Differential Diagnosis

The differential diagnosis of localized acute cutaneous LE is listed in Table 30–3 under the malar erythema section. Dermatomyositis is the non-LE rheumatic disorder that most frequently mimics acute cutaneous LE on the face. However, the absence of the other characteristic features of dermatomyositis (periorbital violaceous erythema, Gottron's sign, Gottron's papules, pruritus, and myositis) can serve to distinguish this entity from acute cutaneous LE.

Subacute cutaneous LE, when it does affect the face, presents with annular or papulosquamous lesions that are distinct from acute cutaneous LE. It should be remembered that some SCLE patients will develop typical acute cutaneous LE lesions during their disease course, often in association with the development of more aggressive underlying SLE (see Chap. 31). The presence of follicular involvement and scarring allows DLE lesions to be easily distinguished from those of acute cutaneous LE.

The dermatologic conditions that can be confused with acute cutaneous LE along with their distinguishing features are also listed in the first section of Table 30–3. The erythemato-telangiectatic type of acne rosacea is often the dermatologic condition that causes the greatest degree of confusion[A34] The histopathologic changes found in this disorder—vascular dilatation with an associated nonspecific perivascular dermal inflammatory cell infiltrate—is distinctly different from those changes found in LE-specific skin lesions. One of the dermatologic entities listed in Table 30–3 should be strongly suspected with any facial butterfly erythema reaction that has a markedly protracted course and that is not associated with clinical or specific laboratory evidence of underlying SLE.

Disease Course and Prognosis

Acute cutaneous LE skin disease activity usually waxes and wanes in parallel with SLE disease activity, and the prognosis of patients with this form of LE-specific skin disease is usually dominated by the pattern of their underlying systemic disease. These issues and other aspects of the relationships that exist between acute cutaneous LE, photosensitivity, and SLE are further discussed in Chapter 37.

Treatment

Acute cutaneous LE lesions usually respond to the more aggressive regimens of systemic corticosteroids and other immunosuppressive agents that are often required to quell the associated systemic manifestations of LE that usually accompany this form of LE-specific skin disease. The aminoquinoline antimalarial agents such as hydroxychloroquine and quinacrine that can have a steroid-sparing effect in the systemic manifestations of LE[C56] can also favorably impact acute cutaneous LE.

Subacute Cutaneous LE

The clinical and laboratory manifestations of patients who develop SCLE skin lesions are presented in depth in Chapter 31.

Chronic Cutaneous LE

The author's view of the relationship that exists between the cutaneous and systemic manifestations of LE is based upon the following assumption—isolated DLE lesions represent a manifestation of the same disease process that produces SLE disease activity. In support of this hypothesis are the following observations: 1) there are no clinical, histopathologic, or immunopathologic differences between the DLE lesions that occur as an isolated clinical phenomenon and those that develop in patients with preexisting SLE; 2) antinuclear antibodies are often present in patients who clinically have only DLE lesions;[M413,O71] and 3) B-cell abnormalities similar to those present in SLE patients also can be found in DLE patients.[K231]

Epidemiology

There are no reliable data pertaining to the true prevalence or incidence of classic DLE (the most common form of chronic cutaneous LE) presenting in the absence of systemic LE activity. This results from the fact that prior to 1979, investigators did not distinguish between DLE and SCLE, usually lumping these two varieties of cutaneous LE together under the generic designations of DLE or disseminated DLE. Thus, the data presented in LE population studies prior to that time cannot be used to gain an accurate view of the overall prevalence of chronic cutaneous LE. It is the author's opinion that a considerable percentage of the overall U.S. LE population are not seen by rheumatologists and internists, since they are patients who suffer only from chronic cutaneous LE clinically and who are managed throughout their illness by dermatologists. Population-based studies are needed to determine the overall frequency with which LE manifests itself only as skin disease.

Based upon data from the older LE population studies,

the following points can be made that are likely to be generally reflective of the true epidemiology of DLE, as distinguished from SCLE. The most common age of onset of DLE is between 20 and 40 years in both males and females;[C19,D29,M155,P326,R352,S226,S397] however, DLE lesions can appear in infancy and childhood as well as in individuals beyond 70 years of age. The female:male ratio for DLE has been reported to be between 3:2 to 3:1.[D19,H445,M155,R352,S226,S397] Any race can be affected, including African-Americans,[C19,P326,R352] who were erroneously felt in earlier times to be relatively protected from DLE. In fact, Hochberg and co-workers have presented data that suggest that DLE is actually more prevalent in African-Americans.[H347]

All forms of cutaneous LE together have a significant socioeconomic impact in the United States. One study suggests that cutaneous LE is the third most common cause of industrial disability from dermatologic disease, with 45% of cutaneous LE patients experiencing some form of vocational handicap.[O91]

Classic DLE

Lupus erythematosus was originally described by Cazanave in the mid-nineteenth century on the basis of the striking clinical lesions of classic DLE.

Clinical Features

The most common form of chronic cutaneous LE is classic DLE (hereafter, the unqualified term DLE will be used to refer to this form of DLE). DLE lesions of this type begin as flat or slightly elevated, well-demarcated, red-purple macules or papules with a scaly surface. These early DLE lesions most commonly evolve into larger discrete, coin-shaped (i.e., discoid) erythematous plaques covered by a prominent, adherent scale that extends into dilated hair follicles (Figs. 30-3-30-5). These discoid-shaped plaques can enlarge and merge to form even larger, confluent, disfiguring plaques (Figs. 30-6-30-8).

Involvement of the hair follicle is a prominent clinical feature with scales accumulating in dilated follicular openings from which the hair is lost. When the adherent scale is peeled back from more advanced lesions, follicle-sized keratotic spikes similar in appearance to carpet tacks can be seen to project from the undersurface of the scale (the carpet tack sign). Erythema and hyperpigmentation is present during the initial phase of lesions. The lesions slowly expand with active inflammation at the periphery leaving depressed central scarring, telangiectasia, and depigmentation. The central atrophic scarring is highly characteristic. Pigment changes alone are not sufficient to qualify as a form of scarring as this term is used in describing LE skin lesions.

The more typical larger DLE lesions occur most often on the face, scalp, ears, V-area of the neck, and extensor aspects of the arms. Any area of the face can be involved, including the eyebrows, eyelids, nose, chin, and malar areas. Occasionally, a classic, symmetric butterfly shaped DLE plaque is present over the malar areas and bridge of the nose. Such DLE lesions should not be confused with the more transient, edematous erythema reactions that

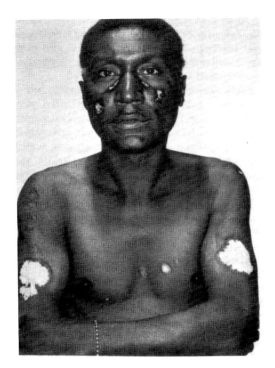

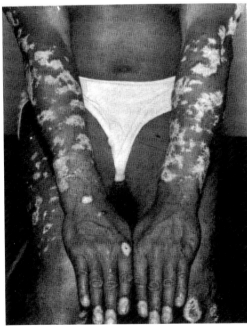

Figs. 30-3 and 30-4. Clinical varieties of the distribution of DLE.

occur over the same distribution in acute cutaneous LE lesions. As with acute cutaneous LE, the nasolabial folds are usually spared by DLE. Perioral DLE lesions often resolve with a striking acneiform pattern of pitted scarring. DLE often involves the external ear including the outer portion of the external auditory canal, with the earliest lesions in this area presenting as dilated, hyperpigmented follicles (Fig. 30-9).

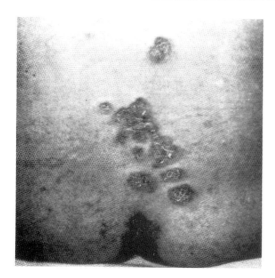

Fig. 30–5. Classic plaques of DLE.

Scalp involvement occurs in 60% of DLE patients, and is the only area involved in approximately 10%.[P326] Irreversible scarring alopecia can result from the permanent follicular destruction that often occurs early in the course of active DLE. The irreversible, scarring alopecia that occurs as the result of persistent DLE activity in a localized area differs from the more widespread, reversible, nonscarring alopecia that SLE patients often develop during periods of disease activity.

The term localized DLE is used to describe those patients who have lesions only on the head or neck. The occurrence of DLE lesions both above and below the neck is referred to as generalized DLE. The presence of DLE lesions below the neck only is distinctly uncommon. When DLE lesions are present below the neck, they are most commonly found on the extensor aspect of the arms, forearms, and hands (Figs. 30–3 and 30–4), although DLE lesions can occur at virtually any site on the body, including completely sun-protected sites (Fig. 30–5). Unusual locations can at times reflect the fact that DLE skin disease activity can follow in the wake of any form of trauma to the skin (i.e., the Koebner or isomorphic response). Painful palmar-plantar DLE involvement can predominate in some cases, producing significant disability and presenting an especially difficult management problem.[A345,P56] On occasion, DLE lesions can remain as small discrete, follicular-based papules having a diameter of less than 1 cm or less. Such lesions are often seen around the elbow, but can occur elsewhere as well.

In some patients DLE lesions are clearly precipitated or exacerbated by sunlight exposure. It is predominantly the UVB portion of the solar spectrum (the same wavelengths that cause sunburn) that aggravates DLE lesions, although increasing evidence suggests that the longer UVA wavelengths can also be deleterious in some LE patients. In as many as 50% of patients, however, sun exposure does not appear to be related to the cause of their DLE lesions. DLE lesions that begin in the scalp or ears (both being anatomic locations that receive virtually no direct sunlight exposure) are examples where this form of cutaneous LE is not related to light exposure. In addition, as noted elsewhere, nonspecific trauma to the skin can precipitate or exacerbate all forms of LE-specific skin disease, including DLE.

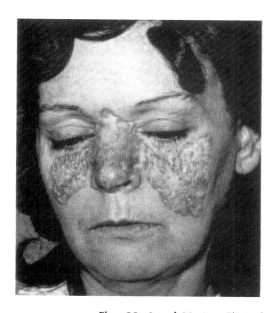

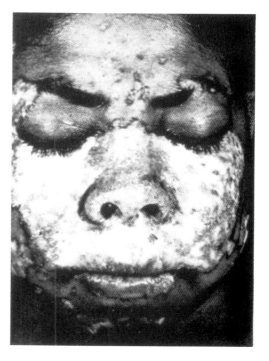

Figs. 30–6 and 30–7. Clinical varieties of the distribution of DLE.

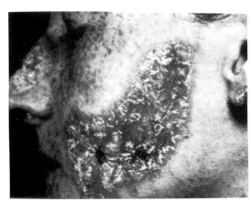

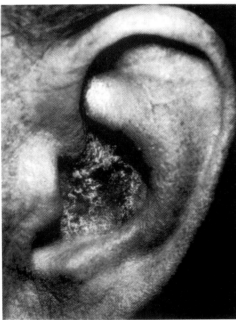

Figs. 30–8 and 30–9.   Classic plaques of DLE.

Histopathology

The basal (or germinal) cell layer of the epidermis is the principal site of injury in all three forms of LE-specific skin disease[B76] (Table 30–2). In chronic cutaneous LE (DLE), there is also prominent hyperkeratosis and follicular plugging (Fig. 30–10). The nucleated layer of the epidermis is generally not thickened and may be somewhat atrophic. Epidermal basal layer changes include loss of the normal organization and orientation of basal cells, edema with vacuole formation between and sometimes within basal cells (i.e., liquefaction or vacuolar degeneration), partial obliteration of the dermal-epidermal junction by a mononuclear cell infiltrate, thickening of the epidermal basement membrane, increased melanin pigment formation, and interruption of pigment transfer between melanocytes and keratinocytes leading to the accumulation of melanin by phagocytosis in dermal macrophages.

The dermal histopathologic changes are less specific. A mononuclear cell infiltrate composed predominantly of activated T lymphocytes (CD4 and CD8) and macrophages is present most predominantly in the periappendageal and perivascular areas. Plasma cells are occasionally seen in the more chronic lesions, and dermal mucin deposition can at times be prominent. It should be emphasized that the only histologic difference between the acute, subacute, and chronic cutaneous LE lesions is in the degree or extent of the pathologic alteration in the skin (Table 30–2). The chronic scarring DLE lesions more often have a denser inflammatory cell infiltrate that extends well into the deeper reticular dermis and/or subcutis. In contrast, the acute and subacute cutaneous LE lesions contain a less dense inflammatory infiltrate that is confined to the upper dermis but still shows the distinctive pattern of injury along the dermal-epidermal junction.[B76] The periappendageal inflammation that is characteristic of DLE is less prominent in SCLE and acute cutaneous LE.

Immunopathology

A thick continuous band of immunoreactants is commonly found along the dermal-epidermal junction upon direct immunofluorescence examination of biopsy specimens taken from DLE lesions[D12,W127] (Fig. 30–11). This band also extends along the basement membrane of the hair follicle, a finding that is not often seen in those other disorders that have been reported to have similar dermal-epidermal junction immunoreactants deposited in a band-like pattern. Multiple immunoglobulin classes (IgG, IgA, IgM) are usually present within this band and various complement components (C3, C4, Clq, properdin, factor B, and the membrane attack complex, C5b–C9) can also be present in many of these lesions.[D12,W127]

Early reports suggested that over 90% of DLE lesions had lesional immunoreactants at the dermal-epidermal junction[P229] however, subsequent studies have reported somewhat lower frequencies.[D12,W127] The frequency with which immunoreactants are found in DLE lesions also appears to vary with the anatomic region from which the biopsy is taken. In one study, lesions on the head, neck, and arms were more often positive (80%) than were those below on the trunk (20%).[W126] The frequency of band-like immunoreactant deposition at the dermal-epidermal junction appears also to be a function of the age of the lesion being examined with older lesions (i.e., >3 months) being more often positive than younger ones (i.e., <1 month).[D10] Ultrastructural localization of immunoglobulin at the dermal-epidermal junction has confirmed that these proteins are deposited on the upper dermal collagen fibers and along the lamina densa of the epidermal basement membrane zone.[U6] There is, however, little evidence that these immune deposits are primarily involved in the pathogenesis of the LE-specific pattern of cutaneous inflammation.

Laboratory Findings

Only a small percentage of patients with classic DLE who have no historical or physical evidence of systemic disease will have detectable immunologic abnormalities.[M413,P326] Antinuclear antibodies may be detected in low titer in as many as 30 to 40% of DLE patients; how-

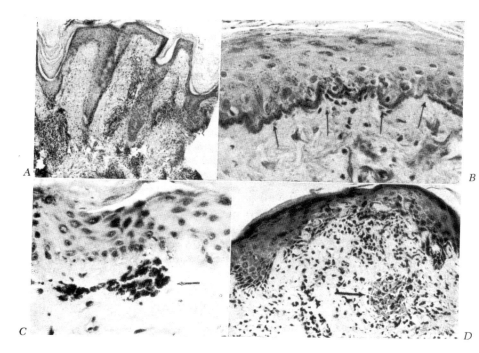

Fig. 30–10. *A*, DLE showing hyperkeratosis, keratotic plugging, epidermal atrophy with some areas of acanthosis, dissolution of the basal cell layer, and the dermal perivascular and periappendageal infiltrate of mononuclear cells (H&E; ×19). *B*, DLE, PAS stain, showing the thickened "basement membrane" (×127). *C*, DLE showing incontinence of pigment with collection of melanin below areas of liquefaction degeneration (×100). *D*, SLE showing changes similar to DLE but with more edema and the presence of red cell extravasation (arrow) (H&E; ×50).

ever, less than 5% will have the higher levels that are characteristic of severe SLE. While antibodies to single-stranded DNA are not uncommon in DLE, antibodies to double-stranded DNA are distinctly uncommon.[C19,C22] Precipitating antibodies to U1-RNP are sometimes found in patients whose disease course is dominated by DLE lesions; however, such patients usually have evidence of mild SLE or overlapping connective tissue disease.[C19] Ro/SSA precipitins can also occasionally be seen in DLE patients.[P310] The presence of precipitating Sm and La/SSB antibodies are, however, distinctly unusual in patients with isolated DLE lesions.[P310] It has been our experience that antiphospholipid antibodies are also uncommon in uncomplicated DLE patients. Fewer than 10% of our patients have had IgG anticardiolipin antibodies (personal unpublished observation) and that has been the experience of others as well.[M221]

A small percentage of DLE patients will have a biologic false-positive serologic test for syphilis (VDRL), positive rheumatoid factor tests, slight depressions in serum complement levels, modest elevations in gamma globulin, and modest leukopenia. However, unexplained anemia, marked leukopenia, a persistently positive high-titer antinuclear antibody assay, hypergammaglobulinemia, an elevated erythrocyte sedimentation rate (especially >50 mm/hr), and immune deposits at the dermal-epidermal junction of nonlesional skin (i.e., a positive lupus band test) should raise concern for the possibility of impending systemic LE disease activity.[M413,O71,P324]

Differential Diagnosis

With respect to diagnosis, discoid-shaped skin lesions that have erythema and hyperpigmentation at their active borders and depigmentation, telangiectasia, and atrophy at the centers are unlikely to result from dermatologic disorders other than cutaneous LE. However, there are other dermatoses that can produce persistent red plaques on the face that at times can be confused with DLE (see persistent red plaques section of Table 30–3).

Polymorphous light eruption (PMLE), as the name implies, is an exclusively phototriggered dermatosis that can be expressed in several clinical forms, including succulent red plaques that can occasionally mimic the earlier phases of evolving DLE lesions. PMLE lesions, however, clinically lack the keratinaceous follicular plugging, telangiectasia, and atrophy that are characteristic of DLE lesions. Histopathologically, PMLE lacks the prominent liquefaction degeneration of the epidermal basal cell layer and basement membrane thickening that is characteristic of DLE lesions. In the dermis, the lymphoid cell infiltrate is predominantly perivascular in PMLE and does not involve the cutaneous appendages as in DLE. Immunoglobulins and complement components are not deposited at the dermal-

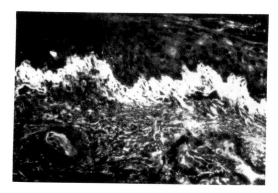

Fig. 30–11. Biopsy taken from a chronic plaque of DLE stained with fluorescein-labeled anti-IgG.

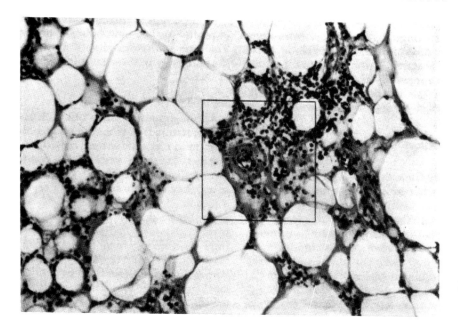

Fig. 30–15. Vasculitis and panniculitis in lupus erythematosus profundus. (Courtesy of Dr. C. G. Schirrer, University of Munich.)

Approximately 70% of the patients with this type of chronic cutaneous LE also have typical DLE lesions often overlying the panniculitis lesions or on other parts of the body,[T261] and half have a relatively mild form of SLE.[172,P143,T261,W301] The term LE profundus is used by some to designate those patients who have both LE panniculitis and DLE lesions.

LE panniculitis is the only LE-specific skin lesion that spares the epidermis. Absence of the characteristic epidermal changes of LE can make the histologic diagnosis difficult, and controversy has existed in the past as to the specificity of the histopathologic changes of LE panniculitis when overlying changes of DLE are not present at the dermal-epidermal junction. The histologic features are that of a lobular lymphocytic panniculitis: insignificant epidermal involvement; perivascular infiltration with lymphocytes, plasma cells, and histiocytes in the deep dermis and subcutaneous fat (including lymphoid nodule formation); vessel wall thickening and invasion by mononuclear cells (lymphocytic vasculitis); absence of polymorphonuclear leukocytes; hyaline fat necrosis, prominent fibrinoid degeneration of collagen; as well as mucinous degeneration and calcification in old established lesions (Figs. 30–15 and 30–16).[P143,S64] Immunoglobulin and complement deposits are usually found in blood vessel walls of the deep dermis and subcutis by direct immunofluorescence staining of biopsy specimens.[T261] Immunoglobulin deposits at the dermal-epidermal junction may or may not be present depending on the site biopsied, the presence or absence of SLE, and the presence or absence of overlying changes of DLE at the dermal-epidermal junction.

The differential diagnosis of patients with lupus panniculitis includes Weber-Christian panniculitis, factitial panniculitis, pentazocine- (Talwin) induced panniculitis, pancreatic panniculitis, traumatic panniculitis, morphea profundus, eosinophilic fasciitis, sarcoidosis, subcutaneous granuloma annulare, and rheumatoid nodules. Deep excisional biopsy is often required to distinguish LE panniculitis from these other disorders, particularly when classic DLE lesions are not present.

The systemic features of patients with LE panniculitis (profundus) tend to be relatively mild, similar to those in SLE patients who have DLE skin lesions.[172,P143,T261,W301]

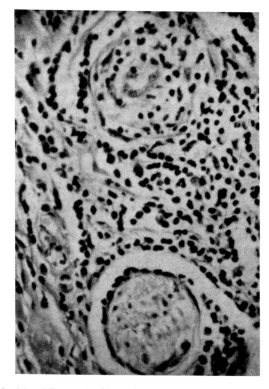

Fig. 30–16. LE panniculitis. There is a lymphocytic infiltrate around a vessel and a nerve (H&E; ×160).

Antinuclear antibodies are present in 70 to 75%, but anti–double-stranded DNA antibodies are uncommon.[P143,T261,W301] Musculoskeletal complaints, fever, and fatigue are common, and vasculitis may occur. Severe nephritis is an uncommon complication in SLE patients with LE panniculitis. Untreated, LE panniculitis (profundus) is indolently progressive with ulceration often eventually supervening. Intralesional corticosteroid therapy should be approached with great caution since even this minimal form of trauma can cause LE panniculitis lesions to break down and ulcerate. Even a carefully executed diagnostic skin biopsy can at times produce chronic ulceration in these lesions. Most cases can be managed successfully with single-agent or combined antimalarial therapy; however, some will require more aggressive treatment with systemic corticosteroids.[W301] The relationship between LE panniculitis and SLE is further addressed in Chapter 37.

Mucosal DLE

Earlier reports had documented that mucosal membrane involvement can occur in chronic cutaneous LE patients.[J123,S144,T264] Work by Burge and co-workers has confirmed that the prevalence of mucous membrane involvement in chronic cutaneous LE (DLE) is about 25%.[B574] While the oral mucosa is most frequently involved, nasal, conjunctival, and genital mucosal surfaces can also be affected (Table 30–4).

Within the oral mucosa, the buccal mucosal surfaces are most commonly involved, with the palate, alveolar processes, and tongue being less frequently affected sites. Individual lesions begin as rather painless, erythematous patches later maturing to a chronic plaque stage that can have an appearance similar to that of lichen planus. The chronic buccal mucosal plaques have a sharply marginated, irregularly scalloped white border with radiating white striae and telangiectasia.[B574] When overlying the palatal mucosa, the surface of these plaques often has a well-defined meshwork of raised hyperkeratotic white strands that encircle zones of punctate erythema, which gives a honeycomb appearance.[B574] The center of older

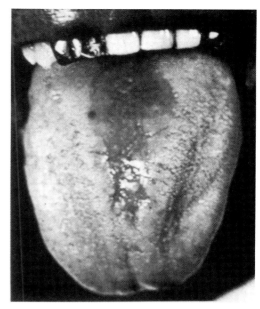

Fig. 30–17.   DLE involving the tongue.

lesions can become depressed and occasionally undergoes painful ulceration. Well-defined chronic DLE plaques can also appear on the vermillion border of the lips. At times LE involvement of the lips can present as a diffuse cheilitis, especially on the more sun-exposed lower lip. Although lesions can appear on the tongue (Fig. 30–17), this location is rare.[B574]

Chronic oral mucosal DLE can occasionally degenerate into squamous cell carcinoma,[A219] as can cutaneous DLE lesions. Any area of asymmetric nodular induration within a mucosal DLE lesion should be carefully evaluated for the possibility of malignant degeneration. With respect to differential diagnosis, oral lichen planus presents the closest clinical appearance to that of oral mucosal DLE.

Discrete DLE plaques can also develop on the nasal, conjunctival, and genital mucosa.[B574] Nasal septum perforation is more often associated with SLE than DLE.[A125,R348,V2] Conjunctival DLE lesions also begin as small areas of nondescript inflammation most commonly affecting the palpebral conjunctivae or the margin of the eyelid. However, as these early lesions progress, scarring becomes evident which can produce permanent loss of eyelashes and ectropion. Although rare, anogenital mucosal DLE lesions have also been observed.[B574] It has been suggested that corneal stromal keratitis can also occur as a result of DLE ocular involvement.[R15]

The clinical diagnosis of mucosal DLE can be confirmed by histopathologic examination of a biopsy from an active mucosal lesion or a concomitant cutaneous DLE lesion that is often present. Except for the differences related to the absence of hair follicles and stratum corneum in mucous membranes, the microscopic changes are highly reminiscent of those seen in cutaneous DLE lesions.[B574]

The associated risk for systemic disease in LE patients with mucosal involvement is a function of the type of mucosal lesion that is present. Superficial, transient oral

Table 30–4.   Prevalence of Mucosal Involvement in LE

	% CCLE (n = 68)	% SLE (n = 53)
Overall prevalence of mucosal involvement	24	21
Pattern of mucosal involvement		
Oral		
Acute ulcers	0	36
Chronic plaques	9	4
Cheilitis	6	
Nasal	9	2
Ocular		
Episcleritis	0	9
Conjunctival scarring	3	0
Lid margin plaque	6	0
Genital	5	0

Data adapted from Burge, S.M., Frith, P.A., Juniper, R.P. et al.: Mucosal involvement in systemic and chronic cutaneous lupus erythematosus. Br. J. Dermatol., *121*:727, 1989.

or nasal mucosal ulcerations are commonly seen in patients with active SLE (such mucosal lesions represent 1 of the 11 American College of Rheumatology's revised classification criteria for SLE). Chronic mucosal LE plaques, however, are seen most commonly in LE patients who do not have life-threatening SLE. The more severe manifestations of SLE such as renal disease appears to be rather uncommon in SLE patients who develop mucosal membrane involvement, especially chronic mucosal plaques.[B574] Mucosal membrane involvement in SLE is also discussed in Chapter 37.

Other Rare Clinical Variants of Chronic Cutaneous LE

The accumulation of prominent amounts of dermal mucin early in the course of DLE skin lesions can result in the succulent, edematous, urticaria-appearing plaques of LE tumidus.[K230] The characteristic epidermal histological changes of DLE are often not as prominent in lupus tumidus lesions. When this occurs, confusion can arise concerning the diagnosis.

Some LE patients develop red-purple patches and plaques on their face and hands that are precipitated by cold, damp climates. Such lesions are highly reminiscent of simple chilblains or pernio lesions.[M412] As these lesions evolve, however, they take on the typical appearance of DLE lesions. The terms chilblains lupus and perniotic LE have been used to describe such lesions. Unfortunately, the term lupus pernio has also been used for such lesions; however, this term is more properly used to designate a form of cutaneous sarcoidosis.[J40]

BULLOUS SKIN LESIONS IN LE

The different varieties of bullous skin lesions that can occur in LE patients can also be divided into those that do and do not have a LE-specific histopathology (Table 30–5).

Bullae may develop in LE-specific skin lesions such as acute and subacute cutaneous LE lesions as an extension of the liquefaction injury pattern that is focused at the epidermal basal layer. Skin cleavage occurs as a result of hyperacute basal cell injury and failure, resulting in a subepidermal cleavage plane. In both acute[G145] and subacute[B296] cutaneous LE, large areas of sheet-like cleavage occasionally develop, resulting in the clinical appearance of toxic epidermal necrolysis. Since such patients are also frequently on systemic medication, documentation of LE

Table 30–5.   Bullous Skin Lesions in LE Patients

LE Specific (Classic Bullous LE)
  Toxic epidermal necrolysis-like acute and subacute cutaneous LE
  Vesiculobullous subacute cutaneous LE
  Bullous DLE
LE Nonspecific
  Bullous pemphigoid
  Pemphigus erythematosus
  Bullous SLE
    Dermatitis herpetiformis-like cutaneous LE
    Epidermolysis bullosa acquisita
  Porphyria cutanea tarda

as the causal factor in this type of bullous skin change can be difficult, as toxic epidermal necrolysis most often develops as a drug hypersensitivity reaction. In some SCLE patients, vesiculobullous changes develop at the active advancing edge of annular SCLE lesions.[W119] Subepidermal bullous changes have also rarely been reported to occur in DLE lesions.[N14]

Examples of LE-nonspecific bullous skin lesions would include the case reports of bullous pemphigoid,[M423] dermatitis herpetiformis,[D75] acquired epidermolysis bullosa,[B278,B382] and porphyria cutanea tarda[W114] that have occurred in both DLE and SLE patients. In these cases, the histopathologic and immunopathologic changes were not those of LE-specific skin disease but rather the same as those changes that occur in patients who develop these blistering disorders but who never acquire any other evidence of LE. In many of these reports, it is not clear whether the bullous skin changes are the result of the LE autoimmune process or develop as a mere chance occurrence in patients who also have LE.

Pemphigus erythematosus is a photosensitive form of acantholytic skin disease that is associated with circulating autoantibodies that bind to determinants within the hemidesmosome of epidermal keratinocytes.[M170] Considerable evidence indicates that dissolution of the intercellular attachments within the epidermis with resultant intraepidermal bulla formation (acantholysis) is directly mediated by the binding of these autoantibodies. Patients with this form of pemphigus often have immunologic evidence of LE-like autoimmunity—circulating antinuclear antibodies and immunoglobulin/complement deposition at the dermal-epidermal junction (i.e., the Senear-Usher syndrome.[C249] However, such patients rarely develop significant clinical manifestations of SLE.

Active SLE patients will occasionally develop a severe generalized vesiculobullous eruption that resembles dermatitis herpetiformis (DH) or epidermolysis bullosa acquisita (EBA).[H58] The histology of these lesions shows marked neutrophilic infiltration with papillary microabscess formation similar to DH and the inflammatory variant of EBA. The direct immunofluorescence findings, however, are more consistent with those seen in SLE. Autoantibodies against type VII collagen (the EBA antigen), a normal constituent of anchoring fibrils of the sublamina densa zone, are present in some such patients.[B110] This type of lesion can occasionally represent the initial manifestation of SLE.[B382] Some workers have used the rather vague term bullous SLE to describe such lesions;[B110] however, we prefer the more descriptive terms DH-like cutaneous LE or EBA-like cutaneous LE since other forms of bullous skin lesions can occur in SLE patients. Bullous skin disease occurring in the context of SLE is further addressed in Chapter 37.

PHOTOSENSITIVITY IN LE

The issues related to photosensitivity and photoprotection as discussed in Chapters 31 and 37 also apply to chronic cutaneous LE, with the exception that sun exposure is less frequently an exacerbating factor in all forms of chronic cutaneous LE compared to acute and subacute cutaneous LE.

THE LUPUS BAND TEST

The clinical and immunologic significance of the lupus band test has been a point of controversy since its initial description in the early 1960s.

Definition

Burnham and co-workers[B589] first identified by direct immunofluorescence microscopy the presence of immunoglobulins and complement components in a continuous band-like array at the dermal-epidermal junction of lesional skin biopsies in LE patients. This phenomenon, subsequently referred to as the lupus band,[B587] was initially felt to be specific for LE. Later studies, however, have documented that the lupus band can be found in a number of skin disorders other than those caused by LE.[D12]

Cormane[C387] later described similar findings in biopsies from clinically normal skin of SLE patients in the complete absence of any signs of cutaneous inflammation (Fig. 30–18). Since DLE patients did not have this finding in their nonlesional skin, it was initially felt that such results might have diagnostic specificity for SLE. The search for immunoreactant deposition in nonlesional skin of LE patients has subsequently been referred to by many as the lupus band test (LBT).

Controversies concerning terminology have clouded this field since its inception, stemming in large part from the fact that the readout end point of immunofluorescence microscopy that has been employed in virtually all LBT studies published to date has been the subjective, qualitative end point of verbal description by a human observer. Even the meaning of the term LBT has been a point of contention. While some workers use this term to refer to LE lesional as well as nonlesional immunopathologic findings,[W127] others reserve this appellation for reference only to the results of immunopathologic examination of nonlesional skin.[D11] In the author's estimation, less confusion might exist in this area if the terms lesional LBT and nonlesional LBT were conventionally employed by those working in this area.

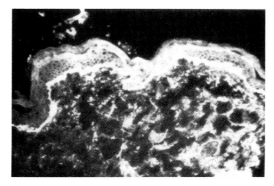

Fig. 30–18. Uninvolved skin from a patient with SLE stained with fluorescein-labeled antisera to IgG.

Table 30–6. The Lupus Band in Various Subgroups of LE Patients

	% Lesional	% Nonlesional	References
Systemic LE	90	50–60	P229
Cutaneous LE			
Acute cutaneous LE	90 (?)	50–60	B588,G141,P229
Subacute cutaneous LE	60	25	S568
Chronic cutaneous LE			
Classic DLE		0*	P326
Above neck	80–90		W126
Arms	80		W126
Trunk	20		W126
Hypertrophic DLE	100	?	U12
LE panniculitis	80	50	T261
Normal controls			
Sun-exposed skin	NA	20	F5
Non sun-exposed skin	NA	0	F5

* Non sun-exposed skin.
NA = Not applicable.

The immunopathologic findings in nonlesional skin of LE patients must be distinguished from those present in LE lesional skin biopsies. Issues related to immunopathologic findings in LE-specific skin lesions have been discussed in the relevant sections above and in Chapter 31. The results of lesional and nonlesional immunofluorescence testing in different LE subgroups are summarized in Table 30–6. The remainder of this discussion will be limited to the presence or absence of immunoreactants at the dermal-epidermal junction of nonlesional skin (i.e., the nonlesional LBT).

All three major immunoglobulin classes (IgG, IgM, and IgA) and a variety of complement components including constituents of the membrane attack complex have been identified in these subepidermal deposits.[D12] The immunoglobulin staining pattern under low power is generally described as being granular. Upon high power magnification, the pattern of fluorescence has been variously described as appearing stippled, fibrillar, shaggy, lumpy-bumpy, linear, or thready. Ultrastructurally, these immunoreactants are seen to be deposited on and below the lamina densa of the dermal-epidermal junction.[U6] The intensity of the staining and the number of immunoreactants present in these deposits can vary considerably.[D12,W127] Most authorities require a continuous pattern of immunoreactant deposition along the dermal-epidermal junction for a positive nonlesional LBT. Numerous studies have suggested that a discontinuous or interrupted nonlesional LBT can be seen in a number of other disorders and thus is much less specific for SLE.[D12] In addition, the presence of IgM alone appears to be nonspecific.[D12]

The clinical significance of the nonlesional LBT has been the subject of much controversy over the past two decades, especially with respect to both its diagnostic and prognostic significance. In-depth analyses of these issues are available elsewhere,[D12,D78,W127] however, this is beyond the scope of the current discussion. The following summary points can serve to acquaint the reader with the clinically relevant issues pertaining to the nonlesional LBT.

Standardization

It is somewhat disturbing that a test such as this, which has been used clinically for well over two decades, has been so poorly standardized. Only recently have large numbers of clinically normal individuals been studied to determine the incidence of a false-positive nonlesional LBT in both sun-exposed and nonexposed skin regions. It has been suggested that as many as 20% of healthy young adults have a positive LBT in sun-exposed nonlesional skin regions such as the lateral aspect of the neck, whereas virtually none are positive in sun-protected nonlesional sites such as the buttocks.[F5] Thus, great care must be taken when interpreting the results of immunopathologic findings in both lesional and nonlesional biopsies taken from fully sun-exposed skin sites (e.g., face, neck, extensor aspect of forearm and hand) or partially sun-exposed skin sites (flexor aspect of the forearm, deltoid region) with respect to the diagnosis of cutaneous or systemic LE.

Autofluorescence of dermal collagen and elastin fibers that at low power can give the appearance of a positive LBT has been described as the fibrillar pseudoband.[B587] At high power, the artifactual nature of this false-positive finding becomes apparent. A false-negative LBT can occur when high levels of unbound extravascular IgG are present in the upper dermis (a correlate of hypergammaglobulinemia), that can obscure the distinctness of the lupus band at the dermal-epidermal junction.[B514]

It is also important to understand that considerable anatomic regional variation exists with respect to the nonlesional LBT. It has been suggested that there is a cephalocaudal gradient in the frequency of a positive lupus band in DLE lesions, with lesions on the head more often being positive than those on the trunk.[W127] There are indications that a similar phenomenon might exist with the LBT in nonlesional skin of NZB/NZW mice, a murine model of SLE.[S564] Firm data addressing this issue have not yet been presented in human LE patients.

Diagnostic Specificity

Since the strongest clinical association of the nonlesional LBT has been with SLE, it is not surprising that chronic cutaneous LE (DLE) patients without laboratory or clinical evidence of extracutaneous disease have been uniformly nonlesional LBT negative.[P326] Only about 25% of SLE patients who have DLE lesions have a positive nonlesional LBT.[P326] Approximately 25% of SCLE patients (an LE subset that frequently has mild symptoms of SLE) are nonlesional LBT positive in relatively sun-protected flexor forearm skin.[S568]

As noted earlier, the diagnostic specificity of the nonlesional LBT for SLE has become a point of controversy. Taking into account the profile of immunoreactants present in a positive nonlesional LBT has been suggested to be one approach to enhancing the specificity of this test. Smith and Rothfield have suggested that when three or more immunoreactants are present in the nonlesional LBT, the diagnostic specificity for SLE is high.[S502] This observation, taken together with the fact that actinically damaged skin can often yield false-positive nonlesional LBT results,[F5] would suggest that a positive nonlesional LBT (confirmed under high-power observation to exclude the artifacts such as the fibrillar pseudoband) in fully sun-protected skin from the buttock or inner aspect of the upper arm that consists of three or more immunoglobulin or complement components might have the greatest specificity for SLE. Under these conditions, a positive nonlesional LBT can serve as a useful piece of additional diagnostic information in those difficult cases of SLE where the clinical and laboratory manifestations of this disorder are being expressed atypically.

Prognostic Significance

While the nonlesional LBT was initially adopted because of its perceived diagnostic specificity for SLE, subsequent work suggested that it also correlated positively with a more aggressive course of systemic disease including the development of lupus nephritis.[B588,G141,P307,R344] The presence of IgG in the nonlesional LBT was suggested to be more indicative of severe SLE than the presence of IgM alone.[P105] The idea that the nonlesional LBT had prognostic value also became a point of contention. However, prospectively ascertained followup studies have now confirmed the predictive value of a positive nonlesional LBT.[D78] It is not clear, however, that the nonlesional LBT provides incremental value over more generally available, less invasive, and less expensive tests such as circulating double-stranded DNA antibody levels in prognosis assessment. It is the author's opinion that the nonlesional LBT has its greatest utility as an additional diagnostic maneuver in patients with atypical clinical presentations of SLE. The significance of both the lesional and nonlesional LBT is further discussed in Chapter 37.

CONCLUSIONS

The highly diverse and often confusing group of skin lesions that can accompany LE can be rationally divided into two broad groups—those that have a pattern of histopathologic changes upon skin biopsy that is seen only in LE patients (i.e., LE-specific skin lesions) and those that do not have this pattern (i.e., LE-nonspecific skin lesions).

Each of the three major types of LE-specific skin disease (acute cutaneous LE, subacute cutaneous LE, and chronic cutaneous LE [discoid LE]) have different relationships with SLE. The presence of acute cutaneous LE in the large majority of cases correlates positively with the more severe systemic manifestations of SLE while chronic cutaneous LE is often inversely related. Subacute cutaneous LE represents an intermediate risk category.

The LE-nonspecific skin disorders are a clinically and histopathologically diverse group of skin lesions clinically and histopathologically that are most commonly seen in patient with SLE and are in some way associated with the underlying autoimmune abnormalities that are present in SLE patients.

Classic discoid LE (DLE) is by far the most common form of chronic cutaneous LE. Classic DLE most often occurs in patients who have relatively little underlying systemic disease activity, its persistent nature and proclivity for producing dystrophic scarring can result in considerable psychosocial and occupational disability. Single agent or combined aminoquinoline antimalarial therapy will control skin disease activity in a large majority of patients with classical DLE as well as the other clinical forms of chronic cutaneous LE. No form of medical therapy, however, will correct the disfiguring scarring produced by unchecked disease activity.

Variant clinical form of chronic cutaneous LE such as hypertrophic discoid LE, lupus panniculitis (profundus), mucosal discoid LE, lupus timidus, and chilblains lupus are differentially associated with SLE and can present diagnostic challenges.

The various forms of blistering skin lesions that can occur in LE patients can also be classified according to the presence or absence of the LE-specific histopathological pattern.

Considerable controversy has surrounded the nonlesional lupus band test since its initial description almost three decades ago and debates continue concerning both its diagnostic and prognostic significance. Recent data have suggested that false positives occur in biopsies from sun-exposed skin sites more frequently than was previously recognized. A positive nonlesional lupus band test in fully sun-protected skin such as that from the buttock or inner aspect of the upper arm that consists of three or more immunoglobulin classes or complement components has the greatest specificity for SLE. Under these conditions, a positive nonlesional LBT can provide additional valuable diagnostic information in those atypical clinical and laboratory presentations of SLE.

Chapter 31

SUBACUTE CUTANEOUS LUPUS ERYTHEMATOSUS

DANIEL P. McCAULIFFE
RICHARD D. SONTHEIMER

The concept of subacute cutaneous lupus erythematosus (SCLE) was first presented by Gilliam in 1977[G140] and expanded in 1981.[G144] The first series of SCLE patients was presented by Sontheimer et al. in 1979[S568] (see Chap. 30). This description and the others that have followed indicate that SCLE is a distinct subset of cutaneous LE, with certain clinical, serologic, and genetic characteristics.[B295, B341, C24, C25, D61, H280, H524, J86, M291, M523, M555, N90, P312, P313, R367, S396, S566, S567, W143] In the past decade, additional insight into the pathogenesis of this disease has been gained, more sensitive laboratory tests to aid in its diagnosis have been developed, and a number of agents for the treatment of this disorder have been identified.[S561]

SCLE consists of nonscarring, papulosquamous or annular skin lesions (or both) that have an LE-specific histopathology[B76] and that occur in a characteristic photo-distribution[S568] (Fig. 31–1). Although the presence of circulating Ro/SSA autoantibodies supports this diagnosis,[S566] their presence is not required.

EPIDEMIOLOGY

We have found SCLE lesions in approximately 9% of our entire LE patient population.[S568] Others have found SCLE lesions in 7 to 21% of their LE patients.[H280, K230, M523, M555, W143] SCLE, like systemic LE, is primarily a disease of Caucasian females. Of our SCLE patients, 70% have been female and 85% have been Caucasian.[S568] Only 15% of our SCLE patients are black or hispanic, although at our institution these two groups represent at least 50% of our total patient population. The mean age of our original 27 patients was 43.3 years, with a range of 17 to 67 years. Others have reported similar racial and sexual demographic data.[C24, H280, J86, M523, S396]

CLINICAL FEATURES

Cutaneous Findings

SCLE patients present initially with red macules or papules that develop into scaly, papulosquamous, or annular-polycyclic plaques (Fig. 31–1). Approximately 50% of patients have papulosquamous (psoriasiform) lesions (Fig. 31–2), and the other half have the annular-polycyclic form (Fig. 31–3), although a few patients may develop both types of lesions. Others have found varying percentages, with either a predominance of papu-

losquamous lesions[C24, M523] or the annular-polycyclic form.[B295, H280, S396] SCLE lesions occur predominantly on sun-exposed areas (i.e., upper back, shoulders, extensor aspects of the arms, V area of the neck and, less commonly, on the face; Fig. 31–2), and are frequently precipitated or exacerbated by ultraviolet (UV) light exposure.

Rarely, the lesions may initially present with an appearance of erythema multiforme[S565] with vesiculobullous changes[G337] and, on at least one occasion, have progressed to mimic toxic epidermal necrolysis.[B296] One SCLE patient initially presented with exfoliative erythroderma.[D180]

Lesions typically heal without scarring but can leave long-lasting and sometimes permanent vitiligo-like leukoderma and telangiectasias. In one patient, annular SCLE lesions were observed to progress to plaque-type morphea lesions.[R41]

Patients with SCLE lesions may also have, have had, or later develop the other two major types of LE-specific skin disease: acute cutaneous LE (ACLE) and chronic cutaneous LE (discoid LE, DLE; Fig. 31–4). Localized ACLE lesions (e.g., malar erythema reactions) have been reported to occur in 7 to 100% of SCLE patients.[D61, M523, S396, S558] Approximately 15% of our SCLE patients have developed ACLE lesions that generally occur in the setting of active systemic LE, and these patients are more ill-appearing and more apt to manifest lupus nephritis.[D61, S557, S558] ACLE skin lesions tend to be more transient and heal without scarring or pigmentation change. They are generally more edematous and less scaly than those of SCLE. ACLE more commonly affects the malar areas of the face, whereas in our SCLE patients the face has often been spared.

Various reports have noted that 0 to 29% of SCLE patients manifest discoid LE lesions at some time during their clinical course.[C24, D61, M523, S396, S557, S568] Of our original cohort of SCLE patients, 19% had typical DLE lesions (Fig. 31–4). DLE lesions may actually predate SCLE lesions. DLE lesions are usually confined to the head and neck, but may be more widely distributed. They are generally associated with greater degrees of hyper-pigmentation and hypopigmentation, may display atrophic scarring, and are more characteristically associated with follicular plugging and adherent scale. If the scale of a DLE lesion is physically removed, the underlying attached follicular keratinaceous plug can be extracted, and resembles a carpet tack. This has thus been referred to as the "carpet tack sign."

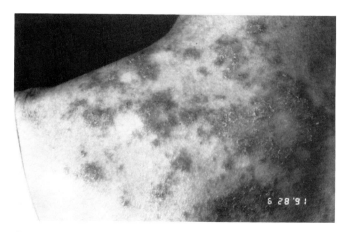

Fig. 31–1. Primary lesions of subacute cutaneous LE. Note the red, scaly macules and papules that are evolving into both papulosquamous and annular SCLE lesions in this patient.

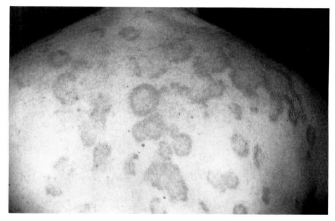

Fig. 31–3. Annular subacute cutaneous LE. The red rings of annular SCLE on this middle-aged man's back are merging to produce a polycyclic array.

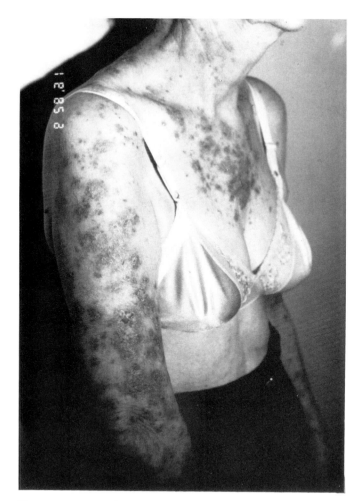

Fig. 31–2. Papulosquamous subacute cutaneous LE. The prominent, photoexposed distribution in this elderly woman also suggests the possibility of photosensitive psoriasis.

Other LE-nonspecific skin lesions may be present or develop later in SCLE patients.[S561] The most frequently encountered of these include alopecia, mucous membrane lesions (often painless), livedo reticularis (a red to blue net-like, nonpalpable, pigmentation pattern), periungual telangiectasias, vasculitis, and Raynaud's phenomenon.[C24,C25,D61,H280,M523,S558,S568] Cutaneous sclerosis and calcinosis have rarely been reported in SCLE patients.

Systemic Findings

Approximately half of SCLE patients meet the revised criteria of the American College of Rheumatology (ACR) for the classification of SLE (Fig. 31–4). It has been the experience of most observers, however, that severe SLE (i.e., glomerulonephritis, central nervous system disease) develops in only 10% of SCLE patients (Fig. 31–4). Al-

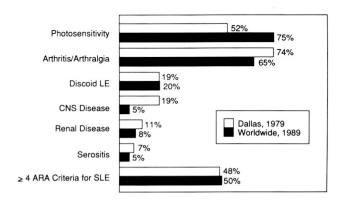

Fig. 31–4. Clinical manifestations of subacute cutaneous LE. The open bars represent the results of the initial analysis of our original cohort of 27 subacute cutaneous LE patients examined in Dallas in 1979,[S568] and the solid bars indicate extrapolated mean frequencies for the same findings from studies of over 200 SCLE patients during the next decade[B341,C24,C25,D61,H280,H524,J86, M291,M555,N90,P312,P313,R367,S396,S566,S567,W143] (data reviewed and summarized in[S561]).

though most SCLE patients who develop SLE tend to have a relatively mild course, SCLE patients have had severe and sometimes fatal outcomes, usually from renal and central nervous system involvement.[C24,H280,P313,W144] Some reports have indicated that patients with the papulosquamous variety of SCLE are more likely to develop renal involvement.[D61,S557,S558] We have identified 5 patients in a cohort of 47 individuals with SCLE that had renal disease. All 5 of these patients had the papulosquamous type of SCLE, leukopenia, high-titer antinuclear antibodies (ANAs. <1.640) and anti-ds (double-stranded) DNA antibodies. All 5 also developed ACLE lesions at some point during their disease course, and had been refractory to antimalarial treatment.[D61,S557,S558] Another report noted that SCLE patients with renal disease were more likely to have the papulosquamous type of lesions.[C25] It has been suggested that the presence of annular lesions marks the most homogeneous subgroup of SCLE patients immunogenetically.[B295]

DIFFERENTIAL DIAGNOSIS

The cutaneous lesions of papulosquamous SCLE are most closely mimicked by those of psoriasis, particularly photosensitive psoriasis. Seborrheic dermatitis, polymorphous light eruption, dermatophyte infections, nummular eczema, contact dermatitis, dermatomyositis, and cutaneous T-cell lymphoma—mycosis fungoides can also occasionally be confused with SCLE. Annular SCLE lesions are more apt to be misdiagnosed as granuloma annulare, erythema multiforme, or types of figurate erythemas, such as erythema annulare centrifigum. The photodistribution of SCLE lesions and the characteristic histopathologic findings are often crucial in helping the clinician differentiate SCLE from these other skin diseases. The presence of circulating Ro/SSA autoantibodies can further support a diagnosis of SCLE.

Overlap With Other Autoimmune Disorders

Several groups have noted patients with SCLE who later manifest Sjögren's syndrome, or patients with Sjögren's syndrome who later develop SCLE. The percentage of SCLE patients who later developed Sjögren's syndrome has ranged from 3 to 12%.[C24,P313,S396,S567] It is interesting to note that both groups frequently have circulating Ro/SSA and La/SSB autoantibodies, and both have been associated with the HLA-DR3 phenotype. A group of Japanese workers has reported four patient's with Sjögren's syndrome, Ro/SSA autoantibodies, and an annular erythema reaction that clinically resembled annular SCLE, although biopsies of the lesions revealed histopathologic findings somewhat distinct from those of SCLE.[N127]

We have found that as many as one-third of our SCLE patients produce rheumatoid factor. It is therefore not surprising that SCLE patients have sometimes developed rheumatoid arthritis (RA).[C336] We have also noted some RA patients who developed SCLE lesions. One group reported that, of 12 RA patients with Ro/SSA autoantibodies, 2 had SCLE skin lesions.[B386]

Possible Disease Associations

Several case reports have suggested an occasional association between SCLE and malignancy (breast, lung, and gastric),[B335,K446,N69,S129] Sweet's syndrome,[G215] porphyria cutanea tarda,[C26] and gluten-sensitive enteropathy.[M369,R236] The infrequency of these associated conditions mitigates against extensive evaluation to rule them out in SCLE patients whose history, review of systems, and physical examination do not suggest their presence. The clinician needs to be aware, however, that the usual dose of aminoquinoline antimalarial agents used in the management of SCLE can cause significant hepatotoxicity in patients who might have underlying subclinical porphyria cutanea tarda.

LABORATORY FINDINGS

Microscopic Findings

Although the histopathologic findings of SCLE (Fig. 31–5) can be pathognomonic for LE-specific skin disease, it may be impossible to differentiate SCLE from ACLE and DLE clearly (see Table 30–2). Characteristically, ACLE, SCLE, and DLE have variable degrees of hyperkeratosis, basal cell degeneration, dermal edema, and mononuclear cell infiltrates around the dermal-epidermal junction, extending into the dermis. In SCLE, focal basal cell injury and disorientation with liquefaction degeneration, sparse upper dermal mononuclear cell infiltrate, which may partially obscure the dermal-epidermal junction, dermal edema and, rarely, epidermal necrosis may occur.[B76] The mononuclear infiltrate is usually limited to perivascular and adnexal structures in the upper third of the dermis, and the epidermis may be mildly atrophic. Vesicular changes can occur in SCLE lesions, particularly at the active border of annular SCLE lesions.[H280,W119] These pa-

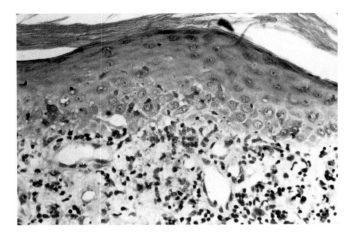

Fig. 31–5. Histopathology of subacute cutaneous LE lesions. Note the epidermal basal cell injury pattern of disorientation and liquefaction degeneration. In this biopsy, a prominent, mononuclear cell infiltrate in the upper dermis partially obscures the dermal-epidermal junction. The mononuclear infiltrate is often less prominent than in this particular biopsy, and is generally most noticeable in the perivascular areas, (stain: H&E).

tients may more likely be HLA-DR3—positive and have Ro/SSA autoantibodies.[H280]

SCLE lesions generally have less hyperkeratosis, less follicular plugging, less mononuclear cell infiltration of adnexal structures, and fewer dermal melanophages than DLE lesions. We and others have noted qualitative differences among the pathologic changes in SCLE versus DLE,[B76,M555] although another group has not been able to make this histopathologic distinction.[H408]

We have been unable to differentiate papulosquamous from annular SCLE by blinded histopathologic examination.[B76]

Immunofluorescence Staining

As in other LE-specific lesions, immune deposits can be frequently detected at the dermal-epidermal junction (DEJ) by immunofluorescence staining in SCLE skin lesions.[S568] These deposits consist of immunoglobulin (IgM, IgG, and/or IgA) and complement components arranged in a granular, band-like pattern. Approximately 60% of SCLE lesions from our patients have these deposits, compared to higher percentages for ACLE and DLE lesions (see Table 30–6). Others have found similar results in SCLE skin lesions.[H280,H524,S396,W143] Thus, the presence of immune deposits can help confirm a diagnosis of SCLE, but its absence does not necessarily rule it out. These immune deposits are not specific for LE, because similar deposits can be found in normal or sun-damaged skin and in other non-LE dermatologic conditions.[D12,F5]

Nieboer et al. have reported finding a "dust-like particle" pattern of IgG deposition in and around the epidermal basal keratinocytes and subepidermal regions in 30% of SCLE lesional skin biopsies.[N90] They have suggested that this pattern of immunoglobulin deposition is specific for SCLE, although its presence did not correlate with the presence of circulating Ro/SSA. The pattern is similar to that found in human skin explants grafted onto nude mice that resulted from an intravenous infusion of human Ro/SSA autoimmune sera.[L135] We have found a similar pattern of IgG and IgM deposition in guinea pig skin resulting from intradermal injections of human Ro/SSA autoimmune sera.

Lupus Band Test

The lupus band test consists of direct immunofluorescence examination of *nonlesional* skin to detect immunoglobulin deposition in patients with or suspected of having SLE. Approximately 50% of patients with SLE have immune deposits at the DEJ of nonlesional, normal skin.[G141] Nonlesional deltoid and flexor forearm skin biopsies from SCLE patients have revealed immune deposits in 46% and 26%, respectively.[S568] In patients with cutaneous LE, a positive lupus band test can indicate which patients are at risk for developing more severe disease, particularly if the immune deposits contain IgG, IgM, and IgA.[D78,G141,S562] Deposits with IgM alone are found in patients with more benign disease.[P105]

Serologic Findings

Antinuclear antibodies (ANAs) have been detected in 60 to 81% of SCLE patients when human tissue substrate

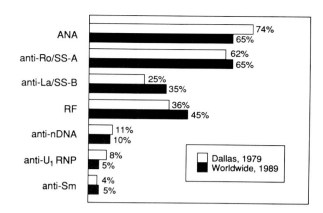

Fig. 31–6. Laboratory findings in subacute cutaneous LE patients. (The open and solid bars are the same as those in Fig. 31–4.)

was used,[C24,D61,H524,S396,S558,S566,S567,S568] but in only 49 to 55% of patients when mouse or rat substrates were used[C25,H280,M523] (Fig. 31–6). Ro/SSA antibodies have been observed in 40 to 80% of patients using immunodiffusion techniques, and in higher percentages of patients by use of the more sensitive enzyme-linked immunosorbent assay (ELISA); (Fig. 31–6).[Y10] Some have suggested that anti-Ro/SSA precipitins are only associated with annular SCLE patients,[B295] although this has not been our experience. Most SCLE series have reported finding La/SSB antibodies in 12 to 42% of their SCLE patients,[C24,C25,H280, J86,M291,P313] but two other reports (not from the United States) found that 71% of their patients had these antibodies.[B341,S396] The mean age of our original 27 SCLE patients was 43.3 years, with a range of 17 to 67 years.[S568]

False-positive Venereal Disease Research Laboratories (VDRL) reactions, indicative of the presence of antiphospholipid antibodies, have been detected in 7 to 33% of patients.[S559] Anticardiolipin antibodies have been detected by the use of ELISA in approximately 10% of patients.[S561] Rheumatoid factor was present in approximately one-third of our patients, but relatively few developed rheumatoid arthritis.[C336] Sm, dsDNA, and ribonucleoprotein (RNP) antibodies have been found in approximately 10% of SCLE patients (Fig. 31–6). One report found anti-RNP antibodies in 8 of 15 patients (53%),[M149] although others have noted a lower incidence.[C25,H280,S396,S566] Antilymphocyte antibodies were found in 33% of patients,[S566] and antithyroid antibodies in 18%.[C25]

Other Findings

Patients with SCLE, particularly those with systemic involvement, may have a number of laboratory abnormalities. Various studies have found the following: anemia, leukopenia, thrombocytopenia, an elevated erythrocyte sedimentation rate, hypergammaglobulinemia, proteinuria, hematuria, urine casts, elevated serum creatine and blood urea nitrogen (BUN) levels, and depressed complement levels.[S561] Elevated prothrombin and partial thromboplastin times can result from anti-phospholipid-anticardiolipin antibodies ("circulating anticoagulant").

Preliminary data suggest that SCLE patients with high-titer ANA, leukopenia, and/or anti-dsDNA may be at a higher risk of developing complications of systemic disease.[S557,S558]

PATHOGENIC MECHANISMS

Photosensitivity

Approximately 85% of our SCLE patients report photosensitivity, and this figure approximates those reported by others,[C24,D61,H280,H524] although one group noted that only 27% of their Chinese SCLE patients experienced photosensitivity.[S396] Wolska et al. induced SCLE lesions in 15 of 24 SCLE patients (63%) after a single exposure to UVB light.[W331] Lehmann et al. induced SCLE lesions in 14 of 22 SCLE patients (64%) with UVA and/or UVB irradiation.[L178] They induced lesions in 6 of 22 patients (27%) with UVB, in 2 of 22 patients (9%) with UVA, and in 6 of 22 patients (27%) with combined UVA and UVB irradiation.

The pathogenic effects of UV light are poorly understood. Several mechanisms have been proposed.

1. UV light may cause keratinocyte injury that exposes normally concealed intracellular antigens or induces the expression of "neoantigens."[N41] Investigators have demonstrated that UVB can displace Ro/SSA antigens from within keratinocytes to the cell surface.[F320,F321,L154] This displacement would allow the Ro/SSA autoantibodies to have access to the normally sequestered Ro/SSA autoantigens. Antibody binding to the exposed antigens could result in tissue injury through complement-mediated lysis or antibody-dependent, cell-mediated cytotoxicity.
2. UV light may cause an exaggerated release of immune mediators in LE skin, such as interleukin-1, α-tumor necrosis factor, prostaglandin E, proteases, and histamine.[B325,G7,G128,K469,P109,U28]
3. UV light may directly affect immunoregulatory cells, such as cutaneous T cells, which normally help suppress "abnormal" cutaneous inflammation.[C449]

Autoantibody Production

Autoantibodies are a hallmark of any LE-related disease process. Although Ro/SSA autoantibodies are common in SCLE, they are also found in a number of other autoimmune disorders and in some normal individuals.[Y10] Whether these autoantibodies play a direct role in the pathogenesis of skin disease, or represent merely an epiphenomenon, has not been determined. The most compelling evidence that these antibodies play a major role in the pathogenesis of disease comes from neonatal LE patients. These infants acquire maternal Ro/SSA antibodies transplacentally and develop skin lesions not unlike those of SCLE, typically within the first few days or weeks after delivery. Several months later, as the maternally acquired Ro/SSA antibodies are cleared from the infants' circulation, the skin lesions resolve spontaneously.[L134] These antibodies are probably also responsible for the congenital heart block, transient hematologic abnormalities, and hepatic injury that may occur in these infants.[L134] The mere presence of the Ro/SSA antibodies, however, is not sufficient to induce disease, because many neonates who are exposed to Ro/SSA antibodies from their mother's circulation never develop skin, heart, hepatic, or hematologic disease. This suggests that the presence of some cofactor (e.g., congenital viral infection) might be necessary for the full expression of this syndrome.

HLA Type

Most SCLE series have noted that at least half of the patients have the HLA-DR3 phenotype,[H280,J86,P312,S567] although one group found a lower frequency of the DR3 haplotype in their patient population.[C24] This phenotype is found in approximately 25% of the normal United States' population.[A66] Another group has suggested that the HLA-DR3 phenotype is most strongly associated with annular SCLE.[B295] Patients with the extended haplotype B8, DR3, DRW6, DQ2, and DRW52 have been reported to produce high levels of Ro/SSA autoantibodies.[B184,H137] Patients with signs and symptoms of both SCLE and Sjögren's syndrome are more likely to have this extended haplotype.[P312] High Ro/SSA antibody titers have been associated in individuals with HLA-DQw1/DQw2.[H137] Although no apparent correlation between infant HLA type and the development of neonatal LE has been found, one report has indicated that mothers who are HLA-DR2–positive are less likely to have affected infants than are mothers who are HLA-DR3–positive.[H132]

Basal Keratinocyte Injury

Basal keratinocyte injury, with immune deposits in the basement membrane zone and lymphohistiocytic infiltration of the dermis and basal epidermis, is a common element in the histopathologic features of SCLE, ACLE, and DLE. Whether basal cell injury occurs before or after immune deposition and (or) mononuclear cell infiltration is not certain. The predominance of T cells in the skin lesions, as well as histopathologic similarities with graft-versus-host disease and lichen planus (both T-cell–mediated disorders), suggest that cell injury in SCLE may arise from cell-mediated immunity.[C210,S366,S797]

Complement Deficiency States

Genetic deficiency of C2 or C4 has been associated with both SCLE and SLE.[P57,P308] It is interesting to note that the vast majority of patients with homozygous C2 or C4 complement deficiency have circulating Ro/SSA autoantibodies.[M381,P308] Both the C2 and the C4 genes lie on chromosome 6, within the HLA locus. It has therefore been proposed that the association with complement deficiency states and SCLE may arise from a genetic linkage to the HLA locus.[H455] One group of investigators has found that C4 deficiency can arise from chromosomal deletions that frequently include the 21-hydroxylase A gene.[P57] They speculated that such deletions might predispose an individual to the development of LE by impairing the clearance of immune complexes (complement deficiency) and by alterating steroid homeostasis (21-hydroxylase A gene deficiency).

It may be difficult to determine whether a low C2 or C4 complement level is a result of an absence or defect in an individual's C2 or C4 genes, or is secondary to complement consumption resulting from systemic disease activity. An individual with homozygous C2 or C4 deficiency can more easily be diagnosed, because their total hemolytic complement activity is zero.

Drugs

Hydrochlorothiazide, procainamide, penicillamine, sulfonylureas, oxprenolol, and griseofulvin may induce SCLE skin disease.[B229,D45,F96,G31,M499,R96,S351] These cases of drug-induced SCLE are frequently associated with Ro/SSA autoantibodies. Reed et al. have reported 5 patients with hydrochlorothiazide-induced SCLE in whom both psoriasiform and annular skin lesions were found.[R96] Of the 5 patients, 3 were HLA-typed and were found to be positive for either HLA-DR2 or HLA-DR3 (expected frequency of 50%.[A66]) In all patients the SCLE lesions promptly resolved after discontinuance of the hydrochlorothiazide. Ro/SSA autoantibodies were found in all 5 and persisted after discontinuation of the hydrochlorothiazide at 9 months in 1 patient and at 3 years in another patient. Reed et al. did not detect Ro/SSA autoantibodies in any of 16 patients without SCLE on longterm hydrochlorothiazide therapy.[R96]

The pathogenic mechanisms of drug-induced SCLE are unknown. The prompt resolution of SCLE lesions after the discontinuation of hydrochlorothiazide-induced lesions led Reed and coworkers to hypothesize that this drug is directly involved in the development of SCLE lesions by the potentiation of keratinocyte cytotoxicity.[R96]

Estrogens have also been reported to exacerbate both SLE and SCLE. Estrogen, when added to cultured human keratinocytes, may increase the amount of Ro/SSA antigens on the cell surface.[F321]

TREATMENT

The management of any patient diagnosed with SCLE should include evaluation to rule out underlying systemic disease at diagnosis and at 6- to 12-month intervals, unless the patient develops symptoms that dictate an earlier reassessment.[S560] This should include a history, review of systems, and physical examination to elicit symptoms and signs of underlying systemic disease (i.e., arthritis, serositis, CNS disease, renal disease) and a laboratory evaluation that should at least include a CBC with differential and platelet counts, erythrocyte sedimentation rate, urinalysis, and blood chemistry profile. The initial management of all SCLE patients should include education regarding protection from sunlight and other UV light sources, and the elimination of potentially provocative drugs such as hydrochlorothiazide.

Local Therapy

Sun Protection. Patients should be advised to avoid direct sun exposure, particularly during the midday hours and during the summer months, when UV light is least attenuated by the atmosphere. Tightly woven clothing and hats should be worn in conjunction with broad-spectrum sunscreens to achieve maximal shielding from sunlight. Patients should select sunscreens containing agents that block both UVA and UVB light, with a sun protection factor (SPF) of 15 or greater. Preparations containing Parsol 1789, such as Photoplex and Filteray, provide the greatest degree of UVA protection.[A240,L395] Products should also be selected that are most resistant to washing off by sweating or bathing. Sunscreens should be applied at least 30 minutes before sun exposure, and reapplied after swimming or appreciable perspiration. Sunscreen agents have been reviewed in two reports,[L395,P65] and an excellent consumer comparison of sunscreen products has been presented.[A240] To block UV light transmission, films can be applied to home and plastic shields can be placed over automobile windows, and fluorescent light bulbs.

Corrective camouflage cosmetics such as Dermablend and Covermark offer the dual benefit of being highly effective physical sunscreens and esthetically pleasing cosmetic masking agents for patients suffering from chronic, disfiguring skin disease.

Local Corticosteroids. Initial treatment usually includes a potent topical corticosteroid, such as clobetasol propionate 0.05% ointment (Temovate) or betamethasone dipropionate 0.05% ointment (Diprolene). We prefer the following regimen: twice daily application to lesional skin only for 2 weeks, followed by a 2-week rest period. This cycle can then be repeated. Such a cyclical regimen is necessary to minimize the risk of side effects, such as cutaneous atrophy and telangiectasia. Cutaneous LE represents one of the few clinical situations in which potent topical fluorinated corticosteroids can be recommended for atrophy-prone areas such as the face, because the alternatives are unchecked, disfiguring skin disease or the potential for more harmful side effects from systemic therapy. Unfortunately, topical corticosteroids alone do not provide adequate improvement for the large majority of SCLE patients. Most of their lesions are too numerous to be amenable to intralesional corticosteroid injections, and oral corticosteroids should be avoided if possible when treating this chronic cutaneous condition.

Conventional Systemic Agents

Antimalarials. Although various systemic medications have been reported to be of benefit to SCLE patients (Table 31–1), the most useful are the aminoquinoline antimalarial agents. We and others[F317] have found that 80% of SCLE patients respond to single-agent or combined antimalarial therapy. The three agents most frequently prescribed for SCLE patients are hydroxychloroquine sulfate (Plaquenil), chloroquine phosphate (Aralen), and quinacrine hydrochloride (Atabrine). In general, hydroxychloroquine is best tolerated, with the lowest incidence of side effects.

The need for ophthalmologic examination to rule out retinal toxicity from hydroxychloroquine and chloroquine (quinacrine has not been confirmed to be retino-

Table 31–1. Beneficial Systemic Medications in the Management of SCLE

Aminoquinoline antimalarials
   Hydroxychloroquine sulfate (Plaquenil)
   Chloroquine phosphate (Aralen)
   Quinacrine hydrochloride (Atabrine)
Dapsone
Gold (auranofin, Ridaura; aurothiomaleate, Myochrysine)
Retinoids
   Isotretinoin (Accutane)
   Etretinate (Tegison)
   Acitretin (Etretin)
Clofazamine (Lamprene)
Thalidomide
Interferon-α2A
Systemic corticosteroids, cytotoxic immunosuppressives

---

pathic) makes this therapy more costly. A baseline ophthalmologic evaluation is required before starting antimalarial therapy, and should be done at 6-month intervals while the patient is on therapy. This evaluation should include a fundoscopic examination, visual field testing (including central fields with a red object), and visual acuity testing. Retinal changes can be irreversible, if not detected early. It has been suggested that the risk of retinal toxicity is minimized when the total daily dose of hydroxychloroquine does not exceed 6 mg/kg/day, or the chloroquine dosage does not exceed 4 mg/kg/day.[L55]

Glucose-6-phosphate dehydrogenase (G6PD) deficiency should also be checked before starting therapy with these agents, particularly in black patients, because antimalarials may cause hemolytic anemia (rarely). Quinacrine hydrochloride (Atabrine) is more likely to induce hemolysis in G6PD-deficient patients than is hydroxychloroquine or chloroquine.[T212] In addition to following patients for antimalarial-induced retinal and hematologic toxicity, patients should also be checked periodically for the development of muscle weakness and hypoactive deep tendon reflexes.

Antimalarial agents can induce a number of dermatologic changes. All can cause a blue-black pigmentation of the skin (particularly in sun-exposed areas), the palate, and the nails. Rarely, they can also cause bleaching of lightly pigmented hair. Quinacrine frequently causes diffuse yellowing of the skin, sclera, and bodily secretions that is fully reversible on discontinuation of the drug. Occasionally, quinacrine produces a lichenoid drug reaction that can be the harbinger of severe bone marrow toxicity.[W24]

We begin therapy with hydroxychloroquine alone, 400 mg/day, for 6 weeks, followed by 200 mg/day. If no significant improvement is seen to 2 to 3 months, we add quinacrine, 100 mg/day. Hydroxychloroquine alone or in combination with quinacrine controlled cutaneous lesions in approximately 80% of our patients, although it sometimes takes 6 to 8 weeks to see the full effects of this medication.

If the response is inadequate after 1 to 2 months of hydroxychloroquine plus quinacrine, we substitute chloroquine, 250 mg/day, for hydroxychloroquine while continuing the quinacrine, because some cutaneous LE pa-

tients appear to respond better to chloroquine than to hydroxychloroquine.

We have observed several patients whose previously refractory cutaneous LE improved dramatically following the cessation of cigarette smoking, without any other change in their treatment regimen. Perhaps the effects of cigarette smoking on hepatic microsomal enzyme induction[M426] can alter the metabolism of the aminoquinoline antimalarials so that their effect on cutaneous LE is blunted.

Dapsone. Dapsone is best for treating the rare patient with the LE-nonspecific vesiculobullous skin lesions that can occur in those with SLE.[H58,R439] Within days, 100 mg/day may provide significant improvement in vesiculobullous SCLE.[H58,R439] Hematologic, renal, neurologic, and hepatic toxicity can occur with this drug, however, so its use requires frequent monitoring. We have had little positive experience in treating SCLE patients with this agent, although others have reported benefit in isolated cases within a few weeks after starting therapy.[F61,H400,M244]

Gold. Oral gold (auranofin; Ridaura) or parenteral gold (aurothiomaleate; Myochrysine) therapy has been successfully used in those cutaneous LE patients whose disease is resistant to the less toxic forms of therapy.[D21] Gold frequently has mucocutaneous toxicity and, less commonly, has hematologic, renal, and pulmonary toxicity, which may require its discontinuance.

Newer Systemic Agents

During the past several years, other medications have shown promise in treating SCLE patients. These include the oral retinoids (isotretinoin, etretinate, and acitretin), clofazimine (an antileprosy agent now available in the United States), thalidomide (currently available in the United States for research purposes only) and recombinant interferon-α2A.

Retinoids. The synthetic retinoids isotretinoin (Accutane), etritinate (Tegison), and acitretin (Etretin; not yet approved for use in the United States, at dosages of approximately 1 mg/kg/day, have been shown to improve SCLE lesions.[N78,R440,R441] The dose may be adjusted downward as necessary to lessen side effects. The teratogenic effects of the retinoids makes it imperative that fertile women use contraceptive techniques, according to guidelines set forth specifically for patients on retinoids. A common dose-related side effect is mucocutaneous dryness. It is advisable to have patients use sunscreens judiciously while being treated with these agents to minimize their tendency to aggravate photosensitivity. Drug-induced hepatitis and hypertriglyceridemia can occur with these agents, and patients require periodic laboratory evaluation. Occasionally, these drugs can also induce bony changes consistent with the diffuse idiopathic skeletal hyperostosis (DISH) syndrome.

Clofazimine. Crovoto has reported the successful use of clofazimine (Lamprene) in a patient with annular SCLE in 1981.[C444] He used 100 mg/day and noted clearing of the lesions within a few weeks. At this dosage clofazimine is generally well tolerated, although gastrointestinal intolerance can be a problem. At higher doses, clofazimine has rarely been reported to precipitate in mesenteric arteries, resulting in major abdominal catastrophes, such as splenic infarction.[M271] A pink to brownish-black skin pigmentation develops in most patients on longterm clofazimine therapy. This resolves over months to years after discontinuing the drug. Similar discoloration of bodily secretions also frequently occurs.

Thalidomide. Thalidomide, 100 mg/day, can be effective, although it is seldom used because of difficulties in procuring it in the United States and because of its neurotoxicity.[K323,N1,V100]

α-Interferon. Earlier clinical observations had suggested that endogenously produced interferon might be of benefit in SCLE.[C211] Recombinant interferon-α-2A (Roferon-A) has been used to treat four SCLE patients.[N89] The dosage ranged from 18 to 120 × 10⁶ units injected weekly for 4 to 13 weeks. Two patients had a complete response, one had a partial response, and one patient had no response to treatment. All three patients that responded to treatment later relapsed 4 to 12 weeks after treatment was stopped.

Systemic Corticosteroids and Cytotoxic Agents

Systemic corticosteroids and cytotoxic agents are reserved for patients with more severe disease who have not responded to the less toxic forms of therapy discussed above. A patient may occasionally be encountered whose disease is so severe that these more potent agents may be used earlier in the disease course, even before the patient is given a complete trial of the less toxic agents.

Methylprednisolone given in "pulse doses" (1 g intravenously for 3 consecutive days) has been reported to provide improvement in SCLE patients with systemic LE.[G238] Anecdotally, cyclophosphamide and methotrexate,[F317] as well as azathioprine,[C27] have been suggested to be of benefit in refractory SCLE. Because of the potential for severe immunosuppression, risk of cancer induction, and bone marrow and mucous membrane toxicity, these agents

should be reserved for patients with severe SLE, and should be used only as a last resort in patients with severe cutaneous LE alone. The overlap between Sjögren's syndrome and SCLE should cause us to question whether certain SCLE patients might also be susceptible to developing malignant B-cell lymphomas, and whether the use of immunosuppressive therapy might increase this risk.

SUMMARY

SCLE is now a well-established subset of LE skin disease that occurs in a relatively homogeneous group of patients who are frequently of the DR3 haplotype and have circulating Ro/SSA autoantibodies. The hallmarks of SCLE lesions are papulosquamous or annular lesions in a photodistribution with characteristic LE-specific histopathologic findings.

In general, SCLE is a recurring or persistent disease, and 50% of patients meet the ACR criteria for systemic LE. Although most SCLE patients have relatively mild disease, these patients require careful follow-up, because a small percentage of patients goes on to develop life-threatening complications, such as renal and central nervous system disease. Also, small percentages of patients may develop signs of other autoimmune diseases, such as Sjögren's syndrome or rheumatoid arthritis. Several reports have suggested an association between SCLE and an underlying malignancy. The number of cases, however, seems too small to consider SCLE as a paraneoplastic syndrome.

Sunlight (UV light) can induce SCLE lesions, and thus UV light avoidance measures must be emphasized to LE patients. The vast majority of patients improves with sun avoidance and antimalarial therapy alone. Several drugs have been reported to induce SCLE, and such agents should be discontinued. Almost all patients with drug-induced SCLE clear promptly once the offending agent is discontinued. A number of agents are available for the treatment of SCLE, but many of these have potentially serious side effects and their use requires close monitoring.

Chapter 32

THE RELATIONSHIP BETWEEN DISCOID AND SYSTEMIC LUPUS ERYTHEMATOSUS

DANIEL J. WALLACE

The relationship between discoid (cutaneous) and systemic lupus erythematosus has been a subject of debate for over a century. Because SLE patients may develop discoid skin lesions and DLE patients sometimes evolve systemic complications, they probably represent poles of a "lupus" spectrum. Despite this, both syndromes are often mutually exclusive. This chapter addresses these issues. See Chapter 30 for a discussion of the descriptive features of DLE, and Chapter 37 for a description of the skin lesions of SLE.

The concept of a relationship between DLE and SLE was pointed out as early as 1872 by Kaposi, who first noted that in some cases chronic DLE may disseminate:

> Lupus erythematosus discoides is confined, with scarcely any exception to the face and head, has a regular and chronic course, and is unattended by any severe complications, but may, nevertheless, now and then be complicated with erysipelas, or with the aggregated form (SLE) and its acute symptoms.
>
> [That] the two forms of lupus, are, however, intimately related to one another is apparent from the fact that the primary "eruptive spots" are the same for each.[H237]

Early investigators were hampered by the lack of clinical and laboratory criteria for differentiating SLE from pure cutaneous disease.[B194,K144,M550,S343,S714,W255] This led to a mistaken notion that SLE and DLE were unrelated. As recently as 1951, Baehr[B16] stated that "in spite of its name this disease (discoid lupus) bears no relation whatsoever to systemic lupus." The pervasiveness of this idea into teaching internal medicine was emphasized by the results of a questionnaire sent out by Reiches[R111] to 100 board-certified internists in 1957: 61% replied that no relationship existed between the two diseases.

In 1963, Tuffanelli and Dubois observed chronic discoid skin lesions in 149 (28.7%) of 520 SLE patients, and it was the initial presentation of the disease in 56 (10.8%) of them.[T264] Other reports have since confirmed this observation, noting that about 5% of cases evolve from DLE to SLE.[B152,B376,C59,G231,H44,H281,R377,S226,S721] Clinicians became aware that DLE afflicts a lower percentage of females and blacks than SLE, as well as having an older age of onset.[C246,D29,D334,M154,M550,059,R135,R352,S226,W13] For the purpose of this review, only studies published after 1971 are considered, because the advent of the American

Rheumatology Association (ARA) criteria for SLE and the availability of antinuclear antibody (ANA) testing have provided the requisites for any comparative analysis.

EVIDENCE FOR "SYSTEMIC" ABNORMALITIES IN DLE PATIENTS

Clinical Evidence

Since 1971, only a handful of studies have evaluated DLE patients for evidence of systemic abnormalities; these are summarized in Table 32-1. Our series, shown in Table 32-1, compares patients with DLE to those with SLE. Prystowsky, in Gilliam's group,[P326] excluded patients with systemic symptoms from their DLE group, which skewed their cohort toward those with milder disease. Our DLE patients were defined as those with characteristic biopsy-documented skin lesions who did not fulfill the ARA criteria for SLE. The data demonstrate that constitutional symptoms (e.g., fever, aching) are present in a minority of patients with DLE, but organ-threatening disease rarely, if ever, occurs. Tebbe's group in Berlin followed 97 patients with cutaneous lupus and associated disseminated skin lesions with more systemic symptoms in the absence of SLE.[T91] This confirms the validity of O'Leary's 1934 Mayo Clinic classification of discoid lupus into local and generalized types, which was also supported by O'Laughlin et al.'s 1978 Mayo Clinic follow-up.[059,P326] Dubois labeled the latter grouping as "discoid lupus with mild systemic dissemination." The authors reviewed 67 of their DLE patients seen between 1980 and 1989 and compared them with 464 SLE patients seen during the same period[W18] (Tables 32-1 and 32-2). We concluded the following: (1) a 1:7 DLE:SLE prevalence ratio is likely; (2) DLE is noted in fewer females, more Caucasians, and has no older age of onset than SLE;[W255] (3) the frequency of cutaneous subsets (bullous LE, panniculitis, SCLE) is similar in DLE and SLE; and (4) DLE patients have a strong family history for SLE, but not for DLE.

Serologic and Laboratory Abnormalities

Table 32-2 summarizes the principal laboratory abnormalities in DLE. Prystowski et al.'s data suggested that abnormal findings can be present, even if no systemic symptoms are present. All the studies documented that active cutaneous lesions alone can be associated with an elevated sedimentation rate. Our group found a higher preva-

Table 32–1. Clinical Features of DLE Compared With SLE (%)

Parameter	Prystowsky	O'Laughlin	Callen	Wallace	Wallace	p < .05
Number of cases	80 DLE	69 DLE	56 DLE	67 DLE	464 SLE	DLE versus SLE
Year (reference)	1975[P326]	1978[059]	1982[C19]	1992[W18]	1991[P216]	1991[P216,W18]
Females	65	57	66	81	93	.05
Caucasian	55	100	—	82	72	—
Family history of LE	4	7	7	8	16	—
Hospitalized, 1980–1989	—	—	—	15	48	.000
Mean age at diagnosis	—	33	39	37	34	.05
Fever	0	3	—	15	41	.000
Arthritis, arthralgia	0	10	12	49	91	.000
Pericarditis	0	0	—	0	12	.006
Hypertension	—	—	—	9	25	.006
Pleurisy	0	0	—	6	31	.000
Skin lesions	75	100	—	100	55	.000
Malar rash	—	—	—	36	34	—
Alopecia	60	4	—	27	31	—
Oral ulcers	4	3	4	8	19	—
Photosensitivity	60	84	84	37	37	—
Raynaud's phenomenon	—	6	4	6	24	.001
Severe headache	—	—	—	12	31	.002
Cerebritis	—	—	—	1	11	—
Fibrositis	—	—	—	12	22	—
Nephritis	—	—	0	0	28	.000
Thromboemboli	—	—	—	1	8	—
Adenopathy	—	—	—	3	10	—

lence of ANA compared to the results of earlier studies; this probably reflects the use of the more sensitive Hep-2 ANA substrate, which may explain why most patients tested positive. All three of our patients who were anti–Ro/SSA-positive had subacute cutaneous LE lesions. Aside from leukopenia, the only other common abnormality was the presence of anticardiolipin antibodies. Even though anticardiolipin antibody was seen in 30 to 40% of patients with both DLE and SLE, it was not associated with any complications in DLE. This finding has been confirmed in another report.[M221] In addition to the findings presented in Table 32–2, many other studies have looked for

anti-DNA in DLE. Although most studies confirmed the absence of anti–double-stranded DNA, anti–single-stranded (SS) DNA was frequently present.[B203,D90,G389, H191,K451,M88,S795] Callen followed seven patients with anti-ss DNA (out of 40 with DLE) for 3 years, and found that this subgroup had more systemic symptoms, higher erythrocyte sedimentation rates, and a greater probability of evolving into SLE.[C22]

CAN DLE EVOLVE TO SLE?

As mentioned above, numerous studies in the 1950s and 1960s reported that 5% of DLE cases disseminate to

Table 32–2. Laboratory Data Comparing DLE and SLE (%)

Parameter	Prystowski	O'Laughlin	Millard	Callen	Wallace	Wallace	p Value
Number of cases	80 DLE	69 DLE	92 DLE	56 DLE	67 DLE	464 SLE	DLE versus SLE
Year (reference)	1975[P326]	1978[059]	1979[M413]	1982[C19]	1990[W18]	1992[P216]	1991[P216,W18]
Anemia	2	10	27	0	7	30	.000
Hemolytic anemia	—	—	—	0	0	8	.009
Leukopenia	0	14	12	10	30	51	.002
Thrombocytopenia	—	—	4	—	2	16	.000
Positive ANA	4	49	25	22	63	96	.000
Low C3	8	—	—	0	10	39	.000
High anti-ds DNA	0	0	—	4	8	40	.000
Positive anti-RNP	—	—	—	5	2	14	.000
Positive RA latex	1	6	13	21	9	23	.02
Positive Ro SSA	—	—	—	—	4	18	.003
Positive anti-cardiolipin antibody	—	—	—	—	31	38	.53
High sedimentation rate	56	45	20	43	31	54	.001
Therapy							
NSAIDs	—	—	—	—	31	72	—
Aspirin	—	—	—	—	16	27	—
Antimalarials	—	—	—	55	75	70	—
Oral steroids	—	—	—	40	33	77	—
Cytotoxics	—	—	—	—	1	30	—

SLE. Few investigations have addressed this issue using currently acceptable classification criteria. Millard and Rowell followed 150 British patients with DLE for a mean of 16 years. In 1984, they reported a 5.5% SLE conversion rate.[R377] Over this period, 52% of the localized DLE patients (confined to the head) remitted. In 1984, Shiodt[S142] also reported that 8% of 56 DLE patients followed for a mean of 6 years developed SLE. Analysis of these studies reveals that localized DLE rarely, if ever, evolves to SLE; non-localized DLE can evolve into SLE, however, particularly if systemic symptoms or anti-ss DNA are present.

Our DLE patients often ask, "If I have a 5 to 10% chance of developing SLE, what can I do to prevent this from occurring?" Even though no study has addressed this issue, we advise such patients to avoid the sun if they are photosensitive, avoid stress, try to prevent physical or emotional trauma, get plenty of rest along with modest exercise, eat a well-balanced diet, and bring any fever or signs of infection to their doctor's attention. A yearly physical examination is advisable. If lesions are controlled by local steroids, patients should have a complete blood count and urinalysis every 6 months. If antimalarials are necessary, routine blood counts should be done at 3-month intervals.

CAN THE LUPUS BAND TEST DISTINGUISH DLE FROM SLE?

The use of the lupus band test (LBT) in diagnosing SLE and DLE is discussed in Chapters 30 and 37. To summarize briefly, a patient with DLE usually has a negative biopsy in a nonlesional, nonsun-exposed area (e.g., the buttocks) and a positive biopsy in a lesional, sun-exposed area. DLE patients should have a negative LBT in light-exposed normal skin. SLE patients have a positive LBT in active lesional areas and may have positive LBT in both uninvolved sun-exposed and nonsun-exposed areas. The interpretation of what is a positive test depends on how many immunoreactants (immunoglobulin or protein components) are present, as well as on the amount and degree of confluence of the deposits. The results of Tuffanelli's comparative study of 348 SLE and 286 DLE biopsies have been confirmed by many other, smaller scale investigations (Table 32–3; summarized in reference[W127]). It can therefore be concluded that, if the LBT is positive in uninvolved, non-exposed skin, the presence of SLE is likely.

RELATIONSHIP OF SUBACUTE CUTANEOUS LUPUS ERYTHEMATOSUS TO DLE AND SLE

Subacute cutaneous lupus erythematosus (SCLE) is a relatively new term for previously known cutaneous variants of lupus erythematosus (see Chapter 31). It is considered to be present in 5 to 10% of all patients with LE. It can be differentiated from DLE by its nonscarring, nonatrophic, follicle-sparing papulosquamous or polycyclic appearance. SCLE has several distinct associations. Anti-Ro/SSA antibody and HLA-DR3 are found in most patients in this subgroup (Table 32–4), and half of cases fulfill the ARA criteria for SLE. Systemic symptoms are usually mild and organ-threatening disease is uncommon. SCLE can also be drug-induced, appear as a paraneoplastic phenomenon, and has been reported in patients with rheumatoid arthritis and primary Sjögren's syndrome. Even though SCLE is considered to be a distinct subset of LE, blinded reviews of SCLE biopsies cannot always be distinguished from DLE lesions.[J71] DLE does not evolve into SCLE, which in turn probably does not evolve into SLE. SCLE is simply a descriptive term for a skin lesion that has several associations. Its prognosis and longterm outcome may be elucidated when longterm prospective studies (in progress) delineate its natural history.

SUMMARY

DLE is a mild form of LE that rarely disseminates to frank SLE or to life-threatening disease. Between 10 and 50% of patients may display other cutaneous manifestations, constitutional symptoms, aching, and/or laboratory abnormalities (e.g., ANA, anticardiolipin antibody, elevated sedimentation rate, leukopenia). Aggressive therapy is rarely necessary. The factors that differentiate DLE from patients with SLE having identical cutaneous features remain poorly elucidated, and are not ascertainable by current serologic and/or histologic techniques.

Table 32–4.   Relationship Among DLE, SLE, and SCLE

1. DLE is characterized by the presence of typical skin lesions, confirmed by biopsy if necessary, in a patient with none or few mild systemic complaints. These patients do not fulfill the ARA criteria for SLE.
2. About 25% of DLE patients may have constitutional symptoms during the course of the disease, and 5 to 10% may evolve into SLE.
3. ANAs are positive in 22 to 62% of patients with DLE. High sedimentation rates and anticardiolipin antibody are not uncommon; the presence of anti–single-stranded DNA may indicate more severe disease.
4. Skin biopsies of nonlesional areas studied by immunofluorescence may help distinguish between DLE and SLE.
5. SCLE is a nonscarring form of cutaneous lupus seen in 5 to 10% of patients with LE. Half have SLE; most have HLA-DR3 and are anti-Ro/SSA antibody-positive. Its prognostic implications are uncertain.

Table 32–3.   Direct Immunofluorescence in LE[T258]

Clinical Diagnosis	Biopsies	No. Positive	% Positive
Systemic LE			
Involved skin	150	135	90
Uninvolved skin	198	108	54
Discoid LE			
Involved skin	234	216	90
Uninvolved skin	52	0	0

Section VI

SYSTEMIC LUPUS ERYTHEMATOSUS

PART A

CLINICAL AND LABORATORY FEATURES

Chapter 33

THE CLINICAL PRESENTATION OF SLE

DANIEL J. WALLACE

Prior to the description of the LE cell by Hargraves[H129] in 1948, SLE was considered to be a rare fulminant disease occurring in young women, with classic rash and a fatal termination in months. The illness is now conceptualized as a chronic disorder of a pleomorphic nature. No classic pattern exists, and the diagnosis must be based on an overall view of the clinical picture with the aid of serologic and laboratory studies and, if required, biopsies or other diagnostic procedures. The "typical" case, with the classic butterfly area eruption, is only seen occasionally. This chapter presents an overview of the clinical presentation of SLE, and the following chapters detail its involvement in various organ systems.

HISTORY

The most important part of the examination of a patient suspected of having this disorder is the history; it must be obtained in painstaking detail, along with a review of systems. Earlier, seemingly unimportant events often provide clues to the correct diagnosis. It is best to take a chronologic history of all possible pertinent events and to carry out a complete systems review. The family history is also important, because between 10 and 20% of patients have a relative with SLE, from first cousin to grandparent.[B552,P216]

All the items in Table 33–1 and Fig. 33–1 should be covered. The physician should inquire specifically about the effects of sun exposure on the patient's skin and their general sense of well-being. Other important questions concern hair loss, fracturing of frontal hair, positive serologic tests for syphilis, seizures, blood clots, miscarriage(s), adenopathy, dry eyes or mouth, anemia, leukopenia, thrombocytopenia, pleuritis, pleural effusion, pericariditis, myalgia and arthralgia with or without overt joint swelling, diffuse puffiness of the hands without localization to joints, Raynaud's phenomenon, and leg ulcers.

The transitory nature of the polyarthralgia and arthritis during the early phases of SLE should be emphasized. Patients frequently complain of morning stiffness, with diffuse puffiness of the fingers and dorsa of the hands. These conditions may subside in 10 minutes to several hours after awakening. Fleeting pains may be present in both joints and muscles. At the time of physical examination, usually later in the day, no objective abnormalities are seen. Early in the course of the disease, although the sedimentation rate and other routine laboratory tests may be normal, antinuclear antibody (ANA) may be positive. Consequently, it is important that SLE be considered in equiv-

ocal cases, and that further studies be performed. (Caution must be exercised in interpreting previously positive ANA tests. The test is performed on various substrates and is positive in low titers in 2 to 5% of healthy persons, especially in older individuals.) Difficulties in early diagnosis were summarized in a review of 40 cases,[C96] in which patients presented problems in the diagnosis of migratory polyarthralgia, "functional illness," or mild illness with nonspecific, systemic symptoms.

Sometimes it is useful to have patients fill out a detailed medical history questionnaire during their first visit, which should take less than 30 minutes to complete. This allows detection of subtle pyschosocial or sensitive issues that would otherwise not be found. Having patients write down what bothers them, in their own words, can be revealing. Filling out a questionnaire also decreases the possibility that important information might be inadvertently omitted.

CHIEF COMPLAINT

Many variations are seen in the presenting complaint that brings the patient to the physician. Diagnosis is rendered difficult by the protean manifestations of the disease. The classic presentation of butterfly rash and arthritis in a young woman occurs in a minority of patients. Initially, any system may be affected and heal; months or years later, the same or another system may become involved. Table 33–2 lists the chief complaints noted with a diagnosis of SLE in several large studies. The two major areas of involvement are joint and cutaneous systems, followed by the nonspecific complaints of fatigue, fever, and malaise. The presentation of 101 children followed at the Mayo clinic was similar to that of adults.[N131] In addition, Ropes[R294] found that joints were the first system involved in 27% of 142 patients, followed by fever, weight loss, and malaise (25%), and skin rash (20%). Grigor et al.[G385] followed 50 lupus patients. The initial manifestations were arthritis or arthralgia (62%), cutaneous (20%), fever and malaise, thrombocytopenia, hemolytic anemia, and neuropsychiatric symptoms (4% each), and recurrent thrombophlebitis (2%).

Variations in Clinical Presentation

The presentation and clinical characteristics of SLE are presented in detail in the following chapters. Age and sex may result in variations in the appearance of the disease. These distinctions are summarized here.

Table 33–1. Cumulative Percentage Incidence of SLE Manifestations

Manifestations	Harvey[M280] (105 cases) 1956	Dubois[D340] (520 cases) 1963	Estes[E147] (140 cases) 1970	Fries[F256] (193 cases) 1975	Tan[T46] (177 cases) 1982	Hochberg[H347] (150 cases) 1985	Worrall[W352] (100 cases) 1990	Wallace[P216] (464 cases) 1991
I. Systemic Sx								
A. Fever	86	84	—	55	—	—	—	41
B. Weight loss	71	51	—	31	—	—	—	—
II. Musculoskeletal								
A. Arthritis and arthralgia	90	92	95	53	86	76	94	91
B. Subcutaneous nodules	10	5	11	—	—	12	—	—
C. Myalgias	—	48	—	42	—	—	—	79
D. Aseptic bone necrosis	—	5	—	—	—	24	—	5
III. Cardiorespiratory								
A. Cardiomegaly	15	16	—	10	—	—	—	—
B. Pericarditis	45	31	19	6	18	23	—	2
C. Myocarditis	40	8	8	—	—	—	—	12
D. Cardiac failure	8	5	11	—	—	—	—	3
E. Systolic heart murmur	44	20	—	38	—	—	—	12
F. Diastolic heart murmur	—	1	—	2	—	—	—	1
G. Libman-Sacks valvulitis	32	—	—	—	—	—	—	1
H. Hypertension	14	25	46	—	—	—	—	25
I. Pleurisy	56	45	48	41	52	57	—	31
J. Pleural effusion	16	30	40	16	—	—	—	12
K. Lupus pneumonia	22	1	9	—	—	—	—	6
IV. Cutaneous-vascular								
A. Skin lesions, all types	85	72	81	67	—	—	90	55
B. Butterfly area lesions	39	57	39	10	57	61	—	34
C. Alopecia	3	21	39	45	26	45	27	31
D. Oral nasal ulcers	14	9	7	18	27	23	36	19
E. Photosensitivity	11	33	—	—	43	45	48	37
F. Urticaria	7	7	13	—	—	—	—	4
G. Raynaud's	10	18	21	17	29	44	—	25
H. Discoid lesions	—	29	9	10	18	15	—	23
V. Nervous system								
A. CNS damage, all types	—	26	59	—	12	39	45	—
B. Peripheral neuritis	—	12	7	—	—	21	2	5
C. Psychosis	19	12	37	—	13	16	12	5
D. Seizures	17	14	26	8	—	13	9	6
VI. Ocular lesions								
A. Cytoid bodies	24	10	—	—	—	—	—	4
B. Uveitis	—	1	—	2	—	—	—	1
VII. Genitourinary								
A. Proteinuria/abnormal sediment	65	46	53	47	60	—	29	31
B. Nephrotic syndrome	—	23	26	—	—	13	—	14
VIII. Gastrointestinal								
A. Dysphagia	6	2	—	—	—	—	—	8
B. Severe nausea	14	53	—	36	—	—	—	7
C. Diarrhea	8	6	—	25	—	—	—	8
D. Ascites	—	11	9	—	—	—	—	—
E. Abdominal pain	10	19	16	34	—	—	—	8
F. Bowel hemorrhage	5	6	—	6	—	—	—	1
IX. Hemic-lymphatic								
A. Adenopathy	34	59	36	23	—	—	—	10
B. Anemia (<11 g)	78	57	73	38	—	57	—	30
C. Hemolytic anemia	—	—	12	—	18	—	2	8
D. Leukopenia (<4500)	—	43	66	35	46	41	57	51
E. Thrombocytopenia (<100,000)	26	7	19	—	21	30	21	16
X. Serologic								
A. Hypoalbuminemia	58	32	77	—	—	30	—	—
B. False + VDRL	15	11	29	—	15	26	3	—
C. ⊕ LE PREP	82	82	78	—	73	71	—	42
D. ⊕ ANA	—	—	87	95	99	—	99	96
E. Low C3	—	—	—	40	64	59	—	39
F. ⊕ Anti-DNA	—	—	—	39	67	28	55	40
G. ⊕ Anti-Sm	—	—	—	26	31	17	7	6
H. ⊕ Anti-SSA (Ro)	—	—	—	—	—	32	39	19
I. ⊕ Anti-RNP	—	—	—	—	—	34	19	14
J. ⊕ Anticardiolipin	—	—	—	—	—	—	32	38

"Proto" or Latent Lupus

When does lupus begin? A 1981 survey of our 609 private patients diagnosed between 1950 and 1980 revealed a 4.1-year interval between the onset of symptoms and the diagnosis of SLE.[W39] Our survey of 464 patients with idiopathic SLE seen between 1980 and 1989 documented a 2.1-year interval.[P216] Is the disease changing, or has increased physician awareness and newer diagnostic and serologic testing made it possible to diagnose SLE earlier? In the 0- to 19-year–age group, it took only a mean of 3 months to make the diagnosis; in patients over 60 years

Table 33–2. First System Involved as Determined by History (%)

Manifestation	Dubois[D340] (520 cases)	McGehee-Harvey[M280] (105 cases)	Haserick[H179] (275 cases)	Larson[L75] (200 cases)	Children[N131] (101 cases)
Arthritis and arthralgia	46	47	55	59	48
Discoid lupus	11	0	4	0	13
Butterfly area eruptions and blush	6 }	20	17 }	14	—
Eruptions on other parts of body (nonspecific dermatitis)	2		0		—
Fever	4	2	0	1 }	24
Fatigue, malaise, weakness	4	17	0	0	
Renal involvement	3	5	3	6	—
Pleurisy	3	5	2	2	—
Edema and anasarca	1	0	0	0	2
Positive STS	2	5	8	4	—
Cervical adenopathy	2	0	0	0	—
Anemia	2	4	0	0	—
Raynaud's phenomenon	2	3	5	1	—
Myalgia	2	0	0	0	—
Photosensitivity reaction	1	4	4	0	—
Pericarditis	1	1	0	2	—
Pleural effusion	1	0	2	0	—
Epilepsy	1	0	3	0	—
Generalized adenopathy	1	2	0	1	—
Purpura	—	—	—	—	9
Mouth ulcers	—	—	—	—	3

the more subtle presentation of idiopathic SLE took 3.2 years to detect, on average. Hochberg's John Hopkins-based group reported a 1-year interval among 150 patients seen between 1980 and 1984.[H347] Urowitz's group identified 22 patients with a constellation of features suggestive of SLE who did not fulfill American Rheumatology Association (ARA) criteria.[G29] Over a 5-year observation period, 7 patients (32%) evolved into SLE. Few had organ-threatening disease, and no predictive factors distinguished the 7 who developed SLE from the 15 who did not. In summary, nonorgan-threatening lupus, especially in older patients, can be difficult to diagnose initially. In addition, it may be difficult to determine when SLE started.

Lupus in Children

See Chapter 44.

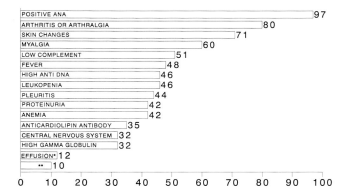

Fig. 33–1. Cumulative percentage incidence of 16 clinical and laboratory manifestations of SLE based on the five studies (1084 cases) in Table 33–1 published since 1975 (*,pleural or pericardial; **,adenopathy).

Late-Onset Lupus

Defined as when the disease appears in patients over the age of 50 years, late-onset lupus is often insidious, with a polymyalgia-like or rheumatoid arthritis-like pattern,[M121] and may be difficult to distinguish from primary Sjögren's syndrome.[B181] It comprises 6 to 20% of all cases,[S679] and includes more men than any other group except young children (Table 33–3). The clinical course is generally benign, and the disease is more easily controlled with medication. The relatively small number of patients with late-onset lupus in large published series led Ward and Pollison to perform a meta-analysis of its clinical and laboratory features based on nine studies.[W75] Their 1989 effort compared 170 late-onset patients with 1612 younger onset patients. They concluded that the older onset subset had more serositis, interstitial lung disease, Sjögren's syndrome, and anti-La/SSB. A significantly lower incidence of alopecia, Raynaud's phenomenon, fever, lymphadenopathy, hypocomplementemia, and neuropsychiatric disease was present (see also reference[W78]). Only one of the studies reviewed was population-based.[J119] Addi-

Table 33–3. Sex Ratios by Age at Age of Onset or First Diagnosis of SLE

Age at Onset or First Diagnosis (years)	Female:Male Ratio
0–4	1.4:1
5–9	2.3:1
10–14	5.8:1
15–19	5.4:1
20–29	7.5:1
30–39	8.1:1
40–49	5.2:1
50–59	3.9:1
60 and above	2.2:1

tional reports have suggested that HLA-DR3 is more common in whites with late-onset lupus,[H347] autoantibodies other than ANA are much less common,[W367] serositis is the most frequent presenting feature,[B36,D219] lupus appears in proportionally more younger than older blacks compared to whites[B58], and blacks with late-onset lupus have a worse prognosis than whites with late-onset disease.[S742] Braunstein et al.[B463] evaluated joint films of 24 patients with SLE onset over the age of 50 years. No differences were noted in the amount of osteoporosis, erosions, or soft tissue calcification, but soft tissue swelling was significantly increased in the older group. In summary, most studies have shown that patients with SLE onset after the age of 50 years have more serositis, pulmonary parenchymal disease, and Sjögren's syndrome, less CNS involvement, and a better prognosis.

Male Lupus

Even though males constitute only 4 to 18% of those with SLE, their clinical presentation is similar to that observed in women. Hochberg et al. noted a mean age of onset in men of 40.4 years (versus 31.8 in women) among a 150-patient cohort. Except for a statistically significant increase in peripheral neuropathy, no other clinical, laboratory, or HLA phenotypic differences could be found.[H347] Similarly, Ward and Studenski[W77] compared 62 men with 299 women followed at Duke University between 1969 and 1983; 23 clinical and laboratory variables were analyzed. The only significant differences were more seizures and renal disease in the men. Wallace compared 125 clinical and laboratory parameters among 30 men and 434 women seen in his office between 1980 and 1989.[P216] Only four significant differences were observed (p < .01): men had less alopecia and fibrositis, but more nephritis and hypocomplementemia. Two other controlled studies have evaluated acceptably large numbers of males to make their data relevant. Fries and Holman observed that men had more anti-DNA and skin disease;[F256] Urowitz's group[M433] found that men had more pleuritis but less photosensitivity, alopecia, and thrombocytopenia. Thus, each study comparing men with SLE to women with the disease reached different conclusions, so a typical "male" pattern cannot be defined.

Constitutional Symptoms

The generalized symptoms of fever, weight loss, malaise, and fatigue do not fit into any organ system classification, and are therefore discussed here.

Fever

Fever secondary to active disease was recorded at some time in 86% of Harvey's patients seen in the early 1950s,[M280] in 84% of Dubois' 520 patients between 1950 and 1963,[D340] in 55% of 193 patients at Stanford University in the 1960s and 1970s,[F256] and in 41% of Wallace's 464 patients seen between 1980 and 1989.[P216] This consistent, decreasing trend probably reflects better understanding of the disease and the greater availability of nonsteroidal anti-inflammatory drugs (NSAIDs). No fever

curve or pattern is characteristic. SLE can present with fever as its sole manifestation.[P144] Active SLE can result in temperatures as high as 106° F (41° C). It can be difficult to distinguish the fever of SLE from fever caused by complicating infections.

Stahl and associates at the National Institutes of Health[S608] studied 106 SLE-hospitalized patients. In 63 patients (38%) 83 febrile episodes were recorded; 60% resulted from SLE activity, 23% from infection (bacteremia was present in half of these and fatal in one-third), and 17% from other causes (primarily postoperative fevers and drug reactions). The single most useful feature identifying infection was the presence of shaking chills. Leukocytosis (especially in the absence of steroid therapy), neutrophilia, and normal anti-DNA levels were also helpful. The SLE components associated with fever were dermatitis, arthritis, and pleuropericarditis. Although often associated with SLE, a daily low-grade fever, up to 100° F (37.8° C), may be overlooked unless patients are specifically asked to check their temperatures daily. Inoue et al. followed 49 SLE patients through 74 febrile episodes,[126] and found that 25 episodes were secondary to infection. Discriminant analysis showed that 95% of 74 febrile episodes could be correctly classified as to the cause of fever when a combination of white blood count (low with SLE, normal to high with infection) and α_2-globulin levels (high with SLE, normal with infection) are used as variables. A close correlation between α-interferon (but not interleukin-1 or tumor necrosis factor) and degree of fever was observed in 25 untreated SLE patients.[K49]

Temperature elevation in an illness characterized by a high incidence of this finding should not prevent the physician from carefully searching for other causes. The frequent occurrence of infection in patients with SLE often warrants blood cultures, urine cultures, and chest roentgenograms. Urinary tract infections are common in young women, who may be asymptomatic. Opportunistic infections should be considered. The cause of the temperature elevation should be investigated before suppressing this helpful clinical finding by administering or increasing the dose of salicylates, NSAIDs, or corticosteroids.

Anorexia and Weight Loss

Anorexia and an insidious onset of weight loss over a period of months were noted in 51% of patients in the Dubois series,[D340] in 71% of patients in Harvey's group,[M280] in 31% of 193 patients followed by Fries and Holman,[F256] in 63% of Rothfield's 209 patients,[R340] and in 35% of children with SLE.[S800] The degree of weight loss is almost always less than 10%, and most immediately precedes the diagnosis of SLE.

Malaise and Fatigue

A sense of malaise and fatigue is common in SLE patients, especially during periods of disease activity. They feel tired and achy but initially find difficulty in pinpointing the problem. Low-grade fevers, anemia, or any source of inflammation can result in fatigue, as can emotional stress or depression. Rothfield noted moderate to severe fatigue in 81% of 209 patients,[R340] and Fries and Holman noted fatigue in 82% of 193 patients[F256]. Recently, 59 patients followed by Steinberg's group at the National Institutes of Health filled out a fatigue questionnaire.[K435]

Their mean fatigue severity (on a scale of 1 to 7) was 4.6. Of these, 53% reported fatigue to be their most disabling symptom, even though it did not correlate with any laboratory measure.

See Chapter 56 for a discussion of the management of fatigue.

Chapter 34

THE MUSCULOSKELETAL SYSTEM

DANIEL J. WALLACE

Joints, muscles, and their supporting structures are the most commonly involved system in SLE, affecting 53 to 95% of patients (see Table 33–1). Kaposi, in 1872, first described the joint manifestations.[K65] Musculoskeletal symptoms are the most common chief complaint in lupus (see Table 33–2), and articular pain is the initial symptom in 50% of patients.[S680] The biochemical mediators of joint inflammation in SLE and the pathophysiology of the arthritis have not been studied, which probably contributes to our poor understanding of its joint manifestations.

JOINTS: SYMPTOMS, SIGNS, DEFORMITY, AND X-RAY FINDINGS

The chief joint manifestations are stiffness, pain, and inflammation. The pattern of arthritis is recurrent, often evanescent, and can be deforming. Morning stiffness occurs in 46 to 73% of patients.[D340,R294] Fries and Holman[F256] found arthritis in 53%, nodules in 3%, wrist swelling in 31%, metacarpophalangeal (MCP) swelling in 31%, and proximal interphalangeal (PIP) swelling in 40% at any point in a sizable proportion of their 193 patients. Grigor et al.[G385] described nondeforming arthritis or arthralgia in 88%, deforming arthritis in 10%, erosions in 6%, avascular necrosis in 6%, myalgias or myositis in 32%, and tendon contractures in 12% of their patients.

Areas Affected

All the major and minor joints may be affected, including the wrists, knees, ankles, elbows, and shoulders, in that order. Most SLE patients eventually develop some PIP and MCP involvement. Complaints of joint pain without objective physical findings for long periods may be noted. Once symptoms of discomfort became objectively apparent, morning stiffness characteristic of typical rheumatoid arthritis is usually seen. Marked, diffuse puffiness of the hands often occurs. Stress fractures caused by corticosteroid-induced osteoporosis can produce swelling and mimic synovitis.[B593]

Hand

Persistent, rheumatoid-like deformities may occur, as they did in 35% of Dubois' 520 patients,[D340] with thickening of the PIP joints, ulnar deviation, and subluxation. Armas-Cruz[A289] found similar changes in 22% of 108 patients. Those changes often may appear insidiously over the course of many years while the patient is in an apparent clinical remission. The primary lesion appears to be inflammation involving synovial tissues, with minimal or belated destruction of cartilage and bone. Bywaters[B614] taught that whenever a patient with "rheumatoid-like arthritis" remained free of erosions for 2 or more years, the diagnosis of SLE was more likely, although this concept does not necessarily apply to children.[M169] He was the first to emphasize the similarity between the fibrosing synovitis of SLE and that reported by Jaccoud in recurrent rheumatic fever.[B615] Silver and Steinbrocker[S438] noted that when synovial swelling persisted, a lessened tendency toward destruction of the cartilage occurred, compared to that seen in rheumatoid arthritis (RA).

Hand deformities can include ulnar deviation and subluxation, Swan-neck deformities (in 3 to 38%), and subluxation of the thumb interphalangeal joints.[A93,B342,D290,E139,K16,R294] Erosions are rare (seen in about 4%). Some authors have noted positive correlations among deforming arthritis, Sjögren's syndrome, and the presence of rheumatoid factor.[A93,E159,G168,K279,K407,L3,M115,N121] Jaccoud's reversible subluxing nondeforming arthropathy is seen in 3 to 14% of patients with SLE.[B342,D290,K16] Table 34–1 summarizes the differential diagnosis between SLE and RA of the hand. Figs. 34–1 to 34–4 demonstrate some of the above-mentioned abnormalities. Jaccoud's arthropathy does not require treatment, because grip strength is usually intact. In 1981, Dray et al.[D133] treated 10 patients with subluxation excision, MCP arthroplasties, and joint stabilization by ligamentous reconstruction. Unfortunately, 70% of the tendon relocations failed to maintain correction.

Several reports have examined the x-ray findings of the lupus hand in detail. Weissman et al.[W164] evaluated 59 patients, and 34 demonstrated abnormalities. Of these, 10 had acral sclerosis (these probably had mixed connective tissue disease), seven had alignment abnormalities, and 1 showed an erosion. Leskinen's group reviewed joint radiographs of 124 SLE patients.[L1,L199] Cystic bone lesions were found in 51 (41%). Most were subchondral, located in the small joints of the hands and feet, and a vasculitic cause was proposed.

A resorptive arthropathy resembling the opera-glass hand has rarely been reported,[M658,S792] as has periosteal elevation secondary to ischemic bone disease or perhaps vasculitis.[M166]

Knees

Jaccoud-like arthropathy (reversible subluxation) has been observed in the knees.[D132,D133,G196] Deep venous

Table 34–1. Comparison of Hand Involvement in SLE and RA Patients

Parameter	Systemic Lupus Erythematosus	Rheumatoid Arthritis
Raynaud's phenomenon	About 30%	Less than 10%
Joint pain	Mild	May be severe
Recurrent synovitis	Not common; evanescent when it occurs	Common
Joint deformity	Caused by loss of soft tissue support	Caused by loss of soft tissue support and articular surface destruction
Thumb IP joint hyperextension	Not associated with MP joint flexion contracture	Often associated with thumb MP joint flexion contracture
Ulnar drift of fingers	Almost always reversible	Often irreversible, with subluxed MP joints
Wrist	May be lax; normal function	Often subluxed, with carpal bone destruction
Erosive changes seen on roentgenograms	Rare	Common
Cause of deformity	Uncertain; occurs after supporting soft tissue structures are weakened	Synovitis, pannus formation; cartilage and bone destruction

Adapted from Bleifeld, C.J. and Inglis, A.E.:[B342] The hand in systemic lupus erythematosus. J. Bone Joint Surg. 56-A:1207, (Sept.) 1974.

thrombosis in a patient with anticardiolipin antibodies may be difficult to differentiate from a Baker's cyst, both of which are observed in SLE.[R132] At least one case of chrondrocalcinosis involving the knee joint associated with SLE has been reported,[M624] and it is certainly more common.

Feet

Mizutani and Quismorio[M492] noted hallux valgus, metatarsophalangeal subluxation, hammertoes, and forefoot widening without erosions or cystic changes in patients with SLE. This is similar to the Jaccoud type of arthropathy in the hands. Other studies have confirmed these findings.[M591] The deformities result in painful bunions and callosities. Several podiatry publications have reviewed the issues of proper foot care in those with SLE.[B171,L13]

Neck

Several cases of atlantoaxial subluxation have been reported.[B5,K280] One report postulated that patients treated with corticosteroids have increased ligamentous laxity, which promotes the rupture of ligamentous and capsular supporting structures,[K280] but it seems equally likely that laxity of ligaments in the neck have the same physiologic bond as laxity in any other joint. In the other report, 5 of 59 patients with lupus had atlantoaxial subluxation, and all were asymptomatic. Subluxation was associated with longer disease duration, Jaccoud's arthropathy, and chronic renal failure.[B5]

Sacroiliac Joint

Several studies of almost 100 patients suggested that over half of all active SLE patients have radiographic sacroiliitis or increased uptake on joint scanning. Seronegative spondyloarthropathies were excluded, and most had no sacroiliac symptoms.[D178,G310,N37,V94,V95] I believe this figure is too high.

Temporomandibular Joint

Jonsson et al.[J124] evaluated temporomandibular (TMJ) joint involvement in 37 SLE patients and compared them to a control group of 37 healthy age- and sex-matched individuals. Of those referred to an oral surgeon with SLE, 59% had severe past TMJ symptoms (versus 14% of con-

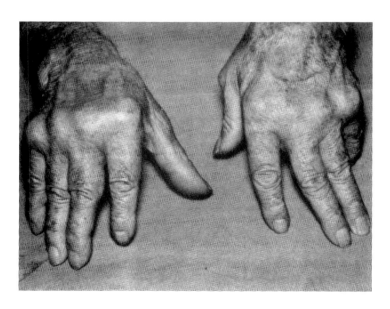

Fig. 34–1. SLE of 10 years' duration in a 70-year-old male. Note Jaccoud-type deformity, voluntarily correctable by patient.

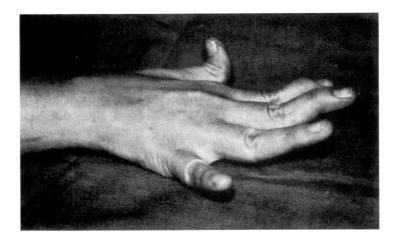

Fig. 34–2. Hyperextension of the hand, with characteristic PIP subluxation and hyperextension of thumb.

trols) and 14% had present severe symptoms (versus 3% of controls). Clinical examination revealed TMJ signs, such as clicking, crepitation, jaw fatigue or stiffness, facial pain, tenderness to palpation, pain on movement of the mandible, locking, or dislocation to be present in 41% (versus none of the controls). Of the SLE patients, 30% had abnormal roentgenograms (versus 9% of controls) that included condyle flattening and osteophytes, 11% had erosion, confirming other reports,[G81,L278] and 72% had renal disease (versus only 27% of the non–TMJ-involved SLE patients). Although symptoms may be referred to this joint, limitation of the ability to open the jaw is rare unless coexistent scleroderma is present.[D328]

Synovial Histopathology

SLE is characterized by a mild to moderate inflammatory synovitis similar in character but less "angry"-appearing than that seen in RA.[A289,C447] Bywaters[B614,B615] reported the presence of chronic synovitis with a fibrotic process in SLE in patients with Jaccoud-type deformities.

Only three studies have examined the synovial histopathology of SLE in any detail. Goldenberg and Cohen[G248] studied 13 lupus patients: 92% had synovial membrane hyperplasia, all had microvascular changes, 83% had surface fibrin deposits, and most had a perivascular infiltrate.

Several of the biopsies were indistinguishable from those of RA. Labowitz and Schumacher[L3] studied synovial biopsies from seven patients; superficial fibrin-like material was seen in four, and focal or diffuse synovial lining proliferation in six. Five had a primary perivascular inflammatory reaction with predominantly mononuclear cells. Vasculitis was noted in only one patient. Synovial and vascular lesions were found in two patients, who had no objective signs of joint inflammation. On electron microscopy, fibrin was noted in three of four specimens. Type A (phagocytic), type B (synthetic), and intermediate cells were seen, without any clear predominance. Two patients had platelets and fibrin-like material obliterating small-vessel lumens. Vascular endothelial inclusions of a virus-like type were observed in two patients.

Natour et al.[N46] reviewed 30 knee synovial biopsies. The most frequent findings were synoviocyte hyperplasia, minimal inflammation, edema, congestion, vascular proliferation, fibrinoid necrosis, intimal fibrous hyperplasia, and fibrin on the synovial surface.

In conclusion, the synovial histopathology of SLE does not appear to be specific, and cannot clearly be differentiated from that of RA. Despite the extensive connective tissue change, little cartilage and bone destruction seems to occur. This gross finding tends to separate the de-

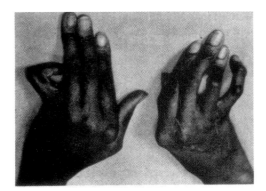

Fig. 34–3. Ulnar deviation and contractures in a patient with SLE.

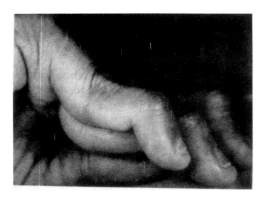

Fig. 34–4. Subluxation deformity that appeared insidiously over a period of years in a patient with classic, multisystem SLE.

forming arthritis associated with SLE from that typically seen in RA.

Subcutaneous Nodules

Described by Hebra[H235] and Kaposi in 1872, subcutaneous nodules are present in 5 to 12% of the large series listed in Table 33–1 and in 2 to 10% of other series.[G283,M556,R328] Most occur in small joints of the hand, but nodules as large as 2 cm in diameter occur frequently on the extensor tendons of the hand and wrist. They may be exceedingly tender, and are often transitory. Hoarseness secondary to rheumatoid-like vocal cord nodules has been described.[S210] The nodules are associated with SLE patients who have rheumatoid-like arthritis and positive rheumatoid factor, and are rarely seen without these features.[A152a,F251a,Z27]

Subcutaneous nodules are histologically granulomas and need to be differentiated from lupus panniculitis (profundus),[T261] erythema nodosum, and a benign mesenchymoma. In children, it is important to distinguish them from granuloma annulare. Several reviews of the histology of the nodules in SLE have appeared.[D323,G283,L75] Vascular damage, with structural disarray in areas with collagen degeneration, is found, along with fibrinoid deposits and lymphocytic infiltrates in vessel walls. This microvasculopathy is similar to that observed in rheumatoid nodules.

Tendinitis, Tendon Rupture, and Carpal Tunnel Syndrome

Synovitis can induce a carpal tunnel syndrome, which may be the initial manifestation of idiopathic SLE or drug-induced lupus.[D319,S409] Numerous reports and reviews have been published regarding tendon ruptures in SLE, the most important of which are cited here.[F316,H73,K188,P300,P374] The following conclusions can be derived: (1) almost all occur in weight-bearing areas, especially in tendons about the knee (65%; most are infrapatellar); and ankle (Achilles tendon; 27%); (2) an increased association with trauma, males, longterm oral steroid administration, intra-articular injections, Jaccoud's deformity, and/or long disease duration is noted; and (3) most patients are in clinical remission at the time of rupture.

A definitive diagnosis can be made by the use of magnetic resonance imaging (MRI).[G325] Tendon biopsy specimens reveal degeneration, mononuclear infiltration, neovascularization, and vacuolar myopathy.[P274] One group has correlated hyperparathyroidism (especially in patients with severe renal disease) and hydroxyapatite and urate crystal deposition in the knee tendons, with resulting ligamentous laxity.[B4,B6] Pritchard and Berney observed four cases of tendon rupture (all patellar) in 180 patients followed over a 10-year period.[P300] Carpal tunnel syndrome was found in 48 (11%) of 436 SLE patients seen at the University of Pittsburgh between 1972 and 1990.[M333]

Synovial Cysts

Large synovial cysts are uncommonly reported in SLE patients.[D331,H178,P17] Our group has observed soft synovial cysts several millimeters in diameter appearing in the dorsum of PIP joints in SLE patients following years of localized inflammation. These should be differentiated from rheumatoid nodules.

Calcinosis

Commonly observed in scleroderma, dermatomyositis, and cross-over syndromes, soft tissue calcifications are rarely seen in SLE.[C82,L106] They were observed radiographically in 9 of 130 patients in one study in which SLE was not adequately defined.[B554] Otherwise, about 30 case reports have appeared in the literature. Calcinosis universalis has been noted.[W131] Deposits in muscle, subcutaneous nodules, and periarthritis can occur in those with discoid or systemic lupus.[G393,J83,N119]

Osteoporosis

See Chapter 61.

Chondritis

See Chapter 40.

Costochondritis

Patients with SLE frequently complain of discomfort at the costochondral junctions. Esophageal spasm, angina pectoris, and pericarditis must be ruled out.

Synovial Fluid

Ropes[R249] found that the volume of accessible synovial joint fluid (Table 34–2) ranged from 5 to 1500 ml in 133 patients. It was unusually clear, but occasionally hemorrhagic, and could be a transudate or an exudate. Pekin and Zvaifler[P95] reported synovial fluid findings in 26 patients with SLE. Viscosity was uniformly good. The white count was less than 2000/mm³ in 19 and exceeded 10,000/mm³ in only 2 patients. Granulocytes were always less than 50%, and the synovial fluid complement level was normal in 11. Of the 26, 10 were classified as having noninflammatory transudates. Most had nephrotic syndrome. The exudates had a high protein content but variable complement levels. Serum: synovial fluid complement ratios were generally elevated in contrast to the total protein or IgG ratios, suggesting consumption of complement at the synovial level. Schumacher[S187] examined 17 SLE synovial fluids. All had a white count lower than 15,000/mm³. In comparing SLE with rheumatoid arthritis, Hollander[H381] reported a mean white count of 5,000/mm³ for SLE (versus 15,000 for RA) with 10% neutrophils (versus 50% for

Table 34–2. Characteristics of Synovial Fluid in SLE

Clear, yellow, normal viscosity, good mucin clot
White blood cell count: 2,000 to 15,000/mm³, with primarily lymphocytic predominance
Low-titer ANA may be present; LE cells are occasionally seen
Glucose level normal
Protein levels normal or increased
Complement levels normal or decreased

RA) and a good mucin clot and high viscosity (versus a poor mucin clot and low viscosity for RA). Hesselbacher[H202] confirmed the increased viscosity in SLE synovial fluid, and found generally low C3 complement levels. Cell counts in joint fluids must be interpreted cautiously, because analysis of the same fluid is subject to a great deal of variability among laboratories.[S188]

Secondary joint infection or avascular necrosis of bone may occur infrequently in SLE, and should be suspected when a localized effusion persists, despite anti-inflammatory therapy.[B95,E28,M595,Q16]

LE cells can be found in vivo in synovial fluid.[B95] They were present in 6 of 9 patients in one report,[H501] in 8 of 17 fluids examined by Schumacher[S187] with electron microscopy, in 45% of 18 patients,[F229] and in 2 of 3 patients with drug-induced lupus.[V97] Rarely, RA cells (ragocytes) may be found in SLE synovial fluid.[S552,W252]

Antinuclear antibodies are difficult to measure in synovial fluid, which must be treated with hyalurinadase prior to analysis. ANA is present in about 20% of synovial fluid samples from both RA and SLE patients,[L3,M38,M39,P248] irrespective of serum levels. The synovial fluid of those with drug-induced lupus is similar to that reported for idiopathic SLE.[V97] Lipid synovial effusions rarely occur.[R443] These observations are summarized in Table 34–2.

MYALGIA, MYOSITIS, AND MYOPATHY

Generalized myalgia and muscle tenderness (Table 34–3), most marked in the deltoid areas and quadriceps (proximal muscles), are common during exacerbations of the disease, and were observed in 40 to 48% of patients.[D340,F256,I38] Inflammatory myositis involving the proximal musculature occurs in 5 to 11% of patients,[E147,F46,I38,K9] and can be confirmed by muscle biopsy, electromyographic studies, and elevation of the serum creatine phosphokinase (CPK) or aldolase levels. Myoglobin levels may also be increased.[K9] The myositis responds to steroid therapy.

The differential diagnosis of proximal muscle weakness is a common problem in the management of patients with SLE. An inflammatory myositis must be differentiated from a drug-induced myopathy (glucocorticoid or antimalarial). Muscle enzyme levels are only elevated in the former group, but many untreated SLE patients with myalgias have normal muscle enzyme levels. Frequently, generalized weakness is so prominent that some patients are initially diagnosed as having dermatomyositis.[M240] Inflammatory myositis can develop at any time during the course of the disease.[D119,G328,G329,K145,K146,P9,T277,W2069] Three large groups of dermatomyositis-polymyositis patients demonstrated a 7%, 4%, and 1% concurrence of SLE.[D186,P226,R382] The skin lesions of dermatomyositis-polymyositis can also appear in SLE patients.[K145,K146]

Tsokos et al.[T243] evaluated 228 SLE patients at the NIH. Of these, 18 (8%) had prominent muscle disease. The CPK level was elevated in 1 patient and the aldolase level was higher in 11. In 72%, myositis was concomitant with disease onset. No evidence of myocarditis was found, and all responded to 20 mg of prednisone daily or less.

Foote et al.[F159] followed 276 SLE patients at the Mayo Clinic, and 11 met the diagnostic criteria for dermatomyositis-polymyositis. All were female, with a mean age of 29 years. In contrast to the NIH findings, the onset of myositis in their patients occurred 13 years after the onset of SLE. Also, Raynaud's phenomenon was more prevalent in this group. The patients were treated with 30 to 60 mg of prednisone daily, and 1 was given azathioprine. After 4 years, 2 were dead and 6 were asymptomatic.

Electromyography

The principal electromyography (EMG) findings in polymyositis and dermatomyositis are the following: (1) spontaneous fibrillation; (2) positive or sawtooth potentials; (3) small-amplitude, complex, polyphasic, or short-duration potentials; and (4) salvos of repetitive, high-frequency potentials. In SLE patients, the EMG findings range from normal to those of classic dermatomyositis-polymyositis. Only three studies, however, have examined EMG findings in SLE patients. O'Leary et al.[O61] found nonspecific EMG abnormalities in 2 of 9 patients with SLE but in all with dermatomyositis. Erbsloh and Baedeker[E127] performed EMGs on 15 patients with muscle symptoms. Their main findings were a decrease in mean potential duration to only 54% of normal, an increase in the mean phase frequency, and a corresponding decrease in the phase quotient; in only 1 patient were the findings normal. Tsokos et al.[T243] performed EMGs on 8 of their 18 patients with SLE and myopathy; of these, 5 had normal findings neuropathy was demonstrated in 1, and the classic polyphasic peaks seen in polymyositis were noted in 2. In a study of 35 unselected SLE patients, EMGs were suggestive of a myopathy in 23.[V84]

Depending on various parameters, such as observer interpretation, whether an outpatient or inpatient population was used, and whether they had muscle symptoms, between 22 and 90% of patients with SLE have abnormal EMGs.[E127,O61,S680,T243,V84]

Muscle Biopsies

Muscle biopsy findings (Figs. 34–5 and 34–6). range from normal to interstitial inflammation, fibrillar necrosis, degeneration, and vacuolization with fibrosis as a late occurrence seen with polymyositis-dermatomyositis. First used in the 1930s,[K284,O61] muscle biopsies can be helpful in distinguishing inflammatory from drug-induced myopa-

Table 34–3. Lupus Myositis and Myopathy in SLE

1. Myalgias occur in 40 to 80% of SLE patients, and are most marked in proximal muscles. Weakness is a common symptom.
2. Inflammatory myositis (often with an increased CPK level) has a cumulative incidence of 5 to 11%.
3. Steroid-induced and antimalarial-induced myopathies must be excluded.
4. EMG and muscle biopsy findings range from the normal to classic patterns seen in dermato/polymyositis.
5. Myalgias without myositis may respond to salicylates, NSAIDS, antimalarials, or 20 mg/day of prednisone, or less.
6. If diagnostic criteria are met for both SLE and dermato/polymyositis, treatment with 1 mg/kg/day of prednisone should be initiated.

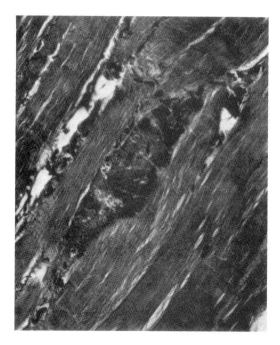

Fig. 34–5. Muscle biopsy from patient with SLE and proximal muscle weakness. Note focal necrosis (H & E stain; × 225).

thies, as well as in determining reversibility based on the degree of fibrotic changes.

Klemperer[K284] noted an inflammatory infiltrate in 5 of 30 cases of SLE, and Madden[M41] in 6 of 21 biopsies. The changes were nonspecific. Erbsloh and Baedecker[E127] biopsied 16 patients; 2 demonstrated impressive round cell infiltration, and 12 had parenchymal damage that occasionally included necrosis, along with a sparse interstitial infiltrate. Tsokos et al. biopsied 11 of 18 patients with SLE

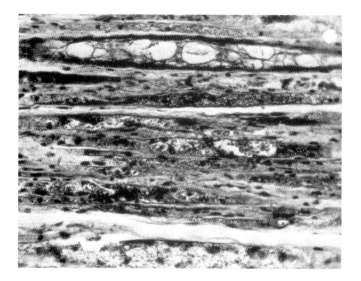

Fig. 34–6. Vacuolar myopathy caused by SLE. Note marked muscle degeneration with loss of striation, vacuolization, and fine pigmentary degeneration (H & E stain; × 800).

and myopathy.[T243] A mixed cellular, perivascular, inflammatory reaction with interstitial inflammation without much muscle fiber degeneration was noted in 6 patients, and 5 had nonspecific changes or atrophy without inflammation.

Pearson[P85] described muscle biopsies in 20 patients with various forms of SLE and noted rare, nonspecific fiber degeneration and interstitial myositis in 10 patients, no change in 3 patients, and 7 with minor or insignificant muscle fiber vacuolization (4 taking steroids and 2 antimalarials). The vacuolar lesions were variable in extent and degree, sometimes being focal and scanty and on other occasions appearing widespread and extensive in individual fibers. These changes did not correlate with CPK levels, clinical measures of strength, or steroid administration. No vacuolar myopathy was noted among 16 biopsies at the University of Toronto,[R431] and was seen in only 1 of 12 cases in another report.[F101] One case of inclusion body myositis has been observed in SLE.[Y47]

Three studies have included ultrastructural examinations. Oxenhandler et al.[O133] evaluated the immunopathologic characteristics of lupus myopathy in 19 patients. Type I fibers predominated in 44%, and type II fiber atrophy was seen in 33%. Of the 19, 8 had an inflammatory myositis. Immunoglobulin or complement staining was seen in 13 patients in sarcolemmal-basement membrane areas, 5 had myofibrillar IgG, 5 showed vascular immunoglobulin or complement deposits, and IgG-containing globules were seen in 10. The University of Toronto group[R431] emphasized the universality of immunoglobulin deposition in 16 SLE muscle biopsies, despite the rarity of concurrent inflammation. Finol et al. emphasized the presence of muscle atrophy, microtubular inclusions, and a bland mononuclear cell infiltrate in 12 biopsy specimens.[F101] Necrotic changes were only present in the one patient, who had an elevated CPK level. Their group confirmed earlier suggestions by Norton et al.[N134,N135] that the microvascular circulation of skeletal muscle is decreased because of capillary basement membrane thickening.

AVASCULAR NECROSIS OF BONE

First reported in SLE by Dubois and Cozen in 1960,[D330] avascular necrosis (AVN; also known as aseptic necrosis or ischemic necrosis of bone) was observed in 26 of Dubois' 520 patients (5%),[D340] in 5% of Wallace's 464 patients,[W18] and in 24% of Hochberg's 150 patients at Johns Hopkins, which is an AVN referral center.[H347] Other studies noted AVN in 4 to 9% of SLE patients.[A10,D198,D218,K25, K310,L298,S504,U30,V117,Z34] AVN is a major source of morbidity and alteration in the quality of life in young women with lupus. This section reviews the pathophysiology, diagnostic testing, clinical presentation, and associations of AVN, as well as its treatment (Table 34–4).

Pathophysiology and Classification

The usual mechanism is death of subchondral bone, resulting in osseocartilaginous sequestration with adjacent secondary osteosclerosis. The name "osteochondritis dissecans" has been used to refer to small areas of this

Table 34–4. Avascular Necrosis of Bone in SLE

1. AVN occurs in 5 to 10% of patients.
2. Most cases are associated with corticosteroid administration; the remainder are probably induced by Raynaud's phenomenon, a small-vessel vasculitis, fat emboli, or the antiphospholipid syndrome.
3. MRI scanning is the diagnostic method of choice; CT scanning and bone scans are less accurate and do not pick up preradiographic lesions as well. The roentgenographic appearance can be classified into four stages.
4. Multiple sites can be affected; the femoral head, tibial plateaus, and humeral head are the most common.
5. An association exists between AVN and Raynaud's phenomenon, increased steroid dosage, and duration of treatment.
6. Treatment includes limiting weight-bearing, anti-inflammatory analgesics, and core decompression for stage I and II lesions; reconstructive surgery is usually required for stage III and IV disease.

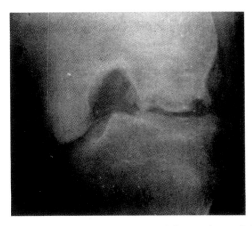

Fig. 34–8. Aseptic necrosis of lateral femoral condyle, right knee.

process, such as disease involving a segment of femoral head or condyle.

The initial pathologic lesion is probably obliteration of the blood supply of the epiphysis, followed by reactive hyperemia, which is seen on the roentgenogram as osteoporosis. At this stage, the necrotic bone is roentgenographically demarcated from viable bone because the dead tissue does not take part in the decalcification (Figs. 34–7 to 34–10). By contrast, the necrotic area appears increased in density compared to the osteoporotic bone around it. During the healing stage, as new blood vessels grow in and bone repair occurs, the newly formed bone is soft. With continued pressure on the surface flattening may occur as, for example, on the medial and superior aspects of the femoral head. These irregularities in the contour of the articular surfaces cause definite and consistent adaptive changes that are manifested later as degenerative arthritis.

AVN can have various types of causes[G383]—post-traumatic, nontraumatic or idiopathic. Fractures, microfractures, or dislocations may cause AVN. Nontraumatic

causes include embolic factors (e.g., as in sickle cell anemia, thalassemia, alcoholism, pancreatitis, and decompression states), small-vessel changes (e.g., as in SLE, polyarteritis, or Fabry's disease), and deposition ischemic necrosis (e.g., increased lipocytes caused by steroid therapy, Gaucher's disease, Cushing's disease). Renal transplant patients who receive pulse steroids and high doses of steroids are especially susceptible. Conditions associated with idiopathic AVN include gout, pregnancy, prolonged immobilization, cytotoxic therapy, hyperparathyroidism, familial tendencies, lymphoma, metastatic carcinoma, and degenerative arthritis.

In SLE, Raynaud's phenomenon, vasculitis,[M409,S421,V59] fat emboli,[F113,F114,J109] the antiphospholipid syndrome,[N5] and corticosteroids can induce ischemia that results in bony necrosis. The fact that no cases of AVN were recorded prior to 1960 indicates the importance of the introduction of corticosteroids in the 1950s in regard to our perception of this entity.

Arlet and Ficat have classified AVN using a radiographic scale.[F81] In stage 0, only hemodynamic changes have taken place. The patient is asymptomatic and routine roentgenograms are normal. In stage I, minimal pain with mild restriction of motion may be present. Stage II is characterized by a dull, aching pain on weight-bearing, decreased range of motion, and a slight limp. Roentgenograms demonstrate diffuse osteoporosis, sclerosis, or cyst formation. By the time stage III is reached advanced radiographic changes are evident, and the patient has taken a quantum leap in restricted movement and pain. Subchondral bone collapse (the crescent sign), with normal joint space, is present radiographically. Stage IV represents end stage disease with osteoarthritis, as seen on the roentgenogram. Most patients are symptomatic and require surgery.

Diagnostic Techniques and Hemodynamic Studies

Magnetic resonance imaging (MRI) can detect AVN months to years before it is evident on routine roentgenograms (Fig. 34–11). This has made earlier, noninvasive methods of detecting AVN obsolete. The test should be

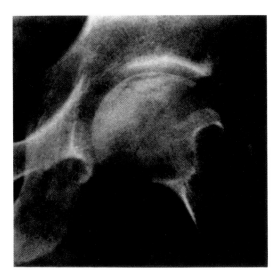

Fig. 34–7. Early aseptic necrosis of femoral head (frog-leg view). Note subcortical necrosis.

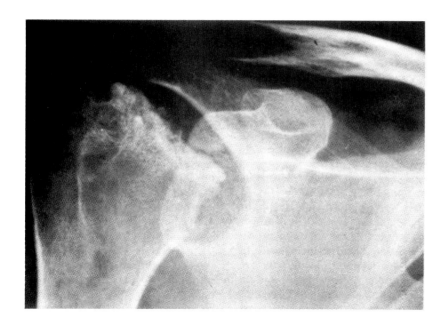

Fig. 34–9. Aseptic necrosis of right humeral head in a patient with SLE who was receiving steroids.

ordered for a patient with SLE who has hip pain and a normal roentgenogram if glucocorticoid therapy is being given. Gallium scans[M219] and technetium scans with pertechnetate or sulfur colloid[D22,L429,S223,Z37] are accurate, but can be subject to false-positive or false negative interpretation. Scintigraphic images of radiographically negative osteonecrosis tend to contain a photopenic zone, whereas more advanced lesions have increased uptake.[M480] Several studies have compared bone scanning with MRI[B195,G88,K40,R252,S743]—the latter has better speci-

ficity and sensitivity, but both procedures can yield false-positive findings. Even though computerized tomography (CT) with multiplanar reformation[S82] can be useful, MRI derives the same or more information with less effort and without exposing the patient to radiation. On MRI, the reactive interface between live and dead bone at the periphery of AVN lesions has a characteristic double-line sign on T2-weighted images.[M481] Early changes at the femoral head can demonstrate bone marrow edema,[T275] and premature conversion to fatty marrow is evident in

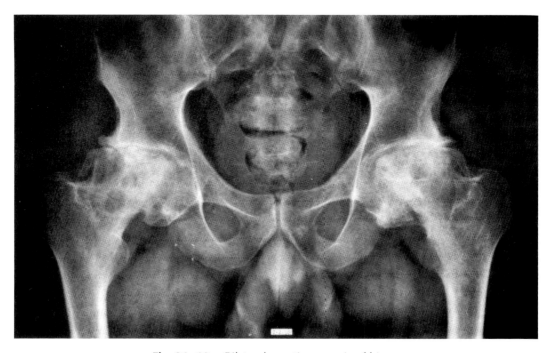

Fig. 34–10. Bilateral aseptic necrosis of hips.

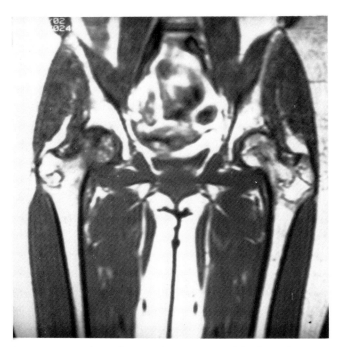

Fig. 34–11. Bilateral avascular necrosis of the hips shown on an MRI scan. (Courtesy of Dr. J. Mink.)

younger patients. In AVN, the femoral neck is usually surrounded by joint fluid. These findings have been confirmed in SLE patients[G30,K40,S223,Z33] (Fig. 34–11).

Zizic and colleagues at Johns Hopkins[Z38a,Z38b] have used invasive techniques to obtain more information about the hemodynamics of AVN. They found increased baseline bone marrow pressure in most SLE patients after carrying out a stress test (a greater than 10 mm Hg elevation after instillation of 5 ml of physiologic saline into the femoral head). Almost 90% of patients had abnormal intraosseous venography, as characterized by incomplete filling of the main extraosseous veins, diaphyseal reflux, and stasis of contrast material. Venography was abnormal in all stages of AVN, including preradiologic ones. In a follow-up study, bone marrow pressure, saline stress test, and/or ischemic intraosseous venography results were abnormal in 254 (94%) of 259 ischemic bones so evaluated, and AVN was detected in 93% of 55 radiologically normal bones.[Z41] Using these parameters, 36 of 48 joints on the contralateral asymptomatic side had abnormalities, and 15 patients (42%) developed AVN over a 47-month follow-up period. Thus, hemodynamic measurements are of predictive value in identifying the joints at risk,[Z39] but this procedure is not widely available.

Clinical Associations in SLE

In SLE, AVN tends to occur at multiple sites. At the NIH, 90% of 31 cases were polyarticular and 83% were symmetric.[K310] Of Dubois' 26 patients, 22 had bilateral femoral head involvement, 1 was unilateral, and 3 affected the knee.[D340] Zizic's group[K313,Z38,Z40] reported that 91%

of cases involved the femoral head and 83% occurred in multiple sites. Reports have appeared of 6, 8, 13, and even 17 different sites in a single patient.[F117,L286,N99,R408] Although the hip is the most common site, AVN can involve other joints and often results in a delay in diagnosis. Three of Urman's 11 University of Connecticut patients had AVN of the wrist.[U30] Most studies have recorded a mean onset of AVN in the fourth decade, with an average SLE disease duration of 4 to 7 years.[D218,D323]

The diagnosis of AVN should be considered in any patient with SLE who has persistent pain in one or a few joints without evidence of disease activity in other systems, especially if glucocorticoids have been given. The association between vasculitis and AVN in the absence of steroid administration is well documented.[M409,S421,V59] Many studies have addressed the role of corticosteroids in inducing AVN in those with SLE. Early studies were hampered by control groups in which AVN was excluded on the basis of normal roentgenograms.[D218,K310] Abeles et al. and Zizic et al.[K313,W136,Z38,Z40] have suggested that increased doses of steroids (especially in the first year of treatment) and the duration of steroid therapy are correlated with a greater risk of AVN in SLE patients. Bolus steroids were not similarly associated.[W240] These dose-time relationships were confirmed in a meta-analysis of 22 papers (most patients without SLE) by Felson et al.[F57]

SLE also has additional unique features that might predispose a patient to the development of AVN. Zizic has commented[Z35] on the comparative rarity of AVN in steroid-dependent populations of asthma, dermatologic, and inflammatory bowel disease patients. AVN was found to be associated with Raynaud's phenomenon, central nervous system lupus, vasculitis, myositis, peripheral neuropathy, and elevated sedimentation rates.[K313,Z38] Although others have only been able to confirm the association with Raynaud's phenomenon,[K25,S504] two reports noted an increased incidence of the antiphospholipid syndrome in AVN patients.[A11,S223] This reinforces the importance of thromboembolic considerations in the etiopathogenesis of AVN.

Treatment

Small areas of AVN can remain asymptomatic, or can heal spontaneously. Rare reports of spontaneous regression have appeared,[L128] but most patients with a clearly established diagnosis experience progressive disease if treated nonoperatively. Conservative management is usually a holding action and consists of analgesics, nonsteroidal anti-inflammatory drugs (NSAIDs) and limited or non–weight-bearing for several months.[L388] Alcohol use should be discouraged, and efforts to decrease steroid doses should be attempted.

A number of surgical techniques have been successfully used with AVN of the femoral head, including drilling or core decompression, free bone grafts (cortical or osteochondral allograft), vascularized bone grafts (muscle pedicle graft, vascular anastomosis), osteotomy (varus or valgus angulation, rotation), and joint reconstruction (femoral head or total hip replacement).[L388] Other joints are approached in a conceptually similar manner. The discussion here is limited to results reported for SLE.

Early series documented excellent results with total hip replacements.[B24,P321] Between 1971 and 1982, 39 of 43 prosthetic hip replacements performed at the Mayo Clinic on SLE patients were for stage III or IV AVN.[H114] Of these, 29 patients had conventional hip replacements and 14 had bipolar endoprosthetic replacements. Over a 66-month follow-up period, all were rated as having good or excellent results. Complications included delayed wound healing (15%) and superficial wound infection (10%).

Whereas few disagree regarding the management of stages III and IV AVN, the indications for core decompression in earlier stages are controversial. First reported by Zizic et al.[Z38b,Z42] as removal of an 11-mm diameter core of bone from the central axis of the femoral head, success was claimed in treating stages I, II, and III disease. Two studies of SLE failed to confirm these findings,[G30,K25] and our results at UCLA Medical Center have been mixed. Zizic's review[Z35] of the literature (including other diseases) suggests a 77% success rate for preradiologic disease and a 52% success rate for stage II AVN. The coring procedure is probably not indicated for patients with stage III or IV disease.

Chapter 35

CARDIAC ABNORMALITIES IN SYSTEMIC LUPUS ERYTHEMATOSUS

FRANCISCO P. QUISMORIO, Jr.

Cardiac abnormalities are one of the most important clinical manifestations of SLE, contributing significantly to the morbidity and mortality of the disease. Cardiac involvement, including arterial hypertension, has been reported in from 52 to 89% of patients.[A289,B490,J75,M280,S339] The pathologic picture is that of a pancarditis affecting the pericardium, myocardium, endocardium, and coronary arteries. Involvement of one layer of the heart, such as a pericarditis, may predominate the clinical picture in one patient, whereas in another the heart may be diffusely affected.

At times, it is difficult to differentiate between primary cardiac changes caused by SLE and those resulting from complicating conditions. Symptoms referable to the heart and the cardiovascular system that occur frequently must be carefully evaluated and differentiated from noncardiac symptoms, which they can mimic. Symptoms of angina pectoris, hypertension, cardiac failure, and pericarditis frequently mimic those of esophageal spasm, reflux esophagitis, pleurisy, pneumonitis, and costochondritis. The concurrence of costochondritis and musculoskeletal chest pains with SLE has received little attention, despite the apparent high frequency (33%) noted by Ropes.[R294]

PERICARDITIS

"Pericarditis is diagnosed in proportion to the care of the examination."[B137]

Prevalence

Involvement of the pericardium in SLE, first recognized by Keefer and Felty[K140] in 1924, is a common feature, and is the most common cardiac abnormality in this disease. In several reported series, the prevalence of pericarditis ranges from 6 to 45%. Godeau et al.[G207] diagnosed pericarditis in 27% of 112 patients and Rothfield[R341] in 25% of over 200 patients. Doherty and Seigel[D249] found the prevalence of pericarditis to be 25.6% among 1,194 SLE patients collected from several clinical series in the literature. In contrast, they found a prevalence of 62.1% among 254 autopsy cases, indicating that asymptomatic pericardial involvement is common. Moreover, the diagnosis may be missed unless the patient is specifically questioned about its clinical manifestations. The introduction of echocardiography as a diagnostic modality has confirmed the high frequency of asymptomatic pericardial effusion and thickening in SLE patients (see Table 35–1).

Clinical Presentation

Acute pericarditis may occur as an isolated finding or as part of a generalized serositis. Estes and Christian[E147] noted cardiac manifestations in 38% of their 150 patients. Pericarditis occurred in 29 patients and was associated with pleural effusions in all but 7.

The clinical picture of lupus pericarditis is usually typical, with complaints of substernal or pericardial pain, aggravated by motion such as breathing, coughing, swallowing, twisting, and bending forward. At times, a pericardial rub may be heard in an asymptomatic patient. Symptoms may either be severe and persistent or mild and transitory. Complaints may last for hours or weeks, and often recur over a period of years. Pericarditis usually develops during the subacute or chronic period.

The typical pericardial friction rub was heard at any one time in only 8% of 520 cases of Dubois[D340] and in 29% of 142 patients of Ropes.[R294] The rub is often confused with a coarse systolic murmur, but the former tends to become louder, rougher, and more superficial on expiration, usually disappearing and recurring erratically.

Electrocardiographic changes may confirm the clinical diagnosis of lupus pericarditis, with typical tall T waves and elevated ST segments characteristic of the disorder in the acute phase. Routine electrocardiograms (ECGs) of patients with SLE who do not have cardiac symptoms may show typical ECG changes that indicate asymptomatic pericarditis. If myocarditis is present concomitantly, ST-segment elevation may occur with T-wave inversion. Brigden et al.[B490] noted that 52 of 60 patients had ECG abnormalities consistent with pericarditis at some stage of their illness.

Pericarditis with or without effusion may be the initial manifestation of SLE. Of the 520 cases of Dubois, 6 (1.2%) presented with pericarditis.[D340] When pericarditis is the presenting feature of SLE, it may be mistaken for acute idiopathic pericarditis, which is assumed to have a viral cause. McCuiston and Moser[M253] emphasized contrasting features of the two conditions. Precordial or substernal chest pain and antecedent respiratory infection are more frequently seen in acute idiopathic pericarditis, whereas relapses are more common in lupus pericarditis. In contrast to the female predominance in SLE, males outnumber

Table 35–1. Selected Echocardiographic Studies of Cardiac Functions in SLE

Source	No. of Patients	Modalities Used	Pericardial Abnormalities	Valvular Defects	Myocardial Function
I. Uncontrolled Studies					
Elkayam et al. (1977)[E75]	32	M-mode	2 with effusion	Mitral valve (MV) thickening in 1 patient	Not tested
Doherty et al. (1988)[C248a]	50	M-mode, 2-D	21 (42%) effusion	MV thickening in 6 (12%); MV prolapse in 3 (6%)	4 with decreased left ventricular (LV) contractility; 4 with global hypokinesis
Chia et al. (1981)[C232]	21	M-mode	5 (24%) with effusion; 6 (29%) thickening	None	71% with LV dysfunction
II. Controlled studies					
Klinkoff et al. (1985)[K290]	47 SLE, 46 controls	M-mode, 2-D	10 (21%) SLE; none in control	10 (21%) in SLE and 7 (15%) in controls	2 (4%) of SLE patients with wall motion abnormalities
Crozier et al. (1990)[C445]	50 SLE, 50 healthy controls	M-mode, 2-D, Doppler	27 (54%) SLE; 5 (10%) of controls with effusion	High frequency of valvular regurgitation in SLE	LV dysfunction more common in SLE
Enomoto et al. (1991)[E112]	43 SLE, 93 healthy females	M-mode, 2-D, color Doppler	No data	Regurgitation (SLE versus controls): mitral—54 versus 31%; tricuspid—74 versus 25%; pulmonary—79 versus 18%; aortic—7 versus 0	No data
Galve et al. (1988)[G23]	74 SLE, 60 controls	M-mode, 2-D	No data	Libman-Sacks in 7; valve dysfunction in 6 SLE; valve abnormality, no dysfunction in 5 SLE and 4 controls	Normal LV systolic function
Comens et al. (1989)[C357]	21 SLE, 31 PSS, 18 MCTD, 88 normals*	M-mode, 2-D	No data	Mitral prolapse; SLE—8 (36%); PSS—10 (32%); MCTD—12 (32%); normals—9 (10%)	No data

* PSS, progressive systemic sclerosis; MCTD, mixed connective tissue disease.

females in the former condition. Thus, SLE should always be considered in the differential diagnosis of acute pericarditis, especially in women.

Echocardiography

M-mode and two-dimensional (2-D) echocardiography are currently the methods of choice for diagnosing pericardial effusions. In 1977, Elkayam et al.[E75] described asymptomatic effusions in 2 of 32 SLE patients. Other uncontrolled and retrospective studies using M-mode echocardiography have found varying frequencies of pericardial effusion. Ito et al.[K219] found effusions in 46% of 48 unselected SLE patients undergoing echocardiography. Bomaski et al.[B395] noted effusions in 49% of 47 patients, and Chia et al.[C232] described effusions in 24% of 21 unselected patients. Using both M-mode and 2-D echocardiography, Doherty et al.[C248a] found pericardial effusion in 42% of 50 SLE patients studied retrospectively. Two studies have compared the echocardiographic findings in unselected SLE patients and in age- and sex-matched healthy controls. Klinkoff et al.[K290] found pericardial involvement in 10 of 47 SLE patients and in 0 of 46 healthy controls. Effusion was present in 4 patients and pericardial thickening in 6. Crozier et al.[C445] found pericardial effusion in 27 of 50 Chinese SLE patients and in 5 of 50 matched controls, with the effusions significantly larger in the SLE patients (Table 35–1).

Cardiac Tamponade

Despite the high frequency of pericarditis and effusion, cardiac tamponade occurs rarely in SLE. Of 150 SLE patients followed prospectively by Estes and Christian,[E147] 29 developed pericarditis, and only 2 of these developed cardiac tamponade that required pericardial fenestration. The prevalence of cardiac tamponade was 0.8% in a combined series of 15 studies consisting of 1,332 SLE patients.[D249]

Cardiac tamponade has been reported as the initial manifestation of the disease in a few pediatric and adult cases, as well as late-onset SLE.[B236,C112,K158,L193,O78,P26,Z15] Fatal cardiac tamponade has also developed as a complication of heparin anticoagulation in an SLE patient undergoing hemodialysis.[L204]

Constrictive Pericarditis

Few cases of constrictive pericarditis resulting from SLE have been reported.[H247,J32,M433,Y65] All the reported cases were males; interestingly, the condition developed while the patients were on systemic corticosteroids. Pathologic findings included hyalinized fibrotic thickening of the pericardium and perivascular mononuclear infiltrates.[J32] Constrictive pericarditis has also been seen in patients with procainamide- and hydralazine-induced LE.[B527,R194]

Pathologic and Histologic Findings

The pathologic picture of the pericardium in SLE is affected by steroid therapy. Prior to the advent of corticosteroid therapy, autopsy cases showed focal or diffuse fibrinous pericarditis. Following the widespread use of steroids for treatment, a predominantly fibrous pericarditis has been observed more frequently.[B563]

The pericardial fluid in SLE is straw-colored to serosanguinous, exudative, and has a high leukocyte cell count, with a predominance of polymorphonuclear cells. Occasionally, the fluid may be hemorrhagic.[A348] Typical LE cells may be seen in the centrifuged cell sediment; their presence is helpful in diagnosing SLE as the cause of the pericarditis.[A348,S237,W328]

Pathogenesis

The pathogenesis of pericarditis in SLE probably involves the deposition of immune complexes, with activation of the complement system. Evidence supporting this includes the low concentration of whole hemolytic complement, the presence of C1q, C4, and C3 in the pericardial fluid,[G249,H500] and in vivo activation of the classic and alternative complement pathways.[H500] I have also mixed cryoglobulins and immune complexes containing antinuclear antibody (ANA), including anti-DNA antibodies in SLE pericardial fluid.[Q12] Furthermore, vascular deposits of immunoglobulins and complement have been described in the parietal pericardium of a lupus patient with constrictive pericarditis.[J32]

Treatment

The treatment of lupus pericarditis depends partly on the severity of the condition. Asymptomatic, small pericardial effusions do not necessarily require specific therapy.

Drug Therapy

Patients with mild symptoms and with small or no pericardial effusions can be treated with salicylates pushed to therapeutic levels (20 to 30 mg/dl) or preferably other nonsteroidal antiinflammatory drugs (NSAIDs), such as indomethacin (150 to 200 mg per day). An antimalarial agent can also be added to the regimen. If these measures fail, or in more severe cases, 20 to 40 mg of prednisone/day are usually beneficial. If the diagnosis of SLE is proven, it is not necessary to perform a pericardiocentesis. If the patient appears critically ill, high-dose steroids given parenterally promptly relieve symptoms and gradually reduce the size of the effusion. High-dose immunoglobulin has also been used to treat severe, life-threatening lupus pericarditis.[P145]

Septic Pericarditis and Pericardiocentesis

Septic pericarditis caused by Staphylococcus aureus, Salmonella, Mycobacterium tuberculosis, or Candida albicans have been reported, but is uncommon in SLE patients.[D271,K322,S66] Lupus pericarditis may predispose to seeding by a bloodborne pathogenic organism. If the index of suspicion of an infectious process is high pericardiocentesis is indicated, because the mortality is high if the condition is inadequately treated. Pericardiocentesis should preferably be done in an operating room with a chest surgeon and anesthetist available, because SLE patients tolerate pericardiocentesis poorly. Berbir et al.[B228] have reviewed the literature, and found that 5 of 24 procedures were complicated by death resulting from myocardial or coronary artery lacerations. At our medical center, 1 such patient had a small laceration in the ventricle discovered at autopsy. The pericardium was normal but the myocardium was flabby secondary to myocarditis. In view of the high risk of these aspirations, it seems that, during life, the pericardial lining must be extremely vascular. Furthermore, in the presence of myocarditis, the flabby myocardium is readily penetrated during the procedure and does not contract adequately to close a small puncture. Pericardial drainage should be reserved for life-threatening tamponade and for the resolution of serious diagnostic dilemmas, such as in patients with a rapidly enlarging effusion (despite high doses of systemic corticosteroids) and the need to exclude an infectious pericarditis. Following pericardiocentesis in those patients with tamponade, an indwelling catheter is placed in the pericardial space to monitor reaccumulation of fluid. It may be safer and therapeutically more beneficial to perform a pericardial fenestration or window in other patients. Pericardiectomy is rarely required.[J32,P278]

MYOCARDITIS

Primary myocardial involvement in SLE is uncommon (see Table 33–1). Myocarditis was diagnosed clinically in 8% of 520 patients by Dubois,[D340] in 8% of 150 patients by Estes and Christian,[E147] and in 10% of 128 patients by Ropes. Borenstein et al.[B418] found 5 cases of myocarditis in 140 SLE patients reviewed retrospectively for myocardial disease. In a prospective study of 100 SLE patients for cardiovascular manifestations, myocarditis was diagnosed in 14%.[B17]

Clinical Presentation

The clinical picture of SLE myocarditis is similar to that of myocarditis resulting from viral infection or some other cause. The earliest change is usually tachycardia, which is disproportional to the fever. The heart becomes diffusely enlarged, often with the point of maximal impulse at the anterior axillary line. The patient may have dyspnea, palpitations, heart murmurs, sinus tachycardia, ventricular arrhythmias, gallop rhythm, and/or congestive heart failure. The diagnosis of SLE myocarditis is often difficult to make clinically because other factors that can lead to congestive heart failure may be present, such as anemia, uncontrolled hypertension, systemic infection, valvular disease, or fluid and salt retention resulting from renal disease or systemic corticosteroid use.

Pathology

At autopsy, SLE myocarditis is diagnosed more frequently than is reported in clinical series. Among 236

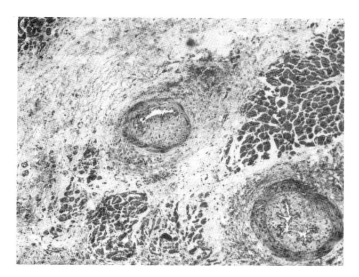

Fig. 35–1. Arteritis and scarring in the myocardium of a 9-year-old girl with SLE (H & E stain; ×85).

autopsied SLE cases collected by Doherty and Siegel[D249] from eight separate reports, myocarditis was found in 100 (40%). The pathologic abnormalities vary in severity, usually consisting of small foci of interstitial plasma cell and lymphocyte infiltrates, and, rarely, of a widespread diffuse interstitial inflammation. Fibrinoid change and hematoxylin bodies are seen.[B490] Small foci of patchy myocardial fibrosis are common in corticosteroid-treated patients.[B564] (Fig. 35–1).

Endomyocardial Biopsy

Percutaneous endomyocardial biopsy has been used for the diagnosis of myocarditis in a small number of SLE patients. Fairfax et al.[F9] found the results of the endomyocardial biopsy helpful, not only in establishing the diagnosis but also in determining the extent of the myocarditis. Cardiomyopathy secondary to chloroquine was also diagnosed in SLE patients by endomyocardial biopsy.[R55] Although the specificity and sensitivity of the endomyocardial biopsy in SLE myocarditis remains to be determined, a positive result should be helpful clinical information.

Pathogenesis

The pathogenesis of the myocardial lesion in SLE is thought to be mediated by immune complex deposition disease with complement activation. Bidani and associates[B194] found granular deposits of immunoglobulins and complement components in the walls of myocardial blood vessels, as well as along or within muscle bundles. In contrast to the extensive immune deposits, the histopathologic changes in the myocardium were more focal and less impressive, and the immune deposits did not always correlate with the site of inflammatory focus. Conversely, the intensity and extent of the immune deposits were greater in those patients who had evidence of increased serologic and clinical activity during life.

Borenstein et al.[B418] found an association between myocarditis in SLE and the presence of skeletal myositis, suggesting the possibility of a generalized process directed against striated muscles. In addition, antibodies to nuclear RNP were found uniformly in these patients, suggesting that this may define a subset of SLE patients with myositis. This is noteworthy because we have reported myocarditis in patients with mixed connective tissue disease (MCTD),[L81] an entity characterized by skeletal myositis and an elevated serum titer of antibodies to U1RNP.

The antibody activity of the immune deposits in the myocardium in SLE is not entirely clear. Antimyocardial antibodies have been found to be prevalent in SLE, but the presence of these antibodies did not correlate with cardiac involvement. We have also observed the absence of correlation with heart disease in MCTD.[L81]

Treatment

SLE patients with acute myocarditis are treated with prednisone, at least 1 mg/kg daily. In Harvey's series,[M280] 8 of 9 patients with good renal function, in whom myocarditis appeared to be the main factor contributing to heart failure, responded to cortisone therapy. This resulted in cessation of gallop rhythm, decrease in heart size, and reversion of abnormal T waves to normal configuration. In 3 patients with severe cardiac failure, the clinical response was dramatic. Cytotoxic agents such as azathioprine and cyclophosphamide have also been used in few patients.[B418,F9] Skeletal myositis responded more rapidly to systemic corticosteroids than did myocarditis in those SLE patients who had both disease processes.[B418]

MYOCARDIAL FUNCTION ABNORMALITIES AND CONGESTIVE HEART FAILURE

Myocardial Function

Myocardial function abnormalities have been found frequently in SLE patients, even in those without cardiac symptoms.

Noninvasive Studies

Strauer et al.[S726] studied cardiac hemodynamics during right and left heart catheterization in 5 young, female, SLE patients without clinical symptoms and signs of cardiac disease. Evidence of impaired pump function, reduced contractility, increased myocardial wall stiffness, and decreased coronary artery reserves were found. It was suggested that lupus cardiomyopathy may affect intrinsic contractile properties of the myocardium, and frequently may occur subclinically.

Del Rio and associates[D145] compared systolic time intervals, a noninvasive method helpful in assessing myocardial function, in 25 SLE patients and 22 healthy controls. The SLE patients had shorter left ventricular ejection times and longer pre-ejection periods than the controls, suggesting impaired left ventricular systolic function. These abnormalities were found to be independent of age, duration of SLE, blood pressure, anemia, renal disease, steroid treatment, and immunologic activity.

Two independent controlled studies from Hong Kong using full echocardiography and pulse Doppler studies found a high frequency of subclinical myocardial involvement in SLE (see Table 35–1). Crozier et al.[C445] reported that SLE patients, compared to healthy controls, have a significantly decreased left ventricular ejection fraction and diastolic compliance and an increased left ventricular systolic dimension. These abnormalities were not explained on the basis of hypertension or coronary artery disease, suggesting primary myocardial involvement. Leung et al.[L206] described an abnormal pattern of left ventricular diastolic filling dynamics characterized by prolongation of isovolumic relaxation, reduction in the rate of early diastolic filling, and reduced deceleration rate of early peak filling velocity. These abnormalities were present in patients with clinical symptoms of cardiac disease, and were more pronounced in those with active disease.

Effect of Treatment

Myocardial function in a group of SLE patients with active disease was assessed before the initiation of corticosteroid therapy and when the illness became inactive following steroid therapy. Using computer-assisted analysis of digitized echocardiograms, Murai et al.[M661] found evidence of left ventricular systolic and diastolic dysfunction that reversed with treatment. Moreover, these cardiac abnormalities were correlated with increased serum titer of anti-DS DNA antibodies as a parameter of disease activity. Been et al.[B164] detected evidence of myocardial abnormalities in SLE patients with active disease but without cardiac symptoms by magnetic resonance imaging, even though the results of other noninvasive cardiac investigations were negative.

Thus, data from various noninvasive studies (Table 35–1) consistently indicate that abnormalities in myocardial function are common in SLE patients with active disease, even in the absence of overt cardiac symptoms. That these abnormalities reverse with steroid therapy supports the immunologic basis of myocardial disease.

Congestive Heart Failure

Causes

The clinical diagnosis of congestive heart failure in SLE is often difficult because manifestations of activity of the underlying disease can mimic symptoms of cardiac failure. Failure is often preceded by fever, tachycardia, hepatomegaly, and hypertension associated with nephropathy. Corticosteroid therapy can aggravate these processes. Dyspnea resulting from pleuritis and pleural effusions is often present. In addition, the diaphragm may be elevated because of splinting from pleuritis, ascites, or primary diaphragmatic dysfunction. Other factors that may contribute and aggravate congestive heart failure are often present, such as valvulitis, myocarditis, pericarditis with effusion, and anemia. Because these may coexist, it is often difficult to ascertain how much of the patient's dyspnea and other symptoms are the result of cardiac decompensation and how much results from other manifestations of the disease.

Prevalence

Congestive heart failure was diagnosed clinically in 5% of Dubois's patient[D340] and in 11% of Estes and Christian's patients.[E147] Of 100 SLE patients followed prospectively by Badui et al.[B17] for cardiovascular manifestations, 10 developed congestive heart failure. This was associated with myocarditis in 5 patients, hypertension in 4, and valvular heart disease in 1. Congestive heart failure occurred in 10 of 142 patients (7%) reported by Hejtmancik et al.[H247] Myocarditis was the major cause of the heart failure in 6 patients. All 5 patients who succumbed to congestive heart failure had pathologic evidence of myocarditis at autopsy. In contrast, Brigden et al.[B490] diagnosed cardiac failure in 22 of 60 SLE patients and hypertension was the major cause, although rarely was it the sole responsible factor. Decompensation with a low or normal blood pressure developed in 5 patients, 3 of whom had pericarditis and 1 of whom had bacterial endocarditis. Myocarditis as the sole cause of cardiac failure was not seen in any of their patients.

Treatment

The mainstay of treatment of congestive heart failure in SLE is the suppression of the underlying process by the use of corticosteroids during the active phase of myocarditis and pericarditis, and the correction of other factors such as hypertension and anemia.

LIBMAN-SACKS ENDOCARDITIS AND VALVULAR HEART DISEASE

Libman-Sacks Endocarditis

Gross Morphology

Libman-Sacks "atypical verrucous endocarditis," the most characteristic and classic cardiac lesion of SLE, is comprised of verrucous vegetations that range from 1 to 4 mm in diameter. Grossly, the verrucae appear as "granular, tawny or pinkish, pea-sized masses densely adherent to the underlying endocardium and formed single or conglomerate and sometimes mulberry-like clusters."[B389] The lesions are found near the edge of the valve, on both surfaces of the valves, on the rings and commissures and, less frequently, on the chordae tendinea, papillary muscles, and atrial and ventricular mural endocardium.[D249] The vegetations can develop in any valve and are often multivalvular. Libman and Sacks[L269] and Gross[G405] noted the verrucae most commonly in the tricuspid valve, but more recent studies have found a higher frequency on the mitral valve,[B564,M280] especially in the recess between the posterior valve leaflet and the ventricular wall.[D249]

Histopathology

The histopathology of the vegetations is considered characteristic and differs from the lesions of rheumatic fever and bacterial endocarditis. Libman-Sacks vegetations consist of proliferating and degenerating cells, fibrin, fibrous tissues, and hematoxylin bodies. The involved leaflet contains granulation tissue, fibrin, and necrotic foci. Variable amounts of lymphocytes and plasma cells are seen. Shapiro et al.[S322] described three zones in the verrucous lesions: 1) an outer exudative zone of fibrin, nuclear debris, and hematoxylin bodies; 2) a middle zone of proliferating capillaries and fibroblasts; and 3) an inner zone of neovascularization, with thin-walled junctional blood vessels. Vascular deposits of immunoglobulins and complement have been identified in the inner zone. Bidani et al.[B294] found granular immune deposits in the endocardial stroma at the base of the valve, along the valve leaflet, and in the vegetation. These deposits are probably immune complexes, which may be important in the pathogenesis of the verrucous lesions.[B294,S322]

Diagnosis

The diagnosis of Libman-Sacks endocarditis can only be made with certainty at autopsy or at surgery. The prevalence of these lesions varies greatly among autopsy series, ranging from 13 to 74%.[B490,B564,D340,G406,H247,H497,J75, K284,K366,L174,M280,R294,S339] Prior to the availability of steroids, Doherty and Siegel[D249] found a prevalence of 59% among 86 autopsy cases reported in the literature. In contrast, 35% of 236 autopsy cases reported after 1953 who had received steroids had Libman-Sacks verrucous lesions.

Another explanation for the decreasing prevalence may be that the endocardial lesions were formerly considered a requisite to the diagnosis, because these constituted the most specific gross postmortem findings, whereas the diagnosis of SLE is now made primarily on clinical grounds. Thus, the latter series would not be weighted in favor of endocardial involvement.

The clinical diagnosis of Libman-Sacks endocarditis is difficult. The physical findings and echocardiographic abnormalities may suggest the diagnosis, but are not diagnostic. Many patients with active SLE have tachycardia, anemia, and fever, all of which may be associated with a cardiac murmur. Thus, it is often difficult to interpret the significance of murmurs, even if they are of greater intensity. Griffith and Vural[G378] demonstrated that the diagnosis of verrucous endocarditis cannot be made on the basis of systolic murmurs. They heard systolic murmurs in only 2 of 6 patients with Libman-Sacks endocarditis at autopsy. Kong et al.[K366] noted systolic murmurs in 13 of 30 autopsied cases, but Libman-Sacks endocarditis was found in only 4.

Complications

Libman-Sacks endocarditis rarely produces hemodynamic changes, but it has been associated with ruptured chordae tendineae,[K238] aortic stenosis,[P302] thromboembolic disease,[P302] and cerebral emboli.[F181]

Valvular Heart Disease

It is now recognized that hemodynamically and clinically significant valvular disease occurs in SLE patients, and may require prosthetic valve replacement. Aortic insufficiency represents the most commonly reported lesions.[B222,B248,E72,I30,S399] Doherty and Siegel[D249] collected 36 cases in the English literature and concluded that the insufficiency is probably a result of multiple factors, including Libman-Sacks endocarditis, fibrinoid degeneration causing thinning and fenestration of the valve cusps, distortion of the valve tissue by fibrosis, valvulitis, bacterial endocarditis, aortitis, and aortic dissection. They identified systemic hypertension, steroid therapy, bicuspid aortic valves, and rheumatic fever as risk factors in some of the patients.

Few cases of significant isolated mitral insufficiency or of combined mitral and aortic insufficiency have been described in SLE patients.[B307,M673,R75] Bulkley and Roberts[B161] have suggested that steroid therapy leads to the healing of verrucae and fibrous scarring. The posterior mitral leaflet and its chordae tendineae become shortened and adhere to the underlying mural endocardium, causing mitral regurgitation. Other causes include fibrinoid necrosis of the papillary muscles and rupture of the chordae tendineae.[D249] Color Doppler echocardiography has shown a high frequency of valvular regurgitation in SLE, with right-sided regurgitation more common than left-sided regurgitation. Right-sided regurgitation may be related to pulmonary vascular lesions causing increased pulmonary artery pressure.[E112] Massive thrombotic deposits on the valve causing isolated aortic stenosis[P302] and isolated mitral stenosis[V53] have also been reported.

Surgery for Valvular Disease

Dajee et al.[D15] summarized findings on 15 valve replacements in 12 SLE patients. Of these, 7 were aortic and 8 were mitral. Although the overall surgical mortality rate was 25%, it was shown that valve replacement can be successful in selected SLE patients; also, 2 patients required repeat valve surgery.[M626,R75] Walts and Dubois[W64] reported a case of a fatal acute dissecting aneurysm of the aorta that complicated an aortic valve replacement procedure. Marked mucoid degeneration of the aorta was found.

Two studies have suggested that valvular heart disease is becoming a significant cause of morbidity and mortality in SLE patients. In a retrospective analysis of 421 SLE patients, Straaton et al.[S718] found 14 patients with clinically significant valvular heart disease. Of these, 6 patients had anatomic features of SLE valvular disease, such as verrucous vegetations or valvulitis with necrosis and valvulitis. Successful valve replacement was done in 2 patients, but 4 died from cardiac complications. Thus, 1 to 2% of SLE patients develop hemodynamically significant valve disease. Galve and associates[G23] studied a group of 74 SLE patients and 60 matched healthy controls prospectively for 5 years for valvular heart disease using echocardiography. Four groups were identified: 7 patients had Libman-Sacks verrucous vegetations (group 1); 6 had rigid and thickened valves with stenosis, regurgitation, or both (group 2); 5 had miscellaneous valvular abnormalities without significant dysfunction (group 3); and 56 had normal findings (group 4). Valve surgery was required for 1 patient in group 1 and for 5 in group 2. Thus, the overall prevalence of clinically important valvular disease in this study was 18%. The chronic valvular lesions seen in group 2 patients probably represents the healed stage of Libman-Sacks endocarditis. Indirect evidence for this is that these patients were older, had SLE for a longer period, and had received greater amounts of corticosteroids than those with verrucous vegetations.

Association with Antiphospholipid Antibodies

Valvular heart disease, particularly affecting the mitral valve in SLE patients, appears to correlate with the presence of antiphospholipid antibodies. In 1988, Ford et al.[F163] described two SLE patients with clinically significant mitral insufficiency and associated lupus anticoagulant. Both patients underwent prosthetic valve replacement, and both had thrombus formation on the mitral valve. Chartash et al.[C214] described a syndrome in 11 patients characterized by a tetrad of recurrent thrombotic disease, valvulitis, thrombocytopenia, and antiphospholipid antibodies. Of these, 8 had aortic insufficiency, 3 had isolated mitral regurgitation, and 2 had combined lesions. One multicenter prospective study undertaken on 132 consecutive SLE patients and 68 healthy controls using echocardiography has confirmed this association.[K185] Valvular lesions were found in 22.7% of patients and in 2.9% of controls. Antiphospholipid antibodies were present in 50 patients (38%). The prevalence of valve vegetations (16%) and of mitral regurgitation (38%) was significantly higher in SLE patients with antiphospholipid antibodies than in those without (1.2 and 12%, respectively). Clinically significant valvular disease developed in 6 patients, although only 1 required surgery. In a controlled study using M-mode, 2-D, and Doppler echocardiography, Leung et al.[L206] found a positive correlation between antiphospholipid antibodies and valvular abnormalities, and with isolated left ventricular dysfunction.

The significance of antiphospholipid antibodies in the pathogenesis of valvular lesions in SLE patients is not clear. The vascular deposits of immunoglobulins and complement in the valve lesions[B294,S322] suggest that antigen-antibody complexes may be important in the growth and proliferation of the vegetations. Whether antiphospholipid antibodies participate in the formation of pathogenic immune complexes remains to be determined. Antiphospholipid antibodies may only play a secondary (but important) role in lupus valvular disease. The thrombotic tendency associated with antiphospholipid antibodies may contribute to the thrombosis on the cardiac valves, which are primarily damaged by other processes. One review of neuropathologic findings in SLE showed a high frequency of brain infarcts caused by cardiac emboli from Libman-Sacks endocarditis, chronic valvulitis, and mural thrombus.[D188]

Infective Endocarditis

Libman-Sacks endocarditis may be complicated by infective endocarditis. An analysis of 15 reports by Doherty and Siegel[D249] showed that 4.9% of Libman-Sacks endocarditis cases diagnosed at autopsy and 1.3% of clinically diagnosed cases were complicated by infective endocarditis. Bacterial endocarditis was diagnosed in 6 of 571 SLE patients admitted to the National Institutes of Health (NIH) and in 2 of 142 patients of Ropes.[L174,R294] In the NIH study, all 6 patients were treated with corticosteroids, and 4 had pre-existing heart murmurs. Endocarditis occurred after dental procedures in 2 subjects and for no known cause in 4 patients. Endocarditis was diagnosed in 1% of SLE patients, a greater percentage than in any other connective tissue disease seen at the NIH. Antibiotic prophylaxis is recommended prior to operative dental and other surgical procedures in all SLE patients. The need for prophylaxis is further supported by the disproportionately high frequency of mitral valve prolapse in SLE diagnosed by echocardiography.[C357,K290]

CORONARY ARTERY DISEASE AND MYOCARDIAL INFARCTION

Frequency

The incidence of coronary artery disease and myocardial infarction in SLE patients appears to be increasing. The occurrence of myocardial infarction in female lupus patients below the age of 35 years has been reported.[D249] Two mechanisms are implicated in the pathogenesis of coronary artery disease in SLE patients. Atherosclerosis, a pathologic process that is accelerated by long-term corticosteroid use, is the most common. Vasculitis involving the extramural coronary arteries and resulting in luminal occlusion is the other cause, although rare.

In 1964, Dubois described a 35-year-old white female with classic ECG changes who died of acute myocardial infarction.[D340] At autopsy, vasculitis of the extramural coronary artery with acute hemorrhage was found (Fig. 35–2) In the same year, Bonfiglio et al.[B404] described four women with coronary artery disease and SLE. One patient died as a result of coronary arteritis at the age of 16 years. Three patients had angina pectoris, and coronary angiography demonstrated severe focal stenosis. The first established occurrence of coronary arteritis in a live patient was reported by Heibel et al. in 1976.[H243] Saccular aneu-

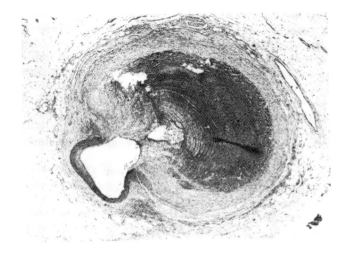

Fig. 35–2. Coronary artery from a 35-year-old woman who had acute myocardial infarction secondary to vasculitis of the extramural coronary artery with acute hemorrhage (H & E stain; ×35).

rysms were found on angiography, producing significant obstruction in what had been a normal vessel 18 days earlier.

Myocardial Infarction

Myocardial infarctions have been reported in SLE patients below the age of 35 years, even as young as 5 years old.[147] In 1982, Homcy et al.[H401] described 6 cases of ischemic heart disease in SLE patients aged 15 to 29 years. Of these, 3 patients had atherosclerotic lesions, and 1 was helped by coronary artery bypass surgery. Coronary arteritis was found in 3 patients; 1 of these was diagnosed during life and benefited from systemic corticosteroids.

In 1983, Spiera and Rothenberg[S582] described 4 other relatively young patients with premature coronary artery disease caused by atherosclerosis. They were 22 to 34 years old, and all had lupus nephritis and hypertension. All had been on long-term steroid therapy, with a mean duration of 9 years. Severe coronary atherosclerosis rather than vasculitis was seen at autopsy.

Doherty and Siegel[D249] analyzed the features of 33 SLE patients younger than 35 years of age with coronary artery disease reported in the literature. The vessel lesion was atherosclerosis in 12 patients, arteritis in 7, and stenosis in 6. It is unclear whether the latter was a result of atherosclerosis or vasculitis. The most common presenting manifestation was myocardial infarction, followed by congestive heart failure and sudden death. The left anterior descending artery was involved in most cases, and thrombosis was frequently noted.

Pathology

Immunoglobulins and complement components have been identified in the walls of inflamed and non-inflamed extramural coronary arteries in SLE patients with coronary vasculitis.[K382] The deposition of immune complexes may lead to arteritis, luminal narrowing, and tissue ischemia. In addition, the immunologically mediated vascular damage predisposes to the development of atherosclerosis, which further narrows the vessel and produces occlusion by intimal thickening. Fukumoto et al.[F304] found that the thickness of the intima of coronary arteries in SLE patients measured at autopsy is greater compared to non-SLE controls. Interestingly, the intimal thickening was significantly greater in 4 SLE patients who had not been treated with corticosteroids during life than in those who had received steroids. Although the number of patients in the former group was small, the data suggest that the underlying inflammatory process resulting from SLE promotes atherosclerosis.

Haider and Roberts[H42] measured the degree of coronary artery narrowing in 22 SLE patients at autopsy. Of these, 10 patients had at least one major coronary artery narrowed by more than 76%. These patients had higher mean blood pressures, higher serum cholesterol levels, and an increased frequency of mitral valve disease and pericardial adhesions. Thus, hypertension and hypercholesterolemia may contribute to the accelerated coronary atherosclerosis. The higher frequency of pericardial and

valvular involvement suggests the possible role of immunologic factors.

Differential Diagnosis and Treatment

Coronary artery disease in a young SLE patient may pose a problem in clinical management. Homcy et al.[H401] reported that, in the presence of concomitant extracardiac involvement, medical treatment was determined by the underlying disease rather than by the cardiac status. Conversely, in the absence of extracardiac involvement, management was primarily determined by the heart condition. The latter patient underwent aggressive cardiac evaluation and intervention, including angiography.

The differentiation between atherosclerosis and arteritis in a lupus patient with coronary artery disease is clinically important. Coronary angiography in patients with vasculitis have shown smooth focal lesions, aneurysmal dilation, and an abrupt change from normal to severe obstruction of a coronary artery on serial studies.[H243,H401] The presence of these abnormalities can, at best, only provide a presumptive diagnosis of vasculitis, but it is the only method of evaluation currently available.[K382] A therapeutic decision can then be made to institute high-dose steroid and/or cytotoxic therapy or to consider surgery.

ELECTROCARDIOGRAPHIC CHANGES AND CONDUCTION DEFECTS

The electrocardiographic record can be useful in the diagnosis and treatment of SLE patients. It is of particular value in equivocal cases in whom the tracing shows changes suggestive of pericarditis or myocarditis that are not apparent by history and physical examination, thereby alerting the clinician to evaluate carefully for evidence of multisystem disease. The electrocardiogram may show abnormalities caused by electrolyte imbalance, which are not uncommon in patients with renal or cardiac disease who are receiving corticosteroids and/or diuretics.

Frequency of Abnormalities

Abnormal electrocardiograms are often found in SLE patients, but no changes are actually considered characteristic of the disease.[S339] Abnormal tracings were found in 34% of 291 patients by Dubois[D340] and in 74% of 100 female SLE patients followed by Badui et al.[B17] specifically for cardiovascular disease. Differences in patient selection, frequency of obtaining an electrocardiogram, and other factors probably account for the wide variation in the prevalence of abnormalities.

Kong et al.[K366] correlated electrocardiograms with the findings at autopsy in 30 SLE patients. Low voltage was noted in 10 patients and, at autopsy, 5 had pericarditis, 1 had pericardial effusion, and 3 had myocarditis. Nonspecific T-wave changes and RST depression interpreted as indicative of myocardial dysfunction were recorded in 5 patients. Cardiac lesions were found in 4 patients, pericarditis in 1, myocarditis in 2, and left ventricular hypertrophy in 1. Of 9 patients with normal electrocardiograms, 4 had cardiac lesions at postmortem examination, including adhesive pericarditis, mild focal myocarditis, and left ventricular hypertrophy. Thus, electrocardiographic findings in SLE correlated poorly with the pathologic lesions in the heart seen at autopsy.

Conduction Defects

Conduction defects and rhythm disturbances are not uncommon in SLE patients. The prevalence is not known, although it has seldom been reported to be more than 10%.[J38] Studies using constant electrocardiographic monitoring are not available. Different types of abnormalities have been described, including bundle branch block, atrioventricular block, complete heart block, and atrial premature contraction.[B17,H247,I54J75,M380,S339] First-degree heart block is uncommon in SLE patients; it is more characteristic of acute rheumatic fever. Occasional patients with first-degree block in SLE, however, have been reported.[B17J75,M280]

Pathology of the Conduction System

James et al.[J38] examined the cardiac conduction system in eight SLE patients who had an arrhythmia or conduction disturbance prior to death, three of whom died suddenly. One patient had sudden onset of complete heart block followed by cardiac arrest. Focal degeneration and fibrosis of the sinus node caused by arteritis and occlusion of the central sinus node artery were found. Damage to the atrioventricular node was less extensive but showed focal degeneration secondary to small artery pathology. Bharati et al.[B283] studied the cardiac conduction system in a 12-year-old girl with complete heart block, lupus nephritis, and renal failure. The sinoatrial and atrioventricular nodes were completely replaced by fibroblastic and mononuclear cells. Degenerative and necrotic changes in the small blood vessels and capillaries had occurred. Thus, disturbances in cardiac rhythm and in conduction in SLE patients may be associated with structural damage to the conduction system.

The prevalence of coronary atherosclerosis is increasing in SLE patients. Ischemic heart disease should therefore be considered as a cause of electrocardiographic abnormalities in this disease.

Persistent Tachycardia

Estes and Christian[E147] observed persistent sinus tachycardia in the absence of fever or other manifestations of heart disease in 19 of 150 patients. We have also seen similar cases, and this often presents a clinical problem in management if the patient is otherwise asymptomatic. Echocardiography and other noninvasive cardiac laboratory tests are indicated to exclude myocardial dysfunction. Increasing the dosage of steroids may suppress the tachycardia in some patients. In the absence of other evidence of cardiac disease, however, it may be necessary to use a steroid dose that partially controls the tachycardia but that has no excessive side effects. β-blockers such as propranolol may be helpful in patients with symptomatic sinus tachycardia.

HYPERTENSION

Prevalence

Arterial hypertension is a common feature of SLE (see Table 33–1). Blood pressure readings over 140/90 mm of Hg were found at some time in the clinical course in 25% of Dubois' 520 patients.[D340] The mean prevalence of hypertension in nine published series of SLE patients is 28.8% (range, 12 to 49%).

Causes

Hypertension in SLE is related to the development of nephropathy and to the use of systemic corticosteroids. In 1948, Humphreys[H497] suggested that, in the absence of renal disease, the blood pressure in SLE patients is normal or, more often, low. Subsequent investigators have confirmed the frequent association between hypertension and renal disease in SLE. Brigden and associates[B490] reported that, of 26 hypertensive SLE patients in their series, 20 had renal disease, 2 had incidental essential hypertension, and the remaining 4 developed hypertension while on systemic corticosteroids. Kong et al.[K366] found hypertension in 16 of 30 SLE patients at autopsy, and all had evidence of nephropathy. An additional 9 patients with renal involvement had normal blood pressure. In contrast to these findings, a retrospective analysis of 232 SLE patients at the NIH revealed that hypertension occurs early in the course of SLE in many patients, and that it is not necessarily associated with clinically severe renal disease.[B558] Two-thirds of the hypertensive SLE patients had a creatinine clearance greater than 60 ml/minute and nonnephrotic–range proteinuria. Moreover, only 60% of their patients with biopsy-proven diffuse glomerulonephritis were hypertensive. Normotensive SLE patients tended to be on a lower dosage of corticosteroids than the hypertensive patients, but considerable overlap occurred between the two groups.

Complications

Long-standing hypertension can lead to the development of myocardial hypertrophy in SLE patients. Although hypertension is a major factor in the pathogenesis of congestive heart failure in SLE, it is rarely the only cause. Other predisposing factors are often present, such as anemia, myocarditis, pericarditis, infection, and corticosteroid use.

Effect of Corticosteroids

In 1952, Sofer and Bader[S535] noted the development of hypertension in 9 of 18 SLE patients receiving steroid therapy, although it was initially present in 1. In 5 patients, blood pressure returned to normal as the steroid dosage was reduced. Approximately 10 to 19% of patients developed a significant rise in blood pressure following steroid therapy.[D309] Hypertension developed in 10% of 32 patients treated with prednisone or prednisolone,[D309] in 13% of 40 patients on methylprednisolone,[D312,D314] in 17% of 29 patients on triamcinolone,[D311] and in 19% of 50 patients treated with dexamethasone.[D315] Increases in blood pressure as high as 60 mm Hg systolic and 30 mm

Hg diastolic occurred with steroids alone in patients without renal disease. Severe hypertension may occur as a complication of high-dose pulse methylprednisolone.

Treatment

Hypertension in SLE usually responds to drug therapy, and the general outlook does not appear to be as poor as previously believed. The dosage of corticosteroids should be reduced, if feasible, in those with poorly controlled hypertension. It is sometimes necessary to add a steroid-sparing agent such as azathioprine to the regimen to allow the reduction of steroid dose in such patients. Occasionally, severe, uncontrollable hypertension may occur in SLE patients with nephritis and, in a few such patients, generalized vasculitis involving the renal arteries has been found at autopsy.[R294] Malignant hypertension with papilledema may occur. Of 31 hypertensive SLE patients of Hejtmanck,[H247] 2 developed malignant hypertension.

Various agents can be used to treat hypertension in SLE patients. Although certain antihypertensive agents such as hydralazine, methyldopa, and β blockers can cause lupus-like syndrome, they have been used safely in idiopathic SLE without exacerbating the disease.[R184] Calcium channel blockers such as nifedipine are effective and are generally safe in SLE patients.[B592] I have also found angiotensin I-converting enzyme inhibitors such as enalapril to be effective and well tolerated in SLE, although a few of our patients, especially those with lupus nephritis, developed mild hyperkalemia, which necessitated discontinuation of the drug.

EFFECT OF CORTICOSTEROIDS ON THE HEART IN SLE

The longterm use of systemic corticosteroids for the treatment of SLE can result not only in an increased prevalence of hypertension, left ventricular hypertrophy, and congestive heart failure, but also in other important changes in the heart. Bulkley and Roberts[B564] have compared the pathologic findings in the hearts of 36 autopsied SLE patients who were treated with systemic corticosteroids to those of patients studied before systemic corticosteroids were used for treatment. They found that the frequency of lupus carditis was the same in the two groups, but the morphology of the endocardial and pericardial lesions differed. In the steroid-treated patients, the Libman-Sacks endocardial lesions were smaller, fewer in number, and involved single rather than multiple valves. The mitral valve was most commonly involved in the steroid-treated patients, and the lesions showed evidence of partial or complete healing. The lesions consisted of deposits of fibrin on the surfaces, with focal fibrosis and necrosis. Proliferation of vascularized fibrous tissue (healing) uniformly occurred at the periphery of the active lesion. Calcification of the mitral annular and subannular regions also occurred. The scarring led to variable thickening of the leaflet tissue and to adherence of the leaflet to the mural endocardium. In 1 patient, the scarring led to severe mitral regurgitation and, in 2, to aortic insufficiency. The change in valve lesions may "cure" the noninfective endocarditis of SLE, analogous to the cure of infective endocarditis by antibiotics. The pericardium in nonsteroid-treated patients showed active fibrinous changes. In contrast, steroid-treated patients most commonly showed a fibrous (healed) pericarditis and, occasionally, infective pericarditis. The focal lesions of lupus myocarditis were found less frequently in steroid-treated patients. Steroid-treated SLE patients showed increased amounts of epicardial fat and intramyocardial fat, especially in the right ventricle, probably analogous to the deposition of subcutaneous adipose tissue in the face and upper back. Finally, steroid-treated patients showed a greater degree and frequency of narrowing of extramural coronary arteries by atherosclerotic plaques, leading to significant ischemic heart disease.

CHEST PAIN

Chest pain is a frequent complaint of SLE patients. The evaluation of such a patient is based on the same general principles followed for any patient presenting with acute or chronic chest pain. A thorough clinical history and careful physical examination are the cornerstone of the diagnostic process. Certain clinical entities, however, should be remembered when formulating the differential diagnosis of chest pain in SLE, because these conditions may be relatively more prevalent in these patients.

Causes

Cardiac Causes

Acute lupus pericarditis is probably the most common cause of chest pain of cardiac origin in SLE patients. The patient may present with the typical retrosternal pain, which builds in intensity, is aggravated by lying down, swallowing, and/or inspiration, and eases with sitting and leaning forward. Concomitant pleurisy is often present. Angina pectoris should be considered, even in a young female, because longterm steroid therapy can lead to accelerated atherosclerosis and coronary artery disease. Although rare, arteritis of the extramural coronary arteries can develop, resulting in myocardial infarction. Other cardiac causes include chest pain associated with mitral valve prolapse, which appears to be more prevalent among SLE patients.[C357,K290]

Extracardiac Causes

Pleurisy with or without effusion is one of the most common intrathoracic causes of chest pain in SLE patients. Pleurisy may not necessarily be a result of the underlying disease, but of tuberculosis or other infections. Bacterial pneumonia can present with pleuritic or nonpleuritic chest pain. Pulmonary embolism should be considered in the differential diagnosis of acute chest pain, particularly in those with antiphospholipid antibody syndrome. It must be stressed that pulmonary embolism may occur even in patients who test negative for anticardiolipin antibodies or lupus anticoagulant. Less frequent causes of chest pain include diffuse spasm and other esophageal abnormalities,[P111] and pulmonary arterial hypertension.[Q21] Patients on aspirin or other NSAIDs and corticosteroids are prone to gastritis and peptic ulcer disease and, when complicated by esophageal reflux, epigastric and retrosternal pain may develop.

Pain arising from musculoskeletal structures should be specifically sought. Costochondritis and fibromyalgia are not uncommon in SLE patients, and both conditions are characterized by thoracic or chest wall pain.[R294] The examiner should palpate for tender points in the upper chest, trapezius, and infrascapular regions. Osteoporosis complicating chronic steroid therapy predisposes to rib fractures and vertebral body collapse.

Renal vein thrombosis in a patient with lupus nephritis and nephrotic syndrome may present with pleuritic chest pain.[A270]

Laboratory Evaluation

In choosing the laboratory investigations needed to evaluate the individual patient, the clinician should be guided by the clinical history and physical findings. A chest roentgenogram, ECG, and echocardiogram are helpful when intrathoracic causes of chest pain are being considered. The laboratory diagnoses of acute pulmonary embolism, angina pectoris, myocardial infarction, and chronic pain associated with esophageal abnormalities are basically the same in lupus and in non-SLE patients. When exacerbation of the underlying disease is suspected, serologic markers of disease activity, such as anti-dsDNA and serum complement levels, should be obtained. Evidence of other organ involvement should be sought. Tests for anticardiolipin antibodies and lupus anticoagulant are helpful in those patients with thromboembolic disease and valvular heart disease.

SUMMARY

1. Chest and cardiac complaints in SLE patients related to ischemic heart disease, hypertension, arrhythmias, heart failure, or pericarditis must be differentiated from pulmonary complaints and esophageal and musculoskeletal abnormalities.

2. Pericarditis is present in 6 to 45% of SLE patients; pericardial effusions are identified by echocardiograms in 21 to 49%. Pericardial lesions are found in 60 to 80% of cases at autopsy.

3. Most SLE patients with small pericardial effusions do not require specific drug therapy. Mild to moderate pericarditis can be treated with salicylates or with other NSAIDs. Moderate to severe symptoms respond to 20 to 80 mg of prednisone daily. Rare instances of cardiac tamponade can be relieved, preferably by fenestration.

4. Acute myocarditis occurs in 8 to 10% of patients, and usually responds to steroid therapy. Evidence of myocardial dysfunction by the use of noninvasive studies is common, even in patients without cardiac symptoms.

5. Libman-Sacks endocarditis is not uncommon in SLE patients, but it rarely causes significant hemodynamic changes. Steroids may lead to healing and fibrosis of verrucous endocarditis, resulting in chronic valve dysfunction. Clinically significant valvular disease is associated with the presence of antiphospholipid antibodies.

6. Young, hypertensive, hypercholesterolemic, steroid-treated SLE patients have accelerated atherosclerosis, and may develop coronary artery disease. Coronary arteritis is rare and may coexist with atherosclerotic heart disease, but, unlike the latter, may respond to steroid therapy.

7. All SLE patients should receive antimicrobial prophylaxis prior to and during surgery, including dental procedures.

Chapter 36

PULMONARY MANIFESTATIONS

FRANCISCO P. QUISMORIO, JR.

Primary involvement of the lungs and pleurae is common in SLE. The clinical manifestations are protean, and can sometimes become the presenting feature of the disease. Subclinical involvement is also prevalent, as evident from the high frequency of abnormal pulmonary function test results in patients free of respiratory complaints. The pulmonary disease in some patients, as in those with lung hemorrhage, predominates the clinical picture and determines the overall prognosis. Table 33–1 lists the cumulative percentages of pleurisy, pleural effusion, and lupus pneumonitis in large series of patients. This chapter discusses the clinical and pathologic features of specific entities affecting the pleura, lung parenchyma, airways, pulmonary vasculature and respiratory muscles in SLE patients.

HISTORICAL PERSPECTIVE

In 1904, Osler[O107] remarked on the frequency of pneumonia in SLE, and suggested that the "recurring skin lesions, the pleuropneumonia, the phlebitis, the general glandular enlargement and the fatal nephritis were due to one and the same poison." In 1934, Tremaine[T211] reported two young females with polyserositis and patchy lung consolidation who were probably SLE patients. Rakov and Taylor[R20] in 1942 and Foldes[F137] in 1946 focused attention on the pulmonary changes, describing isolated cases of SLE with "atelectising pneumonitis" leading to respiratory failure. At autopsy, diffuse consolidation of the lungs was seen, with hyaline thickening of the alveoli and marked cellular infiltration obliterating normal landmarks. Baggentoss[B25] noted this type of pneumonitis and observed a peculiar basophilic, mucinous edema of the alveolar walls and the peribronchial and perivascular tissues in association with interstitial pneumonitis and alveolar hemorrhage. These pathologic changes were distinct from the ordinary pyogenic and fibrinous bronchopneumonia that frequently complicates the terminal stages of SLE, but were not pathognomonic of SLE.[P336] In "atelectising pneumonitis," the alveolar walls and peribronchial and perivascular connective tissues were apparently the primary sites of an inflammatory process that obliterated alveolar spaces.

In 1953 and 1954, two reports of roentgenographic studies in SLE emphasized the high frequency of pulmonary involvement. Israel[I51] showed that nonspecific pneumonia occurred frequently, not only during the terminal stages of SLE but throughout the course of the disease. Garland and Sisson[G51] reported lung parenchymal changes in one-third of their patients, and observed pleural and cardiac abnormalities to be prevalent.

Comprehensive reviews of pulmonary manifestations of SLE in adults[Q13,S248] and in children[D141] have appeared.

PATHOLOGY

Various types of gross and histologic lesions have been described in the lungs, but none of these changes is considered specific for SLE. A pathologic study of the lungs of 54 cases at autopsy by Purnell et al.[P336] showed the following abnormalities in more than 50%: bronchopneumonia, hemorrhage, pleural effusion, edema, interstitial pneumonia, and congestion. Fibrinoid necrosis and hematoxylin bodies were seen occasionally,[Q72] whereas bronchiolar dilatation and foci of panacinar emphysema were often found.[G408] Fayemi[F34] noted the high frequency of occlusive vascular changes of varying severity in the lungs of 8 of 20 SLE patients; these affected arterioles, arteries, and veins. The acute lesions consisted of fibrinoid necrosis and vasculitis, and the chronic lesions included intimal fibrosis, medial hypertrophy, alteration of the elastic laminae, and periadventitial fibrosis.

Haupt and associates[H207] examined the pathologic changes in the lungs of 120 patients seen at autopsy and correlated these with their clinical features. In contrast to the high frequency of lung involvement in clinical series,[Q13] they showed that many of the pathologic lesions were not caused by SLE itself but by secondary factors, such as congestive heart failure, infection, aspiration, and oxygen toxicity. Only 18% of the lung parenchymal lesions were found to be directly attributable to SLE.

Analyses of autopsy cases, although informative, do not necessarily represent a cross section of the general SLE population. Moreover, in the clinical setting, pulmonary abnormalities can change rapidly and can subside spontaneously or with drug therapy, so anatomic lesions may not be evident later, at autopsy.

PLEURISY

Prevalence

Pleurisy is the most common manifestation of the respiratory involvement in SLE (see Table 33–1). Recurrent pleuritic pain was noted in 45% of 520 patients of Dubois,[D340] and pleural effusion was detected in 30.3%. Harvey et al.[M280] reported pleurisy in 56% of their patients, and 16% had associated pleural effusion. Recurrent

343

episodes of pleuritis were noted in 13% of their patients. The high frequency of pleurisy has been reported by other investigators, ranging from 41 to 56%,[E147,G385,R294] but a definitive diagnosis of pleurisy in clinical series has not been well defined.

Radiographic and autopsy studies have confirmed the high prevalence of pleurisy. In a retrospective analysis of the chest roentgenograms of 111 SLE patients, Levin[L214] found pleural effusion in 33 patients. No effusion was seen in 5 patients with pleurisy diagnosed clinically. Ropes described pleural changes in 93% of 58 SLE patients at autopsy, with fluid in the pleural cavity in 33.

Clinical Features of Pleurisy

Pleuritic chest pain may be unilateral or bilateral and is usually located at the costophrenic margins, either anteriorly or posteriorly. Attacks of pleuritis pain often last for several days and, when associated with effusions, the pain may persist for weeks. The effusion generally occurs on the side of the chest pain. It must be noted that pleural effusions may occur in SLE patients with nephrotic syndrome as part of the anasarca and, in these patients, may be asymptomatic.[L214] Pleural effusion may also be the result of an infectious process, such as tuberculosis.

Pleurisy as the initial manifestation of SLE was noted by Dubois in 13 of 520 patients.[D306] Pleural symptoms may antedate other manifestations by months or years, resulting in a delay in the diagnosis of SLE. Winslow et al.[W307] emphasized this type of presentation and reported three cases. In addition, they noted that pleural involvement was among the earliest symptoms in 16 of 57 patients.

Pleural Fluid

The volume of pleural effusions is usually low to moderate (400 to 1000 ml); (Table 36–1).[G286,Q13] Large pleural effusions are uncommon. The effusion may be unilateral (right- or left-sided) or bilateral. Thoracentesis is often not necessary in lupus pleuritis unless the cause of the pleural effusion is uncertain. The pleural fluid in SLE is exudative in character, although transudative pleural fluids have also been reported.[Q13] The fluid can be yellow, amber, or slightly turbid in color. In a study of 14 patients with lupus pleuritis,[G286] the white cell count in the pleural fluids ranged from 325 to 14,950 cells/mm³ (mean, 4,895 cells/mm³). Half of the specimens showed a predominance of polymorphonuclear leukocytes, with cell counts ranging from 10 to 100% (mean, 57%). The pleural fluid of one lupus patient showed a predominance

Table 36–1.   Characteristics of Pleural Fluid in SLE

Color: yellow to amber
Protein: >3 g/dl
White blood cells: 3,000 to 5,000/mm³, with mononuclear and lymphocyte predominance
Glucose: near serum levels
C3 and C4: decreased
ANA titer: ≥serum titer
Cell sediment: contains typical LE cells
pH: usually >7.35

of T lymphocytes (70%) in contrast to that of peripheral blood (28%).[M390] Kelly et al.[K150] examined pleural effusions from 10 SLE patients and found atypical cells resembling plasma cells. The presence of these cells with other inflammatory cells, fibrinoid debris erythrocytes, and few mesothelial cells, and in the absence of pathogenic organisms or malignant cells, constituted a pattern characteristic of SLE in 8 of 10 patients studied.

In most patients with lupus pleuritis, the pleural fluid glucose concentration is greater than 60 mg/dl, with a pleural fluid:serum glucose ratio greater than 0.5. Good et al.[G286] found the mean pleural fluid:serum glucose ratio to be 0.3 or lower. This contrasts with the finding of low glucose levels in the pleural fluid of rheumatoid arthritis patients with pleurisy, in whom the glucose concentration is less than 30 mg/dl in 75% of patients.[S306] Low glucose concentrations or a low pleural fluid:serum glucose ratio may also occur in those with malignant effusions,[M390] empyema (80%), or tuberculosis (20%).[S306]

The pH of SLE pleural fluid is usually greater than 7.35. A few patients have a pH less than 7.3 associated with a low pleural fluid glucose level.[S306,G286]

Pandya and associates[P25] were the first to document the presence of classic LE cells in smears of SLE pleural fluids, indicative of an in vivo LE cell phenomenon. This finding has been confirmed by other investigators.[G286,R91] In a series of eight SLE patients who had pleural fluids examined for LE cells, seven were found to have at least one typical LE cell.[G286] The yield of LE cells can be increased by incubating the pleural fluid at room temperature for a few hours before examination.[R91] LE cells have been found in cytocentrifuge preparations of lupus pleural fluid.[K179] It has been suggested that the presence of in vivo LE cells in the pleural fluid is highly characteristic of SLE, and has not been described in other conditions except in drug-induced LE.[C78] It must be emphasized, however, that a positive LE cell test in blood is not diagnostic of SLE, and currently no information is available as to whether LE cells are present in pleural fluid in those with rheumatoid arthritis or other conditions in which LE cell tests of the blood can be positive.[Q13]

The presence of antinuclear antibodies (ANA) in the pleural fluid as a diagnostic test for lupus pleuritis has been studied. Leechawengwong and colleagues[L151] tested pleural fluid from 100 consecutive patients with pleural effusion and found positive ANA in all 7 patients with SLE and in 1 patient with drug-induced LE, but not in patients with other diagnoses. Conversely, Small and associates[S495] found that a positive ANA in the pleural fluid was not specific for SLE, but was also found in non-SLE patients with pleural effusions who tested positive for ANA in the blood. Good and co-workers[G286] measured the ANA titer in paired samples of pleural fluid and serum of SLE patients. In lupus pleuritis, the pleural fluid:serum ANA ratio was greater than 1. In contrast, the ratio was less than one in SLE patients who had pleural effusions from other causes, such as congestive heart failure. Moreover, none of 67 patients with pleural effusions of different causes had a positive ANA. To establish the clinical usefulness of the pleural fluid:serum ANA ratio further studies are needed to examine this parameter in other conditions, such as cancer and other systemic rheumatic diseases.

In 1972, Hunder and associates[H501] found significantly reduced levels of hemolytic complement, C1q, C4, and C3 in SLE pleural fluids when compared to the pleural fluids of patients with cancer, heart failure, and other conditions. Low levels of pleural fluid complement are not specific for SLE, but have been found in those with rheumatoid arthritis (RA)[G200,H501,P150] and empyema.[A224,P150] The reduction in complement level in SLE pleural fluid is evident, even after an adjustment is made for the total protein content of the pleural fluid.[G200]

Several lines of evidence have shown that the reduction of pleural fluid complement level in SLE is a result of activation by immune complexes. Conversion products generated by the activation of complement-cascade are present in SLE pleural fluid.[A224,H499] Immune complexes abound in SLE pleural fluid.[A224,H63,H499] Immune complexes are detected primarily by the Raji cell test and, less frequently, by the C1q binding and monoclonal rheumatoid factor tests.[A224,H63] Perivascular deposits of immunoglobulins and complement components in the parietal pleura are seen in those with lupus pleuritis.[A224]

The nature of the immune complexes in SLE pleural fluid is not clear. Riska and associates[R216] observed that enzymatic digestion of SLE pleural fluid results in an increase in anti-DNA titer, suggesting that DNA–anti-DNA complexes are present in pleural fluid.

None of the immunologic abnormalities described in SLE pleural fluid is diagnostic of lupus pleuritis. Thus, the presence of immune complexes, complement activation products, and immune deposits in the parietal pleurae have all been reported, not only in pleurisy associated with other rheumatic diseases such as RA but also in nonrheumatic conditions, including cancer and empyema.[A224,S495] This suggests that an immune-mediated mechanism(s) is a common pathway by which SLE and other diseases can cause pleurisy.

At autopsy, 54 of 58 patients (93%) in Ropes' series showed pleural involvement.[R294] Fluid was found in the pleural space in 33 patients and adhesions were seen in 63%. Microscopic changes of varying degrees were observed in 24%; these consisted of accumulations of lymphocytes and macrophages, pleural thickening, perivascular fibrinoid necrosis with neutrophilic and mononuclear infiltrates, fibrinous exudate, and rare hematoxylin bodies. Pleural biopsy in 1 SLE patient with bilateral effusions revealed noncaseating pleural granulomas.[D47]

Treatment of Pleurisy

Analgesics and nonsteroidal anti-inflammatory drugs (NSAIDs) are used to treat mild cases of lupus pleurisy. If the patient fails to improve, or if the symptoms are severe, systemic corticosteroids, 10 to 40 mg of prednisone daily, are indicated. Hydroxychloroquine may be added. Most patients respond promptly to this regimen. The effusion, when present, begins to clear within days of beginning steroid therapy. It may take several weeks for the roentgenographic changes to clear up completely. In rare cases of chronic, unremitting, lupus pleurisy, refractory to med-

ical therapy, pleurectomy,[B190] talc poudrage,[K16] and tetracycline pleurodesis[G137] may be used.

ACUTE LUPUS PNEUMONITIS

Clinical Presentation

Acute lupus pneumonitis is an uncommon clinical manifestation of SLE. In Estes and Christian's[E147] series of 150 patients, 48% had evidence of pulmonary involvement at some time during the course of their illness, but only 14 (9.3%) had acute lupus pneumonitis. Two of 50 (4%) SLE patients followed prospectively by Grigor et al.[G385] developed acute lupus pneumonitis. Two retrospective studies correlating clinical features and radiographic abnormalities in SLE patients found a low frequency of acute lupus pneumonitis. Levin[L214] reported that 3 of 207 patients (1.4%) developed acute lupus pneumonitis.

Mathay and co-workers[M205] described the clinical presentation and course of 12 patients with acute lupus pneumonitis. The patients presented with fever, dyspnea, cough productive of scanty sputum, hemoptysis, tachypnea, and pleuritic chest pain. Physical findings included cyanosis and basilar rales. The chest roentgenograms demonstrated diffuse acinar infiltrates with a predilection for the bases in 100% and pleural effusion in 50% of patients. All patients had arterial hypoxemia. The white cell count was usually normal, and anti-DNA antibodies were positive in all subjects tested. Most patients had multisystem involvement from the SLE. Multiple cultures and investigations for bacteria, fungi, and viruses failed to reveal an infectious cause of the pulmonary disease.

Pathology

The histopathology of the lung in acute lupus pneumonitis has been examined in a few untreated patients; the light microscopic changes are variable and nonspecific. An open lung biopsy obtained prior to therapy in a patient of Mathay et al.[M205] showed a diffuse, interstitial, lymphocytic infiltrate with prominent lymphoid nodules and bronchiolitis. Despite therapy, the patient died 5 months later and, at autopsy, alveolar hyaline membranes and persistent cell infiltrates were found. Other findings found at autopsy of 4 patients included acute alveolitis, interstitial edema, hyaline membranes, and arteriolar thrombosis. Of 8 SLE patients of Pertschuk et al.[P137] who presented with a clinical diagnosis of acute lupus pneumonitis, 50% had changes of interstitial pneumonia. The pathologic picture was considered nonspecific, similar to that seen in those with oxygen toxicity, viral pneumonia, or uremia. The remaining four patients showed other pathologic changes: bronchiolitis, pulmonary infarction, focal atelectasis, and cytomegalovirus pneumonia, respectively. Vasculitis was not observed in any patient in either study.[M205,P137] Widespread thrombosis was found in the lungs and other organs at autopsy of a patient with acute lupus pneumonitis and disseminated intravascular coagulation.[C179]

The wide variety of histologic changes in the lungs suggests that acute lupus pneumonitis may be the result of different pathologic processes.[Q13] Many of the patients studied had received prior treatment, however, including oxygen therapy, high-dose steroids, or cytotoxic agents, which can affect lung pathology directly or indirectly. Thus, some of the pathologic abnormalities in the lungs may be secondary changes, rather than resulting directly from SLE.

Inoue and co-workers[125a] reported the presence of granular deposits of IgG, C3, and DNA antigen in the alveolar septae of two patients with acute lupus pneumonitis. Electron microscopy revealed electron-dense deposits in the septal interstitium and in the walls of alveolar capillaries. Immunoglobulin eluted from the lung tissue had ANA activity, including IgG anti-DNA antibody. Pertschuk et al.[P137] described deposits of immunoglobulin within the nuclei of alveolar lining cells and pleural mesothelial cells rather than in the septal interstitium in acute lupus pneumonitis. The concomitant presence of C3 within the nuclei suggests that this is an in vivo rather than an artifactual phenomenon. These immunopathologic observations are consistent with the deposition of antigen-antibody complexes, and may be important in the pathogenesis of the lung injury.

Parenchymal pulmonary infiltrates developing acutely in a patient with SLE should not be considered to be acute lupus pneumonitis unless infectious processes such as viral pneumonia, tuberculosis and other bacterial pneumonias, and fungal and Pneumocystis carinii infections have been excluded.[Q13]

Treatment

High-dose corticosteroids remain the mainstay of drug therapy of acute lupus pneumonitis, although no controlled trials have established their efficacy.[125a,Q13] Cytotoxic agents such as azathioprine are added to the regimen in patients who fail to respond to the steroid therapy.[M205] Acute lupus pneumonitis carries a poor prognosis. Of 12 patients of Mathay et al.,[M205] 6 died during the acute episode from respiratory failure, opportunistic infection, and thromboembolism. All 6 surviving patients remained relatively well after more than a year of follow-up but 3 patients developed residual interstitial infiltrates with abnormal pulmonary function tests, indicating that the acute process can progress to chronic interstitial lung disease.[Q13] Adult respiratory distress syndrome developed in 1 patient with acute lupus pneumonitis.[D252]

PULMONARY HEMORRHAGE

Clinical Presentation

Pulmonary hemorrhage is a rare but often fatal manifestation of SLE. Abud-Mendoza and associates[A23] found 12 cases of massive pulmonary hemorrhage among 750 SLE patients (1.6%) whose clinical course was followed for at least a year. It was the primary cause of death, however, in 14.4% of their 76 autopsy cases of SLE collected over a period of 20 years, with an exceedingly high case: fatality ratio of 9.6%.[A23] Similarly, Mintz et al.[M470] reported pulmonary hemorrhage to be the cause of death in 6 of 57 SLE cases (10.5%) at autopsy.

The mode of presentation is similar to that of acute lupus pneumonitis, with a sudden onset of fever, dyspnea, cough, and blood-tinged sputum. The course is rapidly progressive, with increasing tachypnea, arterial hypoxemia, tachycardia, acute respiratory distress, and frank hemoptysis. The hemoglobin and hematocrit drop suddenly and chest roentgenograms show bilateral pulmonary infiltrates, with a predominantly alveolar pattern. The infiltrates are coarsely nodular, fluffy, or homogeneous in pattern, often extending to the bases, but occasionally unilateral in distribution. Patients usually have clinical and laboratory evidence of multisystem involvement, including positive anti-DNA antibodies and hypocomplementemia.

Frank hemoptysis does not always occur, even with massive intra-alveolar hemorrhage, so the clinical diagnosis is often delayed in some patients.[A23,M470] Over a 2-year period, 3 of 140 SLE patients studied by Marino et al.[M133] developed pulmonary hemorrhage and, in 2 of these patients, the diagnosis was made only at autopsy. In the absence of hemoptysis, a rapidly falling hematocrit in a SLE patient with diffuse lung infiltrates should alert the clinician to the possibility of lung hemorrhage.[A23] A lung biopsy sample, obtained by the transbronchial approach or open thoracotomy should be examined.[Q13]

Pulmonary hemosiderosis with recurrent hemoptysis has been reported as the initial presentation of SLE, antedating the onset of multisystem disease.[B609] In most patients, however, pulmonary hemorrhage occurred in those with established disease, often with multisystem involvement. Mintz et al.[M470] found a mean disease duration of 3.2 years in their patients with lung hemorrhage. Several cases of pediatric SLE patients with lung hemorrhage have been reported.[M437,R18]

Pathology

The histopathology of the lung is that of diffuse, intra-alveolar hemorrhage with intact erythrocytes and hemosiderin-laden macrophages in the alveoli.[E1,M470] Other microscopic findings include thickening of the alveolar septae, hyaline membrane formation, and fibrin deposits within the alveolar cavities. Evidence of vasculitis is usually not seen. A distinctive microangiitis characterized by acute inflammation and necrosis of alveolar capillaries, arterioles, and small muscular arteries has also been described in four patients.[M682]

Electron microscopic studies in a small number of cases have shown type II alveolar lining cell hyperplasia and electron-dense deposits in the alveolar septae within the basement membrane of alveolar capillaries and in the walls of small arteries.[C148,C263,E1,G323] Direct immunofluorescence studies have demonstrated the presence of granular deposits of immunoglobulin, principally IgG, and complement components in the alveolar septae and in the walls of small blood vessels.[C148,C263,E1,R265] Other investigators, however, have failed to find immune deposits in the alveolar septae in SLE patients with pulmonary hemorrhage.[D179,E1]

Pathogenesis

The pathogenesis of pulmonary hemorrhage in SLE is not known. Deposition of immune complexes in the alveolar septae and in blood vessels, with activation of the complement system, has been proposed as the major mechanism, analogous to the lung changes seen in experimental models of chronic serum sickness. Brentjens et al.[B476] described changes of interstitial pneumonitis, with proliferation of septal cells, thickening of the alveolar septae, accumulation of leukocytes in capillaries, and alveolar hemorrhages in rabbits hyperimmunized with foreign serum protein. Conversely, Eagen and associates[E1] identified several factors that potentially contributed to the pathogenesis of lung hemorrhage in their SLE patients. These factors included bleeding diathesis, oxygen toxicity, infection, uremia, and "shock lung." Desnoyer et al.[D179] described a SLE patient with cutaneous vasculitis, nephritis, and pulmonary hemorrhage without the complicating factors described above that could cause nonspecific alveolar damage. No immune deposits were found in the alveolar septae, although they were present in the renal glomeruli. They suggested that pulmonary hemorrhage can occur in SLE by mechanism(s) other than immune complex deposition, such as vascular injury with disruption of the alveolar capillary membrane.

Treatment and Prognosis

The prognosis of massive pulmonary hemorrhage in SLE patients is grave, despite treatment with high-dose systemic corticosteroids combined with a cytotoxic agent. Our clinical experience is similar to that reported by others in that most of the patients succumbed to the lung disease, which progressively worsens and is frequently complicated by opportunistic infection, oxygen toxicity, and other problems.[A23,E1,M205,Q13] The mortality rate of pediatric cases with lung hemorrhage has been reported to be 50%.[M437] Millman et al.[M440] have described a patient who recovered following treatment with plasmapheresis and cyclophosphamide. Because of the poor prognosis in these patients, it may be advisable to employ a regimen of high-dose corticosteroids, cyclophosphamide, and perhaps plasmapheresis.

Carette et al.[C81] reviewed the 10-year study at the National Institutes of Health of SLE patients with severe and acute pulmonary disease. Out of more than 400 SLE patients followed during this period, 8 became acutely ill, with diffuse lung infiltrates on chest roentgenography. Pulmonary hemorrhage was eventually diagnosed in 6 patients, congestive heart failure in 1, and Pneumocystis carinii infection in another. Of the 6 patients with lung hemorrhage, 4 had other complicating factors including uremia, coagulopathy, and infection. Based on their experience, a practical approach to such a patient was outlined by the authors. Four major conditions should be considered in the differential diagnosis: congestive heart failure, noncardiogenic pulmonary edema, infection, and pulmonary hemorrhage. A careful clinical history is taken and a thorough physical examination performed. Evidence of lupus activity in other organ systems should also be investigated. If the diagnosis of congestive heart failure is unclear on clinical grounds, a Swan-Ganz catheter should be inserted. Infection and factors associated with noncardiogenic pulmonary edema, including uremia, pancreatitis,

and side effects to drugs, should be aggressively excluded. If a definite diagnosis is not reached at this point, broad-spectrum antibiotics and high-dose corticosteroids are administered while transbronchial lung biopsy and brushing are being prepared to rule out infection. If pathogenic organisms are not found after appropriate stains and cultures, antibiotics should be discontinued. Systemic corticosteroids are continued until clinical improvement occurs but, if the patient fails to respond, an open lung biopsy sample should be obtained and examined.

DIFFUSE INTERSTITIAL LUNG DISEASE

Clinical Presentation

Diffuse interstitial lung disease (ILD) is a well-recognized pulmonary manifestation of systemic rheumatic diseases, particularly systemic sclerosis and rheumatoid arthritis. ILD may be the dominant clinical feature in some patients. The occurrence of ILD in SLE was recognized in 1973, when Eisenberg and colleagues[E57] reviewed 18 cases from our clinic. We have studied the longterm clinical course of SLE patients with ILD.[W138]

The prevalence of symptomatic ILD in SLE has not been systematically examined in large series of patients. Our experience is similar to that of other investigators, in that ILD is relatively uncommon. Eisenberg et al.[E57] calculated the prevalence to be about 3% of SLE patients. In 1973, Holden[H378] described an elderly woman with SLE who presented with severe ILD and, at that time, found only two other cases of ILD in SLE in the medical literature. Of the 150 patients studied prospectively by Estes and Christian,[E147] 9 developed roentgenographic changes of pulmonary fibrosis, but it is unclear from their report whether the patients were symptomatic and how severe were the pulmonary functional abnormalities. In a retrospective study of 63 SLE patients Boulware et al.,[B431] looking for interstitial pneumonitis, found 16 patients (25.4%) with ILD. The high prevalence is partly a result of the inclusion of severely ill hospitalized SLE patients in their series.

The initial presentation of diffuse ILD in SLE can be one of two types. The more common presentation is an insidious onset of chronic, nonproductive cough, dyspnea on exertion, and a history of recurrent pleuritic chest pain. Less commonly, ILD may develop in a patient following a bout of acute lupus pneumonitis. Of Mathay et al.'s[M599] patients who survived the acute episode, 50% developed diffuse ILD. Of 16 SLE patients with ILD reported by Boulware et al.,[B431] 7 (43%) presented initially with acute lupus pneumonitis.

The clinical manifestations of ILD in SLE are similar to those of systemic sclerosis and RA. Persistent dyspnea on exertion, pleuritic chest pains, and nonproductive cough are the most common. ILD can occur at any time during the course of SLE, but most cases developed in those with long-standing disease. Most patients have multisystem involvement and test positive for ANA and anti-DNA antibodies.

In the study of Eisenberg et al.[E57] the mean age of their 18 SLE patients with ILD was 45.7 years, with a mean disease duration of 10.3 years. Pulmonary manifestations

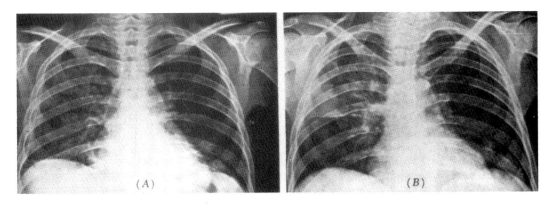

Fig. 36–1. Lupus pneumonitis. *A,* Infiltrations in right upper and left lower lobes, nonspecific in appearance. *B,* Infiltration in the right upper lobe has progressed during the subsequent 2.5 months. Persistent but less marked changes in the left lower lobe infiltrate can be noted.

were present for a mean of 6 years. Initially, 7 patients presented with pulmonary symptoms. All had dyspnea on exertion and 3 subjects were dyspneic, even at rest; 12 complained of cough with scanty sputum, and a similar number had pleuritic chest pain. All patients had poor diaphragmatic movement, with diminished resonance to percussion over the lung bases. Cyanosis and clubbing were present in 1 patient; 12 had basilar rales. Only 1

patient had an elevated rheumatoid factor titer. All 18 had persistent diffuse interstitial infiltrates on chest roentgenography that could not be attributed to any secondary complication (Figs. 36–1, 36–2, and 36–3). Markedly elevated diaphragms were seen in 8 patients. Diaphragmatic excursion was decreased in 6 patients as evaluated by chest roentgenography on deep inspiration and expiration. A pleural reaction was present in 9 patients and plate-

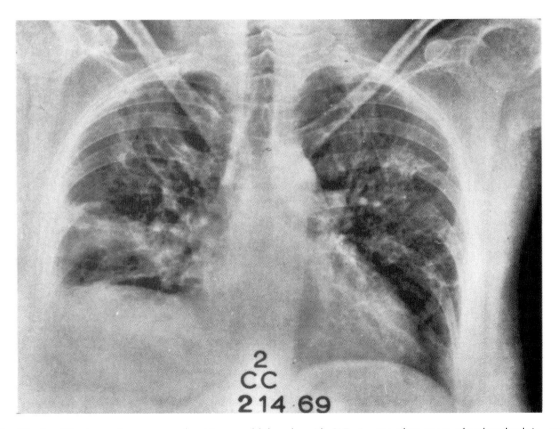

Fig. 36–2. Chest roentgenogram of a 48-year-old female with SLE, 1 year after onset of polyarthralgia, and before the start of steroid treatment. These are diffuse reticulonodular infiltrates, elevated right diaphragm, and a small right pleural effusion, with a large patchy infiltrate in the right lower lung field.

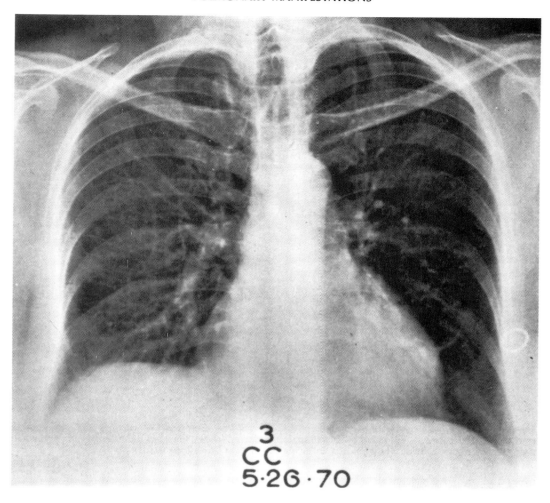

Fig. 36–3. Chest roentgenogram 15 months after the onset of steroid therapy (prednisone, 35 mg/day, for 4 months, followed by gradual tapering to cessation at 15 months).

like atelectasis in 6; this was usually situated above the diaphragm, and persisted for several months to years. The diffusing capacity of the lung, as measured by the carbon monoxide method, was decreased below predicted normal values in all but 1 patient.

Laboratory Evaluation

To investigate the possibility of pulmonary infarction, ventilation-perfusion lung scans were obtained in 13 patients. Of these, 8 had both ventilation and perfusion defects occurring at the same site. In 7 of 13 patients, ventilation-perfusion defects were noted in areas other than those occupied by long line shadows, effusions, or atelectasis.

Spirometry and lung volume measurements were consistent with a "restrictive defect" or loss of ventilable lung volume without obstruction to air flow. Diffuse pulmonary interstitial infiltration typically results in this type of ventilatory defect. Infiltrated lung areas are less elastic and change their volume less with each breath. Underventilation results in underoxygenation of blood perfusing these regions. Such ventilation-perfusion mismatching is the major cause of arterial hypoxemia. Obstruction to air flow was not demonstrated in any patient. The diminution of flow rate was proportional to and consistent with the loss of vital capacity, and did not signify an obstructive airway process.

The arterial blood oxygen tension (Pao_2) was diminished in all patients, and the alveolar-arterial difference for oxygen ($PAo_2 - Pao_2$) increased significantly. The Pao_2 was lowest and the $PAo_2 - Pao_2$ difference was greatest in patients with the most extensive pulmonary involvement, as noted in their roentgenograms. The oxyhemoglobin saturation, however, was above 94% in all but 4 patients. Ventilation-perfusion mismatching was responsible for these changes. Thickening and fibrosis of the interstitial wall and microinfarcts in the lung alter the elastic properties of the ventilatory lung units, leading to underventilation relative to perfusion. Lung biopsy in 4 patients showed nonspecific interstitial fibrosis, with chronic inflammation in 2 (Fig. 36–4).

Boulware and Hedgpeth[B431] found a higher frequency of precipitating anti-Ro/SSA antibodies (81%) in SLE pa-

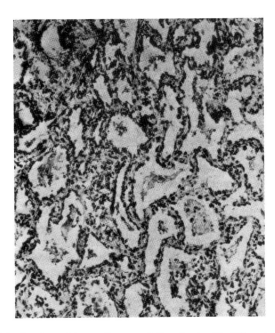

Fig. 36–4. Lung biopsy from an SLE patient with diffuse interstitial lung disease. Note the relatively uniform thickening of the alveolar walls by loose fibrous tissue, lymphocyte and plasma cell infiltrate, and minimal collagen. Some alveolar spaces contain fibrinous proteinaceous deposits (H & E stain; ×125).

tients with ILD compared to that seen in their general SLE population (38%). In contrast, the frequency of other specific types of ANA, such as anti-U1RNP, and anti-La/SSB, was not significantly increased. We have not observed an increased prevalence of anti-Ro/SSA antibodies in our SLE patients with ILD,[W138] and the discrepancy may be a result of differences in patient selection.

Treatment and Prognosis

We have analyzed the longterm clinical course (mean duration of follow-up, 7.3 years) of 14 SLE patients with diffuse ILD.[W138] All patients presented with dyspnea on exertion, pleuritic chest pain, chronic cough, and basilar rales. The diffusing capacity for carbon monoxide (Dco) was impaired in 10 patients, with a mean value of 57% of the predicted value. Lung biopsy in 4 patients showed alveolar septal thickening, interstitial fibrosis, lymphocytic infiltrates, and type II pneumocytic hyperplasia. Deposits of immunoglobulin and complement components were found in the alveolar septae and within cell nuclei. All patients received high-dose prednisone (60 mg daily) for at least 4 weeks early in the course of the pulmonary disease. The Dco and inspiratory vital capacity (IVC) improved or remained unchanged in most patients. Respiratory complaints decreased in all patients, but 2 died of progressive pulmonary fibrosis and another succumbed to bacterial pneumonia. Our study showed that the clinical course of chronic ILD is variable in individual patients, but in most patients it follows a slow course and tends to improve or stabilize with time. Thus, the clinical course

is similar to that of ILD associated with systemic sclerosis or rheumatoid arthritis.[Q13,W138]

SLE patients with symptomatic, chronic, and progressive ILD should undergo assessment of the extent and activity of the lung disease by the use of pulmonary function tests, gallium lung scan, bronchoalveolar lavage (BAL), and/or transbronchial biopsy. An open lung biopsy is usually not indicated. Pulmonary function tests, Dco and IVC, are useful in following the course of and response to therapy.[Q13] In the presence of an active inflammatory process in the lung, the patient is treated with high-dose prednisone (40 to 60 mg daily) for at least 6 to 8 weeks. The dose is tapered depending on the clinical and laboratory responses of the patient. The use of immunosuppressive agents such as azathioprine and cyclophosphamide should be considered in patients who fail to respond satisfactorily to steroids.

The corticosteroid therapy of interstitial lung disease associated with connective tissue disease, including SLE, has been found to cause a decrease in total cell count, immune complexes, and levels of immunoglobulins in BAL fluid.[J48] The efficacy of systemic corticosteroid and immunosuppressive agents in the treatment of ILD and SLE has not been validated by well-designed controlled trials.

PULMONARY EMBOLISM

Pulmonary embolism (PE) is frequently suspected in SLE patients with respiratory symptoms, especially pleuritic chest pain and dyspnea. We have seen several cases of PE documented by angiography, but most patients presenting with these symptoms usually have pleurisy or pneumonitis. Lung scans demonstrating abnormal perfusion may be obtained from those with active lung disease in the absence of PE. Nevertheless, if PE is suspected clinically in a patient with an abnormal scan, angiography should be performed. The lung scan accurately designates the areas of absent or reduced perfusion but does not diagnose the cause.

Thrombophlebitis is not uncommon in SLE patients. Dubois[D340] described thrombophlebitis in 24 of 520 patients (5%), and Estes and Christian[E147] observed it in 9% of 150 patients. Gladman and Urowitz[G176] observed 21 episodes of deep vein thrombosis or pulmonary emboli in 17 of 180 SLE patients (11%). No association between the thromboembolic event and the presence of hyperlipidemia, oral contraceptive use, or smoking was found. Peck et al.[89] reported that thrombophlebitis developed in 12.2% of 114 SLE patients and pulmonary emboli in 6%. Of the 14 episodes, 10 occurred within a year after the diagnosis of SLE. Thrombocytopenia and an abnormal partial thromboplastin time were found to be common among the patients who developed thrombophlebitis. Several factors that predispose SLE patients to thrombophlebitis were postulated, including chronic, low-grade disseminated intravascular coagulation, small vessel angiitis, prolonged bed rest, and increased thromboplastic generation. Pulmonary embolism in SLE has been associated with pulmonary arterial hypertension, along with lupus anticoagulant.[A208]

Angles-Cano et al.[A233] evaluated 28 SLE patients for predisposing factors to thrombosis. An increase in von Willebrand factor activity and decreased plasminogen activator release after venous occlusion correlated with the occurrence of thrombosis. Both proteins are synthesized by endothelial cells, so it was postulated that damage to the vascular endothelium mediated by immune complexes may be responsible for these abnormalities.

It is now recognized that venous and arterial thromboses are associated paradoxically with circulating lupus anticoagulants and other antiphospholipid antibodies.[B379,H152] A case-control study of 72 SLE patients showed that the presence of lupus anticoagulant, positive IgG anticardiolipin antibodies, decreased protein S, and a mild thrombocytopenia are significantly associated with history of thrombosis.[H200] (See Chapter 24 for a further discussion of thrombosis and antiphospholipid antibodies.)

Reversible Hypoxemia

Abrahamson et al.[A13] have described a syndrome of reversible hypoxemia in acutely ill SLE patients without evidence of parenchymal lung involvement. Among 22 patients hospitalized for acute disease exacerbation, 6 (27%) had this syndrome. Although some patients had mild pleuropulmonary symptoms, chest roentgenograms and lung scans were normal. The patients had hypoxemia and hypocapnia with a wide alveolar-arterial gradient, which reversed with corticosteroid therapy. The pathogenesis of the syndrome is unclear, but a correlation between hypoxemia and the level of complement split product was noted. Complement activation may lead to diffuse pulmonary injury by the aggregation of neutrophils in the lungs, as has been observed in cardiopulmonary bypass, hemodialysis with cuprophane membranes, and adult respiratory distress syndrome.

Pulmonary Hypertension

Clinical Presentation

Severe symptomatic pulmonary hypertension (PH) is a rare manifestation of lung involvement in SLE, but mild subclinical cases are probably not uncommon. Perez and Kramer[P121] collected four cases of severe PH in a group of 43 SLE patients over a period of 2 years, but we could identify two symptomatic cases of PH in a clinic population of approximately 400 SLE patients.[Q21] The clinical diagnosis of PH is difficult to make in early and mild cases, and only the severe cases with right ventricular hypertrophy and/or congestive heart failure have been reported in the literature. A study of the prevalence and severity of PH in a group of 36 SLE patients and healthy controls was undertaken by Simonson et al.[S458] using two-dimensional and Doppler echocardiographic data to calculate pulmonary artery systolic pressure. Five patients (14%) and none of the controls had PH, defined by a pulmonary artery pressure of greater than 30 mm Hg. The results of this study suggest that PH is common in SLE, but usually mild in degree. Conceivably, mild cases of PH in SLE may improve with systemic corticosteroid and/or cytotoxic

drug therapy that is given for other organ involvement, so that PH remains unrecognized. Badui et al.[B17] identified 9 PH patients out of 100 consecutive SLE patients (9%) who were examined specifically for cardiovascular manifestations.

We have reviewed the clinical features of our SLE patients with PH and those of 20 other patients reported in the literature.[Q21] The symptoms of PH in SLE were similar to those of patients with idiopathic or primary PH. In most of the reported cases, the symptoms of PH occurred within a few years after the onset of the multisystem disease, with a mean duration of approximately 2.3 years.[Q21] The most common complaints were dyspnea on exertion, chest pain, and chronic, nonproductive cough. Chronic fatigue, weakness, palpitations, edema, and/or ascites also occurred. Symptoms developed insidiously and progressed gradually. The physical findings included a loud second pulmonic heart sound, systolic murmur, and right ventricular lift. Chest roentgenography revealed cardiomegaly with a prominent pulmonary artery segment and clear lung fields. Electrocardiography revealed changes of right ventricular hypertrophy. Although pulmonary function tests (PFT) showed restrictive abnormalities, these were mild in degree and disproportionate to the severity of the PH. Pulmonary angiograms, which were obtained from a number of patients, demonstrated symmetric dilatation of the central pulmonary artery trunk, with pruning of the peripheral blood vessels. Cardiac catheterization confirmed the diagnosis with the characteristic elevation of the pulmonary artery pressure and normal wedge pressure; no evidence of intracardiac or extracardiac shunting was found.

Pathology

The histopathology of the lung in SLE patients with PH is that of "plexiform" lesions similar to those seen in primary PH.[Q21] Medial hypertrophy and intimal fibrosis of the branches of the pulmonary artery can be noted. Thrombosis and vasculitis have also been reported in few patients.[Q21] We found deposits of IgG, IgM, and C3 in the walls of the pulmonary blood vessels. The immunoglobulin deposits were eluted with acidic buffer and showed antinuclear antibody activity, including anti-DNA antibody and rheumatoid factor activity.[Q21] The putative antigen DNA was also found in the walls of blood vessels, indicating the deposition of immune complexes.

Pathogenesis

The pathogenesis of PH is not well understood. Although we found evidence of immune deposits in the large pulmonary vessels, it is not clear whether this is important in the pathogenesis or merely represents a secondary phenomenon. Vasculitis affecting the pulmonary artery is rarely seen, and is thus unlikely to be a major cause of PH.[S458] PH can occasionally develop as a complication of diffuse pulmonary fibrosis. Asherson et al.[A326] reported a high frequency of anticardiolipin antibodies in SLE patients with PH, indicating the possible causative role of recurrent thromboembolic phenomena, but we and others[S458] have not observed this association. Moreover, other features of antiphospholipid syndrome are uncommon in SLE patients with PH,[A326] and thrombosis is not commonly seen in autopsied cases.[Q21] The high frequency of Raynaud's phenomenon in this group of patients suggests that PH may be a complication of pulmonary arterial vasospasm.[A326,S458]

Prognosis and Treatment

The overall outcome of PH in SLE is poor. Of patients reported in the literature, 50% were dead at the time of the report because of cardiac failure or the sudden onset of arrhythmia. Most patients reported were treated with various vasodilator agents, anticoagulants, systemic corticosteroids, or cytotoxic agents. Some patients have experienced symptomatic improvement, although hemodynamic abnormalities remained unchanged with drug therapy.[G174,M67,Q21] Despite combinations of these drugs, most of Asherson et al.'s patients died within 5 years after diagnosis of PH; 2 of their patients underwent heart-lung transplantation, with satisfactory results in 1 but poor results in the other because of the chronic rejection.[A326]

"Shrinking Lung Syndrome"

In 1965, Hoffbrand and Beck[H360] described a group of 8 SLE patients who complained of breathlessness and had reduced chest expansion, but with no cyanosis, clubbing, or abnormal auscultatory findings. Many patients had a previous history of pleurisy. Chest roentgenography revealed a clear lung field, but an elevated diaphragm, which moved sluggishly but not paradoxically. The vital capacity was extremely reduced. They coined the term "shrinking lung syndrome," and suggested that the main pathologic lesion is that of alveolar atelectasis secondary to deficiency of the surface tension-reducing film that lines the normal alveoli. Gibson and associates[G123] measured diaphragmatic function in these patients by determining the transdiaphragmatic pressure using a double-balloon technique, and found it to be grossly abnormal. This finding led them to suggest that diaphragmatic dysfunction rather than parenchymal or pleural disease accounts for the unexplained dyspnea in these patients. Marten et al.[M157] concluded that the restrictive ventilatory defect in these patients is primarily a result of the weakness of expiratory and inspiratory muscles. Diaphragmatic dysfunction correlated with the degree of dyspnea but not with overall disease activity, proximal muscle weakness, or serologic markers.[M157] Contrary to these reports, Laroche and colleagues,[L68] using a wide range of tests for determining respiratory muscle strength, found no evidence of isolated weakness of the diaphragm in 12 SLE patients with this syndrome. The discrepancy with their results from previous studies is not entirely clear, but may partly be caused by patient selection and differences in methods used to assess diaphragmatic function.

The pathogenesis of the diaphragmatic weakness in SLE patients is not well understood. Wilcox et al.[W226] found no evidence of phrenic nerve neuropathy as the cause of the weakness. Diffuse fibrosis of the diaphragm without evidence of acute inflammatory infiltrates was observed in one patient examined at autopsy,[R385] supporting an extrapulmonary, restrictive cause of this unusual syndrome. An electromyographic study of the diaphragm and external intercostal muscles demonstrated that fatigue of the respiratory muscles occurs at lower loads in SLE patients compared to healthy controls.[W353] Whether myopathy is an isolated process affecting primarily the diaphragm and other respiratory muscles or is a part of a generalized muscle disease in SLE is not entirely clear. When the diagnosis of shrinking lung syndrome is suspected, transdiaphragmatic pressures and elastic recoil of the respiratory system should be measured.

The clinical course of the syndrome is that of a chronic, low-grade, restrictive defect. Follow-up of some patients over a period of several years has shown that the volume restriction is not progressive.[G123,M157] In symptomatic patients, prednisone therapy, 30 to 60 mg daily, for several weeks is clinically beneficial and tends to stabilize the PFT abnormalities.[S684] β-Agonist agents may also be useful in the treatment of this syndrome.[T156]

Airway Obstruction

Severe airway obstruction has been reported in a small number of SLE patients.[K31,K239] Lung biopsy in one patient showed obliterative bronchiolitis and an acute inflammatory process that affected small bronchi and bronchioles, resulting in necrosis and eventual endobronchiolar proliferation of epithelial cells and peribronchial infiltration by lymphocytes. Dense plugs composed of alveolar debris and fibrin strands within the bronchioles caused partial or complete obstruction.

Evidence of airway obstruction has been described in several controlled studies of PFT in SLE patients.[C236,C352, G232,H464,W321] The effect of cigarette smoking was not taken into consideration in some series but, in those that did, it was evident that airway obstruction occurred, even in nonsmoking SLE patients. The frequency of airway obstruction is variable, primarily because of differences in the criteria used to define the abnormality and in the selection of patients. In the only controlled study of lifelong, nonsmoking, SLE patients, Andonopoulos et al.[A216] observed a high prevalence (24%) of isolated small airway disease in SLE patients. The clinical significance of this observation remains unclear, however, because a similarly high frequency (17%) of small airway disease was found in their healthy, nonsmoking subjects matched for age and sex.

CHEST ROENTGENOGRAPHY IN SLE

Prevalence of Abnormalities

Abnormalities in chest roentgenograms are not uncommon in SLE patients. In a prospective study of 50 unselected patients, abnormalities were found in 38%[G385] and, in a study of 43 patients specifically examined for pulmonary dysfunction, 23% had abnormal chest radiographs.[S430] In contrast, none of 70 nonsmoking SLE patients free of respiratory complaints enrolled in a study of pulmonary function had abnormal chest roentgenograms.[A216] Several factors can account for the wide variability in the prevalence of abnormalities found in clinical series, including patient selection, the protean manifestations of the disease, the transitory nature of lung lesions, and the timing of the radiographic study.

Roentgenographic Findings

A wide array of abnormalities can be seen in the chest roentgenograms. Early studies thoroughly and meticulously documented the radiographic changes in the pleura, lung parenchyma, and heart.[B561,M279,M515] None of the abnormalities is considered specific or diagnostic of SLE and may be seen in other conditions, such as rheumatoid arthritis and systemic sclerosis.

Pleural changes as an isolated abnormality or in combination with cardiac or parenchymal lesions are the most common radiographic changes.[B561] The pleura may appear as a shaggy thickening of the pleural surface. Pleural effusions are small, and in 50% of patients are bilateral.[M279] With clearing of the effusion, residual pleural thickening may be seen. Parenchymal lesions are characterized by ill-defined focal patches, linear bands, infiltrates, small nodules, or plaques in the bases.[G324] Diffuse granular, reticular, or reticulonodular lesions throughout the lung fields, but more prominent at the bases, are found in a small number of SLE patients with chronic interstitial fibrosis.[Q13] Cardiomegaly, with a nondistinct enlargement of the heart, is usually minimal to moderate.[B561] Isolated cardiac enlargement is almost as frequent as isolated pleural disease. Multiple factors can usually be identified in an individual patient to account for cardiomegaly, such as hypertension, pericarditis, myocardial involvement, and anemia.[B561] Elevated diaphragms are found in 5 to 18% of patients.[G385,S430]

Early workers often ascribed parenchymal changes in chest roentgenograms to primary lung involvement caused by SLE. The term "lupus pneumonitis" was used indiscriminately to encompass various types of pulmonary lesions, and has been reported in 15 to 50% of patients.[L214,M279] In a retrospective but careful study of 111 SLE patients, Levin[L214] found that radiographic parenchymal changes (infiltrates or small nodules) were mostly the result of secondary complications, such as infections, uremic pulmonary edema, and basilar atelectasis. Primary lupus pneumonitis was relatively rare, found in only 3 patients (2.7%), and the diagnosis therefore became one of exclusion.

PULMONARY FUNCTION TEST ABNORMALITIES

PFT abnormalities are exceedingly common in SLE patients, even in those without an active or past history of respiratory complaints, and with normal chest roentgenographic findings (Table 36–2).[C352,G385,S430] In 1965, Huang et al.[H465] studied 28 consecutive SLE patients, 20 of whom had a history of pleurisy and/or pneumonitis, and 8 patients without pleuropulmonary involvement. They found a high prevalence of physiologic abnormalities, with a restrictive pattern. Reduction of the diffusing capacity was the most common finding, seen in 16 patients, and with a mean value of 65% of the predicted value. More importantly, they observed a disparity among clinical and chest roentgenographic findings and PFT abnormalities.

In 1966, Gold and Jennings[G233] carried out PFT in 20 SLE patients with respiratory symptoms and found evidence for three major changes: restrictive disease, airway obstruction, and pulmonary vascular obstruction. Twelve of the patients had evidence of restrictive disease, 3 had severe airway obstruction without pulmonary restriction, and 5 had pulmonary vascular obstruction. Three patients died, and the pathologic findings in the lungs correlated with the physiologic abnormalities observed during life.

Wohlgelernter et al.[W321] found PFT abnormalities in 90% of SLE patients with a previous history of pleuritis

Table 36–2. Summary of Selected Studies of Pulmonary Function in SLE

Source	No. of Patients in Study	Major Findings and Comments
Uncontrolled studies		
Huang and Lyons (1965)[H465]	20 patients with and 8 without history of lung disease	↓ Dco in 16 (57%); ↓ lung volumes in 14 (61%); no correlation among PFT changes and clinical or roentgenographic findings
Gold and Jennings (1966)[G233]	20 patients, 5 with pulmonary complaints	Restrictive lung changes in 12 (60%); obstructive changes in 2 (10%); ↓ Dco most common abnormality
Wohlgelernter et al. (1978)[W321]	10 patients with (group I) and 14 without (group II) pulmonary symptoms or findings	↓ Dco, arterial hypoxemia, and/or restrictive lung changes present in 90% of group I and 71% of group II; small airway disease in 10 patients
Silberstein et al. (1980)[S430]	43 patients; only 11 were not on steroids or cytotoxic agents, 15 had history of cigarette smoking	88% with abnormalities—↓ Dco (72%), ↓ lung volumes (44%), airway obstruction (7%); no correlation among PFT and other measures of disease activity
Longitudinal study		
Eichacker et al. (1988)[E45]	Serial PFT on 25 unselected SLE patients followed 2–7 years	No significant changes in Dco, forced vital capacity, and total lung volumes; reduction in small airway function was significant, but unrelated to smoking
Controlled studies		
Chick et al. (1976)[C236]	28 patients with no pulmonary findings, 13 smokers, 26 age- and sex-matched controls, 13 smokers	SLE group had lower total lung capacity, functional residual volume, and Dco than controls, effect of smoking on airway function similar for SLE and controls
Andronopoulos et al. (1988)	70 nonsmoking patients; 70 nonsmoking, age- and sex-matched controls	Isolated ↓ Dco in 31% of SLE patients and none in controls; small airway disease seen in 24% and 17%, respectively; only 37% of SLE patients but 83% of controls had normal PFT

and/or pneumonitis, and in 71% of patients without pulmonary complaints. The most common abnormalities were a decreased DLCO, lack of response to breathing helium, restrictive ventilatory defect, and arterial hypoxemia. None of their patients with chronic discoid LE had abnormal PFT, a finding consistent with the limited disease process in this condition.

In a prospective study of 43 ambulatory consecutive SLE patients, Silberstein et al.[S430] attempted to correlate PFT abnormalities with other measures of lupus activity. Pulmonary dysfunction was noted in 88% of patients. An impaired DLCO (72%), reduction in lung volume (49%), and hypoxia (44%) were the most common abnormalities found. No correlation was found among the type and severity of the abnormality and serum complement levels, anti-DNA antibody, lupus band test, and nephritis. SLE patients with abnormal PFT results did not differ from those with normal PFT results in regard to their clinical features and immunologic findings. In contrast, Holgate et al.[H380] reported that SLE patients with prominent pleuropulmonary disease had a lower prevalence of lupus nephritis, suggesting that this is partly a result of the low frequency of anti-DNA antibodies in this group of patients. These two studies are not comparable, however, because the latter included only SLE patients with pleuropulmonary disease.

Most studies of PFT in SLE patients summarized above were uncontrolled, and did not consider the effects of cigarette smoking. Although no correlation was seen between PFT abnormalities and lupus activity at a single point in time, no systematic serial PFT studies were available until relatively recently.

Chick and co-workers[C236] compared PFT findings in 28 SLE patients without pulmonary involvement and healthy individuals matched for age, gender, and height. A restrictive pattern with reduced lung volume and vital capacity was seen in the SLE group. DLCO was reduced in SLE patients in proportion to the reduction in lung volume, suggesting that this is a result of pleural thickening rather than parenchymal disease causing the impaired lung expansion. Cigarette smoking caused a reduction in flow at low lung volumes in both SLE patients and normal controls.

Andronopoulos et al.[A216] have conducted the largest controlled study of PFT in SLE patients to date. They studied 70 lifelong, nonsmoking SLE patients and an equal number of age- and sex-matched nonsmoking healthy subjects. None of the patients had active pulmonary disease, and all had normal chest roentgenograms at the time of the study. An isolated reduction in the DLCO was the most prevalent abnormality found in the SLE patients (31%), but was not found in the controls. Isolated small airway disease, defined as less than 60% of the predicted value of the maximal flow at 25% of vital capacity, was common in both SLE patients (24%) and controls (17%). Restrictive and obstructive patterns were uncommon in SLE, seen in 5.7% of SLE patients. Overall, only 33% of the SLE patients had normal PFT results, compared to 83% of the controls.

Eichacker and associates[E45] evaluated the PFT of 25 SLE patients serially over a period of 2 to 7 years. Reduction in diffusing capacity, forced vital capacity, and total lung capacity did not change significantly with time. In contrast, small airway function decreased significantly with time, and appeared not to be related to smoking history. The significance of this finding is not clear, however, in view of the finding of Andronopoulos et al.[A216] that the prevalence of small airway disease in SLE patients is the same as in healthy controls.

In the absence of respiratory symptoms, isolated abnormalities in PFT, such as a reduced DLCO, do not require treatment. Longterm longitudinal studies correlating serial PFT abnormalities with bronchoalveolar lavage or with histologic findings are not available.

BRONCHOALVEOLAR LAVAGE

The technique of bronchoalveolar lavage (BAL) allows the recovery of cellular and soluble components from the epithelial surface of the lower respiratory tract. BAL has yielded valuable information about the immune responses of the host and the pathogenesis of lung injury in various diseases, including connective tissue diseases (especially systemic sclerosis and RA). BAL findings may be diagnostic in some diseases, such as infections; in others, however, the findings are nonspecific but may contribute to the management of these diseases. For example, an increased number of BAL eosinophils was found to be associated with progressive lung disease in idiopathic interstitial pulmonary fibrosis, RA, and scleroderma.[P147] Unfortunately, BAL has yet to find wider application in SLE.

In a multicenter study designed to standardize the test procedure, BAL was carried out in 24 patients with diffuse interstitial lung disease secondary to rheumatic disorders, including SLE.[B41] The total number of cells in the BAL fluid was increased with the percentage increase in neutrophils and decrease in macrophages. Total protein, IgM, IgG, and IgA, but not albumin, increased in concentration in the BAL fluid. Wallaert et al.[W10] studied BAL fluid in 61 patients with collagen vascular disease without respiratory symptoms. Included in their study were 11 patients with SLE, all of whom had normal PFT results. An abnormal differential count of BAL fluid leukocytes was found in 48% of patients, including 3 with SLE. In contrast to patients with RA and systemic sclerosis, who had a predominant polymorphonuclear alveolitis, SLE patients showed a lymphocytic predominance. An increased percentage of BAL fluid eosinophils was found in 2 SLE patients with interstitial lung disease.[P147]

Alveolar macrophages obtained by BAL from 17 SLE patients without evidence of active disease were found to be normal in numbers, viability, and respiratory burst activity, but had severely impaired antibacterial function.[W10] This dysfunction, which was observed in both steroid-treated and untreated patients, may contribute to the increased frequency of pulmonary infections in this disease.

The concentration of soluble immune complexes was found to be higher in BAL fluid than in the corresponding serum specimen of patients with interstitial lung disease associated with rheumatic diseases, including SLE.[J48] Immune complexes were also seen within the cytoplasm of BAL neutrophils, indicating that locally formed immune complexes may induce an inflammatory response in the lungs in these patients.

Further studies are needed to evaluate the usefulness of BAL in the assessment and follow-up of SLE patients with pulmonary involvement, especially those with acute lupus pneumonitis and chronic diffuse interstitial lung disease.

SUMMARY

1. Pleuritis is present in 42 to 60% and effusions in 16 to 40% of patients during the course of SLE. Depending on the severity, treatment consists of aspirin, NSAIDs, and systemic corticosteroids.
2. The most common cause of an infiltrate seen in a chest roentgenogram is an infection. Lupus pneumonitis is relatively uncommon.
3. Acute lupus pneumonitis and diffuse interstitial lung disease probably represent immune complex-mediated lung disorders. These may respond to steroid therapy.
4. Symptomatic pulmonary arterial hypertension is uncommon, and may occur in the absence of significant interstitial fibrosis. The prognosis is poor, despite high-dose steroid therapy.
5. Pulmonary hemorrhage is a rare and life-threatening event that may occur in the absence of frank hemoptysis. The prognosis is generally poor, despite high-dose steroid therapy.
6. Chest roentgenography, pulmonary function tests, lung scans, bronchoscopy (including bronchoalveolar lavage), and hemodynamic monitoring are useful for assessing disease activity. Chest radiographic abnormalities are seen in 50 to 70% of SLE patients.
7. Most patients have mild abnormalities in PFT, but do not require specific therapy. Impairment of the diffusing capacity (DLCO) is the most common; also, lung volume may be decreased and hypoxia may be present.
8. BAL fluid in SLE patients shows a lymphocytic predominance. In patients with interstitial lung disease, BAL fluid may show increased neutrophils, eosinophils, and immune complexes.

Chapter 37

CUTANEOUS MANIFESTATIONS OF SLE

DANIEL J. WALLACE

Skin manifestations represent some of the most common symptoms, signs, and pathologies noted in SLE. The lesions are pleomorphic, running the entire gamut of the dermatologic field from erythema to bullae. Cutaneous involvement does not always occur in SLE; it was present in 55 to 85% of patients in the large series detailed in Table 33–1. The skin presentation can often be subtle. A typical history is that of a persistent or recurrent sunburn, butterfly area flush, or discoid lesions appearing years prior to any other manifestation of SLE. Harvey noted that 28% of patients in his series had cutaneous manifestations of SLE prior to systemic spread, with intervals as long as 14 years.[M280] Many patients first seek out a dermatologist and, if no systemic complaints are expressed, necessary laboratory evaluations are often delayed. Years later, when the disease disseminates and the patient seeks the aid of an internist, the skin lesions may no longer be present.

The immunopathogenesis of cutaneous lupus is discussed in Chapter 29; clinical and pathologic aspects of chronic cutaneous (discoid) lupus and subacute cutaneous lupus are reviewed in Chapters 30 and 31. The relationship between DLE and SLE is presented in Chapter 32. This chapter is limited to a discussion of cutaneous features found in SLE.

Table 37–1 lists the incidence of specific skin manifestations of SLE observed in several large studies. Much of the variation was a result of patient selection. For example, Grigor et al.[G385] evaluated a subgroup of patients with known SLE who had severe enough disease to warrant treatment at a tertiary referral center in Great Britain. As a result, the incidence of dermal vasculitis was 70%. All the data on patients in these reports were derived by rheumatologists, not dermatologists. In the only study of its type, published in 1987, an Australian group had a dermatologist examine 84 consecutive patients attending a university SLE clinic.[W143] Cutaneous features attributable to SLE were mucous membrane lesions (35%), malar erythema (22%), subacute cutaneous LE (22%), moderate or severe livedo reticularis (18%), vasculitis (palpable purpura or infarction; 18%), diffuse palmar erythema (17%), nail fold erythema (16%), nail fold telangiectasia (11%), discoid lesions (11%), lupus pernio (5%), and sclerodactyly (4%). These results differ considerably from those in Table 37–1, and indicate the importance of taking into account the specific skills of different observers. The incidence of dermal pathologies in SLE is not age-related. A review of the pediatric literature[N66] and studies

in elderly patients with SLE[B36,D219] described similar distributions to those in Table 37–1.

HISTORICAL CONSIDERATIONS

The first modern description of cutaneous lupus was by Biett's student, Cazenave,[C168] who distinguished it from lupus vulgaris (a form of tuberculosis) in 1833. The systemic nature of lupus was first reported by Kaposi. In 1869, he wrote an excellent description of the initial papular lesion in LE, which he referred to as a "primary eruptive spot," and noted that it was identical in both discoid and systemic LE:[H237]

Lupus erythematosus always becomes developed in the form of slightly elevated spots, which are of the size of pins' heads or of lentils, isolated or arranged in groups, are of a bright or dark-red color, and pale slightly on pressure with the finger, but do not wholly disappear. The center appears slightly depressed and paler, almost cicatricial, or is covered by an adherent, thin scale, which is greasy to the touch. The central scale with the red border at the periphery gives the spot an appearance somewhat resembling ... a favus cup. As the small spots described always have the same characters and are always present where lupus erythematosus is commencing, we may designate them as "primary eruptive spots." They make their appearance, first of all, almost without exception, on the face, and mostly on the skin of the nose, of the cheeks, of the eyelids, or of the ears. Now and then only one such spot may be present; at other times there may be several, isolated and scattered irregularly; frequently there are many of them from the very commencement. By close inspection it is easily seen that the center of each spot corresponds to the mouth of a follicle, and the red areola to the part immediately surrounding it. The development of the primary eruptive spots is not as a rule attended by any local or constitutional symptoms. Occasionally, however the eruption is associated with very remarkable secondary, local, and constitutional symptoms ... *From this stage of primary efflorescence, lupus erythematosus may be further divided in a two-fold manner. First, as characteristic large discs, which I shall call the discoid form. Secondly, as disseminated and aggregated small spots, of the character described, which I shall call lupus erythematosus disseminatosus et aggregatus* [editor's italics].

Finally, the historically oriented reader is referred to a classic review of 265 cases of SLE compiled by Wilson and

Table 37–1. Cutaneous Manifestations of SLE (%)

Parameter	Dubois[D340] 1963	Estes[E147] 1970	Lee[L140] 1977	Grigor[G385] 1978	Rothfield[R30] 1982	Wallace[P216] 1990
No. of cases	520	150	110	50	375	464
Butterfly blush	37	39	36	68	52	34
Photosensitivity	33	—	50	28	71	37
Alopecia	21	37	38	64	74	—
Raynaud's phenomenon	18	21	46	32	20	24
Mouth ulcers	9	7	—	34	40	19
Urticaria	7	13	—	—	10	4
Dermal vasculitis	—	21	—	70	20	—
Hyperpigmentation	8	—	—	—	—	—
Leg ulcers	6	—	—	—	—	—
Gangrene	1	1	—	—	—	—
Bullae	1	2	—	—	—	—
Panniculitis	—	2	—	—	—	1

Jordan[W255] in 1950 from the dermatologic literature. This impressive summary of the state of the art in the presteroid and pre-LE preparation era provides vivid descriptions of the various lesions associated with the disease and their natural course.

SPECIFIC PRESENTATION AND FEATURES

Butterfly Area Lesions (Malar Rash)

The "butterfly area" consists of the malar region and bridge of the nose. Lesions in this zone were noted in 22 to 68% of patients in various series (Table 37–1). Three basic changes are observed. The most common is an erythematous (butterfly) blush (Fig. 37–1), either transitory or relatively permanent, which occurred in 37% of Dubois' 520 patients.[D340] The second type is a discrete maculopapular eruption with fine scaling (butterfly eruption) that appeared in 21% of his patients. The third variety is chronic discoid lupus, which was seen at some time in 29% of patients.

The classic butterfly rash is a scaly, erythematous, papular facial lesion in the butterfly and V areas; it may be precipitated by sun exposure. It appears either as a confluent erythema involving the cheeks and extending toward the bridge of the nose, or as a series of erythematous macular or papular lesions that become confluent in the same area. Periorbital edema and edema of the involved skin[B253,D329] may occur. Sometimes a transient erythema of the malar area may last a few days during an illness extending over a period of years. These lesions must be differentiated from acne rosacea, photosensitive eczema, contact dermatitis, polymorphous light eruption, erysipelas, and rashes associated with steroid administration. Persistent rashes are associated with the elevation and follicular plugging characteristic of discoid lupus. Ropes[R294] correlated malar rashes with disease activity. Most lesions can heal without scarring if present for a short time; atrophic, cigarette paper thinning may be noted at the site of old lesions, especially if the patient has had prolonged treatment with topical fluorinated steroids.

Discoid Lesions

Discoid lesions (Fig. 37–2) were observed in 14 to 29% of the SLE patients reported in Table 37–1. They represent the initial presentation of SLE in 10 to 12% of all cases.[H179,T264] Discoid rashes can antedate, coincide with, or follow the diagnosis of SLE. The histopathology of these

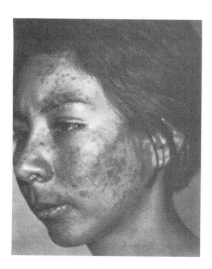

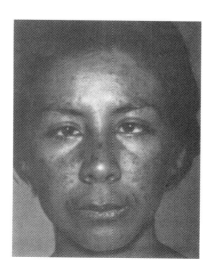

Fig. 37–1. Acute butterfly area scaly maculopapular eruption in a patient with acute SLE.

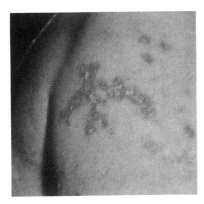

Fig. 37–2. Discoid-type lesions in a patient with SLE.

lesions is discussed in Chapters 29 and 30, and the relationship between DLE and SLE is described in Chapter 32. Hochberg et al. reported that blacks have a greater prevalence of discoid lesions than Caucasians.[H347] Callen evaluated 17 SLE patients[C20a] with discoid rashes. Except for milder renal lesions, the patients had no unique features separating them from the other SLE patients. Discoid lesions rarely appear on the palms; if they do, this may portend disease dissemination.[P56] Calcification can occur in discoid lesions associated with SLE.[K3a]

Alopecia

Alopecia is a common and characteristic finding in SLE. Some loss of hair was noted by 24 and 70% of the same group of patients, depending on whether the information was derived by chart review or detailed interview.[D306] This range reflects that shown in Table 37–1. The wide latitudes of interpretation and reporting of alopecia, and its resulting nonspecificity, caused it to be deleted from the 1982 revised ARA criteria for SLE after appearing in the 1971 preliminary classification. Nonetheless, it is still a prominent feature of SLE.

Alopecia can be classified into several categories: patchy, diffuse, scarring, or nonscarring. Discoid lesions are usually associated with scarring; they were observed in 4% of Dubois 520 patients.[D340] At times, extensive alopecia may be noted over localized zones of the scalp, either with minimal erythema in the involved area or no overt changes. Fortunately, the most common sites are toward the vertex, where it is easily covered. Franks' group at New York University found alopecia areata in 7% of 56 patients with SLE.[W183] The lesions were nonscarring, and all responded to intralesional steroids.

The most frequent type of alopecia is the diffuse type, which can be noted following combing of the hair. At times it is so marked that the scalp is readily visible through the sparse hairs. Armas-Cruz et al.[A289] noted that one-third to one-half of patients with SLE have fracturing of their frontal hair, especially in acute cases. In addition to the thinning described above, these patients often note that the frontal hairs tend to break off, leaving hairs several millimeters to 3 cm long, which tend to stand forth in an unruly fashion. They do not comb together with the rest of the hair, and produce a disheveled appearance. This has been referred to as "lupus hair," which was also noted in 6% of Dubois' patients.[D340]

Hair loss in an SLE patient must be differentiated from that induced by corticosteroids or infection. In the former case, alopecia is noted in the male pattern of baldness (e.g., in the temporal and parietal-occipital borders). An increased incidence of universal alopecia, SLE, and papular mucinosis has been reported.[L8]

Discoid-type scalp lesions should be treated with antimalarials or intralesional injections, because the persistence of such lesions leads to atrophic scarring with the destruction of hair follicles and permanent hair loss at these sites (Fig. 37–3). The other forms of hair loss respond to antimalarial and oral steroid therapy, because these treat local inflammation near the hair follicles. I have had some favorable results with minoxidil solution (Rogaine), used in the same doses as those prescribed for male baldness.

Mucous Membrane Lesions and Oral Hygiene

Mucous membrane involvement of the nose or mouth occurs in 7 to 40% of patients (Table 37–1; also see Table 33–1). Several good literature reviews and papers with excellent illustrations have appeared.[A219,A220,B574,K400, S144,V10] The lesions are most prominent during exacerbations of the systemic disorder. Typical lesions begin as a petechia on the buccal mucosa, palate, or gum, developing into a shallow, painful ulcer, perhaps becoming 1 to 2 cm in diameter, covered with a dirty grayish base, and surrounded by an erythematous areola (Fig. 37–4). They are often so painful that the patient has difficulty swallowing, and SLE may even initially present with complaints of recurrent sore throat.[G197,O81] When present on the lips, lesions are associated with fissuring, oozing blood, and edema. Ulcers can occasionally appear as a cheilitis.[C411]

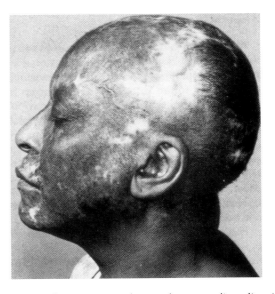

Fig. 37–3. Alopecia secondary to long-standing discoid-type lesions in a patient who initially developed discoid lupus, followed by dissemination with renal involvement.

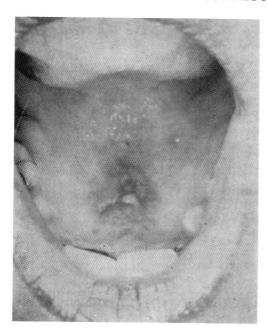

Fig. 37–4. Mucous membrane lesion in SLE. (Courtesy of Dr. R. Kitridou.)

Erythema, petechiae, and acute ulceration of the hard palate (especially at the midline) may occur frequently, particularly during systemic exacerbations. Gingivitis (tender, erythematous swollen gums) can be seen.[E147] Many patients with this manifestation have had local dental therapy for years, with no improvement until SLE was diagnosed. The epithelium over this area is easily traumatized.[M530] After the erythema persists for some time, many whitish lines appear on an erythematous background. Subsequently, the lager zones show deep fissures or ulcers. The buccal mucous membrane is also frequently involved when palate and gum lesions are present. Estes and Christian[E147] also noted that the most common site of these lesions is the central posterior part of the hard palate. Urman et al.[U31] noted ulcers in 47 of 182 SLE patients (25%). Of these, 82% were painless, and 89% were on the hard palate. The ulcers were associated with increased clinical activity but not with elevated serologies. On biopsy, immune deposits were present. Jonsson et al.[J123] noted that 23 of 51 SLE patients (45%) had oral mucosal lesions. They appeared primarily on the hard palate, buccal mucosa, and vermilion border. Oral ulcers were only seen in patients with active disease.

Superficial ulceration with recurrent oozing from lesions in the anterior nasal septum is not uncommon,[A125,V2] and may be asymptomatic. Whenever a patient complains of hemoptysis, the nasal mucous membrane should be examined carefully. A history of cocaine abuse needs to be considered. Nasal ulcerations respond well to antimalarial and topical steroid therapy. Their persistence and coalescence can lead to perforation of the nasal septum; this occurred in 3 of my 464 patients.

Perianal mucous membrane involvement may also be seen.[R369] Ulcerative lesions of the type described above appear on the vaginal mucosa concurrent with oral lesions, and result in dyspareunia.[B574]

Mucous membrane lesions must be distinguished from herpes stomatitis, methotrexate-induced ulcers, oral moniliasis, lichen planus, and leukoplakia, all of which can coexist with lupus.[G17,K72,S65,V33,Y62] One case of lingual infarct in a patient with positive anticardiolipin antibodies has been reported.[K384] A review of 17 cases reported the most common histopathologic findings as vacuolization of keratinocytes, patchy PAS-positive deposits subepithelially, lamina propria edema, PAS-positive thickening of blood vessel walls, and severe or perivascular inflammatory cell infiltrates.[K72] Immunocytochemical studies demonstrate DR antigen expression associated with active T-helper cells and macrophages in the lesions. B cells and Langerhans' cells are usually sparse or absent.[S65,V33] Increased β_2-microglobulin expression is present, but fewer than 5% of the inflammatory cells stain for interleukin-2 or transferrin receptors. All these findings are typical for SLE lesions, but are not specific for the disease.

Mucous membrane ulcers may be treated symptomatically with a hydrogen peroxide gargle, buttermilk gargle, or a steroid-impregnated dental gel (triamcinolone dental paste; Kenalog in Orabase). Antimalarials alone may heal all mucosal lesions; the healing with scarring often resembles leukoplakia with whitish strands throughout the zone, resulting from areas of increased fibrosis.

Dental problems are common in SLE, and dental work should be postponed during a lupus flare.[R188] When mouth sores are present, toothpaste should be avoided and the teeth cleaned with baking soda on a moist, soft toothbrush. NIH investigators reported that the administration of steroids to children with SLE can result in delayed primary and permanent tooth eruption and twisted roots. Steroids have been hypothesized to inhibit fibroblast contraction.[V39] Sjögren's syndrome can make oral hygiene more difficult and predispose a patient to infection. Antibiotic prophylaxis is discussed in Chapter 62.

Photosensitivity of the Eruption

Exposure to sunlight may precede or aggravate an eruption in 11 to 58% of patients.[M280,S340,T264] Photosensitivity was present in 11 to 45% of patients in the series listed in Table 33–2. In another report, 73% of 125 SLE patients claimed to be photosensitive.[W365] In 42% it exacerbated symptoms on at least one occasion, and 35% thought it had a significant impact on their lifestyle.

In one study, 128 lupus patients voluntarily underwent ultraviolet A and B light treatments. Skin lesions were induced in 42% of 86 with discoid lupus, in 64% of 22 with subacute cutaneous lupus, and in 25% of 20 SLE patients.[L178] Tuffanelli and Dubois demonstrated that white females with SLE are the most photosensitive, and Hispanic males the least,[T264] (Table 37–2). Another study repeated their experiment but focused on the role of anti-Ro/SSA antibody.[S768] The results indicated that 71% of 56 whites were photosensitive; this included 87% of those who were antibody-positive and 54% who were antibody-negative. Only 19% of blacks were photosensitive; anti-Ro/SSA did not influence photosensitivity in this group.

Table 37–2. Sex and Racial Incidence of Photosensitivity in SLE

Group	No. Photosensitive	Total in Group	% of Total
White male	5	29	17
White female	109	270	40
Black male	4	17	24
Black female	37	130	29
Hispanic male	1	11	9
Hispanic female	12	51	24
Asian female	2	12	17
Total	170	520	33

Source: Tuffanelli et al.[T264]

The effect of ultraviolet light on the eruption may be detected only by the distribution of skin lesions in light-exposed areas (Fig. 37–5). Chapter 55 discusses the management of sun sensitivity. The mechanisms by which ultraviolet light flares lupus has been a subject of controversy. In controlled settings, both ultraviolet A and B can induce skin eruptions in established lupus patients.[V62,L178] Patients may not notice erythema but may complain of increased arthralgia, malaise, and fever hours to days later. Much attention has focused on the observation that anti–double-stranded DNA becomes immunogenic after exposure to 254-nm ultraviolet radiation. It has been hypothesized that this induces a disease flare, decreases DNA repair, and results in increased in vitro release of DNA from lymphocytes.[G221,G224] Other studies, however, have disputed many of these claims.[B157,Z3,Z4] Infusion of ultraviolet-irradiated blood (e.g., photopheresis) can induce a flare of LE,[R185] as can exposure to fluorescent lights.[M160] Lupus patients run the gamut from no sun sensitivity to solar urticaria[D144] to intravascular hemolysis after ultraviolet light exposure.[W258] Lupus serum in the presence of ultraviolet light (but not without) can induce skin lesions in guinea pigs, implying that photosensitivity can be transferred passively.[11] Several reports have suggested that the increase in skin prostaglandin E reported in SLE results in an increased inflammatory response to ultraviolet light. Lupus patients may have a serum factor that blocks normal phospholipase A2 inhibition. Indomethacin can block this reaction and decrease ultraviolet light-induced erythema.[G345,G353,S528]

It is often difficult to distinguish lupus photosensitivity from a light-sensitive dermatitis. SLE lesions can be clinically identical in appearance to those of polymorphous light eruption, characterized by eczematous, papular, and plaque-like lesions that appear several hours to days after sun exposure. Polymorphous light eruptions demonstrate impressive CD1 + (Langerhans') cell infiltrates that are usually sparse in lupus,[V62] appear different under light microscopy,[W354] and yield a negative lupus band test result.[F112,V62] Therefore, it is useful to perform a skin biopsy when these two conditions cannot be distinguished.

Pigmentary Changes

Diffuse hyperpigmentation was noted in 8% of Dubois' 520 patients,[D340] 5% had localized areas of hyperpigmentation, and another 5% had small zones of depigmentation. Armas-Cruz[A289] observed hyperpigmented areas in 38% of patients and hypopigmentation in 10%. More than 20 years have elapsed since the last article that addressed pigment abnormalities in SLE. Pigmentary changes most commonly occur as postinflammatory residuals of active skin lesions of all types.[D304,D306] These changes gradually appear several months following the healing of lesions. Figure 36–6A shows a patient who had postinflammatory hyperpigmentation, and Figure 37–6B demonstrates its disappearance 11 years later. Localized, increased pigmentation following skin lesions is most common in blacks.

Diffuse hyperpigmentation is more prominent on the light-exposed and extensor surfaces of the body. The generalized increase in pigmentation usually persists and the skin gradually darkens over the years, even with treatment. Localized increases in color frequently fade slowly during the course of years. At times, insidious pigmentary changes may be noted when patients are apparently in remission (Fig. 37–7). Occasionally, areas of hypopigmentation may be the only clue to the prior existence of any type of skin lesions. Antimalarial and corticosteroid therapy can induce pigment changes and should be differentiated from abnormalities caused by the underlying disease (see Chaps. 57 and 58).

Purpura

Ecchymoses and petechiae may be noted, depending on the platelet count and whether the patient has received steroid therapy. Cutaneous hemorrhages were seen in 9 to 21% of patients in various series.[D340,E147,H179,M280] The most common cause of hemorrhagic lesions was steroid therapy, although salicylates and nonsteroidal anti-in-

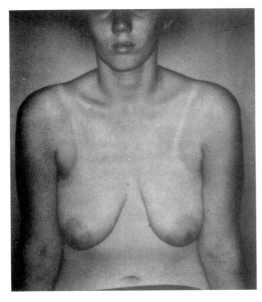

Fig. 37–5. Persistent erythema of light-exposed areas that lasted for weeks in a 20-year-old woman with SLE. She developed joint pain, fever, and pleurisy following sun exposure.

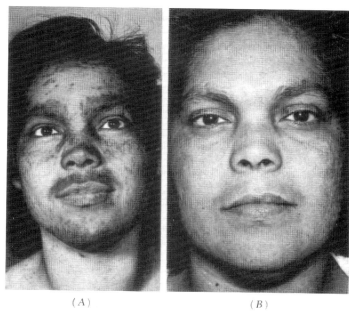

Fig. 37–6. A, Hyperpigmentation following the facial lesions of SLE. Note increased pigment supraorbitally, in the mustache area, and on the chin of this 30-year-old Mexican woman. B, Same patient 11 years later.

flammatory drugs (NSAIDs) can also induce them. NSAIDs can induce ecchymoses as a result of their antiplatelet actions, and longterm steroid administration is associated with skin atrophy. Untreated SLE patients occasionally report that they bruise easily, many are thrombocytopenic. Occasionally, petechiae may occur because of active cuta-

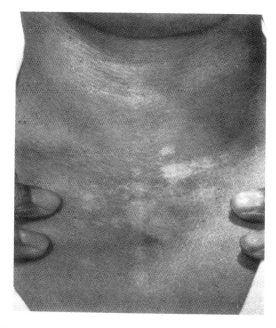

Fig. 37–7. Hypopigmentation at the site of a former erythematous macular eruption caused by SLE.

neous vasculitis. Purpuric leg lesions should be differentiated from pigmentary changes resulting from longterm antimalarial therapy. Thrombotic thrombocytopenic purpura, idiopathic thrombocytopenic purpura, cryoglobulinemia, and other dysproteinemias may be seen in SLE, and need to be ruled out.

Hives and Urticaria

Urticaria and angioneurotic edema were noted in 4 to 13% of patients in the large series shown in Table 37–1 (also see Table 33–1). In my experience, although these findings were common, it is unclear whether their occurrence in SLE is more frequent than in allergic patients who do not have this disease. On the other hand, urticarial vasculitis can be a specific skin finding in SLE.[A319] Zone and Provost[Z44] were able to associate elevated levels of circulating immune complexes and active systemic disease in 7 patients with urticarial vasculitis. Similar findings were noted by O'Loughlin et al.[O70] in 12 patients with urticaria, and biopsy documented necrotizing vasculitis.

SLE usually involved the small- and medium-caliber arteries and arterioles, and urticaria can be a manifestation of a leukocytocylastic angiitis of the smallest arteries and capillaries. Amano et al. reviewed the literature in 1989 and reported that 49 concurrent cases of SLE and hypocomplementemia with cutaneous vasculitis, arthritis, and urticaria had appeared.[A177] Skin pathology demonstrated polymorphonuclear and mononuclear leukocyte infiltration, nuclear dust, extravasation of red blood cells, and fibrinoid necrosis of small vessels. About 50% of the 49 cases met the ARA criteria for SLE. Wisnieski and Naff[W309] noted that patients with hypocomplementemic urticarial vasculitis syndrome (HUVS) have serum IgG antibodies to C1q, and that these are probably identical to C1q precipitins (C1q-P). The clinical feature of HUVS and the presence of anti-C1q antibodies in SLE suggest that HUVS is a syndrome related to SLE, (see Chap. 13). Organ-threatening SLE is frequently seen in patients with urticarial vasculitis, even without hypocomplementemia.[A319]

Bullous Lupus Erythematosus

The occurrence of bullous skin lesions is a rare but well-recognized manifestation of SLE.[L40] These were noted in 0.4% of Dubois' 520 patients in 1963[D340] and in 2 of Wallace's 464 patients with idiopathic SLE. The widespread skin lesions are chronic, recurrent, vesiculobullous eruptions with a special predilection for the face, neck, and upper extremities. They may develop in association with a generalized flare of the disease, or may occur without evidence of visceral involvement.[H58] Bullous LE must be differentiated from other primary vesiculobullous diseases that have been reported in association with SLE, including bullous pemphigoid,[J128,S702] porphyria cutanea tarda,[R300] epidermolysis bullosa,[D278,L34] herpes simplex or zoster,[F27] dermatitis herpetiformis,[B110,D13,L34] and infection.[T223] It can occur in children with SLE,[K181] be induced by hydralazine,[F129] or appear concurrently with urticaria.[F24]

In 1983, Camisa and Sharma[C44] described vesiculobullous lesions in two SLE patients. Biopsy revealed subepidermal vesicles containing neutrophils with microabscesses, nuclear dust, and fibrin at the tips of the dermal papillae; these resembled the histopathologic features of dermatitis herpetiformis. After a careful analysis of previously reported cases, they concluded that these patients comprise a unique and distinct subset of cutaneous lupus, not merely a coexistence of SLE and another primary bullous disease. They formulated the following diagnostic criteria for bullous LE: (1) a diagnosis of SLE based on ARA criteria; (2) vesicles and bullae arising but not limited to the sun-exposed areas; (3) histopathology compatible with that of dermatitis herpetiformis and leukocytoclastic vasculitis in the superficial dermis and mid-dermis; (4) positive direct immunofluorescent test showing granular-linear deposition of IgG, IgM, and often IgA at the basement membrane zone; and (5) negative result for circulating antibodies at the basement membrane zone. Subsequently, the last criterion was modified to include some patients with detectable serum antibasement membrane antibodies.[C43]

The direct immunofluorescent pattern in bullous LE is often difficult to differentiate from that of bullous pemphigoid because, in both conditions, a continuous deposit of IgG and complement components are present in the basement membrane zone.[C42,D13,F147,J128,O52,R47] Gammon et al.[G27] demonstrated for the first time in 1985 the presence of serum antibasement membrane zone antibodies in some bullous LE patients. Previous studies had been uniformly negative but, by using human skin that was split at the dermal-epidermal junction as a substrate, they found two types of serum antibodies. In bullous LE, the antibasement membrane zone antibodies reacted only with the dermal side of the separated skin, whereas in bullous pemphigoid, antibasement membrane antibodies reacted with the epidermal side alone or with both the epidermal and dermal sides of the split. Bullous LE antibodies were found to react with epidermolysis bullosa acquisita (EBA) antigen, a major component of the basement membrane. This has been identified as the carboxyl terminus of type VII procollagen.[W344]

Serum antibodies to basement membrane are not detectable in all cases of bullous LE tested. Fleming et al.[F129] found that only 4 of 32 patients reported in the literature tested positive for these antibodies, but the low prevalence may just be a reflection of the low sensitivity of the indirect immunofluorescent test. In two of three patients with bullous SLE, with characteristic linear-granular immune deposits at the dermal-epidermal junction, serum antibodies to basement membrane were found.[T157] The antibodies differed in specificity in the two patients—one reacted to the EBA antigen, whereas the other reacted to the bullous pemphigoid antigen. Thus, vesiculobullous skin lesions in SLE can be a manifestation of bullous LE or a co-occurrence of a primary bullous skin disease such as bullous pemphigoid, and the mechanisms of skin injury may differ.[G25,R47] Immunopathologic studies on the skin and serum are important in the evaluation of these patients.

Systemic corticosteroids are often not effective for the treatment of bullous LE, even in high doses. Clinical response is slow or incomplete. In some cases, the bullous

LE lesions may develop while the patient is already on corticosteroids for other organ involvement. Various drugs used in combination with systemic corticosteroids, including azathioprine, antimalarials, and cyclophosphamide, gave varying results,[F129] although the number of cases treated are too small to make any definitive conclusions. Dapsone was reported to be effective in several patients, although in an occasional patient the drug could not be tapered and discontinued without recurrence of the lesions.[C42,H58,K131] (See Chap. 61.) Bullous LE frequently recurs, and occasionally may go into spontaneous remission. Recurrence of the skin lesions might be associated with a generalized exacerbation of the disease.[H255] Bullous lupus is generally mild, but serious cases associated with organ-threatening disease have been described.[F147] (See Chap. 30.)

Pemphigus Erythematosus ("Senear-Usher" Syndrome)

In 1926, Senear and Usher described a group of patients with clinical features of both pemphigus and lupus erythematosus.[S277] These patients presented with lupus facial skin rash and bullous lesions on the chest, upper back, and intertriginous areas, which resembled pemphigus. The histopathology was similar to that of pemphigus foliaceus with subcorneal blister with acantholysis. Controversy as to whether the disease was a clinical variant of lupus or pemphigus followed the initial description. In 1968, Chorzelski and associates[C249] found immunopathologic features of both diseases in these patients by confirming the presence of immunoglobulin and complement deposits at the dermal-epidermal junction and in epidermal intercellular areas, as well as circulating antinuclear antibody (ANA) and antibodies to intercellular substance. Other investigators have corroborated these findings, suggesting that Senear-Usher syndrome represents coexistence of the two diseases.[A182,B138] The lupus band test has been shown to be positive in uninvolved nonexposed and sun-exposed skin.[J1]

Most patients reported with pemphigus erythematosus do not have multisystem involvement, nor do they meet the ARA criteria for the classification of SLE. ANAs are present in 30 to 80% of patients.[F147] Antibodies to DNA and ENA are negative.[A182] Rare cases of true co-occurrence of pemphigus and classic, multisystem SLE have, however, been reported.[F147,N83] Pemphigus erythematosus may be induced by drugs, including D-penicillamine, which is used in the treatment of rheumatoid arthritis.[K64] (See Chap. 30.)

Lupus Panniculitis (Profundus)

This entity is covered in detail in Chapter 30 in the discussion of cutaneous (discoid) lupus; this section briefly discusses its relationship to SLE. Panniculitis (lupus profundus) occurs in 2 to 3% of patients with SLE.[D304,D340,E147,K230,T261] Wallace observed panniculitis in 6 of his 464 idiopathic SLE patients. Of 34 patients with lupus panniculitis reported by Izumi and Takiguchi[172] 12 met the ARA criteria for SLE. Of 27 patients followed at the Mayo Clinic, 18 had a positive ANA test result.[W298]

Clinically, lupus profundus presents as multiple, indurated, deep subcutaneous nodules and/or plaques. They can be painful or tender and usually involve the proximal extremities and/or trunk head, or neck. Ulceration, lipoatrophy, calcification, and scarring may complicate the lesions.[P143]

Histopathologic analysis demonstrates hyaline necrosis of fat, lymphocytic aggregates, and nodules, periseptal or lobular panniculitis, and calcification. Changes of discoid lupus, lymphocytic vasculitis, hyalinization of subepidermal papillary zones, and mucin deposition may also be seen. The reader is referred to an excellent clinicopathologic review for more details.[P143]

The lesions are difficult to clinically differentiate from those of Weber-Christian disease, morphea, linear scleroderma, and eosinophilic fasciitis, and from subcutaneous nodules. Lupus profundus can occur in children,[K376,T6] and one case of an anti-Ro/SSA–positive mother and neonate, both with panniculitis, has been reported.[G401] An association has also been made with C2 and C4a null alleles.[T6]

Lupus panniculitis generally responds to antimalarial drugs,[M567,P143,W297] and systemic steroids are usually effective.

Hand and Nail Changes

The principal changes in the hands include periungual erythema, Gottron-like lesions, nail fold capillary alterations, nail changes, Raynaud's phenomenon, cutaneous vasculitis, and palmar erythema. Most of these are vascular changes, and are discussed later in this chapter.

One characteristic change is the appearance of periungual erythema and edema. Initially, erythematous papules may appear in this area.[R413] With severe exacerbations, these occasionally ulcerate. Erythematous macules may be scattered on the palmar surface with a tendency to localize either near the fingertips or in the thenar and hypothenar eminences, and resemble "liver palms." Sometimes these lesions, particularly when adjacent to the fingertips, have a purplish hue as a result of ischemia; they may progress to infarction (Fig. 37–8).

Papular lesions, when present on the dorsum of the fingers, often with scaling and erythema, are most prominent between the joints. In contrast, the scaly Gottron's lesion of dermatomyositis is found on the skin, over the joints.[K144,K146]

Nail Fold Microcapillaroscopy

In 1935, Baehr et al.[B18] noted that the involved skin about the nail bed, when viewed under the capillary microscope, contained many more patent and dilated capillaries than normal. In 1968, Buchanan and Humpston[B549] observed hemorrhage in 62% of 29 patients and abnormal capillary loops in 93%. These findings were confirmed by others.[M459,R94] Maricq and colleagues have studied these phenomena extensively in connective tissue diseases.[M130,K168] Capillary loops in SLE (independent of coexistent Raynaud's) appear meandering and tortuous, with most having some disorganization and glomerulization (Fig. 37–9).[C141] They claimed that a trained, blinded observer cold identify SLE 75% of the time. Three independent studies have given photomicrographs of patients with scleroderma, rheumatoid arthritis, SLE, and mixed connective tissue diseases to blinded observers. Lefford and Edwards could not find any relation between capillary morphology and those clinical diagnoses,[L155] Granier et al. noted that 64% of patients with mixed connective tissue disease had a scleroderma pattern, and only 23% an SLE pattern,[G336] and McGill and Gow found an 89% specificity and 80% sensitivity in selecting the correct diagnosis.[M284]

Dermatoglyphics

Whether the study of dermatoglyphics in SLE patients is useful is undecided. Dermatoglyphic (hand print and fingerprint) patterns are genetically controlled. Statistically significant differences were observed between SLE patients and sex- and race-matched controls.[D343] Vormittag et al.[V114] found no association with HLA phenotypes in 37 SLE patients and 100 controls, but those in the former group had an increased incidence of a low ending line A and a pattern in interdigitum IV of the left hand. Fraga et al.[F188] claimed that 28 Mexican patients with SLE

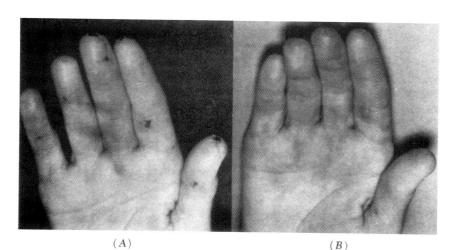

(A) (B)

Fig. 37–8. A, Cutaneous infarcts caused by the vasculitis of acute SLE. B, Same patient after 2 weeks of prednisone, 40 mg/day.

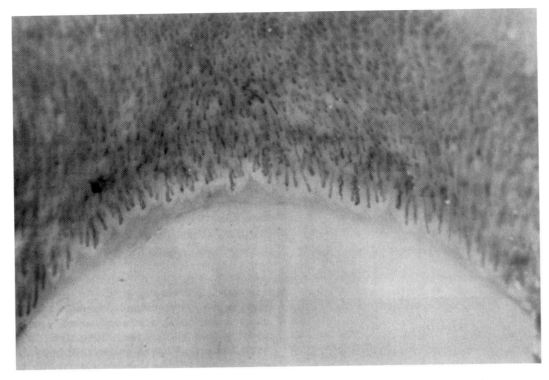

Fig. 37–9. Nail fold microcapillaroscopy in SLE. See text for details. (Courtesy of Dr. J. Kenik.)

differed from controls, and those with increased fetal wastage had higher total crease counts and ridges. Schur examined patterns in 18 SLE patients, 14 controls, and 33 relatives.[S202] Even though significant differences of the palmar patterns of the right hand and right medial and left lateral triradius displacements were found among all three groups, no clinical, immunologic, or genetic marker associations were noted.

Nails

Urowitz et al.[U37] observed nail lesions in 42 of 165 SLE patients (25%). Onycholysis was seen in 36 of 42 patients with lesions. Those with nail pathology had more active disease and Raynaud's phenomenon than those without. Illustrations in that report revealed nonspecific changes and possibly fungal infections. Color changes in nails can result from antimalarial drug therapy, especially with quinacrine. Other distinctive nail changes described in SLE patients include pitting, ridging, leukonychia, splinter hemorrhages, telangiectasia, proximal nail fold atrophy, onychomadesis, and diffuse redness of the lunula.[F189,F252,V52] Vaughn et al.[V52] reported that half of 33 blacks with SLE, but no Caucasians or blacks without lupus, had diffuse, dark, blue-black chromonychic changes. No clinical or laboratory variables identified those with as opposed to those without the dyschromic markers. Weinstein et al. found nail fold erythema in 13 and nail fold telangiectasia in 9 of 84 subjects with SLE.[W143] One patient with congenital ischemic onychodystrophy (Iso-Kikuchi syndrome) and lupus has been described.[B317]

Cutaneous Vasculitis, Ulceration, and Gangrene

Patients with active vasculitis may manifest necrotic ulcerations, digital and peripheral gangrene, and/or cutaneous infarctions (Figs. 37–8, 37–10, and 37–11). They frequently have a high-titer ANA, elevated levels of serum anti-DNA and IgG, and reduced serum complement levels.[K249,T266] Direct immunofluorescence has demonstrated IgG, complement, and fibrinogen with fibrin in the vessel walls surrounding the involved tissue.[A254,B1,H189,K218,T266]

Vasculitic leg ulcers were found in 29 of Dubois' 520 patients in 1963,[D340] and in 3% of Brogadin and Meyers' patients.[B503] Dermal vasculitis was present in 18 to 70% of the patients in the series listed in Table 37–1. Of Dubois' 520 patients, developed peripheral gangrene, as did 3 of Estes and Christian's 150 patients.[E147]

Ulcerations and gangrene can occur as a result of active vasculitis, the antiphospholipid syndrome, or both.[A99,A320,J78,J84a] Asherson et al. followed six patients with gangrene of the extremities; three had the antiphospholipid syndrome with no vasculitis, two had a classic immune complex-mediated vasculitis without evidence of a lupus anticoagulant, and one had both.[A320] Similar findings were reported by Alarcon-Segovia et al.[A99] and by Lockshin's group.[G365,H149a] Additionally, the lupus anticoagulant is rarely associated with a syndrome of cutaneous necrosis, not unlike what has been reported in protein C deficiency states.[A131,F196] Cutaneous necrosis, antiphospholipid antibodies, livedo reticularis, and central nervous system findings have been termed "Sneddon's syn-

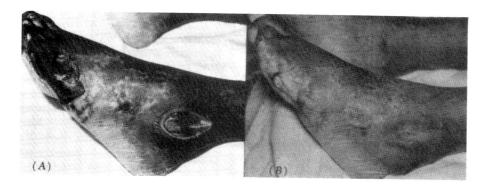

Fig. 37–10. A, Exposed tendons over the external malleolus. Extensive gangrene of the fifth toe is evident. B, Following steroid therapy, autoamputation of several toes and healing of the ulcers occurred.

drome." (See Chapter 24.) The differential diagnosis of cutaneous ulcerations requires ruling out ischemia from degenerative arterial disease, venous stasis, cryoglobulinemia, hyperviscosity syndrome, cholesterol emboli, and other hypercoagulable states.

The optimal treatment of peripheral vasculitis includes systemic corticosteroids, cyclophosphamide and, if necessary, plasmapheresis.[F291,G365,J79] If the antiphospholipid syndrome is present, anticoagulation is advised.[G365,H149a]

Raynaud's Phenomenon

Paroxysmal vasospasm of the fingers, or Raynaud's phenomenon, is a frequent abnormality in SLE. Here again, as with examples of alopecia and fractured frontal hair, the

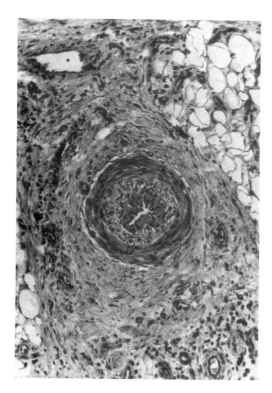

Fig. 37–11. Arteritis at base of amputated finger (H & E stain; ×150).

incidence varies with the observer's specific questioning of the patient. Raynaud's phenomenon was present at some time in 10 to 45% of the patients listed in Table 33–1. Because a history of Raynaud's phenomenon may be vague, nonspecific, and difficult to document, it was deleted from the 1982 revised ARA criteria for SLE. Its prevalence takes the middle range between the 95% found in scleroderma[R259] and the 3% seen with rheumatoid arthritis.[C107] Cholesterol emboli, cryoglobulinemia, digital infarcts from the lupus anticoagulant, and reflex sympathetic dystrophy can mimic Raynaud's phenomenon, and must be excluded.

Raynaud's phenomenon is nonspecific and may be present years prior to the development of other changes caused by SLE, scleroderma, or dermatomyositis. De Takats and Fowler[D184] reviewed 66 patients with Raynaud's phenomenon with follow-up for 1 to 25 years, and observed that 32 subsequently developed scleroderma, 2 developed SLE, and 1 developed dermatomyositis. Three later reports repeated their survey and found that 0 of 96, 0 of 85, and 0 of 87 patients with Raynaud's phenomenon carried a diagnosis of SLE, with a mean 5-, 6-, and 9-year follow-up.[G94,K34,P299] Studies of patients referred to rheumatologists because of Raynaud's phenomenon that revealed 5 to 9% had SLE.[B367,K35,M280,V60] Raynaud's phenomenon was the first manifestation of SLE in 2% of Dubois' patients (see Table 33–2).

Dimant et al.[D220] compared 91 of their 276 patients with Raynaud's phenomenon to those without it. Those in the Raynaud's group had significantly more arthritis, malar rash, and photosensitivity, less renal disease, lower steroid requirements, and fewer deaths than those in the unaffected group. The Raynaud's phenomenon associated with SLE is similar to that seen in Raynaud's disease, and is less severe than in scleroderma.[R298] The vasospasm rarely leads to permanent damage; small ulcers on the fingers can occur following prolonged and frequent attacks. Raynaud's phenomenon usually operates independently of disease activity, and is not steroid-responsive. Arteriograms on 10 Raynaud's phenomenon patients with SLE showed severe vasospasm and severe digital artery involvement that did not correlate with disease activity.[P266] Evaluation of two studies[F7,W308] leads to the conclusion that cold pressor testing improved or did not change diffusing capacities in SLE-Raynaud's phenomenon patients, but worsened it in those with primary Raynaud's phenomenon. One report was able to document a "renal Raynaud's" after cold exposure with 99m-technetium scanning.[Y25] Another demonstrated Raynaud's phenomenon of the tongue.[B75]

The treatment of Raynaud's phenomenon is not different in those with concurrent SLE. Avoidance of cold or inciting drugs (e.g., beta blockers, ergot alkaloids) along with wearing gloves, biofeedback,[M418] and vasodilators (e.g., nifedipine, nicardipine, nitroglycerin paste)[S79,S766] is advised. Pentoxifylline[G236] may be useful. Prostaglandin E1 infusions[L49,R245] improve digital ulcers and early gangrene in severe cases.

ADDITIONAL SKIN ABNORMALITIES

Atrophy and Scarring

Atrophy and scarring occur fairly often with the lesions of SLE, and are usually a function of the age of the lesions or of prolonged therapy with potent topical steroids. If persistent for months, permanent damage appears. It is therefore important to use all available modes of therapy to heal extensive cutaneous lesions in patients with SLE as rapidly as possible.[W255] Pseudoatrophy resulting from thinning of the epidermis and stretching resulting from underlying edema might occur.

Epitheliomas and Dermatofibromas

Epitheliomatous changes in lupus lesions have been reported.[M549] Dermatofibromas (histiocytoma cutis) are firm, reddish-brown cutaneous nodules with a specific histologic appearance. Two studies have associated these nodules with steroid therapy.[L297,N74]

Livedo Reticularis

Livedo reticularis occurs as a result of disordered blood flow through subpapillary and dermal blood vessels. It can be brought on by cold, connective tissue diseases, cold agglutinins, and cryoglobulinemia. In SLE, it presents as a reticulated poikiloderma, most often occurring on the arms and legs. Usually painless, livedo can rarely appear as a cutaneous vasculitis known as "livedoid vasculitis." This reddish-purplish mottling on the skin blanches on pressure, is independent of temperature changes, and represents a vasospastic phenomenon of dermal ascending arterioles.[A101,A111,G247,T267,W296] In the last decade, livedo reticularis has been shown in case-controlled studies to be unequivocally associated with cutaneous necrosis, central nervous disease, and the antiphospholipid syndrome.[A130,E110,F195,M292,W142,V38] Livedo was observed in 11 of 66 patients with SLE in one report,[Y38] and anticardiolipin antibodies were found in 81% of patients with SLE and livedo.

Erythromelalgia

Erythromelalgia consists of burning distress of the extremities accompanied by increased redness and increased skin temperature, initiated by an increase in environmental skin temperature, and diminished by measures that cool the skin.[M392] Mostly seen in myelodysplastic dis-

orders with thrombocytosis, erythromelalgia can occur in SLE patients with normal platelet counts.[A96,A101,D183,K409] It is usually treated with antiplatelet agents (e.g., low-dose aspirin, dipyrimadole) or corticosteroids, but one report documented a dramatic response to clonazepam.[K409]

Chilblain Lupus (Lupus Pernio)

Lupus pernio consists of cold-induced vessel damage that leads to a secondary dermopathy. Patients present with painful, purplish acral swellings after exposure to cold weather (see Chap. 30 for a more complete discussion). In one study, it was seen in 17 of 150 patients with cutaneous lupus; 3 of the 17 met the ARA criteria for SLE. All were mild cases.[M412] This has been confirmed by other studies,[J18,P251,U38] although the reported incidence is probably too high. Pathologically a vasculitis, it must be differentiated from cholesterol emboli. One case of lupus pernio concurrent with the antiphospholipid syndrome has been documented.[A146]

Miscellaneous Problems

Several patients with cutaneous mucinosis coexisting with SLE have been reported.[F177,R287,L8,R286] In the acutely ill, highly febrile patient, miliary vesicles may appear over the trunk and neck, suggestive of malaria.[D306,R346]

CUTANEOUS FEATURES NOT ATTRIBUTABLE TO SLE

Lupus patients can have nondisease-related rashes. Weinstein et al. compiled their experience with 84 patients (Table 37–3). A total of 119 nonlupus dermatoses was observed. The most common lesion was seborrheic dermatitis. Some of these rashes were related to lupus treatment (e.g., acne, drug eruption, malar telangiectasias secondary to fluorinated steroid overuse). Others were found to coexist with the disease, including tinea,[D205,G132,S321] acanthosis[B519,T259] pityriasis rosea,[S252] ichthyosis,[D369,F150] erythema multiforme[C433,R150,R380] (which in several early reports was actually subacute cutaneous lupus), rosacea-like lesions secondary to fluorinated steroid abuse,[M127] veruccae,[T60,E105] malignant

Table 37–3. Cutaneous Features Not Directly Attributable to SLE in 84 Lupus Patients

Lesions	Occurrence (%)
Any lesion	69
Seborrheic dermatitis	41
Essential telangiectasia, malar area	23
Severe xerosis	18
Nonvasculitic urticaria	11
Eczema	9
Acne	9
Drug eruption	8
Infection	6
Psoriasis	4
Nevi	2
Purpura	1
Solar keratoses, ichthyosis, leg ulcer	1
Other	12

Adapted from reference.[W143]

atrophic papulosis,[D282] erythema nodosum[D2] Stevens-Johnson syndrome,[B573] mulluscum contagiosum[S538] lipodystrophy[F154] and erythema elevatum diutinum.[S186] Lichen planus "overlaps" can be seen in SLE, and can mimic the disease.[A70,M549,N96,P223] A literature review found 35 reported concurrent cases.[S618] Chapter 49 discusses the relationship between psoriasis and SLE.

DIAGNOSTIC CONSIDERATIONS

Skin Biopsy

Prior to the availability of tests for ANA, skin biopsy was often helpful in the diagnosis of SLE, particularly when the LE cell tests were negative and compatible skin lesions were present. Biopsy was confirmatory in 91% of 74 patients in Dubois' series.[D310] A discussion of the histopathology of acute and chronic cutaneous and subacute cutaneous lesions is presented in Chapters 29–31; all these can be observed in SLE patients.

Because SLE may present with skin manifestations that antedate serologic abnormalities, lesional skin biopsy is still useful. LE cells and hematoxylin bodies characteristic of SLE are not usually found in the skin biopsy material, but rare reports of its presence have been made.[V73,W271]

Grishman and Churg[G395] studied the ultrastructure of SLE biopsies. Electron microscopy indicated electron-dense deposits at the dermoepidermal junction, in vessel walls, or among collagen fibers. These deposits morphologically resembled those found in the "wire loop" lesions of lupus nephritis as a result of circulating immune complexes being trapped and deposited in tissues. In addition, nuclear breakdown, fibrin, fibrillar bodies, and elastic fiber changes were noted. Halevy et al.[H50] also found these deposits in the same distribution in 18 patients. Of these, 90% had a positive lupus band test.

Evaluations for immunocytochemical markers have produced contradictory results. Langerhans' cells, the antigen-presenting cells of the skin, have been reported to be decreased overall,[A226] increased in early lesions only,[B240,K48] and decreased in central lesional sites only.[K48] Even though the cellular infiltrates are predominantly T cells, reports have suggested high suppressor cell levels[B240] or high helper and low suppressor cell levels,[A226] or equal amounts.[Y83] Infiltrating cells are usually DR (Ia-like) antigen-positive.[B240,K118]

Lupus Band Test

The landmark demonstration by Burnham et al. in 1963[B589] of immunoglobulin deposition at the dermoepidermal junction (DEJ) of patients with discoid lupus and SLE is called the lupus band test (LBT). It is still an important procedural test in establishing the diagnosis of questionable lupus.[W245] A discussion of the pathogenesis of this finding, its technical methologies, and its interpretation in DLE and subacute cutaneous lupus can be found in Chapters 29, 30, and 31.

Use of the LBT in SLE

LBTs on lesional skin are positive in most patients, but a negative result by no means rules out SLE.[B522] LBTs can be positive with negative light microscopy findings.[W220] Discoid lupus is never positive in nonlesional areas, so the LBT is usually also performed there. Many large-scale studies have been undertaken, but only the most important are cited here. The reader is referred to an excellent review of the subject.[W219]

Provost's group performed biopsies on untreated SLE patients at the extensor surface of the forearm (sun-exposed) and buttocks area (nonsun-exposed).[A69] LBTs were positive in 87% at the former site and 37% at the latter (p < .025). Therefore, in suspected SLE patients, the site chosen should be the extensor surface of the forearm. The use of certain medications, such as topical or systemic corticosteroids, can also alter the results of the LBT[H169] by making it negative. A French group noted a positive LBT in 95 of 100 lesions in SLE patients and in 47 of 100 nonlesional biopsies.[L211] Tuffanelli's large study gave similar results (see Table 32–3).[T265] Uninvolved oral mucosa yielded a positive LBT in 45% of 42 patients.[J125]

Rothfield and colleagues[S502] performed nonlesional, normal, deltoid skin area biopsies from 102 SLE patients and from 151 patients with other connective tissue diseases. One or more immunoreactants were present at the DEJ in 73% with lupus, 35% with rheumatoid arthritis, 43% with progressive systemic sclerosis, 12% with CREST syndrome, 34% with Raynaud's phenomenon, 41% with inflammatory myositis, and 44% with Sjögren's syndrome. These nonspecific-appearing results became more specific when adjusted for protein content. The predictive value for SLE was greatest with C4 (100%), properdin (91%), and IgA (86%), and lowest with IgM (59%). The specificity for the diagnosis of SLE was 64% if the presence of one or more proteins was used as the criteria, 80% if two or more proteins were present, 94% if three or more proteins, and 99% if four or more.

LBTs on drug-induced lupus patients are usually negative or weakly positive.[C363,W213] Neonatal LE LBTs are positive in 50%.[W219]

Clinical Correlates

Rothfield and Marino[R344] studied repeat skin biopsies of nonlesional skin in 31 SLE patients. Those with less active disease had fewer deposits. Staining with IgG, C3, and IgA indicated increased clinical activity, whereas IgM, C4, or C1q staining did not correlate with changes in disease activity. Other studies have confirmed these findings.[G11,W245] Davis and Gilliam[D78] followed 51 biopsied SLE patients from their series of 241 patients for 10 years, and generally found no change. Those whose LBTs remained positive had a poorer prognosis.

An LBT can be positive with immune reactants to IgG, IgM, IgA, complement components, or fibrinogen. Properdin and fibrin have been seen at the dermoepidermal junction.[R345,S55] β_{1H}-Globulin, protein S, and late complement components (C5, C7, and C9) have also been observed.[C85,M392,O19] If anti-DNA of the IgM class was prominent, an improved prognosis was postulated by Pennebaker and colleagues.[P105] Bresnihan et al.[B479] noted that prominent IgM staining had a better prognosis than prominent IgG staining. Sontheimer and Gilliam[S563] found that the intensity of the immunofluorescence correlated with the presence and amount of anti-DNA in 66 patients. In another study, patients with the most active disease had staining with IgG, IgA, and IgM.[S563] Of 60 patients with positive LBTs, 91% had active disease, as opposed to 33% of 30 patients with inactive disease.[H48] Leibowich et al.[L181] found C1q deposits at the DEJ in 90% of SLE patients but in only 29% of those with discoid LE, and its presence correlated with disease activity.[T66] Another study associated positive LBTs with increased C1q binding activity, low serum complement levels, and decreased ability to solubilize preformed immune complexes.[G5]

Whether renal disease activity correlates with skin biopsy patterns is a subject of controversy.[B2,B586,C72,G142] Some investigators have reported significant positive correlations between large quantities of IgM at the DEJ and severe renal disease, others have reported negative associations, and still others have found no correlation.[A310,B2, B260,B409,B479,B586,C72,G142,L281,M600,N114,P307,S569]

Differential Diagnosis of a Positive LBT

DEJ immune deposits have been found in many other disorders. In RA, deposits are present in 0 to 50% of patients, and are usually IgM alone in a discontinuous pattern.[B43,D109,F122,M1,P129] Positive findings were noted in 0 to 40% of patients,[B1,C227,W298,W299] with patchy uptakes of a single immunoglobulin in scleroderma and dermatomyositis. Occasional reports have appeared of similar findings in patients with Berger's disease (IgA nephropathy),[C130] postobesity bowel bypass syndrome,[A68] primary biliary cirrhosis,[N67,R39] vasculitis, porphyria, lichen planus, psoriasis,[B277] and Sjögren's syndrome.[O134] One study found a positive LBT to be of no predictive value in distinguishing undifferentiated connective tissue disease from SLE.[G274]

Prystowski et al.[P325,P327] observed epidermal nucleolar IgG deposition in normal skin from patients with sclerodactyly and speckled ANAs. Epidermal nuclear immunoglobulin deposits (in vivo ANA) are usually IgG.[K32] One abstract reported that 20% of 50 healthy controls had positive LBTs in sun-exposed areas but none in nonsun-exposed areas.[F4]

A review of these studies shows that, except in rare circumstances, no disease other than SLE can produce a continuous, confluent, intense immunofluorescent pattern at the DEJ. When such a pattern is seen with more than one immune reactant, a diagnosis of SLE is almost certain. Scattered or threaded patterns are often seen in those with other immune-mediated disorders.

Immunofluorescence of Non-DEJ Areas

Some observers have studied areas of skin other than the DEJ. Igarashi et al.[I2] found staining with IgM and fibrin at intramural and perivascular sites (especially in small-caliber vessels and capillaries) more often than in the intima. The intima is the main site of immune reactant deposition only in large-caliber arteries. Others have noted scattered deposits.[S282] O'Loughlin et al.[O71] noted vessel wall deposition about half as often as at the DEJ. A French group reported vascular fluorescence in LBTs in 57 of 100 lesional SLE biopsies and in 38 of 100 nonlesional biopsies.[L211] In vivo fluorescent staining of epidermal ANA was found to be predictive of a connective tissue disease 88% of the time. The antibody was detected against non-histone nucleoprotein that was not anti-DNA. It was present in 66, 55, and 28% of 63 patients with SLE, DLE, and subacute cutaneous lupus, respectively.[V61]

Conclusion

Almost all SLE patients with active disease have a positive LBT in skin lesion tissue, and half are positive in nonlesional areas. Almost all DLE patients have a positive lesional LBT; nonlesional areas are negative. I believe that patients with nonspecific symptoms, a low-titer, positive ANA, and marginal fulfillment of the ARA criteria for systemic lupus can often be definitively diagnosed and treated if an LBT is positive. Therefore, performing an LBT may be an extremely useful diagnostic procedure in the differential diagnosis of SLE. A negative nonlesional LBT, however, does not rule out lupus.

SKIN TESTING AND DELAYED HYPERSENSITIVITY

The status of cellular immunity in SLE has been assessed by in vivo skin testing with ubiquitous antigens and sensitization with dinitrochlorobenzene (DNCB). The reactivity of SLE patients with ubiquitous fungal and bacterial antigens has been studied by various investigators (Table 37–4).

The only significant finding in the study by Block et al.[B345] was a total anergy to intermediate-strength purified protein derivative (PPD) in the SLE group. Of the 20 in this group, 12 were steroid-treated. Only 20% manifested positive responses to intradermal calf thymus DNA, which was not significant, and had no clinical correlations. Dubois and co-workers found total anergy in 10 consecutive active untreated patients with SLE to bacterial, fungal, and mumps antigens.[B318] Reduced, delayed hypersensitivity to PPD and Trichophyton was also found by Hahn et al.[H26] in 39 patients with SLE, as compared with 30 controls.

Goldman et al. (Table 37–4)[G260]; noted no significant differences with matched controls, but Isobe found increased anergy to PPD and streptokinase-streptodornase (SKSD) in an uncontrolled study.[I49] Niwa and Kahon[N113] could not sensitize 18 of 22 SLE patents with DNCB. Of the 10 who were sensitized, 8 lost immunologic memory for DNCB 6 to 12 months later. Macrophage primary antibody responses were decreased in 14 of 22 patients, 18 had negative PPDs, and 2 of 13 had no response to typhoid or diphtheria testing. Most of the discrepancies in these studies can be accounted for by differences in therapy for those in the tested groups, which can alter the results.

RNA skin testing is probably of no diagnostic value.[J84,K372] Calf thymus DNA skin testing, however, produces a leukocytoclastic angiitis in the deep dermis of most SLE patients, but not in controls.[K372] Azoury et al.[A380] found positive skin reactions to leukocyte suspensions from normal blood donors (96%), calf thymus nucleoprotein (84%), calf thymus histone (92%), and calf thymus DNA (48%) among 25 SLE patients. Other small-

Table 37–4. Skin Testing of SLE Patients and Controls with Five Ubiquitous Antigens

Antigen	Block et al.[B345] 1968		Goldman[G260] 1972		Abe et al.[A7] 1971		Horwitz[H428] 1972		Isobe[I49] 1978
	SLE	Controls	SLE	Controls	SLE	Controls	SLE	Controls	SLE
Candida	14/20	78/112	19/23	22/23	—	—	1/14	7/12	10/16
Trichophyton	19/20	106/112	3/9	9/13	—	—	0/14	8/12	—
PPD	0/20	37/112	8/23	5/24	4/20	15/20	—	—	2/16
Histoplasmin	1/20	17/112	3/7	8/14	—	—	—	—	—
Streptokinase-streptodornase	7/20	43/112	—	—	—	—	3/14	11/11	2/15

scale studies have confirmed these percentages,[B211,O97] but Hahn observed no significant differences.[H26]

In summary, many SLE patients with active disease have impaired delayed hypersensitivity reactions. Therefore, negative skin tests to antigens such as tuberculin cannot be used as evidence against infection. Because systemic glucocorticoid therapy also impairs delayed hypersensitivity, skin testing is often of little clinical usefulness in SLE.

SUMMARY

1. Skin changes are present in 55 to 80% of SLE patients of all age groups.
2. The "butterfly" rash or flush is pleomorphic, and is present in 50% of patients at some time during the disease.
3. Discoid lesions are seen in 8 to 22% of patients with SLE.
4. The incidence of alopecia varies greatly, depending on definition and history. It can also be secondary to medication, infection, or any severe systemic disease.
5. Mucous membrane lesions, usually painful, occur in 9 to 45% of patients, and correlate with active disease. Anterior nasal mucous membrane ulcerations occur on the septum.
6. Approximately 28 to 76% of SLE patients especially Pwhites, are photosensitive.
7. Hyperpigmentation and hypopigmentation, urticaria, livedo reticularis, purpura, bullae, and panniculitis are seen in 1 to 10% of SLE patients; other skin lesions are rarer.
8. Raynaud's phenomenon is noted in 18 to 46% of patients with SLE, and is treated similarly to idiopathic Raynaud's.
9. Dermal vasculitis is seen in 20 to 70% of patients. If inflammatory, it is usually steroid-responsive. Dermal or peripheral vasculitis rarely induces gangrene; before steroids are given, the antiphospholipid syndrome needs to be ruled out.
10. Skin biopsy may identify lupus rashes, and may antedate positive serologies.
11. The lupus band test (LBT) is positive in light-exposed areas in most patients with SLE. It is positive in other disorders.
12. Biopsy of normal, sun-exposed sites helps distinguish SLE from DLE. LBT may change with medication or remission, but is only a rough guide to disease activity. The test is more than 90% specific if three or more immunoreactants in the DEJ are used as criteria for the diagnosis of LE.

Chapter 38

SYSTEMIC LUPUS ERYTHEMATOSUS AND THE NERVOUS SYSTEM

DANIEL J. WALLACE
ALLAN L. METZGER

Neurologic manifestations of SLE are frequent, vary from mild to severe, and are often difficult to diagnose and distinguish from other diseases. All portions of the nervous system may be affected, with symptoms and signs ranging from fatigue and decreased concentrating ability to seizures, stroke, and coma. At the initial development of neurologic manifestations, many patients are receiving drugs such as antimalarials or steroids, which can affect the central nervous system; thus, it is important to understand the character of the disease process unmodified by medication, and to be aware of the toxic potential of several therapeutic agents. This chapter describes the symptoms, signs, laboratory findings, differential diagnosis, and treatment of lupus involving the nervous system. (Chapter 27 discusses the etiopathogenesis of CNS lupus and the immunology of various antineuronal antibodies.) The discussion here has been developed in the context of a pathologic and clinical classification system that we believe allows the reader to grasp important concepts more easily.

HISTORICAL CONSIDERATIONS

Neurologic involvement of SLE was first mentioned by Kaposi in 1875, who described stupor and coma as terminal manifestations of the disease.[H96] Osler, in several papers on the systemic effects of the erythema group of skin diseases, discussed associated cerebral changes and presented a patient who "imagines all sorts of things."[O107,O108,O110] In 1904, Baum[B128] related active delerium, aphasia, and hemiparesis to probable disseminated lupus erythematosus. During the next 40 years, the psychiatric and neurologic correlates of SLE were recognized but seldom discussed.

The first modern study of central nervous system (CNS) lupus was by Daly in 1945.[D19] He correlated clinical symptoms with abnormal spinal fluid findings and with the pathologic finding of vasculitis. In 1948, Sedgwick and Von Hagen[S247] discussed five cases in detail. Dubois in 1953 described clinical neurologic subsets among 62 cases,[D306] and Lewis in 1954[L239] was the first to focus on the importance of electroencephalographic findings and psychometric testing in CNS lupus patients.[L239]

From the 1950s through the 1970s, hundreds of reports delineated the various manifestations of CNS involvement in SLE. Over the last decade, however, appreciation of the clinical significance of anticardiolipin, antiribosomal P,

and antineuronal antibodies, as well as advances in brain imaging, have again altered our concepts of CNS lupus.

CLINICAL PRESENTATION: AN OVERVIEW

The incidence of CNS involvement in SLE ranges from 24 to 51%, depending on ascertainment methodology. It is often impossible to compare studies of CNS lupus, because no standardized definition or classification system is used. Some reports include patients who have minimal nonspecific symptoms, and others restrict themselves to those with objective neurologic findings. Attempts to derive diagnostic criteria are in the formative stage.[S463] Clinicians are often confused and misled by the imposing array of inconsistencies in the symptoms, signs, and laboratory findings that CNS lupus patients can exhibit.

The symptoms and signs of CNS lupus are protean (Table 38–1); they include headache, confusion, seizures, myelopathy, papilledema, focal or generalized neurologic deficits, psychosis, severe depression, and organic brain syndrome (OBS). The pathologic abnormalities observed in the nervous system are also diverse (Table 38–2); furthermore, often no clear-cut clinicoanatomic relationship between CNS signs and localized CNS lesions can be noted. This section discusses the prevalence and focus of CNS lupus as described in some of the principal surveys of the last 40 years. Because the prevalence and features of CNS lupus might be changing, these surveys are categorized by decade, and are summarized in Table 38–3.

CNS Lupus in the 1950s

Of Dubois' 520 patients[D340] followed between 1950 and 1963, 25% had some type of central or peripheral nervous system damage. In a 1956 review of the clinico-neurologic changes observed in 24 of 100 patients with SLE followed at the Mayo Clinic, Clark and Bailey[C276] reported changes that varied from convulsive seizures to monoplegia, and revealed an entire gamut of neurologic damage. Signs and symptoms of neurologic disease alone were noted in 11 patients, and neurologic and psychiatric disease together were present in 13.

CNS Lupus in the 1960s

In 1966, O'Connor and Musher[O11] reviewed 150 SLE patients followed at Columbia Presbyterian Medical Cen-

Table 38–1. Major Clinical Neurologic Manifestations of SLE

Cognitive dysfunction
Headache
Seizure
Altered consciousness (stupor, somnolence, coma)
Aseptic meningitis
Cerebral hemorrhage, infarction
Paresis, myelopathy
Peripheral neuropathy (cranial neuropathy, polyneuritis)
Movement disorder (chorea, ataxia, tremor)
Altered behavior (psychosis, organic brain syndrome, depression, confusion, affective disorder)
Stroke
Optic neuritis
Pseudotumor cerebri

Table 38–2. Pathologic Classification of Central Nervous System Changes Observed in SLE

Vasculopathy
  Hyalinization
  Perivascular inflammation without infection
  Endothelial proliferation without infection
  Thrombosis
  Vasculitis
Infarction
  Microinfarcts
  Large infarcts
Hemorrhage
  Subarachnoid
  Microhemorrhages
  Subdural
  Intracerebral
Infection
  Meningitis
  Perivascular inflammation with infection
  Septic hemorrhages
  Focal cerebritis
  Vasculitis with infection

Adapted from Ellis, S.G., and Verity, M.A. Sem Arth Rheum 8:212, 1979.

ter. Of these, 4 presented with CNS lupus. CNS disturbances were more frequent among patients followed through terminal illness; 67% of the 150 had psychiatric disorders and 43% had neurologic disorders. Neurologic signs were seen at one time or another in 46 of 150 patients.

In 1971, Estes and Christian[E147] observed neuropsychiatric manifestations of SLE in 59% of 150 patients followed mostly in the 1960s. Disorders of mental function were found in 42% and grand mal seizures in 26%. The neurologic manifestations were cranial nerve involvement (7 patients), oculomotor signs (6), and optic atrophy and blindness (3). Intention tremor was observed in 8 patients and was associated with cogwheel rigidity in 2. Hemiparesis occurred in 8 patients, 6 of whom had chronic renal disease with hypertension and/or uremia. Peripheral neuropathy with predominantly sensory deficits developed in 10 patients.

CNS Lupus in the 1970s

In 1975, Sergent et al.[S287] reported on 52 episodes in 28 SLE patients; 10 had seizures, 9 had organic brain syndrome, 4 had aseptic meningitis, 7 had focal neurologic deficits, 15 had psychiatric abnormalities, and 1 had chorea. They found no evidence that large doses of steroids were helpful in treating these patients. Also in 1975, Klippel and Zvaifler[K312] compiled a literature review of CNS abnormalities in 995 reported SLE patients. Half were Dubois' 520 cases. Overall, neuropsychiatric abnormalities were found in 33%, 16% had seizures, 10% had neuropathy, 18% had psychopathology, and 4% each had myelopathy and chorea.

In 1976, a review of 140 SLE patients at the Johns Hopkins Hospital revealed neuropsychiatric changes in 52%; [F46] 63% of these had episodes in the first year of disease. Only two instances of documented steroid-induced psychosis occurred. Of the 140 patients, 84% improved with SLE treatment. A striking positive correlation was noted among CNS involvement, vasculitis, and thrombocytopenia. Five- and 10-year survival rates of those in the CNS group were 94 and 82%, respectively.

Urowitz's group at the University of Toronto[A8,L140] published two large SLE studies that emphasized CNS findings; the group with CNS disease had lower serum complement levels and more disease manifestations than those without CNS pathology. Grigor et al.[G385] found neuropsychiatric symptoms in 50% of 50 patients. No correlations could be found with any other SLE manifestations, including vasculitis and thrombocytopenia.

Gibson and Myers[G124] noted CNS episodes in 41 of 80 patients (51%) followed before 1976. More episodes were noted in blacks, and an increased incidence of renal failure as well a poorer survival was seen in this group, as

Table 38–3. Neurologic Manifestations of SLE in Selected Large Series (%)

Parameter	Clark & Bailey[C276] 1956	Estes & Christian[E147] 1971	Ropes[R294] 1976	Gibson & Myers[G124] 1976	Feinglass[F46] 1976	Lee[L140] 1977	Hochberg[H347] 1985	Wallace[P216] 1990
No. of cases	100	150	150	81	140	110	150	464
CNS Manifestations	24	59	—	51	52	40	55	50
Seizures	14	26	11	20	17	8	13	6
Cranial neuropathy	—	7	—	4	16	3	—	—
Vasculopathy	8	8	15	10	16	3	—	11
Peripheral neuropathy	3	7	5	2	15	8	21	5
Psychosis	17	16	28	27	14	16	16	5

opposed to the non-CNS group. In contrast to most of the preceding reports, Seibold et al.[S255] calculated that CNS involvement occurred 4.3 years (mean) after disease onset in 26 patients.

CNS Lupus in the 1980s

The 1980s saw a continuing decline in the reported frequency of classic CNS lupus. Our group observed 49 cases of cerebritis and, comparing patients evaluated from 1950 to 1963 with those evaluated between 1980 and 1989 this represents a decrease from 26 to 11%.[P216] Using the American College of Rheumatology definition for CNS lupus as a criterion (seizures or psychosis), 30 patients (6%) had seizures and 24 (5%) had psychotic episodes. Severe headaches are now the most common neuropsychiatric abnormality in SLE patients; we have observed it in 144 (31%) of our patients. Antiribosomal P antibodies became recognized in the 1980s, and were associated with psychosis.[B401] A Norwegian study observed migraine headaches in 40% of patients with additional CNS manifestations and severe protracted headache in another 20% without other CNS symptoms or signs.[O79] West et al. noted CNS lupus in 50 of 184 patients (28%) in Colorado, and others noted CNS disease in 40 of 188 patients (21%) in Saskatchewan, in 35 of 222 (16%) in Australia, and in 22 of 53 (42%) in Italy.[B551,M402,O77,W188]

The recognition of anticardiolipin antibodies affirmed the usefulness of classifying CNS episodes into "diffuse" and "focal," with the latter usually reflecting lupus anticoagulant-mediated thromboembolic episodes.[F86,K72] These surveys confirmed the early presentation of CNS involvement,[F324,G399] its association with generally active lupus,[K7] and the rarity of steroid-induced psychosis necessitating hospitalization.[B551,W188] A survey of strokes in SLE found a 15% incidence among 105 patients.[F324] The major risk factors were the circulating lupus anticoagulant and a patient age of more than 60 years. Of 184 SLE patients followed by West et al. between 1980 and 1989, 50 (28%) had 52 CNS episodes; 32 episodes were diffuse, 10 were focal, and 10 had features of both. CSF abnormalities were associated with diffuse episodes, anticardiolipin antibody was associated with focal episodes. Of the 42 patients with diffuse CNS manifestations, 6 succumbed.[W188] In the only published analysis of the genetics of CNS lupus, a Japanese group reported an increased association with CNS episodes and HLA-Bw61.[K127]

Studies by the Denburgs[D152,H100,K156] have established cognitive dysfunction as a subset of CNS lupus; this was often present in the absence of objective neurologic, clinical, or laboratory abnormalities.

CNS Disease in Children and the Elderly

Several groups have examined CNS lupus in children. Cassidy[C147] noted a 31% incidence in 58 children. Yancey et al.[Y29] found a 43% incidence in 37 children, and her literature review of 11 pediatric studies found a 33% incidence in 353 children. CNS involvement was less frequent in older age groups (more than 50 years old)—19% and 6% in two studies[B36,D219]—and it was generally milder.[M267] In one report, however, 9 of 10 patients diagnosed with SLE at an age over 50 had neuropsychiatric manifestations. of these, 5 had peripheral neuritis, 3 had cerebellar ataxia,[M267] and nearly all were steroid-responsive.

Summary

SLE can involve the nervous system in many ways. No exact definition of "CNS lupus" has been established. Until recently, the presence of specific neuropathology (e.g., seizures, stroke, paresis) was considered to constitute CNS lupus, and was found in about 25% of patients with SLE. Over the last three decades, the incidence of these features has decreased as early intervention in the diagnosis and treatment of active SLE became more common. Over the last decade, however, the recognition of lupus headache and cognitive dysfunction as distinct "vasculopathies" (as evidenced by flow abnormalities on positron emission tomography [PET] scanning), in the absence of specific neuropathology, has resulted in a net *increase* in the incidence of what many rheumatologists call "CNS lupus." CNS lupus as now defined is present in most SLE patients at some point during the course of their disease; specific neuropathology is seen in a minority, is usually of short-term duration, and may lead to a chronic organic brain syndrome.

CEREBRAL VASCULITIS, VASULOPATHY, AND ITS CLINICOPATHOLOGIC CORRELATIONS

The cause of CNS lupus was formerly thought to be cerebral vasculitis. Although this entity exists, it is less common than initially believed. Cerebral vasculitis is noted in 8 to 16% of patients with CNS manifestations (Table 38–3). It is likely that the etiopathogenesis of CNS vasculitis is similar to the immune dysfunction that produces vasculitis elsewhere in the body, and probably includes immune complex trapping, in situ immune complex formation, and/or T-cell—mediated damage. Currently, most experts believe that the majority of CNS manifestations are mediated by a few autoantibodies. Chapters 18 to 28 review some autoantibody system specificities that may be relevant to CNS disease in SLE, including antibodies to neuronal tissues, cardiolipin and other phospholipids, antiribosomal P, and lymphocytotoxic antibodies, as well as immune complexes or fragments thereof deposited in the choroid plexus. Additionally, cytokines can affect mood and behavior, and many of these may be abnormal in SLE. Neurotransmitter dysfunction levels have also been associated with antireceptor antibodies (e.g., myasthenia gravis), and these autoimmune disorders are seen in association with SLE.

Clinicopathologic Studies

Most of our knowledge in this area is derived from the results of three groups that carried out detailed studies of the neuropathology of SLE. Johnson and Richardson[J95,J96] reviewed the brain sections of 24 patients observed at Massachusetts General Hospital in the 1960s. Neurologic and psychiatric manifestations were found in 18 patients (75%). In 9 of these 18, neurologic involvement occurred during the last 6 weeks of life. Death was attributable to CNS disease in 6 patients (4 intracerebral hemorrhage in 4, 2 status epilepticus in 2). Seizures were present in 54%, cranial nerve disorders in 42%, hemiparesis in 12%, paresis in 4%, peripheral neuropathy in 8%, and mental disorders in 33%. Significant gross abnormalities were found in 10 of the 24 patients, including large intracerebral hemorrhages (3), multiple pontine hemorrhages (1), fresh hemorrhages (2), small areas of old infarction (4), and a small, subapical hemorrhage (1). Microscopic lesions were more common than macroscopic; microinfarcts with increased pericapillary microglia were found in 20 of the 24 patients. Johnson and Richardson concluded that nervous system involvement of SLE was caused primarily by vascular disease affecting small vessels and producing microinfarcts with hemorrhages. True vasculitis was rare; inflammatory cells within the vessel wall were found in only 3 of the 24 patients. In contrast, perivascular inflammation was more common. Destructive lesions in the walls of small vessels, described as fibrinoid degeneration, were found in 5 patients. No distinct typical or pathognomonic lesion in the brain was documented to be comparable to the "wire loop" lesion of the kidney, or to the "onion skin" lesion of the spleen. The degenerative and proliferative changes observed in the small cerebral vessels were not distinct from the vascular changes found in hypertensive encephalopathy. The neuropathologic lesions of SLE, however, were characterized as more focal or more scattered, and by the fact that they varied in age from region to region, rather than appearing to have occurred simultaneously.

Funata[F311] performed detailed neuropathologic evaluations on 26 SLE patients; 12 died as a result of uremia, and half had perivascular inflammation in the brain. Thrombi associated with endothelial swelling and proliferation and fibrinoid degeneration were noted in 5 patients.

Ellis and Verity[E85] reviewed 57 autopsied SLE cases at UCLA Medical Center. Vasculopathy was observed in 65%, infarction in 44%, hemorrhage in 42%, and infection in 28%. In the vasculopathy group, hyalinization (54%), perivascular inflammation (28%), endothelial proliferation (21%), thrombosis (7%), and vasculitis (8%) were found. The infarctions consisted mostly of microinfarcts. Hemorrhages included subarachnoid (30%), intracerebral (10%), and subdural (4%) hemorrhages, and microhemorrhages (19%). In those with infections, meningitis (18%), perivascular inflammation (14%), septic hemorrhages (5%), and focal cerebritis (3%) were seen. Many patients in this group had received combined corticosteroid and azathioprine therapy. All these studies antedated anticardiolipin antibody availability.

Some evidence indicates that the prolonged use of corticosteroids may accelerate the onset of cerebrovascular and cardiac atherosclerotic disease. Several cases of subarachnoid hemorrhage caused by berry aneurysm have been described in SLE. It is not known, whether these lesions are more common in those with SLE than in the general population.[H192,N11,S99] One survey of 500 SLE patients treated at the National Institutes of Health revealed evidence for cerebrovascular disease in 15, occlusive in 11 and hemorrhagic in 4.[T246] CNS lupus can also involve the small arachnoid arteries of the spinal cord, causing transverse myelitis. In addition, a nondrug-related aseptic meningitis can occur.[K149,L41,N24] CNS vasculitis can develop during pregnancy.[S774]

Clinical Manifestations

Nonthrombotic CNS Lupus (Including Cerebral Vasculitis)

Cerebral vasculitis is a dramatic process that presents with fever, confusion, and headache followed within hours to days by seizures, psychosis, and encephalomyelitis. If untreated, it can lead to coma and death. Cerebral changes are usually generalized. Laboratory investigation often reveals active multisystem SLE with elevated serologies and decreased serum complement components. The cerebrospinal fluid (CSF) usually demonstrates pleocytosis, an elevated protein level, and increased IgG, along with an elevated IgG:albumin ratio. At least 80% of patients have antineuronal antibodies in the CSF. Cultures are negative. Magnetic resonance imaging (MRI) and CT scanning are not usually helpful at first; positron emission tomography (PET) reveals hypoperfusion. The key to establishing CNS vasculitis involves its generalized features. Cerebral vasculitis is used in a clinical context, and does not necessarily imply that the pathologic lesion is a "true" vasculitis in the brain (Fig. 38–1).

Vasculopathy: Thromboemboli Produced by the Circulating Lupus Anticoagulant

Harris and colleagues increased our understanding of the antiphospholipid syndrome in several reports published in the 1980s. They were the first to relate many focal neurologic complications of SLE to the syndrome.[H151,H156] The most common clinical features are transient ischemic attacks or paresis. The antiphospholipid syndrome may be associated with as many as 40%

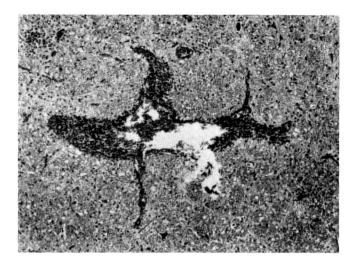

Fig. 38–1. Periphlebitis in the floor of the third ventricle of the brain of a 13-year-old girl with convulsions caused by SLE (H & E stain; ×85).

of all CNS-SLE complications that necessitate admission to a hospital, and partly explains the rarity of vasculitis observed at pathology.[L224] It is not proven, however, whether the presence of circulating antiphospholipid antibodies is associated with most thrombotic lesions in the brain in CNS lupus. In 1989, 13 strokes occurring among 234 SLE patients were analyzed; cerebral infarction was noted in 8, cerebral hemorrhage in 2, and subarachnoid hemorrhage in 3.[K255] Hypertension was the most common cause of stroke, but only 3 had the lupus anticoagulant. None had cerebral angiitis. A brain biopsy of a patient with SLE, stroke, and the lupus anticoagulant demonstrated multiple infarcts, fibrosis, thrombosis, and intimal proliferation.[W196]

Other studies have shown that cerebral artery embolization with fragments from a Libman-Sacks–like endocarditis is associated with the presence of antiphospholipid antibodies.[A322,A338,Y59] In addition to arterial cerebral emboli, venulitis, cerebral venous thrombosis, lupus cerebral phlebitis, and anterior spinal artery syndrome with paresis have been reported and confirmed angiographically.[L224,M142,V80] Chorea is not uncommonly seen (see below).

Although most clinical presentations are focal, they can occasionally be generalized.[L11] Anticardiolipin antibody is not found in cerebrospinal fluid, and is not associated with serum antineurofilament antibodies.[B179,F86] A small percentage of the normal population has anticardiolipin antibodies. Most of these individuals are asymptomatic, but an increased stroke risk is present.[A26,T217] Steroids are generally not helpful for the treatment of thrombotic CNS lupus. Minimum treatment requires platelet antagonists for prophylaxis, and more aggressive treatment centers around anticoagulation in the face of multiple, cerebrovascular events.

Hemorrhagic Complications of Lupus Coagulopathy Including Thrombotic Thrombocytopenic Purpura and ITP

A small subset of SLE patients with the antiphospholipid antibody has an increased bleeding tendency with neurologic consequences, but this group usually has the associated thrombocytopenia or hypoprothrombinemia (see Chap. 24 and 25). Other causes of cerebral hemorrhage such as hypertension, which may occur in SLE, must be excluded.

Lupus patients with or without the antiphospholipid syndrome may develop immune thrombocytopenic purpura (ITP) and/or low platelet counts secondary to uremia, drugs, or chemotherapy, and present a bleeding risk. Of our 464 patients with idiopathic SLE, 4 had thrombotic thrombocytopenic purpura (TTP), which by definition has neurologic sequelae (see Chap. 43). A literature review of 50 patients with TTP in SLE determined that 25 had CNS lesions, 10 had embolic brain infarcts, and 8 had CNS infections.[D188]

Lupus Headache

Headaches are relatively common in SLE. Even if headaches caused by hypertension, nonsteroidal anti-inflammatory drug (NSAID) use, and infection are excluded, the incidence is still high. King et al.[K232] reported headaches in 16% of 108 children with SLE and Rothfield described "severe" headache in 21 of her 209 patients.[R339] A chart review of our 464 patients with idiopathic SLE revealed significant headache symptomatology in 144 (31%).

Despite its frequency, the nature of headache in lupus was not addressed until 1975. At that time, Atkinson and Applenzeller[A355] described a headache syndrome distinct for SLE that was independent of hypertension, renal disease, steroid therapy, and active CNS lupus. They implied that a group of SLE patients had severe headaches in the absence of other CNS findings. Brandt and Lesser[B459] studied what they called the "migrainous phenomenon" in SLE. Eleven patients had detailed evaluations. Headache tended to be associated with disease activity, and usually responded to corticosteroid treatment. Most patients had abnormal cerebrospinal fluid findings, and all had abnormal electroencephalograms. Isenberg et al.[134] found significantly more headaches in SLE patients than in a control group, but could not relate its occurrence to Raynaud's phenomenon. One group, however, could correlate these events in SLE, and another noted an increased association between classic migraine headaches and Raynaud's phenomenon in Sjögren's syndrome, scleroderma, and rheumatoid arthritis with Sjögren's syndrome.[M508,P12] Two studies that attempted to characterize the headaches as vascular (migrainous) or of the muscular contraction type determined that each make up about 50%.[O79,V55]

Over the last decade, attention has been focused on the role of the lupus anticoagulant and migraine. Levine et al. presented 2 cases in detail and reviewed 8 others in the literature.[L222] Migraine was associated with the lupus anticoagulant and thrombotic events. It was postulated that the ability of the lupus anticoagulant to alter prostaglandin and platelet activity also results in interactions with the neuronal phospholipids that lead to headache and ultimately to thrombosis. In another review, 15 patients with SLE and the lupus anticoagulant referred for neurologic consultation were analyzed. Of these, 10 (67%) had migraine and 9 (60%) had thrombotic complications.[H370] Controlled studies are needed to confirm this important observation.

Seizures

Fortunately, seizures are less common than in the 1950s because of the prompt recognition of lupus symptoms that warrant definitive treatment, improved anticonvulsive drugs, and lower doses of antimalarials. Despite the incidence of seizures, a lack of scientific interest prevails; the topic of seizures in SLE has not been reviewed in detail since 1954.

Dubois treated 520 patients with SLE between 1950 and 1963,[D340] 13.8% had grand mal seizures—six episodes were disease-related for every one that was treatment-related.[D306] Most patients who died in the hospital had seizures 48 to 72 hours antemortem. Table 38–3 indicates that the frequency of seizures in numerous large series is between 6 and 26%. Comprehensive reviews of seizures in SLE appeared in 1941, 1951, and

1954.[K284,L239,R433] About 25% of these were grand mal, many were preterminal, and others were associated with hypertension, uremia, and CNS "vasculitis." A brief 1987 report analyzed seizures in six patients.[H20] No CT scan correlates were found; most convulsions were partial tonic-clonic events. Electroencephalography revealed slow background activity and a few paroxysms, suggesting diffuse brain dysfunction. One report associated seizures with the lupus anticoagulant.[V57]

Differentiation of seizures caused by disease from those induced by therapy may be difficult. Seizures caused by CNS lupus usually respond to steroid treatment, and may never recur after the acute episode has subsided.[P288,R433] Steroid withdrawal, intravenous pulse steroids, scar foci from prior vasculitis, infection, nitrogen mustard, and high doses of the antimalarials quinacrine and chloroquine (mostly used in the 1950s) are also associated with epileptic events. Even though some anticonvulsants may induce a positive ANA and rarely clinical SLE, this is no reason to withhold these agents when indicated for patients with established lupus.

Movement Disorders: Chorea, Ballismus and Ataxia

Chorea has been observed in 1 to 4% of SLE patients. In 1971, Donaldson and Espiner[D261] reviewed 22 patients and described a patient presenting as chorea gravidarum. The mean age of onset was 18 years. Chorea was the initial presentation of SLE in 8 patients, and preceded other manifestations of SLE by up to 7 years. Additional neurologic symptoms were present in most. Spinal fluid findings were abnormal in a minority. Groothuis et al.[G403] analyzed 29 cases in the literature in 1977. The overwhelming majority were children, with a 6:1 female-to-male ratio. Of these 29, 85% had an elevated sedimentation rate and the average duration of the chorea was 12 weeks. Arteritis was never found at autopsy; only widespread infarcts were observed, which always included the basal ganglia. Bruyn and Padberg reviewed 52 cases in the literature in 1984.[B546] Chorea did not correlate with any other neurologic symptoms, occurred early in the disease course, and never lasted longer than 3 years. Several patients had chorea gravidarum. Syndenham's chorea secondary to rheumatic fever can be ruled out by obtaining antistreptolysin titers. Steroids and haloperidol were of variable benefit in the above cases.

The availability of antiphospholipid antibodies explains many of the puzzling conclusions of these reviews. In 1986, Hadron et al. reanalyzed the cited cases and determined that at least 20 of the patients had spontaneous abortions, false-positive serologic test results for syphilis, or evidence for the circulating lupus anticoagulant.[H15] Asherson's group observed chorea in 12 of 500 subjects with SLE (2.4%). Of these 12, nine had antiphospholipid antibodies, and 7 of the 12 also had transient ischemic attacks or cerebral infarcts.[A321,A328,K186] Anticoagulation was recommended. Lafeuillade et al. confirmed these findings but cautioned in one literature survey that not all cases are a result of the antiphospholipid syndrome.[L11] Chorea did not adversely affect prognosis, and no other CNS clinicopathologic correlations were found. Two case reports have claimed an association among chorea, the

antiphospholipid syndrome, SLE, and oral contraceptive use.[148,M187] Infarction of the subthalamic nucleus can result in ballismus. Rarely has it been reported in SLE, and it may be steroid-responsive.[T158]

Cerebellar ataxia is noted in fewer than 1% of patients with SLE.[S470] The cause is uncertain, but some cases may be produced by the antiphospholipid syndrome.

Paralysis: Myelopathy and Guillain-Barré Syndrome

Myelopathy is a rare but distinct abnormality in SLE. First reported in 1959,[G241] it is characterized by flaccid paralysis. Dubois found lupus myelopathy in 2 of his 520 patients between 1950 and 1963,[D340] and Wallace found myelopathy in 2 of his 464 SLE cohort followed between 1980 and 1989.[P216] Penn and Rowan reviewed 9 cases in 1968.[P103] They noted rapid onset of an ascending paralysis that correlated with inflammatory infiltrates without vasculitis at autopsy. Extensive necrotizing myelitis may be present, but arteritis is rarely observed (Fig. 38–2).[A229]

Kewalramani et al. found SLE myelopathy to the cause of 2 of 1350 admissions to a spinal cord injury unit, and reviewed 26 cases in the literature in 1979.[K183] Of these, 83% were female, ranging in age from 20 to 40 years. The following features were noted: myelopathy was the initial manifestation in 3, and 11 had no prior diagnosis of SLE; 2 were quadraplegic, 7 paraparetic, and 19 paraplegic (4 of whom subsequently became quadraplegic); the spinal fluid protein level was elevated in 14 of 16 evaluated, and the CSF glucose level decreased in 7 of 12; 15 survived the episode, and only 4 had considerable improvement; 13 died between day 2 and month 34 (most from sepsis or pulmonary compromise); and 2 had spinal cord vasculitis by pathologic evaluation. Steroids were claimed not to alter prognosis, a claim disputed in a review that reanalyzed the data.[P305] Werner and Kredich[W85] reviewed 31 cases and noted weakness and sensory loss in 100% of

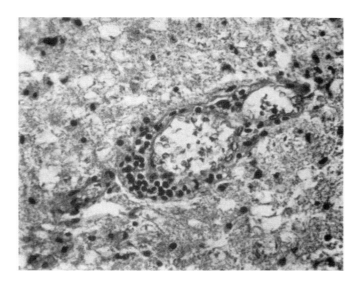

Fig. 38–2. Acute arteritis and edema of surrounding tissue in the spinal cord of a 22-year-old patient with paraplegia caused by lupus vasculitis (H & E stain; ×750).

patients reporting the finding, impaired sphincter control in 100%, and hyperreflexia in 22%. Laboratory abnormalities included elevated CSF protein level (82%), decreased CSF glucose level (50%), and pleocytosis (70%). Of 9 patients who underwent myelography, 8 had normal studies. Another good literature review of 34 cases appeared at the same time and reinforced these findings.[A141]

Alarcon-Segovia's group reported four cases of myelopathy among 500 SLE patients (0.8%). All had antiphospholipid antibodies.[L96] Other reports have appeared supporting this association.[H119,M120] Chang and Quismorio[C204] found anticardiolipin antibodies in 8 of 17 patients who experienced 27 episodes of transverse myelopathy at Los Angeles County-University of Southern California Medical Center. Their subjects had a mean age of 39.8 years at presentation, and it was the initial manifestation of SLE in 8 (47%). Of their 17 patients, 4 developed paraplegia, 2 quadraplegia, 12 paraparesis, and 1 hemiparesis. MRI scans were normal in all 5 patients tested. Over the short term, 13 patients improved in neurologic function and 4 showed no change (2 of these died).

In 1989, a report that emphasized treatment and prognosis was published. Of 26 patients, 7 had a full recovery, 9 had a static or slowly deteriorating course, and 10 died. Of 8 patients who promptly received high-dose corticosteroids, 5 recovered, versus only 2 of 18 who did not receive steroids.[P305] Conversely, Hachen and Chantraine[H11] reviewed 28 cases and showed that steroids can worsen myelomalacia, which can lead to further motor and sensory losses. Cyclophosphamide may be useful.

The cause of lupus myelopathy is unknown. Harris et al. have related it to the presence of antiphospholipid antibodies,[H156] and Daras et al.[D41] correlated it with elevated CSF myelin basic protein levels (a nonspecific finding in the presence of spinal cord injury). Lupus myelopathy has also been associated with neonatal lupus,[K135] pulmonary hypertension,[H119] optic neuritis,[K167] aseptic meningitis,[S68] and pregnancy.[M120]

The differential diagnosis of lupus myelopathy can be confusing. A case of lupus myelitis was presented in the context of showing that accepted criteria for Guillain-Barré syndrome, which only involves peripheral nerves, were also fulfilled, even though the patient clearly had extraneural SLE.[M439] Lupus has rarely been claimed to be independently associated with Guillain-Barré syndrome.[C18,G47,M572,S425] Patients with SLE have also presented with myelopathy that has been shown to be secondary to vertebral compression fractures,[H267] herpes zoster,[B21] tuberculosis,[D294] and the polyoma (JC) virus.[S711] The value of MRI is debatable. A group at the National Institutes of Health presented a patient with lupus myelitis whose MRI scan revealed increased signal intensity and diffuse edema of the cord acutely, which was gone at day 12.[S434] They concluded that early abnormal findings can be helpful, if present, and thus urge early scanning.

In summary, acute lupus myelopathy should be treated with high-dose corticosteroids. If the patient has evidence of antiphospholipid antibodies, heparin therapy should be initiated. The treatment is modified once the results of blood tests and cultures become available.

Psychosis

See Chapter 39.

Organic Brain Syndrome

Any CNS manifestation of SLE that can damage brain tissue—infection, thromboembolic phenomenon, or vasculitis—ultimately heals and scars. This can leave patients with significant cognitive, mood, personality, and seizure disorders, functional impairment, and dementia. These patients have the organic brain syndrome (OBS), which is observed in 3 to 30% of patients with SLE (see Table 39-1). This group only develops more cortical atrophy and behaves more inappropriately if given corticosteroids, so their use is contraindicated unless extracranial lupus activity can be documented. Conversely, acute organic brain syndrome is usually a manifestation of active SLE, is sometimes the only symptom, and may respond to a short course of high-dose glucocorticoids. Chronic OBS is usually nonprogressive but irreversible, and is extremely difficult to treat other than with palliative support measures. See Chapter 39 for a more detailed discussion.

CNS Symptoms Induced by Circulating Factors

A large percentage of patients with mild to moderate SLE complain of nonspecific CNS symptoms. These include difficulty concentrating, mild confusion, depression, loss of stamina, and headache.[K436] Circulating factors such as autoantibodies or perhaps cytokines (without evidence for CNS vasculitis) might be responsible. The neurologic examination is usually unremarkable, but neurodiagnostic testing may indicate cognitive dysfunction (see below). Many of these individuals have high-titer antinuclear antibodies, elevated anti-DNA antibody levels and sedimentation rates, and low C3 or C4 serum complement levels.[S253,S655] Serum and CSF antineuronal antibodies and antilymphocyte antibodies are sometimes present.[K156] In fact, high-titer IgG antineuronal antibodies are highly associated with active CNS lupus. Some reports have suggested that psychosis or severe depression, with or without cerebral vasculitis, is associated with the presence of antibodies to antiribosomal P.[B401,S472] Abnormalities in interleukins (IL), IL-1 and IL-2, IL-2 receptor, and interferon have been reported in SLE patients (see Chap. 9 and 10). Additionally, α-interferon and IL-2 administration have been associated with fibrositis-like symptoms.[M265,W34] The patient's cognitive complaints are usually chronic in nature and rarely evolve into life-threatening CNS lupus. Subacute flares may respond to a short course of 20 mg of prednisone a day or less, but some patients also experience ameliorative results with antimalarials.

Pseudotumor Cerebri and Hydrocephalus

Pseudotumor cerebri is a form of benign intracranial hypertension without focal neurologic dysfunction. Patients complain of headache, and may have swollen optic disks. Spinal fluid is biochemically and immunologically normal. Pseudotumor cerebri in SLE patients has been the subject of eight papers describing a total of 12 patients.[D143,K63,L256,L257,P54,S429,S719,W154] Nearly all the individuals were young girls or adolescents. About half had dural venous sinus thromboses; in others, the pseudotumor was associated with corticosteroid treatment, especially during periods of rapid taper. None of those tested had the lupus anticoagulant, but this has not been adequately studied. Treatment consists of corticosteroids in some cases, and anticoagulation or antiplatelet agents in others. One case of normal pressure hydrocephalus in an elderly female with SLE has been reported.[U11]

PERIPHERAL, CRANIAL, AND AUTONOMIC NEUROPATHIES

Peripheral Neuropathies

Peripheral neuritis of varying degrees has been observed in 2 to 21% of patients in various series (Table 38–3). Mononeuritis multiplex may be the initial presentation of SLE.[B235] A Norwegian lupus clinic asked their 57 patients to undergo voluntary, extensive, neuromuscular testing.[O79] Of the 30 who complied, 7 patients (23%) were found to have carpal tunnel syndrome and 2 had a peripheral polyneuritis on a vasculitic, nonradicular basis. Patients with peripheral neuritis may complain of numbness and tingling.

Vasculitis of the peripheral nerves was established clinicopathologically by Sedgwick and von Hagen in 1948,[S247] and confirmed in numerous reports.[B28,C276,L239,S119] These patients were characterized by a high degree of CNS abnormalities, in addition to frequent elevations in spinal fluid protein levels. The diagnosis was often established by nerve conduction times or nerve biopsy. Of Estes and Christian's 150 patients, 7% had peripheral neuropathies. Most were of a sensory nature, but 1 had bilateral wristdrop and another had bilateral footdrop (Fig. 38–3).[E147] Most patients in these studies were steroid-responsive, but refractory patients have responded to cyclophosphamide and plasma exchange.[H482] Some patients, however, do not respond to any current therapies. Fibromyalgia and radiculopathies must be ruled out as a cause of numbness and tingling. A case of sensory ataxia as the initial presentation of SLE has been documented.[S12]

McCombe et al. performed detailed pathologic analyses of seven connective tissue disease patients (four had SLE) who underwent sural nerve biopsy.[M239] Chronic sensorimotor peripheral nerve changes were clinically evident, with predominantly sensory features and gradual onset. The pathologic findings were those of axonal degeneration and vasculitis. Of the seven patients, six had increased Ia antigen expression within the nerve fascicle, perineurium, and endothelial cells.

Cranial Neuropathies

Cranial neuropathies are present in 3 to 16% of lupus patients (Table 38–3) during the course of their disease. They are usually transient and steroid-responsive, and consist primarily of ophthalmoplegias, trigeminal neuralgia, or facial palsy.

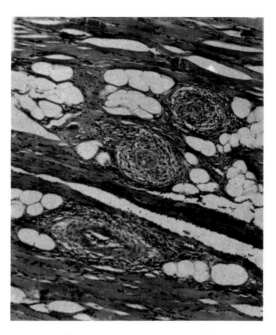

Fig. 38–3. Vasculitis in gastrocnemius muscle biopsy of patient with severe peripheral neuritis of legs and bilateral footdrop (H & E stain; ×150).

Lundberg and Werner[L420] described five SLE patients who had unilateral or bilateral trigeminal sensory neuropathy. The lesions did not correspond to the trigeminal branches, and it was postulated that the changes are caused by vascular lesions in the medulla oblongata. Another report on this subject has also been published.[G45] A definite association exists between this entity and mixed connective tissue disease.[C321] Carbamazepine (Tegretol) is helpful in some patients.

Internuclear ophthalmoplegias result in paresis of the medial rectus muscle. Generally associated with multiple sclerosis, seven documented reports in SLE patients have been published. The reader is referred to a recent case presentation, with an excellent literature review.[S241] Ptosis and third and sixth cranial nerve palsies have been reported. The lesions are usually a result of vasculitis or infarction.[A275,R189,R310] One case of bilateral facial nerve palsy caused by angioedema has been reported in an SLE patient.[C452]

Autonomic Neuropathies

Acute autonomic dysfunction, as defined by severe sympathetic and parasympathetic impairment, with preservation of somatic sensory and motor functions, rarely occurs in those with autoimmune disorders, but has been reported in one case of SLE and one case of mixed connective tissue disease.[H462] Gastrointestinal, cardiovascular, genitourinary, sweating, and pupillary abnormalities are evident; these responded to corticosteroids. A South African group performed a battery of sophisticated autonomic tests on 15 patients with SLE and Raynaud's phenomenon.[G189] Of these, 13 had at least one abnormal evaluation. This implies that subtle autonomic dysfunction is present more often than is clinically appreciated. Maddison's group evaluated 23 outpatients with mild SLE using standardized autonomic testing. Mild abnormalities were found in 3 (13%) with SLE but in no controls.[T185]

MECHANICAL SLUDGING—CRYOGLOBULINS OR HYPERVISCOSITY

Circulating cryoglobulins are found in 5 to 90% of SLE patients, but clinically significant cryocrits (greater than 8%) are rare (Chap. 28). Nevertheless, an infrequent patient with cryoglobulinemia who complains of mental clouding, dizziness, and confusion requires intervention with α-interferon, plasmapheresis, and/or cytotoxic drugs in preference to corticosteroids. Hyperviscosity syndrome is also rarely seen; if identified, it is readily treatable with plasmapheresis.[A46,F302,J50,S341]

DIFFERENTIAL DIAGNOSIS OF SECONDARY CNS DISORDERS IN SLE PATIENTS

The presence of antinuclear antibodies in a patient with neurologic symptoms does not imply that the patient has CNS lupus or, for that matter, lupus at all.[M143] Many other possibilities need to be considered in the differential diagnosis; these are discussed in this section.

Effects of Medication for SLE

Lupus patients often take medications known to have CNS effects. Corticosteroids can induce psychosis, euphoria, altered moods, and helplessness.[H56,J81,J82,L241] Psychosis resulting from corticosteroids can be difficult to differentiate from CNS vasculitis lupus-induced psychosis (see Chaps. 39 and 58). In a fascinating case presentation, both were shown to coexist in one patient.[H321] Progressive, multifocal leukoencephalopathy may be drug-induced, has been seen in SLE, and can mimic the disease.[N77] Antimalarial administration is rarely associated with hyperirritability and seizures (see Chap. 57). Indolacetic acid derivatives (indomethacin, tolmetin, and sulindac) may induce headache; ibuprofen can cause an aseptic, meningitis-like syndrome virtually peculiar to SLE patients.[A65,W37] Tinnitus and confusion have resulted from salicylism, especially in the elderly. SLE patients have an increased incidence of hypertension, and certain antihypertensive agents may induce fatigue and depression. All treating physicians must obtain a careful drug history from their patients. Nearly all these medications (including steroids) can be withheld for brief periods to determine causation.

Fibromyalgia (Fibrositis)

Of our 464 idiopathic SLE patients, 20% fulfilled established criteria for fibromyalgia (fibrositis).[P216] Fatigue, myalgias, paresthesias, insomnia, and headache, as well as complaints of confusion and depression, may be reported. It is often impossible to differentiate fibrositis in SLE from CNS symptoms. Corticosteroids may alleviate fibrositis temporarily, worsening this diagnostic dilemma. Fibrositis can also be induced by tapering steroid doses ("steroid withdrawal syndrome"). Physicians must resist the temptation to raise the steroid dose, because this is a self-limited process that can go on for several weeks. The use of pain-modulating agents (e.g., tricyclic antidepressants), physical measures (e.g., physical therapy, conditioning, tender point injections), and reassurance with counseling often relieve these secondary fibrositis symptoms.

Central Nervous System Infections

SLE patients have decreased chemotaxis and ability to kill bacteria, and are thus more susceptible to infections.[C282,P120] In addition, corticosteroids and cytotoxic agents have multiple immunosuppresive effects, and their use increases the risk of bacterial, viral, and fungal infections and parasitic infestations in SLE patients.[G159] The neurologic manifestations of CNS infection can include confusion, lethargy, headache, neck pain, seizures, psychosis, and fever, with or without focal or generalized sensory and motor deficits. Nearly every organism has been reported to infect SLE patients (this is discussed in detail in Chap. 46). Tuberculosis,[R145] bacterial endocarditis,[D81] and meningitis[C339,P18] have been mistaken for CNS lupus. The most critical step is a lumbar puncture: although CSF pleocytosis can be also seen in cerebral vasculitis, a low glucose level and positive Gram's stain and/or culture are diagnostic of CNS infection. CT scans with contrast or MRI may help locate an abscess or focal area of involvement. Whenever infection is likely, it is advisable to introduce broad-spectrum and/or multiple antibiotics that cross the blood-brain barrier. After that, glucocorticoid doses can be increased (if considered advisable) to treat CNS lupus when cultures are pending, or to prevent addisonian crisis during stress.

Emotional Adjustments Involved in Coping with SLE

Living with SLE involves lifestyle adjustments and creates its own stresses. Reactive depression with or without anxiety and functional symptoms such as sweating, palpitation, diarrhea, and hyperventilation are observed with increased frequency in SLE patients.[W22] It is imperative not to confuse these symptoms with active disease. Chapter 39 outlines various methods of dealing with these problems.

Nonlupus-Related CNS Symptoms

Patients with SLE can develop non-SLE–related CNS complications of vascular, metabolic, oncologic, neurologic, and psychiatric disturbances that can mimic or aggravate those of CNS-SLE. Any disorder can coexist with SLE and produce neurologic compromise. For example, extreme hypertension can mimic angiitis at arteriography.[G54] Subdural hematomas can present as headache in SLE patients.[B440] In a review of 8 patients that appeared in the literature,[F323] Urowitz's group associated some with an increased bleeding tendency seen in lupus and others with trauma or other causes. Physicians need to keep an open mind and should not treat a putative CNS lupus manifestation incorrectly. Some of the more difficult diagnostic dilemmas are detailed below.

Multiple Sclerosis or Lupoid Sclerosis

Multiple sclerosis is a chronic, relapsing, demyelinating disorder with an autoimmune cause. Some of its neurologic manifestations, such as fatigue, weakness, and transverse myelitis, may be difficult to differentiate from those of SLE.[A147,F307,H522,K62,M588] Overlapping features of both disorders has been termed "lupoid sclerosis."[D192,P99] The advent of MRI has helped to elucidate the diagnosis in most disputed cases, but true coexistence of these diseases has been reported.[B244,L381] and families have been known to have histories of both disorders.[M238,S492] A survey of multiple sclerosis patients showing that 81% have positive antinuclear antibodies further clouds the issue.[D266]

Fluid and Electrolyte Imbalances

Psychosis can be induced by hypokalemia, water intoxication, hyponatremia, and the syndrome of inappropriate antidiuretic hormone (SIADH). Reports have appeared of SLE patients presenting with these abnormalities, especially those with nephropathy who are taking diuretics.[B336,D111,K57,W364] Blood chemistries should be checked in patients with CNS symptoms.

Factitious Illness and Positive ANA Without Lupus

Cases of young women with factitious illness claiming to have SLE have been reported.[L235] Secondary gain and/or the search for an all-encompassing disease entity have led many patients with low-titer, positive ANAs and nonspecific complaints such as fatigue and headache to seek rheumatologic consultation, and become disappointed when told they do not have lupus. Patients in psychiatric facilities have an increased incidence of positive ANAs,[V105] and a small percentage have undiagnosed lupus.[P141] Phenothiazine derivatives, which are given to most institutionalized patients, may induce positive serologies (e.g., ANA antilymphocyte antibody, antierythrocyte antibody, low-titer ds-DNA),[D105,M37,P220,Q15] but rarely clinical SLE.

Myasthenia Gravis

See Chapter 43.

CLINICAL AND LABORATORY EVALUATION OF NEUROPSYCHIATRIC LUPUS

A methodical work-up is essential for the lupus patient who presents with any suspicion of neuropsychiatric disease. A thorough history must include inquiring about medications, headaches, fever, stamina, altered behavior, cognition, and may require interviewing family members. The physical examination must include complete neurologic and mental status evaluations. In addition to baseline laboratory evaluations and serologies, obtaining a lupus anticoagulant profile and carrying out tests for PTT, VDRL, and anticardiolipin antibody are important. Under certain circumstances, viscosity and levels of serum cryoglobulin, protein C, protein S, antiribosomal P antibodies, and antineuronal antibodies should be measured, a two-dimen-

Table 38–4. CNS Involvement in Patients with SLE

Nonthrombotic CNS disease—probably mediated by antineuronal antibodies and other autoantibodies, and/or by immune complexes; includes vasculopathies, vasculitis, and nonvascular lesions
    Cognitive defects
    Seizures
    Organic brain syndromes
    Behavioral disorders
    Psychoses
    Myelopathy
    Peripheral neuropathies
    Headache
Thrombotic CNS disease—often mediated by the lupus anticoagulant or by antibodies to phospholipids; can include vasculitis
    Strokes
    Chorea
    Behavioral disorders related to strokes
    Some cases of myelopathy
CNS disease caused by factors other than SLE
    Side effects of drugs
    Electrolyte abnormalities
    Inherent behavioral or cognitive defects
    Infection
    Complications of hypertension

sional echocardiogram obtained, and a CSF sample tested with appropriate chemistries and immune studies, Gram's stains, and cultures. Routine CSF evaluation and cultures can be augmented by CSF (and serum) antineuronal antibody tests, a search for oligoclonal bands, and determination of IgG:albumin ratios (the albumin quotient). Occasionally, LE cells can be seen in vivo in the CSF.[N137] Neurodiagnostic testing procedures including MRI, CT scanning, evoked response testing, and psychologic testing for cognitive disorders or organic brain syndrome are often useful. Investigational tests such as those for antiglial antibodies, antisphingomyelin antibodies, and antineurofilament antibodies, and CSF measurements of complement components, lactic acid, cyclic GMP, and β_2-microglobulin, may be clinically relevant in the future, as may PET and SPECT scanning (see below). Tables 38–4 and 38–5 outline the diverse subclasses of CNS-SLE and diagnostic studies, and suggests pertinent clinically accepted treatment regimens. This paradigm allows the clinician to carry out a logical approach to what is often a difficult and serious diagnostic and therapeutic dilemma. Figure 38–4 provides an algorithm for working up an SLE patient with potential neurologic disease.

Other Clinical Laboratory Studies in CNS Lupus

No serologic or blood determinations specific for CNS lupus are in general use. Seibold et al.[S253] found elevated anti-DNA levels in 55% of patients, decreased C3 levels in 43%, circulating immune complexes in 30%, and a positive anti-Sm in 46% of 34 patients. Steinman[S655] demonstrated increased anti–ds-DNA in the form of circulating immune complexes in 16 of 20 patients with CNS lupus and/or systemic vasculitis by use of a counterimmunoelectrophoretic assay. Lee et al.[L140] noted that total hemolytic complement and C3 complement are lower in a CNS lupus group than in those SLE patients without CNS involvement. Seibold et al.[S255] and Winfield et al.[W284]

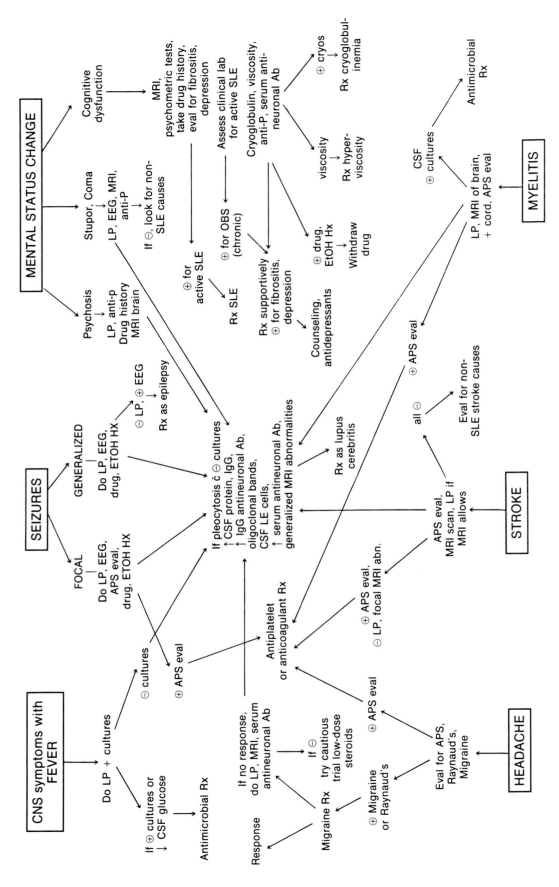

Fig. 38–4. Algorithm for determining whether CNS lupus cerebritis is present (APS, antiphospholipid syndrome; OBS, organic brain syndrome).

could not find this association with complement, anti-DNA, or anti-RNP. In the latter study, an increased incidence of anti-Sm was noted in those with CNS lupus. It is also likely that anaphalotoxins C3a and C5a mediate the CNS effects of immune complexes by eliciting vascular injury.[H414]

Antiribosomal P

Antibodies to the C-terminal region of ribosomal P proteins are found in 12 to 28% of SLE patients.[B401,B402,Q10, S152,S590,T96] Bonfa et al.[B401,B402] first observed it in 18 of 20 individuals with SLE-induced psychosis, and its activity was said to correlate with the clinical course. In addition, blacks, males, and anti-Ro/SSA positivity were associated with the antibody. Two other groups have related anti-P to psychosis,[S152,S590] but others have failed to confirm this association.[Q10,T15] Anti-P is probably less specific for CNS lupus than antineuronal antibodies,[T96] and is usually not found in the CSF.[G276] Levels of the antibody may correlate with the level of psychosis is selected patients.[D168] See Chapter 27 for an immunologic description of the antibody.

Antilymphocyte Antibodies

Antilymphocyte antibodies are not specific for SLE and can occur in other illnesses, including infections, malignancy, inflammatory bowel disease, and multiple sclerosis.[D99,D123] A subset of antilymphocyte antibodies, however, cross reacts with neurons. Fever, neuropsychiatric symptoms, skin lesions, and hematologic abnormalities are the most common manifestations in SLE patients with serum lymphocytotoxic antibodies.[B598,N94] Denburg's group has related cognitive dysfunction to the presence of serum IgM lymphocytotoxic antibodies in over 445 patients evaluated.[D151,D154,L371] This may reflect the presence of the antineuronal subset. In a prospective study, Temesvari and associates[T102] found a correlation between fluctuations of serum lymphocytotoxicity and relapses or remission of neuropsychiatric involvement in individual SLE patients (also see Chaps. 26 and 27).

Serum Antineuronal Antibodies

Serum antineuronal antibodies are neither as sensitive nor as specific as CSF antibody measurements. Nevertheless, 80% of patients with CNS lupus have serum IgG antineuronal antibodies, as compared to 5% of those with SLE without CNS involvement.[B359,B361] Cognitive impairment in children was not related to these antibodies in one survey.[P36] IgG antineuronal antibodies in the CSF correlate well with active CNS lupus. Serum antineurofilament antibodies react against cytoskeletal neurofilament protein antigens; antibody is present in 18% of controls, 20% with focal CNS lupus, and 58% with diffuse CNS disease.[R233] Horowitz et al. have associated a brain synaptic plasma membrane antigen (known as Lp50) with neuropsychiatric lupus.[H423] See Chapter 27 for a full discussion of antineuronal antibodies.

Miscellaneous Antibodies

A Brazilian study of 66 patients correlated CNS lupus with the presence of IgM antiganglioside and IgM antigalactocerebroside antibodies.[C404]

Cerebrospinal Fluid Findings

The results of a lumbar puncture are often unremarkable, but the procedure may be worthwhile because any abnormalities found are helpful in guiding management. The CSF should always be examined in acutely ill lupus patients to exclude secondary infections, because many SLE patients are receiving steroids and immunosuppressives that can mask infection.

Cell Count, Protein and Glucose Levels, and LE Cells

Pleocytosis and elevated protein levels are found in some patients with active CNS lupus. Protein abnormalities are more common (range, 22 to 50%) than pleocytosis (range, 6 to 34%) in CNS lupus in 10 studies analyzing spinal fluid findings in 250 patients.[A8,D340,F46,G124, S253,S255,S497,W295,Y29] Feinglass[F46] noted a worse prognosis in those who had a lumbar puncture evaluation, but related this to a more critical presentation in this group.

The CSF glucose level is rarely decreased in CNS lupus. It was reported as low by Seibold et al.[S253] in 4% of 28 patients, by Gibson and Myers[G124] in 8%, and by Abel et al.[A8] in 3%.

The occasional presence of in vivo LE cells in the CSF is rarely looked for and documented, but can be a helpful indicator of active CNS disease.[N137]

Complement

In 1971, Petz et al.[P167] showed that the C4 level in CSF decreases in those with acute CNS lupus. The C4 level turned out to be unstable in the CSF, and difficult to measure, and its value largely unconfirmed in other reports.[B35,H113,S286,S497] Intrathecal C4 synthesis may be increased in those with diffuse CNS lupus.[J118] Six of seven patients with CNS lupus (and none of two without CNS disease) had CSF fluid phase terminal complement complexes SC5b, as compared to nine patients demonstrating intrathecal complement activation.[S67] (See Chapter 13.)

Immunoglobulins and Immune Complexes

In 1972, Levin et al. reported that IgG levels in the CSF were decreased in 12 patients with CNS lupus.[L213] Subsequent studies revealed opposite results. Seibold et al.[S253] evaluated 34 patients with active CNS lupus. Of these, 96% had elevated CSF immune complexes, in comparison to 4% without CNS disease. The IgG level in the CSF was also elevated in 96%, but the IgM and IgA levels were not. Circulating immune complexes were present in 30%. Small et al.[S497] noted elevated CSF IgG levels in 69%. Bluestein et al.[B361] found that a CSF IgG level greater than 6 mg/dl almost always indicated CNS lupus, but it was present in only 40% of their patients. An IgG:albumin ratio greater than 0.3 was positive in 60% of CNS lupus patients. It is less specific however, because it is present in 20% of all SLE patients. Winfield[W289] reported CSF Ig-G: albumin ratios (also known as the albumin quotient) to be elevated in one-third of patients with SLE, especially those with progressive encephalopathy, transverse myelitis, and paraparesis. A smaller scale study has confirmed these findings.[W187] Winfield's group[W295] also found oligoclonal IgG in the CSF accompanied by an elevated IgG index, indicating a persistent antibody response in the CNS to a putative autogenous or exogenous antigen.

Hirohata and colleagues published several reports reinforcing the valve of determining CSF immunoglobulin indices to monitor CNS lupus.[H320,H323,H325] Increased IgG, IgA, and IgM indices reflected polyclonal B cell activation in neuropsychiatric lupus, and decreased with treatment. IgG: albumin ratios were not helpful. Light chains (κ and λ) could also be detected.

Lymphocytotoxic Antibodies

Cold reactive lymphocytotoxic antibodies have been found in the CSF in higher titers in those with CNS involvement than in those without.[W237] Winfield and colleagues correlated CSF elevations with CNS manifestations better than serum levels, although another group was unable to confirm this.[H507] See Chapters 26 and 27.

Antineuronal Antibodies

Bluestein et al. found serum IgG antibodies to neurons in 74% of SLE patients with CNS involvement, compared to only 11% of SLE patients without CNS disease. Moreover, the antineuron antibody was concentrated eightfold in the CSF relative to its concentration in paired serum specimens.[B359,B361] The Denburgs and their colleagues have evaluated the significance of antineuronal antibodies in several reports on at least 36 lupus patients and 98 controls.[D152,H100,K156] Even though only 14% of lupus CSF samples had IgG antineuronal antibody, it correlated with abnormal albumin quotients, anti-DNA, disease activity, cognitive dysfunction, and nonfocal CNS-SLE. The evolution of improved methodologies for detecting neuronal reactive antibodies is discussed in Chapter 27.

Miscellaneous Determinations

Brook et al.[B505] found CSF lactic acid levels to be normal in those with CNS lupus. Because this value is increased in those with bacterial meningitis, it may be helpful in the differential diagnosis.

Kassan and Kagen[K98,K99] noted that CSF guanosine 3'5'-cyclic monophosphate (cyclic GMP) levels are elevated in CNS lupus. This correlated with pleocytosis and was not present in patients with lupus psychosis alone. It is nonspecifically elevated in other neurologic disorders.

One study reported that most patients with CNS lupus have increased CSF anti-DNA and DNA–anti-DNA complexes.[S497] An elevated CSF β_2-microglobulin level may be specific for CNS lupus.[G277] Substance P levels were higher in those with CNS-SLE, especially with myelitis and seizures, as compared to a control group.[K383] Lipsky's group observed polyclonal T cells to be increased in the CSF, most of which were CD4 +.[C459] Interleukin-6 may also be elevated in those with neuropsychiatric lupus.[H324]

Summary

When a lumbar puncture is performed in a patient with suspected SLE, or in a lupus patient with possible CNS lupus or infection, the following should be determined: cell count, glucose and protein level, cultures, Gram's stain, in vivo LE cells, "multiple sclerosis panel," which includes oligoclonal bands, protein electrophoresis, and immunoglobulin synthesis indices, and antineuronal antibodies. Pleocytosis and an elevated protein level are present in about one-third and suggest acute inflammation; a positive multiple sclerosis panel implies immunologic activity but does not necessarily mean active CNS vasculitis; and high titers of IgG antineuronal antibody strongly suggest active CNS lupus.

Brain Imaging

Technetium Static Scans and Xenon Flow Studies

Technetium brain scans are not usually helpful. They were abnormal in 8% of 37 patients presented by Grigor,[G385] in 9% of Seibold's 34 patients,[S253] in 19% of Gibson and Myers' patients,[G124] and in 2 of 23 patients at Johns Hopkins Hospital[F46] with CNS lupus. On occasion, abnormalities may correlate with clinical findings,[B207] but it is generally not a sensitive tool.[D336] Only the University of Toronto group advocated its use, and consistently obtained excellent sensitivity and specificity with this method.[A8,K449,T55]

Xenon-133 is an outdated means of evaluating cerebral blood flow (e.g., Medicare has stopped reimbursement), whose usefulness will surely be superceded by the use of PET and SPECT scanning.[A369,K482,K483]

Computed Tomography

The advent of CT scanning has enabled rheumatologists to establish the high incidence of steroid-induced cortical atrophy in SLE. Two large studies have noted atrophy in 27%[S253] and 71%[O80] of 64 subjects. It is perisulcal in 50%.[C83,G77,R146] CT scanning can also detect basal ganglia and paraventricular calcification[D54,N124] and subdural collections of fluid.[R146] Even though CT scans may locate sites of infarction,[W153] at least 20% of patients with clear-cut CNS episodes have normal findings[K7] (Fig. 38–5).

Magnetic Resonance Imaging and Comparisons to CT

McCune and colleagues first described three MRI patterns in patients with neuropsychiatric lupus: areas of large infarction, small microinfarcts, and increased intensity in gray matter that resolved 2 to 3 weeks after the acute event.[A77,M259] MRI was the most sensitive in picking up focal deficits,[A77,B179,C362,M259,M260,S692] and can be normal in diffuse CNS disease.

Six groups subjected a total of 92 SLE patients to concurrent CT and MR scanning.[J30,S296,S407,S692,S771,V70] MRI is clearly superior for detecting edema, infarction, and hemorrhage, whereas CT has an edge for detecting cortical atrophy and skull fractures. Of great importance, between 25 and 80% of those with neuropsychiatric symptoms of SLE and a normal CT scan have abnormal MRI results (Fig. 38–6). In a prospective study of the useful-

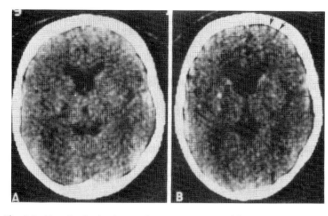

Fig. 38–5. Perisulcal atrophy in a 27-year-old woman with psychosis. A, A CT scan shows top normal lateral ventricles. B, After 1 year, a CT scan shows enlargement of the ventricles, sulci (*arrows*), and fissures (*open arrows*) caused by atrophy. (From Bilaniuk, L. T., Patel, S., and Zimmerman, R. A.: Computed tomography of systemic lupus erythematosus. Radiology, *124*:119, 1977.)

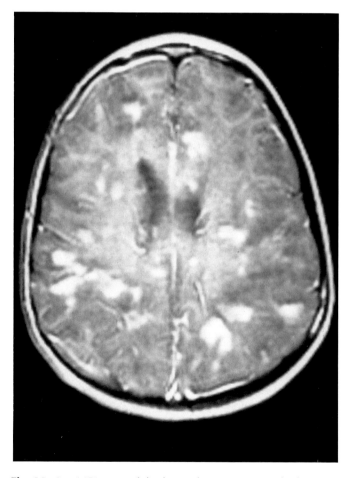

Fig. 38–6. MRI scan of the brain documenting multiple areas of infarction caused by generalized cerebral vasculitis. (Courtesy of Dr. J. Mink.)

ness of MRI in CNS lupus, we found that SLE patients who had CNS findings produced by other causes exhibited similar MRi abnormalities to those with CNS lupus, thus limiting the diagnostic specificity of MRI.[S692]

Nuclear magnetic resonance (NMR) spectroscopy using phosphorus-31 can detect decreased ATP and phosphocreatine levels in patients with CNS-SLE that improves with therapy.[G373]

Angiography

Cerebral angiograms are helpful in identifying angiitis and the vascularity of lesions when noninvasive methods are not definitive.[S37,T216,W135] Angiitis caused by SLE usually involves the small and middle-sized vessels, and rarely large ones.[W135] One report of an exacerbation of CNS lupus following metrizamide dye administration has appeared.[G86] MR angiography can also show vasculitic lesions.

Positron Emission Tomography

In 1978, Pinching et al.[P192,T209] demonstrated $^{15}O_2/C^{15}O_2$ perfusion deficits in CNS lupus patients. The current availability of positron emission tomography (PET) scanners has produced scattered reports of its promise in CNS-SLE.[G437,H319,Y102] Stoppe et al.[M378,S712,S713] obtained CT, MRI, and PET scans from 13 lupus patients who had evidence of CNS involvement. The most common abnormalities included hypometabolism to the temporal and parietal regions; many of these had normal CT or MRI scans. Abnormalities in PET scans improved with therapy.[C76] Because PET scanners require a cyclotron and are restricted to university centers, the availability of community-based single-photon emission computed tomography (SPECT) imaging has piqued interest in its applications for CNS-SLE. Stimmler et al.[S691] studied 9 hospitalized individuals with neuropsychiatric lupus using isopropyl-L-1,2,3-iodoamphetamine. Of these, 8 had SPECT findings, the most common being hypoperfusion of the cerebellar and parietal lobes.

Summary

CT and MRI scanning define anatomic pathology. Both are useful but MRI is superior for localizing infarcts and hemorrhage, whereas CT is superior for identifying cerebral atrophy. The abnormalities seen on the MRI and CT scans are not specific for SLE, and the results should be interpreted along with the clinical and other laboratory findings in establishing the diagnosis of CNS lupus. PET and SPECT imaging can detect perfusion abnormalities, but their promise has not been adequately assessed.

Electrical Studies

Electroencephalography

Abnormal electroencephalography (EEG) patterns are common in SLE patients, with or without overt neurologic changes. Unfortunately, often little correlation exists between the clinical picture and the brain wave changes. Patients with diffuse organic brain disease and psychoses caused by SLE may show normal EEG tracings. At other times, routine EEGs in SLE patients without CNS symptoms may show diffuse abnormalities.

Russell first explored the use of EEG in SLE patients in 1951.[R433] Feinglass et al. observed abnormalities in 71% of 52 patients, most of whom had a seizure disorder.[F46] Gibson and Myers[G124] noted changes in 84% of 41 subjects. Slow waves were seen in most. Focal changes, lateral slowing, or discharges were seen in 43%. Grigor reported that 24 of 39 CNS lupus patients showed EEG abnormalities; most had diffuse slow waves, but a few showed focal changes.[G385] Abel et al.[A8] found focal changes in 15 of 25 patients (out of 46 with CNS-SLE) who had EEGs. Bourke and Rudolf[B437] performed EEG on 67 SLE patients; 68% were abnormal. The best correlates with CNS lupus were increased θ and δ background activity. In those without apparent CNS lupus, 48% of the EEGs showed changes. Yancey et al.[Y29] noted abnormalities in 12 of 15 children tested, most were characterized by diffuse slowing. Other smaller reports have confirmed the above findings.[L239,S253,S287,S497,T55]

Quantitative EEGs

Quantitative EEGs (QEEGs) may detect evidence of cortical dysfunction not present on EEG.[R198] Serial QEEGs may improve quickly with therapy.

Evoked Potentials

Since 1985, two uncontrolled reports[B309,M544] and one controlled[F187] report have evaluated the role of visual, brain stem auditory, and somatosensory evoked potentials in SLE. They may be useful in detecting subclinical disease and in differentiating old from new areas of involvement.

Summary

The EEG is a nonspecific test that is abnormal in most patients with CNS lupus and in many patients without CNS symptoms. It may demonstrate diffuse slow wave or definite focal patterns. Some of these patients have seizure disorders, and others who have extensive CNS disease may have a normal EEG. EEGs might be able to distinguish steroid-induced psychosis from CNS lupus.[F100] QEEGs and evoked potentials deserve further study.

Cognitive Dysfunction

Psychologic profiles such as the MMPI and Wechsler Adult Intelligence Scale are often helpful in SLE, but results can be altered by concurrent medication. These tests by themselves do not provide an optimal assessment of cognitive function. Goodwin and Goodwin[E147] first noted decreased cognitive capabilities in SLE patients in 1979. They related this not to cerebritis, but to disease duration. A National Institutes of Health analysis first outlined that a high percentage (40%) of patients with SLE have impaired ability to focus, maintain attention, and persist in task completion.[R294]

The Denburg Papers

Judah Denburg, Susan Denburg, and their colleagues in Ontario have been exploring this area since the mid-1980s. Their numerous peer-reviewed publications have helped define the role of cognitive impairment in those with SLE.[C75,D150,D151,D152,D153,D154,H100,K156,L371,S463,T102] Their subjects undergo a 3-hour, comprehensive battery of psychologic tests that assess a wide range of cognitive functions, including attention, psychomotor speed, memory, and problem solving. The major points of their work are the following:

1. Up to two-thirds of patients with SLE have cognitive dysfunction, compared to less than 20% of those in control or other rheumatic disease groups.
2. Various deficits are present.
3. Cognitive dysfunction is not necessarily or usually related to emotional stress or medication.
4. Prior CNS-SLE is associated with cognitive impairment, suggesting residual CNS scarring or damage.
5. SLE patients who have never been diagnosed as having CNS lupus demonstrate significantly more cognitive deficits than controls.
6. These deficits correlate with active disease, anti-DNA, lymphocytotoxic antibodies, nonfocal CNS-SLE, and CSF IgG antineuronal antibodies.

Other Studies

Other smaller scale studies and abstracts have confirmed some of these findings in children[P36] and adults.[G153,H102,K485] See also Chapter 39.

TREATMENT

The therapeutic approaches to CNS lupus are reviewed in Table 38–5. Acute, inflammatory, diffuse processes should be managed with at least 1 mg/kg/day of prednisone equivalent. This regimen was first outlined by Dubois in 1956,[D310] who used hydrocortisone and doubled its dose every 24 hours until the patient responded. His 1973 survey documented decreased mortality from CNS disease after this protocol was instituted.[D342] Intravenous pulse methylprednisolone may be required for some patients.[L328,P293] About 25% of CNS vasculitis episodes are not steroid-responsive. Pulse intravenous doses (0.75–1 g/m²) of cyclophosphamide given every 3 to 6 weeks for several months resulted in eight of nine CNS episodes having a favorable outcome at the National Institutes of Health.[B436] All six patients at the University of Pennsylvania treated similarly also improved. Two other reports totaling ten patients[L69,V109] demonstrated only modest improvements and several serious infections. Refractory cases may be ameliorated quickly by plasmapheresis if

Table 38–5. Neuropsychiatric Clinical Subsets of SLE—Diagnosis and Treatment

Subset	Incidence in SLE (%)	Typical Abnormal Laboratory Test Results	Treatment
Cerebral vasculitis	10	CSF pleocytosis; increased protein levels, IgG, IgG: albumin ratio, and antineuronal antibodies; low C3, C4; high anti-DNA	High-dose IV steroids; immunosuppressants may be needed
Antiphospholipid syndrome (APS) with thromboemboli	10–20	Normal CSF; MRI focal infarct; +BFP, +APS work-up; rare, 2-D echo vegetation; occasional thrombocytopenia	Platelet antagonists, anticoagulation
APS with bleeding	2	+APS work-up; abnormal MRI; hypoprothrombinemia, thrombocytopenia	Corticosteroids; factor replacement, transfusion
Thrombotic thrombocytopenic purpura (TTP)	<1	Hemolytic anemia; classic smear; low platelets; azotemia	Corticosteroids; factor infusion, apheresis
Lupus headache	15	Increased incidence of APS; Raynaud's?	Migraine therapy; steroids; platelet antagonists
Secondary to circulating factors, including "cognitive dysfunction"	50	Antiribosomal P (15%); anti-DNA, low C3, C4 (50%); CSF antineuronal antibodies or +CSF LE prep; high sedimentation rate; or all can be normal (50%); neuropsychologic tests abnormal (80%)	Steroids; antimalarials; rarely, cytotoxics
Organic brain syndrome (chronic)	10	CT and MRI show cortical atrophy; neurodiagnostic psychologic tests abnormal	Emotional support; rule out drug toxicity or other CNS disease
Cryoglobulinemia	<1	Cryocrit > 8%	Steroids; apheresis; α-interferon; cytotoxics
Hyperviscosity	<1	Serum viscosity > 4	Steroids; apheresis; cytotoxics
Fibrositis	10–20	Elevated CSF substance P (?)	NSAIDS; counseling; antidepressants; physical therapy
CNS infection	1	+CSF cultures, Gram's stain; pleocytosis; increased CSF protein and/or decreased glucose levels	Antimicrobial Rx

given early in the course.[B439,S507,U23] In the largest reported series, six CNS lupus patients in France had dramatic improvements with plasma exchange.[T64]

When the antiphospholipid syndrome is suspected as the source of thrombotic episodes (e.g., Libman-Sacks endocarditis), antiplatelet drugs or anticoagulation may be indicated. One report suggests using intravenous gamma globulin.[S746] Supportive psychotherapy offering reassurance, and helping patients develop better coping mechanisms, are also useful measures (see Chap. 39). One study suggested that aerobic conditioning decreases the fatigue of SLE.[R229]

Chapter 39

PSYCHOPATHOLOGY IN THE LUPUS PATIENT

HOWARD SHAPIRO

Abnormal behavior patterns were first described in lupus patients by Hebra and Kaposi[H237] in 1875 and by Osler[O108] at the turn of the century (stupor and recurrent coma). Daly[D19] contributed the first detailed modern description of psychotic behavior in central nervous system lupus in 1945. Within 5 years of that time, the introduction of the LE-cell test by Hargraves[H129] and the availability of corticosteroids considerably altered our understanding and approach to neuropsychiatric disorders in systemic lupus erythematosus. This chapter describes the highly variable psychopathologies (including the cognitive dysfunction and deficits) seen with SLE and their differential diagnosis, addresses the special concerns of lupus sufferers, and outlines a rational treatment program.

Psychologic and neurobehavioral difficulties encountered in lupus can be classified as psychoses, mood disorders, specific organic brain syndromes, cognitive impairment, drug reactions (particularly to corticosteroids), functional disorders, and disruptions in circadian biorhythms. Although certain descriptive overlapping is present, the cause and pathogenesis of each of these entities are generally mutually exclusive, and are discussed separately. These conditions must be distinguished and recognized as distinct from the inevitable and ongoing unpleasant "adjustment reactions" that occur and recur during the life of the lupus patient.

INCIDENCE

The incidence of psychiatric symptoms in several series of lupus patients is shown in Table 39–1. The range in various reports is from 12 to 71%. This large variation in results is partly a result of who defined the psychopathology (psychiatrist, neurologist, or internist), whether a hospitalized or outpatient group was used, criteria for defining lupus, and the ethnic, sex, age, and socioeconomic status of the study group. In 1975, Klippel and Zwaifler[K312] reviewed the literature and, in a total of 995 SLE patients, reported that 18% had disturbances in mental function. This is inclusive of Dubois' 520 patients, in whom a 12% incidence of psychosis was reported,[D340] when in fact the incidence of "minor disturbances in mental function" was not reported and was certainly much higher.

Typically, neuropsychiatric lupus (NPL) in the literature is a heterogeneous alloy of neurologic *and* psychiatric symptoms, including seizures, vertigo, headaches, organic brain syndromes, neuropathies, psychosis, depression, and unusual adjustment reactions that cannot be attributed to any other cause. Failure to distinguish "psychiatric" from clearly organic brain syndromes contributes to this large variation.[R212] For example, in 1985, Nollet and Herreman[N117] reported an overall incidence of psychiatric symptoms in 54% of a prospective study of 35 patients with SLE. Abel and Gladman[A8] followed 66 SLE patients (prospectively) who had 77 episodes of NPL. In 1980, they reported that patients with NPL had more SLE manifestations than patients without NPL. (Serologic data and cerebrospinal fluid analysis were not helpful in identifying an episode of NPL, whereas the electroencephalogram was abnormal in more than 50% and brain scans were abnormal in more than 75% of patients.) In 74 episodes with a known outcome, 54 improved, 44 having been treated with increased doses of corticosteroids. Patients with NPL had a higher incidence of deaths compared to patients without NPL.

In 1988, Lim et al.[L290] reported on the frequency and type of psychiatric disease in 40 patients suffering from SLE and 27 control subjects with rheumatoid arthritis or inflammatory bowel disease. The psychiatric morbidity at the time of interview was the same in the two groups, but the patients with SLE had experienced more episodes of psychiatric illness in the past, and psychotic symptoms occurred only in this group. Half of the patients with SLE had previous or current evidence of neurologic involvement. An association was found between neurologic disease and psychotic symptoms in SLE patients whereas anxiety and affective disturbances appeared to be closely related to environmental factors in both patients with SLE and in controls. No correlation was found between psychiatric and neurologic disease and clinical or laboratory indices of disease activity.

In 1988, Darby[D43] reported on 100 psychiatric consultations in a rheumatology unit. Of these, 80% consisted of patients with SLE (36%), rheumatoid arthritis (29%), and fibrositis (15%). Most SLE patients had organic brain syndromes related to central nervous system involvement or corticosteroids, and most rheumatoid arthritis patients had a depressive diagnosis. Fibrositis patients showed no specific psychiatric diagnosis.

Omdal and Mellgren,[O79] in 1988, reported an 83% incidence of NPL in 25 patients, but subdivided psychiatric problems to 17%. It is believed that SLE patients have more psychiatric symptoms than patients with most other medical illnesses, and that they often are as psychiatrically disturbed as psychiatric patient groups. In 1990, Mitchell and Thompson[M489] reported that these beliefs did not

Table 39–1. Incidence of Psychiatric Symptoms in Lupus Patients (%)

Parameter	O'Connor[O10] 1959	Stern & Robbins[S667] 1960	Estes & Christian[E147] 1960	Guze[G440] 1967	Ganz[G34] 1972	Baker[B34] 1973	Ropes[R294] 1976	Feinglass et al.[F46] 1976	Grigor et al.[G384] 1978	Hall et al.[H54] 1981
No. of patients in study	40	53	150	101	68	17	142	150	50	50
Psychiatric symptoms	65	64	42	12	71	41	28	16	40	44
Psychosis	55	52	16	5	15	15	8	14	0	25
Schizophrenia	17	12	10	5	7	9	8	6	0	2
Organic brain syndrome	28	30	21	9	22	15	3	14	18	10
Functional disorders	12	30	5	10	51	36	20	2	22	25

prove to be true for SLE outpatients. In their study, 22 outpatients with SLE, 81 general medical outpatients, and 40 psychiatric outpatients were screened with psychometric tests designed to access psychiatric symptoms and stress. The SLE outpatients' psychiatric symptoms and stresses were more similar to those reported by general medical outpatients, rather than by psychiatric outpatients, except in a few areas, and SLE patients were significantly less distressed than psychiatric patients in all areas, except those relating directly to their SLE.

The exhaustive studies of the Denburgs and Carbotte[C75] in the 1980s clearly and consistently showed, with great objectivity, the unexpectedly high incidence of cognitive impairment in SLE patients with inactive or absent neuropsychiatric symptomatology. By administering a battery of neuropsychologic tests to 62 female patients with SLE (and to controls), an overall incidence of cognitive impairment of 66% was obtained in the SLE patient sample. Neither steroid medication nor psychologic distress could account for these findings.

Several reports in the literature[L54,M37] have emphasized that psychiatric and/or psychologic distress (as contrasted with classic neurologic symptoms) may be the presenting symptoms of SLE.[V13]

Acute psychotic manifestations in SLE have usually been considered to occur early in the course of illness, although these findings are primarily based on studies with few patients and limited lengths of observation. Ward and Stupenski investigated the chronology of acute psychiatric disturbances in SLE. The time course of these episodes was examined in 36 patients over a median duration of observation of 72 months. Of 36 initial psychiatric episodes, 22 (61.1%) occurred within the first year of diagnosis of SLE, although several patients experienced the initial onset of psychiatric manifestations several years after the onset of SLE. Recurrent episodes occurred in 10 of 36 patients at a median of 8 months after the initial episode. Although tending to occur early in SLE, primary acute psychiatric events may first occur in patients with long durations of illness, and the time of onset of these episodes does not appear helpful in their differential diagnosis.[A237,L54,M37]

Clinicians and staff who work with mentally handicapped and with communication impaired patients should be especially sensitive to the possibility of cerebral involvement in SLE patients. CNS complications in a mentally handicapped woman were not recognized early because of impaired communication.[W257] Although routine testing for SLE in psychiatric populations has consistently proved nonproductive,[C400] wherever a large aggregate of younger women patients exists, one must be alert to the possibility of SLE with the development of sudden, unexplained psychiatric symptoms.

PREDISPOSING FACTORS AND THE ROLE OF STRESS

A combination of physical, environmental, biosocial, iatrogenic, and drug-related factors place lupus patients at a greater risk for developing psychologic disorders. Hypertension and uremia were noted by Heine[H245] to be implicated with more psychopathology. Various antihypertensive drugs, corticosteroids, digitalis, and antimalarial agents, among others, can alter mood and behavior patterns. The last two decades have witnessed an exponential rise in the use of various psychotropic agents (e.g., anxiolytics, benzodiazepines, tricyclic antidepressants). These agents may impair cognition, alter impulse control, potentiate an unrecognized but pre-existing deficit in cognition[R418] and amplify pre-existing neurotic and personality problems.

McLeary[M231] observed that, in 13 of 14 patients studied, significant crises in interpersonal relationships preceded the onset of symptoms. Ropes[R294] reported that disease flares in 41 of 45 patients were precipitated by psychogenic or environmental factors. Emotional disturbance, stress, and personality disorder were investigated in the genesis of SLE in 20 women compared to matched controls who had suffered a severe accidental hemorrhage in late pregnancy.[O121] Emotional deprivation in childhood was reported more frequently by patients than by controls. Both mothers and fathers were perceived as unsatisfactory by more patients than by controls. All patients (and 12 controls) reported that the onset of illness was preceded by stresses, particularly relating to marriage and other interpersonal relationships; pregnancy and childbirth, although not always perceived as stressful, were associated with exacerbations of SLE. Patients under 20 years of age reported a considerably lower incidence of emotional deprivation in childhood, and antecedent stress appeared less significant. It is evident that patients frequently try to attribute the onset of physical illness to some type of trauma.[W22]

Blumenfield[B366] questioned 36 patients, and 50% were certain that psychologic factors triggered disease onset and an additional 25% felt it was possible. Once lupus is diagnosed, various factors increase the risk of neuropsychiatric impairment. In one study, only 3% of 140 patients had neuropsychiatric symptoms at diagnosis, but eventually a 37% incidence was observed.[F46]

Ever since Solomon and Moos[S546] first proposed that mental stress flares autoimmune disease, in 1964, a flurry of activity has indirectly confirmed much of their hypothesis, despite a few negative reports. Rogers[R272] summarized a series of studies suggesting that stress can exacerbate rheumatoid arthritis; decreased lymphocyte cytotoxicity, natural killer activity, and mitogenic responsiveness were seen in response to stress, along with diminished lymphocyte response to antigenic stimulation, skin homograft rejection, graft-versus-host response, and delayed hypersensitivity. It has been suggested that right cerebral laterality (left-handedness) is increased in SLE patients.[L24,S43] Satz and Soper[S94] analyzed the claims of an association among left-handedness, dyslexia, migraine, and autoimmune disease. They found that results and theories in various studies offered misleading implications about left-handedness, and contained only minimal support for their conclusions.[S94] Geschwind's[G105-109] pioneering studies, along with Schur's[S199] findings, implicated cerebral lateralization, immune disease, hormonal influences,[V68] biologic mechanisms, and developmental learning disorders. Salcedo et al. disputed any association of SLE with left-handedness.[H238,P259,S43,S594]

Wallace,[W22] in his extensive review of the evidence for the role of stress and trauma in rheumatoid arthritis (RA) and SLE, concluded that stress can depress immune responsiveness, but the result of this (e.g., increased susceptibility to infection, increased disease activity) is not known. It is uncertain how much or what type of stress is required to depress responsiveness, or even how differing degrees of stress can be quantitated or reduced. Even though 8,000,000 Americans have RA and SLE, we still know little about the influences of stress and trauma on these disorders.

The weight of evidence from various studies strongly suggests a role for psychologic stress in inducing, exacerbating, and affecting the ultimate outcome of SLE. Wallace argued convincingly about the need for well-designed controlled trials aimed specifically at deciding these issues. The role of physical trauma has never been investigated, and disease exacerbation induced by emotional stress has been strongly suggested but not yet verified in a scientifically acceptable fashion.

Lupus experts such as Schur,[S197] Dubois and Rothfield have stated that emotional stress can aggravate disease activity, but only Ropes backed up this contention with any data by relating that 41 of 45 lupus flares observed in her 160 patient cohort were precipitated by emotional stress.[R342] Pamphlets distributed by the Arthritis Foundation, the American Lupus Society, and the Lupus Foundation of America reinforce this viewpoint with patients, who are cautioned to develop serious coping mechanisms and to take care of themselves so that their disease activity has less chance of flaring. Many patients who develop serious infections, experience major trauma, and have emotional crises do not experience a flare of the disease. Furthermore, SLE may be exacerbated in the absence of provocative circumstances. The true frequency or probability of disease aggravation following stressful incidents is not known.

A few important points regarding differential diagnosis are noteworthy. Many SLE patients have a secondary fibromyalgia.[S43] Fibromyalgia can produce symptoms of joint pains and stiffness.[D323] Emotional stress[A67,P82] is a well-known provocateur of fibrositis symptoms.[R295,S523] Similarly, reductions in corticosteroid dosages can cause "withdrawal" symptoms of joint pains, and may produce a more labile emotional state. The clinician must be careful to distinguish SLE flares from active fibromyalgia or corticosteroid withdrawal (see Chap. 49).

The effects of psychosocial stress or physical trauma on the immune system have been the subject of extensive study.[A40,C382,S545] Correlations among laboratory data and physical and psychosocial aspects reveal enormous individual differences in SLE patients, especially in their self-reported, subjective ratings of their physical symptoms and well-being.[W167] Except for the studies mentioned, above this has not been investigated in humans. Most SLE patients have depressed immune responsiveness to begin with. That stress induces further depressed immune responsiveness in SLE, and that this results in more active disease, remains a tenable but untested hypothesis (see Chap. 55).

PSYCHOSIS

Psychosis is defined as a gross impairment in reality testing with disordered thinking and bizarre ideation, often including delusions and hallucinations, which usually result in the inability to carry out the ordinary demands of living. As noted in Table 39–1, the incidence of psychosis ranges from 0 to 55%. More common in hospitalized patients, its incidence has probably decreased over the last 30 years as more rapid diagnosis and effective treatment of SLE have become possible. For example, in evolving the preliminary ARA criteria for SLE in 1971, 19% of 245 patients were psychotic compared with only 13% of 176 patients used for the revised criteria in 1982.[T46] Wallace noted psychosis in only 5% of 464 SLE patients seen between 1980 and 1989.[S43]

Literature Review

Comparisons of studies from different decades are clouded by changes in definitions and by criteria for the psychoses (thought and mood disorders), as reflected in DSM-II, DSM-III, DSM-III-R and DSM-IV of the American Psychiatric Association. Brody's pioneer report[B502] included 42 patients, many of whom were seen initially in the last year of the presteroid era (1949) and interviewed by them pretreatment. Of these, 52% were judged to be psychotic (most probably, these were "organic psychoses"). Clark and Bailey[C276] reviewed the records of 100 patients with SLE at the Mayo Clinic from 1948 and found severe psychiatric disturbances in 17%.

O'Connor[O10] studied 40 unselected patients with SLE admitted to Columbia Presbyterian Medical Center between 1950 and 1954. Of these, 21 patients had overt psychotic episodes during their hospitalizations; 7 were schizophrenic in type. In general, these showed paranoid ideation, hallucinations, fear, mutism, and withdrawal from environment. Also, 3 had psychotic depressions. The remaining 11 psychotic patients were given a diagnosis of acute brain syndrome; 5 were intermittently comatose, usually in the terminal phase of the disease. The others showed the classic symptoms of an organic psychosis with disorientation, confabulation, and visual and auditory hallucinations. The length of the psychosis ranged from hours to 4 months. No correlation could be established between the individual psychiatric syndrome and the postmortem findings. Although 18 of the 21 psychotic patients were receiving cortisone at the time of development of this reaction, I believe that organic brain disease resulting from SLE and not steroids caused the psychosis in almost all these patients.

Psychosis of all types occurred in 12% of 520 of Dubois' patients from 1950 to 1963.[D340] Almost all resulted from cerebral vasculitis, and responded to an initiation or increase in the dose of corticoids. A true steroid-induced psychosis was less frequent than the organic form. These hormones frequently produce euphoria or anxiety, insomnia, and restlessness, but rarely a true psychosis. Ropes[R294] reported that only 11 of 40 SLE patients who developed psychiatric problems were taking steroids at the time. The usual error made in therapy is to ascribe the psychosis or severe neurosis to medication, and to withhold corticoid therapy. In Harvey's 1954 study, 19% of patients[H142] also were psychotic. In 13% of them, SLE was the only demonstrable cause.

In 1960, Stern and Robbins[S667] similarly reviewed 53 patients at Bellevue Hospital, primarily cases referred from the medical to the psychiatric service. Half the patients were psychotic, 15 with manifestations of organic brain disease; 6 had schizophrenia and unclassified psychosis, and 2 had psychotic depressions. In only 3 patients was it believed that steroids caused the psychosis. Mild to moderate depressions occurred in 8 additional patients. Again, it was emphasized that the prime cause of the psychosis was organic brain disease, and not steroid therapy.

Fessel[F79] reviewed the literature on the problem of psychoses and SLE. Out of 227 patients, information was given about steroid therapy in 97, and in only 25% of these had there been coincident steroid treatment, again emphasizing the primary organic nature of the psychosis. Tumulty[T270] and others[G188,H108] noted that central nervous system changes were seen frequently, even before the advent of steroids.

In the 1960s, Estes and Christian[E147] observed organic mental symptoms in 21% of 150 patients, evidenced by disorientation, hallucinations, or deterioration of mental function. Of these, 16% had functional psychoses, such as schizophrenia and affective reactions.

In 1967, Guze[G440] reviewed the occurrence of psychiatric illness in 101 consecutive patients with SLE admitted to a university hospital, and found 12 who had significant difficulties. The psychiatric diagnoses varied in different admissions of the same patients and were organic brain syndrome in 9, affective illnesses in 10, and schizophreniform disorders in 5. In patients with the organic brain syndrome, marked fluctuations in both disorientation and degree of memory impairment were frequent. Guze suggested that mental disturbances were more common in black women (25% versus 12% overall). I and others[B10] have noted that organic psychiatric symptoms usually improve following steroid therapy.

Baker's experience with 17 patients was similar to the above findings.[B34] Heine's group[H245] in Scandinavia noted a 24% incidence of psychoses, primarily on a toxic, organic basis. Those with hypertension and renal disease had a worse prognosis. In 1976, Feinglass[F46] observed psychosis to be an early feature of SLE, short-lived in duration and associated with a good prognosis. Its principal manifestations were hallucinations, autism, and paranoia. Steroid psychosis occurred rarely (in 2 of 140 patients) and all other patients responded to increases in steroid doses.

Steroids, Mood, Cognition, and Behavior

Hall et al.[H54] followed 56 SLE patients, 44% of whom had psychiatric symptoms. Of these, 14 patients (25%) had a psychotic episode; 10 were associated with specific neurologic symptoms (including peripheral neuropathy in 4 and seizures in 3), and 3 patients had a steroid psychosis. Of the 14 patients, 10 improved with increases in their steroid doses and, by the time of publication, psychosis had resolved in all 14 patients.

In his literature review, Rogers[R271] estimated the incidence of steroid psychosis as 5% of all psychoses in SLE.

In 1990, Reckart and Eisendrath[R90] reported on eight patients who had undergone more than 5 years of intermittent treatments with corticosteroids and then volunteered to be interviewed about their experiences. Seven patients stated that they were not warned by their physicians of the possible psychiatric side effects. Five patients did not inform their physicians when symptoms did occur. The patients complained of insomnia, depression, hypomania or euphoria, confusion, and memory problems. Based on these reports, the frequency of affective and cognitive side effects of exogenous corticosteroids may be much higher than has been previously reported.

Joffe et al.[J81,J82] assessed mood and cognition on consecutive days in 18 women with systemic lupus erythematosus on alternate-day corticosteroid therapy. No overall differences were observed between the on and off medication days, but 10 patients showed marked worsening or improvement of either depression or anxiety on their off medication day. After 2 weeks of prospective behavioral ratings, the observed mood changes in several women were confirmed.

Because several monoamines (especially dopamine) have been implicated in the regulation of mood, Joffe et al. examined the relationship between alterations in mood and plasma homovanillic acid (HVA) levels in patients on alternate-day corticosteroid treatment. Although several patients had substantial alterations in mood, no significant differences in plasma HVA levels between the on and off medication days were found. Furthermore, alterations in depression and anxiety levels were not related to plasma HVA levels.

In a 1979 study, Hall[H56] defined the symptoms of steroid psychosis in 14 patients who had no central nervous system lesions. This study suggested that patients receiving daily doses of greater than 40 mg of prednisone or its equivalent are at greater risk for developing a steroid psychosis. These reactions are twice as likely to occur during the first 5 days of treatment than subsequently. Premorbid personality, a history of a previous psychiatric disorder, or a history of a previous steroid psychosis do not clearly increase the patient's risk of developing a psychotic reaction during any given course of subsequent therapy.

The steroid psychosis observed by Hall presented as a spectrum psychosis, with symptoms ranging from affective through schizophreniform to those of organic brain syndrome. No characteristic stable presentation was observed in these 14 patients. The most prominent symptom constellation noted during the course of the illness consisted of emotional lability, anxiety, distractibility, pressured speech, sensory flooding insomnia, depression, perplexity, agitation, auditory and visual hallucinations, intermittent memory impairment, mutism, disturbances of body image, delusions, apathy, and hypomania.

Several other critical literature reviews[H53,L241] and newer studies have provided longitudinal insights into the nature of steroid-induced mental changes. The incidence of steroid psychosis varies widely in the literature, ranging from 13 to 62%, with a weighted average of 27.6% for some steroid-induced mental changes, the vast majority of which are mild to moderate and do not herald the development of a full-blown psychosis or affective syndrome. The incidence of a severe psychiatric syndrome in the over 2,500 patients reported in the literature has ranged from 1.6 to 50%, with a weighted average of 5.7%. The incidence of steroid psychoses in patients with lymphoma, multiple sclerosis, severe intractable asthma, ulcerative colitis, regional enteritis, idiopathic thrombocytopenic purpura, rheumatoid arthritis, and severe poison ivy or poison oak was estimated at between 3 and 6%. The patients most at risk for developing steroid psychosis are those with systemic lupus erythematosus (39%) and pemphigus (21%).

The type of psychiatric disturbance seen is difficult to classify, because symptoms tend to change radically during the course of the illness. Overall, approximately 40% of patients present predominantly with a depressive disorder, 25% with mania, 5% with bipolar disorder, cyclical form, 15% with an agitated schizophreniform or paranoid psychosis, and 10% as an acute progressive delirium. Three-quarters of all patients with steroid psychosis evidence affective symptoms at some time during the course of their illness. A frank psychotic state without mood disturbance occurs in 10 to 15% of patients, and some psychotic features (i.e., marked impairment of reality testing) associated with affective symptoms occur in 70% of patients.

The dose of steroid administered has a clear relationship to the likelihood of the patient developing a subsequent steroid psychosis. A statistically significant increase in the incidence of psychiatric disturbances with increasing daily doses of steroid has been found. Patients treated with a mean daily dose of prednisone below 40 mg/day in the Boston Collaborative Drug Surveillance Study[H53a] had an incidence of psychotic symptoms of 1.3%, whereas patients treated with doses between 41 and 80 mg/day had an incidence of 4.6%. Patients receiving more than 80 mg/day of prednisone or its equivalent had an incidence of steroid psychosis of 18.4%. The average daily dose of steroids for patients who developed psychosis was 59.5 mg/day of prednisone or equivalent, as compared with 31.1 mg/day for patients who did not develop adverse psychiatric effects.

Several studies have shown that no relationship exists between the response to the first course of steroid treatment and the response to a subsequent course of treatment. Litz[H54] noted that even the most "highly unstable" patients do not experience any untoward emotional reaction after ACTH or cortisone therapy when compared with their more emotionally mature counterparts. Therefore, a patient's past psychiatric history is not a reliable predictor of developing a future steroid psychosis. The most frequent initial presentation of an impending steroid psychosis is a state of cerebral hyperexcitability, clearly perceived and reported by the patient.[H54] Patients characterize these states as being marked by increased irritability, lability of mood, profound dysphoria, hyperacusis, and pressured thought processes. These changes often antecede other, more serious disturbances of cognition by 72 to 96 hours.

Once a steroid psychosis has been fully defined, it is likely to present as a spectrum psychosis, with the most prominent symptoms consisting of profound distractibility, pressured speech, anxiety, emotional lability, severe insomnia, sensory flooding, depression, perplexity, auditory and visual hallucinations, agitation, intermittent memory impairment, mutism, delusions, disturbances of body image, apathy, and hypomania. Prior to the advent of treatment with phenothiazines, it was noted that these conditions spontaneously remitted between 2 weeks and 7 months after the discontinuance of steroids, with 80% of the cases reported in the literature having remitted untreated by the sixth week. Administration of phenothiazines dramatically reduces this period. The current duration of psychiatric symptoms in patients who develop a steroid psychosis and who are treated with phenothiazines ranges in the literature from 1 to 150 days, with a mean duration until total recovery of 22 days.

According to Hall,[H54] 92% of patients who have steroids tapered fully recover, and 84% of patients who are maintained on steroids but treated with antipsychotic medicines show full recovery from symptoms. In the 11 cases reported in the literature, electroconvulsive therapy (ECT) has been universally effective in reversing the course of steroid psychosis.

Several studies have shown that patients, even those with affective disorder produced by steroids, tend to do poorly when treated concurrently with tricyclic antidepressants and steroids. These patients may also show an exacerbation of symptoms, even after the tapering of steroids, when tricyclics are used. Therefore, it is recommended that tricyclic and other antidepressant medications be withheld until after the patient's steroid psychosis has been appropriately treated with neuroleptics.

Various treatment approaches are available for steroid psychosis. The most widely used and effective treatment strategy is to discontinue steroids, where possible, and to treat the patient with phenothiazines or other antipsychotic medications. Tricyclic antidepressants are usually avoided. The most frequently used drug regimens include the following: thioridazine hydrochloride, 50 to 200 mg daily;[H55] chlorpromazine hydrochloride, 50 to 200 mg orally, daily; or haloperidol, 2 to 10 mg orally, daily.[R271]

Falk et al.[H55] have shown that prophylactic treatment with lithium carbonate may be useful to prevent the development of ACTH-induced psychosis. Excitement, hyperstimulation, and overstimulation should be kept to a minimum and anxiety reduced, if possible. Anxiolytic agents, if tolerated, may be helpful.

If a steroid psychosis exists, Rogers[R271] has advised judicious but rapid tapering of corticosteroids to adrenal replacement levels (7.5 mg of prednisone equivalent daily). Unfortunately, some patients have multisystem disease that requires corticosteroids, and a compromise must be reached and alternative therapies considered. If it was difficult to determine whether the psychosis was steroid-induced, Dubois acutely stopped steroids in hospitalized patients. If the psychosis was steroid-induced, dramatic clearing usually occurred in 48 to 72 hours.

Manic-depressive psychosis is rare in SLE patients but may sometimes be mimicked by corticosteroid administration. Catatonia has also been reported. Psychotic depression in SLE may be helped by shock therapy when all other modalities fail.[C392,K433,K476,L54,R294]

Wysenbeeck et al.[W366] described two patients with SLE who developed an acute psychosis and a cerebrovascular accident after pulse methylprednisolone therapy. A literature review revealed 8 additional patients with SLE with acute central nervous system complications after pulse therapy.

ORGANIC BRAIN SYNDROMES

Several nonpsychotic organic brain syndrome manifestations may occur in SLE patients. Most obvious organic brain syndromes present as a toxic, psychotic type, as noted in the preceding section. Psychosis, in the absence of signs of organic brain impairment, is uncommon in SLE patients.

Impairment in Cognition (Organic Amnestic Syndrome)

More common than previously recognized is organic mental syndrome, whose essential requirement is impairment of cognitive function. This can be expressed as defective short-term memory, diminished attention, and diminution or impairment of the following: concentration, capability for abstraction, problem solving, and visual-spatial functioning. Subtle changes in memory, concentration, and other cognitive functions often do not come to clinical attention unless formal mental status testing is done. Thus, it is difficult to estimate the incidence of nonpsychotic organic mental involvement.

The studies of Carbotte et al.[C75] identified the unexpectedly high incidence of cognitive impairment in SLE patients with either inactive or absent neuropsychiatric (NP) symptomatology. In their study, 86 women with SLE were grouped according to present or past history of NP symptomatology (active, inactive, or never). Performance of these three groups was compared to that of 35 normal women on an extensive battery of neuropsychologic tests that sampled a wide range of cognitive functions. In addition to making group comparisons, they also devised a system for identifying individual impairment using decision rules for both quantitative and qualitative data. Results indicated that various cognitive deficits are present in SLE patients taken together as a group; that no significant association between cognitive impairment and emotional disturbance is present; that patients with resolved NP symptomatology are as impaired as patients with active NP symptoms, suggesting residual CNS involvement, in spite of no significant difference emerging on direct group comparisons; and that significantly more never NP-SLE patients are impaired than are controls on several summary scores, suggesting subclinical CNS involvement.

The major difficulty in determining the significance of antineuronal antibodies in NP-SLE had been lack of consistent clinical diagnostic approaches. In 1987, by using a new clinical classification of NP-SLE, neuropsychologic assessments, and an assay for IgG antineuronal antibodies, the same authors found a significant association between antibody positivity and cognitive impairment or nonfocal NP-SLE. These observations indicate that antineuronal antibodies may play a role in NP-SLE and emphasize the clinical importance of cognitive function in patients with SLE.

In 1990, the Denburg group[L371] re-evaluated the hypothesis that lymphocytotoxic antibodies are associated with neuropsychiatric involvement in SLE. In an unselected cohort of 98 women with SLE, a cross-sectional study was performed to analyze associations among standardized clinical, neurologic, and neuropsychologic assessments and lymphocytotoxic antibodies measured by microcytotoxic assay. Of these, 50 patients showed objective clinical evidence of continuing or past NP-SLE and 54 patients had cognitive impairment. In accordance with previous observations 44% (24 of 54) of the cognitively impaired group did not have clinically detectable evidence of NP-SLE. Although lymphocytotoxic antibodies were found to be only marginally more prevalent in those patients with a clinical diagnosis of NP-SLE than in those without (32 versus 23%), these antibodies were significantly associated with cognitive impairment ($\chi^2 = 5.42$; $p < 0.02$). No association was detected between lymphocytotoxic antibodies and overall systemic disease activity or other organ system involvement, suggesting that the association between lymphocytotoxic antibodies and cognitive dysfunction in SLE is specific.

In another report[D154] by the same authors, 98 consecutive female SLE patients underwent extensive standardized neuropsychologic testing to evaluate central nervous system functioning in relation to serum lymphocyte antibodies, which are measured at the time of neuropsychologic testing by a microcytotoxicity test. A significant association was observed between the presence of serum lymphocytotoxic antibodies (LCAs) and cognitive impairment in patients with SLE. The pattern of impairment that predominated in the LCA-positive patients involved deficits in anteriorly associated, primarily visual-spatial, functions. These findings support the hypothesis of localization of a particular antigen-antibody interaction in the brain in SLE, suggesting the existence of immunologic control mechanisms for normal brain functioning.

One group of lupus patients has organic brain syndrome because of scarring from previously active CNS disease or from multiple infarctions resulting from the lupus anticogulant. Wallace reported[W19] several situations in which these patients were treated with steroid for "CNS lupus," when in fact no active disease was present that could be treated. Giving steroids often worsens the clinical picture, because it produces cortical atrophy.[W20]

Application of Neuropsychologic Testing

The aforementioned studies were done as a result of the application of special neuropsychologic tests (NPTs), which use selected parameters to evaluate the behavioral expression of organic brain injury. Prior to the studies of the Denburgs et al., NPTs were not used widely or routinely with SLE patients.

Neuropsychologic testing has the unique capability of assessing functional deficits irrespective of their origin, functional (no demonstrable lesion) or organic. According to Koffler,[K342] the major behavioral functions studied are cognitive and intellectual abilities, sensory and perceptual functions, motor and psychomotor abilities, language skills, spatial skills, and academic skills. Each sensory modality (auditory, tactile, visual) and each response mode (oral, written, motor) are tested, where applicable, in the examination of these functions.

The results of neuropsychologic tests are used to assess the presence of neural injury and to determine the site, type, and duration of CNS dysfunction. They are derived from studying four major parameters; the expected level of performance, specific pathognomonic signs, comparison of right and left brain function, and pattern analysis.

The two most widely used neuropsychologic test batteries are the Halsted-Reitan and Luria Nebraska neuropsychologic batteries.[B392,R149] Both are reported to detect the presence of organic brain damage with 80 to 90% accuracy.[G245] Their ability to assess CNS dysfunction in patients with ambiguous physical or psychologic signs and to quantitate functional deficits has resulted in their increased use in clinical medicine.

The results of the Luria-Nebraska test have been closely correlated with those of the Halsted-Reitan test when used for the detection of brain injury.[V85] The Luria-Nebraska requires a relatively short period of testing time and minor equipment, and may be administered to both hospitalized patients and outpatients. The Boston Processing Approach developed by Kaplan et al.[K61] may also become an instrument of choice.

In 1990, Papero et al.[P36] reported having studied 21 pediatric patients who met SLE criteria (12 moderate, 9 mild disease activity) and who had no history of CNS damage unrelated to lupus. Comparison of these SLE patients to a contrast group of 11 patients with juvenile rheumatoid arthritis (JRA) revealed decreased complex problem-solving ability for the SLE group. Individual, IQ-adjusted neuropsychologic profile analysis yielded a significant difference in the number of specific neuropsychologic deficits for the two groups, with impairment rates of 43% for SLE and 18% for JRA. A longer duration of lupus was associated with a lower cognitive status. Neuron-reactive antibody studies for IgG and IgM were negative. Results suggest that the incidence of higher cortical impairment may be as great for younger individuals with lupus as has been documented for older populations.

Neuropsychologic testing of SLE patients has shown consistent abnormalities in the four clinical scales (visual, arithmetic, writing, intelligence). This pattern is different than that found in patients with diffuse cerebral dysfunction (e.g., Alzheimer's disease), which typically includes elevations on multiple scales, particularly those measuring memory and language. Diffuse disturbance secondary to metabolic disorders is often reflected in scales sensitive to attentional deficits, such as memory and acoustic discrimination. The pattern for patients with focal lesions varies, depending on the site of the lesion. The functional deficits suggested by the pattern of elevated scales for CNS lupus patients in analogous to the pattern of abnormal scales found in patients with lesions occurring in the parietal-occipital regions or their associated tracts.

Koffler[K342] and Rogers[R271] advocated the assessment of neuropsychologic functioning in SLE patients. Further impetus for the documentation of cognitive changes was provided by a single case study of serial neuropsychologic testing with an SLE patient.[S534] This patient was also evaluated using regional cerebral blood flow CT scanning; each test demonstrated diffuse cortical dysfunction associated with the exacerbation of CNS symptoms.

Wekking et al.,[W166] argued that it has not convincingly been proven that the occurrence of cognitive impairment is uniquely related to SLE patients compared with RA patients. In his opinion, the interpretation of cognitive disturbances in relation to the total clinical picture is not clear, especially in SLE patients without overt CNS disease. Moreover, Wekking stated that the effects of cognitive dysfunction on treatment or prognosis in these patients have not been reported.

Organic affective syndromes and organic personality syndromes are often difficult to differentiate from functional disorders, and could reflect low-grade central nervous system lupus activity, hypertension, uremia, or lower dose corticosteroid effects. Their true incidence is difficult to estimate, but is probably high. Treatment involves managing lupus activity and providing the support mechanisms discussed elsewhere in this chapter.

Functional Disorders

Ever since 1956, when Clark and Bailey[C276] identified depression and anxiety as the most common personality changes in SLE patients, studies have been performed to characterize and classify these disorders in a way that could optimize management. The incidence of functional disorders in SLE is shown in Table 39–1. It ranges from 2 to 51%, and is probably an underestimate. Only a few of the studies included detailed interviewing and diligent searches for subtle functional problems.

Depression is particularly common in SLE patients.[S313] Most is reactive, although "endogenous" and psychotic depression occur. Often it is uncertain as to whether depression is "to be expected" because of the stresses, strains, continuous adjustments, and frequent sacrifices imposed by the illness. The person with lupus is often aware that states of depression may be induced by the lupus or by various factors and forces in the patient's life that are unrelated to lupus.

Depression can be understood as a natural although unpleasant experience that can vary in intensity, duration, and the degree that it is tolerated by the individual but, most important, in the degree to which it interferes with the patient's ability to function and maintain a reasonable sense of well-being. Therapeutic assistance and intervention are indicated when the degree and duration of the depression are disruptive to the individual's well-being and interfere with overall functioning and adjustment.[S314]

The medical condition that we refer to as depression is not to be confused with the transitory, everyday mild mood swing that everyone experiences during a difficult time. Although depressive illness is more common in people with chronic medical illness than in the general population, not everyone with a chronic medical illness (e.g., lupus) suffers from clinical depression.[S43] Clinical depression is characterized by physical and psychologic symptoms: sadness and gloom, spells of crying (often with provocation), insomnia or restless sleep (or sleeping too much), loss of appetite (or eating too much), uneasiness or anxiety, irritability, feelings of guilt and remorse, lowered self-esteem, inability to concentrate, diminished memory and recall, indecisiveness, loss of interest in things one formerly enjoyed, fatigue, and various physical symptoms, such as headache, palpitation, diminished sexual interest and/or performance, other body aches and pains, indigestion, and constipation or diarrhea.

Two of the most common psychologic signs of clinical depression are hopelessness and helplessness. People who feel hopeless believe that their distressing symptoms may never get better, whereas people who feel helpless think they are beyond help, that no one cares enough to help them or could succeed in helping even if they tried.

Not all depressed people have all these symptoms. Someone is considered to be clinically depressed, however, if he or she experiences a depressed mood, disturbance in sleep and appetite, and at least one or two related symptoms that persist for several weeks and are severe enough to disrupt normal daily life. Many people who come for treatment have been depressed for a good deal longer than this; some people stay depressed for years, and life seems flat and meaningless. Thoughts of death and deformity are often present, and occasionally turn into self-destructive urges.

Although many symptoms are associated with depression, seven indicate the depth and degree of depression. These are a sense of failure, loss of social interest, sense of

punishment, suicidal thoughts, dissatisfaction, indecision, and crying.

Depressive illness in the medically ill often goes unrecognized because it presents symptoms similar to those of the underlying medical condition. In lupus (SLE), depressive symptoms such as lethargy, loss of energy and interest, insomnia, pain intensification, and diminished libido can be attributed to the lupus condition. Unfortunately, many people with lupus refuse to acknowledge themselves to be in a depressed state; in fact, most depressive illness goes unrecognized and untreated until later stages, when the severity becomes unbearable to the patient and/or until the family or physician can no longer ignore it. In fact, several studies have indicated that between 30 and 50% of major depressive illness goes undiagnosed in medical settings. Perhaps more disturbing is the fact that many studies indicate that major depressive disorders in the medically ill are undertreated and/or inadequately treated, even when recognized.

Physicians who are familiar with their patients' usual mood and personality, as well as their lifestyle and situation, are more likely to recognize changes associated with depressive illness. Similarly, patients are more apt to open up about their feelings when they are encouraged to do so by a physician they trust and with whom they are familiar. This is especially important for that group of depressed individuals without subjective complaints of unhappy mood, who often deny or resist the notion of emotional distress, and who substitute various physical complaints. Physicians suspect masked depression in such patients, especially when they appear with a saddened facial expression, have lost interest in and are withdrawn from their usual activities, and are preoccupied with painful somatic complaints.

Failure to recognize and diagnose depression in the medically ill reinforces patients' belief that they have reason to feel depressed because they are sick, and therefore discourage appropriate help. This error ignores the fact that clinical depression in the physically ill generally responds well to standard psychiatric treatment, and that patients treated only for their physical illness suffer the effects of depression needlessly. Depression should not be used as a symptom for "sadness."

Effective treatment is available for depressive illness and usually consists of psychotropic medication, psychotherapy and, most often, a combination of both. Antidepressant medication is the major class of drugs used; the four categories are tricyclics, newer generation nontricyclic antidepressants, MAO inhibitors, and lithium. The effectiveness of these medications may be increased by using them in combination or by adding other medications. Not infrequently, depressed patients are undertreated and/or inadequately treated, reflecting therapeutic uncertainty and pessimism.

Adequate and aggressive treatment is vigilant and involves the cooperation of the patient. Such treatment may involve blood tests to determine the appropriate dosages of medication, open communication, trial and error, and a large ration of optimistic support in the form of encouragement, patience, availability, and perseverance. Any underlying organic factors that contribute to the depressive state must be identified and addressed. Antidepressant medications are associated with symptoms associated with various side effects, and may intensify certain symptoms associated with lupus (e.g., increase in the drying of mucous membranes in Sjögren's syndrome).[S316] When antidepressant medications are effective, a welcome improvement is noted in the patient's sense of well-being and overall attitude and adjustment.

Recovery from depression is usually a gradual process. Dramatic improvements cannot be expected in a few days; however, one begins to see some progress after a few weeks. Even when depression seems to clear quickly, it is not unusual to relapse when the medication is stopped. Therefore, medication should be continued for approximately 6 months or longer and dosage should be tapered slowly over a 3- or 4-week period when treatment is discontinued. Patients who are resistant to those treatments mentioned above have several other effective options.

Often, depressive illness involves a general slowing and clouding of mental functions (cognition), and many people with lupus worry about changes in their alertness, attention span, capability for concentration, orientation, memory and recall, reasoning abilities, and use of language and calculations. These troublesome and not infrequent disruptions in mental functioning tend to go underreported to their physicians and are rarely confirmed to be the result of any specific structural change. Transient alterations in mental functioning improve as the depressive condition improves.

Psychotherapy can be helpful in assisting depressed people to work through and understand their feelings, their illness, and their relationships, and to cope more effectively with stress and their life situation. The benefits to the patient are best served when the primary care physician maintains a close relationship with a psychiatrist or psychologist for consultation about and referral of depressed patients who present difficult diagnostic and treatment problems. Such a working relationship maximizes the quality of patient care and provides the most powerful approach to the management of depression.

In addition to the physical and organic aspects of the disease, this chronic illness so alters the life of these women that the incidence of divorce is well over 50%. Estes and Christian[G440] found that 8 patients had anxiety or depressive neurosis. These conditions were severe enough in 2 to require electroshock therapy. Psychiatric disturbances were observed in the absence of other neurologic manifestations in 27 patients. Fries and Holman[B10] noted depression in half of their 193 patients at any time in their disease course, but it was labeled as "severe" in only 10%.

Hall et al.[H56] evaluated 56 patients. Of 25 psychiatric symptoms, 19 had no set of single longterm symptoms but 23 complained of insomnia, 21 of depressed mood, 18 of emotional lability, 18 of nervousness, 17 of confusion, and 16 of a decrease in concentration. Patients who were socially active and not isolated did better. Later in this chapter (see Special Concerns), it is noted that depression is treated with tricyclic or related antidepressants and anxiety is treated with anxiolytics such as diazepam. Temes-

vari et al.[T102] noted depression in 16 of 34 SLE outpatients; 3 had made suicide attempts.

Liang et al.[L260] administered the Minnesota Multiphasic Personality Inventory (MMPI) to 76 SLE patients and to 23 rheumatoid arthritis in patients and outpatients. Despite these numbers, the study was admittedly biased: only 15 to 20% of those followed with these disorders were represented, and consisted of volunteers who generally had multiple complaints. A statistically significant increase in hypochondriasis, hysteria, and depression scales was noted in those with SLE and rheumatoid arthritis. Those with SLE had a marked increase in fear of death compared to the RA group. A sense of fatigue and complaints of loss of independence were common. Nevertheless, 50% stated that at times they thought that their disease had been a positive experience. Kremer et al.[K433] evaluated 37 SLE in patients and outpatients at the Albany Medical Center. Of these, 46% had current psychopathology; 41% were diagnosed as having nonorganic, nonpsychotic psychopathology; and only 2 were believed to be psychotic. Anxiety, tension, depression, and somatic concerns dominated. Abnormal MMPI test results were seen in 61%. Hysteria, depression, and hypochondriasis indices were abnormally high, but only to a small extent. No correlation was found among psychopathology, neurologic evaluations, and clinical activity.

According to Engle et al.,[E108] the Rheumatology Attitudes Index (RAI) is of proven reliability and usefulness with SLE patients. In 1990, Engle reported that all three components of the learned helplessness construct (motivational, cognitive, and emotional deficits) are likely to influence psychosocial adjustments in SLE patients. This correlation was found across all domains, except health care orientation and sexual adjustment. Thus, assessment of patients' efforts to engage in activities of daily living and to develop *new* coping behaviors is associated with, any may be predictive of, their overall psychosocial adjustment. Engle's data correlated perceived helplessness and longer duration of disease.[L382]

Factitious Illness and Positive ANA Without Lupus

Levy[L235] presented two cases of young women with factitious illness who claimed to have SLE. Secondary gain and/or the search for an all-encompassing disease entity have led many patients with borderline positive. ANA and nonspecific complaints to seek rheumatologic consultation and to become disappointed when told they do not have lupus. The overwhelming majority of these patients have fibromyalgia—a somatization disorder that is poorly understood, especially by nonrheumatologists. It represents 15% of "lupus" referrals. The picture is further complicated by the high incidence of secondary fibromyalgia seen in established SLE patients who have difficulty coping with the stress of their disease.

Von Brauchitsch[V105] observed that patients in psychiatric facilities have an increased incidence of positive ANA and proposed that SLE is more common in this group. Two other studies noted the same finding; the issue was resolved when Dubois' group[Q15] found that this phenomenon is secondary to psychotropic therapy, especially with phenothiazine administration for abnormal behavior states. Conversely, the diagnosis of SLE may be missed, resulting in phenothiazine administration for abnormal behavior states. In addition to steroid withdrawal, narcotic withdrawal can produce arthralgias, fevers, and behavior disorders that sometimes may be mistaken for lupus in young women. This is primarily seen in large, urban, public hospital settings.

Organic Versus Functional Disease

According to Bluestein,[B356] the medical (rather than psychiatric) orientation of investigators accounts for the limited analysis of functional psychiatric illness in SLE. Organic brain syndromes and functional disorders have a significant amount of overlap, and are often difficult to differentiate. Patients who manifest seizures, fever, emotional lability, personality changes, impairment of judgment, and focal neurologic abnormalities tend to have more organicity.

Jacobs[J25] has devised a questionnaire and scale to differentiate between organic syndrome and functional disorders. Andrew[A223] noted in a literature review that patients with organic complaints have a much poorer prognosis than those with only functional problems.

In 1982, Kremer et al.[K418] reported a high incidence of patients with nonorganic, nonpsychotic psychopathology (NONPP). Diagnoses of depression, anxiety, mania, and conversion reactions have been made in up to 50% of patients. Adding standardized psychologic tests, such as the MMPI and the Brief Psychiatric Rating Scale to the psychiatric interview, identifies an even higher incidence of NONPP in lupus. In contrast to analyses of organic psychiatric illness, no significant correlation has been found between functional psychiatric disturbances affecting SLE patients and their disease activity, either systemically or in the nervous system. Chronic illness is often accompanied by depression and other NONPP. Its frequency and perhaps its severity, however, may be markedly increased in SLE. Perhaps being told that you have lupus is more stressful than being labeled with some other chronic illness, or the disease process of SLE, itself, makes the patient more susceptible to the stresses of being chronically ill.

Certainly, the represented prognosis was thought to be much worse in the presteroid era, when study subjects often represented the "sickest" and most advanced cases of SLE, usually hospitalized with years of multisystem illness. With the advent of corticosteroids, earlier diagnosis, and earlier therapeutic intervention, the prognosis improved substantially. The recognition of the relatively benign course of ANA-positive cases did not discourage a therapeutic pessimism in some health care professionals, who probably reinforced (inadvertently) the worst fears in their newly diagnosed lupus patients.

In 1960, Stern and Robbins[S667] pointedly stated that "one great problem in managing these patients is the evaluation of how much of an emotional response is reactive." In understanding the psychiatric responses to lupus, both the nature of the disease, and the premorbid personality characteristics of the patients must be considered. SLE has devastating systemic effects; there is no definitive treatment, and the prognosis is poor. These features are anxiety-provoking and at least one third of the nonpsychotic patients have had a depressive reaction.[A152]

Not infrequently, patients report intense anxiety and despair after reading about the prognosis and outcome of SLE in an outdated medical text, or after speaking with some well-meaning but uninformed "expert." To avoid such reactions, as well as to establish a better rapport and cooperation with a naively diagnosed SLE patient (often a new patient of the rheumatologist), it is essential during the initial medical counseling to educate the patient and family (when appropriate) with current and accurate information, and to reassure them and allay their many unstated fears.[L246]

MEDICATION-INDUCED MENTAL CHANGES IN SLE

Behavioral and cognitive disturbances may be associated with the use of barbiturates, anticonvulsant agents, long- and short-acting benzodiazepines, and other psychotropic and psychoactive substances.[R268,S110,S111,S300] Motor function may also be affected,[H313] noncompliance, underreporting, self-medication and overmedication abuse, nonmedically supervised use, and medication withdrawal have all been reported to be associated with a myriad or psychiatric syndromes,[C203,P215] have produced lingering or residual cognitive impairment recognition defects,[B518,L228] and have significantly influenced neuropsychologic test performances.[B507,L330,R267]

Commonly reported adverse reactions[S317] are hyperactivity, disturbed sleep, irritability, and emotional lability. Subtle behavioral disturbances, however, may also adversely affect performance and learning. Behavioral changes resulting from therapy with barbiturates and benzodiazepines tend to be idiosyncratic, as opposed to the dose-related effects seen with phenytoin and valproate therapy. Carbamazepine and valproate can affect mood and behavior negatively, but generally this occurs less frequently than when other anticonvulsants are used; this is especially true in patients without CNS damage. The suspicion of a causal relationship between anticonvulsant therapy and impairment of cognitive skills in nontoxicated patients is gaining increasing support. Neuropsychologic studies in acutely exposed normal volunteers, studies in epileptic patients receiving monotherapy, and cross-over studies between drugs have incriminated barbiturates and hydantoin drugs. Memory and cognitive dysfunction, although affected to a greater extent with higher drug dosages, has been reported with levels within the therapeutic range. Thus, serum drug levels cannot be considered good predictors of which patients have subtle side effects. Carbamazepine and valproate seem to be relatively free of many adverse neuropsychologic effects; anterograde amnesia,[J140] retrograde amnesia,[L336] and toxic "ictal" confusion[V40,M5,S69] have been reported following benzodiazepine use.

Studies of substance abuse have not been specific to SLE but, by extrapolation, it is reasonable to assume that substance abuse occurs in lupus patients. Experience with numerous patients has revealed the excessive use of alcohol and nicotine products, poor dietary practices, and various dependencies on analgesics (included opiates), prescribed and proprietary sleeping products and hypnotics, and an assortment of so-called psychic energizers. A small percentage of lupus patients subjects themselves to unnecessary expense and possible harm by the ingestion of a vast array of health food products and substances labeled "orthomolecular vitamins" and "homeopathic herbs." I have seen at least four patients on 10 g of vitamin C.[S312] These patients customarily do not report the ingestion of such products to their physician.

DIFFERENTIAL DIAGNOSIS OF PSYCHOSES

Although the prime cause of psychotic episodes in SLE is organic brain disease, approximately 5% of cases may be a result of other factors, such as hypokalemia, water intoxication with hyponatremia, steroids themselves, and, occasionally, unusual reactions to antimalarial therapy. Due consideration must be given to each of these additional problems in the evaluation of every case. Complete blood chemistry profiles should be obtained in all patients.

Several patients have had water intoxication with psychosis varying from hallucinations to catatonia, associated with advanced lupus nephropathy.[B336,D111,W364] Hyponatremia and water intoxication (inappropriate ADH secretion) remain a relatively frequent cause of mental disturbance, especially in patients with lupus nephropathy. Central hyperventilation and inadequate antidiuretic hormone secretion[K57] may develop (see Chap. 41).

Although they usually decrease emotional lability, improve depression, and increase energy levels, antimalarials may produce personality changes, convulsive seizures, nightmares, and psychoses (see Chap. 57). Usually these were associated with large doses, and often other side effects were prominent prior to the mental ones.[D303]

Rudin[H453] hypothesized that the choroid plexus in SLE represents a combined transport dysfunction model for schizophrenia, as part of the blood-brain barrier guarding the periventricular primary personality brain or limbic system. This unlikely theory has not been subject to testing, and patients without SLE may have choroid plexus immune complex deposition.

From the preceding, it is clear that the diagnosis of NPL is clinical, and one of exclusion. Brain cross-reactive lymphocytotoxins and various neuronal antibodies may be measured; using a panel of substrates, one can identify a significant proportion of patients who are independently defined as having NPL and who demonstrate specific serum neuronal antibodies.[H453] (See Chapters 27 and 38 for a detailed discussion of the role of neuroimmunologic and neuroradiologic testing in SLE.)

The use of newer imaging techniques, such as magnetic resonance imaging (MRI), and of positron emission tomography (PET) and brain electric activity monitoring (BEAM), for metabolic assessment of the CNS hold great promise. In 1990, Stoppe, Wildhagen et al.[S713] reported that they performed PET using ^{18}F-labeled 2-F-2-desoxyglucose in 13 patients with SLE; 10 of them had clinical signs of central nervous system involvement (NPL). All patients with neurologic symptoms showed pathologic

changes on PET, always in accordance with their clinical state, and 3 patients without neuropsychiatric manifestations had normal PETs. Computed tomography (CT) of the brain and MRI proved to be less sensitive to both the presence and localization of CNS lesions. They concluded that the combination of PET and MRI constitutes the most useful diagnostic procedure for NPL. Reports from Sibbitt et al.[S407] concluded that, for the evaluation of acute NPL, MRI is useful and provides more information than cranial CT.

Kushnermu et al.[K483] studied the patterns of cerebral blood flow (CBF) over time in patients with SLE and varying neurologic manifestations, including headache, stroke, psychosis, and encephalopathy. CBF was least affected in patients with nonspecific symptoms, such as headache or malaise, whereas patients with encephalopathy or psychosis exhibited the greatest reduction in CBF. Reports from Japan, Great Britain, and Scandinavia[B149,M259,M588,S296] have reflected intense interest in the application and correlation of neuropsychiatric disorders in SLE with developments in imaging systems, neuroimmunology, neuroendocrinology, neuropsychologic function assessment, and PET scanning.

Several important reports of rather uncommon and atypical clinical pictures in NPL have appeared. In 1981, Bambery et al.[B70] described one case of a patient with SLE who developed the classic features of anorexia nervosa.

Bovin and Schrader[B441] suggested that the reported low incidence of subdural symptoms in SLE may be more apparent than real. They cited the case history of an SLE patient who presented with headaches, psychiatric disturbances, and increasing pain paraparesis. With surgical evacuation, the NP symptoms and headaches disappeared.

Gossat and Walls[G309] reported on 14 patients in whom SLE was diagnosed for the first time after the age of 45 years. The onset was insidious and diagnosis was delayed in most patients, with the mean duration of symptoms before diagnosis being 5 years. Clinical features in this group of patients differed from classic descriptions of SLE in regard to an unusually high incidence of neuropsychiatric disturbances and a low incidence of serositis. Diagnosis in this age group is difficult, and SLE probably goes unrecognized in a number of older patients with nonspecific complaints.

CLINICAL AND LABORATORY EVALUATION

A well-designed mental status examination is imperative.[N59] It should include evaluation of orientation, recent and remote memory, and level of consciousness, reality testing, and a neurologic examination.[S725] Psychologic profiles such as the MMPI and the Wechsler Adult Intelligence Scale (WAIS) are often helpful, but can be masked by the concurrent administration of medication.

The neuropsychologic testing described earlier in this chapter can be a useful and highly sensitive instrument for identifying and monitoring cognitive function impairment and its progression or improvement for clinical, investigative, and legal purposes.

Neuroendocrine testing, such as the dexamethasone suppression test (DMST) and the measurement of 24-catecholamine breakdown in homovanillic acid (HVA) studies, has led to an impressive body of research on biologic markers of depressive illness. The evidence suggests that abnormalities of the hypothalamic-pituitary-adrenal-IPA axis in depression (resistance of dexamethasone suppression, spontaneous plasma cortisol secretion, abnormal metyrapone responses, β-endorphin and β-lipotropin secretion, and corticotropin-releasing factor [CRF] challenge) tend to subside on clinical recovery.[F31] In particular, abnormal DMST results tend to normalize on antidepressant treatment; failure to do so is often associated with a poor prognosis, indicating that full recovery from depression should include normalization of the HPA axis.[B443,C208,H397,H398,S220,T71,Y41] As a result, persistent nonsuppression, despite antidepressant treatment, or reversion to abnormal DMST results, may be a prodromal signs of relapse in unipolar depression. Specific applications of these neuroendocrine tests to NPL have not been studied to any signification extent.

Thyroid testing, including thyroid-stimulating and thyroid-releasing hormone studies, may unmask a subclinical hypothyroidism. Typically, these patients are refractory to tricyclic antidepressants, but respond favorably with the addition of thyroid products.

The use of lumbar puncture, neuroradiologic testing, electroencephalography, and BEAM, and further details about neuroimmunologic subjects, are discussed in Chapters 27 and 38.

SPECIAL CONCERNS, CHALLENGES, AND ADJUSTMENTS

From the onset of symptoms, the lupus patient must adapt to a continuous series of unexpected physical, psychosocial, and emotional stresses and challenges. Usually, a person with SLE must adjust to a *chronic illness* with no cure, to an illness with a pattern of remissions and flares, often of brief duration, that generally occurs early in life, commonly after a prolonged period of elusive symptoms that have gone undiagnosed for some time. Often, prior to a specific diagnosis of lupus, the undiagnosed person and family and friends even begin to wonder about the validity of the patient's actual complaints. A transient sense of elation and relief is often experienced when a specific diagnosis, is finally established.

A common and problematic aspect of SLE is that the patient often doesn't "look sick," and often tries to conceal symptomatic complaints. This discourages support and empathy from those unfamiliar with the disease, even though the patient is exhausted and feels terrible.[S315] Life's stresses often serve as explanations to the patient and family for all the fatigue and emotional instability. Unexpressed, but commonly felt by the lupus patient, is the fear of death, disfigurement, and disability; perhaps most often feared is being an invalid, unable to care for oneself and thereby dependent on others. These common feelings in the lupus patient are certainly factors in the high incidence of depression, anxiety, and insomnia that are seen but other factors seem to be at work, because other types of chronic illness seem to be associated with depression and insomnia, to a lesser degree.

The lupus patient needs to cope with all aspects of modification in their goals and lifestyle dictated by their illness. The personality type seen so frequently in lupus—namely, a person who is outgoing, self-reliant, independent, and not given to complaint or passivity—can interfere with this. Unfortunately, such a person has a particularly difficult time in adjusting to the specific requirements of this illness—namely, frequent and careful medical monitoring, openness and honesty with the rheumologist, and careful self-scrutiny and limit setting on oneself. The struggle with self-esteem and depression can be and often is complicated by self-image and body image problems.[L54] The stress of accepting this illness is followed by new challenges; the use of steroids often produces added physical changes and imposes limitations on an already fatigued patient. Fatigue, physical pain, and decreased muscle and joint mobility can lead to depression and withdrawal from normal activities, resulting in social isolation and personal disintegration, with loss of hope and suicidal despair.

During the prediagnosis phase of their illness, some younger patients try to cope with all these stresses and tensions by doing what had worked so well for them before, prior to the onset of symptoms—actively pushing on even harder. This is common with the first abatement of symptoms when they push on gain, until they burn out and drop. This can erode their self-confidence and self-image, intensify their anxiety and uncertainty, and often cloud their confidence in the physician's inability to "make the diagnosis."

The return of symptoms begins to overcome any thoughts they might have about being just "stressed out," or that their symptoms are a result of psychologic forces. It ushers in the deep and growing conviction that, despite what their physician cannot find, something is seriously and organically wrong. All this commonly occurs in the prediagnosis phase. Most demoralizing after the uncertainty of the condition is the patient's loss of energy and fatigue, which leads to reduced and limited productivity.

Rogers[R271] has noted that for many patients the perceived injustice of an early recommendation for psychiatric treatment prior to the diagnosis of SLE may create wariness and resistance, suspicion, and even hostility about later (in the illness), more appropriate and needed psychiatric intervention. As with any chronic illness, the relationship established with the primary physician is crucial in managing the patient's illness properly. The physician treating a patient with lupus can benefit by knowing about the patient's earlier treatment experience, including psychiatric experience. Patients often believe that their physician is not really listening in a nonjudgmental way. Often, patients report thinking that their physician ignores them as people. Because of the relative obscurity of SLE, family and friends are generally unfamiliar with it, and are less able to relate to the patient. This leads to a sense of loss of independence and of control of their own lives and, when coupled with varying types and degrees of pain and marked fatigue, can lead to an increasing sense of emotional distance and isolation.

The stress early in the illness, especially that of accepting the illness, is followed by a series of new and unexpected challenges and impositions, such as the growing recognition that for the rest of their lives they need to see doctors on a frequent and regular basis. This involves careful and frequent monitoring, incurs a substantial amount of medical expenses, and most likely requires steroids, with their associated physical and functional changes. More importantly, patients must modify many of their dreams and expectations, and must begin to accept increasing responsibility for a lifetime of limitations and financial burdens. The lupus patient needs to cope, sooner or later, with all aspects of modifications in their lifestyle dictated by their particular illness, and this process takes time, work, and practice. As mentioned above, this can be interfered with by the premorbid personality type often observed in lupus, a person who tends to be somewhat outgoing, self-controlled, achievement-oriented, self-reliant, independent, rather physical in their discharges of emotional tension, and not given to complaint or passivity, and who unfortunately has a particularly difficult time in adjusting to an illness that reduces mobility, motor activity, attention span, and energy level, while simultaneously contributing to a greater degree of dependency on others.[M422] This perceived dependency frequently induces guilt, anxiety, and depression, and can lead to acting out, which translates into noncompliance and treatment defiance. All this is occurring at a time in their lives when their healthy peers can anticipate such activities as exposure to the sun, uncomplicated pregnancies, substantially less need for rest, and relative freedom to explore their social and vocational interests and potentials; they tend to withdraw from the lupus patient. Lupus patients are generally ambivalent and hesitant to vocalize their fears, worries, and complaints to their physicians, families, and friends.

Adolescents, in particular, are frequently noncompliant. It is often difficult for them to fulfill these demands. Nashel and Ulmer[N33] have noted that many do not take corticosteroids as advised because of their effects of weight gain fluid retention, promotion of facial hair, acne, and easy bruisability. Fragile social relationships with friends can be altered by sun avoidance, hair loss, a skin rash, and fatigability.[S428] They often have special concerns and questions when confronted with issues of dating, marriage, or childbearing. Compliance improves with a good physician-patient relationship and when the side effects of prescribed drugs (especially steroids) are discussed in detail beforehand.[A311] Changing the lifestyle of the lupus patient is difficult. Often, physicians see their role as entirely treatment-oriented, and minimize the emotional component.

Because the time from onset of symptoms to diagnosis averages 3 years, many patients are already frustrated by the time they are told they have lupus. Their relationships with physicians are strained. Initial feelings of relief, euphoria, and hopes for a quick cure occur after the diagnosis is made. A brief "honeymoon" with the diagnosing physician occurs and is often followed by a letdown as it becomes apparent that no quick fix is available. Some patients, particularly adolescents, try to deny that they have the disease, while others try to control their management by learning everything about it. They pressure the treating physician into therapeutic courses that they might not otherwise undertake. It is especially important, then, that the lines of communication be kept open between patients and physician to avoid irreparable damage. Appropriate relationships, according to Pincus, can reverse the course of the illness, and can promote compliance and positive thinking and enhance the patient's satisfaction in activities of daily living (modified Stanford Health Assessment Questionnaire, HAQ).[P197]

Crisis intervention becomes important when a sense of isolation, fear of death, and loss of independence occur. At this point, patients may feel that they are losing their minds and cannot control mood swings, and may become unable to hold a job. Often they are told they do not look sick when they feel exhausted and terrible. Those who retain their socialization skills, and especially those who attend group rap sessions sponsored by the various lupus societies (see below), tend to cope better. Such group discussions can dispel negative self-images and self-defeating attitudes, and can improve self-esteem. In addition, they facilitate the healthy release of feelings and emotions, encourage participants to confront and resolve their problems, and assist in consolidating and maintaining therapeutic gains. On the other hand, many patients leading a normal life find it depressing to hear of others' bad experiences with the illness. Unconscious guilt feelings that lupus is a punishment meted out be a supreme force must be abolished.

Despite these problems, most lupus patients are outgoing, self-reliant, and independent. Most can handle their imposed handicaps well, maintain their jobs, and live fairly normal family lives. Some patients, however, box themselves into a corner with their defense mechanisms.[S633] Goodwin et al.[G295] studied 25 SLE patients treated by a group of four physicians and had the physicians rate those whom they liked the least. Of the 25 patients, 10 were ranked by three physicians as most disliked. They had more anxiety, hostility, and depression than the others, and were generally immature and uncooperative. An increased incidence of organic brain syndrome and suicidal ideation was noted in this group.

A chief compliant of SLE patients is chronic fatigue.[K436] Periods of activity alternating with periods of rest often result in more being accomplished in a day than working continuously.[J138] Self-employed individuals or those who can set their own pace (e.g., those who work out of their own home) are often the most productive. Demands for resolution of this problem results in patients being given thyroid preparations, iron, and sometimes amphetamines. Substance abuse may be a problem, but is not as common as might be expected. Several pain management centers surveyed in Los Angeles related that SLE patients comprise a small percentage of their practice.

The patient with minimal organic brain disease represents a serious problem in management. Often, because of newly developing personality quirks, home life becomes intolerable. Because the course of the illness is physically exhausting and produces personality changes, the incidence of divorce is exceedingly high. Judgment is often impaired. Patients may be in a state of limbo—not psychotic enough to be declared mentally incompetent, and yet not really able to handle their own affairs effectively. Fruitlessly, many seek the help of psychoanalysts, especially prior to a definitive diagnosis. The physician managing the patient has a difficult time trying to decide how much is reaction to a chronic illness and what to tell the patient and the family. At times, the role of a functional overlay and organic process is so intertwined that it is impossible to be certain.[H354] Many of these patients appear physically well while receiving steroid therapy, with relatively normal laboratory findings, but complain of extreme lethargy and myalgia to the point of invalidism. Although extensive organic disease can be present with minimal findings, the evaluation and management of such problems can be trying to all concerned. Hochberg and Sutton studied 106 ambulatory outpatients with SLE during 1985. The patients completed the Stanford HAQ and the Psychosocial Adjustment to Illness Scale (PAIS). Mean HAQ disability pain and global scores indicated a mild amount of impairment. Significant correlations were observed among increased disability, increased pain, worse global assessment, and poor psychosocial adjustment.[H354]

Marriage, Family, and Sexuality

In dealing with a patient population consisting primarily of women of childbearing age, problems of marriage and pregnancy arise frequently for the physician called on for advice. In general, I have adopted a course of being frank with the patient in discussing the variability of the disease, with emphasis on the optimistic side.

Concerning marriage, it is advisable to review privately with the patient the limitations placed on her by the illness. These restrictions may vary from essentially none to tiring easily, which may interfere with a normal home life, and can progress to the point of longterm expensive medication, repeated hospitalizations, and the need for continuous medical care. The chance of a spontaneous remission occurring at any time should be emphasized repeatedly, because these patients are usually depressed by the chronic nature of the disease, and frightened by the little information they have gathered from medical dictionaries and outdated medical texts.[E141] The risk of recurrences of a serious nature should be mentioned. If it is apparent that the patient is determined to marry, the fiancé, if the patient desires it, is invited to enter the consultation room and the matter is again reviewed with both present. To avoid obvious problems, I never discuss prognosis with the fiancé alone or give him a worse outlook than that given the patient. Otherwise, if the engagement is broken, as often happens, the patient may develop a mistrustful attitude toward the physician, which can interfere with future therapy.

Lupus is a family affair; it is important that the physician inquire about the patient's family life and background. Family members must learn to walk the fine line between encouraging patients to become invalids and pushing them beyond their limitations. They must be informed about the nature of the disease, be able to anticipate physical and emotional changes, and respond in a supportive manner. Pfeiffer has clearly and concisely described the various stages of development in women, along with the coping responses.[P172]

Sexual changes often occur during the course of SLE patients' lives. The disease, side effects of medications, and/or depressions that many lupus patients experience can contribute to a breakdown in sexual relationships. Patients are often reluctant to discuss these problems with their partner or physician, further contributing to the 50% divorce rate among SLE patients. Antihypertensive medications can decrease libido; corticosteroids alter appearance and may interfere with menstruation patterns, as well as affecting mood. Nonsteroidal drugs may cause edema; tranquilizers and psychotropic drugs have more far-reaching effects.

The social functioning of 120 patients (114 women) with SLE was studied in British Columbia. Of these, 61 had 76 pregnancies after the onset of SLE; although fetal wastage was common, outcomes were otherwise satisfactory. Social difficulties worsened with disease exacerbations, drug reactions, and delay in diagnosis. After the onset of SLE, 33% completed their educations; 63% with a work history were employed, and 52% were totally or partially self-supporting. Patients experienced problems with self-image (20%), sexual functioning (4%), and lifestyle (17%). SLE was not a barrier to marriage or a primary cause of divorce; 40% married after the onset of SLE, and 12.5% had a history of divorce. Stein et al.[S633] concluded that SLE patients can function well socially, notwithstanding many varied limitations and readjustments, provided that these difficulties are recognized and accepted and that emotional support is provided. The authors emphasized the importance of psychologic support and referral for counseling as factors in optimal psychosocial adjustment outcomes.

Patients' Rap (Self-Help Groups)

Patients' self-help groups have become a national movement, and are now common with local and national SLE organization.[S319] Patient rap groups are an adjunct to the total psychosocial and medical care of the person with lupus. Rap groups provide all sorts of intrinsic support, including emotional warmth, friendly commiseration, and a sense of closeness with other patients. These groups provide for the transmission of accurate and current medical information, an opportunity for venting one's feelings, and the inevitable selection of "kindred spirits" for friends, along with much more that contributes to the individual's welfare.

Group leaders guide the patients actively in an attempt to restore hope and enhance their cooperation with physicians. Most importantly, perhaps, the group process seems to dispel and reverse negative self-images and self-defeating attitudes and behaviors. Regressive, noncompliant, and treatment-resisting behaviors are often modified or overcome.

Rap group participation seems to promote a greater sense of social involvement and self-control in the patient's mind. It contributes to greater hope, self-esteem, and intelligent and active redirection of energies into appropriate activities. The rap group promotes the acceptance of limitations without despair and fosters greater appreciation for and cooperation with the medical team.

In addition, the participants tend to develop more tolerance and acceptance of their friends, family, and themselves. They feel like they are more active participants in their own care and are contributing to the "lupus cause" by helping other members, usually the newer ones.

Recognizing common psychologic fears and mechanisms so that they can be understood and shared, and their energies redirected into more realistic and appropriate attitudes and behavior, is essential to assisting the lupus patient to cope and contribute constructively. Patient rap groups have proven to be effective.

THERAPEUTIC CONSIDERATIONS

Goals and Attitudes in Adjusting to SLE

The physician and family must recognize and understand that adjustment to a chronic illness is a gradual adaptation process, much like the emotional, psychosocial, and maturation aspects of the developmental process, with various phases, inevitable challenges, opportunities and pitfalls. This adjustment is similar to the way in which good parents assist their child toward optimal growth. An open, relatively relaxed and trusting relationship with the physician contributes directly toward a positive outcome. The adjustment capability and ego strength of the patient are enhanced by increased knowledge and education about their own condition. Toward this end, the physician's knowledge of the disease process and of all aspects of the SLE illness experience, as well as an understanding of adjustment to chronic illness, are essential in assisting the patient.[S318] The physician should understand and transmit the following to the patient and to the important people in the patient's life:

1. Almost all SLE patients experience intermittent periods of anxiety and depression, of varying intensity and duration, during the course of their illness.
2. If patients are to reach and maintain a comfortable emotional equilibrium, with a satisfactory self-image and sense of hope, they must tolerate and understand these powerful emotions and develop a sense of control over their condition and over their life.
3. Cure is not a goal worth pursuing; rather, the patient must learn to gain control of their condition, and of their life.
4. Self-monitoring of the condition is essential, and represents an important step by patients toward contributing and participating in their own medical care. This is important, because they are in a cooperative relationship with their primary care physician.
5. Illness is the best teacher, provided that it is listened to.
6. Pain is natural, inevitable, and tolerable, as long as it is controlled.
7. Families should be encouraged *not* to give advice, but rather to hear and understand the emotional concerns and feelings of the patient.

8. Patients must monitor their emotions as well as their body sensations.
9. Stress of all types exacerbates lupus. Stress is inevitable, so it cannot be avoided totally, but the various stressors should be anticipated, identified, and controlled, to whatever degree is possible.
10. Hope, sublimations, and substitutions help attenuate the continuous series of losses that occur with lupus.

Role of Psychotherapy in SLE

In most cases of lupus, relapse is the rule, and that includes occasional psychologic slips. Physicians, patients, and family must recognize that the value of psychotherapy in chronic illness is well established. The goals of psychotherapy remain the same, whether or not the person has an illness. The goals are simply to encourage greater self-awareness, insight, and coping ability; to alleviate intrapsychic and interpersonal conflict; and to develop health-enhancing attitudes and behaviors.

Understanding the Chronically Ill

As a general rule, obvious neuropsychiatric manifestations in someone with chronic illness are treated in much the same way as in a person without a chronic illness, with regard to the various chemical and physiologic limitations of the underlying physical condition and consideration for the use of concurrent medications. An organic basis for any neuropsychiatric manifestations must first be ruled out; this requires a careful medical and neurologic history and examination, with an emphasis on medication history, appropriate and through laboratory studies, and being prepared for the emergence of some new condition. One must be aware of drug dependency—"masked depression, masked suicide." Even when a definitive organic factor has been identified that contributes to the neuropsychiatric condition, psychologic intervention is usually necessary and helpful, and a visit with the patient's family or even a visit to the home can prove illuminating. One must not be timid or conservative, or use subclinical doses of psychopharmacologic agents if results are desired. Undertreatment can be more destructive than no treatment. Substance abuse, especially of alcohol, is more common than recognized. Liaison with the family is tricky but may prove helpful, especially if it can reinforce or establish support for the patient.

The therapeutic goal with the SLE patient is to increase the sense of self-control and independence, and to promote participation with the health care team. I believe that the following contributes constructively and positively to therapeutic effectiveness with all patients:

1. The quality of life is a worthwhile goal, and the physician's therapeutic focus should be on that quality, now and in the future.
2. Each inevitable loss or sense of loss by the patient should be neutralized in part by some replacement.
3. The process of medical treatment of the lupus patient requires greater patience, tolerance, flexibility, and creativity from the physician than the treat-

ment of other patients. It requires more common sense and acceptance of various, even strange parameters than the more short-term conditions.

4. The physician and the patient must develop a mutual honesty, respect, understanding of one another, and openness of communication to tolerate those aspects of the condition that are unclear, unpredictable, and often intolerable (but important).

5. Somatization and occasional opportunism with the use of illness is a human trait, and inevitable, but by no means unforgivable or insurmountable.

6. Unpleasant emotional responses and mental distortions are an acceptable adaptation, and will pass.

7. Despite incredible disruptions in one's lifestyle and existence, many patients recover their mental, emotional, and spiritual (and often sexual) sense of well-being; they then want to continue living, and to live well.

8. Realistic limit setting is essential, both for the patient and psychotherapist.

9. Many chronically ill patients with severe, neuropsychiatric pathology have been neglected and essentially rejected by a therapeutic pessimism that has led to undertreatment, therapeutic and familial abandonment, and deepening psychopathology and maladaptation.

10. Hopelessness is pathogenic.

11. Each medical condition has its own set of preconditions; these are as important to recognize as the ego strength, premorbid personality, and resources of the individual with a chronic illness.

12. Sexual libido and general aggressiveness are greatly reduced ("tired").

13. A series of *somatopsychic* consequences of a specific condition is almost inevitable, and must be respected.

14. Terms and words mean different things to different patients.

15. Pain and immobility may be more stressful to the physician than to the patient, and patients tend to be highly sensitive to their physician's emotional responses.

16. Rarely should the physician attempt to deny or dispute the truth of a patient's accurate perception of their attitudes, feelings, or behavior.

17. The cornerstone of any good relationship is honest and open communication. The patient has the responsibility to tell the physician what really troubles them, and the physician has the responsibility not only to listen, but to hear. The physician must inquire about the physical condition but, perhaps more importantly, about their inner feelings, relationships, and life situation. Communication is always a two-way street.

18. Physicians should not view psychotherapy as a substitute for vocational or social rehabilitation.

A summary of the psychopathology of the lupus patient is presented in Table 39–2.

Table 39–2. Summary: Psychopathology of the Lupus Patient

1. Historical: psychiatric manifestations in SLE
2. Incidence of psychiatric symptoms in SLE; stage of emergence
3. Predisposing factors; role of stress and drugs
4. Classification
   Psychosis
   1) Schizophreniform illness
   2) Toxic organic psychosis
   3) Steroid-induced psychosis
   4) Affective (mood) psychosis
   5) Steroids, mood, cognition, and behavior
   Organic brain syndromes
   1) Organic personality syndromes
   Impairment in cognition (organic amnestic syndrome)
   Functional disorders, primary depression, and anxiety
5. Application of neuropsychologic testing
6. Factitious illness and positive ANA without lupus
7. Organic versus functional disease
8. Medication-induced mental changes in SLE
9. Differential diagnosis of neuropsychiatric lupus
10. Clinical and laboratory evaluation
11. Special concerns, challenges, and adjustments
    a. Marriage, family, and sexuality
    b. Patient rap (self-help groups)
12. Therapeutic goals and attitudes in adjusting to SLE
13. Role of psychotherapy in SLE
14. General suggestions in the understanding and psychotherapeutic management of the chronically ill
15. "Recipe For Survival" (patient handout)

DR. SHAPIRO'S RECIPE FOR SURVIVAL

The following "recipe for survival" for lupus patients has been widely circulated and reprinted in the newsletters of the Lupus Foundation of America, The American Lupus Society, and other organizations devoted to issues concerning patients' coping with chronic illness. It concisely embodies my suggestions.*

To avoid: FATIGUE
           LONESOMENESS AND LONELINESS
           ALCOHOL AND DRUGS
           RUMINATIONS (*repetitive worrisome ideas*)
           EXHAUSTION
           SELF-ABSORPTION AND SELF-PITY

To seek out: REST, RELAX, RECREATE, AND RAP REGULARLY
              EXERCISE
              LAUGHTER AS OFTEN AS POSSIBLE
              AFFECTION, GIVEN AND RECEIVED
              XCHANGES OF POSITIVE THOUGHTS FOR NEGATIVE THOUGHTS
              EDUCATE YOURSELF ON YOUR CONDITION
              SOCIALIZE WITH AND OFFER SUPPORT TO OTHERS AS MUCH AS YOUR CONDITION ALLOWS AND THEN A LITTLE MORE

R: Rest, relax, and recreate regularly . . . this does not mean just on weekends or holidays, but all the time, as a new life pattern, Now is the time to drop your workaholic tendencies. If you have neglected to incor-

---

* It first appeared in *We Are Not Alone*, by Sefra Pitzek (Minneapolis, Thompson Publishing, 1984).

porate "**R**" into your life so far, it is essential now that chronic illness has entered the picture.

E: Exercise! Not all of you can get out and jog or play tennis, but you should do what you can, at least several times a week, even if you are bound to a bed or wheelchair. Ask your doctor to help you develop an exercise plan suited to your illness. Activity is important, even if it is just range of motion exercises.

L: Laughter can be crucial for your survival. You may be familiar with Norman Cousins, former editor of *Saturday Review,* who used laughter as a key part of his successful attempt to reach a remission of his illness. The same treatment can help us deal with our chronic illness. Laughter does not just make you feel good; it also causes you to take deep, relaxing breaths and, for a short time, it clears your mind of other thoughts and emotions. And laughter begets laughter. What a wonderful habit to develop!

A: Affection, both given and received … SHARE YOURSELF … pet a puppy, hug a child, love your spouse. Equally important, learn to ask for and receive affection in whatever way you feel comfortable. Don't be shy … make it a constant in your life.

X: Exhange negative thoughts for positive thoughts, dwell on what you can change, not on what you can't. Think about how well you can be instead of how ill you might be.

E: Educate yourself about your chronic illness, and not only yourself. Take it upon yourself to gently and slowly educate those around you who care about your well-being.

S: Socialize with and offer support to others as much as your condition allows, plus a little more. If you keep yourself busy, you'll have less time to dwell on your pain and illness. It is hard to concentrate on two things at once. A particularly good way of keeping busy is to use your experiences to provide encouragement and support to others with a similar condition. By helping others, you help yourself even more.

READINGS FOR PATIENTS

A Decade of Lupus by Henrietta Aladjem; Acme Printing, Medford, MA., under the auspices of The Lupus Foundation of America.

Beyond Rage: the Emotional Impact of Chronic Physical Illness by JoAnn LeMaistre, PhD; Alpine Guild, Oak Park, IL (1985).

Coping with Lupus by Robert Phillips, PhD.

Lupus Erythematosus by Ronald Carr, MD, PhD.; available through the Lupus Foundation of America, Washington DC.

Lupus Erythematosus: A Handbook for Nurses by Terri Nass, RN (1984)

Lupus: Hope Through Understanding by Henrietta Aladjem; Acme Printing, Medford, MA. (1982).

So Now You Have Lupus, by Leslie Epstein and Bonnie Romoff; The American Lupus Society (1985).

Successful Living with Chronic Illness by Kathleen Lewis; Avery Publishing Group, NJ, (1985).

The Sun is My Enemy by Henrietta Aladjem; Beacon Press, Boston, MA. (1976)

Understanding Lupus by Henrietta Aladjem; Scribners Publishing, NY, NY (1982)

We Are Not Alone-Learning to Live with Chronic Illness, by Sefra K. Pitzele; Thompson Publishing, Minn, MN (1984).

Winners and Losers by Sydney J. Harris; Argus Communication, Niles, IL (1964).

Chapter 40

HEAD AND NECK FINDINGS IN SLE: SJÖGREN'S SYNDROME AND THE EYE, EAR, AND LARYNX

DANIEL J. WALLACE

SJÖGREN'S SYNDROME

Overview

Sjögren's syndrome (Table 40–1) is a triad of dry eyes (keratoconjunctivitis sicca), dry mouth (xerostomia), and an underlying connective tissue disease such as SLE, rheumatoid arthritis, or scleroderma. The sicca complex may exist alone without any underlying disease (sicca syndrome or primary Sjögren's syndrome). Of those afflicted, 90% are females, with a mean age of 50 years; 50% have an autoimmune disorder, and 20% have Raynaud's phenomenon. Renal tubular acidosis (proximal), bronchitis sicca, cryoglobulinemia, Mikulicz's disease, and hyperviscosity may be seen with Sjögren's syndrome. An increased association with HLA-B8 and HLA-DR3 exists. Serologically, 70% have a positive ANA, 70% have anti-Ro/SSA, 50% have hypergammaglobulinemia, 50% have salivary duct epithelium antibodies, 50% have anti-La/SSB, and 35% have antithyroglobulin antibodies.

Sjögren's syndrome can best be diagnosed by a biopsy of the minor salivary glands in the lower lip.[D39] Other diagnostic modalities that have been used include technetium parotid scanning (80% of SLE patients with Sjögren's syndrome have an abnormal scan),[K117] sialograms (SLE patients show atrophy, strictures, and sialectasis),[K117] Schirmer's test, rose bengal eye staining, and parotid saliva flow rate studies. Sjögren's patients have a 44-fold increase in the risk of developing lymphoproliferative malignancies, such as lymphoma or Waldenström's macroglobulinemia.

Sjögren's syndrome is usually treated symptomatically. Artificial tears are used for dry eyes, and various secretagogues from sour lemon drops to artificial saliva are used to treat xerostomia. Several excellent reviews have provided more detailed descriptions of this entity.[A137,K97, S604,T26] This section emphasizes the association between SLE and Sjögren's Syndrome.

Incidence of SLE in Sjögren's Syndrome

The concurrence of Sjögren's syndrome and SLE was first described by Morgan in 1954,[M573] and numerous investigators in the 1950s and 1960s observed LE cells in Sjögren's patients with lupus-like features.[B30,B344,B568, H229,M36,M573] The incidence of SLE in Sjögren's patients has been estimated to be 4 to 13%.[K97,M168,S340,V8] Of 44 patients seen in an ophthalmology clinic for a chief complaint of dry eyes, 86% had keratoconjunctivitis sicca,

56% had a positive ANA, and 20% had a known connective tissue disease.[M469] Only 2 had SLE. Rheumatoid arthritis (RA) is associated with Sjögren's syndrome more frequently than is SLE. Branson-Geokas et al.[B461] reviewed 300 rheumatology clinic patients at our hospital and found 45 who fulfilled at least three criteria for Sjögren's: 33 (74%) had RA, 2 had progressive systemic sclerosis, 1 had Sjögren's syndrome alone, and 1 had SLE. Mackenzie et al.[M23] reviewed 93 patients with Sjögren's syndrome studied with sialography; 8 had normal parotid sialograms. Of the 93 patients, 65% had RA, 13% had scleroderma, 11% had vasculitis, 10% had polymyositis, 9% had fibrositis, 6% had Mikulicz's syndrome alone, and 4% had SLE. Sylvester et al.[S794] analyzed 28 patients with Sjögren's syndrome using labial gland biopsy, measurement of stimulated parotid secretion, salivary gland scintigraphy, and ophthalmology evaluation. Of these, 7 had RA and 3 had SLE; no associated connective tissue disease was found in 14.

Steinberg and Talal[S653] reported 8 patients with features of Sjögren's syndrome and SLE in a group of 14 with Sjögren's syndrome. Interestingly, 4 of these 8 patients had chronic joint deformities.

Incidence and Features of Sjögren's in SLE

The incidence of Sjögren's syndrome in patients with SLE varies from 1 to 98%, depending on the methods used to make the diagnosis.[A87,B308a,F263,G366,G367,J29,K5,K96,M118, M636,R29,R294,V92,W181] Of Dubois' 520 patients, 7 (1.4%) had keratoconjunctivitis sicca in addition to the usual manifestations of SLE. Rothfield[B308a] reported parotid enlargement in 8% of her 365 patients; only some were related to Sjögren's syndrome. Ropes[R294] identified Sjögren's syndrome in only 2 of her 150 patients, and Wallace in 11 of his 503 patients.[W18] Kaden studied the incidence of Sjögren's syndrome in 194 lupus patients attending Dubois' outpatient clinic at LAC-USC Medical Center.[K5] Schirmer's test, revealed diminished secretion, below 10 mm, in 94 patients (48%), and between 0 and 5 mm in 54 patients (28%). Positive fluorescein staining without a specific pattern was found in 84 (43%). Corneal sensitivity was found to be reduced in 49%. The incidence of Sjögren's syndrome was even higher in those with SLE and deforming nonerosive arthritis.

Grennan et al.[G366,G367] performed similar studies on their patients in New Zealand and Scotland. At least one Sjögren's symptom was identified in 31% of 32 patients

Table 40–1. Features of Sjögren's Syndrome (SS) and SLE

1. SS consists of keratoconjunctivitis sicca (dry eyes) and xerostomia (dry mouth) in association with autoimmunity.
2. SLE patients with SS have multiple autoantibodies (especially anti-Ro/SSA and La/SSB), are often middle-aged women, and are likely to have deforming arthritis and an increased associaton with HLA-B8, DR3, and lymphoproliferative disorders.
3. Depending on patient selection and methods of evaluation, the incidence of clinical SS in SLE patients is from 1 to 10%.
4. Anti-Ro/SSA antibody is associated with "ANA-negative" lupus (on animal substrates), neonatal lupus syndrome, subacute cutaneous lupus, and photosensitivity.
5. Mikulicz's syndrome (salivary gland inflammation and enlargement) may be seen in SLE patients, with or without SS.

in the former group; 8 had dry eyes and dry mouth. In comparison with those without Sjögren's symptoms and SLE, an increased incidence of erosive arthritis, but no difference in renal disease and Raynaud's phenomenon, was found. The Scottish group found a 24% incidence of Sjögren's syndrome among 25 SLE patients, and the same association with erosive arthritis was seen. The highest incidence was reported by Alarcon-Segovia and colleagues: 23 of 50 SLE patients had sicca symptoms, and 49 of the 50 had at least two abnormal Sjögren's test results.[A87,R29] Five years later, 25 of the 30 original patients who were re-evaluated had sicca symptoms, and 8 new cases of xerostomia were found. This group used multiple studies to diagnose Sjögren's syndrome; patients with one positive test were included as having Sjögren's syndrome. This approach raises the question of test validity. It is likely that many patients with SLE have inflammation in their salivary glands; approximately 1 to 10% are symptomatic. Those with deforming arthritis are most likely to develop sicca symptoms.

Genetic Predisposition to Sjögren's Syndrome and Autoantibody Associations

HLA-DR3–positive SLE patients with Ro/SSA antibodies are more likely to have Sjögren's syndrome than DR3-negative–Ro/SSA-positive SLE patients.[P312,P313] This group also has an increased incidence of subacute cutaneous lupus, neonatal lupus, and HLA-B8, DQW2, and DRw52 phenotypes.[A136]

In one report, anti-La/SSB was present in 73% of 11 patients with Sjögren's syndrome and SLE, but in only 2% of 46 patients with SLE alone.[K96] SLE patients with Sjögren's syndrome may have higher anti-La/SSB values than those with Sjögren's syndrome secondary to RA or SLE alone. IgG, IgM, and IgA antibody isotypes were all elevated.[M118]

Histopathology of Sjögren's Syndrome

The results of histopathologic investigation of the labial glands of patients with SLE and Sjögren's syndrome are no different from those who have Sjögren's syndrome without SLE. Lymphocyte tissue subsets reveal CD4 + (helper) cell prominence.[J44,M207,M208] This is in contrast to patients with Sjögren's syndrome caused by human immunodeficiency virus infection; in those cases, the infiltrating lymphocytes have the CD8 + phenotype. Asymptomatic SLE patients have been reported to have positive lip biopsies for Sjögren's syndrome.[L299] Moutsopoulus' group performed lip biopsies on 60 SLE patients in Greece, and 11 were positive. Only 5 complained of dry eyes, resulting in a Sjögren's syndrome incidence of 8.3%. It was noted that Sjögren's syndrome in SLE is usually mild, and has a good outcome.[A217]

SLE with Sjögren's syndrome has an increased association with autoimmune thyroid disease (see Chap. 41).

Mikulicz's Syndrome

Mikulicz's syndrome is visible enlargement and inflammation of the salivary glands with or without symptoms of Sjögren's syndrome. These syndromes are closely related.[M573] Of Dubois' 520 patients, 6 (1.1%) and 2 of Wallace's 503 patients showed extreme enlargement of the parotid, submaxillary, and lacrimal glands (Fig. 40–1).

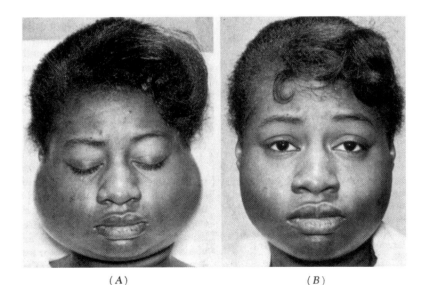

(A)   *(B)*

Fig. 40–1. *A,* Mikulicz's syndrome, caused by SLE, before steroid treatment. *B,* Same patient after 17 days of steroid therapy.

Shearn and Pirofsky[S343] first reported parotid enlargement in 7% of 83 patients with SLE. Futcher[F322] reported 10 patients with Mikulicz's syndrome whose biopsies showed round cell infiltration and reduction in the acini; 5 had SLE.

The initial presentation of Mikulicz's syndrome may antedate the diagnosis of SLE.[R284] Katz and Ehrlich[K116] reported three patients with SLE who developed acute sialoadenitis during active phases of the disease. Bilateral involvement of the parotid and submandibular glands occurred. They were enlarged and exquisitely tender, and, in two patients, were red and hot. All responded dramatically to corticosteroid treatment.

OCULAR LESIONS

Active lupus, antiphospholipid antibody syndrome, and medications used to treat LE can cause ocular pathology (Table 40–2). Immune complex deposition has been found in the blood vessels of the conjunctiva, retina, choroid, sclera, and ciliary body, in the basement membranes of the ciliary body and cornea, and in the peripheral nerves of the ciliary body and conjunctiva.[K82] This may be manifested clinically as vasculitis. Retinal occlusive disease in association with the lupus anticoagulant is important to identify, because it is treated with antiplatelet therapy and anticoagulation as opposed to anti-inflammatory therapies. Medication may affect the eyes, and these changes must be differentiated from those induced by the disease process. Corticosteroids may induce blurred vision and cataracts. Furthermore, they can raise intraocular pressure, which can cause glaucoma. Antimalarials may cause retinotoxic changes, (especially maculopathy), and occasionally deposit in the cornea. Antihypertensive agents can also alter ocular pressures.

Cutaneous Eye Lesions, Conjunctivitis, Corneal Lesions, and Orbital Myopathies

Although the literature emphasizes fundic lesions, changes may be seen from the periorbital tissues back to the retina. Lupus skin lesions have a propensity to appear about the eyelids. Several 1-mm diameter, slightly scaly, erythematous papules caused by LE may resemble those

Table 40–2. Ocular Manifestations of SLE

1. Conjunctivitis occurs in 10% of patients during the disease course.
2. Iritis occurs in 1 to 2% of patients during the disease course. It is more common in children.
3. Choroidal and/or retinal vasculitis can occur.
   a. It can occur as part of an immune complex-mediated process; patients are usually acutely ill.
   b. It can occur as part of the antiphospholipid syndrome.
   c. Cytoid bodies or white patches are seen in 8 to 24% of patients with SLE; these represent infarction from vasculitis or thromboemboli.
4. Macular degeneration may occur as a result of aging or antimalarial therapy.
5. Glaucoma or cataracts are often a result of corticosteroid therapy.
6. Optic or retrobulbar neuritis can be caused by vasculitis or infarction.
7. Infrequent complications include orbital myositis and ophthalmoplegia.

of eczema or infection about the lid. During acute phases of the disease, with extensive cutaneous involvement in the periorbital area, it is common to have periorbital edema. Recurrent conjunctivitis of viral, bacterial, or autoimmune origin is a frequent finding (10% of Dubois' 520 patients). In Harvey's series,[M280] 5 patients out of 105 had conjunctivitis, 2 of the follicular type; 2 also had episcleritis. Conjunctivitis was noted in 8% of 193 patients at Stanford University at any time during the disease course.[F263] A bulbar conjunctival biopsy with positive immunofluorescence (indicative of active SLE) may be useful.[F274]

At least eight cases of orbital inflammation associated with myositis and proptosis have been reported in SLE. Extraocular muscle swelling can be marked. Exophthalmos has rarely been observed.[B77,F45,F172,G371,M277, S402,S502]

Cranial neuropathies can present as ophthalmoplegias and can be difficult to differentiate from multiple sclerosis.[E160,J8] Adie's tonic pupil and blephorospasm have been noted during disease exacerbations.[H286,J45,R16]

Sjögren's syndrome's effects on the eye are discussed above, but corneal infiltration and edema can occur in its absence.[H172,R15,R101,W234] Spaeth[S576] reviewed ocular findings in 24 patients with SLE. Corneal staining with fluorescein was present in 88% of the group, although Schirmer's test was negative in all. Most characteristically, it was just inside the limbus, where the upper lid lay on the cornea. In most cases, staining was limited to three or four punctate spots in a line near the limbus. Only 5 of 100 normal controls showed similar involvement. Gold et al.[G227] observed similar findings in only 6.5% of 61 SLE outpatients.

Uveitis and the Choroid

Many patients with uveitis have circulating autoantibodies and are referred to rheumatologists to rule out an underlying autoimmune disease. Iritis was found in only 0.8% of Dubois' 520 SLE patients, in 2% of 193 patients with SLE at Stanford University,[F263] and in 2 of Moutsopoulos' 112 patients,[D293] and recurrent iritis was found in 4 of Wallace's 503 patients. The incidence of uveitis may be higher in childhood SLE, in which ocular findings of some type are found in 30%. In contrast, Sjögren's syndrome is rare in children.[S108]

Jabs' group at Johns Hopkins presented six cases of choroidal vascular disease and reviewed the literature.[J6] Involvement can lead to multifocal, serous elevations of retinal pigment epithelium and adjacent retinal sensory tissue, with resulting macular pathology and retinal detachment. Lupus arteritis of the eye is an immune complex-mediated disorder, as documented by choroidal vasculitis, cellular infiltrates, and deposits of IgG prominence. Immune complex deposition occurs primarily in the basement membrane and the pars plana of the choroid.[A303] Involved vessels correspond to sites of choroidal fluorescein leakage. This vasculitis is steroid-responsive,[D203] but can lead to rapid visual loss if untreated.

Glaucoma is a known complication of steroid therapy, and is occasionally observed in nonsteroid-treated LE.[W5]

Retinopathy and Optic Neuropathy

For over 50 years, ophthalmologists have recognized the white patches or "cytoid bodies" in lupus patients[B18,C304,H383,K480,M279,W187] that Roth first described in 1872.[R335] Cytoid bodies are characterized histologically by hypertrophy or ganglioform degeneration of the nerve fibers. They occur in 5 to 15% of patients with SLE.[B308a,C325,H179,J75,M280,R294] Significant retinal vascular narrowing was recorded in 13% of Dubois' patients, with and without hypertension. Rothfield[R308a] found conjunctivitis, episcleritis, or cytoid bodies at some time in 15% of her 375 patients. Ropes described blurred vision in 26% of her 150 patients[R294] and cytoid bodies in 9% (which correlated with disease activity).

Urowitz's group commented that 41 of 550 SLE patients (7%) had retinopathy, of whom 5 had significant visual loss. This cohort was associated with active disease and a poor prognosis. Of these 41 patients, 34 had microangiopathy, 3 had papilledema, 2 had ischemic neuritis, 2 had occlusive disease, and 1 had retinal detachment.[S606] Alarcon-Segovia performed fluorescein angiography on 50 SLE patients. Abnormalities were found in 13—9 had microaneurysms, 6 had capillary lesions, and 1 had drusen.[K410] Jabs' group studied 11 patients with retinal occlusive disease in detail; 55% had some visual loss, and most had a history of central nervous system lupus.[J4]

Retinal vasculitis may antedate the diagnosis of SLE,[S702] and visual loss may be the initial presentation of the disease.[S766] Vasculitis of the retinal capillaries, with local microinfarction of the superficial nerve fiber layers of the retina, is usually found.[H111] Severe, occlusive, retinal vascular disease is associated with extensive peripheral nonperfusion of the retina, secondary neovascularization, vitreous hemorrhage, and active CNS lupus.[H159,J5,V86]

Optic neuritis can present as an ischemic neuropathy, retrobulbar neuritis, or both. Over 30 cases have been described in the literature,[J7] with a variable visual outcome. It is usually treated with systemic glucorticoids.

A case of infectious retinitis in a compromised lupus patient indicates the need for careful eye evaluations before pushing high-dose corticosteroids.[C408] Conversely, the case of a psychiatric patient with presumed hysteric blindness who had lupus retinitis emphasizes other important concerns.[S266]

The eye toxicity of antimalarials and steroids is discussed in Chapters 57 and 58. Retinal vasculitis has been observed in both hydralazine- and procainamide-induced lupus.[D248,N85]

In summary, patients with SLE who present with acute visual loss may have retinal or choroidal ischemia (from vasculitis or occlusion), retinal tears, glaucoma, optic or retrobulbar neuritis, or even cortical infarcts of the brain.[R384,V12,W368] In some patients, the manifestations are associated with immune complex deposition in tissue. In others, they are associated with antiphospholipid antibodies; these have been reported in cases of retinal artery occlusion, diplopia, and ischemic neuropathy.[A340,B497,D182,F123,K275,L220,O90,R148,S529] Asherson et al. observed 7 cases of occlusive vascular disease affecting retinal and choroidal vessels among 84 SLE patients with anticardiolipin antibody (9%).[A340] Physicians frequently cannot distinguish these. Because the therapies are different (immunosuppression versus anticoagulation), it is useful to distinguish the two "syndromes," when possible.[B497,D182,K275,L220,O90,R148]

THE EAR: HEARING DEFICITS, AUTOIMMUNE VESTIBULITIS, AND CHONDRITIS

Involvement of the auditory organs in patients with SLE is uncommon, but it does occur. Serous otitis media was found in 2 of 100 consecutive SLE patient admissions in one study.[J5] Autoimmune vestibulitis has been reported;[C16,H76,K400,S344] I found it in 1 of 503 cases. Some have reported that vestibulitis responds to steroid therapy or plasmapheresis.[H76,L411] Otitis or auditory nerve disease can be associated with severe hearing loss. Two studies performed audiometry in SLE patients; in one study, no abnormalities were found in 20 patients.[N32] We prospectively studied 30 hospitalized SLE patients by audiometry and found 5 with moderate to severe sensorineural hearing loss. In 2 patients, the hearing loss was caused by SLE and the remaining 3 had other causes.[B444] Fries and Holman reported that 20% of SLE patients had tinnitus.[F263] Even though it is usually secondary to medication (e.g., salicylates, nonsteroidal anti-inflammatory drugs, antimalarials), dizziness resulting from vestibulitis can be excluded by special testing.[M460]

Kitridou et al. reported that 4 of 400 SLE patients treated at LAC-USC Medical Center had relapsing auricular and nasal polychondritis that was steroid-responsive.[K263] This supports occasional case reports of the concurrence of both diseases.[S496,J80]

THE LARYNX

Laryngeal involvement caused by SLE is rare, but ranges from hoarseness[R294] to airway obstruction.[T186] The cricoarytenoid joint is lined with synovium and can become inflamed, even in the absence of active disease elsewhere.[C458,K379,S505] Glottic stenosis needing surgical repair has occurred.[B576] Laryngeal involvement resulting from SLE caused the death of two patients by asphyxia.[C244,S104] In one, histologic sections revealed extensive edema, inflammation, and fibrinoid degeneration of collagen. Hughes and Asherson[A327] observed two patients with left recurrent laryngeal nerve abnormalities associated with vocal cord paralysis. Both had pulmonary hypertension, which placed direct pressure on the nerve. Right recurrent laryngeal nerve palsy without pulmonary hypertension may be seen.[E144,G303]

Chapter 41

THE ENDOCRINE SYSTEM AND UROGENITAL TRACT

DANIEL J. WALLACE

THE ENDOCRINE SYSTEM

The overwhelming preponderance of SLE in women of child-bearing years has prompted numerous investigations into the disorder's hormonal effects and interactions. Complex interactions occur among neurotransmitters, sex hormones, and immune functions. The potential role of estrogenic hormones in "permitting" SLE to occur, and the role of androgenic hormones in "protecting" against it, are discussed in Chapter 16. The clinical effects of some of these abnormalities on human endocrine pathology in SLE are detailed below. Hormonal therapy in SLE is discussed in Chapter 61.

Menstrual Irregularities and Antiovarian and Antiestrogen Antibodies

Menstrual irregularities are common, and range from menorrhagia to amenorrhea. Menorrhagia was found in 16 of Harvey's 105 patients, and was the initial manifestation of SLE in 3.[M280] Dubois observed menorrhagia in 12% of his 520 cases and associated it with thrombocytopenia or the presence of the circulating lupus anticoagulant.[W28] Salicylate and nonsteroidal anti-inflammatory drugs (NSAIDs) can also increase menstrual flow.

Amenorrhea is associated with SLE disease activity and immunosuppressive (both glucocorticoid and cytotoxic) therapy.[R339] Schaller reported that 24% of females with childhood lupus had amenorrhea, and it was noted in 27 of Fries' 160 women with SLE.[F263,S108] Steroid administration can induce secondary menorrhagia or amenorrhea, the latter of which is seen in the overwhelming majority of patients with spontaneous Cushing's syndrome.[P225] Glucocorticoid therapy suppresses prolactin and FSH and LH release, thus reducing estrogen and progesterone release and regular menstruation.

Steinberg and Steinberg followed 28 menstruating females with SLE through 991 cycles. Increased signs or symptoms of disease activity were observed in 172 (18%); in 140 (81%), these occurred in the 2 weeks prior to menstruation.[S651] Lahita observed that premenstrual flares of lupus symptomatology are noted in 60%, with resolution when menses begins.[L19]

The cause of amenorrhea in SLE patients is complex. In one study, 84% of 16 SLE patients had antiovarian antibodies. With an enzyme-linked immunosorbent assay, (ELISA) which uses a soluble and extractable corpus luteum antigen, none of 30 controls were found to have the antibody.[M531] The relationship of such antibodies to idiopathic autoimmune oophoritis (which is associated with amenorrhea) is uncertain.[C135] Lahita's group observed antiestrogen antibody in 26% of 34 lupus patients, which correlated with elevated plasma levels of 16α-hydroxyestrone and active disease. Of 52 controls, however, 25% also had the antibody, which on further analysis turned out to be those taking oral contraceptive preparations.[B548] Beaumont et al. detected antiethinylestradiol antibodies in 30% of 123 disease-free oral contraceptive users and in 57% of 23 SLE users.[B146] Estrogen receptors are autoantigenic, and one group has hypothesized that lupus is an antireceptor antibody disease.[K157]

Fertility and issues related to pregnancy outcome are discussed in Chapter 50 to 52.

Thyroid Disease

In 1956, Roitt et al.[R274] first demonstrated that antibody to thyroglobulin is present in the serum of patients with Hashimoto's disease. Of their 27 patients, 3 had rheumatoid arthritis, and considerable interest was generated concerning the association of thyroiditis and other autoimmune disorders. White et al. and Hijmans et al. presented the first cases of concomitant thyroiditis and SLE in 1961.[H301,W206] The presentation of additional case reports prompted two large-scale, controlled studies at Johns Hopkins in the 1960s, which demonstrated 2 and 4 cases of SLE out of 100 and 170 patients, respectively, with Hashimoto's disease.[M176,M645] Subsequently, 74 autopsy-proven cases of Hashimoto's disease were matched with a control group—2 thyroiditis patients were found to have SLE, but none of the controls. This slightly increased incidence of concurrence is of greater statistical significance if *all* autoimmune disorders are considered.[F319]

Detailed evaluations of thyroid function in SLE patients have been the focus of eight major studies, and are summarized in Table 41–1.[B612,G217,G304,L201,M49,R294,W122] Salient observations from these reports also suggest the following:

1. Hyperthyroidism usually antedates lupus, and the subsequent development of SLE may occasionally be induced by antithyroid medication.[B612,H427,S35,T23]
2. The incidence of hypothyroidism is greater than that shown in Table 41–1, because SLE patients have a greater incidence of elevated TSH levels but are rarely tested for it.[M419,W122]
3. The incidence of all thyroid disorders is probably

Table 41–1. Thyroid Function and Antibody Studies in SLE (%)

Parameter	Gordon[G304] 1987	Rodriguez[R262] 1989	Lesser[L201] 1988	Westman[W122] 1987	Byron[B612] 1977	Goh[G217] 1986	Miller[M419] 1987	Ropes[R294] 1976
No. of cases	41	93	149	41	64	319	332	142
Low T4	9.8	—	15.3	—	4.7	0.9	6.6	0.7
High T4	2.4	6.5	—	—	10.9	2.8	5	—
Hashimoto's disease	—	—	5.9	—	—	0.6	—	2.1
Thyroid antibodies	—	—	11.8	51	—	—	20	—

greater in SLE patients than in the general population when compared with the British National Health Service's estimate of the incidence of hyperthyroidism as 1.9% and of hypothyroidism as 1.0%.[B612]

4. Symptoms of thyroid disease can be confused with those of lupus.

These findings also apply to children with SLE.[E14] The only consistent additional clinical association in those with SLE and thyroid disease is Sjögren's syndrome. After several case reports noted concurrent SLE, Sjögren's syndrome, and Hashimoto's thyroiditis,[F50,G21] a Scandinavian group evaluated 77 lupus patients. Of these, 8 of 10 who had thyroid disease also had Sjögren's syndrome, compared with 6 of 67 without thyroid disorders (p < .01).[J120] A new antimicrosomal antigen-antibody system known as anti-Mic-1 has been described in patients with SLE and hyperthyroidism. Anti-Mic-1 was not present in patients with Hashimoto's disease or rheumatoid arthritis, but its clinical appearance is still controversial.[K351,S42] In addition to this "head and neck" association, three of the nine published reports of SLE patients with red cell aplasia also noted an association with hypothyroidism.[F198,F219] A case of an SLE patient with anti-TSH antibodies has been reported.[S36]

It is likely that the thyroid (and lacrimal and salivary glands) can be targets of the same autoimmune abnormalities that result in SLE.

Diabetes

Type I diabetes mellitus is an autoimmune disorder caused largely by cytotoxic T cells that destroy pancreatic islet cells. Genetic predisposition has been defined, and anti-islet antibodies occur. One survey found that 92 of 222 (41%) type I diabetics have a positive ANA.[H256] An atypical, mild, nonorgan-threatening SLE has been reported in up to 30% of patients with type I diabetes and insulin receptor antibodies.[B23,D225,H457,K148,T242] Occasionally, patients with insulin receptor antibodies may present with severe hypoglycemia and require steroid therapy.[M528,V45] Of our patients with idiopathic SLE, 357 were treated with corticosteroids for more than 1 month, and steroid-induced diabetes developed in 10.[W18] Some of these patients might be more prone to developing anti-insulin antibodies.[T147]

Adrenal Insufficiency

The most common cause of adrenal insufficiency in SLE patients is abrupt cessation of steroid therapy, but adrenal insufficiency secondary to cortical infarction in patients with the lupus anticoagulant can occur.[A157,C79,C88,G414,W65] Rarely, adrenal failure has also been associated with amyloid and adrenal hemorrhage in lupus patients.[E47,L229,O128,T137] Cortisol levels are not elevated in nonsteroid-treated SLE, but the corticosterone level is increased.[H473,L129] Cortisol is rapidly metabolized in patients with active disease.[K272] One patient with androgenital syndrome secondary to adrenal hyperplasia who developed SLE has been reported.[M518] No cases of autoimmune adrenalitis and SLE have appeared.

Parathyroid Gland

Renal dialysis patients develop secondary hyperparathyroidism, and this has been associated with an increased incidence of Jaccoud's arthropathy in those with SLE.[B6] Two reports of concurrent lupus and hypoparathyroidism have appeared.[H45,H115]

Hyperprolactinemia

A subset with SLE might have hyperprolactinemia; its levels may correlate with clinical activity.[J51]

Fluid and Electrolyte Abnormalities

Antidiuretic Hormone

Scattered reports describing patients who had the syndrome of inappropriate antidiuretic hormone (ADH) and SLE[A64,D111,K57,L210] prompted Ginzler's group to perform an in-depth study of 36 stable SLE patients.[T202] The mean ADH level was elevated at 11.4 ± 1.0 μU/ml (normal, 0.4 to 1.4). High levels were associated with disease duration of more than 2 years, but not with clinical or serologic disease activity. A paradoxic increase in plasma ADH levels was noted in 50% of those who underwent a standard water load challenge. It was concluded that SLE is associated with a state of primary neurohypophyseal hypersecretion of ADH.

Renal Tubular Acidosis

Tu and Shearn[T255] observed latent renal tubular acidosis (RTA) in 12 patients with SLE without clinical renal tubular dysfunction, as well in patients with Sjögren's syndrome. RTA has also been reported in those with other autoimmune disorders.[C121,C124,M598] In RTA, impairment or renal acid secretion occurs out of proportion to reduction of glomerular filtration rate. Clinically, it is manifested by hyperchloremic acidosis and an inability to excrete highly acid urine, and it is often associated with impaired renal concentrating ability. Subclinical cases are detected by an acid loading test designed to detect acid excretion inappropriate to the induced metabolic acidosis. Ropes found RTA in 2 of her 150 SLE patients.[R294]

Hyporeninemic Hypoaldosteronism

Relatively few of our lupus nephritis patients on diuretics require potassium replacement. De Fronzo[D333] first noted this, and determined that a primary defect in renal tubular potassium secretion secondary to an immune complex-mediated interstitial nephritis might be responsible. Four case reports confirmed the existence of a relative hyporeninemic hypoaldosteronism state in SLE patients.[A63,G333,K402,L291] These observations led Quismorio's group to study 142 patients with SLE; almost 10% had unexplained hyperkalemia.[L129] Most of the hyperkalemic group had impaired renin and aldosterone responses to stimulation.

THE UROGENITAL TRACT

Lupus Cystitis

Interstitial cystitis is an uncommon but important manifestation of SLE. First described in SLE patients in 1965,[S368] it is probably an immune complex-mediated disorder associated with bladder vasculitis, a secretory diarrhea with malabsorption, and high titers of ANA.[B448,D131, E13,K460,M587,V77] Patients with idiopathic interstitial cystitis have an increased incidence of antinuclear antibodies.[J99] Isenberg's group performed serologic profiles on 34 patients with idiopathic interstitial cystitis. Antinuclear antibodies were positive in 25 (56.8%), and 7 had SLE.[C256]

Weisman et al.[W158] located immune deposits in the vessel walls of both the small intestine and urinary bladder. His group later examined six patients in detail. Decreased bladder capacities, with thickened and irregular walls, were found. Five had abdominal symptoms. In all patients, symptoms improved with high-dose steroid treatment. Others reported neurogenic bladders associated with interstitial cystitis in patients with SLE.[A178,S759]

Alarcon-Segovia et al.[A94] found bladder abnormalities in 16 of 35 SLE necropsies; interstitial cystitis was found in 11, hemorrhage in 9, congestion in 7, vasculitis in 5, and a perivascular infiltrate in 4. Interestingly, 7 patients had pulmonary hemorrhages. Other causes of bladder pathology in SLE patients include myelopathy, cyclophosphamide administration, and inflammatory polyneuropathies. Intravesical instillation of dimethylsulfoxide (DMSO) is the probable treatment of choice for isolated lupus cystitis.[S571]

Jokinen et al.[J101] performed immunofluorescence tests for tissue-bound immunoglobulin on urinary bladder biopsies from 11 patients with discoid LE and from 14 patients with interstitial cystitis. Of the 11 with discoid LE, 9 had immune deposits at the bladder basement membrane; none with interstitial cystitis had similar changes.

Rarely, vasculitis can induce ureteral obstruction.[B113]

Antisperm Antibodies and Male Sexual Dysfunction

Antisperm antibodies represent a heterogeneous grouping that, when present in women, inhibits conception to varying degrees. In men, these antibodies are present in high levels after a vasectomy.[T271] Marcus and Hess[M125] reported that 14 of 15 serum samples from female SLE patients contained antisperm antibodies with a titer of greater than 1:8. Reichlin and Maas[R117] found these antibodies in 10 of 24 SLE patients. The incidence of the antisperm antibodies in males and females was the same. The presence of the antibody correlated with anti-DNA and increased disease activity.

Sexual dysfunction (decreased libido, erectile incompetence, or failure to ejaculate) has been reported in 19 to 35% of a total of 64 males with SLE in two uncontrolled preliminary studies.[F140,I21,M428] One case report of testicular vasculitis in SLE has appeared.[K110]

HYPOTHERMIA

Four cases of severe hypothermia (temperature < 95° F or 35° C) have been described in SLE patients. All occurred within 48 hours of corticosteroid therapy institution.[C451,J96,K94,K444]

SUMMARY

1. Most female hormones increase and male hormones decrease immune reactivity. This may be partly responsible for the female predominance in SLE.
2. Women with SLE have a low plasma androgen levels and an increased 16α-hydroxyestrone level. Males with lupus have increased estrogen and prolactin levels.
3. Menstrual irregularity is common in women with SLE; amenorrhea is associated with disease activity, steroid administration, and chemotherapy.
4. The incidence of all major thyroid disorders (hyperthyroidism, hypothyroidism, autoimmune thyroiditis) is increased in SLE.
5. Patients taking steroids have an increased risk of developing diabetes. Type I autoimmune diabetes has an increased association with antinuclear antibody, and may display some lupus-like features.
6. Adrenal insufficiency in SLE is usually secondary to abrupt cessation of steroid therapy or infarction in patients with the antiphospholipid syndrome.
7. A small but significant number of lupus patients have renal tubular acidosis, hyporeninemic hypoaldosteronism with resulting hyperkalemia, or clinically relevant complications of antidiuretic hormone hypersecretion.
8. Lupus cystitis is noted infrequently; it is a classic immune complex-mediated vasculitis, and is associated with diarrhea.
9. Antisperm antibodies are found in most women with SLE.

Chapter 42

GASTROINTESTINAL MANIFESTATIONS AND RELATED LIVER AND BILIARY DISORDERS

DANIEL J. WALLACE

GASTROINTESTINAL COMPLICATIONS

Although gastrointestinal (GI) manifestations are common in SLE patients (Table 42–1), their incidence varies with the interest and methods of the observer studying the illness. For example, two major studies failed to mention GI complications,[G385,L140] and another made only a brief reference to it.[E14] GI symptoms can be part of the basic disease, or represent intercurrent process. Nearly all medications used to treat lupus have gastrointestinal side effects.

Osler[O107] was impressed with the frequency of gastrointestinal manifestations, or "gastrointestinal crises," as he called them. He believed that they might mimic any type of abdominal condition. In 1939, Reiferstein et al.[R130] found evidence of peritonitis in 13 of 18 autopsied SLE cases, with perihepatitis and enlargement of the liver in one-third. The most feared GI complication of SLE is lupus enteritis caused by vascular involvement of the bowel wall, with infarction or hemorrhage. The first modern description of this was by Klemperer,[K284] in 1942.

GI complaints were the initial presentation in 10% of Dubois' patients;[D340] 25 to 40% had protracted symptoms. Haserick's group divided the GI symptoms of SLE into 3 groupings among 87 patients: none (63%), minor (29%), and major (8%).[B517] I have found this breakdown to be clinically useful. Subclinical involvement of the GI tract is common. For example, Landing's group at Children's Hospital of Los Angeles found chronic mucosal infiltration in 96% of 26 autopsied children with SLE.[N4]

Pharyngitis, Dysphagia, and Esophagitis

Persistent sore throat is not an infreuent finding, especially in children.[K232] Mucous membrane lesions and other features of oral pathology are discussed in Chapters 37 and 40.

Dysphagia occurs in 1 to 6%[D340,F256,M280,R294,W18,Z33] and heartburn in 11 to 50% of patients.[C151,F256] In a literature review Zizic[Z33] related that, although only 5% of SLE patients complained of dysphagia, 25% had impaired esophageal peristalsis, compared with 67% of scleroderma patients. Several studies using esophageal manometry noted aperistalsis or hypoperistalsis of the esophagus in approximately 10% of patients with SLE.[C279,S681,T74,T278] Aperistalsis sometimes correlated with the presence of Raynaud's phenomenon. Gutierrez

et al.[G434] compared esophageal motility in 14 SLE and 17 mixed connective tissue disease (MCTD) patients. A definite correlation was found between Raynaud's phenomenon and hypoperistalsis, with the latter being more common in MCTD. The SLE group had only a slightly decreased lower esophageal sphincter pressure. Esophageal motor dysfunction in SLE can also produce diffuse spasm and result in symptoms of chest pain.[P111]

The aperistaltic group can show atony and dilatation of the esophagus on upper GI radiography.[K139]

Ramierz-Mata et al.[R26] performed esophageal manometric studies in a group of unselected SLE patients and noted abnormalities in 16. Absent or abnormally low contractions were found at the upper third in 7, at the lower two-thirds in 3, in the entire esophagus in 2, at the lower esophageal sphincter in 2, and at the lower two-thirds plus the lower sphincter in the other 2. They found no relationship among the presence of esophageal dysfunction and activity, duration, or therapy of SLE. Interestingly, 5 of the 34 patients who had normal studies complained of dysphagia and heartburn. Upper esophageal skeletal muscle fiber atrophy was found in 2 of 26 autopsies on children with SLE[N4] One report confirmed these findings, and suggested that hypoperistalsis or aperistalsis may be caused by an inflammatory reaction in the esophageal muscles or by ischemic or vasculitic damage to Auerbach's plexus.[C151]

The treatment of esophageal symptoms is the same as that of "Raynaud's esophagus." Small, frequent meals, avoidance of postprandial recumbency, and the administration of antacids, omeprazole, H2 antagonists, or parasympathomimetic agents play a therapeutic role.

Anorexia, Nausea, Vomiting, and Diarrhea

The most common cause of anorexia, nausea, vomiting, and diarrhea in SLE is related to the use of salicylates, nonsteroidal anti-inflammatory drugs (NSAIDs), antimalarial drugs, corticosteroids, and cytotoxic agents. These symptoms can even occur for weeks after therapy is stopped. When caused by the disease, the manifestations are persistent, and are not explained by other factors.

Anorexia occurs in 49 to 82% of patients,[D306,D340,F256] especially if untreated. Nausea has been reported in 11 to 38%.[D306,D340,F126,F256,H179,M280] When medications are excluded as a cause, however, the incidence is about 8%.[W18] Vomiting can be prominent;[B517,D306,D340,]

Table 42–1. SLE and the Gastrointestinal Tract

1. GI symptoms are common in SLE. Secondary causes such as concurrent disease, stress, and medication must be ruled out.
2. Sore throat is common.
3. Dysphagia is present in 2 to 6% of patients, especially in association with Raynaud's phenomenon
4. Anorexia, nausea, vomiting, or diarrhea may be prominent in one-third of patients when the disease is active. Inflammatory bowel disease, infection, and concomitant drug administration must be ruled out as causes.
5. The incidence of peptic ulcer disease is not known; it is usually caused by anti-inflammatory medication.
6. Ascites is found in 8 to 11% of patients. If a result of nephrosis, cirrhosis, or congestive heart failure, it is a painless transudate. Exudative causes might be painful, and include serosal inflammation. Patients with lupus peritonitis are often steroid-responsive.
7. Pancreatitis is a serious complication of SLE. It is associated with pancreatic vasculitis, activity of SLE in other systems and, rarely, with subcutaneous fat necrosis. Mild elevation of pancreatic enzyme levels may occur in SLE without pancreatitis; high levels suggest pancreatitis. Steroids are the treatment of choice, but they (along with thiazide diuretics and azathioprine) can induce pancreatitis.
8. Abdominal pain and tenderness warrant a search for ischemia or bowel ulceration.
9. Malabsorption syndromes are rare, but do occur.
10. Mesenteric or intestinal vasculitis is a life-threatening complication of SLE, usually associated with multisystem activity. High doses of steroids are required, and surgical intervention is indicated if extensive bowel infarction (with hemorrhage) and/or large intestinal perforations occur. Patients succumb from complications of obstruction, perforation, or infarction.

[F126,F256,F256,H179,M280] we observed it as a symptom in 7% of patients.[W18] Diarrhea occurs in 4 to 21% of patients.[D306,D340,F126,F256,H179,M280] Children have an increased incidence of all these symptoms.[G197]

Abdominal Pain, Acute Abdomens, and the Surgeon*

Abdominal pain is found in 8 to 37% of SLE patients,[D306,D340,F256,K232,M280,W18] with the lowest incidence in series that exclude medication-related symptoms. In 412 consecutive admissions to Cleveland hospitals for collagen vascular diseases,[F126] 63 patients had abdominal complaints; of these, 48 had SLE. Pain was present in 85%, and fever was noted on examination in 76% of patients and peritoneal signs in 10%; corticosteroids were being given to 64%. An acute cause was determined in 33 patients, including duodenal or gastric ulcer, gastritis, and pancreatitis. Mesenteric vasculitis was present in 3 patients; in 16 the pain was of undetermined cause. Surgery was performed on 21 patients; in 11 patients it was exploratory.

Abdominal pain and tenderness in patients with SLE can be the first manifestations of an intra-abdominal disaster. Many episodes, however, are trivial and self-limited. The problem of differentiating between these two scenarios can be excruciatingly difficult. Patients are often on steroids and immunocompromised, masking physical find-

* This section on abdominal pain was contributed by Edward H. Phillips, Jr., M.D., General Surgeon, Cedars-Sinai Medical Center, Los Angeles, CA

ings of bowel perforations and ischemia. Patients with the lupus anticoagulant are especially susceptible to bowel infarction. Also, the disease process itself can cause serositis or pancreatitis without bowel ischemia or perforation. Both these conditions can mimic an acute abdomen. Certainly, celiotomy is associated with significant morbidity in these patients, and it has been found that 20% of exploratory laparotomies reveal serositis with ischemia or perforation.

Patients presenting with abdominal pain, even without tenderness, need an aggressive and comprehensive evaluation, including a complete blood count, amylase level determination, blood chemistry profiles, and abdominal roentgenography. If free air is seen, emergency surgery is indicated. If pseudo-obstruction and/or thumbprinting of the bowel is seen without free peritoneal fluid, observation is in order. If a moderate amount of free fluid, acidosis, or hyperamylasemia without pancreatitis is present, diagnostic laparoscopy should be performed. Specialized tests, such as an upper GI, barium enema, CT, MRI, gallium and indium white cell scanning, and visceral angiography, may be helpful in specific cases.

Patients suspected of having an intra-abdominal crisis should be placed on nothing by mouth and supported with intravenous fluids while undergoing these initial diagnostic evaluations. If peritonitis is suspected, broad-spectrum antibiotics should be administered. Urine output is watched closely and, if third spacing is evident, a urinary catheter should be placed. If hypotension occurs and is unresponsive to a fluid challenge, a central venous catheter or pulmonary artery catheter is required. Aggressive fluid replacement, antibiotics, and steroid stress dose coverage precedes laparascopic or "open" surgical exploration. A low threshold of suspicion should be present for recommending diagnostic laparoscopy for these patients. It is less invasive and is followed by fewer complications than open laparotomy. Also, an increasing number of therapeutic procedures can be performed laparascopically (e.g., perforated ulcers in the bowel can now be sutured laparoscopically). The best application of diagnostic laparoscopy is in the evaluation of the patient with equivocal findings. It can avoid an unnecessary laparotomy and offer an aggressive diagnostic approach in the evaluation of bowel ischemia and perforated bowel in patients who might otherwise go undiagnosed because of their steroid suppression.

Peptic Ulcer Disease

The incidence of peptic ulcers in SLE has been reported as 4 to 21%,[D326,D327,N4,R294] but these studies antedated the endoscopy and gastroprotective therapy era. Perforated ulcers have been reported.[B517,D326,D327,N4] Therapy with acetylated salicylates and NSAIDs is probably a more frequent cause of peptic ulcer disease than is active SLE. Siurala et al.[S484] performed gastric biopsies on 17 SLE patients; 4 had superficial gastritis and 8 had atrophic gastritis in this 1965 report. Twenty-five years and ten gastroprotective agents later, this area is overdue for a re-examination.

Inflammatory Bowel Disease

Ulcerative Colitis

Persistent diarrhea may result from ulcerative colitis associated with SLE. Dubois noted concurrent disease in 2 of his 520 patients,[D340] and Wallace in 2 of his 464 patients with idiopathic SLE.[W18] Kurlander and Kirsner[K474] elegantly documented the clinicopathologic correlations, and remarked that lupus colitis and ulcerative colitis can be indistinguishable. Lupus colitis can be focalized to a single, small area.[P22] In 1965, Alarcon-Segovia reviewed the literature extensively and collected 19 cases of concomitant SLE and ulcerative colitis. He presented 8 additional patients in detail from his Mayo Clinic experience, which accounted for 4% of their SLE cases.[A109] Also, 100 ulcerative colitis patients were evaluated for SLE, which was found in 3 patients. In most, colitis preceded the onset of lupus. In this and other reports, lupus symptoms and signs frequently began after the administration of sulfasalazine for the treatment of inflammatory bowel disease.[A97,F149]

Regional Ileitis

Concurrence of SLE and regional ileitis (Crohn's disease) is surprisingly rare, and has been reported in only 8 patients (Fig. 42–1).[D302,G256,J90,K319,N8,S301,S756] Evidence that inflammatory bowel disease may respond to methotrexate therapy and to antimalarial drugs is intriguing, and emphasizes the importance of initiating studies to delineate the relationship between inflammatory bowel disease and SLE.

One case of Canada-Cronkhite syndrome associated with SLE has appeared.[K441]

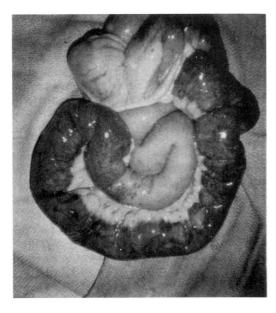

Fig. 42–1. Lupus vasculitis involving distal 2 feet of ileum. The bowel was grossly injected and friable, with edema of the wall and the mesentery. Multiple palpable lymph nodes in the mesentery supplied the involved area.

Protein-Losing Enteropathy and Malabsorption

The presence of severe diarrhea and marked hypoalbuminemia (reported as low as 0.8 g/dl) without proteinuria should raise the suspicion of a protein-losing enteropathy. About 17 reports of clinically evident protein-losing enteropathy have been published, along with several literature reviews.[A97,A379,B453,P113,S484] Siurala[S484] studied the small intestine in SLE patients with diarrhea. Among small intestinal biopsies in 19 cases, 12 were normal and villous atrophy was noted in 2. Roentgenographic signs and signs of intestinal malabsorption were found in 7 patients. Subclinical cases can occur. In patients with protein-losing enteropathy, roentgenography demonstrates spiculation, fragmentation, and clumping of barium. Pathologically, villous atrophy, inflammatory infiltrates, and submucosal edema without vasculitis are evident.[B135,C149,K326,K474] The villi can be lustrous and swollen, and may be of various sizes.[K326] Increased fecal excretion of intravenous radiolabelled albumin is the best quantitative study for following disease activity, although a one report has suggested that α_1-antitrypsin clearance can also monitor response to therapy.[B209]

The cause of protein-losing enteropathy is unknown, but several theories have cited vascular damage, bacterial overgrowth, fat malabsorption, abnormalities in bile salt metabolism, thrombosis, and mesenteric venulitis as possibilities.[B135,K326]

Most patients have abdominal pain, and this can be the initial manifestation of their SLE.[C149] Cases have been reported of protein-losing enteropathy in association with Sjögren's[P98] syndrome and red blood cell aplasia.[H240] It may occur more often in children than in adults.[H276,S108] Laboratory investigation may reveal normal lymphocyte counts, elevated serum cholesterol levels, low serum complement levels, anti-RNP antibody,[E32] and sterile paracentesis fluid with low white counts.[M678] Lymphangiectasia is uncommon.

Response to corticosteroids is nearly universal, but some patients may also require a gluten-free diet.[B453,R436]

Ascites

Ascites can be the initial presentation of SLE. It occurs in 8 to 11% of patients, often as a manifestation of the nephrotic syndrome.[A218,A364,D340,E147,H179,R294] In an excellent review of ascites in SLE, Schousboe et al. classified it as acute or chronic.[S168] Acute causes include lupus peritonitis, infarction, perforated viscus, pancreatitis, and hemorrhagic and bacterial peritonitis. Chronic causes of ascites include lupus peritonitis, congestive heart failure, pericarditis, nephrotic syndrome, Budd-Chiari syndrome, protein-losing enteropathy, underlying malignancy, cirrhosis, and tuberculosis. Ascitic fluid can be inflammatory or noninflammatory. Noninflammatory lesions are always painless and associated with transudative fluid; most patients have nephrotic syndrome. Peritonitis is usually inflammatory and exudative. It is generally painful, but not always.[A364,M395,W230] Peritoneal tissue can contain immune complex deposits and inflammatory infiltrates.[B316,J46] ANA, anti-DNA, and low complement levels, can be present in peritoneal fluid.[B316,J117,S157] Reports have also appeared of concurrent familial Mediterranean fever,[B38] and of oligoclonal protein bands[M420] inducing ascites in SLE patients. Fetal ascites in babies with Ro/SSA-positive mothers may result from congestive heart failure or from various immune mechanisms.[R193]

Ascites caused by lupus peritonitis is usually steroid-responsive. Other causes may require additional interventions.[S168] Gentle diuresis is an important adjunctive measure that often provides symptomatic relief, provided that renal function is not impaired by this approach.

Pancreatitis

Pancreatitis can be a manifestation of SLE. First reported by Dubois in 1953,[D306] it presents with severe epigastric pain radiating to the back, nausea, vomiting, an elevated serum amylase level, and dehydration. Neither Fries and Holman[F256] nor Ropes[R294] noted pancreatitis in any of their combined experience with 350 patients. Ropes attributed this to the sparing use of steroids. Rothfield,[R339] however, observed pancreatitis in 8% of 365 patients. Of 168 consecutive SLE admissions to the University of Alabama Medical Center, 7 (4%) had pancreatitis; 5 of the 7 succumbed.[D230]

Pancreatitis can be the initial presentation of SLE, and can appear in childhood.[G164,M345,R425] Several cases of panniculitis and subcutaneous fat necrosis have been reported with SLE and pancreatitis,[S457] as has type I hyperlipidemia[G202] with increased levels of chylomicrons.

Corticosteroids, azathioprine, and thiazide diuretics are used in the treatment of SLE, and may induce attacks of pancreatitis independent of the disease.[H83,O89,P21,P73] Cases of pancreatic vasculitis were documented in the presteroid era.[R130] In 25 lupus necropsies, 8 cases of pancreatitis were found; 4 had pancreatitic vasculitis and 4 were thought to have steroid-induced disease.[B100] Pancreatitis can also be caused by hypovolemia, ischemia, cholecystitis, alcoholism, carcinoma, and viral infections, all of which can occur in SLE.

Mild elevations of serum amylase levels may be noted in patients with SLE in the absence of pancreatitis. Hasselbacher et al.[H204] studied 25 SLE patients without pancreatitis and 15 non-SLE controls. Amylase levels were elevated in 5 patients, and 6 had macroamylasemia, compared to none of the controls. The mean amylase level in the SLE group was 161.7 mg/dl versus 116.4 mg/dl in the control group, which was statistically significant. Macroamylasemia results from decreased renal clearance of an immunoglobulin-amylase complex. The presence of a pathogenic autoantibody to amylase was proposed. Tsianos et al.[T235] found elevated pancreatic and salivary amylase components in 11 of 36 unselected SLE patients. These reports associated active SLE with elevated amylase levels without abdominal pain.

Reynolds et al.,[R182] in their definitive study on lupus pancreatitis, combined a literature survey with a review of 20 patients (75% were female). The mean age of their group was 34 years, and the mean disease duration was 3.75 years. The mean prednisone dose was 11 mg, and 5 patients were also taking azathioprine. Of the 20 patients, 8 had recurrent attacks of pancreatitis, and amylase levels

did not correlate with renal function or steroid doses. The mean duration of each episode was 15.5 days. The chief clue to the cause (lupus versus drug-induced) was that most of the patients with SLE-induced pancreatitis had multisystem SLE involvement (an average of 6.2 organ systems were involved), and responded well to increased steroid administration.

Two literature reviews subsequently appeared.[E2,W107] One reported on 66 patients, 26 of whom were not taking steroids.[E2] Nearly 75% had a fatal outcome.

Treatment includes immediate discontinuation of nonessential drugs that can induce pancreatitis (e.g., azathioprine, diuretics), intravenous hydration, nothing by mouth, antibiotics if needed, and sparing use of analgesics. The decision on whether to use corticosteroids is difficult if the patient has evidence of active SLE and is on high-dose glucorticoid therapy. Careful observation is essential. Pancreatitis may induce diabetes. (See page 408.)

Mesenteric and Intestinal Vasculitis, Melena, and Bowel Hemorrhage

Mesenteric vasculitis with or without infarction is one of the most serious complications of SLE. Even though Ropes[R294] found peritoneal involvement (from serositis) at autopsy in 63% of patients, with adhesion being common, only a small percentage had mesenteric vasculitis or acute abdomen. Conversely, Landing's group noted ischemic bowel in 60% of 26 necropsies on children.[N4] Melena was observed in 1 to 6% of SLE patients.[D340,F256,M280,W181]

Most mesenteric vasculitis presents with cramping or with constant abdominal pain, vomiting, and fever. Diffuse direct and rebound tenderness are usually present.

Zizic and colleagues have published four detailed and authoritative studies of lupus enteritis and other abdominal complications.[C215,Z33,Z36,Z38] Their 1975 report[Z38] detailed five patients with large bowel perforation. All had active SLE and mesenteric or intestinal vasculitis. The presentation was insidious, with lower abdominal pain. Abdominal rigidity was present in only one patient. Most had nausea, vomiting, diarrhea, and bloody stools. All had tenderness, and most had rebound tenderness and distention. Bowel sounds were diminished or absent. Prior or concurrent administration of steroids masked symptoms in some, and may have promoted the bowel wall thinning that led to perforation.

A 1982 review[C215] recounted 15 cases of acute surgical abdomen in 140 SLE patients. An increased incidence of peripheral vasculitis, central nervous system disease activity, ischemic necrosis of bone, thrombocytopenia, and rheumatoid factor was present. Of the 15 patients, 11 underwent exploratory laporatomies, and 9 were found to have vasculitis and 2 polyserositis. Of the 15, 8 died, primarily from complications of infarction or perforation.

Shapeero et al.[S310] reviewed hospital records on 141 SLE patients admitted to the University of Pennsylvania over a 20-year period. Of these, 68 had abdominal symptoms, and 20 were thought to have ischemic abdominal disease. In 9 patients this was confirmed radiographically by pseudo-obstruction of the gastric outlet, duodenal stasis, effacement of mucosal folds, spasticity, and thumb-printing. Of the 20 patients, most had anorexia, nausea, vomiting, postprandial fullness, and abdominal pain. Only 10% had melena, 35% had fevers, and 50% had guarding; also, 20% had leukocytosis and 65% were anemic. All responded to steroid therapy.

Lupus enteritis can produce gastritis, mucosal ulceration, bowel edema with ileus, hemorrhagic ileitis, intus-susception, perforation, and/or infarction.[B516,B517,B529, F98,H361,M280] Spontaneous hemoperitoneum can be secondary to thrombocytopenia[S556] or to ruptured aneurysms.[K380,Y11] Colonic diverticula[K380] and mesenteric vasculitis[H332,M527] may induce perforation. Intestinal infarction has been associated with the lupus anticoagulant.[A341,S88]

Laboratory evaluations are not particularly helpful. Acute phase reactants and general indicators of active SLE are usually present. Paracentesis may be useful in ruling out pancreatitis or infection.

Roentgenographic changes include pseudo-obstruction of the gastric outlet, duodenal stasis, effacement of the mucosal folds and thumbprinting. Thumbprinting represents bowel submucosal edema or hemorrhage on a barium or Gastrografin enema; this finding is relatively specific for ischemic bowel disease. Similar findings can be found by CT scanning with contrast. CT scans of the abdomen have identified intra-abdominal abscesses, lymphadenopathy, serositis, bowel wall thickening, edematous and distended loops of bowel, pancreatic pseudocysts, and enlarged liver and spleens in SLE patients.[B430,H244] Gallium scans and indium-111 white cell scans can light up areas of inflammation and sepsis.[S586]

The histologic characteristics and distribution of mesenteric vasculitis are similar to those seen in polyarteritis nodosa.[S236,Z36] The colon and small bowel are often involved with vasculitis in the submucosa. This results in ulcerated mucosa, submucosal edema, necrosis, and infarction.[H253] Two cases of appendiceal arteriolitis[D165] have been documented. Pneumatosis cystoides intestinalis may coexist with necrotizing vasculitis.[D117,G235,K277, L29,P320] Although usually benign, it can occasionally cause perforation.

The treatment of choice for lupus enteritis is 1 to 2 mg/kg/day of parenteral prednisolone[B517,E55,H361,K253,M619, T204] or its equivalent, in addition to complete bowel rest. If a rapid response is not noted, surgical intervention may become necessary in cases of perforation or large areas of ischemia.[H361,K253,S310] Mesenteric vasculitis has a high mortality rate. One survey of SLE patients undergoing surgery documented the widely held belief that steroid therapy in and of itself increases the risk of postoperative complications.[P35] A summary of SLE and the gastrointestinal tract is presented in Table 42–1.

LIVER ABNORMALITIES

Hepatomegaly

Enlargement of the liver was present in 10 to 32% of patients in the series listed in Table 33–1, with decreasing frequency over the last three decades. An enlarged liver was present in 28 of 108 children with SLE studied by King et al.[K232] Ropes reported a palpable liver in half of her patients.[R294] The liver usually extends 2 to 3 cm

below the costal margin, but can occasionally reach the iliac crest. Tenderness is uncommon unless viral hepatitis or peritonitis is present. Hepatomegaly and tenderness may be present with normal liver function tests. An enlarged liver can be histologically normal.[K285,L75]

Jaundice

Jaundice was present in 1 to 4% of patients in Table 33–1, and in 9 of Rothfield's 375 patients (3%).[R339] The most common causes of jaundice in SLE are hemolytic anemia and viral hepatitis; Cirrhosis and obstructive jaundice from a biliary or pancreatic mass are responsible for the remainder.

Vascular Lesions: Hepatic Vasculitis, Portal Hypertension and the Budd-Chiari Syndrome

Dubois described the first case of hepatic arteritis in 1953.[D306] It was found in 1 of 58 necropsies reported by Ropes[R294] (Fig. 42–2). This rare complication of SLE can be associated with ruptured hepatic aneurysms.[M237,T205]

The Budd-Chiari syndrome is occlusion of the hepatic veins with secondary cirrhosis and ascites. It is almost always caused by thromboses in patients with the lupus anticoagulant.[D227,H477,K281,N23,O93,P250,R366,V38] This usually leads to portal hypertension, which is rarely seen by itself.[D295,K108] In one study, this disease was associated with antibody to proliferating cell nuclear antigen.[D295]

Liver Function Test Abnormalities: Clinicopathologic Correlates

Only a few considered testing in SLE. It was concluded that nonspecific enzyme elevations are seen in a minority of patients and are usually of little significance. In our experience, most liver function test abnormalities in SLE are a result of the administration of NSAIDs or methotrexate, or are elevated because of increased muscle enzyme levels. Pathologic changes are also nonspecific and mild.

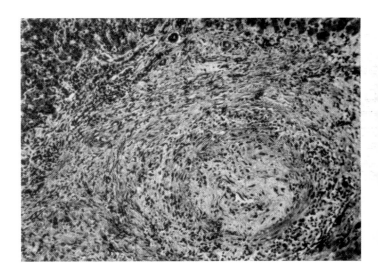

Fig. 42–2. Arteritis in the liver of a 9-year-old girl with classic SLE. The lumen is almost completely obliterated, (H & E stain; ×80).

Rothfield et al.[R339] found elevated liver enzyme levels at diagnosis in 30% of SLE patients. Gibson and Myers[G125] reviewed liver disease in 81 SLE patients; of these, 45 (55%) had abnormal liver function tests at some point, and 27% had enlarged livers. These abnormalities were accounted for by nonhepatic sources in 9 patients, drug-induced in 14, and congestive heart failure in 3. Of 19 biopsies reviewed, 7 were normal, 5 had portal inflammatory infiltrates, 1 had a fatty liver, and 1 had chronic active hepatitis. Only 3 of 81 patients ever had transaminase levels exceeding 100 mg/dl. In one survey, elevations in liver function tests were associated with disease activity and liver membrane autoantibodies.[K481]

Altomonte et al.[A167] compared 18 SLE females without known liver disease with 20 healthy controls. Significant differences included the following: delayed Bromsulphalein (BSP) excretion (27%), elevated fasting serum bile acid levels (50%), and increased γ-glutamyl transpeptidase (GGT) levels (38%). Miller et al.[M431] followed 260 SLE patients and 100 controls for 12 months. Of the 60 SLE patients with abnormal liver function testing, 41 could be traced to an identifiable cause (aspirin, 27; alcohol, 6; others, 7). In 12 of 15 patients with elevated transaminase levels, subclinical liver disease was a probable cause.

Runyon et al.[R422] noted that 124 of 206 SLE patients tested had abnormal liver enzyme values; liver disease was identified in 43. Biopsies were performed on 33—3 died in hepatic failure. The ultimate diagnosis was steatosis in 12 patients, cirrhosis in 4, chronic active hepatitis in 3, chronic granulomatous hepatitis in 3, centrilobular necrosis in 3, chronic persistent hepatitis in 2, and microabscesses in 2. None were hepatitis B antigen-positive. The pathology was thought to be drug-induced in 21% of patients. Corticosteroids were beneficial in 8 of the 12 patients who received them.

Ropes[R294] reported on 58 necropsies in SLE. Of these, 50% had an enlarged liver, moderate to marked fatty infiltration was observed in 44%, and portal congestion was noted in 47%. Hematoxylin bodies were seen in three, arteritis in one, and hemosiderosis in one. Several reports have commented on the presence of nodular regeneration and hyperplasia in SLE.[H472,K281] The patients had normal liver function test results, and this underdiagnosed finding could be secondary to steroid or danazol administration. Concentric membranous bodies in hepatocytes are found in hepatomas, but are occasionally seen in lupus, and reflect increased protein synthesis during regeneration.[S323] Neonatal lupus can present with hepatic fibrosis. This surprising finding was reported in a series of four cases, along with giant cell transformation, ductal obstruction, extramedullary hematopoiesis, and cholestasis.[L108]

In summary, most patients with SLE and elevated liver function tests have liver biopsies that reveal nodules, mild fatty changes, or mild fibrosis. Rarely, features of chronic active hepatitis are found.

Lupoid Hepatitis

In 1955, Joske and King[J134] first called attention to the coexistence of LE cells in patients who had apparent viral hepatitis. Mackay et al.[M15] continued their studies and, in 1956, coined the term "lupoid hepatitis," believing it to be a manifestation of SLE. In spite of steroid treatment, these patients all succumbed from liver failure an average of 3 years after presentation.[M17,M19] Many early studies were conducted before the availability of ANA, smooth muscle antibody, antimitochondrial antibody, or hepatitis virus serologic tests. These reports are of historic interest, and have been reviewed on pages 91 to 93 of the second revised edition of this text.[D323]

Definition and Clinical Features

Lupoid hepatitis is defined serologically and histologically, and is a subset of chronic active hepatitis. Histologic hepatic changes include periportal piecemeal necrosis, dense lymphoid infiltrates, and prominence of plasma cells (Fig. 42–3). Serologically, patients have a positive

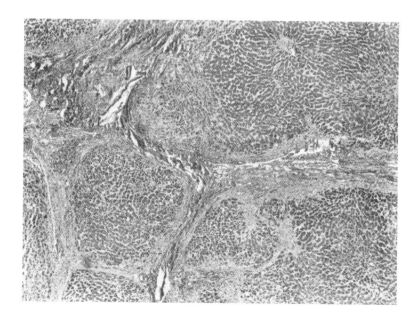

Fig. 42–3. Nodular cirrhosis of the postnecrotic type, which occurs in advanced "lupoid hepatitis." This autopsy specimen is from a patient who died in hepatic coma, (H & E stain; ×30).

Chapter 43

HEMIC AND LYMPHATIC ABNORMALITIES IN SLE

FRANCISCO P. QUISMORIO, JR.

LYMPHADENOPATHY

Lymphadenopathy, a common clinical manifestation of SLE, can be generalized or regional in distribution, especially in the cervical and axillary regions. Hilar adenopathy is rarely seen in SLE.[T73] In his series of 520 patients, Dubois observed adenopathy in 59%,[D340] with axillary adenopathy in 42% and cervical adenopathy in 24%. Cervical adenopathy was an initial manifestation in 2% and generalized adenopathy in 1% of patients. The nodes were usually nontender and discrete, and varied in size from shotty to 3 to 4 cm in diameter. The glandular enlargement was so pronounced in some patients that malignant lymphoma was suspected. Adenopathy was more common in children than in adults, and most marked among black patients. Meislin and Rothfield[M341] reported similar findings, reporting lymphadenopathy or hepatosplenomegaly in 69% of children, compared to 35% in adults with SLE. Among 698 adult SLE patients collected from six large series in the literature, the frequency of regional and generalized lymphadenopathy ranged from 30 to 78%, with a mean prevalence of 50% (see Table 33–1).[A289,E147,G386,L140,M280,R294]

HISTOPATHOLOGY OF THE LYMPH NODE

The characteristic finding in the lymph nodes in SLE patients is a diffuse, reactive hyperplasia.[C133,F184,K282] Varying degrees of coagulative necrosis and lymphoid follicular hyperplasia are seen. Hyperplastic germinal centers with plasmacytosis and varying number of immunoblasts in the interfollicular areas are found. In the necrotic areas and within the sinuses are occasional extracellular amorphous bodies, 5 to 12 μ in diameter, which stain intensely with hematoxylin. These "hematoxylin bodies" contain aggregates of DNA, immunoglobulins, and polysaccharides[C133] and, when present, are considered characteristic of lupus lymphadenitis.[S156] Cells resembling Reed-Sternberg cells have been described in SLE patients.[E95]

Medeiros et al.[M323] examined the immunohistologic features of the lymph node in SLE and found both follicular and paracortical hyperplasia, with paracortical foci of necrosis. Two predominant cell populations within and surrounding the necrotic areas were identified: CD11b+CD15+ histiocytes and CD8+CD3+ cytotoxic-suppressor lymphocytes. The interfollicular regions in the non-necrotic areas were populated by T cells and the lymphoid follicles were composed of polytypic B cells. CD4+/CD3+ helper-inducer T lymphocytes out-number CD8+/CD3+ cytotoxic-suppressor cells by a 3:1 ratio. The immunohistologic characteristics are similar to those of the necrotizing lymphadenitis of Kikuchi and Fujimoto, a self-limited illness of unknown cause in young women characterized by cervical adenopathy, fever, weight loss, and a prodrome of upper respiratory tract infection. Other than a mild leukopenia in 50% of patients, laboratory investigations are generally unremarkable. The disease may be confused clinically with SLE and histologically with malignant lymphoma.[D268] Coexistent Kikuchi's disease and SLE has been described.[T269]

Lymphography of the lower extremities was performed in eight adults with SLE.[W228] Enlarged paraortic lymph nodes were seen in all patients, with a fine or coarse, evenly distributed granulated appearance resembling that observed in the early stage of malignant lymphoma. Following prednisone therapy and clinical improvement, the lymphographic changes decreased. Similar lymphographic findings have been described in rheumatoid arthritis (RA), ankylosing spondylitis, and sarcoidosis, although the granulation in these disorders tends to be coarser and more heterogeneous.

Spleen and Splenic Function

Splenomegaly is not an uncommon finding in SLE patients. In large series, the frequency of splenic enlargement ranges from 9% to as high as 46%.[D340,E147,H179,J75,L75,M280,R349] Dubois found splenic enlargement in 9% of 520 patients.[D340] Splenomegaly, when present, is often associated with hepatomegaly. In some patients, the spleen is so large that it can extend to the iliac crest.[A89]

The characteristic histopathologic picture of the spleen in SLE is periarterial fibrosis or "onionskin lesion." First described in 1924 by Libman and Sacks,[L269] the lesion is defined as the presence of at least 3 to as many as 20 separated layers of the normally densely packed periarterial collagen of the penicillary or follicular arteries, producing the appearance of concentric rings. Larson[L75] found the lesion in 40 of 51 SLE spleens (78%) examined at autopsy. Calcified fibrous nodules continuous to the onionskin lesions have been described.[K257]

Although considered highly characteristic of SLE, periarterial fibrosis may be seen in a few other diseases. Kaiser[K17] examined the specificity of the splenic lesion in 18 SLE patients and 1,679 control cases at autopsy. Of these, 15 SLE patients (83%) and 53 of the control subjects (3.2%) with various diagnoses were positive. In addition to SLE, the only group of patients in whom the lesion was found to be significantly more prevalent than the rest of the controls was comprised of those with essential thrombocytopenic purpura (ITP), with a frequency of 4 in 13 (31%).

Isolated infarction of the spleen associated with circulating lupus anticoagulant and thrombosis may occur.[O2] Spontaneous rupture of the splenic artery in the absence of vasculitis has been reported.[R327]

Functional asplenia is a condition characterized by the failure of splenic uptake of radiolabelled sulfur colloid and the presence of Howell-Jolly bodies, Pappenheimer bodies, spherocytes, and poikilocytes in the peripheral blood smear. Functional asplenia is associated with a number of diseases, including sickle cell anemia, and predisposes to infections, especially by pneumococci or other encapsulated organisms. In 1977, Dillon and co-workers[D216] described its occurrence in a lupus patient, and since then several other cases have been reported.[P189] Most SLE patients with functional asplenia who develop pneumococcal or salmonella infection die.[P189] The condition is relatively uncommon in SLE. Of 70 SLE patients screened by peripheral blood smear, 5 showed changes suggestive of functional hyposplenia; however, only 3 patients had no splenic uptake of the radiolabelled sulfur colloid, yielding a frequency of 4.3%.[D216] In another study, functional asplenia was found in 2 of 44 SLE patients (4.6%) studied by determining the presence of vacuolated red blood cells using phase contrast microscopy, a method more reliable than examination of the peripheral blood smear for assessing splenic function.[N54]

The mechanism of functional hyposplenia in SLE is unclear. In those patients who died, the spleen showed atrophy without evidence of vasculitis.[P189] Functional hyposplenia can also be transient and reversible.[M84,P189] It does not seem to be related to disease activity in SLE, and may manifest clinically as an overwhelming infection in a patient who is in disease remission.

Because of the apparent high risk for pneumococcal infection, the peripheral blood smear of SLE patients should be screened routinely for Howell-Jolly bodies. Polyvalent pneumococcal vaccine should be considered in patients with functional asplenia because, despite the splenic dysfunction, they can still mount an antibody response.[P189,P232] In general, however, the anti-pneumococcal antibody titer is lower in SLE patients than in vaccinated healthy subjects,[J58] and whether the antibody response is protective or not remains to be established.

Thymus Gland, Myasthenia Gravis, and Their Relationships

Structure of the Thymus in SLE

The thymus gland, a central lymphoid organ, is critical in the development and differentiation of T cells and the induction of autoimmunity. Lymphocytes originate in the bone marrow, and must migrate to the thymus to acquire immunocompetence. Microscopically, the thymus gland is comprised of several lobules; each lobule consists of a lighter staining medulla populated predominantly by epithelial cells and a darker staining cortex populated by lymphocytes. Hassall's corpuscles in the thymic medulla

are mature epithelial cells that form concentric layers and become keratinized. Myoid cells with cross-striations are located adjacent to Hassall's corpuscles.

At puberty, when the thymus has reached its maximum size, the organ begins to undergo gradual physiologic involution characterized by the loss of cortical thymocytes, spindling of epithelial cells, and an increase in adipose tissues. During periods of acute stress, cortical lymphocytes are rapidly depleted ("stress" involution).[M16]

The size of the thymus in SLE, as assessed by pneumomediastinography, was found to be small, even in patients who had not received corticosteroids.[S767a] Serial measurements in patients receiving prednisone showed a significant reduction in thymic size following steroid therapy. Most of the information on the histology of the thymus in SLE comes from early studies in 13 SLE patients, before thymic functions were fully understood.[H518,M16] The changes associated with stress involution included a pronounced depletion of lymphocytes, resulting in cortical atrophy and disorganization of the medulla. Aggregates of epithelial cells and cystic Hassall's corpuscles were seen in the medulla. These abnormalities were not specific for SLE, and were also seen in patients with long-standing terminal illness. An increased number of plasma cells, Russell bodies, and germinal centers in the thymus, similar to those found in patients with myasthenia gravis, were present, suggesting an immunologic reaction within the thymus.[G266]

The activity of thymic hormone decreases in SLE patients, especially in those with clinically active disease.[H305,L253] This decreased activity is a result of its low serum concentration, rather than to the presence of a circulating inhibitor.

Thymectomy has been performed in a small number of SLE patients. No significant clinical improvement was noted, and the titer of the antinuclear antibodies remained unchanged.[M16,M444]

Myasthenia Gravis and SLE

Myasthenia gravis (MG) is a neuromuscular disorder characterized by a fluctuating weakness of the skeletal, bulbar, and respiratory muscles. Like SLE, MG has a predilection for young adults, with a female predominance. In MG, however, neuromuscular fatigue and an inability to sustain repeated muscular contractions, are present. The basic defect is the reduction of available acetylcholine receptors (AChRs) at the neuromuscular junction because of an autoimmune process. IgG antibodies to AChRs are present in 85% of patients.

The association between MG and SLE has fascinated investigators for some time. In 1963, Alarcon-Segovia et al.[A107] reported the appearance of SLE in 2 patients several years after thymectomy for the treatment of MG, and collected 9 other patients from the literature. Since then, several reports of coexistent SLE and MG have appeared, although it is questionable whether some of the reported cases had definite SLE. Of 20 cases reviewed by Killian and Hoffman in 1980,[A200] only 10 fulfilled the 1973 ARA criteria for the classification of SLE. More recently, Ciaccio et al.[C268] reported 2 patients with coexistent SLE and MG, and found an additional 42 in the literature. Most of the 24 patients reported prior to 1972 failed to meet at least four of the 1982 ARA criteria, whereas 12 of the 20 patients reported after 1972 fulfilled the criteria.

Of the 44 reported patients with coexistent MG and SLE, MG preceded SLE in 32 (72%) and, in the remaining 12, MG followed SLE. In 13 patients, SLE developed following thymectomy for the treatment of MG.[C268] Polyarthritis and serositis were the most common presenting features of SLE. Malar skin rash was present in 20%, discoid LE lesions in 11%, and photosensitivity in 7%. The disease that develops later tends to dominate the clinical picture and prognosis. A patient with widespread cutaneous and mucosal eruption following MG, and thymoma with features of cutaneous LE and pemphigus erythematosus, has been described.[C450]

Both SLE and MG are characterized by the presence of autoantibodies. Antinuclear antibodies are found in 30% of patients with MG. In addition, antibodies to organ-specific antigens, such as skeletal muscle, thyroid, and thymic cells, about.[L209] The most characteristic serologic abnormality in MG is the presence of IgG antibodies to AChRs. No cross-reactivity between anti-DNA and AChRs antibody was noted.[B200] SLE and MG differ in regard to certain cell-mediated immune functions. Whereas SLE patients have decreased cellular immunity, as measured by skin testing, migratory inhibition factor production by mononuclear cells, and peripheral blood lymphocyte response to mitogens, MG patients have a normal lymphocyte response to mitogens.[D201] Enumeration of lymphocyte subsets yielded normal to abnormal numbers.[L209] Diaz-Juanen[D201] suggested that SLE and MG represent opposite extremes in the spectrum of abnormalities and modulations of the immune response by the thymus that may lead to autoimmunity.

Osterhuis and de Hass[O86] found a 1% prevalence of SLE in a large series of MG patients. Of their 142 MG patients, 2 had SLE and 7 had RA, suggesting that RA and not SLE was more frequently associated with MG. Killian and Hoffman[A200] found 5 SLE cases among 1,604 cases of MG collated from five large series. Taking the prevalence rate of SLE as between 1/2,000 and 1/25,000 and that of MG as 1/20,000, they concluded that the 5 SLE patients in the population of 1,604 MG patients occurred other than by chance. These numbers would be even more significant if the SLE patients who did not fulfill the ARA criteria were included in the computation.

Thymoma is an uncommon epithelial neoplasm largely found in adults, and has no sex predilection. Of patients with thymoma, 40% have parathymic syndromes,[R309] the most common being MG, pure red cell aplasia, and adult-onset acquired hypogammaglobulinemia. Thymomas are found in 15% of MG patients and have also been described in those with connective tissue diseases, including SLE, polymyositis, Sjögren's syndrome, and scleroderma. Of 598 patients with thymomas collected from the literature, 8 had SLE.[S572] In some cases, thymoma and SLE have been associated with another disorder, such as progressive multifocal leukoencephalopathy,[M76] vacuolar myopathy,[M181] or red cell aplasia.[C129] The effect of removal of the thymoma on the clinical course of SLE is variable. Larsson[L78]

Table 43–1. Lymphoid and Thymic Abnormalities in SLE

1. Lymphadenopathy is seen in 30 to 78% of SLE patients. The nodes are discrete and nontender. Massive enlargement of the lymph nodes may develop, particularly in children and blacks.
2. The spleen is palpable in 9 to 46% of patients. An enlarged spleen is present in 67% of autopsy cases. Hyposplenism is noted in 5%. The onionskin lesion in the splenic arterioles is a characteristic finding.
3. Germinal centers consisting of focal collections of lymphocytes are noted in the thymic medulla in SLE patients. Myasthenia gravis and SLE occasionally coexist.

described a 62-year-old woman with SLE and coexistent thymoma. The tumor enlarged while the SLE improved. In contrast, a thymectomy in another patient temporarily reduced the clinical and laboratory manifestations of the SLE.[S451]

In summary, SLE and MG may occasionally coexist, with the MG preceding SLE in 75% of patients. Thymectomy for MG appears to be the precipitating factor in some patients. Whether the association between the two diseases is real, remains controversial and unproven. No controlled epidemiologic studies are available.

Table 43–1 summarizes the lymphoid and thymic abnormalities seen in SLE patients.

HEMATOLOGIC CHANGES

Hematologic abnormalities are exceedingly common in SLE, and often are presenting manifestations of the disease. Sometimes their features may mimic those of primary blood dyscrasias, and the nature of the underlying disorder can be completely overlooked unless SLE is considered in the differential diagnosis and specific diagnostic studies are performed.

Anemia

Prevalence

Most patients with SLE develop anemia at some time during the course of their disease. Michael and colleagues[M387] reported that 87 of 111 SLE patients (78%) had a hemoglobin level lower than 12 g/dl at diagnosis. Subsequently, 15 of 24 patients who had a normal hemoglobin level on presentation developed anemia. In general, anemia was moderate, but was severe in some patients. Of 24 patients, 29% had a hemoglobin level between 10.0 and 11.9 g/dl, 33% had between 8 and 9.9 g/dl; 10% had between 6.0 and 7.9 g/dl, and 5% had below 6 g/dl. The anemia was usually normochromic and normocytic and appeared to depend partly on the severity and duration of the illness. Three of their patients had autoimmune hemolytic anemia.

The experience of other investigators has been similar to that of Michael et al. (see Table 33–1).[M387] Hemoglobin below 11 g/dl was present in 51% of 520 patients of Dubois,[D340] in 73% of 150 patients of Estes and Christian,[E147] and in 98% of 275 patients of Haserick.[H179]

Classification

The causes of anemia in SLE can be classified into two major categories according to putative mechanisms—nonimmune and immune. The former group includes anemia of chronic disease, iron deficiency anemia, sideroblastic anemia, anemia of renal disease, drug-induced anemia, and anemia secondary to another disorder (e.g., sickle cell anemia). Immune-mediated anemias in SLE include autoimmune hemolytic anemia, drug-induced hemolytic anemia, aplastic anemia, pure red cell aplasia, and pernicious anemia.

NONIMMUNE-MEDIATED ANEMIAS

Anemia of Chronic Disease. The most common type of anemia in SLE is anemia of chronic disease. The red cells on the peripheral blood smear are normochromic and normocytic. The serum iron concentration is reduced and the total iron-binding capacity is unchanged or slightly low. A decrease in the iron saturation of transferrin is present. The bone marrow examination is usually normal, with adequate iron stores.[M387] The anemia develops slowly unless it becomes complicated by other factors, such as blood loss. The reticulocyte count is low for the degree of anemia.[U116]

Iron Metabolism. SLE patients taking NSAIDS or those with heavy menses can be iron deficient. Iron metabolism was investigated by Burger et al.[B575] in 11 SLE patients using ^{59}Fe. Iron utilization was decreased in seven patients. Radioactivity over various organs differed from normal, with increased levels of radioactivity over the spleen and liver. The increased amount of absorbed iron did not appear to serve the purpose of hemoglobin synthesis but was stored. Plasma iron turnover, on the other hand, was elevated in most patients. The life span of erythrocytes was reduced in the absence of hemolysis. It was concluded that the anemia of chronic disease in SLE patients may be attributed to insufficient bone marrow activity, shortened red cell life span, and possibly poor uptake of iron.

Whittingham et al.[W212] studied the serum iron levels of six patients with SLE. The mean serum iron level was 59 μg/dl (normal, 40 to 60 μg/dl). Following the administration of prednisolone, a two- to fourfold rise in the serum iron level occurred. The increase in the serum iron concentration was not sustained, however, and the effect of the hemoglobin concentration was not examined.

The mechanism of anemia of chronic disease is not well understood. Results of investigations on its pathogenesis in rheumatoid arthritis[V116] indicate that multiple factors are involved, including impairment of iron release by the mononuclear phagocytic system, iron trapping by binding proteins, decreased erythropoietin responsiveness, and suppressive effects of interleukins on erythropoiesis.

The treatment of anemia of chronic disease in SLE is directed at the disease process, and does not warrant iron therapy or any specific intervention.

Sickle Cell Anemia. Sickle cell anemia and SLE share common clinical manifestations, including arthralgias, chest pain, pleural effusion, cardiomegaly, nephropathy, strokes, and seizures. In addition, we found that patients with sickle cell hemoglinopathies have an increased prev-

alence of autoantibodies, including ANA.[Q19] The coexistence of SLE and sickle cell anemia has been reported[G146,K88,L398,Q19,W86,W132,W133] and, in some of these patients, the recognition of SLE was delayed because of the similarities in clinical features of the two conditions.[K109] Wilson et al.[W133] postulated that abnormalities in the alternative pathway of complement in sickle cell hemoglinopathy may predispose patients to immune complex disorders, including SLE, but no evidence has been found to show that SLE is more prevalent in those with sickle cell hemoglobinopathies.

Sideroblastic Anemia. A few cases of sideroblastic refractory anemia in SLE have been reported, including one terminating in erythroleukemia.[B55,N79] Another patient with refractory anemia with excess of blasts, a myelodysplastic syndrome, developed SLE.[L208] These cases are probably incidental, and do not represent a true association with SLE.

IMMUNE-MEDIATED ANEMIAS

The inhibition of erythropoiesis by cellular and serum factors may be important in the pathogenesis of chronic anemia in SLE patients. The number of erythroid colony-forming units (CFU-E), the late erythropoietic precursors, has been found to be significantly reduced in the bone marrow of anemic SLE patients.[Y20] Moreover, the formation of CFU-E was inhibited in vitro by autologous and allogeneic T lymphocytes from untreated subjects, but not from steroid-treated SLE patients.[Y20] Circulating inhibitors of erythropoiesis have also been described.[C163,D14,F120,K30,M384] Sera from SLE patients with anemia of chronic disease suppressed CFU-E formation.[K30] Dainiak et al.[D14] characterized the serum inhibitor as having the physical properties of an immunoglobulin, and its presence was associated with disease activity. The inhibitor was removed by plasma exchange and by steroid therapy. Whether the inhibitor is an autoantibody to marrow erythroid progenitor cells remains to be established.

Pure Red Cell Aplasia. Pure red cell aplasia (PRCA) is an autoimmune condition characterized by severe normochromic normocytic anemia, reticulocytopenia, and absence of red cell precursors in the bone marrow. Different pathogenetic mechanisms have been proposed in PRCA, including suppression of erythropoiesis by serum antibodies to erythroblasts, to CFU-Es or to erythropoietin and T-cell suppression of erythropoiesis. PRCA is associated with a number of autoimmune conditions and a few cases of coexistent PRCA and SLE, and procainamide-induced LE, have been reported.[A62,F198,F219,K408] Serum IgG from an SLE patient with PRCA inhibited the growth of red cell precursors.[C163] Anticardiolipin antibodies have also been described in SLE patients with PRCA.[A62]

Aplastic Anemia. Aplastic anemia occurs rarely in SLE secondary to the use of nitrogen mustard derivatives, azathioprine, antimalarials, or other agents, such as chloramphenicol.[N148] In a few published cases, the aplastic anemia was considered to be primarily caused by the underlying disease; however, the role of drugs cannot be completely excluded.[A4,F120] The presence of circulating antibodies to precursor bone marrow cells suggests that some cases of aplastic anemia may be the result of an autoimmune process. Brooks et al.[B508] identified a complement-dependent IgG antibody that suppressed the growth of allogeneic granulocyte-macrophage progenitor cells in vitro. Bailey and colleagues[B28a] found a noncomplement IgG antibody that inhibited in vitro granulocyte-macrophage progenitor cells and erythroid blast-forming units in an SLE patient with aplastic anemia. The IgG antibody disappeared on recovery of the patient. Various regimens have been used successfully for the treatment of aplastic anemia associated with SLE, including androgens, cyclophosphamide, and plasmapheresis in conjunction with systemic corticosteroids.[B28a,S732,W50]

Bone Marrow Findings

Michael and co-workers[M387] examined the bone marrow aspirates of 32 SLE patients and found it to be normal in most patients. Plasma cells were increased (greater than 2%) in 13 patients; 1 patient had a hypoplastic marrow, and 2 patients with autoimmune hemolytic anemia had a hypercellular marrow. Similar findings have been reported by others.[Y2]

Careful studies by Burkhardt[B578] of bone marrow biopsies in 21 SLE patients have shown significant alterations in the blood vessels, cellular elements, and intercellular substance. Compared to control subjects, an increased frequency of the following changes in SLE was found:

1. Subintimal swelling of the arteries and arterioles, with evidence of deposition of proteins in the vessel wall, was seen.
2. Endothelial swelling and dissociation were found in the sinusoids.
3. The ground substance was edematous, with fibrinoid and sclerosing changes.
4. A proliferation of histiocytes bearing cytoplasmic inclusions of iron-positive protein material was noted.
5. Diffuse plasma cell proliferation occurred, with the formation of Russell bodies.
6. In the myelocytic parenchyma, a reduction of granulopoiesis with predominantly immature forms and necrobioses with opal nuclei were observed.

It should be noted that these changes are not specific for SLE, but may be seen in those RA and other diseases.[B578] Nevertheless, these findings, as well as the presence of autoantibodies and cellular factors that inhibit the growth of bone marrow precursor cells, suggest that the bone marrow is a "target organ" in this disease.

Myelofibrosis. Myelofibrosis is frequently associated with various benign and malignant disorders, and in some patients, appears to be a primary condition without an underlying disorder. Myelofibrosis occurring in the setting of SLE has been described in a few cases.[C163,E90,K6,L88,M194] The patients presented with pancytopenia, and bone marrow biopsy showed fibrosis with increased fibrillar reticulin, collagen, and fibroblasts. Half of patients had splenomegaly. Treatment with systemic corticosteroids led to regression of the myelofibrosis in 50% of patients. Compared to patients with idiopathic

myelofibrosis with myeloid metaplasia, the SLE patients were younger. It is noteworthy that Rosen et al.[R301] described a group of 5 patients with chronic myelofibrosis with myeloid metaplasia and serologic abnormalities, including a positive LE cell test, antinuclear antibodies, and positive Coombs' test. Other than arthralgia, none of their patients developed other features of SLE. Immunologic factors may be important in the pathogenesis of some cases of idiopathic chronic myelofibrosis.

Gelatinous transformation of the bone marrow, a rare condition associated with cachexia caused by cancer, anorexia nervosa, tuberculosis, and other chronic illnesses, has been reported in 3 of 30 SLE patients who had pancytopenia.[N80] Also, 2 SLE patients were cachectic. Hyaluronic acid, a mucopolysaccharide, was present in the ground substance of the marrow, associated with fat atrophy and cellular hypoplasia.

Acute Hemophagocytic Syndrome. SLE has been added to the list of diseases associated with acute hemophagocytic syndrome. Wong and associates[W334] described 6 SLE patients who presented with fever and severe pancytopenia related to reactive hemophagocytosis. This is a rare condition associated with various infections and neoplasms, especially lymphomas. It is characterized by pancytopenia and a bone marrow picture showing mature-looking histiocytes, many of which have phagocytosed erythrocytes, platelets, granulocytes, and erythroblasts.

Pernicious Anemia and SLE. Pernicious anemia is often associated with other autoimmune disorders, such as Sjögren's syndrome and Hashimoto's thyroiditis, yet only a few cases of coexistent SLE and pernicious anemia have been reported.[C405,F50,K38,L207] Molad and associates[M522] found that 18.6% of 43 female SLE patients had abnormally low serum cobalamin levels, but none of the patients had evidence of pernicious anemia. As a group, SLE patients had lower mean levels of cobalamin than controls. Low serum levels of transcobalamin II and unsaturated vitamin B_{12} capacity correlated with lupus disease activity, a finding also observed in other autoimmune diseases.[L80]

Autoimmune Hemolytic Anemia (AIHA)

Autoimmune hemolytic anemia (AIHA) is not an uncommon cause of anemia in SLE patients. Approximately 7 to 15% of those in large series developed AIHA (see Table 33–1).[A139,C325,R349] Among a group of 186 SLE patients studied by Alger et al.,[A139] 17 (7%) had Coombs'-positive hemolytic anemia. Of the 17 patients, 6 had Evan's syndrome (the concurrence of AIHA and immune thrombocytopenic purpura).

AIHA may be the initial manifestation of SLE, occurring in 2 to 6% of patients.[D305,H179] In 50% of ten patients studied by Videbaek,[V81] AIHA was the initial and dominant clinical feature of the disease for several months, and even years, before other manifestations of SLE appeared. In the remaining five patients, AIHA developed during the course of SLE.

Classification

AIHA can be classified into two major types with respect to the antibody involved in red cell destruction and the optimal temperature of antibody reactivity with antigens on the red cell surface. The warm type of AIHA is mediated by IgG antibodies capable of reacting with antigens optimally at 37° C. Cold agglutinin AIHA is mediated by IgM complement-fixing antibody, which binds optimally to red cell antigens at 4° C. (See Chapter 28 for the immunology of antierythrocyte antibodies in SLE.)

Warm AIHA. Warm AIHA is the predominant type in SLE patients. Red blood cells coated by the warm IgG antibodies are removed from the circulation, primarily by sequestration in the spleen. The antibody-coated red blood cells undergo membrane alteration in vivo, resulting in the formation of spherocytes. Matsumoto et al.[M192] examined the fine structure of the spleen in AIHA in SLE and found that erythrocytes coated with IgG and complement were phagocytosed completely by splenic macrophages and, to a lesser extent, by sinus endothelial cells. In contrast, in the liver, only evidence of occasional phagocytosis of sensitized erythrocytes by the Kupffer cells was found, confirming that the spleen is the major site of red blood cell destruction.

The symptoms and clinical findings in AIHA are variable. Symptoms referable to the anemic state, such as weakness, dizziness, and fever, are common. Evidence of hemolysis, including jaundice and dark urine, may be found. AIHA in the setting of SLE develops gradually in most patients but, occasionally may present as a rapidly progressive hemolytic crisis.[D305,V81]

With a significant degree of hemolysis, anisocytosis and macrocytosis are often noted in the peripheral blood smear. Nucleated red blood cells are seen in patients with marked hemolysis. Occasionally, polychromatophilic red cells, stippled cells, and Howell-Jolly bodies are found. The bone marrow is hyperplastic, frequently with a shift to the left in the myeloid series.[D305] Reticulocyte counts are elevated in association with a significant degree of hemolysis after hemorrhage and during systemic corticosteroid therapy.

The serum haptoglobin level is usually reduced during active phases of hemolysis in SLE, as well as in other diseases.[B544,L389,O128] In the presence of infection, cancer, or steroid treatment, the serum haptoglobin level rises; consequently, if hemolysis coexists with these factors, the result may be normal.[B544,O128] This is also observed when bone marrow function is impaired.

Tan and Chaplin[T45] found low-titer ANA in 39% of patients with idiopathic AIHA who did not have evidence of an underlying systemic connective tissue disease or lymphoproliferative disorder. No correlation was found among ANA and various clinical or serologic parameters. Favre et al.[F32] described 3 patients with AIHA and one with immune thrombocytopenic purpura with positive ANA and anti-dsDNA, who did not develop the full clinical picture of SLE after longterm follow-up. None had evidence of clinical renal disease but, on kidney biopsy, all had mild mesangial proliferation of focal glomerulonephritis. These patients probably had SLE manifesting predominantly with immunohematologic features. Alger et al.[A376] compared the features of 31 SLE patients who had AIHA and/or immune thrombocytopenia to a group of 62 SLE patients without hematologic manifestations. The former group, who were younger and included a greater percentage of females, had a lower prevalence of fever, polyarthritis, serositis, cutaneous vasculitis, nephropathy, and central nervous system disease, and fewer complement abnormalities. It was suggested that SLE patients who develop AIHA and/or immune thrombocytopenia constitute two related subsets of SLE patients. The high frequency of antiphospholipid antibodies in SLE patients with hemocytopenia further supports this concept.[D138]

Combined Warm and Cold AIHA. Sokol and associates[S537] found that 7% of 865 patients with AIHA referred to a blood transfusion center had warm IgG and cold IgM anti-red cell antibodies, and both antibodies contributed to the hemolysis. Of the patients in this group, 20% had SLE.[S537] The high frequency of SLE was confirmed by Shulman et al.[S400] who found that 5 of 12 patients (42%) with combined warm and cold AIHA had SLE.

IgG and C3d are usually present on the patient's red blood cells. In the serum, both IgG warm antibodies and high thermal amplitude cold IgM autoagglutinins are detectable. The IgM antibodies are reactive over a broad temperature range from 0° to 30° C or higher.[S400] Patients with this type of AIHA have severe hemolysis but are generally responsive to corticosteroid therapy.[S400]

Treatment

Medical Therapy. Systemic corticosteroids, 1 to 1.5 mg/kg of prednisone daily, or its equivalent, are efficacious, and are the mainstay of the treatment for AIHA in SLE patients. It is preferable to administer steroids parenterally to the symptomatic and acutely ill patient and later to switch to an oral preparation when the patient has stabilized and improved. The dose is maintained for at least 4 to 6 weeks and gradually tapered, provided a continued and/or sustained response occurs. No controlled trials have been reported on the use of corticosteroids in the treatment of AIHA in SLE, but our clinical experience and that of others indicate that approximately 75% of patients respond satisfactorily to steroid therapy.[P298] The response rate is similar to the 76% reported in patients with idiopathic warm AIHA.[P298]

In steroid-responsive patients studied by Pirofsky,[P298] the clinical response was evident within a week. Stabilization of the hematocrit occurred within 30 to 90 days after the initiation of therapy.

In patients with severe and rapidly progressive hemolytic anemia, pulse methylprednisolone should be tried, 1 g IV for 3 consecutive days, followed by the conventional steroid dose.[J17] The reticulocyte count can be used to monitor the response to treatment and to detect any relapse as the steroid dose is tapered. A drop in the reticulocyte count is associated with a relapse in the hemolytic process.

Various treatment measures have been tried in patients who fail to respond to systemic corticosteroids or in those who continue to require a moderate to high dose of prednisone to control hemolysis. Most of the experiences come from uncontrolled clinical studies. Pirofsky[P298] used azathioprine, 2 to 2.5 mg/kg, in conjunction with prednisone, 10 to 20 mg/day, in AIHA patients who failed to respond to full therapeutic doses of prednisone. Danazol in conjunction with high-dose corticosteroids has been reported to be useful in the treatment of warm AIHA, including that associated with SLE.[A72] Plasmapheresis,[V111] high-dose intravenous gamma globulin,[M69] and vincaladen platelets[A71] have been used with some success in a small number of patients with idiopathic AIHA refractory to conventional therapy. The application of these measures in the treatment of AIHA associated with SLE needs further study.

Splenectomy. Splenectomy is used to treat patients with idiopathic warm AIHA who require a high maintenance dose of prednisone (20 mg/day or more), patients who have frequent relapses, or those with serious side effects to steroid therapy. In general, splenectomy as a treatment measure is less effective for warm AIHA than for immune thrombocytopenia. The response rate to splenectomy in those with idiopathic warm AIHA is 50 to 60%,[M671] with reduction in the steroid maintenance dose or amelioration of the hemolysis.

It was suggested by early workers that splenectomy for idiopathic immune thrombocytopenia or for idiopathic AIHA can, somehow unmasks occult or latent lupus, thus causing a dissemination of the disease. Best and Darling[B272] reviewed the pertinent evidence for and against this controversial issue and concluded that splenectomy does not lead to dissemination of SLE but, on the contrary, has a beneficial effect for many patients.

Early studies on a small number of cases suggested that splenectomy is not efficacious in the treatment of warm AIHA associated with SLE.[D340,V81] More recent studies have shown that splenectomy is of some value in the treatment of selected cases, but the benefit may not be long-lasting. Of 7 SLE patients with warm AIHA (5 had concomitant immune thrombopenia) who underwent splenectomy, 6 patients showed a sustained increase in hematocrit of greater than 20%.[C379] Rivero et al.[R226] compared the clinical course of 15 SLE patients with AIHA and/or immune thrombocytopenia who underwent splenectomy and 15 SLE patients who were treated medically for the hemocytopenia. Splenectomy produced short-term benefit but, at follow-up, no clear cut difference in the clinical course of the two groups was seen. The splenectomy group had a significantly higher frequency of cutaneous vasculitis and serious infections after surgery. More of the splenectomized patients eventually required immunosuppressive therapy than those in the medically treated group at follow-up.

SLE patients with AIHA who fail to respond to systemic corticosteroids should be tried first with immunosuppressive agents. The role of newer measures, in these patients, including gamma globulin, plasmapheresis, or cyclosporin, remains to be defined. Splenectomy should probably be reserved for the patient with acute fulminant AIHA who fails to respond to aggressive medical treatment.[R226] Polyvalent pneumococcal vaccine should be given to splenectomized patients, such as those with functional asplenenia (see above).

Blood Groups and Transfusions in SLE

The distribution of ABO and Rh blood types of 138 SLE patients studied by Dubois[D340] was normal; 86% of the patients were Rh positive. Similar results were obtained by Leonhardt,[L22] who found no differences in the major blood groups of 54 SLE patients, 221 of their relatives, and 5,668 healthy blood donors.

The prevalence of adverse reactions to blood transfusion has been low. In 82 patients (16%) of Dubois who received one or more blood transfusions, only 3 developed reactions, urticaria in 1 and fever in 2. Of Harvey's patients, 39 (35%) received one or more blood transfusions.[H262] Over 200 blood transfusions were administered, and the frequency of untoward reactions was low. Occasionally, a brief febrile response or urticaria occurred, but these patients were subsequently transfused without recurrence of the reaction. In contrast, Michael et al.[M387] commented that, in their experience, transfusion reactions appeared more common in SLE patients than in the general hospital population, but no statistical data were presented.

Blood transfusions should be avoided whenever possible, not only because of the risk of hepatitis and other infectious diseases, but also because of the observation that SLE patients develop isoantibodies against red cell antigens. Callender et al.[C28,C29] reported an SLE patient who, in response to multiple blood transfusions, developed isoagglutinins to five different red cell antigens that are usually ignored by most individuals. Multiple types of isoagglutinins were found in the serum of another transfused patient with probable SLE.[W46] An SLE patient developed hemolytic anemia following multiple blood transfusions, with the appearance of three atypical hemagglutinins.[K448] A hemoglobinuric transfusion reaction resulting from Rh isosensitization has been described.[B52]

The antibody response of SLE patients to blood group antigens has been examined following experimental immunization. The intravenous injection of 1 ml of incompatible whole blood led to the appearance of an unusually high isoagglutinin titer in an SLE patient.[G358] Zingale and associates[Z31] immunized 15 SLE patients and matched controls with incompatible blood group substances. SLE patients developed higher titers of isohemagglutinin antibodies than the controls, as well as the transient appearance of a false-positive test for syphilis, circulating anticoagulants, antithryroglobulin, and antikidney antibodies. In contrast, the antibody production to various exogenous antigens following immunization in SLE has been either normal or depressed.[L142,M677]

The few indications for blood transfusions in SLE patients include those with acute massive bleeding, a symptomatic patient with severe anemia with a hemoglobin level falling to less than 6 g/dl, or those with concomitant severe heart disease or cerebrovascular ischemia. The response of SLE patients with autoimmune hemolytic anemia to systemic corticosteroids is generally prompt and favorable, so that blood transfusion is usually unnecessary. Circulating antierythrocyte antibodies makes blood crossmatching difficult.[P166]

The anemia associated with chronic renal failure can now be treated effectively with recombinant human erythropoietin, provided sufficient iron stores are available.[A35] Used mainly for patients with end-stage kidney disease on maintenance hemodialysis, it is well tolerated except for the development or aggravation of hypertension in 25% and seizures in 2% of patients.[W335] The mechanisms underlying these adverse reactions are not clear. Whether SLE patients on hemodialysis with anemia respond to erythropoietin therapy differently from non-SLE patients has not been specifically investigated. We have treated a SLE patient on chronic hemodialysis prior to renal transplantation, with good results. Lim et al.[L292] have shown that erythropoietin is also effective in ameliorating the anemia in a group of predialysis patients with chronic renal failure that included a lupus patient. Erythropoietin has also been found to be useful in rheumatoid arthritis patients with anemia of chronic disease.[P195] It remains to be determined whether it can be used similarly in SLE patients.

Thrombocytopenia and Platelet Disorders

Frequency and Significance

Thrombocytopenia, defined as a platelet count of less than 150,000/mm^3, is not an uncommon finding in SLE. The prevalence in seven large series in the literature has ranged from 7 to 52%, with a mean cumulative percentage of 14.5% (see Table 33–1).[D340,E147,G170,L75,M280,M387, R294]

The degree of thrombocytopenia is variable, but profound thrombocytopenia is uncommon. Mild thrombocytopenia often appears during an exacerbation of SLE without causing bleeding tendency. Platelet counts were available in 86 patients in Harvey's series[M280] and, in 23 patients, they were definitely depressed. Of the 12 who had platelet counts of less than 50,000/mm^3, patients were included in whom thrombocytopenia purpura was a predominant feature of their disease. Also, 7 had counts between 50,000 and 100,000/mm^3, and 4 patients had counts between 100,000 and 150,000/mm^3. None of these patients had abnormal bleeding. In Larson's series[L75] of 196 patients, 15 (8%) had platelet counts below 100,000/mm^3 on at least two occasions; 9 had purpuric lesions at the time platelet counts were depressed, but 6 patients did not. An additional group of 9 patients had purpuric skin rash as a prominent feature of their illness, but the platelet count was never found to be below 100,000/mm^3. In 112 SLE patients studied for hemostatic functions, Gladman et al.[G170] found 18 patients with a platet count of less than 150,000/mm^3. In this group, 10 patients had counts below 100,000/mm^3, yet only 1 subject developed petechiae.

In association with thrombocytopenia, the usual coexistent laboratory abnormalities are noted, such as a prolonged bleeding time and diminished clot retraction when the platelet count is below 50,000/mm^3. A positive tourniquet test, may be present without any platelet deficit, however, and may merely reflect vascular fragility resulting from SLE or prolonged steroid therapy.[D329] Coexistent hemostatic defects are often observed in SLE patients with low platelet counts.[G170] A correlation between the presence of anticardiolipin and other antiphospholipid antibodies and thrombocytopenia in SLE, as well as in chronic

immune thrombocytopenic purpura, has been recognized (see Chaps. 24 and 25).

The clinical significance of thrombocytopenia in SLE has been examined. A prospective study of 19 patients with platelet counts of less than 100,000/mm^3 revealed two distinct clinical groups: patients who were thrombocytopenic only during severe multisystem disease flares, and those with a chronic low platelet count with intermittent mild flares in other systems. None of the patients in either group developed severe bleeding. Whether acute or chronic, thrombocytopenia itself did not determine the subsequent course and prognosis of the patient.[M430] In two large studies on survivorship, the presence of thrombocytopenia appeared to be a significant risk factor for a worse prognosis in SLE.[P216,R173] When the significance of thrombocytopenia was examined in a highly selective subset of SLE patients with biopsy-proven nephritis, Clark et al.[C287] found that thrombocytopenia is a useful index of disease activity.

Immune Thrombocytopenic Purpura

A special relationship exists between SLE and autoimmune thrombocytopenic purpura (ATP; also referred to as idiopathic or immune thrombocytopenic purpura, ITP), both of which primarily afflict young females. Some patients with ITP who are initially considered as idiopathic may later develop a classic clinical picture of SLE. Furthermore, a thrombocytopenic purpura, clinically indistinguishable from ITP, may occur along the course of SLE.

Three to 15% of ITP patients go on to develop SLE.[K75] Of a group of 62 adults with chronic ITP studied by DiFino et al.,[D207] 3 patients (4.8%) developed SLE. Perez and associates[P119] found that 6 of 18 patients with ITP (33%) tested positive for ANA at presentation, and 4 of these developed classic SLE, within a mean duration of 2.3 years. A retrospective study of 117 ITP patients showed a positive ANA in 24 patients, and 4 of these developed SLE.[D25] Patients with high-titer ANA tested positive for anti-Ro/SSA and anti-La/SSA antibody. Thus, ITP patients with high-titer ANA and precipitating antibodies to Ro/SSA may develop later SLE.[A207] It is noteworthy that anti-Ro/SSA antibody is associated with thrombocytopenia in SLE.[M590] Firkin et al.[F102] coined the term "lupoid thrombocytopenia" to refer to a group of patients with chronic ITP who were ANA-positive but did not have other clinical or laboratory findings of SLE. None had anti-DNA, anti-Sm, or anti-Ro/SSA. The value of using this label is questionable, however, because the ANA-positive patients were similar in every other respect to those in the ANA-negative group.

In 1956, Dameshek[D25] emphasized the high frequency of SLE that occurs following splenectomy for apparent ITP. In a series of 51 consecutive cases, 8 patients subsequently developed definite SLE, 2 probable, and 6 possible. Thus, at least 31% of the patients in this group eventually developed clinical manifestations of SLE, and 15% had definite SLE.[R4] Other investigators have since disputed this claim, and found that splenectomy in ITP does not lead to the development of SLE.[B272,B572,D241,M386] In 1960, Doan et al.[D241] reviewed their experience with 381 cases of thrombocytopenic purpura over a 28-year period, and found that SLE caused the syndrome in 2.0% of patients. After splenectomy, the prevalance of new cases of SLE was 1.2%. Splenectomy did not precipitate or disseminate the symptoms or signs of SLE in any patient, and the investigators believed that the hazards to life during acute hypersplenic thrombocytopenic crises outweigh the danger of developing subsequent SLE. Best and Darling[B272] undertook a critical analysis of the existing data on this issue, and concluded that splenectomy does not lead to dissemination of "latent" SLE but is actually beneficial to some patients with drug-resistant cytopenias.

Clinical Presentation. The clinical manifestations of thrombocytopenia in SLE are generally similar to those seen in patients with ITP or other causes of thrombocytopenia, and depend on the platelet count. When the platelet count is below 50,000/mm^3, spontaneous bleeding or purpura may occur. In addition to the platelet count, however, other factors, including qualitative platelet defects and platelet age, are important in the development of spontaneous bleeding.[K76] Bleeding usually presents as petechiae and/or ecchymoses, especially in the lower limbs, which experience increased capillary pressure. Nasal and buccal mucosal hemorrhage, heavy menstrual blood flow, epistaxis, and gum bleeding may also be present. Spontaneous bleeding into the brain is the most feared complication, and can be fatal.

The immunologic properties of antiplatelet antibodies in ITP and SLE are discussed in Chapter 28.

Treatment. The mainstay of drug therapy is systemic corticosteroids, 1 to 1.5 mg/kg/day of prednisone equivalent. Corticosteroid therapy is considered to be the equivalent of "medical splenectomy" because it prevents the sequestration of antibody-coated platelets in the spleen.[K76] In most patients, a clinical response is seen within 1 to 8 weeks. High-dose intravenous pulse methylprednisolone has also been used for profound thrombocytopenia in SLE, but its superiority over conventional steroid therapy has not been established.[E163] Moreover, repeated courses may result in a diminished platelet response.[M35]

In idiopathic ITP, splenectomy is generally recommended for patients who fail to respond to systemic corticosteroids or for those who require moderate doses of steroids to maintain the platelet count.[K76] Splenectomy removes the major site of destruction of damaged platelets and the source of antiplatelet antibodies. In SLE patients it is preferable to try other agents before recommending splenectomy for steroid-resistant thrombocytopenia, however, because of the increased risk of severe infections following splenectomy and the apparent efficacy of other agents.[R226] Danazol an androgenic steroid with few virilizing effects, has been shown to be effective in some SLE patients with thrombocytopenia refractory to steroids, cytotoxic drugs, and/or splenectomy, and is given at an average dose of 200 mg, tid or qid times a day. Often, though, danazol cannot be discontinued without recurrence of the thrombocytopenia.[M134,W189] Intermittent intravenous cyclophosphamide was shown to be effective in the treatment of thrombocytopenia in 7 SLE patients refractory to splenectomy or steroids or requiring excessive doses of ste-

roids.[B433] Other agents reported to be useful in the treatment of thrombocytopenia, although in a limited number of SLE patients, include azathioprine,[G214] cyclosporine,[M193] dapsone,[M625] and vincristine.[A73] Intravenous gamma globulin is also effective, but its effect may not be long-lasting. As in idiopathic ITP, gamma globulin is most useful in the treatment of life-threatening bleeding or in preparing the patient for urgent surgery.[N73] We have also used gamma globulin successfully as an adjunctive measure in an SLE patient with thrombocytopenia who was not responding optimally to corticosteroids and who had a concomitant serious bacterial infection.

The effectiveness of splenectomy in the treatment of steroid-resistant thrombocytopenia in SLE is controversial. Holman and Dineen[H391] followed 10 patients who underwent splenectomy for thrombocytopenia; 2 died postoperatively and 8 had excellent results, with up to a 30-year follow-up. Brackenridge et al.[B469] reported that 9 of 16 SLE patients had normal platelet counts without medications a year after splenectomy. A similar experience was reported by others.[J31] In contrast, Hall and coworkers[H191] found that only 2 of 14 splenectomized thrombocytopenic SLE patients refractory to drug therapy went into remission at a mean follow-up of 6 years. Rivero et al.[R226] found that splenectomy does not prevent recurrent episodes of thrombocytopenia in SLE.

In summary, profound immune thrombocytopenia (less than 50,000/mm^3) in SLE patients should be treated with systemic corticosteroids. Patients who become refractory to steroids or those who experience undesirable side effects should be given a trial of azathioprine or danazol. Monthly intravenous cyclophosphamide therapy is probably preferable for patients with multisystem involvement, especially nephritis. Splenectomy may be necessary. The longterm effect of this regimen has not been adequately examined.

AMEGAKARYOCYTIC THROMBOCYTOPENIA

Acquired thrombocytopenia associated with decreased numbers of megakaryocytes in the bone marrow, amegakaryocytic thrombocytopenia (AMT), is a rare disorder with different causes and pathogenetic mechanisms. A few cases of AMT associated with SLE have been reported.[G392,M107] In a well-studied SLE patient, peripheral T lymphocytes but not serum inhibited autologous colony-forming megakaryocytes in vitro, suggesting an underlying cell-medicated pathogenetic mechanism.[N7]

ACQUIRED ABNORMALITIES OF PLATELET FUNCTION

Acquired abnormalities of platelet function include disorders of platelet adhesiveness to the vessel wall and subendothelial matrix, platelet aggregation, and platelet secretion. Platelet function, as measured by in vitro qualitative tests and by bleeding time, is affected by a number of factors, including drugs such as aspirin and NSAIDs, common foods, spices, the presence of systemic conditions, including SLE and chronic renal failure, lymphoproliferative diseases and other hematologic disorders, and circulating antiplatelet antibodies.[G90] These factors should be considered when interpreting the results of qualitative tests of platelet function in an individual patient. Disturbances of hemostasis and circulating antico-agulants are discussed in Chapters 24 and 25.

Activation of normal platelets can be induced by adhesion to collagen and by soluble agonists such as epinephrine and adenosine diphosphate (ADP). The activation process involves a complex system of metabolic reactions acting in concert to stimulate platelet aggregation and granule secretion. Regan and associates[R109] found that platelets from 12 of 21 SLE patients studied failed to aggregate in response to collagen, and showed impaired aggregation with ADP and epinephrine. These abnormalities are similar to those induced by aspirin, but none of their patients were on aspirin or any drug known to affect platelet function. Others have confirmed these abnormalities in SLE patients.[D273,K47]

In 1980, Parbtani and co-workers[P40] found that the concentration of serotonin and adenine nucleotides, are stored in the dense granules of platelets, was reduced in patients with acquired platelet function defects, including SLE. Weiss et al.[W160] extended this observation and reported that levels of substances stored in platelet-dense granules and in α granules, including β-thromboglobulin, were decreased in SLE. Because these findings were similar to those observed in patients with congenital storage pool deficiency, it has been suggested that the platelet defect in SLE represents an acquired storage pool disease. The reduction of the intraplatelet concentration of serotonin in SLE has been confirmed by other investigators.[D273,G152,K47,M385,P40,Z19] Although the concentration of plasma serotonin is normal in SLE patients, the urinary excretion of serotonin is increased.[K47]

The low concentration of intraplatelet serotonin has been shown to correlate with disease activity, and has been taken to indicate in vivo platelet activation in SLE.[K47,Z19] This is further supported by the findings of elevated levels of plasma β-thromboglobulin and decreased amounts of platelet factors 3 and 4.[D272,G170,W340] β-Thromboglobulin, a specific constituent of α granules, is released on stimulation of platelets.

The mechanism of in vivo platelet activation in SLE is not known. Parbtani et al.[P40] suggested that the functional platelet defects are a result of the circulation of "exhausted" platelets following their in vivo exposure to factors that induce a release reaction, such as damaged endothelium, thrombin, and immune complexes. The globulin fraction of SLE sera has been shown to contain factors that cause the release of serotonin from normal platelets.[G152] These plasma factors probably include circulating immune complexes and specific antiplatelet antibodies. In addition, the level of platelet-activating factor (PAF), a mediator of inflammation with a wide range of biologic activities, including platelet activation, is increased in the plasma of SLE patients with active disease.[T124] PAF, which is synthesized by a number of cell types, after immunologic stimulation, including monocytes, macrophages, granulocytes, platelets, and endothelial cells, may be involved in SLE.[C54]

Studies in experimental models of immune complex glomerulonephritis have established that platelets participate in the pathogenesis of renal injury. Platelets can facilitate the deposition of immune complexes and augment the subsequent inflammatory response. The involvement of platelets in SLE nephritis has been examined. By infusing radiolabeled autologous platelets to patients with diffuse lupus nephritis, Clark et al.[C284] found the sequestration of platelets not only in the spleen and liver, but also in the kidneys, suggesting intrarenal platelet consumption. Complexes of DNA and specific anti-DNA that are important in lupus glomerulonephritis, have been identified on the surface of platelets of SLE patients.[F193] Moreover, Duffus et al.[D349] have localized platelet surface antigens and platelet factor 4 at sites of glomerular injury in SLE

THROMBOTIC THROMBOCYTOPENIC PURPURA

Thrombotic thrombocytopenic purpura (TTP) is a diffuse disorder of the microcirculation of unknown cause characterizd by a pentad of fever, thrombocytopenic purpura, microangiopathic hemolytic anemia (MAHA), fluctuating neurologic findings, and renal dysfunction. It is a rare disorder, usually seen in women aged 10 to 40 years, and may follow a prodrome of upper respiratory tract symptoms or arthralgias and myalgias.[R204] Patients present with nonspecific constitutional symptoms, including malaise, fatigue, weakness, and fever. Therefore, the other manifestations appear in rapid sequence, often baffling the clinician by the subtle appearance and diversity of features. Delays in establishing a correct diagnosis are not uncommon. Half of patients experience neurologic symptoms at presentation, most commonly headaches, confusion, and paresis. MAHA is diagnosed by the presence of fragmented red blood cells (schizocytes), nucleated red blood cells, an elevated LDH level, reticulocytosis, negative Coombs' test, indirect hyperbilirubinemia, and hemoglobulinuria. Severe thrombocytopenia is a characteristic finding. Coagulation parameters are generally normal or shown only mild abnormalities, such as elevation of fibrin split products. Pathologically, intravascular microthrombi consisting of fibrin and platelet aggregates in capillaries and precapillary arterioles in several organs are found. No histologic evidence of vasculitis is seen. Systemic corticosteroids, antiplatelet agents, splenectomy, plasma infusions, and plasmapheresis are among the therapies used. Despite this, the mortality rate of TTP remains high, about 50%, but this is significantly better than the cumulative experience prior to 1965,[R204] when over 90% of patients succumbed to their disease.

The association between TTP and SLE has been debated for years.[G65] In 1964, Levine and Shearn[L219] reviewed the English literature, emphasizing the possible relationship to SLE. They presented 2 cases of their own showing overlapping features and analyzed 147 cases reported with adequate autopsy protocols. In 34 cases, (23%) evidence of concomitant SLE was found. Libman-Sacks endocarditis was noted in 25 patients, onion ring changes in the spleen in 8, wire loop glomeruli in 7, and positive LE cell test in 5. Patients with features of both SLE and TTP appeared to constitute a clinical variant, and had a higher female predominance, a higher frequency of biologic false-positive tests for syphilis, elevated serum globulin levels, splenomegaly, arthritis and arthralgia, and pleuritis. Amorosi and Ulman[A187] found 13 cases of SLE among 271 cases of

TTP reviewed. In contrast, other investigators concluded that the combination of SLE and TTP is rare.[F179,R204] When prior reports were reviewed using the 1982 SLE criteria, Fox et al.[F214] found 4 unequivocal SLE patients who developed TTP along the course of the illness and 1 who developed both SLE and TTP concurrently.[A158,C176,D128,O14] TTP can antedate the onset of SLE, and can also occur as a terminal event in SLE.[A158,C176,G65,R27,R147] Dixit et al. reported a patient with probable SLE, C2 deficiency, and chronic relapsing TTP.[D231]

The treatment of TTP associated with SLE is similar to that for ITP. Systemic corticosteroids[159] and plasma infusion, with or without plasmapheresis,[G84] have been used successfully in a few cases. A Canadian study of 102 patients has shown that plasma exchange alone with fresh-frozen plasma is more effective than infusion in the treatment of TTP.[R254]

The cause of TTP is not known. Several mechanisms have been proposed to explain the microvascular thrombosis, including the presence of serum platelet-aggregating factor, circulating immune complexes, endothelial injury, defects in the fibrinoloytic system, and prostacyclin abnormalities.[S408] TTP may be caused by a number of different factors. In SLE, Itoh et al.[159] suggested the role of antiplatelet antibodies in the development of TTP in some patients. The importance of antiphospholipid antibodies has yet to be examined.

White Blood Cell Disorders

White Cell Count and Leukopenia. The characteristic change in the leukocyte count in SLE, first observed in 1923 by Goeckerman,[G213] is a depression of the white blood cells to 2,000 to 4,500/mm^3. In large series of SLE patients reported in the literature, leukopenia was observed in over 50%.[D340,E147,G386,L75,M280]

Leukopenia, defined as a white blood cell count of below 4,500/mm^3 was noted in 43% of Dubois's 520 patients and in 66% of Estes and Christian's 150 patients (see Table 33–1).[D340,E147] Severe leukopenia, with counts below 2,000/mm^3, was uncommon. Of 122 SLE patients of Harvey et al.[M280] who had blood count determinations done at frequent intervals, 75 patients and counts below 5,000/mm^3, but in only 4 was the count below 2,000/mm^3. Larson[L75] found 18% of 200 patients had leukocyte counts below, 4,500/mm^3 on two or more occasions, and the usual range of leukopenia was 2,500 to 3,500/mm^3. Among 111 hospitalized SLE patients, Michael et al.[M280] found a white blood cell below 500/mm^3 in 66 patients at some time, so that 60% of the total patient group had leukopenia. In Ropes' series[R294] of 142 patients, a white cell count less than 4,000/mm^3 was found in 67%, but in 12% of patients, the white cell count was always normal.

Leukopenia in SLE has been shown to be significantly associated with a high frequency of skin rash, lymphopenia, and elevated anti-DNA titer. Anemia, fatigue, arthritis, anemia, and elevated sedimentation rate were also more common in leukopenic patients.[F263] A leukocyte count of 4,000/mm^3, occasionally as low as 2,500 mm^3, may occur in patients with active and untreated discoid LE. This may rise after treatment of the skin lesions with antimalarials.

Differential White Cell Count. An increase of non-segmented neutrophils in SLE patients was first reported by Rose and Pillsbury.[R299] This increase was observed in patients with normal as well as elevated total white cell count.[M387] Estes and Christian[E147] noted a normal differential count in 50% of their leukopenic patients. These data are similar to the findings of other investigators.

Of 111 patients studied by Michael and associates,[M387] 64 had an increase in nonsegmented neutrophils, together with an increase in mature granulocytes. Also, 14 patients had 1 to 7% myelocytes when first seen, and a few others showed a similar increase in later counts. This occurred more frequently in patients with normal or low white cell counts than in those with elevated total leukocyte counts. Prior to the institution of therapy, 24% of 105 patients of Harvey et al.[M280] had neutrophilic granulocyte counts of 80 to 89%, and 5% of patients had counts over 90%. More than 5% juvenile forms were noted in 30% of patients.

Eosinophilia. In our experience, eosinophilia is uncommon in SLE patients without concomitant parasite infection, allergic reaction, or some other known cause. Eosinophilia is not mentioned in several series of patients in the literature.[E147,F263,G386,L140] In contrast, earlier workers observed that eosinophilia is not rare in SLE. In Larson's series[L75] of 200, 10% had counts of 3% or more and 5 patients had persistent eosinophilia in excess of 10%. Harvey et al.[232] found eosinophilia of 3% or more in 15 of 46 patients studied prior to therapy. Of these, 2 had counts of 17 and 24%, respectively, associated with extensive skin lesions and not attributable to causes other than SLE. Direct eosinophil counts were done in 60 patients. Counts of less than 50/mm^3 were found in 31 patients, between 50 and 100/mm^3 in 11, between 100 and 200/mm^3 in 10, between 200 and 400/mm^3 in 6, and more than 400/mm^3 in only 2. Ropes[R294] observed a high prevalence of eosinophilia—eosinophil count of more than 5% was seen in 21% of 142 patients at some time along the course of the illness. Michael et al.[M387] noted an eosinophil count of over 3% in 6 of 111 untreated patients (14%).

Basophils. Hunsiker and Brun[H197] enumerated basophils in patients with various skin disorders and found a moderate reduction of basophils in those with discoid LE and a marked diminution in SLE patients. Egido et al.[E41] found the absolute basophil counts in SLE to be inversely related to anti-DNA antibodies and the level of circulating immune complexes and to be directly related to serum complement level. Basophils and tissue mast cells possess receptors specific to the Fc fragment of IgE antibodies. If such antibodies are cross linked by binding to antigen, basophils and mast cells degranulate releasing granules that contain vasoactive substances, producing a hypersensitivity allergic reaction. High levels of IgE have been found on the surface of basophils in SLE patients. More importantly, SLE basophils underwent degranulation when incubated with soluble DNA antigen, suggesting the presence of cell-bound, specific IgE anti-DNA antibodies. Although renal deposits of IgE have been reported in SLE patients, the pathogenic role of these antibodies remains to be established.

Granulocytopenia. This occurs infrequently in SLE patients, and can have a number of causes, including drug reaction, severe infection, decreased bone marrow production, and destruction mediated by antigranulocyte antibodies. At times, the total white blood cell count may decrease to levels as low as 1,000/mm^3 without any other apparent cause than SLE. Nevertheless, in this situation, the physician should always be aware of the possibility that the granulocytopenia may be a result of medications used in SLE, such as antimalarials.[D310,M280] We have observed agranulocytosis in SLE caused by atabrine, levamisole, and triethylenemelamine.[D307] Agranulocytosis in SLE has occurred as a result of reaction to sulfadiazine.[A50] McDuffie[M272] reported three SLE patients who developed agranulocytosis secondary to medications that are not commonly associated with blood dyscrasias—hydroxychloroquine, dextropropoxyphene, and nitrofurantoin. Bone marrow examination showed the absence of myeloid precursors in two patients and aplastic changes in the third patient.

Both humoral and cell-mediated immune mechanisms have been shown to be important in the pathogenesis of neutropenia in SLE. Starkebaum et al.[S617] examined the in vivo neutrophil kinetics of a lupus patient with severe neutropenia and found changes indicative of increased peripheral destruction of granulocytes combined with ineffective granulocytopoiesis by the bone marrow. Elevated levels of surface-bound IgG were detected on the patient's neutrophils. Monomeric IgG antibodies, but not immune complexes, isolated from the serum of the patient opsonized normal neutrophils for in vitro ingestion by other phagocytic cells. These observations provide the basis for the role of humoral factors in some cases of neutropenia. In addition, Hadley et al.[H114] found an inverse correlation between the neutrophil count and the ability of SLE sera to opsonize granulocytes for recognition and clearance by human monocytes. Impairment of reticuloendothelial system function in SLE[F213] may allow antibody-sensitized granulocytes to remain in the circulation. The number of progenitor cells of granulocyte and monocytes in the bone marrow (colony-forming unit–culture, CFU-C) has been found to be reduced in SLE patients, and this correlated with the peripheral granulocyte and monocyte counts.[Y20] Moreover, T lymphocytes suppressed the generation of autologous bone marrow CFU-C in vitro, suggesting a role of cell-mediated mechanisms in the impairment of granulopoiesis in SLE.

In the presence of infection in the patient who is not receiving systemic corticosteroids, leukocyte counts may often rise to 15,000 to 20,000/mm^3. Unfortunately, other SLE patients may have intercurrent infections without a demonstrable rise in the white cell count, so this valuable guide cannot be depended on. Marked leukocytosis with counts above 30,000/mm^3 has been observed by us and others in the presence of concomitant infections. During treatment with corticosteroids, the usual range of leukocytosis is 15,000 to 25,000/mm^3, regardless of the initial white blood cell count.

Bone Marrow Granulocyte Reserve. The leukocytosis that occurs following the administration of endotoxin, etiocholanolone, or glucocorticoids is primarily caused by the release of polymorphonuclear neutrophils (PMN) from bone marrow reserves.[D16] The amount of PMN reserve is considered to be important in the host defense against infections, and also serves as a guide in predicting the ability of the patient to tolerate a myelotoxic drug. Paulus et al.[P78] found the granulocyte reserve measured by etiocholanolone injection in SLE patients with nephritis was higher in those on azathioprine than in those on no medications or in patients on combined prednisone and azathioprine therapy. Kimball et al.[K209] found that 62% of 59 SLE patients had an abnormally low granulocyte reserve when challenged with etiocholanolone. No correlation among deficient granulocyte reserve and other clinical or laboratory parameters was found. Most of their patients were on corticosteroids, however, which are now known to challenge the bone marrow reserves,[D16] so that possibly the administration of etiocholanolone did not augment the maximally stimulated bone marrow, resulting in a "subnormal" response.[B556] This subnormal response of untreated SLE patients to etiocholanolone suggests that the disease itself can suppress bone marrow reserves. Evidence suggesting the role of circulating humoral factor(s) for this abnormality has been described.[K209]

The number of bisegmented neutrophils (Pelger's anomaly) was significantly higher and lymphocyte count lower in patients with leukopenia associated with SLE and other autoimmune disorders.[R225]

Lymphocyte Counts. It is now recognized that lymphopenia is one of the most common hematologic findings in SLE.[G386,R227] Early investigators noted lymphopenia but failed to emphasize it, probably because relative percentages rather than absolute numbers of lymphocytes in the peripheral blood were used.[M280,M387] The mechanism of lymphopenia in SLE is not clear. The role of antilymphocyte antibodies, the distribution of lymphocyte subsets, and abnormalities of lymphocyte functions are discussed in Chapter 26.

Debarre et al.[D112] followed lymphocyte counts in 19 SLE patients and noted that lymphopenia developed in 84% during the acute stage, and was associated with an increased sedimentation rate. At remission the number of lymphocytes increased and the sedimentation rate fell. Grigor et al. found absolute lymphopenia to be more common than leukopenia.[G386]

Rivero et al.[R227] examined the occurrence and significance of lymphopenia in 158 SLE patients. At diagnosis, 75% of patients had a significantly reduced absolute lymphocyte count but, on follow-up, additional patients became lymphopenic, so the total cumulative frequency of absolute lymphopenia was 93%. Lymphopenia was found to be independent of, although contributory, to leukopenia, so these two findings were not primarily interrelated. Absolute lymphopenia was correlated with disease activity, and patients with an absolute lymphocyte count of less than 1,500 cells/mm^3 at diagnosis had a higher frequency of fever, polyarthritis, and central nervous system involvement, but a lower prevalence of thrombocytopenia and/or hemolytic anemia.

Table 43–2 summarizes the changes in red cells, platelets, and white cells in SLE patients.

Table 43–2. Red Cells, White Blood Cells, and
Platelets in SLE

1. Anemia occurs in over 50% of all patients at some time during the
   course of the disease. Anemia can result from one or a combination
   of factors, including chronic disease, autoimmune hemolysis, iron
   deficiency, and chronic renal failure.
2. Autoimmune hemolytic anemia caused by the presence of warm-
   reacting IgG antibodies to red blood cells develops in up to 16% of
   patients, and may be the presenting manifestation of the disease. The
   anemia responds to steroid therapy. A combined warm and cold
   antibody type of autoimmune hemolytic anemia occasionally occurs.
3. Leukopenia is common, and may be the result of active disease or a
   drug reaction. Lymphopenia is a characteristic finding in patients
   with untreated and active SLE. In vitro studies of granulocyte function
   are generally abnormal in SLE.
4. Leukocytosis in SLE is associated with a concurrent infection or corticosteroid therapy.
5. A platelet count lower than 150,000/mm^3 is seen in 7 to 52% of
   patients (mean, 14%). In vitro platelet functions, including aggregation in response to collagen, are frequently abnormal in SLE.
6. Autoimmune thrombocytopenic purpura is not uncommon in SLE.
   Three to 15% of patients diagnosed as having idiopathic autoimmune
   hemolytic anemia go on to develop classic SLE.
7. Thrombotic thrombocytopenic purpura is a rare, life-threatening
   complication of SLE. It is characterized by fever, renal dysfunction,
   microangiopathic hemolytic anemia, thrombocytopenia, and neurologic abnormalities.

Granulocyte Function in SLE

To understand the importance of granulocyte function
as a factor in the susceptibility of SLE patients to infections, studies have been undertaken to examine the phagocytic, opsonizing, chemotactic, and oxidative functions
of neutrophils and monocytes. Most of these studies concluded that, in general, granulocyte function in SLE is abnormal, but the specific qualitative and quantitative abnormalities reported were inconsistent or contradictory. (See
also Chapter 14.)

Phagocytosis and Opsonization. Brandt and
Hedberg[B460] reported that the ability of neutrophils of
SLE patients to ingest yeast particles is significantly lower
than that of normal subjects or of rheumatoid arthritis
patients. Phagocytic activity was not reduced when normal granulocytes were suspended in normal plasma. The
lowest phagocytic activity tended to be associated with
neutropenia. Orozco et al.[O98] confirmed this observation,
and found that the phagocytosis of Escherichia coli by SLE
leukocytes decreased by 62% in those with active disease.
In contrast to Brandt et al.,[B460] they observed that the
phagocytic activity normalized if the SLE granulocytes
were incubated with fresh normal serum rather than with
SLE serum. The presence of serum factor(s) that inhibits
phagocytosis in SLE has also been reported by others,[H66,Z55] although the nature of this factor is not known.
Sera from SLE patients with active disease failed to support
normal granulocytes in phagocytosis, indicating a defect
in opsonic capability. The low serum complement level,
rather than a deficiency in "natural" antibodies, was the
limiting factor in the deficient serum opsonic activity of
SLE sera.[O98] The initial rate of phagocytosis of lipopolysac-
charide-coated paraffin droplets by neutrophils from untreated active SLE patients was significantly lower than
that in normal subjects.[L44] In contrast to the above results,

Al-Hadithy and associates[A140] found the phagocytosis of
Candida by neutrophils of SLE patients to be normal when
the patients were considered as a group, but, 20% of their
patients had impaired phagocytic values. In addition, Hal-
gren et al.[H66] described an increased ability of SLE granulocytes to phagocytose IgG-coated latex particles in a ser-
um-free system to exclude the effects of circulating
inhibitors.

Chemotaxis and Migration. The in vitro chemotactic response of neutrophils of SLE patients when compared as a group to that of healthy subjects has been observed to be normal.[A170,C282] Clark et al.[C282] noted that
the generation of chemotactic factors in SLE serum was
clearly depressed, and that the defect correlated with an
elevated titer of anti-DNA antibodies, low serum immunoglobulin level, and high frequency of infections. Alvarez et
al.[A170] showed that the generation of serum chemotactic
activity by the classic pathway of complement, but not
by the alternative pathway, was impaired in SLE patients.
Serum inhibitors of chemotaxis, including a specific inhibitor of C5-derived chemotactic activity, have also been
found in SLE patients.[A170]

Oxidative Functions. Wenger and Bole[W176] investigated the reduction of nitroblue tetrazolium (NBT) dye
by peripheral blood leukocytes of SLE patients, and found
the activity to be low in resting leukocytes. When the
leukocytes were stimulated by allowing them to phagocytose latex particles, an incremental increase in NBT dye
reduction comparable to that seen in healthy individuals
was noted. On the other hand, neutrophils from SLE patients who were infected failed to demonstrate the anticipated increase in NBT dye reduction. Others have confirmed the abnormal NBT dye reduction test results in SLE
patients.[B268,L44] This test is considered to be a measure
of the oxidative events associated with phagocytosis and
intracellular killings, so it futher supports the role of abnormal granulocyte function in the increased incidence
of infection in those with SLE.

The apparent inconsistencies in the studies of in vitro
SLE grandulocyte function by various investigators probably reflect differences in methodology and in the selection
of patients. This also emphasizes the importance of other
factors that affect these tests, such as the use of steroids
and other drugs, activity of SLE, and the presence of inhibitory factors in the serum. The clinical significance of in
vitro functional abnormalities is not entirely clear, but in
vivo studies in SLE by the Rebuck skin window technique
have shown abnormalities in granulocyte functions.[G112]
Whether the observed abnormalities in granulocyte function are primary cellular defects or are secondary to the
disease process is not completely clear. Hurd et al.[H508]
have postulated that the ingestion of immune complexes
by SLE neutrophils can alter their functions. In vitro exposure of normal granulocytes to SLE sera, especially those
from patients with active disease, resulted in increased
adhesiveness, aggregation, and oxygenation activity.[A14,H194,V74] Activated granulocytes can then contribute
to the development of vasculitis, central nervous system
involvement, and leukopenia, as well as to increased susceptibility to infection.

Chapter 44

SYSTEMIC LUPUS ERYTHEMATOSUS IN CHILDHOOD AND ADOLESCENCE

THOMAS J. A. LEHMAN

Children and adolescents with systemic lupus erythematosus (SLE) represent both a special challenge and a special opportunity. Early onset allows observation of the natural history of SLE, free from the confounding factors that are present in older patients, and demonstrates its diversity. The impact of SLE on children and adolescents, however, is often profound. Special considerations related to ongoing physical and emotional growth directly influence the choice of medications and their likelihood of success.

Success in caring for children and adolescents with SLE requires awareness of the complex interaction between the child's illness and the needs of the family. Children and adolescents are emotionally immature individuals, just beginning to formulate their concept of "self." They are extremely vulnerable to the psychologic impact of chronic illness and to medications that can dramatically alter appearance (Fig. 44–1). Family and peer group pressures, which are difficult for normal children, may be overwhelming for the child or adolescent with SLE. For optimal results, excellent medical care must be coupled with multidisciplinary patient and family education and support. It is these special needs that make caring for children and adolescents with SLE distinct.

Childhood-onset SLE is often described as more severe[M341] than adult-onset disease, and early age of onset has been correlated with a worse prognosis.[G162] Some studies, however, have suggested an improved prognosis for children and adolescents with SLE.[A10,L173] In published series, a large proportion of children and adolescents with SLE have significant renal or central nervous system involvement,[C2,C147,C375,F105,G49,G197,J26,K232,M341,W54] but mild SLE may be underrepresented. The most important risk of early onset is delayed diagnosis. Damage to the evolving self-image of children and adolescents with chronic disease may significantly effect the prognosis.

English language reports of children with SLE appeared as early as 1892.[S717] Sequeira and Balean, writing from the London Hospital in 1902,[S284] noted, that "the disease commences early in life in a much larger proportion of cases than is commonly believed." Eight children with SLE were among 71 cases they reported. Reports of SLE in childhood continued to appear throughout the 1920s, 1930s, and 1940s.[D164,D285,J24,L434,P94,S688]

The modern era began in the 1950s and 1960s with reports of series of children with SLE. Zetterstrom and Berglund described 10 patients in 1956,[Z21] and Gribetz and Henley described an additional 15 in 1959.[G372] Between 1960 and 1968, more than 150 additional children with SLE were described.[C375,J26,M341,P149] The total number of children with SLE in published series now exceeds 500.[C2,C147,C346,F105,G197,G226,K232,L173,N131,W54]

In the presteroid era, childhood-onset SLE was a rapidly evolving and usually fatal multisystem disease. From the 1960s onward, corticosteroids and improved pediatric care have resulted in enhanced survival.[A10,P221] SLE is now a common diagnosis in every large pediatric rheumatology program. With proper care, most children and adolescents with SLE have an excellent prognosis. Systematic management and vigorous treatment protocols are rapidly improving the outlook, even for children with the most severe disease.

EPIDEMIOLOGY

Despite the many published cases of children SLE, its true incidence and prevalence are unknown.[S473] Fessel's 1973 survey of 126,000 members of the Kaiser Permanente plan did not report any patients with onset before 15 years of age.[F74] Siegel and Lee estimated the annual incidence of SLE in childhood to be 0.6/100,000.[S416] Hochberg found a similar incidence in Baltimore.[H340] Efforts to develop a central registry for children with SLE to provide demographically diverse information are underway.

The prevalence of childhood SLE can only be estimated. Figures from the regional referral center in Los Angeles suggest about 5,000 to 10,000 children with SLE in the United States.[L173] A similar estimate arises from the assumption that children with SLE are 10% as common as children with juvenile rheumatoid arthritis (JRA).[S473] (The corresponding prevalence of SLE is 5 to 10/100,000 children,[B125,G46,G110,T197] again suggesting 5,000 to 10,000 children with SLE in the US.) Unfortunately, these figures represent only a first approximation of SLE's true prevalence in children and adolescents.

The influences of sex and racial origin on the occurrence of SLE are widely recognized.[L173,S286,S416] In childhood, the influence of race is striking. The age- and sex-adjusted prevalences of SLE in black, Oriental, and Hispanic children were more than threefold that of white children[L173] at one large center. The influences of female sex, age, and race were even more striking when the inci-

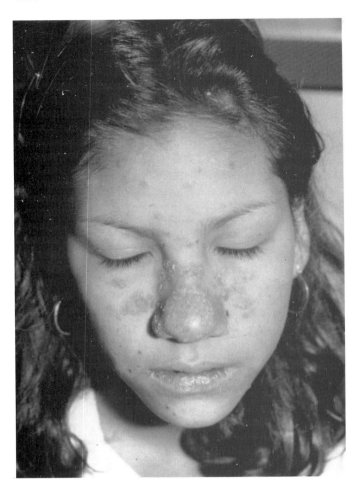

Fig. 44–1. Markedly altered facial appearance resulting from skin manifestations in a teenage female with SLE.

dence of SLE among prepubertal and postpubertal children of various races was considered. For all male children, the frequency of SLE rose from 1/100,000 male children, aged 1 through 9 years, to 1.61/100,000 male children, aged 10 through 19 years (thus, a 60% increase with puberty). For white females, the increase with puberty was from 1.27 to 4.40/100,000 (246%); for black females, the increase was 3.72 to 19.86/100,000 (434%); and for Oriental females, it was 6.16 to 31.14/100,000 (406%). In contrast, the increase for Hispanic females was only 4.62 to 13.00/100,000 (181%).[L173] These data (based on a limited sample) suggest that the relative influence of sex hormones in predisposition to SLE varies among races.

CAUSATIVE FACTORS

The cause of SLE remains unknown. The availability of parents and siblings who live in the same household as children with SLE provides a unique opportunity to evaluate environmental and genetic hypotheses. Many studies have demonstrated an increased frequency of immunologic abnormalities in first-degree relatives of both adults

and children with SLE.[C296,L70,L71,L72,L74,L169,L171,L176,L189, L396,M173,M614,P237,S540] These studies have been interpreted both as evidence of an infectious cause and of a genetic predisposition. These theories are discussed in detail in other chapters.

Much of the evidence for a genetic predisposition to SLE has come from studies of twin and sibling pairs. Many twin pairs have the onset of SLE in childhood or adolescence. Identical twins with the onset of SLE as early as 3 years of age have been reported.[L275] The percentage of identical twins concordant for lupus may be as high as 70%,[B347] but this figure has been challenged. When twins both develop SLE, they typically have the onset of disease at a closer and earlier age than do siblings who develop SLE (16.5 ± 7.9 versus 26.2 ± 20.5 years).[K59]

Additional evidence of a genetic component for SLE has arisen from the study of immunologic abnormalities in family members of children with SLE. Expression of this genetic component appears to be promoted by female sex hormones. In a study of 34 families containing children with SLE, it was found that Ro/SSA–antibody-positive mothers were more likely to have Ro/SSA–antibody-positive daughters than Ro/SSA–negative-mothers (7/11 versus 4/18, p < .05—probands excluded). This was not true for sons or for fathers. Ro/SSA–antibody-positive fathers, however, had fewer male children than expected (5 sons/12 daughters versus 19 sons/19 daughters, p < .05).[L175]

Children with SLE represent a unique contribution to the "supergene" hypothesis. Formulated in response to the occurrence of multiple autoimmune diseases within some families,[H343] this hypothesis proposes the existence of a single gene that predisposes to autoimmune disease. Autoimmune disease in carriers of the gene is determined by its interaction with the remainder of the genome and environmental events. Efforts to evaluate this hypothesis require a means of identifying carriers of the supergene. The increased frequency and amount of antibodies to Ro/SSA in the mothers of children with SLE may be the necessary evidence of gene expression in otherwise well individuals.[L176] Ro/SSA antibody expression is linked to histocompatibility antigens in patients with SLE and Sjögren's syndrome.[H137] Efforts to link Ro/SSA expression to a specific haplotype in children with SLE and their families are underway.

An increased frequency of SLE in childhood occurs in children with defects of the immune system. This is especially true of genetic defects in the complement system (most often C2 or C4 deficiency).[A57,D281,F82,G111,G183,O8, S107,S670] Such an association may occur because the genes controlling C4 synthesis are closely linked to the HLA histocompatibility complex.[F82,S109] HLA linkages in this region have been demonstrated for adults with SLE, but have not been independently evaluated in children.[N94,W170]

IgA deficiency is another defect of immune function that occurs more frequently than expected among children with SLE.[C2,C144,C438] IgA deficiency was found in only 0.03% of the normal population, but in 4.6% of children with SLE.[C144] The association of SLE in childhood with defects in the immune system may indicate that defective antigen processing predisposes to the development of

SLE. The development of discoid lupus and, in one case, SLE in children with chronic granulomatous disease and their mothers, is another observation suggesting that defective antigen processing may predispose to the development of SLE.[B111,M119,S107]

Despite the association between defective immunoglobulin or complement function and SLE, treatment with intravenous immunoglobulin therapy has not been of convincing benefit. Most patients with SLE are hypergammaglobulinemic, even if IgA-deficient. Furthermore, because IgA is a secretory immunoglobulin, intravenous immunoglobulin therapy is unlikely to result in the restoration of effective mucosal immunity in IgA-deficient individuals.

Children and adolescents with SLE are a valuable resource for large-scale efforts to understand its genetics and molecular biology. The opportunity to study SLE in populations such as young white males (who lack the known predisposing factors) may result in the identification of new risk factors. Each risk factor is a piece in the puzzle that might ultimately lead to the understanding of SLE's pathogenesis.[L176]

CLINICAL MANIFESTATIONS

Unexplained fever, malaise, and weight loss are the most common manifestations of SLE in children and adolescents. Because these symptoms may be associated with many chronic illnesses, the physician should seek evidence of the following: arthritis or a photosensitive rash; hematuria or proteinuria; and hypocomplementemia. Any of these findings should prompt consideration of SLE, but their presence cannot be relied on. On initial evaluation, the patient and family often do not describe findings such as alopecia or photosensitivity unless specifically questioned, because they do not relate them to the presenting complaint. The reported frequency of many complaints varies widely among series, reflecting selection and referral criteria (Table 44–1).

In contrast to children who present with chronic illness, some children and adolescents with SLE are acutely ill at presentation. These children may present with seizures, psychosis, uremia, profound anemia, pulmonary hemorrhage, or sepsis as their initial manifestation.[P170]

The diagnosis of SLE in children and adolescents is based on criteria developed by the American Rheumatism Association (ARA) for use in adults.[T46] Classification as "definite" SLE is based on the fulfillment of four criteria, but SLE should not be automatically discarded in children who meet only three. The ARA criteria are useful guidelines, but fulfillment of four does not exclude other diagnoses, and failure to fulfill four does not definitely exclude SLE. Antinuclear antibody (ANA) testing is useful, but a positive test is not sufficient for the diagnosis of SLE in childhood.

Renal Disease

Renal disease is evident in approximately two-thirds of children and adolescents with SLE.[C2,C147,C375,F105,G49, G197,J26,K232,M341,M596,W54] Renal manifestations range from mild glomerulitis with a normal urine sediment to sudden renal failure.[F157,P170] The most common signs of renal involvement are hematuria, proteinuria, and hypertension. Although children and their families may complain of malaise, headache, swollen feet, and/or swollen eyelids (if nephrotic syndrome is present), the signs of renal involvement are commonly silent in childhood.

Renal biopsy of children and adolescents with SLE without regard to clinical manifestations demonstrates varying degrees of renal involvement in nearly every case.[F157,O12,S609] Although most children with a normal urine sediment have only mild glomerulitis, diffuse proliferative glomerulonephritis (DPGN) may be present. The significance of silent DPGN is uncertain. Series reporting follow-up of silent nephritis in SLE have described a benign prognosis.[F157,O12,S609] Most centers agree that renal biopsy may be deferred if the creatinine clearance and urinalysis are normal. Renal biopsy should be performed to investigate unexplained changes in renal function, and when considering or monitoring the effects of aggressive therapy.[M85]

Renal involvement in childhood SLE is categorized according to the World Health Organization (WHO) criteria.[M263] Mild glomerulitis is the most benign form, followed by focal segmental glomerulonephritis and membranous glomerulonephritis. DPGN carries the greatest risk of chronic renal failure. DPGN was found in 54% of children who were biopsied because of abnormal urine sediment, but only 20% of children had DPGN in a series in which all children with SLE were biopsied.[A10,C147,G197, K232,L152,P221] Combining the data from several large series, 42% of children (108 in 256) had DPGN at the time of initial biopsy, 26% had either mild glomerulitis or no abnormality, 25% had focal glomerulitis, and 6% had membranous glomerulonephritis.

Focal glomerulonephritis and membranous glomerulonephritis are generally benign, but either may progress to DPGN, with ultimate renal failure.[A10,D351,G49,K232,M263, M429,P221,R426] Repeat renal biopsy should be performed in these patients if renal function continues to deteriorate. Longterm studies indicate that renal scarring (chronicity

Table 44–1. Clinical Manifestations of SLE in Children and Adults*

Parameter	Cassidy[C147] 1977	King[K232] 1977	Wallace[P216] 1991
No. of cases			
Renal involvement	86	61	28
Hypertension	28	—	25
Musculoskeletal findings	76	79	91
Cutaneous	76	70	55
Photosensitivity	16	—	37
Hair loss	20	—	31
Oral, nasal ulceration	16	—	19
Cardiac involvement	47	17	12
Pulmonary involvement	36	19	12
CNS involvement	31	13	11
Anemia	47	—	30
Leukopenia	71	—	51
Thrombocytopenia	24	—	16

* The findings from Cassidy and King represent two large pediatric series; those from Wallace represent a large adult series.

index) is a better predictor of ultimate outcome than the WHO classification.[A362,M263,R426] In the absence of scarring active disease, including glomerular crescents, is not automatically associated with a poor prognosis.[M429,R426] Most children with SLE do not develop renal disease more than 2 years following diagnosis,[C147,M341] but one-third of those with significant renal disease lack evidence of renal involvement at presentation.

The sudden onset of renal failure in a child with SLE may be a result of active nephritis,[P170] but alternative explanations must be appropriately excluded. Renal vein thrombosis and renal artery thrombosis are other causes of sudden renal deterioration in children with SLE. Both are more frequent in association with anticardiolipin antibodies.[A337,O116] Drugs that interfere with glomerular filtration or are directly nephrotoxic must be considered. A mild rise in the blood urea nitrogen level usually follows the initiation of acetylsalicylic acid or other nonsteroidal anti-inflammatory drugs (NSAIDs) in patients with renal involvement.

Mild clinical manifestations of renal involvement are usually well controlled with corticosteroids and diuretics. Persistent renal disease may require immunsuppressive therapy.[L177] Chronic glomerular scarring is retarded by the use of cyclophosphamide, but it is not known if it is stopped.[B64] The major concern of the physician caring for a child with lupus nephritis is the preservation of sufficient renal function to support normal growth and development. For adolescent females, this includes preservation of adequate renal function to support pregnancy.

Current treatment regimens for children and adolescents with SLE have led to a steady improvement in 5- and 10-year renal function survival. It is not clear whether these improvements result in significantly enhanced survival at 20 and 30 years. Maintaining adequate renal function is important for children and adolescents with SLE. In contrast to adults, they do poorly on longterm dialysis.[M263] Children with SLE coming to dialysis often die of sepsis or other complications within the first year.

Children whose proteinuria and hematuria improve with corticosteroid therapy but whose creatinine clearance slowly deteriorates are of particular concern. Often, these children do well over a 5-year period, but progress to renal failure between 5 and 10 years following diagnosis. Routine monitoring of creatinine clearance and early intervention if deterioration is evident are important. If chronic deterioration is evident, the clinician should intervene aggressively while adequate function to support growth development can be preserved. Adult series suggest that maintaining a creatinine clearance of 70 ml/min/ 1.75 m^2 is adequate,[A360,B64] but intervention at this point may not preserve sufficient renal function for the satisfactory growth and development of children and adolescents.

Optimal therapy for children and adolescents with lupus nephritis remains uncertain. The systematic use of intermittent intravenous cyclophosphamide has been successful for children with DPGN, and useful for children with membranous glomerulonephritis.[L177] Others have reported excellent results with the combined use of large doses of prednisone and, when necessary, azathio-prine.[F105,P221,U29] Routine use of intravenous cyclophosphamide has the advantage of allowing accurate assessment of patient compliance, because the patient must be evaluated before each dose of cyclophosphamide. This allows the physician to monitor renal function status and clinical status, minimizing complications.

All recommended regimens for the treatment of lupus nephritis fail in some patients. Continued efforts to improve care are necessary for these children and adolescents, who may relentlessly progress to renal failure and often death. Systematic therapy modeled on the oncologic experience may hold the key to enhanced survival for children and adolescents with severe lupus nephritis.[L167,L168] Evolution of current therapeutic regimens to include multiple agents given at fixed intervals is under investigation.

Central Nervous System Manifestations

Psychosis, sudden personality change, seizures, chorea, transverse myelitis, peripheral neuropathy, and pseudotumor cerebri may all be presenting manifestations of SLE in childhood.[C447,D143,D206,F46,G124,H274,L319,L371,P36,W85,W148,Y29] Most series have reported CNS involvement in 20 to 30% of children.[C2,G197,K232,M341,P221] Mild evidence of central nervous system involvement is present in up to 45% of children and adolescents, if carefully sought.[Y29,Z21]

Subtle CNS changes, including impaired judgment and poor short-term memory, are the most common CNS manifestations of SLE.[C75,D206,L371] These alterations are often ascribed to steroid therapy or situational stress, but occur with greater frequency in SLE than other childhood rheumatic diseases that require similar corticosteroid therapy. Adolescents with SLE often have difficulty complying with their medications or appointments, and alienate their friends and family in ways that are inconsistent with their prior behavior. Physicians must be acutely aware of these changes because they may have disastrous consequences. A trial of increased corticosteroids may be beneficial in children with SLE whose behavior has become erratic or uncharacteristic, even in the absence of objective findings.

Delirium, hallucinations, seizures, and coma are the most common objective neurologic signs in childhood. Psychosis unrelated to corticosteroids typically occurs in 4 to 10% of children,[C147,K232,M341,N131,P221,Y29] Caeiro reported significant neuropsychiatric findings in 30% of children in an English series.[C2] The reported frequency of neuropsychiatric manifestations in children and adolescents with SLE is lower than in adults.[S781] This may be a true finding, or may represent a decreased appreciation of neuropsychiatric involvement in childhood.

Chorea is more frequent in children than in adults with SLE.[S781] Although it is infrequent, it has been documented as the initial manifestation of childhood SLE in multiple reports,[A287,B546,G403,H274,W148] perhaps because it is such a striking finding. Of children with SLE, 4 to 10% are affected by chorea at some point.[C147,M341,N131,P221,Y29,Z21] This increased incidence may reflect an increased sensitivity of the basal ganglia to damage by autoreactive antibodies or vascular events accompanying SLE in childhood.[A321]

Most often, acute central nervous system involvement occurs early in the natural history of childhood SLE.[B551] Frequently, it first becomes evident or worsens immediately after initiation of corticosteroid therapy. The explanation for this is uncertain. These symptoms frequently resolve with pulse methylprednisolone therapy. Late-onset CNS involvement is more often the result of stroke, uremia, or an infectious process.[L165]

The most striking consequences of CNS involvement in children and adolescents with SLE are the residua of seizures and strokes. Cognitive defects and aberrant behavior, however, present a difficult management problem. Aberrant behavior may have dramatic effects on social acceptance, grades, and compliance, thereby directly affecting both self-image and longterm prognosis. Efforts to ascribe behavioral change to a single cause are rarely successful.[C75,D206,L371] Nonspecific problems in children with diffuse CNS involvement most likely represent the combined effects of SLE, situational factors, and corticosteroid therapy. When such symptoms are present, increasing the corticosteroid dosage is more often successful than a dramatic reduction.

No single objective test for the presence of CNS-SLE is accurate in childhood. Computerized tomography (CT) scans of children and adolescents with SLE who have received longterm corticosteroids commonly demonstrate diffuse cortical atrophy.[B227,C83,G285] Alterations in cerebrospinal fluid protein or sugar levels or cell count cannot be relied on,[B551,D206,Y29] but these studies are often necessary to exclude infection and other explanations for altered CNS function.[L165] Antibodies to ribosomal P have been found to correlate with CNS manifestations of SLE in adults, but have not been comparably studied in children and adolescents.[B402]

Treatment of CNS manifestations in children and adolescents with SLE is a challenge to the physician. Because the manifestations may result from corticosteroid therapy, physicians frequently hesitate to increase the dosage. Nonetheless, this is often the most effective therapy. For severe CNS manifestations pulse methylprednisolone therapy is often effective. When these measures fail, intravenous cyclophosphamide may be beneficial. Children with short-term psychosis or coma often respond to therapy but, when significant impairment has been present for long periods, the prognosis is guarded.

Pulmonary Manifestations

Pleurisy and pleural effusions are the most common pulmonary manifestations.[D141,P230] Severe manifestations, including pneumothorax, pneumonia, chronic restrictive lung disease, pulmonary hypertension, and acute pulmonary hemorrhage may occur.[D127,D141,M205,N3,N437,P230,R18,R25,S477] Pleuritic chest pain, pleural effusions, and chronic interstitial infiltrates affect from 10 to 30% of children with SLE.[C2,G197,K232,M341,N131,P221,W54] When a series of Canadian children with SLE was reviewed for manifestations of respiratory involvement, 17 of 24 patients (77%) had evidence of pulmonary involvement.[D141]

Chronic pulmonary involvement may result in slowly progressive diaphragmatic dysfunction and restrictive lung disease. These changes appear as malaise and dyspnea on exertion.[D127,D141,M437,R25] Diaphragmatic dysfunction may contribute to frequent infection.[D127,D141] Diaphragmatic involvement, ranging from wide variation in fiber size to calcinosis, was common in autopsy specimens of children dying from SLE, and may be more common than recognized.[N3]

Significant restrictive lung disease may be present in children with normal chest roentgenograms. Children with dyspnea or tachypnea at rest should be monitored with periodic pulmonary function testing. As the ability to ameliorate the renal and CNS manifestations of SLE in children and adolescents improves, chronic pulmonary involvement is becoming an increasing concern.

The most common fatal complication of pulmonary involvement in children and adolescents with SLE is pneumonia.[N3] Pneumonia was the primary cause of death for 9 of 26 children with SLE coming to autopsy in a reported series. Pulmonary hemorrhage contributed to the death of 5 others. In contrast, renal failure and CNS involvement were the primary causes of death in only 4 and 3 children, respectively.[N3]

Pulmonary hypertension denoted by accentuation of the second heart sound is an ominous finding in children and adolescents with SLE. Once established, pulmonary hypertension progresses steadily to right-sided heart failure and death.[D127] Pulmonary hemorrhage may occur in the setting of pre-existing pulmonary hypertension or in isolation.[D127,M437,R18,R25] Sudden, unexplained pallor and tachypnea often indicate the onset of pulmonary hemorrhage.[M437] Untreated, it is rapidly fatal.

Minor manifestations of pulmonary involvement normally respond to corticosteroids.[D141,P230,S582] Deaths from pneumonia, in which Escherichia coli, Klebsiella, or Staphylococcus aureus were the predominant organisms, illustrate the need for broad-spectrum antibiotic coverage.[N3] Pneumocystis carinii and other nonbacterial organisms may be present.[G59] When pneumonia is superimposed on active pulmonary SLE or the contributions of infection and active SLE cannot be differentiated with certainty, both antibiotics and increased doses of corticosteroids may be appropriate.

Children with pulmonary hypertension may benefit symptomatically from the addition of nifedipine to reduce pulmonary vascular resistance. No therapy is known to reverse the course of this complication. Cytotoxic drugs have been ineffective. Pneumonia is a frequent complication in children with established pulmonary hypertension, and may progress rapidly to sepsis. Massive pulmonary hemorrhage may respond to large doses of corticosteroids with ventilator support and perhaps plasmapheresis or extracorporeal membrane oxygenation (ECMO).[M437,R18]

Musculoskeletal Manifestations

The arthritis of SLE is generally nondeforming and responds well to anti-inflammatory medications. Significant arthritis at presentation is found in 40 to 60% of children and adolescents. It occurs in over 80% of children at some point.[C2,C147,G110,G197,K232,M341,P221,W54] Usually, the arthritis affects the small joints of the hands and feet, with swelling and pain on motion. Asymptomatic knee effusions are frequently present in children with active disease who may not have arthritis elsewhere.

Rarely, children with well-documented juvenile rheumatoid arthritis and erosive changes develop definite SLE.[R10] These children appear to have two independent diseases. The frequency of this occurrence suggests that SLE and JRA share a common predisposition.

Avascular necrosis is the most significant musculoskeletal complication of SLE in children and adolescents. Avascular necrosis may result from SLE alone, corticosteroid therapy, or their interaction. A cross-sectional radiographic study of 35 children with SLE found evidence of avascular necrosis in 40%. These children, however, were drawn from a program that routinely uses high-dose corticosteroids (2 mg/kg/day).[B241] The frequency of avascular necrosis in a general population of children and adolescents with SLE is unknown.

Avascular necrosis usually affects the hips and knees in children with SLE. Children report the gradual onset of progressive discomfort in the affected joints. Initial evaluation may prove negative. Magnetic resonance imaging (MRI) and, later, routine roentgenography, ultimately reveal evidence of osteonecrosis. Although no clear association of avascular necrosis with total dosage of corticosteroids or mode of administration has been found, the incidence of avascular necrosis is far higher in children who have received corticosteroids.[B241,D218]

Meaningful muscle involvement is rare in children with SLE. Diffuse weakness may be the result of steroid myopathy.[138] Mild elevations of serum creatinine phosphokinase levels are often seen, but are rarely associated with clinical weakness. Antibodies to the acetylcholinesterase receptor may produce a myasthenia gravis-like picture. Transplacental passage of antibodies to this receptor is reported to have caused weakness in the child of a mother with SLE.[R202] Dermatomyositis, which may be associated with a positive ANA, arthritis, a heliotropic rash, and significant proximal muscle weakness, must be excluded if significant weakness is present.

Dermatologic Manifestations

Rashes occur frequently in children with SLE,[C2,C147,G197,K232,M341,N131,P221,W54] but only 30 to 50% ever manifest the typical butterfly rash[G197,N131] (Fig. 44-2). Vasculitis involvement of the hard palate frequently accompanies the facial rash of SLE. These lesions are a useful confirmatory sign if the cause of the facial rash is in question. Cutaneous lesions may take the form of recurrent urticaria, bullae, vasculitis nodules, or chronic ulceration. "Vasculitis" lesions are frequently a manifestation of active disease. Other dermatologic manifestations may wax and wane without exacerbations of systemic disease.

Bullous lesions resembling bullous pemphigoid are the predominant manifestations of SLE in some children.[L40] Boys with this manifestation predominant often have mild systemic disease, but little information is available about these children in the literature. Dapsone is often helpful, but has not been uniformly useful.[A87]

Dermatologic manifestations are usually not of long-

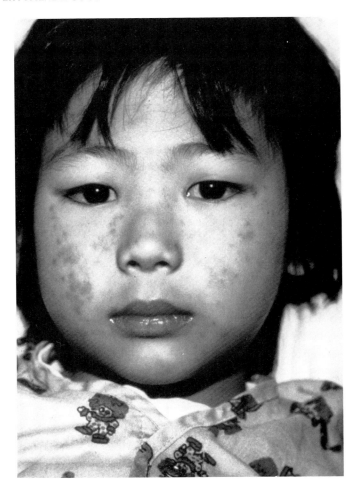

Fig. 44-2. Typical bilateral malar rash in a young oriental female with SLE.

term significance. Most respond to treatment, without significant scarring. All the dermatologic lesions of SLE may be aggravated by sun exposure. Children with SLE should be counseled to use sun-blocking agents and to avoid unnecessary sun exposure, which may provoke increased systemic disease activity. Definite photosensitivity occurs in 16% of children.[C147]

Discoid lupus erythematosus is unusual in childhood. Most children referred for DLE have systemic manifestations. Some children with DLE progress to SLE, but this is rare.[C146] Isolated DLE is of concern because of the associated disfigurement and psychologic effects.

Cardiac Manifestations

Cardiac manifestations are not prominent in children and adolescents with SLE, but occasionally they are catastrophic. Pericarditis, myocarditis, and mild valvular involvement are common.[C2,C147,K232,W54,W131,W341] Clinically evident pericarditis or myocarditis occurs in 10% of children,[G197,K232,N131,W54] but occasional series report a higher frequency.[C147,M341,N3] Rarely, children with SLE develop cardiac tamponade.[L193]

Many children with SLE are anemic and develop flow murmurs. Libman-Sacks endocarditis may occur in childhood, however, and predisposes to bacterial endocarditis. In large series of patients with SLE, bacterial endocarditis occurs with a greater than expected frequency.[L174,N3,S582] All children with significant valvular lesions must receive antibiotic coverage for dentistry and other invasive procedures. Some recommend routine bacterial endocarditis prophylaxis for all SLE patients.

Premature myocardial infarctions occur in the setting of coronary arteritis, septic thrombosis, and prolonged corticosteroid therapy.[B413,D351,E111,F250,H401,I47,S582] The association of prolonged corticosteroid therapy with premature myocardial infarction raises significant questions about the longterm safety of high-dose corticosteroid regimens.

Gastrointestinal Manifestations

Mild gastrointestinal involvement is common in children and adolescents with SLE; 30 to 40% manifest hepatomegaly or splenomegaly at diagnosis.[C147,K232,W54] Chronic abdominal pain, anorexia, weight loss, and malaise are frequent presenting complaints.[C147,G197,K232,M341,P221,W54] They often resolve with corticosteroid therapy. Abdominal pain unresponsive to corticosteroids may be the result of small-vessel vasculitis that cannot be detected by routine testing. These children may respond to a further increase in their corticosteroid dosage.[W54] Abdominal pain, however, may be the result of pancreatitis induced either by SLE, corticosteroids, or both.[B571,F148,K232,M341,N4,S454] Fulminant pancreatitis resulting in death has occurred.

Pneumatosis cystoides intestinalis may be discovered radiographically in patients who have complained of abdominal pain without evident explanation for weeks or months.[B310,K232,N4] This may be the result of chronic ischemia. Frank bowel ischemia is often found at autopsy.[N4] Although severe ischemia is probably a terminal event, its frequency suggests that bowel compromise is often present during life.

Less frequent gastrointestinal manifestations of SLE include hepatitis and ileitis.[M341,N4] Protein-losing enteropathy and marked hyperlipoproteinemia[A171,T252] have been reported. The relationship of these manifestations to SLE is uncertain. Gastrointestinal irritation is frequently secondary to drugs used in treating SLE. Aspirin-induced hepatotoxicity is common. Severe gastritis and ulcers may occur.

Although infarction of the spleen may produce acute abdominal pain, splenic involvement in SLE is usually asymptomatic. Functional asplenia is a worrisome complication because it is associated with increased susceptibility to infection.[M84] The presence of Howell-Jolly bodies on the peripheral smear should alert the clinician to the possibility of functional asplenia and prompt hospitalization if the child is febrile.

Infection

Infection is a major cause of both morbidity and mortality for children and adolescents with SLE.[C2,G197,K232,M341,P221] Platt documented 55 separate infections occur-

ring in 70 patients over a mean of 9 years of follow-up.[P221] Sepsis was a contributing cause of death in 25 to 85% of deaths in various series.[C2,G197,K232,M341,P221] It was a factor cited in 35 of 83 deaths (42%) occurring in 374 children collected from six large studies.[C2,G197,K232,M341,P221]

The increased frequency of sepsis is most likely a result of the combined effects of SLE and the drugs used to mediate it.[G159,S612] The frequency of infection increases with increasing steroid dosage.[G159] Not only bacterial infections increased, but opportunistic infections and infections caused by viruses, fungi, and related organisms were more common in children with SLE.[N3,P221] Potentially fatal infections, including both bacterial endocarditis and meningitis, occurred with a greater than expected frequency.[L165,L174] Functional asplenia, decreased phagocytosis, poor complement metabolism, and corticosteroid effects may all contribute to this problem.

Hematologic Manifestations

The most common hematologic manifestation of SLE in children and adolescents is anemia. Usually, this is not a Coombs'-positive hemolytic anemia with a reticulocytosis, but is a microcytic anemia of chronic disease. Leukopenia and thrombocytopenia are common, but are not invariably present. Sickle cell anemia is not directly associated with SLE, but is common in blacks, who have an increased incidence of SLE. When SLE and sickle cell disease occur together, the similarity of symptoms of the two illnesses may produce confusion.

Children are often seen who have antinuclear antibodies and thrombocytopenia, which has been labeled idiopathic thrombocytopenic purpura (ITP). A false-positive biologic test result for syphilis or prolonged partial thromboplastin time (PTT) may suggest SLE. Other children with ITP may have antibodies to Sm, Ro, La, or RNP, and some of these children ultimately develop SLE (Table 44–2). In the absence of other manifestations of SLE, therapy for these children is similar to that for ITP alone.

Menorrhagia may be the presenting feature of SLE in teenage females. Prolonged bleeding or a prolonged PTT resulting from the lupus anticoagulant may be the initial manifestation of SLE in a patient being screened for other reasons. These findings alone, however, do not establish the diagnosis of SLE. The management of these complications is the same for children and adolescents as for adults.

Table 44–2. Incidence of Serologic Antibodies in 92 Children with SLE (%)*

Antibody	Test Used	
	Ochterlony	ELISA
Ro/SSA	16	46
La/SSB	11	17
Sm (RNP)	27	58

* The presence of these antibodies did not correlate with disease activity, except that Ro/SSA antibodies by Ouchterlony were significantly more common in children younger than 10 years of age (11 of 28 versus 4 of 64, p < .001). Children younger than 10 years of age also had a significantly higher mean ELISA titer of Ro/SSA antibodies.

Studies of older patients with SLE indicate that the risk of sterility following cytotoxic drug therapy increases with increasing age. Premenarchal children may have some protection. In children with amenorrhea secondary to active SLE, menses often return during cyclophosphamide therapy. Several successful pregnancies have been reported following cyclophosphamide therapy. One pregnancy that originated during cyclophosphamide therapy (despite counselling) was successfully carried to term without difficulty (no further cytotoxics were given after the pregnancy was discovered). No definitive data about the risks of infertility or neoplasia are available, however, for children with SLE. Both have occurred in children who received cyclophosphamide as part of multiple drug regimens for neoplastic disease. Families should be warned about these concerns before therapy is begun, and patients selected accordingly.

The ratio of risk to benefit for cytotoxic drugs in children and adolescents with SLE is minimized by appropriate patient selection. Progressively deteriorating creatinine clearance, prolonged hypertension (greater than 6 months), and significant nonhemolytic anemia identify children at high risk of ultimate renal failure.[M263] These findings may occur without significant evidence of extrarenal disease activity. Such children should be aggressively treated. With corticosteroid therapy alone, many children progress inexorably to renal failure. Controlled studies at the NIH have indicated that routine use of intravenous cyclophosphamide prevents or retards this deterioration.[A360,B62,B64,C80]

Methotrexate, cyclosporine, and intravenous gamma globulin have all been used in small numbers of children with SLE.[A82,R337] Sufficient data have not been obtained to judge their efficacy. It is increasingly recognized that SLE is a chronic, recurrent disease that may require prolonged therapy, even in the absence of active disease. Significant improvements in the therapy of children with SLE require careful collaborative studies.

PROGNOSIS

The prognosis for children and adolescent with SLE has improved dramatically over the past 20 years.[L168] With improved anti-inflammatory therapy and improved pediatric care, 10-year survival rates are over 80%.[G197,P221] Nonetheless, significant numbers of children continue to progress to chronic renal failure and/or death (Tables 44–4 and 44–5).[M263]

Often, children and adolescents with SLE do poorly because of the child's and family's inability to cope with the

Table 44–4. Incidence of Adverse Outcomes in 72 Children with SLE (%)

Outcome	Incidence
Renal failure	15
Severe central nervous system disease	11
Stroke	1
Chronic thrombocytopenia	7
Chronic active disease	56
Death	18

Table 44–5. Predictors of Poor Prognosis in Childhood SLE

1. Persistent anemia: Hb <10 gm for >6 months
2. Persistent hypertension: diastolic BP > 90 mmηHg for >6 months
3. Persistent hematuria: >20 RBC/HPF* for >6 months
4. Pulmonary hypertension
5. Recurrent emergency admissions

* HPF = high powered field.

chronic, relapsing nature of the disease. Success requires a sustained relationship among the child, family, and treating facility. Institutions serving socioeconomically stable populations consistently report superior survival to those serving disadvantaged populations.[G197,M263,P155,P221] Poor understanding of the importance of medications for silent manifestations of SLE, such as hypertension, remains a familiar cause of morbidity. These preventable deaths have become increasingly frustrating as the ability to control the manifestations of SLE has improved.

The quality of survival must be addressed in efforts to improve the outcome for children and adolescents with SLE. Longterm survival of a cushingoid adolescent with aseptic necrosis who requires dialysis may not be satisfactory to the patient. Platt has described three young adults who died more than 10 years following diagnosis.[P221] Two of the three died after they had discontinued their medications against medical advice.

Although end stage renal failure and dialysis have been associated with decreased SLE activity in some reports,[C384,K215] children and adolescents requiring chronic dialysis often fare poorly. In one series, 9 of 16 children with SLE succumbed within 5 years of beginning dialysis.[M263]

For children and adolescents with SLE, a satisfactory outcome is measured in decades. Children without renal disease who have survived 5 years are at low risk. Children with renal disease of any type however, remain at risk. Gradual progression to renal failure over 5 to 10 years or more, despite clinically inactive disease, has been reported in both children and adults with SLE.[A360,C80,P221] Health care professionals dealing with children and adolescents with SLE must strive to aid patients and their families through a normally difficult period under even more difficult circumstances. Every effort must be made to guarantee the availability of appropriate services. Not only must medical therapy be aggressive, but so should patient and family education to ensure their compliance. With the increasing presence of specialized pediatric centers for children with rheumatic diseases, and growing numbers of collaborative studies to determine optimal therapy, survival measured in decades should become the norm.

SUMMARY

1. Children and adolescents represent both a special challenge and opportunity. Success in caring for this group requires awareness of the complex interactions among the child's illness, the needs of their families, and their own needs as developing individuals.

2. Childhood onset SLE has been recognized since the early 1900s. Although it is frequently described as a more severe disease than adult SLE, this may be the result of failure to diagnose many mild cases properly.

3. No thorough studies of the epidemiology of SLE in childhood have been completed. It is estimated that the annual incidence is about 0.6/100,000 and that between 5,000 and 10,000 children with SLE are in the United States today. The incidence of SLE is much higher in females than in males and in nonwhites than in caucasians.

4. The cause of SLE remains unknown, but the high frequency of immunologic abnormalities among family members of children with SLE suggests that a combination of genetic and environmental factors play an important role. The presence of Ro/SSA in a large proportion of the mothers of young children with SLE may indicate predisposing genetic factors in the family. SLE is also more frequent in children with defects of the immune system, suggesting that defective antigen processing may predispose to the development of SLE.

5. The most common clinical manifestations of SLE are fever, malaise, and weight loss, but these are nonspecific manifestations of many chronic ailments. The typical butterfly rash is present in only about one-third of children. The diagnosis is based on fulfillment of the ARA criteria, just as in adults.

6. Renal disease occurs in two-thirds of children with SLE in most reported series. Although the renal disease may be mild, severe, diffuse, proliferative glomerulonephritis remains a leading cause of morbidity in childhood SLE. Mild renal disease can often be controlled with corticosteroids, but active renal disease that does not respond fully to corticosteroids, and diffuse proliferative glomerulonephritis with a falling creatinine clearance, require therapy with cytotoxic agents. Children with active SLE do poorly on dialysis.

7. All the central nervous system manifestations described in adults with SLE also occur in children. Behavioral disturbances, which may be ascribed to acting out by an adolescent with SLE, often represent CNS disease, which may respond to increased therapy. Chorea is also seen more commonly among children with SLE.

8. Pulmonary involvement in childhood SLE takes many forms, including pleurisy, pleural effusions, pulmonary fibrosis, and pulmonary hemorrhage. Diaphragmatic dysfunction is common, and may be the underlying factor predisposing to recurrent episodes of pneumonia. Pulmonary hypertension is often a life-threatening complication. Abnormal pulmonary function may be present, despite a normal chest roentgenogram.

9. Musculoskeletal manifestations of SLE include arthritis and mild inflammatory myopathy, and are often predominant at presentation. Both are responsive to corticosteroid therapy, however and rarely contribute to longterm morbidity. The exception is avascular necrosis, which may occur as a complication of SLE with or without corticosteroid therapy, and requires ultimate joint replacement.

10. Dermatologic involvement is common in childhood SLE but is rarely a significant problem except when the face is prominently disfigured, causing psychologic problems (Fig. 1). Discoid lupus is unusual in childhood.

11. Cardiac manifestations of SLE include pericarditis and myocarditis, sometimes with recurrent effusions. These can usually be controlled with NSAIDs or low-dose corticosteroids. Valvular involvement is common, and may predispose to bacterial endocarditis. Careful consideration should be given to antibiotic prophylaxis whenever bacteremia is expected. Premature myocardial infarctions have occurred in young adults, with significant atherosclerosis following prolonged corticosteroid therapy.

12. Gastrointestinal manifestations of childhood SLE are varied. Nonspecific findings such as chronic abdominal pain and anorexia are frequent. Significant bowel infarction may occur. Pneumatosis intestinalis may be the result of recurrent microvascular insults.

13. Infection is a major cause of morbidity and mortality in children and adolescents with SLE. Active SLE predisposes to infection. Often, it is unclear whether a child's rapid deterioration is the result of infection or of active SLE. In this setting, increased doses of both corticosteroids and antibiotics may be necessary. Reticuloendothelial system overload and functional asplenia may predispose to rapid progression of sepsis in children with active SLE.

14. Hematologic manifestations are common in children and adolescents with SLE. Most are nonspecific. Thrombocytopenia is a frequent presenting complaint, particularly in young males. Menorrhagia may also be a significant problem in adolescent females. The presence of anticardiolipin antibodies predispose to clotting dysfunction and stroke in children, as in adults.

15. Laboratory manifestations of childhood SLE are identical to those of adults. A unique concern is awareness that a positive serologic result for syphilis in a child or adolescent is reported to the school district, and warrants prompt investigation by public welfare authorities. Families should be warned about this possibility, and inquiries should be promptly diverted to the physician.

16. Therapy for childhood-onset SLE is similar to that for adults. Because of the increased burdens of growth and development on renal function, it may be important to institute aggressive intervention earlier in children with diffuse proliferative glomerulonephritis. The goal must be to develop therapies that provide acceptable 50-year survival, not 5-year or 10-year survival, for children and adolescents with SLE. The systematic administration of cytotoxic drugs may provide superior quality of life and longterm survival.

Chapter 45

DRUG-INDUCED LUPUS

MARVIN J. FRITZLER
ROBERT L. RUBIN

In 1945, Hoffman described a 19-year-old army recruit who developed cutaneous, hematologic, and renal disease with features resembling those of systemic lupus erythematosus (SLE) after treatment with topical and oral sulfadiazine.[G230] In the next decade, after the description of the LE cell test, case reports of drug-induced lupus (DIL) became more common. In 1953, Morrow and colleagues were the first to report a lupus-like disease in patients on hydralazine therapy.[M630] Two reports of hydralazine-induced lupus characterized by fever, rash, arthralgia, abnormal liver function, and LE cells followed in the next year.[D365,P133] Although procainamide was introduced for the treatment of cardiac arrhythmias at about the same time, it was not until 1962 that Ladd reported a patient who developed lupus-like features after 6 months of procainamide therapy.[B350] Since these initial reports, it has become widely appreciated that patients on various drugs (Table 45–1) can develop autoantibodies and other clinical features similar to those seen in patients with idiopathic SLE. Reports of autoimmune features expressed after patients are treated with biologic materials, such as recombinant interleukin and other cytokines, suggest that the spectrum of drug-induced lupus will continue to increase.

Because such a large number of drugs have been implicated in DIL, the distinction between drug-induced autoimmunity and drug-induced disease is important. When patients receiving drug therapy develop autoantibodies or other laboratory features of autoimmunity, such as elevated immunoglobulin levels,[R388] the term "drug-induced autoimmunity" (DIA) or "drug-related autoimmunity" is used. A relatively minority of these patients, including those who have circulating autoantibodies, develop clinical and serologic features indistinguishable from those seen in idiopathic SLE. This syndrome is referred to as drug-related lupus or drug-induced lupus (DIL).

DRUGS IMPLICATED IN DIL AND DIA

Although approximately 60 drugs have been implicated in DIA, only 8 are thought to have a clear association with DIL (Table 45–1). The drugs commonly implicated in DIL include procainamide and hydralazine, with quinidine, chlorpromazine, isoniazid, and acebutolol being distinctly less common.[H290,R388,S541] The interpretation of many other reports of drugs responsible for the induction of a lupus-like illness is difficult because of their potential use in preclinical or unrecognized cases of idiopathic SLE.

The drugs reported to induce lupus can be categorized as anti-arrhythmics, antihypertensives, anticonvulsants, β-adrenergic blocking agents, phenothiazines, sulfonamides, antithyroidals, estrogen preparations, and various other agents (Table 45–1). Although these drugs represent wide chemical heterogeneity, the drugs associated with the highest frequency of DIL are the arylamines and hydrazines (Fig. 45–1). This is noteworthy because related environmental agents have been implicated in DIL. For example, lupus-like illness has been reported in association with hydrazines,[R126] compounds found in mushrooms and other fungi, tobacco and tobacco smoke, and certain industrial reagents. Aromatic amines, such as the eosin in lipstick, have been implicated in lupus.[B107] The association of L-canavanine, an amino acid present in relative abundance in bean sprouts, alfalfa seeds, and other legumes, has gained some interest because of its association with a lupus-like illness in monkeys.[P290] (See Chapter 3.)

Extensive studies on how lupus-inducing drugs alter the immune response are essentially limited to hydralazine and procainamide. The amino group of procainamide, and hydrazine group on hydralazine and isoniazid, and the sulfhydryl group on propylthiouracil are required for the induction of autoimmunity.[B583a] Because hydralazine-induced lupus (HIL) and procainamide-induced lupus (PIL) are the best studied, the major part of this chapter is devoted to the clinical and pathogenic mechanisms of these two drugs.

Drugs That May Exacerbate SLE

Treatment of a number of diseases with various drugs has been noted to have a temporal relationship with the onset or aggravation of SLE.[W26] These drugs can be classified as antibiotics, hormones, nonsteroidal anti-inflammatory drugs (NSAIDs), hormones, dermatologic agents, and gold salts. As noted in the introduction to this chapter, sulfonamide derivatives have a historical association with the onset of lupus-like features.[G230,G231] This drug and tetracyclines,[D254] griseofulvin,[A138a,A213,W96] piroxicam,[B302] and benoxaprofen[S524] are reported to be photosensitizers of varying frequency. Other drugs, such as sulfonamides, penicillin,[G230,L75] hydrochlorothiazide,[R96] hair dyes and permanent wave preparations,[P117,P227] cimetidine,[D69] gold salts,[L75] phenylbutazone,[C106,F18,F271,H96,O22] salicylates,[S62,S554] and other NSAIDs[W26] have been associated with hypersensitivity reactions that have been interpreted as initiating or aggravating factors in SLE. Ibupro-

Table 45–1. Drugs Implicated in Drug-Induced Autoimmunity (DIA), Drug-Induced Lupus (DIL), or Exacerbation of Lupus*

Anticonvulsants[A88,A106,A192,A307,B274,G191,L146,L305,R438]	*Antibiotics*[L75,W26]
Mephenytoin (Mesantoin)[L146]	Penicillin[G230]
Diphenylhydantoin (Dilantin)[A112,A176,G190,L146,R21,B583a]	Tetracycline[D254]
Trimethadione (Tridone)[B276,J26,L146]	Sulfamethoxypyridazine (Kynex)[G230]
Primidone (Mysoline)[A76,C316,D29]	Sulfadimethoxine (Madribon)
Ethosuximide (Zarontin)[A164,D1,D41,G413]	Griseofulvin (Fulvisin)[A138a,M53,W96]
Carbamazepine (Tegretol)[A121,B120,D118,J65,K361,P5,T48]	Nalidixic acid (NegGram)
Phenylethacetylurea (Pheneturide)[D269]	Nitrofurantoin (Macrodantin)
	Antiarrhythmics
Antituberculous Drugs[D107,D367,E157,G206,G352,L109,R350,S134]	**Procainamide (Pronestyl)**[H291,R388,R390,S541]
Isoniazid (INH)[A104,B293,C57]	Quinidine[A114,A175,A201,B81,B105,B583a,C332,D360,K406,L99,M242,W191,C329,G318]
Para-aminosalicylic acid (PAS)[L146,S460]	Disopyramide (Norpace)[I141,W70]
Streptomycin[L109]	
	Anti-Inflammatories and Antirheumatics[B302,W36]
Psychotropics[A105,G419,O11,Q15,S460]	
Chlorpromazine (Thorazine)[A124,A189,B238,D339,Z7,Z14]	D-**Penicillamine***[C191,C239,E115,K49,L116,T232,V32]
Perphenazine (Trilafon[G229]	Sulfasalazine (Azulfidine)[C106,D248,G381,O67,R8,V32]
Promethazine (Phenergan)	Phenylbutazone[F18,H96]
Perazine[G229]	Benoxaprofen (Oraflex)[S524]
Thioridazide (Mellaril)[G18]	Gold salts
Levomeprazone (Levoprome)	Ibuprofen (Motrin)[S62,S158,S524,Q8a,W92,W218]
Phenelzine[S788]	Sulindac[B56]
Chlorprothixene (Taractan)[M317]	Diclofenac[C318]
Lithium carbonate (Eskalith)[G118,P287,S398,W201]	Tolmetin[R424]
	Pyrithoxine[L66]
Antithyroidal and Hormonal Drugs	
Propylthiouracil (PTU)[A188,B245,B271,M501,P146]	*Miscellaneous*[L146,W26]
Thionamide[S242,T23]	
Methimazole (Tapazole)[H318]	Amoproxan
Danazol (Danocrine)	Methysergide (Sansert)
Methylthiouracil[V1]	L-Dopa[H269]
Oral contraceptives[B104,B390,K130,M471]	Psoralen[M275]
	Metrizamide[G86]
Antihypertensives[W26,W262]	Minoxidil[T272]
Hydralazine (Apresoline)*[H291,R388,S134,S541]	Aminoglutethimide[M250]
Methyldopa (Aldomet)[D361,H175,M12,N125,R390,S355]	Cinnarazine
Guanoxan (Envocar)[B369]	Oxyphenisatin[R183]
Prazosin (Minipress)[M151,M346,W261]	Hydrazine[P115,R128]
Captopril (Capoten)[C128,P66,P188,R127,S411]	Nomifensine[G42,M342,S164]
Clonidine (Catapres)[W311]	Alpha interferon[C369,O1,S362]
Practolol[B167,M445,S448]	Tolazamide (Tolinase)
Acebutolol (Sectral)[B306,H447]	Anthiomaline
Atenolol,[G319] labetalol,[B523] Pindolol[B223]	Phenopyrazone
Spironolactone (Aldactone)[U4]	L-Canavanine[P290]
	Timolol eye drops[M156]

* Drugs in boldface type are those with good evidence supporting induction of DIL.

fen- and other NSAID-induced (e.g., sulindac, tolmetin, diclofenac) aseptic meningitis in SLE patients is an important consideration for the physician involved in the care of SLE patients who present with signs of meningeal irritation.[B56,C318,Q89,R424,S62,S554,W92,W218] A critical appraisal of the literature suggests that, rather than inducing lupus, these agents may unmask incipient lupus or aggravate lupus disease activity. Last, some reports have suggested that the incidence of SLE is increased after taking oral contraceptives, and that remissions often follow cessation of their use.[B390] Dubois and colleagues[W26] and others[G56,G134,K130,M471,T208] were unable to substantiate these findings.

By definition, symptoms of DIL invariably resolve after discontinuation of therapy, although in severe cases full recovery may require up to 1 year. A well-entrenched view that some cases of idiopathic SLE were "unmasked" during drug therapy in patients with a lupus diathesis is

difficult to discount or prove. The possibility that unknown environmental "chemicals" might induce a lupus-like syndrome by a mechanism analogous to that of DIL appears unlikely, because DIL requires months to years of frequent exposure (i.e., medications two to six times daily) to a xenobiotic. In addition to the exposure factor, it appears that sustained, elevated, steady-state blood levels of the implicated agents are required for DIA and DIL.

EPIDEMIOLOGY

The incidence of DIL is 15,000 to 20,000 new cases annually in the United States, and PIL accounts for the vast majority of these cases.[H290] In the United Kingdom, the incidence of HIL was 6.7% after 3 years of treatment[C35] and 4.3% after 13 years.[R430] A similar incidence of PIL was reported in Australia.[H413] The incidence of DIL in other countries is unknown, but it has been estimated that

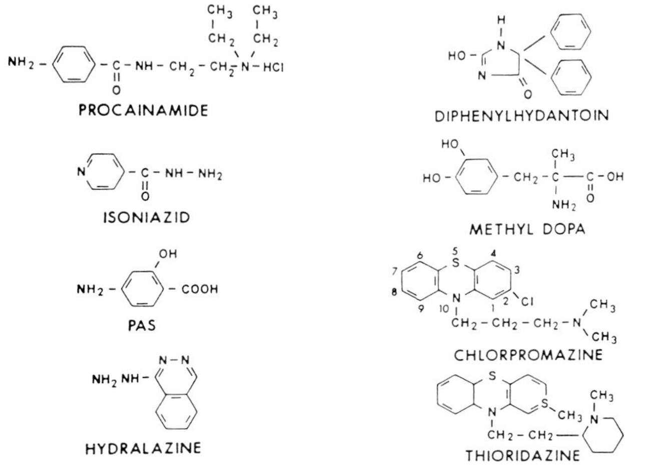

Fig. 45–1. Structural formulas of drugs that may induce lupus-like syndromes. Procainamide and para-aminosalicylic acid (PAS) are examples of arylamines, and hydralazine and isoniazid (INH) are examples of hydrazines.

it is 10% that of idiopathic SLE.[W26] Lee et al.[L146] reviewed the medical histories of 285 consecutive SLE case records and found that drugs were a possible causative factor in 12.4%. Fries and Holman identified only 12 DIL cases in a population of 198 lupus patients.[F263] The frequency of DIL might be much higher than most reports indicate because most cases are mild, and only a small proportion are correctly diagnosed or seen by a rheumatologist. Because drugs such as isoniazid are more frequently administered in certain countries, studies in such countries are important to provide a more thorough epidemiologic picture of DIL. The age of patients developing DIL reflects the age of the population at risk, because these drugs, especially procainamide and hydralazine, tend to be administered to the older population.

Two epidemiologic features distinguish DIL from SLE. First, the high female-to-male predominance seen in SLE (9:1 to 7:1), is not seen in DIL, although PIL appears to be disproportionately more common in females.[C35,H266, M112,R430,S555,T193] This is in contrast to DIA, in which the female-to-male ratio is almost 1:1.[M112,R388] Second, unlike SLE, the frequency of DIL in blacks is four-[C364] to six-fold[P130] lower than in whites. Whether this reflects an effect of genetic factors or other demographic features is not known.

Studies of patients receiving procainamide therapy have shown that 75% of patients develop antinuclear antibodies (ANA) within 1 year of treatment[B349,H266] and almost 100% develop ANA after 2 years.[K388,W348] Most of these patients remain asymptomatic, but 10 to 30% of patients on therapy with procainamide and hydralazine, respectively, go on to develop symptoms of SLE.[B350,H266, S555,W348]

The onset of symptoms can be slow or acute, although an interval of 1 to 2 months typically passes before the diagnosis is made.[B349,H266,S555,W348] Linkage of these observations to a single inciting agent holds promise that a thorough study of DIL can elucidate the mechanisms that underlie autoimmunity.

CLINICAL AND LABORATORY FEATURES

The clinical and laboratory features of PIL and HIL are shown in Table 45–2. Musculoskeletal complaints are commonly observed, with arthralgia heading the list for both drugs. Arthritis is a less common (~20%) feature of PIL than HIL (50 to 100%), whereas pericarditis is a common presenting feature of PIL. By contrast, HIL is associated with a higher frequency of skin rashes than PIL. Otherwise, the observed frequency of clinical symptoms suggests that clinical features alone do not distinguish PIL from HIL patients.

Because arthralgia is such a common feature of patients in the age group at risk, the presence of other features, such as pleuritis, pleural effusion, fever, splenomegaly, skin rash, and pericarditis should lead the clinician to consider the diagnosis of DIL when these are also present. Approximately 50% of patients have constitutional symptoms of fever and weight loss. Three reports have indicated that HIL is associated with acute neutrophilic dermatosis (Sweet's syndrome).[R33,S285,S293] The signs and symptoms of DIL usually resolve within days to weeks of discontinuing the offending drug. The mechanisms underlying the clinical manifestations of DIL are unknown.

With a few exceptions, the frequency of serologic abnormalities in HIL and PIL is also similar (Table 45–2). The immune response in this setting is characteristic and restricted. The most commonly observed abnormality is a positive ANA. Like the clinical features, these autoantibodies are truly drug-induced, and they gradually subside after drug therapy is discontinued.

Table 45–2. Incidence of Clinical and Laboratory Features of HIL and PIL (%)

Feature	PIL	HIL
Arthralgia	85	80
Arthritis	20	50–100
Pleuritis, pleural effusion	50	Uncommon
Fever, weight loss	45	40–50
Myalgia	35	Uncommon
Splenomegaly	25	15
Pericarditis	15	Uncommon
Rash	Uncommon	25
Glomerulonephritis	Rare	5
ANA	>95	>95
LE cell	80	50
Antihistone	>95	>95
Anti-dDNA	50	50–90
Anti-nDNA	Rare	Rare
Anticardiolipin	Uncommon	Uncommon
Rheumatoid factor	30	20
Anemia	20	35
Leukopenia	15	Uncommon
Elevated gamma globulin levels	25	10–50
Immune complexes	Normal	Normal

Data from Rubin RL, Burlingame RW, Bell SA.[R390] Specific antihistone antibody common to lupus induced by diverse drugs [abstract]. Arthritis Rheum 1991; 34 Suppl:S104. Solinger AM.[S554] Drug-related lupus. Clinical and etiological considerations. Rheum Dis Clinics North Am 1988; 14:187–202.

Other laboratory features noted in a minority of patients include a mild anemia, leukopenia, and thrombocytopenia,[B350,D319,E87,H290,K278,R388,S541] a hypergammaglobulinemia that is not as frequent as in SLE,[B350,D319,H266, K265,S541,W285] and an elevated erythrocyte sedimentation rate (ESR), which commonly reverts toward normal as symptoms resolve.[S541] In centers in which it is still done, a positive LE cell preparation is generally noted. Pancytopenia has been reported in association with procainamide therapy,[G135,S361] and, although one patient had a positive ANA, it is unlikely that these patients had PIL. More uncommon laboratory features include rheumatoid factor (procainamide),[K278] circulating immune complexes (hydralazine),[S134] positive Coombs' test (methyldopa,[P131] chlorpromazine,[Z7] and procainamide),[K278] hypocomplementemia (procainamide),[B458] and a positive lupus band test.[K246] Antibodies to the neutrophil components myeloperoxidase (MPO) and elastase have been described in six of six HIL patients.[N36] After 2 years of follow-up the elastase antibodies were eliminated, but the MPO antibodies persisted. Phospholipid and cardiolipin antibodies, circulating anticoagulant activity, and biologic false-positive serologic test for syphilis (STS) results are discussed later in this chapter.

Histone Autoantibodies

In 1978, Fritzler and Tan were the first to report that histone antibodies are a common and predominant serologic feature of DIL.[F280] Since then, numerous studies have confirmed and refined this observation,[C427,D346,E117, G218,P262] and it is now accepted that autoantibodies directed against histones are associated with various drugs implicated in DIL (Table 45–3). Also, histone antibodies are probably responsible for positive LE cell test results and a positive anti-deoxyribonucleoprotein (DNP) response,[B350,K265,M526] so that earlier studies describing these features in DIL are congruous with the observation that histone antibodies are common in DIL.

In addition, the histone moieties and major histone determinants that react with DIL antibodies are known.[C427,G218,G219,P262,P265,T193] In one study, ELISA (enzyme-linked immunosorbent assay) and immunoblotting techniques were used to show that antibodies from both DIL and SLE bound all classes of histones: H1 > H2B > H2A > H3 > H4.[G218] Furthermore, when epitope analysis

was conducted using peptide fragments of the purified histones, 10 of 11 DIL sera and 11 of 12 SLE sera bound only the amino terminal and carboxyl terminal peptides.[G218] Only one serum in each patient group bound to the central trypsin-resistant domain of histones. Using chromatin rather than purified histones as the antigen source, Portanova and colleagues[P262] showed that most SLE antibodies bind to the protease-sensitive regions, but that DIL sera bind to the trypsin-resistant regions. These data suggest that some epitopes in PIL are more closely associated with the macromolecular form of the histones that are complexed in the nucleosome. Unlike PIL sera, HIL sera react primarily with H3 and H4,[P262,P265] although one report demonstrated predominant reactivity with H3, H2B, and H2A,[C427] and another study reported no particular pattern of histone reactivity.[H336] The reactivity of histone antibodies in DIL is summarized in Table 45–3. It appears that the reactivity with different classes of histones varies among the drugs. Some of these patterns of reactivity were based on a single case of DIL, so generalizations are therefore not possible.

The data demonstrating epitope reactivity in the carboxyl and/or amino termini of purified histones,[G218,G219] and other observations that PIL sera bind to protease-resistant regions on nucleosomes and chromatin,[P262] have been interpreted as being incompatible. It is important to appreciate, however, that these studies used different procedures and reagents. It is generally agreed that the autoimmune response in both DIL and SLE points to the nucleosome rather than to isolated histones or molecular mimics of histones as the immunogen that drives the autoimmune response in both DIL and SLE.[D346,P262,R388, T193,W26]

Denatured DNA Autoantibodies

The other autoantibody found in up to 50% of DIL sera is directed against denatured DNA (dDNA).[A114,B350,H38, K266,K339,L334,R394,W285] These autoantibodies probably have multiple reactivities, which have also been identified as reactivity with the nucleoside guanosine[W152] and the phospholipid cardiolipin.[L10] Even antibodies directed to lymphocytes described in HIL[R442] and PIL[B358,B363] may be related to the dDNA reactivity, because it is known that the surfaces of lymphocytes bear DNA.[B2126] The clinical significance of dDNA antibodies is not clear, because they are commonly seen in asymptomatic patients and in those with a wide variety of rheumatic and inflammatory conditions.[T43]

Antibodies to Drugs

Antibodies to the offending drugs have been reported in PIL[R429] and HIL patients,[B257,H38] and in those with amiodarone-induced autoimmunity.[P180] Other studies[K265,K266,R397] have been unable to confirm the observations of drug antibodies in HIL and DIL. One study of HIL demonstrated that only 1 of 27 sera bound to the drug.[L334] The significance of antibodies to the drugs themselves is unclear, because they are present in varying amounts in asymptomatic and symptomatic patients. In addition, it

Table 45–3. Histone Antibodies Reported in DIL

Drug	Histone Antibody	Reference
Procainamide	(H2A-H2B)-DNA, H1, H5, H2B, H2A, H3, H4	B583a,C364,G218,P76, P262,T193
Hydralazine	H3, H4, H2B, H2A	C427,P265
α-Methyldopa	H1	N125
D-Penicillamine	(H2A-H2B)-DNA	E115
Quinidine	H1, (H2A-H2B)-DNA, H3, H4, H2B	B583a,C329,W191
Carbamazepine	Total histone*	A121
Timolol eye drops	(H2A-H2B)-DNA	M156

* Class of histone not characterized.

is unlikely that drug-binding antibodies represent cross reactions between DNA or DNP antibodies.[C95,H38,M273]

Phospholipid Antibodies

The observation that up to 75% of DIA patients can have phospholipid (cardiolipin) antibodies, circulating anticoagulants, or a biologic false-positive STS result is noteworthy, because much attention has focused on the clinical and pathogenic features of these autoantibodies. The presence of the lupus anticoagulant or of cardiolipin antibodies has been described in patients on hydralazine,[M545] procainamide,[A344,C243,D95,E36,L329,T221] and chlorpromazine[C63,C65,D171,L288,T177,Z14,Z49] therapy.[M312] In one study, up to 75% of patients treated with chlorpromazine for up to 2.5 years developed a lupus anticoagulant.[Z14] Canoso et al.[C63] reported that 54 of 93 chlorpromazine-treated psychiatric patients had IgM lupus anticoagulant (LAC) activity. Of the 54 LAC-positive patients, 31 also had IgM cardiolipin antibodies (ACA), 4 also had IgG cardiolipin antibodies, and 5 had cardiolipin antibodies alone. During a mean follow-up period of 5 years, thrombotic events occurred in 3 patients (1 with LAC, 2 with IgM cardiolipin antibodies). In a Canadian study, Lillicrap et al.[L288] evaluated 97 psychotic patients treated with chlorpromazine, fluphenazine, or promazine. Of these, 25% developed a positive ANA, 4% had elevated titers of antibodies to cardiolipin and phosphatidyl serine, and 5% had elevated titers of antibodies to phosphatidyl inositol. None of the patients developed features of SLE or evidence of thrombotic events. These observations and others[C65] suggest that no increased risk of thrombotic events is present in those with chlorpromazine-induced LAC and cardiolipin antibodies. The antibody isotype in almost all these patients is IgM,[C63,C65,Z14] as are the associated antinuclear antibodies.[C62] It is likely that these observations also apply to procainamide and hydralazine, because thrombosis appears to be a rare clinical event in HIL and PIL. The clinician should be cautious, however, because recurrent thrombotic events have been reported in phenothiazine-induced[S631] and procainamide-induced[A344,L329] lupus patients.

It is not known why patients on various drugs, especially those in the phenothiazine group, develop lupus anticoagulants and cardiolipin antibodies during therapy. Because chlorpromazine is amphophilic (Fig. 45–1), it can interact with phospholipids, intercalate into plasma membranes, and bind to plasma lipoproteins.[B595,M312,M574] Based on these features, it has been postulated that the binding of the drug lipid moieties exposes cryptic epitopes or creates neoantigens that then serve as the stimulus for the production of autoantibodies.[M312]

Other Autoantibodies

Rheumatoid factor has been reported in PIL patients.[B350] Prospective studies suggest that it is not actually drug-induced, and might merely reflect the increased prevalence of this autoantibody in the population treated with the drug.[R397] One study has reported antibodies in DIL sera directed against poly(adeno-

sine diphosphate-ribose).[H336] Another study demonstrated neutrophil myeloperoxidase antibodies in HIL patients.[N35,N36] This antibody system is one of several antineutrophil cytoplasmic antibodies (ANCAs) associated with Wegener's granulomatosis and other vasculitides.[R24,V25] Other antibodies reported in PIL and HIL patients include those directed against U1RNP,[C189] lymphocytes,[R442] and other unidentified autoantigens.[L99] Some studies have not confirmed the presence of RNP (ribonucleoprotein) antibodies in DIL.[F280,K265,K266,R397]

DIAGNOSIS

The diagnosis of DIL should be considered when certain clinical and serologic markers are present. One concern of clinicians is how to differentiate DIL from SLE, and from other systemic rheumatic diseases. The reasons for this concern are threefold. First, the elderly SLE patient does not often present with the classic features of SLE (e.g., butterfly rash, glomerulonephritis).[C158,W75] Indeed, the clinical features of SLE in the elderly and DIL have significant overlap. Second, the treatment of DIL is generally straightforward, requiring only withdrawal of the drug and short-term anti-inflammatory therapy, whereas the treatment of SLE can involve the prolonged use of corticosteroids or other immune modulators. Third, the outcome of DIL is better than SLE because these patients rarely, if ever, develop renal or neurologic disease.

Guidelines

Some studies have shown that most patients fulfill at least four of the American College of Rheumatology (ACR) criteria for the classification of SLE.[T46] Therefore, these criteria are not reliable for distinguishing these two syndromes. Guidelines for the diagnosis of DIL, based on those suggested by Hess,[H290] can be summarized as follows:

1. Presence of signs or symptoms of SLE in a patient taking a lupus-inducing drug
2. Absence of multisystem involvement and serious CNS or autoimmune renal disease
3. Improvement and resolution of symptoms within days or weeks of discontinuing therapy
4. Presence of antihistone antibodies, especially to the (H2A-H2B)-DNA complex
5. Absence of antibodies to dsDNA, Sm, RNP, Ro/SSA, and La/SSB
6. Absence of hypocomplementemia
7. Decreasing titer of histone antibodies after discontinuation of the drug

These guidelines, of overlapping and contrasting clinical and serologic features of DIL and SLE, are based on a number of reports, but they have not been rigorously tested in a multicenter study. Central nervous system disease is distinctly uncommon in DIL[R388,S541] but, because of potentially toxic reactions to drugs and other causes of stroke, convulsions, and dementia syndromes in the elderly, this feature is not included in the exclusion guidelines. Because glomerulonephritis has been reported in

HIL,[I4,N31,P265] it is also not included as an exclusion guideline. The clinician should appreciate, however, that glomerulonephritis is rare in DIL. A positive ANA in a patient on drug therapy should not be taken as sufficient evidence for a diagnosis of DIL. Supporting evidence of antibodies to histones and other nuclear antigens (e.g., Sm, dsDNA, RNP, SSA) should be requested, if the test is available, but the presence of antihistone antibodies without clinical features of SLE should not be sufficient reason for discontinuing therapy because some drugs, especially procainamide, isoniazid, and chlorpromazine, can induce histone antibodies in patients who remain asymptomatic. Based on observations that 20% of symptomatic DIL patients had one symptom, 25% had two symptoms, and 55% had three or more symptoms,[T193] the presence of three clinical features and the serologic marker of histone antibodies would provide a high diagnostic specificity for the diagnosis of DIL.

Discriminating Serologic Features

As described above, a common serologic feature of DIL is the presence of histone antibodies. Because histone antibodies are seen in most SLE patients, and with lesser frequency in those with other rheumatic diseases,[T43] it is clear that this autoantibody does not serve as a serologic marker for DIL. A striking feature of DIL is the absence of autoantibodies to certain other nuclear antigens seen in patients with idiopathic SLE and other systemic rheumatic diseases.[T43] SLE is characterized by autoantibodies that are often associated as "linked sets."[C426] For example, in SLE, histone antibodies are frequently accompanied by dsDNA antibodies, Ro/SSA antibodies by La/SSB antibodies, and Sm antibodies by U1RNP antibodies.[C426,T43] This is not the case in DIL, in which the antibody response to histone is rarely accompanied by dsDNA antibodies or other ANAs. Only a few SLE patients with monospecific histone antibody responses have been described.[F278] These patients clinically resembled DIL patients in that arthralgia and arthritis were common features, but glomerulonephritis was uncommon. Therefore, in the clinical setting, in which the diagnosis of SLE or DIL cannot be clearly distinguished on clinical grounds, the presence of antibodies to dsDNA, Sm, RNP, Ro/SSA, La/SSB, proliferating cell nuclear antigen (PCNA)/cyclin, and other nuclear antigens should be considered as evidence against a diagnosis of DIL.

The absence of antibodies to other nonhistone nuclear antigens in DIL was demonstrated by Fritzler and Tan,[F280] Meyer and colleagues,[M379] and Barland and Epstein.[E117] Using the relatively insensitive indirect immunofluorescence reconstitution assay for histone antibodies, Barland and Epstein showed that more than 80% of patients with symptomatic PIL had histone antibodies, compared to approximately 30% of those with asymptomatic disease. The study by Meyer et al.[M379] showed a correlation in those with idiopathic SLE between histone IgG and dsDNA antibodies, as assessed by the Farr assay. Histone antibodies were found, however, in the absence of high titers of dsDNA antibodies in DIL. The ANA in PIL can be accounted for by histone-reactive antibodies, because native nucleosomes can absorb essentially all the ANA activity in these sera.[R397] Since these early reports, other studies of PIL and HIL have noted a relative absence of antibodies directed against the nonhistone antigens Sm, U1RNP, Ro/SSA, La/SSB, and Scl70.[R388,T50]

Differential Diagnosis

Because the clinical features of DIL are protean, a differential diagnosis should be considered.[S541] Viral syndromes and infectious diseases may present with arthralgia, fever, and pleuropericarditis. Dressler's syndrome should be considered in a patient with a previous myocardial infarction. An additional ischemic myocardial event may present with fever and pericarditis. The postpericardiotomy syndrome, which may present after cardiac surgery and is similar to Dressler's syndrome, can be confused with drug-induced lupus because these patients are often treated with antiarrhythmics, such as procainamide. Other diagnoses to be considered in the appropriate setting are underlying malignancy, adverse or hypersensitive drug reactions, and graft-versus-host disease.

TREATMENT

Once the diagnosis of DIL has been established, the first step is discontinuation of the offending drug. Treatment with anti-inflammatory agents, including corticosteroids, may be indicated for those with or severe manifestations of the disease (e.g., pericarditis with tamponade). The judicious use of NSAIDs and corticosteroids in the elderly is important because of potential side effects. The prolonged use of high doses of corticosteroids, or the use of chloroquine, hydroxychloroquine, or immunosuppressive agents, is not indicated in the treatment of DIL. If DIL is associated with the rare feature of glomerulonephritis, as reported with hydralazine-induced[I4,N31,S320] and D-penicillamine-induced[C239] lupus, corticosteroids can be used. Although some DIL patients have been restarted on procainamide or hydralazine without incident, this is usually not advisable because accelerated recurrence of the disease has been reported in this setting.[S541]

Clinicians are often consulted to consider the safety of drugs associated with DIL in the treatment of idiopathic SLE. The use of hydralazine to treat hypertension in SLE patients has not been associated with exacerbations of the disease.[W26] Procainamide or N-acetylprocainamide has been used to treat cardiac arrhythmias, but the patient should have trough levels of the drug monitored to prevent toxicity. The use of anticonvulsants to treat seizure disorders in SLE patients has not been associated with flares or acceleration of disease activity. Isoniazid has been given to SLE patients on corticosteroids without aggravating lupus.[S541] Despite the apparent safety of these drugs in the setting of SLE, the clinician should use the drugs judiciously and carefully document the clinical and serologic status of the patient being considered for treatment.

OTHER DRUGS IMPLICATED IN DIA AND DIL

Only selected drugs are considered in this section. The reader wishing a comprehensive review of drugs reported to be associated with DIA and DIL should see Table 45–1 and other reviews.[R388,S541,W26]

Methyldopa

Several cases of DIL associated with methyldopa therapy have been reported.[D361,N125,S355] More commonly, methyldopa (Aldomet) was reported to induce an autoimmune hemolytic anemia, and serologic findings identical to those of idiopathic autoimmune hemolytic anemia with a positive direct Coombs' test have been seen.[S347] In another study, when 38 patients being administered the drug for the first time were followed for 3 to 6 months, 10 (24%) developed a positive direct Coombs' test. The ANA was positive in 14.6% of 158 patients already taking methyldopa, compared to only 3% of 82 patients receiving other antihypertensive medications. The studies of Hunter et al.[H356] demonstrated a dose-related, transitory positive Coombs' test in 98 patients receiving this drug for several years. Of these, 5 patients had positive LE cell tests and 11 had a positive ANA. Routine VDRL and rheumatoid factor (latex agglutination) tests were negative. None of the patients were symptomatic.

Methyldopa-induced hemolytic anemia associated with positive LE cell tests has been reported.[H175,M12,S355] Because LE cell phenomenon is associated with antihistone antibody activity,[R388] it is assumed that these patients had histone antibodies, similar to the findings in one case report.[N125] All these patients responded to cessation of methyldopa therapy. In a group of 2,470 hypertensive patients who had received methyldopa therapy (at any time), 13% had a positive ANA, versus 3.8% in a group of patients who had not taken methyldopa.[W262]

β-Blockers and Other Antihypertensive Drugs

Although longterm therapy with acebutolol (Sectral) has been associated with a 15 to 89% incidence of ANA,[B412,C319,H439,W262] only a few cases of clinical lupus have been reported.[B523,G382,P187] In the latter report, the clinical features of 11 patients were similar to those seen in PIL. A well-documented case of captopril-induced lupus has been reported.[S411] Practolol, no longer available for use by clinicians, is of historical interest because of a high frequency of ANA (45%) and a wide variety of features, including oculomucocutaneous involvement, sclerosing periarteritis, cutaneous anergy, decreased mitogenic responses of lymphocytes, antibodies that bind intracellular epithelial cell antigens, and the production of circulating anticoagulants and inhibitors of factor XIII.[B167,E36,M445,P329]

Cases of DIL have been reported to follow therapy with guanoxan (Envocar),[G191] clonidine,[C6] and spironolactone.[U4] Despite its chemical similarity to D-penicillamine, captopril (Capoten) was not associated with DIL in 100,000 patients receiving the drug[P188] although a relationship with positive ANAs was observed.[C128,P188,R127] The ANAs were not correlated with clinical symptoms or acetylator phenotype. Neither clinical disease nor increased frequencies of ANAs have been associated with prazocin (Minipress).[M346,W261] In those in whom ANA

positivity was noted,[M151] the patients were also on diuretics and β-blockers.

Quinidine

Five cases of quinidine-induced lupus were reported by Lavie et al. in 1985.[L99] All these patients had polyarthritis, an elevated erythrocyte sedimentation rate (ESR), high-titer ANAs, and negative anti-DNA. A literature review and an additional case was reported by West et al.[W191] Of interest, histone antibodies directed to H1 and H2B were noted in this patient. In a study of seven patients with a quinidine-induced rheumatic syndrome, Cohen et al.[C329] identified four patients with clinical and serologic features similar to those of PIL including the presence of IgG antibodies to histone H1 and H2A-H2B complex, and IgG antibodies to the (H2A-H2B)-DNA complex were reported in seven of twelve patient with quinidine-induced lupus.[R388] Antibodies to individual core histones were not detected. The other three patients, who had negative ANAs, had milder symptoms, which returned after rechallenge with the drug.

Anticonvulsant Drugs

As early as 1957, it was recognized that anticonvulsants induced lupus-like features.[L305] One difficulty with studies implicating these drugs as unequivocal inducers of lupus is the observation that the effects of convulsive disorders may precede those of typical SLE by many years.[R438] Furthermore, some anticonvulsants induce renal and cutaneous disease on their own.[W26] Second, it is difficult to identify the drug responsible for DIL or DIA reactions because many of the patients are on more than one drug, including an additional anticonvulsant medication. Dubois and Wallace[W26] have suggested that the association of DIL with anticonvulsants is "rare" and "their role as causative agents doubtful." The best evidence of DIL is associated with the use of diphenylhydantoin[A88,A106,L146] and carbamazepine,[A121,B276,D118,K361,P5,P13] although other longterm follow-up studies have disputed these observations.[B274,W26,W254] In studies of lymphocyte function, Gleichman[G190] proposed that diphenylhydantoin promotes polyclonal B-cell activation, although other studies of diphenylhydantoin-related lupus patients showed normal lymphocyte mitogenic responses, T-cell surface markers, and T-cell suppressor function.[A307] One interesting conclusion of studies on anticonvulsants and their relation to DIA and DIL is that the administration of phenobarbital does not correlate with an increased incidence of autoimmune reactions.[W26]

Antituberculous Drugs

As with anticonvulsant therapy, patients who develop DIL or DIA associated with antituberculous drugs are on more than one medication. Triple therapy with isoniazid (INH), para-aminosalicylic acid (PAS), and streptomycin was once standard practice. The best evidence, however, points to INH as the drug most likely to cause DIA or DIL.[R350] This is noteworthy because INH, like hydralazine, is a substituted hydrazine, and both compounds are metabolized by the same hepatic acetyltransferase.[P134] Nevertheless, Alarcon-Segovia et al.[A104] could find no difference in the development of ANA in fast and slow acetylators on INH therapy. The major manifestation of DIA in patients on INH appears to be the development of ANA, and clinically diagnosed DIL is rare.[W26]

Psychotropic Drugs

The major effect of psychotropic drugs appears to be the induction of ANA. In prospective studies of 177 female patients receiving chlorpromazine,[B238] 26% developed a positive ANA, versus 2.5% of controls. None of these patients reported symptoms of SLE.

The interest in chlorpromazine as an inducer of DIL and DIA has been fostered by two observations. First, phenothiazine derivatives are associated with light-sensitive eruptions.[G363,P134] Second, in vitro studies have shown that chlorpromazine reacts with single-stranded DNA (ssDNA) in the presence of ultraviolet light.[K12] The latter observation raises the possibility that, if this reaction occurs in vivo, the DNA might become immunogenic. Evidence supporting this notion is that patients treated with chlorpromazine showed a dose-related appearance of ssDNA antibodies.[Q15] As noted earlier, in the discussion of PIL and HIL, however, the mechanisms leading to the appearance of ssDNA or dDNA antibodies may not require binding of the drug to nucleic acids. Of further interest, patients taking chlorpromazine have been reported to develop circulating anticoagulants,[C63,C65,S631,T177,Z14,Z49] which may represent cross-reactivity with ssDNA.[L10]

Antithyroid Drugs

Patients with lupus-like features have been reported with a number of agents used to treat thyrotoxicosis.[A188,B271,H318,M501,R146,S242,T23] Methimazole, which is not commonly associated with DIL in most countries, was associated with hypoglycemia and insulin antibodies in 17% of Japanese patients treated for Graves' disease.[H318]

INDUCTION OF DIL

Humoral Responses

Involvement of the immune system in DIL (Table 45–4) is suggested by a number of factors.[B583a,R388] The

Table 45–4. Possible Mechanisms Underlying Autoantibody Responses in DIA and DIL

1. Drug binds to and alters self-macromolecule; immune response to drug-altered macromolecule includes antibodies that react with native macromolecule
2. Drug binds to self-material or foreign material, resulting in immune response to altered site; drug-altered epitope possesses antigenic mimicry with nonhomologous self-macromolecule, resulting in cross-reacting antibodies
3. Drug alters degradation or clearance of self-material, resulting in elevated levels of unusual forms of self-macromolecule, which then elicit autoimmune response
4. Drug nonspecifically activates T and/or B cells by direct mitogenic stimulation; this requires drug-specific T-cell response and bystander lymphocyte activation

delay of weeks to months from the onset of drug therapy to the development of autoantibodies and clinical symptoms suggests an immune reaction, rather than drug hypersensitivity. The slow kinetics and dose dependency of autoimmune phenomena elicited by procainamide and hydralazine imply that a sequence of two or more events or a coincidence of events occurs before autoimmune disease is manifested. As discussed above, the autoantibody response in DIL is largely restricted to histones and dDNA.[F280,P265] In addition, anti-DNA antibodies bearing the 16/6 and 32/15 idiotypes have been reported in one-third of DIL patients.[S160] This finding is noteworthy because these anti-DNA idiotypes are also commonly expressed in idiopathic SLE. Therefore, both the DNA and histone antibody responses in DIL and SLE appear to be similar, and are no less restricted in DIL.

The kinetics of the appearance of serum autoantibodies after procainamide therapy indicates that both IgG and IgM dDNA responses occur almost simultaneously.[R388] Histone antibodies appear in the serum at about the same time, but are restricted to IgM. This is especially true of patients who remain asymptomatic during drug therapy. The sine qua non of DIL is the appearance of histone and dDNA antibodies in the absence of other ANAs, and their disappearance after the drug is discontinued. The rather slow development of autoantibodies and the apparent concordance of IgG and IgM antibodies suggest that the drug reaction is not a classic immune phenomenon. Furthermore, the perpetuation of the IgM response is also not a feature of a typical, T-cell–dependent response.

Histones as Antigens

To understand the predominant autoantibody response to histone, it is important to appreciate some of the techniques used to study histone antibodies. Mammalian histones consist of five major proteins, which are separable by physicochemical methods and by polyacrylamide gel electrophoresis. ELISA, radioimmunoassay, or Western immunoblotting techniques can be used to demonstrate various patterns of reactivity with purified histones and chromatin components.[B582,C427,G218,P262,R393] The apparent lack of agreement on the predominant histone antigens in these reports is probably because of technical factors, such as antigen purification, blotting procedures, and differences in reagents used. Exclusive reliance on immunoblotting to detect antigenic reactivity is fraught with potentially false-negative observations, because epitopes or determinants expressed as higher order protein structures may not be available for binding using this technique. Thus, the use of purified histones, histone complexes, nucleosomes, and other chromatin fractions in an ELISA or other immunoassay is essential for histone antibody determination.

The use of chromatin fractions has provided important insights into the pathogenesis of DIL.[B583a,P262,R394,T193] Although considerable variation in the reactivity of PIL patients with individual histone has been observed, a common denominator was the presence of IgG and IgM antibodies directed against the H2A-H2B complex (Table 45–3). These sera also showed reactivity with H2B and

H2A consistent with the immunoblotting data. By comparison, the magnitude of the autoantibody reactivity with H2A-H2B complexes is often fivefold greater than the reactivity with individual histones. In addition, H2A-H2B antibodies bind to native chromatin[B583a,P265] and to protease-digested chromatin.[P262] In contrast, only 6% of patients treated with an average dose of 2.5 g of procainamide for an average of 31 months developed IgG histone antibodies. Because most patients with only IgM antibodies are asymptomatic, it is assumed that the IgM histone and dDNA antibodies are not pathogenic. These observations indicate that the key epitopes are present in the native conformation of histones, and that chromatin components such as the nucleosome may be driving the autoimmune response in DIL.

The reactivity of histone antibodies with native conformations of histones has received indirect support using a different approach. In one study, purified histones, nucleosomes, and reconstituted nucleosomes were used to study the mitogenic responses of lymphocytes.[F263] The results essentially parallel observations on DIL antibody reactivity: the most significant proliferative responses were observed when the intact nucleosomes were added to lymphocyte cultures, whereas purified histone components and nucleosomal DNA did not produce observable proliferative responses. In this study, the proliferative responses of lymphocytes appeared to be dependent on the presence of monocytes.

The interaction of procainamide and hydralazine with DNP has been inferred from various studies. Hydralazine has been shown to increase the viscosity of DNP and its resistance to protease degradation.[T40] Hydralazine has been shown to bind covalently to pyrimidines, thymidine, and deoxycytidine.[D345] At concentrations of greater than 50 mM, hydralazine induced initiation of DNA repair in primary cultures of rat hepatocytes and, at concentrations of 6 mM, was mutagenic, suggesting an interaction with DNA.[W236] Therapeutically relevant concentrations of hydralazine, however, are less than 10 μM.

Procainamide has an even lower propensity to develop stable interactions with DNA,[B350,G228,U7] and has been shown to complex with denatured DNA only under conditions of photo-oxidation.[B350,T180] A direct interaction of procainamide and DNA has been suggested by an increased thermal stability of DNA and an altered optical rotation and structure of supercoiled circular DNA in the presence of the drug.[E71,Z1] Procainamide has also been shown to destabilize dsDNA, and facilitates the transition from the B to Z conformation of synthetic polynucleotides having a propensity for Z conformations.[T153] Hydralazine has similar effects,[E71,T153] but N-acetylprocainamide (NAPA) does not. In addition, DNA damage in kidney and liver nuclei was observed after hydralazine was administered to rats.[J64] Procainamide was only weakly mutagenic in the microsome-facilitated Ames test,[F228] however, and did not bind to microsomal proteins.[F227]

Although covalent complexes of drugs with DNA can be obtained by several methods, no evidence has shown that these adducts have increased immunogenicity.[B350] Antibodies directed against hydralazine have been reported,[H38] but none were detected in a prospective study.[H293] Complexes of DNA and nucleoproteins with procainamide induced antibodies to procainamide and transient reactivity with DNA.[G228] Immunization of rabbits with covalent complexes between hydralazine and albumin elicited hydralazine antibodies and antibodies to dDNA if the drug was conjugated to human but not rabbit albumin.[Y26] These studies also suggested that antibodies to hydralazine and DNA represent cross-reacting antibodies. The importance of this observation is not clear, because dDNA antibodies that cross-react with hydralazine or other drugs have not been demonstrated in human DIL.[C95,H138,M273] Hydralazine is reported to cause nonspecific binding of antibodies to lymphocytes in vitro.[K445] A drawback of many of these investigations is the need to induce artificial complexes in vitro and/or the use of adjuvants to elicit the observed responses. Thus, the relevance of these findings in human DIL is not clear.

Cellular Immune Responses

The effects of hydralazine and procainamide on cellular immune function has not been studied as widely as autoantibody and humoral changes. Procainamide has been shown to enhance both pokeweed mitogen[B358,D108] and phytohemagglutinin[O7] stimulation of peripheral blood lymphocytes. In one study,[D108] procainamide inhibited the immunoglobulin secretion of lymphocytes in vitro.[D108] Procainamide-hydroxylamine, an important metabolite of procainamide (see below), enhances mitogen-mediated lymphocyte proliferation and IgM secretion in vitro.[A32] Studies of in vivo cellular immunity of procainamide-treated patients have led to differing results. In one study, normal numbers and ratios of T helper and T suppressor cells were reported.[Y60] Concanavalin A-induced T suppressor cell function was also normal, but pokeweed mitogen-induced immunoglobulin secretion was reduced. In the same study, T helper cell and B-cell activities were decreased in approximately 50% of patients and B-cell activity alone was decreased in 25%. These studies are in contrast to in vivo studies by the same group, who demonstrated an enhancing effect of procainamide on immunoglobulin secretion.[O7] This observation, attributed to the inhibition of T suppressor cell activity, was supported by other investigators,[G347,M424] who noted an increase of immunoglobulin secretion in the presence of pokeweed mitogen in patients treated with procainamide. These observations agree with the report of B-cell activation in PIL patients.[F168] In a more recent study, procainamide did not augment the proliferative effects induced by pokeweed mitogen, concanavalin A, or nucleosomes.[F231] N-acetylprocainamide (NAPA), which has been used as a safe alternative to procainamide to avoid DIL, was shown to be a less potent inducer of T-cell autoreactivity in a cloned T-cell assay.[R195] This effect may be related to decreased T-cell DNA methylation[C388] and to DNA methyltransferase inhibition[S118] in the presence of these drugs. The importance of these observations is based on evidence that inhibition of DNA methylation is associated with the development of CD4 + T-cell autoreactivity in vitro.[C388,R195]

Cellular dysregulation by hydralazine has been even less thoroughly studied. When patients treated with hydralazine were subjected to a battery of skin tests for delayed hypersensitivity, the responses were normal.[L334] In other studies, lymphocytes from patients with symptomatic HIL were shown to have a decreased stimulation index when incubated with hydralazine.[H138] In another study, 50% of asymptomatic hydralazine-treated patients showed a 3- to 4-fold increase in stimulation when peripheral blood lymphocytes were incubated with hydralazine-albumin conjugates.[L334] Finally, peripheral blood lymphocytes from HIL patients responded to dDNA in a proliferation assay.[H138]

It is not clear whether the increased responsiveness of patients to procainamide and hydralazine represents hypersensitivity, a nonspecific reaction, or an important mechanism underlying autoimmunity that has yet to be determined. The lack of toxicity in most animals and humans at high dosage levels suggests that the mechanism underlying DIL is not direct cytotoxicity. Carefully designed studies of the cellular responses in patients undergoing therapy with these drugs are required.

In the autoimmune state, it is assumed that an endogenous antigen drives host B cells and that T helper cells contribute to the growth and differentiation of clonally expanded, antigen-activated B cells.[R388] In DIL, the drug, or a metabolite of the drug, might bind to and alter surface antigens, such as Ia on non-T cells. The altered Ia may then be recognized as foreign by T helper cells, with resulting B-cell activation against an immunogen such as the histones and DNA on nucleosomes.[G192,R281]

Genetic Factors

Five features of DIL have suggested that genetic factors are important in the expression of DIL: 1) HLA phenotypes; 2) low hepatic acetyltransferase activity; 3) gender; 4) race; and 5) complement.

HLA Phenotypes

Interest in the immunogenetic factors that underlie DIL is based on observations that only a few people develop symptomatic disease, and that the immune response is restricted to a relatively narrow range of autoantigens. One feature is class II antigens, which control T-cell—dependent antibody responses. A study of 25 HIL patients by Batchelor et al.[B118,S581] showed a 73% frequency of HLA-DR4 versus a frequency of 25% in asymptomatic patients, representing a relative risk of 8.1. Another study using some of the same patients as in the Batchelor study found a 70% frequency of HLA-DR4 in HIL patients.[R430] A study of other HIL patients[B457] and of PIL patients,[T193] however, failed to find a significantly increased incidence of major histocompatibility complex (MHC) markers. Reexamination of HIL patients in the English study for complement protein phenotypes demonstrated a significant increase in C4 null alleles compared to normal controls.[S583] The genes encoding the C4 complement proteins are situated between HLA-B and HLA-DR loci, and the C4 null-DR4 haplotype displays linkage disequilibrium in Caucasians. Therefore, the reported association of HIL with HLA-DR4 is probably a result of the C4 null trait, and

linkage disequilibrium between HLA-DR4 and C4 may not occur in the Australian study group.[B457]

HLA-DR4 has been reported in those with penicillamine-induced lupus[C191,C239] and hydralazine-induced Sweet's syndrome.[R33] HLA-Dw44 was suggested as a significant risk factor (relative risk, 3.6) in the induction of ANA by chlorpromazine.[C64] More controlled studies are required to determine whether MHC genes are important in the development of DIL. Because most patients treated with hydralazine or procainamide develop ANA, it is unlikely that specific MHC factors are active in this phase of development of the disease.

Acetylator Phenotypes

The importance of the acetylator phenotype in DIL has been recognized.[H290,R388] The studies of Perry and colleagues demonstrated for the first time that levels of hepatic acetyltransferase activity and the "acetylator phenotype" of individuals were associated with the development of DIL.[P134] These studies were based on the knowledge that the acetyl group on procainamide and the hydralazine group of hydralazine and isoniazid is central to the pathogenesis of DIL. Based on the activity of acetyltransferase, North American Caucasian and black populations can be almost evenly divided into slow or fast acetylators. The acetylator phenotype can be determined by administering a tablet of dapsone, isoniazid, or caffeine to a patient and testing the serum or urine suing chromatography.[H122,R129] Slow acetylators are homozygous for a recessive gene that controls hepatic acetyltransferase activity, and they have a twofold higher serum level of unacetylated drugs at equivalent therapeutic doses.

During the treatment of slow acetylator patients with hydralazine[B118,P134] and procainamide,[W348] autoantibodies and clinical symptoms develop more quickly and in higher frequency than in rapid acetylators. It should be noted, however, that the development of clinical symptoms can occur in up to 20% of rapid acetylators,[R430] but both the dose and duration of drug administration are generally higher in these patients.[W348] These studies support the hypothesis that the steady-state concentration of procainamide and hydralazine and the cumulative duration of exposure are important elements in the development of DIL. Also, these studies indicate that the primary amino or hydrazine group on these drugs is a key to the autoimmune state.[L14,R257] Such observations have led to the successful use of N-acetylprocainamide to treat patients who had previously developed DIL or to avoid the development of DIL. Another approach has been to continue procainamide therapy and adjust the dosage by monitoring trough levels of the drug.[S555]

The importance of the primary amino or hydrazine group on these drugs in the development of DIA has been interpreted in two ways. A commonly held view is that these chemical moieties play a direct role in the induction of autoimmunity. Another explanation is that in vivo metabolism of the drug generates an active compound, and that N-acetylation blocks further drug metabolism. These putative reactive metabolites, rather than the parent molecule, would interact with a key immune target, leading to induction of autoimmunity. The association of the slow acetylator phenotype with symptomatic DIL can then be explained by a higher steady-state concentration of the metabolizable form of the drug. The lack of an association between acetylator phenotype and induction of ANA by isoniazid[A104] or by captopril,[R127] as well as idiopathic SLE,[B19] indicates that the slow acetylator phenotype is not a general predisposing factor for the autoimmune state, nor is it genetically linked to a putative autoimmunity-inducing or autoimmunity-accelerating gene.

Some studies have identified metabolic products of these drugs that may be more closely related to immune dysregulation. For example, the incubation of procainamide with human or rat liver microsomes under appropriate conditions results in the formation of an unstable product, procainamide hydroxylamine (PAHA).[B555,U9] This metabolite readily forms covalent bonds with a number of proteins in an oxidizing environment[U7] and is cytotoxic to various cell types.[R402] Cytotoxicity and covalent binding require further nonenzymatic oxidation to a nitroso compound, a hypothetic intermediate with a relatively low redox potential. Rapidly dividing cells with a high intrinsic biochemical-reducing ability are the most sensitive to the toxic effects of PAHA, suggesting that redox cycling between PAHA and the intermediate nitroso compound within the cell may deplete intracellular reducing potential and enhance cytotoxicity. In the resulting NADPH-depleted state, resting lymphocytes are slowly killed by PAHA, either because of depleted energy stores or because the single-stranded DNA breaks[R402] and cannot be repaired. In vitro procainamide hydroxylamine-nitroso cytotoxicity[R402] and hyperimmune effects[A32] may reflect their profound biochemical and biologic properties, implicating these metabolites as key factors in the induction of autoimmunity.

PAHA can be detected after the perfusion of rat liver with procainamide,[R244] supporting the view that hepatic "mixed function oxidases" may be an important site for generation of this reactive metabolite.[B555,U9] PAHA is taken up by erythrocytes and oxyhemoglobin enhances its functional effects,[A32,R244] presumably by converting PAHA to nitroso-procainamide. The PAHA generated in the liver might be transported by erythrocytes to lymphoid compartments. In addition, peripheral blood neutrophils activated with opsonized zymosan readily metabolize procainamide to the cytotoxic PAHA product.[R391a,U8] Metabolism of drugs by activated neutrophils provides a mechanism for generating highly reactive drug metabolites directly within lymphoid tissue, where autoimmunity presumably develops.

Gender

The role of gender in the development of ANA or DIL during drug therapy is not clear-cut. The best evidence is based on studies of HIL patients in which a 2- to 4-fold greater prevalence of women was observed.[B118,C35,R430] A 4-year study of the incidence of HIL demonstrated a disease rate of 11.6% in women and 2.8% in men.[C35] In this same study, women treated with a daily dose of 200 mg hydralazine had a 19.4% incidence of HIL over a 3-

year period. This is in contrast to the development of ANA in patients treated with hydralazine over a 3-year period, during which no gender differences were noted.[M112]

The effects of gender in the development of PIL are less dramatic. Some studies have suggested a disproportionate increase of PIL in women,[H266,S555,T193] but some of these results failed to reach statistical significance. Therefore, the role of gender and presumably sex hormones on the development of DIL is not clearly established. Studies of HIL, however, suggest that, similar to idiopathic SLE, hormonal effects may play a modulating or accelerating role in the expression of disease.

Race

Symptomatic DIL is rare in blacks. The frequency of HIL is 4-fold[C364] to 6-fold[P132] lower in blacks than in whites.

Complement

Hydralazine, cadralazine, isoniazid,[S447] and metabolites of procainamide and practolol,[S448] have been shown to inhibit C4 binding activity in vitro. It has been suggested, therefore, that these drugs may interfere with immune complex clearance.[R127] The C4a isotype is particularly reactive, so patients with the C4b null allele would be most vulnerable to drug-compromised immune clearance. Although these effects were observed at drug concentrations that were 10- to 100-fold higher than therapeutic plasma levels in humans, penicillamine inhibition of C4A binding falls within therapeutically relevant concentrations.[S446] Individuals with deficiencies in one, and especially both, C4 genes have increased susceptibility to SLE (see Chap. 2). It is possible that an acquired C4 deficiency may precede DIL through the inhibition of C4 by drugs. Patients carrying the C4 null allele (i.e., a deleted or nonfunctioning C4 gene) would be most susceptible to the induction of lupus, presumably because of lowered steady-state levels of C4. It is of considerable interest, therefore, that 76% of HIL patients had one or more absent C4 alleles, compared to 43% of controls.[S583] Another study has also identified C4 null alleles in HIL.[S583] It has not been determined, however, whether patients treated with hydralazine who remain asymptomatic have a low frequency of C4 null alleles. Similarly, it is not clear whether the hypocomplementemia associated with PIL reported in 1976 by Utsinger et al.[U40] was related to C4 deficiency. In most patients with PIL, serum complement levels are normal.

Another study of HIL patients showed a reduction of erythrocyte C3b receptors, CR1, but normal restriction fragment length polymorphism (RFLP) patterns of the CR1 gene.[M486] Because CR1 plays an important role in immune complex clearance, and abnormalities of CR1 have been documented in SLE, low levels of CR1 expression in HIL may be a factor in disease expression.

PATHOGENESIS

The observation that the symptoms and serologic features of DIL patients overlap with those of idiopathic SLE suggests that similar pathogenetic factors are present in these two syndromes. Immune complex formation and deposition in vital organs, one of the mechanisms shown to operate in SLE, does not appear to be a predominant feature of DIL. Evidence supporting the involvement of immune complexes is based on observations that complement breakdown products (e.g., C4d), theoretically resulting from activation of the classic pathway of complement by immune complexes, increase in symptomatic DIL and fluctuate with exacerbations of the disease.[R388,R395] As discussed above, other studies have implicated abnormalities in complement and immune complex clearance in DIL.[M486,S447,S448,S583] High levels of circulating immune complexes in DIL, however, have not been consistently observed.[S446] Because symptomatic DIL is related to the appearance of H2A-H2B antibodies, H2A-H2B—antibody complexes might be mediators of the disease, responsible for complement activation. Support for this theory is based on observations that antibodies directed against H2A-H2B during active disease are the complement-fixing IgG1 and IgG3 classes of IgG,[E87] but circulating histone-antihistone complexes in DIL have yet to be identified. If histone-antihistone complexes are found in DIL, it would be difficult to explain why DIL patients rarely develop renal disease, whereas idiopathic SLE patients do. A possible explanation is that DNA—anti-DNA complexes in SLE are pathogenic and are targeted to certain organs, but histone-antihistone complexes are not.

One study of complement binding by histone and dsDNA antibodies using indirect immunofluorescence has suggested that histone antibodies do not bind complement.[F278] Another study used a more sensitive ELISA technique to show that histone antibodies can fix complement,[K50] and that patients with active DIL have complement-split products in their serum.[B458,R395] It is difficult to prove that histones or other autoantibodies in DIL are pathogenic, and are not merely part of a specific autoimmune response directed against altered or native antigens.

Another hypothesis regarding the pathogenesis of DIL is based on the concept of molecular mimicry. One observation on which this theory is based is that some autoantibodies observed in SLE cross-react with bacterial cell walls.[S218] This suggests that autoantibodies in lupus may be primarily directed against a pathogen but can also cross-react with self-antigens, such as DNA. At present, little evidence supports this hypothesis in DIL. The nitroso derivative of procainamide reacts with many proteins in vitro, including histones.[U8] Thus, because the most common antibody in DIL is directed against histones, the nitroso derivative or some other metabolite of the drug might bind to histone and serve as a hapten to induce autoantibody production. Histone is an intranuclear protein, so it would be more likely that cell surface or cytoplasmic proteins are exposed to high concentrations of this metabolite. Although peripheral blood lymphocytes (PBL) do not metabolize procainamide,[U7,U8] other mechanisms involving drug metabolism by neutrophils and monocytes[R391a,U8] (see above) might lead to the induction of autoimmunity in lymphoid tissues.

An attractive alternative to histones as the target of drug binding is the myeloperoxidase system found in neutrophils and monocytes. It has been shown that, when procainamide is incubated with phorbol or zymosan-activated neutrophils, the hydroxylamine derivative and nitroso analogue of procainamide are produced.[R391a,U8] Furthermore, like histones, myeloperoxidase is a highly basic protein. ($pI > 11$). This suggests that myeloperoxidase antibodies may cross-react with histone, and vice versa. Antibodies to neutrophil myeloperoxidase, an antigen in the neutrophil cytoplasm recognized by antineutrophil antibodies,[R24,V25] have been reported in patients on hydralazine.[N35] Myeloperoxidase or other intracellular, cell surface, or environmental agents might share epitopes with histones. As noted above, studies of the autoantibody response and epitope analysis have indicated the nucleosome as the immunogen in DIL.

Chapter 46

INFECTIONS IN SYSTEMIC LUPUS ERYTHEMATOSUS

DANIEL J. WALLACE

Infection is a major source of morbidity and mortality in SLE patients. In 1987, Hellmann et al. reviewed mortality studies over a 40-year period.[H254] They compiled 3175 patients included in the largest series: of these 641 died, 170 from infection (27%). This percentage has not changed over the last 40 years, but the types of infective organisms have changed. The addition of corticosteroids to the therapeutic regimen further increases infection risk. At times, the actions of microbial agents on the host are difficult to differentiate from those of a lupus flare, and, by themselves, may aggravate the disease. Lupus patients are also susceptible to infection by opportunistic organisms. This chapter reviews infections in SLE, discusses differential diagnosis, and describes the infectious agents found most frequently in these patients.

FACTORS INFLUENCING SUSCEPTIBILITY OF LUPUS PATIENTS TO INFECTION

Even in the absence of corticosteroid treatment, infections are common in patients with SLE. Ropes used steroids sparingly, and rarely, if ever, gave immunosuppressives, yet 108 of 137 patients (79%) had serious infections during their disease course.[R294] These infections were usually associated with disease exacerbations. Several abnormalities may account for this susceptibility to infection, including immunoglobulin deficiency, defects in chemotaxis, phagocytic activity, and delayed hypersensitivity. Perez et al.[P118] associated an increased incidence of infections in SLE patients to the presence of a serum inhibitor of C5 complement-derived chemotactic activity. When levels of this inhibitor decreased as disease activity lessened, the incidence of infection dropped in the 16 patients followed. A National Institutes of Health report also correlated a decrease in serum generation of chemotactic factors with infection in 23 SLE patients.[C282]

Other studies have found impaired in vitro antibacterial activity from alveolar macrophages obtained at bronchioalveolar lavage,[W42] decreased staphylococcus aureus intracellular destruction capability,[M165] impaired opsonic capability,[D167] and defective degradation of bacterial DNA by phagocytes in patients with both discoid and systemic lupus,[R243] independent of steroid therapy. Abnormal cell-mediated immunity with delayed hypersensitivity responses is characteristic of SLE patients; this defect can improve after steroid therapy.[R312]

Because serum C-reactive protein levels are not helpful in diagnosing infection in SLE (see Chap. 47), some investigators have evaluated other markers. One group reported that levels of con A-bound serum α_1-acid glycoprotein predicted infection in 18 patients with SLE, as opposed to disease activity in 42 noninfected patients.[M27] Although superior to C-reactive protein, it was not 100% accurate. In another study,[T173] IgG3 and IgG4 isotypes were abnormally low in 15 infected patients but not in 33 noninfected patients with SLE. Neither of these tests is practical with regard to making clinical decisions about acutely ill patients.

SLE patients show signs of greater microbe exposure than control groups. Of 56 patients with SLE, 45% (versus 12% of controls) had elevated wart-virus titers, although the titers, when present, were lower than in control patients.[J85] Antibodies to varicella zoster were found in 43% of 92 patients with SLE, compared to 30% of controls,[N6] and the titers were higher in SLE. Of those with SLE, 30% also had defective delayed hypersensitivity skin reactions to varicella. Toxoplasmosis antibody titers were examined in 50 SLE patients and in 50 controls. The SLE group had significantly higher titers.[W225]

INCIDENCE OF INFECTION IN SLE AND THE ROLE OF STEROIDS

Steroid therapy clearly increases the incidence of infection in patients with SLE. Frenkel[F236] reviewed the role of corticosteroids as predisposing factors in fungal diseases and concluded that the mechanism is inhibition of cellular host responses. Proliferation of epithelioid and giant cells was impaired, and the digestive capability of these cells and macrophages was decreased.

Ginzler et al.[G159] followed 223 SLE patients for 655 patient-years. During this time, 163 bacterial, 183 viral (excluding herpes zoster), 12 herpes zoster, and 28 opportunistic infections (15 were Candida) were noted. In those not steroid-treated, 35 infections/100 patient-years were noted, compared to 179 who were. One opportunistic infection/100 patient-years was seen in the nonsteroid-treated group versus 42 for the treated group. The results for bacterial (10 without versus 87 with) and viral (23 without versus 39 with) infection groups are of interest. Steroids represent a significant risk factor for the development of infection of any type, and the risk for invasion by opportunistic organisms in steroid-treated patients is particularly high. The only nondrug-related predisposing factor is active renal disease, with abnormal urinary sediment.

The role of opportunistic infections has been studied at the New York University hospitals (Bellevue Hospital and the Hospital for Joint Diseases).[R217,R218] Between 1977 and 1987, 797 patients were admitted with SLE. Of these, 26 SLE patients with opportunistic infections were compared in a case-control study with SLE patients without opportunistic infections. Prednisone was a major risk factor for the development of opportunistic infection. The most common opportunistic organisms included Salmonella, Nocardia, Strongyloides, and Aspergillus monocytes. Patients with active disease and opportunistic infection had a 75% mortality rate; if the disease was inactive, the mortality rate was lower than 10%. Hellmann et al.[H254] reviewed 44 lupus-related deaths at Moffitt Hospital in San Francisco between 1969 and 1986. Opportunistic infections occurred in 15 of patients (35%) and caused death in 10. Antemortem diagnosis was only made in only 3 of 15. Candida and Pneumocystis were the most common organisms.

Gerding et al.[G96] compared the occurrence of infection during chronic hospitalization in 23 patients with SLE; 20 had rheumatoid arthritis (RA) and 11 had idiopathic nephrotic syndrome. Most patients were receiving steroids. The infection rate was 1.64/100 days of observation for SLE and 0.16/100 days of observation for non-SLE. In SLE patients, infections increased in proportion to the steroid dosage. For each 100 days of observation, the incidence of infections was the following: without steroids, 0.43%; 1 to 20 mg/day prednisone (or equivalent), 0.92; 21 to 50 mg/day, 2.17; 51 to 80 mg/day, 2.2; and over 80 mg/day, 4.00. The infection rate also increased with greater SLE disease activity and with azotemia.

At a center in Buenos Aires, 126 lupus patients were followed between 1976 and 1982.[D134] Of these, 52 developed serious infections, 28 required admission to a hospital, and 5 died. The most common outpatient infections were in the urinary tract and respiratory tract. Staphylococcus aureus, Proteus mirabilis, and Escherichia coli accounted for 31 of the 52 infections; also 2 had tuberculosis. A survey of 96 Spanish patients with SLE reported 0.17 infections/year. Of the 102 infections in 55 patients, 31% were urinary tract, 25% respiratory, 17% skin, and 16% bacteremia. Only 4 had opportunistic infections; 12 died from septicemia.[D146]

Lee et al.[L140] followed 110 patients for a mean of 4.5 years and observed 49 infections in 29 patients; 12 were judged to be serious, resulting in 4 deaths. Cohen et al.[C31] compared the incidence of infection in 19 SLE patients treated with azathioprine or cyclophosphamide with 56 others with immunologic disorders treated with the same drugs. No statistically significant differences were noted. In a Scandinavian study, 60 relatively stable SLE patients (mean prednisone dose, 2 to 8 mg) were compared to an RA control group, and no increase in opportunistic infections was found. Infections were more common during disease flares, and mucocutaneous S. aureus lesions were frequently seen.[N112]

SPECIFIC TYPES OF INFECTION

Bacterial Infections

In addition to respiratory tract and urinary infections, septic bacterial arthritis is occasionally seen. In a 1980 literature review, Hunter et al.[H506] collected 25 cases. The mean age was 33.6 years, with a mean disease duration of 6.4 years. Of the 21, 20 were receiving steroids and 3 were on azathioprine. Prior intra-articular injections and genitourinary infections were the chief predisposing factors. The most common organisms were Neisseria gonorrhoeae,[C320,M488] Staphylococcus, Tuberculosis, Salmonella, and Proteus mirabilis. Quismorio and Dubois[Q16] found three cases of septic arthritis in SLE patients at the LAC-USC Medical Center over a 5-year period. Abscesses of various bursae can mimic those of phlebitis and sciatica.[S304,L38]

Among the most common opportunistic bacterial infections seen in SLE are those caused by Salmonella,[A18,F221, G421,G432,H92,L4a,L393,M595,S305,S450] especially S. typhimurium and S. enteritidis. Occasionally, Salmonella infection can coincide with the initial presentation of the disease, and aspects of the infection can mimic those of SLE.[L4a] Hospitalized lupus versus nonlupus patients have an increased risk for Salmonella infections.[A18] In addition to diarrheal illnesses, it can manifest as gas-producing leg abscesses[S305] and septic arthritis.[C253,V16] Patients with glomerulonephritis may have an increased susceptibility to becoming chronic Salmonella carriers.[M325]

Tuberculosis can mimic the presentation of SLE. Feng and Tan[F60] found concurrent tuberculosis in 16 of 311 SLE patients (5%) seen in Singapore between 1963 and 1979. Atypical mycobacterial infections are rarely observed in SLE patients.[E114,L2]

Meningococcal infections can also mimic SLE.[C102,D243, L165,M487,S122] Mitchell et al. presented two cases and reviewed nine in the literature. Patients with complement deficiencies did better; six of nine survived.[M488] Five cases of Legionnaire's disease complicating steroid therapy have been reported.[E29,J33,S278,W174] Two splenectomized patients who received pneumococcal vaccination nevertheless developed Streptococcal pneumoniae infections.[V18,W117] Other unusual bacterial infections reported in SLE patients include Campylobacter endocarditis,[D381] toxic shock syndrome (we have had three cases of this),[F94] pneumococcal epiglottitis,[S303] urosepsis from Escherichia coli with resulting jaundice secondary to an α-hemolysin,[E103] Pseudomonas pseudomallei meningitis,[C254] and a documented tick bite with high antibody levels against Borrelia burgdorferi that coincided with the initial presentation of lupus.[F40]

Viral Infection

The most common viral infection seen in SLE patients is herpes zoster. Its incidence is high in steroid-treated SLE patients, ranging from 3.2 to 21%.[B21,D342,H180, K11,M635] The addition of cytotoxic drugs to prednisone therapy greatly increases the risk of herpes zoster. Of 83 patients entered into the National Institutes of Health lupus nephritis study, 21% developed herpes zoster.[M635] Of the 18, 3 were on prednisone alone and 15 were also given cytotoxic therapies. Generalized herpes zoster was seen in only 2 patients. It resolved in all. Kahl and Sheetz observed herpes zoster in 47 of 348 patients (13.5%) that was associated with severe disease, but not necessarily with disease flares or immunosuppressive therapy. Of the 47 patients, 3 died during the episode. One report of herpes zoster myelitis that mimicked central nervous system lupus has appeared.[B21]

Herpes simplex is not uncommon in SLE, and is particularly associated with perianal lesions.[B163,K23] Cytomegalovirus is observed rarely, but may have unusual presentations.[B566,K493,S291] It is responsive to gancyclovir.[B484,E129] See the differential diagnosis section (Chap. 49) for a discussion of human immunodeficiency virus infection and SLE.

Fungal Infections

Candidal infections are a common complication. Peripheral blood lymphocytes from patients who received high doses of prednisone had markedly depressed in vitro lymphocyte transformation to antigenic stimulation by Candida.[F136] Half of patients who have esophageal moniliasis do not have the oral disease.[G234,S345] Candida may coexist with herpes simplex.[B163]

In 1975, Sieving et al.[S424] presented 3 patients with deep fungal infections in SLE and reviewed 30 in the literature. Of these, 14 patients had Candida and 11 had cryptococcus. Of the 33, 28 were receiving corticosteroids; 27 died. Cryptococcal infection is not uncommon, and usually produces a terminal meningitis with or without pulmonary changes.[A160,C349,C351,F146,K189,K226,K438,S190,S584] An insidious onset of persistent headache is often the earliest manifestation. Zygomycosis (formerly known as mucormycosis) is a severe infection that has been associated with central nervous system complications, thrombotic thrombocytopenic purpura, and a high mortality.[B353,F97,W337] Coccidioidomycosis has been reported in 4 patients as a complication of steroid-treated lupus,[A190,B264,C365,J107] and was the cause of death in 2 of our patients.

Less common fungal infections in SLE patients include Nocardia pneumonitis, laryngitis and encephalitis,[G305,G410,I42,L408,W68,P154,S73] disseminated histoplasmosis,[D301] maduromycosis,[L325] and aspergillosis.[K110,Q2]

Parasitic Infestations

Hyperinfection with Strongyloides stercoralis may occur in immunosuppressed patients. The syndrome is characterized by profound malabsorption, diarrhea, electrolyte disturbance, gram-negative or opportunistic fungal sepsis, coma, and death. It can mimic an SLE flare, and eosinophilia may be absent as a result of steroid treatment.[L337,R221] Visceral leishmaniasis has been reported in one patient,[W47] as has paragonimiasis.[K411]

Protozoan Infections

Pneumocystis carinii pneumonia has been noted in SLE in three reports.[F171,R427,R428] Toxoplasmosis is especially prominent in neonates with SLE[W118] and in lymphopenic patients,[P261] and may be difficult to identify, because false-positive antibody titers can be seen in patients with SLE.[F97,K273,W99,W225] (Antinuclear antibodies bind to some antigens used in assays for toxoplasmosis.)

IMMUNIZATION AND ANTIBIOTICS

See chapter 61.

SUMMARY

1. Infections are a major source of morbidity and mortality in SLE patients.
2. Patients with SLE are susceptible to infection; treatment with corticosteroids increases this susceptibility in a dose-dependent fashion.
3. The respiratory and urinary tracts are the most common sites of infection in outpatients.
4. Patients on steroids are at a particularly increased risk for opportunistic infections. The most common organisms include herpes, Candida, Salmonella, Cryptococcus, and Toxoplasma.
5. Presentations of SLE are often difficult to differentiate from those of infection. The most helpful clues to infection are the presence of shaking chills, leukocytosis (unless steroids are being given), and the absence of active SLE in multiple systems.

Chapter 47

SERUM AND PLASMA PROTEIN ABNORMALITIES AND OTHER CLINICAL LABORATORY DETERMINATIONS IN SLE

DANIEL J. WALLACE

Abnormalities in plasma proteins are observed in most SLE patients. Certain clinical manifestations of the disease, such as edema secondary to hypoalbuminemia, can be attributed directly to these aberrations. The following sections review nonserologic laboratory abnormalities and discuss their clinical relationships and importance.

HYPOALBUMINEMIA

In 1943, Coburn and Moore[C314] first reported on the determination of proteins in SLE and found a low albumin and high globulin fraction in 17 patients. Scores of other reports have confirmed these findings. Albumin levels lower than 3.5 g/dl were found in 50% of Dubois' 398 patients,[D340] in 50% of Harvey's 105 patients,[M280] in 47% of Ogryzlo's 36 patients[O24] and in 34% of Ropes' 106 patients.[R294] In 29 of Dubois' patients, the albumin level was less than 2 g/dl; all were nephrotic. Pollak[P241] was able to correlate albumin levels with disease activity. Fries and Holman found a mean serum albumin level of 3.4 g/dl in 193 patients.[F256] Low serum albumin levels are observed in those with SLE complicated by nephrotic syndrome, protein-losing enteropathies, malnutrition, and chronic disease.

SERUM GLOBULINS

SLE is characterized by a polyclonal gammopathy representing a nonspecific, immunologic, antibody response. Hyperglobulinemia was found in 32% of Dubois' 398 patients,[D340] in 58% of Harvey's 105 patients,[M280] in 76% of Ropes' 106 patients,[R294] and in 30% of Hochberg's 150 patients.[H347] Certain globulin fractions that exhibit specific abnormalities are described below. Elevated serum globulin levels may be present with (as in lupus nephritis) or without (as in Sjögren's syndrome) low serum albumin levels.

α-Globulins: Alpha 1-Acid Glycoproteins, Alpha 1-Antitrypsin and Alpha 1-Antichymotrypsin

Pollak et al.[P241] noted the mean level of α_1-globulin to be in the upper limits of the normal range. Patients with the highest levels had proteinuria, regardless of disease activity. α_1-Globulin levels were elevated in 19 of Dubois' 110 patients (17%),[D323] and in 8% of Ropes' 106 patients.[R294] α_1-Globulins are often acute phase reactants, which are glycoproteins made in the liver that defend

against cellular injury. Others function as carriers and are decreased with cellular injury.

Denko and Gabriel found α_1-glycoprotein levels to be increased by 69 to 90% in 48 patients,[D157] and another group has confirmed this.[B233] They also observed a 25% increase (mean) in α_1-antitrypsin levels in their patients. Gladman et al.[G170] noted elevated levels in 5% and decreased amounts in 11% of 112 patients. A Chinese and a Swedish group were unable to find any significant differences.[D18,Z23] α_1-Antitrypsin is the dominant protease inhibitor in plasma. SLE is not associated with any specific α_1-antitrypsin phenotype.[B470,K87,R335] One study evaluated 33 SLE patients and found that α_1-chymotrypsin and α_1-antitrypsin levels are higher in those with inactive disease,[S747] but another study found no abnormalities.[D18] Plasma neutrophil elastase and lactoferrin levels may be slightly elevated in SLE patients.[A41]

α2-Globulins: Ceruloplasmin, Haptoglobin, and Alpha-2 Macroglobulin, HS Glycoprotein

Elevations in the α_2-globulin fractions were noted in 19 of Dubois' 110 patients,[D323] in 19 of Ropes' 73 patients,[R294] and in 33% of Ogryzlo's patients.[O24] Pollak et al.[P241] found the highest levels in patients with active disease and considerable proteinuria. In contrast, the mean level was not elevated in patients with inactive disease and no proteinuria. This may represent selective retention by a damaged kidney of the high-molecular-weight α_2-globulin. Ogryzlo's group confirmed this,[O24] but these findings have been challenged.[R99] Serum α_2-HA-glycoprotein is a negative acute phase reactant that is active in bone mineralization and resorption. Its levels are probably decreased in active SLE.[K22]

Ceruloplasmin, which is both an acute phase reactant and carrier protein, is increased by 20 to 40% in SLE.[D157] α_2-Macroglobulin is a protease inhibitor and is elevated in SLE.[B470,M7] In one study, SLE patients had a significant increase in haptoglobin type 2-2.[D18] See Chapters 24 and 25 for a discussion of antithrombin 3.

β-Globulins: Transferrin and Serum Lipids

β-Globulin levels were elevated in 18% of Dubois' 110 patients.[D323] Pollak's group found that mean levels were not different than those of controls, but those with active disease had significantly decreased values.[P241,R99] Transferrin, a β-globulin carrier molecule, was decreased in 20% in one report[D157] and normal in another.[D18] See Chapters 13, 24, 25, and 43 for a discussion of complement components, prothrombin, fibrinogen, plasminogen, and other clotting factors in the β-globulin region.

β-Lipoproteins comprise a sizable component of the β-globulin fraction. Wallace found significant hypercholesterolemia (>240 mg/dl) in 88 of 434 idiopathic SLE patients (21%) and hypertriglyceridemia (>200 mg/dl) in 17.6%.[W18] The hyperlipidemic effect of corticosteroids has long been recognized and documented in rheumatic disease patients. Ettinger et al.[E154,E155] reported that female patients with SLE who were not taking steroids have lipid levels similar to those of a control group; however, the administration of steroids led to significant increases in triglyceride, cholesterol, apolipoprotein B, and low-density lipoprotein cholesterol (LDL-C) levels. Others have confirmed this.[A278] Wallace et al.[W38] reported that hydroxychloroquine can decrease LDL-C, cholesterol, and triglyceride levels in SLE patients by 15 to 20%. Two other preliminary reports confirmed our findings.[H359,M56] Because most patients with organ-threatening lupus are taking corticosteroids, and most without organ-threatening disease are on antimalarials, these agents often interfere with baseline lipid determinations. Reports of types I, III, and V hyperlipidemia in SLE patients have appeared.[A119,B668,P71] Nephrotic syndrome is associated with extremely high levels of cholesterol (especially high LDL), low high-density lipoprotein-2, and triglycerides.[K138] Ginzler's group evaluated 10 children with SLE and identified two distinct patterns of dyslipoproteinemia.[18] Active disease was associated with a depressed HDL level and apoprotein A-1 was associated with elevated very low-density lipoprotein cholesterol (VLDL-C) and triglyceride levels. After corticosteroid therapy, total cholesterol, VLDL-C, and triglyceride levels were increased. Corticosteroid therapy of SLE is associated with accelerated atherosclerosis with resulting increased mortality.[U34]

Gamma Globulins

A broad polyclonal elevation of the gamma globulin fraction was observed in 61% of Dubois' 110 patients,[D323] in 77% of Estes and Christian's 150 patients,[E147] but in only 29% of Ropes' 73 patients[R294] and in 8% of Rothfield's 365 patients.[R339] Although associated with active disease and proteinuria, gamma globulin levels can be normal, even with significant disease activity.[F51,O24,P241,R99,S266]

Marked acquired hypogammaglobulinemia in SLE has been noted in 14 case reports, usually following high-dose corticosteroid and immunosuppressive therapy.[A346,B124,E120,G270,H180,S632,S767,W147] This group is especially susceptible to recurrent infections.

SERUM IMMUNOGLOBULINS

Immunoglobulin G and Its Subclasses

Mean serum levels of immunoglobulin G (IgG) are increased in SLE patients compared with healthy controls.[A103] Evidence that this increase is polyclonal stems from the observation that isolated IgG elevation occurs in only 9% of SLE patients.[C142] The IgG level tends to be elevated at diagnosis, but normalizes with therapy. At any time, IgG was increased in 22% of 39 patients followed serially.[S159] Levy et al.[L231] studied the mean survival half-life for IgG in patients with SLE. It averaged 8.2 days, compared to an average of 28 days in normal controls. An average of 10.1% of total body IgG was catabolized daily, compared to a mean of 3.9% in normals. Despite normal serum IgG concentrations in SLE patients, their synthetic rates were as much as four to five times normal, revealing far greater IgG antibody production in SLE than suggested merely by serum concentration. In a longterm serial study at the NIH, 18 patients developed low IgG levels during the course of their disease, but it was transient in 10; also, 4 developed recurrent infections. Excessive T-cell suppressor and decreased B-cell activity characterized this subset.[C438] Ward et al. were unable to correlate IgG levels with age, sex, race, or duration of disease.[W73]

Several centers have evaluated SLE patients for IgG subclasses. Among 20 children, significantly increased IgG1 and IgG3 subclasses were present along with decreased IgG4;[O76] 48 adults with SLE had decreased IgG2 and IgG4 levels. Low IgG3 and IgG4 levels correlated with an increased rate of infection.[T173] In another report, an increased IgG1 level was associated with a subgroup of patients with high-titer rheumatoid factor, antinuclear antibody, and low levels of anti-dsDNA.[K133]

Immunoglobulin M

Elevated mean immunoglobulin M (IgM) levels were found by Alarcon-Segovia and Fishbein[A103] in 481 serum samples from 106 patients compared with 106 controls. Schoenfeld et al.[C142] noted that the IgM level was often decreased at diagnosis but normalized later. In 39 patients followed serially, the IgM level was elevated at any time in 18%. Two other large-scale studies found that very low IgM levels (> 2 standard deviations below the mean) can be found in 20% of over 150 SLE patients.[S16,S274] Low IgM levels tended to correlate with disease duration, but not with activity.[W73] Survival studies of IgM in SLE show a normal half-life.[L231]

A 7S γM-globulin occurs in SLE, rheumatoid arthritis, and in the cord blood of apparently normal infants, but is absent in normal human adult sera.[S607] This fraction was found by Rothfield et al. in 8 of 53 patients with SLE, 4 of whom were males[R349] and in 32% of 31 men with SLE by Kaufman et al.[K121] Low-molecular-weight IgM as a monomeric subunit probably comprises about 15% of the total IgM seen in SLE patients.[R246]

Immunoglobulin A

Immunoglobulin A (IgA) deficiency is found in 1/400 to 1/3800 adults. It has been observed in 3 of 96 and 3 of 72 SLE patients in two reports,[K484,R209] which suggests an increased incidence of this uncommon finding. Men may have an increased incidence of IgA deficiency in SLE.[K121] Although the serum IgA level is usually normal or slightly elevated in SLE,[A103,C142,S274] elevations of IgA were found in 30% of patients during the course of the disease in one study.[S159] Saliva gamma A or secretory IgA levels may be reduced in patients with SLE and frequent attacks of respiratory disease.[T179] Blacks with SLE may have a higher IgA2 level than Caucasians.[C368]

Immunoglobulin E

Increases in immunoglobulin E (IgE) levels may correlate roughly with disease activity in LE.[G259,M406,R384a] Two cases of "hyper-IgE" syndrome, one following carbamazepine administration, have been reported in SLE patients.[L255,S161] A hyperimmunization phenomenon might by contributory.

Paraproteinemia and Paraproteinuria

Of 415 SLE patients followed in Toronto, 9 (2.2%) had evidence of paraproteinemia.[R89] The monoclonal proteins were IgG (6), IgA (2), and IgM (1). None had myeloma, and no consistent patterns could be discerned. About 30 cases have appeared in the literature.[F152] Characterized as either transient, stable, or increasing, they are almost always benign. The large number of patients in this group treated with corticosteroids has led to the hypothesis that these agents might enhance production of immunoglobulin.

Unbound free urinary light chains are increased in lupus nephritis, and represent quantitative markers of concurrent, in vivo immunoglobulin synthesis and secretion.[E123,H410]

SEDIMENTATION RATE

Elevation of the sedimentation rate occurred in 84% of 463 of Dubois' patients between 1950 and 1963,[D323] and in 94% of Armas-Cruz's 108 patients,[A289] and Wallace observed Westergren sedimentation rates to be greater than 30 mm/hr in 236 of 434 patients (54%) tested.[W18] The mean Wintrobe sedimentation rate of Fries and Holman's 193 patients was 39 mm/hr.[F256] It was significantly associated with fevers, fatigue, alopecia, myalgias, and greater disease activity when elevated. Sedimentation rates can be high with no obvious clinical activity, and normal with active disease. They are usually helpful in following the subset of patients in whom its rise and fall reflect other clinical and laboratory parameters.

The rapid sedimentation rate is partially attributable to the tendency of red cells to clump and form rouleaux, often because of the associated abnormal antibodies in SLE. When the Wintrobe method is used, rapid falling occasionally occurred, and the final value was often limited by the hematocrit; the Westergren method is more precise. An excellent review of the subject can be found in reference B161.

C-REACTIVE PROTEIN

C-reactive protein (CRP) is a serum component that binds to pneumococcal C-polysaccharide. It activates complement, inhibits cytokine production, and generates T-suppressor cells. It is composed of five identical, nonglycosylated, polypeptide units of 187 amino acid residues each that are noncovalently associated in a disk-like configuration. CRP is synthesized by hepatic parenchymal cells, weighs 120,000 daltons, and circulates in the gamma globulin fraction. It can act as an opsonin or agglutinin and mediates phagocytic activities while inhibiting immune responses. A putative evolutionary homology with immunoglobulin, complement, and HLA has been suggested.[K242]

First described as being elevated in SLE patients with infection by Hill[H302] in 1951, other reports suggested that it was an accurate test for active SLE.[B154,B464,H405,S358] Enthusiasm peaked in 1980 when an Arthritis and Rheumatism editorial suggested that it might be a good ARA classification criterion for SLE.[D177] Other studies, however, found the CRP level useful neither for SLE nor infection.[L92,R356] It soon became apparent that older methods for determining the CRP level were not accurate when rheumatoid factor was also present. Using the more reliable radioimmunodiffusion assay, Rothschild[R356] noted it to be elevated in 56% of 52 SLE patients, with or without infection. It vaguely correlated with clinical activity, but not with any organ system involvement, except leukopenia. Bertouch et al.[B265] observed elevated CRP levels in 55 of 70 SLE patients. It was very high in 13, none of whom had infection. Morrow et al.[M607] noted that CRP was present in 60% of 27 patients, especially in those with active disease. Zein et al.[Z21] found it in some patients without obvious explanation, and observed numerous disease exacerbations in patients without any CRP changes. In a more recent study, only 9% of 34 SLE patients had an elevated CRP level.[S483]

Pepys et al.[P112] reviewed the subject at length. One of the strong advocates of its use, his group followed sedimentation rates and CRP binding in 429 measurements involving 124 patients with inactive, mildly active, and active SLE, and in SLE with infection. If one evaluates their data (as opposed to their conclusions), it is clear that the *mean* CRP level is not elevated or only slightly elevated in the first three categories, but is high with infection. Mean CRP levels were significantly greater than sedimentation rates with infection, but significantly less with active disease. The CRP levels in *individual* patients, with active disease or infection, however, ranged from absent to high. In other words, CRP was not useful in individual cases, even though the mean values in patient groups were significantly elevated. The only positive conclusion that can be reached is that, if the CRP level is very high (greater than 60 mg/L), the chances of infection are greater.[H311,T110] CRP values are high in those with rheumatoid arthritis and the seronegative spondyloarthropathies, but only modestly elevated in systemic vasculitis.

In conclusion, CRP is a misunderstood test of disease activity that is neither sensitive nor specific in SLE. It may be of some value, however, in ruling in infection and may be of some hitherto undescribed value in following SLE patients.

β₂-MICROGLOBULIN

β_2-microglobulin is a single-chain polypeptide (molecular weight 11,800 daltons) found on the surface of most nucleated cells, especially T and B lymphocytes. A normal constituent of serum that is catabolized by the kidney, it is associated with the light chains of class I HLA antigens. Its serum values increase slightly with age and are elevated with decreased glomerular filtration rates and various rheumatic diseases. In SLE sera, anti−β_2-microglobulin antibodies inhibit in vitro mitogenic stimulation and lymphocyte proliferation.[M368] Seven well-designed studies have evaluated its clinical importance in SLE,[E136,F14, F153,K364,V4,W163,Y43] and all came to similar conclusions. Overall, it has a 64% sensitivity and 87% specificity for assessing disease activity when compared to healthy controls. β_2-Microglobulin levels are increased with active disease, nephropathy, low C3 complement levels, elevated sedimentation rates, and anti-DNA. Its highest levels are seen in lupus nephritis, although azotemia with inactive disease can also result in larger values.

VISCOSITY

Viscosity is an important determinant of blood flow. Plasma viscosity can be increased by elevations of high-molecular-weight globulins, such as fibrinogen and immunoglobulin. Three studies have shown that SLE patients have slightly increased levels when compared to control groups.[H226,S483] Rarely, complexes of IgG, and especially IgM rheumatoid factor, produce high levels of plasma viscosity and a clinical syndrome resembling that found in Waldenström's macroglobulinemia. This so-called "hyperviscosity syndrome" has been observed infrequently in SLE, and is an indication for emergency plasmapheresis and steroid therapy.[A46,F302,J50]

MISCELLANEOUS LABORATORY ABNORMALITIES: CONNECTIVE TISSUE COMPONENTS AND TRACE METALS

SLE is characterized by striking changes in the amorphous ground substance of tissues. Consisting largely of hyaluronic acid and chondroitin sulfuric acid, hexosamine constitutes about 40% of each of these mucopolysaccharides, and human serum contains definite amounts of bound hexosamine as glucose and galactosamine. Serum levels of hexosamine were increased in active disease in one report that followed 19 patients serially.[B370] Free and bound glycosaminoglycans (which consist mostly of slow

sulfated chondroitin 4-sulfate) is also elevated with active disease.[F269] Serum immunoreactive prolyl hydroxylase is also an acute phase reactant in SLE, and its increased levels may reflect greater connective tissue disease metabolism.[K487] On the other hand, serum sulfhydryl and serum histidine levels decrease in active disease.[L380,S483] Urinary sialyated saccharides, serum sialic acid, and serum amyloid A protein may also act as acute phase reactants in SLE.[M218,O118] Serum laminin P1—one of the glycoproteins of basement membranes—is found in high amounts with active disease.[S155] Seromucoid levels may reflect connective tissue destruction and are probably higher in SLE.[G356,P29,S747]

Zinc and selenium levels are normal in SLE.[A153] Single reports have claimed that cathepsin D activity,[P173] and plasma neopterin[H119] and plasma thrombospondin levels[H466] are increased in SLE.

SUMMARY

1. Hypoalbuminemia occurs in SLE patients with active disease, particularly nephrosis. Following its level serially is of prognostic value.
2. α_1- and α_2-globulins include acute phase reactants that are increased and carrier proteins that are decreased in active SLE. β-Lipoprotein levels are elevated with nephrosis and corticosteroid therapy, and decreased by antimalarial agents.
3. The IgG level is elevated with disease activity in patients not on steroids or immunosuppressive drugs. Its turnover is greatly increased. No IgG subclass is characteristic. The IgM level is consistently decreased in 20% of patients.
4. Sedimentation rates are elevated with active SLE; disease activity can thus be followed in a subset of patients. In some patients, the sedimentation rate does not correlate with disease activity. The C-reactive protein level is usually normal or slightly elevated in SLE; high levels should raise suspicions of infection.
5. β_2-Microglobulin levels are generally increased in active SLE, especially if renal disease is present.
6. Although plasma viscosity is slightly increased in SLE, hyperviscosity syndrome is an extreme rarity.

Chapter 48

CLINICAL APPLICATION OF SEROLOGIC ABNORMALITIES IN SLE

FRANCISCO P. QUISMORIO, Jr.

One hallmark of SLE is the wide array of serologic abnormalities, including a polyclonal increase in serum gamma globulins, the presence of antinuclear antibodies and various serum organ-specific and nonorgan-specific autoantibodies, circulating immune complexes, and serum complement changes. The presence of some of these abnormalities is important in corroborating the clinical diagnosis of SLE, whereas others are useful in monitoring disease activity. Each abnormality is discussed in a separate chapter (see Chaps. 11, 13, 19, 20, 21, 22, and 23). This section focuses on the clinical application of selected serologic abnormalities in establishing the diagnosis, in assessing disease activity, and in predicting specific organ system involvement and overall prognosis of the patient. Serologic tests that are generally available in most clinical laboratories are included.

SEROLOGIC TESTS

Diagnosis of SLE

When the diagnosis of SLE is suspected or made on clinical grounds, the following serologic tests are considered helpful in corroborating the diagnosis (Table 48–1): fluorescent antinuclear antibody (ANA) test, ANA panel, serum complement level, and VDRL or other comparable serologic test for syphilis. In certain situations other serologic tests are also applicable, such as Coombs' test in a patient presenting with hemolytic anemia, lupus anticoagulant, test and anticardiolipin antibody test in a patient with a history of thrombosis or multiple fetal loss.

Virtually all SLE patients with active and untreated disease test positive for ANA. Nevertheless, ANA is also prevalent in other rheumatic and nonrheumatic disorders, including some conditions that may mimic the clinical picture of SLE. Thus, by itself, a positive ANA has a low diagnostic specificity for the disease, but its value increases when the patient meets the clinical criteria for SLE. The indirect immunofluorescent test is the most commonly used method for detecting ANA, and the choice of substrate in this test is important. Sections of rodent liver or kidney and tissue culture cell lines (Hep-2 or KB cells) are used in most clinical laboratories. Certain types of ANA, such as anti-Ro/SSa and anticentromere antibodies, can be detected with these cell lines but not with rodent tissues.[H140] A positive serum should be titered to give a semiquantitative value to the antibody level. The fluores-

cent staining pattern should also be included, but, in the presence of multiple types of ANA, the staining pattern may change as the serum is titered (see Chap. 19).

The "ANA panel" available in clinical laboratories includes ANA of defined specificity: anti-dsDNA, anti-Sm, anti-U1RNP, anti-Ro/SSA, and anti-La/SSB. Some laboratories include antinucleoprotein, anticentromere, antihistone, and/or anti-ssDNA in their panel. When the fluorescent ANA is positive in a patient suspected of having SLE, an ANA panel should be obtained. Anti-dsDNA and anti-Sm antibodies are considered highly diagnostic, and their presence almost confirms the clinical diagnosis. The other types of ANA in the panel have lesser value as diagnostic markers for SLE, except in special situations such as the presence of anti-Ro/SSa antibody in a patient with subacute cutaneous lupus erythematosus (see below for a discussion of individual ANA types).

The serum complement level is generally measured as concentration of C3 or C4, or as $C'H50$ hemolytic units. Although used more commonly in assessing disease activity, the presence of both hypocomplementemia and high titers of anti-dsDNA in a patient suspected of having SLE almost confirms diagnosis of the disease.[W141] In addition, a genetic deficiency of C2 or C4 may present clinically with an LE-like syndrome, and the combination of a low or absent $C'H50$ and normal C3 level should raise the possibility of this diagnosis.[S195]

A biologic false-positive test for syphilis is one of the four immunologic abnormalities included in the ACR criteria for the diagnosis of SLE. Other antiphospholipid antibodies, such as lupus anticoagulant and anticardiolipin antibodies, are helpful in delineating subsets of SLE patients, such as those who are prone to recurrent arterial or venous thrombosis and fetal loss (see Chap. 24).

Monitoring Disease Activity in SLE

Serologic tests are widely used for assessing disease activity and predicting exacerbations (Table 48–2). Determination's of the serum titer of anti-dsDNA and of the complement level are the most common and probably the most useful tests that are readily available to the clinician. Although applicable to most patients, both tests have limitations. Anti-dsDNA antibodies and hypocomplementemia do not occur in all patients, and their correlation with disease activity is not absolute. A few patients can have persistently elevated anti-dsDNA antibody titers without

Table 48–1. Serologic Tests Useful in the Diagnosis of SLE

1. Fluorescent ANA
2. ANA panel: anti-DNA, anti-Sm, anti-U1RNP, anti-Ro/SSA, anti-La/SSB
3. Serum complement level
4. VDRL
5. Anticardiolipin antibodies
6. Coombs' test

developing evidence of clinical disease, even when followed for several months.[G28,W66] Serial measurement of the serum titer of anti-Sm and anti-Ro/SSA antibodies can be useful, particularly in those who test negative for anti-dsDNA antibodies (see below).

In analyzing reports about the predictive value of various serologic tests in SLE, the following points should be remembered. The selection of patients varies widely, and the clinical criteria used to define "active SLE" are not uniform. The effect of previous drug therapy is frequently not addressed. Most studies compare groups of patients, and only few are well-designed, longterm, prospective studies. Conclusions are often derived from a single serum determination rather than from multiple specimens over a period of time. Different test systems are used by various investigators to measure a given serologic parameter. Thus, comparison of the results of various studies is not always feasible and appropriate.

We and others have found the concentration of serum cryoglobulins to be a useful parameter that correlates with disease activity, especially in those with nephritis.[S623,W282,H458,Q20] Although technically simple, the measurement of cryoglobulins requires careful handling of the specimen for proper interpretation of the results. Venous blood is allowed to clot at 37° C immediately after venipuncture. Following incubation at 4° C for 48 hours, the specimen is centrifuged in the cold and the precipitate is saved. The precipitate is washed carefully with a low ionic phosphate buffer, and the protein concentration is measured by standard methods.

The role of circulating immune complexes in monitoring disease activity in SLE remains controversial and unproven.[E104] The lack of a widely accepted standardized test system, the heterogeneity of immune complexes in SLE sera,[K201,V5] and the imprecise and inconsistent correlation with disease activity limit the application of circulating immune complexes in following the clinical course of the disease in individual patients (see Chap. 11). Of the

Table 48–2. Serologic Tests for Assessing Disease Activity in SLE

1. Anti-DNA antibodies
2. Serum complement level: C3, C4, C'H50
3. Anti-Sm and other specific types of ANA
4. Circulating immune complexes
5. Serum cryoglobulin levels
6. Split products of complement
7. Serum level of sIL-2R

numerous serologic tests for circulating immune complexes, the C1q solid phase binding assay appears to be the most frequently used method in SLE patients.[A20,L341,V6,W175]

Two serologic tests with promising value are the measurements of products of complement activation and of soluble interleukin-2 receptors (sIL-2R).[A19,C52]

CLINICAL SIGNIFICANCE OF THE ANTI-DNA ANTIBODY

Diagnostic Value

Antibodies to DNA are classified according to their reactivity to native or double-stranded (anti-dsDNA) or to denatured or single-stranded DNA (anti-ssDNA). The presence of anti-dsDNA is highly characteristic of idiopathic SLE and is rarely seen in other rheumatic conditions, including drug-induced LE.[T43,M543] One of the four immunologic criteria for the classification of SLE by the ACR is the presence of anti-dsDNA. In contrast, anti-ssDNA antibodies, although prevalent in SLE, are found in those with many other disorders, including rheumatic and nonrheumatic conditions.[K339] Thus, in the clinical laboratory, anti-dsDNA but not anti-ssDNA antibodies are tested for routinely in the ANA panel.

In a large cohort prospective study, Weinstein et al.[W141] found that high titers of anti-dsDNA and a low serum C3 are sensitive and that each test had a high predictive value (94%) for the diagnosis of SLE when applied to a patient population in which the diagnosis was clinically suspected. Moreover, the predictive value was even higher when both serologic abnormalities were present in an individual patient.

Clinical Tests for Anti-dsDNA

The four most commonly available tests for anti-dsDNA antibodies in the clinical laboratory are radioimmunoassay using either the Farr or the millipore filter binding technique, enzyme-linked immunosorbent assay (ELISA), and the Crithidia luciliae immunofluorescence test. The radioimmunoassay is a sensitive technique, and approximately 60 to 70% of SLE patients test positive for anti-dsDNA by use of this methods.[T43,M543] False-positive results are occasionally seen with this test because of the contamination of the DNA substrate with single-stranded forms. The ELISA test for anti-dsDNA is technically easy to perform, and is the least labor-intensive. The serum titer can be readily measured and, more importantly, both high- and low-avidity anti-dsDNA antibodies can be detected. The immunofluorescence test uses fixed smears of Crithidia luciliae, a nonpathogenic hemoflagellate that contains a circular cytoplasmic organelle called a kinetoplast, which consists of dsDNA. Serum anti-dsDNA, but not anti-ssDNA antibodies, bind to the kinetoplast. We have used this method to measure not only the titer of the antibody but also the immunoglobulin class and complement-fixing property of anti-dsDNA.[B143]

Qualitative properties of anti-dsDNA antibodies, including avidity, Ig class, and complement-fixing property, may affect the pathogenicity of the antibodies (see Chap. 20).

Because the three available tests for anti-dsDNA preferentially measure antibodies of different properties, some controversy has arisen as to which test yields the most useful information in assessing disease activity.

Ward et al.[W76] compared the ELISA, Crithidia luciliae immunofluorescence test, and filter binding radioimmunoassay in SLE patients followed over a period of time. They found that, in most patients, the changes in anti-dsDNA antibody levels measured over time parallel each other, and that the anti-dsDNA titer measured by each assay is inversely correlated to the serum C3 concentration. The data from this study indicated that the repertoire of anti-dsDNA antibodies detected in an individual patient remains relatively constant over time, confirming the observation that high- and low-avidity anti-DNA antibodies do not move independently in an individual patient, but rise and fall in a parallel pattern.[M286]

In summary, the most commonly available tests for anti-dsDNA antibodies yield comparable results over time in individual patients. In clinical practice, any of these tests can be used to follow the antibody titer sequentially in most SLE patients. If a lupus patient with clinically active disease has repeatedly low serum levels of anti-dsDNA antibodies with one test, use of a different test system should be considered.

Assessment of Disease Activity

A number of studies, most retrospective, but a few prospective, have examined the value of anti-dsDNA antibodies in predicting disease exacerbations and response to drug therapy. Table 48–3 summarizes the results of selected studies.[A44,D92,I32,L341,M456,S782,S784,T108]

Retrospective Studies

Davis et al.[D92] described a fairly good correlation between disease activity and anti-dsDNA antibodies measured by a millipore radioassay. Several patients in clinical remission, however, had a mild to moderate elevation of anti-dsDNA antibody levels. Swaak and associates[S782] found a sharp drop in anti-dsDNA antibody titer, usually preceded by a rise, that correlated with lupus nephritis and other major organ involvement. In contrast, a continuously high antibody titer was not predictive of disease flare. Isenberg et al.[132] reported that severe lupus nephritis, but not central nervous system and other extrarenal involvement, correlated with anti-dsDNA antibodies, especially with antipoly (dT) antibodies. Measurement of antibodies to different synthetic polynucleotides did not significantly add to the routine determination of anti-dsDNA antibodies. Lloyd and Schur[L341] observed that anti-dsDNA antibody measured by the Crithidia luciliae test correlates only fairly with disease activity. A rising antibody titer correlated with 75% of renal, 60% of extrarenal, and 30 to 50% of combined renal and extrarenal flares. In a study of patients with lupus nephritis treated with azathioprine and steroids Adler et al.,[A44] using the Farr assay, found a persistently elevated anti-dsDNA to be predictive of a poor renal outcome.

Prospective Studies

A few longterm prospective studies have evaluated the clinical significance of anti-dsDNA antibodies and of these in combination with serum complement level and other

Table 48–3. Association of Anti-dsDNA and Disease Activity

Source	No. of Patients in Study	Method Used	Results and Comments
Retrospective studies			
Davis et al. (1977)[D92]	23	Radioassay	Good correlation between disease activity, but positive sera were seen in several patients in remission
Swaak et al. (1979)[S782]	78	Farr assay	Sharp drop in anti-dsDNA titer, especially if combined with low C3 and C1q; predictive of nephritis or major organ flare; persistently high titer was not predictive of flare
Isenberg et al. (1988)[132]	39	ELISA	Severe lupus nephritis but not extrarenal involvement correlated with anti-dsDNA, and especially with antipoly (dT); antibodies to synthetic polynucleotides did not add significantly to routine measurement of anti-dsDNA antibodies
Lloyd and Schur (1981)[L341]	27, with 47 flares	Crithidia luciliae test	Anti-dsDNA showed only fair association with disease activity; rising titer coincided with 75% of renal, 60% of extrarenal and 30 to 50% of combined renal and extrarenal flare; combination of C'H50, C4, C3, and C1qBA most useful test for predicting disease activity
Adler et al. (1975)[A44]	21 (diffuse lupus nephritis)	Farr assay	Persistently high anti-dsDNA despite drug therapy correlated with poor renal outcome; an initial high titer had no prognostic value; all received azathioprine and steroids
Swaak et al. (1986)[S784]	143, with 33 flares	Farr assay	All 33 flares preceded by a progressive rise and sharp drop in antibody titer; 20 to 25 weeks prior to onset of nephritis, serum C4 decreased, followed by C1q and C3
Ter Borg et al. (1990)[T108]	72, with 27 flares	Farr assay, Crithidia luciliae test, and ELISA	24 of 27 flares (89%) preceded by a rise in antibody titer by 8 to 10 weeks; anti-dsDNA was more predictive than C3 or C4; Farr assay was the most sensitive test; no qualitative changes in anti-dsDNA prior to exacerbation were observed
Miniter et al. (1979)[M456]	70	Radioassay, filter	Half of active episodes associated with low C'H50 and high anti-dsDNA; isolated high anti-dsDNA or low C'H50 occurred significantly in inactive disease; most CNS episodes occurred without low C'H50 or high anti-dsDNA; C'H50 correlated with disease activity better than anti-dsDNA

serologic parameters. Minter et al.[M456] studied 70 patients longitudinally over 3 years. Only slightly more than half of the active disease episodes were associated with both a low C'H50 and a high anti-dsDNA level, as measured by the Farr assay. Many patients with clinically inactive disease had isolated elevated anti-dsDNA titers or low C'H50 levels. Active lupus nephritis was associated with complement-fixing anti-dsDNA or a low C'H50. In contrast, most episodes of central nervous system disease occurred without significant changes in the C'H50 level and anti-dsDNA antibody titer. Overall, the C'H50 parameter correlated better than anti-dsDNA antibodies with disease activity. In a longitudinal study of 143 SLE patients, Swaak et al.[S784] found that a progressive rise followed by a sharp drop in anti-dsDNA titer, as measured by the Farr assay, preceded all 33 major disease flares. A drop in the serum C4 level followed by a decrease in the serum C1q and C3 levels occurred 20 to 25 weeks prior to the onset of lupus nephritis. Ter Borg et al.[T108] reported that 89% of all disease flares that occurred in 72 SLE patients studied serially were preceded by a rise in anti-dsDNA titer by 8 to 10 weeks. The anti-dsDNA antibody titer was more sensitive in predicting exacerbations than serum C3 or C4 levels. The Farr assay was superior to the Crithidia luciliae or ELISA test for the determination of anti-dsDNA antibodies.

Summary

The quantitative determination of anti-dsDNA antibodies alone does not adequately predict disease flares in every patient. This is not unexpected, considering the heterogeneity of the clinical disease and of the anti-dsDNA antibodies. Several investigators have proposed that the qualitative properties of the anti-dsDNA antibodies, such as the complement-fixing property, avidity, dissociation constant, and immunoglobulin class are more important determinants than total antibody content in regard to pathogenicity and correlation with disease activity.[B144,C440,M28,P88,S562] The data from these studies are inconsistent, however, and qualitative tests are not readily available to the practicing clinician. Meanwhile, the anti-dsDNA antibody titer continues to be used widely as a serologic parameter for assessing disease activity. Combined with serum complement values, it is valuable in patients with lupus nephritis. In our experience, it is especially useful if the patient in question had a high anti-dsDNA titer and a low serum complement level in previous exacerbations of the disease. Isolated and continuous elevation of the anti-dsDNA titer is not an indication of steroid or cytotoxic drug therapy (see also Chap. 20).

CLINICAL SIGNIFICANCE OF THE ANTI-Sm ANTIBODY

Diagnostic Value

Anti-Sm antibody is present in only approximately 30% of SLE patients, but it has considerable diagnostic value because it is rarely found in other rheumatic diseases, such as mixed connective tissue disease, systemic sclerosis, and rheumatoid arthritis.[M51,M660] Anti-Sm is included in the ACR criteria for the classification of SLE and,

as an immunologic parameter, it carries the same weight as anti-dsDNA, positive LE cell test, and false-positive serologic test for syphilis.

The anti-Sm antibody is usually measured in the clinical laboratory by immunodiffusion, counterimmunoelectrophoresis (CIE), ELISA, and hemagglutination methods. The ELISA test, using purified antigens, is more sensitive but less specific than immunodiffusion and CIE.[A297,M51] The lower specificity of the former is partly a result of the difficulty in preparing pure Sm antigen.[F82] The ELISA test is superior to other methods, however, in measuring the serum titer of the antibody (see Chap. 22).

Prevalence

Studies have shown that the prevalence of anti-Sm antibody in SLE varies among different ethnic groups. In the United States, Arnett et al.[A297] found anti-Sm and anti-U1RNP to be more common in Afro-Americans (25% and 40%, respectively) than in whites (10% and 24%, respectively). Antibodies to Ro/SSA and La/SSB, however, occurred in equal frequencies in the two racial groups. The higher prevalence of anti-Sm and anti-U1RNP in Afro-Americans has been confirmed by others.[R173,W248] The frequency of anti-Sm antibody in SLE appears to be lower in France than in the United States.[A22] Anti-Sm was present in 12% (by immunodiffusion) and in 17% (by immunoblotting) of French SLE patients. In contrast, the prevalence among French West Indies patients was five times higher—39% by immunodiffusion and 50% by immunoblotting. In a smaller study, Field et al.[F84] found a higher frequency of the antibody among SLE patients originally from West Africa, the Caribbean Islands, and Asia than local whites in England.

Association with Organ Involvement

Whether the presence of anti-Sm antibodies defines a clinical subset of SLE patients or whether it carries a prognostic value in SLE remains controversial. Winfield et al.[W305] found a higher frequency of anti-Sm antibodies among SLE patients with central nervous system dysfunction. Winn et al.[W282] reported anti-Sm antibodies to be associated with milder central nervous system and renal disease. Other investigators, however, could not confirm these associations.[B82,R144] Yasuma et al.[Y37] found a positive correlation among serositis, interstitial pulmonary fibrosis, and IgG anti-Sm antibodies in a large cohort of Japanese patients. The discrepancies in the results may be caused by the variation in prevalence among various ethnic groups and by differences in the sensitivity of the test system. More importantly, conclusions were based on a single serum specimen rather than on a sequential determination of the anti-Sm antibody.

Antibody Titer and Disease Activity

Few longitudinal studies have been done on the usefulness of anti-Sm antibody titers in monitoring disease activity in SLE patients. A prospective study of 14 SLE patients with anti-Sm antibodies, over a period of 7 to 30 months, showed fluctuations in serum titer. A 4-fold rise in titer predicted disease flare in 50% of patients (but in only 28% of episodes), and correlated with exacerbation of the disease in 60%. The rise in titer occurred within 2 to 12 weeks preceding a major disease flare (nephritis and CNS disease), but not in milder flares (arthritis, rash, or serositis).[Y37]

Summary

The anti-Sm antibody is considered specific for SLE, so it is a valuable serologic marker for diagnosis. It should be tested in all patients suspected of having SLE. Further studies are needed to evaluate the value of anti-Sm antibody titer in monitoring disease activity, to determine whether it adds to the measurement of anti-DNA antibodies and other serologic tests, and to ascertain whether it may be more useful in blacks and other ethnic groups, in whom the antibody is more prevalent.

SIGNIFICANCE OF ANTI-U1RNP ANTIBODY

Prevalence and Diagnostic Significance

Arnett et al.[A297] found that the prevalence of anti-U1RNP, tested by immunodiffusion and counterimmunoelectrophoresis, is higher in black (40%) than in white patients with SLE (23%). Using immunoprecipitation and autoradiography, Williamson et al.[W248] found a higher frequency of anti-Sm (34% versus 15%) but not anti-U1RNP (36% versus 27%) in black patients compared to whites. The ELISA test is a sensitive test for anti-U1RNP, showing a prevalence of the antibody as high as 55% in SLE patients,[M51] (see Chap. 22).

Unlike anti-Sm antibodies, anti-U1RNP antibodies are not considered specific for SLE. They may be found in patients with other systemic rheumatic conditions, such as mixed connective tissue disease, rheumatoid arthritis, Sjögren's syndrome, systemic sclerosis, and polymyositis.

Clinical Association of Anti-U1RNP

The presence of high titers of anti-U1RNP antibodies is associated with mixed connective tissue disease (MCTD), an entity characterized by overlapping features of SLE, scleroderma, and polymyositis.[M543,T43] Some have proposed that, in MCTD, anti-U1RNP should occur in the absence of other autoantibodies, such as anti-Sm and anti-DNA,[S336] and that the occurrence of multiple types of ANA in an individual patient is more indicative of SLE. The issue of whether MCTD is a distinct rheumatic disease or is merely a syndrome that may occur during the course of SLE or systemic sclerosis remains controversial (see Chap. 33). Some patients with MCTD eventually evolve into a more distinct rheumatic disease, such as clear-cut systemic sclerosis.[G338,N101]

In 1972, Reichlin et al.[R120] found that anti-U1RNP antibody is prevalent in SLE, and is associated with more benign disease. A cross-sectional study of 49 SLE patients revealed that patients with anti-U1RNP and/or anti-Sm antibodies have a higher frequency of scleroderma-associated features, such as Raynaud's phenomenon, sclerodactyly, interstitial changes in the chest roentgenogram, and nail fold capillary abnormalities,[T107] Vasculitis and de-

forming, nonerosive Jaccoud-type arthropathy of the hands have also been reported to be associated with anti-U1RNP in SLE patients.[R131,W248]

Serum Antibody Titer

A few reports of longitudinal measurements of the serum titer of anti-U1RNP among SLE patients have appeared. Nishikai et al.[N102] showed that in some but not all SLE patients the anti-U1RNP titer appeared to fluctuate with disease activity. A prospective study of 71 SLE patients with 40 separate clinical exacerbations has shown that the measurement of antibodies to 70-kD and A polypeptides of the U1RNP complex was not useful in monitoring disease activity or in predicting disease exacerbations.[T104] The presence of anti-U1RNP and/or anti-Sm did not appear to affect survivorship in SLE.[H348] A prospective study of patients with anti-U1RNP antibodies showed that most patients with a persistently high serum titer evolve into a clinical picture of mixed connective tissue.[L419]

Summary

Anti-U1RNP and anti-Sm antibodies are commonly found together in the sera of SLE patients. Anti-U1RNP antibodies are not considered diagnostic of SLE; when present alone in a patient with systemic rheumatic disease (especially in a high titer), the possibility of MCTD should be considered. Although the serum titer of anti-U1RNP may fluctuate in some patients, the determination of anti-dsDNA and complement are more useful in monitoring disease activity in SLE patients.

ANTI-Ro/SSA AND ANTI-La/SSB

Diagnostic Specificity

Anti-Ro/SSA antibodies are most commonly found in the sera of patients with primary Sjögren's syndrome and SLE, although they also occur in some patients with other systemic rheumatic diseases, including systemic sclerosis, rheumatoid arthritis, and polymyositis.[T43] In the clinical laboratory, anti-Ro/SSA antibodies are determined by double-diffusion in agarose or by counterimmunoelectrophoresis (CIE). They are present in 30 to 40% of SLE and in 40 to 70% of primary Sjögren's syndrome patients.[M543] Immunoblotting, RNA precipitation, and ELISA tests have been developed to measure anti-Ro/SSA and anti-La/SSB antibodies. A comparative study of these methods[M338] has shown that, although the RNA precipitation test has the highest sensitivity and specificity, the most convenient and practical clinical test is CIE for anti-Ro/SSA and immunoblotting for anti-La/SSB. The use of highly purified antigens or recombinant protein as a substrate in the ELISA test should improve the laboratory measurement of these antibodies (see Chap. 23).[S20]

Like anti-Ro/SSA antibodies, anti-La/SSB antibodies are found predominantly in patients with primary Sjögren's syndrome and SLE. Precipitating anti-La/SSB antibodies are found in 12% of unselected SLE patients.[H347]

Using various test systems, anti-Ro/SSA antibodies have been reported to occur in low titers in 15% of normal individuals, especially those who are HLA-DR3–positive, and anti-La/SSB antibodies have been detected in 7.5% of normal subjects.[G8,G9,H139,M51]

Disease Associations

Although anti-Ro/SSA antibodies do not have a high diagnostic specificity for SLE, their presence is associated with a number of clinical conditions, including subacute cutaneous lupus erythematosus (SCLE), neonatal lupus syndrome, homozygous C2 and C4 deficiency with SLE-like disease, "ANA-negative" SLE, photosensitivity in SLE, and interstitial pneumonitis.

SCLE is a distinct clinical subset of SLE. It is characterized by recurrent, erythematous, photosensitive, nonscarring skin lesions in a characteristic distribution involving the face, trunk, and arms and by mild systemic disease. Anti-Ro/SSA antibodies are found in 63 to 90% of patients with SCLE (see Chap. 31).[G144,H524,S566]

Neonatal lupus syndrome is an uncommon condition in infants born of SLE mothers. It is characterized by photosensitive, annular, discoid or erythematous skin lesions of the face and trunk, which appear at or before 2 months of age and disappear by 6 to 12 months of age. Congenital heart block with or without structural cardiac defects is seen in 50% of patients. Almost all afflicted infants and their mothers have anti-Ro/SSA and/or anti-La/SSB antibodies.[F204,L45,W103] The frequency of anti-Ro/SSA antibodies is increased in mothers of male children with SLE and in mothers of children with SLE that develops before the age of 10 years (see Chaps. 50–52).[L176]

Homozygous C2 deficiency is characterized by a lupus-like illness, with photosensitive cutaneous lesions reminiscent of those of SCLE and arthralgia, but rare central nervous system and renal involvement. Anti-Ro/SSA antibodies are present in 50 to 75% of these patients.[H524,M381] A genetic deficiency of C4, which may manifest clinically as SLE or a lupus-like syndrome, is also associated with anti-Ro/SSA antibodies.[M381] In one study, one of four patients with a genetic deficiency of C1q had anti-Ro/SSA antibodies (see Chap. 11).[M381]

ANA-negative SLE, first described by Fessel[F105] and by Gladman et al.[G171] refers to patients with clinical features compatible with those of SLE, except that their sera test negative for ANA by immunofluorescence using sections of rodent liver or kidney. In a study of 66 patients, Madison et al.[M48] found that most patients presented with photosensitive dermatitis, and many of them probably had SCLE. Precipitating anti-Ro/SSA antibodies were found in 41 patients and anti-ssDNA antibodies were present in 18. Moreover, 66% of patients actually had a positive fluorescent ANA (FANA) when KB epithelial tissue culture cells rather than mouse kidney sections were used as substrate. The Ro/SSA antigen appears to have a variable species distribution with significant amounts in certain cells, including a concentration in mouse, rat, and rabbit tissues.[H140]

The presence of anti-Ro/SSA antibodies has been reported to correlate positively with photosensitivity in white SLE patients.[M533] In contrast, among blacks, anti-Ro/SSA antibodies appear to be inversely associated with photosensitivity.[S768] A probable relationship between anti-Ro/SSA antibodies and interstitial pneumonitis in SLE has been described.[H242]

SLE patients with anti-La/SSB antibodies usually have anti-Ro/SSA antibodies concomitantly, and tend to be older at diagnosis.[C158,H347] While lupus nephritis is positively associated with anti-dsDNA, it is inversely related with anti-La/SSB antibodies.[H138]

Hochberg and associates[H87,H347,W91] suggested two serologic genetic subsets of SLE in whites but not in blacks, with different ages of onset. White SLE patients with anti-Ro/SSA antibodies alone differ from those with both anti-Ro/SSA and anti-La/SSB antibodies. Those in the former group have a lower titer of anti-Ro/SSA antibodies, a younger age of onset, and a higher frequency of anti-dsDNA and significant renal disease, and are strongly associated with DR2 and DQw1. In contrast, those in the latter group are associated with an older age of onset, sicca complex, less renal involvement, and HLA-B8, Dr3, Drw52, and DQW2.

Serial Measurement of Antibody Titer

Scopelitis et al.[S225] reported fluctuating titers of anti-Ro/SSA antibodies in SLE patients that appeared to correlate with disease activity and anti-dsDNA antibody levels. Moreover, some episodes of acute exacerbation were characterized by a rising titer in anti-Ro/SSA antibody in the absence of detectable anti-dsDNA antibodies.

Summary

Anti-Ro/SSA antibodies are strongly correlated with the clinical subsets of SCLE, ANA-negative SLE, and lupus-like syndrome associated with a genetic deficiency of complement. Infants of SLE mothers with anti-Ro/SSB and anti-La/SSB antibodies have an increased risk of neonatal lupus syndrome, so pregnant SLE patients should be tested for these antibodies.

ANTIHISTONE ANTIBODIES IN SLE

Prevalence and Diagnostic Specificity

Antihistone antibodies comprise a heterogeneous group of antibodies reactive with various subfractions or complexes. Although found mainly in patients with SLE, drug-induced LE, or rheumatoid arthritis, these antibodies have been described in those with other rheumatic conditions, malignancy, and liver disease (see Chap. 21). In SLE, these antibodies are directed against H1, H2B, H3, and H2A-H2B complex,[R396] although other specificities can occur.

Several methods have been devised to measure antihistone antibodies, including ELISA, immunoblotting, complement fixation, and immunofluorescence.[C402] Depending on the method, substrate, and patient selection, the prevalence of antihistone antibodies in SLE has been reported to be from 21 to 90%.[C402]

Antihistone antibodies have limited diagnostic specificity for idiopathic SLE. The presence of these antibodies does not appear to be any more significant that that of anti-dsDNA or anti-Sm antibodies in corroborating the clinical diagnosis of the disease. (The diagnostic value of antihistone antibodies for drug-induced LE is discussed in Chapters 21 and 45).

Clinical Association

Few published studies have examined the relationship between the presence of antihistone antibodies and the clinical features of SLE. In a small number of lupus patients, Fishbein et al.[F107] found a significantly lower prevalence of central nervous system involvement among those with antihistone antibodies. Fritzler et al.[F278] confirmed the lower frequency of neuropsychiatric disease and the lower prevalence of nephritis, alopecia, anemia, and hypocomplementemia in SLE patients with antihistone antibodies, suggesting a milder form of the disease. In contrast, other investigators have failed to find any positive or negative correlation with specific clinical manifestations of the disease.[G165,K423]

Similarly, the available data on the association between antihistone antibodies and disease activity are few and inconclusive. Fishbein et al.[F107] found a significant drop in the serum antibody titer within a month after the initiation of steroid therapy of active SLE. Gioud et al.[G165] reported a higher frequency of antihistone antibodies in patients with active disease (87%) than in those in remission (18%). A serial study in a small number of patients showed a correlation with disease activity. In untreated patients with lupus nephritis, antibodies to H2B correlated with renal, histologic, and clinical activity of the disease.[K346] Other investigators, however, have found no correlation among antihistone antibodies, disease activity, or activity index in the renal biopsy.[F278,G279,K423,N147]

The discrepancies in the results of the various studies have several causes, mainly differences in patient selection, test system used, histone preparation, and inadequate study design.

Association With Anti-DNA Antibodies

Antihistone antibodies have been shown to correlate with the presence of anti-DNA antibodies[G165,K423] and circulating immune complexes.[K346] Subiza et al.[S752] have established that some of the antihistone activity measured in SLE sera is a result of complexes of dsDNA–anti-dsDNA, which bind to the histone substrate used in the assay.

Summary

Antihistone antibodies are of limited value in corroborating the clinical diagnosis of SLE. Serial determinations of these antibodies do not add significantly to measurement of anti-dsDNA and other serologic parameters in assessing disease activity in SLE patients. Well-designed prospective studies are needed to understand fully the clinicopathogenetic significance of these antibodies in SLE.

SEROLOGIC PARAMETERS AND RENAL BIOPSY FINDINGS IN LUPUS NEPHRITIS

A number of studies (Table 48–4) have examined the relationship between renal biopsy findings and the serologic data obtained at biopsy.[C310,E140,F53,H190,H239,H305, H440,N147,P190] Could the histologic type of lupus nephritis, histologic activity, and chronicity indices be predicted by anti-dsDNA, C3, and/or serologic parameters? The results of various studies are not necessarily comparable because of differences in morphologic classification, in parameters measured, and in patient selection, including consideration of the effects of previous or current drug therapy. All studies except two[H239,P190] were based on a single kidney biopsy, performed within a few months after the onset of the renal abnormality. (See Chapters 53 and 54.)

Hill et al.[H305] found an excellent correlation between

Table 48–4. Correlation of Serologic Changes and Renal Histology

Source	No. of Patients in Study	Results and Comments
Hill (1978)[H305]	59, with 77 biopsies	Excellent correlation between anti-dsDNA and C3 with overall amount and distribution of immune deposits; rheumatoid factor was found in those with milder lesions, whereas cryoglobulins correlated with more severe changes
Hossiau (1990)[H440]	50	High anti-dsDNA titer and low C3 correlated with nephrotic syndrome, with or without renal failure; class IV nephritis patients had higher anti-dsDNA titer than those with class III or V lupus nephritis
Nossent (1991)[N147]	35	High histologic activity index correlated with IgM ANA and IgM anti-dsDNA; histologic type of lupus nephritis showed no correlation with serologic parameters
Clough (1980)[C310]	11	IgM anti-dsDNA was higher than IgG anti-dsDNA in patients with diffuse (class IV) lupus nephritis; in contrast, IgG anti-dsDNA was higher than IgM anti-dsDNA in those with focal (class III) lupus nephritis
Hashimoto et al. (1983)[H190]	20	Histologically active lesions, especially in class IV lupus nephritis, were associated with high-titer and complement-fixing IgG anti-dsDNA; glomerular C3 deposits correlated with complement-fixing anti-dsDNA
Feldman et al. (1982)[F53]	34	Renal activity index but not chronicity index correlated with anti-dsDNA (Farr) and IgG anti-dsDNA (ELISA); serum IgM concentration inversely correlated with chronicity index; effect of serum complement was not examined
Esdaile et al. (1989)[E140]	87	Low C3 was predictive of renal insufficiency, renal death, and total SLE death; high anti-dsDNA was related with renal death and inversely associated with nonrenal death
Hecht et al. (1976)[H239]	31, all with repeat biopsy	Persistently normal C3 was associated with stability or improvement of renal lesion of repeat biopsy in some but not all patients; anti-dsDNA serum level showed better correlation with clinical histologic improvement
Pillemer et al. (1988)[P190]	55, all with repeat biopsy	Normalization of C3 correlated better than decrease in anti-dsDNA titer with activity index during repeat biopsy

serum levels of anti-dsDNA and C3 with the overall amount and distribution of immune deposits in the renal biopsy, as assessed by immunofluorescence. In contrast, a poor association between the degree of epithelial proliferation and the histologic type of lupus nephritis, using the Baldwin classification system, was noted.[B50]

Houssiau et al.[H440] reported a good correlation among the anti-dsDNA titer and the serum C3 (but not C4) level with the functional severity of the renal disease and the WHO histologic classification of lupus nephritis. Patients with nephrotic syndrome or with renal failure had a higher anti-dsDNA titer and a lower C3 level than those presenting with proteinuria alone and a normal serum creatinine level. Patients with class IV nephritis had a higher anti-dsDNA level than those with class III or V nephritis. In contrast, the serum C3 level did not correlate with the histologic type. Considerable overlap in values among the various clinical or histologic groups was found, however, so that these associations are not applicable to the individual patient.

Nossent et al.[N147] observed no correlation among the WHO histologic classification and various serologic parameters (anti-dsDNA, other types of ANA, C3, C4, C1q, immune complexes, and anticardiolipin antibodies [ACA]) in 35 patients with lupus nephritis. Conversely, the activity index, using the National Institutes of Health renal histology index, correlated with serum titers of IgM ANA and IgM anti-dsDNA. Glomerular proliferation showed the best overall correlation with serologic parameters. Clough[C310] described a similar correlation between IgM anti-dsDNA and diffuse lupus nephritis.

Hashimoto et al.[H190] reported a good correlation between histologically active lesions, especially in diffuse lupus nephritis, and high titers of IgG complement-fixing anti-dsDNA. Feldman et al.[F53] obtained similar results, and noted a good correlation between anti-dsDNA using the Farr binding assay and IgG anti-dsDNA using ELISA and renal activity, but not with the chronicity index.

In contrast to the above studies, Pillemer et al.[P190] correlated serologic tests and histologic changes over time in 55 patients who had initial and repeat renal biopsies. All patients received various immunosuppressive drugs for nephritis during the interval. At the time of the second biopsy, the serum C3 level improved in 78% and the anti-dsDNA level decreased in 85% of patients. Patients with a normal C3 level at the time of the second biopsy had a significantly lower activity index than those with a low C3 level. The activity index was not significantly affected by a decrease in anti-dsDNA antibody titer. The duration of hypocomplementemia was less consistent as a prognostic indicator. Esdaile and associates[E140] also found a low serum C3 level to be a valuable predictor of renal insufficiency, renal death, and total SLE death in a study of the longterm outcome of 87 patients with lupus nephritis. In a similar study of 31 SLE patients with serial kidney biopsies, Hech et al.[H239] showed that normalization of the serum C3 level and a drop in the anti-dsDNA titer following drug therapy are associated with stabilization or improvement of the renal disease.

Summary

Kidney biopsy is useful in the management of patients with lupus nephritis. The histologic type of lupus nephritis and the severity of renal damage as assessed by the activity and chronicity of the lesions are predictive of the outcome of lupus nephritis in most patients. None of the serologic parameters at the time of biopsy, either singly or in combination, can adequately and satisfactorily predict the histologic type or severity of the renal lesion in an individual patient. During drug therapy, a persistently low serum C3 level appears to be a better measure of active glomerular disease than an elevated anti-dsDNA antibody titer. Corollary to this, the normalization of a previously low serum complement level is frequently associated with improvement or stabilization of the renal disease.

ACTIVATION PRODUCTS OF COMPLEMENT IN SLE

The in vivo activation of the complement system by complexes of anti-DNA and DNA antigen and other autoantibodies is central to the pathogenesis of the glomerular injury, and possibly to other tissue damage, in SLE patients. Acute exacerbations of the disease are often associated with hypocomplementemia. Serial measurements of total hemolytic activity ($C'H50$) and the serum concentrations of C3, C4, and C1q are widely used to assess disease activity (see Chap. 13).

Some studies have postulated that small-vessel injury in SLE may occur without evidence of immune complex mediation by the release of split products of complement activation, such as anaphylatoxins. These activation products, such as C3a and C5a, can activate and attract inflammatory cells. This can lead to cell aggregation and vascular adherence, resulting in an occlusive vasculopathy and ischemia.[A19]

Correlation With Disease Activity

A number of studies have shown that the measurement of the plasma concentration of activation products of complement, including iC3b neoantigen, C3a, C4a, C3d, C4d, and the terminal complex, C5b-9, can be useful in assessing disease activity and predicting exacerbations (Table 48–5).[H414,H420,G60,K176,N53,S275,W227] The consensus of the various studies is that measurement of the activation products is superior to the determination of serum C3 or C4 values. Many patients with clinically active disease and normal serum C3 or C4 levels have elevated activation products of complement. Nevertheless, except for a few,[G60,H414] most of these studies emphasized differences between patient groups (active versus inactive) rather than longitudinal determinations in individual patients. Further prospective studies are needed to compare the relative value of the various complement activation products in assessing disease activity, and to determine the possible effects of comorbid conditions, such as infections. The measurement of activation products of complement may be particularly useful in patients with isolated central nervous system involvement, who frequently do not exhibit hypocomplementemia.[H414]

Table 48–5. Activation of Complement as Measure of Disease Activity in SLE

Source	Activation Product	No. of Patients in Study	Results and Comments
Negoro et al. (1989)[N53]	iC3b neoantigen	40 untreated clinically active	Plasma levels elevated in 83% of patients; highly correlated with disease activity and renal histologic activity index
Hopkins et al. (1988)[H414]	C3a and C5a anaphylatoxins	40	C3a level increased in all patients, occurring 1–2 months prior to exacerbation; marked elevation in cerebritis; C5a levels were less sensitive
Wild et al. (1990)[W227]	C4a and C3a anaphylatoxins	24	C4a levels higher in patients with severe disease than in those with mild disease; C4a correlated with anti-dsDNA and C1q test for immune complexes; C4a superior to C3a measurements
Senaldi et al. (1988)[S275]	C4d and C3d	48	C4d correlated better than C3d with disease activity; serum C3 and C4 levels were not associated with disease activity
Horigome et al. (1987)[H420]	Terminal complement attack complex (TCC)	54	TCC correlated with circulating immune complexes, C'H50, C4, C3, C5, and alternate pathway activity
Garwryl et al. (1988)[G60]	Terminal complement complex (C5b-9)	22	Elevated TCC level correlated with 89% of disease exacerbations
Kerr et al. (1989)[K176]	Factor B activation product (Ba)	51	53% of patients with Ba had severe multisystem disease, associated with cutaneous vasculitis; Ba correlated better than C4a and C3d with disease severity

SOLUBLE INTERLEUKIN-2 RECEPTORS IN SLE

Following activation, resting T lymphocytes express receptors for interleukin-2 (IL-2R) on the cell surface, and a high-affinity IL-2R enables T lymphocytes to proliferate in response to the cytokine. The receptor can be shed or released in vitro, or physiologically in vivo, and can be detected in supernatants of cell cultures, in blood, and in body fluids. Elevated serum concentrations of soluble IL-2R (sIL-2R) have been found in patients with conditions characterized by immune system activation, including SLE, RA, chronic infections, and malignancies.

Association With Disease Activity

We have found a positive correlation between serum levels of sIL-2R and immunologic markers of disease activity in SLE, including reduced serum C3 and high cryoglobulin levels.[C52] Sequential studies in SLE patients with active disease have revealed a decrease in serum sIL-2R levels concomitant with a clinical response to steroid therapy. Our findings have been confirmed and extended by other investigators.[S271,T109,W18,W74,W323]

A prospective study of 71 unselected SLE patients by Ter Borg and associates[T109] showed an elevation of sIL-2R in 18 of 21 patients who developed clinical exacerbations, and correlated with changes in anti-dsDNA antibodies and with C3 and C4 values. Of these exacerbations, 75% were preceded by a rise in sIL-2R levels, but changes in anti-dsDNA and C3 levels tended to precede the increase in sIL-2R. The serum concentrations of sIL-2R in SLE patients with inactive disease were higher than those of healthy individuals, suggesting that an ongoing T-cell activation process was occurring in SLE, even during periods of clinical quiescence. The sIL-2R level increased further prior to disease exacerbation.

Summary

The serial measurement of sIL-2R is a sensitive test for assessing disease activity and for predicting exacerbations of SLE. It is probably at least as sensitive as determination of the serum C3 level and anti-dsDNA titer, and may be particularly valuable in SLE patients who test negative for anti-dsDNA antibodies. Additional prospective studies are needed to confirm these results, to determine whether the sIL-2R measurement has an additive value with other serologic parameters, and to examine the effects of infections and other comorbid conditions in SLE patients.

APPLICATION OF MULTIPLE SEROLOGIC MEASUREMENTS IN SLE

It is clear that no single serologic test can adequately assess or predict the clinical course of SLE in individual patients. A few studies have examined the application of a panel of serologic reactions in an attempt to improve sensitivity and correlation with disease activity.

In an early study, Schur and Sandson[S207] concluded that a combination of complement-fixing anti-dsDNA and C'H50 correlated better with active disease, especially lupus nephritis, than either of the serologic test alones. In a more recent study, Lloyd and Schur[L341] found that the serial measurement of a combination of C'H50, C3, C4, and circulating immune complexes by C1q binding assay appears to be the most useful. Anti-dsDNA antibodies did not significantly increase the usefulness of the panel (see Chap. 13).

In a prospective study of 48 unselected SLE patients, Abrass et al.[A20] found that circulating immune complexes, as determined by a solid phase C1q binding assay, correlate with active disease manifestations, particularly nephritis or arthritis, but not with skin or other organ involvement. A change in disease activity, prompting the physician to make a change in management, was predicted by the results of solid C1q binding test. Neither C3 nor anti-dsDNA correlated with disease activity, and neither gave additional information when combined with that obtained by use of the solid phase C1q binding test.

Using a battery of laboratory tests, Morrow et al.[M608] failed to identify a single test that reliably distinguished severely active, moderately active, and inactive disease groups of SLE patients. Determination of circulating immune complexes by polyethylene glycol precipitation, platelet count, and erythrocyte sedimentation rate (ESR) distinguished the active from the inactive disease group. Patients with severely active disease with involvement of three or more systems were different from the less active group by C1q solid phase binding assay for immune complexes, anti-dsDNA, C′H50, and lymphocyte count, but patients with neuropsychiatric involvement and those with thrombocytopenia were the most difficult to sort out. Only 44% of patients could be classified accordingly into clinical grades when combinations of four out of five laboratory tests were used. Isenberg et al.[136] were unable to find a correlation between clinical disease activity and multiple serologic reactions to dsDNA, ssDNA, RNA, synthetic polynucleotides, and cardiolipin. In a retrospective study of complement and circulating immune complexes (tested by five different assays) in 33 patients, Valentijn et al.[V6] concluded that, although disease activity correlates with serum levels of C′H50, C3, or C1q (by binding assay), the sensitivity and predictive value of the serologic parameters are low. In 20% of patients, one or more parameters was constantly abnormal, regardless of disease activity. On the other hand, in a small subset of patients, a patient-specific activity parameter could be identified.

CONCLUSION AND RECOMMENDATIONS

Many reports evaluating the application of serologic tests in the assessment and prediction of disease activity have been rife with shortcomings. No uniform index of clinical disease activity has been used, and certain groups of patients (such as those with nephritis) were either overrepresented or underrepresented in the test populations. Conclusions were often based on a single test sample and the length of the follow-up period was too short. Serologic tests were not standardized, so the comparison of various studies is not feasible. Despite these obvious faults, it is clear that no single serologic test available today is ideal and applicable to all lupus patients. Considering the heterogeneity of the clinical disease, it is unlikely that single such test will be found. Serologic abnormalities in a patient with active lupus nephritis are not necessarily the same as those in another patient with skin rash, fever, hematologic changes, and/or serositis.

Table 48–6. Summary of Serologic Abnormalities in SLE

1. Anti-dsDNA and anti-Sm antibodies are serologic markers of idiopathic SLE. Their presence in patients suspected of the disease on clinical grounds confirms the diagnosis.
2. Mixed connective tissue disease should be considered in a patient with overlapping features of SLE, polymyositis, and scleroderma in the presence of a high titer of anti-U1RNP and the absence of anti-dsDNA and other specific types of ANA.
3. Pregnant SLE patients should be tested for anti-Ro/SSA antibodies because their presence indicates a risk for neonatal lupus syndrome.
4. Anti-Ro/SSA antibodies are associated with SCLE, ANA-negative SLE, and genetic deficiency of complement with LE-like clinical features.
5. Antihistone antibodies have limited diagnostic value for idiopathic SLE but are considered characteristic of drug-induced LE.
6. No single serologic test is predictive of disease exacerbation in SLE. The most useful parameters for assessing disease activity are anti-dsDNA and serum complement levels. Circulating immune complexes may be helpful in some patients.
7. Measurements of the activation products of complement and sIL-2R are promising serologic markers predictive of disease severity and exacerbation.

Newer serologic tests such as determination of sIL-2R serum levels and complement split products are undergoing further evaluation, and a combination of anti-dsDNA and serum complement is now generally used in clinical practice. The Farr binding test for anti-dsDNA is probably the most widely available test. As emphasized in Chapter 20, the clinician should become familiar with the advantages and limitations of the assay used in the laboratory to which specimens are sent. In patients who continually do not have anti-dsDNA antibodies (even after using different assay methods), measurement of the serum titer of some other ANA, such as anti-Sm or anti-Ro/SSa, may be useful.[Y37] The serum C3 concentration is more frequently measured than C′H50, although the latter is probably more a more sensitive parameter.[L341,M608] In our experience serial measurement of serum cryoglobulins is a useful parameter, but others may use a specific test for circulating immune complexes, such as the C1q solid phase binding assay.[A20,L341]

It must be remembered that some patients in clinical remission have persistently abnormal serologic findings.[G28,W66] Careful monitoring of specific organ functions, such as renal function, remains an important aspect in the assessment of disease activity and response to therapy.

Part B

Differential Diagnosis

Chapter 49

DIFFERENTIAL DIAGNOSIS AND DISEASE ASSOCIATIONS

DANIEL J. WALLACE

Systemic lupus erythematosus has replaced syphilis as the great imitator. Osler's classic remarks concerning the disease might now be paraphrased to include SLE: "Know syphilis and all its manifestations and relations and all things clinical will be added unto you .... Syphilis simulates every other disease. It is the only disease necessary to know. One then becomes an expert dermatologist, an expert laryngologist, an expert alienist [psychiatrist], an expert oculist, and expert diagnostician."[B137]

SLE's mimicry of other diseases was noted by Harvey,[M280] who listed 24 different diagnoses made on his patients during the early stages of their disease. Usually the greatest difficulty is the separation of SLE from closely related connective tissue disorders. To make these differences readily apparent, the clinical data are summarized in Table 49–1.

In addition to obtaining a detailed history, attempting to correlate any past features that might have been manifestations of SLE with the current illness, the physician must perform a thorough physical examination (see Chap. 33) and make a careful laboratory survey. This should include determination of the presence of antinuclear antibody (ANA), rheumatoid factor, creatine phosphokinase (CPK), C3 complement, and Westergren sedimentation rate, and a complete blood count (with differential and platelet counts), blood chemistry profile, VDRL test, partial thromboplastin time, urinalysis, chest roentgenogram, and electrocardiogram. If these tests are not diagnostic and SLE is strongly suspected, assays for anticardiolipin antibody, anti-Ro/SSA, anti-La/SSB, anti-DNA, anti-Sm, and anti-RNP should be done, as well as a serum protein electrophoresis. Along with a thorough clinical evaluation, a diagnosis can be derived 90% of the time.

The differential diagnosis of connective tissue disorders is complicated by the overlapping of coexisting rheumatic syndromes. Two large clinics have reported that 25% and 33% of their patients, respectively, had features of two connective tissue disorders.[B203,W27] Coexisting SLE and scleroderma, as well as SLE and polymyositis, have been found in a number of patients. If a positive anti-RNP is present, the "overlap" syndrome represents a distinct entity known as mixed connective tissue disease (MCTD).

Complicating these issues is the recognition that autoimmune hemolytic anemia, idiopathic thrombocytopenic purpura, Sjögren's syndrome, or Raynaud's phenomenon can be isolated processes for years before evolving into an established connective tissue disease. As early as 1956, Talbott and Ferrandis[T34] observed frequent transition

forms from one rheumatic disease to another. Some patients, who appear to have fulfilled all or most of the clinical criteria for a diagnosis of active rheumatoid arthritis, lose the exclusive features of this malady at some future time and manifest unmistakable SLE, polyarteritis, polymyositis, or scleroderma. Currently, it is not possible to determine whether the disorder was present from the beginning of symptoms and subsequently changed into another disorder.

Why is it necessary to differentiate among these conditions? Arriving at a specific diagnosis is necessary to understand the course and prognosis of the illness and to treat it effectively. For example, if gold therapy had been instituted in a patient thought to have rheumatoid arthritis, and if urinary or hematologic abnormalities developed, it would be assumed that they were a reaction to the treatment; however, if ANA had been initially sought and found, gold therapy might not have been used, and the changes noted would have been recognized as evidence of progression of the underlying disease.

ANA-NEGATIVE LUPUS

Positive ANA is only one of 11 criteria used to define SLE, according to the 1982 American Rheumatism Association (ARA) classification. As noted in Chapter 5, 4 of the 11 criteria must be present to make a diagnosis, but the ANA is so central to current concepts of SLE that many rheumatologists find it inconceivable that SLE can be present without it.

Several reports have documented the delayed appearance of ANA in patients suspected of having SLE. In view of our studies,[W39,W40] documenting a mean of 3 to 4 years between onset of symptoms and time of diagnosis, this is not surprising. Cairns[C11] reported 11 patients with lupus nephritis in whom a negative ANA persisted for years before becoming positive. Bohan[B383] and Enriquez et al.[E113] presented several well-documented cases. Persillin and Takeuchi[P136] found ANA in the urine and pleural fluid of a patient with diffuse proliferative nephritis and nephrotic syndrome for some time before serum ANA was present. Low antibody concentrations in the serum secondary to loss in body fluids can be present, as also noted by Ferreiro et al.[F71]

Numerous reports in the 1960s and 1970s examined the ANA-negative lupus subgroup, but only animal substrates for ANA were considered reliable at the time.[D265,F76,M48,P311,W90] Many patients actually had discoid or subacute cutaneous lupus and did not meet ARA

Table 49–1. Differential Diagnosis of Connective Tissue Disorders

Parameter	SLE	RA	Progressive Systemic Sclerosis	MCTD
Sex incidence	90% female	75% female	66% female	80% female
Age of majority	10–50 yr	20–40 yr	20–50 yr	All ages
Family history	+ for LE or RA in 12% or more	Often +	0	Rarely +
Disease duration	Mo–yr	Mo–yr	Mo–yr	Variable
First changes	Arthritis, rash	Arthritis	Skin	Arthritis, Raynaud's phenomenon
Cardiac involvement (clinical)	33%	65% at autopsy; clinically rare	+; perfusion and conduction abnormalities seen	Myocarditis in children
Skin and mucous membranes	Alopecia, butterfly erythema, scaling erythematous papules, ulcers	Subcutaneous nodules	Tightness of skin of hands, face, neck; hyperpigmentation of involved skin	Rashes of SLE, PSS, and dermatomyositis
Ocular	Iritis, retinal vasculitis or infarcts; Sjögren's syndrome	Scleritis, Sjögren's syndrome	Sjögren's syndrome	Rare; Sjögren's syndrome
Adenopathy	Moderate	Minimal	0	Minimal
Pleurisy or lung disease	Most cases	Rare	Interstitial fibrosis common	30%
Pericarditis	30%	Clinically rare	Rare	25%
Generalized abdominal pain and tenderness	Often	0	Dysphagia common; bowel motility decreased	Dysphagia common
Hepatomegaly	Occasional	0	0	0
Splenomegaly	10%	Rare	0	0
Joints involved	All joints, esp. minor	All joints	Minor	Erosive arthritis in 30%
Arthritic deformity	Frequent, nonerosive	Often erosive	Often	20%
Myalgia	48%	Frequent	+20%	50%
Raynaud's phenomenon	26%	Occasional	Common	80%
CNS involvement	Personality changes, convulsions and localized deficits, fatigue	Rare	Rare	10%
Laboratory:				
Urine abnormalities	46% at some time	0	Creatinuria	Lupus nephritis in 10–40%
WBC and differential	Leukopenia in 43%	Leukocytosis, acute phase	Normal	Leukopenia in 35%
Anemia	10% hemolytic; 56% < 11.0 g Hb	Normocytic	0	41%
Uremia	5–10%	0	Occasional	0
Hyperglobulinemia	Common	Frequent	40%	80%
LE cells	+ in 75%	+9% only	+5%	14%
ANA	+95%	+25%	+50% speckled, nucleolar	+100% speckled
Muscle biopsy	Usually 0	Usually 0	Myositis uncommon	Often positive
Skin biopsy	Suggestive +	0	Diagnostic	+ lupus band test or PSS
Remarks	No classic course; pattern of symptoms and findings suggest diagnosis; anti-DNA and low complement levels indicate systemic disease	RA-latex + in 80%	Progressive over years; may spontaneously remit	Swollen hands; anti-RNP

criteria, but the remainder of ANA-negative lupus patients were larger than necessary. This became documented when human cell line ANA substrates were introduced. Pollak et al.[P245] observed ANA-negative lupus in 9 of 112 patients and Leonhardt[L191] in 3 of 71 patients in 1964, Zweiman[Z68] in 2 of 28 nephritis patients in 1968, Estes and Christian[E147] in 13% of their 150 patients in 1971, Bartholemew[B108] in 5 of 121 patients in 1974, Fries and Holman[F256] in 2% of 193 patients in 1975, and Lee et al.[L140] in 5 of 110 patients in 1977.

Provost's group evaluated 28 patients with SLE who had titers of 1:20 or less with a mouse liver substrate.[D265]

Dermatomyositis and Polymositis	Polyarteritis Nodosa	Rheumatic Fever	Serum Sickness	Behçet's Syndrome
66% female	40% female	Equal	Equal	Mostly female
10–50 yr	All ages	2–19 yr	All ages	10–50 yr
0	0	0	0	0
Mo–yr	Variable	Mo–yr	Weeks	Mo–yr
Myalgia, skin changes, or weakness	Asthma, polyneuritis, abdominal pain, or fever	Arthritis	Urticaria	Orogenital ulcers
Occasional	Occasional	Most in acute phase	0	0
Periorbital edema, dusky erythema, Gottron's nodes	Hives, necrotic ulcertations, cutaneous and subcutaneous nodules	Erythema marginata, subcutaneous nodule	Hives, angioneurotic edema	Recurrent aphthous stomatitis, cutaneous vasculitis
0	Rarely, retinal hemorrhages and exudates	0	0	Uveitis in 66%
Rare	Minimal	Minimal	Minimal	0
Rare	0	0	0	0
Rare	0	Often	0	0
0	Often	Occasionally	Occasionally	Inflammatory bowel disease, occasionally
0	20%	+ with failure	0	0
Occasional	0	Rare without subacute bacterial endocarditis	0	0
Rare	Major	Major	All	55%
0	0	0	0	Rare
Marked	Common	Frequent	Rare	0
Common	Rare	0	0	0
0	25%	Chorea	0	22%
Creatinuria	Hematuria and red cell casts	0	0	0
Normal; eosinophila occasionally	Leukocytosis, eosinophilia in 18%	Leukocytosis	Leukocytosis, eosinophilia	0
Uncommon	50%	Normocytic	?	0
0	Common	0	0	0
0	Occasionally	0	0	Occasional
0	0	0	0	0
+30%	+20%	0	0	0
Usually +	Suggestive if +	0	0	0
Suggestive	Suggestive	0	Suggestive	0
20% of dermatomyositis cases associated with malignancy; proximal muscles involved; EMG may be diagnostic, CPK level elevations common	Association of asthma, eosinophilia, hypertension and polyneuritis suggests diagnosis; Biopsy + in only 50%	Preceding streptococcal infection. Diastolic heart murmur almost pathognomonic; elevated antistreptolysin titer		HLA-B5 associations, antibody to human mucosal cells

Using a rat liver substrate, 3 (11%) had a positive ANA. With human spleen imprints, 16 (57%) were positive, 9 (32%) were positive on a KB cell line substrate, and 8 (28%) were positive with an Hep-2 cell line. These results emphasize how a negative ANA can become positive merely by using another substrate, thereby converting ANA-negative lupus to ANA-positive lupus. Reichlin[R113] has stated that, with a KB or Hep-2 substrate, 98% of all SLE patients are ANA-positive, because non-DNA–containing antigens such as Ro/SSA are better represented when these cell lines are studied. Unfortunately, human cell lines are less specific, although they are more sensitive.

Larger numbers of healthy people have positive ANAs when human cell lines are used. Only 17 of 447 patients (3.8%) with idiopathic SLE tested between 1980 and 1989 on Hep-2 substrate were ANA-negative.[P216] They were evenly divided into three groups: 1) antiphospholipid syndrome; 2) renal biopsy-documented lupus in patients who had received steroids and chemotherapy; and 3) skin biopsy-positive patients who also fulfilled ARA criteria. Several reports have documented patients with high-titer cardiolipin antibody, recurrent thromboses, and negative ANAs who fulfilled the ARA criteria for SLE.[C136,M382]

Rothschild[R357] compared 10 seronegative SLE patients who met the ARA criteria with 42 seropositive patients. The former group included more whites and men. They were more leukopenic and had higher complement levels and less anti-DNA than the ANA-positive group.

Technical inaccuracy, prozone phenomenon, variations in microscope quality, ANA hidden within circulating immune complexes, in vivo binding of ANA by tissues, substrate specificity, low cutoff dilutions, and the use of monospecific antisera are other causes of negative ANAs in SLE patients. Occasionally, patients with positive LE cell preparations and negative ANAs have been observed.[K359] Wide variations in the reproducibility of ANA tests and difficulties in standardization are also problems that have not yet been overcome.[B278,C190]

A positive ANA is often found in patients with other disorders, even in seemingly healthy patients. A suburban rheumatology group studied 276 patients referred for a positive ANA without a diagnosis.[S360] After a comprehensive evaluation, 52 (18.8%) were diagnosed with SLE, 44 (15.9%) had an organ-specific autoimmune disease, 8.3% had an infectious disease, and 2.9% had neoplasia. No diagnosis was made in 13.4%.

In summary, if a KB or Hep-2 cell line substrate is used to detect ANA, 90% of the "ANA-negative" patients who meet ARA criteria can be shown to be ANA-positive. If these substrates are not available, specific tests for anti-Ro/SSA may be useful. Other ANA-negative lupus patients may fulfill discoid LE, subacute cutaneous LE, or juvenile rheumatoid arthritis definitions without fulfilling ARA criteria. ANA-negative lupus patients usually fall into several categories: antiphospholipid syndrome, early disease, and previously positive ANA made negative by steroids, cytotoxic drugs, or uremia. True ANA-negative lupus probably comprises less than 2% of all SLE cases. Many patients who claim to have ANA-negative lupus do not have SLE.

CROSS-OVER SYNDROMES: AN OVERVIEW

It has long been recognized that patients with SLE, rheumatoid arthritis, scleroderma, and dermatopolymyositis have overlapping features, and that the disease may occasionally evolve from one entity into another. On clinical services in which large numbers of patients with various rheumatic disorders are seen, it soon becomes evident that many patients do not fit into typical nosologic classifications. In 1969, Sabo[S8] used the term "lanthanic" or "undifferentiated collagen disease" for this group. As a result, the categorization of MCTD as a distinct disorder on the basis of a single serologic finding (anti-ribonucleo-

protein (RNP− or anti-U1RNP) present in other disorders has been controversial.

For example, Hess's group[G338] followed 23 patients with MCTD. Of these, 4 had a negative ANA initially, which became positive, anti-Sm antibody was transiently present in 3, and anti-ENA levels underwent as much as 10-fold titer fluctuations in 9 patients. In addition, 9 evolved into a more or less pure SLE, polymyositis, rheumatoid arthritis, or scleroderma. Ginsberg et al.[G154] compared 83 SLE patients with 71 who had overlap disease. The overlap group had a higher frequency of arthritis and Raynaud's phenomenon but a lower incidence of renal disease compared with the SLE group. The association was evident regardless of antibody patterns. Anti-U1RNP and anti-Sm were not predictive of the diagnosis or prognosis.

LeRoy et al.[L197] rejected the notion of MCTD and, in an excellent review and editorial, advocated the use of "undifferentiated connective tissue disease syndrome" for cases that were difficult to define. Fessel[F75] also observed that definitions of MCTD overlapped those of SLE, and anti-U1RNP was found in 25% of his SLE patients. He was unable to distinguish clinically between the two groups with anti-U1RNP antibodies. Reichlin[M47] considered MCTD to be SLE modified by anti-RNP. Other noted rheumatologists have put forth a strong case for the existence of MCTD as a distinct entity; these are discussed in the next section.

MIXED CONNECTIVE TISSUE DISEASE

In 1971, Sharp et al.[S333,S336] described an antibody to extractable nuclear antigen (ENA) whose presence appeared to correlate either with a benign form of SLE nephritis or MCTD. ENA was prepared from calf thymus nuclei, and presence of the antibody was determined by hemagglutination.[H386,S333] Because patients with SLE frequently had similar ENA titers, attempts were made to differentiate between the two groups by enzymatic treatment of the tanned red cells with ribonuclease (RNase). In those with MCTD, the titers were reduced or abolished by treatment of ENA with RNase, whereas in SLE the antibody titer was unaffected. This antibody, called antiribonucleoprotein (anti-RNP), was further defined by immunoblotting, ELISA, and immunoprecipitation techniques in the 1980s.[K37] In 1986, Sharp's group reported that antibodies reacting with a 68K protein were associated with the anti-RNP specificity in MCTD and rarely occurred in SLE sera.[P162] This pattern persisted for years, and only disappeared with a prolonged remission. Their work has been independently confirmed[N52] and challenged.[M288]

Clinical Features

Table 49−2 delineates the clinical and laboratory features described in six of the most detailed studies of MCTD.[B218,K262,P216,P327,R315,S334] Because an in-depth analysis of these features is beyond our scope here, these papers (as well as several other reports)[K101,M42,P323, S329,S332] are recommended. Articles cited in the following sections are also useful studies for review. The wide divergences noted in Table 49-2 for certain MCTD features can be explained by the inclusion in some studies of almost

Table 49-2. Comparison of Clinical and Laboratory Features of MCTD Patients (%)

Parameter	Sharp et al.[S334] 1976	Prystowsky[P327] and Tuffanelli 1978	Rosenthal[R315] 1979	Bennett[B218] and O'Connell 1980	Kitridou et al.[K262] 1986	Wallace[P216] 1990
No. of cases	100	46	40	20	30	23
Arthralgia/arthritis	95	91	95	100	97	96
Raynaud's phenomenon	85	81	75	75	83	70
Swollen hands	66	45	88	75	60	—
Myalgia	70	57	48	35	53	90
Lymphadenopathy	40	30	30	50	17	17
Cutaneous LE	38	51	50	5	83	39
Alopecia	—	42	8	50	67	30
Fever	33	—	55	45	—	57
Serositis	27	32	23	50	53	26
Sjögren's syndrome	7	19	10	20	23	—
Vascular headaches	—	30	—	10	—	17
Neurologic lesions	10	6	13	55	20	22
Nephritis	10	21	10	20	40	13
Positive ANA	100	98	100	100	—	96
Hyperglobulinemia	80	72	95	75	—	—
Anemia	41	20	85	75	53	39
Leukopenia	35	18	68	75	30	41
LE cells	14	46	3	—	—	44
Positive rheumatoid factor	55	48	93	2	—	22
Esophageal dysfunction	73	58	15	47	60	22
Anti-nDNA	12	24	13	100	10	40
Low serum complement level	4	39	3	30	23	25
Positive lupus band test	—	34	—	—	—	—

all patients with anti-RNP as having MCTD and others that excluded patients with obvious SLE. Fig. 49-1 compares the incidence of some of the signs, symptoms, and laboratory findings of patients with scleroderma, lupus, and MCTD. In most categories, MCTD occupies a middle ground between progressive systemic sclerosis (PSS) and SLE, except for a 100% incidence of ANA by definition and a greater incidence of myositis and Raynaud's phenomenon.

Of those with MCTD, 80% are female; their mean age at onset is 37 years. Familial aggregations have been reported.[H422,R28] No HLA specificity has been confirmed. Children with MCTD have more nephritis, deforming arthritis, and central nervous system involvement and a worse prognosis than their adult counterparts.[S475,S478,S740]

Skin

Cutaneous lesions are found in most MCTD patients. Sclerodermatous changes are seen in the hand, but rarely extend beyond the wrist. Cutaneous LE changes are present in up to 50% of patients. Alopecia, pigment changes, telangiectasias, and cutaneous vasculitis may be present. Raynaud's phenomenon, noted in 85%, is usually one of the most prominent features of MCTD. Speckled (particulate) epidermal nuclear IgG deposition was seen in normal skin in 70% of 46 patients with MCTD, and in 28% with SLE.[P327] Positive lupus band test results may be found. Nail fold capillaroscopy shows increased dilatation and dropout.

Joints and Muscles

Inflammatory arthritis is almost always seen; erosive arthritis is present radiographically in 25 to 60% of pa-

tients.[H63,R30] Among the most common findings are swollen hands, seen in 45 to 88%. Diffuse soft tissue finger swelling without sclerodactyly, especially in the morning, is common in SLE. Many patients initially present with rheumatoid arthritis-like picture. Deforming arthritis is more common than in SLE.[A92] Over 50% of patients with MCTD have elevated muscle enzyme levels at some point. Electromyographic and muscle biopsy findings range from SLE to polymyositis.[O132]

Cardiopulmonary System

Pericarditis has been described in one-third of patients, but it is apparently more common in children. Myocarditis is rare in adults.[A159] Pulmonary disease is evident in 80%, most of whom may be asymptomatic. Interstitial fibrosis, dyspnea, and decreased diffusing capability are common. In contrast to scleroderma, lung involvement of MCTD is usually steroid-responsive.[L287] Pulmonary hypertension is rare in adults but, unfortunately, is not uncommon in children.[J116,R304,W221]

Gastrointestinal System

Esophageal hypomotility is common, but dysphagia is not always evident.[D270,M152] Changes similar to those of scleroderma bowel have been reported, along with mesenteric vasculitis.[C378,N129]

Nervous System

Neurologic lesions, usually minor, are seen in 10% of patients. The most common abnormality is trigeminal neuralgia. Changes identical to those seen in central nervous system SLE may occur.[B213] Vascular headaches may be pronounced.[B504]

SYSTEMIC LE

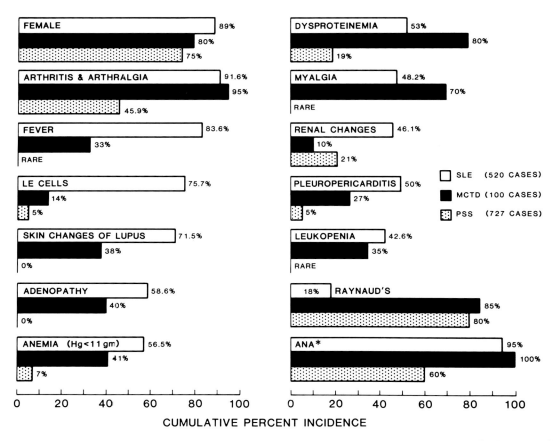

Fig. 49–1. Cumulative incidence (%) of the most common clinical manifestations. SLE,[D240] MCTD,[S186] PSS.[T137,T138]

Hematologic Disorders

Moderate anemia and leukopenia are common; thrombocytopenia is rare in adults, but uncommon in children. Only 2 of our 23 patients had antiphospholipid antibodies. Hemolytic anemia is rare.

Renal Disease

Immune complex-mediated nephritis has been described in 10 to 40% of adults and 40% of children with MCTD. In most series, it is usually clinically inapparent in adults. Most lesions are mesangial or membranous,[B219,G186,K262] but these findings are not universal.[K261] Kitridou et al. followed 11 nephritis patients (of 30 with MCTD) for a mean of 10 years.[K262] Of these, 9 were nephrotic, and most were steroid-responsive. Only 3 required dialysis.

Pregnancy

Normal fertility rates, decreased parity, increased fetal wastage, and a tendency toward postpartum disease exacerbation characterizes MCTD.[K128] These findings are similar to those observed in SLE.

Pathologic Lesions

Pathologic lesions are less inflammatory than in SLE. Intimal proliferation and medial hypertrophy of arteries and arterioles are evident.

Serologic and Immunologic Studies

By definition, almost all patients with MCTD are ANA-positive, usually with a speckled pattern, and have anti-RNP antibody. If anti-Sm are also present, SLE is the probable diagnosis. Rheumatoid factor is seen to 22 to 93%, anti-nDNA (native DNA) in 12 to 100%, and low serum complement in 3 to 39%. These widely divergent figures point out different selection criteria used to define MCTD. Alarcon-Segovia and Cardiel[A98] tested 593 patients with connective tissue disease for three proposed criteria for MCTD (Table 49–3). Using their criteria, 80 patients with putative MCTD had a 99.6% specificity rate.

Several studies have evaluated the importance of anti-RNP. One group correlated anti-RNP levels with disease activity and polyclonal B-cell responses.[H452] McCain[M226] screened 284 patients with rheumatic diseases; 2 had anti-RNP, both had known MCTD, and no new cases were uncovered. Reichlin's group evaluated 43 patients[M48]

Table 49–3. Diagnostic Criteria for MCTD

Sharp[S331]	Kasukawa, et al.[K102]	Alarcón-Segovia and Villarreal[A117]

A. Major criteria
  1. Myositis, severe
  2. Pulmonary involvement
    a. CO diffusing capacity < 70%nl
    b. Pulmonary hypertension
    c. Proliferative vascular lesion or lung biopsy
  3. Raynaud's phenomenon or esophageal hypomotility
  4. Swollen hands observed, or sclerodactyly
  5. Highest observed anti-ENA $\geq 1{:}10{,}000$ and anti-U1RNP + and anti-Sm −
B. Minor criteria
  1. Alopecia
  2. Leukopenia
  3. Anemia
  4. Pleuritis
  5. Pericarditis
  6. Arthritis
  7. Trigeminal neuropathy
  8. Malar rash
  9. Thrombocytopenia
  10. Myositis, mild
  11. Swollen hands
	A. Common symptoms
	  1. Raynaud's phenomenon
	  2. Swollen fingers or hands
	B. Anti-nRNP antibody
	C. Mixed findings
	  1. SLE-like findings
	    a. Polyarthritis
	    b. Lymphadenopathy
	    c. Facial erythema
	    d. Pericarditis or pleuritis
	    e. Leukopenia or thrombocytopenia
	  2. PSS-like findings
	    a. Sclerodactyly
	    b. Pulmonary fibrosis, restrictive change of lung, or reduced diffusion capacity
	    c. Hypomotility or dilatation of esophagus
	  3. PM-like findings
	    a. Muscle weakness
	    b. Increased serum levels of myogenic enzymes (CPK)
	    c. Myogenic pattern in EMG
		A. Serologic: positive anti-RNP at a hemagglutination titer of 1 : 1,600 or higher
		B. Clinical
		  Edema of the hands
		  Synovitis
		  Myositis
		  Raynaud's phenomenon
		  Acrosclerosis

	Requirements for Diagnosis of MCTD	

Four major criteria: anti-U1RNP $\geq 1{:}4{,}000$; exclusions; anti-Sm +
     or
Three major criteria; two major criteria from 1, 2, and 3 and two minor criteria with anti-U1RNP $\geq 1{:}1{,}000$
     or
Three major without anti-U1RNP; two majors, one major, and three minors with anti-U1RNP ≥ 100
	A. Positive in either one of two common symptoms
	B. Positive anti-nRNP antibody
	C. Positive in one or more findings in two or three disease categories or 1, 2, and 3
		A. Serologic
		B. At least three clinical findings
		C. Association of edema of the hands, Raynaud's phenomenon, and acrosclerosis requires at least one of the other two criteria

Modified from Alarcón-Segovia, D., and Cardiel, M.: Comparison between three diagnostic criteria for mixed connective tissue disease. Study of 593 patients. J. Rheumatol. 16:328, 1989.[A98]

with anti-RNP. Of these, 30 met the ARA criteria for SLE; 15 had both anti-RNP and anti-Sm, and only 5 had MCTD. Jonsson and Norberg[J122] proposed that anti-RNP provides prophylaxis against serious vasculitis and nephropathy. Hamburger screened 378 sera[H77] and noted that 100% with MCTD, 15% with SLE, and 9% with PSS had anti-RNP. Two other reports have suggested that slightly under 50% of those with anti-RNP have MCTD.[L110,R51]

Munves and Schur[M660] evaluated 1,115 patients with positive ANA test results; 150 had anti-Sm and/or anti-RNP. None of the 42 with anti-Sm alone had MCTD, and 3% of the 76 patients with both antibodies had MCTD. Of the 150 patients, 66% were believed to have SLE. Similarly, only 1 of 25 patients followed by Clotet et al.[C307] with anti-RNP alone failed to meet the ARA criteria for SLE.

Levels of circulating immune complexes (CICs), as measured by the Raji cell assay, were elevated in 88% of 72 sera in 20 MCTD patients, and these correlated with disease activity.[H64] A smaller scale study reached similar conclusions.[C456] Reticuloendothelial system clearance of CICs is probably normal if anti-Sm is not present.[H81] Alar-con-Segovia's group found free RNP in 10% of 299 MCTD sera at any time, but cumulatively present in 44% of 25 MCTD patients, in comparison to 7% of 72 SLE patients and 5% of 230 PSS patients. Free RNP was found, usually when anti-RNP titers fell or with steroid therapy.[F108]

Course and Prognosis

Most MCTD patients are responsive to nonsteroidal anti-inflammatory drugs (NSAIDs), antimalarials, and salicylates and those with systemic involvement are usually steroid-responsive. Despite widespread acceptance of this statement, no controlled studies have been performed. MCTD is a dynamic, changing syndrome. Cases of discoid LE[G143] or idiopathic Raynaud's phenomenon[E86] evolving into MCTD are not uncommon. Alarcon-Segovia[A128] commented that 9 of his 40 MCTD patients also met the criteria for four different connective tissue diseases, and that 14 met the criteria for two connective tissue diseases. Wolfe et al.[W324] used the American College of Rheumatology data base (ARAMIS) to compare 308 MCTD patients with 262 SLE patients. Significant differences ($p < 0.01$)

demonstrated in MCTD patients were a negative LE cell test result, absent renal disease, and the presence of myositis and Raynaud's phenomenon.

Nimelstein et al.[N101] re-evaluated 22 of Sharp's original MCTD patients 5 years later. Of these, 8 had died—only 2 from disease-related problems—but this is still a much worse 5-year survival than in any SLE subset. Of the 14 patients who were alive, 5 had almost no symptoms, 6 evolved into prominent PSS, and 1 evolved into prominent RA. Fever, rashes, hepatosplenomegaly, adeonopathy, renal disease, and myositis were rare. Raynaud's phenomenon was universally present, and inflammatory arthritis was still seen in only 3 patients. Serum complement was normal in all patients, and anti-DNA was present in 2. Anti-RNP titers varied greatly, with levels independent of disease activity. Thus, those who survived generally improved, and their disease took on the appearance of a mild, chronic scleroderma.

The trend of MCTD to evolve into PSS has been observed for others.[M118] De Clerk et al. followed 18 MCTD patients for a mean of 4.6 years.[D116] Of these, 6 evolved into SLE, 5 into scleroderma, and 1 into rheumatoid arthritis. Of 44 patients followed by Lemmer et al., 7 died in a 5-year follow-up.[L184] Sharp's group has cited a 7% mortality in 300 patients followed for a mean of 7 years.[S330] These discrepancies in life table findings emphasize the problems of following a disease that lacks precise definition.

RHEUMATOID ARTHRITIS AND SLE

Differentiation

Rheumatoid arthritis (RA) and SLE share many clinical and serologic features, an overlapping that was recognized in the 1950s and 1960s by the publication of hundreds of papers on "RA with LE cells." (See pages 464 to 476 of the second edition of this monograph for an extensive review of them.) RA and SLE can usually be distinguished from each other easily, especially if the former is ANA-negative or erosive. When RA displays extra-articular involvement or is ANA-positive, however, it is occasionally difficult to differentiate from SLE. When a patient presents with a new inflammatory arthritis, with overlapping features of both diseases, it may take 6 to 12 months of clinical observation before a definitive diagnosis can be made.

Extra-articular RA may include serositis, Sjögren's syndrome, subcutaneous nodules, cutaneous vasculitis, anemia, and other features observed in SLE. Ropes[R294] compared 142 SLE patients with a cohort of RA patients. The latter had a 6% incidence of LE cells, 1% sun sensitivity (versus 34% in SLE), and 4% alopecia (versus 46% in SLE). The incidence of thyroid antibodies is increased in both disorders;[H301] 4% of 250 and 365 RA patients in two reports had reduced complement levels.[F203,H498] Felty's syndrome consists of a positive ANA, splenomegaly, arthritis, leukopenia, and an increased incidence of cutaneous vasculitis. I have had a few Felty's syndrome patients who were misdiagnosed as having lupus. Felty's syndrome is characterized by antigranulocyte (as opposed to antilymphocyte antibodies), and elevated complement levels.[D158] Close examination, however, reveals that the

overwhelming majority of those with Felty's syndrome are middle-aged men, anti-DNA is never present, and most have circulating cryoglobulins.[G237,R409,W156] Central nervous system involvement and renal disease are absent.

Another differentiating feature between RA and SLE is the lack of kidney involvement in those with rheumatoid arthritis. In what might be *the* definitive study, Davis et al.[D80] reviewed the records of 5,232 RA patients followed at UCLA between 1955 and 1977. Of these, 28 (0.5%) had renal disease of all types, only 4 of whom (0.1%) had glomerulonephritis. Also, 3 of the 4 met the ARA criteria for SLE, and 1 had MCTD. Davis et al.'s literature review of glomerulonephritis in RA[D80] demonstrated that most of the cases could be accounted for by gold- or penicillamine-induced nephropathy, interstitial nephritis, amyloid, or diabetes. Rheumatoid factor (RF) was present in 15 of 166 SLE patients studied in Ginzler's group in detail,[F52] and in 22.7% of 365 patients tested with idiopathic SLE followed by Wallace. Its presence is associated with milder disease.

Numerous investigators have looked for ANA in RA, and its incidence has ranged from 3 to 88%, with an average of 25%.[B98,E83,P237] A subset of RF-negative, ANA-positive RA has been described.[G204,L318] Many of these patients have juvenile RA (JRA); most have erosive disease and a good prognosis.

Coexistence of SLE and RA

Do these disorders coexist? It has long been known that patients may start with a diagnosis of RA or SLE, which becomes SLE or RA over a period of years. Assuming that MCTD is not present, however, the true coexistence of these conditions is rare. Despite the frequent clinical overlap between RA and SLE features, the combination of advanced, deforming, erosive RA and a significant degree of biopsy-proven SLE is an extremely unusual finding.

Occasional case reports have appeared documenting a true coexistence.[B97,C130,D323,F104,K55,P252,T187,V17,V65] Of our 464 idiopathic SLE patients, 1 had classic seropositive, erosive, nodular RA with biopsy-documented proliferative SLE nephritis and nephrotic syndrome. The concurrence of subacute cutaneous LE in RA patients who are Ro/SSA-positive is more common.[C336,M352] Cohen and Webb[C330] reported the development of SLE in 11 Australian patients with typical RA observed over a 17-year period, but the total number of RA patients followed was not stated. Panush et al.[P52] have identified a true coexistence in 6 of 7,000 RA patients evaluated over an 11-year period. It was concluded that "rhupus" did not occur more frequently (0.09%) than expected from the chance concurrence of SLE and RA (1.2%).

Juvenile RA (JRA) and SLE

JRA has been classified into systemic (Still's disease), oligoarticular, and polyarthritis subsets. Several large-scale studies have observed ANA in about 60% of patients with JRA, particularly oligoarticular disease in young girls with uveitis.[C145,C260,L113,M563,O104] One study has determined that ANA in this subset is directed against a ribonucleoprotein that requires both RNA and protein moieties for antigenic integrity.[S96] Despite the high frequency of ANA, other antibody systems such as anti-RNP, anti-Sm, anti-Ro/SSA, anti-La/SSB, anti-nDNA, and anti-PM1 are rarely found.

About 2.5% of patients with classic deforming polyarthritis originally diagnosed as JRA later develop multisystem lupus.[N66,R10,S97] In one study, 2 of 85 JRA patients evolved into SLE—both had anti-DNA while still carrying a JRA diagnosis.[R303] These distinctions are often clouded by the high incidence of ANA and relatively low incidence of rheumatoid factor in JRA. ANA-negative childhood SLE has also been reported.[G138]

RELATIONSHIP OF SLE TO OTHER AUTOIMMUNE AND RHEUMATIC DISEASES

Scleroderma and Other Fibrosing Syndromes

Even though ANA is present in most scleroderma patients, other serologies associated with SLE are observed in a small minority with scleroderma. These include LE cell preparations,[D328] antiphospholipid antibodies,[R381,S254] and other nuclear antigens.[B212] Anticentromere antibodies are usually associated with the CREST (Calcinosis, Raynaud's, Esophagitis, Sclerodactyly, Telangiectasias) syndrome, but can be found in up to 5% of patients with pure SLE.[W1] In contrast to SLE, familial occurrence of scleroderma is rare. Clinically, sclerodactyly, telangiectasias, calcinosis, and malignant hypertension with acute renal failure are almost unheard of in SLE patients. It is important to differentiate among SLE, MCTD and scleroderma, because the latter is rarely responsive to steroids or cytotoxic agents. Conversely, one would not attempt to treat SLE or MCTD with penicillamine or colchicine.

Features relatively unique to both scleroderma and SLE are infrequently observed in patients who do not have MCTD. Dubois reviewed 14 cases of coexistent scleroderma and SLE in detail in 1971 and summarized the literature to date.[D328] Unfortunately, his work was hampered by the lack of accepted criteria for scleroderma, SLE or MCTD. Since then, case reports have appeared of autoimmune hemolytic anemia,[I63,R314] high levels of anti-nDNA,[H113] lupus nephritis,[K14,M479] and discoid lupus[R379,U15] occurring in scleroderma patients. Scleroderma may evolve into SLE, and vice versa.[A317] Linear scleroderma can be seen with SLE.[G251]

One case of neonatal LE with morphea[O35] and two of eosinophilic fasciitis with SLE have been presented.[G43,S434] The extreme rarity of retroperitoneal fibrosis in SLE has been noted.[G43,L270,U3]

Polymyositis and Dermatomyositis

In contrast to SLE, polydermatomyositis patients are less often women, (66%) and rarely have an autoimmune family history. Also, different skin lesions are present (Gottron's nodules and heliotrope rashes), a coexisting malignancy may occur, serositis is rare, and nephritis, liver inflammation, and hematologic abnormalities are absent. Rarely, MCTD may evolve into a pure polydermatomyositis. A low-grade myositis with muscle enzyme levels two

to three times normal may be seen in lupus that responds to low doses of corticosteroids. (Refer to Chap. 34 for a detailed discussion of lupus myopathy and its comparison with other inflammatory myopathies.)

Systemic Vasculitis

Although polyarteritis nodosa is relatively rare, it can be mistaken for SLE. In contrast to SLE, polyarteritis nodosa patients are usually men, and include all age groups equally. Cutaneous vasculitis may be more prominent, as may eosinophilia, wheezing, nerve and bowel symptoms. The ANA is often negative; LE cells are rarely seen. Hypersensitivity angiitis and serum sickness may mimic SLE at first, but can ultimately be distinguished by a self-limited course, an absence of ANA, and rarity of severe visceral involvement.

Behçet's syndrome can mimic SLE with its uveitis, oral and genital ulcers, central nervous system involvement, and frank synovitis, but in Behçet's syndrome the ANA is negative and certain ethnic predispositions (Japanese and Turkish), as well as HLA proclivity (the B5 haplotypes), can be observed. I have little doubt that some "ANA-negative" lupus patients actually have Behçet's syndrome. The lack of any diagnostic test for Behçet's syndrome further complicates the picture.

One case of SLE in a child with Kawasaki disease has been reported.[L107]

Large-Vessel Vasculitis

SLE is a disease of the small arteries and medium-sized arterioles, and does not affect larger caliber vessels. Large-vessel vasculitis is not associated with autoantibody formation. Elderly people more commonly develop polymyalgia rheumatica and giant cell arteritis, however, and SLE is occasionally included in the differential diagnosis, because musculoskeletal symptoms are present and an age-related positive ANA may be found.[F138,M121] A true concurrence of giant cell arteritis and SLE has been reported twice.[B569,S112] Takayasu's "pulseless' arteritis is found in young women, mostly Japanese, but also in other Asiatic and Hispanic women. One Japanese literature review described 10 cases of Takayasu's arteritis with coexistent SLE.[I3] The coexistence of large-vessel vasculitis with SLE is coincidental, possible, and rare.[S101]

Crystal-induced Arthropathies

Even though 29% of SLE patients are hyperuricemic (usually secondary to nephritis, diuretics, or chemotherapy), clinical gout is rare.[F283] This could be the result of the predominance of menstruating females among those with active SLE. Fewer than 20 cases have been described in the literature;[D110,G354,H252,K471,M266,M521,T250] most were males taking diuretics. Wallace has reviewed the negative association between gout and RA.[W33] Only 3 of his 464 idiopathic SLE patients had clinical gout, including a 25-year-old woman with nephritis who had tophaceous deposits. It has been proposed that SLE patients (who often have decreased synovial fluid complement levels) have a natural barrier to gout because urate requires the presence of near-normal synovial fluid complement levels to induce inflammation.[W41]

The rarity of pseudogout in SLE patients has been reviewed.[R263]

Fibromyalgia (Fibrositis) Syndrome

A secondary fibromyalgia fulfilling Wolfe's criteria was found in 22% of Wallace's 464 idiopathic SLE patients.[P216] Brought on by inadequate coping mechanisms, emotional stress, physical trauma, and abrupt changes in steroid doses, the resulting fatigue, tender points, aching, and nonrestorative sleep can be difficult to differentiate from those of a lupus flare. In the absence of abnormal laboratory test results (e.g., Westergren sedimentation rate, C3 complement, and bone scan, if necessary, to rule out inflammatory arthritis), physicians must reassure the patient, promote the use of physical measure (e.g., moist heat, gentle massage), and prescribe mild sedatives (particularly tricyclic antidepressants) to be taken at bedtime, but should not increase steroid doses (as they are often tempted to do).

Because the diagnosis of primary fibromyalgia is frequently missed or misunderstood by internists, patients with severe symptoms sometimes believe that they have a serious, undiagnosed disorder. When confronted with normal laboratory results and an otherwise normal physical examination, a desperate physician might latch onto a low-titer, positive ANA (e.g., 1:10, 1:20) as evidence of early lupus. Their patients might then read SLE literature and become certain that they have SLE. Convincing this group that they do not have SLE is extremely difficult.[L342]

Rheumatoid nodules can occasionally be mistaken for fibrositic nodules.[Z50] Some groups have found discontinuous IgG deposits in the dermal-epidermal junction of nonlesional skin[C92,D223] and have suggested that fibrositis might be immune-mediated. This can be differentiated from a positive lupus band test in SLE, which generally shows continuous deposits of at least two proteins (IgG, IgM, IgA, C3, C4, C1q, fibrinogen) on immunofluorescence.

Dermatitis Herpetiformis

Thomas and Su[T146] found nine patients with concomitant dermatitis herpetiformis and SLE followed at the Mayo Clinic from 1950 to 1981, and reviewed the literature. Five other reports have appeared, the most important of which are cited here.[A304,D75]

Primary Biliary Cirrhosis and Pseudolupus

Patients with primary biliary cirrhosis are usually females, and often have a positive ANA.[M510] An autoimmune basis is probable, and high titers of antimitochondrial antibodies are found. Only a handful of cases of coexistence with SLE have been reported,[C280,17,K434,S38] of which only two were well documented.[C280,17]

During the mid-1970s, a series of articles appeared on a bizarre, SLE-like syndrome among Western Europeans. Maas and Schubothe[M2] described 21 patients who showed only antimitochondrial antibodies without evidence of liver disease, antinuclear antibodies, or LE cells. The primary manifestation was chronic, recurrent attacks of pyrexia. In addition, varying combinations of polyarthritis, muscle aching, pericarditis and myocarditis, pleural effusions, and pulmonary infiltrates occurred. In this and other reports,[G402,G420] the "pseudolupus syndrome" was found to occur in patients taking Venocuran, an extract of phenopyrazone, horse chestnut extract, and cardiac glycosides for venous disease. Maas et al.[M179] analyzed the medication intake in 58 patients with this entity, and found that 45 were taking Venocuran. None subsequently developed SLE.

Sarcoidosis

SLE and sarcoidosis share many immunologic features.[H505,17] Both manifest hyperglobulinemia, decreased skin test and lymphocyte responsiveness, lymphopenia, impaired antibody-dependent cellular cytotoxicity, and increased levels of circulating immune complexes. Cryoglobulins and antilymphocyte antibodies may be present in both disorders, and up to 32% of patients with sarcoidosis may have a positive ANA. Differential diagnosis can be a problem[S570] but, despite these similarities, only four cases of coexistence have been reported in the English language literature.[H167,H505,N50]

Amyloid

It would be expected that SLE patients have an increased incidence of amyloid, as do those with RA or ankylosing spondylitis. Cathcart and Scheinberg[C156] enumerated many reasons why SLE and amyloid should coexist. For example, both have a common pathogenetic pathway, and polyclonal B-cell proliferation is seen in both. Benson and Cohen[B224] found serum levels of amyloid protein A to be elevated in 25 cases of active SLE (although these were half the levels seen in an RA group). This α-globulin is a precursor of the major protein constituent of secondary amyloid fibrils. Serum amyloid P component can also be deposited in lupus tissues without evidence of clinical amyloid.[B468] Despite this, only 13 cases of the coexistence of SLE and amyloidosis have been reported.[A154,C117,C198,D40,K233,N120,P163,S147,S791,T111,W115,W123]

Seronegative Spondyloarthropathies

Nashel et al.[N34] estimated that 500 concurrent cases of ankylosing spondylitis (AS) and SLE should be present in the United States, but this figure does not take into account the differences in catchment groups (AS—white males, SLE—females, especially nonwhites). They presented the first true case of coexistence, and reviewed three cases reported earlier. None of these met both AS and SLE criteria, but one has since appeared.[O68] Kappes et al.[K67] noted the difficulty in differential diagnosis because SLE patients may have sacroiliitis by bone scan, and may be HLA-B27 positive. Only one case of SLE and Reiter's syndrome and one case of discoid lupus in AS has been reported.[A78,M509]

Several reviews have drawn attention to the coexistence of psoriasis and SLE.[E174,K450,M442,S791] A 1980 report presented 23 cases of coexistence at the Mayo Clinic (10 met ARA criteria for SLE and 13 had DLE) between 1950 and 1975, and reviewed 15 reports of 33 cases (11 of which antedated 1960).[M442] Of these, 63% were female, SLE and psoriasis each appeared first half of the time, and 80% had discoid lesions that were usually distinct from psoriatic patches (appearing and disappearing independently), but 7 of 27 biopsied lesions had pathologic features of both disorders. Discoid LE may flare with ultraviolet B or psoralen-ultraviolet A (PUVA) therapy,[E174,K450] and subacute cutaneous lupus can be induced during PUVA treatments in patients who are Ro/SSA-positive.[D284,M287] Despite the not uncommon concurrence of LE and psoriasis, only one case of psoriatic arthritis and SLE has been reported, and no HLA studies were cited in any of these reports.[O28]

ASSOCIATION OF SLE WITH OTHER DISORDERS

Several disorders have increased or decreased associations with SLE, and others can mimic its presentation and must be considered in the differential diagnosis. The relationship among Raynaud's phenomenon, multiple sclerosis, myasthenia gravis, thyroiditis, inflammatory bowel disease, syphilis, Klinefelter's syndrome, sickle cell anemia, autoimmune hemolytic anemia, Sjögren's syndrome, thrombocytopenic purpura, pemphigus, chronic active hepatitis, and SLE are discussed in other chapters (see the index for specific listings). Additional associations and differential diagnostic considerations are reviewed here.

Porphyria

Both porphyria and SLE are characterized by fever, rash, sun sensitivity, leukopenia, anemia, arthralgias, and central nervous system abnormalities. Although almost 50 concurrent cases have been reported, many of these patients did not fulfill established criteria for SLE, and almost all of their symptoms could be explained by porphyria alone.[H294,L93,N114,R300,S329] Two comprehensive evaluations of 55 and 158 porphyria cutanea tarda patients[C301,G398] found that none met the ARA criteria for SLE, even though 12% were ANA-positive. One review of 38 patients with porphyria[A145] found that 8 of 15 with acute intermittent porphyria were ANA-positive; 1 had SLE.

Angioimmunoblastic Lymphadenopathy with Dysproteinemia

Angioimmunoblastic lymphadenopathy with dysproteinemia (AILD) is a hyperimmune state that presents with rash, polyclonal gammopathy, Coombs'-positive hemolytic anemia, hepatosplenomegaly, anergy, and decreased T-cell suppressor levels. It is fatal within months without treatment. AILD can resemble SLE[B156,G194,G431,P184,R311] in that sicca syndrome, symmetric peripheral polyarthritis, and positive serologies can be observed.[B305,M289,R311] In their literature review, Rosenstein et al.[R311] discussed several patients who followed the pattern of having an established autoimmune disease terminate with AILD, and speculated that it represents a "malignant" transformation of immune-mediated disorders.

Carcinoma

The occurrence of malignancies in those with SLE is discussed in Chapter 62. The initial presentation of a patient with fevers, weight loss, adenopathy, and joint pains requires consideration of autoimmune and malignant disorders. Hypernephromas can present with necrotizing vasculitis, Raynaud's phenomenon, cryoglobulinemia, positive ANA, false-positive syphilis serologies, and elevated levels of circulating immune complexes.[H131,M124] Resection of the tumor usually reverses these findings. A case of a woman with breast carcinoma and postradiation pneumonitis and serositis with a positive ANA and LE cell preparation that disappeared after corticosteroid therapy has also been reported.[W41] Patients with immunoblastic sarcoma,[S677] lymphoma,[A318] Burkitt's lymphoma,[P271] hairy cell leukemia,[S733] and ovarian carcinoma[F242] were thought to have SLE on initial presentation. Tumor-associated antigen CA 19-9, a fairly specific marker for gastrointestinal adenocarcinomas, was positive in 6 of 19 patients with SLE in one report.[S364]

Infectious Diseases

The propensity of SLE patients to develop infections, and specific infectious associations with the disease, are discussed in Chapter 46. Problems relating to differential diagnosis, are presented here.

Leprosy

Leprosy rarely occurs in association with SLE,[O27,P270] but the presence of deforming arthritis, alopecia, rash, and neuropathy in both conditions can make the differential diagnosis confusing.[B403,C219,K259,L32,M436] A positive ANA or rheumatoid factor is found in 3 to 36% of leprosy cohorts, but other antibody systems are absent.[B403,C219,L32,M436] Mackworth-Young et al. have found a common idiotypic determinant shared by patients with SLE and lepromatous leprosy.[M34]

Tuberculosis

Tuberculosis and SLE have overlapping chest and central nervous system features, as well as symptoms of fever, malaise, and weight loss. Feng and Tan[F60] found concurrent tuberculosis in 16 of 311 SLE patients (5%) seen in Singapore between 1963 and 1979.

Viral Infections

Viral infections may display overlapping features with those of lupus on initial presentation, including intense fatigue. The chronicity of certain viral infections, such as the Epstein-Barr virus, cytomegalovirus, and viral hepatitis in young women, as well as the tendency of SLE patients to develop infections, makes this a complex issue.[B566,J108] Infections with these viruses can induce a low-titer ANA. A study of 44 patients with parvovirus B12 infection demonstrated an association with a transient, subclinical autoimmune state, complete with expression of anti-nDNA and antilymphocyte antibodies in most patients.[S547] Increased antibody titers to Epstein-Barr viral capsid antigen, early antigen, and nuclear antigen, compared to controls, have been noted in SLE patients,[K254,N10,S235] and false-positive Monospot test results have been reported.[A143] Winfield's group reported that the IgM in sera from children with acute infectious mononucleosis and hepatitis A is reactive with different antibody epitopes than from those with SLE.[C34]

AIDS

The presentation of human immunodeficiency virus (HIV) infection can mimic that of autoimmune phenomena.[D115,K375] Fevers, lymphadenopathy, rash, renal dysfunction, neurologic and hematologic disorders, sicca syndrome, and polyarthralgias can be observed. HIV positivity is associated with the presence of the lupus circulating anticoagulant (although thrombosis does not occur), hemolytic anemia, ANA, rheumatoid factor, CICs, immune thrombocytopenia, polyclonal hyperglobulinemia, and leukopenia. Anti-Ro/SSA and anti-La/SSB are not seen.[C14,C323,S693] Despite this, four reports representing a total of 6 cases of coexistence have been presented; 3 of the 6 had congenital AIDS, and SLE developed.[D7,F315,] [K375,S727] Kaye[K134] hypothesized that SLE may somehow be protective of AIDS. Assuming that 500,000 Americans have SLE and that 150,000 have AIDS, at least 400 concurrent cases would be expected. This negative correlation becomes more impressive when one considers that, if 10% of SLE patients had autoimmune hemolytic anemia or other complications that required transfusions (e.g., uremia, surgery) between 1978 and 1983, when the United States blood supply was unsafe, up to 50,000 should have been at risk of becoming infected with HIV[W25] but not a single report has stated that any converted to HIV seropositivity. One case of thrombotic thrombocytopenic purpura, HTLV-1 infection, and probable SLE, however, has appeared.[S232]

Miscellaneous Disorders

Skin lesions of chronic granulomatous disease can mimic those of discoid lupus[B543,S722] and coexist with SLE;[M119] thallium poisoning can result in ANA formation and mimic SLE.[A95] Down's syndrome is associated with an inflammatory arthropathy that sometimes resembles SLE,[F217,Y30] and one case of Hunter's syndrome with SLE has appeared.[Z29]

Part C

Pregnancy

Chapter 50

THE MOTHER IN SLE

RODANTHI C. KITRIDOU
GREGORIO MINTZ

Systemic lupus erythematosus (SLE) is primarily a disease of young women who are perfectly capable of having children, and pregnancy is a frequent occurrence in these patients. The course of pregnancy in systemic lupus has changed materially in the last 40 years: In the 1950s, pregnancy in lupus was frequently fraught with serious disease exacerbations, fetal death, and even maternal death. More recently, and especially over the last decade or so, pregnancy in lupus patients has become commonplace, and the outcome has improved remarkably. Before addressing lupus and pregnancy, we examine the available evidence for immunologic mechanisms in pregnancy, which seem intimately linked to the survival of the fetus, and briefly review sex hormone metabolism in SLE patients.

IMMUNOLOGY OF NORMAL PREGNANCY

Maternal tolerance to the fetus has been the subject of extensive research. Pertinent questions include the following:

1. Is the maternal immune response decreased during pregnancy?
2. Is the fetal immune response capable of suppressing the maternal immune response?
3. Is there a maternal immune response against fetal (paternal) antigens?
4. Are the humoral factors generated during pregnancy responsible for fetal tolerance?
5. Is the uterus an immunologically privileged site?
6. Is the maternal-fetal interface immunogenic?
7. Do steroid hormones have immunomodulatory activity?

Several studies relative to these issues are worth mentioning.

One review has critically examined the precepts of the immunology of pregnancy.[F44] In pregnant women, numbers of T and B lymphocytes are normal.[D244,H316] In contrast to prior conflicting reports about T-cell subset alterations in pregnancy, studies with monoclonal antibodies and flow cytometric techniques have shown normal results.[C409,G185] Although there are reports of depressed lymphocyte responses to antigens and mitogens in pregnancy,[P160] marked fluctuations of such responses in normal, nonpregnant individuals have also been demonstrated.[D224,G136,G343,O102] A longitudinal study of normal pregnant and nonpregnant women showed normal lymphocyte proliferative responses to mitogens in both groups.[G80] Cell-mediated cytotoxicity is maintained during pregnancy, and there is in vivo normal cellular reaction to tuberculin.[B8,P286] However, it has been suggested that soluble factors induce selective suppression of maternal cellular immunity: Depressed responses to purified protein derivative (PPD) and phytohemagglutinin (PHA) have been attributed to a serum factor, potentially an α_2-macroglobulin, which increases in pregnancy and decreases to normal during postpartum.[S514,Y63] Lymphocytes from nonpregnant women incubated in pregnancy or fetal serum showed a decreased response to PHA, and vice versa.[S23] Immediately after delivery there was a marked reduction in maternal T helper cells and a high suppressor activity when added to normal lymphocytes; cord blood contained a lower number and percentage of T suppressor cells which, however, had high suppressor activity on maternal and normal lymphocytes.[S390] Suppression of maternal lymphocyte proliferation was shown to occur across a cell-impermeable membrane, suggesting that a soluble factor elaborated by newborn suppressor lymphocytes may be responsible.[O54] A potential activator of fetal suppressor cells is alpha-fetoprotein, which in purified preparations is not capable of immunosuppression by itself.[B78,F284,G205]

The ability to produce lymphokines is generally normal; in vitro production of interleukin 1 (IL-1),[B270] IL-2,[H208] IL-1β, IL-6, and tumor necrosis factor (TNF) are normal throughout pregnancy.[F44] However, there was reduced stimulatory activity for IL-2 production in maternal serum at delivery and higher activity in cord serum; the same study showed an inhibitory activity on the two-way allogeneic mixed lymphocyte reaction in almost all maternal sera and in 70% of the cord sera.[B269] Maternal serum also has a lower stimulatory activity for IL-1 production.[B270] Normal primiparae and pregnant recurrent spontaneous aborters had no evidence of maternal cell-mediated reactivity to paternal antigens, although one-third of the latter had circulating cytotoxic cells at miscarriage.[S81]

During pregnancy, there are normal numbers of maternal natural killer (NK) cells with depressed NK activity[G362,T170] which is reconstituted in vitro by IL-2.[V43]

IgG from normal pregnancy serum blocks maternal lymphocytotoxicity against cultured monolayer trophoblasts.[T83] Women with recurrent spontaneous abortions lack this antibody.[R255,S696] The induction of blocking antibody by immunization with paternal leukocytes prevents recurrent spontaneous abortions.[C94] There is an abundance of maternal immunoglobulins of all classes bound to the placenta. Eluates of such immunoglobulins, especially IgG, inhibit T-cell blastogenesis by mixed lymphocyte reaction or by T-cell mitogens.[B406,F29,J146]

Perhaps the most important aspect of fetal tolerance is whether the fetoplacental unit is immunogenic. There is ample evidence that transplacental traffic allows the passage of cells and proteins between mother and fetus.[A42] The layer of trophoblast cells surrounding the chorionic villi of the placenta (villous syncytiotrophoblast), which is in direct contact with maternal blood, does not exhibit any major histocompatibility complex (MHC) antigens.[G326,L366] Thus, the trophoblast may be "invisible" to the maternal immune system. It has been suggested that trophoblastic HLA antigens are masked by transferrin.[F28,F30] The villous trophoblast shares an antigen with certain lymphocytes, called trophoblast-lymphocyte cross-reactive (TLX) antigen, which has a degree of polymorphism and may be coded by a gene locus in the vicinity of the MHC.[M297,M298] It has been suggested that immunity to TLX antigens is regulated through a TLX idiotype network,[T191] and that antibodies to TLX antigens may be beneficial to pregnancy by acting as "blocking" antibodies. Another area of maternal-trophoblast contact, the migrating extravillous trophoblast, seems to express an MHC class I-like molecule. It differs from typical class I MHC antigens by being smaller (40 kD instead of 45), by lacking in polymorphism, and by being mainly intracellular, with only sparse cell surface expression.[L367] Its function is not yet clear. Noncytotoxic IgG antibodies to paternal lymphocytes were found in 30% of primiparae and 46% of multiparae, but not in nulliparae; these antibodies were directed to HLA-linked antigens, but not to known A, B, C, or DR specificities.[123] Circulating immune complexes with IgG antitrophoblast antibody were found in normal pregnancy sera by some authors and not by others.[D23,M180]

An interesting area concerns maternal and fetal serum factors that may have immunomodulating properties. Early pregnancy factor (EPF) is found 48 hours after fertilization as a high- (180 kD) and a low-molecular-weight fraction (40 kD) and is heat-stable, low pH-resistant, and not species-specific.[M616] Pregnancy-associated α_2-glyco-protein (PAG, pregnancy zone protein) has a molecular weight of 364 kD, increases during gestation in 75% of women, and in women on oral contraceptives, may be produced by maternal leukocytes and has various immunosuppressive properties.[T154] Pregnancy-specific β_1-glycoprotein is produced by the placenta and fibroblasts, has a molecular weight of about 90 kD, and greatly reduces PHA-induced blastogenesis.[B166,C251] In the process of in vitro fertilization, an embryo-associated immunosuppressor factor (EASF), which is produced and released in the embryo growth medium, has been associated with success of the pregnancy.[B420] Furthermore, a heat-resistant protein produced by human placental chorion causes reversible inhibition of in vitro processes associated with early lymphocyte triggering; specifically, it prevents expression of IL-2 receptors and of class II MHC glycoproteins (HLA-DR).[S485]

The notion that the uterus may be an immunologically privileged site has been dispelled.[B165] Of interest are the lymphocyte populations found in the pregnant uterus; most are large granular lymphocytes (LGLs) with natural killer cell activity, approximately 10% are mature lymphocytes, and virtually no B lymphocytes or plasma cells are present.[L366] The recruitment of LGLs appears to be under hormonal control, with peak numbers at the proliferative phase of the menstrual cycle and during pregnancy, but their function is not clear.[L366]

Estrogens, progestins, androgens, and corticosteroids are produced at a 4- to 100-fold greater-than-normal rate during pregnancy, and fall abruptly to normal within 2 days postpartum (Table 50–1).[P135] Estrogens and progesterone are present at concentrations 50- to 100-fold in the third trimester. Pharmacologic doses of either suppress inflammation, delay allograft rejection, and decrease in vitro blastogenic responses.[C298,S697] Pregnancy serum concentrations are not adequate for immunosuppression, but the action of progesterone is evident within areas of high *local* concentration, and such levels are achieved in placental tissue.[S426] Cortisol is present at a 4 fold concentration in the third trimester, and the free cortisol index is elevated.[N118,P135] Again, local events at the maternal-fetal interface may be more important than serum levels.[W184] Human chorionic gonadotropin and somatotropin appear to suppress in vitro T-cell functions.[C374,P135] It would appear, then, that various immuno-

Table 50–1. Plasma Steroid Hormone Levels in Nonpregnant and Pregnant Women

| Hormone (ng/ml) | Nonpregnant | Trimester | | | Postpartum |
		1	2	3	Day 2
Estrone	0.1–0.3	1–2	3–8	5–20	0.5
Estradiol	0.2–0.5	2–4	5–10	10–30	0.5
Estriol	<0.1	0.2–1	2–4	5–15	<0.1
Progesterone	1–10	20–40	50–80	100–200	1
12α-hydroxyprogesterone	0.1–0.2	2–6	2	3–5	<0.5
Testosterone	0.4	1	1–2	3	1
Androstenedione	1–2	3	4	5–6	2
Cortisol	120	180	300	400–500	150

Persellin, R.H.: The effect of pregnancy on rheumatoid arthritis. Bull Rheum Dis 27:922, 1977.[P135]

modulatory events occur during pregnancy, especially at the maternal-fetal interface, which regulate the maternal immune response and result in tolerance of the embryo.

In summary, the following immunologic mechanisms appear to operate in normal pregnancy, with the net result being the survival and growth of the fetoplacental graft:

1. Maternal lymphocyte response to antigens and mitogens and lymphocyte-mediated cytotoxicity appear normal, while NK cell reactivity is depressed. In vitro lymphokine production (IL-1, IL-1β, IL-2, and TNF) by maternal cells is normal.
2. Cord lymphocytes have increased suppressor activity on maternal and nonpregnancy lymphocytes, most probably through elaboration of soluble factors.
3. An IgG from pregnancy serum blocks maternal lymphocytotoxicity against trophoblast monolayers. Maternal IgG from placental eluates depresses T-cell reactions in vitro.
4. The layer of villous trophoblast in direct contact with maternal blood lacks any class I or II MHC determinants, therefore, the fetoplacental unit evades recognition as "foreign." The role of trophoblast-lymphocyte cross-reacting antigens and of the MHC class I-like antigen present on extravillous trophoblast has yet to be clarified.
5. The role of uterine large granular lymphocytes with NK activity, which are under hormonal control, is unclear.
6. Several pregnancy-associated serum factors, some of which are elaborated by the embryo (alpha-fetoprotein, early pregnancy factor, pregnancy-associated α_2-glycoprotein, pregnancy-specific β_1-glycoprotein, embryo-associated immunosuppressor factor) appear to have immunomodulatory effects on the maternal response, especially at the maternal-fetal interface.
7. Greatly increased levels of hormones such as progesterone, estrogen, cortisol, chorionic gonadotropin, and somatotropin may depress cellular immunity at the maternal-fetal interface.

SEX HORMONE METABOLISM IN SYSTEMIC LUPUS ERYTHEMATOSUS

As mentioned, gonadal hormones modulate the immune response. There is suggestive evidence that these effects occur through a thymus-hypothalamus-pituitary-gonadal axis.[G275] Thymic secretion of thymosin-β_4, and possibly other factors, affects the release of gonadotropin-releasing hormone (GnRH), which regulates the release of luteinizing hormone, resulting in ovarian development. Levels of thymosin-β_4 decrease in postmenopausal and ovariectomized women, suggesting possible modulation of thymic function by gonadal steroids. The hypothalamic-pituitary-ovarian axis in SLE is normal.[L94] Abnormalities in the metabolism of sex hormones in SLE have been extensively studied and are discussed in detail in Chapter 16. To summarize, women and men with lupus, and their first-degree relatives, have a higher rate of C16 hydroxyla-

tion of estradiol to metabolites with estrogenic activity, decreased C2 hydroxylation of estrogen, and increased C17 oxidation of testosterone, resulting in inactive metabolites.[L17] Women with lupus have decreased androgen levels, with the lowest levels found in women with active SLE.[L21] The net effect would seem to be an overall increased estrogenic effect. During lupus pregnancy, prolactin levels are significantly higher than in control pregnant women, are highest late in pregnancy, and in active lupus patients.[J52,J54] Prolactin is considered necessary for immunocompetence. In the same study, serum estradiol and testosterone levels in pregnant SLE women were significantly lower than those of controls during the 10th to 30th weeks of gestation.

DEFINITION OF TERMS

The following terms are used in this and Chapters 51 and 52:[C175,K122,K260,M473]

Fertility rate   Average number of pregnancies per pregnant woman

Parity rate   Average number of viable infants per pregnant woman.

Adjusted fertility or **parity rate**   Corrected for years at risk for pregnancy (10-year intervals)[B140]

Success rate or **percentage**   Expresses the percentage of viable infants per group of patients (live births per total pregnancies × 100)

Spontaneous abortion   Spontaneous termination of pregnancy prior to 20 weeks' gestation

Elective or **induced ("therapeutic") abortion** Voluntarily induced termination of pregnancy

Stillbirth   Spontaneous termination of pregnancy after 20 weeks' gestation

Fetal wastage   Sum of spontaneous abortions and stillbirths; Cecere and Persellin have also defined it as the sum of spontaneous abortions, stillbirths, and perinatal deaths divided by the number of pregnancies minus elective abortions and expressed as a percentage[C175]

Total fetal loss   Sum of abortions and perinatal deaths

Neonatal death   Death of a newborn within 30 days of birth

Perinatal mortality   Sum of stillbirths and neonatal deaths

Recurrent fetal loss (habitual abortion)   Three or more,[C430,M472] or two or more,[L392] consecutive spontaneous abortions

Recurrent (habitual) aborter   A woman with recurrent fetal loss

Premature birth   Spontaneous termination of pregnancy with a live birth between weeks 21 and 37

Full-term or **term birth**   Spontaneous termination of pregnancy with a live birth between weeks 38 and 40

Pregnancy-induced hypertension (PIH)   Presence of diastolic blood pressure ≥ 95 mm Hg on at least two occasions, 6 or more hours apart[W43]

Pre-eclampsia   Variously defined, as PIH and concomittant proteinuria of > 0.5 g/L in the absence of urinary tract infection[W43] or abrupt onset of hypertension and proteinuria after 24 weeks of gestation[D162,G379]

Severe pre-eclampsia Characterized by one or more of the following: blood pressure of at least 160 mm Hg systolic, or 110 mm Hg diastolic on two readings 6 hours apart; proteinuria $\geq$ 5 g/24 hr, oliguria (<400 ml/24 hr), cerebral or visual disturbances, pulmonary edema, or cyanosis[W145]

Eclampsia Severe pre-eclampsia with malignant hypertension, seizures, and renal failure

PREGNANCY AND LUPUS INTERACTIONS—THE CONTROVERSY

Since the earliest studies, the effect of pregnancy on SLE activity, and vice versa, has been the subject of controversy and contradiction. If no interactions had been noted, the reports would have been scarce and unanimous in their conclusions. However, many reports, both by rheumatologists and by obstetricians, have described the reciprocal relationship of these conditions.

Early reports from the 1950s recommended against pregnancy and implied that it was not advisable, or that termination should be offered.[E84,T279] These studies have been followed by a massive collection of data which now indicate that, if well managed, pregnancy in lupus patients can often be associated with a successful, if not completely normal, outcome. Nevertheless, controversy is still apparent, and probably arises from the following:

1. Study design: There are a few prospective controlled studies,[L356,M472,W336] but many retrospective studies;[B371,F95,F190,H205,H224,H448,I11,K122,M334,N144,P216,S633,T200,V47] (the latter include some by patient questionnaire[K122,S633] and some by questionnaires to physicians)[H224]
2. The great variability of SLE severity in general
3. Variability in definition of flare or exacerbation, which ranges from complicated analysis of laboratory data, to the use of clinical indices of signs and symptoms, the functional class of the patient, or the physician's decision to increase prednisone dosage[L262]
4. The frequency of flares within the "natural history" of SLE has only recently been defined.[M472,W336]
5. Variability of patient population in each report in terms of disease severity and educational-socioeconomic background, ranging from private office patients to university, tertiary level hospitals with economically deprived patients.[W39]

A comprehensive review was published in 1981[C175] comparing the reports from 1950 to 1980. This showed a relative decrease in maternal disease exacerbation rates during these decades, from 60% between 1950 and 1960 to 48% between 1970 and 1980. However, fetal wastage remained at 27% and 28%, respectively, without variation during these three decades. Subsequent reviews[B577,G63,O127] also showed substantial agreement among authors regarding the high fetal morbidity and mortality, as a varying frequency of maternal morbidity. Prospective studies of controlled populations have begun to be published,[L356,M472,W336] and the long-held concept

of increased SLE flares related to pregnancy has been challenged as data on the frequency of exacerbations in nonpregnant patients begin to emerge.

When analyzing this mass of new data, consideration should be given to the fact that patients diagnosed as having SLE in studies reported since 1980 are different from those diagnosed 20 to 40 years ago, for three reasons:

1. The availability of sophisticated antinuclear antibody (ANA) testing has allowed the diagnosis of patients with very mild disease; such patients would not have been diagnosed as having SLE in 1950.
2. The application of the SLE classification criteria, preliminary and revised, since 1971 and 1982, respectively, has provided relative diagnostic uniformity.[C325,T46]
3. Three decades of experience with the treatment of SLE patients in the poststeroid era have resulted in increased survival, a large patient population with controlled SLE and, indeed, a modification of the "natural history" of the disease.[P216,R173,S741]

EFFECT OF PREGNANCY ON SYSTEMIC LUPUS ACTIVITY

During menses, a number of women with lupus complain of increased symptoms, and some have menstrual irregularities; amenorrhea can be present, with inability to conceive during periods of severe disease activity, or during high-dose steroid therapy.[D323,R340] Pregnancy in SLE patients has become a frequent event since the prognosis has greatly improved by proper management, and patients function well within society and their families.[S633] Their fertility is normal, at 2 to 2.4 pregnancies per patient[F190,F251,G387,H205,K122,N144] not only in quiescent periods of the disease, but also during active episodes, when approximately 10% of total reported pregnancies occur.

The early reports established several points (Table 50–2). In the presteroid era, conception was considered rare and exacerbations and remissions occurred almost equally during pregnancy, but severe postpartum exacerbations were seen in virtually all patients.[F251] The course of pregnancy tended to be smoother in patients who conceived during a period of inactive lupus.[E148] An early report of the value of steroid therapy in decreasing relapses during pregnancy and the postpartum period appeared in 1962: 16 of 33 patients on prednisone for at least part of the pregnancy had 8 flares during pregnancy and 5 flares during the 8 weeks postpartum; the remaining 17 patients, who did not receive steroids, had 15 exacerbations during gestation and 11 flares postpartum.[G58] A sizeable proportion of patients developed pre-eclampsia (1.8 to 20%).[D262,D323,M57] It is still debated whether hypertension alone or with proteinuria during pregnancy represents pregnancy-induced hypertension, pre-eclampsia, or active lupus nephritis.[G387,L356,Z52] The more acute the lupus, the worse was the outcome, with maternal death occurring in 10 to 25% of patients.[D262,E84] In general, the earlier the report, the more dire the course of pregnancy and the postpartum period. The abundant, uncontrolled

Table 50–2. Effect of Pregnancy on Systemic Lupus Erythematosus

Source	No. of Pregnancies	No Change (%)	Intrapartum or Postpartum Flare (%)	Postpartum Flare (%)	Improved or Remission (%)	Onset in Pregnancy
Retrospective studies						
Ellis and Bereston (1952)[E84]	69	25	50	—	25	—
Friedman and Rutherford (1956)[F251]	42	40	75	50	10	10
Donaldson and de Alvarez (1962)[D262]	153	56	30	26	26	—
Estes and Larson (1965)[E148]	68	52	24	—	13	10
Fraga et al. (1974)[F190]	225	57	27	5	0	28
Dubois (1976)[D323]	217	37	27	—	6	—
Tozman et al. (1980)[T200]	24	62	25	13	8	0
Varner et al. (1983)[V47]	38	55	35	8	—	21
Meehan and Dorsey (1987)[M334]	22	55	45	42	—	—
Nossent and Swaak (1990)[N144]	39	26	74	63	—	—
Prospective studies						
Lockshin et al. (1984)[L356]	33	43	28	—	—	—
Mintz et al. (1986)[M472]	102	40	60	20	—	—
Wong et al. (1991)[W336]	29	42	58	0	—	—

retrospective studies since the early 1950s have been analyzed in several reviews,[C175,G63,O127,W39] which reported frequent exacerbations of SLE during pregnancy and postpartum.

In the mid-1960s to mid-1970s, three major studies were published: Dubois reported 217 pregnancies in 112 patients, Estes and Larson reported 79 pregnancies in 36 patients, and Fraga et al. reported 225 pregnancies in 53 patients, from Los Angeles, New York, and Mexico City, respectively.[D323,E148,F190] In these patients, the appropriate use of corticosteroids decreased pregnancy and postpartum flares to half of those in the 1950s, and maternal mortality was very rare. The study by Fraga et al. from Mexico City[109] was followed up by a prospective study by Mintz et al. (see below).[M472]

It seems then, that exacerbations have become milder over the last 30 years, with the exception of patients in whom disease began during pregnancy or postpartum. Associated maternal mortality has also been reported with lesser frequency. In the excellent review by Cecere and Persellin of 688 SLE pregnancies from 1950 to 1980, maternal exacerbation occurred in 360 (52%), remission in 132 (19%), and maternal death in 48 (7%).[C175] Data comparison between the first and last decades indicates that disease exacerbations decreased from 60% (1950 to 1960) to 48% (1970 to 1980), remissions decreased from 35 to 8%, and maternal deaths decreased from 17 to 1%. In 272 pregnancies reported between 1970 and 1980, 142 exacerbations occurred (48%), of which one-third were in the postpartum period and the rest were equally divided among trimesters. Patients whose SLE was inactive at conception had a 35% likelihood of experiencing a disease flare. Table 50–2 summarizes the major reports that have examined the effects of pregnancy on women with lupus.

Six studies, spanning from 1962 to 1991, have examined the question of whether pregnancy induces lupus exacerbations.[B58,L356,M472,P135a,W336,Z52] Two studies used the patients as their own controls[G58,Z52] and three used case-controlled observations (Table 50–3).[L356,M472,W336] Garsenstein et al.[G58] noted a clear-cut increase in exacerbations during the first 20 weeks of pregnancy (3.04/100 weeks at risk versus 0.91/100 weeks for the 32 weeks prepregnancy), a small increase during the second half of pregnancy (1.62/100 weeks), a 7-fold increase during the 2 months postpartum (6.31/100 weeks), and a return to baseline in the 9 to 40 weeks postpartum. Zulman et al.[Z52] expressed the number of exacerbations per number of pregnancies as a percentage during the 6 months preceding pregnancy (4%), each trimester of pregnancy (13, 14, and 55%, respectively), and during 6 months postpartum (23%). The flow rate during the 3rd trimester and postpartum appears extensive. Results of the three case-control studies are as follows. Lockshin et al.[L356] reported similar flares in 28 pregnant and 21 nonpregnant patients, with the exception of greater thrombocytopenia in the pregnant patients. Mintz et al.[M472] reported 55 exacerbations in 909 months at risk in their pregnant patients, which were not significantly different from the 19 exacerbations in 468 months of their nonpregnant patients ($p = NS$). Wong et al., however,[W336] noted 13 exacerbations in 155 patient-months in their pregnant patients, twice the rate found in their nonpregnant patients (218 per 5,202 patient-months; $p < 0.02$).

Petri et al., in a prospective study of 40 pregnancies in 37 women, noted 27 exacerbations in 24 pregnancies, or 60% flares. Flare was defined as a change of over 1.0 in the physician's global assessment (scale of 0–3) since the preceding visit or during the previous 93 days. The intrapregnancy flare rate of 1.6337 ± 0.30087 per person-year was significantly greater than the flare rate after delivery (0.6392, $p < 0.001$), and the rate in nonpregnant patients (0.6518, $p < 0.0001$).

Therefore, four studies have suggested increased exacerbations during pregnancy and postpartum,[G58,P135a,W336,Z52] and two, a similar risk of exacerbation, regardless of pregnancy status.[L356,M472] Interestingly, when the data in the Garsenstein et al. Mintz et al., Petri et al., and Wong et al. studies are expressed as an index of exacerbations

Table 50–3. Exacerbations of SLE in Pregnant and Nonpregnant Patients

Study	Exacerbations	
	(Per 100 weeks at risk)	(Per patient-month)
Garsenstein et al.[121]		
32 weeks before pregnancy	0.91	0.04
0–20 weeks of pregnancy	3.04	0.13
21–40 weeks of pregnancy	1.62	0.07
0–8 weeks postpartum	6.31	0.27
9–40 weeks postpartum	0.84	0.04
Zulman et al.[368]		
Exacerbations/pregnancies		
6 months before pregnancy	4%	
1st trimester	13%	
2nd trimester	14%	
3rd trimester	55%	
6 months postpartum	23%	

Study	Pregnant	Nonpregnant
	(Per patient-month)	
Wong et al.[365]		
Pregnant: 13 in 155 patient-months	0.08	0.04 (p < 0.02)
Nonpregnant: 218 in 5202 patient-months		
Petri et al.[274a]		
Pregnant: 1.6337/patient-year	0.14	0.05 (p < 0.0001)
After delivery: 0.6392/patient-year	0.05	
Nonpregnant: 0.6518/patient-year		
Mintz et al.[240]		
Pregnant: 55 in 909 patient-months	0.06	0.04 (p = NS)
Nonpregnant: 19 in 468 patient-months		
Lockshin et al.[211]		
Similar in 28 pregnant and 21 nonpregnant patients		
Greater thrombocytopenia in pregnant patients		

per patient-month, these indices are remarkably similar for the nonpregnant patients, at 0.04 to 0.05 (0.039565, 0.040598, 0.054316, and 0.041907, respectively). This suggests that over the last 30 years the rate of exacerbation in systemic lupus over time has not changed, but the severity of exacerbations appears to have lessened. The differences in flares during pregnancy in these five studies may be explained by differences in patient populations and therapeutic strategies over three decades.

In the last 12 years several retrospective reports[F95,H205,M334,N144,P216,T200,V47] and three prospective studies with control groups have appeared[L356,M472,W336] in an attempt to define the influence of pregnancy on the evolution of maternal SLE. Studies which specifically addressed a minimum of 10 lupus pregnancies are reviewed here. Fetal effects are reviewed in Chapter 51.

Tozman et al.[T200] reviewed 24 pregnancies. Of these, 7 had elective abortions and had active SLE. Of the 17 completed pregnancies, 7 had active disease at conception, and 5 of 7 remained active; in the 10 pregnancies with inactive disease at conception, only 1 woman flared. The episodes of SLE activity were judged to be mild with less central nervous system involvement, pericarditis, and pleuritis than those in the nonpregnant population studied. Only 8 of 17 patients received prednisone during pregnancy, which indicates a group of patients with mild disease.

Varner et al.[V47] analyzed retrospectively 34 pregnancies from the University of Iowa Hospitals; 8 of them con-

ceived with active SLE. Of the 26 pregnancies that began with inactive disease, 9 exacerbated (35%), with one maternal death. The remaining 17 patients had inactive disease throughout pregnancy and postpartum: 7 were receiving corticosteroids, and 10 were on no treatment.

Meehan et al.[M334] reported, from the same institution, a retrospective evaluation of the effect of pregnancy on the course of SLE in patients receiving corticosteroids or azathioprine at conception, and compared them to a matched group of nonpregnant patients receiving the same therapy. There were 10 exacerbations in 22 pregnancies (45%), and 12 in 22 nonpregnant patients (54%). In patients constantly receiving less than 15 mg of prednisone daily, 10 of 19 experienced exacerbations in pregnancy (53%), and 7 of 11 (64%) nonpregnant patients. However, when the prednisone or azathioprine dosage was reduced, a flare occurred in all 7 pregnant patients, and in 5 of 13 nonpregnant patients (38%). As a further comparison, the authors analyzed disease behavior from 3 to 15 months postpartum) and found an exacerbation rate of 42%, similar to intrapregnancy rates.

Nossent and Swaak reported a retrospective Dutch study of 39 pregnancies in 19 patients, and found that 74% had exacerbations during pregnancy. Six patients had active SLE at conception; 9 (47%) with previously inactive disease had a flare during pregnancy, and 12 (63%) during puerperium.[N144] These episodes of active SLE included mostly skin and joint manifestations and were considered mild; however, during pregnancy, 2 patients developed new kidney disease with diffuse proliferative nephritis (class IV by WHO classification on biopsy).[M232] 2 developed serositis, and 4 developed thrombocytopenia. During the postpartum period, 2 patients developed serositis, 1 had convulsions with normal blood pressure, and 4 had thrombocytopenia without bleeding.

The largest retrospective series of lupus pregnancy was reported by Pistiner et al. in a cohort of 570 private patients followed during the 1980s.[P216] Of 307 women with lupus, 227 (74%) had 634 pregnancies, with 439 live births (69%), 106 elective abortions (17%), and 95 spontaneous abortions (18%). There were 29 women with recurrent abortion (13%), and most of those tested for anticardiolipin antibodies were positive. About half of the elective abortions were performed to protect the health of the mother. Pregnancy outcome in these patients was similar to that in 40 women with discoid lupus reported in the same article. These SLE patients had well controlled lupus, with relatively less organ-threatening disease than most university clinic patients: 54% overall, with 28% nephritis and 11% neuropsychiatric disease. In the same metropolitan area, the indigent lupus population at the Los Angeles County-University of Southern California Medical Center had more than a 50% prevalence of nephritis.

Three prospective studies on lupus pregnancy, starting in 1984, Lockshin et al. reported on a multicenter study in New York City with 33 pregnancies compared to a matched group of nonpregnant patients.[L356] Three criteria for the definition of a flare were used: new signs from a previously inactive organ system, increase in corticosteroid dosage, or the treating physician's statement that a flare was present. Of the 33 pregnancies, 8 were terminated by elective abortion in the first trimester; in the remaining 21 pregnancies there were 8 instances of thrombocytopenia, 5 of which (24%) were considered to be caused by SLE, 4 patients developed new proteinuria which subsided after delivery (no renal biopsy), and corticosteroid dosage was increased in 7 patients (28%). The authors further analyzed laboratory values (ESR, anti-DNA antibody, serum complement), dosage of prednisone, and number of patients treated, and found no statistically significant differences between the pregnant and nonpregnant groups. They concluded that pregnancy does not cause SLE exacerbations. It is important to note that 40% of these patients, both pregnant and nonpregnant, did not receive corticosteroids during the observation period, which suggests a population with mild SLE. In 1989, Lockshin et al. reported on 80 pregnancies, including 16 of the 33 in the 1984 study, without a control group.[L348] A smaller proportion of patients was on steroids at the time of pregnancy (33%), which defines them as having mild disease and, by global criteria, 26% had clinical evidence of active SLE during pregnancy.

In a 9-year prospective study in Mexico City, Mintz et al.[M472] reported 102 consecutive pregnancies in 75 patients. All patients were closely followed by a team consisting of a rheumatologist, obstetrician, and neonatologist. No elective abortions were performed, and all patients received a minimum of 10 mg of prednisone daily

from the time pregnancy was diagnosed. Of the 102 pregnancies studied, 10 started with active maternal disease and, in the remaining 92, which began with inactive SLE, a 60% exacerbation rate was noted; over half of these flares (54%) occurred during the first trimester and 20% occurred in the postpartum and postabortion periods. This exacerbation rate was compared to that of a similar group of young women with SLE who were in a parallel study of progestogens as contraceptives during the same 9 years. The progestogen study had a control group, and all patients were followed with the same criteria for SLE activity as the pregnant patients.[M471] The pregnant patients had 55 exacerbations in 909 patient-months and the contraceptive study group had 19 exacerbations in 468 patient-months, which is not statistically different. The authors concluded that the exacerbation rate during pregnancy is not increased. The most frequent SLE flares were mucocutaneous and articular, while fever, serositis, and thrombophlebitis were mild; however, 9 patients had episodes of nephritis activity and 8 had central nervous system manifestations consisting of headache of varying severity with EEG changes in 5 patients and grand mal seizures, chorea, and transient episodes of memory loss with dyslalia in 1 each of the remaining 3 patients. These bouts of active disease were controlled by increasing prednisone to 15 to 45 mg daily, with the exception of 7 patients: 5 patients with severe kidney disease were given 60 mg daily, 1 very ill patient with high fever, cutaneous vasculitis, and pericarditis required up to 300 mg daily, and 1 patient with thrombocytopenic purpura and hemolytic anemia was controlled with 200 mg of prednisone daily. No maternal deaths occurred in this study.

Wong et al. reported a prospective study of 29 pregnancies in 22 patients from Hong Kong.[W336] There were 12 abortions, 2 spontaneous and 10 elective. The remaining 15 patients had 17 successful pregnancies. In 11 of 19 pregnant patients, 13 SLE relapses occurred (58%); these included 6 episodes of renal disease, 5 of arthritis, and 2 of vasculitis. In their study protocol the steroid dosage was maintained as needed until the 30th week of pregnancy, when it was increased to 10, 20, or 30 mg if the patients were taking less than 10, 10, or more than 10 mg daily, respectively. If disease activity required higher dosages, it was adjusted accordingly, and that dose was maintained until 4 weeks after delivery. No postpartum flares or maternal deaths occurred. The exacerbation rate during pregnancy, 13 per 155 patient months, was significantly higher than that of Wong et al.'s nonpregnant patients (218 per 5,202 patient-months, p < 0.02).

Comparison of these reports emphasizes the variability of definition of exacerbation and disease severity in different studies. Lupus appeared mild in the New York reports[L348,L356] in which 67% of patients and 40% of controls did not need steroids prior to conception, and 30% did not need corticosteroids during pregnancy. The patient population in the report from Mexico City[M472] had moderately severe SLE, with 50% of patients having had a previous episode of kidney involvement that required a renal biopsy and, although 90 of 102 pregnancies started with inactive SLE, all patients required therapy. The Hong

Kong patients also appeared to have moderately severe disease.[W336]

Many reports have described severe SLE associated with pregnancy or the postpartum period, particularly in previously undiagnosed or untreated patients, with a catastrophic illness frequently terminating in maternal death.[E147,F190,F251] This is why certain authors[M472,W336] have recommended steroid administration at the time pregnancy is diagnosed, and others have strongly suggested that medications not be decreased during pregnancy and postpartum.[M334,L348] In a population with benign disease, no retrospective evidence that steroid-treated patients did better than untreated patients was found; however, some patients from the original study were selected and included, new ones were added, and the controls were excluded. Lockshin arrived at his conclusion in a retrospective fashion, with a study protocol that was not designed and was not suitable to answer this question. Several authors have shown that mild or quiescent SLE rarely flares during pregnancy or nonpregnant periods, and may not need specific therapy.[F95,H224,S799,W39,Z52]

A special area of concern, onset of lupus during pregnancy or postpartum, has been described in approximately 20% of patients, with a range from 13 to 50%.[F251,G151,H224,I11,J142,K105,K122,M657] Maternal outcome in these patients may be dire, especially if SLE is not suspected and there is a delay in diagnosis and appropriate management. Any organ system may be involved, but the potentially most ominous problem is lupus nephritis (see below).

The effects of pregnancy on SLE activity can be summarized as follows:

1. Fertility in women with lupus is normal, except for amenorrhea and infertility during periods of severe disease activity.
2. The average probability of exacerbation during pregnancy and postpartum in SLE patients is 50%; however, in contrast with early studies of the 1950s and 1960s most exacerbations are minor, with arthritis and cutaneous manifestations being most prevalent. Nevertheless, severe exacerbations occur in approximately 20% of pregnancies and, for this reason, this should be treated as a *high-risk pregnancy*.
3. Risk factors for exacerbation include disease activity during the 3 to 6 months preceding conception and pre-existing renal disease (see below). Conversely, conception during quiescence or remission is associated with a lesser risk for exacerbation. Mild lupus rarely exacerbates during pregnancy.
4. Postpartum exacerbations may be prevented by increasing the corticosteroid dosage during late pregnancy and up to 2 months postpartum, or by watching the patient very carefully and raising steroid doses at the slightest indication of flare.
5. There is a chance for lupus onset during pregnancy in as many as 20% of patients. A high index of suspicion for SLE should prevail when a young woman, during pregnancy or the early postpartum period,

has a combination of unexplained rashes, arthritis, alopecia, proteinuria with active urine sediment, psychosis, chorea, pleuropericarditis, and/or vasculitis.
6. There is a greater prevalence of pre-eclampsia or pregnancy-induced hypertension in lupus patients (see below).

EFFECT OF PREGNANCY ON LUPUS NEPHRITIS

Several early reports on lupus and pregnancy mentioned a few patients with nephritis, usually in the context of severe exacerbation, renal deterioration, onset of nephritis during pregnancy, and even maternal death.[E148,F251,G58,M278,M672] Increased intra-partum and postpartum nephritis activity, manifested by proteinuria, hypertension, and azotemia, occurs mostly in patients with active kidney disease at conception and in patients without adequate therapy. In the presteroid era, Friedman and Rutherford's 1956 report mentioned 6 patients with nephritis, 2 of whom had severe postpartum exacerbation, with 1 death.[F251] Garsenstein's 8 patients with severe lupus nephritis had progression of renal disease during pregnancy and active SLE during the postpartum period, including 2 patients with spontaneous and therapeutic abortion, and 4 maternal deaths.[G58] Estes and Larson had 10 patients with renal disease and 8 with hypertension among their 68 pregnancies.[E148] Nephritis worsened during pregnancy in the 10 patients and, after delivery, it returned to prepregnancy status in 4 and stabilized in 3 patients, 2 of whom died within a year.[E148] A few early reports mentioned a better outcome, with 3 patients whose nephrotic syndrome improved during pregnancy[D262] and 6 with proteinuria, edema, and hypertension who did not have exacerbations or develop eclampsia;[D382] 3 of the latter 6 patients had overt nephritis.

On the other hand, in the 1970s and 1980s, several papers reported an uneventful course of pregnancy when renal function is normal or SLE is inactive;[E148,F95,T200] lupus nephritis seems to have a better prognosis if it has been inactive for 3 to 6 months before conception.[B371,H224,I11,J142] Again, studies that have specifically addressed a minimum of 10 pregnancies in lupus nephritis are reviewed here. Fetal effects are reviewed in Chapter 51.

Among relatively recent retrospective studies Thomas et al., in 1978, reported 13 pregnancies in 11 women, 8 with normal renal function at onset of pregnancy, 7 with diffuse proliferative nephritis on biopsy, 4 of whom had nephrotic syndrome.[T150] Of these, 6 had SLE exacerbations and 3 progressed to renal failure. Devoe and Taylor reported 13 pregnancies in 8 women, 5 of whom had biopsy-proven nephritis (2 with mild focal, 1 with mild diffuse, and 2 with moderately active diffuse glomerulonephritis).[D191] All nephritis patients were on prednisone and had disease remission from 3 months to 10 years at conception, but 2 had exacerbations, 1 with decreased renal function and pre-eclampsia. This latter patient had the stormiest course and the poorest renal histology. The authors credited serum complement C3 and C4 levels with prognostication of SLE exacerbation. In a subsequent

Table 50—4. Effect of Pregnancy on Lupus Nephritis

Study	No. Pregnancies	Proliferative Nephritis (%)	Intra/postpartum %			Renal Failure (%)*
			Nephrotic syndrome	Flare	Pre-eclampsia	
Thomas 1978	13	64	31	55		23
Devoe 1979	13	25		15	8	15
Houser 1980	18					
	10 inactive			0	0	0
	8 active			13	38	
Hayslett 1980	65	77	25	39		
	25 active			48		
Zulman 1980	24					
	16 nephritis			63	25*	
Fine 1981	45					32 (14)
Gimovsky 1984	46			35	25	21 (16)
Imbasciati 1984	26	58		54		27 (15)
Bobrie 1987	53			34		
	26 active			62		
	27 inactive			7.4		5
Lockshin 1984	33			15	31	
	11 no nephritis				18	
	11 nephritis				64	
Mintz 1986	58 inact.	40		10		
Wong 1991	29	42		21		

* Numbers in parentheses indicate irreversible renal failure.

report of 18 pregnancies in 15 women with lupus and renal biopsies prior to conception, Devoe et al. found that decreased renal function, rather than severity of renal biopsy class, correlates with abnormal fetal outcome.[D190] In 1980, Houser et al.[H448] reported a retrospective analysis of 11 patients with 18 pregnancies and documented lupus nephritis; 10 pregnancies in 5 patients with inactive SLE were uneventful, while 8 pregnancies in 6 women with active disease included 3 with pre-eclampsia, severe in 2 and mild pre-eclampsia in 1 and disease exacerbation in a patient who developed class III lupus nephritis. All patients were receiving prednisone, and no maternal deaths occurred.

Also in 1980, Hayslett and Lynn published the results of a questionnaire of 13 nephrology centers and individual nephrologists.[H224] The report included 47 patients with 65 pregnancies, with renal biopsies in 36 of the patients, which showed focal or diffuse proliferative nephritis. In 9 instances (14%) SLE began during pregnancy and, in the remaining 56 pregnancies, manifestations of lupus nephritis preceded conception in 80%; 61% were not adversely influenced by pregnancy, and a relapse or worsening of kidney disease was found in 39% of the mothers, 16 during pregnancy and 6 in the postpartum period. Of 25 pregnancies with active renal disease at conception, 12% improved, 48% worsened, and 40% remained unchanged. Pregnancy in patients with ongoing activity of SLE was associated with a more hectic course, and successful outcome was reduced by 25%. Only 9 of 16 patients with nephrotic syndrome had successful deliveries. When the serum creatinine level was lower than 1.5 mg/dl, 9 of 10 pregnancies resulted in live births, but in 10 pregnancies with serum creatinine above 1.5 mg/dl, fetal loss was 50%. In 4 patients, however, with serum creatinine of 4 mg/dl or higher, pregnancies resulted in live births, indicating

that a successful outcome is still possible despite severe renal failure.

Among the patients of Zulman et al., 10 of 16 (62.5%) with prior nephritis had exacerbations during pregnancy.[Z52] In 25% of patients, differentiation of acute presentation of lupus nephritis from toxemia was necessary. The authors suggested that the pre-eclamptic picture was a result of lupus nephritis. Fine et al., in 1981, observed that nearly one-third of pregnancies (12 of 37) resulted in worsened renal function, 5 of them irreversibly.[F95] No conception occurred in patients with even moderate renal function impairment. The authors presented an excellent literature review of 20 patients who needed hemodialysis during pregnancy; 1 of the 20 patients had lupus and, despite requiring dialysis in the latter part of pregnancy, delivered a normal child, and her renal function normalized in the postpartum period. The authors formulated a hemodialysis strategy for pregnant patients based on the physiology of pregnancy. Dialysis is indicated for a maternal blood urea nitrogen (BUN) of 50 mg/dl or greater and should maintain BUN under that level. Volume removal should be done through isolated ultrafiltration, blood pressure should be supported with albumin, the dialysate should contain glucose and bicarbonate, low-dose heparin should be used, and progesterone should be administered, because the endogenous progesterone is lost in the dialysate.

From Paris, Jungers et al.[J142] reported on a retrospective study of 36 patients with 104 pregnancies seen between 1962 and 1980 at the Hospital Necker. Of these, 78 pregnancies began before SLE onset (24 women) and 26 after SLE onset (14 women) and, in 9 patients, onset of lupus and nephritis occurred during pregnancy or postpartum (25% of patients, 8% of pregnancies). All patients had clinical renal disease and 31 had biopsies: 5 with mesangial or minimal disease, 8 with focal proliferative, 6 with diffuse proliferative nephritis, and 2 with membranous nephropathy. Overall exacerbations occurred in 12 of 26 pregnancies after SLE onset (46%), 2 of which (8%) progressed to irreversible deterioration of kidney function. A full 66% of patients with active nephritis at the time of conception had a flare; in contrast, only 9% of patients with inactive disease during the 5 months before conception had an exacerbation.

Gimovsky et al.[G151] reviewed retrospectively 39 patients seen between 1973 and 1982 in the Department of Obstetrics and the Rheumatology Section at the University of Southern California; 46 pregnancies occurred in 19 SLE patients with nephritis, confirmed by renal biopsy in 15 (79%). Onset of lupus during pregnancy or postpartum occurred in 8 of 39 patients (20%). Hospitalization was required because of flare in 9, 8, 14, and 4% of patients at risk during the three trimesters and postpartum, respectively. Of the 10 cases of pre-eclampsia, 6 occurred in the patients with nephritis; this represents 25% of 24 pregnancies, after 6 elective, and 16 spontaneous abortions are subtracted from the 46 pregnancies. Of 19 patients, 4 (21%) developed a decrease in renal function within 2 years of delivery, and 3 required chronic hemodialysis (16%). Only 18 of 40 pregnancies (excluding induced abortions) were successful, with a total fetal loss of 55% in the renal group.

Imbasciati et al.[111] from the University of Milan reported 19 SLE nephritis patients with 26 pregnancies and repeated kidney biopsies; 4 had minimal lesions, 7 had focal proliferative, 11 had diffuse proliferative glomerulonephritis, and 5 had membranous nephropathy. During 8 pregnancies (4 patients) there was no change in renal function, although extrarenal flares occurred in 3 pregnancies; 6 patients with previously diagnosed renal disease had a flare in 7 pregnancies, without decrease in kidney function; 3 patients had moderate deterioration of renal function, hypertension, and proteinuria during pregnancy, reversed in 2 by steroid therapy. Seven patients had onset of SLE with nephritis during pregnancy; of these 7, 4 patients had mild nephritis but 3, along with a fourth who had SLE for 1 year, developed anuric renal failure, with 2 maternal deaths. It is important to note that, in all but 2 pregnancies, SLE was active and, by current standards, steroid dosage was low or of short duration, with inadequate control of maternal disease. Only in 7 instances, mainly in postpartum, did exacerbating patients receive high-dose steroid therapy (50 mg prednisone daily or more), which controlled SLE activity in most patients. This suggests that earlier therapeutic intervention was indicated. Multiple renal biopsies performed in 7 patients showed that the majority (4 patients) showed progression of a minimal, focal proliferative, or membranous lesion to a diffuse proliferative nephritis. The converse occurred in 2 patients, in whom diffuse proliferative disease regressed to focal proliferative in 1 and to minimal lesion in the other patient. This implies that careful assessment of renal function and general SLE activity may predict histologic deterioration. Fetal outcome was poor, with 61% live births (corrected for induced abortions).

In 1987, Bobrie et al.[B371] again reviewed the patient population at the Hospital Necker in Paris and added 32 more pregnancies to their previous report.[J142] Of the 73 patients reviewed, 8 developed SLE manifestations during pregnancy, and 6 during the postpartum or postabortion periods, for a 19% prevalence of SLE onset; nephrotic syndrome with increased serum creatinine levels was seen in 7 of these 14 patients. Subsequent kidney biopsies showed proliferative glomerulonephritis in all 14 patients (diffuse in 11); high-dose steroid therapy was followed by improvement in all but 1 patient, who progressed to renal failure in 2 years. In 35 women with 53 pregnancies after the onset of SLE, nephritis exacerbation occurred in 18 (34%), either during pregnancy or during postpartum (10 and 8 cases, respectively). These exacerbations were more frequent in patients whose SLE was active at conception (16 of 26—61.5%), than in patients with stable remissions (2 of 27—7.4%). Corticosteroid therapy failed to reverse the course in 4 patients, who rapidly progressed to end-stage renal failure.

The largest prospective study was conducted in Mexico City, where 58 of 102 pregnancies occurred in patients with known SLE nephritis, and all but 3 had previous renal biopsies.[M472,M473] Of 58 patients, 27 had mesangial lesions (46%), 13 had diffuse (22%) and 9 had focal (15%) proliferative glomerulonephritis,[M232] 5 had membranous nephropathy (9%), 1 had membranoproliferative (1.7%), and 3 were undetermined.[M473] They were treated with 30 to 60 mg of prednisone daily, and were well 4 years later. The rate at which patients with SLE without renal disease develop it is not known; in this study 3 cases occurred in 472 patient-months at risk during pregnancy and postpartum (0.006 new cases of nephritis/patient-month). The authors compared it with patients in the same study followed further for 1,537 patient/months, during which another 5 cases developed new nephritis (0.003/patient-month; p = NS). Of these 58 pregnancies in patients with known SLE nephritis, 6 exacerbations occurred (10.3%), evenly distributed by trimester and postpartum period, and all responded to increases in prednisone dosage. These 6 patients had inactive renal disease for 2 to 5 years before pregnancy. On longterm follow-up of 75 total patients (40 to 65 months), renal function deterioration occurred in 2 of 8 with diffuse proliferative and in 1 of 7 with focal proliferative nephritis; 5 deaths occurred, only 1 from renal disease, 49 months after pregnancy. Of the remaining 44 pregnancies without previous kidney disease, renal involvement appeared for the first time in 3 patients (6.8%) during the second and third trimesters; subsequent biopsies showed 2 with mesangial and 1 with diffuse proliferative glomerulonephritis. All patients in this study had been previously diagnosed and were treated with at least 10 mg of prednisone daily during the entire pregnancy; also, all had mild, inactive kidney disease at the time of conception. Of these patients, 6 had experienced a bout of nephritis within 1 year of conception, but none exacerbated during pregnancy. The exacerbations were not related to the histologic biopsy class. The outcome of pregnancy in this study was not different for patients with or without kidney disease, and the authors related a better fetal outcome to inactive, well-controlled SLE, rather than to the absence of kidney disease.

In the prospective study from Hong Kong,[W336] 6 nephritis relapses occurred in 13 patients, with increasing proteinuria in 3 and nephrotic syndrome in 3. Two of the nephrotic patients, remitted within 4 weeks after elective abortion and increased steroids and the other 4 remitted with only increased dosages of prednisone. Eight women with a history of pre-existing diffuse proliferative renal disease had successful pregnancies, and it was suggested that this was possible because of proper prednisone therapy. The study noted a good maternal outcome in patients with severe disease, perhaps because of their treatment protocol with increasing doses of prednisone as pregnancy progressed.

Reports by Lockshin[L346,L348,L349,L350,L351,L352,L353,L354,L356] have added an overly optimistic view to this problem. His group of patients with very mild disease seem to have had high incidence of pre-eclampsia and pregnancy-induced hypertension (PIH), 30.5%, along with few SLE exacerbations (10 to 15%). Most cases of PIH occurred in patients with prior lupus nephritis, however, (7 of 11; 63.6%), with only 2 of 11 (18%) with PIH and no nephritis (in the remaining 2 patients the nephritis status was unknown). The same is true in the report from Rotterdam,[N144] in which 23% of the SLE patients had PIH, or pre-eclampsia, compared to 5 to 10% in the general Dutch population. As noted earlier, these authors also had a group of patients with benign disease.

Opinions have varied widely as to whether hypertension and proteinuria during pregnancy represent pre-eclampsia or active lupus nephritis.[G387,L356,Z52] Pre-eclampsia, defined as the abrupt onset of hypertension and proteinuria after 24 weeks of gestation, is found in 0.5 to 10% of all pregnancies, and is by far more common in the primigravida.[D162,G379] In lupus pregnancy, up to 25% of patients develop significant proteinuria in the second half of pregnancy. This is variably associated with hypertension, edema, low complement levels, and no hyperuricemia. Some authors have interpreted this as evidence of SLE nephritis flare;[H224,I11,J142,Z52] however, Lockshin et al.[L356] noted no improvement with corticosteroids and spontaneous improvement over several months postpartum, regarded it as a "variant" of PIH. Although the issue of increased prevalence of pre-eclampsia versus nephritis flare in pregnant SLE patients has not been fully resolved,[B577,N144] it is worthwhile to examine the frequency with which pre-eclampsia occurs in women with nephritis of other types.

Experience in pregnancy with maternal renal disease causes other than lupus has established that hypertension develops in 41%, with a higher risk for severe hypertension in women with diffuse proliferative nephritis or with nephrosclerosis.[H443,K111] In these women, too, hypertension occurs most frequently during the third trimester.[H443,H444] Fisher et al., in a renal biopsy study of 176 women without lupus and with the clinical diagnosis of pre-eclampsia, found the typical histologic picture of glomerular endotheliosis in 96 of 176 patients (54.5%), 79 of whom (82%) were primigravidae, thus confirming that pre-eclampsia is uncommon in the multipara.[F116] Furthermore, the clinical diagnosis of pre-eclampsia was confirmed by the biopsy picture in 50% of primigravidae but only in 25% of multigravid women. Of the remaining patients, 10% had a mixed picture of glomerular endotheliosis plus nephrosclerosis, other renal disease, or both, 14% had nephrosclerosis with or without other renal disease, 17.6% had renal disease alone, and 4.5% had normal histology. Therefore, a clinical pre-eclamptic picture does not necessarily mean pre-eclampsia by histology.

A further cause for potential confusion of pre-eclampsia with a lupus exacerbation is the HELLP syndrome (*h*emolysis, *e*levated *l*iver enzymes, *l*ow *p*latelets), which may complicate the course of severe pre-eclampsia in a minority of patients.[W145] Hemolysis and thrombocytopenia are due to microangiopathic hemolytic anemia; 28 of 29 (97%) of Weinstein's patients with HELLP had characteristic blood smears with burr cells and schistocytes, and all had platelet counts under 100,000/mm^3. Elevated liver enzyme levels (SGOT and SGPT) were found in all 29 patients and an increased bilirubin level in 57%. The liver dysfunction is attributed to fibrin deposition with obstruction of the hepatic sinusoids, resulting in liver distention, subcapsular hematomas, and even rupture.[M299] Treatment of pre-eclampsia and prompt delivery by cesarean section is advocated because of grave danger to the mother and fetus (perinatal mortality, 9 to 60%).

Serum complement levels (C3) and anti-double-stranded (ds) DNA can help differentiate between active lupus nephritis and pre-eclampsia. The C3 level is generally low in active nephritis, but normal in pre-eclampsia;[B603] anti-dsDNA is strongly positive, with complement-fixing activity, in active nephritis, and was negative in 40 patients with toxemia, even in 6 of 40 with a positive ANA.[G40] Renal biopsies before conception and postpartum in these patients may provide the definitive answer.

Three pregnancies have been reported in 3 lupus patients who underwent kidney transplantation.[G150,R224] Two were successful, and one terminated in spontaneous abortion; 1 patient had an episode of acute rejection of her kidney 5 months postpartum, but this was reversed by massive doses of corticosteroids.[G150]

Proteinuria, with severe flank pain and hematuria, especially in the presence of membranous nephropathy, a history of deep vein thrombosis, and positive antiphospholipid antibodies, should raise the possibility of renal vein thrombosis. Venography is contraindicated in a pregnant woman; a Doppler ultrasound examination of the renal veins can detect abnormal turbulence in the renal veins. The value of magnetic resonance imaging (MRI) has not been fully evaluated in this area.

The effects of pregnancy on lupus nephritis can be summarized as follows:

1. Patients with SLE nephritis have a 50 to 60% chance of nephritis exacerbation during pregnancy or postpartum if they conceive during a period of active SLE. In contrast, patients with well-controlled SLE, who conceive after a 3- to 6-month period of remission, have only a 7 to 10% chance of nephritis exacerbation.
2. Nephritis exacerbations during pregnancy and postpartum can be very severe, with anuric renal failure and even maternal death, or chronic renal failure;

Vigilance for early detection and vigorous treatment of exacerbations is required.

3. No definitive relationship between the histologic class of lupus nephritis and the severity of flare during pregnancy has been established, but there seems to be a tendency for more severe exacerbations in patients with proliferative nephritis, WHO classes IV and III. Limited information on repeat kidney biopsies before and after SLE pregnancy has shown progression in 4 patients and regression in 2.

4. Women with lupus nephritis are prone to pre-eclampsia, with the prevalence of a pre-eclampsia–like picture during SLE pregnancy being much greater than in normal pregnancy (1.8 to 30.5% versus 0.5 to 10%); up to 18% of these cases occur in women without and up to 64% in those with SLE nephritis. This clinical picture should be viewed as a possible nephritis exacerbation until proven otherwise because of the possibility of acute anuric or chronic renal failure that may follow an exacerbation, and of the distinctly different therapeutic management indicated.

5. The onset of lupus with nephritis during pregnancy is often associated with a stormy course and acute anuric renal failure, and should be suspected in any young woman with a multisystem presentation that includes rashes, arthritis, and alopecia.

6. Renal vein thrombosis should be suspected, detected, and treated, especially in patients with antiphospholipid antibodies and/or membranous nephropathy.

7. Hemodialysis should be instituted during lupus pregnancy in patients with BUN levels of 50 mg/dl or greater.

8. In the presence of active lupus nephritis, especially diffuse proliferative, nephrotic syndrome, moderate to severe hypertension, and a serum creatinine level of 2 mg/dl or greater, pregnancy is contraindicated.

LABORATORY FINDINGS, SEROLOGIC MARKERS, AND ANTIPHOSPHOLIPID ANTIBODIES

When used judiciously and in the context of the patient's clinical picture, certain laboratory tests in pregnant lupus patients can be useful in predicting disease exacerbation, or potential fetal problems. Monitoring of disease activity can be achieved by the determination of complement levels, anti-dsDNA antibodies, and circulating immune complexes. Fetal wastage is high in patients with antiphospholipid antibodies, and neonatal lupus erythematosus is associated with anti-Ro/SSA, anti-La/SSB and, rarely, with anti-U1RNP antibodies.

Pregnancy test results may be false-positive in SLE. A lupus patient with nephrotic syndrome and a false-positive radioimmunoassay pregnancy test was described by Regeste and Painter in 1981.[R110] False-positive urine pregnancy tests occur in about 10% of nonpregnant lupus patients, especially those with nephritis.[W125] Wei et al. at the National Institutes of Health reported this in 14 of 140 nonpregnant lupus patients, including 1 male; 11 of the 14 had renal disease, 8 with the nephrotic syndrome. The false-positive test presents as an atypical ring pattern and reflects a nonimmunologic interference with agglutination of human chorionic gonadotropin (HCG) by anti-HCG serum. Urine gamma globulins in concentrations of 1.7 to 16.6 mg/ml produced this phenomenon. Serum radioimmunoassay for β-HCG gives no false-positive results.

Certain laboratory values change in normal pregnancy. The sedimentation rate increases and is not generally relied on for predicting disease activity;[Z57] average values by the Westergren method are 29 mm/hr in the first, 42 mm/hr in the second, and 36 mm/hr in the third trimester. Nonetheless, in 1956, Friedman and Rutherford reported a high incidence of postpartum exacerbations in lupus patients with Westergren sedimentation rates in excess of 100 mm/hr.[F251] In addition, creatinine clearance increases, immunoglobulin levels decrease but are still within normal limits, and the hemoglobin decreases; the latter two are attributed to hemodilution.

Several studies have shown that the C3 complement level rises in normal pregnancy but little, if at all, in SLE;[C229,Z57] failure of C3 to rise, or declining levels, have been associated with SLE exacerbation, with or without fetal morbidity. Zurier et al. noted a 30% mean rise of C3 level in 20 normal pregnant women and concluded that a declining C3 during pregnancy was a valuable indicator of increased SLE activity.[Z57] Zulman reached similar conclusions.[Z52] Chetlin et al. found that the C3 level rose by 25% in a control group of normal pregnant women, while it only increased by 10% in a group of pregnant SLE patients.[C229] Ziegler and Medsger confirmed the above findings at the same center, with a larger series; 87 of their patients who had a flat or declining C3 level had a significant increase in maternal problems, and in fetal morbidity and mortality.[Z26] Devoe et al. also noted that a falling C3 level was associated with increased SLE activity in the mother and with an increased risk of abortions.[D189,D191] It has been suggested that hypocomplementemia in the pregnant lupus patient may be the result of a different mechanism than in the nonpregnant patient.[L353]

Antinuclear antibody (ANA) tests are not particularly specific for determining disease activity in the pregnant lupus patient. On the other hand, most studies of ANA in normal pregnant women have shown a similar prevalence as in the general population, between 1 and 5% (mean, 2.3%).[H292,H312,R179] One report of 52% ANA positivity in normal pregnant patients[P234] has been refuted by the above studies. A subsequent report by Farnam in 1984 compared 214 normal pregnant women with 50 age-matched controls and found 11 and 2% ANA positivity, respectively, which was significantly higher in pregnancy (p < 0.05).[F21] Most positive ANAs were found in the third trimester. None of the ANA-positive subjects were symptomatic, or took lupus-inducing drugs, and only 2 had anti-dsDNA. In an interesting study from Mexico, Garcia-de la Torre et al. found a positive ANA in 6 of 20 habitual (recurrent) aborters (30%), in 6 of 40 toxemic patients (15%), and in 2 of 30 normal pregnant women (6.6%).[G40] Of the 2 ANA-positive habitual aborters with anti-dsDNA, 1 fulfilled four criteria for SLE; three more in this group had one to three criteria. Of the 6 pre-eclamptic patients with a positive ANA, 3 patients had one and 1 patient had two criteria. The authors concluded that the high prevalence of ANA in women with recurrent abortion can help identify patients who will eventually develop lupus. We concur that ANA does not appear in pregnancy unless the patient is developing lupus.

Anti-dsDNA, especially the complement-fixing variety, has been recognized as a helpful marker for assessing the activity of lupus and lupus nephritis,[B144,R354,T51] and increasing anti-dsDNA levels or titers or finding predict disease exacerbation.[T108] When present in the mother's serum, anti-DNA may or may not be present in cord blood: Grennan et al. followed 4 systemic and 1 discoid lupus patients through pregnancy; they found anti-dsDNA in the 4 SLE patients and in the cord blood of the neonate whose mother had the highest DNA binding.[G368] In this baby, the DNA binding capacity fell from 96% in the cord blood to 52% at 2 weeks and to 9% (negative) at 8 weeks of age. Zulman et al., however, did not detect anti-dsDNA in the cord blood of 6 neonates whose mothers had it.[Z52] The appearance of complement-fixing anti-dsDNA, or an increase during pregnancy, should alert the physician to the possibility of new onset or exacerbation of lupus nephritis.

It has been well established that cold-insoluble complexes (mixed cryoglobulins) are present in up to 30% of lupus patients' sera, and represent immune complexes. They are associated with decreased serum complement levels and with evidence of active lupus, especially nephritis.[S623] We have also found that increased levels of cryoglobulins correlate with disease activity.

Cold-reactive lymphocytotoxic antibodies, known to occur in lupus patients and their relatives, have been shown to cross-react with the trophoblast in certain pregnant lupus patients.[B478] Such antibodies were found in 3 of 4 SLE patients with spontaneous abortions, in 17% of 12 SLE patients with live births and in 10% of 46 controls. Thus, lymphocytotoxic antibodies were proposed as a potential mechanism of fetal loss. On the other hand, Lom-Orta et al., in a report of 19 pregnancies in 27 SLE women, concluded that lymphocytotoxic antibodies were not associated with spontaneous abortions but with third trimester exacerbations in 7 of 11 patients.[L369]

One of the most important laboratory tests in lupus pregnancy is the determination of antiphospholipid antibodies, the most common of which are anticardiolipin (ACL) antibody and lupus anticoagulant.[H150,L392] Although separate and distinct, these antibodies to negatively charged membrane phospholipids frequently coexist. Antiphospholipid antibodies have been linked to intravascular clotting, arterial or venous, recurrent fetal loss, livedo reticularis, immune thrombocytopenia, Coombs'-positive autoimmune hemolytic anemia, and false-positive tests for syphilis.[A314] In a review of 21 studies comprising over 1,000 lupus patients, circulating anticoagulant was found in 34% (7 to 73%), and anticardiolipin antibody in 44% (21 to 63%).[L392] Patients with circulating anticoagulant have a prolonged activated partial thromboplastin time (APTT), which does not correct with a 1 : 1 dilution with normal serum. A quantitative determination is performed using the Exner test or the kaolin clotting time.[E170,G11] The Russel viper venom time

(RVVT) has also been used.[S324] Anticardiolipin antibody can be detected by ELISA or radioimmunoassay.[H150]

The literature now contains many reports of the association of recurrent spontaneous abortion, fetal loss, and fetal distress with antiphospholipid antibodies in patients with and without lupus. It should be remembered that thrombotic events have also been described with a functional or quantitative deficiency of protein C or protein S in association with antiphospholipid antibodies.[R416] In eight retrospective studies of nearly 400 pregnant patients with lupus or lupus-like illness, one or more fetal losses occurred in 13 to 68% of antiphospholipid-positive women and in 3 to 42% of antibody-negative women.[B379,C337,E74,F170,G115,H150,K42,P157] The difference showed a trend but was not statistically significant. In five prospective studies of 160 patients with lupus or lupus-like disease, those with lupus anticoagulant or anticardiolipin antibody had significantly higher fetal loss (60%) than those without these antibodies (13 and 5% fetal loss, respectively).[E109,H101,K386,L350,L354] In a prospective study of lupus pregnancy, 9 patients with midpregnancy fetal distress, manifested by abnormal fetal heart deceleration or fetal death, had anticardiolipin levels over 7-fold higher than 12 patients without fetal distress.[L350] Among 30 pregnancies in 25 asymptomatic women with a high ACL titer, 21 pregnancies with a history of prior fetal death resulted in 67% fetal loss, whereas 9 pregnancies without such a history had half as much fetal loss, 33%.[L351]

Studies of women with recurrent fetal loss and of general obstetric patients provide insight from a different viewpoint. Among 35 women without lupus and with recurrent fetal loss, defined as three or more consecutive spontaneous abortions, antiphospholipid antibodies were found in 11 (31.4%): lupus anticoagulant was found in 7 (20%), anticardiolipin antibody in 6 (17%), and both in 2 (5.7%).[C430] These 11 patients had a total of 54 pregnancies with only 7 live births, for a success rate of 13%. In the same study, of 31 women with one or two episodes of fetal loss, only 1 had lupus anticoagulant and none had anticardiolipin antibody. The difference between the two groups was significant ($p < 0.05$). In a study by Parke et al., three groups of women without lupus were evaluated for lupus anticoagulant, IgG and IgM anticardiolipin, and false-positive VDRL.[P51] Antiphospholipid antibodies were significantly more prevalent in 81 women with recurrent spontaneous abortion (three or more), at 16%, versus 7% in 88 women with successful pregnancies, and 3% in 64 women who had never been pregnant. Almost half of those with recurrent fetal loss, 46%, had two or more positive test results. The authors found that VDRL and IgG anticardiolipin are more specific for fetal wastage. In a study of 737 low-risk pregnant women, Lockwood et al.[L358] found lupus anticoagulant in 2 (0.27%) and anticardiolipin antibodies in 16 (2.2%) patients. Both pregnancies with lupus anticoagulant ended in mid-pregnancy fetal loss; the 16 patients with anticardiolipin had only 4 live births and a total fetal loss rate of 50% (25% spontaneous abortions, 12% stillbirth, and 12% neonatal death), compared with only 7% fetal loss in the anticardiolipin-negative patients. Low-birth weight was present in 60% of the live births of ACL-positive mothers compared to

11% of ACL-negative mothers. In all, 12 of 16 ACL-positive patients (75%) had adverse perinatal outcomes (fetal loss, prematurity, and intrauterine growth retardation). A case-control study of 256 pregnant women, 207 nonpregnant women, and 229 women with recurrent fetal loss[H214] compared the presence of anticardiolipin, antilymphocyte, ANA, and anti-dsDNA antibodies: the third group had more positive autoantibody tests than the other two (51.6 versus 23.9 versus 36.7%), and the likelihood of having a history of recurrent fetal loss was 2.9 if two autoantibodies (ACL, antilymphocyte, or anti-dsDNA) were present. In 350 women studied prospectively for several antiphospholipid antibodies (PTT, RVVT, VDRL, and IgG, IgM, and IgA ACL), the risk of fetal loss was increased with increased levels of antiphospholipid antibody, although no single test showed a statistically significant increased risk.[L432] As a group, however, women with elevated antiphospholipid levels by any test had a 2.6-fold increase in fetal loss, which was statistically significant.

A study from Japan is noteworthy in that Ishii et al. described two subsets of lupus patients with IgG ACL antibodies. They found that 39 patients who were persistently positive for ACL, whether lupus was active or inactive, had the following significant differences from 29 patients who were positive only during active lupus:[146] higher titers of ACL, more thromboses (33 versus 3%), spontaneous abortions (41 versus 7%), and lupus anticoagulant (45 versus 8%), less nephritis (44 versus 72%), and less anti-dsDNA positivity (72 versus 97%). It may prove that fine differences within patients positive for ACL, as above, are important markers for ACL-associated morbidity.

IgG antiphospholipid antibody appears to be responsible for recurrent fetal loss,[H150] but no specific pathogenic subclass has been incriminated.[Q1] The mechanism invoked for fetal loss is intravascular clotting, possibly through interference with endothelial prostacyclin production, which results in a small placenta with infarcts.[H101]

Two studies of antiphospholipid antibodies in pre-eclamptic women have reported disparate results, which may be explained on the basis of relatively small numbers of patients. None of 15 patients reported by Scott had anticardiolipin antibodies,[S231] but 7 of 43 pre-eclamptic women (16%) studied by Branch et al. had elevated levels of anticardiolipin antibodies, and 6 of 7 had evidence for lupus anticoagulant.[B454] Of these 7 women, 3 had peripartum episodes of intravascular clotting that necessitated anticoagulant therapy; no information was provided about renal disease, antinuclear antibody, or complement determination in these patients.

The determination of anti-Ro/SSA and anti-La/SSB antibodies in the pregnant lupus patient is highly recommended because of their link to the neonatal lupus erythematosus syndrome (see Chap. 52).[F204,M43] Anti-Ro/SSA is found in 25 to 40% of lupus patients and anti-La/SSB in 10 to 15% (see Chap. 52). The proportion of children with neonatal lupus in mothers positive for anti-Ro/SSA and/or anti-La/SSB is small, up to 8.8%, but it is worth looking for these ANAs, so as to counsel the patient appropriately. Anti-U1RNP antibody is detected in 40 to 45% of lupus

patients and is rarely associated with the neonatal lupus syndrome.[P315]

Lockshin et al. have proposed that thrombocytopenia during lupus pregnancy may not be the result of exacerbation but of association with antiphospholipid antibodies, and that accompanying hypocomplementemia may be caused by decreased synthesis rather than increased activation of the classical pathway.[L353] No studies of antiplatelet antibodies were performed. Thrombocytopenia in the presence of pre-eclampsia should suggest the previously mentioned HELLP syndrome,[W145] which needs to be differentiated from lupus exacerbation.

Recommendations for laboratory monitoring in SLE pregnancy can be summarized as follows:

1. Initial laboratory assessment of the pregnant lupus patient should include a complete blood count (CBC), platelets, urinalysis, chemistry panel inclusive of BUN, creatinine, and blood glucose, Coombs' test, VDRL, APTT, anticardiolipin, anti-dsDNA, anti-Ro/SSA, anti-La/SSB, anti-U1RNP, and complement C3 and C4. Highly positive levels of antiphospholipid antibodies should alert the rheumatologist and obstetrician to the possibility spontaneous abortion or stillbirth, fetal distress, or pre-eclampsia. Positive anti-Ro/SSA and/or anti-La/SSB and, to a lesser extent, a positive anti-U1RNP, should alert these physicians to the possibility of neonatal lupus erythematosus. If the patient is nephrotic, or on corticosteroids, serum lipid tests are also indicated. At the University of Southern California we also obtain quantitative serum cryoglobulin levels as an indicator of circulatory immune complexes. Patients with known nephritis should have frequent monitoring of blood pressure and an initial 24-hour urine collection for protein, creatinine, and creatinine clearance.
2. Monthly laboratory assessment during lupus pregnancy should include CBC, platelets, urinalysis, chemistry panel (as above), anti-dsDNA, C3, and cryoglobulins or other measures of immune complexes. Patients with known lupus nephritis should also have 24-hour urine collections for protein, creatinine, and creatinine clearance.
3. In the event of a hematocrit decrease, the Coombs' test should be repeated. Increasing antibodies to dsDNA, especially if they are complement-fixing, decreasing complement C3 and C4, and increasing immune complexes, indicate active lupus or impending flare in over 80% of patients.

MANAGEMENT DURING PREGNANCY, DELIVERY AND POSTPARTUM PERIOD

General Principles

The pregnant woman with lupus requires special conjoint attention by the rheumatologist and obstetrician, who should have experience in systemic lupus and high-risk pregnancy, respectively. At the onset of pregnancy, a thorough assessment of system involvement and disease severity and activity should be made. The pregnant woman, her husband or mate, and other family members should be counselled with regard to the pregnancy (see below). During the first half of pregnancy, the woman with SLE under control should be followed every month, with increased frequency of visits (every 2 to 3 weeks), if necessary, during the second half. Laboratory evaluation and monitoring should be performed, as recommended above. Blood pressure should be monitored at every visit in every patient, and even more frequently, at home, in patients with known nephritis. Follow-up should be geared toward early detection, and aggressive therapy of lupus exacerbations during pregnancy and the postpartum period.

Follow-up of fetal development includes repeated ultrasound evaluation of growth of the fetal pole and fetal heart monitoring, including repeated nonstress test (see also Chap. 51 and 52).[D299,E165]

Women with nephritis, with or without a history of hypertension, should be considered for low-dose daily aspirin till week 36 of gestation, for prevention of preeclampsia.

Patients with high levels of antiphospholipid antibodies, and especially those with recurrent abortions, should be considered for treatment protocols that enhance the possibility of live births (see below). Cytotoxic drugs should be avoided during the first trimester and full doses of prostaglandin inhibitors should be used sparingly. Steroid preparation for the stress of delivery is needed for patients on steroids up to 2 years before. Cesarean section should be considered for certain maternal or fetal indications, such as maternal aseptic necrosis of the hips with inadequate hip abduction, fetal distress, abnormal nonstress test, and the usual obstetric indications (e.g., cephalopelvic disproportion, transverse presentation). Ideally, a neonatologist should be available at delivery.

During the immediate postpartum period, the mother should be watched carefully for development of infection at the site of episiotomy or cesarean incision, endometritis, urinary tract infection, pneumonia, and disease exacerbation. Infection and exacerbation should be treated promptly and aggressively.

Use of Medications during Pregnancy

The major drugs used to treat lupus are corticosteroids, nonsteroidal anti-inflammatory drugs (NSAIDs, including salicylates), antimalarials, and immunosuppressives. There is a justifiable tendency to use as few drugs as possible during gestation, but a smooth course for mother and fetus might dictate their use. The major concerns about medication use in pregnancy are the pharmacologic effects on the mother and fetus, effects on the length of gestation and labor, and developmental effects on the fetus (intrauterine growth, malformations, and survival). Books by Briggs[B492] and Niebyl[N91] have addressed the use of drugs in pregnancy in general, as have two other reports.[B512,G3]

Corticosteroids

In 1962, Donaldson and de Alvarez observed that the steroid requirement in pregnant lupus patients decreased during the second trimester and was often not needed during the third trimester, in contrast to the first 2 weeks postpartum, when steroid was again required.[D262] Garsenstein et al. noted that prednisone therapy seemed to decrease exacerbations during pregnancy and the postpartum period.[G58] This finding was confirmed in subsequent decades by McGee and Makowski[M278] and by Fine et al.[F95] A plethora of more recent reports further asserts that, if the patient has active lupus or exacerbates during pregnancy or postpartum, aggressive therapy with steroids should be used to control disease activity.[M472,M473,W336,Z52,Z57] Dose selection depends on the extent and severity of system involvement. Nephritis of the more severe types (diffuse and focal proliferative), neuropsychiatric manifestations, autoimmune hemolytic anemia, thrombocytopenia, and extensive, severe vasculitis, cutaneous or visceral, require doses greater than or equal to 1 mg/kg/day of prednisone, or equivalent. Pleuropericarditis usually requires less, 0.5 to 0.8 mg/kg/day, while skin rashes and arthritis require 5 to 20 mg of prednisone daily, and/or antimalarials and NSAIDs.

Mintz et al. decided to put all their pregnant patients on 10 mg of prednisone per day, even with inactive lupus.[M472] The majority of their patients did well, with mostly mild exacerbations. Wong et al. decided on a protocol in which the steroid dosage was maintained as needed until the 30th week of pregnancy, when it was increased to 10, 20, or 30 mg if the patients were taking less than 10, 10, or more than 10 mg per day respectively.[W336] If disease activity required a higher dosage, it was adjusted accordingly, and that dose was maintained until 4 weeks after delivery. No postpartum maternal exacerbations or deaths occurred in this study.

Any woman treated with systemic steroids within 2 years of the anticipated delivery should be considered as potentially adrenal-insufficient, and should be given steroid stress coverage (steroid prep) during delivery. The most usual form consists of 100 mg hydrocortisone IV just prior to onset of delivery, followed by the same dose every 8 hours for the first day. During the next day the dose can be reduced to 50 mg every 8 hours and then adjusted to the patient's previous oral dose. If the patient is receiving more than 75 mg of prednisone daily, the appropriate hydrocortisone equivalent should be used in the first 2 days, and then the patient's steroid dose resumed.

Cortisol,[B174] prednisone,[B173] prednisolone,[B173] methylprednisolone,[A202] betamethasone,[B54] and dexamethasone[F314,O103] have all been shown to cross the placenta. With maternal administration of prednisone or prednisolone, fetal blood levels are approximately 10% of the mother's level; with methylprednisolone hemisuccinate, cord levels are 18 to 45% of the mother's, with a large standard deviation; with betamethasone, cord levels are approximately 33% and, with dexamethasone, are similar to the maternal level. Therefore, the use of prednisone or prednisolone to treat the mother is least likely to affect the fetus; conversely, if steroid therapy of the fetus is indicated, dexamethasone is the appropriate choice.[B605] There is evidence that placental oxidative enzymes inactivate in vitro cortisol and prednisolone, but not betamethasone or dexamethasone.[B252,B338] Therefore, one should not hesitate to use appropriate doses of corticosteroid whenever warranted by maternal disease.

Furthermore, there is a paucity of evidence for corticosteroid induction of fetal abnormalities, so that concern about teratogenic or other untoward effects on the fetus seems unwarranted. Despite reports of corticosteroids causing cleft palate in rabbits and mice,[F220,K38] such congenital abnormalities are extremely rare in humans. Bongiovanni and McPadden reviewed 260 pregnancies in the literature, during which the mothers received pharmacologic doses of steroids.[B246] There was 1 spontaneous abortion, 8 stillbirths (3%), and 15 premature infants (5.8%). These figures are comparable to those in the general, non-steroid-treated population,[K122] and the role of steroid was not clear. There were 2 infants with cleft palates (0.77%) and 1 with adrenocortical failure of 3 days' duration, who recovered. The prevalence of cleft lip with or without cleft palate in the United States varies, depending on race: It is 1:300 in the Navajo, 1:400 to 600 in Asians, 1:750 to 800 in whites, and 1:1,500 to 2,000 in blacks.[C261] The authors concluded that no fetal injury resulted from maternal steroid therapy. Oppenheimer reported a premature newborn who died of adrenal failure born to a mother receiving large doses of prednisone for sarcoidosis 24 days prior to delivery.[O88] The neonate had evidence of degeneration of the adrenal cortex with cystic changes, hemorrhage, and necrosis.

Intrauterine growth retardation (IUGR), with low birth weight, has been reported with maternal steroid therapy.[R142] In the large prospective study by Mintz et al.,[M472] however, it seemed that IUGR was more a function of active maternal SLE than of steroid dose.[M473] Hodgman et al. reviewed the growth and development of 23 infants whose 19 mothers received 7.5 to 22.5 mg of prednisone daily during pregnancy.[H357] Sixteen of the mothers had lupus (19 infants) and 3 had rheumatoid arthritis. Two of 20 children whose mothers received steroid during the first trimester had major congenital defects without clefts. Gestational age was small and prematurity higher than in normal populations; the birth weight was below the 50th percentile in 14 of 19 infants (73.7%) and below the tenth percentile for 5 of them (26%). Follow-up at 6 months to 8 years showed normal height, weight, and developmental progress for 22 of 23, with the sole exception of 1 child with a major congenital defect, whose development was below the 3rd percentile.

Two studies of steroid-treated patients without lupus are worth mentioning. Schatz et al. reported 70 pregnancies in 55 asthmatic patients on an average dose of 8.2 mg of prednisone daily and found no increase in spontaneous abortion, congenital malformation, stillbirth, neonatal death, toxemia, or bleeding, but found an increase in prematurity, which they did not attribute to steroids.[S115] Similar results were noted in 287 patients with steroid- or Azulfidine-dependent inflammatory bowel disease.[M517] In the authors' large experience with lupus pregnancies under substantial steroid therapy, no clefts have been observed.

Overall, corticosteroid therapy seems innocuous in terms of fetal effects. It is the major factor in improved maternal survival between 1950 and 1980, with maternal mortality decreasing from 24 to 3%.[C175]

Salicylates and Other NSAIDs

Salicylates and the newer NSAIDs have in common the capacity to interfere with prostaglandin formation through variable inhibition of cyclo-oxygenase. This inhibition includes prostaglandin action anywhere in the body, including uterine, platelet, renal, and other prostaglandins. Thus, aspirin and NSAIDs inhibit uterine contractility and prolong labor and gestation. Aspirin irreversibly inhibits platelet aggregation, and the other NSAIDs have a reversible effect; however, they can cause bleeding during delivery.[B343] Given the immaturity of hepatic enzyme systems in the fetus and newborn, transplacentally delivered drugs may persist much longer. Several animal and human studies have shown aspirin teratogenicity with clefts and skeletal and vascular malformations.[K225,L77,T206]

There is extensive experience with the use of salicylates in human pregnancy. Lewis and Schulman linked high-dose aspirin therapy (greater than or equal to 3 g daily for 6 months) to prolonged gestation and labor and increased blood loss at delivery.[L249] Turner[T276] and Collins[C350] followed 144 pregnant women who took aspirin regularly during pregnancy and noted lower birth weights and increased perinatal mortality, but no increased fetal bleeding or congenital abnormalities. The mothers were more anemic, had a prolonged gestation, more complicated deliveries, and an increased incidence of antepartum and postpartum hemorrhage. Other reports have confirmed this.[S739] Slone et al. examined data on 50,282 mother-child pairs; 35,418 of the mothers had not taken aspirin during pregnancy. Of 14,864 who had taken aspirin, 9,736 had intermediate exposure and 5,128 were heavily exposed during the first 16 weeks of pregnancy. The observed and expected numbers of malformations were similar in the three groups.[S493] Jick et al. reached similar conclusions, with absence of increased incidence of congenital abnormalities in 6,837 pregnant women enrolled in a Seattle health plan.[J76]

Other NSAIDs have, to varying degrees, similar effects to those of aspirin in pregnancy. They readily cross the placenta, potentiate vasoconstriction under conditions of hypoxia, raise systemic vascular resistance, and have profound effects on fetal and neonatal circulation.[L215] Aspirin ingestion during pregnancy has been incriminated as the cause of in utero closure of the ductus arteriosus,[A282] with severe heart failure, tricuspid insufficiency, and acidosis, all of which disappeared the day after birth. Maternal indomethacin therapy was considered the cause of primary pulmonary hypertension in a newborn.[M87] Transient neonatal renal failure and oligohydramnios have also been described.[C69]

On the other hand, the pharmacologic actions of prostaglandin inhibitors can be used to therapeutic advantage. For example, indomethacin has been successfully used to inhibit premature labor,[N92] and for the closure of patent ductus arteriosus.[F254]

The capacity of low aspirin doses (0.45 mg/kg/day) to inhibit thromboxane synthesis by platelets, while prostacyclin production by endothelium is unaffected,[P67] has some promising applications in situations encountered in lupus pregnancy—pre-eclampsia and recurrent fetal loss. Pre-eclampsia seems to occur as a consequence of exaggerated placental production of thromboxane A_2, with normal or deficient prostacyclin production.[M70,W57] In a double-blind, placebo-controlled study, 46 primigravidas at risk for development of pre-eclampsia, as determined by angiotensin-sensitivity at 28 weeks' gestation, were divided into two groups. Twenty-three women were given 60 mg of aspirin daily, a dose that causes 90% inhibition of platelet thromboxane synthesis, and the 23 remaining, placebo.[W43] Only 2 of 21 patients (9.5%) in the aspirin group developed mild pregnancy-induced hypertension, while 12 of 23 women in the placebo group (52%) developed hypertension (PIH in 4, pre-eclampsia in 7, and eclampsia in 1). The necessity for cesarean sections was significantly greater in the placebo group. In a study of mostly multiparous women, 52 at high-risk for pre-eclampsia were treated with aspirin, 150 mg/day, and dipyridamole, 300 mg/day, and 50 women with similar risks received no treatment.[B142] Uncomplicated hypertension was similar in both groups (40 and 49%, respectively), but pre-eclampsia, fetal and neonatal loss, and severe intrauterine growth retardation (IUGR) occurred only in the untreated group (13, 11, and 9%, respectively). There is further evidence of low-dose aspirin for prevention of IUGR: A good review on the subject has appeared.[L399]

Wallenburg and Rotmans treated 24 women with prior fetal growth retardation with low-dose aspirin and dipyridamole after 16 weeks' gestation, with reduction of fetal growth retardation to 13% in treated versus 61% in untreated pregnancies.[W45] Two mothers had lupus anticoagulant.

Several reports and a review have addressed the prevention of recurrent fetal loss in patients with antiphospholipid antibodies.[B456,B550,G64,L351,L401,L400,O92,R322C,S273,S437,R95] Combinations of low-dose aspirin, 75, 81, or 150 mg/day, and 20 to 60 mg/day of prednisone,[B456,B550,G64,L351,L400,L401,O92,S437] heparin alone, heparin and prednisone, or heparin and aspirin have been used. With the exception of one study in which fetal loss continued unabated on prednisone and aspirin, the remainder of the studies reported an overall increase in the proportion of live births. (See also table 51–2.) Rosove et al. treated 14 patients during 15 pregnancies with subcutaneous heparin to achieve prolongation of the thrombin time to more than 100 seconds, with the prothrombin time permitted to rise by 1.5 seconds. The mean heparin dose was 24,700 ± 7,400 units/day. The 14 patients had 28 prior fetal losses and 1 live birth (3.4% success rate); after heparin therapy, there were 14 live births out of 15 pregnancies (93.3% success rate). Semprini et al. treated 14 women with heparin and prednisone: prior to treatment, only 1 of 27 pregnancies was successful (3.7%), but after therapy, success rate rose to 64%.[S273] Low birth weight was reduced from 44 to 12%. Lubbe[L400,L401] and Branch[B456] treated 18 women with lupus anticoagulant and recurrent fetal loss with prednisone, 40 to 60 mg/day, and aspirin, 75 or 81 mg/day; the live birth rate increased to 86 and 63%, from 10.7 and 3%, but pre-eclampsia, fetal growth

retardation, distress, prematurity, and steroid complications were common. Gatenby et al., using aspirin and prednisone, reduced fetal loss in 15 SLE patients from 88 to 55% and, in 22 patients without definite SLE, from 79 to 25%.[G64] Ordi et al. treated 7 women with 0% live births with prednisone and aspirin and achieved 78% fetal survival.[O92]

In a prospective study by Silveira et al., 12 patient with a history of 33 pregnancies and 5 live births (13.2% success rate) were treated with prednisone, 40 mg/day for 4 weeks, and then tapered to 5 mg/day till delivery, and 81 mg aspirin/day, during 13 pregnancies.[S437] All pregnancies resulted in live births, and the mean level of IgG and IgM anticardiolipin was reduced. In a prospective study from the United Kingdom, 87 pregnant women with lupus and antiphospholipid syndrome had 101 prior pregnancies and 81.3% fetal loss (18.7% success rate); those with prior thrombotic events were treated with 75 mg of aspirin and 10,000 units of heparin/day, and those without prior thromboses were treated with aspirin only.[B550] Lupus flares were treated with low-dose prednisone, azathioprine, or hydroxychloroquine. Live births in these 87 pregnancies increased, to a success rate of 63.2%. Cowchock et al. conducted a multicenter randomized study of 20 women with 2 to 4 consecutive fetal losses, and positive antiphospholipid antibodies (IgG anticardiolipin in 100%, lupus anticoagulant in 35%).[C418a] None of these patients had 3 or more criteria for lupus. None had had an uncomplicated live birth without treatment during the 5 years prior to the study. All women were treated with aspirin, 80 mg per day, in addition to heparin, 10,000 units every 12 hours (12 women), or prednisone, 20 mg BID (8 women). The heparin-treated patients also received calcium and vitamin D supplements. Live births after both treatment regimens were 75%, but maternal and fetal complications were greater in the prednisone-treated group. Maternal complications in the prednisone group (75% versus 40% in the heparin group) included pre-eclampsia in 3, cataracts in 1, and diabetes mellitus in 3 of 8 pregnancies (0, 0, and 1 of 10 with heparin, respectively). All live births in the prednisone group were premature (6 of 6, versus 2 of 8 in the heparin group), with premature rupture of membranes in half (3 of 6, versus 0 of 9 with heparin). It should be noted that not all pregnancies in mothers with antiphospholipid antibodies are doomed; 4 patients had uncomplicated pregnancies and delivered at term.[S605] A prospective multicenter study sponsored by the National Institutes of Health is ongoing, with treatment of low-risk patients (1 fetal loss or less, and positive antiphospholipid) with usual care versus low-dose aspirin, and of high-risk patients (2 fetal losses or more, and positive antiphospholipid) with aspirin plus heparin, or aspirin plus prednisone.[R95]

It can be concluded that large, anti-inflammatory doses of aspirin and NSAIDs should be avoided during the last 2 to 4 weeks of pregnancy for fear of prolonging gestation and labor, increased maternal and fetal bleeding during delivery, and possible premature closure of ductus arteriosus. However, a great deal of possibilities are open, for low-dose aspirin therapy in susceptible patients, to prevent recurrent fetal loss, pre-eclampsia and, perhaps, intrauterine growth retardation.

Antimalarial Drugs

Antimalarial drugs have been used by pregnant women for years as prophylaxis in large-scale malaria eradication programs in Africa and Asia, mostly without problems.[B550,L246a] Several reports have asserted that maternal malaria prophylaxis with chloroquine is safe in pregnancy.[A233a,B512,B550] Antimalarials do not appear to induce premature labor or abortions.[B530] Chloroquine (Aralen) has been found to cross the placenta and accumulate in the eyes of fetal mice, with uncertain results.[U14] In vitro chromosomal damage has been shown in rheumatoid arthritis patients on chloroquine.[N55] Even if the patient discontinues antimalarials early in the pregnancy, there are deposits in the liver and other organs, from which the drug is slowly excreted.[M21,R387]

One report of retinal degeneration in two infants as a consequence of malaria prophylaxis in the mother has appeared.[P27] Wolfe and Cordero reported 2 infants (1.2%) with birth defects (tetralogy of Fallot and congenital hypothyroidism) in 169 women who took chloroquine weekly for malaria prophylaxis.[W325] In a control group, however, 4 infants (0.9%) had microcephaly, congenital heart disease, clubfoot, and hematoma. In view of the similar prevalence of malformations in these two groups, and the small dose of chloroquine (300 mg base weekly), it is difficult to incriminate antimalarials for these malformations. No reports of fetal malformations associated with hydroxychloroquine (Plaquenil) per se have appeared.

Most of the admonitions against the use of antimalarials during pregnancy have cited a report of a woman with discoid lupus who intermittently took 500 mg of chloroquine daily.[H170] Of her 7 pregnancies, 3 were conceived off the drug, and these children had no congenital defects; of 4 pregnancies conceived while on chloroquine, 1 child had hemihypertrophy of the body and a Wilms' tumor, 1 had neonatal seizures, deafness, ataxia, and vestibular paresis, 1 had mental retardation, deafness, ataxia, and vestibular paresis, and a fourth pregnancy ended in spontaneous abortion at 3 months. However, in 14 pregnancies among 8 women with SLE who continued chloroquine or hydroxychloroquine during pregnancy, there were 6 normal full-term babies and 8 fetal losses, the latter in patients with active disease and a false-positive VDRL.[P47] Similarly, Levy et al. reported their experience with 24 women who took chloroquine or hydroxychloroquine during the first trimester of 27 pregnancies, and reviewed the literature.[L233] Data were given for 18 women who took antimalarials for a mean of 32 months before pregnancy (1 to 172 months), and for 21 pregnancies. Of the 18, 11 women had SLE, 3 had rheumatoid arthritis, and 4 took malaria prophylaxis. Six elective abortions were performed for severe disease activity or social conditions. Of the 21 pregnancies, 14 resulted in normal full-term births, 4 in spontaneous abortion, and 3 in stillbirths. No congenital malformations or developmental problems occurred in these children, who were followed up for a mean of 5.3 years (9 months to 19 years). In their litera-

ture review, 215 pregnancies were reported under first trimester antimalarial exposure, with 7 cases of congenital malformations (3.3%), as detailed above.

Fetal loss occurs frequently in SLE patients, and it would be difficult to evaluate the contribution of antimalarials, especially when other factors, such as antiphospholipid antibodies, are not determined. In a prospective study of 87 SLE pregnancies with prior fetal loss, hydroxychloroquine was used in 15 women, without any resultant fetal malformations.[B550] At any rate, the patient should be informed about the few reports of congenital anomalies, and about the antimalarial deposits in the liver, when deciding about the use of antimalarials during pregnancy. In our experience, most patients opt to discontinue medications during gestation.

Immunosuppressive-Cytotoxic Drugs

The most commonly used immunosuppressive drugs in SLE are azathioprine, cyclophosphamide, nitrogen mustard, methotrexate, chlorambucil, and cyclosporin. The first four are known to induce fetal malformations in animals. Cyclophosphamide, azathioprine, methotrexate, and chlorambucil have reportedly shown potential for human teratogenesis.[B94,S666] Use of these drugs during fetal organogenesis (the first trimester) has the greatest potential for causing fetal demise or malformation. Azathioprine crosses the placenta,[S2] decreases thymic shadow size, lymphocyte count, and IgG and IgM in the neonate,[C407] and can cause neonatal chromosomal abnormalities that may persist for up to a year.[O115] Cyclophosphamide is highly teratogenic in experimental animals, but its effects are species-specific. Nitrogen mustard induces skeletal, limb, palate, and central nervous system abnormalities in animals. Methotrexate is also associated with skeletal and limb defects and, in high doses, is embryolethal in animals. The experience with cyclosporin in pregnancy is almost entirely in renal transplant recipients.

In humans the teratogenic effects of cytotoxic drugs do not appear to be as common. Among 50 pregnancies exposed to cytotoxic agents, there were 36 normal children (72%).[S536] Stern and Johnson have culled the experience of several authors with cytotoxic drugs given for neoplasias, transplants, or systemic lupus, alone or in combination.[S666] A total of 145 pregnancies occurred in women receiving single cytotoxic drugs, which included azathioprine, cyclophosphamide, 6-mercaptopurine, methotrexate, nitrogen mustard, and chlorambucil. In 83 of the pregnancies (57%) these drugs were administered during the first trimester (group 1), and, in the remaining 62 (43%), after the first trimester (group 2). Fetal morbidity and mortality were far greater in group 1: spontaneous abortions occurred in 23% versus 1.6% of group 2, total fetal loss was 36% in group 1 versus 8% in group 2, premature births were 6% and 0%, respectively, malformations were noted in 13% of group 1, and none in group 2. Overall, a normal live birth occurred in 47% of group 1 pregnancies and in 92% of group 2.

Azathioprine therapy in the first trimester was followed by the birth of 1 normal infant, 1 spontaneous abortion, and 1 ectopic pregnancy. Outcome in 42 women treated throughout pregnancy, included 39 normal infants, 5 spontaneous and 5 induced abortions, 3 premature births, and 3 abnormal infants (2 with lymphopenia and adrenal insufficiency and 1 with IUGR and abnormal chromosomes).[S666] Another infant had polydactyly.[W250] A review of three reports on the offspring of renal transplant recipients on azathioprine shows that the majority of the infants were normal, although fetal wastage was rather high. Of 36 pregnancies in mothers with renal transplants, 20 infants were normal, 5 were premature (4 died of respiratory distress syndrome) and there were 6 spontaneous and 5 elective abortions. Of 57 pregnancies with fathers with renal transplants 56 infants were normal, with 3 spontaneous abortions and 1 infant with a neural tube defect, perhaps attributable to paternal mutagenicity with thalidomide.[W250] Several additional reports of normal pregnancies and neonates in lupus and renal transplant patients who received azathioprine and prednisone have appeared.[D97,F95,H224,M36,M334,S326]

Meehan and Dorsey reported on 22 lupus pregnancies, during 7 of which azathioprine was given, with 3 elective and 2 spontaneous abortions, and 2 normal infants.[M334] Sharon et al. presented their experience with 5 SLE patients on azathioprine at conception; of these, 2 patients discontinued azathioprine and subsequently aborted, but 3 patients continued it and delivered 4 normal, albeit small babies, who had no malformations or karyotype abnormalities.[S326] Ramsey-Goldman et al. reported on 23 lupus pregnancies with azathioprine, cyclophosphamide, both, or methotrexate (2 during and 21 before pregnancy). They found that 10 of 23 had an adverse outcome, similar to pregnancy outcomes before SLE diagnosis.[M36] Adverse outcomes included miscarriage (spontaneous abortion), stillbirth, prematurity, or neonatal complications, including miscarriage (spontaneous abortion), stillbirth, prematurity, or neonatal complications, including congenital defects. No difference in neonatal complications was observed among 519 pregnancies before SLE, 117 pregnancies after SLE on no immunosuppressives, and 23 pregnancies on immunosuppressive therapy.

Daily oral cyclophosphamide causes amenorrhea within a year, usually with permanent ovarian failure (71%), and monthly intravenous "pulse" cyclophosphamide can also cause amenorrhea (45%), depending on the dose.[K306] It has been suggested that the administration of monthly IV cyclophosphamide be timed during menses, when the ovarian follicles are quiescent. Maternal therapy with cyclophosphamide only in the first trimester was associated in 3 pregnancies, with multiple abnormalities of the toes and extremities, palatine grooves, and hernias in one infant, a small hemangioma in another, and absent digits in one induced abortion. One pregnancy with cyclophosphamide late in the first trimester, and (4) pregnancies with chemotherapy including cyclophosphamide beyond the first trimester had a normal outcome.[S666] At the Los Angeles County-University of Southern California Medical Center, two of our lupus patients on monthly IV cyclophosphamide became pregnant: cyclophosphamide was immediately stopped on both. One woman proceeded with a normal pregnancy and had a normal infant at term. The other patient had a first-trimester sponta-

neous abortion but conceived two more times, after cessation of cyclophosphamide therapy and, despite a mild exacerbation during both pregnancies, carried to term and had two healthy infants. It is virtually impossible to foretell any risk of oncogenesis among such children.

Nitrogen mustard has been used for the treatment of lupus nephritis.[W39] In a report of 250 patients with nephritis, 18 of 44 women who had at least one course of nitrogen mustard had 11 successful pregnancies.[W39] Among the patients reviewed by Stern and Johnson, 6 pregnancies had exposure during the first trimester; there were 2 normal infants, 3 spontaneous abortions and 1 elective abortion with a normal fetus, while 4 women treated after the first trimester had normal infants.[S666] Combination therapy with nitrogen mustard during the first trimester resulted in 1 normal infant, 1 preterm infant with IUGR, 1 infant with digital, ear, and lower extremity anomalies and 1 spontaneous abortion with a normal fetus. Combination therapy with mustard after the first trimester resulted in 3 normal infants.[S666]

Two infants exposed to methotrexate in the first trimester had multiple cranial defects, malformed extremities, IUGR, and poor neonatal growth.[S666] Exposure after the first trimester in combination with other drugs resulted in 8 normal infants. Methotrexate-induced malformations can reportedly be prevented by simultaneous treatment with citrovorum factor (folinic acid). Kozlowski et al. reported 8 women with rheumatoid arthritis who conceived during weekly methotrexate, 7.5 mg.[K404] All except one stopped methotrexate within the first trimester. Of the 10 pregnancies, 5 resulted in full-term normal infants, with 3 spontaneous and 2 elective abortions. Most of their patients received folate supplements.

Cyclosporin has been widely used to prevent rejection in organ transplantation; it can cross the placenta, and is excreted in milk. A total of 51 pregnancies in 48 women treated with cyclosporin during pregnancy have been reported, and 11 pregnancies have been conceived from men receiving the drug.[G346] Most of the women, 43 of 48, received cyclosporin after transplantation, especially of the kidney (39 of 43). Only 1 patient had systemic lupus. In these high-risk pregnancies, a number of antenatal maternal complications arose in 20 of 41 mothers (48.8%), including hypertension, pyelonephritis, uterine dystonia, diabetes mellitus, seizures, encephalopathy, and secondary hyperparathyroidism. Also, 2 spontaneous and 6 elective abortions occurred, 1 for fetal anencephaly. Of the 43 deliveries (95.6% live births), 15 were premature (34.9%), and 17 required forceps or cesarean section (39.5%). The mean birth weight for 29 of the babies was low (2,093 g). Of the 43 newborn, 34 were healthy (79%), 2 had birth defects, including absence of the corpus callosum, with seizures and death in 1, and 7 had various problems—neonatal jaundice, thrombocytopenia, leukopenia, or hypoglycemia with mild disseminated intravascular coagulation, asphyxia with intracerebral bleeding, oxygen dependence for 2 days, with subsequent cataracts, and mild hypoparathyroidism. On follow-up, 1 of 20 babies had slight growth retardation. Overall, 38 of the 43 liveborn who were exposed to cyclosporin throughout pregnancy did not have birth defects. Of the 11 pregnancies fathered by 9 men on cyclosporin, 2 resulted in spontaneous abortions, and 2 pairs of twins were born. The 11 neonates were healthy. The fathers of the twins were being treated with cyclosporin for infertility resulting from an autoimmune disorder, and the remaining 7 men were receiving it for renal transplantation.

The decision to continue cytotoxic drugs during pregnancy depends on the need for disease control, and should be made jointly with the patient, while weighing the potential risks versus benefits. If continuation of pregnancy under cytotoxic therapy is desired, it is wise to have an amniocentesis done and the karyotype determined.

Miscellaneous Therapeutic Measures

Plasmapheresis

Plasmapheresis can be safely performed during pregnancy and has been used for years in Rh-incompatible pregnancies.[R253] It has been used for treating severe preeclampsia with HELLP syndrome during pregnancy, with success in four of five patients;[A264,C3,G429] with postpartum HELLP persistence beyond 3 days, with success in seven of seven patients,[M159] and in eclampsia.[K424] Three lupus patients have been treated during pregnancy. In one patient, plasmapheresis improved vasculitis, and decreased steroid requirement;[H469] in a second, extremely ill woman, striking improvement of myositis and overall disease occurred;[T154a] and, in the third patient plasmapheresis failed to reverse thrombocytopenia, with subsequent fetal demise.[P301] Two patients with recurrent fetal loss and anticardiolipin antibody were given plasmapheresis. In one, a dramatic reduction of antiphospholipid antibody with a successful pregnancy outcome;[F192] in the other, who had a multisystem disease with myositis, plasmapheresis was given because of fetal distress. The authors believed that they gained 2 more weeks of gestation, during which further fetal maturation occurred, which allowed fetal survival after cesarean section at 29 weeks.[F306] A good review on plasmapheresis in pregnancy has appeared.[W105]

Intravenous Immunoglobulin Therapy

Five papers have reported 7 women with 4 to 9 fetal losses each, positive anticardiolipin antibodies and lupus anticoagulant, and pre-eclampsia in 3.[C103,K115,P46,S229,W72] Treatment with IV immunoglobulin, at times with the addition of low-dose aspirin, heparin, and steroids, resulted in live births. Immunoglobulin was given monthly, or in 5-day courses. This expensive treatment seems worth considering in such difficult clinical situations.

BREAST FEEDING

All drugs are excreted in human milk, usually in trace but variable amounts.[B512,B530,N51] Factors influencing drug concentrations derived from milk in the infant have been delineated by Needs and Brooks.[N51] Maternal factors include fat and protein concentrations in milk, milk pH, mammary blood flow, and maternal drug metabolism (e.g., absorption, protein binding, and plasma clearance). Drug-

related factors include molecular weight, lipid solubility, pK_a, elimination half-life, pharmacokinetics, dose amount and interval. Infant factors include volume of milk consumed, feeding intervals relative to maternal drug intake, absorptive capability, and metabolic and deconjugating ability of the infant.

After a single dose of 5 mg of prednisolone, 0.07 to 0.23% of the dose was found in maternal milk.[M304] Katz and Duncan calculated that a child drinking 1 L of milk daily would receive 0.028 mg of prednisolone with a maternal dose of 7.5 mg (0.33%).[K112] Longterm treatment of the mother with 10 to 80 mg/day of prednisolone produces milk concentrations 5 to 25% of those in serum.[O112,T77] The mild:plasma ratio increases with increasing serum concentrations and it has been calculated that, at a maternal dose of 80 mg/day, the infant would be exposed to less than 0.1% of the maternal dose.[O112,S423a] The peak plasma level after oral intake is attained at 1.1 ± 0.7 hours, therefore, the exposure of the infant can be minimized by appropriate timing of nursing. No untoward effects in nursing infants have been reported,[L104,O112] and maternal doses of up to 30 mg/day are probably safe.

Cyclophosphamide is found in substantial concentrations in human breast milk,[W222] thus, nursing is contraindicated in a mother who required this drug. The milk level of methotrexate in a woman with choriocarcinoma of the uterus was 8% of the plasma level.[J87] With small weekly doses, such as those used in rheumatic diseases, there may be a greater measure of safety. Only small amounts of azathioprine have been detected in breast milk.[A212] Overall, a great deal of good judgment and caution should be exercised. In our opinion, the need for cytotoxic drug therapy would preclude breast feeding.

Antimalarials are also found in small amounts in human milk.[S531] Nation et al. have calculated that the infant would be exposed to about 2% of the maternal daily dose.[N45] Although there are very few problems with malaria prophylaxis in nursing mothers, doses used in lupus could expose the child to the risk of retinopathy.

In general, NSAIDs are weak acids and achieve low concentrations in the acidic pH of milk. After a single aspirin dose of 450 to 650 mg, 0.1 to 21% reaches the infant over a 24-hour period.[B246] Peak salicylate concentrations in milk occur about 2 hours after peak serum levels.[F93] However, with maternal intake of anti-inflammatory doses, and immature neonatal metabolic processes, the infant may develop acidosis and bleeding diathesis. Furthermore, the infant can absorb free salicylic acid from the cleavage of salicylphenolic glucuronide in the milk.[L230] Trace amounts of naproxen, piroxicam, ibuprofen, and diclofenac have been reported in milk. Some of the NSAIDs have the enterohepatic circulation (e.g., indomethacin, sulindac), and are not recommended during lactation.

CONTRACEPTION

Uncontrolled and anecdotal reports have suggested that oral contraceptives containing estrogens cause SLE exacerbations.[C205,G56] In a study by Jungers et al. of 20 women with SLE nephritis,[J141] the use of preparations containing ethinyl estradiol was associated with exacerbation of disease in 43% within 3 months of beginning oral contraceptives. Nevertheless, many patients are reported to tolerate small-dose estrogen contraceptives ("mini-pills") without adverse effects.[L346,W21] An important complication is that thromboembolic phenomena have been associated with estrogen and anticardiolipin antibodies.[A324] In contrast to estrogen-containing oral contraceptives, lupus flares did not occur in 11 patients receiving pure progestogens during a 30-month period. In a controlled study with progestogens[M471] using either oral levonorgestrel 0.03 mg daily, or norethisterone enanthate 200 mg IM every 3 months, the authors found no increase in exacerbation rate when compared to a control group. Commercially available progestational agents include oral norethindrone (norethisterone), norgestrel, levonorgestrel, ethynodiol diacetate, and lynestrenol.[A240b] If longterm contraception (up to 5 years) is desired, a subdermal progestin implant (levonorgestrel) may be considered.[A239] In a lupus patient, the site of implantation should be carefully watched for any infection. Menstrual irregularity for 6 to 12 months from onset of use is common, and bleeding, amenorrhea and, rarely, ectopic pregnancy may occur.

Mechanical barrier methods, such as the diaphragm or condom with spermicide cream or jelly, although considered cumbersome by some, are safe and effective. Intrauterine devices are associated with more frequent local infections[D323] and menorrhage.

FAMILY PLANNING AND COUNSELLING

The patient with SLE and her partner must understand that she is just as fertile as any other woman in the general population,[F190,F251,M472] and that she is capable of having children. Ample evidence in the literature has shown that, even during active periods of SLE, patients do become pregnant. The pregnant SLE patient must know, however, that she has an increased likelihood of a high-risk pregnancy.[M472]

The woman with lupus should ideally plan her pregnancy during a period of disease remission or relative inactivity sustained for several months. She, her partner, and the physician should assess her functional limitations and explore her emotional motivation prior to undertaking pregnancy and the responsibilities of raising a child.[D323] Her socioeconomic setting and spouse (mate) relationship are no less important. Because of the chance of a 20 to 60% exacerbation associated with pregnancy, fetal wastage, newborn prematurity, and IUGR, the rheumatologist and obstetrician should counsel the patient and family honestly about these possibilities, and prepare her to cooperate with the rigorous follow-up necessary. Only in the event of severe renal, myocardial, or pulmonary compromise should elective abortion be considered. The patient and husband should be cautioned, however, about the possibility of exacerbation after elective abortion.

Couples should be made aware of the following points:

1. The normal fertility of women with lupus—and therefore the need for family planning, just as in individuals without lupus.

2. The best time to plan a pregnancy—during an inactive period of SLE, even though there is no guarantee that the disease will remain inactive. It should be emphasized that the chance of a flare with conception after 5 to 6 months of remission is 10% or less.

3. The probability of a flare—varies among series and depends on the severity of disease. The milder the disease, the lesser the chance of a flare.

4. The probability of hypertension or pre-eclampsia—especially in SLE nephritis patients, and particularly in patients conceiving with active disease.

5. Increased abortion rates—double or triple that of the general population; In women with two or more abortions and the presence of antiphospholipid antibodies, the use of prednisone plus small doses of aspirin,[B456,L400,L401,P285] or heparin with or without prednisone,[B550,R322c] improve remarkably the possibilities of a successful pregnancy.

6. The risk of a stillbirth should be explained. The methods for monitoring fetal growth need to be clearly understood (see Chap. 51 and 52).

7. The potential necessity of and indications for cesarean section—should be outlined (maternal aseptic necrosis of the hips with inadequate hip abduction, pre-eclampsia, fetal distress, abnormal nonstress test, and usual obstetric indications, including cephalopelvic disproportion, transverse presentation, and others).

8. The risk of prematurity—may be as high as 60% in those with active disease—and the risk of intrauterine growth retardation—which may reach 30% of premature deliveries has to be explained. The need for proper care of the newborn in adequate intensive care units should be stressed.

9. Women positive for anti-Ro/SSA and/or anti-La/SSB should be aware of the small risk of congenital heart block in the child, up to 8.8%.[D292] The general lupus population seems to have a 1% probability of congenital heart block in live births (in studies of Mexican[M472] and Japanese[H205] patients). Because this is related to the presence of these maternal antibodies, the 1% probability may not be applicable to other ethnic groups. (See also Chap. 52.)

10. No risk of congenital malformations caused by prednisone has been noted, but cytotoxic drugs taken during the first trimester carry a potential risk of congenital anomalies.

11. With close monitoring and aggressive treatment during pregnancy and the postpartum period, no long-term worsening of the SLE should occur.

In the poststeroid era, the early diagnosis and appropriate therapy of lupus have led to tremendously increased survival rates of SLE patients—up to 97% for 5 years, 93% for 10 years, and 83% for 15 years.[P216] Similarly, with increased awareness of the potential problems for the mother and fetus, meticulous multidisciplinary follow-up, and effective disease control, most women with lupus can and do achieve motherhood.

Chapter 51

PREGNANCY IN LUPUS: THE FETUS IN SLE

RODANTHI C. KITRIDOU
GREGORIO MINTZ

There is a variety of fetal and neonatal problems associated with lupus. Certain facts emerge through a plethora of studies over the last four decades, although the populations studied may lack homogeneity, the study designs differ, and our practices have evolved toward earlier disease detection and aggressive therapy. In the series antedating 1980, the outcome of pregnancy in patients with SLE was clearly unsatisfactory. The total fetal loss was generally triple the usual prevalence for normal populations, and there is ample record of increase in spontaneous abortions, stillbirths, and prematurity. As analyzed by Cecere and Persellin,[C175] there had been little change in the 30 years between 1950 and 1980 (Table 51–1). For a definition of terms used, please see Chapter 50.

SPONTANEOUS ABORTIONS

The prevalence of spontaneous abortions in pregnant SLE mothers (Table 51–1) in the previous decades was 11.6% for 1950 to 1959, 19.5% for the years 1960 to 1969, and 19.4% for the period 1970 to 1981. All these figures are derived from retrospective studies with no particular therapeutic intervention.

In most studies that compare pregnancy outcome before and after lupus onset, fetal loss was found to be increased in lupus patients even before disease onset.[E148,F190,G151,J142,K122,M657] Spontaneous abortions ranged from 14 to 35%, with rates in normal general population reported at 7 to 12.5%. Full-term deliveries ranged from 64 to 86% (average 78%). After onset of SLE, there is generally an increase in spontaneous abortions, reported in 4 to 40% of women with known SLE, or SLE onset during pregnancy. In a study of 183 pregnancies before SLE onset by Fraga et al., 23.1% ended in spontaneous abortion, with 12.5% in 288 control pregnancies.[F190] After SLE onset, spontaneous abortions rose to 40.5%. An exception is a study from Greece, where no increased fetal loss prior to disease onset was found.[S403]

In the 14 reports published after 1980, which have specific information on total numbers of pregnancies excluding elective abortions,[B371,F95,G151,H224,H448,I11,M334,M472,N144,P216,S633,T200,V47,W336,Z52] the prevalence of spontaneous abortions is 17.5% (194 in 1109 pregnancies) (Table 51–1). The highest prevalence is 35% in a retrospective study,[128] followed by 30% in a patient questionnaire study from Vancouver,[S633] while the lowest rate is 6%, in a retrospective records review.[F95] In the prospective studies, the frequency of spontaneous abortions was 16.6% (17 of 102) in Mexico City,[M472] and 10.5% (2 of 19) in Hong Kong.[W336] In most reports the spontaneous abortion rate seems independent of lupus activity or inactivity—for example, there is no statistical difference between spontaneous abortions in active SLE (7 of 51 pregnancies, 13.7%) versus inactive lupus (10 of 51 pregnancies, 19.6%) in the largest prospective study.[M472]

Some data, however, suggest that SLE activity and active lupus nephritis contribute to fetal wastage. In women with lupus nephritis, Gimovsky et al.[G151] reported 40% spontaneous abortions (16 of 40 pregnancies), with 28% occurring in women without nephritis (7 of 25). It should be noted that these patients are socioeconomically disadvantaged with a great proportion (as much as 60 to 70%) being illegal aliens. In the report by Imbasciati et al. on pregnancy in lupus nephritis,[I11] there were 25% spontaneous abortions (6 of 24 pregnancies). Houser et al. reported that 10 pregnancies in the absence of SLE nephritis or exacerbation resulted in full-term births, while 3 of 7 pregnancies with nephritis or active lupus ended in spontaneous abortions.[H448] In Jungers' report of 104 pregnancies with lupus nephropathy, there were 3 fetal deaths in 12 pregnancies with active nephritis (25%), while all 11 pregnancies with inactive nephritis resulted in live births.[J142]

The proportion of recurrent (habitual) abortions among lupus patients according to the classic definition (three or more consecutive fetal losses) has not been determined; however, in the last 7 to 9 years, it has been intimately linked to the presence of antiphospholipid antibodies in the mother.[A314] In five prospective studies of 160 patients with lupus or lupus-like disease, those with lupus anticoagulant or anticardiolipin antibody had significantly higher fetal loss (60%) versus those without these antibodies, who had 13 and 5% fetal loss, respectively.[E109,H101,K386,L350,L354] The mechanisms of fetal wastage are examined later in this chapter.

STILLBIRTHS

The frequency of stillbirths in the previous decades (Table 51–1) was 10.3% from 1950 to 1959, 6.8% between 1960 and 1969, and 8.5% in the years 1970 to 1981.[C175] In the 14 series reported from 1980 on with information on fetal outcome, the following data are derived: of a total number of 581 pregnancies, excluding elective abortions, there were 40 (6.9%) still

Table 51–1. Effects of SLE on the Fetus

Decade	Spontaneous Abortions		Stillbirths		Prematurity		Fetal Wastage* (%)
	No.	(%)					
1950–1959	18/155	(11.6)	16/155	(10.3)	—		(27.5)
1960–1969	60/307	(19.5)	21/307	(6.8)	before 1980:		(27.0)
1970–1981	98/505	(19.4)	43/505	(8.5)	119/775	(15)	(27.9)
1980–1991	194/1109	(17.5)	40/581	(6.9)	126/35	(29)	146/581 (25.1)

Author	No. of Pregnancies				
Tozman et al.[T200] 1980	18	(6)	(6)	(11)	(11)
Houser et al.[H448] 1980	17	(18)	0	(21)	(18)
Zulman et al.[Z52] 1980	24	(8)	(4)	(4)	(17)
Hayslett et al.[H224] 1980	55	(15)	(9)	(5)	(25)
Fine et al.[F95] 1981	45	(7)	(22)	(31)	(29)
Varner et al.[V47] 1982	34	(9)	(6)	(10)	(17)
Gimovsky et al.[G151] 1984	65	(35)	(11)	(22)	(52)
Imbasciati et al.[I11] 1984	24	(25)	(8)	(42)	(33)
Stein et al.[S633] 1984	54	(30)	(7)	—	(37)
Mintz et al.[M472] 1986	102	(17)	(5)	(63)	(23)
Meehan and Dorsey[M334] 1987	18	(17)	0	(17)	(17)
Bobrie et al.[B371] 1987	67	(16)	(4)	(12)	(20)
Nossent and Swaak[N144] 1990	39	(10)	(5)	(18)	(15)
Wong et al.[W336] 1991	19	(11)	0	(47)	(11)
Pistiner et al.[P216]	528	(18)	—	—	(18)

* Includes 9, 2, 0, and 7 neonatal deaths, respectively. Pregnancy numbers exclude elective abortions. Decimal numbers in quoted series are rounded.

births.[B371,F95,G151,H224,H448,I11,M334,M472,N144,S633,T200,V47,W336,Z52]

There was 1 stillbirth in 18 pregnancies (5.6%) reported by Tozman,[T200] and none in 17 reported by Houser,[H448] or in 24 reported by Zulman.[Z52] Hayslett and Lynn found 5 stillbirths in 55 pregnancies (9.1%), all of which occurred with active maternal lupus nephritis.[H224] Fine et al. had 10 stillbirths in 45 pregnancies (22%); however, these data may be biased, because the pregnancies retrospectively selected made mention of fetal outcome.[F95] In the retrospective study by Varner et al. there were 2 stillbirths in 34 pregnancies (6%): both were in acutely ill mothers.[V47] In the study from the University of Southern California[G151] there were 7 stillbirths in 65 pregnancies (10.8%); 5 of 7 occurred in patients with nephropathy, 2 of whom had hypertension. Imbasciati et al. reported 2 stillbirths in 24 pregnancies (8.3%) with lupus nephritis:[M334] both mothers had exacerbations. Stein et al. found 7.4% of stillbirths (4 of 54 pregnancies) in a patient questionnaire study.[S633] In a prospective study of 102 consecutive pregnancies, Mintz et al.[M472] reported 5 stillbirths (5%), 4 of which had intrauterine growth retardation as well: 3 of the mothers had active SLE, and 2 had inactive disease. Bobrie and collaborators[B371] found 2 stillbirths in 67 pregnancies (4%). Nossent and Swaak found a stillbirth prevalence of 5.1% (2 of 39 pregnancies), which is significantly higher than 0.6%, the rate for the Dutch population.[N144] Wong et al. had no stillbirths among 19 uninterrupted pregnancies.[W336]

The rate of stillbirths in SLE seems to be relatively stable and is significantly higher than in normal populations. Stillbirths seem to be associated with more severe maternal disease or the presence of lupus nephritis, as above, or with anticardiolipin antibodies. Ever since the observa-

tions of Firkin et al. and Soulier and Boffa,[F103,S573] suggesting a link between lupus anticoagulant and recurrent abortions, a tremendous collection of data has been amassed. Briefly, in eight retrospective studies of nearly 400 pregnant patients with lupus or lupus-like illness, one or more fetal losses occurred in 13 to 68% of antiphospholipid-positive women, and in 3 to 42% of antibody-negative women.[B379,C337,E74,F170,G115,H150,K42,P157] The difference showed a trend, but was not statistically significant. As mentioned above, in five prospective studies of 160 patients with lupus or lupus-like disease, those with lupus anticoagulant or anticardiolipin antibody had over fourfold fetal loss (60%) compared to those without these antibodies, who had 13 and 5% fetal loss, respectively.[E109,H101,K386,L350,L354] In a prospective study of lupus pregnancy by Lockshin et al., 9 patients with mid-pregnancy fetal distress, manifested by abnormal fetal heart deceleration or fetal death, had over sevenfold anticardiolipin levels compared to 12 patients without fetal distress.[L350] In addition, these authors determined, in 50 pregnant women with lupus, the sensitivity and specificity of antiphospholipid antibody tests for predicting fetal death, and concluded that anticardiolipin was superior to activated partial thromboplastin time (APTT, a test for lupus anticoagulant): sensitivity was 0.55 for APTT, and 0.85 for anticardiolipin antibody, and specificity was 0.81 and 0.92, respectively.[L354] For more extensive information see Chapter 50.

NEONATAL DEATHS

Neonatal deaths have been reported in systemic lupus pregnancies; however, there is no suggestion of excessive prevalence, with the exception of the 1965 study by Estes and Larson, where neonatal deaths were 20%,[E148] and the 1978 study by Thomas et al. with 25% perinatal mortality rate.[T150]

In 1950 to 1959 there were 5.8% neonatal deaths (9 of 155 uninterrupted pregnancies), in 1960 to 1969, 0.7% (2 of 307), and in 1970 to 1981, zero of 505 pregnancies.[C175] Among the 14 detailed series published between 1980 to 1991, there were only 7 neonatal deaths in 581 pregnancies (1.2%): 4 of 65 pregnancies in the University of Southern California series,[G151] and 1 each in the Hayslett, Mintz, and Zulman publications.[H224,M472,Z52] It would seem then, that there is a trend toward reduction of the neonatal death rate in lupus pregnancies.

FETAL WASTAGE

Fetal wastage has been defined as the sum of spontaneous abortions and stillbirths. Cecere and Persellin have also defined it as the sum of spontaneous abortions, stillbirths, and perinatal deaths divided by the number of pregnancies minus elective abortions and expressed as a percentage.[C175] In Table 51–1, fetal wastage includes neonatal deaths.

Excluding elective (induced, therapeutic) abortions, the prevalence of fetal wastage in lupus patients has remained stable in the three decades between 1950 and 1980, at 27 to 28% (Table 51–1). The reported figures since 1980 have an overall fetal wastage prevalence of 25.1%, and seven series show, for the first time, a decrease in fetal wastage to under 20%.[H448,M334,N144,T200,V47, W336,Z52] The other seven series in Table 51–1 show fetal wastage exceeding 20%; in the three remaining series of the dodecade 1980 to 1991, fetal wastage was 20, 24, and 32%, respectively.[H205,L348,L356]

That activity of lupus, and specifically of lupus nephritis before conception and during pregnancy, may adversely affect pregnancy outcome has been mentioned above under spontaneous abortions and stillbirths. Hayslett and Lynn specifically state that pregnancy in patients with ongoing activity of SLE was associated with a more hectic course; successful outcome was reduced by 25%, and only 9 of 16 patients with nephrotic syndrome had successful deliveries.[H224] When serum creatinine was less than 1.5 mg/dl, 9 of 10 pregnancies resulted in live births, while in 10 pregnancies with serum creatinine above 1.5 mg/dl, fetal loss was 50%. There was an exception of 4 patients, however, with serum creatinine of 4 mg/dl or higher and live births, indicating that a successful outcome may occur despite severe renal failure. In the retrospective study by Gimovsky et al., fetal wastage in 40 pregnancies in nephritis patients was 55%, not unlike the 48% in those without nephritis.[G151]

It is of interest that in the Dutch study the male:female sex ratio of offspring of lupus patients (male babies per 100 female babies) was 72.7 and 78.9 before and after onset of SLE, respectively: this is decreased compared to the normal of 105 for the Dutch population.[N144] This would imply greater fetal wastage of male offspring. In an attempt to explain the high female:male ratio in SLE, Oleinick examined the family histories of 198 lupus patients and their 581 siblings. He found that the ratio of

male to total siblings born within 4 years of the birth of lupus patients was lower and suggested that excessive male fetal wastage may explain, in part, the female preponderance in SLE.[O65] In a further investigation, Oleinick found that there was no excess mortality risk early in life for male siblings or offspring of lupus patients.[O66]

Of the three prospective studies in lupus pregnancy, the one by Lockshin et al.[L356] did not utilize any specific intervention methods and has the highest fetal wastage, 32% (8 of 25 pregnancies). Of special interest are two studies from the same center in Mexico City.[F190,M472] In the retrospective study, fetal loss amounted to 40.5%.[F190] In the prospective study of 102 pregnancies, Mintz et al.[M472] used maternal disease surveillance with appropriate therapeutic intervention, treatment of every pregnant woman with a minimum of 10 mg of prednisone per day, frequent obstetric followup of fetal development, early detection of fetal distress with immediate cesarean section, and utilization of newborn intensive care units: fetal wastage diminished to almost half, 22.5%.[M472] Interestingly, in the prospective study by Wong et al.,[W336] with similar procedures, but with higher doses of prednisone than Mintz et al.,[M472] fetal wastage was only 10.5% (2 of 19). However, the number of pregnancies is small, and there were many therapeutic abortions.

Another area of great interest is the prevention of fetal wastage associated with antiphospolipid antibodies. In 11 studies, low-dose aspirin with or without corticosteroids,[B456,B550,G64,L351,L401,L400,092,S403] heparin alone,[R322c] heparin and prednisone,[S273] or heparin and aspirin,[B550] have resulted in reduction of fetal wastage from 81 to 100%, to 0 to 55% (Table 51–2). For more details see below under management, and Chapter 50.

In summary, there is a substantial prevalence of spontaneous abortion, stillbirth, and overall fetal wastage in lupus patients. Fetal wastage tended to be constant during 1950 to 1980, but there are recent trends toward diminution. The decreased fetal wastage evident in two prospective studies that utilized steroid treatment protocols still remains significantly higher than that of normal populations, which varies from 6.7% in the Mexico City study controls[M472] to 15%.[S461]

ELECTIVE (INDUCED, THERAPEUTIC) ABORTIONS

Elective, induced, or therapeutic abortions in lupus pregnancies are reported as high as 34% from Hong Kong,[W336] 25% from Toronto,[T200] 21% from Vancouver,[S633] and as low as 0% from Mexico City.[M472] In the U.S. series the prevalence ranges from 10[V47] to 24%.[L356] These worldwide variations are probably a result of different local legislation regarding elective abortion, patient attitudes and socioeconomic setting, and physician attitudes, sophistication, and level of comfort with lupus pregnancy. Patient and physician attitudes toward the activity or severity of maternal disease probably play a role.

In some reports[D262,F95,F251] therapeutic abortion was followed by severe exacerbation of SLE and, not uncommonly, by death of the mother, or it failed to induce remission. Other experience has been that patients tolerate the procedure, and that disease activity improves in direct

Table 51–2. Outcome of Treatment in Antiphospholipid-associated Fetal Loss

Author	Daily Therapy Used	No. of Pregnancies		Live Births (%)	
		Before Therapy	After Therapy	Before Therapy	After Therapy
Branch et al.[B456]	Aspirin 81 mg + Prednisone 40–60 mg	31	8	3.2	62.5
Lubbe et al.[L400,L401]	Aspirin 75 mg + Prednisone 40–60 mg	28	6	10.7	85.7
Gatenby et al.[G64]	Aspirin 75–150 mg + Prednisone 30–50 or Prednisone 10–60 mg	145	27	17.2	63
Ordi et al.[O92]	Aspirin 50 mg + Prednisone 20 mg	18	9	0	78
Silveira et al.[S437]	Aspirin 81 mg + Prednisone 40 mg	33	13	13.2	100
Buchanan et al.[B550]	Aspirin 75 mg, or ASA + Heparin 10,000u	101	87	18.7	63.2
Rosove et al.[R322c]	Heparin 24,700u	29	15	3.4	93.3
Semprini et al.[S273]	Heparin + Prednisone	27	14	3.7	64
Cowchock[C418A]	Aspirin 80 mg + Heparin 20,000u, or ASA + Prednisone 40 mg	*	12	0	75
		*	8	0	75

* Unspecified

relation to corticosteroid administration. Pistiner et al. reported 106 elective abortions in 634 pregnancies among 227 women with lupus, without ill effects.[P216] Wong et al.[W336] reported 10 elective abortions in 29 pregnancies—in 3, the indication was active SLE; in 2, nephrotic syndrome relapse; in 3, fear of teratogenicity; and 2 were unwanted pregnancies. In the last 5 patients there was no postabortion flare, and the 2 patients with nephrotic relapse had a remission in 4 weeks. However, all of these patients were on a minimum of 30 mg of prednisone daily.

It appears, then, that appropriate, vigorous steroid treatment, rather than induced abortion is medically indicated for suppression of disease activity during pregnancy. If an elective abortion is indicated for psychologic or social reasons, a careful evaluation of SLE activity should be undertaken, and steroid dosage adjusted accordingly before the procedure.

PREMATURITY

Prematurity is generally defined as birth before week 37 of gestation. Before 1980 the prematurity rate, defined as the percentage of premature infants among total neonates, was 15.3%, or 119 premature and 656 term births. The lowest rate was 6%,[D323] and the highest, 31 and 30%.[F95,G387] After 1980 there are 14 reports with adequate data, with a total of 435 neonates, 126 (29%) of whom were premature (Table 51–1). Houser et al.[H448] report 21%, 3 in 14 pregnancies—in 10 pregnancies with no evidence of active renal disease or active SLE there were 10 term deliveries, in contrast to 8 pregnancies with active renal disease or active SLE, where there was only 1 term newborn, 3 premature infants, and 4 abortions. In Devoe and Loy's patients, low maternal C3 and C4 levels correlated with premature delivery and spontaneous abortion, while in 11 of 12 term deliveries complement was normal.[D189]

Varner et al.[V47] also showed that prematurity and decreased birth weight were associated with increased severity and activity of maternal disease: there were 10 premature infants out of 17 newborns from mothers with active disease (59%), and only 2 premature infants out of

17 pregnancies with inactive or controlled disease (12%). This is a fivefold increase in prematurity with active maternal lupus. In contrast, in Dutch lupus patients, the prematurity rate of 18.9% was not significantly greater than that of the Dutch population (13.2%) or of the rate before lupus onset (16.7%).[N144] It is of note that these patients appeared to have mild lupus. In the study by Gimovsky et al.[G151] there were 14 premature births out of a total of 65 deliveries (21.5%) after the onset of SLE, equally divided between renal and nonrenal patients; three of four neonatal deaths were a result of prematurity. In the same group there had been no premature newborns in 22 deliveries before the diagnosis of SLE.

The decrease in fetal wastage evident in two prospective studies from 1986 and 1991 is accompanied by an increase in premature births.[M472,W336] In the prospective study from Mexico City,[M472] there were 50 premature births out of the total 85 deliveries (62.5%) compared to 8.9% in the control group. With active disease during pregnancy there were 30 premature births in 44 deliveries (68.1%), and with inactive disease there were 20 premature births in 41 deliveries (48.7%). Although not deemed statistically significant, there was a 20% increase in frequency of prematurity with active maternal disease. A full 30% of the premature infants had intrauterine growth retardation. Moreover, of the 10 pregnancies that were conceived during active SLE, 7 were delivered prematurely and only 2 were term births. In the study by Wong et al.[W336] 47% of births were premature (8 of 17), and 2 of these had intrauterine growth retardation. There was no apparent relation to SLE activity, but the number of pregnancies is small; the prematurity rate for the general population of a university hospital in Hong Kong was reported at 5.7%. All of these patients were receiving at least 10 mg prednisone daily during pregnancy. In a prospective study, Lockshin et al.[L356] reported 64.7% premature births (11 of 17 deliveries) in a population considered to have mild disease and several patients not requiring corticosteroids. There is no control group to compare frequency of prematurity in this study.

In summary, although there is no complete unanimity in the reported series, premature births are commonplace in lupus and tend to be associated with active maternal disease during pregnancy.

INTRAUTERINE GROWTH RETARDATION

Birth and fetal weight is normally a function of the gestational age of the newborn or fetus, and growth curves have been developed to show this relationship.[D344] When weight is below the norm for gestational age, the condition has been alternatively called intrauterine growth retardation, small newborn for gestational age, or intrauterine malnutrition.

Few reports have this information. In the retrospective study from UCLA,[F95] 32% of prematures were below the tenth percentile. It is important to note that all newborns delivered to mothers with no evidence of active disease, and who were not receiving medication, were above the tenth percentile, in contrast to 5 of 14 born to mothers with active disease that required treatment, who were below the tenth percentile for birth weight as a function of gestational age. Varner et al.[V47] found that 3 of 31 neonates (10%) were small for gestational age. The study by Gimovsky et al.[G151] showed that 66% of premature neonates (8 of 14) were small for gestational age, compared to 28% (6 of 21) of the term neonates; there was no apparent relationship to maternal disease activity. Imbasciati et al.[111] reported 2 of 10 premature infants (20%) with intrauterine growth retardation, one of whom died with respiratory distress syndrome. On the other hand, 11 term babies had adequate weight.

Of the 86 newborns (85 pregnancies, 1 twin birth) reported by Mintz et al.,[M472] 20 (23%) were small for gestational age, including 4 stillbirths, 1 neonatal death, and 1 with complete atrioventricular heart block. In contrast, only 5 (14%) of the term neonates had low weight for gestational age, and all survived. This difference is statistically significant. In the prospective study by Wong et al.,[W336] 2 of 17 (12%) newborns were small for gestational age. There seems to be a clear trend toward greater intrauterine growth retardation in premature newborns, which tends to be associated with active maternal lupus. It is of interest that when Semprini et al. treated 14 habitual aborters with heparin and prednisone, achieving a 64% rate of live births compared to 3.7% before treatment,[S273] the prevalence of low birth weight was reduced from 44 to 12%. Wallenburg and Rotmans treated 24 women with prior fetal growth retardation with low-dose aspirin and dipyridamole after 16 weeks' gestation, with resultant reduction of fetal growth retardation to 13% in treated versus 61% in untreated pregnancies.[W45] Two mothers had the lupus anticoagulant.

LIVE BIRTHS

Depending on the number of spontaneous and elective abortions, stillbirths, and neonatal deaths, the proportion of live births in systemic lupus varies from a low of 48% to a high of 89%.[B371,F95,G151,H224,H448,I11,M334,M472,N144,P216, S633,T200,V47,W336,Z52]

PATHOGENESIS OF FETAL WASTAGE

The nearly triple than normal prevalence of fetal wastage in systemic lupus has puzzled clinicians and investigators alike. Several findings from serologic and placental studies have been reported, and mechanisms have been proposed. Grennan et al. in 1978 examined the placentas of four mothers with SLE and one with discoid lupus and positive ANA:[G368] macroscopically the placentas were normal. By immunohistology all had granular IgG, C3, and fibrinogen deposits on placental vessels and stroma, and linear and "tramline" IgG deposits on trophoblast basement membranes, as described in normal placentas.[F29,M247] In addition, there were granular deposits of IgG and C3 on the trophoblast membrane of one patient with lupus nephritis and high DNA binding in the serum, which diminished appreciably after incubation with deoxyribonuclease (DNAse); on placental elution, IgG with DNA-binding activity was obtained, which produced peripheral nuclear fluorescence. These findings are highly suggestive of DNA–antiDNA immune complex deposits in the trophoblast membrane. It is of interest that the child of this patient, who had high DNA binding in cord blood, which diminished to negative by 8 weeks' age, was healthy. In another SLE placenta there was IgG-speckled nuclear fluorescence in cytotrophoblast cells, and the respective eluate contained antinuclear antibody which produced speckled fluorescence.[G368]

Abramowsky et al. studied the placentas of 10 women with systemic lupus and 1 with discoid lupus.[A15,A16] Of the 11 women, 6 had at least one fetal loss, including two spontaneous abortions and four stillbirths during the index pregnancy. No studies of antiphospholipid antibodies were performed in these patients. Two placentas had extensive infarcts (>25%), one from a patient with preeclampsia and one from the DLE patient, who both had stillbirths. The other placentas showed focal hemorrhages. Microscopically, the most prominent change was decidual vasculopathy in five multigravidas, who had spontaneous abortion or stillbirth: the affected vessels showed fibrinoid necrosis, at time to the point of vessel wall dissolution, occasionally with a mono- or polymorphonuclear infiltrate, dilatation, or aneurysmal appearance, and atherosis (infiltration of the vascular wall by foamy cells). Rupture of damaged blood vessels resulted in hemorrhage. Changes of placental vasculopathy and atherosis have been described in pre-eclampsia.[F180,K264] Of the five patients with necrotizing decidual vasculopathy, three had nephritis (two with pre-eclampsia and one with antepartum flare), and two were stable, including the patient with DLE, who was hypertensive. Immunopathology in the patients with decidual vasculopathy showed massive vascular deposits of IgM and lesser of C3 in two, one of whom had large IgG deposits in the decidual intercellular space. In two other patients there were IgG and IgA deposits in trophoblast nuclei.

De Wolf et al. also found decidual vasculopathy and massive placental infarction in a woman with lupus anticoagulant, recurrent fetal loss, recurrent venous and arterial thromboses, whose platelet-poor plasma inhibited the production of prostacyclin by rat aorta.[D194] Small-diameter decidual vessels showed intimal thickening, fibrinoid necrosis, acute atherosis, and intraluminal thrombosis. The same group of authors had described a similar patient with lupus anticoagulant, whose platelet-poor plasma and, specifically, the IgG fraction, inhibited the generation of prostacyclin by rat aorta and by pregnant human myometrium.[C104] The authors suggested that the lupus anticoagulant may interfere with the release of arachidonic acid (prostacyclin precursor) from cell membrane phospholipids.

In a study of 5 placentas from four lupus patients and 20 from healthy women with term pregnancies, Guzman et al. found the former to be significantly smaller in size and weight;[G441] 2 of 5 lupus placentas and 1 of 20 normals had large infarcts; findings seen only in lupus placentas included focal infarcts, "onionskin"-like proliferation of the media of vessels, mononuclear cells in decidual vessels, villi and trophoblast, ANA-like nuclear staining by IgG in 5, and by C3 in 2, and IgG deposits along the amniotic membranes in a lupus band-like pattern. The predominant T-cell subset in SLE and normal placentas was OKT8, about 75%.[G441] In a fifth study of lupus placentas, Hanly et al.[H101] also found low placental weight as compared to healthy women and diabetic controls. As in the previous studies, massive infarcts and hematomas were found in two patients each, three of whom had antiphospholipid antibodies. Deposition of IgG and C3 was found in one SLE patient and in a woman with positive ANA, anti-Ro/SSA, and anti-La/SSB, whose both pregnancies resulted in children with complete heart block. Electron microscopy showed trophoblast basement membrane thickening in three of eight lupus patients, in the woman with positive serology, and in two diabetic controls: such thickening is a nonspecific finding. These authors suggested that the small size of the placenta in lupus patients may impair the capacity to tolerate additional insults, such as a clotting tendency. In the report by Lubbe et al.,[L401] 9 of 16 placentas from intermediate and late fetal deaths had multiple scattered infarcts as the major histologic finding.

As mentioned previously, antiphospholipid antibodies have been widely associated with fetal wastage[L392] (Table 51–2). To repeat the most compelling evidence, in five prospective studies of 160 patients with lupus or lupus-like disease, those with lupus anticoagulant or anticardiolipin antibody had significantly higher fetal loss (60%) versus those without these antibodies, who had 13 and 5% fetal loss, respectively.[E109,H101,K386,L350,L354] It is thought that antiphospholipid antibodies, probably in association with additional factors, interfere with the production or release of prostacyclin (PGI$_2$),[C103,D194] and thus can promote intravascular clotting. Prostacyclin is a potent inhibitor of platelet aggregation, is produced by placental endothelium and human pregnant myometrium, is increased in human fetal vessels, and is considered an important regulator of fetal circulation. A balance in placental production of prostacyclin and thromboxane is considered essential for the changes in placental vessels necessary to allow trophoblast ingrowth. Indeed, preeclampsia seems to occur as a response to placental ischemia, as a consequence of exaggerated placental production of thromboxane A2, with normal or deficient prostacyclin production.[M70,W57]

Other autoantibodies incriminated in fetal loss include lymphocytotoxic antibodies[B478] and anti-Ro/SSA antibodies.[H495,W101] Cold-reactive lymphocytotoxic antibodies were present in 65% of nonpregnant SLE patients, 3 of 4 of pregnant SLE patients with spontaneous abortions, 17% of 12 SLE patients with live births, 10% of 46 healthy pregnant women, and 1 of 6 healthy women with fetal loss; the antibodies could be absorbed out by purified trophoblast antigens.[B478] No information about antiphospholipid antibodies was available. Thus, lymphocytotoxic antibodies were proposed as a potential mechanism of fetal loss. Conversely, Lom-Orta et al., in a report of 27 pregnancies in 19 SLE women, concluded that lymphocytotoxic antibodies were not associated with spontaneous abortions, but with third-trimester exacerbations in 7 of 11 patients.[L369] Hull et al. and Watson et al. have implied a possible role for anti-Ro/SSA antibodies in fetal wastage in SLE.[H495,W101] In a retrospective study of 50 anti-Ro/SSA–positive and 47 anti–U$_1$-RNP–positive women, 20 of the former and 33 of the latter fulfilled criteria for SLE.[W101] Of the anti-Ro/SSA–positive women, 34 had 84 pregnancies with 28% fetal wastage, which was similar to that of the anti–U$_1$-RNP group (19%). However, black (Afro-American) women with anti-Ro/SSA had a much higher fetal loss (71%). Unfortunately, no information is given about the antiphospholipid status of these patients.

In summary, fetal wastage in lupus patients is strongly related to maternal antiphospholipid antibodies, and to associated placental changes of small size with infarcts, hematomas, decidual vasculopathy with thrombosis, thickened trophoblast membrane, and immune deposits. The exact mechanisms are not fully understood, and autoantibodies as anti-DNA and anti-Ro/SSA may be contributing factors. It seems that the fetus in certain lupus pregnancies is subject to conditions of relative ischemia; perhaps this can in part explain the intrauterine growth retardation so common in this disease.

PREGNANCY MANAGEMENT FOR OPTIMAL FETAL SURVIVAL

The value of multidisciplinary care, careful maternal and fetal monitoring, and judicious use of surgical delivery were demonstrated in the retrospective and prospective studies from Mexico City, where fetal wastage was reduced by almost half from 40.5 to 22.5%.[F190,M472] The following are recommendations for management of lupus pregnancy in order to optimize fetal survival and diminish loss.

1. As recommended in Chapter 50, maternal disease should be assessed carefully for activity and severity at the outset of pregnancy, which should be planned after several months of remission. The mother should be watched carefully for exacerbations.
2. The mother's status in terms of antiphospholipid antibody and anti-Ro/SSA, anti-La/SSB positivity should be known: the former, because of predisposition to fetal loss, and the latter two because of the small risk for congenital heart block in the child (see also Chap. 52).
3. Joint followup by the rheumatologist and obstetrician should be done every month for the first half

of pregnancy, and more frequently thereafter, with repeat of CBC, urine, chemistry, quantitation of proteinuria in patients with nephritis, complement C3 and C4 levels, anti-dsDNA, and a measure of circulating immune complexes.

4. In the event of positive antiphospholipid antibody, especially with a history of intravascular thrombosis, or recurrent fetal loss, the patient should be enrolled in an effective antithrombotic protocol (low-dose aspirin with or without prednisone, heparin alone, with low-dose aspirin, or with prednisone).

5. Ultrasound evaluation of the growth of the fetal pole and placental size should be done monthly. Failure of normal growth should alert to the possibility of impending spontaneous abortion.

6. Accurate gestational dating is important because of the frequent IUGR and premature births in SLE. Menstrual dating should be confirmed by ultrasonography at the first prenatal visit.[S61] Attention should be paid to the amount of amniotic fluid, which, if decreased, may presage IUGR or cord accidents leading to stillbirth.

7. In the event of positive anti-Ro/SSA and/or anti-La/SSB, fetal cardiac monitoring and echocardiography should be done periodically starting the sixteenth to twentieth week of gestation. The mainstay of antepartum fetal heart testing is the nonstress test.[D297,D298,D299] During normal intrauterine fetal movement, the fetal heart accelerates. Failure to accelerate constitutes a nonreactive, or abnormal nonstress test. Fetal bradycardia during the nonstress test is associated with the risk of fetal distress during labor,[D298] and nonperiodic fetal heart decelerations at 20 to 28 weeks may detect the fetus at risk for intrauterine death.[D299]

8. An abnormal nonstress test (NST) should be followed by a contraction stress test (CST), or a biophysical profile.[S61] The contraction stress test is performed with the patient receiving oxytocin and by monitoring of the fetal heart rate during contractions. The biophysical profile consists of real-time ultrasonography, during which the fetal tone, movements, breathing movements, and amniotic fluid volume are scored; a nonstress test follows and a score of 0 to 10 is assigned. From 28 to 34 weeks the NST/CST should be performed every week, and then twice weekly.

9. In the event of fetal distress, if the fetus is viable, cesarean section should be promptly performed. If the fetus is considered immature, precesarean and intraoperative betamethasone or dexamethasone therapy can promote lung maturation and prevent respiratory distress syndrome.[D299]

10. Maternal exacerbation should be diagnosed early and treated aggressively with appropriate steroid dose. Unless there is a dire emergency, i.e., acute anuric renal failure, cytotoxic drugs should be avoided during the first trimester. Mothers with nephritis at risk for hypertension and pre-eclampsia should be treated with low-dose aspirin (60–81

mg/day) until the thirty-sixth week of gestation. See Chapter 50 for details.

11. While we are not fully justified to advocate the routine use of corticosteroids during pregnancy, because of lack of controlled data, in two prospective series the following protocols were used: 10 mg prednisone per day in all pregnant lupus patients cared for by Mintz et al. may have contributed to a smoother course.[M472] Wong et al. maintained the steroid dosage as needed until week 30 of pregnancy, when it was increased to 10, 20, or 30 mg, if the patients were taking less than 10 mg, 10 mg, or more than 10 mg per day, respectively.[W336] If disease activity required higher doses, it was adjusted accordingly, and that dose was maintained until 4 weeks after delivery. There were no postpartum exacerbations in this study.

Other drugs should be used with great care. Maternal thiazide diuretic therapy has been associated with severe, at times fatal, neonatal thrombocytopenia.[R264] Disseminated ectopic calcifications were described in a newborn whose mother with SLE received furosemide and prednisolone for SLE nephritis; the infant died and might have suffered pancreatitis in utero.[L52] Neonatal renal failure with death occurred in the infant of a lupus patient whose severe hypertension necessitated aggressive antihypertensive therapy, including the angiotensin inhibitor enalapril.[S227] (The Food and Drug Administration has authorized a warning against the use of all ACE-inhibitors in pregnancy.[A240c]) These drugs have been found to cause fetal and neonatal hypotension, anuria, reversible or irreversible renal failure, oligohydramnios with limb contractures, craniofacial deformation, skull hypoplasia, and hypoplastic lung development. Prematurity, IUGR and patent ductus arteriosus have been also found, but the causative relationship is not clear. For more information on antirheumatic drugs in pregnancy and lactation, see the section on use of medications in Chapter 50. As mentioned in the above chapter, prednisone, prednisolone, and methylprednisolone are oxidized by placental enzymes, while dexamethasone and betamethasone are not.[B54,B338] In fact, this principle was utilized to treat in utero a fetus with pericarditis, presumed myocarditis, and congenital heart block.[B605]

Under dire circumstances, unusual and unconventional therapeutic interventions may be appropriate. Plasmapheresis, for example, can be safely performed during pregnancy, and has been used for years in Rh-incompatible pregnancies.[R253] Two patients with recurrent fetal loss and anticardiolipin antibody were given plasmapheresis—in one, there was a dramatic reduction of antiphospholipid antibody and successful pregnancy outcome,[F192] in the other one, who had a multisystem disease with myositis, plasmapheresis was given because of fetal distress. The authors felt that they gained 2 more weeks of gestation, during which there was further fetal maturation, which allowed fetal survival after cesarean section at 29 weeks.[F306] A good review on plasmapheresis in pregnancy has appeared. Five papers have reported seven women with four to nine fetal losses each, positive anticardiolipin antibodies and lupus anticoagulant, and pre-eclampsia in three.[C103,K115,P46,S229,W72] Treatment with intravenous gamma globulin, at times with addition of low-dose aspirin, heparin, and steroids resulted in live births. Immunoglobulin was given monthly, or in 5-day courses. This expensive treatment seems worth considering in such difficult clinical situations.

It is reassuring to note that in over 1000 lupus pregnancies reported in the last 40 years (Table 51–1), there were only four cases of congenital malformations, with the exception of congenital heart block (see Chapter 52). These figures include infants whose mothers were on cytotoxic medications, mainly azathioprine and cyclophosphamide. Details are mentioned in Chapter 50 and in references.[B405,M334,W250]

Chapter 52

THE NEONATAL LUPUS SYNDROME

RODANTHI C. KITRIDOU
GREGORIO MINTZ

Neonatal lupus erythematosus (NLE) is a syndrome of cutaneous lupus, or congenital complete heart block, or both, and/or other systemic manifestations, which appears in children of women with systemic lupus, Sjögren's syndrome, other systemic rheumatic diseases, or asymptomatic mothers with anti-Ro/SSA, anti-La/SSB, and, rarely, anti–U1-RNP. The first description of congenital heart block was in 1901 by Morquio,[M594] the association with SLE was first recognized by Hogg,[H372] and the first description of cutaneous neonatal lupus and association with maternal SLE was made by McCuistion and Schoch.[M254] Among the earliest authors to describe congenital complete heart block were Aylward in 1928,[A375] in two infants of a woman with Mikulicz's (Sjögren) syndrome, and Plant and Steven, in an infant of a mother with SLE in 1945.[P219] In the last 14 years there has been tremendous interest in neonatal lupus, and a voluminous literature has been amassed, including two excellent reviews.[M43,P158]

PREVALENCE

Franco et al.[F204] at first, then Kephart et al.,[K173] and Miyagawa et al.[M498] suggested in 1981 that maternal anti-Ro/SSA antibody, perhaps through transplacental passage, was responsible for the development of neonatal lupus. Evidence for the association of NLE with anti-Ro/SSA and anti-La/SSB has been mounting during the last 10 years. For this reason, it is important to review the prevalence not only of the neonatal lupus erythematosus syndrome, but also of the anti-Ro/SSA and anti-La/SSB in mothers with SLE and their offspring. In 12 studies of 11,895 normal individuals, including blood donors, pregnant women, and mother-infant pairs, a prevalence of 0 to 11%.[C30,F277, G9,G41,H87,H139,H141,M46,M51,S476,T85] The prevalence of anti-Ro/SSA by immunodiffusion or counterimmunoelectrophoresis varies from 0.1 to 2%, whereas by ELISA it is found in 2.3 to 11% of normals. Anti-La/SSB is even more rare, found in 0 to 1.8% of normals by immunodiffusion or counterimmunoelectrophoresis, and in 0 to 12.5% by ELISA.[F277,G9,H87,H139,M51,T85] The prevalence of anti-Ro/SSA in normal pregnant women is 0.4 to 1%,[C30,H141,T85] and that of anti-La antibody, 0.7% of 445 normal pregnant women.[T85] In 16 studies of 1,874 systemic lupus patients, anti-Ro/SSA was found by the two former methods in 14 to 52%, and by the more sensitive ELISA in 39 to 87%; an average, well-accepted prevalence is 40%.[B183,B184,D163, D217,G41,H87,M45,M46,M51,M534,P50,R34,R118,S225,S798,W276] Miyagawa et al. determined the frequency of anti-Ro/SSA anti-

bodies in 825 patients with systemic rheumatic diseases and found it significantly greater in women (74 of 670, 11%) than in men (5 of 155, 3.2%).[M497] The frequency of anti-La/SSB in SLE by immunodiffusion has been reported from 1.2 to 24% and by ELISA from 21 to 38%.[D217,H87, M45,M51,R118,S225,S798] A generally accepted prevalence of anti-La/SSB in SLE is 15 to 20%. In Sjögren's syndrome patients, anti-Ro/SSA prevalence is 40 to 45%, and anti-La/SSB, 15 to 20%.[A135]

It should be noted that anti-La/SSB is associated with anti-Ro/SSA in 99% or more of cases,[R118] whereas anti-Ro can be found alone. Rarely, cutaneous neonatal lupus has been associated with anti–U1-RNP.[G263,P315,R202]

The prevalence of congenital complete heart block is estimated at 1 in 20,000 births, or 0.005%[M388] (Table 52–1). The overall prevalence of neonatal lupus in live births of SLE mothers, derived from the largest prospective study, is 1 in 86, or 1.2%.[M472] Ramsey-Golman et al. reported 7 infants with NLE in 259 (2.7%) of lupus pregnancies:[R34] there was 1 NLE in 180 births without anti-Ro/SSA (0.6%) and 6 in 79 (7.6%) with anti-Ro, and the occurrence of heart block correlated with high titer of the antibody. These authors estimated the overall risk of a woman with lupus having a child with congenital heart block as 1:60, which increases to 1:20 in the presence of anti-Ro/SSA. In other series of lupus patients positive for anti-Ro/SSA, the prevalence of neonatal lupus has been reported as 1 in 67 births (1.5%) in the retrospective study by Watson et al.,[W101] 1 in 28 (3.6%) by McHugh et al.,[M293] 1 in 26 (3.8%) by Maddison,[M43] 4 in 38 (10.5%) by Lockshin et al.,[L349,L352] 3 of 34 (8.8%) in mothers with lupus and Sjögren's syndrome, in a prospective study by Drosos et al.,[D292] and in 5 of 20 (25%) by Nossent and Swaak.[N144] In all, there were 21 children with neonatal lupus in 292 live births in women with lupus or Sjögren's syndrome positive for anti-Ro/SSA, for an overall prevalence of 7.2%.

CLINICAL MANIFESTATIONS

A total of 294 babies with neonatal lupus have been described to date, barring any duplication (Table 52–2).
[A375,B85,B267,B284,B471,B605,C23,C196,D228,D276,D286 D292,E6, E119,E146,F124,F182,F183,F186,F197,F204,G76,G79,H124,H135,H372, H407,H451,H494,J9,J127,K91,K105,K136,K173,K182,K387,L56,L108, L111,L117,L125,L132,L138,L238,L266,L296,L332,L349,L352,L416,L422, M52,M243,M252,M254,M255,M293,M472,M498,M561,M629,N84,N108, N115,N144,O35,P41,P50,P315,R97,R98,R160,R202,R283,S117,S260,S363,]

Table 52–1. Neonatal Lupus Erythematosus—Prevalence of Congenital Heart Block: 1 : 20,000 Births

	No.	%
In unselected SLE births		
Mintz et al.[M472]	1/86	1.2
Ramsey-Goldman et al.[R34]	7/259	2.7
overall	8/345	2.3
In SLE Births without anti-Ro/SSA		
Ramsey-Goldman et al.[R34]	1/180	0.6
In Anti-Ro/SSA–positive SLE		
Watson et al.[W101]	1/67	1.5
McHugh et al.[M293]	1/28	3.6
Maddison[M43]	1/26	3.8
Ramsey-Goldman et al.[R34]	6/79	7.6
Drosos et al.[D292]	3/34	8.8
Lockshin[L348]	4/38	10.5
Nossent and Swaak[N144]	5/20	25.0
Overall	21/292	7.2

Table 52–3. Maternal Diagnosis in Neonatal Lupus

	No.	%
Systemic lupus	111	39.5
Asymptomatic	107	38.0
Sjögren's syndrome	37	13.2
Miscellaneous rheumatic disease	26	9.3
Total	281	

[S440,S551,S665,S793,T85,V58,W103,W199,W303,W355] Of these 294 babies, 160 (54.4%) had congenital heart block, 109 (37.1%) had cutaneous NLE, 21 (7.1%) had both, and 4 (1.4%) had other manifestations. There is adequate information on 281 mothers: 111 (39.5%) had systemic lupus, 37 (13.2%) had Sjögren's syndrome, 26 (9.3%) had other rheumatic diseases (undifferentiated, mixed connective tissue disease, hypocomplementemic vasculitis, and rheumatoid arthritis), and 107 (38.%) were asymptomatic (Table 52–3).

Congenital Heart Block

One-half to nearly two-thirds of complete heart block babies are female, and the remainder, male. In Esscher and Scott's study of 67 children, 42 were female (62.7%) and 25 were male (37.3%);[E146] in McCue and coauthors' study of 22 children, there were 12 female (54.5%) and 10 male (45.5%);[M252] and of the 14 children reported by McCune et al., 9 were female (64%) and 5 were male (36%).[M255] The congenital heart block is complete in over 90% of reported cases. Other types of conduction defects described include second-degree atrioventricular block,[F204,G76] 2:1 AV block,[R97] transient AV block,[B471,M252] right bundle-branch block,[K173,S665,W103]

Table 52–2. Manifestations of Neonatal Lupus

	No.	%
Congenital heart block	160	54.4
Cutaneous NLE	109	37.1
CHB and cutaneous NLE	21	7.1
Other manifestations	4	1.4
Manifestations in addition to CHB and cutaneous NLE		
Hepatic/gastrointestinal	23	7.8
Hematologic	19	6.5
Neurologic	4	1.4
Pulmonary	3	1.0
Total infants reported	294	

and sinus bradycardia.[F183] Two fascinating reports of postnatal progression of second- to third-degree AV block have appeared.[G79,G263] Goldsmith[G263] reported a male infant of an asymptomatic mother with arrhythmia and documentation of second-degree AV block at 10 weeks; at 7 months of age, an episode of tachycardia to 200 beats per minute with diaphoresis, unresponsiveness and pulselessness, was followed by development of complete heart block necessitating pacemaker implantation. In the report by McCue, Mantakas et al., transient arrhythmias and varying block were noted by electrocardiography.[M252] These changes and the evolution of complete heart block in the two infants suggest that the process of myocarditis, or other insult to the conducting system, can be active after birth, and that efforts should be aimed at early detection and effective therapy. In addition to conduction defects, a variety of other cardiac anomalies have been described in neonatal lupus, usually in association with congenital heart block, in approximately 30% of the babies. These defects include, in order of approximate frequency, patent ductus arteriosus,[C196,E146,K91,M255,S665] ventricular septal defect,[E146,H451,M252] corrected transposition,[B284,E146,M252] atrial septal defect,[C196,L111] patent foramen ovale,[K387] coarctation,[M252] possible tetralogy,[E6] hypoplastic right ventricle,[M252] dysplastic pulmonic valve,[C196] pulmonary regurgitation,[L56] anomalous pulmonary venous drainage,[E146] tricuspid insufficiency,[M252] and mitral insufficiency.[M252] It is of note that complete heart block alone does not cause heart failure and death in utero, which tend to occur if there is an associated serious defect. Aside from structural defects, inflammatory processes have been described in babies with neonatal lupus, usually with congenital heart block: pericarditis with effusion,[B605,D276,F182,J127,L349] with pericardial tamponade,[N115] myocarditis,[B284,B605,H278,L349] or cardiomyopathy.[C196] In one instance, a girl with congenital complete heart block went on to develop almost immediately severe systemic lupus with Libman-Sacks endocarditis and died.[F182] Presumed viral myocarditis developed in a child with congenital heart block.[R162]

Not all instances of congenital heart block are associated with maternal rheumatic disease and anti-Ro/SSA and anti-La/SSB antibodies—in particular, congenital heart block with atrioventricular canal defects and atrial isomerism seems to occur independently of the above autoantibodies.[G87,S350] Gembruch et al. diagnosed complete heart block prenatally in 21 fetuses, 18 (85.7%) of whom had associated cardiac defects, especially complete atrioventricular canal with atrial isomerism in 5, and "corrected" great vessel transposition in 4, with only one mother with SLE.[G87] In 11 fetuses, all of whom had cardiac defects, there was evidence of intrauterine congestive heart failure and nonimmune hydrops fetalis.

Heart block in neonatal lupus usually occurs abruptly during the few weeks prior to term, although it has been noted as early as week 22 of gestation, or postnatally, as late as 7 months of age.[G263] As mentioned in Chapter 51, fetal monitoring with the nonstress test and contraction stress test[D297,D298,D299] can detect fetal bradycardia; two-dimensional M-mode echocardiography can detect abnormal atrial and ventricular function, chamber enlargement, decreased cardiac output, and fetal pericardial effusion.[B605,M43,P222] Both major varieties of neonatal lupus, complete heart block and cutaneous eruption, have been described in siblings and in successive pregnancies.[E146,L137,M23,M252,P158,S117] Among 172 siblings in 65 families with 2 or more siblings reported in the above publications, 100 (58%) had NLE. A full 29 of the 65 families (44.6%) had 2 or more affected siblings, well above the prevalence in the general population. Of two sets of twins, one was discordant for congenital heart block,[H135] and the other concordant.[M252]

An interesting report has appeared of a photosensitive, but otherwise asymptomatic woman with high antinuclear antibody and nine spontaneous abortions, who, after therapy with 5 to 10 mg prednisolone per day during her tenth pregnancy, gave birth to a female infant with complete heart block. Anti-Ro/SSA, anti-La/SSB, and antiphospholipid antibodies were not reported.[H176]

In the largest series, mortality in babies with congenital heart block was from 15[M252] to 21[M255] or 22%[E146] occurred mostly in the neonatal period, and was associated with severe cardiac anomalies, cardiomyopathy,[C196] or myocarditis.[H278] The most common cause is congestive heart failure or Adams-Stokes attack. Pacemakers are needed in 20 to 45% of the children, with the majority implanted between 10 and 49 years of age.[R124] In the review by Reid et al.,[R124] only 2 patients reached age 50 without need of a pacemaker. Among the 22 children with heart block reported by McCue et al., 6 (27%) needed pacemakers;[M252] 5 of 24 (20.8%) reported by Esscher and Scott,[E146] and 5 of 11 (45.5%) reviewed by McCune et al.[M255] A substantial proportion (20 to 30%) of these children undergo cardiac catheterization as a preamble to corrective cardiac surgery. The longterm outlook, especially past the immediate postnatal period, is generally good.

Although not an example of neonatal lupus, a report by Yemini et al.[Y40] is of great interest: a very low birth weight infant born to a woman with hydralazine-induced lupus died of pericardial effusion with tamponade, confirmed by autopsy. The mother had pregnancy-induced hypertension.

Autopsy studies of infants with complete heart block have almost uniformly shown dense connective tissue enveloping the conducting system, including the sinoatrial and atrioventricular nodes and bundle of His, and endocardial fibroelastosis.[B284,C119,C196,E146,H494,S476] At times there is a fibrous body around the AV bundle,[C196] epicarditis near the SA node,[B284] microcrystalline structures in the conducting system,[C119,R162] and calcification of the heart, the conducting system, and valves.[L108,L332] Inflammatory infiltrates are conspicuously absent,[S476] or occasionally seen.[L133,L332]

Cutaneous Neonatal Lupus

As stated above, 37% of the reported neonatal lupus patients have cutaneous NLE, and the majority (70 to 75%) are females.[D286,M255,V107] There may be under-reporting of cutaneous NLE as compared to congenital heart block, because it is transient and a great proportion of mothers are asymptomatic. It is likely that annular erythema of newborn,[M498] and annular eruptions of infancy[K182] represent cutaneous NLE. Cutaneous neonatal lupus was first described in 1954 by McCuistion and Schoch in a 6-week-old daughter of a lupus patient,[M254] as possible discoid lupus. A biopsy of the child's rash indeed showed findings similar to those seen in SLE and DLE (hyperkeratosis, follicular plugging, areas of acanthosis and atrophy, liquefactive degeneration of the basal layer, and perivascular lymphocytic infiltrate). Since then 109 cases of cutaneous neonatal lupus have been described (see above for references). Skin biopsies in subsequent patients showed findings similar to those mentioned above.[D286,R98,S551,V107,W103] An interesting finding of microtubular structures in the endothelial vessels of cutaneous NLE biopsy, and in the labial salivary gland biopsy of the infant's mother, was reported by Nitta and Ohashi,[N108] and tuboreticular structures were found by Levy et al.[L238]

The skin rash of cutaneous NLE consists of transient, annular, occasionally scaly, erythematous lesions of the face, scalp, trunk, and extremities. Vonderheid et al. described a tendency of greater concentration of the lesions around the eyes, with telangiectasia.[V107] When the rash is annular, it resembles that of subacute cutaneous lupus erythematosus,[S568] and that of lupus with C2 complement component deficiency. Both of these variants of lupus have a high prevalence of anti-Ro/SSA. The rash usually appears shortly after birth, probably as a result of skin exposure to ultraviolet light, or as late as 5 months of age (mean, 7 weeks); The rash is found on sun-exposed areas, and is strongly photosensitive.[B85,L45,L132,L422,W103] In a report from Taiwan, an infant girl born to a mother with lupus developed cutaneous NLE after phototherapy for hyperbilirubinemia.[L422] Severe, generalized relapse of the NLE rash after an upper respiratory infection was described in a 50-day-old girl born to a mother with SLE.[L266] Cutaneous NLE typically lasts for 2 to 6 months and disappears without leaving a scar, or with minimal atrophy. The disappearance of the rash about the sixth month of age is consistent with the half-life of transplacentally acquired maternal IgG. However, there are reports of NLE skin lesions persisting for up to 15,[L45] 28,[B545] and 36 months.[O35]

Data on the occurrence of neonatal lupus, cutaneous and cardiac, in siblings, have been reviewed under congenital heart block. Suffice it to say that 29 of 65 reported families (44.6%) had two or more siblings affected.[E146,L137,M252,M255,P158,S117] A set of dizygous twins concordant for cutaneous NLE was born to an asymptomatic mother.[L103] Mother and twins were positive for anti-Ro/SSA and anti-La/SSB. Another set of dizygotic twins born to an asymptomatic, anti-Ro–positive mother was discordant for cutaneous NLE with negative anti-Ro antibody in the twins at 4 months of age.[C23] The coexistence of congenital heart block and cutaneous NLE is not common, encountered only in 21 of the reported 294 cases (7.1%).[E146,G76,H124,L352,M252,M255,N115,S440,W103]

As mentioned, cutaneous NLE has been reported in three male infants and one female infant in association with maternal anti–U1-RNP antibodies, in the absence of anti-Ro/SSA and anti-La/SSB.[G263,P315,R202] To these we would like to add a fifth (male) infant born to a systemic lupus patient at the Los Angeles County–University of Southern California Medical Center. The infant developed a few erythematous, macular, and annular lesions on the face and trunk shortly after birth, which disappeared over the ensuing month. Both mother and child had anti–U1-RNP antibody and no anti-Ro/SSA or anti-La/SSB. It may be purely coincidental that four of the five infants were black males.

Katayama et al. reported an infant with cutaneous NLE and severe gastrointestinal hemorrhage who had a positive anticardiolipin antibody for more than 6 months. Her mother was asymptomatic, with anticardiolipin and anti-Ro/SSA antibodies.[K105] It is possible that when the infant was seen at age 4 months, maternal anti-Ro had already been catabolized.

Other Manifestations of Neonatal Lupus

The first description of Coombs-positive hemolytic anemia, leukopenia, and thrombocytopenia in an infant born to a lupus patient with the same manifestations was reported by Seip in 1960.[S260] Since then hepatic, hematologic, neurologic, and pulmonary manifestations have been reported and reviewed in neonates, usually in association with congenital heart block, or cutaneous NLE.[B471,D286,E6,F204,H124,H407,H494,K105,K136,K173,L108,L215,L238,L296,M252,M255,M629,N84,R98,R160,R202,V107,W102,W103,W303]

Hepatic and gastrointestinal involvement was seen in 23 of 294 infants (7.8%), hematologic involvement in 19 (6.5%), neurologic involvement in 4 (1.4%), and pulmonary involvement in 3 (1%). Anti-Ro/SSA and anti-La/SSB antibodies are commonly found in these infants and their mothers. Hepatic manifestations, in order of frequency, included hepatomegaly, often accompanied by splenomegaly,[F204,K105,L108,L238,L296,M629,R98,R160] transiently increased liver function tests, icterus,[L108] noninfectious hepatitis, cholestasis,[L108] cirrhosis,[L108,M255] and severe gastrointestinal hemorrhage.[K105,L108] Liver biopsies and autopsies in some of the infants revealed noninfectious hepatitis, neonatal giant cell hepatitis, intra- and extracellular cholestasis, ductal and ductular hyperplasia, portal septal fibrosis, cirrhosis, and excessive extramedullary hematopoesis.[L108,M255]

Hematologic manifestations in NLE include thrombocytopenia, immune hemolytic anemia with Coombs' test positivity in mother and infant, and leukopenia. Thrombocytopenia has been reviewed by Watson et al.:[W102] it is frequently accompanied by splenomegaly. One infant had microangiopathic hemolytic anemia. Antiplatelet antibodies were negative in the mother-infant pair reported by Seip.[S260] At times, hemolytic anemia and thrombocytopenia were severe enough to require transfusions and steroid therapy of the infant.[S260] Neurologic manifestations have been described in four infants: one developed a myelopathy with residua at 16 months of age, in addition to cutaneous NLE and anti-Ro/SSA antibody,[K136] another had aseptic meningitis with congenital heart block and anti-La/SSB;[B604] a third had seizures and hypocalcemia, in addition to rash, hemolytic anemia, and hepatosplenomegaly;[M629] a fourth infant, whose mother had lupus and acetylcholine receptor antibodies, had transient myasthenia gravis, confirmed by electromyography, cutaneous NLE, and the mother's acetylcholine receptor and anti–U1-RNP antibodies;[R202] there were no anti-Ro or anti-La antibodies. Pneumonitis was present in three infants,[B471,L238,W103] in addition to cutaneous NLE and hemolytic anemia.

PATHOGENETIC MECHANISMS

The transplacental passage of maternal IgG is well known. In 1954 and 1957 such passage of the LE-cell factor (anti-DNP antibody) was reported, producing positive LE cells in healthy infants of lupus mothers up to the seventh week of age.[B248,F488] Seip found an equivocal Coombs' test in a child with hemolytic anemia, whose mother also had it.[S260] At first Franco et al.,[F204] the Kephart et al.,[K173] and Miyagawa et al.[M498] suggested in 1981 that maternal anti-Ro/SSA antibody may be causally linked to neonatal lupus erythematosus. Substantial accumulated evidence shows that transplacental passage of anti-Ro/SSA and/or anti-La/SSB, and, rarely, anti–U1-RNP, possibly in concert with other factors, results in neonatal lupus erythematosus.[S230] In the previously mentioned reports and series, with an aggregate of 294 children and 281 mothers, information on antibody status is available as follows. Of 148 infants tested for anti-Ro/SSA, 125 (84.5%) were positive, 65 of 131 (49.6%) tested for anti-La/SSB were positive, and 4 of 148 (2.7%) were positive for anti–U1-RNP. Of 190 mothers tested for anti-Ro/SSA, 171 (90%) were positive, 69 of 129 (53.5%) tested for anti-La/SSB were positive, and 4 of 190 (2.1%) had anti–U1-RNP. In all infants tested serially for anti-Ro and anti-La, the antibodies tended to disappear in 3 to 8 months' time, consistent with catabolism of transplacentally transmitted maternal IgG.[L132,S230,T85] Anti-Ro/SSA and anti-La/SSB are IgG antibodies. Several instances of NLE with anti-La/SSB alone have been reported, suggesting that this antibody may also be responsible pathogenetically.[B605,F197,F204,L117,L138,L266,T85,W199] Silverman et al. consider the presence of both anti-Ro and anti-La important in the development of neonatal lupus:[S440] all of their 15 infants with congenital heart block and 6 of 8 infants with cutaneous NLE were positive for both antibodies, with only 2 cutaneous NLE infants positive only for anti-Ro/SSA. Some of the earlier studies did not test for anti-La/SSB, and it is possible that available methodology in the past was less sensitive. The exact function of Ro/SSA and La/SSB is not known; Bachmann et al. have found that Ro/SSA and La/SSB are associated with a fibrous network akin to cytokeratin, an intermediate filament system.[B13] La/SSB is intriguing in that it probably is a cofactor for RNA polymerase III[R213] and binds adenoviral and EB viral RNA.[M316] Ben-Chetrit et al. have described a 52 kD component of the Ro/SSA particle;[B197] Buyon et al. have found antibodies to the 52 kD Ro/SSA, and to the 48 kD La/SSB component in 75 and 90%, respectively, of mothers of children with congenital heart block;[B602,B606] the authors suggested that the presence of both these antibodies confers an odds ratio of 35. These peptides were also found in fetal cardiac tissues aged 18 to 24 weeks.

Several lines of evidence have accumulated incriminating anti-Ro/SSA, and less so, anti-La/SSB, in the genesis of NLE:

1. Harley et al. described HLA-identical twins discordant for congenital complete heart block, with anti-Ro/SSA titers in the affected twin thirteenfold less than the normal twin,[H135] implying that it was bound to cardiac tissue. They also showed that Ro/SSA antigen is present in fetal heart aged 18 to 23 weeks and in adult heart.

2. Deng et al.[D155] identified Ro/SSA in nuclei of conduction system cells and cardiac myofibers in hearts of 9 to 10 weeks' gestation. Ro/SSA antigen was also found by Lee et al. in fetal myocardium, kidney, liver, and spleen, and in neonatal and adult, but not in fetal epidermis.[L136] The latter finding may explain why cutaneous NLE appears after birth and not in utero. These authors also identified Ro/SSA on the surface of cultured keratinocytes.

3. Taylor et al. demonstrated IgG antibodies against cardiac tissue in the sera of 51% of mothers of children with CHB, in three of eight CHB babies under 3 months old, and in none of normal controls.[T84] Eighty-one percent of the mothers with anticardiac antibodies were positive for anti-Ro/SSA. She also found that anti-Ro/SSA titers in infants with NLE were less than the mothers, whereas unaffected infants had titers similar to the mothers.[T85]

4. Litsey et al.,[L332] Taylor et al.,[T84] and Lee et al.[L133] demonstrated immunoglobulin and complement component deposition in a total of four hearts from congenital heart block. Litsey et al. showed diffuse staining for IgG in the epicardium, and for IgG and IgA in the endo- and myocardium of the right atrial appendage. Taylor et al. found diffuse cytoplasmic staining for IgG, IgM, IgA, and complement components in all cardiac tissue examined, including nodal tissue, bundle of His, Purkinje fibers, and myocardium at large. Lee et al. found particulate staining for IgG and C3 in all sections, but most intense and extensive in the atria.

5. Alexander et al. showed that anti-Ro/SSA and anti-La/SSB–containing sera of mothers with congenital heart block children preferentially inhibited in vitro the repolarization of neonatal, but not adult rabbit cardiac cells.[A134]

6. Lee et al. grafted nude athymic, and SCID mice with normal human skin, injected anti-Ro/SSA in the peritoneal cavity,[L135] and showed particulate cytoplasmic deposition of IgG in the epidermis, and occasionally at the dermo-epidermal junction, similar to that seen in patients with NLE or SCLE. Absorption of the anti-Ro–containing serum with Ro/SSA antigen resulted in marked diminution of fluorescence. Anti-Ro/SSA from NLE mothers bound to skin grafts is predominantly of the IgG1 subclass.[B221]

7. Low-dose UV irradiation induces cultured keratinocytes and fibroblasts to express Ro antigen.[L154,W327] UV-induced microvascular flow rates of skin test sites in guinea pigs were greatest with injections of anti-Ro/SSA–containing SCLE sera.[D96] These data suggest a mechanism of induction of photosensitivity by anti-Ro/SSA.

8. Furukawa et al. showed that estradiol enhances binding of anti-Ro and anti-La antibodies to cultured human keratinocytes, implying that estrogen may promote the expression of Ro and La antigens on keratinocytes.[F321] This could perhaps be significant for the greater expression of cutaneous NLE in females.

In summary, it appears that maternal antibodies to Ro/SSA and La/SSB recognize cytoskeletal or other antigens present in the immature cardiac conduction system and, alone or in concert with other factors, cause an inflammatory reaction in utero, resulting in fibrosis of the conduction system, heart block, and myocarditis. Similarly, the same maternal antibodies may recognize antigens present in neonatal skin, which are expressed in greater density upon UV light exposure, and cause the dermal inflammation of cutaneous NLE.

Another area of apparent significance of anti-Ro/SSA antibody is the reported association of maternal anti-Ro/SSA with the development of SLE in male children younger than 18, and in all children younger than 10 years at the time of diagnosis.[L176]

HEALTH AND GENETICS OF THE MOTHER

We previously mentioned that to date, of 281 mothers of NLE infants, 111 (39.5%) had systemic lupus, 37 (13.2%) had Sjögren's syndrome, 26 (9.3%) had other rheumatic diseases (undifferentiated, mixed connective tissue disease, hypocomplementemic vasculitis, and rheumatoid arthritis), and 107 (38.%) were asymptomatic with positive antibodies to Ro/SSA and La/SSB (Table 52–3). This last group of mothers is interesting in that they may have none or minimal problems, such as photosensitive rash after oral contraceptives,[J127] Raynaud's phenomenon,[M497] or subclinical Sjögren's syndrome;[N108] however, it appears that the majority of these women, given a long enough followup, will eventually develop a rheumatic disease, usually systemic lupus or Sjögren's syndrome. In the longterm study by McCune et al., 8 of the 11 asymptomatic mothers (73%) developed a systemic rheumatic disease in a span of 5 years.[M255] In Esscher and Scott's series, which included NLE children as old as 30 years of age, 64% of mothers had a systemic rheumatic disease. The time interval to development of maternal disease was as long as 14 years in Kasinath and Katz's report,[K91] and 26 years in Reichlin's patient.[R114]

Lee et al. first studied the genetic makeup of mothers with NLE children,[L132] and found HLA-DR3 positive in 5 of 6 tested (83%), with a relative risk of 32. All were positive for HLA-B8, 6 for MT2, and 5 for MB2 (the terminology has now changed, see below). Watson et al. found HLA-DR3 in 5 of 10 mothers, with a relative risk of 8, and confirmed the other findings.[W103] Vazquez-Rodriguez et al. also found a 50% prevalence of DR3 in Madrid.[V56] A study by Alexander et al.[A136] examined 21 mothers of NLE infants and compared them to 17 patients with Sjögren's syndrome—lupus overlap: 17 of 21 women (81%) had HLA-DR3, with a relative risk of 13.8; HLA-DQw2 was present in 95%, for the highest relative risk of 26.4; B8 was found in 81% with a relative risk of 12.2; and DRw52 was seen in 95%, with relative risk of 11.7. The extended haplotype HLA-B8, DR3, DQw2, DRw52 was present in 15 of 20 NLE mothers (75%) and conferred a relative risk of 11.3. similar findings were noted in the Sjögren's syndrome—lupus overlap patients, and the authors concluded that these two groups were closely related immunogenetically. It is well known that DR3 and DR2 are associated with the ability to produce antibody to Ro/SSA.[A66,A169,H87] Hamilton et al. showed that patients with anti-Ro/SSA alone have a strong association with the linked HLA alleles DR2 and DQw1, and have lower levels of anti-Ro;[H87] patients with both anti-Ro and anti/La are associated with the linked alleles B8, DR3, DRw52, and DQw2, have higher levels of anti-Ro, more sicca complex, and less renal involvement. In a study of 31 women (7 with CHB children and anti-Ro/SSA antibodies, 15 with anti-Ro but no CHB births, and 9 without anti-Ro but with CHB births) Arnaiz-Villena et al.[A290] confirmed the striking prevalence of DR3 in CHB mothers (100%), and suggested that class III antigens, (complement genes), such as BfS and/or C4AQ0B1, are increased in Ro-positive mothers of infants with heart block. In all, of 59 NLE mothers with HLA typing, 48 (81.4%) were positive for HLA-DR3 (31 mothers summarized by Petri et al.[A136,A290,P158]) There is no particular HLA association in children with NLE; the prevalence of DR3 is approximately 43% and can be explained on the basis of the high prevalence in the mother.

TREATMENT OF NEONATAL LUPUS

It would seem that the best treatment for congenital heart block is prevention, because attempts of treatment, once it is diagnosed, are to no avail.[B605,H278,L108,P158] Prenatal testing for anti-Ro/SSA and anti-La/SSB should probably be restricted to the population at risk, that is, women with SLE, Sjögren's syndrome, and other systemic rheumatic diseases. As mentioned, a previous child with NLE puts future pregnancies at risk. A positive anti-Ro and anti-La would suggest a potential risk of 2 to 9% of neonatal lupus, as stated in greater detail under prevalence. In the prospective study of pregnancies in SLE and Sjögren's syndrome patients with anti-Ro and anti-La by Drosos et al., the prevalence of CHB was 8.8%.[D292] Careful monitoring during gestation with the nonstress test and M-mode

echocardiography should be instituted from the sixteenth to eighteenth week of pregnancy.

Therapy in utero has been attempted in seven instances, four times with established heart block, and three as prophylaxis. Buyon et al. treated a lupus patient with anti-La/SSB antibodies, whose fetus showed evidence of heart block, presumed myocarditis, and pericardial and pleural effusion at 24 weeks of gestation.[B605] Plasmapheresis and dexamethasone, 9 mg/day, were used, followed by cesarean section at 31 weeks. There were no effusions or myocarditis evident at birth, but heart block persisted. Herreman et al. used prednisone and plasmapheresis from the twenty-third week, but, again the heart block went unabated.[H278] Laxer et al. treated a fetus at 31 weeks with digoxin and dexamethasone for severe fetal hydrops and bradycardia at 35 beats per minute; despite cesarean section and insertion of a pacemaker, the fetus died 3 hours later.[L108] Petri treated a woman with fetal heart block diagnosed at 22 weeks' gestation with dexamethasone, 8 mg/day—the patient refused plasmapheresis; the heart block persisted.[P158]

The following three patients were treated prophylactically. An ANA-positive woman with nine prior spontaneous abortions was treated with 5 to 10 mg/day of prednisone and delivered a child with complete heart block.[H176] A woman with pericarditis, polyarthralgia, anti-Ro/SSA, and anti-La/SSB had four unsuccessful pregnancies, including one with heart block and fetal bradycardia. She was given 25 mg prednisolone per day from the twelfth week of gestation and plasmapheresis, with reduction in anti-Ro titers;[B90] placenta previa caused interruption of plasmapheresis at 28 weeks and a live infant with transient bradycardia was delivered at 31 weeks, with anti-Ro in the cord blood. Buyon et al. treated a woman with Sjögren's syndrome, who had a prior child with heart block who had died, with plasmapheresis from week 19, prednisone at 23 weeks, changed to dexamethasone at 35 weeks;[B604] she had a live healthy baby through planned cesarean section. There was anti-Ro and anti-La in the cord blood. It is difficult to make any firm recommendations from these heroic efforts to save a much-threatened pregnancy; however, under the preceding circumstances, therapeutic heroism seems justified. Cutaneous NLE alone does not require much therapy beyond avoidance of sun exposure, sunblock, and hydrocortisone cream.[L45]

It is self-evident that rigorous followup of such a high-risk pregnancy by the obstetrician and rheumatologist, and the presence of a neonatologist at delivery, are essential. A report of anesthetic problems with complete fetal heart block has appeared.[P279]

LONGTERM PROGNOSIS OF THE CHILD WITH NLE

Early, perinatal mortality in congenital heart block has been mentioned under that segment. Late mortality may occur from arrhythmia,[C196,E146] pacemaker failure,[B604] or congestive heart failure.[M243,R97] A fascinating outcome is the occurrence of systemic rheumatic disease in adulthood or adolescence in children with neonatal lupus. Seven such children have been reported, two with cutaneous NLE and five with CHB.

1. The original patient of McCuistion and Schoch,[M254] who had cutaneous NLE, presented at age 19 with hair loss, weight loss, malar rash, leukopenia, positive ANA, membranous nephropathy, and oral ulcers.[F186] She did well on high doses of prednisone. Her mother had died of severe SLE.

2. A female infant with cutaneous NLE was born to a woman diagnosed with SLE at age 13 who died of SLE postpartum.[J9] At age 13 the child developed SLE with polyarthritis, a subcutaneous nodule, Coombs-positive hemolytic anemia, leukopenia, and nephritis, and required steroid therapy.[J10]

3. A 23-year-old woman with congenital heart block developed Adams-Stokes attacks and was given a permanent pacemaker. During the operation, pericarditis with effusion was noted, and she further developed noninfectious pneumonitis, anemia, positive ANA, Raynaud's phenomenon, and polyarthritis. She was diagnosed with SLE and responded to prednisone and azathioprine.[W95]

4. A fourth female, born to a mother with SLE, had congenital heart block, and at 23 years of age developed anemia, positive ANA, purpura, polyarthritis, dry eyes, and had a lip biopsy compatible with Sjögren's syndrome.[L56]

5. A fifth female with CHB and pulmonary regurgitation was born to a mother with SLE who died of a cerebrovascular accident at age 38.[L56] At age 19 the patient developed arthritis and, after a spontaneous abortion, vasculitis, positive LE cells, ANA, and anti-DNA.

6. A female with CHB, reported by Esscher and Scott, developed SLE at age 15.

7. A boy with CHB, reported by McCue et al., developed juvenile rheumatoid arthritis at age four and a half.[M252]

As a footnote we mention a report by Reichlin et al. of a fascinating family.[R114] An asymptomatic woman gave birth to a male infant with complete heart block. Antibodies to Ro/SSA and La/SSB have developed in the son, now age 33, and his mother developed features of SLE and Sjögren's syndrome 26 years after the birth of her son. Neonatal lupus erythematosus is a capricious experiment of nature that, hopefully, will be soon elucidated.

Part D

Lupus Nephritis

Chapter 53

LUPUS NEPHRITIS

Pathology, Pathogenesis, Clinicopathologic Correlations and Prognosis

VICTOR E. POLLAK
CONRAD L. PIRANI

PREVALENCE OF LUPUS NEPHRITIS

The classic studies of Klemperer et al., in 1941, based on autopsy material,[K284] and the observations of Muehrcke et al. in 1957, based on percutaneous kidney biopsies,[M642] showed that renal involvement is a frequent and serious feature of SLE. Clinically, renal disease is reported in about 50% of patients during the first year from the clinical diagnosis of SLE. The prevalence appears to increase in subsequent years.[B49,C130,E147,F105,G162,P245,R353,W39,W40] Furthermore, numerous kidney biopsy studies of SLE patients without clinical evidence of renal involvement have clearly shown that lesions of varying severity may occur in almost all patients.[B220,C164,H382,L152,M236,M642,W149] On the other hand, severe renal disease leading to death or the need for renal replacement therapy occurs in a much smaller percentage of all patients with SLE, probably about 15 to 20%.[B540,N107] A higher percentage of deaths from lupus nephritis (30% or more) has been reported from several nephrology centers, but this is probably because of the referral of patients with more severe renal disease.[A269,B48,C39,P245]

PATHOLOGY

The pleomorphic character of the lesions that may develop in the kidneys of SLE patients and the lack of uniformity in their interpretation has led to confusion and misunderstanding, but this has been greatly clarified in recent years. These lesions, which may involve both the glomeruli and other renal structures, have now been defined by the use of light microscopy (LM), immunofluorescence (IF), and electron microscopy (EM) (Table 53–1).[A269,A362,B49,B350,P204,S480,S659,T75]

Morphologic Classification

A simple classification of the various morphologic patterns of lupus nephritis proposed under the auspices of the World Health Organization (WHO)[P203] is based primarily on the characteristics of the glomerular lesions (Table 53–2). The great majority of cases can be entered into this classification scheme, which has been in general use for over almost 15 years. A more detailed classification, with many subclasses, was originally developed for the International Study of Kidney Diseases in Children,[C264] but has yet to be applied to large series of cases.

Class I. In this class, the kidneys are shown to be normal by LM, IF, and EM.

Class II. Mild to moderate mesangial changes can be noted (Fig. 53–1).

Class IIA. Lesions are normal by LM, but the presence of immune deposits is limited to the mesangium as revealed by IF and/or EM.

Class IIB. Lesions are characterized by mesangial hypercellularity and/or sclerosis with deposits. Immune deposits limited to the mesangium are shown by IF and/or EM.

In both class IIA and IIB lesions, no deposits in the periphery of the capillary wall are seen. Tubules, interstitium, and blood vessels are essentially normal by LM; in a small percentage of cases, immune deposits can be found by EM and/or IF in the tubular basement membranes and in the wall of small vessels.

Class III. Focal and segmental proliferative and/or necrotizing glomerulonephritis (GN; Fig. 53–2). The active form of class III lesions is characterized by focal and segmental mesangial and endocapillary hypercellularity, with associated narrowing of capillary lumens involving less than 50% of the total surface area of the glomeruli or tufts (WHO definition).[P203] As in other classes of lupus nephritis, mesangial hypercellularity may be the result of an increased number of mesangial type I (contractile) or type II (monocytic-phagocytic) cells.[M541,S180] In the more severe active and necrotizing forms, inflammatory cells, karyorrhexis (nuclear dust), "fibrinoid," destruction of basement membranes (glomerular basement membrane, GBM), capillary thrombi, and generally small epithelial crescents are present in various combinations. Hematoxyphil bodies are rare. By the use of IF and EM, immune deposits are found in the mesangium and along the peripheral capillary wall in a subendothelial position. Focal interstitial inflammation and tubular changes are almost always present. Deposits are detected in the tubular basement membranes, interstitium, and small vessels in about 50% of the biopsies.

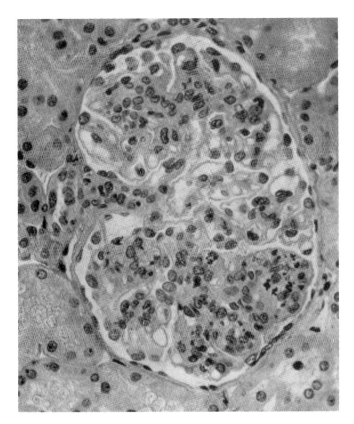

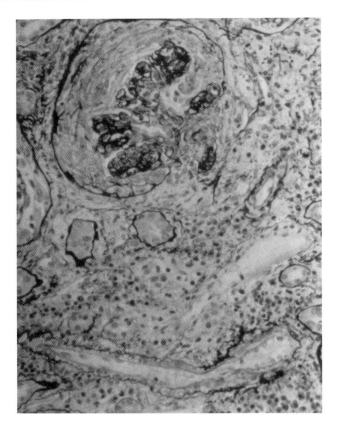

Fig. 53–3. Representative glomeruli s in active global and diffuse lupus glomerulonephritis (class IV). Prominent endocapillary hypercellularity involves practically the entire tuft. In two segmental areas, inflammatory cells and karyorrhexis are also present (H & E stain; ×400).

Fig. 53–4. Active severe global and diffuse lupus glomerulonephritis (class IV). In this glomerulus, a large fibro-epithelial crescent is seen compressing the tuft, which is partially sclerotic. In this biopsy, large and small crescents involved about 30% of the glomeruli. Most of the others were globally hypercellular. Moderate tubular atrophy and interstitial fibrosis indicate some degree of chronicity (silver-methenamine stain; ×240).

sional sparse, subepithelial deposits may be seen in other classes of lupus nephritis, but the term "membranous glomerulonephritis" should be reserved for those with numerous, regularly distributed, subepithelial deposits.

Mixed Forms. It is not uncommon to find segmental or global proliferative and/or necrotizing lesions of the type seen in class III and IV lesions associated with a diffuse membraneous lupus nephritis (class V). In this type of histologic lesion, class III and IV lesions often appear to be of more recent development than those of class V. Clinically, these patients should be considered to have a

more active form of lupus nephritis (class III or IV), and should be treated accordingly.[D256,K54,P238]

Prevalence of Different Classes

The prevalence of different patterns of lupus nephritis is summarized in Table 53–3. Most cases (between 43 and 62% in the several series) fall into classes III and IV. The five series summarized are from centers in which renal biopsies were being done systematically in all SLE

Table 53–3. Prevalence of Histologic Findings in Five Series of SLE Patients

Class	Feature(s)	Mery 1973[M362]	Baldwin 1977[B49]	Appel 1978[A269]	Kant 1981[K54]	Tateno 1983[T75]	Total
I	Normal kidney		0	0	1	0	1
IIA, IIB	Mild to moderate mesangial changes	25	12	22	22	17	98
III	Focal, segmental, proliferative GN	20	12	15	5	16	68
IV	Diffuse, proliferative GN	34	38	9	34	27	142
V	Membranous GN	8	20	10	8	14	60
	Chronic sclerosing GN	0	6	0	1	0	7
	Total	87	88	56	71	74	376

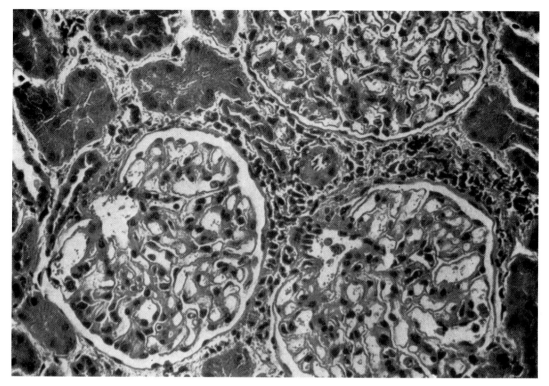

Fig. 53–5. Membranous lupus glomerulonephritis (class V). Mild, diffuse thickening of the capillary basement membrane occurs in all glomeruli, but no significant hypercellularity or necrosis. Note that the interstitial tissue between the glomeruli is infiltrated by numerous lymphocytes and plasma cells (H & E stain; ×200).

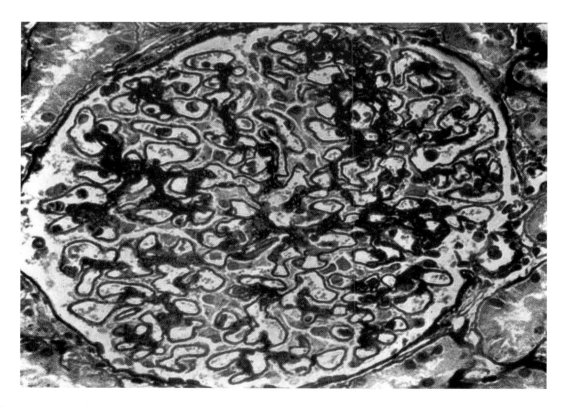

Fig. 53–6. Membranous lupus glomerulonephritis (class V). Diffuse, mild thickening of the glomerular capillary basement membrane is present, but no other significant changes (2-μ section; silver-methenamine stain; ×370).

patients, whether or not obvious clinical evidence of renal involvement was present. Because such centers serve as referral centers for both renal disease and SLE patients, lesser degrees of involvement (classes I and II) are probably underrepresented.

Comments on the WHO Classification System

The major advantage of the use of the WHO classification system over previously used classifications is the recognition of a strictly mesangial pattern (class II) and its separation from the focal and segmental pattern (class III), in which the lesions may involve only a few glomeruli but affect the peripheral portion of the glomerular capillary wall.[A269,B49,P238] Previously, many investigators considered class II and III lupus nephritis, at least in their mild forms, to be a single pattern,[B50,M642,P245] although their clinical evolution is often different.

Several features of the WHO classification require clarification. Class IIB lesions mild to moderate mesangial changes, can have a segmental or global distribution, and can be focal or diffuse if all glomeruli are considered. In some patients, the mesangial hypercellularity of class IIB lesions may extend for a short distance to the peripheral capillary wall, with mesangial cell interposition. When this process is more pronounced, and glomeruli have the features of membranoproliferative glomerulonephritis, these patients should be considered as having a form of diffuse proliferative lupus glomerulonephritis (class IV). Classes III and IV are characterized by the same type of lesions, varying only in severity and distribution, and progression from class III to IV is common. The clinical features and evolution of these two classes tend to be similar. Therefore, it might be preferable to combine the focal (class III) and diffuse (class IV) forms of proliferative and necrotizing GN in a single class, and to indicate whether the glomerular lesions are mild, moderate, or severe, depending on the percentage of involved glomeruli.[H304,K53,P204,T75] A possible source of confusion is that mild to moderate mesangial hypercellularity characteristic of class IIB is also almost invariably present in classes III, IV, and V, even in those glomeruli or segments of glomeruli that are not involved by more severe lesions. Finally, definite "mixed" forms, such as class III or IV associated with class V (diffuse membranous glomerulonephritis), can be present. From a clinical view-point, it is prudent to regard these patients as behaving like those in class III or IV. Inactive glomerular lesions, such as sclerosing changes and thickening of the GBM, with or without associated immune deposits and/or residual proliferative or necrotizing changes, tend to have the same distribution as the active lesions, (i.e., mesangial segmental or global).

The WHO classification system is based primarily on the glomerular changes. It should be emphasized, however, that tubular, interstitial, and vascular lesions may be a prominent feature of lupus nephritis, especially in classes III, IV, and V. From a renal functional standpoint, these lesions may be of considerable importance.[M61,P44,R215,S211] Interstitial and vascular changes in lupus nephritis may to a large extent be secondary to and reflect the activity, severity, and chronicity of glomerular lesions, as is the case in many other glomerular diseases. It is well known, however, that immune deposits may be present in tubular basement membranes, interstitium, and arterial wall in about 50% of biopsies from patients with lupus nephritis, a prevalence considerably higher than that observed in any other form of immune-mediated renal disease, with the exception of anti-GBM disease.

Interstitial inflammation, consisting primarily of lymphocytes and plasma cells, may be prominent, and is usually associated with a comparable degree of interstitial edema and eventually fibrosis. Interstitial inflammatory cell infiltrates tend to be located predominantly around involved glomeruli in class III and are more diffuse in classes IV and V; they are also often seen around small veins. Generally, a good correlation is noted between the degree of glomerular and interstitial changes and that of degenerative and/or atrophic lesions of the tubules.

Interstitial inflammatory cell infiltrates, especially when plasma cells are numerous, must be considered an active type of lesions and treated accordingly. In lupus nephritis, interstitial inflammation is considered by many[B299,L163,P44,S211] to be caused by deposits of immune complexes in the tubular basement membranes, in the interstitium proper, or in the walls of the small blood vessels. Interstitial inflammation in lupus nephritis, however, may be present even in the absence of tubulointerstitial immune complex deposits, a finding that is also common in other renal diseases of nonimmune pathogenesis, such as arteriolar nephrosclerosis. Using monoclonal antibodies, it was found that the T4:T8 cell ratio is significantly lower in lupus nephritis than in other renal diseases.[D8] Whatever their pathogenesis, tubulointerstitial lesions contribute significantly to the degree of renal insufficiency that might occur in lupus nephritis. Only in rare instances, however, does the renal insufficiency appear to be caused predominantly or exclusively by the presence of interstitial nephritis in the absence of significant glomerular lesions.[C130,C455,T225] In these cases, the possibility that the tubulointerstitial lesions are caused by drug toxicity or infection must be carefully excluded.

Arterial and arteriolar lesions have not been taken into consideration, either in the WHO classification or in activity and chronicity indices, even though they may influence the prognosis significantly. Vascular lesions are not rare, and involve almost exclusively intralobular arteries and arterioles with different morphologic features, which probably have a diverse pathogenesis. Larger vessels are usually spared. The most common type of lupus vasculopathy is the presence of large or small immune complex deposits in the intima and media (Fig. 53–7). This change, best defined by immunofluorescence and electron microscopy, should not be confused with the much less common lesion, frank necrosis of the vessel wall, in which fibrin-related antigens (FRAs) are invariably present in the mural deposits, together with immunoglobulins and complement fractions, and might or might not be associated with fibrin-platelet thrombi in the arterial lumen.

Fibrin-platelet thrombi, particularly in afferent arterioles (as well as in glomerular capillaries), are especially common in renal biopsies from patients with circulating anticardiolipin antibodies, the so-called lupus anticoagulant.[B289,D6,D170,G62,G203,K54,K229] Similar arterial changes

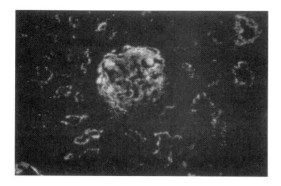

Fig. 53–7. Active, diffuse, proliferative lupus glomerulonephritis (class IV). Glomerular IgG granular deposits occur along the capillary walls and in the mesangial areas. Similar deposits are also present along the tubular basement membranes (IF; frozen section; × 200.)

are also found in a relatively rare clinical entity in which SLE is associated with severe thrombocytopenia (Fig. 53–8).[G84] These three types of arterial lesions are not associated with arterial or periarterial inflammatory cell infiltrates, and differ completely from the lesions of polyarteritis nodosa and hypersensitivity angiitis. They should be referred to as a lupus vasculopathy rather than a lupus vasculitis.[A268,B286,G397] If true arteritic lesions occur in patients with apparent lupus nephritis, they should probably be interpreted as part of a mixed connective tissue disease, rather than as a feature or complication of lupus nephritis.

Renal vein thrombosis is another vascular complication of lupus nephritis. It occurs almost exclusively in patients with the membranous form of lupus glomerulonephritis (WHO class V) and the nephrotic syndrome. It is still not clear why renal vein thrombosis should occur preferentially with the membranous rather than with the other

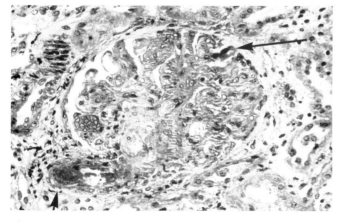

Fig. 53-8. Renal biopsy from a 50-year-old woman with a 12-year history of active serology, circulating lupus anticoagulant, and mild renal disease. Following corticosteroid therapy, she developed thrombocytopenia and renal failure. Renal biopsy disclosed lupus nephritis, WHO class IIB, with recent thrombi in afferent arterioles and glomerular capillaries (arrows) (trichrome stain; × 250).

forms of lupus nephritis, even when associated with the nephrotic syndrome.[A270,B452]

All classifications are somewhat arbitrary and rigid, but they are necessary to enhance our understanding and as a general outline. In SLE the lesions are pleomorphic, and overlap between classes is common. Most important clinically, for the prognostic and therapeutic implications, is recognition of active lesions, even in a few glomeruli and of relatively minor degree. These active lesions should be considered to be clinically important, whatever the histologic class or clinical and laboratory features of the disease.

Immunopathologic and Electron Microscopic Studies

Immunopathologic and electronmicroscopic studies have contributed significantly to the understanding of lupus nephritis lesions. Using IF and immunoperoxidase methods (Figs. 53–9, 53–10) glomerular, tubulointerstitial, and arterial immune deposits are almost invariably granular, and have been shown to consist of immunoglobulins (IgG, IgA, and IgM) and complement fractions (C1q, C3, and C4).[B477,D236,K336,M455] The membrane attack complex (C5–C9) has also been detected within deposits in a large proportion of cases.[B299,K204] Fibrin-related antigens are frequently found along the glomerular capillary wall in a subendothelial position, especially in those with the active and severe forms of lupus nephritis (classes III and IV); they have been reported in about half of all renal biopsies from those with class IV nephritis.[B73,K54] The presence of FRA is most unusual when the disease and the deposits are limited to the mesangium (class II). FRA is uncommon, but does appear in a few cases in which the deposits occur in the subepithelial areas (class V). The so-called hyaline thrombi present within glomerular capillaries have usually been shown to contain FRA, which is often admixed with immunoglobulins and complement fractions.[K204] Histochemical methods for fibrin (PTAH and Lendrum) often stain these thrombi only in part, or occasionally not at all. Properdin is frequently present in the glomeruli, especially in classes III and IV, which indicates that the complement system may be activated by the alternate and by the classic pathway.[M233] DNA antigens and anti-DNA antibodies have also been detected in immune deposits, or after elution of immunoglobulins from renal biopsies.[A221] Immune deposits are more abundant in the active glomerular lesions but tend to persist, although in much smaller amounts, even in the more chronic sclerotic lesions. Immune deposits in tubular basement membranes, interstitium, and arterial walls appear to have a similar but more variable composition than that of the glomerular deposits.

More recently, the use of immunopathologic and histochemical methods, particularly those using monoclonal antibodies for the identification of surface antigens, has revealed increased numbers of monocytes in the glomeruli, especially in class IV lupus nephritis.[J135,M541] Also, in the active forms of lupus nephritis, these methods have shown a relative increase in T8 (suppressor-cytotoxic)

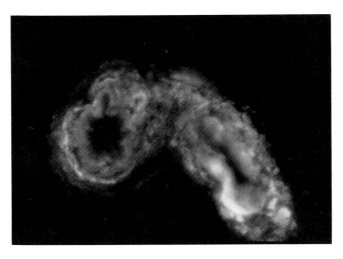

Fig. 53-9. Lupus nephritis, WHO class III. This renal interlobular artery contains segmental intimal and medial deposits of complement (immunofluorescence; × 540).

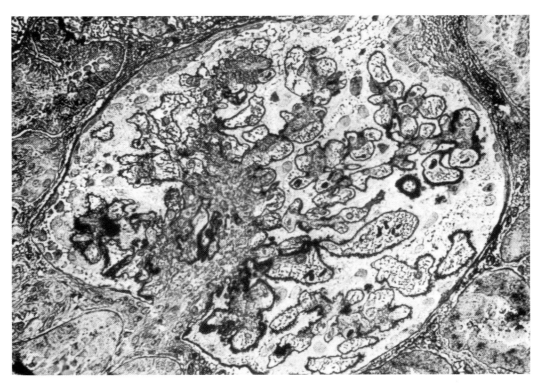

Fig. 53–10. Diffuse lupus glomerulonephritis. The distribution of IgG (γ chain) is shown. An area of sclerosis from previous active disease is present. IgG is segmentally distributed in the subepithelial and intramembranous positions. A single subendothelial deposit can be identified slightly to the left of center in the lower portion of this photomicrograph. The patent glomerular capillaries contain IgG, as demonstrated by the immunoperoxidase technique with PAS-hematoxylin stain. (From Dujovne, I., et al.: The distribution and character of glomerular deposits in systemic lupus erythematosus. Kidney Int. 2:33, 1972.)

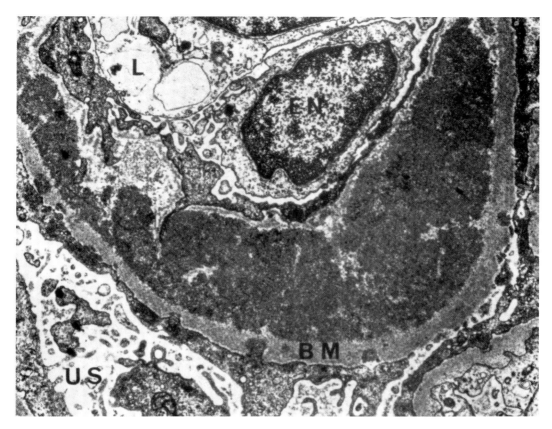

Fig. 53–11. Active lupus glomerulonephritis. The lumen (L) of this segment of glomerular capillary is almost completely filled by swollen endothelial cells (EN). Between the endothelium and the basement membrane (BM) is a large, semicircular, electron-dense deposit. Bowman's space (US) contains many elongated foot processes, which are almost completely fused along the basement membrane. This electron microscopic picture corresponds to the wire loop lesion of light microscopy (×6,200).

cells, with a resulting low T4 (helper):T8 ratio in the interstitial inflammatory cell infiltrates.[D8]

Ultrastructural studies can further delineate the character of the immune deposits in lupus nephritis (Figs. 53-11 through 53-15). They are usually well defined, electron-dense, and finely granular. In epimembranous and intramembranous areas, these can have a "washed out" or electron-lucent appearance, presumably representing their solubilization and gradual elimination. High-magnification EM often reveals, especially in subendothelial deposits, a substructure characterized by parallel arrays of curved or straight lines that frequently assume a fingerprint-like appearance (Fig. 53–13). This feature appears to be highly characteristic of lupus nephritis, because it is exceptionally rare in the deposits in other glomerular diseases.[G396,P202] Cryoglobulins, not infrequently elevated in the serum of SLE patients, can rarely be detected in the glomeruli by their typical microtubular substructure, usually within subendothelial deposits. Although FRAs are frequently found by IF in the more active glomerular lesions, fibrillar fibrin and fibrin-platelet thrombi are not often detected by EM. Indeed, EM has shown that "thrombi" thought to be free within the lumen of the capillaries by LM are usually intraluminal projections of massive subendothelial deposits containing immunoglobulins, complement fractions, and other serum proteins, as well as FRA. In a high proportion of cases, EM reveals the presence of membrane-bound tubular arrays, most frequently within the cytoplasm of glomerular endothelial cells; these are usually referred to as myxovirus-like aggregates (Fig. 53–12). Their presence is not related to the class or activity of lupus nephritis, but their high frequency can be of diagnostic value.[G36,H304,K284] These structures are not considered to represent viral particles, but rather are a form of cellular response to injury probably related to interferon ("interferon footprints"). Myxovirus-like particles are also found frequently in other immune-mediated renal diseases, including allograft rejection, and also in the acquired immunodeficiency syndrome (AIDS), a condition of viral origin.[G390,O96,R191,S105]

The most important contribution of EM in lupus nephritis is the precise localization of immune deposits (Fig. 53–16). This is impossible using LM and, even by IF, localization is often inaccurate. Deposits restricted to the mesangium and to subepithelial areas, (i.e., not directly in contact with the bloodstream) are associated with a less pronounced cellular reaction and, generally, with less activity and severity of the glomerular disease.[D350,P202] Con-

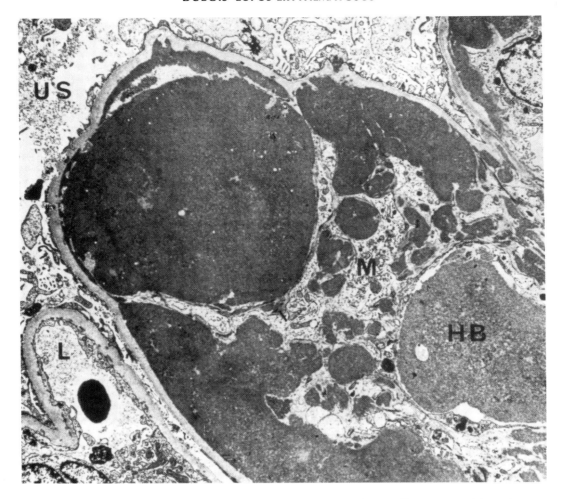

Fig. 53–12. Active lupus glomerulonephritis, segment of two glomerular capillaries. One of them has a patent lumen (L) containing a red blood cell. The other is markedly distended because of massive electron-dense desposits in the mesangium (M) and between the mesangium and the basement membrane. The lumen of this capillary is almost completely filled by a structure (HB) consistent with that of a degenerated nucleus, or hematox-yphil body (×4,800).

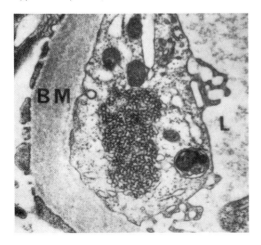

Fig. 53–13. Active lupus glomerulonephritis, segment of a glo-merular capillary. Within the cytoplasm of the endothelial cell is an accumulation of microtubular structures, considered by some to be of viral origin (×12,400).

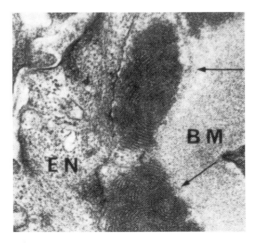

Fig. 53–14. Active lupus glomerulonephritis, segment of a glo-merular capillary. Between the basement membrane (BM) and the endothelium (EN) are several electron-dense deposits (ar-rows) with an organized fingerprint pattern (×15,200).

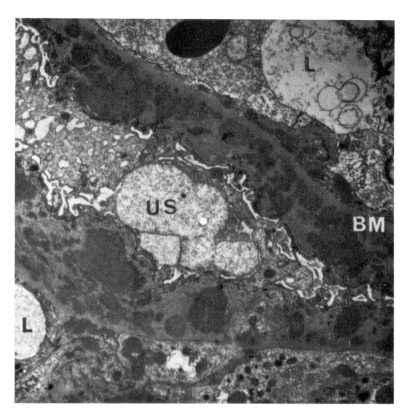

Fig. 53–15. Membranous form of lupus nephritis. This segment of two capillaries (L) is separated by a urinary space (US) that is almost completely filled by swollen epithelial cells. Between the basement membrane (BM) and the fused foot processes of the visceral epithelium are numerous electron-dense deposits, separated and often surrounded by protrusions (spikes) of basement membrane (× 6,240).

versely, subendothelial deposits are likely to be associated with endocapillary and extracapillary proliferative and inflammatory changes, including intravascular coagulation,[D215,D253,D350,T75] features that are all characteristic of active class III and IV lupus nephritis. Changes of the glomerular basement membrane, best seen by EM, include intramembranous, electron-dense deposits, intramembranous extensions of endothelial or epithelial cell cytoplasm, and actual gaps of the GBM.[P202,S659]

Differentiation of idiopathic membranous glomerulonephropathy from class V (membranous) lupus nephritis is also best achieved by EM. In the latter, the frequent transmembranous and intramembranous character of subepithelial deposits and the high prevalence of associated mesangial deposits and of myxovirus-like reticular structures in endothelial cells, are all strongly indicative of SLE.[J60,S212,S342]

PATHOGENESIS

Lupus nephritis is generally considered to be an autoimmune disease of chronic immune complex pathogenesis. This conclusion is based on several observations:

1. Presence of granular deposits of Ig and C components in glomeruli and other renal sites
2. Deposits of autologous DNA in glomeruli, in small arteries, and along the TBM
3. Glomerular eluates containing antibody of high specific activity to dsDNA
4. Circulating dsDNA–anti-dsDNA immune complexes
5. Decreased serum complement fractions and related fragments consistent with increased complement consumption
6. Correlation among activity and severity of renal lesions, increased levels of circulating immune com-

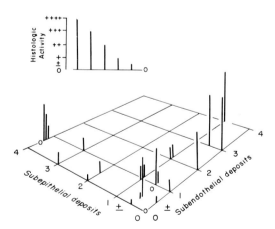

Fig. 53–16. Three-dimensional representation of the interrelationship among subendothelial deposits, subepithelial deposits, and histologic activity in biopsies from patients with lupus nephritis. These studies were made by electron microscopy, using ultrathin sections from three to four glomeruli per biopsy and a semiquantitative method to examine the site and extent of the deposits. Note that, with a single exception, either fairly extensive subendothelial or subepithelial deposits are present. (From Dujovne, I. et al.: The distribution and character of glomerular deposits in systemic lupus erythematosus. Kidney Int. 2:33, 1972.)

plexes, and greater decrease of serum complement levels.[A53,A221,C416,S217,S650]

Some patients with SLE and lupus nephritis may have no detectable antinuclear antibody (ANA) in the serum. In some cases of severe lupus nephritis, dsDNA—anti-dsDNA complexes are deposited extensively in the kidney and in other vessels, but no dsDNA antibody or ANA can be detected in the serum. Swaak and colleagues, in serial studies on patients with SLE, clearly showed that exacerbations of lupus nephritis are accompanied by a fall in the serum levels of both dsDNA antibody, measured quantitatively, and complement.[S782]

Some patients with clinical manifestations compatible with those of SLE have a persistently negative test for antinuclear antibodies.[H479,M48] These patients, who seem to comprise less than 5% of the total SLE population, frequently produce anticytoplasmic (anti-Ro and anti-La) rather than antinuclear antibodies. Clinically significant renal involvement has been reported in about 12% of these patients.[M48]

Cell-mediated mechanisms and an imbalance between B and T cells, as well as between T4 (helper) and T8 (suppressor) lymphocytes, may also play a role in the pathogenesis of lupus nephritis in general,[C217,D126,H86,M235,O84,W243] and in determining the development of different patterns of renal involvement.[D8,S519]

FACTORS AFFECTING THE PATTERN OF GLOMERULAR AND TUBULOINTERSTITIAL LESIONS

Immune Complexes

Size. In experimental animals, immune complexes may be deposited in glomeruli. If circulating immune complexes are deposited in the glomeruli in human SLE, complexes of intermediate size tend to be deposited predominantly in the glomeruli; their level in the blood might determine whether localization is limited to the mesangium (class II) or extends to the subendothelial areas (classes III and IV). Smaller complexes would localize preferentially in the subepithelial areas (class V).[G97,L225,O85] Large immune complexes tend to localize predominantly in the walls of small arteries and, passing into the postglomerular circulation, to be deposited along the tubular basement membranes and in the renal interstitium. Because larger immune complexes are probably in antibody excess, reduction in antibody production by corticosteroids and immunosuppressive therapy might explain the reported transformation of the proliferative to the membranous forms of lupus nephritis in treated patients.[H223a,L187,P204] Circulating dsDNA—anti-dsDNA immune complexes have been detected rarely,[168] however, and with difficulty.[B535] Conversely, evidence has shown that local formation of immune complexes ("planted" antigen) may be responsible for the epimembranous location of immune complexes in class V lupus nephritis.[C416,167] The affinity of DNA for glomerular basement membrane has been clearly shown,[167] and in SLE might provide a mechanism for in situ immune complex formation. One analysis has concluded that most studies that show cross-reactivity between anti-DNA antibody

and non-DNA targets used low-avidity IgM class antibody molecules, which are the least likely to be of pathogenic significance.[B496] The role of C1q may also be important. DNA binds to C1q, and it has been reported that renal disease is more likely to occur in SLE when the complexes contain C1q.[G364] On balance, the evidence seems increasingly to favor the importance of in situ immune complex formation.[C416]

Avidity. Immune complexes of high avidity tend to localize in the mesangial-subendothelial areas, and those of low avidity tend to localize in the subepithelial region[G98] or remain in the circulation.[W286] The finding that those with the proliferative form of lupus nephritis usually have precipitating antibodies and those with the membranous form have nonprecipitating antibodies is in accord with the importance of avidity of immune complexes in different types of lupus nephritis.[F255,G284]

Electrical Charge. Cationic immune complexes have been shown experimentally[G19] to localize along either side of the GBM and on the outer aspect of the tubular basement membrane (TBM), whereas anionic complexes localize preferentially in the mesangium.

Rate of Delivery and Production. In chronic serum sickness in the rabbit, increasing the rate of antigen administration and of delivery of complexes to the glomeruli may "transform" a membranous into a proliferative form of glomerulonephritis.[G97] Such a transformation (activation of membranous GN) has been observed in lupus nephritis.[A269,H305,S212]

Complement Activation. Complexes containing immunoglobulins that have low or no complement-activating properties cause less proliferative or inflammatory response (class V) than complexes with strongly reactive globulins.[L225] This might explain why comparable amounts of electron-dense deposits in classes IIA and IIB are sometimes associated with glomerular hypercellularity. Also, complement receptor is detectable in the podocytes of the membranous form but is absent in proliferative lupus nephritis.[E94] The possible role of altered expression of complement receptors and of inherited abnormalities of the complement system in the pathogenesis of SLE have been reviewed.[K137,P281,W264] In general, complement or receptor deficiencies appear to be associated predominantly with the milder mesangial (class II) or membranoproliferative (class IV) patterns of lupus nephritis.

Cellular Factors

Inflammatory cells, predominantly monocytes, are present in varying numbers in the glomeruli of those with proliferative forms of lupus nephritis (classes III and IV) and are almost absent in classes II and V. Polymorphonuclear leukocytes are usually present only in association with necrotizing lesions. Monocytes probably contribute in a significant manner not only to the hypercellularity of the proliferative forms of lupus nephritis but also to the severity of glomerular capillary lesions through the release of proteolytic enzymes[D74] and procoagulant factors,[C341] which have been detected using immunohistologic methods.[C55]

T cells are present only in small numbers within the glomerular tuft, whereas they are predominant in the interstitial inflammatory cellular infiltrates. The T4:T8 cell ratio varies greatly in the interstitial cell infiltrates but tends to be higher in those with more active glomerular lesions. Conversely, the T4:T8 ratio in the circulating blood does not correlate with either the type or activity of glomerular lesions.[D8]

Coagulation

Fibrin-related antigens (FRAs) are often demonstrated in those with the active forms of lupus nephritis (classes III and IV), especially in the subendothelial position in segmental and diffuse proliferative and/or necrotizing lesions.[K53,K204] True fibrin-platelet thrombi are less common, and are not necessarily associated with proliferative and/or necrotizing lesions. It is not clear whether the presence of FRA and/or true thrombi is the cause or the consequence of the presence of more severe glomerular capillary lesions. Immune complexes per se can activate the coagulation system. Levels of antibodies to Ia determinants, a normal antigenic component of glomerular endothelial cells,[N39] are elevated in the circulating blood of some patients with SLE.[O47] Endothelial cell damage produced by immune complexes, by anti-Ia antibodies, or by one or more of the many mediators of inflammation may be responsible for activation of the coagulation system in patients with lupus nephritis. Other evidence for activation of the coagulation system includes increases in serum and urine levels of fibrin(ogen) degradation products,[K89,M122] fibrinogen catabolism,[S288] and plasma levels of fibrinopeptide A.[C441] Monocyte infiltration in glomeruli and the consequent activation of the coagulation system has been thought to be a potentially important mechanism of damage. In patients with focal and diffuse proliferative lupus nephritis, Cole and colleagues demonstrated a marked increase in monocyte procoagulant activity, an active principle that can activate prothrombin directly.[C341] The prothrombinase activity was shown not to be factor Xa. This observation provides further evidence for a correlation between direct prothrombinase and endocapillary proliferation in lupus nephritis, and for a potential mechanism of injury.

Platelet involvement has also been shown by decreased numbers of circulating platelets,[C284,K54] an association of decreased circulating platelet levels with intraglomerular fibrin and thrombi,[K54] decreased levels of platelet serotonin,[P40] and the presence of high titers of platelet aggregating material.[K56] Platelet-related antigens have been demonstrated by immunofluorescence in kidney biopsy specimens of patients with lupus nephritis.[D5] Although many of the studies cited show correlations between platelet and coagulation abnormalities and activity of SLE and lupus nephritis, this has not been the universal experience.[G170] The occurrence of systemic venous and arteriolar and of glomerular capillary thrombosis in patients with the circulating anticoagulant has been emphasized.[G203,K54]

Only recently have abnormalities of fibrinolysis been described. A decreased fibrinolytic capability was suggested by studies of euglobulin lysis times at rest and after forearm venous occlusion.[A233] Decreased levels of vascular plasminogen activator were found in about 60%, elevated levels of an inhibitor of plasminogen activator in about 90%, and increased levels of α2-antiplasmin in about 25% of patients with SLE.[G181]

CLINICOPATHOLOGIC CORRELATIONS[A269,B49,C39,K54,M608,P243,P246,S734,T75]

Class I. The number of SLE patients reported in the literature in whom renal biopsy studied by LM, EM, and IF demonstrated neither glomerular nor other abnormalities is extremely small. This precludes any reliable correlation with clinical and laboratory features. Rare cases of SLE patients with entirely normal renal biopsies have occurred; these presented with microscopic hematuria and mild proteinuria. Some may be explained by the extreme focality of glomerular lesions, which may have been missed because of the limitations of renal sampling.

Class IIA. Only about one-third of patients with mesangial deposits but no hypercellularity have leukocyturia, hematuria, and mild proteinuria; most of these were associated with normal renal function. Serum DNA binding and complement levels may be slightly abnormal.

Class IIB. About half of patients with mild to moderate mesangial hypercellularity have mild hematuria and proteinuria, usually less than 1 g/24 hr. Nephrotic range proteinuria is most unusual. Mild renal insufficiency is present in less than 30% of patients. About one-third of these patients have elevated DNA binding and decreased serum complement levels.

Class III. Almost all patients in this group have proteinuria, usually 1 g/24 hr or more, and about 20 to 30% of them have the nephrotic syndrome. Hematuria and leukocyturia are more pronounced than in classes IIA and IIB, and appear to be related to the degree of activity of the glomerular lesions. A decreased glomerular filtration rate (GFR), mild to moderate renal insufficiency, and diastolic hypertension, are present in about one-third of patients. Abnormal serum DNA binding and complement levels are detected in about 80% of patients.

Class IV. Hematuria, leukocyturia, and proteinuria are more pronounced than in class III, and are present in almost all patients. The nephrotic syndrome is present in about 60% and hypertension in 40% of patients. The GFR is moderately to markedly decreased in most patients. Renal insufficiency appears to be the result, not only of the more diffuse and severe glomerular lesions but, to a considerable extent, also of the invariably associated and often prominent tubulointerstitial changes.[P44,S211] Serum DNA binding levels are increased and serum complement fractions decreased in almost all patients.

Class V. The clinical hallmark of membranous lupus nephritis is severe proteinuria; about 50% of patients develop the nephrotic syndrome. The urinary sediment is active in less than one-third of patients. Decreased renal function and hypertension are unusual, but may develop in those with the more chronic forms. Serologic findings are variable; often dsDNA antibody levels are not elevated, and serum complement (C3 and C4) levels have been found by many (but not all) to be within normal limits. Serum antibodies are often of the nonprecipitating type.

In trying to interpret the relationship of certain clinical findings to the renal histology, it is important to keep several points in mind:

1. No test or combination of tests—whether the results are positive or negative—correlates so well with the underlying renal histology that it can be used uncritically to predict the presence or absence of certain types of renal injury.
2. Although serum complement, ANA, and anti-dsDNA levels are helpful in the diagnosis of SLE, their determination can be used with less assurance to diagnose the presence of certain types of histologic changes in the kidney in SLE patients.
3. The fact that these tests are helpful in the diagnosis of SLE and of renal involvement does not necessarily mean that they are important for the longterm follow-up of patients with SLE and renal disease, nor does it mean that they can be used reliably to predict whether new episodes of renal involvement have occurred.

Unfortunately, little correlation has been found between various types of extrarenal organ system involvement in patients with SLE and the nature of the renal disease, with perhaps, one exception. A high incidence of venous and/or arteriocapillary thrombotic events in patients with circulating anticoagulant has been noted. Circulating anticoagulant is often but not invariably associated with class IV and V disease, in which thrombosis in the glomeruli and renal arterioles is the dominant pathology.[G203,K54] In such patients the anti-dsDNA antibody is frequently undetectable.

Urinalysis should be done carefully in SLE patients. Microscopic hematuria and microscopic pyuria without infection, or both, with or without occasional casts, is a frequent indication of glomerular inflammatory change. These abnormalities are present in most but not all patients with proliferative GN (classes III and IV), in about 25% of those with mesangial lupus (class II), and in 50% or more of those with membranous GN (class V). Significant numbers of casts are found, predominantly in the urine of patients with proliferative GN. Proteinuria occurs in almost all patients with proliferative and with membranous GN, and is seen in about 50% of patients with mesangial lupus. Massive proteinuria and nephrotic syndrome does not occur in mesangial lupus, is relatively uncommon in focal proliferative GN, and occurs in about 70% or more of patients with diffuse proliferative GN (class IV) and membranous GN (class V). Because we believe that the early detection of new glomerular change is important, we have found it useful for patients to test their urine regularly using a dipstick to detect a recurrence of or increase in hematuria and/or proteinuria.

When interpreting data on renal function in SLE patients, it is important to recall that the glomerular lesions may be strictly mesangial and progress rarely, or that the lesions may initially be focal and segmental proliferative and later progress to severe involvement of most glomerular capillary loops. Thus, the GFR may be relatively well maintained, and the flow of blood from the glomerulus into the peritubular capillary system intact, until advanced, severe, glomerular changes occur. Also, most patients with SLE and lupus nephritis are relatively young women who often have only a modest muscle mass, and whose normal serum creatinine values generally cluster around or just above the lower limits prescribed by the clinical laboratory. In these patients, therefore, any serum creatinine values of 1 mg/dl or greater should be considered as probably abnormal, perhaps even significantly abnormal. Elevated levels of creatinine and urea nitrogen are found in many patients with diffuse proliferative GN (class IV) and in a lesser number of patients with membranous GN (class V). Elevated creatinine and urea nitrogen levels are rare in patients with mesangial lupus (class II); any disturbance of renal function should raise the question of whether more serious renal disease is present.

A decrease in the serum hemolytic complement or C3 level is found in most patients with proliferative GN. This has little diagnostic predictive value, however, because the level is decreased in a significant proportion of patients with mesangial lupus (class II) or membranous GN (class V). The proportion of patients with focal and diffuse proliferative GN (classes III and IV) is higher than that of patients with mesangial lupus (class II) or membranous GN (class IV) in whom the LE test is positive, and in whom increased levels of anti-dsDNA antibody and of antinuclear antibody are present. Similarly, they appear to have limited value in predicting whether an exacerbation of underlying glomerular nephritis has occurred. The combination of low complement levels and elevated levels of anti-dsDNA antibody is a better predictor of proliferative forms of glomerular nephritis, but does not distinguish them in absolute terms from mesangial lupus and membranous glomerular nephritis. Several authors have drawn attention to platelet behavior in those with lupus nephritis. Evidence is emerging that decreased platelet counts may be helpful in predicting the proliferative forms of glomerulonephritis.

NATURAL HISTORY AND TRANSFORMATION FROM ONE HISTOLOGIC PATTERN TO ANOTHER

The "true" natural history of renal involvement in SLE is poorly understood, primarily because almost every patient has, during the last 35 years or so, been treated with corticosteroids and/or immunosuppressive drugs. It was once thought[G163] that the spectrum of glomerular lesions in SLE represents a continuum in the evolution of the renal disease, but experience is not consistent with this view. Progression of the renal histologic changes from class II to classes III, IV, or V appears to be uncommon. Most patients with mesangial hypercellularity only do not subsequently develop the proliferative forms of lupus glomerulonephritis. In literature review, Silva found that 24 of 74 patients with class II lupus nephritis had transformed, on serial biopsy, to class III, IV, or V.[S435] Because most patients with class II lesions have little clinical evidence of progressive disease, serial renal biopsies are probably done less frequently than in those with any other class of involvement, and serial renal biopsies are more likely to be done when clinical evidence of progression is present. The 28% incidence of transformation from class II to classes III and IV seems to be a gross overestimate. Transformation from class II to the more serious classes III and IV probably occurs in no more than 5% of patients. Transformation of histologic class III to IV occurred in 27 of 66 patients (41%) summarized by Silva.[S435] As indicated earlier, class III should be regarded simply as a milder and earlier stage of proliferative glomerulonephritis. Thus, this should be regarded not as a transformation, but rather as an expression of more severe involvement of the same type of disease process.[Z30] The actual incidence of change from class III (focal) to class IV (diffuse) may be lower because of the tendency to select patients with class III lesions who have later evidence of clinical deterioration for biopsy. Transformation from class III or IV to class V has been reported in 19 of 169 biopsies, and appears to be associated with relatively successful treatment of focal or diffuse proliferative glomerulonephritis with corticosteroids and immunosuppressives. Successful treatment of patients in class IV with these agents has long been known to result in considerable improvement in renal histologic findings, and therefore to produce a transformation "from class IV to classes II, III, or V.[C264,H305,M568]

Several studies have shown that subendothelial immune deposits tend to decrease or disappear totally following therapy, except when they are extensive[D350,K204,M362] (Fig. 53–16). Deposits in mesangial and subepithelial locations may decrease in amount but are less likely to disappear completely. Glomerular hypercellularity, whether resulting from proliferation or inflammation, may also be markedly reduced by therapy. This has been shown with prednisone treatment,[O38,P245] probably occurs somewhat more rapidly when alkylating agents are given in addition to prednisone,[D214] and has also been shown to occur after treatment with the defibrinogenating agent ancrod.[K53,K204] The extent of the interstitial inflammatory cell infiltrates is usually also reduced. Varying degrees of segmental or global glomerular sclerosis, interstitial fibrosis, and tubular atrophy may develop, depending on the severity of the changes, the presence or absence of glomerular necrotizing lesions, and of capillary thrombi, and the adequacy of treatment.[A362,K54,P245] In other words, "active" lesions are transformed into inactive, irreversible changes that slowly progress probably because of factors unrelated to SLE (e.g., hypertension and functional overload on residual functioning nephrons).[D47,H441] An elevated chronicity index, based on the degree of glomerular sclerosis, fibrotic crescents, and interstitial fibrosis, has been shown to be a more reliable index of poor prognosis than the activity index. The arrest of progression of less severe active lesions and the prevention of the development of new ones are probably the important elements in the clinical and functional improvement of patients following therapy. Lack of or inadequate treatment, according to older studies,[K284,M642] was associated with the development of more diffuse active lesions and more rapid progression of the renal injury.

PROGNOSIS

The different WHO classes of lupus nephritis, when determined at the time of clinical onset of renal disease, have different prognostic implications (Fig. 53–17). Data from several large series of patients studied in the 1950s and 1960s[B50,C220,H239,P245,Z68] indicated that patient survival at 4 years was about 65% for class III, 25% for class IV, and 85% for class V. The existence of class II (exclusively mesangial disease) was not clearly recognized at that time. The relatively good prognosis assigned to class III was probably the result, least in part, of the inclusion of class II patients in class III. When these data were reanalyzed, taking the WHO classification into account, the 4-year survival of patients with exclusively mesangial disease (class II) was about 84% and that of patients with focal GN (class III) was about 45%[P238] In the 1950s and 1960s, most patients were treated with corticosteroids in moderate or

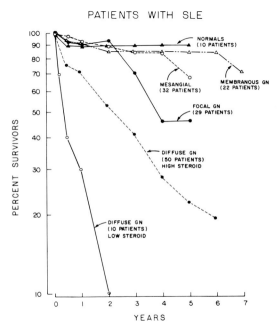

Fig. 53–17. Survival, calculated by life table analysis from the time of the initial renal biopsy, in two series of patients with SLE. Patients were divided into groups according to the findings of the initial biopsy. The histologic classification in the original papers has been reclassified using the WHO terminology. These results are for patients studied and treated 35 to 50 years ago. The 5-year survival was good in patients with normal kidneys, with mesangial lupus (class II), and with membranous lupus nephritis (class V). Survival of patients with focal glomerulonephritis (class III) was better than that of patients with diffuse glomerulonephritis (class IV). The mortality in class III patients began about 2 to 3 years after the initial study, but thereafter the curve parallels that of class IV patients. The 5-year survival of patients with diffuse glomerulonephritis was about 25%. In patients studied and reported since 1970, the major difference is the improvement in survival of patients with diffuse glomerulonephritis (class IV); the 5-year survival is now about 45 to 70%. (Modified from Pollak V. E., and Dosekun, A. K.: Evaluation of treatment in lupus nephritis: Effects of prednisone. Am. J. Kidney Dis., 2, Suppl. 1:70, 1972.)

high dosage, but relatively few were given immunosuppressive agents.

More recent studies[A266,A269,A362,C39,D114,D214,D259,G161,H130,M60,P255,R321,,R426,T75,W12,W39] have shown a significant improvement in prognosis. The survival of patients in classes III and IV now appears to be 65 to 75% or better at 4 years. Most investigators[B48,P238,R321,T75,W39] have found that the prognosis for class III is considerably better than that for class IV. The shape of the survival curve (Fig. 53–17) suggests that, in class IV patients, death starts early, whereas in class III patients a delay of about 2 years occurs before death; thereafter, the survival curves for classes III and IV patients are parallel.[P238] This is consistent with the belief that classes III and IV represent different degrees of severity of the same disease process.

The prognosis for patients with mesangial disease alone (class II) and membranous disease (class V) has been shown to be relatively good; the 4-year survival of series published in the 1960s was about 85%.[P238] The prognosis for these two groups of patients has not improved significantly until now. It seems that many deaths, especially in patients with class II disease, were caused not by renal disease but by infectious and cardiovascular and cerebral complications, generally attributable to corticosteroid treatment.[P240] Large doses of corticosteroids are inappropriate for patients in classes II and V.

The improvement in the prognosis of lupus nephritis can be attributed to several factors. These include the following: 1) a greater awareness of the importance of renal involvement in SLE among rheumatologists and internists; 2) earlier and more precise diagnosis of the type and severity of renal lesions through a more liberal use of renal biopsy, even when the clinical renal disease is mild; 3) more appropriate use of corticosteroids and immunosuppressive agents, and particularly of alkylating agents; 4) better control of nonrenal complications, either of those that are part of the SLE syndrome or those that are related to therapy. Nevertheless, large doses of prednisone are now used commonly in treatment, and are often given over long periods, without knowledge of the nature and severity of the renal disease. Relatively few longterm studies of patients followed for 8 to 15 years after diagnosis of the type of renal involvement have been done.[A266,C39,D256,H130,P221,P255]

Several studies of lupus nephritis, noted an obvious clustering of some patients who presented with or rapidly progressed to extremely severe renal involvement, with a rapidly progressive renal failure, within 2 to 3 years from onset ("malignant lupus nephritis").[A266,P245] These were predominantly class IV patients. Early identification of these patients, their possible differentiation from others with class IV disease by clinical and laboratory means, and the selection of more appropriate treatment might lead to a better prognosis, even in this group.

Activity and Chronicity Indices

Individual histopathologic features, such as subendothelial deposits, glomerular sclerosis, and interstitial inflammation, graded appropriately by severity and analyzed individually or in clusters (e.g., activity index, chronicity index) have also been used for prognosis.[A362,B73,D214,D350,H130,H304,K54,K204,M60,M568,R240,R426,T75,W208] Of those with active lesions, the presence and abundance of subendothelial deposits, the presence of numerous epithelial crescents, and the degree of interstitial inflammation at the onset of renal disease appear to be reasonably accurate indicators of a poor short-term prognosis, especially if the patient has been inadequately treated. A high chronicity index (glomerular sclerosis, fibrotic crescents, interstitial fibrosis) has been emphasized as a most accurate indication of a poor prognosis.[A362,O38] This is not surprising, because the lesions that comprise this index represent evidence of previous damage, and are generally considered to be slowly progressive and unresponsive to treatment. Whereas the value of the activity index has long been recognized, the importance of thrombosis as a predictor of progressive glomerular sclerosis was only shown more recently.[B73,H130,K53,K54,K204] A microvascular thrombosis index[K53] comprised of glomerular thrombi, subendothelial deposits, fibrinoid, and arteriolar fibrinoid also seems valuable. In future studies it would seem appropriate to include microvascular thrombosis in the activity index and arteriolar sclerosis in the chronicity index.

In the interpretation of biopsies taken early in the clinical course, sclerotic and fibrotic lesions are likely to be absent or mild, and the chronicity index is therefore likely to be low.[P255] Here, the prognosis probably depends on the extent and precise nature of the lesions, and extensive evidence of thrombosis may be the forerunner of later sclerosis and fibrosis.

Clinical Correlates

The clinical features that appear to be important in predicting the evolution of renal disease and in determining prognosis have been reviewed.[P240] Younger age (<23 years), male sex, and elevated serum creatinine levels (>1.3 mg/dl) were the only findings clearly identified as being associated with a bad prognosis in one study;[A362] in another, the longterm survival in children was excellent.[P221] Nephrotic syndrome occurs commonly in patients with class V lesions in whom the prognosis is relatively good, and in those with class III and IV, in whom it is probably associated with a somewhat worse prognosis. None of the nonrenal systemic manifestations of SLE, including cutaneous, cardiac, central nervous system, and pulmonary, nor such widely used serologic findings as complement and anti-DNA levels, seem to correlate with severity or prognosis.[A269,A362,K204,R426]

ROLE OF RENAL BIOPSY

The clinical value of renal biopsy in lupus nephritis is controversial. Some question its usefulness,[F262,M239,W208,W209] whereas others recommend its use for every SLE patient, even in the absence of clinical and laboratory data indicating renal involvement.[A362,B47,B64,M64] Most investigators agree that it is impossible to predict the type, severity, and activity of renal lesions from any combination of clinical and laboratory findings. Therefore, the question should properly be asked whether a patient with SLE should be treated with potentially dangerous drugs[A233,C327,E153,E155,G159,H130,O38,P240,R386] without knowing the type of pathologic process present in the kidney with reasonable precision.[P201] The type of treatment required to control or reverse certain immunologic or renal function manifestations might be different from that needed to arrest the progression of or reverse the different types of renal lesions that may be present in the kidneys. Class IIA, class V, and perhaps class IIB lupus nephritis might be a result of pathogenic mechanisms different from those involved in classes III and IV. Also, because of the relatively high incidence of nonrenal deaths in class II patients, less aggressive treatment appears to be indicated for this group and for class V patients, for different reasons (see above).

In view of the importance of glomerular and arteriolar thrombi as predictors of later glomerular sclerosis, it is important to assess the relative contributions of inflammatory and necrotic changes on the one hand and of microvascular thrombosis on the other. Also, in a subset of patients with circulating anticoagulants, the renal pathology may be dominated by microvascular thrombosis.[G203,K54] Corticosteroid treatment does not appear to have favorable effects, and might have adverse effects in these patients. No general guidelines can be established, however, and every patient must be evaluated individually. A close collaboration between the clinical nephrologist and renal pathologist is most important before making a decision about the therapeutic approach most appropriate for each patient.[P201] The value of renal biopsy is greater if obtained early in the course of the renal disease, when appropriate therapy is more likely to halt or slow progression of the active lesions and prevent their transformation to irreversible changes.

Chapter 54

LUPUS NEPHRITIS

DANIEL J. WALLACE
BEVRA H. HAHN
JOHN H. KLIPPEL

Renal involvement in SLE is one of the most serious complications of the disorder. Virtually all studies of prognosis have identified lupus nephritis as a predictor of a poor outcome.

Chronic glomerulonephritis was first described in 4 SLE patients in 1922.[K147] Baehr, Klemperer, and Schifrin observed "wire loop" lesions at autopsy in 13 of 23 lupus patients in 1935 and associated it with the disease.[B18] In the late 1950s, pioneers in rheumatology including Dixon, Holman, Mellors, Kunkel, and Muller-Eberhard among others[F225,F273,L6,M350,V54] noted that positive LE-cell preps were often found in patients who had immune deposits in renal tissue. The introduction of the LE-cell prep in 1948[H129] allowed investigators to evaluate the prevalence of SLE in patients with idiopathic nephritis. Its bleak prognosis was improved by the availability of corticosteroids and nitrogen mustard in 1949 and hemodialysis in 1960.

The immunopathogenesis, pathology, and clinicopathologic correlates of lupus nephritis are covered in Chapter 53. Detailed discussions of specific treatment modalities being employed for renal disease are covered separately. The reader is referred to Chapter 58 (corticosteroids and pulse steroids), Chapter 59 (cyclophosphamide, nitrogen mustard, azathioprine, chlorambucil, and methotrexate), Chapter 60 (apheresis, total lymphoid irradiation, hemodialysis, and transplantation), and Chapter 61 (gamma globulin). This chapter discusses the epidemiology, incidence, clinical features, natural course, and reviews the general management concepts of renal lupus.

DEFINITION, EPIDEMIOLOGY, AND PREVALENCE

On renal biopsy, nearly all patients with SLE will have histologic evidence of renal pathology, even though many patients have entirely normal clinical findings. Although urine sediment and protein measurements along with serum creatinine, C3 complement, and anti–double-stranded DNA determinations are useful in analyzing the prognosis, course and projected treatment, nephritis can be present even if all these parameters are normal. Renal biopsies have shown early changes of SLE with normal urinalyses.[B220,E68,F157,H382,K73,L152,M64,M642,R275,W347] This has been termed "silent lupus nephropathy" and is usually nonprogressive.[F157,R275] Although these instances generally represent minimal disease histologically, diffuse proliferative lesions have occasionally been found.

We recommend the following definition of lupus nephritis, which has identified over 95% of clinically relevant nephritis[P216,W39,W40] One of the following must be present: 1) a renal biopsy showing mesangial, focal proliferative, diffuse proliferative, or membranous glomerulonephritis; 2) a 30% decrease in creatinine clearance over a 1-year period; 3) greater than 1 g of urine protein in a 24-hour urine specimen. If none of these features are present, at least three of the following are required in a 12-month period: 1) serum albumin level of less than 3 g/dl; 2) 2 to 4+ proteinuria; 3) oval fat bodies; granular, hyaline, or red cells casts in the urine; 4) persistent hematuria of greater than five red cells per high-power field in the urine. Finally, other etiologies of genitourinary disease (e.g., diabetes, hypertension, drug-induced nephropathies, infection) must be excluded.

With these or similar criteria, the prevalence of renal involvement varied from 29 to 65% in the eight series compiled in Table 33–1. Tertiary referral centers tended to have higher percentages of renal disease patients, as did studies published before 1965 (when ANAs became widely available and identified more mild cases of SLE). The true prevalence is probably about 40%. Nephritis is present in most children (see Chap. 44) and is rare in the elderly[B36,D219] Nephrotic syndrome (defined as a serum albumin <2.8 g/dl with >3.5 g of urine protein per 24 hours) was observed in 13 to 26% of all SLE cases in eight well-detailed series shown in Table 33–1; we found (as have others) that about half of our 128 nephritis patients were nephrotic at some time in their disease course.[W39]

The mean age at disease onset in patients with nephritis in the Wallace series was 4 years less than in those with SLE without nephritis (27 versus 31 years of age; 230 versus 379 patients)[W40] Nossent et al. also observed a similar difference in 110 Dutch patients.[N146] Smaller-scale surveys have suggested that males have a relative increased incidence of renal disease.[B364,D371,W12] We observed proportionately more men than women had renal disease among our 464 SLE patients seen between 1980 and 1989, but it did not achieve statistical significance.[P216] Orientals may have more nephritis than other racial groupings.[L131,P216] Inheritance of the DR2 gene is associated with an increased risk of developing nephritis, in some populations, and this risk is amplified if certain DQβ genes are also present (see Chap. 2).

CLINICAL AND LABORATORY PRESENTATION

In 3 to 6% of cases, renal disease manifestations constitute the initial presentation of SLE.[E147,H179,L75,M280] This may occur before clinical lupus is apparent. Cairns et al.[C11] reported 11 ANA-negative patients whose onset of SLE began with clinical glomerulonephritis as the initial manifestation. All became ANA positive over a 6-year period. A similar group of 17 patients was described by Adu et al.[A49] ACR criteria may not be fulfilled at first even if the ANA is positive.[F109] Our group reviewed the literature and concluded that the overwhelming majority of clinically relevant nephritis is evident within 5 years of the diagnosis of SLE.[A36] Only 5 of our 230 lupus nephritis patients seen between 1950 and 1980 had the onset of renal disease after 10 years. Others have confirmed this.[N146]

Klippel has described five clinical types of lupus nephritis:[K307] occult (or silent), chronic active nephritis, rapidly progressive (fulminant course) nephritis, nephrotic syndrome, and progressive renal insufficiency in patients with normal urinalysis results. Drugs (especially nonsteroidal), hypertension, and glomerulosclerosis probably cause renal insufficiency in most of the latter group. Patients in this group, along with those with occult disease and chronic active nephritis are often asymptomatic. Acute deterioration in renal function was observed in 36 of 196 (18.4%) SLE hospital admissions in the group followed by Yeung et al.[Y42] Infection and active central nervous system disease were frequent precipitating events, and recovery of renal function with aggressive management was reported in 76%. Others have confirmed these findings.[H268] Mildly nephrotic subjects may only have ankle edema on examination. Frankly nephrotic states are associated with ascites, pre-sacral edema, pleural and pericardial effusions. Physical examinations are often deceptively normal except for blood pressure measurements in patients with isolated lupus nephritis. SLE patients have an increased incidence of renal tubular dysfunction clinically characterized by a proximal or distal renal tubular acidosis.[K401] This is particularly evident in patients with Sjögren's syndrome. See Chapters 41 and 53 for a discussion of renal physiology abnormalities in SLE.

Numerous surveys have evaluated the prognostic importance of a variety of laboratory and serologic parameters; these are discussed later in this chapter. No published surveys have studied the prevalence of these parameters in nephritis versus no nephritis subsets. Our group recorded 125 parameters and compared 128 nephritis patients with 336 without renal disease seen between 1980 and 1989 (data in preparation; only parameters with p values <.01 shown). Table 54–1 summarizes the findings. Some investigators proposed that rheumatoid-like arthritis is protective of renal disease, especially if rheumatoid factor is present and the patient possesses the HLA-DR4 haplotype.[H249,H458,K601] We found no differences in the prevalence of rheumatoid factor in the nephritis versus no nephritis groups (21 versus 23%). Walker et al. noted that arthritis and arthralgia was the most common symptom in a group of 45 lupus nephritis patients followed in New Zealand.[W12] Usually, elevated

Table 54–1. Findings in SLE Patients With Nephritis (n = 128) Compared to Those Without Nephritis (n = 336); p < .01

More Frequent	Less Frequent
Family history of SLE	Cerebritis
Anemia	Seizures
High sedimentation rate	Thrombocytopenia
High serum cholesterol	Fibrositis
High serum triglycerides	
Positive ANA	
High anti-dsDNA	
Low C3 complement	
Low C4 complement	
Positive LE-cell prep	

Westergren sedimentation rates, low C3 complement, elevated anti-dsDNA levels, and low serum albumin levels are associated with more active nephritis. Gallium scans demonstrate increased renal uptake with active disease.[B37]

Measurements of Renal Function

The principal tests used to evaluate renal function are blood urea nitrogen (BUN), serum creatinine, and creatinine clearance. The utility of the BUN is limited by its alteration with hydration status, bleeding, hepatic and dietary conditions. Serum creatinine level can vary with body weight, muscle mass, and tends to overestimate renal function by as much as 20% since it does not take into account proximal tubular creatinine secretion. Creatinine is hypersected by injured tubules in patients with glomerulopathy. Since creatinine is calculated on a logarithmic scale (a rise from 1 to 2 mg/dl represents a 50% change, while a rise from 6 to 7 mg/dl reflects a 3% change), the test value is often difficult to conceptualize. For example, investigative studies comparing creatinine with arithmetically derived parameters must obtain a 1/creatinine value in order to perform any statistical analysis. Since determining a true, reliable renal function is vital in SLE, glomerular filtration rate (GFR) measurements have become the gold standard. Calculated by the standard formula (U × V)/P, GFRs derived by inulin clearance, iothalamate clearance, iothalamate clearance, and Tc99-DTPA clearance have proven to be reliable but expensive and inconvenient.[P151,R54,R359] Creatinine clearance, which is inexpensive and convenient to obtain, overestimates true GFR.[P151,R54,R359] One study suggests that giving cimetidine (400 mg) tablets four times a day for 2 days blocks tubular secretion of creatinine and provides a reliable measure of GFR.[R54]

Urinary Proteins and Sediment

Ropes was the first to attach importance to following urinary sediment and protein level.[R293] In a survey that will never be repeated, she noted that 15 of 68 who had proteinuria and were not given corticosteroids had spon-

Table 54–2. Abnormal Urinary Findings in 520 Cases of SLE

	No. of Cases	%
Albuminuria	240	46.1
WBCs in urine (more than 6/HPF in clean specimen)	185	35.5
Hematuria	170	32.6
Granular casts	164	31.5
Hyaline casts	148	28.4
RBC casts	39	7.5
Fatty casts	32	6.1
Oval fat bodies	23	4.4
Double refractile bodies	10	1.9
Waxy casts	9	1.7
Mixed fatty casts	6	1.2

taneous disappearance of it up to 14 years later. In the most thorough study to date, Dubois' 520 patients seen between 1950 and 1963 had multiple urine evaluations, and his findings are summarized in Table 54–2.[D323] Other reports have found microscopic hematuria in 33 to 78%;[A269,A362,E140,F256,P216,W272] fat bodies in 33 to 48% with nephritis;[W39,W272] cellular casts were observed in 34 to 40%;[E140,R349] greater than 1 g of urinary protein per 24 hours in 26 to 87%. One report has suggested that a random spot urine collection protein: creatinine ratio[S294] is just as reliable as a 24-urine collection.

Even though the urinalysis may be normal despite abnormal findings on a renal biopsy, nearly all patients with clinically important renal disease have microscopic urine findings. The appearance of five leukocytes or red cells in a clean midstream urine specimen, especially with at least a trace of albumin suggests active nephritis. As the process progresses, the amount of albumin gradually increases as do the numbers of leukocytes and erythrocytes. Often at this point many patients are considered to have urinary tract infections and are frequently given multiple courses of antibiotics, although the pyuria results from renal damage and not primary infection. Dubois observed cystitis or pyelonephritis in 22.5% of his 520 patients. Fries and Holman reported dysuria in 14 of their 193 patients[F256] but stones or urethral discharge in only 1. Ropes reported urinary tract infections in 47% of her 150 patients.[R294]

As lupus damage advances, hyaline and fine granular casts may appear. Later in the disease process, coarse granular casts, red cell casts, and white cell casts are found. If nephrotic syndrome is present, urinary protein may be as high as 30 g per 24 hours with good renal function. The other classic findings of nephrosis—such as oval fat bodies in the urine, hypoalbuminemia, hyperlipidemia, and anasarca—may also be present.

With further progression of renal disease, the numbers of all types of casts increase, broad renal failure casts appear, and a telescoped sediment becomes evident.

Analysis of Urine Protein Components

Albumin

Urine protein can be separated into albumin and gamma globulin fractions, whose features have been studied. Mea-

surements of urinary albumin excretion by radioimmunoassay can pick up larger amounts than would normally be detected, and diminution in albumin excretion correlates with clinical response to treatment.[T114]

Gamma Globulins

Urinary protein electrophoresis demonstrates increased gamma globulin levels with active disease that decreases with therapeutic response.[B89,S682] No specific patterns are observed in SLE. Quantitative urine protein analysis with SDS-PAGE can detect glomerular versus nonglomerular proteinuria.[B78] Epstein's group studied serial determinations of free light polypeptide chains of immunoglobulins in the urine.[E122,E124,S600] They and others[C381] showed increased levels correlated with active disease, but methodologic flaws hampered progress in this area for 20 years. Hopper et al. associated clinical relapse with an antecedent elevation of urinary free light-chain immunoglobulin levels using improved techniques.[H415]

Other Urinary Findings

Meryhew, Messner, and Tan studied urinary antinuclear antibodies (ANAs).[M551] Positive tests were found in 4 of 25 (16%) of SLE patients as measured by incubating mouse kidney substrates with concentrated urine. Thirty-two percent of patients were positive with Hep-2 substrate. IgG ANA was most frequently seen; half had more than one immunoglobulin class detected. Anti-Sm, anti-RNP, anti-Ro/SSA, and anti-dsDNA were also detected. The presence of anti-dsDNA and ANA correlated with increased clinical severity. ANA might appear in the urine as a result of decreased tubular reabsorption, antigen deposition, or genitourinary tract inflammation, but is probably representative of glomerular leakage. It appears with inact immunoglobulin molecules and not with heavy or light chain molecules. The significance of urinary ANA is unknown.

Nephrotic syndrome is associated with false-positive urine pregnancy tests.[K398] Unconfirmed reports have suggested that numerous urinary measurements are increased with active lupus nephritis and are good markers of clinical activity. These include urinary ferritin,[N104] urinary anti-RNA polymerase I antibodies,[P182] urinary neopterin,[L188] urinary acid mucopolysaccharides,[B319] histuria,[A261] fibrin degradation products,[K56,S683] and a panel of gastrointestinal enzymes.[D135]

Urinary prostaglandins, renal tubular acidosis, aldosterone, the syndrome of inappropriate antidiuretic hormone, and renin activity measurements are discussed in Chapters 41 and 53.

Renal Vein and Arterial Thrombosis

Thrombosis of the renal veins was first reported in 1968[H84] and has been described in numerous cases since. It should be strongly considered in patients with nephrotic syndrome and/or the lupus anticoagulant who present with flank pain and fever, thrombophlebitis, or pulmonary emboli.[K54,L339,M438,M469] Kant et al.[K54] reviewed 105 renal biopsies in 71 SLE patients with nephritis. Glomerular thrombi were found in none of 25 with mesangial disease, 3 of 15 with membranous and 31 of 63 with proliferative patterns. Although associated with thrombocytopenia and circulating anticoagulants, no correlations with C3, anti-DNA, or fibrinogen levels were noted. Twenty-four patients who underwent a second biopsy after having thrombosis in the first had a pattern of accelerated glomerulosclerosis. The same investigators also suggested that patients with an antibody to a synthetic single-stranded RNA analog (Poly A) of native DNA had fewer thrombotic episodes.[G339] Bradley et al.[B452] found renal vein thrombosis in 11 of 280 patients with membranous glomerulonephritis or lupus glomerulonephritis. All 11 (3 of whom have SLE) had nephrotic syndrome and 10 had pulmonary emboli.

Mintz et al.[M469] performed inferior vena cava phlebography in 43 SLE patients. Inferior vena cava or renal vein thrombosis was found in 27% of 11 nephrotic syndrome patients, 62% of 13 with a history of thrombophlebitis, and none of 20 controls with SLE. A hypercoagulable state is thus a greater risk factor than the presence of nephrotic syndrome. Even though the circulating lupus anticoagulants predispose one to renal vein thrombosis, their presence is not mandatory.[C4,T112] Renal vein thrombosis has also been reported in SLE patients who have received renal allografts.[L265] Kincaid-Smith et al. reported a series of 12 pregnant women with SLE who had biopsy-documented thromboses.[K229]

If reasonable clinical suspicions are aroused, a MR angiogram or venogram should be performed. Renal vein thrombosis must be treated promptly with anticoagulants. Renal failure and pulmonary emboli are its most serious complications. Purified Malayian pit viper venom (ancrod) may be useful as a defibrinator,[D227] but is not generally available.

Several case reports have appeared of renal artery thrombosis associated with the antiphospholipid syndrome[B451,O116] (see also Chap. 53).

MANAGEMENT OF LUPUS NEPHRITIS

The management of lupus nephritis is controversial. The principal goals of therapy are first, to improve or prevent the progressive loss of renal function, and second, since end-stage renal failure may be managed by dialysis or transplantation, treatment must do the patient as little harm as possible (Table 54–3 lists toxicities of various therapies).

The general concepts and specific therapies outlined below have evolved over a 20 to 30-year period. We have been able to achieve over 80% 10-year survivals with our approach. The guidelines are by no means absolute. Many highly qualified rheumatologists and nephrologists would treat lupus nephritis differently. General concepts:

1. All patients who present with lupus nephritis as defined earlier in this chapter should have a renal biopsy if there are no contraindications and a physician expert in biopsy is available. Since therapy differs greatly between biopsy patterns, tissue evaluation is desirable. If possible, activity and chronicity

Table 54–3. Toxicities of Aggressive Regimens Used to Treat Proliferative Nephritis That May Occur >5% of the Time

I. Prolonged high-dose oral prednisone therapy (1 mg/kg/day equivalent >6 weeks)
   Accelerated development of cataracts, glaucoma, hypertension, osteoporosis
   Diabetes mellitus
   Avascular necrosis of bone
   Diffuse ecchymoses
   Weight gain and marked cushingoid appearance
   Diplopia
   Emotional lability, mood changes
   Dyspepsia, ulcer risk
   Increased infection risk
   Menstrual irrgularities
II. Cyclophosphamide (more common in oral doses)
   Alopecia
   Amenorrhea, infertility
   Hemorrhagic cystitis
   Risk of malignancy
   Severe nausea and vomiting
   Increased risk of infection
   Teratogenicity
   Anemia, leukopenia, thrombocytopenia
III. Azathioprine
   Nausea and vomiting
   Abnormal liver function tests
   Increased risk of infection
   Anemia, leukopenia, thrombocytopenia

indices should be assessed from the histology. A renal biopsy may need to be repeated in patients with persistent nephritis in whom additional more aggressive therapy is being considered.

2. Salt intake is restricted if blood pressures are elevated, fat intake is restricted if hyperlipidemia is present or the patient is nephrotic, protein intake is restricted if renal function is impaired by over 40%. Calcium supplementation is given to minimize corticosteroid-induced osteoporosis.

3. Loop diuretics are used to diminish edema when necessary, but if the creatinine level is greater than 3 mg%, they should be used with caution.

4. The authors place in order of importance the following parameters in evaluating renal activity: urine sediment appearance, serum creatinine, creatinine clearance, blood pressure, serum albumin, 24-hour urine protein, C3 complement, anti-DNA, proteinuria estimated by urine dipstick. These may be monitored as the clinical situation dictates. Daily measurement of serum creatinine may be useful in rapidly progressive disease; other parameters require 1 to 2 weeks to change.

5. The authors place in order of importance the following parameters in monitoring toxicity of corticosteroids, diuretics, and cytotoxic agents: complete blood count, platelet count, potassium, glucose, cholesterol, liver function tests. These are closely monitored as the clinical situation requires.

6. Patients are instructed to avoid therapeutic doses of salicylates and nonsteroidal anti-inflammatory agents since they may impair renal function unless

used for short periods at low doses with careful supervision.

7. Hypertension must be aggressively treated.
8. Pregnancy should be discouraged in patients with active nephritis, since it is associated with a greatly increased risk of renal failure.
9. Antimalarials may be given if there is active skin disease; baby aspirin may be given if the patient has the lupus circulating anticoagulant. Neither of these interventions will benefit lupus nephritis per se.

The following therapies are advised for specific biopsy patterns (see Fig. 54–1):

I. Class I—no specific therapy is necessary.
II. Class II—some mesangial lesions do not need therapy. In patients with class IIb patterns and over 1 g proteinuria, high anti-dsDNA, and low C3 complement, we usually administer 20 mg of prednisone equivalent daily for 6 weeks to 3 months followed by tapering and adjustment in accordance with the degree of clinical activity. Extrarenal lupus is commonly present and is treated as is necessary.
III. Class III and class IV are treated similarly and have the same prognosis. (see Fig. 54–1). Since the risk of end-stage renal disease in 10 years may exceed 50%, aggressive management is advised. We recommend the following:
   A. Administration of 1 mg/kg/day of prednisone equivalent for at least 6 weeks and up to 26 weeks, depending on clinical response. Cytotoxic drugs often take 3 to 4 months to become effective, and glucocorticoids stabilize the patient in the interim. Prednisone is tapered to alternate-day therapy as soon as feasible. When a level of 40 mg of prednisone daily equivalent dose is achieved, doses are then decreased by 10% a week to a maintenance of 10 to 20 mg of prednisone equivalent daily for at least 2 years.
   B. Prednisone is capable of treating proliferative disease by itself and cytotoxic drugs are not always needed. Depending on the clinical situation, cytotoxic drugs might be added at the onset of therapy

or later if there is a suboptimal response to glucocorticoids alone. Some published evidence suggests that the addition of cytotoxic drugs might be associated with an increased probability of a good response, as well as being steroid sparing. Intravenous administration of 750 mg/M^2 of cyclophosphamide is given monthly for 6 months, and tapered to every 2 to 3 months thereafter, depending upon clinical response. We currently do not administer this therapy consecutively for more than 3 years. Mesna can be given with each infusion to minimize bladder toxicity.

   C. Somewhere between 30 and 50% will be refractory to prednisone with intravenous cyclophosphamide, especially those who are nephrotic. Most of these patients will respond by the fourth to sixth month but begin to worsen at 9 to 15 months. In this subset the following options are available:
      1. Repeating cycle of monthly intravenous cyclophosphamide for 6 months. Pulse doses of methylprednisolone may be added to the intravenous cyclophosphamide.
      2. Adding oral azathioprine to prednisone and monthly IV cyclophosphamide. Consider changing from parenteral to daily low-dose oral cyclophosphamide.
      3. Adding apheresis, especially in a pulse/synchronization fashion with cyclophosphamide (see Chap. 60).
      4. Raising corticosteroid doses.
   D. Acute flares with renal deterioration can be managed with pulse methylprednisolone or apheresis. The latter is especially useful if the patient has cryoglobulinemia, hyperviscosity, or thrombotic thrombocytopenic purpura.
   E. Special circumstances may warrant adjustments or changes in the above regimen. These include:
      1. Corticosteroids: uncontrollable diabetes or hypertension, multiple sites of painful avascular necrosis, severe osteoporosis, steroid psychosis, life-threatening infection, severe myopathy.
      2. Cyclophosphamide: refractory hemorrhagic cystitis in spite of Mesna therapy, severe nausea and/or vomiting, refusal to accept the possibility of infertility, prior radiation therapy, history of malignancy, cytopenia as a result of marrow suppression (cytopenias as a result of peripheral destruction are not contraindications).
   F. Azathioprine is usually the second line agent of choice. Rarely, chlorambucil or nitrogen mustard may be advised.
IV. Class V—patients are treated with 1 mg/kg/day of prednisone equivalent for 6 to 12 weeks followed by its discontinuation or tapering to a maintenance of 10 mg prednisone equivalent a day for 1 to 2 years. Cytotoxic drugs are generally not used unless a proliferative component is present. Pure membranous lesions are uncommon, comprising less than 15% of all biopsies.

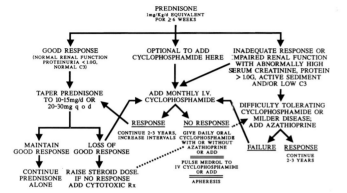

Fig. 54–1. Algorithm for the treatment of proliferative (class III or IV) nephritis.

V. Patients with a long-standing creatinine level over 3 mg/dl and/or a high chronicity index.
   A. Aggressive management is usually not advised unless a high activity index is also present or extrarenal disease warranting cytotoxic therapy is evident.
   B. Patients are usually maintained on 5 to 10 mg of prednisone equivalent daily if needed to control extrarenal lupus.
   C. Salt and protein restrictions are carefully enforced. Blood pressure is closely monitored.

The reader is referred to Chapter 60 for a discussion of the management of lupus patients with end stage renal disease; specifically dialysis and transplantation.

WHEN SHOULD A RENAL BIOPSY BE PERFORMED?

Dubois felt that there were only two undisputed reasons to obtain a renal biopsy: confirmation of diagnosis in equivocal cases and determination in advanced cases, when azotemia was present, as to whether further treatment was indicated. If diffuse scarring was present with little or no inflammation, conservative management would be the course of action. This view was upheld in 1978 by Fries, who summarized the literature up to that date, examining 177 renal biopsies from several studies in detail.[F262] He concluded that biopsy information provided certain prognostic information but added little relevant clinical information. It was not cost effective and had some inherent risks. Other reports appearing between 1978 and 1985 questioned the reliability of two observers coming to the same conclusion about a specific biopsy,[W209] failed to correlate a clinical nephritis index with histologic patterns,[S494] and showed that the World Health Organization histologic classification was not a predictor of results of therapy at rebiopsy 12 months later.[W208] Smeeton et al. concluded that there was "a small but definite risk of missing significant renal disease if a biopsy is not performed."[S501] Chapter 53 reviews the various patterns and their clinicopathologic significance.

Several advances have resulted in the authors' current enthusiasm for renal biopsy in most patients:

1. The development of Activity and Chronicity Indices by the National Institutes of Health.[A361,B64] Increased chronicity is clearly associated with a poorer outcome.[M305,N142] Higher activity indices are also associated with poor outcomes, but are reversible[E140,M60] with aggressive treatment (see Table 54–4).
2. Availability of an improved renal biopsy needle, which decreases the risk of significant bleeding.
3. Evidence that tubulointerstitial disease, which can be only diagnosed at biopsy, is of prognostic importance.[P44]
4. Documentation that mesangial disease can clinically present identically to proliferative disease. Since the therapies are different and only biopsy can distinguish the two, biopsy is desirable. Mesangial disease does not require cytotoxic therapy.[G178,M305]
5. Documentation that pure membranous disease has

Table 54–4. Renal Pathology Scoring System*

Activity Index	Chronicity Index
Glomerular abnormalities	
1. Cellular proliferation	1. Glomerular sclerosis
2. Fibrinoid necrosis, karyorrhexis	2. Fibrous crescents
3. Cellular crescents	
4. Hyaline thrombi, wire loops	
5. Leukocyte infiltration	
Tubulointerstitial abnormalities	
1. Mononuclear cell infiltration	1. Interstitial fibrosis
	2. Tubular atrophy

From Austin, H.A., Muenz, L.R., Joyce, K.M., et al.: Prognostic factors in lupus nephritis: Contribution of renal histologic data. Am. J. Med. 75:383, 1983.
* Fibrinoid necrosis and cellular crescents are weighted by a factor of 2. The maximum score of the activity index is 24; that of the chronicity index is 12.

a different treatment and outcome than proliferative disease and can only be diagnosed by biopsy.[A45,M305]

We now recommend that all patients who fulfill the definition of lupus nephritis undergo an initial biopsy. Followup biopsies are indicated if therapy would be significantly altered as a result of the findings. As reviewed in Chapter 53, up to 30% of patients undergoing second biopsies transform to different patterns.

CLINICOPATHOLOGIC LABORATORY CORRELATES

The six major parameters used to follow lupus nephritis disease activity are serum creatinine, 24-hour urine for protein, creatinine clearance, C3 complement, urine sediment, and anti-dsDNA. Each of these tests tells the clinician different things; therapeutic decisions are based on considering the results of all of these values.

Serum creatinine, or creatinine clearance, reflects the level of renal function. It tells us little about disease activity. A persistent elevation in the serum creatinine to the abnormal range (>1.4 mg/dl) implies that at least 40% of glomeruli are damaged. Normalization of the creatinine level is associated with a favorable prognosis.[E38,E140] A creatinine clearance less than 10 ml/hr or a serum creatinine over 7 mg/dl is usually an indication for dialysis. As mentioned earlier, hydration status, severe infection, and certain medications (especially nonsteroidal anti-inflammatory agents) can temporarily raise serum creatinine levels without glomerular injury being present.

Twenty-four-hour urine proteins are valuable to follow only if they are elevated.[E38,E140,W39] Levels below 200 mg per 24 hours are normal; values up to 1000 mg do not usually provide an indication for significant interventions and can be seen in healthy subjects after vigorous exercise. When more than 3500 mg per 24 hours is recorded, the patient usually has nephrotic syndrome and ankle edema is present; anasarca can be observed in patients who have more than 7000 mg per 24 hours. Twenty-four-hour urine proteins tend to correlate with disease activity, though this is not always the case.[E140] We have had patients with membranous disease who have had nephrotic range proteinuria continuously for more than 20 years and still have normal serum creatinines! Decreases in 24-hour urine protein values usually correlate with clinical improvement unless the serum creatinines are above 5 mg/dl; in this circumstance dropping levels are a sign of renal failure.

Complement is a protein whose levels are reduced with inflammation. Various tests of complement are available in the clinical laboratory that are relevant to lupus nephritis: C3, C4, total hemolytic complement, C3d:C4d ratios. Chapters 13 and 48 review the biology and clinical importance of complement. Low complement levels are associated with greater renal disease activity.[A269,C39,D92,D93, E140,G314,G369,H450,L30,L285,M60,S207] Falls in complement usually predict disease exacerbation.[E140,G50,H305,H450,L30, L285,L435,M60,S783] The above cited studies suggest that the most specific test is C3, followed by total hemolytic complement, and then C4. C3 correlates with activity indices on biopsy,[P190] and longterm normalization of complement is associated with a better prognosis.[L30] Conversely, low complement levels may also denote congenital or acquired deficiencies of various components, and many patients have persistently low complement levels with no clinical evidence of disease activity. Gladman et al.[G179] found 14 such patients in a group of 180 with SLE. Followed for a mean of 4.25 years, they had no symptoms and were on no medications and none developed any evidence of lupus activity. Also, complement levels tend to normalize or only be slightly decreased in advanced renal failure.

Anti-dsDNA is elevated in patients with active nephritis.[A265,B60,C39,D92,D93,G369,H190,H305,H450,L308,M456,S782, S786,T224] Enzyme immunoassays or the Farr assay allow one to quantitate its presence; the Crithidia luciliae test simply tells one whether or not it was found since its titers are of no value in following disease activity. Anti-DNA is found in 50 to 75% of patients with active nephritis; its levels are often normal in patients with pure membranous disease. Chapters 20 and 48 review the biology and clinical importance of anti-DNA. Anti-DNA is not as reliable as C3 complement in assessing renal disease activity,[C308,M60] and it may be elevated if extrarenal lupus activity is evident.

Other clinical correlates have been sought that might be useful in following renal disease activity. These include cryoglobulins,[H458,R237] autoantibodies to poly(ADP)ribose,[M606] circulating immune complexes,[D92,L225,W175] interleukin-2 receptor levels,[L91] ANA patterns,[A84] antiendothelial cell antibody levels,[D101] and measurement of activation and degradation components of complement (see Chap. 13). These tests are either not universally available or are less reliable than those discussed in the preceding paragraphs. No one test (except for a dramatic change in serum creatinine or C3 complement) usually allows the practitioner to take any particular course of action unless it is consistently abnormal or supported by other confirmatory laboratory tests and the clinical picture.

In summary, laboratory testing with serum creatinine, 24-hour urine protein and creatinine clearance, C3 complement levels, urine sediment abnormalities, and anti-dsDNA provide extremely useful information when used adjunctively with a careful history and physical examination, knowledge of the patient's disease, and clinical experience. No one test usually allows the practitioner to take any particular course of action unless it is supported by other confirmatory laboratory tests and the clinical picture.

Patients who should not be treated include those who have significant renal scarring or evidence of irreversible disease. There is little benefit in aggressively managing patients with a stable creatinine level above 5 mg/dl, and frequently produces more harm than good.

COURSE OF LUPUS NEPHRITIS

Over the last four decades, a tremendous change has evolved in the approach to lupus nephritis which has greatly altered its outcome.[C322] In the early 1950s, low-dose corticosteroids were used with 5-year survival rates close to zero.[D329] By the late 1950s and early 1960s, prolonged high-dose corticosteroids were employed (with a few centers using nitrogen mustard). The overall 5-year survival was 25%.[B196] The mid to late 1960s were characterized by the availability of hemodialysis, moderate-dose steroid usage, and widespread use of high doses of azathioprine and oral cyclophosphamide. The overall 5-year survival was 40 to 70%. By the early 1970s, physicians temporized their use of cytotoxic drugs and took advantage of newer antibiotics and antihypertensive agents, resulting in 60 to 80% 5-year survivals. (In the Dubois/Wallace series, 10-year survivals for patients diagnosed in the decades beginning of 1950 were 65%; 1960, 60%; and 1970, 76%).[W39] The WHO classification system helped stratify renal disease into pathologic subsets that helped tailor therapy. The 1980s saw the introduction of intermittent, parenteral cyclophosphamide combined with corticosteroids. Activity and chronicity indices were described, and interventions with pulse-dose corticosteroids and apheresis became more common. In 1989, Esdaile et al. were able to document 85 and 73% 5- and 10-year survivals among 87 patients followed for a mean of 8.4 years.[E140]

Along the way, new insights were derived that allowed investigators to determine prognostic subsets and assess the impact of various therapies. Associated with a poorer outcome were nephrotic syndrome, class IV lesions, high chronicity indices, hypertension, and childhood onset of nephritis.[E140,W39] The National Institutes of Health group correlated corticosteroid therapy with progressive renal scarring and a worse prognosis than those given corticosteroids plus cytotoxic treatments.[A360,S652] Efforts were made to correlate prognosis with biopsy pattern. McClusky[M232] in 1975 and Pollak and Kant in 1981[P239] summarized several studies and found the 5-year survival of patients with minimal lesions to be 80 to 90%, mesangial 68%, mild proliferative 40 to 80%, severe proliferative 25 to 40%, and membranous 60 to 80%. The worst prognostic subset of lupus nephritis is nephrotic syndrome, where half are dead within 10 years.[A266,W39] The most common causes of death were complications of renal disease and sepsis. Papers in the last few years for the first time have mentioned discontinuing therapy after successful treatment.[P253,S184] More emphasis is now being placed on decreasing the risk of evolving end-stage renal disease. Despite all these advances, certain subsets of patients with focal or diffuse proliferative lesions and scarring glomerular and tubulointerstitial regions still have a 50% chance of evolving into end-stage renal disease within 5 years, and aggressive management appears to be warranted.

In summary, lupus nephritis has evolved from a frequently terminal process to one in which a fairly normal quality of life and good outcome are possible. First, the treating physician must accurately stage the disease with laboratory and tissue evaluations. Next, therapy is fashioned for the specific disease subsets involved. Third, the side effects and complications of treatment must be managed along with frequent assessments and modifications of therapy depending upon the patient's response. Hopefully, the 1990s will see further advances in this difficult aspect of SLE.

Section VII

MANAGEMENT AND PROGNOSIS

Chapter 55

PRINCIPLES OF THERAPY AND LOCAL MEASURES

DANIEL J. WALLACE

Take pneumonia. It has been treated by bleeding, and got well. It has been treated by brandy and got well. It has been left to itself and got well. And the bleeders, the brandy givers, and the doers of nothing at all, respectively, have had a vast deal to say for themselves and against their rivals. And which of them are to be our guides and masters in the treatment of pneumonia? None of them for a single day, much less for always.

Latham[B139]

Formulation Overview

One of the most difficult and misunderstood aspects of lupus is its management. Before therapy is initiated, the practitioner must determine the type of lupus and, on this basis, formulate a treatment program. Because the prognosis of each clinical subset differs widely, it is essential that the patient data base be completed before an educational session is initiated. Have all blood tests, roentgenographic measures, biopsies, and scans, which provide information that can affect treatment, been performed? Once these prerequisites have been met, the physician should be able to answer the following questions:

1. Does the patient meet the American College of Rheumatology criteria for SLE?
   a. If not, does the patient meet biopsy criteria for discoid lupus or subacute cutaneous lupus? If not, is the physician satisfied that the patient has SLE, in spite of lacking four criteria? (This distinction is a matter of clinical judgment.)
   b. If so, are related disorders such as mixed connective tissue disease, scleroderma, and dermatopolymyositis excluded?
2. If the patient has SLE, is life-threatening organ involvement present? If not, does the patient have "mild SLE?"
3. Which subset best describes their disease? Does a particular aspect of the patient's disease require specific considerations, intervention, or counseling (e.g., antiphospholipid syndrome, Ro(SSA) positivity, seizures, inappropriate behavior, concurrent fibromyalgia)?

The Educational Session

All newly diagnosed patients, as well as those new to the treating physician, deserve an educational session that includes concerned family members and loved ones. The session is supervised by the physician and may involve other health professionals or use audiovisual aids. Several studies have demonstrated that socioeconomic differences account for widely divergent outcomes in those with SLE.[G162,W39] It is critical that the patient establish a relationship and rapport with the physician, keep appointments, take medication as prescribed, and be able to have access to medical assistance or advice 24 hours a day. Educational and informational literature relating to various aspects of the disease, including therapy, are available from organizations such as the Arthritis Foundation, Lupus Foundation of America, and The American Lupus Society (see App. 2 for additional resource information).

The treatment of LE is divided into three categories: physical and psychologic measures, drug therapy, and surgery. The latter is rarely employed, and the first is infrequently discussed. Table 55–1 summarizes the issues that should be discussed with the patient, and family during the educational session.

GENERAL THERAPEUTIC CONSIDERATIONS

Rest and the Treatment of Fatigue

In discoid LE, rest may be necessary only if the patient complains of tiring easily and arthralgias. Many patients with transition forms, however, complain of fatiguing easily and, in such individuals, a nap in the afternoon and adequate sleep at night are recommended.

Rest is important in the therapy of SLE. It is essential during the early phases of remission. Tiring easily, one of the earliest manifestations of SLE, is also one of the most persistent and difficult features to evaluate. Because some patients may initially appear to be in good health, the physician is apt to label them as "neurotic" before the diagnosis of SLE is made, and may consider persistence of easy fatigability as a recurrence of a similar reaction. This is a characteristic complaint, however, caused by low-grade activity of the underlying disease. Massive doses of steroids mask this symptom, but are neither advisable nor safe for the longterm therapy of fatigue. As the dosage is reduced, the symptom becomes more evident, and increased rest is necessary to control its rebound.

A typical complaint during periods of mild disease activity is that the patient feels fine in the morning but "collapses" after lunch. During such times, which often occur following a reduction in steroid dosage or induction of a remission, a few hours' rest after breakfast and lunch is advisable. The morning rest period may be abolished grad-

Table 55–1. Issues to be Covered in the Educational Session

1. What is lupus and what are its causes?
2. Many types of lupus exist. You have (discoid, mild, organ-threatening) LE, which has a (fair, good, excellent) prognosis with treatment.
3. Physical measures include the use of heat, exercise, diet. Physical, occupational, or vocational therapy, favorable climate, and sun avoidance are also helpful.
4. Psychologic measures include dealing with fatigue, emotional stress (in appropriate cases), physical trauma, family and job problems, and pain. Genetic counseling and a discussion of lupus and pregnancy may be needed.
5. Medication includes salicylates, NSAIDs, antimalarials, corticosteroids, cytotoxic drugs, and investigational measures. Adjunctive measures may be helpful, such as vitamins, birth control, immunizations, and the prevention of phospholipid syndrome complications.
6. Resource information includes patient education materials, counseling availability, self-help and exercise groups, and useful telephone numbers.

ually and, when the patient feels well in the evening, the afternoon rest periods can also be eliminated.

Following a severe exacerbation, these patients often require several weeks of sick leave before they can return to work—preferably half-time at first. Patients with active disease who must work an 8-hour day should take two to three 20-minute rest periods during the day to prevent excessive fatigue and to allow them to perform quality work. They may need to rest all evening. Total bed rest is inadvisable because it promotes osteoporosis, muscle disuse, and atrophy, and is unnecessary unless the patient is critically ill.[A312]

If patients overexert themselves from too much work or too vigorous a social life, they can experience minor disease exacerbations that require a few days of increased rest. Often, during active phases, patients learn resting for much of the afternoon is essential if they want to go out in the evening. The homemaker with chronically active disease may lead a semblance of normal life if she rests regularly during the afternoons so that she can carry on her regular household activities in the evening.

Treatment of fatigue requires consideration of the source and of contributory factors. Iron deficiency anemia is common because of dietary deficiency, heavy menstrual periods, and/or blood loss resulting from the use of salicylates and nonsteroidal anti-inflammatory drugs (NSAIDs). If the fatigue is caused by parenchymal pulmonary disease, oxygen may be helpful; if secondary to inflammation, anti-inflammatory drugs are used. In addition to corticosteroids, quinacrine (Atabrine) and hydroxychloroquine (Plaquenil) are cortical stimulants, and may decrease fatigue in patients without organ-threatening involvement.[D325,W24] Many SLE patients who have minimal disease activity and normal blood work (other than a positive antinuclear antibody, ANA) complain of profound fatigue. Depression and emotional stress must be excluded as causes. An organic is probably the basis for at least some of the fatigue, which may be mediated by cytokines (e.g., interleukin-1 or α-interferon) or by neurotransmitter and hormonal deficiencies (see Chap. 38). Secondary fibromyalgia with a concomitant sleep disorder is not uncommon. Some physicians empirically prescribe low doses of thyroid or amphetamines for the nonspecific fatigue of SLE. The routine use of these agents should be discouraged. In contrast, the use of agents that promote restorative sleep should be considered.

Exercise, Physical Therapy, and Rehabilitation

The SLE patient should remain physically active and avoid excessive bed rest. Exercises that strengthen muscles and improve endurance while avoiding undue stresses to inflamed joints are desirable. Activities such as swimming, walking, and bicycling should be encouraged. Recreational activities involving fine motor movements and placing stress on certain ligamentous and other supporting structures (e.g., bowling, rowing, weight lifting, golf, tennis, jogging) should be considered on an individual basis. Exercises involving sustained isometric contractions increase muscle strength more than isotonic exercises. Physical measures, such as the use of local moist heat or cold, decrease joint pain and inflammation. Many patients benefit from a whirlpool bath (Jacuzzi), hot tub, or therapy pool, or from merely soaking in a tub of hot water.

Physical therapists instruct patients in strengthening and toning exercises, improved body mechanics, and gait training. No specific measures or treatment approaches are unique for lupus patients. Joint deformities develop in about 10% of patients; physical and occupational therapies to minimize deformities are desirable in that group. Splints are useful for most patients with carpal tunnel syndrome related to SLE. Corrective tendon surgery and joint replacement are helpful in advanced cases.

Occupational therapists instruct patients in the principles of energy conservation and joint protection. They evaluate activities of daily living and advise on the use of devices or aids, such as wrist splints, comb handles, and raised toilet seats, when needed.

Vocational rehabilitation may be important in retraining an SLE patient who can no longer work in the sun (e.g., farmer, construction worker, fisherman) or perform tasks requiring fine hand motor function (e.g., typist).

Pain Management

Patients with inflammatory arthritis respond poorly to analgesics with no anti-inflammatory effects. The use of propoxyphene, codeine, or pentazocine in SLE should be limited to postoperative management and other situations. These drugs can induce dependence, have short-lived effects, and do not affect the underlying problem. inflammatory drugs (e.g., salicylates, NSAIDs, corticosteroids) are therefore more effective in treating pain symptoms in SLE. Some patients with chronic pain problems who are unresponsive to simple measures should be referred to pain management centers. These centers use such measures as acupuncture, transcutaneous electrical nerve stimulation (TENS) units, biofeedback, psychologic counseling, and physical therapy to alleviate pain and eliminate narcotic dependence.

Role of Stress and Trauma

Many studies have shown that certain forms of emotional stress, including depression and bereavement, and physical trauma, can affect the immune system—for example, causing decreased lymphocyte mitogenic responsiveness, lymphocyte cytotoxicity, increased natural killer cell activity, skin homograft rejection, graft-versus-host response, and delayed hypersensitivity.[A236,C13,W22] Stress, unfortunately, is difficult to quantitate for evaluation of its clinical effects. Could the impairment in T-cell immune functions be responsible for a clinical flare of lupus mediated by B-cell hyperreactivity? Have these immune abnormalities been reproduced in lupus patients? Can the neuroendocrine axis influence immune responses? The results of animal studies in this area have been inconsistent. Few human studies have been attempted.

In 1955, McLeary et al.[M231] related the onset of disease to significant crises in interpersonal relationships in 13 of 14 SLE patients. In 1967, Otto and Mackay[O121] compared 20 SLE patients with 20 controls. The SLE-hospitalized group experienced significantly more stress before the onset of disease than other hospitalized, seriously ill controls. All patients thought that stress provoked their illness. In another study, 18 of 36 SLE patients (50%) interviewed believed that psychologic factors triggered disease onset, and an additional 25% thought it was possible.[B366]

Can stress exacerbate pre-existing SLE? Ropes observed 45 serious disease flares in her 160-patient cohort over a 40-year period. Of the 45 patients, 41 believed that emotional stress precipitated their flare.[R294] In 1989, Hinrichsen et al. exposed 14 women with SLE, 14 healthy controls, and 12 sarcoidosis patients to acoustic stress.[H314] Significant increases in polymorphonuclear leukocyte and lymphocyte counts and significant elevations of circulating B and CD8+ T lymphocytes, with a relative reduction in CD4+ T lymphocytes, were noted in the healthy controls but not in the SLE or sarcoid patients. The difference in effects was not steroid-related.

Most SLE patients already have abnormal immune function, but it has not been proven that stress further impairs these functions and results in a disease exacerbation. Nevertheless, I believe that stress reduction is a helpful measure in the overall management of SLE.

No evidence has shown that physical trauma is related to the causation or exacerbation of SLE. I have had many patients, however, whose condition appeared to worsen after major vehicular accidents. Discoid LE (DLE) can develop as a result of physical trauma; King-Smith first observed this in 1926.[K234] In 1956, Kern and Schiff reported on 5 well-documented cases and sent a questionnaire to 400 dermatologists. Of these, 54 reported having treated 78 patients.[K174] The most common causes of DLE were blows from various objects, lacerations, and scars. In 1963, Lodin confirmed these findings and noted that 10 of 458 Swedish patients (2.2%) with DLE had a documented preceding trauma.[L360] These observations were reinforced by Eskreis in 1988.[E143]

In summary, several authors have implicated stress as a factor that can induce or exacerbate SLE. A definitive study using large numbers of patients and controls with a similar chronic illness is needed before the association is considered established. Until then, I believe that stress reduction is prudent and important.

Diet and Vitamins

Patients with SLE should eat three well-balanced, nutritious meals daily. Animal studies suggesting that fish oil intake might be beneficial in the treatment of autoimmune diseases have led to several human clinical trials based on the findings that eicosapentanoic acid and docosahexanoic acid inhibit platelet aggregation, leukotriene B_4 production by polymorphs, and 5-lipoxygenase products in polymorphs and monocytes.[H403,L147,R248] In contrast to rheumatoid arthritis, three double-blind placebo studies of SLE failed to show any anti-inflammatory actions or any other clinical benefits, except for a slight lowering in plasma triglyceride and an elevation of high-density lipoprotein levels.[C288,K417,W61,W193] Substituting dietary polyunsaturated fatty acids with saturated fats (which I do not recommend) was suggested in one uncontrolled study.[T162] In some animal studies, caloric restriction was found to suppress autoimmune diseases,[H403,L370] but three clinical reports showed that reduced caloric intake has no effect on parameters such as hemoglobin, serum IgG levels, or antibody titers.[C386,F65,Y56] The ingestion of alfalfa sprouts can induce lupus in primates and might exacerbate human SLE; thus, it should be avoided.[A127,M80, M548,M585,P291,R238] The offending agent is probably an amino acid, L-canavanine, which has been shown to alter both T- and B-cell responses.[A127,P29] Two controlled studies have found SLE patients to have increased food allergies,[C101,D229] but the clinical significance of this observation is uncertain.

Patients taking large doses of corticosteroids and those who are hypertensive should restrict their salt intake. Some nephritis patients need to be salt-, potassium-, and protein-restricted. Potassium supplementation may be needed for some patients on diuretics. Anemic patients often benefit from foods with a high iron content (e.g., red meat). Steroids can increase lipid levels and induce a chemical diabetes, and a low-fat or diabetic diet should be implemented if this occurs.

Almost all of our patients have asked us about the efficacy of vitamins in SLE. No controlled studies have been published demonstrating any clear-cut benefits from their use. Vitamin B_{12} and folic acid can be used to treat specific types of anemias. Vitamin E may improve wound healing. Vitamin B_6 (pyridoxine) is a diuretic and has been used in carpal tunnel syndrome as an adjunctive agent. Vitamin D, with calcium supplementation, may retard osteoporosis induced by corticosteroids. Other than these nonspecific measures, the judicious use of vitamins by lupus patients is probably harmless and often has a placebo effect, as long as intake is not excessive.

Sun Avoidance and Sunscreens

One study of 125 SLE patients noted that 73% are sunsensitive. In 42% of patients, sun exposure exacerbated systemic symptoms and, in 35%, it had a significant effect on lifestyle.[W365] The mechanism by which this occurs is controversial but it is probably related to the action of ultraviolet light on epidermal DNA, which enhances its antigenicity. This could lead to the formation of immune complexes in situ at the dermal-epidermal junction, or perhaps delay normal DNA repair[T17,Z2] (see Chaps. 29, 30, and 37).

Ultraviolet (UV) light consists of three bands, two of which are important in SLE. UVA light (320- to 400-nm wavelength) is responsible for drug-induced photosensitivity (photoallergic reactions) and delayed tanning, and is constant during the day. It takes about 1 hour of UVA exposure to induce a sunburn. UVB light (290 to 320 nm) is more significant in SLE. It is more pronounced during midday (10 A.M. to 3 P.M.) and causes sunburn readily (phototoxic reactions).

Hundred of prescription drugs can cause photoallergic and/or phototoxic reactions. The most common are phenothiazines, tetracyclines, nalidixic acid, sulfa-containing agents, piroxicam, methotrexate, amiodarone, psoralens, phenytoin, and carprofen.[A235] Photosensitizing chemicals are found in certain perfumes, mercury vapor lamps, xenon arc lamps, tungsten iodide light sources, discotheques, color television sets, and photocopy machines. The presence of anti-Ro/SSA antibody is associated with photosensitivity in more than 90% of white SLE patients.[M533] Fluorescent lights are a source of UVA and only rarely might its avoidance be beneficial.[M160] Clear jacket and bulk covers that control UV emanation without reducing visibility are available.*

Although the ultraviolet end of the spectrum is the most damaging to lupus skin lesions, heat and infrared exposure can also cause exacerbations. The flares produced by infrared exposure are characterized by a marked increase in erythema of short duration. These are frequently experienced by SLE patients who work near a hot stove, oven, or furnace for any length of time. One characteristic of DLE and SLE is that skin burns and scalds can produce localized lesions of DLE at the site of trauma, the Koebner phenomenon, even in apparently normal skin.[K174,K234, L360]

Sunscreens are ultraviolet light-absorbing chemical agents in a cream, oil, lotion, alcohol, or gel vehicle. These chemicals can block UVA, UVB, or both. They include aminobenzoic acid esters (UVB), cinnamates (UVB), salicylates (UVB), benzophenones (UVA, UVB), anthralites (UVA, UVB), and butylmethoxydibenzomethanes (UVA, UVB). Physical sunblocks containing titanium dioxide and zinc oxide scatter light. A sun protection factor (SPF) value is the ratio of the time required to produce erythema through a UVB sunscreen product to the time required to produce the same degree of erythema without it. The SPF ranges from 2 (minimal protection) to 50 (highest protection). We advise outpatients to use agents with a high SPF (at least 15); unfortunately, because of irritation, contact dermatitis, and occasional photosensitivity, patient compliance is poor, and it may be necessary to try several compounds before an acceptable block is

Table 55–2. Examples of Sunscreen Products for Lupus Patients

Product	SPF*	Active Ingredients
Total Eclipse	15	Glyceryl aminobenzoate; padimate O; oxybenzone
PreSun	15	p-Aminobenzoic acid;† padimate O; oxybenzone
Coppertone Sunshade	15	Padimate O; oxybenzone
Ti Screen	15, 30	Ethylhexyl-p-methoxycinnamate; oxybenzone
Bull Frog	36	Benzophenone-3; octocrylene; octyl methoxycinnamate
Clinique Sunblock	19	Padimate O; benzophenone-3; octyl methoxycinnamate
Sundown Sunblock	20	Octyl dimethyl PABA; titanium dioxide; oxybenzone; octyl methoxycinnamate
Photoplex	15	Padimate O; butylmethoxybenzomethane

* SPF of 15 or high; protects against UVA and UVB.
† PABA.

found. In particular, the alcohol base in PABA and PABA esters may sting and dry the skin. Some available sunscreens are listed in Table 55-2.

Sunscreens should be applied about 30 minutes prior to sun exposure over active and healed lesions and to areas that may burn, including the cheeks, nose, lips, and arms. They can be applied over the scalp hair before going outdoors. Cosmetics may be applied over sunscreens.

Two forms of UV exposure are often overlooked. Skin lesions are frequently more intense on the left cheek and on the lateral aspect of the left arm because of UVA exposure while driving a car. If the lesions are primarily distributed in these areas, the physician should inquire whether such exposure might be responsible, and advise the patient on avoiding it. Merely keeping the window closed or tinting the window may filter the sunlight sufficiently. Another unnoticed source of exposure is UV light that is reflected off the surface of sand, water, cement, or snow. UV radiation is greater at higher altitudes. For example, the intensity at 5,000 feet is 20% higher than that at sea level. Patients should be cautioned about these sources of danger. A cloudy day only decreases UV exposure by 20 to 40%.

Sunscreens block vitamin D activation in the skin, and oral supplementation may be required. An occasional patient develops eye sensitivity to UV light that is not responsive to wearing ordinary sunglasses. Special coated lenses to protect the eyes are available.**

In LE patients with definite UV sensitivity, walking a few blocks without any protection is usually permitted. If further exposure is necessary, general measures such as wearing a broad-brimmed hat and long-sleeves and using an umbrella can be used; these decrease exposure by 30 to 50%.

When a remission occurs, either spontaneously or induced, greater freedom of sun exposure is permitted. Frequently, otherwise asymptomatic patients have a persis-

---

* From the Solar Screen Company, 53-11 105th Street, Corona, NY 11368, (212)592-8222.

** From Suntiger Biomedical Optics, 12423 Gladstone Ave, No. 21, Sylmar, CA 91342.

tent butterfly erythema aggravated by sun exposure. The use of antimalarials and local sunscreens usually controls this if it is severe enough to warrant therapy.

Avoidance of UV exposure has been so overemphasized that many patients are irrational about going out during the day. Unless definite evidence of exacerbations provoked by such exposure is noted, normal activities need not be restricted or curtailed. Although it is advisable to caution the patient that sun exposure may result in an increase in local erythema or in the development of new skin lesions, the physician should avoid causing a sunlight phobia. The average patient, even one who is photosensitive, can usually walk a few blocks at midday without protection and experience no ill effects. The question of how much light exposure should be limited must be determined on an individual basis. The physician must use judgment so that the patient's way of life is interrupted as little as possible.

Antimalarial therapy increases the patient's tolerance to sun exposure, even in those who were extremely sensitive to UV light prior to taking them.[L53,M230,P8] The degree of limitation must frequently be re-evaluated, because the tendency to sunlight-induced exacerbation of skin lesions can subside, particularly with disease remission, either spontaneous or drug-induced.

LOCAL THERAPY FOR DLE AND SLE

Local treatment is used for isolated lesions of DLE or for refractory skin lesions in patients with DLE or SLE. The most effective, safest, and least scarring type of local therapy is the use of various steroid preparations. These can be fluorinated or nonfluorinated and may be of low, intermediate, or high potency (Table 55–3). Most nonfluorinated steroids include hydrocortisone cream or ointment and are now available as over-the-counter preparations in strengths of less than 1%. These agents are cheaper but less potent than the fluorinated preparations, which produce more stinging, dermal atrophy, depigmentation, striae, acne, folliculitis, and Candida superinfection.[W198] Fluorinated steroids cannot be applied to the face for more than 2 weeks at a time without expecting cutaneous side effects. I have found betamethasone dipropionate 0.05% (Diprosone) and fluocinonide 0.05% (Lidex) creams or ointments to be the most effective dermatologic agents for the short-term treatment of discoid lesions, especially in conjunction with antimalarials. Other studies also support this.[B176] The most potent steroids, betamethasone dipropionate 0.05% (Diprolene) and clobetasol proprionate 0.05% (Temovate),[A234] should never be used for more than 2 weeks at a time unless to avoid the use of medications with even more side effects.

The preparations should be used three or four times daily for optimal effectiveness and only applied directly over the lesions. Patients should be warned not to use them on normal skin because they induce atrophy. Improvement is usually noted within a few days. Unfortunately, recurrences frequently appear within a few days to weeks after cessation of treatment, but small lesions can be controlled adequately and indefinitely by the inter-mittent use of this method. Old, indurated, and chronically scaling lesions respond poorly to this form of treatment alone and require occlusive therapy (see below), intracutaneous injection, and/or antimalarials. We usually start patients on an intermediate-strength steroid cream or ointment and move up to high-potency agents for resistant lesions. Ointments are generally used for dry skin and creams for oily skin, but the ointment form is more effective than a cream, gel, or lotion; fluorocarbon-propelled sprays are the least effective. Thin skin is more permeable to topical steroids.

The introduction of Actiderm patches allows for the improved absorption of high-potency steroids with less irritation. This should replace the use of translucent plastic, steroid-impregnated tape (Cordran Tape) and occlusive dressings such as Saran Wrap, which increase percutaneous absorption by a factor of 100 and have been documented to be effective for those with severe DLE.[G38,M303,S162,S761,W312] Airtight occlusion of the skin causes obstruction of the sweat ducts, however, which may exacerbate pruritus and foster bacterial overgrowth on the skin surface.

Jansen et al.[J47] reported that topical fluocinolone acetonide cream 0.025%, (Synalar) when applied by massaging into the lesions four or five times daily or by using an occlusive dressing daily, was effective in 43 of 59 DLE patients. It was necessary to supplement local therapy with antimalarials or corticosteroids in 11 patients. Of the 59 patients, 5 failed to respond. Also, 23 patients who had required antimalarials were able to discontinue them with the consistent use of local medication. All 24 patients who responded well to topical therapy and were followed through two summers did well, except for 3 who relapsed and required retreatment.

The daily application of triamcinolone acetonide 0.5% in a flexible collodion base to recalcitrant DLE lesions was effective in 6 of 7 patients, compared to the use of nonmedicated collodion as a control.[B498] It may be especially helpful in the external ear, where occlusive dressings are impractical.

Intralesional therapy is often helpful when these fail. Several studies have shown the value of intradermal injections of steroids. Callen has documented the superiority of this method to the use of topical or oral steroids in resistant lesions.[C19,C21,J39,W312] Triamcinolone suspensions have been the most widely used; these include triamcinolone diacetate 1.25 or 2.5% suspension (Aristocort Diacetate Parenteral), triamcinolone acetonide 10 mg/ml (Kenalog Parenteral), and 1 or 2.5% aqueous suspension (Meticortelene Acetate Suspension).

Occasionally, acute swelling may occur at the site of injection, but this usually subsides within 24 hours. A local depression may appear because of tissue reabsorption; this may be noted in 5% of patients[J39] and usually disappears within several months. This is probably a pseudoatrophy resulting from true tissue destruction. James[J39] reported the results in 9 DLE patients treated in this manner; five had an excellent response and, in 2, the benefit was satisfactory. Rowell[R375] treated 28 patients with multiple intralesional injections of triamcinolone at 3-week intervals. In 13 patients the injected lesions cleared, and 13

Table 55–3.   Some Topical Steroids

Steroid		Vehicle
Lowest potency		
0.1%	Dexamethasone (*Decadron Phosphate*—Merck)	cream
1.0%	Hydrocortisone	cream, ointment
	(*Cort-Dome*—Miles)	cream
		lotion
2.5%	Hydrocortisone	cream, ointment
Low potency		
0.01%	Betamethasone valerate (*Valisone*—Schering)	cream
0.1%	Clocortotone (*Cloderm*—Hermal)	cream
0.05%	Desonide (*Desowen*—Owen)	cream, ointment
	(*Tridesilon*—Miles)	cream, ointment
0.01%	Fluocinotone acetonide	cream
0.025%	Flurandrenolide (*Cordran, Cordran SP*— Dista)	ointment, cream
0.025%	Triamcinolone acetonide	ointment, cream lotion
	(*Aristocort A*—Lederle)	cream
	(*Kenalog*—Westwood-Squibb)	lotion
Medium potency		
0.025%	Betamethasone benzoate (*Uticort*—Parke Davis)	lotion
0.1%	Betamethasone valerate	cream, ointment
	(*Valisone*—Schering)	lotion
		cream, ointment
0.05%	Desoximetasone	cream
	(*Topicort LP*—Hoechst-Roussel)	
0.025%	Fluocinolone acetonide	cream, ointment
0.2%	Hydrocortisone valerate (*Westcort*—Westwood-Squibb)	cream, ointment
0.1%	Mornetasone furoate (*Elocon*—Schering)	cream, ointment
		lotion
0.05%	Flurandrenolide	lotion
	(*Cordran, Cordran SP*—Dista)	cream, ointment
0.025%	Halcinonide (*Halog*—Westwood/Squibb)	cream
0.1%	Triamcinolone acetonide	cream, ointment lotion
	(*Aristocort*—Lederle)	cream, ointment
	(*Aristocort A*—Lederle)	cream, ointment
	(*Kenalog*–Westwood-Squibb)	cream
0.005%	Fluticasone propionate (*Cutivate*—Glaxo)	ointment
0.05%		cream
High potency		
0.1%	Amcinonide (*Cyclocort*—Lederle)	cream, ointment lotion
0.05%	Betamethasone dipropionate	cream, ointment
		lotion
	(*Diprosono*—Schering)	lotion
0.25%	Desoximetasone	cream, ointment
	(*Topicort*—Hoechst-Roussel)	
0.05%	Diflorasone diacetate	cream, ointment
	(*Florone*—Dermik)	
	(*Maxiflor*—Herbort)	cream, ointment
0.2%	Fluocinolone (*Synalar HP*—Syntex)	cream
0.05%	Fluocinonide	
	(*Lidex, Lidex-E*—Syntex)	cream, ointment
0.1%	Halcinonide (*Halog, Halog-E*—Westwood-Squibb)	cream, ointment
		solution
0.5%	Triamcinolone acetonide	cream, ointment
	(*Aristocort A*—Lederle)	cream
Super-high potency		
0.05%	Betamethasone dipropionate (*Diprolene*—Schering)	cream, ointment
		lotion
0.05%	Clobetasol propionate (*Temovate*—Glaxo)	cream, ointment
0.05%	Diflorasone diacetate (*Psorcon*—Dermik)	ointment
0.05%	Halobetasol propionate (*Ultravate*—Westwood-Squibb)	cream, ointment

Modified from Med. Lett. *28*;58–59, 1986.[A234]

other improved. Only 2 patients did not respond. Smith[S513] also described favorable results in 13 DLE patients. Biopsy studies before and after therapy showed a diminution of follicular plugging and hyperkeratosis in all patients, accompanied by some thinning of the epidermis. Vascular dilatation and cellular infiltration disappeared and skin atrophy was not observed.

Triamcinolone acetonide in an emollient dental paste (Kenalog in Orabase), used two or three times daily and at bedtime, is useful for sensitive lupus mucous membrane lesions. A buttermilk or hydrogen peroxide swish or gargle is also effective as an adjunctive agent. Over the long term, systemic antimalarials are more efficacious for lupus mucous membrane involvement.

The transplantation of normal skin to sites of excised quiescent lesions has been successful in a small number of patients.[F247,F248] The transplantation of 4-mm hair-bearing punch grafts into active plaques of DLE patients, however, showed recipient dominance with a decrease in hair survival and the appearance of discoid lesions in the implanted skin.[N126]

Intralesional administration of quinacrine and chloroquine was used in the 1950s with good results[E164,L53, P97] but was abandoned because of the high incidence of hemorrhagic bullae, local discomfort, erythema, bleeding, and crusting of blood. Caustic acids, intralesional gold, and solid carbon dioxide have also been used.[H237,P97,S762] None of these are currently recommended.

Chapter 56

SALICYLATE AND NONSTEROIDAL THERAPY

DANIEL J. WALLACE

Salicylates and nonsteroidal anti-inflammatory drugs (NSAIDs) are mainstays in the therapy of nonorgan-threatening lupus. A survey at our institution found that 77% of 925 SLE patients were given a therapeutic trial of NSAIDs and 41% were given salicylates.[W37] Medsger's group noted that 73% of 100 SLE patients were taking NSAIDs.[R35] In spite of their widespread use, only few investigations have examined the efficacy of these agents in SLE. No NSAIDs are approved by the Food and Drug Administration for the treatment of SLE. Lupus patients experience more adverse reactions to salicylates and NSAIDs than healthy individuals, and certain lupus subsets (e.g., nephritis with azotemia) present relative contraindications to their use. Acetaminophen (Tylenol) has little anti-inflammatory effect, but it may be helpful as an antipyretic and analgesic in patients who cannot tolerate salicylates or NSAIDs.[B368] This chapter discusses the role of these medications in the management of SLE, but not their general action and toxic effects.

SALICYLATES

Clinical Studies

Aspirin is useful in treating the fever, joint pain, and serositis seen in SLE. Low-dose aspirin may be useful in the management of the antiphospholipid syndrome.

Dubois noted that the incidence of spontaneous remission in SLE patients treated with rest and salicylates was 39% (see Chap. 62 and Table 56–1).[D310] Harvey[M280] observed that 7 of 19 patients experienced dramatic clinical benefit from aspirin and that 4 others defervesced following its administration, but without significant improvement in joint pains. Karsh and colleagues at the National Institutes of Health[K85] studied 19 SLE patients with fever, arthritis, pleuritis, or pericarditis in a blinded fashion. Of these, 9 were randomized to receive 3,600 mg of aspirin daily and 10 received 2,400 mg of ibuprofen. A 3-day placebo washout period was followed by 10 days of treatment. The salicylate group had significant decreases in the number of swollen joints and joint pain as assessed by the physician and patient. Of the 9 in the aspirin group, 7 improved overall, compared to only 2 of 8 on ibuprofen.

Sustained-release preparations (timed-release aspirin; Zorprin) have fewer gastrointestinal side effects and require fewer tablets at longer intervals to achieve therapeutic salicylate levels. Although slightly less effective, nonacetylated salicylates (Disalcid; Trilisate) do not prolong bleeding times and are not ulcerogenic. Salicylates should be given until significant clinical improvement is evident or when symptoms of salicylism appear. Determination of serum salicylate levels can be done to adjust dosage and monitor compliance.

Mechanism of Action, Renal Effects, and Drug Interactions

The mechanism of action of aspirin (i.e., acetylated salicylates) in SLE is most probably related to its antiprostaglandin effects. Kimberly and colleagues[K214,K220,K224] examined the effects of acetylated salicylates on renal function. SLE patients have increased baseline urinary immunoreactive prostaglandin E (PGE) material; its level was reduced by 50% with salicylate therapy.[K214] A reversible decrement in creatinine clearance, from 14 to 29%, was observed. Subsequently, Kimberly et al. noted acute renal failure in an SLE patient taking aspirin and ibuprofen.[K224] In another study, 13 of 23 SLE patients experienced reversible, decreased creatinine clearance.[K220] The greatest changes were seen in those with active nephritis and in those with low serum complement levels. Changes in renal blood flow mediated by prostaglandin inhibition were implicated. Rasmussen et al.[R52] also noted a 50% decreased PGE urinary excretion in 8 patients given 65 mg/kg/day of aspirin for 2 weeks, but no decrease in renal function was observed.

Salicylates have important interactions with other drugs that are sometimes used to treat patients with SLE. Intraarticular injection of steroids in patients with inflammatory arthritis can decrease serum salicylate levels by 50% for up to 36 hours after injection.[B20] Concomitant administration of salicylates with some NSAIDs decreases blood levels of the NSAIDs.[K491] Aspirin inhibits the renal clearance of methotrexate, resulting in higher serum levels and greater potential toxicity of the chemotherapeutic agent.[L282]

Evidence that low-dose aspirin (324 mg/day or less) blocks thromboxane A_2-dependent aggregation but not prostacyclin I_2 biosynthesis indicates that this therapy has potent antiplatelet effects.[P185] Therefore, low-dose aspirin therapy has been advocated by some rheumatologists as a safe and relatively benign way to treat the antiphospholipid syndrome in those who are at risk for developing thromboembolic phenomena. Its use in pregnant patients with a history of recurrent spontaneous abortions has also been explored, and is advocated by some. Also, other evidence has shown that treatment with salicylates during pregnancy can reduce the incidence of pre-eclampsia, to

Table 56–1. Salicylate and Clinical Trials of NSAIDs in SLE

Investigator(s) and Year of Report	Agent	No. of Patients	Controlled Benefit	Found
Harvey and Cochran (1954)[M280]	Aspirin	105	No	Yes
Dubois (1956)[D310]		163	No	Yes
Karsh et al. (1980)[K85]		19	Yes	Yes
Langhof (1953)[L50]	Phenylbutazone	4	No	Yes
Dubois (1966)[D317]		?	No	Yes
Dubois (1966)[D317]	Indomethacin	22	No	Yes
Marmont et al. (1964, 1965)[M145,M146]		10	No	Yes
Dubois (1975)[D322]	Ibuprofen	17	No	Yes
Karsh et al. (1980)[K85]		19	Yes	No
Gergely (1989)[G95]	Piroxicam	30	No	Yes

which patients with lupus nephritis are prone.[E70,G64, L402,O92] Chapters 50 and 51 present further details, and discuss the use of salicylates and NSAIDs during routine pregnancy and lactation.

Adverse Reactions

Acetylated salicylates can reduce the glomerular filtration rate. Several studies have suggested that SLE patients are more susceptible to drug-induced hepatic toxicity than healthy subjects taking the same dose of aspirin. In 1976, Seaman and Plotz gave salicylates in therapeutic doses to SLE patients and to a rheumatoid arthritis and control group.[W198] Of the 16 SLE patients, 7 developed abnormal liver enzyme levels during the 2-week study and, in 6, the transaminase levels exceeded 100 IU/dl. Of the 16 SLE patients, 3 were asymptomatic and all had active disease. The prevalence of hepatotoxicity was greater in SLE patients than in the other patient groups.

Four other reports have confirmed these findings.[F263,K85,P165,T207] Fries and Holman reported that 25% of their 192 lupus patients who received aspirin developed evidence of transaminitis.[F263] I do not discontinue aspirin unless the transaminase levels are higher than 100 IU/dl, or the patient becomes symptomatic. No cases of chronic hepatitis have been described, but one report of Reye's syndrome in a 14-year-old girl with SLE associated with aspirin use has appeared.[H110]

The toxicity of acetylated salicylates in SLE patients may be related to the drug's prolongation of bleeding time, its promotion of erosive gastritis, and the high doses that are often required. The risk of gastrointestinal toxicity is high, and this represents a cogent argument for concomitant gastric cytoprotection. This can be accomplished by in-gesting tablets with meals, antacid administration and, in higher risk patients, by giving H2 blockers, sucralfate, misoprostol omeprazole, and prostaglandin agonists.

Nonacetylated salicylates do not alter bleeding times, and may be useful for patients with coagulation disorders or upcoming surgery. These inhibit prostaglandins less than acetylated salicylates and therefore have substantially fewer gastrointestinal and renal toxic effects. Gastrointestinal blood loss with these agents has been found to be similar to that with placebo. Some physicians therefore use these drugs, rather than any of the acetylated salicylates. The combination of acetylated salicylates and heavy menstrual periods often leads to iron deficiency anemia, which requires iron replacement therapy. In an occasional patient, parenteral iron (Imferon) may be necessary, but it should be noted that iron dextran may temporarily worsen inflammatory synovitis by promoting lipid peroxidation.[B332] Elderly patients have an increased incidence of tinnitus and confusion from salicylates of any type, and should be given lower doses of the drug and monitored carefully.

NONSTEROIDAL ANTI-INFLAMMATORY DRUGS

Clinical Trials (see Table 56–1)

NSAIDs were first used by a German group, which reported phenylbutazone to be of value in the treatment of "subacute" lupus in 1953.[L50] In 1966, Dubois wrote that he had successfully used phenylbutazone in doses up to 300 mg daily.[D317] He also described his experience with indomethacin in 22 patients given 50 to 125 mg daily over a 9-month period.[D317] Even though 18 patients "improved" (especially their arthritis), 17 developed adverse reactions, necessitating that the drug be discontinued in 11. Marmont et al. found steroid-sparing properties of indomethacin in 10 patients.[M145,M146] A case report of cardiac tamponade responding to indomethacin alone has appeared.[P260] Dubois presented data on 17 SLE patients SLE given ibuprofen, 1,200 to 3,200 mg daily (median, 2,400 mg) for an average of 16 weeks.[D322] Clinical improvement was noted in 69%, in 13 patients arthralgias were diminished, and in 1 serositis decreased. Many minor adverse effects were reported. Steroid-sparing properties were reported in 30 Hungarian SLE patients given 20 mg of piroxicam daily for 3 months.[G95]

The only controlled trial of NSAIDs in SLE patients was performed in 1980 by Karsh et al.[K85] (see above for details). Only 2 of the 8 who received 2,400 mg of ibuprofen daily for 10 days benefited, whereas 7 of the 9 patients given aspirin improved. In the ibuprofen group, abnormal liver function developed in 2 patients and transient decrements in creatinine clearance were observed in 2.

Antiprostaglandin Renal Effects and Other Actions

Four controlled studies have examined the interaction between prostaglandins and NSAIDs in over 100 nonuremic lupus patients.[H279,N12,P68,T105] Most patients had elevated baseline urinary prostaglandin E_2 (PGE_2) and thromboxane A_2 levels, decreased urinary 6-ketoprostaglandin F_1 levels, and increased peripheral renin activity.

The administration of ibuprofen or indomethacin decreased the glomerular filtration rate by about 16%, as estimated by creatinine clearance, diminished the urinary excretion of PGE_2, 6-ketoprostaglandin F_1, and thromboxane A_2, and decreased peripheral renin activity. Because renal plasma flow remained constant, these NSAID effects could be a result of mesangial contraction or interference with distal tubular sodium reabsorption. Other studies have also demonstrated that ibuprofen can induce renal function decrement (measured by various methods), but it rarely causes irreversible renal failure in SLE patients. Naproxen and fenoprofen have similar effects.[F145,K211, L309,R368,T106] Sulindac probably impairs renal prostaglandins to a lesser degree than other NSAIDs,[C267] but its use can be associated with a rise in the serum creatinine level. It might be the most effective NSAID in patients with lupus nephritis. The antiplatelet effects of NSAIDs may decrease the incidence of thromboembolic disease in patients with the lupus anticoagulant.[W322]

Other Adverse Reactions

The same precautions apply to all patients on longterm NSAID therapy, whether or not they have lupus. These include knowledge of potential gastrointestinal, dermatologic, hepatic, hematologic, and renal toxic effects. Ramsay-Goldman et al. observed that 36% of 73 SLE patients had a significant adverse reaction to at least one NSAID.[R35]

A distinct hypersensitivity reaction to ibuprofen characterized by hypotension, fever, rigors, conjunctivitis, nausea, arthralgias, transaminitis, and aseptic meningitis has been reported in 25 patients, 18 of whom had documented SLE.[A65,D363,J69,L383,M89] This reaction can occur early, or can be seen even after several years of uncomplicated ibuprofen administration; in several patients, it occurred after drug rechallenge. Schoenfeld et al. demonstrated cell-mediated hypersensitivity to ibuprofen in patients with SLE but not in those with rheumatoid arthritis.[S158] One case of ulcerative proctitis in SLE has been reported after ibuprofen therapy.[K193] Phenylbutazone is associated with a hypersensitivity reaction that can lead to a lupus activity flare.[F18] Hypersensitivity reactions similar to those described with ibuprofen have been observed with sulindac[B56,D195] and tolmetin.[R424] Tolmetin can interfere with urine dipstick readings, resulting in "pseudoproteinuria."[W171] Indoprofen has been associated with a case of aplastic anemia in SLE.[S1]

Three NSAIDs are known photosensitizers and should be avoided or used with caution by SLE patients: benoxaprofen, carprofen, and piroxicam. Benoxaprofen (no longer available in the United States) was associated with a 9% incidence of photosensitivity in the general population.[S524] Of rheumatic disease patients, 6 to 10% given carprofen developed rashes, including serious phototoxic reactions.[O6] Piroxicam can induce a unique photosensitivity response mediated by ultraviolet A light exposure.[S292] The Adverse Drug Reaction Reporting System of the American Academy of Dermatology compiled 29 cases of serious phototoxic reactions resulting from piroxicam in its first year of use.[S671] This has been associated with lupus flares.[R370] Indomethacin, phenylbutazone, and sulindac rarely include photosensitive rashes,[B302] but indomethacin can also decrease erythema induced by ultraviolet light, as documented by epicutaneous xenon-133 flow studies.[G353]

SUMMARY

1. Salicylates and NSAIDs can be useful in treating the fever, arthralgias, serositis, headaches, and soft tissue pain associated with nonorgan-threatening lupus.
2. Only aspirin has been shown to be effective in a controlled trial. Except for ibuprofen, controlled studies on the efficacy of NSAIDs in the treatment of SLE have not been done.
   a. Nonacetylated salicylates are recommended for patients with gastrointestinal symptoms—sulindac for nephritis, and short-term indomethacin to treat acute joint or serositis flares. A minimum 7-day trial is essential.
   b. It is not known whether these agents are steroid-sparing.
3. Complications of salicylate and NSAID therapy occur more frequently in SLE patients than in patients with nonrheumatic diseases.
4. Physicians must be alert to increased risks in SLE patients of NSAID-induced renal impairment, photosensitivity, liver function abnormalities, and hypersensitivity reactions (including aseptic meningitis).
5. All patients on salicylates or NSAID should have a complete blood count and renal and liver function testing at 3- to 4-month intervals. Serum creatinine levels should be measured before and within 2 weeks of institution of aspirin or NSAID therapy in all patients with evidence of nephritis, or in those over 65 years old.

Chapter 57

ANTIMALARIAL THERAPIES

DANIEL J. WALLACE

Antimalarials are effective nonsteroid drugs for some patients with nonorgan-threatening lupus. Unlike other therapeutic agents used to treat SLE, antimalarials are probably underused and their role misunderstood. This chapter attempts to clarify these issues.

HISTORICAL PERSPECTIVE

Antimalarials were first used therapeutically in 1630 as an antipyretic.[L124] They were first used in the treatment of discoid LE in 1894, when Payne tried quinine.[P81] Marstenstein, in 1928, reported good results in 22 of 28 patients with discoid and subacute systemic lupus treated with pamaquine (Plasmachin), which is similar to quinine in that both are substituted 8-aminoquinolines.[M159] Davidson and Birt,[D68] in 1938, reported excellent results in 19 of 29 patients treated with quinine bisulfate. In 1941, Prokoptochouk[P304,P304a] successfully treated 35 patients with discoid LE by giving daily doses of 300 mg of Atabrine (quinacrine, mepacrine), a compound first synthesized by the Germans during the 1920s. During World War II, quinine supplies were cut off by the Japanese, and the Surgeon General of the United States declared Atabrine to be the official drug to treat malaria.[O15] Between 1943 and 1946, 3 million Americans took the drug daily. Anecdotal evidence of its efficacy in treating some skin disorders among British soldiers prompted Page to study the drug for use in the treatment of discoid lupus. Unaware of Prokoptochouk's work, he reported its benefits in an uncontrolled study of 18 lupus and 2 rheumatoid arthritis patients in 1951, and the report received wide attention.[P8] These findings were soon confirmed at the Mayo Clinic by O'Leary et al.[O60]

Subsequently, it was shown that other antimalarials are also effective. Chloroquine and hydroxychloroquine were synthesized in the mid-1940s and shown to be less toxic than Atabrine. In 1953, Goldman et al.[G261] reported that chloroquine was helpful in 21 patients, including 3 with subacute disseminated disease and, in 1954, Pillsbury and Johnson[P191] noted that 15 of 16 patients with SLE taking chloroquine improved. Hydroxychloroquine (Plaquenil) was released in 1955 after it was found to be effective in SLE and rheumatoid arthritis (RA), with fewer adverse reactions than chloroquine.[C391,L245,M654] Amodiaquin (Camoquin) was also efficacious in SLE but it was taken off the market in the United States in the early 1970s because of its propensity to induce agranulocytosis,[L153,M63,P39] although it is still available in many other countries. Finally, an extremely potent antimalarial, Triquin (which contained chloroquine, hydroxychloroquine and Atabrine) took advantage of the synergy between Atabrine and the chloroquines. It was released in 1959 after a report claimed that 44 of 45 lupus patients, mostly antimalarial-resistant, at Boston City Hospital had dramatic responses.[T285] The preparation sold well until it was withdrawn in 1972 as part of a campaign against the use of combination drugs.

PHARMACOLOGY OF THE ANTIMALARIALS

Chloroquine

Chloroquine (7-chloro-4-(4-diethylamino-1-methylbutylamino) quinoline; Aralen; Nivaquine B, Sanoquin, Avlovlor, Bemaphate, Tanakan, Résoquine) is a 4-aminoquinoline available in oral, injectable, suppository, and liquid forms (Fig. 57–1).[C306,G290,O44] Almost completely absorbed by the gastrointestinal tract, only 10% is fecally excreted. Renal excretion (50%) is increased by acidification and decreased by alkalinization. The drug is bound by plasma proteins and is largely deposited into tissues. High concentrations can be found in the liver, spleen, kidney, lung, and all blood elements[F233,N136,P81,R9] as well as in pigmented tissues. Chloroquine is broken down into three N-dealkylated metabolites that are of toxologic and pharmacologic importance.[B247,E152] The drug readily crosses the placenta and is excreted in small amounts in breast milk. A child receives less than 1% of the maternal dose.[A83,E151,L185]

Chloroquine is slowly excreted, with detectable amounts in the urine, red cells, and plasma for as long as 5 years after discontinuation.[R387] The half-life is governed by dose-dependent kinetics, increasing from 3 hours after a single 250-mg dose to 13 days after 1,000 mg. Drug interactions have been reported with ampicillin (chloroquine decreases its bioavailability), but not with aspirin.[A39,A142] It has in vitro synergy with cyclosporine and antagonism with D-penicillamine.[D211]

Hydroxychloroquine

Hydroxychloroquine sulfate (2-[[4-[(7-chloro-4-quinolinyl) amino]pentyl]ethylamino]ethanol sulfate; Plaquenil) is a 4-aminoquinoline that differs from chloroquine by a hydroxyl group at the end of a side chain (Fig. 57–1). The two agents have similar pharmacokinetics. The 200-mg tablets contain 155 mg of hydroxychloroquine base.

Generic name	Synonyms		Structural formulae
1) Quinacrine	1) Atabrine	6) Acriquine	
	2) Mepacrine	7) Acrichine	
	3) Atebrin	8) Palacrin	
	4) Chinacrin	9) Metoquine	
	5) Erion	10) Italchin	
2) Chloroquine	1) Aralen	5) Bemaphate	
	2) Nivaquine B	6) Tanakan	
	3) Sanoquin	7) Resochin	
	4) Avloclor	8) Résoquine	
3) Amodiaquin	1) Camoquin		
	2) Camoquinal		
	3) Miaquin		
	4) CAM-AQ1		
4) Hydroxychloroquine	1) Plaquenil		

Active radical ?

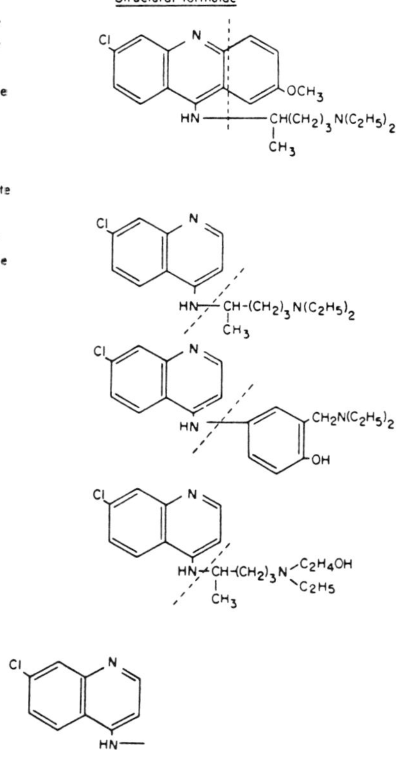

Fig. 57–1. Structural formulas of commonly used antimalarial drugs and their synonyms. (From Merwin, C. F., and Winkelmann, R. K.: Dermatologic clinics. 2. Antimalarial drugs in the therapy of lupus erythematosus. Proc. Mayo Clin. 37:253, 1962.)

Hydroxychloroquine is 75 to 100% absorbed in the gastrointestinal tract and 50% bound by serum proteins.[M21,T123] Some is conjugated with glucuronide and excreted in the bile, but 30 to 60% is biotransformed in the liver. Excretion occurs in two stages—a rapid one, with a half-life of 3 days, and a slower one, with an overall half-life of 40 days; 45% is excreted by the kidney, 3% by the skin, and 20% fecally. It takes 6 months to reach a 96% steady state. Much of the drug is deposited into tissues, with the highest concentrations in the adrenal and pituitary glands. Other areas with high concentrations include melanin-containing tissues, liver, spleen, and leukocytes.

The dosage must be reduced in patients with renal failure; dialysis does not help overdosage, because the agent is extensively sequestered.[T123] Hydroxychloroquine can interact with digoxin and reduce its levels (a quinidine-like effect).[L123] One five-center survey has suggested that hydroxychloroquine administration may decrease the frequency of liver enzyme abnormalities seen in RA patients on methotrexate or salicylate therapy.[F265]

Atabrine

Atabrine (6-chloro-9-(1-methyl-4-diethylamine)butylamine-2-methoxyacridine; quinacrine, mepacrine, Atebrin, chinacrin, Erion, Acriquine, Acrichine, Palacrin, Metoquine, Italchin) differs from chloroquine only in having an acridine nucleus (an extra benzene ring) instead of a quinoline (Fig. 57–1). The drug is rapidly absorbed after oral administration. Plasma levels rise in 2 to 4 hours, reaching a peak in 8 to 12 hours.[J98] Plasma concentration increases rapidly during the first week, and 94% equilibrium is attained by the fourth week. The drug is distributed widely in tissue but is slowly liberated, with the highest concentrations in the liver and spleen and the lowest concentrations in the brain and heart. The liver concentration may be 20,000 that in plasma. Skin deposits are often clearly visible. Atabrine crosses the placenta and reaches the fetus. Spinal fluid levels are 1 to 5% of plasma levels. Eighty to 90% of the drug is bound to plasma proteins in therapeutic doses and slowly excreted from the body. Less than 11% is eliminated in the urine daily.[W24]

Atabrine can also be administered intralesionally,[O122,T141] for discoid lesions, intramuscularly, intravenously, rectally, or transcervically, or delivered through a chest tube for malignant pleural effusions.[W24]

MECHANISMS OF ACTION

Light Filtration

One of the major aggravating factors in SLE patients is ultraviolet (UV) light exposure. More UV radiation is absorbed (Table 57–1) when skin concentrations of antimalarials are higher.[C5,M230,S302] Antimalarials deposited in the skin absorb UV light in a concentration-dependent manner.[C5,M230,S302] Hydroxychloroquine, but not methotrexate, methylprednisolone, or saline, blocked cutaneous reactions induced by UV light.[L202] Atabrine can impede photodynamic actions, inhibit laser-induced photosensi-

Table 57–1. Important Mechanisms of Action of Antimalarial Drugs

Ultraviolet light absorption
Immunologic actions:
    Inhibit natural killer activity, mitogenic stimulation
    Block interleukin-1 and interleukin-2 production
    Impede formation of and help dissolve immune complexes
    Decrease LE cell factor and DNA binding to anti-DNA
Anti-inflammatory effects:
    Prostaglandin antagonization
    Inhibit phospholipase's A_2 and C
    Decrease fibronectin release by macrophages
    Lysosomal actions—result in membrane stabilization and depletes
        cells of their receptor sites
    Block superoxide release at multiple sites
Hormonal actions:
    Chloroquines—hypoglycemic, decreased vitamin D, and are adrenal-
        stimulating and steroid-sparing
    Atabrine—impairs prolactin and insulin release
Antiproliferative activities:
    Intercalation with DNA
    DNA, RNA polymerase inhibition
    Decreased tumor size and chemotherapy resistance
Inhibits platelet aggregation and adhesion
Antimicrobial effects, decrease antibiotic resistance
Anticholinesterase and sympatholytic actions
Quinidine-like cardiac actions, reduction of infarct size
Lowers cholesterol and low-density lipoproteins levels by 15 to 20%

tivity,[F69,R85] and increase UV light tolerance.[P8] Hissung et al.[H330] suggested that, in solutions containing both DNA and quinacrine, mutual radioprotection results from the scavenging of water radicals.

Immunologic Effects

In vitro studies of chloroquine have concluded that the drug can inhibit natural killer cell activity,[A357,P91] phytohemagglutinin (PHA) mitogenic stimulation,[B607,D212,H516] pokeweed mitogen-induced immunoglobulin production by peripheral blood mononuclear cells,[H52,V34] and interleukin-2 production by human lymphocytes.[B608] These actions might result from the stabilization of lysosomal membranes or from the action of complement on autologous cells.[F169,H516] Salmeron and Lipsky[S44] found that chloroquine inhibited tritiated thymidine uptake by lymphocytes in a dose-dependent fashion by interfering with the accessory function of monocytes. The inhibition of monocytes is accomplished through selective interference with the secretion of interleukin-1.

Atabrine inhibits natural killer cell cytotoxicity and enhances the ability of x rays to kill cells.[F69,S41] It blocks the primary but not the secondary proliferative response of cytotoxic T cells to allogeneic non–T-cell antigen and impedes interleukin-2 receptor expression because of its phospholipase A_2 blocking actions. Atabrine does not interfere with the recognition of antigens by cytotoxic T cells but suppresses the mitogenic response of T cells to allogeneic antigen.[N18] It can impair the uptake and incorporation of leucine, thymidine, and uridine in acid-insoluble material in human lymphocytes stimulated by PHA.[T222] In one report, Atabrine was five times more powerful than chloroquine in suppressing in vitro parameters of lymphocyte stimulation.

Chloroquine has opposing actions in that it inhibits the formation of antigen-antibody complexes in vitro and enhances the association of such complexes in a dose-dependent fashion,[S801] or it can split them.[W360] Chloroquine has been used to dissociate antigen-antibody complexes as part of a laboratory technique used in typing red blood cells with a positive direct antiglobulin test;[E35] also, it strips HLA antigens from platelet membranes.[L405] Clinically, it has been shown to decrease circulating immune complex levels in patients with rheumatoid arthritis.[S249]

Chloroquine blocks the DNA–anti-DNA reaction by binding not to the anti-DNA antibody but to the DNA.[S707] Competition for binding sites on DNA among chloroquine, sodium ions, and anti-DNA antibodies occurs only under nonphysiologic conditions.[R139] Work from Dubois' and Kunkel's laboratories documented that the binding of Atabrine to nucleoproteins can block the LE cell factor.[C247,D308,H390]

Anti-Inflammatory Effects

Chloroquine is a strong prostaglandin antagonist and a weak agonist.[E93,H425,M93] The antagonist effect is clearly demonstrable at concentrations reached in human plasma when the drug is used therapeutically.[M93] Chloroquine reduces prostaglandin synthesis through the inhibition of phospholipases A_2 and C.[C262,E93,F88,M201] Antiphospholipase A_2 blockade decreases the actions of bradykinin in synovial fibroblasts, suppresses its algesic effects, and decreases histamine release from basophils.[C443,J139,M484,N15,T176] In vitro hexosamine depletion of intact articular cartilage by E prostaglandins is accomplished through the DNA-dependent RNA synthesis of cathepsin-like proteases.[F308] This can be inhibited by chloroquine through the inhibition of DNA primer.

Chloroquine is concentrated in the nuclear and lysosomal fractions of white blood cells.[J105,Z61] It may also act by stabilizing lysosomes against various injuries.[F158,S661,W159,Z61] Chloroquine becomes trapped in lysosomes and alters their pH, which results in an increase in lysosome number and volume. Inclusion bodies ("myelin bodies") containing plasma membrane phospholipid accumulate because of the reversible inhibition of membrane recycling; this remarkable action leads to decreased phagocytosis, chemotaxis, and cell functioning. More specifically, it substantially depletes the cell of its surface receptors (trapping about 50% of them), which alters the cell's responsiveness to mitogenic stimuli.[F69,F158,L4,M21,S661]

Chloroquine and hydroxychloroquine also exhibit anti-inflammatory actions by decreasing interleukin-1–induced cartilage degeneration,[R14] fibronectin release by macrophages,[S627] and reactions dependent on sulfhydryl-disulfide interaction.[G93]

Atabrine is also a potent inhibitor of phospholipase A_2, which results in decreased leukotriene and prostaglandin release.[A363,C262,D226,E133,E161,F130,F134,H367,H425,H512,L387,R79] It is a nonselective antilipolytic agent that decreases prostaglandin E_2 production in a dose-dependent fashion. Thromboxanes B_2 and A_2 are specifically suppressed. Atabrine also stabilizes cell membranes as a result of its Na-K-adenosine triphosphatase (ATPase) inhibitory effects,[H512] and inhibits lysosomal enzymes involved in phospholipid catabolism. Strongly concentrated in leukocytes and lysosomes, Atabrine has a stabilizing effect.[E133] Phagocytosis, chemotaxis, RNA synthesis, and hexose monophosphate shunt burst activity are inhibited by the drug.[B33,F69,R85,R86,T76] Atabrine is also an antipyrogen.[C428,S577]

Hormonal Effects

Chloroquine may have an adrenal-stimulating effect.[G417] In patients with rheumatoid arthritis and sarcoidosis, it decreases 1,25-hydroxyvitamin D levels.[O62,P15] A major area of interest concerns its applications in diabetes as a result of the agent's hypoglycemic action. This occurs secondary to chloroquine-induced decreased degradation of insulin,[Q4,S506] and possibly decreasing insulin-induced loss of receptors.[M58]

Atabrine accumulates in peptide hormone-producing cells[E69,L421] and can block prolactin[R210,R211] and insulin release. Conflicting reports about its effects on 17-ketosteroids have been published.[N15,P8]

Antioxidant Effects

In high doses, chloroquine can inhibit polymorphonuclear oxidative bursts.[K192] Chloroquine, hydroxychloroquine, and Atabrine block superoxide release by actions at multiple sites on the metabolic pathway.[H512,H513,H514,M495,S45,T76] It is doubtful whether this action occurs at clinically recommended doses.[S45]

Antiproliferative Effects

Chloroquine interferes with protein synthesis in vivo and in vitro.[C269,C367] It blocks DNA and RNA biosynthesis and produces rapid degradation of ribosomes and dissimilation of ribosomal RNA. By intercalation, chloroquine inhibits DNA and RNA polymerase reactions in vitro and DNA replication and RNA transcription in susceptible cells.[B393] Chloroquine does not alter the ability to repair damage from UV light-induced DNA excisions.[H421] It impedes DNA synthesis stimulated by platelet-derived growth factor.[B425] Interest has focused on its anticarcinogenic properties. Chloroquine can inhibit the replication of Moloney leukemia virus and tumor development in newborn mice,[P83] as well as inhibit pancreatic adenocarcinoma cell growth.[Z16] Furthermore, it can potentiate hyperthermia therapies,[M604,T151] block Z-DNA formation,[K490] and enhance chemotherapy cytotoxicity in multiple drug-resistant human leukemic cells.[Z5]

Atabrine also binds to DNA by intercalation between adjacent base pairs.[D247,O5,V98] Atabrine blocks radiation-induced DNA strand breaks and potentiates the antiproliferative effects of radiation.[B308,F303,G119,H307,H330,P168,V98] It reduces the incidence of cancer in rats given nitrosourea,[M245] decreases the number of somatic mutations induced in murine leukemia cells,[B11] and reverses resistance to vincristine.[I12]

Antiplatelet Effects

Hydroxychloroquine and chloroquine can inhibit platelet aggregation and adhesion.[B266,K237,R305] A desludging effect was demonstrated in the retinal veins of 20 patients with rheumatoid arthritis.[C174] Additional studies suggested that hydroxychloroquine reduces the size of thrombi and does not prolong bleeding time.[C118,R305] As a result, the drug has been used for thromboprophylaxis of postoperative pulmonary emboli in orthopedic patients.[L390] Atabrine can also inhibit platelet aggregation, probably as a result of its antiphospholipase actions or its interaction with cyclic GMP.[M195,M251,W306,Y12]

Antimicrobial Effects

The inhibition of DNA replication may be the mechanism of action of the antimicrobial effects of chloroquine. It does not impede the growth of viruses, but protects the cells against virus-induced cell damage.[W97] Atabrine has antiparasitic, antiprotozoan, antibacterial, antiviral, and antifungal actions.[W24] It can prevent resistance to various antibiotics and increase interferon production.[R76]

Muscle and Nerve Effects

Chloroquine is a muscarinic receptor antagonist, which results in an atropine-like effect in humans.[H6,M650,R76] The agent can also block dopamine β-hydroxylase.[S4] Atabrine is a strong inhibitor of cholinesterase because of its inhibition of cyclic GMP.[A168,J139,L387,M458] It can block β agonists, α-adrenergic actions, and norepinephrine.[A168,L386,L387,T188,T189] Atabrine protects mice from lethal amounts of snake venom neurotoxins.[C442]

Cardiac Effects

Both chloroquine and Atabrine possess quinidine-like actions. Chloroquine increases the heart rate and decreases premature ventricular contractions in humans.[H1163,T181] Atabrine's anti-arrhythmic actions occur as a result of slowing inward current and decreasing the automaticity of Purkinje fibers; it can treat atrial fibrillation and prevent ventricular fibrillation.[B114,G289] The antiphospholipase A_2 actions of chloroquine and Atabrine resulted in studies demonstrating that both can decrease acute myocardial ischemic damage in dogs, rats, pigs, and cats.[A179,C234,C235,F35,K228,M516,O120,S251,V103]

Antihyperlipidemic Effects

Animal studies have shown that chloroquine decreases serum bile acid and cholesterol levels by 10 to 20%.[L12,M200,S297] Lysosomotropic agents reduce the proteolysis of many plasma membrane receptors, and chloroquine increases the number of low-density lipoprotein (LDL) receptors.[B282,G267,G268] Alternatively, the inhibition of hydrolysis of internalized cholesterol esters may also lead to increased LDL receptor levels[G267,G268] (see below).

CLINICAL STUDIES

As early as 1956, Ziff et al. noted a favorable response in 11 of 12 SLE patients given antimalarials, and commented on the reduction of steroid requirements (Table

Table 57–2. Major Clinical Trials of Chloroquines in SLE

Source	Findings
Ziff et al.[Z27] (1956)	11 of 12 patients had favorable responses; steroid-sparing properties noted
Dubois[D325,D334] (1950–1985)	90% with nonorgan-threatening disease improved with hydroxychloroquine; over 300 patients treated
Rothfield et al.[R343,R347,R412] (1975)	27 patients who stopped chloroquine because of macular changes had more flares after 1 year than in either of the prior 2 years while taking it
Callen[C19] (1982)	33 of 34 given hydroxychloroquine for cutaneous lupus responded (9, excellent; 15, very good; 6, good; 3, fair; 1 poor)
Esdaile et al.[C56] (1991)	47 patients controlled with hydroxychloroquine were given continued therapy or placebo for 24 weeks; treated group had fewer disease flares and severe disease exacerbations

57–2).[Z27] Dubois claimed that 90 to 95% of patients had a favorable response.[D325] To evaluate the effectiveness of medication for the treatment of discoid LE, it is essential to know the incidence of spontaneous remissions. In Dubois' studies, 10% of patients had a history of spontaneous improvement.[D334] In the series of Herman et al.,[H281] 14% of patients healed spontaneously, compared with 85% or more who improved with antimalarials.[M361,W300] Callen treated 62 discoid lupus patients at the University of Louisville over a 5-year period[C19] and he reported on 34 who were given hydroxychloroquine. Of these, nine patients were said to have an excellent response, 15 were very good, 6 good, 3 fair, and 1 poor.

Rothfield et al.[R343,R347,R412] studied the effects of the discontinuation of antimalarial therapy on SLE activity in 27 patients who had developed maculoretinopathy. Exacerbations during the 2 years prior to and 1 year after discontinuation of antimalarial treatment were compared. On this basis, 10 patients had more exacerbations during the year after antimalarials were stopped than during either of the 2 previous years while receiving these drugs. Of these, 3 had no increase in the number of exacerbations and 4 had fewer exacerbations after the discontinuation of therapy. The maintenance dose of prednisone required was higher after the discontinuance of antimalarial treatment. The data suggested that chloroquine therapy is a factor in the suppression of disease in 10 of 17 patients, and is steroid-sparing. Hughes found hydroxychloroquine to be particularly useful for anti-Ro/SSA–positive disease, confirmed its steroid-sparing properties, and advocated combined antimalarial therapy for resistant cases.[H475] Esdaile et al. studied 47 SLE patients whose disease was controlled with hydroxychloroquine and randomized them either to continued hydroxychloroquine or placebo

for 24 weeks. The hydroxychloroquine group had significantly fewer disease flares and a lower risk of severe disease exacerbation.[C56]

I have examined the effects of two nonimmunologic activities of hydroxychloroquine on SLE patients. In the first study, antiplatelet effects of the drug were associated with a statistically significant decrease in thromboembolic disease among 92 patients evaluated.[W23] In another report, hydroxychloroquine induced a 15 to 20% decrease in serum cholesterol and LDL levels.[W38] These actions might decrease the hyperlipidemic and atherogenic effects of corticosteroids, and suggest a greater adjunctive role for hydroxychloroquine.

The results of the last Atabrine clinical trial was published in 1961, but between 1940 and 1961 20 reports on 771 patients were published (Table 57–3).[W24] Remarkable for the similarity of their findings, 27% of patients had an excellent response, 46% improved, and 27% did not respond. Cutaneous and constitutional symptoms improved first; the chloroquines were superior to Atabrine in treating synovitis. Clearly, additional controlled trials are urgently needed to assess all three antimalarial

Table 57–3. Twenty Clinical Trials of Atabrine in Lupus

Investigator	Year	No. of Patients	Response (%)		
			Excellent*	Improved*	None or Doubtful
Prokoptchouk*	1940	(35)	?	?	?
Sorinson	1941	51	23	33	43
Page	1951	18	50	33	17
Somerville et al.	1952	23	17	66	17
Cramer and Lewis	1952	6	83	0	17
Wells	1952	12	25	50	25
Sawicky et al.	1952	30	20	50	30
Black	1953	60	17	38	45
O'Leary et al.	1953	40	40	36	25
Courville and Perry	1953	13	38	54	8
Kaminsky and Knallinsky	1953	61	16	62	21
Harvey and Cochrane	1953	62	37	23	40
Kierland et al.	1953	52	33	46	21
Rogers and Finn	1954	45	47	38	15
Helanen	1954	36	28	58	14
Christiansen and Nielson	1956	97	32	40	28
Dubois	1956	61	25	56	20
Nielsen	1956	12	17	75	8
Buchanan	1959	25	28	52	20
Winklemann et al.	1961	67	10	75	15
Totals (N)		771	209	352	210
Totals (%)		100	27	46	27

Modified from Wallace, D.J.: The use of quinacrine (Atabrine) in rheumatic diseases: A re-examination. Semin. Arthritis Rheum. *18*:282–296, 1989.
* Excellent or improved response, 73%.[W28]

agents alone and in combination for the treatment of subsets of patients with nonorgan-threatening lupus.

Despite the lack of adequate controlled clinical trials, it seems to be generally agreed that antimalarials are effective for cutaneous manifestations, polyarthralgia, pleuritis, and low-grade pericardial inflammation associated with SLE. In addition, some of the associated malaise and lethargy are ameliorated. Antimalarials are of no effect in seriously ill patients with central nervous system involvement, hematologic changes, or renal disease. They help in withdrawing steroid therapy once remission has been induced by steroids and other agents.[B177,R412]

DOSAGE

The dosing schedule used in the treatment of discoid LE varies with the extent of the skin lesions and the patient's tolerance of the drugs. If one or more lesions several mm to 2 cm in diameter are present, with no evidence of systemic involvement, local measures (e.g., avoidance of UV light, sunscreens, topical corticosteroids) should be tried. If the skin lesions are disfiguring or are refractory to local measures, systemic antimalarials should be instituted. These drugs have no place in patients with organ-threatening disease, but are appropriate therapy for constitutional symptoms (fever, fatigue, malaise), serositis, mucocutaneous ulcers, and arthritis.

Theoretically, it is advisable to begin with a larger initial dosage so that equilibrium can be reached sooner. From a practical point of view, the treatment of discoid LE is not urgent. Although the use of an initial loading dose is advisable for the moderately ill patient with SLE, larger starting doses produce a high incidence of side effects, such as nausea, vomiting, and diarrhea, and therefore discourage the patient from further trials with the drug. Hydroxychloroquine should usually be initiated in a dosage of 400 mg daily (given once daily, or in 200-mg divided doses). This should approximate 5 to 7 mg/kg/day. Responses usually begin in 2 to 3 months but the drug does not reach its peak efficacy for 6 to 12 months. In more urgent situations, 600 mg daily may be given for 1 to 2 months. This is associated with a greater incidence of gastrointestinal complications and retinotoxicity if used for more than a few months. Chloroquine is usually given in a dosage of 250 to 500 mg daily; this should approximate 4 mg/kg/day. Chloroquine works within 1 to 2 months but is associated with a 10% incidence of retinotoxicity, compared with 3% for hydroxychloroquine.[B258] Hence, the eyes should be checked at 3-month intervals for patients on chloroquine and at 6-month intervals for those on hydroxychloroquine. Plasma levels do not correlate with efficacy.[M417]

As little as 1 g of chloroquine can be fatal to a child, and 3 g to an adult. The pills taste bitter, which tends to discourage abuse. Overdoses are managed with mechanical ventilation, epinephrine, and diazepam.[K243,M415,R214,S24]

If additional therapy is required, Atabrine can be added. It has established synergy with the chloroquines.[M230,R134,]

[T285] Usually, 100 mg are given daily (although up to 200 mg daily can be administered), but as little as 25 mg may be effective. Occasionally, therapy can be initiated with Atabrine as opposed to the chloroquines when ophthalmologic considerations contraindicate the latter's use. Also, Atabrine is a much greater cerebral cortical stimulant than the chloroquines, and is used in patients whom fatigue is overwhelming.[E106] Atabrine is not retinotoxic. Its onset of action is 3 to 6 weeks.

In our experience, at least 95% of patients with skin lesions of DLE and SLE show moderate to significant benefit from treatment with antimalarials. The most common cause of failure is the physician's impatience in giving the drugs time to work. After 1 to 2 years of therapy, antimalarials can be tapered. Hydroxychloroquine is decreased to 200 mg daily for 3 to 6 months and then reduced by eliminating days of the week (e.g., the next decrement from 200 mg daily would be 5 days a week for 3 months, then 3 days a week). One or two tablets per week may be all that is required to suppress skin lesions, and this helps minimize toxicity.

ADVERSE REACTIONS

The adverse reactions to antimalarials are listed in Table 57–4 and delineated below.

Table 57–4. Toxic Effects of Chloroquine and Hydroxychloroquine*

Nervous system†	Gastrointestinal system‡
Peripheral neuropathy	Anorexia
Involuntary movements	Abdominal distention
Difficulty in visual	Abdominal cramps
accommodation	Heartburn
Vestibular dysfunction	Nausea
Nerve deafness	Vomiting
Tinnitus	Diarrhea
Migraine-like headache	Weight loss
Lassitude	Eyes
Nervousness	Subjective‡
Insomnia	Impaired reading ability
Mental confusion	Poor distant vision
Toxic psychosis	Scotomas
Convulsive seizures	Night blindness
Skin and hair	Entopic phenomena
Dryness of skin‡	Objective
Pruritus‡	Decreased color vision‡
Urticaria‡	Scotoma with or without
Morbilliform rash‡	pigment changes in
Maculopapular rash‡	fundus‡
Desquamating and exfoliating	Arterial constriction†
lesions†	Retinal edema†
Increased pigmentation of skin‡	Pallor of optic disk†
Bleaching of hair†	Pigmentation about
Hair loss†	macula‡
Blood†	Bull's eye lesion‡
Leukopenia	Loss of corneal reflex‡
Agranulocytosis	Deposits in cornea‡
	Retinopathy‡

Modified from Kelley, W.N., Harris, E.D., Jr., Ruddy, S., and Sledge C.B.: Textbook of Rheumatology. Philadelphia, W.B. Saunders, 1980.
* If given in recommended doses.
† Occurs in less than 1%.
‡ Occurs in 1 to 20% given chloroquine and in 1 to 10% given hydroxychloroquine.

Generalized and Gastrointestinal Reactions

Considering their remittive potential, antimalarial therapies are generally well tolerated when compared to other disease-modifying drugs. About 10% of those receiving hydroxychloroquine and 20% who are given chloroquine complain of anorexia, abdominal distention and cramps, heartburn, nausea, vomiting, diarrhea, and/or weight loss. These symptoms are transient, decrease, or disappear with lower dosing, and do not cause longterm sequelae. Atabrine may create these symptoms in up to 30% of patients, and diarrhea may be particularly pronounced. It can be alleviated with lower doses or by taking a bismuth suspension (e.g., Pepto-Bismol) with Atabrine. The chloroquines are associated with musculoskeletal flu-like symptoms of aching and fatigue in 5 to 10% of patients, but symptoms resolve within 1 to 2 weeks, even if therapy is continued.

Neuromuscular Effects

In 1948, Nelson and Fitzhugh first reported that the chronic administration of chloroquine to rats induces necrosis of cardiac and voluntary muscle.[N60] The term "chloroquine neuromyopathy" has evolved over the years; it is clinically evident in fewer than 1% of those taking chloroquine, and has been the subject of only about a dozen case reports with hydroxychloroquine.[A51,G92,H297,H481, I52,L160,M225,P87,R55,R230,S298,T95,W203] Patients complain of muscle weakness, numbness, and tingling, and sometimes have myasthenic symptoms. Active inflammatory myositis, hypokalemia, and steroid myopathy must be considered in the differential diagnosis. A myasthenia gravis-like picture with ptosis occasionally appears, which is reversible with drug discontinuation.[E149,R445] The patient may present with an acute polyneuropathy. Peripheral nerves may demonstrate segmental demyelination, cytoplasmic inclusions in Schwann cells and in perineural and endothelial cells to a lesser extent. Histopathologic investigation of the muscles reveals a vacuolar myopathy, acid phosphatase-positive vacuoles in type I fibers, and lysosomal hyperreactivity with large secondary lysosomes. Electron microscopy reveals electron-dense curvilinear bodies and concentric and parallel lamellae within the muscle. Both skeletal and cardiac muscle can be involved. Muscle enzyme levels are only occasionally elevated. Electromyography reveals fibrillations, positive sharp waves, complex, repetitive discharges and, sometimes, a myotonia pattern. Dramatic recovery is associated with discontinuation of the drug. Plasma chloroquine levels do not correlate with the clinical or pathologic picture.[G208] Muscle enzyme levels are only occasionally elevated. This syndrome does not occur with Atabrine.

Cutaneous and Pigmentary Changes

Antimalarials can induce skin dryness, pruritus, urticaria, changes in pigment, rashes, and exfoliating lesions. Approximately 3% of patients have to discontinue the drug secondary to adverse cutaneous reactions.[R445] Atabrine is associated with a lichen planus or eczema-like eruption that, if ignored, can be the first sign in a chain of events that ultimately leads to aplastic anemia. *Any rash resulting from Atabrine requires its immediate cessation.*[W24]

Pigment changes occur in 10 to 25% of those receiving longterm chloroquine therapy and in a smaller percentage of those taking hydroxychloroquine.[A172,C45,C46,D310,K494] These adverse effects rarely, if ever, require discontinuing treatment. Grayness at the roots of scalp hair, eyelashes, eyebrows, and beard may be observed, along with gray streaks in the hair. A blue-black discoloration is occasionally noted on the skin (Fig. 57–2). Chloroquine binds with melanin in vivo and in vitro by the electrostatic attraction of positively charged drug molecules to negative groups of the melanin polymer; this is probably supplemented by van der Waals forces or charge transfer complexes. These changes are reversible when chloroquine therapy is stopped. Nail beds can be affected and appear diffusely pigmented (Fig. 57–3) or display transverse bands.

Atabrine also binds to melanin. Membrane-bound intracellular Atabrine granules combined with large amounts of iron and sulfur produce asymptomatic "black-and-blue marks," especially on the shins and hard palate (Fig. 57–4). Atabrine can also induce a yellow stain which, like the pigment, is dose-related and resolves with cessation of therapy or lowering of the dose. The stain may be evident in up to 30% of patients; it sometimes appears as a tan and may enhance the patient's appearance.[W24] All these changes are also reversible.

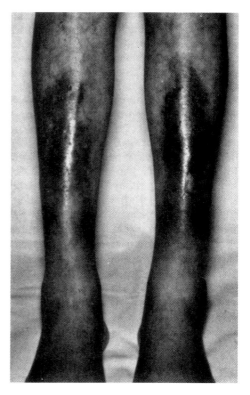

Fig. 57–2. Blue-black pretibial pigmentation from prolonged antimalarial administration.

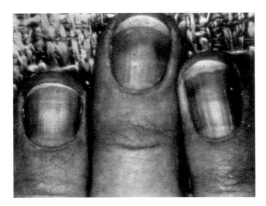

Fig. 57–3. Nail bed pigmentation resulting from antimalarial therapy.

Central Nervous System

Atabrine and, to a lesser extent, chloroquine, are cerebral cortical stimulants. Engel's classic study documented electroencephalographic patterns compatible with pronounced psychic stimulation in a group of healthy volunteers given 200 to 1,200 mg of Atabrine daily for 10 days.[E106] Symptoms of fatigue and mental clouding may be ameliorated. On the other hand, excessive dosing can result in psychosis, seizures, and hyperexcitability.[D325,E106,E162,L301,R197,W24] A 0.4% incidence of reversible, toxic psychosis was reported among 7,604 American soldiers given 100 mg of Atabrine daily in World War II and in 28 patients among 30,000 treated for malaria (0.1%).[G61,L272]

Hematologic Toxicity

Hydroxychloroquine has been associated with only one case of agranulocytosis in a patient given 1,200 mg daily,[P231] which is three to six times the current recommended dose. Chloroquine has been implicated in some reports with glucose-6-phosphatase deficiency hemolysis[C252] and with agranulocytosis.[K178] Toxic granulation

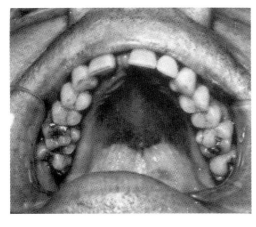

Fig. 57–4. Blue-black pigmentation on the hard palate caused by antimalarial therapy.

has been observed in the leukocytes of patients receiving longterm chloroquine, which represents large, membrane-bound myelin bodies in mature neutrophils and lymphocyte.[F41,R87]

The prevalence of aplastic anemia among American soldiers in the Pacific during World War II increased from 0.66 to 2.84/100,000 after Atabrine's introduction.[C461] This represented 58 patients, 48 of whom received Atabrine. Of these, 16 were associated with overdoses, and 2 received other marrow suppressant drugs concurrently. Of the 48 patients, 25 first developed lichen planus rashes; subsequent experience has indicated that this is a precursor of aplastic anemia, and is reversible if the drug is stopped.[C461,F118] Eleven cases of aplastic anemia in SLE have been published; nearly all were reported in the early 1950s among patients taking 300 mg daily (three to six times the current recommended dose). Bone marrow transplantation was successful in 1 patient who exceeded the recommended doses of Atabrine for discoid lupus.[S150] Wallace estimated the risk of aplastic anemia to be 1/500,000 if patients with SLE are given 100 mg daily and have their blood monitored every 2 to 3 months.[W24]

Miscellaneous Effects

Antimalarials may inhibit gastric motility based on their parasympatholytic effects,[M457] and may induce hypokalemia.[J34] The relationship of pregnancy and antimalarials is discussed in Chapter 50.

Ocular Toxicity

Corneal, Ciliary Body, and Lens Changes

Corneal deposits of chloroquine are observed in 18 to 95% of patients, appear within several weeks, and are symptomatic in 50% of patients.[B162,B258,C17,C453,H335, L397,M75] Keratopathy is limited to the corneal epithelium; the pattern can vary from punctate opacities to whirling lines. Visual acuity is not reduced, but patients may complain of halos around light sources and photophobia. No residual damage occurs, corneal deposits disappear with drug discontinuation, and are usually not a reason to stop therapy. Corneal sensation may be decreased by 50%.[H265] Because chloroquine doses have decreased over the last 30 years, corneal problems occur less frequently.[K5] Two studies were unable to find any corneal changes among 164 patients given hydroxychloroquine for 3 to 7 years.[R446,T166] Easterbrook reported a 5 to 10% incidence of corneal infiltrates with hydroxychloroquine, but none were symptomatic.[E10,E12] A decreased dosage is advised for these patients. Hydroxychloroquine crystals may be seen in the tear film by slit lamp examination.[B162] In doses three to six times greater than those currently recommended, Atabrine can induce corneal edema rarely.[A255,C192]

Alterations in accommodation and induction of cataracts rarely occur with longterm chloroquine therapy, and have not been reported with hydroxychloroquine or Atabrine.[L397]

Retinopathy

Since the first report appeared in 1957,[C33] about 300 cases of chloroquine and hydroxychloroquine retinopathy have been reviewed in the literature. Retinopathy is an often misunderstood problem that needlessly deters patients from initiating antimalarial therapy. Bernstein's thorough analysis concluded: "I would estimate that the risk of retinopathy in patients who are *not* regularly monitored ophthalmologically is 10% for those receiving chloroquine and 3 to 4% for those receiving hydroxychloroquine at presently recommended dosage levels. With regular and accurate observation and testing, these risks might be reduced substantially."[B258]

CLINICAL PRESENTATION AND PATHOPHYSIOLOGY

SLE can induce retinal vascular lesions secondary to disease activity that are unrelated to any form of therapy, and macular degeneration is a common feature of the normal aging process. Thus, it is not always easy to implicate antimalarials as the cause of retinal dysfunction. The chloroquines usually take years to induce pathology, and early retinopathy is asymptomatic. Lupus patients aware of the retinotoxicity of antimalarials often complain of visual symptoms weeks after starting therapy; this can be attributed to corticosteroid or NSAID treatment, or to psychopathology.

The most common presenting symptoms are difficulty in reading, photophobia, blurred distance version, visual field defects, and light flashes. Premaculopathy consists of fine pigmentary stippling of that area. Eventually, it becomes surrounded by a zone of depigmentation encircled by an area of pigment, giving a bull's eye appearance (Fig. 57–5). Rods and cones (which comprise the macula) are particularly sensitive to the chloroquines. With more extensive retinal damage, the arterioles show generalized attenuation and segmental constriction with disk pallor. In the periphery of the fundus, a prominent choroidal pattern and fine granularity of the retina are seen. Many years later, gross pigment changes of hereditary retinal

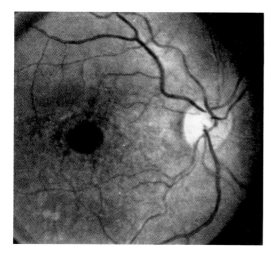

Fig. 57–5. Bull's eye macular pigmentation secondary to hydroxychloroquine (1200 mg/dl for 15 months in a 90-lb woman).

depigmentation may occur, and the foveolar reflex is lost.[B257,K422,L397,M75,V99]

Several theories account for chloroquine retinopathy. Retinal pigmented epithelial cells perform as macrophages and digest the discarded outer segments of photoreceptor cells as they are physiologically shed. Lysosomal accumulation (see above) results in an intracellular buildup of lamellar myelin bodies, which leads to scotoma.[E91] Alternatively, melanin deposits in the retina produce pigmentation of the rods and cones and of the pigmented cells in the outer nuclear and outer plexiform layers, with resulting pathology.[L340,W200] Cases of retinopathy have been reported, however, in the absence of pigment deposition.[B79] Chloroquine, but not hydroxychloroquine, breaks down the blood-retina barrier, as documented by vitreous fluorophotometry.[R13]

IMPORTANT CLINICAL STUDIES

The incidence of retinopathy has decreased over the last 30 years, because currently recommended doses of both chloroquine and hydroxychloroquine are about 50% of the formerly recommended doses. Most clinical studies address issues of cumulative dose and duration of therapy, incidence of lesions, and methods of detection. The latter topic is discussed in the next section.

In 1967, Bernstein[B257] first observed that lower chloroquine doses were associated with a lower incidence of retinopathy. In 1966, Voipio believed that lupus patients are more susceptible to retinopathy than those with rheumatoid arthritis.[V99]

Mackenzie[M22] reviewed experiences with over 900 RA patients. If doses were kept below 5.1 mg/kg/day for chloroquine or 7.8 mg/kg/day for hydroxychloroquine in patients with normal hepatic and renal functions, retinotoxicity did not occur. Marks[M141] followed 222 patients given a mean of 286 g of chloroquine for a mean of 36 months; 22 developed retinal changes, and only 1 had decreased visual acuity. These changes were directly related to age, total dose, and duration of treatment. In another study, Marks[M140] sent questionnaires to 45 rheumatologists in Great Britain; 23 had never had a patient with antimalarial eye toxicity. Mills[M441] reviewed the experience of 347 patients treated with hydroxychloroquine. The chief risk factor was a patient age of more than 70 years (in whom pre-existing macular degeneration is commonly seen) and a cumulative dose of more than 800 g. Of the patients in this subset, 29% had at least a mild pigmentary maculopathy, but none had decreased visual acuity or altered foveolar light thresholds. Macular changes in patients under the age of 40 years, on doses of less than 600 mg a day of hydroxychloroquine, were not seen. Runge[R421] reported no cases of retinopathy among 101 RA patients given hydroxychloroquine for a mean of 20 months. Rynes and colleagues have also carried out a number of studies on the effects of antimalarials.[B109,B398,R446,T166] In 99 patients (31 of whom had SLE) given 400 mg of hydroxychloroquine daily for a mean of 37 months, no retinotoxicity was reported,[R446] but in a follow-up report 4 years later[R444] it was observed in 4 of the RA patients. Elman et al.[E88] studied 270 RA patients given chloroquine for up to 15 years. They noted that senile macular atrophy is seen in 30% of healthy patients over the age of 65, and that chloroquine toxicity is greater in this group and more difficult to evaluate. Only 1 patient had clear-cut, drug-induced retinopathy. Two studies from the National Institutes of Health followed over 100 patients.[F90,F91] No differences in retinopathy between SLE and RA groups were noted, and retinotoxicity from hydroxychloroquine did not occur. Retinotoxicity occurred in 4% of patients with total chloroquine dosages less than 400 g and in 8% with less than 800 g, but in 50% (2 of 4) with greater than 800 g. Frenkel[F237] followed 100 patients for a mean of 3 years on daily dosages of hydroxychloroquine from 200 to 400 mg. No retinopathy was noted. Bell et al. noted retinopathy in 4% of 142 RA patients given hydroxychloroquine but, contrary to previous reports, was unable to relate this to total dose, duration, or age.[B178]

Easterbrook screened 1,500 patients at the University of Toronto for retinopathy over a 15-year period.[E9,E11] Of the 50 cases that were detected, only 1 was on hydroxychloroquine (in a high dosage of 600 mg daily). The chloroquine retinopathy patients were only taking a dose slightly higher than the mean. Chloroquine is associated with progressive visual loss, even after drug discontinuation, because of the long time it is present in tissues.[E9] One report documented the onset of macular changes in a young man with progressive visual impairment 7 years after stopping the drug.[E43] A total of seven such cases has appeared, and interpretation is difficult as a result of poor documentation or the likelihood of the macular degeneration of aging being a factor.[B590,M161,O20,S89] *The onset of retinotoxicity has never been reported after the cessation of hydroxychloroquine.* One large center in Great Britain stopped screening patients taking hydroxychloroquine after failing to find a single case of retinopathy in 73 patients who had taken the drug for more than 18 months.[M613]

Only one case of questionable retinotoxicity has been reported with Atabrine.[C100] Zuelhke et al.[Z51] noted no eye toxicity from Atabrine in 26 patients followed at the University of Iowa over a 30-year period, and reviewed the literature. None of the 200 patients treated with Atabrine by Dubois or those that I have treated have evolved retinopathic changes.[W24]

Once the lesion appears, no specific therapy other than cessation of the antimalarial is required. Although antimalarial excretion can be increased by acidification with ammonium chloride, ascorbic acid, or British antilewisite (BAL), nothing indicates that the ocular lesion is improved.[B257] The best and only treatment is discontinuation of the drug if even equivocal changes of retinopathy occur. Mackenzie and Szilagy[M27] suggested that sunglasses may prevent the retinal lesion. They showed that high-dose chloroquine concentrates in melanin in pigment epithelium, blocking the normal light-absorbing action of melanin and thereby removing its protective mechanism. This has been supported by laboratory studies in rats,[L162] but it is premature to advocate the use of sunglasses in all patients taking antimalarials.

RETINAL TESTING AND CLINICAL CORRELATES

Ophthalmologists have many techniques that purport to evaluate retinal and macular integrity and function, but most agree to disagree about the optimal sequence of testing. Patients taking chloroquine should have an eye examination every 3 months, and every 6 months with hydroxychloroquine. Two helpful reviews of these methods for antimalarial monitoring have been published.[L397,P268]

If color vision is abnormal, testing is inexpensive and reliable; some investigators believe it is the most sensitive method.[C446] The time it takes to recover macular function after illumination of the retina is known as the macular dazzle test. Although it is thought to be prolonged in patients with early antimalarial maculopathy,[C98] Easterbrook found that it is abnormal in almost all patients on antimalarials and does not distinguish those with retinopathy from those without.[E11] Fluorescein angiography shows striking macular uptake. Its sensitivity and specificity ratings are disappointing,[L397] and it was less reliable than color vision testing in a controlled, comparative study.[C446]

Visual field testing, especially if augmented by Amsler grids, are simple and inexpensive screens for paracentral scotomas. Amsler grids can be self-administered and are easily reproducible in cooperative patients.[E8] Electo-oculography (EOG) reflects the metabolic integrity of the retinal pigment epithelium but correlates poorly with the macular changes induced by chloroquines. Electroretinography (ERG) is another technically complex procedure that detects late changes but it is difficult to interpret in early disease, and many nonspecific abnormal readings are noted in normal patients. Dark adaptation testing is probably of little value. One controlled study found contrast sensitivity testing to be superior to pattern visual evoked potentials and EOG.[B315] In a fascinating report, a British survey found that rheumatologists could identify 52 of 65 minor retinal changes in patients on chloroquine and concluded that expensive, frequent eye examinations are generally unnecessary.[F127]

SUMMARY

1. Three antimalarials commercially available in the United States have documented efficacy in the treatment of lupus erythematosus: chloroquine, hydroxychloroquine, and Atabrine.

2. These agents are the safest drugs available and are recommended for patients with nonorgan-threatening lupus who require more than sunscreens, steroid salves, or NSAIDs.

3. Chloroquines are most effective for treatment of the following features of LE (in order): cutaneous lesions, arthritis-arthralgias, fatigue, and serositis. Chloroquine is more powerful than hydroxychloroquine. Atabrine is most effective for the following (in order): cutaneous lesions, fatigue, arthritis-arthralgias, and serositis.

4. Chloroquine and Atabrine are effective in 1 to 2 months; hydroxychloroquine often requires a 3- to 6-month wait. Chloroquines and Atabrine are synergistic and can be combined.

5. Antimalarials work by blocking damaging ultraviolet light, suppressing immune reactivity, inhibiting antibody formation, and blocking prostaglandin and leukotriene synthesis by the inhibition of phospholipase A_2. They also inhibit platelet aggregation and adhesion, decrease membrane receptor sites because of lysosomal membrane accumulation, and are antimicrobial and antiproliferative.
6. Steroid-sparing actions have also been documented.
7. Higher dosing can cause a faster response but also greater toxicity.
8. Generalized gastrointestinal and musculoskeletal complaints are reversible and usually minor. The only serious complication of the chloroquines is retinotoxicity, which is observed in 10% of patients on chloroquine and in 3% of those on hydroxychloroquine. This can be minimized by frequent eye examinations and the use of hydroxychloroquine. *Irreversible retinal changes have never been reported in a patient taking hydroxychloroquine in recommended doses who undergoes eye checks every 6 months.* Atabrine is not retinotoxic but blood counts need to be monitored, because it can cause aplastic anemia (rarely).

Chapter 58

SYSTEMIC CORTICOSTEROID THERAPY IN SYSTEMIC LUPUS ERYTHEMATOSUS

FRANCISCO P. QUISMORIO, Jr.

GENERAL CONSIDERATIONS AND PRINCIPLES OF TREATMENT

Longterm use of systemic corticosteroids constitutes one of the most important issues in the management of SLE because of their potential serious side effects. There are two clinical settings in which these agents are generally employed in SLE. Corticosteroids are prescribed for patients with a mild form of the disease, in whom inflammatory arthritis, mild serositis, or other symptoms are inadequately controlled with salicylates, other NSAIDs and/or antimalarial therapy (see Table 58–1). A small dose, usually 2.5 to 10 mg of prednisone daily, added to the therapeutic regimen frequently results in a prompt favorable response. In the other clinical setting, high doses of corticosteroids are administered to a severely ill patient with a single major organ disease or with multisystem involvement. The patient may have a life-threatening condition such as pulmonary hemorrhage, lupus cerebritis, profound autoimmune thrombocytopenia, or severe hemolytic anemia. Salicylates, NSAIDs, or antimalarial agents are not used in the initial treatment of these patients, but instead, a large dose of prednisone such as 60 to 100 mg/day is used.

Systemic corticosteroids are not the first line of treatment for the fever, fatigue, polyarthritis, serositis, or skin rash of SLE. An isolated laboratory abnormality such as elevated erythrocyte sedimentation rate, positive ANA, anemia of chronic disease, leukopenia, or low serum complement by itself is not an indication for corticosteroids.

CHOICE OF CORTICOSTEROID PREPARATIONS AND PHARMACOLOGY

Adrenal corticosteroids are classified into two major categories: glucocorticoids and mineralocorticoids. Glucocorticoids affect the function of practically every organ system in the body and influence intermediary metabolism, immune functions, and inflammatory processes. Mineralocorticoids are vital to water and salt metabolism. The distinction between glucocorticoid and mineralocorticoid activities of a given adrenocorticoid hormone is relative and frequently depends on the given dosage used.

Adrenal glucocorticoids comprise a heterogeneous group of hormones. Fig. 58–1 shows the molecular structure and points out the significant groups in the currently available glucocorticoids used in the treatment of systemic inflammatory conditions. Table 58–2 lists the standard tablet sizes of the commonly used glucocorticoid preparations that have equivalent therapeutic effects on the average patient.

In 1949, Hench et al.[H261] first described the beneficial effects of cortisone and ACTH on rheumatoid arthritis. Soon thereafter, both hormones were also shown to have beneficial therapeutic effects in SLE.[D329,E75,G327,T161] No clinician doubts the usefulness of corticosteroids in SLE; however, there are major issues that remain controversial including when to start corticosteroids in an individual patient, how much to employ in various phases of the illness, and how long should these agents be administered. It must be recognized that controlled trials of corticosteroid in the management of specific organ involvement in SLE such as central nervous system disease, pneumonitis, autoimmune hemolytic anemia, etc., have not been undertaken. Studies comparing the efficacy of corticosteroids with cytotoxic agents in lupus nephritis are discussed in Chapters 54 and 59. Controlled studies on the use of high-dose "pulse" methylprednisolone are discussed below.

An analysis of the effect of corticosteroid therapy on the survival of SLE patients followed by Ropes was undertaken.[A122] The patients were stratified using a prognostic index. Corticosteroids had a significant effect on the overall survival of the very ill high-risk patients, but not on the less severely affected patients. Steroid use was considered conservative, so that it cannot be ascertained whether the administration of higher doses could have resulted in an even better overall survival.

Several excellent reviews on the physiologic effects and biochemistry of adrenal corticosteroids have appeared.[A372,A373,F24,G39,117]

CHOICE OF CORTICOSTEROID PREPARATION

Prednisone, prednisolone, methylprednisolone, and hydrocortisone are the preparations most commonly used in the treatment of SLE. Hydrocortisone is avoided when significant cardiac or renal disease exists because significant salt and water retention may develop. If there is any doubt on the ability of the patient to absorb orally administered steroids because of vomiting or diarrhea, the medication should be given intravenously. Intermittent intramuscular injections can be given to the less ill patient. There is no evidence to indicate that one corticosteroid preparation is more specific than another in its effect(s)

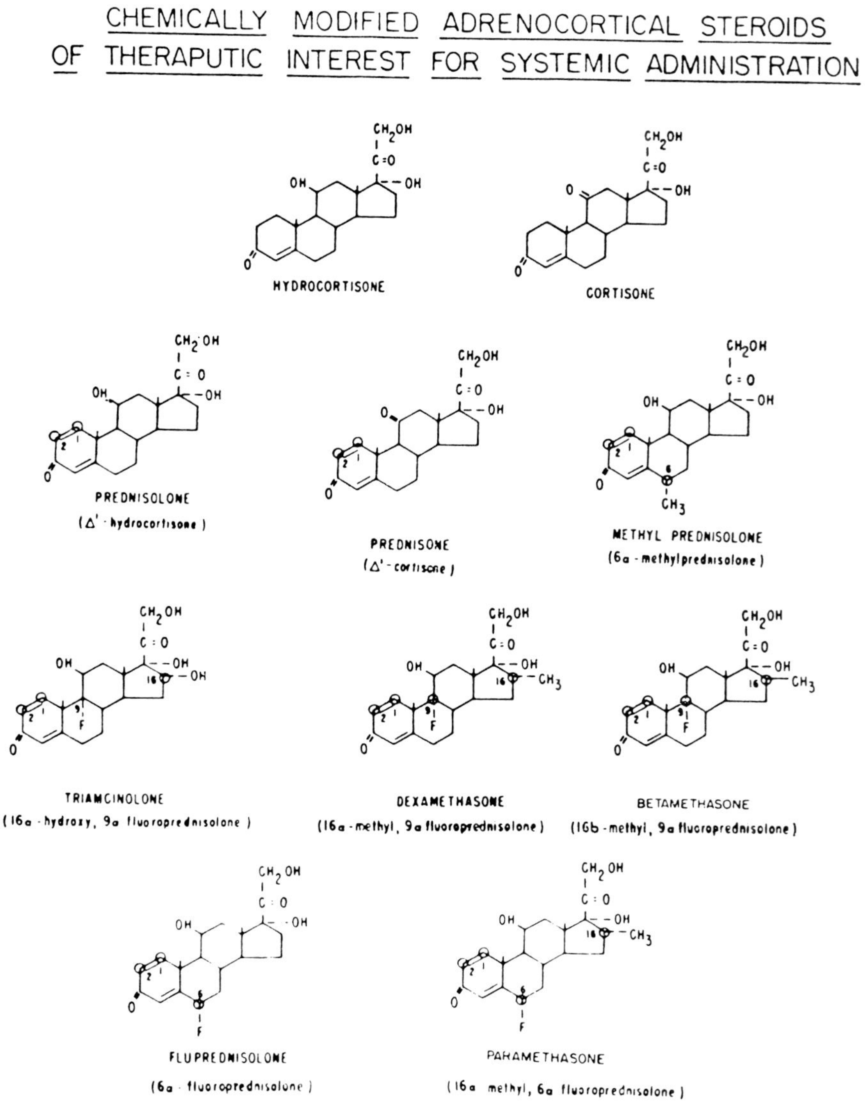

CHEMICALLY MODIFIED ADRENOCORTICAL STEROIDS OF THERAPUTIC INTEREST FOR SYSTEMIC ADMINISTRATION

Fig. 58–1. Structural formulas of the commonly used adrenocortical steroids. (Courtesy of E. W. Boland.)

Table 58–1. Classification of SLE According to Severity of Clinical Status*

Mild Disease	Severe Life- or Organ-Threatening Disease
Fever	Massive pleural and/or pericardial effusions
Arthritis	Significant renal disease
Mild pericarditis	Hemolytic anemia
Small pleural and pericardial effusions	Thrombocytopenic purpura
	CNS involvement
	Acute vasculitis
Rash	Myocarditis
Fatigue	Lupus pneumonitis, lung hemorrhage
Headache	

* Type of treatment depends on the current clinical picture. Clinical course unpredictable. Remissions are frequent.

Table 58–2. Average Equivalent Anti-inflammatory Potencies of Cortisone and its Derivatives Based Upon Tablet Size

Hormone Preparation	Equivalent Commercial Tablet (mg)
Cortisone acetate (Cortone)	25
Hydrocortisone (Hydrocortone, Solu-Cortef)	20
Prednisone (Meticorten, Deltra)	5
Prednisolone (Meticortelone, Hydeltra)	5
Methylprednisolone (Medrol)	4
Triamcinolone (Aristocort, Kenacort)	4
Dexamethasone (Decadron)	0.75
Betamethasone (Celestone)	0.6
Fluprednisolone (Alphadrol)	1.5
Paramethasone (Haldrone)	2

Table 58–3. Corticosteroid Side Effects Observed in Patients with SLE Receiving the Equivalent of 100 mg/Day of Cortisone (%)

Side Effect	Prednisone or Prednisolone 37 Cases	Methylprednisolone 40 Cases	Triamcinolone 29 Cases	Dexamethasone 50 Cases	Paramethasone 51 Cases
Cushingoid features	49	52	45	60	63
Hirsutism, marked	3	8	21	28	12
Acne	16	10	17	10	8
Striae, marked	3	3	14	4	10
Ecchymoses, marked	3	27	14	20	32
Edema	6	5	3	28	6
Diabetes mellitus	6	0	3	4	4
Epigastric distress	33	17	37	30	29
Muscle weakness	0	0	19	0	2
Hot flushes	0	0	0	0	4
Insomnia	0	0	0	8	4
Psychoses	0	0	0	2	0

on the disease process in SLE, when comparable dosage is used. For practical purposes, the physician should become knowledgeable and familiar with two glucocorticoids: a saturated physiologic preparation such as hydrocortisone and an unsaturated synthetic agent such as prednisone or methylprednisolone. All the corticosteroids listed in Table 58–2 have been used by Dubois for the treatment of SLE in open trials with satisfactory results.[D309,D311,D312,D313,D314,D315,D316,D329] Betamethasone and fluprednisolone have less salt-retaining property than prednisone, which may be of theoretic value in the treatment of the edematous patients. Triamcinolone has the least appetite-stimulating effect, whereas dexamethasone has the greatest pantophagic effect. Prednisone must be converted to prednisolone in the liver to become an active hormone. Although prednisolone or methylprednisolone may appear to be preferable to use in the presence of significant hepatocellular disease, the impaired hepatic conversion of prednisone in these patients is compensated for by the decreased rate of elimination of prednisolone from the plasma. Moreover, when the serum albumin is low, a higher proportion of the drug circulates as the free biologically active form.[D85] For these reasons, there is no clear-cut contraindication to the use of prednisone in these patients.[M377]

Table 58–3 summarizes selected clinical and laboratory findings in four comparable groups of SLE patients treated with unsaturated corticosteroids by Dubois.[D311,D314,D315,D316]

Absorption and Metabolism

Absorption of synthetic glucocorticoids takes place in the upper jejunum, and peak plasma levels are attained in 30 to 120 minutes. About 80% of the circulating cortisol is bound to transcortin, a specific corticosteroid-binding α-globulin, and the remainder is bound to albumin. Hypoalbuminemia results in higher level of unbound drug, and increased frequency of steroid toxicity has been observed in patients with liver disease and low serum albumin.[L244]

Glucocorticoids are metabolized in the liver. The plasma half-life of cortisol and its synthetic analogs range from 30 minutes for cortisone and 300 minutes for beta-methasone and dexamethasone. The plasma half-life of a particular glucocorticoid does not necessarily correlate with its potency or its biologic half-life, which reflects the action of the drug at the tissue level. The plasma half-life of prednisolone is comparable to that of dexamethasone, yet the latter is significantly more potent than the former.

Effects on Immune Functions and Inflammatory Responses

Much has been written about the various effects of glucocorticoids on immune functions and inflammatory responses. However in analyzing the published data, one must be cognizant of the fact the effects observed in healthy subjects, or even in other disease states, may not necessarily apply to SLE. The corticosteroid dose used in many in vitro experiments cannot be attained in vivo, or only with the repeated use of megadoses. Early studies have often failed to recognize species variability in cellular sensitivity to glucocorticoids. The subcellular and tissue effects of glucocorticoids are well known, yet the precise mechanism(s) involved in their anti-inflammatory and immunosuppressive properties is not clear. The principal effects of glucocorticoids are summarized below and the reader is referred to several excellent recent reviews for detailed references.[A372,A373,F24,G39]

Glucocorticoids act at different tissue and cellular levels to exert anti-inflammatory effects, affecting the microvasculature, neutrophils, macrophages, lymphocytes, other mononuclear cells, and various soluble mediators. Glucocorticoids decrease capillary permeability and local blood flow in inflammatory sites, limit endothelial cell swelling and the passage of immune complexes through basement membrane. The inhibition of migration and accumulation of leukocytes in inflammatory sites is probably the most important anti-inflammatory effect of glucocorticoids.[P41a] Bactericidal activity, Fc receptor binding, and other functions of monocytes and macrophages are impaired. Glucocorticoids induce eosinopenia, monocytopenia, and lymphocytopenia. Cellular responses to kinins, histamine, prostaglandins, or chemotactic factors are altered and the amount of prostaglandin released from stimulated cells is reduced.[C272a,D40a]

Glucocorticoids affect cell-mediated and humoral antibody immune functions. Lymphocytopenia is caused by redistribution of cells to other lymphoid compartments. T lymphocytes are selectively depleted more than B cells. Lymphocyte proliferation in response to specific antigens is suppressed more easily than to mitogens. IL-2 production by activated lymphocytes is diminished. The effects of glucocorticoids on human B-cell responses are not as pronounced as on T lymphocytes. Patients on pharmacologic doses of glucocorticoids have normal antibody responses to immunization.[K461,M644,T257] Conversely, short-term therapy with high dose of glucocorticoids causes a reduction in serum level of IgG and IgA but not IgM.[P269] Glucocorticoids may affect B-cell function indirectly by their action on accessory cells.[M377] In a study of eight SLE patients treated with a mean dose of 55 mg of prednisone daily for 14 to 30 days, serum IgG level decreased by an average of 22%. More importantly, there was a reduction of IgG ANA including anti-DNA but not of IgG antibodies to viral and bacterial antigens.[W150] The clinical efficacy of corticosteroids in the treatment of SLE may partly be a result of this selective effect on autoantibodies.

The immunosuppressive potency of various glucocorticoid preparations does not necessarily correlate with their anti-inflammatory potency. Methylprednisolone and betamethasone rank the highest in in vitro immunosuppressive activity while dexamethasone, hydrocortisone, and prednisolone are of intermediate potency, and prednisone has the lowest activity.[L51] Moreover, the various lymphocyte subsets differ in their susceptibility to the suppressive effects of glucocorticoids.[L51]

Effect on Lymphocyte Subsets

Tereyeva et al.[T67] enumerated T- and B-cell percentages in 40 SLE patients prior to and after prednisone therapy. No significant changes were noted. Conversely, Bakke et al.[B40] found that high-dose prednisone therapy in SLE resulted in a T-cell lymphopenia with a predominant decrease in CD4 + lymphocytes. In a study of 3 SLE patients, Raziuddin et al.[R83] observed a decrease of CD4 + HLA DR + subset but not CD8 + HLA DR + lymphocytes with prednisone therapy.

Steroid Withdrawal

When the disease activity is adequately controlled, or another agent such as an antimalarial agent with steroid-sparing effects becomes effective, or if the side effects of steroids become intolerable, a tapering regimen is instituted. The rate at which the dosage is tapered depends on how long the patient had been on steroids, the dosage, the method of administration (daily or alternate-day dosing), and how active the disease process is.

In withdrawing steroids, considerable experience is needed to determine the amount and rapidity of reduction. There is no evidence that the concurrent intermittent use of ACTH aids in decreasing the dosage or diminishes the side effects of steroids.[B16,C257] When given after the course of steroids, ACTH does not accelerate the recovery of the pituitary-adrenal axis function, thus the routine use of ACTH is not recommended.[A372] In those patients receiving large doses (50 mg of prednisone daily or more) for several weeks, 10% of the dosage may be reduced at intervals as short as 4 days, whereas if the patient has been taking this dose of several months (e.g., for active nephritis), a 10% reduction at intervals of a few weeks is recommended. This allows time for monitoring renal function as the medication is withdrawn. In patients whose illness is stable and who are receiving smaller doses of steroids (10 to 20 mg of prednisone daily), a reduction of approximately 10% of the dose every 2 weeks can be followed. A few patients may experience worsening of symptoms such as arthralgia and fatigue with a drop of as little as 0.5 mg when they are on 5 mg of prednisone per day. The use of the 1 mg tablet preparation of prednisone helps in careful titration of the dosage.

It must be emphasized that the majority of SLE patients receiving 20 mg of prednisone or less per day will benefit from the addition of an antimalarial agent, which will help reduce the steroid required to control the disease. Azathioprine or other cytotoxic agents may be needed in some patients to reduce the steroid dose.

During remission, attempts should be made to withdraw steroid therapy gradually and completely if possible. The prevalence of coronary atherosclerosis is increased even with maintenance doses of 10 mg of prednisone daily.[B56,U34]

When the prednisone dose is below adrenal replacement levels (7.5 mg/day), tapering should proceed slowly (e.g., 1 mg of prednisone per month), if the patient has been on the drug for a prolonged period. Recovery of the hypothalamic-pituitary axis function varies widely from one individual to another, and complete recovery may take up to 1 year. The cosyntropin stimulation test is helpful in guiding the physician as to when pituitary-adrenal function is completely recovered. After a baseline plasma cortisol determination, 250 μg of synthetic ACTH is administered intramuscularly. An increment of 6 to 20 μg/dl in the plasma cortisol 30 minutes after the injection is taken to indicate pituitary-adrenal recovery.[B616] The metyrapone test has been reported to be more useful in detecting subtle degrees of HPA dysfunction that ACTH stimulation and insulin hypoglycemic tests.[H176a]

If the steroid dose is tapered too fast, the underlying disease can flare or a steroid-withdrawal syndrome may develop. The latter may be difficult at times to distinguish from active SLE and is a form of fibrositis syndrome. The patient may complain of joint pains (although on examination the tender areas are in the soft tissues rather than in the joints), fatigue, malaise, depression, and fever. If the steroid dose is kept at the same level, the withdrawal syndrome will eventually subside, although this can take up to 6 weeks. Physicians must resist the temptation to greatly increase steroid doses in situations in which the underlying disease is not active. Unless steroids are abruptly discontinued, Addisonian crises are extremely rare.

Four types of steroid-withdrawal syndrome have been described in patients who have been on chronic corticosteroid therapy.[D239] In the first type, there is clinical and biochemical evidence of suppression of the hypothalamic-pituitary adrenal function (HPA). The patient's symptoms are relieved promptly with replacement doses of cortisone. In the second type, there is a recrudescence of the symptoms of the underlying disease when the steroids are withdrawn. In our experience, this is the most common type seen among SLE patients. The third type is characterized by corticosteroid dependence. The patient experiences symptoms without clear-cut evidence of recurrence of the underlying disease. The HPA function is normal, but the patient requires supraphysiologic doses of steroids (greater than 5 mg of prednisone daily) to control the symptoms. In the fourth type, there is biochemical evidence of suppression of the HPA axis, although the patient is asymptomatic and with no recurrence of the underlying illness.

DOSAGE OF CORTICOSTEROIDS IN THE TREATMENT OF SLE

To simplify the concept of steroid therapy, we empirically classify the disease into mild or severe (see Table 58–1). The treatment of the individual patient depends primarily on the current clinical picture. The following drug schedule is used for adults.

Mild Disease

Aspirin or other salicylates can be tried initially. The dosage should be gradually increased depending on the clinical response. If arthritis or fever is inadequately controlled, add a nonsteroidal anti-inflammatory drug (NSAID). We have used salicylates and another NSAID concurrently in some patients without diminished therapeutic potency of the latter, and the combination is often beneficial. Many patients, however, are unable to tolerate the combination because of gastrointestinal complaints or other side effects.

In the presence of skin rash or mucous membrane lesions, or if the mild disease is inadequately controlled by NSAIDs, add one of the following antimalarials: hydroxychloroquine sulfate (Plaquenil) 200 mg bid (5 to 7 mg/kg/day), chloroquine phosphate (Aralen) 250 mg daily (for adults weighing over 100 lbs), or quinacrine hydrochloride (Atabrine) 100 mg daily. In an occasional patient, the combination of Atabrine and one of the other two agents can be used if the response to the single preparation is unsatisfactory after several months of therapy. Should these measures fail to control the polyarthritis, myalgia, and/or serositis, add prednisone 2.5 mg or 5 mg daily. Increase the prednisone dose by 20% increments every 1 to 2 weeks depending on the clinical response. Never suppress mild disease with doses larger than absolutely necessary for moderate relief, because then steroid side effects and difficulty of withdrawal pose greater problems.

Severe Disease

NSAIDs and antimalarials are not used in acutely ill patients because their therapeutic potency is weaker than corticosteroids. Prednisone is administered daily to febrile patients before meals in two or three divided doses. To those without fever and severe constitutional symptoms, prednisone can be given as a single dose in the

morning. Alternate-day steroid therapy should be tried in those patients whose predominant clinical problem is active nephritis to minimize side effects. The following suggested dosages are for adults. Children may require almost as much.

Autoimmune Hemolytic Anemia

Administer 60 to 80 mg of prednisone daily. If no improvement in clinical and laboratory features occurs within several days to a week, increase the dose to 100 to 120 mg of prednisone. Full response may take as long as 8 to 12 weeks.

Autoimmune Thrombocytopenia

Administer 60 to 80 mg of prednisone daily. The rise in the platelet count may not be seen until up to 4 weeks of therapy.

Acute Systemic Vasculitis

Use 60 to 100 mg of prednisone per day. Clinical response appears within a few days, except in patients with gangrene of the extremities when improvement may not be evident until after several weeks.

Acute Central Nervous System Involvement

If the patient is critically ill, administer methylprednisolone (Solu-Medrol) intravenously every 8 to 12 hours with a total daily dose ranging from 48 to 80 mg. Hydrocortisone sodium succinate (Solu-Cortef) can also be used at a dose of 250 to 500 mg intravenously every 12 hours. Double the dose every 24 to 48 hours daily up to 3000 mg daily, until therapeutic effects are obtained. We have used the latter agent empirically in an occasional patient who has not responded adequately to methylprednisolone and does not have significant cardiac or renal disease.

Active Lupus Nephritis

Use 50 to 60 mg of prednisone per day (1 to 2 mg/kg/day) for 6 to 12 weeks. If the patient's problem is primarily renal disease and in the absence of fever, constitutional complaints, or other major organ involvement, 100 to 120 mg of prednisone is given every other day.

SINGLE DAILY DOSE ORAL STEROID THERAPY AND GUIDES TO STEROID DOSAGE

The entire dose of steroids can be given at one time, preferably before breakfast, with milk and food.[D325a] If severe morning stiffness is a major complaint of the patient, an evening dose may be tried; however, some patients on this schedule may experience difficulty sleeping.

The entire dose may be given before breakfast to control midday exacerbations or before lunch for relief of maximal discomfort in the late afternoon. Converting patients receiving divided-dose therapy to single-dose therapy has been effective in 85 to 90% of cases in which it was attempted.[D325a]

Epigastric distress was noted in only 13% of the group receiving methylprednisolone as a single daily dose compared with a prevalence of 17 to 33% in patients on divided-dose regimen using equivalent doses of methylprednisolone or other preparations.[D325a]

In the acutely ill and febrile patient, single daily dose administration of large doses of steroids may not result in a satisfactory 24-hour clinical effect. Frequently, a febrile relapse is noted about 16 hours after the oral medication is given. Consequently, it is advisable to administer steroids at least on a 12-hour basis in these patients.

Experimental evidence indicates that single daily dose therapy of corticosteroids should be sufficiently effective. Although the serum levels as determined by plasma half-life persist (a maximum of 200 minutes after administration of dexamethasone and prednisone), it is evident that the tissue anti-inflammatory effect is much longer.[J66] Dougherty[D280] showed that the presence of measurable cortisol in the blood is not necessary for anti-inflammatory action in the tissues. In experimental animals, hydrocortisone tends to be concentrated in areas of inflammation, either within or at the surface of fibroblasts, for as long as 24 hours after intravenous administration of the drug.

When more than 20 mg of prednisone or its equivalent is given to a patient daily, sodium intake usually should be restricted to 2 g or less per day, depending on the clinical situation. Massive doses of corticosteroids frequently cause sodium retention, even with the new preparations. If the daily equivalent of 40 mg or more of prednisone is required, some patients may need supplementary potassium. Frequent determination of blood glucose and electrolytes as well as urinalysis for glycosuria should be performed.

The clinical picture is used as the major guide to steroid therapy, particularly in patients with mild disease. In addition, the temperature curve provides an excellent indicator for dosaging. If concomitant infection is excluded, the dose of steroid should be adequate to produce a normal temperature within a few days in a moderately ill patient requiring massive doses of steroids.

As the steroid dose is reduced, recurrence of fever often precedes a clinical relapse. Consequently, if fever recurs, the interval between reductions of dosage should be lengthened until the temperature curve returns to normal. Renal involvement is assessed by careful urinalysis, serum creatinine level, 24-hour urinary protein excretion, and creatinine clearance. Measurements of serum C3, C4, and anti-dsDNA antibodies are also essential in the overall assessment (see Chap. 48).

Erythrocyte sedimentation rate (ESR) should not be used as the major or sole index of steroid dosage because it does not correlate strongly with disease activity in many patients. The ESR can be persistently elevated in some patients in clinical remission.

The steroid dose must be adjusted for patients undergoing surgery or during periods of major stress, trauma, and severe infections. The hypothalamic-pituitary-adrenal axis is usually suppressed and cannot respond adequately in these situations. If the patient is receiving 10 mg of prednisone daily or less, usually two doses of hydrocortisone sodium succinate (Solu-Cortef), 100 mg IV every 12 hours may be used, starting 12 hours prior to the surgery.

PULSE METHYLPREDNISOLONE THERAPY IN SLE

Impressed by its efficacy in the treatment of acute rejection of renal allografts, Cathcart and associates[C157] in 1976 administered 1 g IV methylprednisolone infusions to seven SLE patients with nephritis and rapidly deteriorating renal function. The treatment was beneficial and, moreover, it made it possible to maintain the inpatients at a lower oral dose of prednisone. Since then, this mode of therapy has been reported in a number of uncontrolled studies in the treatment not only of lupus nephritis but also for other major organ involvement such as CNS disease, bone marrow aplasia, or profound thrombocytopenia.

Effects on Immune Functions and Leukocyte Kinetics

The effects of pulse steroids on immune functions are thought to be quantitatively different from those of conventional doses used in the treatment of SLE and other systemic diseases; however, current experimental data do not firmly establish this.

In healthy individuals, the infusion of high-dose methylprednisolone causes a profound lymphopenia concomitant with neutrophilia, which persists for 24 hours.[W116] The lymphocytopenia is a result of preferential depletion of recirculating T cells.[W116] The response of peripheral blood lymphocytes to stimulation by phytohemagglutinin and allogenic lymphocytes is markedly suppressed within 24 hours, lasting as long as 72 hours in some subjects.

In RA patients, Fan and associates[F16] studied the effects of 1 g doses of methylprednisolone for 1 to 3 days and found that the nadir of lymphopenia and selective depression of T cells occurred at 6 hours. Complete recovery was observed within 24 hours. The degree of lymphopenia and time of recovery were similar when a smaller 50 mg dose was given to the patients. Moreover, both doses produced comparable suppression of proliferation of RA lymphocytes when stimulated with mitogens. The suppressive effects were short-lived, disappearing within 24 hours. The administration of pulse steroids for 3 consecutive days did not alter the observed suppression. Skin test reactivity to recall antigens and humoral antibody response to primary as well as secondary immunization were preserved after pulse steroid therapy.[F16] In contrast, considerable and long-lasting suppression of natural killer cell function followed pulse steroid therapy in RA.[P90] In ankylosing spondylitis, pulse steroids resulted in an immediate anti-inflammatory effect with prompt lowering of acute-phase reactants in the serum but a delayed onset of immunosuppressive effects.[R201] The effect(s) of pulse steroids on various aspects of immune function may depend in part on the underlying immunologic abnormalities in the patient, and the effects observed in other diseases may not necessarily apply to SLE.

Perez and associates[P120] examined the effect of pulse methylprednisolone on polymorphonuclear neutrophil (PMN) functions in SLE. Adhesiveness to plastic surface was consistently and significantly decreased; however, the abnormality was transitory, lasting for less than 24 hours. Other PMN functions including random motility, chemotaxis, superoxide anion generation, and degranulation were either normal or only slightly affected. Boghossian et al.[B381] observed that following pulse steroids in SLE, there was a marked delay in the secretion of lactoferrin by PMNs and significant decrease in their adherence, but more importantly there was an impairment of bacterial killing and digestion. In contrast, SLE patients on maintenance dose of steroids demonstrated no defects in antimicrobial functions of phagocytes except for failure of accumulation of monocytes in Rebuck skin windows and decreased lactoferrin secretion. These abnormalities in PMN function may contribute to susceptibility to infections noted in some patients receiving pulse steroid therapy.[G57]

Clinical Use of Pulse Steroids in SLE

Several reports of open uncontrolled studies on the use of pulse steroids in SLE have appeared. The initial enthusiasm for its use is tempered by the results of controlled trials in SLE that showed only a transitory or small benefit when added to conventional corticosteroid therapy.[E34,M29]

Uncontrolled Studies

In uncontrolled studies of single or small numbers of patients, pulse methylprednisolone has been reported to be beneficial in the treatment of lupus cerebritis,[F77,G175,H89,P293,Y29] refractory subacute cutaneous LE,[G238] lupus pneumonitis,[F77] bone marrow aplasia,[Y24] and refractory thrombocytopenia.[L424] The beneficial effect on thrombocytopenia was also observed to diminish with a repeated course.[M32]

Isenberg et al.[I34a] administered methylprednisolone pulse therapy to 20 SLE patients with a wide variety of clinical manifestations. Arthralgias, pleuritic chest pain, cutaneous vasculitis, fever, and adenopathy were the principal features that responded to treatment. Serum C3 level rose and anti-DNA titers decreased. However, the improvement was generally not sustained. Pulse steroid therapy followed by alternate-day corticosteroid therapy was prospectively evaluated.[B59] Pulse therapy was effective in the initial management; however, alternate-day regimen was ineffective in sustaining disease control for prolonged periods.

Pulse Steroid in Lupus Nephritis

Dosa and associates[D275] used combined pulse steroid and cytotoxic agents in the treatment of acute oliguric renal failure in lupus nephritis. Ponticelli et al.[P254] administered three daily doses of pulse methylprednisolone as initial treatment of 43 patients with diffuse proliferative lupus nephritis, followed by oral prednisone at the lowest dose possible. A cytotoxic agent was added in 31 patients. Extrarenal or renal disease flare-ups were treated with additional methylprednisolone pulse. At 10 years, the actuarial renal survival rate was 91%. Except for one subject, the kidney function remained stable in all patients who had normal function when first seen, and tended to improve in those with impaired function. Four patients failed to respond with progression to end-stage renal failure in

one. Kimberly et al.[K216] treated 34 patients with lupus nephritis. Twelve patients (35%) responded to therapy with a decrease in serum creatinine value by at least 20% within 2 months. Twenty-two patients (65%) failed to respond. Those patients who responded were characterized as a group by a recent deterioration in renal function, more diffuse lesions on renal biopsy, and higher levels of anti-DNA and circulating immune complexes as well as lower serum complement level. Improvement in renal function was sustained in 60% of patients for at least 6 months. This study suggested that pulse therapy may be beneficial in a subset of lupus patients with recent worsening renal function and more severe active histologic changes. In a retrospective study of 36 episodes of acute deterioration in renal function in 34 SLE patients, Yeung et al.[Y42] found that crescentic class IV lupus glomerulonephritis was the most common underlying pathology. Twenty-four patients (67%) had nephrotic syndrome and 11 (31%) had hypertension. In addition, concurrent infections at the onset of the illness were the precipitating factor in 7 episodes (19%). Pulse methylprednisolone combined with either cyclophosphamide or azathioprine was used, and improvement was noted in 28 separate episodes (78%). Eight patients died and 5 developed chronic renal failure. Treatment was complicated by serious infections in 6 patients, 5 of whom received pulse therapy. Four of these patients died.

Controlled Studies

There are few controlled trials on the use of pulse steroid therapy in SLE. Barron et al.[B106] compared 15 SLE children with diffuse proliferative glomerulonephritis treated with 2 mg/kg/day of prednisone with 7 similar patients who received 6 daily pulses of methylprednisolone, 30 mg/kg/day, and followed by prednisone, 2 mg/kg/day. Although the latter group had a more rapid improvement in glomerular filtration rate, the longterm effect on the renal function was similar in the two groups of patients. In a small double-blind trial, Liebling et al.[L279] treated 5 SLE patients with diffuse proliferative nephritis with monthly pulse methylprednisolone for a year and compared them with 4 patients who received placebo pulse. At 1 year, significant improvement in serum creatinine level was noted in the former group but not in the placebo group. Renal function remained stable in the treated group, 2 years after completing the study. The sample size was too small to draw definitive conclusions on the efficacy of pulse steroid therapy for lupus nephritis.

Two double-blind controlled studies concluded that pulse methylprednisolone therapy confers no or some short-term benefit over conventional corticosteroid therapy. Edwards et al.[E34] treated 21 SLE patients with varying multisystem involvement with either 100 mg or 1 g of methylprednisolone for 3 consecutive days in a randomized double-blind study. Using individualized outcome criteria, there was no added benefit obtained from the megadose over and above that achieved by the smaller dose. Mackworth-Young and associates[M29] compared the effect of 1 g dose of methylprednisolone for 3 consecutive days to that of placebo in the treatment of 25 moderately or severely ill SLE patients. All patients concomitantly received conventional oral doses of prednisone and were followed for 6 months. The treatment group showed more consistent clinical improvement than the placebo group in the first 2 weeks; however, the difference between the two groups was not maintained after 1 month.

Adverse Reaction to Pulse Steroids

The administration of pulse steroids is associated with some significant risk. Wollheim[W330] reviewed the complications of pulse therapy when given in a variety of medical disorders. In SLE patients, seizures, hemiplegia, psychoses, hallucinations, fatal cardiac arrhythmias, intractable hiccups, and sudden death have been attributed to pulse steroid therapy.[A376,B22,B373,M622,S753] Garrett and Paulus[G57] noted a 56% complication rate in 50 patients given pulse steroids at UCLA Medical Center, 23 of whom had SLE. Seven developed infections, 7 had nausea and diarrhea, 5 had psychiatric problems, 5 had hypertension, and 4 had hyperglycemia. The complications were judged to be serious in 8 patients, 2 of which were life threatening. In controlled trials, however, pulse steroid therapy in SLE was not associated with increased frequency of adverse reactions.[B106,M29,T161]

Sakemi et al.[S37] observed transient renal failure in 3 of 25 subjects with nephrotic syndrome including SLE patients receiving pulse therapy. The renal failure was more marked in those who were severely nephrotic with highly impaired kidney function. The renal failure was transient, improving with discontinuation of the pulse therapy.

Summary

Over a decade has passed since it was introduced, and yet the role of pulse steroids in the treatment of SLE remains undefined and unsettled because of insufficient data from controlled trials.

Case-control studies in a small number of patients indicate that it has definite beneficial therapeutic effects but are not long lasting and may not be superior to that of conventional steroid dosage. Controlled clinical trials in lupus nephritis are needed. Its current application in life-threatening manifestations such as severe pulmonary hemorrhage, generalized vasculitis, etc., especially in those patients who have not responded to standard steroid dose is empiric and unproven.

INITIAL RESPONSE TO CORTICOSTEROID THERAPY

Shortly after Hench and his associates[H261,H262] reported the beneficial effects of ACTH and cortisone in rheumatoid arthritis and SLE, other workers confirmed their results.[C84,E76,G327,H177,T160] Harvey et al.[M280] reviewed in detail the earlier publications on the response to corticosteroid therapy and analyzed their results in 63 cases. In 1956, Dubois[D310] evaluated the outcome in his first 132 steroid treatment cases.

The efficacy of corticosteroids in the treatment of the various aspects of SLE has not been examined since the pioneering work in the early 1960s, except for work on the use of pulse methylprednisolone therapy. Most of the studies reviewed in this chapter came from this period.

The rapid and often striking improvement in patients with acute SLE treated with ACTH and cortisone has been documented repeatedly in the earlier papers,[B542,C84,D329, E76,G327,H177,H181,I28,T160,T161,S343] and subsequent reviews have confirmed these findings.[D310,D311,D312,D314,D315,D316, K155,M241,P192] Table 58–4 compares the clinical experience of Dubois with 409 SLE patients treated with corticosteroids compared to that of Harvey et al.[M280] In many instances when salicylates or other NSAID alone, or in combination with antimalarial agent was used, improvement occurred after weeks instead of days of therapy.

The frequency and timing of improvement in most of the manifestations listed in Table 58–4 vary greatly with more rapid response; however, as described subsequently, the unfavorable effects of steroids become greater when large doses are employed. Although manifestations such as fever and synovitis can be rapidly controlled within a few days after beginning therapy with high doses, the amount used must be individually determined and excessive doses avoided.

ALTERNATE-DAY CORTICOSTEROID THERAPY IN SLE

During the last decade, considerable interest in single-dose alternate-day corticosteroid therapy has emerged. Physiologic studies have shown evidence of less suppression of the endogenous pituitary adrenal axis and fewer side effects including the frequency of infections and catabolic effects.[A28,C120,H167,H174,M6,W63] Plasma 17-hydroxycorticoid response to hypoglycemic stress and unwanted catabolic steroid effects have been reported to be normal during alternate-day prednisone therapy.[A28]

Immunologic Effects

In a 1974 landmark study, Dale, Fauci, and Wolf[D17] compared the effects of prednisone on leukocyte kinetics in 20 patients with various systemic inflammatory disease including SLE, who were either on daily dose or alternate-day prednisone therapy. Neutrophilia, monocytopenia, prolonged neutrophil half-life, and reduced Rebuck skin window monocyte response were seen during the "on" day, but were normal on the "off" day. Patients taking a daily dose of prednisone had similar abnormalities as the alternate-day therapy tested on the on day. MacGregor et al.[M6] found that delayed hypersensitivity measured by skin testing to recall antigens and sensitization to new antigens remained intact in patients on alternate-day regimen but not in those on daily dosage of prednisone. Thus, the favorable effects on leukocyte kinetics and cell-mediated immunity may in part account for the lower frequency of infections noted in patients on alternate-day steroid therapy.[D17]

Clinical Application in SLE

Uncontrolled studies have shown that alternate-day prednisone therapy was as beneficial as daily dosage in the treatment of non–SLE-related nephrosis in children.[S575] In 1970, Ackerman[A27] treated six SLE patients with nephritis

Table 58–4. Effects of Corticosteroid Therapy on Manifestations of SLE Based on Cases of Dubois and Harvey[D323,M280]

Manifestations	Effects of Therapy
Fever	Subsides within 24–48 hours with oral steroids. In acute lupus crisis, defervescence may take 5 days or more.
Arthritis	Improves within several weeks. Low-grade arthralgia may persist unless excessive doses are used.
Cerebritis	Large doses produce improvement in most cases after several days to 2 weeks of treatment.
Peripheral neuritis	Improves within several days. Advanced changes and footdrop require months. Complete recovery may not occur.
Raynaud's phenomenon	No definite benefit. Improvement may occur during a course of years and be unrelated to steroid therapy.
Pleuritis	Pain gone within 1 week; x-ray changes may persist for months or indefinitely even when asymptomatic.
Pneumonitis	Responds to high doses of steroids after a number of weeks of treatment.
Pericarditis	Pain improves within several days. Effusion decreases within several days but requires several weeks for complete disappearance.
Myocarditis	Chronic type responds slowly and equivocally in most cases. Heart size may decrease, tachycardia, gallop, and ECG changes may improve over several weeks to several months.
Lymphadenopathy	Regresses within 1 week. A moderate degree of enlargement may persist despite clinical improvement.
Parotid enlargement	Regresses within several weeks to normal.
Hepatomegaly	Decreases within several weeks. Enlargement may persist in some asymptomatic patients.
Splenomegaly	Subsides with n several weeks.
Nausea and vomiting	Clears within several days.
Abdominal pain	Clears within several days.
Retinal changes	Hemorrhages and exudates clear within several weeks if patient is normotensive and not uremic.
Anemia	Hemoglobin usually returns to normal within several weeks unless uremia and other factors are present.
Leukopenia	Within 1–2 weeks there is a temporary return to normal or even leukocytosis of up to 25,000 with large doses of steroids. Leukopenia may return during clinical remission with or without steroid maintenance.
Elevated ESR	Tends to return toward normal within several weeks. Persistent elevation may remain despite good clinical remission. Returns to completely normal in 10% of cases.
LE-cell test	Becomes negative in 60% of patients within several weeks to several months. May persist despite clinical remission.
Renal Abnormalities:	
Proteinuria	Improves in those with mild nephropathy and in those with acute glomerulonephritis picture.
Cylindruria	Tends to disappear.
Hypoalbuminemia	Improves within several weeks and often returns to normal values.
Hypergammaglobulinemia	Decreases within several weeks and often returns to within normal limits while receiving maintenance steroid therapy.
False-positive STS	Frequently disappears within several months. May persist despite clinical remission
Abnormal liver function tests	Improve within a few weeks to a few months.

with 100 to 120 mg of prednisone every 48 hours for 6 to 8 months. Improvement in renal status occurred in five. None of his patients developed cushingoid changes. However, there are no controlled trials comparing daily and alternate-day regimens in the treatment of SLE.

Although high-dose alternate-day prednisone therapy may be successful in SLE patients whose only active clinical manifestation is nephropathy, it cannot be used effectively in those patients with multisystem disease, especially in the presence of fever, hemolytic anemia, or cerebritis. In our experience, these patients will experience a flare of arthralgia, fever, pleuritis, or constitutional complaints within 24 to 48 hours after receiving one dose of prednisone. Most patients with active multisystem disease will require at least single daily dose. The febrile patient frequently requires treatment every 8 to 12 hours. An alternative approach is to treat these patients with divided daily dose up to a point when there is significant control of the clinical symptom improvement in laboratory parameters. Thereafter, the steroid therapy is converted to a single alternate-day regimen, doubling the dose.[J28] In some patients, conversion to alternate-day dosage can only be accomplished gradually. These patients require a smaller dose of prednisone and NSAID on the off day to control arthralgias or other mild symptoms. The dose on the off day is then gradually tapered and discontinued. Should there be a recurrence of mild symp-

toms on the off day, the on day dosage can be increased, or a NSAID can be added or antimalarial drug therapy begun. If a major disease relapse occurs, it is necessary to return to the daily dosing of prednisone.

An additional problem with alternate-day therapy is occurrence of marked mood swings. Some patients become hyperactive, euphoric, agitated, or irritable during the on day and become depressed with low self-esteem, poor concentration, and malaise on the off day.[S325]

Dexamethasone has longer half-life than prednisone and induces a more prolonged and a more potent suppression of pituitary adrenal function.[H171,R1] Even when given on alternate-day dosing, dexamethasone produced significant pituitary-adrenal suppression. For this reason, long-acting steroids such as dexamethasone and betamethasone are not used in alternate-day steroid therapy. Instead, short-acting preparations such as cortisone, hydrocortisone, prednisone, prednisolone, and methylprednisolone are preferred.

Intermittent Regimen

For patients who are unable to tolerate alternate-day dosing, a discontinuous intermittent regimen in which the patient takes steroids 3 days out of 4, has been proposed. Beris et al.[B243] have shown that SLE patients on discontinuous but not on daily steroid therapy retained an adequate responsiveness of the adrenal glands to ACTH stimulation.

Moreover, in retrospective and uncontrolled observations, their patients on discontinuous regimen had few complications from the steroid therapy. In yet another approach, Lange et al.[L48] treated SLE patients with large daily doses of prednisone until the serum levels of complement and gamma globulin normalized, irrespective of prior relief from the clinical complaints. Thereafter, the patients were placed on prolonged 2-year intermittent steroid therapy with 48 to 64 mg of triamcinolone per day for 4 successive days of each week and off steroids for the remaining 3 days of the week. Not only was the regimen beneficial but side effects were minimal. However, before intermittent steroid therapy is recommended, controlled studies are clearly needed to establish its efficacy and advantage over alternate-day or daily steroid therapy.

RENAL EFFECTS OF GLUCOCORTICOIDS

Proteinuria may increase within a week after beginning high-dose corticosteroid therapy in patients with lupus nephritis. Treatment with high-dose steroids should be continued for 6 to 12 weeks despite the increase in proteinuria. This is usually transitory and will improve with gradual reduction in dosage and provided that the nephritis is steroid responsive.

Heymann and Grupe[H295] found considerable increase in proteinuria resulting from the administration of corticosteroids in 10 of 21 children with chronic renal disease, treated with alternate-day or on intermittent schedule. Two of their patients had SLE. On the day of steroid administration, proteinuria increased abruptly twofold to tenfold from the off day and promptly decreased within 24 hours after cessation of medication. As the degree of proteinuria is often used as an index in the management of lupus nephropathy and other forms of primary renal disease, it must be recognized that it can be aggravated by systemic steroids. Consequently, the duration of steroid therapy may be prolonged unnecessarily long after the basic lesion has improved.

The mechanism of steroid-induced proteinuria is unknown. Improvement in proteinuria, urinary sediment, and renal function usually occur in lupus nephropathy when the dose of steroid is tapered after several months of treatment. As the dosage is reduced, hypertension frequently becomes easier to control, BUN falls and creatinine clearance improves. When an immunosuppressive agent such as azathioprine is administered coincident with reduction in steroid dosage, the resulting decrease in proteinuria is inappropriately attributed to the newly added agent.

Corticosteroid therapy frequently causes an acute elevation in BUN secondary to its catabolic effect; the creatinine level is usually not affected in the absence of renal disease. A high BUN with normal creatinine level is frequently seen in active SLE with or without urinary abnormalities, even prior to administration of steroids. Dossetor[D277] showed that serum creatinine value correlates much better with renal function than BUN and should always be determined in evaluating patients with early renal disease. Prognosis also is better correlated with creatinine level. The creatinine clearance test is a useful guide to following clinical response and should be done at least twice as a baseline value, because the test may have a day-to-day variation from normal to abnormal in as high as 32% of cases.[K202]

BENEFICIAL EFFECTS OF STEROIDS IN LUPUS NEPHRITIS

The administration of corticosteroids to normal human subjects causes an increase in the glomerular filtration rate (GFR). The mechanism(s) is not clear, but several factors have been proposed including the catabolism of proteins results in the production of amino acids which are known to increase GFR.[B134] The beneficial effects of corticosteroids on lupus nephritis are a result of the modification of cellular and humoral immunologic processes involved in the glomerular injury and to their anti-inflammatory properties. The renal hemodynamic effect of steroids probably plays a minor role;[B134] however, steroids may also preserve glomerular permeability. In the murine model of lupus nephritis, treatment with methylprednisolone has been shown to retard the progression of the renal disease by decreasing the immune deposits in the glomeruli by altering the loss of anionic sites that favor the localization of immune complexes in the glomerular capillaries.[C167]

SIDE EFFECTS OF CORTICOSTEROIDS

The side effects of corticosteroids are protean and well recognized. This topic is the subject of review articles; however, the clinical data are derived mostly from uncontrolled and retrospective studies or from isolated case reports that often emphasize less common complications.[G14,N61,T228] See Table 58–4 for a representative list. This section discusses selected side effects and studies that deal primarily with SLE patients. Table 58–5 lists the commonly observed side effects in SLE based on patients who received an average dose of 20 mg of prednisone per day or equivalent.

Certain factors may influence the development of side effects of glucocorticoids. Kozower et al.[K405] noted that the frequency of hirsutism and obesity was more common in patients who have a slow catabolic rate for prednisolone. Therapeutic response, however, did not correlate drug clearance rate. The prevalence of side effects to prednisone doubled when the serum albumin was less than 2.5 g/100 ml, presumably because of the higher concentration of free unbound prednisolone in hypoalbuminemic states.[L244]

Hypothalamic-Pituitary-Adrenal (HPA) Axis Suppression

Suppression of the HPA axis with glucocorticoids is well known. In patients with rheumatic diseases, Klinefelter et al.[K288] found that none of 42 RA and 2 SLE patients had complete HPA suppression by doses of less than 15 mg of prednisone per day. None of the patients on 7.5 mg of prednisone a day had a blunted response. In contrast, 33% of those above 7.5 to 12.5 mg, and 47% of those on 12.5 to 15 mg of prednisone daily exhibited a blunted response.

Table 58–5. Adverse Effects of Glucocorticoid Therapy

Metabolic
　Central obesity
　Glucose intolerance
　Hyperosmolar nonketotic coma
Endocrine
　Hypothalamic-pituitary-adrenal axis suppression
　Growth failure in children
　Menstrual irregularities
Musculoskeletal
　Osteoporosis
　Aseptic necrosis of bone
　Myopathy
Cutaneous
　Thin fragile skin
　Purpura
　Striae
　Acne
　Hirsutism
　Impaired wound healing
Ocular
　Posterior subcapsular cataracts
　Glaucoma
Central nervous system
　Psychiatric disorders
　Pseudotumor cerebri
Cardiovascular-renal
　Sodium and water retention
　Hypokalemic alkalosis
　Hypertension
Gastrointestinal
　Pancreatitis
　Peptic ulcer
　Intestinal perforation
Impared immune response
　Bacterial, viral, fungal, and parasitic infections

Reprinted from Mayo Clin. Proc., 55:758, 1980.[N61]

Drug Intereaction

Klinenberg and Miller[K289] showed that the simultaneous administration of salicylates and corticosteroids results in lower serum salicylate concentration than expected because the renal clearance of salicylates is increased. In at least two SLE patients who received phenytoin for seizure disorders, marked decrease in dexamethasone levels was observed.[B450,M307] The effects of liver microsomal enzymes in this instance suggests an increase in the dose of dexamethasone.

Osteopenia

Osteoporosis is a major and often a serious complication of longterm corticosteroid therapy. The pathophysiology of the bone loss is poorly understood. Several factors including suppression of intestinal absorption of calcium, decreased renal tubular resorption with increased calcium urinary loss, and suppression of osteoblast function and bone formation are implicated.[H358]

In an overview of their extensive studies in this area, Hahn and colleagues[H40] reported that 83 to 90% of rheumatic disease patients had significant bone loss as measured by several indices. Bone loss can occur early during corticosteroid therapy; however, the degree of bone loss is dependent on the cumulative amount of glucocorticoid

used. Discontinuation of the corticosteroid therapy, if possible, with the addition of NSAIDs, antimalarials, or cytotoxic agents to the regimen is the most important therapeutic measure. Whether the bone loss is reversible or not has not been examined in SLE patients.

Gluck et al.[G201] compared steroid-induced osteopenia in 25 patients with rheumatic diseases on alternate-day dosage and 25 matched patients on daily prednisone therapy. Significant bone loss was noted in 40% of patients in both groups, indicating that alternate-day regimen was not helpful in minimizing osteoporosis. An effective therapy for steroid-induced osteoporosis is yet to be found; however, the available clinical data suggest that calcium and estrogen replacement in estrogen-deficient individuals are useful prophylactic measures.[H40,H358] Good nutrition, low sodium intake (2 to 3 g/day), and maintenance of physical activity are useful measures.[L415a] A controlled trial of oral 1,25-dihydroxyvitamin D, a more potent stimulator of intestinal calcium absorption, concluded that it is not useful in the treatment of steroid-induced osteopenia.[D375] Large doses of vitamin D or its metabolites should not be used routinely in all patients on chronic steroid therapy. Patients with low serum 25-OHD should be given pharmacologic doses of vitamin D and followed closely for toxicity.[L415a] The efficacy and longterm safety of sodium fluoride, biphosphonates, calcitonin, and anabolic steroids in treatment of patients with crush fractures and severe osteoporosis secondary to chronic steroid therapy have not been fully investigated; however, preliminary studies appear promising.[H358,L415a]

Psychosis and Other Mental Changes

Most psychotic episodes that occur in SLE patients are related to active CNS involvement; however, it is possible to have combined organic and steroid psychosis.[H321] Dubois et al.[D320] have observed untreated SLE patients who presented with an organic schizophrenic reaction associated with an exacerbation of SLE. Following institution of high-dose corticosteroid therapy, the psychosis either improved initially, then relapsed or persisted despite treatment for several weeks with 2500 mg of pareteral hydrocortisone daily. When the dose was reduced eventually to as little as 25 mg daily of cortisone or discontinued, without relapse of the underlying disease, the patient's mental status improved.

The temporal onset of corticosteroid-induced mental changes is unpredictable and varies from one patient to another. The Boston Collaborative Drug Surveillance program found a strong correlation between acute psychosis and inappropriate euphoria and the daily dose of prednisone among a large group of hospitalized patients with various diagnoses including rheumatic conditions.[B421] Conversely, the daily dose, the duration of therapy, or a previous history of mental illness does not affect the time of onset, severity, or the type of mental changes.[L310]

The most common manifestations of steroid-induced mental changes are inappropriate euphoria, depression, and psychotic reactions. These abnormalities are not uncommon in SLE. Ten of 62 SLE patients (16%) of Harvey et al.[M280] on corticosteroids developed psychosis, although 3 subjects had a similar episode prior to steroid therapy. Two of 19 patients (10.5%) with lupus nephritis enrolled in treatment protocol of prednisone and azathioprine developed psychosis.[D291] In a study of 50 patients with diffuse lupus nephritis treated with four different regimens, Cade and associates[C1] observed psychotic episodes in 5 of 15 patients (33%) treated with 60 to 100 mg prednisone daily for 6 months and 3 of 13 patients (31%) who received both prednisone and azathioprine. Conversely, none of 13 SLE patients on azathioprine alone and only 1 of 13 patients who received azathioprine had heparin-developed psychosis. In a retrospective analysis of clinical course of 28 SLE patients with 52 episodes of neuropsychiatric events, Sergent et al.[S287] found 15 separate episodes in 14 patients of steroid-induced psychosis. In contrast to these studies, other investigators,[C276,D309, D311,D314,D316,G440] as well as our own experience, have found a lower frequency of steroid-induced psychosis in SLE.

Steroid-induced psychosis generally improves with a reduction in the daily dose. Should the patient require continued drug therapy for a major organ involvement, it may be necessary to add a cytotoxic agent as the prednisone dose is reduced. In an occasional patient, psychosis may not be resolved until total cessation of steroid therapy is possible. Chlorpromazine or haloperidol is effective in managing these episodes. Lithium has been used to prevent steroid-induced psychosis.[G216] On the other hand, tricyclic antidepressants may cause exacerbation or worsening of the clinical state of the patient.[H56] In our experience, phenothiazines and haloperidol do not produce exacerbations of SLE when used for several months. Reinstitution of steroid therapy in a patient with a history of steroid-induced psychosis does not necessarily result in the reappearance of steroid-induced psychosis.

Healthy individuals given a single 1 mg dose of dexamethasone or 80 mg of prednisone daily for 5 days in a controlled study committed significantly more errors in verbal memory tests than subjects receiving placebo.[W329] Thus, corticosteroids can induce impairment of cognitive functions, and this effect should be considered when evaluating mental functions in SLE patients (see also Chap. 39).

Peptic Ulcer Disease and Gastritis

Gastrointestinal complaints such as epigastric distress, abdominal pain, nausea, and vomiting are common in patients on corticosteroids (Table 58–5). Whether corticosteroid use increases the risk to peptic ulcer disease or gastrointestinal hemorrhage remains a controversial issue. Two retrospective analyses of published data have come to divergent conclusions. Conn and Blitzer[C371] reviewed 42 controlled trials and concluded that the association is a myth and that corticosteroids do not cause peptic ulcer unless patients had been on the steroids for longer than 300 days and had taken more than 1000 mg prednisone. In contrast, Messer et al.[M370] pooled data from 71 controlled trials comprising 3064 patients with various medical disorders and concluded that corticosteroids increase the risk to peptic ulcer (relative risk = 2.3) and gastrointestinal hemorrhage (relative risk = 1.5). A case-control study of elderly Medicaid patients has shown that the risk of developing peptic ulcer disease among current users of oral glucocorticoids was increased only in patients who were concurrently receiving aspirin or other NSAIDs. The risk for peptic ulcer disease in this group was 15 times greater than that of nonusers of either drug.[P199a] The discrepant results in the earlier studies may be partly because of the differences in the use of NSAIDs among the study subjects. Whether these findings are applicable to a younger population such as SLE patients remains to be established.

The risk for peptic ulcer disease may be higher in certain patient groups when they are receiving corticosteroids including those with cirrhosis, rheumatoid arthritis, or those who are concurrently taking ulcerogenic medications.[G14] Whether SLE patients have an increased ulcer risk is not definitely established; however, they are often prescribed aspirin or NSAIDs concomitantly with corticosteroids.

Dubois and co-workers[B562,D326,D327] studied 91 patients, 85 with SLE and 7 with other rheumatic diseases, who had upper gastrointestinal roentgenograms. Sixty-four subjects who required high doses of corticosteroids had serial x-ray examinations at 3 months while the remaining 28 had a single examination. The prevalence of peptic ulcer in 52 of these who were treated with salicylates and antimalarials alone was 4%. In contrast, 21 patients (27%) who received steroids had peptic ulcers. The ulcers developed within 2 to 12 months following institution of corticosteroids. In 21 cases in which a definite ulcer crater was seen, 15 were gastric and 6 were duodenal. This ratio of 2.7 gastric to 1 duodenal was the reverse of the usual 1:10 ratio, suggesting the possible role of local factors. The occurrence of a peptic ulcer was related to the dose; however, the corticosteroid preparation used did not appear to be an important factor. It must be emphasized that these studies were undertaken before H2 blockers, misoprostol, and other agents became available and prior to the widespread use of the flexible endoscope. Thus, the figures are not necessarily applicable to current practice.

An active peptic ulcer is not necessarily an indication to stop corticosteroids immediately if the patient's condition requires continued therapy. The risk of perforation or hemorrhage is not significantly higher when compared to ulcer patients not taking corticosteroids; however, these complications may develop silently.[G14] Aspirin and NSAIDs should be discontinued. Antacids, H2 blockers, sucralfate, or omeprazole therapy should be instituted and the response to therapy followed by upper gastrointestinal endoscopy. Whether the risk of peptic ulceration in steroid-treated SLE patients is reduced by the concomitant administration of antacids and/or cimetidine has not been properly investigated. Nevertheless, we prescribe these medications empirically to all patients with a previous ulcer history or to those with dyspepsia while on steroids. We also recommend misoprostol to these patients when they require the longterm use of NSAIDs.

Steroid-Induced Myopathy

Myopathy secondary to longterm corticosteroid therapy should be differentiated from myopathy caused by SLE or the use of antimalarials. In steroid-induced myopathy, serum enzymes are usually normal, and the majority of the patients are receiving either fluorinated preparations or large doses of nonfluorinated derivatives.[A51]

Askari et al.[A347] reviewed the literature on the subject and described 8 patients, 3 of whom had SLE, who developed steroid-induced myopathy. Most patients experience an insidious inset of weakness and myalgias. Weakness was most pronounced in the pelvic girdle muscles with lesser involvement of the shoulder girdle and distal muscles. An elevated urinary creatine excretion was found in most patients. Muscle strength improved and creatinuria decreased following reduction in steroid dose. Kanayama et al.[K51] followed 27 SLE patients for steroid myopathy. LDH but not CPK or SGPT levels were elevated in 15, all of whom were on corticosteroids. Six of the 15 patients developed steroid-induced myopathy. Serum LDH decreased with improvement in muscle strength following reduction in steroid dose.

Myopathy developed in 6 of 29 SLE patients treated with 12 mg or more of triamcinolone daily for 4 to 32 weeks.[D311] Studies of the effect of various glucocorticoids on dog muscle have shown that triamcinolone produced the greatest degree of atrophy.[F13]

A review of the muscle biopsy in 20 subjects with steroid-induced myopathy showed an increase in the number of sarcolemmal nuclei, rowing and centralization of the nuclei, vacuolization and loss of fiber cross-striations and phagocytosis to the most common findings of light microscopy.[A51] Electron microscopy in six cases showed major structural changes in the mitochondria and glycogen aggregates. These pathologic changes in the mitochondria were nonspecific and may occur in other disease states. A study of rheumatoid arthritis patients has shown that prednisone therapy caused atrophy of type I and particularly type II muscle fibers, which may explain muscle wasting often seen in these patients.[D40b]

Other Side Effects

Dyslipoproteinemia

It is now well recognized that longterm corticosteroid therapy in SLE causes dyslipoproteinemia characterized by elevated plasma triglyceride, cholesterol, and low-density lipoprotein cholesterol.[E154,S668,W38] These abnormalities are known to be associated with increased risk for coronary artery disease and may be important in the apparent increase in atherosclerotic heart disease and myocardial infarction in SLE.[H401,R321,S102,U34] Patients should be screened for lipid abnormalities and treated. The observation that hydroxychloroquine improves these steroid-induced lipoprotein abnormalities should be investigated further to determine whether premature atherosclerosis is also prevented.[W38]

Widening of the Superior Mediastinum

This may simulate a mass lesion and can occur during high-dose steroid therapy in SLE.[P294] This is a result of fat accumulation and usually regresses as the steroid dose is reduced.

Diabetes Mellitus

This is a common complication of high-dose steroid therapy; however, ketoacidosis is infrequent. Four SLE patients developed ketoacidoses following treatment with at least 60 mg of prednisone daily for 2 to 8 months.[A120] All responded to insulin and fluid therapy. Hyperosmolar nonketotic coma is rarely seen as a complication of glucocorticoids in SLE.[B449] Corticosteroid-induced pancreatitis appears to be more prevalent in children than in adult patients.[R208] Another cause of abdominal pain in longterm corticosteroid-treated patients is perforation of colonic diverticuli.[C68] Spontaneous colonic perforation may occur in the absence of diverticuli.[Z238a]

Pseudotumor Cerebri

This is a rare complication of corticosteroid therapy in SLE and may be associated with an increase in the steroid dosage.[V119] However, benign intracranial hypertension may also be a manifestation of the central nervous system involvement in this disease.[B275,162] Improvement in the symptoms following a reduction in the steroid dosage will differentiate the former from the latter cause.

Posterior Subcapsular Cataracts

Cataracts as a complication of corticosteroid therapy were first reported in 1960.[B328] Although early studies have failed to consistently demonstrate this association, subsequent investigations especially in RA patients and recipients of renal allografts have convincingly established this association.[B328] The daily and total cumulative dose have been found to be important factors, although cataracts have occurred even in patients on less than 10 mg of prednisone daily over a period of a year.[C432,F318,H210,S585] In a study of adult RA patients, Williamson et al.[W249] found no cataracts in 65 patients who received prednisone for less than 2 years. In contrast, 7 of 52 patients tended to develop cataracts earlier and at a lower steroid dose than older subjects. Certain individuals and ethnic groups appear to have increased susceptibility to steroid-induced cataracts.[U27]

Steroid-induced cataracts are usually bilateral but rarely cause visual impairment until far advanced. Most patients do not volunteer visual impairment until far advanced.[U27] There is no indication that dose reduction or discontinuation of corticosteroids results in regression and disappearance of the cataracts, although reversibility has been described in some early cases.[G14,U27] The severity of visual impairment depends on the extent of the cataracts, and if clinically indicated lens extraction can be performed with excellent results.

Glaucoma

High-dose corticosteroids may cause glaucoma in SLE patients. The intraocular pressure improves with a reduction in the steroid dose.[B259]

Ecchymosis

Ecchymoses on the distal extremities as a result of corticosteroids must be differentiated from pigment deposition caused by antimalarials. The skin is atrophic and friable in steroid-treated individuals, and minimal trauma often results in extensive laceration. Winer et al.[W281] found ecchymoses in one-third of RA patients on longterm steroid therapy and in only 2% of those on no steroids. On biopsy, steroid-induced ecchymoses show perivascular infiltrates of lymphocytes and polymorphonuclear leukocytes and fragmentation of elastic fibers around blood vessels. These changes are similar to those observed in senile purpura.[W281] Ecchymoses caused by steroids or senile purpura persist for periods of several weeks, and longer than those following a bruise in normal skin. Reduction of the dose and discontinuation of the corticosteroids will result in disappearance of the ecchymoses.

Skin Rashes

Maculopapular or urticarial rashes caused by drug hypersensitivity to systemic corticosteroids occur rarely.[C355] In isolated cases, the hypersensitivity may be directed to additives in the tablet formulation.[G14]

Growth Suppression

This is an important complication of longterm administration of corticosteroids in children. This is minimized by alternate-day regimen,[R100] but the precise mechanism of growth suppression is not known.[G14] Corticosteroid therapy may also interfere with the onset and progress of puberty and the growth spurt.[R100]

The relationship between avascular necrosis of bone and corticosteroids is discussed in Chapter 34. Infections in SLE, including the effects of corticosteroids are discussed in Chapter 46.

SUMMARY: SYSTEMIC CORTICOSTEROIDS IN SLE

1. Adrenal glucocorticoids are potent anti-inflammatory and immunosuppressive drugs. Systemic corticosteroids are used for the treatment of active SLE with heart, kidney, hematologic, or central nervous system involvement.

2. Systemic corticosteroids are used in small doses in patients with fever, arthritis, mild serositis, fatigue, or rash only after salicylates, NSAIDs, or antimalarials have failed to provide satisfactory therapeutic effect.

3. For the patient with solely renal or hematologic involvement and without constitutional symptoms, alternate-day steroid therapy is ideal. Single daily dose oral therapy is utilized in most patients with active disease; twice or thrice daily administration is used in those with active CNS and in febrile patients not controlled by less potent measures.

4. Pulse methylprednisolone therapy is of uncertain benefit. It is most commonly used empirically in critically ill patients with active disease who are not responsive to conventional measures.

5. Dosing of systemic corticosteroids varies widely, depending on the organ involved and the severity of the disease. Prednisone and methylprednisolone are the most commonly used preparations; hydrocortisone is given to critically ill patients and when rapid onset of action is required.

6. Side effects of systemic corticosteroids limit their use. Hyperglycemia, cataracts, osteoporosis, pituitary axis depression, edema, psychosis, hypertension, glaucoma, aseptic necrosis of bone, gastric irritation, and increased susceptibility to infections pose the most significant risk of therapy.

Chapter 59

CYTOTOXIC DRUGS

DANIEL J. WALLACE

Cytotoxic or immunosuppressive drugs have been used in the treatment of SLE since 1947. Because adverse side effects are common and potentially life-threatening, their use should be limited to patients with organ-threatening disease who fail to respond to corticosteroids, or when the benefits of introducing a steroid-sparing agent outweigh the risks of administering these drugs. The superiority of cytotoxic drugs plus steroids to steroids alone has been documented in well-designed controlled trials for lupus nephritis and for chronic active "lupoid" hepatitis, but not for any other manifestation of SLE.

Several considerations are in order whenever the use of cytotoxic drugs are contemplated in SLE. None of these agents have been approved by the Food and Drug Administration (FDA) for use in the treatment of SLE, but this should not discourage their use in cases of proven benefit.[A280] Most of these agents introduce a carcinogenic risk to patients with a nonmalignant disease. Also, because 80 to 90% of SLE patients are female, the use of drugs that can decrease fertility, increase teratogenesis, and induce premature menopause is a serious issue.

Our group followed 464 SLE patients between 1980 and 1989. Of the 252 with organ-threatening disease, 64 were given cyclophosphamide (CTX), 58 were given azathioprine (AZA), 13 were given methotrexate (MTX), 13 were given nitrogen mustard (HN2), and 9 were given chlorambucil (CHL).[P216] About 25% with SLE and 50% with organ-threatening disease were thought to have required immunosuppressive therapy.

Several excellent papers have reviewed the mechanisms of action, therapeutic effects, and adverse reactions of cytotoxic drugs. This chapter is limited to a discussion of their efficacy and side effects in the treatment of SLE.

NITROGEN MUSTARD

Methylbis(β-chloroethyl)amine hydrochloride (nitrogen mustard; mechlorethamine hydrochloride; HN2; Mustargen) was the first alkylating agent used in the treatment of SLE. HN2 is rarely employed at present, mainly because of the ease with which cyclophosphamide, a closely related alkylating agent, can be administered. Nevertheless, it has some advantages in specific circumstances.

Clinical Trials

The first report (1947) of the use of HN2 in lupus was for the treatment of severe cutaneous disease.[O105] HN2 ointment is currently used for the treatment of mycoses fungoides and other cutaneous lymphomas.[K489,V108] Unfortunately, few physicians realize that it can be efficacious for refractory discoid lesions.

Chasis et al.,[C216] in 1949, reported on the successful use of intravenous HN2 for glomerulonephritis. Other groups recorded good results in small numbers of patients.[B51,D72, D364,P244,R273,S179,S213,W272] Dubois[D307,D310] and Kellum and Haserick[K154] gave HN2 to over 100 patients in the mid-1950s. The patients were not classified with regard to renal histology. Dubois found the drug to be particularly effective in managing patients with the nephrotic syndrome, accounting for a 78% success rate. Favorable responses persisted for years. Most patients treated had a significant decrease in urine protein levels, steroid requirements, and weight. The best response was observed in nephrotic patients with rapidly advancing disease. The indication for implementing HN2 therapy in these patients was failure to respond to 2 months of high-dose oral steroids. I have summarized the results of giving 74 courses of HN2 to 44 of Dubois' patients (Table 59–1).[W40] A significant improvement in urine sediment and serum creatinine levels occurred in the 30 to 40% of patients. The response of lupus nephritis patients to HN2 can be rapid. Dubois gave 0.3 to 0.4 mg/kg over 1 to 2 days intravenously and observed diuresis as soon as 3 to 14 days later; serum levels of protein, cholesterol, and urea nitrogen improved, and proteinuria diminished within a few weeks. One author[O105] reported a concurrent improvement of skin lesions, but not of arthritis.

In 1973, Dillard et al.[D214] studied the effect of combined initial treatment with high-dose prednisone (60 mg/day) and a single course of HN2 (0.4 mg/kg total, given over 2 to 4 days) in 17 patients with active diffuse proliferative lupus glomerulonephritis. Renal biopsies, before and sequentially after treatment, were analyzed in detail using semiquantitative methods. Patients treated with both drugs had a greater decrease in histologic activity than a previously treated group that received prednisone alone. Of those in the combination therapy group, however, 5 died in renal failure within 6 weeks and 1 died at 17 months. The initial serum creatinine level was over 2.3 mg/dl in only one patient. In this small series the clinical results were not favorable, and were similar to those for patients receiving prednisone alone. No evidence indicated that HN2 was of value for the treatment of nonrenal manifestations of SLE.

In 1982, Cruz et al.[C448] treated 15 patients with SLE and

Table 59–1. Parameters 40 Days after Nitrogen Mustard Administration

Parameter	Incidence No.	Incidence %	Disappeared No.	Disappeared %	Mean Duration of Response (mo)
Hematuria	45/56	80	14/45	31	46
Hyaline casts	28/58	48	11/28	39	33
Granular casts	32/56	57	11/32	34	63
Oval fat bodies	19/56	34	2/19	11	—

Parameter	Decreased No.	Decreased %	Criteria for Decrease	Mean Decrease
Serum creatinine level	13/33	39	≥0.1 mg/dl	0.63 mg/dl
Serum cholesterol level	19/27	70	≥1 mg/dl	99 mg/dl
24-hr urine protein level	31/38	82	100 mg/24	3,595 mg
Prednisone dosage	26/43	60	≥1 mg	19 mg
Weight	39/57	67	≥0.1 kg	2 kg

From Wallace, D.J., Podell, T.E., Weiner, J.M. et al.: Lupus nephritis: Experience with 230 patients in a private practice from 1950 to 1980. Am. J. Med. 72:209, 1982.

biopsy-proven diffuse proliferative nephritis with 0.4 mg/kg of HN2 administered in split doses 2 days apart. The mean serum creatinine level decreased 60 days after treatment, steroid requirements for prednisone decreased from 48 to 19 mg daily, and the 24-hour urine protein decreased from 7,060 mg to 1,930 mg.

Dosage, Administration, and Adverse Effects

Dubois always performed a baseline bone marrow study prior to the use of nitrogen mustard. Despite essentially normal or borderline reduced blood counts, the marrow may show marked hypocellularity, in which case the drug dose should be reduced or not used if severe changes were found. Adults are usually given a single dose of 15 to 20 mg. The drug is diluted with 20 ml of saline and infused with 5% dextrose in water over 1 hour, which approximates 0.3 to 0.4 mg/kg. It is usually administered in the evening after premedication to minimize the nausea and vomiting that occur several hours later in 80% of patients; these effects are generally worse than with cyclophosphamide. Dividing the daily dosage into two parts may reduce the severity of these reactions. Localized phlebitis distal to the needle occurs if it is not well placed intravenously, or when it is withdrawn immediately after infusion.[Q11] Phlebitis can be eliminated by a rapid infusion of 1 L of 5% dextrose with half-normal saline to remove any high local concentrations of the material. Chemical damage to the vascular wall may precipitate thrombosis following IV injection of HN2, especially in thrombosis-prone SLE patients with antiphospholipid syndrome.[Q11]

Seven to 10 days after administration of the nitrogen mustard, a transitory leukopenia appears, usually for about 1 week. In some patients, no appreciable decrease in leukocyte count occurs. Following therapy, the leukocyte count rarely diminishes below 2,500/mm³. In our experience, no patients developed persistent agranulocytosis or had a serious reaction to the medication. If some improvement occurs, treatment can be repeated at intervals of about 6 weeks without any danger of accumulation.[S603] If no response is obtained at all after two courses, this form of therapy should be abandoned.

In contrast to patients whom we have treated with oral cyclophosphamide, HN2 produces more nausea but less alopecia; hemorrhagic cystitis has not occurred. Of 44 patients reviewed in 1982, 10 subsequently had normal babies.[W40] None of these patients developed a malignancy (mean follow-up in 1982, 15 years). Bone marrow suppression was limited to a fixed, 6-week interval, and patient compliance was not a problem. The efficacy of parenteral cyclophosphamide (IVC) is probably similar to that of HN2 but hospitalization is not required, because the medication can be given in a single dose. IVC is usually much better tolerated in terms of nausea and vomiting.

CYCLOPHOSPHAMIDE

Cyclophosphamide (Cytoxan; CTX) is a bifunctionally substituted nitrogen mustard compound that was first synthesized in 1958. It is an alkylating agent that acts throughout the cell cycle by inducing chemical reactivity with the nucleophilic centers of molecules, including DNA, RNA, and proteins. The drug cross links DNA and thus inhibits DNA replication.

The serum half-life of CTX is 2 to 10 hours. Less than 20% is excreted in the kidney; liver microsomal enzymes produce a number of metabolites that are also alkylating agents. The pharmacokinetics of single doses of oral CTX and IVC are similar. Maximum leukopenia occurs at 7 to 14 days, with complete recovery in most patients by 21 to 25 days. Anemia rarely occurs without leukopenia, and thrombocytopenia is uncommon. Stem cell function is spared; thus, marrow aplasia is usually transient. Several good review articles on the use of cyclophosphamide in the treatment of rheumatic diseases have appeared.[C300,K399,L276,M257,S637] This section is limited to the discussion of the application of CTX to SLE.

The immunologic effects of CTX include the following: toxicity to rapidly proliferating lymphoid tissues, induction of immunologic tolerance, inhibition of suppressor cell function, impairment of humoral antibody production, and bone marrow suppression. McCune et al. studied the effects of IVC on lymphocyte subsets in 9 lupus nephritis patients who received 6 monthly IVC doses of 500 mg/m².[M258] CD3+, CD4+, CD8+, and B1+ lymphocytes all decreased after treatment but the B cells soon returned to baseline levels, whereas the T-cell changes persisted. T-cell proliferative responsiveness was not altered.

Clinical Applications

Oral CTX for Nonrenal SLE

Schulz and Menter[S185] reported nine patients with severe discoid and subacute lupus skin lesions treated with oral CTX in doses of 50 to 200 mg daily (for adults) for from 3 to 38 months. Clinical improvement was excellent in five patients, moderate in three, and negligible in one. In two patients in whom cyclophosphamide was stopped, no recurrence of skin lesions was seen after 6 and 23 months.

The effects of IVC ($0.75-1.0$ G/m²) given monthly for 4-6 months have been studied with lupus thrombocytopenia.[B433] The thrombocytopenia was refractory to steroids or required excess amounts. IVC was given in a single monthly infusion of 0.75 to 1.0 g/m² for four to six doses. Five patients had a long-lasting improvement in their platelet count; the remaining two responded initially but experienced recurrences 1 to 3 years later.

Three preliminary studies have reported anecdotal experiences involving 11 patients with central nervous system SLE who were given monthly IVC.[F244,L69,V109] Modest to good improvements were observed, along with two serious infections. Two reports totalling 4 patients have documented the value of IVC in patients with inflammatory myositis associated with SLE.[B432,K369]

Numerous case presentations have attributed the improvement of a nonrenal clinical manifestation of SLE to CTX therapy. Many of these patients received multiple drug therapies, but the studies cited here provide evidence for the interventional efficacy of CTX. In these uncontrolled studies the following SLE manifestations were found to have improved after the introduction of CTX: pulmonary hemorrhage, pulmonary hypertension, lupus pneumonitis, transverse myelopathy, hyperviscosity syndrome, aplastic anemia, autoimmune neutropenia, necrotizing vasculitis, antiphospholipid syndrome with vasculopathy, and inhibitors of specific clotting factors.[B432,C134, E1,J50,K119,L264,P122,P305,Q21,S449,S486,V69,W50,W302] Decker[D112] reviewed several nephritis studies that suggested that concomitant systemic flares decrease in CTX-treated patients.

Oral CTX for Lupus Nephritis

Lupus nephritis is a difficult disease to follow because repeated biopsies are not practical; serologic parameters can be conflicting, and often have no correlation with the results of renal function tests.[M320] Renal disease can also be present with normal urinary sediment. Hundreds of articles have been published, with most being uncontrolled reports of a small number of cases treated with CTX. Selected studies are summarized in Table 59-2 and discussed here.

In 1967, Dubois reported that patients with SLE are extremely sensitive to the side effects of CTX, particularly if they are receiving only minimal amounts of corticosteroids.[D323] Of those in his lupus nephropathy group, 18 patients who had failed to respond to 1 mg/kg/day of prednisone for 2 months were treated with CTX in a median dose of 50 mg daily for 2 months. Of these 18, 3 had definite improvement, with a decrease in proteinuria and better renal function; 2 had some decrease in proteinuria. Leukopenia was induced by this small dose in all but 2 patients for transitory periods, and was severe enough to discontinue medication in 6 patients.

Fries et al.[F263] alternately assigned 14 patients with active multisystem SLE to a treatment group with CTX alone or prednisone alone. Of the 14 patients, 10 had nephropathy. No response to therapy was found in the CTX group compared to a good response in the prednisone-treated group. It was concluded that CTX alone is significantly less useful than prednisone. The difference was most significant with regard to the nonrenal manifestations. Following the failure of CTX alone, the patients responded to prednisone therapy.

Cameron et al.[C37] reported six patients with lupus glomerulitis treated with CTX. The improvement in five of the patients was attributed to CTX. During the initial phase, when being treated with CTX and prednisone, patients could tolerate as much as 200 mg of CTX daily but, if the alkylating agent was used alone, only 50 mg could be taken without the induction of leukopenia.

Garancis and Piering[G37] treated 22 patients with SLE and biopsy-proven membranoproliferative glomerulonephritis with less than 10 mg of prednisone/day to control the extrarenal manifestations and with either cyclophosphamide (2 mg/kg/day) or azathioprine (2 mg/kg/day) for 6 to 36 months. Each group contained 11 patients. No deaths occurred in the CTX series, but 4 in the azathioprine group died. Studies of both renal function and biopsy appearance during therapy showed that CTX was superior to AZA.

Feng et al.[F59] reported 42 patients with SLE treated with CTX and prednisone in varying doses. Of these, 31 patients had renal involvement, 19 of them diffuse prolifera-

Table 59-2. Studies of Cyclophosphamide for the Treatment of Lupus Nephritis

Source	No. of Patients	Study Type	Results*
Dubois[D323] (1967)	18	Uncontrolled	P + CTX > P
Fries[F263] (1973)	14	Controlled	P > CTX alone
Garancis[G37] (1973)	22	Controlled	P + CTX > P + AZA
Feng[F59] (1973)	42	Uncontrolled	P + CTX helpful
Donadio[D256,D257,D259] (1978)	26	Controlled	More recurrences with P; P versus P + CTX = survival, and on dialysis
Ginzler[G158] (1976)	14	Controlled; cross-over	P + AZA = P + CTX
Marmont[M147] (1980)	24	Uncontrolled	P + CTX helpful
Sessoms[S295] (1984)	10	Uncontrolled	P + IVC helpful
NIH[B65] (1987)	111	Controlled	P + IVC > P + AZA + CTX > P + CTX > P + AZA > P
McCune et al.[M258] (1988)	9	Controlled	P + IVC helpful
Lehman[L166] (1989)	16	Uncontrolled	P + IVC helpful in 15 of 16 children
Frutos[F292] (1990)	19	Uncontrolled	P + IVC decreases activity, not chronicity, on second biopsy

* P, prednisone; AZA, azathioprine; CTX, oral cyclophosphamide; IVC, intravenous, intermittent cyclophosphamide.

tive nephritis. Biopsies were reported in 7 1 year later, and 5 were unchanged. Despite this, 3 of 5 patients had no proteinuria or hematuria at the time of repeat biopsy. Not enough follow-up data were obtained to determine whether those in the diffuse nephritis group were significantly helped.

Donadio and colleagues at the Mayo Clinic[D256,D257,D259] compared prednisone with prednisone plus CTX. Prednisone was given to 26 patients, 40 mg daily, for 6 months and compared with 24 patients given 40 mg of prednisone plus CTX (1 to 2 mg/kg/day) for 6 months, followed by tapering doses of prednisone alone. Initial improvement occurred in 84% of all patients. More recurrences were noted in the prednisone alone group 4 years later, but the incidences of patients alive and not requiring dialysis in both groups was the same.

Marmont reported that 24 lupus nephritis patients treated with prednisone plus CTX had a greater than 50% decrease in proteinuria and edema and a mean 70% improvement in glomerular filtration rate.[M147]

A pooled analysis of eight controlled studies suggested that patients receiving CTX or AZA had a lesser chance of renal deterioration and end-stage renal disease than those treated with corticosteroids alone.[F57] The report did not consider wide variations in study designs, toxicity of the agents, or quality of life.[F258] These results are similar, however, to those reported in the long-term NIH study (see below).

NIH 20-Year Study

Since 1969, the National Institutes of Health (NIH) has randomized patients with clinically and histologically active lupus nephritis into the following groups: 1) prednisone (P), 1 mg/kg/day; 2) prednisone plus azathioprine (P + AZA), up to 4 mg/kg/day of AZA; 3) prednisone plus oral cyclophosphamide (P + CTX), up to 4 mg/kg/day of CTX; and 4) prednisone plus the two latter drugs in low doses (P + AZA + CTX), up to 1 mg/kg/day. Several years later, a fifth group consisting of prednisone along with IV, intermittent cyclophosphamide was added (P + IVC), 0.5 to 1 g/m² every 3 months. A total of 111 patients have been entered into the study; follow-ups exceed 7 years in almost all cases, and several articles have reported their findings.[A273,A360,B63,B64,B65,C80,D113,D114,D221,K307,K308,R291,S636,S638] These investigators also devised a "chronicity index" and "activity index" in interpreting the kidney biopsy findings to measure improvement in renal histology, in addition to the usual evaluation of clinical and serologic parameters. The studies cited above summarize their principal conclusions, which are presented below and in Figs. 59–1 and 59–2.

Regarding the efficacy of each regimen, four outcomes were reported:

1. Any regimen containing a cytotoxic drug was superior to prednisone alone in suppressing the development of chronic, irreversible changes in renal biopsies. Most patients, however, showed an increase in their chronicity score.
2. IVC + P was significantly better than P in preventing end-stage renal disease.

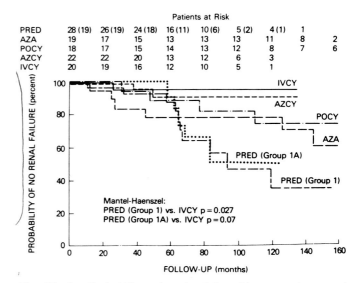

Fig. 59–1. Probability of maintaining life-supporting renal function in 107 patients with active lupus nephritis, according to treatment group (PRED, prednisone; AZA, azathioprine; POCY, oral cyclophosphamide; AZCY, combined oral azathioprine and cyclophosphamide; and IVCY, intravenous cyclophosphamide; PRED (group 1) all patients receiving prednisone; PRED (group 1A), subset of patients receiving prednisone who were randomly assigned concurrently with the groups, AZCY and IVCY. In the table at the top of the figure (Patients at Risk), numbers in parentheses refer to group 1A. (From Balow, J.E., Austin, H.A., Tsokos, G.C., et al.: Lupus nephritis. Ann. Intern. Med. 106:89, 1987.)

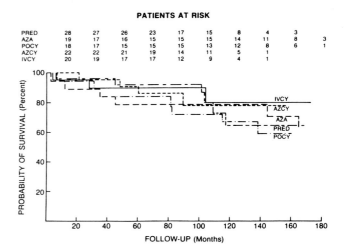

Fig. 59–2. Probability of survival in patients with lupus nephritis by treatment groups, (PRED, prednisone; AZA, azathioprine; POCY, oral cyclophosphamide; AZCY, combined oral azathioprine and cyclophosphamide; IVCY, intravenous cyclophosphamide). (From Balow, J.E., Austin, H.A., Tsokos, G.C., et al.: Lupus nephritis. Ann. Intern. Med. 106:91, 1987.)

3. P + AZA + CTX, P + CTX, and P + AZA appeared to be better than P alone in preventing end-stage renal disease, but differences did not reach statistical significance.

4. Over the 14-year study period, differences in overall survival among the groups were not statistically significant, although survival appeared slightly better for P + IVC and P + AZA + CTX than the other groups.

Overall patient survival was good: the 1-, 5-, and 10-year life table analysis was 95, 87, and 74%, respectively. No significant differences were noted among the groups until 10 years had passed. Regarding toxicity of the regimens, hypertension and major infection (except herpes zoster) were more common in in the P group. Herpes zoster and amenorrhea were more common in groups receiving cytotoxic drugs of any type. Malignancies occurred exclusively in patients receiving AZA, CTX, or both. These included fatal myelocytic leukemia, nonfatal polycythemia vera, carcinoma of the bladder, cervix, bladder, and skin, and acoustic schwannoma. Hemorrhagic cystitis occurred only in groups receiving oral CTX.

The study can be criticized for not including patients with aggressive disease who could not wait to be transferred to a tertiary center that only manages selected patients with established diagnoses of SLE. Moreover, 29 of the patients had membranous or mesangial biopsy patterns, or no biopsy at all. Most rheumatologists would not treat class II or class V lupus nephritis with cytotoxic agents, because they have a more favorable outcome than class III or IV patterns (see also Chaps. 53 and 54).

Parenteral CTX for Lupus Nephritis

McCune et al.[M258] gave 9 patients monthly doses of 500 mg/m[2] IVC for 6 months. Statistically significant improvements in creatinine clearance, 24-hour urine protein, C3, C4, and CH50 complement levels, and Westergren sedimentation rate were noted. The mean daily prednisone dose decreased from 45 to 17 mg. A 2-year follow-up suggested continued improvement.[M256] Sessoms and Kovarsky[S295] treated 10 patients with steroid-resistant lupus nephritis with monthly doses of 0.75 g/m[2] of IVC. Of these, 9 had a favorable response. Two studies examined lupus nephritis in children,[L166,M261,W7] and similar results were obtained in a total of 40 patients. Wagner-Weiner et al.[W7] reported flares with pulse discontinuation but maintenance of improvement if the pulse was given at 3-month intervals. Appel et al.[A267] administered five or six monthly infusions to 20 patients. Most became serologically inactive, but not all responded clinically. Those who were rebiopsied had a lower activity index but a higher chronicity index. Another study has confirmed this.[F292] Schatten et al.[S113] treated 13 patients with severe, diffuse, proliferative nephritis, high chronicity and activity indices, and fibrin thrombi on biopsy. This high-risk group received monthly IVC and pulse IV methylprednisolone. Preliminary results indicated dramatic clinical and serologic improvements. A similar study is in progress at the NIH.[S228]

In addition to the 1- to 3-month IVC cycles discussed,

various other dosing regimens have been studied. Case reports and abstracts suggest that weekly doses, low doses (less than 500 mg at a time), or high-dose oral, intermittent administration is safe and feasible.[H449,K365,S441,S425] Further study is warranted.

Toxic Effects

The toxicity of CTX includes bone marrow suppression, hemorrhagic cystitis, gonadal dysfunction, alopecia, teratogenesis, carcinogenesis, and increased rates of infection. Acrolein, an aldehyde metabolite, has a direct toxic effect on bladder transitional cell epithelium. Bone marrow toxicity is cumulative. The concurrent administration of allopurinol increases the risk of leukopenia. The dose of CTX must be reduced in those with moderate to severe renal insufficiency; only 30 to 60% of an administered dose is removed by hemodialysis.[A272,B25a,C295,F263,K400,L276,M150,M257] Other studies referred to in this section describe these and other side effects of the drug in SLE patients.

Short-term reactions in SLE include nausea and vomiting, which are dose-related, and are most severe 6 to 18 hours after parenteral administration. Fatigue is observed 1 to 3 days later.[L276,M257] McCune and Fox noted diarrhea and alopecia in those who were excessively leukopenic.[M257] Adequate hydration is necessary after oral administration to reduce the concentration of acrolein. Although hemorrhagic cystitis is uncommon with IVC, patients at risk can be protected with a 2-g IV dose of 2-mercaptoethane (Mesna) at the time of infusion.[H23]

McCune's group[M571] related serious infection to prednisone doses above 25 mg daily, and not to CTX doses or blood counts. The NIH experience also bears this out.[K308] Hellman et al. reported that serious infections, however, especially with opportunistic organisms, increased in SLE patients receiving cytotoxic drug.[H254]

Pregnancy should be avoided while on this agent, because the drug is highly teratogenic in SLE patients.[G129,K248] Pregnancy should always be excluded before administration of the drug. CTX produced even more chromosomal damage than chlorambucil in one study that measured sister chromatid exchanges in peripheral lymphocytes of patients with connective tissue diseases.[P20] Amenorrhea was found in 18 of 33 patients given CTX at the NIH.[B65] Klippel has advised administering IVC at the time of menses to minimize the risk of ovarian failure.[K305a]

Malignancy was reported in 3 of 19 patients given azathioprine and in 3 of 18 given oral CTX at the NIH. McCune et al. reported 3 malignancies out of 30 patients receiving IVC,[M257] and another report has appeared.[G120] Skin, urinary bladder, and hematologic neoplastic disorders are the most common.[C420,T61]

Walker et al.[W11] observed a patient treated with CTX who developed prolonged apnea after general anesthesia and the use of suxamethonium, a relaxant. The patient's plasma cholinesterase level was reduced, as it was in seven of eight other patients receiving CTX. Walker et al. suggested that plasma cholinesterase levels be determined if patients receiving CTX require general anesthesia in which a depolarizing relaxant may be used. Levels return to normal 10 days after the cessation of CTX.

Summary and Comment

CTX is effective but not curative in most patients with severe lupus nephritis or thrombocytopenia. It may be effective for other manifestations, but that is unclear. It is probably steroid-sparing. CTX is also relatively toxic. It is not FDA-approved for use in SLE patients, and probably had inadequate efficacy when used as the sole agent in patients with severe disease. Daily, oral CTX is carcinogenic, and teratogenic, and is associated with a high risk of infection, hemorrhagic cystitis, alopecia, and sterility. Low-dose oral or high-dose parenteral cyclophosphamide in combination with prednisone or other agents such as azathioprine is probably effective in SLE, and certainly warrants further study. IVC may be safer than high-dose oral CTX and has a lower incidence of urinary bladder toxicity. Different protocols have used induction schedules of every week to 3 months for IVC, but the greatest benefits have been reported in patients who received the drug monthly for at least 6 months in doses of 0.75 to 1.0 g/m^2. Our experience with 47 patients suggests that it takes three to six cycles to obtain significant benefits, and that relapses are common if cytotoxic therapy is completely discontinued at this point. Additional maintenance treatments at 1- to 3-month intervals are usually required for a few years. About one-third of our nephrotic syndrome patients have had no or limited responses.

AZATHIOPRINE

Azathioprine (Imuran; AZA) is a purine analogue of hypoxanthine. It is readily absorbed after oral administration and is cleared through degradation, urinary excretion, and tissue uptake. The drug acts through suppression of antibody responses. Despite its widespread use, little attention has been given to its immunologic actions in SLE. In one report of 40 lupus nephritis patients,[T67] high-dose AZA decreased B-cell levels more than T-cell levels. Those with the highest initial B-cell levels in peripheral blood appeared to respond better to treatment. Several general reviews of its immunologic activities have appeared.[C300,F6]

Paulus et al.[P79] studied the release of granulocytes from bone marrow that follows the administration of etiocholanolone in patients with SLE compared to non-SLE patients with chronic glomerulonephritis. The increase in granulocytes in those with SLE was smaller, and consequently the dose of AZA tolerated in this group was only half of that tolerated by those with chronic glomerulonephritis. Therefore, leukopenia may occur when prednisone is decreased, even though the dose of cytotoxic drug is constant. This is true with either AZA or CTX. Blood counts should be carefully monitored as the corticosteroid dose level is reduced.

Clinical Trials

Nonrenal Lupus

Azathioprine has been used frequently in patients unresponsive to corticosteroid treatment or as a steroid-sparing agent. Of 352 patients primarily with SLE who responded to a questionnaire from a lay lupus group (Leanon), 14% reported that they were receiving this drug[P280]. Of our 464 SLE patients seen between 1980 and 1989, 61 (13%) were given AZA.

Azathioprine is of proven value in managing lupoid hepatitis (see Chap. 42). This has been documented in several controlled studies.[M10,M478,M674]

Within the last decade, three separate, uncontrolled reports (including one from the National Institutes of Health) have reported improvement in severe cutaneous lesions after treatment with AZA.[S346,T241a,W182]

Several studies have addressed the effects of AZA on active multisystem lupus and survival. In 1971, Sztejnbok et al.[S803] attempted a controlled evaluation of AZA in the management of active, multisystemic SLE patients with good renal function. Alternative patients were assigned to treated groups and control groups (steroid treatment alone) of 21 patients each; the only difference was that the treated group received 2.5 mg/kg/day of AZA in addition to the amount of steroids required. No evidence was found to show that AZA is useful in the management of acute, severe exacerbations, but it was concluded that the AZA-treated group showed a decreased mortality and morbidity and required less prednisone than controls.

In an uncontrolled study, Swaak et al. reported improvement of symptoms, reduction of anti-DNA, and fewer exacerbations in 17 lupus patients given AZA.[S779] One report suggested that improvement occurring with prednisone-AZA therapy would deteriorate when AZA was discontinued.[L227] In the three cases described, however, steroids were also stopped. Sharon et al.[S327] abruptly withdrew AZA in 9 patients with stable SLE receiving combination AZA-prednisone therapy. Combined therapy was continued in 7 similarly treated control patients. Of the 9 patients, 7 had exacerbations within 21 to 200 days after abrupt withdrawal, compared with only one exacerbation in the continuation group. In a subsequent report, 21 of the 28 patients who discontinued AZA for any reason relapsed within an average of 3.6 months. Cameron observed no relapses following abrupt cessation of AZA therapy in 11 patients with glomerulonephritis.[C36]

Lupus Nephritis

Fewer than a dozen groups have seriously studied various combinations of interventions, including AZA, for lupus nephritis over the last 30 years. These observations are summarized in Table 59–3.

Drinkard et al.[D291] in 1970, reported on 20 patients with lupus nephropathy treated with AZA. Of these, 19 were cushingoid and were receiving 15 to 80 mg daily of prednisone when AZA (2 to 4 mg/kg/day) was added to their therapeutic regimen. Little evidence was found to indicate active systemic disease. Serum creatinine levels were normal at the start of therapy in fifteen patients. Prednisone was usually administered in divided doses of at least 30 mg daily for the first 6 months, and then gradually reduced. Of the 20 patients, 5 died (3 from infections), 1 developed hepatotoxicity, and clinical improvement occurred in 12, 10 of whom showed a decrease in proliferation on rebiopsy. Other histologic evidence of progression of renal disease, however, was found in 9 of

Table 59–3.   Studies of Azathioprine for the Treatment of Lupus Nephritis

Source	No. of Patients	Type of Study	Results
Drinkard[D291] (1970)	20	Uncontrolled	10 steroid-resistant patients improved
Donadio[D258] (1972)	15	Controlled	P + AZA and P both improved
Cade[C1] (1973)	50	Controlled	P + AZA > AZA > AZA + P + heparin
Garanois[G37] (1973)	22	Controlled	P + CTX > P + AZA
Hahn[H33] (1975)	24	Controlled	P and P + AZA improved
Lindemann[L300] (1976)	20	Uncontrolled	55% given P + AZA improved
Ginzler[G158] (1976)	14	Cross-over; controlled	P + AZA = P + CTX
NIH[B65] (1987)	111	Controlled	P + IVC > P + AZA + CTX > P + CTX > P
Nossent et al.[N146] (1989)	39	Uncontrolled	P + AZA = P

P, prednisone; AZA, azathioprine; CTX, oral cyclophosphamide; IVC, intravenous, intermittent cyclophosphamide.

these patients. Treatment was ineffective in 2 patients with advanced renal failure. Almost uniform suppression of immunologic manifestations occurred (antinuclear antibody titer, serum IgG), irrespective of clinical response.

A 6-month controlled study of 16 patients with lupus nephritis comparing prednisone (mean dose, 40 mg/day) with the same dose of prednisone plus AZA (2 to 3 mg/kg/day) was done by Donadio et al.[D258] in 1972. Patients were divided into two comparable groups based on renal biopsy (9 controls and 7 in the combined treatment group). Improvements in renal function, proteinuria, and biopsy appearance were identical in each series. Rebiopsy after 6 months therapy showed that both groups had less karyorrhexis, necrosis, and hyaline thrombi, intracapillary and extracapillary proliferation, and fibrinoid deposition. Serologic tests did not reflect renal improvement.

In 1973, Cade et al.[C1] studied 50 patients with proliferative nephritis resulting from SLE, assigning the patients alternately to daily high-dose prednisone (60 to 100 mg) for at least 6 months, AZA alone in a maximum dose of 2 mg/kg/day, prednisone and AZA combined, or combined AZA and heparin. Using this large dose of prednisone over an extended period resulted in a high incidence of side effects and actual worsening of renal function. Only 2 of 15 patients in the prednisone group were alive at the end of the study, with an average survival of 19 months. AZA alone appeared effective, with 9 of 13 patients alive and well (average survival, 38 months). Combinations of AZA and prednisone or AZA and heparin were the most successful; only 2 of 13 in each group died of renal failure. AZA alone was found to be helpful, with or without heparin.

In 1975, Hahn et al.[H33] treating patients with life-threatening SLE in any organ systems, demonstrated no benefits of prednisone plus AZA over prednisone during a 2-year study period. With regard to nephritis, however, only 3 of 13 prednisone patients versus 9 of 11 prednisone plus AZA patients had diffuse proliferative lesions. Lindemann et al.[L300] followed 20 SLE patients treated with AZA and prednisone for a mean of 43 months. Only 11 remitted or improved, 3 had decreased function, and 6 went on to dialysis or death. Ginzler et al.[G158] performed a double-blind cross-over study on 14 patients using prednisone plus AZA versus prednisone plus AZA plus CTX. No differences were noted.

The National Institutes of Health study (see above, Cy-

clophosphamide) included 19 lupus nephritis patients given AZA (4 mg/kg/day) with prednisone and 22 who received low-dose CTX with low-dose AZA (1 mg/kg/day).[A360,B63,B65,K307,K308,S636] Both groups had better results with regard to maintaining renal function than the group on prednisone alone, but differences were not statistically significant (Fig. 59–1).[F56] Hahn has also used a low-dose combined therapy approach, with favorable results.[H23] Swaak's group followed 39 lupus nephritis patients over a 15-year-period. Of these, 19 patients who received AZA with prednisone had identical survival curves to 16 who received prednisone alone[N146] (also see Chaps. 53 and 54).

Toxic Effects

The primary toxicity of AZA in SLE is to the bone marrow. Leukopenia is the most common abnormality, followed by thrombocytopenia and anemia.[N148,R22] Some of these responses can be idiosyncratic.[N148] Stomatitis, nausea, vomiting, hepatitis, fever, rash, and muscle aching can also occur.[N38] AZA can predispose patients to infection.[R157,S619] The NIH trial reported serious infections in 11% receiving AZA, in 14% receiving combined AZA/CTX low-dose therapy, and in 29% of patients receiving prednisone alone.

Longterm prednisone-AZA treatment has been associated with an increased incidence of malignancy in other disorders.[H412,S619] Wessel et al.'s literature review[W185] surveyed 721 patients given AZA for SLE in four reports; 29 (4%) developed cancer. The NIH study found carcinomas in 3 of 19 who received AZA plus prednisone, but in none of the 22 who had low-dose AZA/CTX.[A360,B65,K308] An increased incidence of cervical cell atypia in AZA-treated SLE patients was noted in two reports.[G160,N152]

Summary

Azathioprine appears to have some effectiveness in multisystem, active SLE, but is not curative. It is the cytotoxic agent of choice for the treatment of lupoid hepatitis and can also ameliorate joint and cutaneous manifestations of SLE in some patients. AZA is steroid-sparing. In lupus nephritis, it is probably superior to prednisone alone. It does not suppress immune responses as well as CTX; it is probably less effective but safer than CTX.

METHOTREXATE

In 1965, Miescher and Rietmuller[M401] treated 10 SLE patients with 50 mg IV methotrexate (MTX) weekly or 2.5 mg orally/day. The results were regarded as satisfactory. Also in the 1960s, Dubois gave 7 nephritis patients 7.5 mg daily for 6 weeks. Neither benefit nor toxicity was observed.[D323] The clear-cut ameliorative actions of methotrexate (MTX) in rheumatoid arthritis stimulated new interest regarding its potential use in SLE.

Using standard dosing regimens for rheumatoid arthritis (7.5 to 10 mg weekly), a Wisconsin group reported beneficial results in 1 patient in 1987.[D71] Encouraged by their success, they conducted an open label study on 10 SLE patients.[R337] MTX had to be discontinued in 3 patients because of adverse reactions (2 developed leukopenia), but the remaining 7 had documented improvements in arthritis (5), myositis (1), rash (3), pleurisy (1), and nephritis (2). A Cleveland Clinic group has reviewed their experience with 17 patients.[W229] The drug was clearly steroid-sparing, but only moderately effective in controlling cutaneous, pleuritic, or arthritic symptoms. Of the 17 patients, 70% experienced adverse reactions, including leukopenia in 6, and 36% discontinued MTX because of toxicity. At the University of Connecticut, 6 patients receiving 5 to 10 mg of oral MTX weekly tolerated the drug well. It was steroid-sparing and effective in ameliorating synovitis.[W269] I have given MTX to 22 patients. It has been steroid-sparing in 3 taking the prednisone for arthritis, but did not control any other manifestations of the disease. A high incidence of leukopenia was also found. MTX is also a photosensitizing agent and must be used carefully in SLE patients.[N56]

In summary, MTX is associated with a high incidence of leukopenia and other adverse effects in patients with SLE, and its efficacy has not been proven.

CHLORAMBUCIL

Chlorambucil (Leukeran; CHL) is an alkylating agent that was first reported as useful in 10 lupus nephritis patients in 1962.[M294] Dubois subsequently treated 7 patients with doses of 0.1 mg/kg/day, but without success.[D323] Amor et al.[A186] gave 0.2 mg/kg/day to 12 patients with active SLE for 2 to 21 months, but noted no significant differences compared to 12 prednisone-treated controls. Snaith et al.[S525] treated 5 patients with lupus nephropathy in 1973 using this agent, with favorable results.

Epstein and co-workers[E121-E123] treated 16 of 31 SLE patients with diffuse proliferative nephritis with prednisone and chlorambucil and reported their findings in 1974. Their chlorambucil group had a 78% 5-year survival. Of the 16 chlorambucil patients, however, 5 had serious bone marrow aplasia, enough to discontinue the drug. In 1 patient it was irreversible. Herpes zoster developed in 3 other patients.

In 1981, an international study found chlorambucil to be less effective than CTX but as effective as AZA in the treatment of lupus nephritis.[160,161] This included a Russian randomized, controlled trial in 40 patients. In a large Egyptian study of 163 lupus nephritis patients,[S5] 67 were given prednisone alone, 11 P + AZA, 32 P + CTX, and 53 P + CHL (10 mg/day of CHL). The last group had the best survival curve, but 95 of 163 (58%) died over a 5-year mean follow-up period. One report suggested that chlorambucil should be considered in patients with steroid-resistant nephrotic syndrome.[A7]

Chlorambucil is a potent drug whose efficacy has never been evaluated adequately in SLE. Evidence that it might be less oncogenic than cyclophosphamide warrants further analysis.[P20] It may be somewhat less effective than cyclophosphamide in SLE patients, but it is safer in terms of lack of damage to the urinary bladder. Irreversible bone marrow suppression is more common with CHL than with cyclophosphamide.

ANTIMETABOLITES

Damashek and Schwartz first proposed the use of 6-mercaptopurine (6-MP) and 6-thioguanine (6-TG) in the 1950s, but later reported disappointing results.[D26,S214] Favorable case presentations[E56,L143] led to larger studies, which included a total of 31 patients at four centers.[D149,D323,M401] Using 3 mg/kg/day of 6-MP or 2 mg/kg/day of 6-TG, generally transient initial responses were observed. Most patients developed reversible but significant marrow hypoplasia, and about one-third had no clinical response.

Mackay and Wood[M18,M20] and Page[P8] recorded dramatic improvements in liver function with 6-MP in lupoid hepatitis, even in the absence of corticosteroid therapy. Because 6-MP is a precursor of azathioprine, these observations led to trials with the latter, far safer agent, which clearly showed its efficacy in the treatment of lupoid hepatitis.

FRENTIZOLE

Frentizole (1-(6-methoxy-2-benzothiazolyl)-3-phenylurea); is an immunosuppressive that was used experimentally in the late 1970s to treat SLE. Kay et al.[K131] administered it to nine patients; eight improved serologically, and many had a lower incidence of skin, mucosal, serosal, and joint disease. In three patients, hepatotoxicity was noted. Sabharwal et al.[S6] observed improvements in three of seven patients, but five developed liver toxicity. More ominously, O'Duffy et al.[O13] successfully treated refractory thrombocytopenia associated with SLE but observed infarcts of the large bowel, along with hepatotoxicity. In early 1980, a controlled, double-blind, five-center trial was discontinued because hepatotoxicity and bowel infarcts occurred too frequently.[B75]

Chapter 60

NONPHARMACOLOGIC THERAPEUTIC MODALITIES

DANIEL J. WALLACE

In addition to medication, physical measures, and psychologic support, the treatment of SLE may necessitate the use of other nonpharmacologic modalities. These include dialysis and transplantation for end-stage renal disease, lasers for cutaneous lesions and possibly synovitis, plasmapheresis for life-threatening complications of the disease, and lymphocyte depletion through thoracic duct drainage, total lymphoid irradiation, or lymphapheresis for selected patients with refractory disease.

DIALYSIS

Uremia. Uremia was the major cause of death in SLE patients until the 1960s, when dialysis became available. Only a small percentage of dialysis patients have SLE. Between 1977 and 1985, 5,726 persons in Australia and New Zealand were placed on dialysis; only 63 (1.1%) had SLE.[P249] Despite therapeutic advances, 26 of 128 nephritis patients followed by Wallace between 1980 and 1989 evolved end-stage renal disease that required dialysis.[P216] All but 3 of the 26 had nephrotic syndrome. Uremia and dialysis are both associated with a decrease in the systemic activity of SLE in many, but not all, patients.[B515,W40] Ziff and Helderman[Z28] have speculated that the toxic effects of uremia on the immune system are responsible for its ameliorative effects on extrarenal disease. It is also possible that the disease has run its course in some individuals and subsided, but by that time the chronic renal damage is irreversible.

Reversibility: Some patients who develop renal failure from lupus nephritis can discontinue dialysis. This was true in 41% of Kimberly's 41 patients; 11 were dialyzed for less than 2 months.[K217] On the other hand, 37% died. Five were transplanted successfully. Coplan et al.[C384] reported on their experience with 28 dialysis patients followed between 1969 and 1980. Of these, 8 were dialyzed for a mean of 4.3 months before discontinuing it; 6 deaths occurred in the patients with the highest steroid requirement; 7 were transplanted; and only 3 had extrarenal disease. The first few months on dialysis appear to be critical—a high mortality rate is observed, but many of those who survive can either discontinue dialysis or become candidates for transplantation.[C394] Acute tubular necrosis superimposed on lupus nephritis can induce transient renal failure.[H268]

Prognosis: Survival on dialysis is good. Ziff and Helderman's 30 patients had a 67% 5-year survival,[Z28] Jarrett et al.[J57] had 59%, and Cheigh et al.[C222] had 65% in the late 1970s. These figures compare favorably with those of non-

SLE dialysis patients. Some reports have documented a better survival rate: 71% in Australia and New Zealand at 5 years,[P249] and 89% of 55 Dutch patients at 5 years.[N143] In these studies, nonrenal SLE activity was minimal. Most deaths were related to infection or vascular access problems. At the University of California, only 3 of 12 patients on dialysis for lupus nephritis needed corticosteroids after 31 months' mean observation.[P10] In 1990, Cheigh et al. presented a follow-up of 59 patients with end stage renal disease seen at New York Hospital between 1970 and 1987.[C221] Of these, 86% were female; the mean age was 27.4 years at end-stage renal disease onset, and they were followed for a mean of 6.5 years. SLE disease activity at years 1, 5, and 10 was 55, 6.5, and 0%, respectively. The 5- and 10-year survival rates were 81.1 and 74.6%.

Ginzler's multicenter trial of 1,103 SLE patients[G162] showed that dialysis has little impact in evaluating causes of death in SLE, even though dialysis patients had a much higher rate of infection.[B515,G334] Socioeconomic considerations are also important. In the largely indigent group at Los Angeles Harbor-UCLA Medical Center, 6 of 9 dialysis patients died at 1 to 28 months, and 5 of the 6 had disease flares.[S482]

Hemodialysis Versus Peritoneal Dialysis. The success of hemodialysis in ameliorating disease activity may be a result of its ability to remove circulating pathogenic immune complexes, complement, and other factors.[N81] Hemodialysis also has anti-inflammatory effects, decreases T helper lymphocyte levels, and diminishes mitogenic responsiveness.[R256,W357] In contrast, peritoneal dialysis does not cause these changes. Several studies have documented more reactivation of SLE, higher anti-dsDNA levels, more thrombocytopenia, and higher steroid requirements with peritoneal dialysis.[H268,R256,W357] In one center, 4 of 6 patients who were started on peritoneal dialysis had to be switched to hemodialysis.[K10] *Barring extenuating or unusual circumstances, hemodialysis is preferable to peritoneal dialysis.*

TRANSPLANTATION

Graft and Patient Survival. By 1975, SLE patients in the United States were transplanted, and another 150 between 1975 and 1980.[A180,C159] These studies concluded that allografts from a living related donor have a much better survival—2-year graft survivals averaged 50%. In Australia and New Zealand, 19 transplants performed between 1977 and 1985 were associated with 95- and 83% survivals at 1 and 5 years, and with 75 and 70% 1- and

5-year graft survivals, respectively.[P249] In 1987, Roth et al. reported a 93% patient survival and an 84% graft survival at 6 years among 15 transplants at their institution.[R336] Of 2,510 renal transplants performed at the University of Minnesota between 1969 and 1987, 33 (1%) were for SLE,[B567] as were 20 of 616 (3%) at Albert Einstein College of Medicine.[S116] Of Cheigh et al.'s 59 patients with lupus and end-stage renal disease (see above), 18 were transplanted over a 17-year period.[C221] Currently, 5-year graft survivals average 70%.[B567,C221,K426,N143,S116]

Indigent pediatric populations do not do as well. Among 17 children with SLE transplanted in Brooklyn,[T100] 80 and 45% 1- and 4-year graft survivals were reported. The availability of cyclosporine has resulted in a decreased use of azathioprine to prevent rejection. The only study comparing these two drugs in SLE transplants (19 received azathioprine and 17 cyclosporine) documented the statistically significant superiority of cyclosporine on graft survival.[P130]

Serologic Features and Disease Recurrence. Patients undergoing transplantation may have persistent elevations of antinuclear antibody, anti-DNA antibody titers, and reduced complement levels. These serologic abnormalities are of little importance, and do not affect the outcome of the graft.[A180,B515,R336] They were present in 4 of 7 patients transplanted in our group between 1980 and 1989. Despite this, disease recurrence in the transplanted kidney is rare. Various centers have noted nephritis in 0 of 12,[M344] 0 of 7,[B515] 1 of 17,[T100] 2 of 15,[R336] 1 of 28,[N143] and 1 of 18 patients,[A180] for a total of 5 in 97, or 5%. Isolated case reports of disease recurrence suggest that a disproportionate number of those patients had undergone peritoneal dialysis or had active disease at the time of transplantation.[C67,K458,M564,Y2] Despite this, most of the allografts were still functioning well. Extrarenal lupus activity is usually quiescent after renal transplantation.[S720]

In summary, to achieve the optimal transplant environment, patients should be in remission, not be on dialysis or hemodialysis, and receive an allograft from a living, related donor. Cyclosporine with or without azathioprine and low-dose prednisone constitute the immunosuppressive regimen of choice.

LASER THERAPY

Lasers have been sporadically studied in rheumatoid arthritis since 1980.[G257] Evidence has suggested that Nd:YAG lasers can decrease synovial proliferation,[H275] and that gallium-aluminum-arsenide lasers diminish lymphocyte mitogenic responsiveness.[I24] Carbon dioxide lasers have been used to treat discoid lesions. The lesions can be vaporized, but cellular alterations in nonvaporized cells that are several hundred microns away may be responsible for decreased disease activity.[H263] Laser therapy should be regarded as experimental, and should preferably be used as part of a well-designed research protocol.

LYMPHOCYTE DEPLETION

Basic Principles

Evidence that the lympholytic actions of alkylating agents, corticosteroids, and radiation were responsible for

ameliorating certain disease states has led to investigations of the role of thoracic duct drainage, total lymphoid irradiation, and lymphapheresis in rheumatic diseases. Lymphoid tissue occupies up to 3% of the body weight; this includes 1% lymphocytes, or 10^{12} lymphocytes/70-kg. Lymphocytes are widely distributed and consist of long- and short-lived populations. T cells comprise roughly 90% of the lymphocytes in the thoracic duct lymph, 65% in peripheral blood, 75% in the mesentery, and 25% in the spleen; most of these are long-lived. Therefore, thoracic duct drainage and localized radiation remove lymphocyte populations in a different manner than those removed by lymphapheresis.[W32]

Thoracic Duct Drainage

Pioneered by researchers at UCLA in the early 1970s, cannulation of the thoracic duct followed by removal of billions of lymphocytes clearly improved disease activity in SLE patients.[N155] The procedure is not practical for clinical use, however, because it is technically difficult, expensive, frequently complicated by infection, and can only be done once.

Lymphapheresis

On-line lymphocyte depletion has not been adequately studied as a treatment modality for SLE. No commercially available membranes selectively remove lymphocytes without other leukocytes, so only cell separation by centrifugation methods have been used. Because most SLE patients are lymphopenic, and this is aggravated by the concomitant use of corticosteroids or cytotoxic drugs, it is often difficult to remove the lymphocyte fraction on cell separators. Our studies in rheumatoid arthritis patients have shown that a 5×10^9 lymphapheresis performed three times a week for 6 weeks can induce a significant lymphopenia that persists for 4 to 6 months.[W35] Unlike plasma removal, 15% of the body's blood volume must be extracorporeal to perform a lymphocyte "cut" on centrifugation devices, and this requires a near-normal cardiovascular and pulmonary status. In addition, blood transfusions may be required. Despite these drawbacks, Spiva and Cecere reported that a combination of lymphapheresis and plasmapheresis was clinically beneficial in 16 of 19 SLE patients on concurrent immunosuppression, and that helper:suppressor T-cell ratios were decreased.[S599]

Total Lymphoid Irradiation

During the 1980s, a total of 17 patients with lupus nephritis and nephrotic syndrome refractory to conventional drug therapy received 2,000 rad of total lymphoid irradiation over a 4- to 6-week period at Stanford University.[C188,E37,S548,S735–S737,T121] Clinical responses were seen within 3 months, and sometimes persisted for years. At follow-up, ranging from 12 to 79 months, 7 patients were off corticosteroids and without nephrosis; however, 1 patient died, 1 ultimately required chronic dialysis, and 4 developed neutropenia, 1 thrombocytopenia, 3 bacterial sepsis, and 4 herpes zoster. T helper populations

(CD4 + cells) decreased, and selective B-cell deficits documented by diminished pokeweed mitogen-induced immunoglobulin secretion was observed. Total and serum immunoglobulin-specific IgE levels were not altered. Survivals at 7.5 years were identical to those of a historical control group treated with steroids and immunosuppressives, with an equal prevalence of serious complications.

Trentham's group at Harvard[T213] also used total lymphoid irradiation (for rheumatoid arthritis), but no longer advocates its use. Trentham agrees that, although short-term benefits are apparent, the high probability of disease recurrence after several months to years limits the physician's options in giving alkylating agents to patients who have already been irradiated.[M623] Furthermore, a high infection rate is observed, and newer therapeutic strategies (e.g., parenteral cyclophosphamide) are probably superior to total lymphoid irradiation. An Israeli group noted unsatisfactory results in two patients who underwent total lymphoid irradiation.[B199]

PLASMAPHERESIS

Basic Principles

Apheresis refers to the removal of a blood component (red blood cells, lymphocytes, leukocytes, platelets, or plasma) by centrifugation or a membrane cell separator, with return of the other components to the patient. Removal of 1 L of plasma decreases plasma proteins by 1 g/dl but, because of compartmental equilibration and protein synthesis, 2.5 L of plasma must be exchanged weekly to decrease protein levels. In the intravascular space, 50% of the total IgG and 67% of the total IgM are found. Nine exchanges of 40 ml/kg over 3 weeks leave only 5% native plasma. The removal rate of plasma proteins and components depends on charge, solubility, avidity to other plasma proteins, configuration, synthesis, and uptake rates. In immunologic disorders, the recovery of immunoglobulin levels can be slowed by the concurrent use of immunosuppressive agents. If none are used "antibody rebound," or the tendency of certain antibody levels to rise rapidly above their prepheresis baseline after initially decreasing, is observed; this often correlates with a disease flare.[W32] Plasma is usually replaced with a combination of albumin, salt, and water. Certain complications of lupus (e.g., thrombotic thrombocytopenic purpura) necessitate the use of fresh-frozen plasma replacement, because a plasma factor is deficient When performed by personnel at experienced blood banks or dialysis facilities, plasmapheresis is usually safe; serious complications (e.g., hypotension, arrhythmia, infection) occur less than 3% of the time in this group of sick patients.[P228]

Rationale in SLE

Plasmapheresis can remove circulating immune complexes and immune reactants (e.g., free antibody, complement components), alter the equilibrium between free and bound complexes, and restore reticuloendothelial phagocytic function.[L245] Three different centers have documented the reversal of the reticuloendothelial system blockade by plasmapheresis.[H79,L394,W52] In one report,

plasmapheresis improved suppressor cell functioning[A2] and, in another, selectively removed IgG anti-DNA.[C340] Steven et al.[S678] demonstrated improved bacterial killing by monocytes after plasmapheresis. In patients with mild disease, Tsokos et al. found no changes in proliferative responses to mitogens or lymphocyte subpopulation percentages.[T241] In 17 steroid- and immunosuppressive-resistant lupus nephritis patients, however, Wallace et al. reported normal B- and T-cell counts but diminished mitogenic responsiveness and decreases in CD4 levels (compared to preplasmapheresis values) after 15 exchanges.[W31]

Clinical Studies in SLE

The use of plasmapheresis was first reported by Jones et al. in 1976.[J113] His follow-up observations concluded that patients who are the most seriously ill and have the highest levels of circulating immune complexes respond best.[J110,J111,J112,J115] Patients treated concomitantly with plasmapheresis, prednisone, and cyclophosphamide do better than those treated with prednisone and azathioprine,[H78] and those on prednisone alone may become worse.[W124] The procedure is well tolerated in children and pregnant women with SLE.[J129,W105]

The most impressive results were reported in patients with lupus nephritis who had active disease and minimal scarring. Of 31 Finnish patients in this subset, 24 responded to treatment.[V109] Kincaid-Smith's group rebiopsied 8 patients with acute crescentic proliferative lupus nephritis several weeks after they received prednisone and cyclophosphamide, and underwent plasmapheresis, and found dramatic improvements in 7.[L115] A literature review in 1986 noted that 69% of 42 cases of diffuse proliferative nephritis improved after plasma exchange.[S60] These and other promising reports[L359,S328,W29] led to two controlled trials. Lewis et al. randomized 86 patients with new-onset proliferative nephritis to oral cyclophosphamide and prednisone, with or without plasmapheresis; both groups improved, and no differences in the outcome were noted.[C309,H232,L242] Wallace et al. restricted their study to 27 patients with nephrotic syndrome who were resistant to a minimum 3-month trial of steroids and cytotoxic drugs. Of these, 10 were randomized to continue their therapy, and plasmapheresis was added to 17. After 2 years, 7 had a good outcome (normal serum creatinine level and resolution of nephrotic syndrome), and 7 had a poor outcome (dialysis or death). All 7 who had a good outcome underwent plasmapheresis (p = .026). Of the 7 responders, 5 had undergone pheresis. The poor responders could not be predicted in advance by any of 30 variables used.[W30,W31]

Interest has focused on the removal of anticardiolipin antibody and the lupus anticoagulant by plasmapheresis during pregnancy or in patients who have experienced recurrent thromboembolic episodes. Results have been mixed.[K403,D166,F309,P62,T159] Plasmapheresis is safe in pregnancy,[H469] and can be used weekly for the temporary removal of anticardiolipin; it is especially helpful if large amounts of the IgM isotype are present. Clark et al.[C285,C286] embarked on a study of longterm plasmapheresis in SLE patients and achieved modest but not cost-effective results. Isolated case reports have claimed efficacy for almost every manifestation of SLE; the largest nonrenal series was comprised of 6 French patients with central nervous system lupus who had favorable responses.[T64] The usefulness of plasmapheresis in cryoglobulinemia, thrombotic thrombocytopenic purpura, and hyperviscosity syndrome is well established.[K43] These complications occasionally occur in SLE patients.

Euler's group in Germany has devised an innovative approach for the treatment of seriously ill SLE patients. It involves deliberately inducing antibody rebound with plasmapheresis, followed by high-dose IV cyclophosphamide to eliminate the increased numbers of "malignant clones." Their pulse synchronization technique has resulted in some spectacular successes and is now being studied in an international controlled trial.[B102,C283,C309, D53,E156,S184]

New membrane technologies have enabled selective plasmapheresis to be performed. Membranes that remove cryoproteins,[K373] anti-ssDNA,[T119,T203] and anti-dsDNA by immune adsorption[E73,H117,H187,K240,M308,P16,S154,S772] have been developed. Unfortunately, membranes activate complement, and may present additional risks of hemolysis. In my experience, any theoretic cost saving obtained by avoiding albumin replacement is countered by the frequent clogging of expensive membranes, which necessitates termination of the procedure or the use of a second membrane. Also, many patients with SLE do not have anti-DNA, and it is only one of many putative autoantibodies that may accelerate the disease process. Furthermore, selective membranes remove *fewer* plasma proteins than conventional plasmapheresis; this is not usually the practitioner's intent.

Summary

At this time, plasmapheresis should only be used for patients with renal disease who are resistant to corticosteroid and cytotoxic drug therapy, specific disease subsets in which its efficacy is established (e.g., those with hyperviscosity syndrome, cryoglobulinemia, or thrombotic thrombocytopenic purpura), and in those with acute, life-threatening complications of SLE, in combination with corticosteroids and cytotoxic therapy.

Chapter 61

OTHER MEDICATIONS AND ADJUNCTIVE MEASURES

DANIEL J. WALLACE

The last five chapters have discussed conventional therapies of lupus erythematosus. These include general measures, local applications, nonsteroidal anti-inflammatory drugs, antimalarials, corticosteroids, and immunosuppressive agents. Occasionally, specific subsets of lupus require additional approaches, and some patients with refractory disease benefit from innovative management. This section reviews these and discusses ancillary measures.

MEDICATIONS

Antileprosy Drugs

Dapsone. Dapsone, or 4,4'-diaminodiphenylsulphone, interferes with folate metabolism and inhibits para-aminobenzoic acid. It also blocks the alternate pathway of complement activation and neutrophil cytotoxicity[R143] and inhibits superoxide and hydroxyl generation in rheumatoid arthritis patients.[M494] Its use is limited by its toxicity, which includes sulfhemoglobinemia and methemoglobinemia and a dose-related hemolytic anemia. In a case reported in 1978, it was said to benefit urticaria associated with SLE.[M206] Small series[F61,H58,H400,M625,R439,Y9] have reported that dapsone can ameliorate vasculitis, bullae, urticaria, oral ulcerations, thrombocytopenia, lupus panniculitis, and subacute cutaneous lupus. Dapsone may be steroid-sparing, and can be effective in chloroquine-resistant patients.

Dubois' group found dapsone helpful in 3 of 7 patients, but 3 developed a significant anemia.[J37] Coburn and Shuster[C315] reported that 9 of 11 discoid LE patients improved on 100 mg daily. Lindskov and Reymann gave dapsone to 33 patients with chronic cutaneous LE—8 had excellent and 8 had fair results, but 17 (52%) had no response.[L307] Dapsone can occasionally make rashes worse.[A87]

All patients treated with dapsone should have their baseline glucose-6-phosphate dehydrogenase (G6PD) levels determined; the drug should not be given to individuals with low levels. Complete blood counts should be performed every 2 weeks for the first 3 months, and every 2 months thereafter. Dapsone should be started at a dose of 50 mg daily and eventually raised to 100 mg. Dapsone also interacts with all oxidant drugs, such as phenacetin and furadantoin. Concurrent administration of 800 U of vitamin E daily may decrease the degree of dapsone-induced hemolysis.[B103]

I believe that dapsone has a place in the treatment of cutaneous and musculoskeletal lupus, especially when steroids are ineffective or contraindicated. Hematologic toxicity is high, however, and the drug should be used infrequently and cautiously.

Thalidomide. Also known as α-phthalimidoglutarimide, thalidomide is a highly teratogenic drug with antileprosy and antilupus effects. It has no influence on the complement system, but can stabilize lysosomal membranes, antagonize prostaglandin, inhibit neutrophil chemotaxis, and alter cellular and humeral immunity.[B99,H197] Thalidomide's side effects include teratogenicity, fatigue, dizziness, weight gain, constipation, amenorrhea, dry mouth, and a non–dose-related polyneuropathy associated with chronic administration.[L409] Despite these rather significant drawbacks, Barbra-Rubio et al.[B83,B84] pioneered its use in discoid LE in Mexico in the mid-1970s. Improvement begins within weeks on doses between 100 and 400 mg daily.[L343] Knop et al.[K323] reported that, in 46 patients with antimalarial-resistant discoid LE given 400 mg/day and followed up to 2 years, 90% had complete or marked regression. Also, 71% relapsed on its discontinuation and improved when it was restarted, and 25% developed a polyneuritis. The drug can heal antimalarial-resistant lesions,[H196] and similar favorable responses and toxicity have been noted by others in smaller groups of patients.[H197,K324,L343,S59,S222] Thalidomide has also been used to treat graft-versus-host disease, Behçet's syndrome, and rheumatoid arthritis.[G436,R37] It is not available in the United States. Thalidomide should never be used in women who are pregnant or are contemplating pregnancy.

Clofazimine. In 1976, Krivanek et al.[K427] reported resolution of discoid LE in all 9 patients treated with 100 to 300 mg/day of clofazimine (Lamprene) for 3 months, but a follow-up paper found it to be effective only in early, acute onset lesions.[K428] The drug has antileprosy, antibacterial, and antimalarial activity. It is sequestered in macrophages, stabilizes lysosomal enzymes, and stimulates the production of reactive oxidants.[Z18] Two other favorable studies have appeared,[C444,M26] but Dubois' group had no responses among 8 patients treated.[J37] Longterm use of clofazimine in LE can result in cutaneous pigment deposits.[K389]

Cyclosporin

Cyclosporin is a fungal cyclic polypeptide that interferes with the release of interleukin-2 and inhibits the activation of both T and B lymphocytes. It also blocks certain macrophage functions. Miescher's group[F33,M399,M400] reported an 80% response rate in patients with organ-threatening lupus, and had only minimal toxicity. No other investigators have had these favorable results. Isenberg et al. observed nephrotoxicity in all 5 SLE patients given 10 mg/kg/day, with no clinical benefits.[139] Urowitz's group noted a response in 2 of 7 patients; however, 4 died within 1 year.[H68] Bambauer et al. combined cyclosporin with plasmapheresis; transient improvements were noted, but long-term survival was poor.[B67,B68] Bach's group reported clinical responses in half, but nephrotoxicity and hypertension were seen in most. No changes in ANA titers, anti-DNA, or IgG levels were found.[F80,F295] Zurier's group presented a case of a patient in remission who experienced a well-documented flare after receiving cyclosporin for transplant rejection prophylaxis.[M75]

To summarize, early studies with cyclosporin in lupus nephritis have not been promising, largely because of the nephrotoxicity of the drug.[B69] It may have a role, however, in the therapy of patients with nonrenal lupus who are steroid-resistant and cannot take cytotoxics. Also, lower doses may prove helpful. Even more promising is the advent of similar drugs (e.g., FK 506), which may be equally immunosuppressive but less nephrotoxic.

Gold

In the 1940s and 1950s, gold was frequently used to treat LE. It was thought to be beneficial but toxic.[B148,C435,H216,P59] These reports antedated criteria for defining SLE and rheumatoid arthritis and the introduction of lupus serologies.

In 1983, 16 SLE patients without renal involvement were given oral gold at the University of California, San Diego.[W157] They had fevers, fatigue, arthritis, serositis, vasculitis, rashes, and mouth ulcers. Gold was of modest benefit, with significant improvement noted only in physician assessment and steroid dose reduction. A British group treated 22 patients with biopsy-documented cutaneous lupus with oral gold for up to 1 year. Of these, 12 had dramatic clearing of lesions, and 5 others demonstrated definite improvement.[D20] In another report, 7 of 12 patients who received aurothioglucose (Solagnol) injections had improved arthritis and decreased steroid requirements.[S465] Some are still concerned than gold can flare SLE,[S728] and further studies are needed to define its potential role.

Vitamin A, β-Carotene, and Retinoids

β-Carotene, vitamin A, and retinoids are related compounds that may have antilupus actions because of their sun blocking and antioxidant activities. Skin tests with vitamin A have revealed an increased hyperreactivity in patients with SLE and their relatives compared with controls,[W165] and its oral administration in SLE enhances natural killer cell activity and mitogenic responsiveness.[V82]

β-Carotene has been used to treat polymorphous light eruption, erythrohepatic protoporphyria, and discoid lupus. Of 7 patients with cutaneous lupus, 6 improved in two reports,[H116,N71] but Dubois found beneficial results in only 1 of 26 patients.[D335]

Retinoids inhibit collagenase, prostaglandin E$_2$, and rheumatoid synovial proliferation, interfere with intracel-

lular binding proteins, and interact with kinases, such as cyclic AMP.[B447,H145] In addition, epidermal antibodies can be altered, and an effect on epidermal cell differentiation may be observed.[N78] Three retinoids have been evaluated in cutaneous lupus: isotretinoin (13-cis-retinoic acid; Accutane), etretinate (Tegison), and the aromatic retinoid, acitretin (Etretin). When given in doses of 40 mg twice daily, isotretinoin induced complete resolution of lesions in 8 of 10 patients, including several patients with refractory subacute cutaneous lupus.[N78] Other case reports have confirmed these findings.[F166,G351,R383,S393] In another open trial it was effective in 20 of 24 patients.[L343]

I have had similar success but, unless the patient is kept on a maintenance dose of 10 to 40 mg daily, recurrences are common. Isotretinoin can cause arthralgias and skeletal hyperostoses.[M196] Etretinate may also ameliorate cutaneous lesions,[R378] but extraspinal tendon and ligamentous calcifications have resulted from therapy.[D210] A new aromatic retinoid acitretin, is not yet available in the United States. In one paper, 7 favorable reports were reviewed, and 15 of 20 patients studied had complete clearing of all lesions with acitretin.[R440] This included 5 of 6 patients with refractory subacute cutaneous lupus. The teratogenicity of the retinoids is a major concern in treating females of childbearing age. Topical retinoids with sunscreens may also be useful.[S258]

Danazol

Danazol (Danocrine) is an impeded androgen whose effects in SLE are unclear. It may decrease Fc receptor expression and platelet-associated IgG, and may also have a hormonal down-regulating action. Danazol displaces steroids by binding to steroid-binding globulin, which frees the latter compound. Its most promising use is for the treatment of idiopathic thrombocytopenia, in which steroid-sparing effects are observed, and low doses can be administered as maintenance therapy.[A75] Idiopathic thrombocytopenia caused by SLE responds well in some patients to 800 mg/day of therapy.[M132,W190] Several reports have documented its efficacy in cases of SLE with autoimmune hemolytic anemia.[A277,C197,P217] Danazol has also been reported to help patients with persistent, premenstrual LE flares.[M592] In combination with cyproterone acetate, 11 patients with SLE had fewer exacerbations and persistent, disabling mouth ulcers disappeared in 3 patients.[J144] Danazol may be effective in discoid lupus.[T190] Of 21 patients given danazol in a controlled trial with corticosteroids, all had fewer flares, lower steroid requirements, and higher hemoglobin levels, platelet counts, and C4 complement levels than 20 patients taking steroids alone. Of the 21 in the danazol group, however, 8 withdrew because of hepatotoxicity, gastric symptoms, or asthenia.[D279] Occasionally, danazol can worsen SLE,[G424] and it has been associated with the development of hepatocellular carcinoma in 1 patient[W130] and with hyperglucagonemia in another.[D60]

Danazol has no role in the management of life-threatening non-hematologic manifestations of lupus.

Other Hormones

In 1948, Lamb gave androgens to 5 lupus patients, but without significant improvement.[L33] In 1950, Dubois treated several female patients with massive doses of testosterone, orally and intramuscularly, using as much as 500 to 1,000 mg/day for as long as 5 weeks without benefit.[D329] After a 30-year hiatus, interest in androgen therapy resurfaced. Lahita and Kunkel[L25] treated 4 men and 4 women with 19-nortestosterone (Nandrolene) for 2 months to 2 years. The men got worse, but some women improved. Androgens should probably not be used in men with SLE. Minimal masculinization was noted, sedimentation rates and anti-DNA levels decreased slightly, and hemoglobin and white counts improved. Hazelton et al.[H227] observed no clinical change in 10 patients treated with the drug. A Soviet androgen preparation, Sustanon-250, has been purported to decrease disease activity.[F142,F143,Y61]

A double-blind cross-over trial treating 11 SLE patients with tamoxifen, an antiestrogen, demonstrated no benefits of the drug.[S749] Gonadotropin-releasing hormone reduces estradiol levels. Of 6 young SLE patients with active disease who had never taken oral contraceptives, 4 improved when given the gonadotropin-releasing hormone preparation burselin (Suprefact).[C153] Jungers et al. used the antigonadotropic agent, cyproterone acetate on 7 patients and observed fewer clinical exacerbations.[J143]

Prolactin appears to have proinflammatory effects and interest has centered on the use of prolactin suppression with bromocriptine in SLE.[J53,R2]

Gamma Globulin

Intravenous gamma globulin delays the clearance of antibody-coated autologous red blood cells, competitively inhibits reticuloendothelial Fc receptor blockade, and decreases pokeweed mitogen-induced B-cell differentiation.[S690] Hypogammaglobulinemia with recurrent infections is a rare event in SLE (see Chap. 47), and the use of intramuscular gamma globulin to prevent infection in lupus is not uncommon, even though no controlled studies have documented its efficacy.

Intravenous gamma globulin was first used in a case of lupus nephritis in 1982,[S758] and its use has increased since. It may be helpful for autoimmune thrombocytopenia secondary to SLE[G6,H456,M68] and for the neonatal thrombocytopenia seen in children of SLE mothers.[H93] Gamma globulin is thought to be useful for life-threatening complications (e.g., central nervous system lupus),[C396] lupus nephritis,[A82,L294] pericarditis,[H331] acquired factor VIII deficiency,[P205] pancytopenia,[A82] and preventing recurrent fetal loss in patients with the antiphospholipid syndrome.[C103,K115,P49] Gamma globulin does not lower anticardiolipin levels and, in one case, the patient also received heparin and baby aspirin.[P49] In patients with mild disease, little response to gamma globulin was noted.[B61]

Intravenous gamma globulin is expensive, and indications for its use should be clarified by controlled trials currently in progress.

Levamisole

The T-cell immunostimulant drug levamisole was first noted to be effective for SLE in 1975 in a case report of an ANA-negative patient.[G299] The same group subsequently reported that 16 patients treated with levamisole for a minimum of 4 months[G300] "improved," but no clinical parameters were mentioned. Other groups found the drug not only to be ineffective in a total of 17 patients, but associated it with serious adverse reactions and no discernible immunologic changes.[R5,R319,S125,S517] Rovensky et al.[R373] documented clinical responses in 16 of 20 patients but, in a follow-up report, noted that nearly 50% had significant leukopenia or hepatoxicity that required discontinuation of the drug.[R374] Ogawa et al.[O18] claimed some amelioration of nephritis in 50% of their patients in an uncontrolled study. Feng et al.[E107] treated 17 patients with 150 mg/day for 3 days consecutively every 2 weeks. Of these, 5 had their lupus completely suppressed, and 11 could reduce their steroid doses. Unfortunately, only 8 of 17 patients had a positive LE preparation, ANAs were not reported, and no statistical analyses were used.

The only controlled trial of levamisole was performed by Hadidi and colleagues.[H12] In their study, 26 SLE patients inadequately controlled by up to 30 mg/day of prednisone were given either 150 mg of levamisole or a placebo weekly for 6 months. Most of the patients had to have their steroid doses increased, and no improvements were observed.

Antilymphocyte Globulin

Because antilymphocyte globulin is immunosuppressive, it has been tried experimentally in a number of patients with SLE. Treatment was usually combined with steroids and other agents. Fever and local and hematologic reactions were frequent. The results were generally equivocal.[B472,H277,P207] In the largest and only controlled study, 9 patients given antilymphocyte globulin, azathioprine, and prednisone did no better than those in a prednisone-only treated group.[H385]

Current preliminary studies employ antibodies to T-cell and B-cell subsets (CD4, CD8) and B-cell subsets. No results are available to date, but the idea of depleting pathogenic subsets of B and T cells is appealing.

Antibiotics

Chloramphenicol and its analogues inhibit antibody production by interfering with nucleic acid synthesis or function.[S775] An analogue of chloramphenicol, thiamphenicol was given to 6 patients with lupus nephritis.[W155] Following a 16-day course of 2 g daily, 4 patients had increased complement and decreased anti-DNA levels, lower ANA titers, and disappearance of glomerular-bound gamma globulin. Sustained remissions lasted 9 months to 3 years following a single course of therapy. In 1979, Richmond gave thiamphenicol to 13 lupus nephritis patients for 2 weeks[R199] and reviewed the drug's record in inhibiting cell-mediated immune reactions and prolonging rat renal allograft survival. Symptomatic improvement was noted in only 2 patients, but 6 had serologic improvement.

Chloramphenicol,[J97] penicillin,[M597,S721] sulfonamides,[P236,W134] tetracycline,[B391] and streptomycin[G321,R53] have also been purported to help SLE. The usefulness of these approaches is doubtful, however, and no controlled studies are available.

Antiviral Agents

α-Interferon given for presumed rheumatoid arthritis induced multisystemic SLE in 1 patient,[M8] but α-interferon was effective in managing 10 patients with discoid and subacute cutaneous lupus.[N89,T142] In one case report, isoprinosine given to a lupus patient for a viral infection produced improvement in disease activity.[H43]

Thymosin and Thymectomy

Because the thymus gland is an important lymphoid organ, in which lymphocytes differentiate, proliferate, and mature, experimental thymectomy has been undertaken to treat SLE, but with uniformly negative results.[A107,C248, D3,H518,L77,M14,W253] The administration of thymosin, or thymic hormone, represents the opposite approach. It increases T lymphocyte counts, improves lymphocyte responsiveness, and decreases null cell counts in vitro.[B133,C154,L97,S121] Factor 5 thymosin was given to 4 SLE patients, and improvement was claimed in 3, with no adverse reactions observed.[G265] Unfortunately, improvement was not defined or described, nor was the degree of disease activity in these patients stated. Thymus factor X was thought to be useful in a poorly documented report.[L82]

Vitamin E

In 1979, Ayres and Mihan[A102] reviewed ten papers that evaluated the use of the antioxidant vitamin E for discoid lesions. Nine were published prior to 1955. Mixed results were obtained, but Ayres continued to use this relatively nontoxic vitamin successfully in his active dermatologic practice.[A377]

Vasodilators

Prostaglandin E_1 (PGE_1) is a vasodilator that can suppress effector systems of inflammation and enhance and diminish cellular and immune responses.[Z56] Several case reports have associated PGE_1 infusion with improved renal function in lupus nephritis and decreased levels of circulating immune complexes.[L293,N12,Y55] Renal function also improved in a double-blind cross-over study of 10 patients given a thromboxane inhibitor,[P185] and the angiotensin-converting enzyme inhibitor captopril[S311] may be capable of reducing proteinuria.

Drugs to Avoid

D-Penicillamine and sulfasalazine are clearly effective for rheumatoid arthritis, and D-penicillamine also has antiscleroderma actions. Both drugs have been given to SLE patients who were thought to have rheumatoid arthritis or scleroderma. Because sulfa drugs may exacerbate lupus (and can be photosensitizing), and D-penicillamine can induce lupus, extreme caution is advised if SLE is suspected (see Chap. 45).

Miscellaneous Agents and Therapies

The older literature is replete with references to the successful use of many systemic drugs. Vitamin B_{12} and pantothenic acid, in controlled studies, have been reported to be of benefit.[F287,G243,G244,W172] Authorities such as Sulzberger[S762] recommended the use of vitamin B_{12}, liver extract, and bismuth[B250,P58] for the treatment of discoid lupus. The Soviet literature contains numerous reports of the beneficial effects of methylxanthines, "splenin," lysozyme, and "prospidin."[B206,B312,G187,M212] Other drugs and modalities that have been tried include tuberculin,[C58] Chinese herbs,[T254,W67,W69,W71,Y33,Y64] arsenic,[G239] heliotherapy,[B57,H216] para-aminobenzoic acid,[Z11,Z12] colchicine,[C20] hemotherapy,[K475] transfer factor,[F313] auriculoacupuncture,[C226] and sodium diethyldithiocarbamate.[D136] Routine splenectomy has been advised in patients without significant hematologic complications.[J92] Witchcraft has even been used successfully.[K247] I do not, however, recommend the use of any of these measures.

ADJUNCTIVE MEASURES AND ISSUES
Osteoporosis, SLE, and Its Management

No evidence has shown that SLE per se, induces osteoporosis, but most SLE patients are given steroid therapy, which promotes osteopenia. These mechanisms include increased bone resorption by osteoclasts, decreased bone formation by osteoblasts, decreased calcium absorption by the gastrointestinal tract, increased renal calcium excretion, and decreased osteocalcin release.[M483] Hahn's group correlated corticosteroid administration to SLE patients with elevated diaphyseal:metaphyseal mass ratios, osteoporosis, and increased fractures. They reported that calcium alone increased bone mass slightly, and that the addition of 25-hydroxyvitamin D prevented loss of bone mass.[D374,D375,M639] On the other hand, the administration of 1,25-dihydroxyvitamin D reduced bone formation, and was not useful. A British group performed dual photon densitometry testing on 22 SLE patients (12 on steroids, 10 on no steroids), 14 steroid-dependent patients without lupus, and 10 controls. No differences were noted among the groups, but the cohort was probably too small and the mean steroid dose and duration were not stated.[D196]

Probably all female and most male lupus patients should be given calcium replacement. Vitamin D (50,000 U, one to three times a week) or 25-hydroxyvitamin D (20 µg daily) should be considered in patients with a 24-hour urine calcium lower than 120 mg. If vitamin D therapies are introduced, regular screening for hypercalciuria and hypercalcemia is recommended. Vitamin supplementation should be stopped during intercurrent illnesses that make the patient bedridden. Those taking corticosteroids and maintenance calcium may benefit from additional measures at menopause (e.g., sex hormone replacement, diphosphonates, fluoride, calcitonin). More aggressive measures may be used in those who fracture.

Should SLE Patients Take Hormones?

Several early studies reported an increased incidence of SLE in women taking oral contraceptives, with remissions following cessation of their use.[D390,S145] Dubois disputed these reports.[D338] Two other studies noted that patients purported to have developed SLE from the use of birth control pills had biologic false-positive serologies prior to the initiation of contraceptive therapy.[G56,T208] McKenna et al.[M302] studied the incidence of clinical manifestations and various immunologic tests in 271 women, 176 receiving oral contraceptives (average, 12.4 months) and 95 using intrauterine devices (average, 14.0 months). LE cell tests were negative in all; ANAs were positive in 1 on oral contraceptives and in 2 with an intrauterine device. The authors doubted that anovulatory drugs might activate latent or mild SLE. In another paper, 4 of 82 women started on oral contraceptives developed a positive ANA and 9 developed a positive rheumatoid factor; none had any symptoms.[K130] A prospective controlled trial by Tarzy et al.[T73] of 80 patients and 35 controls showed no evidence that women using these drugs are at a greater risk of developing clinical or serologic changes than nonusers. In a frequently cited study that remains unconfirmed, Jungers et al.[J141] followed 26 lupus patients started on oral contraceptives. Nephritis worsened in 43% of them, but did not become worse in any of 11 patients taking discontinuous or continuous norsteroids or progesterone as contraceptives. No control group was followed.[J141] Mintz et al.[M471] found that progestogens are effective contraceptive agents and do not exacerbate the disease.

Tartrazines are lupogenic chemicals closely related to hydrazines and hydralazine. These aromatic amines are used as preservatives in numerous pharmaceutical preparations, including birth control pills.[P114,R128] Some "flares" noted in patients taking contraceptives might actually result from the preservative rather than the hormone.

Antiestrogen antibodies are found in 26% of men and women with SLE and in 25% of normals taking oral contraceptives, but in 0% of normal men.[B548] One report associated thrombotic episodes in 10 women with SLE receiving oral contraceptive therapy with antiethinylestradiol antibodies; none had anticardiolipin.[B536] Women who have antiphospholipid antibodies are probably at an increased thrombotic risk if they also take oral contraceptives.[A324,A325,M427]

I recommend that women with SLE use a barrier contraceptive method (e.g., diaphragm with contraceptive jelly, foam, sponge) or a progestational agent alone for contraception, or their partner should use a contraceptive device (e.g., condom). Intrauterine devices increase the risk of pelvic infection and probably should be avoided in those with SLE. If oral contraceptives are indicated, the addition of one baby aspirin a day might be advisable for women with hypercoagulable states. If an SLE patient also has antiphospholipid antibodies, hypertension, or severe headaches, oral contraceptives should probably be avoided.

Postmenopausal estrogen replacement therapy is generally safe. Only a single case of SLE flare in a postmenopausal women on estrogen replacement has been reported.[B104]

Should Lupus Patients Be Immunized?

The issue of immunization in lupus is controversial and misunderstood. This section attempts to clarify the misunderstandings and summarize salient points.

1. Infrequent reports have claimed that immunizations induce systemic lupus or rheumatoid arthritis, but the cases were poorly documented.[A378,J59]
2. SLE may present a relative contraindication to allergy shots, because this might induce the formation of antibodies that could flare the disease.[H442]
3. Patients with SLE usually tolerate immunizations well and adverse reactions may be less common than in normals.[T282] Disease flares are no more frequent than the incidence of spontaneous flares.
4. Immunizations are less effective in SLE patients on high doses of corticosteroids. Antibody responses depend on concentration of antigen, HLA type, and concurrent medication.
5. Immunization with killed vaccine (e.g., Pneumococcus, influenza, tetanus) is generally regarded as safe, but the safety of live vaccines (e.g., polio, measles, rubella) has not been established in SLE patients who are on high-dose steroids or cytotoxics.

In 1980, Jarrett et al.[J58] reported on their experience administering pneumococcal vaccine to SLE patients. Mean antibody levels at 1 month and 12 months following vaccination were significantly lower than those in control patients. In follow-up studies,[C437,M264] the persistence of pneumococcal antibodies in immunized patients was found to be protective for a mean of 3 years, and polyclonal B-cell response was restricted. In a double-blind, controlled study, Klippel et al.[K313] obtained similar results. Concurrent immunosuppression did not effect response.[L322] No disease flares or adverse reactions were reported.

In similar studies of influenza vaccination in patients with SLE, Williams et al.[W239] noted no disease flares but decreased antibody titers compared to a control group in a double-blind trial. Two other studies reported similar findings.[B501] Herron et al.[H282] observed that antibody responses are especially decreased in steroid-treated patients. Of 20 immunized patients, 1 experienced a serious disease flare after injection. Mitchell et al.[M482] attempted to study the kinetics of specific antiinfluenzal antibody production by cultured lymphocytes following immunization, but in vitro responses (which have been reported to be decreased)[T280,T281] did not correlate with in vivo changes.

Abe and Homma[A7] administered tetanus toxoid to 200 subjects with SLE and a similar number of controls. No difference in antibody titer existed between the two groups following both primary and secondary immunizations, but a subgroup had lower antibody responses. In one study, the time of appearance of the antibodies and serum titers were normal in SLE patients,[L142] but others have found lower responses[R399] and have documented a restricted IgG1 response.[D187] Nies et al.[N93] studied antitetanus toxoid antibody synthesis after booster immunization in SLE and a control group. The SLE patients had decreased prebooster antibody levels, and one-third had a blunted antibody response. It was shown that the blunted response results from poor B-cell responsiveness and is not related to T helper or suppressor function. In an ominous follow-up report,[L391] this group found increased anti-DNA production in vitro following keyhole limpet hemocyanin (KLH) immunization. This was especially true after secondary immunizations, and might represent a risk of repeated immunization of SLE patients.

Additional reports have examined responses to other bacteria. Antibody responses after immunization with flagellin derived from Salmonella adelaide, Proteus OX-2, and Rickettsia rickettsii were normal,[L126,L142] decreased with antistreptolysin O[C127] Escherichia coli,[B127] and Shigella[B345] and both increased and decreased with Brucella.[B127,M340] In one unit, all 3 SLE pediatric dialysis patients failed to seroconvert after hepatitis B vaccination.[M639]

In summary, I recommend that patients with SLE should receive all appropriate vaccinations, but should first consult their rheumatologist.

Antibiotic Prophylaxis

Only two peer-reviewed publication have addressed this issue.[L407,Z70] It was recommended that, because those with SLE are more susceptible to infections on the basis of the underlying disease and its therapy, antibiotic prophylaxis should be used for most dental and surgical procedures. Only a minority of rheumatologists give antibiotic prophylaxis routinely; however, this should be decided on an individual basis.

Chapter 62

PROGNOSTIC SUBSETS AND MORTALITY IN SYSTEMIC LUPUS ERYTHEMATOSUS

DANIEL J. WALLACE

Our concepts of SLE have changed over the last 50 years. Prior to 1971, no widely accepted criteria for defining SLE were available. The criteria used at present were revised in 1982. Many patients who had been labeled as having "lupus" in the 1950s would not meet the current criteria for the disease, and a positive ANA test was not even a criterion until 1982. Moreover, many patients considered as having lupus in the 1950s would meet current definitions for overlap syndromes, mixed connective tissue disease, rheumatoid arthritis, or even scleroderma. Most mild cases of SLE were overlooked. Until 1948, no blood test was available to diagnose the disease. Survival studies published before the availability of the LE cell test tended to include only those with severe SLE who could be diagnosed by biopsy or at autopsy. After 1948, the introduction of corticosteroids had a tremendous impact on the natural course of SLE.

This chapter examines survival, duration of disease, and causes of death. Studies that deal only with specific groupings (e.g., nephritis, children) are discussed in the section on prognostic subsets. That section also lists prognostic associations by individual parameter (e.g., C3, anti-DNA, age, sex, race, geography, socioeconomic status) and delineates reports that have found correlations among outcome and these characteristics.

OVERALL SURVIVORSHIP AND DURATION OF DISEASE: MAJOR STUDIES

Early Studies: 1939–1964

In 1939, Bywaters and Bauer[P181] reported that 52.3% of 55 SLE patients were dead 2 years after onset of disease. In a group of 103 cases reported by Jessar et al.[J75] in 1953, 50% died within 3 years of onset, and 13 of 44 were alive after 5 years, accounting for a 20% 5-year survival.

The question of duration of disease was analyzed carefully by Merrell and Shulman[M280,M359] using a life table method and time of diagnosis as the first time point (Table 62–1). In their classic 1955 study, data extrapolated from 99 cases of SLE predicted that 78% would be alive 1 year after diagnosis, 67% after 2 years, and 51% after 4 years. Patients who were diagnosed within 2 years of onset of symptoms had a poorer survival.

In 1963, Posnick[P273] noted a mean survival of 2 years in his control group of 39 cases. Kellum and Haserick[K155] used Merrell and Shulman's technique to study their 299-

patient cohort in 1964. Survivals from 1 to 4 years decreased from 89.3 to 70.7%. They reported that male SLE is more severe: 34.5% of men were alive at 8 to 10 years, compared to 56.3% of women.

Ropes published the first of her survival studies in 1964.[R293] Although these figures have been recalculated and reworked several times, with the latest evaluation in 1988,[S444] they primarily involve the approximately 150 patients she treated at Massachusetts General Hospital between 1922 and 1966. In the first report, the 4-year survival rate of 47 patients followed between 1932 and 1944 was 24%, compared with 55% in 25 patients followed from 1945 to 1963. Ropes attributed this improvement mainly to the early use of antibiotics. In 1979, Albert et al.[A122] used these data to claim that improved survival in SLE patients had nothing to do with the introduction of steroids. Of 52 studies reviewed, all showed consistent improvement in survival since 1922 in a linear fashion. Only a slight improvement occurred between 1950 and 1960 life curves—the decade in which steroids became widely available. They concluded that steroids are overused and are only of short-term value in selected, high-risk patients. This conclusion ignored such factors as the sudden, greatly increased detection rate of SLE when the LE cell test became available (ironically, the same year as corticosteroids), increased physician awareness of SLE and its treatment over the years, and the fact that physicians did not know how to use steroids properly for several years after they were introduced. Ropes' early patients (1923 through 1949) had an unusual mortality curve. Most died within 1 year, and those who lived had a prolonged survival (34% 5-year and 24% 15-year survival rates, respectively). Her 1988 study compared these survival rates using both Kaplan-Meier curves and a Markov analysis, and concluded that the latter method is superior.[S444]

Dubois' group pioneered large-scale survival studies with reports in 1956 and 1963[D306,D340,D342] that included 163 and 520 patients, respectively. In the 1956 survey, the 5-year survival was 40%. Of the 60 patients from the presteroid era or those who were "inadequately treated," 50% succumbed within 2 years after diagnosis. Their 1973 report[D342] consisted of a 10-year follow-up of patients diagnosed between 1950 and 1963. Dubois concluded that patients treated in his private practice did better than those treated in publicly-funded clinics where

Table 62–1. Survival in Years After Diagnosis (%)

| Series | No. of Cases | Year Reported | Year | | | | | |
			1	2	3	4	5	10
Merrell and Shulman[M359]	99	1955	78	67	62	51	ND*	ND
Kellum and Haserick[K155]	299	1964	89	80	75	70	69	54
Leonhardt[L191a]	54	1966	81	78	72	72	70	51
Siegel et al.[S414]	292	1969	85	80	70	65	63	50
Estes and Christian[E147]	150	1971	98	92	90	85	77	59
Dubois et al.: Total[D340,D342]	491	1973	90	82	76	71	67	57
LAC/USC	306		86	75	69	62	58	47
Private	133		96	94	91	89	82	75
Consultation	52		96	88	82	82	80	65
Males	56		87	78	73	63	57	46
Females	435		90	82	77	73	68	58
Renal disease	225		77	70	64	59	54	42
Blacks	139		88	79	75	66	62	49
Nonblacks	352		91	83	77	73	69	60
Lee et al.[L140]	110	1977	93	93	91	91	91	ND
Urman and Rothfield[U32]	156	1977	99	98	97	93	93	84
Wallace et al.[W39]	609	1981	98	96	93	92	88	79
No nephritis	379		99	97	96	95	94	87
Nephritis	230		97	94	88	87	80	65
Females	546		98	96	94	93	89	80
Males	63		100	93	87	85	77	75
Blacks	38		97	95	95	95	89	85
Ginzler et al.[G162]	1,103	1982	96	93	90	88	86	76
Reveille et al.[R173]	389	1990	96	ND	ND	ND	89	84
Males	85		96	ND	ND	ND	89	83
No nephritis	174		95	ND	ND	ND	91	89
Nephritis	215		95	ND	ND	ND	87	79
Females	304		96	ND	ND	ND	89	84
Blacks	203		96	ND	ND	ND	82	78
Whites	184		95	ND	ND	ND	92	85
Wallace†[W18]	464	1990	98	98	97	97	97	93

* ND, not determined.
† The 1981 study included approximately 100 patients seen between 1950 and 1980 (included in Wallace et al.[W39]).

he worked; also, whites had a better survival than non-whites, and females had a better prognosis than males. The median interval from onset of first symptom to diagnosis was 5 years. Diagnostic skills have improved since 1963. In 1980, working in the same practice as Dubois, I found a mean interval of 4 years from onset to diagnosis; in 1990, the interval was 2 years.[W18,W39]

The duration of disease from diagnosis to death was divided by Dubois into three periods of observation: 1950–1955, 1956–1962, and 1963–1973. This was not an artificial division; 1956 marked the first time that central nervous system lupus was treated with high doses of steroids, and 1963 marked the general availability of procedures such as the use of potent, nonmercurial diuretics and peritoneal dialysis. The median duration of disease (until death) in the group treated before 1955 was less than 2 years, and by 1973 it had increased to 8.5 years.

Studies From 1965 to 1975

In 1966, Leonhardt[L191a] summarized the estimated prognoses from time of diagnoses in 54 Swedish patients with SLE and obtained survival curves identical to those reported by Kellum and Haserick.[K155] Matched normal individuals had 97 and 94% 5-year and 10-year survivals, respectively.

Siegel et al.[S414,S416] analyzed the relationship between survival and race among a black, Puerto Rican, and white population in a series of 292 cases in the 1960s, and observed no differences. The 5-year survivals by group ranged from 62.7 to 65.1%.

Estes and Christian[E147] used Merrell and Shulman's methods on 150 patients seen between 1962 and 1970, 90% of whom received steroid therapy. The 5-year and 10-year survival rates were 77 and 59%, respectively. Age at onset, sex, and race did not affect overall prognosis. Renal disease had a worse outcome.

Masi et al.[M175] analyzed 158 deaths in SLE patients compared with two sets of controls in Baltimore's 20 hospitals. SLE mortality rates were twice as high in blacks as in nonblacks.

Lee et al.[L140] analyzed 63 patients in Urowitz's Toronto group and, in 1977, reported that 72% were alive 10 years after diagnosis.

Survival Studies: 1975–1986

Tremendous improvements in survival were evident throughout the 1970s. Urman and Rothfield[U32] evaluated the survivorship of 156 patients treated at the University of Connecticut between 1968 and 1976 and compared it with 209 of Rothfield's New York City patients treated

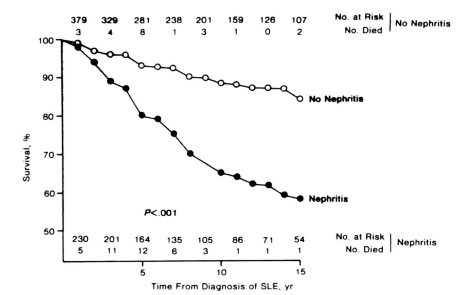

Fig. 62–1. Survival in SLE with nephritis. From Wallace, D.J., Podell, T., Weiner, J., et al.: Systemic lupus erythematous—survival patterns: Experience with 609 patients. JAMA 245:934, 1981.

from 1957 to 1968. Although the validity of comparing two such totally disparate groups has been questioned, the 5-year survival rates were 93 and 70%, respectively. Over 90% received steroids, but fewer than 1% got immunosuppressive drugs. Improved survival was attributed to better disease understanding, newer antibiotics, use of C3 and anti-DNA to monitor activity, and judicious adjustment of steroid doses. The prevalence of central nervous system disease decreased significantly between the two groups.

In 1981, I evaluated the course of 609 patients followed in Dubois' private practice since 1950.[W39] The overall 5-, 10-, and 15-year survivals were 88, 79, and 74%, respectively. Females versus males) and those without nephritis (versus those with nephritis) had significantly improved survival, but no racial differences could be discerned in our middle-class population (Fig. 62–1). Overall survival improved only in those diagnosed since 1970. Patients over 50 years old had a benign course and children did well (100% 10-year survival) only if renal disease was not present. At least 100 of the 609 patients were off all medication and in complete remission for at least 5 years. These findings are consistent with those in a report by Urowitz's group of several patients with severe multisystem disease who were off all medications and asymptomatic a mean of 75 months later.[T201] Dubois' privately treated patients did much better than his publicly treated ones (Fig. 62–1).

Ginzler et al.[G162] reported the results of a nine-center study of 1,103 patients in 1982. The 5- and 10-year survival rates were 86 and 76% respectively, (note the similarity to the Wallace data). No improvement in survival was noted in the patients entered between 1965 and 1970 compared to those entered between 1971 and 1976. Half of the patients received public funding, and they had a significantly lower survival rate. Overall, whites lived longer than blacks, but this difference was not noted in the privately funded patients. A Canadian group followed

110 patients for 4.5 years and found an 88% 5-year survival rate.[L140]

Other investigators reported better survival's of SLE patients than those found in the Wallace and Ginzler studies. In a study at the Johns Hopkins Hospital, 140 subjects had 94 and 82% 5- and 10-year survivals,[F46] respectively. A British group observed a 98% 5-year survival among 50 patients followed for 29 months.[G385] Fries and Holman[F256] reported that more than 90% of their 193 patients survived for 10 years.

Studies Since 1986

The small number of deaths reported in some surveys has led to difficulty in devising survival curves. Jonsson et al.[J121] found 133 patients with SLE out of 158,572 Swedish individuals. Only 9 deaths occurred, and the 5-year survival was 95%. In a large, hospital-based Danish study, 39 deaths occurred between 1965 and 1983.[H46,H47] An 80% 10-year survival was reported, which did not change when divided into those diagnosed before or after 1973. Similarly, a Dutch group that followed 110 patients between 1970 and 1988 noted only 14 deaths.[S785]

Between 1973 and 1985, at the University of Mississippi, 50 deaths occurred in SLE patients. Serositis,[H132] nephritis, central nervous system disease, and leukopenia were associated with a fatal outcome, and the mean interval from diagnosis to death was 4.1 years. Urowitz's[U34] bimodal survival curve (see below, Causes of Death) was not found. Reveille et al. examined survivorship in 389 patients seen at the University of Alabama hospitals between 1975 and 1984.[R173] Blacks, older age at onset, and thrombocytopenia were clearly associated with a poorer outcome, as were factors such as nephritis, central nervous system disease, anemia, and hypertension. The 89 deaths resulted in 89 and 84% 5- and 10-year survival rates, respectively. Blacks with private insurance did better than those without it, but whites with private insurance had a much better outcome. In another southeastern

United States study of largely publicly funded patients, Studenski et al.[S741] reported on the outcome of 411 patients observed between 1969 and 1983 at Duke University hospitals in North Carolina. Only patients seen within 2 years of diagnosis were considered. Blacks and those of lower socioeconomic background had a worse prognosis. (Medicare insurance was considered a marker of low socioeconomic status, which is not necessarily the case in our practice.) The 81 deaths allowed 84% 5-year and 82% 10-year Kaplan-Meier survival curves to be devised. Sex and age did not affect outcome.

Wallace[W18] followed 570 lupus patients between 1980 and 1989; which included those in Dubois' practice after his death in 1985. A 270-patient cohort was identified; this consisted of patients seen at our office between 1970 and 1989 within 1 year of diagnosis. Our largely middle-class (only 9% had Medicaid), privately insured patients had 97 and 93% 5- and 10-year survival's, respectively, which is the best ever reported. Males, those with renal disease, and thrombocytopenia were associated with a poorer outcome. No racial differences were noted.

Summary

The survival of SLE patients has improved from 50% at 2 years in 1939, to 5- and 10-year survivals of 70 and 50% after the introduction of corticosteroids in the 1950s, and to 5- and 10-year survivals of 90 and 80% in the 1980s. Subsets at generally higher mortality risk were blacks, males, those with nephritis or thrombocytopenia, children, and patients from a lower socioeconomic background, especially if they received public funding. It may be concluded that the major contributing factors toward improved survival since 1950 are the availability of dialysis, corticosteroids, and improved antibiotics and antihypertensive agents.

PROGNOSTIC SUBSETS

Some physicians have contended that SLE is a relatively homogeneous disorder, whereas others believe that it represents various disorders that share some common features. The ACR criteria allow us to take a set of signs and symptoms, along with certain laboratory findings, and to state that a combination of these comprise a "disease." Nevertheless, whether a "lumper" or a "splitter," almost every SLE investigator has endeavored to ascribe a particular value to a clinical or laboratory abnormality when following disease activity or assessing prognosis.

A few of those who have studied SLE have gone beyond the relatively simple task of following one or two parameters and describing their relationship to disease activity. Fries and associates at Stanford University[F256,F257,S264] pioneered the use of multivariate analysis in evaluating the significance of combinations of clinical, laboratory, and epidemiologic factors. Alarcon-Segovia[A102] has shown that following the clinical and laboratory abnormalities is not enough—that genetic and epidemiologic considerations must be factored into the prognostic equation. We agree with the foresight of Fries, Alarcon-Segovia, and others, and we have found that their concepts can be ex-

Table 62–2. Prognostic Variables in SLE

1. Method of health care delivery
   Site of delivery
   Source of patient funding
   Specialty and training of treating physician
2. Epidemiologic factors
   Age (special subsets include SLE in children and the elderly)
   Race
   Environment
   Geography
   Socioeconomic status
   Time
3. Genetic factors
   Sex
   Family history
   Genetic traits
4. Clinicopathologic variables
   Symptoms
   Signs
   Organ system involvement
5. Laboratory variables
   Complete blood count
   Blood chemistries
   Urinary findings
   Electrical studies (ECG, EMG, EEG)
   Radiologic studies (roentgenography, nuclear scan, ultrasound, CT, MRI)
6. Serologic and immunologic variables
   Autoantibodies
   Plasma proteins (e.g., immunoglobulins, complement, immune complexes)
   Lymphocyte subsets and function tests
7. Treatment variables
   Drug dose, method of administration, duration of therapy
   Types of treatment
   1) Salicylates, NSAIDs
   2) Antimalarials
   3) Corticosteroids
   4) Immunosuppressives
   5) Biologic modifiers (e.g., cytokines)
   6) External devices (e.g., apheresis, laser, total lymphoid irradiation, dialysis)
   7) Surgery
   8) Adjunctive measures (e.g., antibiotics, diuretics, antihypertensives, hormones, immunizations)

tended further. Table 62–2 lists the general subheadings that must be considered in devising prognostic subsets. Many of these headings are covered elsewhere in the text. The reader is referred to these sections and, if appropriate, previously unreviewed topics are discussed. It is hoped that future studies using sophisticated computer analytic methods can assess the importance of multiple combinations of factors in determining prognostic subsets of greater clinical relevance than those currently available.

Methods of Health Care Delivery

Patients treated in different health care settings (e.g., private practice, university medical center, prepaid health plan, local clinic, or within a government-controlled system, such as the Veterans Administration) are probably different. Therefore, the health care setting from which a series of SLE patients is obtained can influence prognosis indirectly. The availability of services and specialists varies widely. Sicker patients are often funneled into tertiary university centers, thus lowering their reported survival curves for SLE.[H264]

In the United States, health care is funded by private insurance (fee for service, managed care, or prepaid health maintenance plan), Medicare, Medicaid (an extension of the welfare system), cash, or local governments that provide subsidized care to indigent patients. Fessel,[F74] working with middle-class patients with at least one family member employed and therefore enrolled in the Kaiser-Permanente prepaid health plan, reported good survivals in SLE patients. Ginzler et al.[G162] studied 1,103 SLE patients at nine centers and found that privately funded patients had better survival rates than those receiving public funding. Reveille et al.[R173] documented that blacks with private insurance have improved survival compared to those without it. Some reports only surveyed hospitalized patients. Hochberg et al. showed that this group has a decreased survival compared to patients who are never hospitalized, and this can skew survival data.[S770] Reports of patient outcome are probably influenced by the specialty of the physician analyzing the data. For example, Wasner and Fries[W93] found that rheumatologists and nephrologists usually agree with each other on general treatment approaches for SLE, but that nephrologists place more emphasis on renal biopsy and use immunosuppressive drugs more frequently.

Epidemiologic Factors

Age

The incidence, prevalence, and clinical and laboratory features of SLE in various age groups are described in the mortality section (see below). In general, disease in individuals under 30 years of age is associated with a worse prognosis than disease developing in patients over 50.

SLE IN CHILDREN

Childhood SLE is characterized by more organ-threatening disease than adult-onset disease, and has a poorer prognosis. Lupus in children is managed the same way as in adults,[C143,G48] with particular attention being given to their specific psychosocial needs and special problems (Chap. 44). In prepubertal age groups, male SLE occurs in proportionately greater numbers than in adults, but the prognosis may be the same or worse than in their female counterparts.[C178,F298,K232] All studies performed prior to 1977 were associated with a less than 50% 10-year survival.[A10,C346,C375,G49,G287,J27,W54] Because 80% of children with SLE have renal disease, the availability of dialysis was a limiting prognostic factor in early studies. Since the advent of parenteral cyclophosphamide, improved antihypertensive agents, renal transplantation, cyclosporine, and other diagnostic advances, the 10-year survival has improved to an average of 85%[C2,F105,G197,K232,L7,M262,M596,P221,W17] for children treated in optimal settings. A practice containing largely indigent black and Hispanic patients in Brooklyn reported a 25% 5-year mortality and a 25% 5-year renal failure requiring dialysis.[T101] In contrast, Singaporean children had 5- and 10-year mortalities of 20 and

30%, respectively (27 and 41% for nephritis).[L127] Lehman's group in Los Angeles was unable to find any prognostic differences among patients with onset at an age less than 10 years versus 10 to 20 years.[L173] We could not find any differences in survival between 55 patients who survived to adulthood diagnosed at younger than 20 years versus 409 patients diagnosed at a later age.[W39]

In summary, the bleak prognosis for childhood SLE reported in the 1960s and 1970s has improved substantially. Children now have only a slightly worse outcome than adults.

OLDER ADULTS

Idiopathic SLE developing in individuals over the age of 50 years compared to adults with onset before the age of 50 is characterized by a milder serologic picture, infrequent renal disease, and more serositis and arthritis.[W259] These older-onset SLE patients had a 92 and 83% 5- and 10-year survival rates in our 1980 survey.[W39] Fewer elderly patients require corticosteroids and, when they do, lower doses are needed, for shorter durations.[D219] Nephritis does not appear to alter overall survival.[W39] The single exception to these data was contained in Reveille et al.'s survey of 389 patients, in which older age of onset was associated with a poorer outcome.[R173] Our 1990 analysis of 464 patients suggested that the time from onset of symptoms to diagnosis in those over 60 years of age is 3.2 years, the longest of any age group.[P216]

Race

Race distribution and its influence on SLE prognosis is discussed in Chapter 4 and in the previous sections of this chapter. In general, Caucasian's have a better outcome than non-Caucasians. The influence of socioeconomic factors, however, may be as important as race (see below).

Environment

Environmental considerations, such as climate, occupation, exposure to chemicals, diet, lifestyle, exercise, and drug-induced SLE, are described in Chapters 3, 4, and 55. Whether they influence prognosis is uncertain.

Geography

Geography may be a factor in survival patterns. The incidence and prevalence of SLE in various parts of the world are discussed in Chapter 4. Generally, Canadian, Japanese, and European SLE patients have similar outcomes as those in the United States. SLE might present differently in certain locales, which this may alter prognosis. For example, black SLE patients in Zimbabwe have an unusually high incidence of renal disease (71%) and a low incidence of photosensitivity (16%).[T82] In India,[B290] Egypt,[S5] and Thailand,[C241] mortality rates are high.

Socioeconomic Status

Socioeconomic factors have been implicated in the increased mortality rates seen in developing nations (see above). We have observed higher mortality rates in clinic

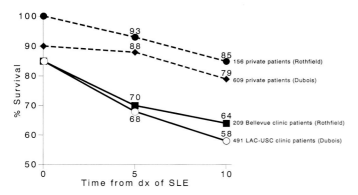

Fig. 62–2. A comparison of survival curves of private and clinic patients treated by the same physician in the 1960s and 1970s.

patients compared to our private practice patients (Fig. 62–2).[W39,W40] Studenski et al. confirmed this observation,[S741] but Esdaile et al. found that socioeconomic status had no correlation with health outcomes among Canadian SLE patients, but all of them had health insurance.[E141]

Time

The year of disease onset is a critical factor in the prognostic equation. As noted above, the overall survival of SLE patients has improved dramatically over the last 40 years. Treatment practice has changed and varied depending on the year, location of treatment, and source of health care delivery. For example, corticosteroids at higher doses were used for longer periods in the 1950s and, similarly, certain immunosuppressive agents were used more extensively in the late 1960s and early 1970s than at present. The advent of steroids, dialysis, newer antihypertensives and antibiotics, and parenteral cyclophosphamide has had an impact on patient survival.[F260]

The other issue is whether the nature of SLE has changed with time. Hashimoto et al.[H185,H186] conducted a comparison by decades of 229 Japanese patients studied since 1955. They concluded that the incidence of Raynaud's phenomenon, alopecia, oral ulcers, and nephritis has increased in the last decade. In contrast, Wallace et al. compared 464 American SLE patients (diagnosed between 1980 and 1989) with the 520 patients seen by Dubois (diagnosed between 1950 and 1963) in the same office.[P216] The percentage of patients with organ-threatening disease decreased from 65 to 52%, and acute central nervous system vasculitis practically disappeared. This might be attributed to earlier recognition and treatment of symptoms and signs of SLE, an evolutionary change in the disease process, changes in referral patterns, and/or the availability of ANA testing and other serologic procedures that can help identify milder cases.

Genetic Factors

Sex

Because 90% of SLE patients are women, and their greatest periods of disease activity often occur during the reproductive years, extensive hormonal investigations

have been conducted (see Chaps. 16 and 41). The effect of male gender on lupus prognosis has been hampered by the small numbers of men in most of the reported series. Our 1980 and 1990 surveys included 90 men with SLE, and it was concluded that they do significantly worse than women with SLE.[P216,W39] Kaufman et al.,[K120] Swaak et al.,[S785] Blum et al.,[B364] and a Soviet group[F141] have confirmed these findings, whereas three other groups found no differences.[H347,J121,W77] No comparative study has demonstrated that men do better than women, and even the three surveys that showed no differences generally noted that men had more organ-threatening disease.

Family History and Genetic Traits

Family history is discussed in Chapters 2 and 4.

The influence of genetic markers, such as HLA haplotypes, acetylation phenotypes, and the presence or absence of certain complement alleles on prognosis, is discussed in Chapter 2.

Clinical, Laboratory, and Serologic Variables

Multivariate Analyses

Fries and Holman[F256] conducted multivariate analyses on their 193 patients to assess the prognostic value of the absence or presence of various parameters. Those with the worst prognosis were anemic, hypoalbuminemic, and on high-dose steroids, and had elevated anti-DNA levels. Factors most likely to be associated with increased serum creatinine levels were oral ulcers, pleurisy, anemia and a 24-hour urinary protein higher than 4 g. The severity of nephritis correlated with alopecia, low hematocrit, elevated sedimentation rate, and elevated creatinine, high anti-DNA, and low C3 complement levels. An elevated anti-DNA titer was associated with anemia, proteinuria, urinary red cell casts, and decreased C3. Patients who did not receive cytotoxic drugs or steroids had a higher survivorship, but were not as ill as those given these medications.

The best predictors of mortality were a platelet count lower than 60,000/mm³, seizures, high fever, and a serum creatinine level greater than 1.5 mg/dl. Organ system correlations were sought. Arthritis was associated with elevated anti-DNA and anti-ENA levels and seizures. Skin exacerbations occurred more frequently with high fever, Raynaud's phenomenon, anti-ENA, normal complement, and a creatinine level above 1.5 mg/dl. Pleurisy was most often seen with high fever, oral ulcers, and elevated anti-DNA, and anti-ENA levels. Increasing proteinuria was associated with high fevers and elevated anti-DNA and decreased C3 levels. In a follow-up report, their group found that the two greatest mortality risks among 310 patients were systolic blood pressure greater than 144 mm Hg and a blood urea nitrogen (BUN) level greater than 39 mg/dl at entry.[S264]

Clinical and Laboratory Correlates

The issue of using various combinations of clinical features and laboratory findings to calculate activity indices has been discussed in Chapter 5. These indices are still too new to reach any conclusions about their impact on outcome, but other limited studies have been performed. Eto et al.[E150] examined skin lesions in 106 SLE subjects and found that those with discoid LE or lupus pernio had a better prognosis than those without it, whereas those who had nodular lesions or cutaneous angiitis had a worse prognosis. Alarcon-Segovia and Diaz-Jouanen[A102] correlated absence of lymphopenia with a more benign course. Hematocytopenias correlated with youth, a greater number of males, and fever.

The multicenter study of 1,103 patients by Ginzler et al.[G162] found that those with a serum creatinine level greater than 3 mg/dl, a low hematocrit, and an elevated 24-hour urinary protein had the lowest survival rates. Survival was poorer in patients who met seven or more ARA criteria.

Feinglass et al.[F46] found that neuropsychiatric findings do not adversely affect survival curves in 140 patients. Bokemeyer and Thiele[B389] followed 109 subjects for a mean of 6.7 years. An elevated serum creatinine level, proteinuria, oral ulcers, and severe anemia correlated with a poorer prognosis than in those without renal involvement, especially those who had Raynaud's phenomenon. Our group found an association among a low serum albumin level, diastolic hypertension, and active urine sediment with significantly poorer survival in 230 nephritis patients.[W40] Reveille et al.[R173] correlated worse survival with central nervous system disease, thrombocytopenia, anemia, and hypertension.

In summary, studies done in the last 15 years have shown that severe nephritis (manifested by an elevated creatinine level or nephrotic syndrome), hypertension, and anemia are predictors of a bad outcome.[B389,F256,G162,R173,S264,W40] Additional data have indicated poor survivals in patients with thrombocytopenia, lymphopenia, vasculitic skin lesions, active central nervous system lupus, elevated sedimentation rate, and oral ulcers,[A102,E150,F256,M608] but these findings have been less uniform than those related to nephritis, hypertension, and anemia.

The foregoing provides examples of how combinations of clinical, laboratory, and serologic parameters may help the clinician assess outcome probabilities. Chapters 34 to 43 discuss the relationship of specific signs and laboratory findings to prognosis by organ system. Clearly, SLE is a complex disorder in which a single index or formula is not going to be particularly useful; only generalized conclusions can result.

The influence of serologic and other immune parameters on prognosis is discussed in Chapter 48.

SPONTANEOUS REMISSIONS

During periods of remission, either no symptoms or minor complaints, such as slight morning stiffness or occasional pleuritic discomfort, may occur. Laboratory abnormalities such as leukopenia, elevated sedimentation rate, and positive ANA may persist or disappear.

SLE can spontaneously improve and remit. Dubois has reported that 35% of 520 patients had multiple spontaneous remissions of varying lengths of time not associated with treatment.[D310] Some were of 10 to 20 years' dura-

tion. Ropes[R293,S444] noted spontaneous remissions of a few months to several years in 70% of 72 patients. Tumulty,[T270] in 1954, observed spontaneous remission in 19 of 34 patients treated symptomatically. Tozman et al.[T201] remarked that 4 of 160 patients with SLE followed for a mean of 75 months with a history of severe organ involvement had no treatment and no disease activity. Gladman et al.,[G179] in 1980, reported that 14 of 140 patients were in complete remission off therapy, with a follow-up range of 2 to 11 years, despite abnormal serologies. Heller and Schur[H250] noted that 13 of their 305 patients (4%) developed clinical and serologic (with ANA becoming negative) remissions between 1967 and 1981, lasting at least 18 months. Only 8 of 13 patients, however, were off all medications.

Overall, it seems that 2 to 10% of patients who fulfill ARA criteria for SLE can enter true disease remissions that can last months to years. That is, they have no symptoms and require no therapy for SLE. This must be remembered when considering therapy for the individual patient or when evaluating the efficacy of treatment. Such remissions might account for reports purporting to show beneficial effects as a result of unusual interventions, such as IM blood injections or vitamins.[K475,W172]

MORTALITY RATES IN LARGE POPULATIONS

Five major reports have appeared that allow trends in overall mortality rates among SLE patients to be interpreted (Table 62–3). All but Siegel's and Hochberg's[H342,S416] studies extrapolated data from the National Center for Health Statistics. See also Chapter 3.

The data of Cobb[C312] and Siegel and Lee's study[S415] demonstrate surprisingly low death rates. These must be interpreted with caution because the definitions of lupus have broadened since the 1950s. Between 1968 and 1972[K93] and 1972 and 1977,[G298] improvements in mortality rates were seen in all subsets. Both studies suggested that mortality in blacks is accentuated in early adulthood and then declines, whereas mortality in whites consistently increases with age. Death rates increased earlier in females than in males. These figures cannot be interpreted to imply a greater incidence of SLE in blacks than whites because socioeconomic differences between the groups are still large, and consequently influence mortality.

Kaslow[K92] also studied mortality patterns in 12 states that include 88% of all Americans of Asian ancestry. Between 1968 and 1976, the mortality rate for Asians was 6.8 million person-years, compared with 8.05 for blacks and 2.8 for whites. Serdula and Rhodes[S286] noted the mortality rate in Hawaii (1970 to 1975) to be 1.89 million person-years for whites and 14.46 for nonwhites who were almost entirely of Asian ancestry. For the same reasons (see above), this finding implies greater disease severity, increased incidence of SLE, or more socioeconomic hardships among Asian-Americans, but these contentions remain to be proven.

Two reports have addressed mortality rates of SLE in Europe. Helve[H257] derived a 4.7 million person-years mortality rate among SLE patients in Finland, but the study considered only hospitalized patients. Hochberg[H342] ac-

Table 62–3. Death Rates from Lupus Erythematosus by Race and Gender in Large Populations (per million person-years)

Gender/Race	Siegel and Lee[S416] 1955–1964	Cobb[C312] 1959–1961	Kaslow and Masi[K93] 1968–1972	Gordon et al.[G298] 1972–1977	Hochberg[H342] 1974–1983
Female	8.3	4.7	6.31	5.41	3.94
White	5.5	4.0	5.42	4.62	—
Black	15.4	10.6	15.10	13.32	—
Male	1.9	1.1	1.6	1.38	1.02
White	0.7	1.1	1.48	1.23	—
Black	6.7	1.8	2.41	1.87	—

*Over 95% in this study were white.

cessed the Office of Population Censuses and Surveys data from 1974 to 1983 for England and Wales. He concluded that females have a 4-fold higher mortality rate than men, and that the highest mortality rates were in the 65- to 74-year age group. The annual mortality rate among females fell from 4.47 to 2.99 million person-years between 1974 and 1983. These mortality patterns are similar to those observed in the United States.

CAUSES OF DEATH

Studies Prior to 1975

The primary cause of death may sometimes be difficult to determine, but early studies followed the detailed protocols given in Klemperer's classic paper[K284] of 1941 (Table 62–4). Before 1962, the most common cause of death was progressive renal failure and its associated complications. Since then, uremic demise has occurred much less frequently as a result of better care of patients with end-stage renal disease, including dialysis and the use of cytotoxic therapy for lupus nephritis. Between 1956 and 1973, it decreased from 36 to 14% for all causes of death.

The second most common clinical pattern was evi-

dence of active central nervous system lupus. With high-dose steroid therapy, central nervous system lupus became a much less frequent cause of death after 1956.[D310] In Dubois' series, it decreased from 26 to 8% between 1956 and 1973. Dubois also found[D342] that the median age at death rose from 30 to 45 years during this period.

Most patients in Klemperer's series died of infections because of low resistance and the unavailability of antibiotics. Common bacterial pathogens and tuberculosis accounted for most of these infections;[D67,D342,H165,H306,K284] opportunistic organisms were rare in the presteroid era. The incidence of uremia increased from 5% of patients treated in the 1930s to as high as 36% in Estes and Christian's[E147] report in the 1960s, before declining in the 1970s. Central nervous system involvement was a major cause of death in 25% of patients in the 1930 series, and has declined continuously since. These early groups averaged a 4% prevalence of death from myocardial infarction and atherosclerotic heart disease, a figure that has risen dramatically over the years. Treatment complications were also unusual causes of death in the early series. Ropes[R294] emphasized that the major causes of death prior to 1949 were infection, active lupus, and uremia but, by

Table 62–4. Causes of Death in SLE Patients (%)

Cause	Klemperer[K284] (20 cases) 1930–1941	Harvey[M280] (38 cases) 1940–1954	Dubois[D340,D342] (57 cases) 1950–1955	Dubois[D340,D342] (100 cases) 1956–1962	Dubois[D340,D342] (92 cases) 1963–1973	Estes and Christian[E147] (53 cases) 1963–1971	Wallace et al.[W39] (128 cases) 1950–1980	Rosner et al.[R321] (222 cases) 1965–1976	Reveille et al.[R173] (89 cases) 1975–1984
Uremia	5	24	26	36	14	36	20	18	4
Central nervous system disease	25	3	26	11	8	19	14	7	ND*
Multiple or unknown	5	16	9	12	10	8	19	13	ND
Bronchopneumonia	40	3	11	5	14	13	10	15	ND
Congestive heart failure	5	0	2	5	5	0	5	0	ND
Malignancy	0	0	2	2	7	0	2	0	8
Myocardial infarction	0	0	2	5	5	4	10	3	9
Miscellaneous	20	54	22	24	37	20	20	44	29
Related to SLE (e.g., uremia, CNS, vascular)	30	39	64†	63†	47†	68	39	31	11
Related to Rx (e.g., peptic ulceration, agranulocytosis)	ND	ND	7	4	2	4	ND	ND	ND
Unrelated to SLE (e.g., myocardial infarction, suicide, cancer)	5	5	4	9	23	7	31	19	ND
Multiple factors or unknown	5	17	9	12	10	8	9	23	ND
Infection	60	39	16	12	18	13	21	33	39

* ND, not determined.
† Comparison of deaths occurring from 1950 to 1962 with those during the 1963–1973 period showing a significant difference (p < 0.007).

1964, they were uremia, infection, and central nervous system disease.

By 1975, the primary cause of death remained progressive renal damage, despite the benefits that may follow steroid or cytotoxic therapy. The second most common cause was infection, particularly bronchopneumonia caused by opportunistic pathogens.

Studies From 1975 to 1986

Urowitz et al., in 1976, demonstrated a bimodal mortality pattern in SLE.[U34] Of 81 patients studied, 11 died; 6 of these died within a year of diagnosis, usually of complications of active lupus or sepsis. All were on high-dose steroids. The remaining 5 patients died a mean of 8.6 years after diagnosis. None had active nephritis or sepsis. The mean dose of steroids was minimal, and 4 patients had myocardial infarctions. Their follow-up paper,[U36] as well as the works of others cited in this section, confirmed these findings. Urman and Rothfield[U32] also demonstrated a change in the causes of death as patients with SLE age. In 209 patients studied in New York City from 1957 to 1968, the main cause of 49 deaths was active lupus (excluding uremia; 39%), lupus nephritis (27%), and infection (22%). In 19 deaths among their 156 Connecticut patients followed from 1968 to 1976, the causes were lupus nephritis (42%), active lupus (excluding uremia; 21%), and infection (16%).

A multicenter study of 1,103 patients conducted by Rosner et al.[W39] reported 222 deaths between 1965 and 1976. As in Urman and Rothfield's report,[R321] none died from a malignancy. The major causes were infection (18%), renal disease (18%), central nervous system disease (7%), and cardiovascular disease (6%). Karsh et al.[K86] reviewed 94 deaths in 428 lupus nephritis patients seen at the National Institutes of Health between 1954 and 1977. The bimodal pattern first reported by Urowitz et al. was observed. The causes of death were renal complications (40%), vascular disease (25%), and infection (16%). Only one death occurred from cancer, even though most of the patients were treated with immunosuppressive drugs. In a similar study, 42 of 138 lupus nephritis patients followed at Guy's Hospital in London between 1964 and 1982 died.[C393] Of these, 12 died within

a month of starting dialysis—usually from active lupus or infection. The bimodal curve with late vascular deaths was borne out.

Wallace and Dubois' group reported their experience with 128 deaths among 609 private patients seen between 1950 and 1980.[W39,W40] Only 38% of those in the group had kidney disease, but they accounted for 67% of the deaths. The most common causes of death without nephritis were cardiovascular disease (primarily atherosclerotic; 30%), central nervous system disease (mostly vasculitis; 24%), and sepsis (17%). We confirmed Urowitz's finding that most early deaths result from active SLE, and that the preponderance of later deaths are a result of cardiovascular complications. The nephritis trend over a 40-year period is shown in Table 62–5.

Studies Since 1986

As noted above, several of the large studies reported few deaths. Only reviews of more than 20 deaths are discussed in this section. Of 148 Danish[H146,H147] patients followed between 1965 and 1983, 39 died. Half were caused by active SLE, with a mean age at death of 20 years, and the other half had a mean age of 38.2 years. Uremia and infections were each responsible for 18% of deaths. Information was available on 55 of 67 SLE patients who died at the university hospital in Jamaica between 1972 and 1985.[H162] Of these, 23 were early demises and 32 were late. Deaths were caused by infection (37%), renal disease (24%), hemorrhage (17%), and central nervous system disease (17%).

Of 167 patients with SLE at the University of Mississippi followed between 1973 and 1985, 50 died.[H132] None had a malignancy; 30% had been ill for less than 2 years. The bimodal curve was not found among this mostly indigent population. Causes of death included infection (28%), renal failure (36%), and active SLE (16%). Of 88 deaths observed in a SLE cohort by Studenski et al. at Duke University, 71 were a result of the disease.[R173] Reveille et al. reviewed the charts of 389 lupus patients at the University of Alabama seen between 1975 and 1984.[S741] Of the 89 who died, 74 had a determinable cause of death. The principal causes of death were infection (39%), active SLE (11%), and cardiovascular disease (9%).

Table 62–5. Causes of Death in Patients with Nephritis (%)

Cause	Before 1961 (n = 22)	1961–1970 (n = 40)	1971–1980 (n = 20)	1981–1990 (n = 18)	Overall (n = 100)
Renal disease	54	30	10	22	30
Infection	23	25	30	17	24
CNS lupus	14	—	10	0	5
Cardiovascular disease	5	10	10	17	10
Pulmonary disease	—	5	—	6	3
GI vasculitis	—	5	5	17	6
Unknown	—	—	15	0	3
Miscellaneous	4	25	20	21	19

Adapted from Wallace, D.J., Podell, T.E., Weiner, J.M., et al.: Lupus nephritis: Experience with 230 patients in a private practice from 1950 to 1980. Am. J. Med. 72:209, 1982.

I have completed a 10-year update of 570 lupus patients seen between 1980 and 1989.[P216] None of the discoid or drug-induced lupus patients died. The most common causes of deaths were active disease (35%), sepsis (19%), stroke (15%), and cardiovascular disease (15%).

In summary, in the 1980s, death resulted from active disease (with a decreasing percentage from renal disease), infection, and cardiovascular disease. Central nervous system disease is rarely fatal. Those who succumb from thromboembolic complications of SLE (e.g., the thrombocytopenic subset with antiphospholipid antibodies) may be decreasing in number, because the prophylactic management of this group in the 1990s may further increase the life span of these patients.

MALIGNANCIES IN SLE

Data concerning the incidence of malignancies in SLE are of great interest because it is believed that the failure of immune surveillance is a cause of induction and spread of tumors. In SLE two reasons for faulty immune mechanisms are known. One involves abnormalities in immune regulation associated with the disease process. The second involves longterm treatment with cytotoxic agents, which increases the risk of developing cancer. In fact, cancer is an extremely infrequent cause of death in SLE. Eight large surveys[H46,K86,R173,R321,S741,U32,U34,W39] were comprised of 3,683 patients. Of the 667 who died, 16 had malignancies, representing 2.5% of patients. About 1,000 of these had received some type of immunosuppressive treatment. Before any conclusions are reached, however, it should be emphasized that this implies only a low mortality rate from cancer but says nothing about the overall incidence of neoplasia in SLE.

Various types of neoplasms have been described in SLE patients.[O64] Malignancies were found in 18 of 484 SLE and in 4 of 253 discoid LE patients seen at the University of Michigan between 1955 and 1974.[L248] Of the 18 malignancies, 6 were cervical or uterine, in women who had been treated with corticosteroids. Ginzler et al. observed an increased incidence of cervical carcinoma in SLE patients, especially in blacks, in those without renal disease, and in individuals who received azathioprine therapy.[G160] Another study found an increased incidence of cervical atypia in azathioprine-treated SLE subjects.[N152] Among 151 SLE patients in Finland, 9 malignancies were found. In the 1,456 person-years at risk, an increased association with lymphoma was observed.[M416]

Miller[M416] reported 17 malignant lymphomas in association with various immune disorders at Sloan-Kettering and analyzed the prevalence of various connective tissue diseases in 1,893 patients with carcinoma and sarcoma and in 4 with lymphoproliferative neoplasms. One patient in each group had SLE. The prevalence of all systemic connective tissue disease in those with solid tumors was 0.58%, and in those with malignant lymphoma it was 1.86%. The difference in prevalence between the groups was statistically significant. In a 1959 report from the same center, no cases of SLE were observed among 1,002 patients with Hodgkin's disease, 2,200 with leukemia, and 1,269 with lymphosarcoma.[R82] SLE usually antedates the lymphoid malignancy.[G349] The Mayo Clinic conducted a similar survey.[B80,C370] In their report, 29 lymphoid neoplasms were seen in rheumatic disease patients between 1965 and 1975; only 1 had SLE. There are 20 single case reports of SLE with lymphoproliferative disorders in the literature, which would make the prevalence of lymphoma in SLE low. These reports add little to our knowledge of the subject, but one paper described the initial presentation of SLE in a patient after receiving total body irradiation for lymphoma.[S598]

Other malignancies seen include sarcoma,[G412,K274,L326] ovarian seminoma,[D300,K15,R356] leukemia,[B93,D104,H333,I53,J131,K286,P34,S106] myeloma,[B597,J126,S276,S539] lung cancer,[M408] adrenocortical carcinoma,[T174] breast cancer,[T35] endometrial carinoma,[S39] cervical carcinoma,[O69] Kaposi's sarcoma,[G355] and hepatocellular carcinoma[M627] (see the section on lupoid hepatitis in Chap. 42). Malignancies can often mimic the initial presentation of SLE, and some patients with cancer can have a positive ANA (see Chap. 49). No evidence has shown that antimalarials, NSAIDs, salicylates, or corticosteroids increase the incidence of malignancies.

Thus, malignancies are rare in SLE, and are no more common than in the general population. The use of cytotoxic drugs might increase the risk of cancer, but this association has not been documented in SLE patients.

SUMMARY

1. Overall survivorship and duration of disease:
   a. Over 90% of SLE patients survive at least 2 years after diagnosis, compared with 50% 30 years ago. More recent surveys reveal an 80 to 90% 10-year survival.
   b. SLE can become inactive for many years; 15 to 20% of our patients have no evidence of clinical activity, and are on minimal or no medication.
   c. Blacks, males, children, patients who receive public funding and those with thrombocytopenia have a poorer prognosis, especially if nephritis is present.
2. Mortality rates and causes of death:
   a. A bimodal mortality curve in SLE is prevalent. Patients who die within 5 years of disease onset usually have active SLE, high steroid requirements, and infections. Patients who die later usually have steroid-complicated cardiovascular disease; in contrast, active SLE, infection, and high steroid requirements are uncommon.
   b. Most SLE patients die from active SLE, nephritis, sepsis, and cardiovascular disease. Mortality from central nervous system disease or malignancies rarely occurs.

Section VIII

APPENDIX

Appendix I

A PATIENT'S GUIDE TO LUPUS ERYTHEMATOSUS

DANIEL J. WALLACE
BEVRA H. HAHN
FRANCISCO P. QUISMORIO JR.

PURPOSE OF THIS SECTION*

When first told they have lupus erythematosus, or LE, many patients have never before heard the term. This appendix is intended to help you understand what lupus is, how it may affect your life, and what you can do to help yourself and your physician in the management of the illness. It will not replace your physician's advice. Because each case of LE is different, only your physician can answer specific questions about individual situations. It is hoped that by providing facts about LE in nontechnical terms, you may increase your knowledge of the disease. In addition to explaining what lupus is, we have tried to answer other questions that you, your relatives, and your friends may have, such as what causes LE, the difference between discoid and systemic LE, how the diagnosis is made, and how the illness is treated.

We have attempted to use easy-to-understand terms throughout and a glossary, or explanation of the more complicated words, is located at the end.

Because many of the most significant studies of LE are fairly recent—indeed, are constantly in various stages of exciting change and medical progress—much of the information available is already out of date. If you look up LE in an encyclopedia or a medical book, you are likely to be confused, maybe even frightened. This is not only unnecessary, but it may interfere with your seeking proper diagnosis and treatment.

BRIEF HISTORY OF LUPUS ERYTHEMATOSUS

Lupus means wolf in Latin and *erythematosus* means redness. The name was first given to the disease because it was thought the skin damage resembled the bite of a wolf.

Lupus erythematosus has been known to physicians since 1828 when it was first described by the French dermatologist, Biett. Early studies were simply descriptions of the disease, with emphasis on the skin changes. A dermatologist named Kaposi, 45 years later, noted that some patients with LE skin lesions showed signs that the disease affected internal organs.

In the 1890s, Sir William Osler, a famed American physician, observed that systemic LE (also called SLE) could affect internal organs without the occurrence of skin changes.

In 1948, Dr. Malcolm Hargraves of the Mayo Clinic described the LE cell, a particular cell found in the blood of patients with SLE. His discovery has enabled physicians to identify many more cases of LE by using a simple blood test. As a result, during the succeeding years, the number of SLE cases diagnosed has steadily risen. Since 1954, various unusual proteins (or antibodies) that act against the patient's own tissues have been found to be associated with systemic LE. Detection of these abnormal proteins has been used to develop more sensitive tests for systemic LE (antinuclear antibody tests). The presence of these antibodies may be the result of factors other than SLE.

WHAT IS LUPUS ERYTHEMATOSUS?

LE usually appears in one of two forms. *Discoid*, or *cutaneous lupus erythematosus* (the skin form, called discoid LE) or *systemic lupus erythematosus* (the internal form, systemic LE or SLE).

Discoid (or chronic cutaneous) LE has a particular type of skin rash with raised, red, scaly areas, often with healing in the centers or with scars. These eruptions are seen most commonly on the face and other light-exposed areas. Usually, patients with discoid LE have normal internal organs. A skin biopsy of the lesion may be helpful in confirming the diagnosis.

Subacute cutaneous lupus erythematosus is a nonscarring subset of lupus that is characterized by distinct immunologic abnormalities and some systemic features.

Systemic lupus erythematosus is classified as one of the autoimmune rheumatic diseases, in the same family as rheumatoid arthritis, and is usually considered a chronic, systemic, inflammatory disease of connective tissue. *Chronic* means that the condition lasts for a long period of time. *Inflammatory* describes the body's reaction to irritation with pain and swelling. LE involves changes in the immune system, so that elements of the system attack the body's own tissues. The organs affected are different in each person. Joints are usually inflamed. Inflammation can also involve the skin, kidney, blood cells, brain, heart, lung, and blood vessels. The inflammation can be controlled by medication.

SLE can be a mild condition but, because it can affect joints, skin, kidneys, blood, heart, lungs, and other internal

* The material in this appendix is revised and adapted from a pamphlet by Dubois, E.L., and Cox, M.B.: Lupus Erythematosus. Torrance, CA, The American Lupus Society, 1983. Copies of this appendix are available from The American Lupus Society.

organs, it can appear in different forms and with different intensities at different times in the same person. A large number of people with SLE have few symptoms and can live a nearly normal life. Therefore, while reading about the symptoms, you should not become unnecessarily worried, because all the symptoms probably do not occur in one person.

How serious lupus is varies greatly from a mild to a life-threatening condition. It depends on what parts of the body are affected. Even a mild case can become more serious if it is not properly treated. (The results are usually good with use of the more recently developed medicines.) The severity of your LE should be discussed with your physician.

LE is not infectious or contagious. It is not a type of cancer or malignancy. LE is not related to acquired immunodeficiency syndrome (AIDS).

FREQUENCY OF LE

No one has made an accurate estimate of the number of patients with discoid LE because many people have mild cases and probably don't know it. There may be as many as 1,000,000 people with systemic LE in the United States.

The number of new cases of systemic LE diagnosed by physicians is definitely increasing, for several reasons. After the LE cell test came into use, physicians were able to diagnose the illness correctly in patients who were believed to have other rheumatic diseases, or who were thought to have "neurotic" complaints. Tests for *antinuclear* and *other antibodies*, which are usually positive in systemic LE, have helped physicians discover even more patients with milder cases, but the test might be positive in patients without SLE. It has also been learned that certain medications, like procainamide (Pronestyl) and number of other drugs, may cause systemic LE. Patients with this type of drug-caused lupus usually improve dramatically after stopping the offending medication. Therefore, some of the increase in the number of cases of LE is the result of better recognition by physicians, and some may be the result of increasing toxic changes in our environment, with greater exposure to drugs, chemicals, and possibly triggering agents.

Many patients have combined symptoms of SLE, scleroderma (thickening and hardening of the skin), and polymyositis (inflammation of muscles). These combinations may be called mixed connective tissue disease (MCTD), or cross-over or overlap syndrome, depending on certain laboratory features.

Seven of ten patients with discoid LE are women, half of them developing their first symptoms between the ages of 15 and 30 years. LE is rare in children under the age of 5. It is found throughout the world, and affects all ethnic groups and religions.

SLE is more common than rheumatic fever, leukemia, cystic fibrosis, muscular dystrophy, multiple sclerosis, hemophilia, and several other well-known diseases.

WHAT CAUSES LE?

The cause of discoid LE is unknown. In most cases, the cause of SLE is also unknown, although it is believed that many factors may be involved, including genetic predisposition and environmental factors such as excessive sun exposure, certain medicines, and infections. In families of SLE patients, it is known that there is an increase in the number of relatives with SLE and rheumatoid arthritis compared with the normal population. Many of the relatives have abnormal proteins in their blood, such as antinuclear antibodies, although they may not have any symptoms of the disease.

Some of the genes that increase a person's risk for SLE are known. For example, in the United States, a gene called DR2 increases a person's risk of developing lupus nephritis, although the vast majority of individuals with the gene are healthy.

Many researchers suspect that a special type of immune reaction causes the disease. It is believed that patients develop antibodies against their own tissues, as if vaccinated against themselves. These antibodies are known as autoantibodies (*auto* means self), and the type of allergy is called *autoimmunity*, or an allergy against oneself. Some of us possess lupus "genes." Certain viruses, drugs, chemicals in the environment, or extreme emotional stress might activate the gene. This gene encodes antibodies and/or other products that damage tissue, the net effect of which results in the white blood cells' (lymphocytes) surveillance system ultimately stimulating the formation of antibodies. Still, the basic question that remains unanswered is what events set off the mechanism that causes antibodies to be produced against one's own tissues. Answering this question may be an important step toward preventing and curing LE.

In perhaps 10% of patients with SLE, the disease may have been caused by medicine. The most common is procainamide (Pronestyl), which is often used to treat heart irregularities. It is essential that your physician be told of all medications you are taking, including birth control pills and estrogens for menopause.

DIAGNOSIS

The skin rash of discoid LE may be so typical that an experienced doctor can make the diagnosis by the history and appearance of the rash. If there is any question, a skin biopsy usually helps. It is essential that each patient with discoid LE have a thorough physical examination, including laboratory tests, to check the possibility of systemic LE being present.

Diagnosing systemic LE is more difficult. Finding a definite answer may take months of observation, many laboratory tests, and sometimes a trial of drugs. Because of many different symptoms, some patients are thought to have another disease, rheumatoid arthritis, with swelling of a few or many joints of the hands, feet, ankles, or wrists. If typical skin lesions are present, they are helpful in making the diagnosis. Other findings, such as fever, pleurisy (painful breathing), or kidney disease also point to the diagnosis of SLE.

In addition to a complete medical history and physical examination, routine tests are done to learn what internal organs are involved—for example, a blood count to see if there are too few red cells, white cells, or platelets (cells that are necessary for clotting). A routine analysis of the urine is always done and often a kidney function test, using all urine passed in a 24-hour period, is necessary. A chest x-ray and electrocardiogram may be recommended if clinical evidence of problems in the lung or heart is found.

Diagnostic Criteria

In 1982, the American College of Rheumatology established new diagnostic criteria for systemic lupus. After excluding rheumatoid arthritis, scleroderma, and polymyositis, a diagnosis of systemic LE can be made if 4 of the following 11 criteria are met:

1. "Butterfly" rash on cheeks
2. Discoid lupus
3. Sensitivity to sunlight
4. Mouth sores
5. Arthritis
6. More than 0.5 g of protein in the urine per day or cellular casts in a urinalysis
7. Seizures or psychosis
8. Pleuritis or pericarditis
9. Low white blood count *or* low platelet count *or* hemolytic anemia
10. Antibody to DNA or to Sm antigen (a fairly specific antibody found in about one-fourth of lupus patients) *or* LE cells *or* false-positive syphilis test
11. Positive antinuclear antibody test

To help confirm the diagnosis, special tests for SLE are performed that measure blood antibodies. These include examinations for antinuclear antibody (ANA), which is the most sensitive test for the disease. Serum complement (a protein that is decreased during active phases of autoimmune illness) is often measured. Anti-DNA antibody is a specific type of antinuclear antibody that is often present in the blood of SLE patients. Its presence is helpful in confirming the diagnosis of SLE. Moreover, when the disease is active, especially if the kidneys are affected in SLE, anti-DNA antibodies are usually present in high amounts in the blood. Thus, tests for anti-DNA antibody can be useful in monitoring disease activity in SLE. Again, none of these tests is specific for SLE. Different medical centers may use other diagnostic tests, depending on their individual experience. For example, the LE cell test is fairly specific for the disease but is technically difficult to perform. A small percentage of people without disease have positive ANA tests; consequently, obtaining such a result does not confirm the diagnosis of SLE. All tests must be evaluated by the physician in regard to the signs and symptoms of the patient.

Some patients with a negative ANA may still have SLE. Usually, these patients have anti-Ro/SSA antibody or a positive, nonlesional skin biopsy using immunofluorescence (lupus band test). Discoid LE patients often have a negative ANA and positive lesional lupus band test or typical light microscopic findings.

Resemblance to Other Diseases

One problem in diagnosis is that there is no single set of symptoms or pattern of disease. Also, SLE can mimic symptoms of many other diseases and can strike many different parts of the body, sometimes confusing even the most experienced physicians. One out of six patients may have a false-positive blood test for syphilis as one of the first symptoms of LE. This is frequently found during a routine premarital examination, but does not mean that the patient has venereal disease or that there is any relationship between syphilis and SLE. This test is associated with the lupus anticoagulant and anticardiolipin antibody.

SYMPTOMS AND COURSE

The patient with systemic LE may have periods of severe illness (flare or exacerbation) with extreme symptoms, intermingled with periods of no illness and complete freedom from symptoms (remission). The illness comes and goes so unpredictably that no two cases are alike. Even before the discovery of corticosteroids, some patients made a full recovery with treatment by aspirin and rest alone. Although causes for disease flare-ups may be recognized and prevented by the patient, at other times their cause is unknown. *Some possibly preventable causes of flare-ups are excessive sun exposure, injuries, insufficient rest, stopping the medications that have been controlling the disorder, irregular living habits, and emotional crises.* It cannot be emphasized too strongly that abruptly stopping medication, particularly large doses of corticosteroid derivatives such as prednisone, can lead to severe flare of the disease or fatal outcome.

Symptoms and Disorder

Symptoms of systemic LE are varied, and no two patients have exactly the same ones. Any part of the body can be involved, so symptoms may include one or more of these in any combination: joint and muscle pain, fever, skin rashes, chest pain, swelling of hands and feet, and hair loss (Fig. AP–1). Joint involvement in SLE is usually less severe than that occurring in rheumatoid arthritis, and is usually nondeforming. You should remember that, in most patients, most of the symptoms disappear. This clearing of symptoms is called a remission. Medications are usually necessary to cause remissions, but sometimes they occur spontaneously—that is without treatment.

Physicians use the term "remission" or "controlled" rather than "cure" in speaking of the periods when pa-

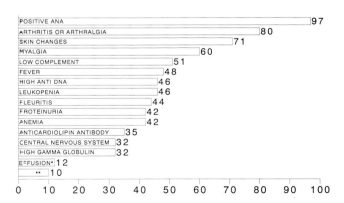

Fig. AP–1. Cumulative percentage incidence of 16 clinical and laboratory manifestations of SLE based on five studies published since 1975 (1,084 cases) (*, pleural or pericardial; **, adenopathy).

tients are free of symptoms because both doctor and patients can then be watchful for signs and symptoms, which may be a warning that a flare is beginning. Treatment can then be started, before unnecessary damage occurs.

General Symptoms

Generalized aching, weakness, tiring easily, low-grade fever, and chills are commonly associated with active SLE. Although these symptoms are usually particularly noticeable during flare-ups of the disease, some patients give a life-long history of low energy, malaise (generalized discomfort), and inability to keep up an active work schedule. A low-grade rise in temperature (99.5 to 100.5°F), usually in the late afternoon, may be a sign of smoldering LE activity, and may appear several days before the patient feels really ill. In the patient with systemic LE, the loss of energy, development of weakness, low-grade fever, or tiring easily are each considered to be danger signs. They may indicate that new activity of the disease is developing. When any of these early warning signs develop, patients should consult their physician immediately, so that examination may be made and further treatment prescribed, if necessary.

The following description of symptoms has been adapted mainly from Haserick and Kellum.*

Skin. A reddish rash or flush may appear involving the cheeks and nose in a so-called butterfly pattern. Other eruptions resembling discoid LE may occur in light-exposed areas of the body. Some patients are particularly sensitive to cold. After exposure to cold, the skin of their hands and feet may show several distinctive changes in color. Other patients may notice red, scaling changes on the back of the hands and on the fingers between the knuckles. Small areas of scarring on the scalp may produce baldness, and small red areas on the lips and the lining of the mouth may be related to SLE. Some patients have a definite sensitivity to ultraviolet rays of the sun, and even small amounts of sunlight may make these patients much worse. Easy bruising or pinpoint bleeding into the skin is sometimes related to SLE.

Chest. Pleurisy, or irritation of the membranes lining the chest, causes painful breathing and is common in SLE patients. Shortness of breath or rapid heartbeat is sometimes a related symptom. There may be accumulation of fluid in the chest cavity from inflammatory changes.

Muscular system. Tiring easily and weakness are often the first symptoms of systemic LE. Indeed, without these complaints, the diagnosis of systemic involvement in LE is open to doubt. Because they are also common in many other diseases and with plain nervous exhaustion, it is best to let your physician decide on their importance. Weakness caused by corticosteroid drugs is more likely than others to cause weakness in certain patients. Often, in these cases, a change to another steroidal drug is all that is necessary to return muscle strength.

Bones and Joints. Arthritis, joint swelling, and stiffness are common signs of SLE activity. These may involve

only one joint, may move from one region to another or, rarely, may progress to a deforming arthritis. This, however, is rarely disabling, and is less frequent than in rheumatoid arthritis.

Blood. Anemia, or a low red blood cell count, is common in patients with LE. There may be a decrease in white blood cells, usually around 2,500 to 4,000 per mm³ (cubic millimeter; normal is 5,000 to 10,000 per mm³). The blood platelets, which are necessary for clotting, may become affected.

Frequently, abnormalities in the proteins in the blood are present. Sometimes, a false-positive reaction for syphilis occurs when the blood is tested. Of course, this does not mean that the patient has syphilis, because this false reaction is only a manifestation of SLE.

Heart. In some patients with SLE, swelling of the feet and ankles may occur, as well as shortness of breath or difficulty in breathing after exertion or when lying down. These symptoms may mean the heart is affected. Fluid may collect in the pericardial sac surrounding the heart. The patient should remember that LE involvement does not always damage the heart permanently, because such changes disappear completely with treatment.

Stomach and Intestinal Tract. Pain in the abdomen, nausea, vomiting, diarrhea, or constipation are sometimes associated with SLE. These symptoms may be so severe as to imitate acute appendicitis, a stone in the kidney, or some other condition requiring surgical treatment. If these symptoms appear, it is important for the patient to tell the surgeon first that he or she has SLE, and second the type of dosage of medication being taken.

Kidney and Bladder. The kidney serves as the filtering plant of the body, filtering out waste products while preserving the many chemical parts of the blood essential for good health. Involvement of the kidney by SLE may cause loss into the urine of some of these essential chemical components, and there may be poor excretion of the waste products usually discarded in the urine. The retention and accumulation of the waste products can produce further symptoms that may require specialized treatment. The development of SLE kidney involvement is painless and should be checked by urinalysis every few months. Kidney biopsy (removal of a bit of tissue for study under the microscope) may be helpful for confirmation of the diagnosis or treatment.

Lymph Glands, Spleen, and Liver. Occasionally, the lymph glands of the neck, under the arms, and in the groin become enlarged. The spleen, an internal organ, may also become enlarged, and sometimes SLE hepatitis (an inflammation of the liver) develops.

Nervous System (brain, spinal cord, and nerves). Temporary seizures that resemble epilepsy may be early evidence of SLE, and the diagnosis of SLE is suggested only after other symptoms appear. Mental depression, excitability, unusual worry, headache, mental confusion, forgetfulness, "nerves," or even a nervous breakdown can be caused by SLE. Some patients have transient paralysis, stroke, neuritic pains, or poor bladder control related to their disease. Cognitive impairment (difficulty in thinking clearly) is common.

---

* Haserick, J.R., and Kellum, R.E.: Primer on Lupus Erythematosus . . . For Patients. Pinehurst, NC, Pinehurst Medical Center, 1973. (no longer in print).

Menstrual Periods. Menstrual periods may become irregular, more or less frequent, or even stop completely for several months. This is usually related to the activity of systemic LE or to side effects of glucocorticosteroids. When the disease is brought under control, menstrual periods may return to normal.

Thus, it is obvious that a wide range and variety of symptoms may announce the onset of SLE. Some patients, through the entire course of their illness, have symptoms involving only one organ, others may have symptoms that come and go, and some may begin with one group of symptoms, and acquire others as new parts of the body become involved with the SLE process. Remember that 40% of patients improved with rest and aspirin alone before the discovery of cortisone derivatives.

Other Considerations

Early warnings that may indicate a flare-up include chills, fatigue, loss of pep, new symptoms, and fever, such as change from the normal daily temperature to a slight afternoon fever of 99.5 to 100.5°F. If any of these changes occur, the physician should be notified.

The patient with systemic LE can generally return to his or her regular occupation. Usually, after the illness is well controlled, it does not interfere with full-time work.

Childbearing. Patients with discoid LE usually have no problems with pregnancy. The safety of many common medicines in pregnancy, however, is not well established. Glucocorticoids (steroids) are generally safe for the fetus and can be continued throughout pregnancy and delivery if needed for disease control. Nonsteroidal anti-inflammatory drugs (NSAIDs) and high-dose aspirin should be stopped. Antimalarials are controversial; it may be safest to discontinue them. Active SLE is associated with fetal loss.

A subset of LE patients with a false-positive syphilis test and/or lupus anticoagulant (especially those with high levels of anticardiolipin antibody) has been shown to have spontaneous recurrent abortions and/or low platelet counts. They may also be at risk for developing blood clots. Children of mothers with SLE who have Ro/SSA antibody are at a slight risk for developing neonatal lupus or congenital heart block.

Patients with systemic LE usually can have successful pregnancies, provided they do not have too much kidney or heart disease. Although many women with systemic LE feel better during pregnancy, an occasional flare-up can occur. Physicians cannot predict the effect of pregnancy on a particular individual. Whether pregnancy is advisable in your case should be discussed with your physician before you become pregnant.

Contraception. The safest methods of contraception are the use of barrier methods such as diaphragm and jelly, foam, sponges, or condoms. Although birth control pills are safely used by many SLE patients, the incidence of pill-related complications appears to be higher in these patients than in the normal user. Intrauterine devices are not advisable because of the high incidence of infections connected with their use.

TREATMENT OF LE

Several effective methods of treatment are available. Unfortunately, all the medications used to treat SLE, including regular aspirin, have some potential dangers but we must use them, hopefully at low levels and for a short time. The one used in a particular individual depends entirely on the type of LE. Patients with discoid LE may be treated with creams or ointments containing corticosteroid medications and sunscreens. With more extensive skin changes, antimalarial or quinine-related drugs are extremely effective.

Treatment is usually required for months. Stopping medication may produce a flare of skin lesions.

Systemic LE is managed by local treatment for any skin eruptions, plus various medications taken by mouth for such symptoms as arthritis, fever, rash, and kidney disease. Aspirin may be the only medicine prescribed by the physician. Because it is a common, well-known, and easily obtained medication, patients sometimes underestimate its usefulness.

Aspirin and NSAIDs. Aspirin is not merely a pain killer. When taken regularly, and as often as prescribed, such as 8 to 16 5-grain tablets daily, for adults, it frequently controls fever, pleurisy (painful breathing), and joint discomfort. Aspirin and the other anti-inflammatory medications discussed below should be used with caution in patients who have had stomach ulcers; rarely, internal bleeding may result. When possible, it is advisable to stop these medications 1 week before surgery because of their tendency to slow down blood clotting. Taking the tables with food or milk often eliminates the stomach upsets experienced by some patients. Antacids and a class of drugs known as H2 blockers (Tagamet, Zantac, Pepcid) or prostaglandins (Cytotec) and others (Prilosec; omeprazole) frequently help protect the stomach lining. NSAIDs, such as indomethacin (Indocin), naproxen (Naprosyn), or ibuprofen (Motrin), are frequently effective for relieving joint pains and pain at other sites of inflammation. Patients with kidney involvement should only take NSAIDs under close medical supervision.

Antimalarial Drugs. This group of medications was first developed during World War II for the treatment of malaria when it became known that quinine, which was then standard treatment for malaria, was in short supply. It was discovered that many patients with LE showed definite improvement after receiving the antimalarial drug atabrine, especially those who had skin changes of discoid LE, although these chemicals are also helpful in systemic types of LE. It should be emphasized that there is no relationship between LE and malaria (which is caused by a small parasite transmitted by mosquitos.) Table AP–1 lists the most commonly used antimalarial drugs.

Table AP–1. Antimalarial Drugs

Generic Name	Trade Name (Manufacturer)	Usual Tablet Size (mg)
Atabrine	Atabrine (Sonofi-Winthrop)	100
Chloroquine	Atalen (Sonofi-Winthrop)	500*
Hydroxychloroquine	Plaquenil (Sonofi-Winthrop)	200

* Also available in 250-mg, tablets from other manufacturers.

The exact mechanism of the antimalarial drugs in LE is not known. In many patients with systemic LE, the antimalarials appear to make it possible to reduce the total daily dose of cortisone drugs. Another advantage of antimalarials is that they increase resistance to sun exposure and block the appearance of SLE rashes on exposure to ultraviolet light. Antimalarials are not used for the management of patients with organ-threatening involvement (e.g., heart, lungs, kidney, liver), but are useful in managing skin, joint, and muscle symptoms as well as fever, fatigue, and pleurisy. These agents often do not take effect for several months.

Side effects of antimalarials in patients with LE do not often occur, but can be important. The most common side effects usually involve the digestive system with mild nausea, occasional vomiting, and diarrhea. Formerly, certain antimalarials, especially chloroquine (Aralen) and hydroxychloroquine (Plaquenil), were found to affect the eyes when used in doses twice as great as those now prescribed. Therefore, to be certain that no such bad effects occur, patients taking these medications must have eye examinations by an ophthalmologist at regular intervals of 4 to 6 months. Atabrine has not been reported to be a cause of eye complications. Any changes in vision should be called to the attention of your physician.

Corticosteroids. The corticosteroid drugs (such as prednisone) are used primarily for treating the internal changes caused by lupus, but they also help to heal the skin.

Cortisone and later hydrocortisone were the first of the corticosteroid family to be used in medicine, and they have been lifesaving in many thousands of patients with many different diseases. They are synthetic forms of hormones normally produced by the adrenal glands, which are the small glands above the kidneys. In addition to the beneficial effects of cortisone and hydrocortisone, however, these drugs have unwanted and undesirable side effects that may produce complications when the drugs are taken for long periods. Over the past half-century, experimental research by pharmaceutical companies has led to the development of a large family of drugs chemically related to cortisone (corticosteroid "cousins"), which has the beneficial effects of cortisone and fewer, less severe undesirable side-effects and complications than those that occur from the long use of cortisone (Table AP–2).

In some cases of systemic LE, the physician may choose to prescribe corticosteroid drugs every other day instead of daily. This method reduces side effects considerably, but may not be satisfactory for active cases.

The chief action of the corticosteroid drugs is to decrease inflammation, so that these drugs control many of the symptoms and signs of SLE that are caused by inflammatory changes, such as arthritis and pleurisy. The drugs may be given by mouth in the form of tablets, or by injection into the muscle or directly into the vein.*

Another effect of the synthetic cortisone drugs is their "shrinking effect" on the adrenal glands. This occurs be-

---

* When taking these hormones, some patients experience temporary personality changes caused by the medication. They should be reassured that they are not "going crazy."

Table AP–2. Average Equivalent Anti-Inflammatory Potencies of Cortisone and its Derivatives Based on Tablet Size*

Generic Name (Trade Name)	Equivalent Tablet Size (mg)
Cortisone acetate (Cortone)	25
Hydrocortisone (Hydrocortone; Cortef)	20
Prednisone (Meticorten; Deltra)	5
Prednisolone (Meticotelone, Hydeltra)	5
Methylprednisolone (Medrol)	4
Triamcinolone (Aristocort, Kenacort)	4
Dexamethasone (Decadron, Deronil)	0.75
Betamethasone (Celestone)	0.60
Fluprednisolone (Alphadrol)	1.5
Paramethasone (Haldrone)	2

* Although the tablet size corresponds to accepted clinical findings, only average individual potencies can be transferred from one steroid to another. These steroids may vary in strength, therefore, and daily clinical observation is necessary.

cause the adrenal glands may stop producing the natural hormone, which is of special importance for two reasons. First, the synthetic hormone should not be stopped suddenly, because the adrenal glands may take several months to start production of natural hormone again. A sudden withdrawal of the synthetic hormone leaves the patient without this support and may cause a serious crisis. Therefore, the dosage of the corticosteroids should be reduced gradually over several weeks or months, so that the patient's adrenal glands may increase their production of the natural hormone gradually over the same period. Second, any physical or mental stress, surgical procedure, dental extraction, or severe illness may increase the patient's need for large amounts of corticosteroids. When patient's have taken corticosteroids for a long time, their own adrenal glands cannot satisfy this increased need, and larger, "booster" doses of the synthetic drug are required.

Persons taking corticosteroid drugs, or those who have taken them during the previous year, should carry with them an identification card stating this fact for emergency use (much like the card carried by the diabetic person who must take insulin, or by a person who is extremely sensitive to penicillin).

These two points must be emphasized to every patient with SLE who is taking the corticosteroid groups of drugs: 1) the drug should never be stopped suddenly, but should gradually be reduced over a long period (this is best done under the direct supervision of a physician); and 2) when any patient is on long-term cortisone therapy, he or she may need increased booster doses of the drug before, during, and after any period of general body stresses (such as surgery), and should tell the physician or dentist of this possibility.

Because corticosteroids have an appetite-stimulating effect, an effort should be made to avoid excessive weight gain. Damage to weight-bearing joints may occur following long-term steroid treatment and occasionally in some patients with untreated SLE. In addition, steroids may induce diabetes, hypertension, cataracts, glaucoma, edema, avascular necrosis, bone demineralization, and ulcers.

Many powerful drugs are used in the treatment of severe SLE, such as immunosuppressives (antibody suppressors); these include azathioprine (Imuran), cyclophosphamide (Cytoxan), and nitrogen mustard. These drugs are most commonly used in those with aggressive kidney disease. Indications for the use of these agents are the subject of great deal of debate because they are toxic and their effectiveness has not always been demonstrated. Evidence from the National Institutes of Health suggests that intravenous, intermittent cyclophosphamide in combination with corticosteroids represents the treatment of choice for severe lupus nephritis. Plasma exchange (plasmapheresis) is a popular experimental procedure, but is very expensive and the results are only of uncertain benefit. Its use is reserved for those with life-threatening complications of lupus. Other agents occasionally used in LE are methotrexate, gamma globulin, danazol, chlorambucil, dapsone, and cyclosporine.

It is essential that once an effective treatment program has been started, the patient should continue the medication faithfully and not change it without the physician's advice. Severe flare-ups may occur suddenly in patients who stop their treatment abruptly.

Rest. This is important during the active phase of systemic LE. It is essential that, following a serious flare-up, patients resume normal activity *slowly* over a period of several months. A full night's sleep is essential, usually at least 8 to 10 hours. A morning and afternoon rest period or nap is helpful for the first few weeks or months after a flare-up. Patients must learn that, if they tire out after some activity, they probably tried to do too much and should have stopped sooner. For example, patients with systemic LE who feel well after 9 holes of golf should stop, rather than exhaust themselves after playing 18 holes.

Women with systemic LE require at least part-time household help for several weeks after leaving the hospital, particularly for heavy work. It is advisable for patients who have regular jobs to return to work on a half-time basis for the first few weeks.

Physicians monitor lupus patients by following their vital signs (pulse, weight, temperature, blood pressure), blood counts, and urine, and by doing a physical examination. In selected patients, following sedimentation rates, complement components, anti-DNA levels, or other autoantibodies may be useful. Physicians do not necessarily treat isolated laboratory abnormalities unless they fit in with the clinical picture.

Should the Patient with LE Avoid Excessive Sunlight?

The danger of sun exposure has been overemphasized in most reports. Newer effective sunscreens, which can be applied to the skin, are available. They should have at least a 15 SPF (sun protection factor). This means that a person is 15 times more protected than if no sunscreen were used. The sunscreens should also block both ultraviolet A and ultraviolet B (UVA and UVB) light (such as Ti-Screen and Photoplex). The average patient with either discoid or systemic LE, however, can go out during midday for 10 to 15 minutes without using sunscreens. The amount of protection necessary depends on whether skin lesions are present, and their location, and whether the patient has had previous sensitivity to sunlight. Excessive exposure, such as sunbathing, sitting for hours by the pool, fishing, or resting at the beach, even in the shade, may produce a mild flare-up, even in the treated patient, and should be avoided. Also to be avoided is reflected sunlight from water, sand, or snow, which may often go unnoticed until the damage has been done.

COPING WITH LE

Goals of this section:

1. To help you understand and accept your illness
2. To emphasize that you are not alone
3. To provide sources of help

When you learned that you had the rather mysterious disease lupus erythematosus you probably experienced feelings of anxiety, fear, and apprehension. You probably have never before even heard of the illness. Because there are many differences in the way the illness affects people, and because people differ in the way they react to problems, one person may be more upset at having lupus than another. Many social and emotional problems are associated with having a chronic disease such as LE. As explained in other sections of this appendix, lupus can be a mild illness, affecting only a small portion of the skin, or can be a more serious form, alternating with periods of feeling well. Therefore, when we discuss some of the emotionally frustrating aspects, remember that not everyone experiences all of these, and that there will be improvement as the disease improves and medication is reduced.

Some persons react to overwhelming fear by pretending that the condition does not exist. To acknowledge it seems impossible. Denial is sometimes thought of as courage, but actually it is unhealthy. To live intelligently with LE, the disease should be accepted, along with its limitations. Such acceptance may take time and perhaps counselling.

You may feel angry and depressed over the loss of your former good health. Along with pain from the illness itself, your appearance may change: skin lesions, weight gain or loss, facial rounding, and mood changes, sometimes aggravated by the medication.

It is important to discuss your doubts and fears with family, friends, or health personnel. The patients who come to our lupus clinics find it helpful to participate in group discussions with other patients and a psychiatric social worker. Feelings of frustration and other problems can be discussed, and possible solutions suggested. Family members can gain a better understanding of the illness when they attend such group sessions.

Several states have local chapters of lupus societies, such as those affiliated with the American Lupus Society (TALS). You may find that joining one of these groups is emotionally supportive. If no local group is in your area, perhaps you and your friends would be interested in forming one. Contact TALS for information.*

---

* 3914 Del Amo Boulevard Suite 922, Torrance, CA 90503. (310) 373-1335, or (800) 331-1802.

Occasionally you may feel discouraged because your family and friends do not understand your feelings of being tired when there may be no outward signs of your illness. At such times you should not try to continue your regular activities. You may find it necessary to drop out of school temporarily or to take a leave of absence from your job, and to obtain help with the housework. Perhaps other members of the family can help more with running the household.

An increased amount of rest is necessary for most lupus patients but rest may not mean complete inactivity, and limited employment is frequently permissible. Your physician should decide how much rest you need, and for how long. As your condition improves, activity can be increased. Just remember to take brief rest periods before you feel tired. Short rest periods are better than long ones. For instance, while doing housework, you could rest 5 minutes every half-hour. Don't do anything standing that you can do sitting. Alternate heavy tasks with light ones. Distribute heavy tasks over several days.

Frequent recreational activities are desirable for everyone, including LE patients. Such activities can include golf, tennis, dancing, and swimming, depending on your physician's evaluation of your current condition, and less strenuous activities, such as needlework, light carpentry, and walks. Whereas the importance of avoiding becoming overtired is emphasized, the opposite extreme—dwelling on your disease to the extend of becoming an emotional cripple—is not desirable either.

In a nutshell, therefore, concentrate on getting the best possible medical treatment. Take medication regularly, and generally follow your physician's recommendations.

Eat a good diet, and keep regular hours.
Have a calm, stable environment, as much as possible.

Be aware that tension affects the disease. Many patients note the beginning of symptoms following events such as a death in the family, a separation, or some other emotional shock.

The following is a partial list of places and people that can help you with various problems connected with your illness:

1. *Your physician.* If you should move to a new area, there are several ways to locate a physician familiar with LE. A rheumatologist is a physician with special training in the diagnosis and treatment of patients with rheumatic conditions, including lupus. Most dermatologists are well trained in managing discoid lupus. If you have the systemic form (SLE), contact the Department of Medicine of your nearest medical school for recommendations. Individual lupus societies may also have lists, as do your local arthritis foundation and The American Lupus Society.
2. *Clergyman.* Religious consolation often means much to those who are depressed and ill.
3. *Social workers.* Hospital and public welfare agencies can help with social problems, living arrangements, and provisions for care and supervision at home.
4. *Vocational rehabilitation counselors.* They have various resources at their command, particularly training for new occupations and location of job openings.
5. *Physical and occupational therapists.* They help the handicapped to learn self-care activities, among other things.
6. *Visiting Nurse Association.* These nurses can help with follow-up health care, checking blood pressure, and giving medications.
7. *City and county parks and recreation departments.* These can provide various recreational activities.
8. *Local chapter of lupus societies.* This consist of lupus patients, their families, friends, and others.

To summarize:

Do:
  Rest.
  Follow your physician's advice.
  Avoid excessive sun exposure.
  When planning surgery or dental procedures, tell your dentist or surgeon that you are taking steroids or aspirin and have them call your treating physician.
  Remember that steroids are as important in lupus as insulin is in diabetes.
  Allow some time for recreation.

Do not:
  Get exhausted.
  Stop medications abruptly, particularly steroids.
  Dwell excessively on your illness to the point of becoming an emotional cripple.
  Believe every "popular" article on LE by the news media.

IS THERE HOPE OF CONQUERING SYSTEMIC LE?

There certainly is! A great deal of fast-moving research is going on throughout the world. Medical scientists are interested in systemic lupus, not only because they want to help those suffering from it, but also because they want to find the key to other closely related rheumatic disorders, such as rheumatoid arthritis. We expect laboratory research to improve methods of treatment and eventually provide a means of prevention and cure. In 1963, a strain of New Zealand mice was found to develop a disease picture resembling that of human systemic LE. Studies on these animals have already shown that certain drugs that prevent antibody formation can arrest the disease. The fact that animals can be used for laboratory experiments allows scientists to test new drugs and theories that medical ethics would prohibit being tried in patients. Thus, mice can serve as "guinea pigs," not the patient. For example, the intermittent multiple drug therapies now used in people with severe lupus nephritis were developed using this mouse model of human disease. Manipulations in steps critical to immune regulation and intervention involving circulating glycoproteins known as cytokines have brought us closer to studying new classes of drugs and developing antilupus vaccines. These and other leads provided by laboratory studies can be translated into better patient care in the future.

COMMON QUESTIONS

Q: Is LE inherited?

A: There is an increased incidence of rheumatoid arthritis and abnormalities of blood proteins in the families of patients with systemic LE. Many relatives have abnormal antibodies with no symptoms of LE. Approximately 8% of sisters and mothers of patients with SLE may also develop the disease. Because SLE in men is rare, the chances are low of a brother or father having the disorder.

Q: Do more females than males have LE?

A: Seventy percent of patients with discoid LE are women, and as are 90% of those with systemic LE. The reason for the high incidence in females is unknown. On the other hand, LE caused by medications occurs with equal frequency in both sexes.

Q: Can women with LE have children?

A: In discoid LE, there should be no problem with pregnancy, provided that the patient is not receiving antimalarial drugs. The effects of these medicines on the unborn child are not well known, so they should be stopped some months prior to beginning pregnancy. Most women with systemic LE can have successful pregnancies, but the occurrence of late complications, such as toxemia and premature births, is somewhat higher than in normal pregnancies. If SLE is in remission and no significant kidney and heart damage is present, pregnancy can be considered. The course of the illness during pregnancy is unpredictable. Many women feel better during pregnancy, and the doses of steroids required may be reduced and even discontinued by the last 3 months. Occasionally, some women become worse during pregnancy. After childbirth mild flares often occur, which may require taking the medication that was used prior to the pregnancy. It is important to consider that having a child to manage may prevent getting adequate rest. The question of pregnancy and additional stress should be discussed frankly with the physician.

Q: Is it advisable to avoid sun exposure?

A: The degree of sun sensitivity has to be evaluated individually. Most patients with discoid and systemic LE can walk several blocks without even using sunscreens. Some patients have no difficulty despite extensive sun exposure, whereas others may note flares of skin lesions or even systemic (overall) complaints after brief periods of exposure to sunlight.

Q: I have always enjoyed outdoor activities, such as tennis and horseback riding. Will I have to give these up?

A: Many patients can enjoy active sports during remissions as long as they do not exercise to the point of exhaustion.

Q: Why has my doctor prescribed only aspirin, up to 20 tablets daily, for my LE?

A: Aspirin is not only a painkiller, but has a direct effect on inflammatory changes in tissues. In large doses it acts similarly to corticosteroids, and reduces the amount of other medications required.

Q: Is it all right for me to have immunizations or vaccinations, such as flu or tetanus shots?

A: When the disease is in remission, there is no reason to avoid necessary immunizations, including live polio vaccine. During active periods of the disease, with such symptoms as fever or joint aches, it is not advisable for the patient to be further stressed by immunizations, particularly if receiving large doses of steroids. Immunizations may be less effective in SLE patients.

Q: Is LE localized to any particular region or country?

A: No. LE occurs worldwide. Because of its well-known flare-ups after sunburn, many patients ask if it safe to move to warmer climates. The answer is that there is no higher incidence of LE occurs in the southern United States, for example, than in the north. We have no evidence for "clusters" of LE patients in one region or another. This applies to all types of LE, according to current information.

Q: After reading some literature on LE, I believe that my daughter might have the disease. Where should I take her for an examination?

A: See Appendix II.

GLOSSARY

Acute   Of short duration

Adrenal glands   small organs, located above the kidney, that produce many hormones, including corticosteroids and epinephrine

Albuminuria   A protein in urine

Analgesic   An agent that alleviates pain

Anemia   Low red blood cell count

Antibodies   Special protein substances made by the body for defense against bacteria and other foreign substances

Antigen   A protein that produces antibodies

Anti-inflammatory   An agent that counteracts or suppresses inflammation

Antimalarial   A drug used for malaria, but also helpful in lupus

Antinuclear antibodies (ANA)   Proteins in the blood that react with nuclei of cells

Arthralgia   Pain in a joint

Arthritis   Inflammation of a joint

Aspirin   An analgesic that in adequate doses controls inflammation (it is more than a painkiller)

Autoimmune   Allergy to one's own tissues

Biopsy   Removal of a bit of tissue for examination under the microscope

Buffered   Neutralized

Butterfly rash   Reddish facial eruption over the

bridge of the nose and cheeks, resembling a butterfly in flight

Chronic   Persisting over a long period of time

Collagen   A series of proteins in the blood that are consumed in antigen-antibody reactions

Complement   A group of proteins that plays a major role in mediating inflammation

Corticosteroid   Any steroid produced by the adrenal cortex; also, a synthetic equivalents

Cortisone   An early synthetic corticosteroid (also called a steroid), including cortisone, hydrocortisone, prednisone, prednisolone, methylprednisone, triamcinolone, dexamethasone, paramethasone, betamethasone, and fluprednisolone

Creatinine clearance test   Test of kidney function

Dermatologist   A physician specializing in skin diseases

Discoid LE   Lupus erythematosus affecting primarily the skin

DNA (deoxyribonucleic acid)   A type of nucleic acid occurring in the cell nuclei

Erythematosus   Red

Exacerbation   Symptoms reappear; another word for flare

False-positive serologic test for syphilis (STS)   A blood test that reveals an antibody that may be found in syphilis; test result may be falsely positive in people with LE

Fibrositis (fibromyalgia)   A pain amplification syndrome characterized by fatigue, a sleep disorder, and tender points in the soft tissues; can be mistaken for lupus, and 20% with lupus have fibrositis

Flare   Symptoms reappear (another word for exacerbation)

FANA test   Fluorescent antinuclear antibody test; method of demonstrating antibodies that might be directed toward the nuclear materials in a patient's own cells in the blood; test is positive in more than 90% of people having SLE, but also may be positive in other diseases, as well as in normal people

Hemoglobin (Hbg)   Oxygen-carrying protein in red blood cells

Inflammation   Swelling, heat, redness

Intern   Medical school graduate serving in a hospital preparatory to being licensed to practice medicine

Kidney biopsy   Removal of a bit of kidney tissue for microscopic analyses

Lupus anticoagulant   With or without the presence of a false-positive syphilis test or cardiolipin antibody, this represents prolonged clotting times caused by an antiphospholipid antibody

LE cell   Specific cell found in blood specimens of 60 to 90% of patients with SLE, but much less often in patients with closely related diseases

Lupus vulgaris   Tuberculosis of the skin; not related to systemic or discoid LE

Plasmapheresis   Filtration of blood plasma by a machine to remove proteins that may aggravate lupus

Pleurisy   Inflammation of the lining of the cavity containing the lungs (also called pleuritis)

Prednisone, prednisolone   Synthetic corticosteroids levels

Proteinuria   Excess serum protein levels in the urine (also called albuminuria)

Pulse steroids   Giving very high doses of corticosteroids intravenously over 1 to 3 days to critically ill patients

RBC   Red blood cell count

Remission   Quiet period, free from symptoms, but not necessarily a cure

Rheumatoid arthritis   Chronic disease of the joints marked by inflammatory changes in the joint-lining membranes, which may have positive and ANA tests

Sedimentation rate   Test that measures the precipitation of red cells in a column of blood; high rate usually indicates increased activity; but in SLE it may be persistently elevated

Serum   Clear liquid portion of the blood

Steroids   Usually, a shortened term for corticosteroids, which are anti-inflammatory hormones (natural or synthetic) produced by the adrenal cortex

STS   Serologic test for syphilis (see above, false-positive STS)

Synthetic   Artificially made

Systemic   Pertaining to or affecting the body as a whole

Titer   Amount of a substance, such as antinuclear antibody or complement

Urinalysis   Analysis of urine

Urine, 24-hour collection   All urine passed in a 24-hour period is collected and examined for protein and creatinine to determine how well kidneys are functioning

WBC   White blood cell count

Appendix II

LUPUS RESOURCE MATERIALS FOR PATIENTS, PHYSICIANS, AND MEDICAL PERSONNEL

LINDA J. ROSINSKY
DANIEL J. WALLACE

Many lupus patients, physicians, and allied health personnel request informational literature about lupus. Today a wide range of publications is available. The variety of this lupus material spans from the personal life story narratives that captivate the lupus patient to the technical treatises of experimental lupus research that intrigue the physician. The quality and accuracy of some publications are questionable. Medical information is always in a changing state. We have sought to present a representative sampling of lupus material in different media as it mirrors our current state of knowledge. The materials listed here can be obtained singly from the sources listed. Unfortunately, space limitations prohibit a complete listing of all available materials. An expanded listing of sources can be found by obtaining the publication Lupus Resource Guide: For Patients and Professionals, available through the Lupus Network. Listings of fact sheets, smaller articles, and copyable pieces can be found in Lupus: Patient Education Materials, and in Lupus: Professional Education Materials, both produced by the AMS Information Clearinghouse (see below).

ORGANIZATIONS (UNITED STATES)

Included are organizations that disseminate lupus literature and/or promote lupus research; publications distributed by such organizations are also listed.

American College of Rheumatology (ACR), 60 Executive Park South, Suite 150, Atlanta, GA 30329, (404) 633-3777. The ACR, formerly called the American Rheumatism Association, is a professional organization comprised of physicians and scientists (rheumatologists, orthopedists, physical medicine specialists) devoted to the study and treatment of rheumatic diseases, including lupus. The ACR publishes Arthritis and Rheumatism (official publication), A & R supplements, special issues, and other professionally oriented publications.

Arthritis Foundation (AF), 1314 Spring Street NW, Atlanta, GA 30309, (404) 872-7100 or 1-800-283-7800. The AF, which has about 72 chapters in the United States, works to help patients with rheumatic diseases and their doctors through programs of research, patient services, health information, and professional education and training. The AHPA (Arthritis Health Professionals Association) and the AJAO (American Juvenile Arthritis Organization) are groups that work as part of the AF. The AF publishes

a 20-page basic information pamphlet on SLE, as well as numerous pamphlets on topics relating to lupus, such as corticosteroid medications, NSAIDs, aspirin, guide to laboratory tests, and others. The AF also publishes Arthritis Today (official magazine) and Bulletin on the Rheumatic Diseases, a professionally oriented newsletter. Individual chapters also publish their own newsletters. The AF also offers a Systemic Lupus Erythematosus Self-Help Course in selected areas of the country. This 7-week education program includes courses that provides information, skills, and support to persons with lupus and their family to help them cope with the disease.

1. Neil, A. J.: Meeting the Challenge: A Young Person's Guide to Living With Lupus, Atlanta, Arthritis Foundation, 1990, 50 pp. This booklet is written in simple terms, and is aimed at the adolescent with lupus. Its purpose is to help teenagers or young adults learn about their illness and how to take care of themselves. Interspersed throughout are quotes from youngsters with lupus, making the booklet more personal.

L. E. Support Club, 8039 Nova Court, North Charleston, SC 29420, (803) 764-1769. The L. E. Support Club is a patient-oriented organization, that publishes the L. E. Beacon (official newsletter), supplies information on drugs, and maintains and distributes a listing of recommended physicians.

Lupus Foundation of America, Inc. (LFA), 4 Research Place, Suite 180, Rockville, MD, 20850-3226, (301) 670-9292 or 1-800-558-0121. The LFA, which has about 100 chapters, provides patient education and public awareness and funds lupus research. The LFA publishes Lupus News (official newsletter) and the individual chapters distribute their own newsletters and often other pieces of literature. The LFA also produces the Facts About Lupus series—a series of pamphlets on individual topics, including neurologic disease and lupus, what is lupus, depression and lupus, and genetic origins of lupus. These are fold-out pamphlets, with variable pages and dates; the entire series, when complete, should number around 15 pamphlets. The following are some publications available through the LFA or its chapters:

1. Aladjem, H.: Understanding Lupus, New York, Charles Scribner's Sons, 1985, 287 pp. Written in conjunction with 30 lupus experts, this book is a comprehensive guide to lupus geared toward the patient.

2. Aladjem, H.: A Patient's Story, Lupus Foundation of America, Rockville, MD, 1986, 15 pp. This booklet presents the fictionalized story of a lupus patient—her symptoms, diagnosis, treatment, emotional reaction, and acceptance of the disease (extremely easy reading).

3. Aladjem, H.: A Decade of Lupus, Lupus Foundation of America, Rockville, MD, 1991, 178 pp. This book is a potpourri of articles on various topics that were originally published in Lupus News over the past 10 years. Topics span psychologic, clinical, and research aspects of lupus, including select pieces and interjections about the work of the LFA and its key personnel.

4. Aladjem, H., and Schur, P.H.: In Search of the Sun: A Woman's Courageous Victory Over Lupus, New York, Charles Scribner's Sons, 1988, 264 pp. This book chronicles the life story of Aladjem, from her first initial symptoms of lupus to her final triumph of remission. Interspersed among the chapters of her personal story are chapters written by Dr. Peter H. Schur, a lupus specialist. These chapters highlight a particular concern in the preceding chapter.

5. Butler, B.: The Monster Under the Bed: Child Rearing When a Parent Is Chronically Ill, 1990, 30 pp. This booklet is geared toward the parent with a chronic illness, with special insight and examples given by the author, a lupus patient with three children. Available from the Missouri Chapter, LFA, Del Crest Plaza Building, 8420 Delmar Boulevard, St. Louis, MO 63124.

6. Carr, R.I.: Lupus Erythematosus: A Handbook for Physicians, Patients, and Their Families, 2nd ed., 1986, 60 pp. This booklet presents an overview of lupus, with emphasis on SLE, in well-delineated sections that are easy to understand for the lupus patient (also available in Spanish).

7. Nass, T.: Lupus Erythematosus: Handbook For Nurses, 2nd Ed., 1985, 54 pp. This looseleaf book provides an overview of lupus, describes nursing care using a systems approach (e.g., blood, eye, kidney), provides an approach to patient teaching records (salicylates, NSAIDs, antimalarials, steroids, cytotoxic drugs, lupus), includes a chapter on laboratory tests used in the diagnosis and evaluation of SLE, and discusses psychologic implications of lupus. Available from the Bay Area Lupus Foundation, LFA, 2635 North First Street, Suite 206, San Jose, CA 95134.

8. Phillips, R.H.: Coping With Lupus, Avery Publishing Group, 1984, 256 pp. This book, written by a psychologist, is a guidebook to coping with lupus. The material is comprehensive, ranging from emotional aspects to medications to interacting with people. Many useful and practical solutions to problems are presented. Wayne, NJ, Avery Publishers.

9. Pitzele, S.K.: We Are Not Alone: Learning To Live With Chronic Illness. New York, Workman Publishing, 1986, 320 pp. This book provides a well-organized compendium of information on dealing with chronic illness, covering a vast array of topics ranging from emotional aspects to practical concerns. A large appendix lists names of contacts that are useful in finding help.

10. Walters, J.M.: Introduction to Lupus and Disability Issues, 1990, 114 pp. This booklet serves as an introduction to the complexities of applying for social security disability income (SSDI) benefits, with an emphasis on lupus. Also covered are appeals and reviews, applying for social security supplemental income (SSI), Medicare, Medicaid, COBRA, Catastrophic Health Insurance, and Americans With Disabilities Act. Available from the LFA, Greater Atlanta Chapter, 2814 New Spring Road, Suite 102, Atlanta, GA 30339-3036.

11. Moore, M.E., McGrory, C.H., Rosenthal, R.S. (editors): Learning About Lupus: A User-Friendly Guide, 1991, 86 pp. This booklet contains 20 chapters covering various aspects of lupus. Especially helpful for the newly diagnosed patient who wants to learn the basics. It is available from the Lupus Foundation of Delaware Valley, Inc., 44 West Lancaster Ave., Ardmore, PA 19003.

Lupus Network, Inc. (LN), 230 Ranch Drive, Bridgeport, CT 06606, (203) 372-5795. The LN is an organization that provides information primarily to patients. It supports the sharing of information, whether unorthodox or orthodox in nature. The LN publishes Heliogram (official newsletter). It also has a large literature list that covers many lupus topics, such as photosensitivity, cyclophosphamide, and pregnancy.

1. Rosinsky, L.J.: Lupus Resource Guide: For Patients and Professionals, Lupus Network, Bridgeport, CT, 1990, 55 pp. This is a comprehensive guidebook to information on lupus (organizations, foreign organizations, foreign language listings, patient- and professional-oriented literature, audio-visual materials, and lupus educational programs). Items listed can be purchased singly from the source listed.

National Arthritis and Musculoskeletal and Skin Diseases Information Clearinghouse (AMS Information Clearinghouse), Box AMS, 9000 Rockville Pike, Bethesda, MD 20892, (301) 495-4484. The AMS Information Clearinghouse Identifies, collects, processes, and disseminates information about print and audio-visual materials concerned with arthritis and musculoskeletal and skin diseases. It is used by physicians, nurses, allied health professionals, health educators, librarians, mental health and social workers, and patients and their families. The AMS Clearinghouse provides a variety of bibliographies, maintains a mailing list for distribution of the Clearinghouse Memo (official newsletter), answers reference questions, and provides information in response to user requests. The AMS Information Clearinghouse also maintains an on-line bibliographic data base of information on CHID (Combined Health Information Database) through BRS, an on-line vendor.

1. AMS Information Clearinghouse: Lupus: Patient Education Materials, Rockville, MD, AMS Information Clearinghouse, 1990. This annotated bibliography contains 148 citations of educational materials for patients and their families about the symptoms, diagnosis, and treatment of lupus. Included in the bibliography are sources of brochures, fact sheets, pamphlets, books, pertinent newsletter and journal articles, and audio-visual materials.

2. AMS Information Clearinghouse: Lupus: Professional Educational Materials, Rockville, MD, AMS Information Clearinghouse, 1990. This annotated bibliography contains citations published since 1985. Its purpose is to provide information sources on lupus for the primary care physician, nurse, or other allied health professional.

National Institute of Arthritis and Musculoskeletal and Skin Diseases (NIAMS), Building 31, Room 4C05, 9000 Rockville Pike, Bethesda, MD 20892, (301) 496-8188. NIAMS is part of the National Institutes of Health (NIH). The NIAMS leads, coordinates, stimulates, conducts, and supports the national biomedical research effort on a broad range of diseases and long-lasting disabling conditions in the field of rheumatology (e.g., systemic lupus erythematosus, rheumatoid arthritis), orthopedics, bone and mineral metabolism, muscle biology, and dermatology. NIAMS publishes reprints and brochures available to the general public. Research Briefings (official publication) is sent to a select "user" group. A listing of NIAMS Multipurpose Arthritis and Musculoskeletal Diseases Centers is also available.

1. NIAMS: Update: Lupus Erythematosus Research, Bethesda, NIAMS, 1986, 45 pp. This booklet contains a report covering lupus research between 1983 and 1986.

2. NIAMS Task Force on Lupus in High-Risk Populations *What Black Women Should Know About Lupus Kit*, Bethesda, MD, NIAMS, not dated.

3. NIAMS: Lupus Resource Kit, Bethesda, NIAMS (in preparation). This two-pocket folder contains information addressed primarily to black women of childbearing age who may have lupus or symptoms of the disease) in an effort to raise their awareness of lupus. It contains a letter of introduction, a clipsheet of the butterfly logo, a basic information brochure, a lupus fact sheet, an article suitable for organizational newsletters, a suggested activities list, and a feedback form.

Terri Gotthelf Lupus Research Institute (TGLRI), 50 Washington Street, South Norwalk, CT 06854, (203) 852-0120 or 1-800-825-8787. The TGLRI promotes research to find the cause and cure for lupus, provides financial support for lupus researchers, and carries out a program of public and professional education on lupus.

Callers are offered assistance in finding treatment or obtaining information on lupus. The TGLRI publishes periodic reports for supporters and scholars.

The American Lupus Society (TALS), 3914 Del Amo Boulevard, Suite 922, Torrance, CA 90503, (310) 542-8891 or 1-800-331-1802. TALS, which has chapters all over the United States, assists lupus patients and their families in coping with the disease, and is involved in programs to foster public awareness of lupus. TALS also obtains funds for lupus research. TALS publishes Lupus Today (official newsletter) and TALS chapters publish their own newsletters. Additional materials from TALS and its chapters include the following:

1. Epstein, L., and Romoff, B.: So Now You Have Lupus, (not dated), 20 pp. This booklet is an aid to understanding the psychologic aspects of lupus. It describes many specific lupus emotional problems and comments on many areas, such as stress, depression, sexuality, adjustment, and family involvement.

2. Hindman, A.: Tell Me About Lupus: A Booklet for Young People, 1991, 8 pp. This booklet, geared toward the young child with lupus, is simply worded and easy to understand. A number of drawings that illustrate the principles accent the booklet.

3. Hughes, G.R.V.: Lupus: A Guide for Patients, Lupus Clinic, Rheumatology Department, St. Thomas Hospital, London (not dated), 24 pp. This booklet offers a wide range of lupus information, including what is lupus, history, clinical features, symptoms, pregnancy, and treatment, presented in an upbeat manner.

4. Wallace, D.J., Quismorio, F.P., and Cox, M.B.: Lupus Erythematosus, 1990, 18 pp. This booklet covers many aspects of lupus and is presented in a simplified, nontechnical way for the lupus patient. It provides a good introduction to lupus (also available in Spanish).

5. The American Lupus Society, San Diego County Chapter. A Rash of Creativity, 1989, 49 pp. This is a booklet of poetry, prose, and drawings by lupus patients, revealing a wide range of feelings about living with lupus. It is available from TALS, San Diego County Chapter, P.O. Box 837, El Cajon, CA 92022.

INTERNATIONAL ORGANIZATIONS

To obtain a complete listing, contact the Lupus Foundation of America, Attn: International Associates.

Lupus Canada, Box 3302, Station B, Calgary, Alberta T2M 4L8, Canada, 1-800-661-1468 (in Canada only). This is an umbrella organization for many Canadian lupus organizations.

1. Senecal, J.: Lupus: The Disease With A Thousand Faces, Alberta, Canada, Lupus Canada, 1990, 56 pp. This booklet answers some basic questions about systemic lupus, particularly its symptoms, treatments, and effects. The information is easy to find and understand.

B.C. Lupus Association, 895 W. 10th Avenue, Vancouver, British Columbia. V5Z 1L7, Canada, (604) 879-7511.

Lupus Society of Quebec, 3575 Boulevard, St. Laurent, Suite 242, Montreal, Quebec H2X 2T7, Canada, (514) 849-0955.

L.E. Society of Saskatchewan, Box 88, University Hospital, Saskatoon, Saskatchewan S7N 0W0, Canada, (306) 922-5272.

Lupus Foundation of Ontario, 289 Ridge Road, North, Box 687, Ridgeway, Ontario L0S 1N0, Canada, (416) 894-4611.

Ontario Lupus Association, 250 Bloor Street East, Suite 401, Toronto, Ontario M4W 3P2, Canada, (416) 967-1414.

Lupus New Brunswick, Box 429, McAdam, New Brunswick E0H 1K0, Canada, (506) 784-3203.

L.E. Society of Alberta, Box 8154, Station F, Calgary, Alberta T2J 2V3, Canada, (403) 233-8696.

Lupus Society of Manitoba, R.R. 3, Carman, Manitoba R0G 0J0, Canada, (204) 745-2447.

Lupus Society of Hamilton, Jackson Station, P.O. Box 57414, Hamilton, Ontario L8P 4X2, Canada, (416) 527-2252.

Lupus Society of Nova Scotia, 71 Penhorne Drive, Dartmouth, Nova Scotia B2W 1K8, Canada, (902) 462-1829.

Lupus Society of Newfoundland, Box 8824, Manuels, Newfoundland. A1X 1C4, Canada.

Lupus Society of Prince Edward Island, 90 Goodwill Avenue, Charlottetown, Prince Edward Island, C1A 3E5, Canada, (902) 894-8213.

British SLE Aid Group, "Rookery Nook," 17 Monkhams Drive, Woodford Green, Essex 1G8 0LG, England, (709) 834-9365.

United Kingdom Lupus Group, 5 Grosvenor Crescent, London, SWIX 7ER, England, 01-235-0902.

Club de Lupus Centro Medico de Occidente, Pedro Buzeta 870-B, 44660 Guadalajara, Jalisco, Mexico, 41.43.05 or 16.01.32.

PATIENT-ORIENTED LUPUS LITERATURE

1. Hicks, R.: Butterflies and Sunshine, 1984, 12 pp. This booklet, written in simple terms, is geared toward teenagers with SLE to help them understand the disease. Hopefully, teenager's can be helped to deal with this condition so that they may live a happy and satisfying life. Available from Kapiolani Women's and Children's Medical Center, 1319 Punahou Street, Honolulu, HI 96826.

2. Permut, J.B.: Embracing the Wolf, Marietta, GA, Cherokee Publishing, 1989, 175 pp. This book is the personal narrative of a lupus patient, with emphasis on the relationship of the patient to her family (primarily the husband) and how lupus intertwines itself intimately into this relationship.

3. Brown, B.D.: I Choose To Live, Nashville, Winston-Derek, 1990, 184 pp. This book is the personal narrative of a healthy, happy woman who, in the prime of her life, is stricken with SLE. The book reveals Brown's insightful account of her struggles with lupus and the compilation of strategies that help her to live and be happy once more.

4. Epstein, W.V., and Clewley, G.: Living With SLE, 1990, 20 pp. This booklet gives an overview of systemic lupus erythematosus that is especially important in acquainting new patients with the disease. Various aspects of lupus are discussed, such as diagnosis, symptoms, medications, and emotional impact. It is clear and easy to read, and has a calm and reassuring tone. Available from Millberry Union Bookstore, University of California, San Francisco, Box 0230, 500 Parnassus Avenue, San Francisco, CA 94143.

5. Reinertsen, J.L.: Lupus and You, 1986, 31 pp. This booklet was written to help people with lupus understand what lupus is, what effects it might have on their lives, and what they can do to help themselves and their physicians manage the disease. It emphasizes a positive approach to lupus management and the important role of patients and their families in that management. Available from the Arthritis Center, Park Nicollet Medical Foundation, 5000 West 39th Street, Minneapolis, MN 55416.

6. Radziunas, E.: Lupus: My Search For A Diagnosis, Claremont, CA, Hunter House, 1989, 128 pp. This book is a personal narrative of one woman's search for a diagnosis of lupus. The book candidly, describes in a friendly and easy-to-read manner, the paths, problems, and emotional turmoil that can go into a obtaining a diagnosis of SLE.

7. Chester, L.: Lupus Novice, Barrytown, NY, Station Hill Press, 1987, 192 pp. This book is a personal narrative of one woman's coping with lupus, both physically and spiritually. It discusses orthodox and unorthodox therapies in the treatment of lupus, with emphasis on homeopathy and its beneficial effect on the disease. The author, a poet, streams long, literary descriptions of feelings and events throughout the book.

8. Duren, J.: My Bout With Lupus: A Healing From The Son, Inglewood, CA, Duren Enterprises, 1985, 97 pp. This book is a personal narrative of one woman's bout with lupus, with emphasis on the involvement of the spiritual side of the author's nature and how it helped her cope not only with lupus, but with much tragedy and adversity in her life.

9. Hamil-Talman, D.: Heartsearch: Toward Healing Lupus, Berkeley, CA, North Atlantic Books, 1991, 231 pp. This book is a personal account of one individual's search to discover why she developed lupus. It is written by a psychotherapist, who describes in great detail her psychologic self-odyssey and the complex relationship between personality and illness.

10. Szasz S. Living With It. Buffalo, NY: Prometheus Books, 1991, 243 pp. This book is a personal narrative of a woman who was diagnosed with systemic lupus at the age of 13. The story revolves around living with a chronic illness with emphasis on tak-

ing responsibility for the management of that illness.

PROFESSIONAL-ORIENTED LUPUS LITERATURE

1. Lahita, R.G. (ed.): Systemic Lupus Erythematosus, New York, 2nd Ed, Churchill-Livingstone, 1992, 1000 pp.
2. Ropes, M.W.: Systemic Lupus Erythematosus, Cambridge, MA, Harvard University Press, 1976, 224 pp.
3. Klippel, J.H. (ed): Systemic Lupus Erythematosus, (Rheumat. Dis. Clin. North Am.), Philadelphia, W.B. Saunders, April 1988, 252 pp.
4. Schur, P.H. (ed): The Clinical Management of Systemic Lupus Erythematosus, Philadelphia, Grune & Stratton, 1983, 304 pp.

Major Rheumatology Textbooks

1. Kelley, W.N., Harris, E.D., Ruddy, S., and Sledge, C.B. (eds.): Textbook of Rheumatology, 3rd ed., Philadelphia, W.B. Saunders, 1989, 2,144 pp.
2. McCarty, D.J. (ed.): Arthritis and Allied Conditions: A Textbook of Rheumatology, 11th ed., Malvern, PA, Lea & Febiger, 1989, 2,045 pp.

AUDIO-VISUAL RESOURCES

1. Cooper, J., MacKallor, M., et al.: Lupus, 1982. This program, for newly diagnosed lupus patients, acquaints them with systemic lupus erythematosus, including symptoms, treatment, and suggestions for adapting their lifestyles. Graphic drawings complement the easy-to-understand language. The format is 52 slides and 1 audiocassette, plus script (11 minutes), or ¾-in. videocassette or ½-in. VHS or Beta videocassette. Available from Therapy Graphics, 1212 Via Coronel, Palos Verdes Estates, CA 90274.
2. Lupus Erythematosus Society of Alberta: Lupus: Disease In Disguise, 1990. This program contains two segments, medical information and patient support. Segment One deals with items such as possible causes, treatment, and research outlook of lupus. Segment Two contains patient vignettes and information on support groups. The format is ½-in. VHS videocassette (23 minutes) and comes in two versions. Available from Lupus Erythematosus Society of Alberta, Box 8154, Station F, Calgary, Alberta T2J 2V3, Canada.

3. Gill, W., and Gill, E.: Lupus: Insights, Emotions, Encouragement, 1987. This program features discussions with physicians, nurses, patients, and families of patients, and focuses on strategies for living and building constructive relationships. The format is ¾-in. videocassette or ½-in. VHS videocassette (54 minutes); a shorter version of this video (14 minutes) is also available. Available from Lupus Video, c/o Betty Goodwin, 2830 Churchill Drive, Columbus, OH 43221.
4. University of Calgary: Systemic Lupus Erythematosus: A Brighter Tomorrow, 1983. This program was produced with the primary objective of educating and informing newly diagnosed lupus patients about the nature of their disease, its varied symptomatic presentations, and the outlook for the future. The program is based of the experiences of a young teacher and housewife. The format is ¾-in. videocassette, or ½-in. VHS or Beta videocassette, or 16-mm film (45 minutes). Available from the University of Calgary, Productions Accounts Coordinator, Department of Communications Media, Mackimmie Library, Room 24, 2500 University Drive NW, Calgary, Alberta T2N 1N4, Canada.
5. Bay Area Lupus Foundation, LFA: SLE: The Great Deceiver, 1986. This program was produced primarily for newly diagnosed patients and their families. It informs patients of the medical facts, potential problems, and management of SLE, as well as how to build better communication with family and significant others. The format is ¾-in. U-Matic, ½-in. VHS or Beta-Max II videocassette, or 110 35-mm slides with audiocassette (30 minutes), color. Available from the Bay Area Lupus Foundation, LFA, 2635 North First Street, Suite 206, San Jose, CA 95134.
6. Dooley, E. J. Bole, G. G., and Edwards, N. L.: Systemic Lupus Erythematosus: It Means Some Changes, 1981. This program provides insight about how four patients have coped with systemic lupus erythematosus. The patients discuss their reactions to the diagnosis, symptoms, medications, and the emotional impact of the illness on themselves and their families. The format is ¾-in. or ½-in. videocassette (plus discussion guide; 26 minutes). Available from the University of Michigan Media Library, University of Michigan Medical Campus, R4440 Kresge I/0518, Ann Arbor, MI 48109.

Section IX

BIBLIOGRAPHY

Separate copies of this bibliography are available from The American Lupus Society.

ALPHABETIZED BIBLIOGRAPHY

A

A1. Aarden LA, de Groot ER, Feltkamp TEW. Immunobiology of DNA. III. Crithidia lucilliae: a simple substrate for the detection of anti-dsDNA with the immunofluorescence technique. Ann N Y Acad Sci 1975;254:505–515.

A2. Abdou NI, Lindsley HB, Pollak A, Stechschulte DJ, Wood G. Plasmapheresis in active systemic lupus erythematosus: effects on clinical, serum and cellular abnormalities [case report]. Clin Immunol Immunopathol 1981 Apr;19:44–54.

A3. Abdou NI, Sagawa A, Pascual E, Herbert J, Sadeghee S. Suppressor T-cell abnormality in idiopathic systemic lupus erythematosus. Clin Immunol Immunopathol 1976 Sep;6: 192–199.

A4. Abdou NI, Verdirame JD, Amare M, Abdou NL. Heterogeneity of pathogenetic mechanisms in aplastic anemia. Efficacy based on in vitro results. Ann Intern Med 1981;95:43–50.

A5. Abdou NI, Wall H, Lindsley HB, Halsey JF, Suzuki T. Network theory in autoimmunity. In vitro suppression of serum anti-DNA antibody binding to DNA by anti-idiotypic antibody in SLE. J Clin Invest 1981 May;67:1297–1304.

A6. Abe R, Vacchio MS, Fox B, Hodes RJ. Preferential expression of the T-cell receptor V-beta-3 gene by Mlsc reactive T cells. Nature 1988;335:827–830.

A7. Abe T, Homma M. Immunological reactivity in patients with systemic lupus erythematosus. Humoral antibody and cellular immune responses. Acta Rheumatol Scand 1971:17:35–46.

A8. Abel T, Gladman DD, Urowitz MB. Neuropsychiatric lupus. J Rheumatol 1980 May–Jun;7(3):325–332.

A9. Abeles M, Urman JD, Rothfield NF. Aseptic necrosis of bone in systemic lupus erythematosus. Relationship to corticosteroid therapy. Arch Intern Med 1978 May;138(5):750–754.

A10. Abeles M, Urman JD, Weinstein A, Lowenstein M, Rothfield NF. Systemic lupus erythematosus in the younger patient: survival studies. J Rheumatol 1980 Jul–Aug;7:515–522.

A11. Abeles M, Weiner ES, Parke A, Wilson D. The association of osteonecrosis in SLE with anticardiolipin antibodies. Arthritis Rheum 1991;34 Suppl:R39.

A12. Abo W, Gray JD, Baake AC, Horwitz DA. Studies on human blood lymphocytes with iC3b (type 3) complement receptors. II Characterization of subsets which regulate pokeweed mitogen-induced lymphocyte proliferation and immunoglobulin synthesis. Clin Exp Immunol 1987;67:554.

A13. Abrahamson SB, Dobro J, Eberle MA, Benton M, Reibman J, Epstein H, Rapoport DM, Belmont HM, Goldring RM. Acute reversible hypoxemia in systemic lupus erythematosus. Ann Intern Med 1911;114:941–947.

A14. Abrahamson SB, Given WP, Edelson HS, Weissmann G. Neurophil aggregation induced by sera from patients with active systemic lupus erythematosus. Arthritis Rheum 1983;26: 630–636.

A15. Abramowsky CR. Lupus erythematosus, the placenta, and pregnancy: A natural experiment in immunologically mediated reproductive failure. Prog Clin Biol Res 1981;70: 309–320.

A16. Abramowsky CR, Vegas ME, Swinehart G, Gyves MT. Decidual vasculopathy of the placenta in lupus erythematosus. N Engl J Med 1980 Sep 18;303:668–672.

A17. Abrams SB, Weissman G. The mechanisms of action of non-steroidal anti-inflammatory drugs. Arthritis Rheum 1989;32: 1–9.

A18. Abramson S, Kramer SB, Radin A, Holzman R. Salmonella bacteremia in systemic lupus erythematosus. Eight-year experience at a municipal hospital. Arthritis Rheum 1985 Jan; 28(1):75–79.

A19. Abramson SB, Weissman G. Complement split products and the pathogenesis of SLE. Hosp Pract 1988;23:45–56.

A20. Abrass CK, Nies KM, Louie JS, Border WA, Glassock RJ. Correlation and predictive accuracy of circulating immune complexes with disease activity in systemic lupus erythematosus. Arthritis Rheum 1980 Mar;23:273–282.

A21. Abruzzo LV, Rawley DA. Homeostasis, of the antibody response: Immunoregulation of NK cells. Science 1983;11: 581–585.

A22. Abuaf N, Johanet C, Chretien P, Absalon BI, Homberg JC, Buri JF. Detection of autoantibodies to Sm antigen in systemic lupus erythematosus but immunodiffusion, ELISA and immunoblotting: variability of incidence related to assays and ethnic origin of patients. Eur J Clin Invest 1990;20:354–359.

A23. Abud-Mendoza C, Diaz-Jouanen E, Alarcon-Segovia D. Fetal pulmonary hemorrhage in systemic lupus erythematosus. Occurrence without hemoptysis. J Rheumatol 1985;12:558–561.

A24. Acha-Orbea H, Mitchell DJ, Timmermann L, Wraith DC, Traush GS, Waldor MK, Zamvil SS, McDevitt HO, Steinman L. Limited heterogeneity of T cell receptors from lymphocytes mediating autoimmune encephalomyelitis allows specific immune intervention. Cell 1988;54:263–273.

A25. Acha-Orbea H, Steinman L, McDevitt HO. T cell receptors in murine autoimmune disease. Annu Rev Immunol 1989;7: 371–405.

A26. Achiron A, Sarova-Pinhas I. Prevention of stroke in patients with systemic lupus erythematosus. Stroke 1990;21:154–155.

A27. Ackerman GL. Alternate-day steroid therapy in lupus nephritis. Ann Intern Med 1970 Apr;72:511–519.

A28. Ackerman GL, Nolan CM. Adrenocortical responsiveness after alternate-day corticosteroid therapy. N Engl J Med 1968 Feb 22;278:405–409.

A29. Adachi M, Mita S, Obana M, Matsuoka Y, Harada K, Irimajiri S. Thrombocytopenia subsequently develops systemic lupus erythematosus—can anti-SSA antibody predict the next event? Jap J Med 1990;29:481–486.

A30. Adams EM, Yocum DE, Bell CL. Hydroxychloroquine in the treatment of rheumatoid arthritis. Am J Med 1983 Aug;75(2): 321–326.

A31. Adams JL. The familial occurrence of lupus erythematosus. N Z Med J 1954 Oct;53:504–507.

A32. Adams LE, Sanders SE, Budinsky RA, Donovan-Brand R, Roberts SM, Hess EV. Immunomodulatory effects of procainamide metabolites: their implications in drug-related lupus. J Lab Clin Med 1989;113:482–492.

A33. Adams S, Zordan T, Sainis K, Datta SK. T cell receptor V beta genes expressed by IgG anti-DNA autoantibody-inducing T cells in lupus nephritis: forbidden receptors and double negative T cells. Eur J Immunol 1990;20:1435–1443.

A34. Adams-Black A, McCauliffe DP, Sontheimer RD. Prevalence of acne rosacea in a rheumatic skin disease subspecialty clinic. [submitted for publication].

A35. Adamson JW, Eschbach JW. Treatment of the anemia of chronic renal failure with recombinant human erythropoietin. Ann Rev Med 1990;41:349–360.

A36. Adelman DC, Wallace DJ, Klinenberg JR. Thirty-four-year delayed-onset lupus nephritis: a case report. Arthritis Rheum 1987;30:479–480.

A37. Adelman NE, Watling DL, McDevitt HO. Treatment of (NZB × NZW) F1 disease with anti-I-A monoclonal antibodies. J Exp Med 1983 Oct 1;158:1350–1355.

A38. Adelstein S, Pritchard-Briscoe H, Anderson TP, Crosbie J, Gammon G, Loblay RH, Basten A, Goodnow CC. Induction of self-tolerance in T cells but not B cells of transgenic mice expressing little self antigen. Science 1991;251:1223–1225.

A39. Adelusi SA, Salako LA. Protein binding of chloroquine in the presence of aspirin. Br J Clin Pharmacol 1982 Mar;13(3): 451–452.

A40. Ader R, editor. Psychoneuroimmunology. New York: Academy, 1981.

A41. Adeyemi EO, Campos LB, Loizou S, Walport MJ, Hodgson HJF. Plasma lactoferrin and neutrophil elastase in rheumatoid arthritis and systemic lupus erythematosus. Br J Rheumatol 1990;29:15–20.

A42. Adinolfi M. The human placenta as a filter for cells and plasma proteins. In: Edwards RG, Howe CWS, Johnson MH, editors. Immunobiology of trophoblast. Cambridge: Cambridge University Press, 1975:193.

A43. Adinolfi M, Haddad SA, Seller MJ. X chromosome, complement and serum levels of IgM in man and mouse. Immunogenetics 1978;5:149–156.

A44. Adler MK, Baumgarten A, Hecht B, Siegel NJ. Prognostic significance of DNA-binding capacity patterns in patients with lupus nephritis. Ann Rheum Dis 1975;34:444–450.

A45. Adler SG, Johnson K, Louie JS, Liebling MR, Cohen AH. Lupus membranous glomerulonephritis: Different prognostic subgroups obscured by imprecise histologic classification. Modern Pathol 1990;3:186–191.

A46. Adoue D, Arlet P, Duffaut M, LeTallec Y, Abbal M. Major hyprotidemia (sic) with serum viscosity in systemic lupus erythematosus. Sem Hop Paris 1986;62:1261–1264.

A47. Adrianakos AA, Duffy J, Suzuki M, Sharp JT. Transverse myelopathy is SLE. Report of 3 cases and review of the literature. Ann Intern Med 1975;83:616–624.

A48. Adu D, Dobson J, Williams DG. DNA-anti-DNA circulating immune complexes in the nephritis of systemic lupus erythematosus. Clin Exp Immunol 1981;43:605–614.

A49. Adu D, Williams DG. Complement activating cryoglobulins in the nephritis of systemic lupus erythematosus. Clin Exp Immunol 1984 Mar;55:495–501.

A50. Aegerter E, Long JH. The collagen diseases. Am J Med Sci 1949 Sep;218:324–337.

A51. Afifi AK, Bergman RA, Harvey JC. Steroid myopathy. Clinical, histologic and cytologic observations. Johns Hopkins Med J 1968 Oct;123:157–173.

A52. Affolter M, Ruiz-Carrillo A. Transcription unit of the chicken histone H5 gene and mapping of H5 pre-mRNA sequences. J Biol Chem 1986;261:11496–11502.

A53. Agnello V. The Immunopathogenesis of lupus nephritis. In: Hamburger J, Crosnier J, Maxwell MH, editors. Advances in Nephrology. Chicago: Year Book, 1976:119–136.

A54. Agnello V. Complement deficiency states. Medicine 1978 Jan;57:1–24.

A55. Agnello V. Complement deficiency and systemic lupus erythematosus. In: Lahita RG, editor. Systemic Lupus Erythematosus. New York: Wiley, 1987:565–592.

A56. Agnello V, Arbetter A, De Kasep GI, Powell R, Tan EM, Joslin F. Evidence for a subset of rheumatoid factors that cross-react with DNA-histone and have a distinct cross-idiotype. J Exp Med 1980 Jun;151:1514–1527.

A57. Agnello V, DeBracco MME, Kunkel HG. Hereditary C2 deficiency with some manifestations of systemic lupus erythematosus. J Immunol 1972;108:837–840.

A58. Agnello V, Koffler D, Eisenberg JW, Winchester RJ, Kunkel HG. Clq precipitins in the sera of patients with systemic lupus erythematosus and other hypocomplementemic states: Characterization of high and low molecular weight types. J Exp Med 1971 Sep 1;134 Suppl:228S–241S.

A59. Agodoa LYC, Gauthier VJ, Mannik M. Antibody localization in the glomerular basement membrane may precede in situ immune deposit formation in rat glomeruli. J Immunol 1985 Feb;134:880–884.

A60. Agopian MS, Boctor FN, Peter JB. False-positive test results

A61. Aguado MT, Balderas RS, Rubin RL, Duchosal MA, Kofler R, Birshtein BK, Secher DS, Dixon FJ, Theofilopoulos AN. Specificity and molecular characteristics of monoclonal IgM rheumatoid factors from arthritic and non-arthritic mice. J Immunol 1987;139:1080–1087.

A62. Agudelo CA, Wise CM, Lyles MF. Pure red cell aplasia in procainamide induced systemic lupus erythematosus: report and review of the literature. J Rheumatol 1988;15:1431–1432.

A63. Aguirre C, Vallo A, Gonzalez de Zarate P, Alberola I, Alvarez A, Rodriguez-Soriano J. Changes in renin-aldosterone axis in systemic lupus erythematosus [English abstract]. Med Clin (Barc) 1988 Jul 2;91(6):206–210.

A64. Agus B, Nayar S, Patel DJ, McGrath M. Inappropriate secretion of ADH in a patient with systemic lupus erythematosus [letter]. Arthritis Rheum. 1983 Feb;26(2):237–238.

A65. Agus B, Nelson J, Kramer N, Mahal SS, Rosenstein ED. Acute central nervous system symptoms caused by ibuprofen in connective tissue disease. J Rheumatol 1990 Aug;17(8):1094–1096.

A66. Ahearn JM, Provost TT, Dorsch CA, Stevens MB, Bias WB, Arnett FC. Interrelationships of HLA-DR, MB and MT phenotypes, autoantibody expression, and clinical features in systemic lupus erythematosus. Arthritis Rheum 1982;25:1031–1040.

A67. Ahles TA, Yunus MB, Riley SD, Bradley JM, Masi AT. Psychological factors associated with primary fibromyalgia syndrome. Arthritis Rheum 1984 Oct;27(10):1101–1106.

A68. Ahmad AR, Drenick E. Immunofluorescent studies of cutaneous lesions in bowel bypass syndrome [abstract]. Clin Res 1980;28:20A.

A69. Ahmad AR, Provost TT. Incidence of a positive lupus band test using sun-exposed and unexposed skin. Arch Dermatol. 1979;115:228–229.

A70. Ahmad AR, Schreiber P, Abramovits W, Ostreicher M, Lowe NJ. Coexistence of lichen planus and systemic lupus erythematosus. J Am Acad Dermatol 1982 Oct;7(4):478–483.

A71. Ahn YS, Harrington WJ, Mylvaganam R, Ayub J, Pall LM. Treatment of autoimmune hemolytic anemia with vinca loaded platelets. JAMA 1983;249:2189–2194.

A72. Ahn YS, Harrington WJ, Mylvaganam RM, Ayub J, Pall LM. Danazol therapy for autoimmune hemolytic anemia. Ann Intern Med 1985;102:298–301.

A73. Ahn YS, Harrington WJ, Seelman RC, Eytel CS. Vincristine therapy of idiopathic and secondary thrombocytopenias. N Engl J Med 1974;291:376–380.

A74. Ahn YS, Harrington WJ, Simon SR, Mylvaganam R, Pall LM, So AG. Danazol for the treatment of idiopathic thrombocytopenic purpura. N Engl J Med 1982;808:1396–1399.

A75. Ahn YS, Rocha R, Mylvaganam R, Garcia R, Duncan R, Harrington WJ. Long-term danazol therapy in autoimmune thrombocytopenia: unmaintained remission and age-dependent response in women. Ann Intern Med 1989 Nov;111(9):723–729.

A76. Ahuja GK, Schumacher GA. Drug-induced systemic lupus erythematosus, primidone as a possible cause. JAMA 1966 Nov 7; 198:669–671.

A77. Aisen AM, Gabrielsen TO, McCune WJ. MR imaging of systemic lupus erythematosus involving the brain. AJR 1985 May; 144(5):1027–1031.

A78. Aisen PS, Cronstein BN, Kramer SB. Systemic lupus erythematosus in a patient with Reiter's syndrome. Arthritis Rheum 1983 Nov;26(11):1405–1408.

A79. Aisenberg AC. Studies on the mechanism of the lupus erythematosus (L.E.) phenomenon. J Clin Invest 1959;38:325–335.

A80. Aitcheson CT, Peebles C, Joslin F, Tan EM. Characteristics of antinuclear antibodies in rheumatoid arthritis. Reactivity of rheumatoid factor with a histone-dependent nuclear antigen. Arthritis Rheum 1980 May;23:528–538.

A81. Ait-kaci A, Monier JC, Mamelle N. Enzyme-linked immunosorbent assay for anti-histone antibodies and their presence in systemic lupus erythematosus sera. J Immunol Methods 1981;44(3):311–322.

A82. Akashi K, Nagasawa K, Mayumi T, Yokota E, Oochi N, Kusaba T. Successful treatment of refractory systemic lupus erythematosus with intravenous immunoglobulins. J Rheumatol 1990;17(3):375–379.

A83. Akbar AN, Terry L, Timms A, Beverley PCL, Janossy G. Loss of CD45R and gain of UCHL1 is a feature of primed T cells. J Immunol 1988;140:2171–2178.

A84. Akbar S, Tello AI, Luvira U, Heinzerling R, Romanski R, Levin NW, Burnham TK. Significance of antinuclear antibody (ANA) immunofluorescent patterns and titers in systemic lupus erythematosus nephritis. Henry Ford Hosp Med J 1988;36:121–129.

A85. Akhanzarova VD, Vasil'eva EG. Aleutian mink disease as an experimental model of systemic lupus erythematosus. Voprosy Revmatizma 1981;1:46.

A86. Akintonwa A, Gbajumo SA, Mabadeje AF. Placental and milk transfer of chloroquine in humans. Ther Drug Monit 1988;10(2):147–149.

A87. Alarcon GS, Sams WM Jr, Barton DD, Reveille J. Bullous lupus erythematosus rash worsened by Dapsone. Arthritis Rheum 1984 Sep;27(9):1072–1072.

A88. Alarcon-Segovia D. Drug induced lupus syndromes. Mayo Clin Proc 1969 Sep;44:664–681.

A89. Alarcon-Segovia D. Gross splenomegaly in SLE. Arthritis Rheum 1978 Sep–Oct;21:866.

A90. Alarcon-Segovia D. Mixed connective tissue disease—decade of growing pains. J Rheumatol 1981 Sep–Oct;8:535–540.

A91. Alarcon-Segovia D. Pathogenetic potential of antiphospholipid antibodies. J Rheumatol 1988 Jun;15(6):890–893.

A92. Alarcon-Segovia D. Deforming arthropathy of the hands in SLE and the growing pains of MCTD. J Rheumatol 1991;18:632.

A93. Alarcon-Segovia D, Abud-Mendoza C, Diaz-Jouanen E, Iglesias A, De os Reyes V, Hernandez-Ortiz J. Deforming arthropathy of the hands in systemic lupus erythematosus. J Rheumatol 1988 Jan;15(1):65–69.

A94. Alarcon-Segovia D, Abud-Mendoza C, Reyes-Gutierrez E, Iglesias-Gamarra A, Diaz-Jouanen E. Involvement of the urinary bladder in systemic lupus erythematosus. A pathologic study. J Rheumatol 1984 Apr;11(2):208–210.

A95. Alarcon-Segovia D, Amigo MC, Reyes PA. Connective tissue disease features after thallium poisoning. J Rheumatol 1989 Feb;16(2):171–174.

A96. Alarcon-Segovia D, Babb RR, Fairbairn JF 2d. Systemic lupus erythematosus with erythromelalgia. Arch Intern Med 1963 Nov;112:688–692.

A97. Alarcon-Segovia D, Cardiel MH. Connective tissue disorders and the bowel. Bailliere's Clin Rheumatol 1989 Aug;3(2):371–392.

A98. Alarcon-Segovia D, Cardiel MH. Comparison between 3 diagnostic criteria for mixed connective tissue disease. Study of 593 patients. J Rheumatol 1989 Mar;16(3):328–334.

A99. Alarcon-Segovia D, Cardiel MH, Reyes E. Antiphospholipid arterial vasculopathy. J Rheumatol 1989 Jun;16(6):762–767.

A100. Alarcon-Segovia D, Deleze M, Oria CV, Sanchez-Guerrero J, Gomez-Pacheco L, Cabiedes J, Fernandez L, Ponce de Leon S. Antiphospholipid antibodies and the antiphospholipid syndrome in systemic lupus erythematosus. A prospective analysis of 500 consecutive patients. Medicine 1989 Nov;68(6):353–365.

A101. Alarcon-Segovia D, Diaz-Jouanen E. Erythromalgia in systemic lupus erythematosus [case report]. Am J Med Sci 1973 Aug;266:149–151.

A102. Alarcon-Segovia D, Diaz-Jouanen E. Lupus subsets: Relationship to genetic and environmental factors. Semin Arthritis Rheum 1980 Aug;10(1):18–24.

A103. Alarcon-Segovia D, Fishbein E. Serum immunoglobulins in systemic lupus erythematosus. Clin Sci 1972 Jul;43:121–131.

A104. Alarcon-Segovia D, Fishbein E, Alcala H. Isoniazid acetylation rate and development of antinuclear antibodies upon isoniazid treatment. Arthritis Rheum 1971 Nov–Dec; 14:748–752.

A105. Alarcon-Segovia D, Fishbein E, Cetina JA, Raya RJ, Barrera E. Antigen specificity of chlorpromazine-induced antinuclear antibodies. Clin Exp Immunol 1973 Dec;15:543–548.

A106. Alarcon-Segovia D, Fishbein E, Reyes PA, Dies H, Shwadsky S. Antinuclear antibodies in patients on anticonvulsant therapy. Clin Exp Immunol 1972 Sep;12:39–47.

A107. Alarcon-Segovia D, Galbraith RF, Maldonado JE, Howard FM Jr. Systemic lupus erythematosus following thymectomy for myasthenia gravis. Report of two cases. Lancet 1963;2:662–665.

A108. Alarcon-Segovia D, Granados J. Immunogenetics of SLE in Mexicans. Proceedings of the Second International Conference on Systemic Lupus Erythematosus;1989; Nov 26–30; Singapore, 1989:50–51.

A109. Alarcon-Segovia D, Herskovic T, Dearing WH, Bartholomew LG, Cain JC, Shorter RG. Lupus erythematosus cell phenomenon in patient with chronic ulcerative colitis. Gut 1965;6:39–47.

A110. Alarcon-Segovia D, Ibanez G, Velazquez-Forero F, Hernandez-Ortiz J, Gonzalez-Jimenez Y. Sjogren's syndrome in systemic lupus erythematosus. Clinical and subclinical manifestations. Ann Intern Med 1974 Nov;81(5):577–583.

A111. Alarcon-Segovia D, Osmundson PJ. Peripheral vascular syndromes associated with systemic lupus erythematosus. Ann Intern Med 1965 May;62:907–919.

A112. Alarcon-Segovia D, Palacios R. Differences in immunoregulatory T cell circuits between diphenylhydantoin-related and spontaneously occurring systemic lupus erythematosus. Arthritis Rheum 1981 Aug;24:1086–1092.

A113. Alarcon-Segovia D, Ruiz-Arguelles A. Decreased circulating thymus-derived cells with receptors for the Fc portion of immunoglobulin G in systemic lupus erythematosus. J Clin Invest 1978;62:1390.

A114. Alarcon-Segovia D, Sakin KG, Worthington JW, Ward LE. Clinical and experimental studies on the hydralazine syndrome and its relationship to systemic lupus erythematosus. Medicine 1967;46:1–33.

A115. Alarcon-Segovia D, Sanchez-Guerrero J. Primary antiphospholipid syndrome. J Rheumatol 1989 Apr;16(4):482–488.

A116. Alarcon-Segovia D, Sanchez-Guerrero J. Correction of thrombocytopenia with small dose aspirin in the primary antiphospholipid syndrome. J Rheumatol 1989 Oct;16(10):1359–1361.

A117. Alarcon-Segovia D, Villarreal M. Classification and diagnostic criteria for mixed connective tissue diseases. In: Kasukawa R, Sharp GC, eds. Mixed Connective Tissue Diseases and Antinuclear antibodies. Amsterdam: Elsevier, 1987:41–47.

A118. Alarif LI, Ruppert GB, Wilson R Jr, Barth WF. HLA-DR antigens in blacks with rheumatoid arthritis and systemic lupus erythematosus. J Rheumatol 1983;10:297–300.

A119. Alaverson DC, Chase HP. Systemic lupus erythematosus in childhood presenting as hyperlipoproteinemia. J Peds 1977 Jul;91:72−75.

A120. Alavi IA, Pillay VKG. Steroid-induced diabetic ketoacidosis [abstract]. Ann Intern Med 1970 May;72:787.

A121. AlBalla S, Fritzler MJ, Davis P. A case of drug-induced lupus due to carbamazepine. J Rheumatol 1987;14:599−600.

A122. Albert DA, Hadler NH, Ropes MW. Does corticosteroid therapy affect the survival of patients with systemic lupus erythematosus? Arthritis Rheum 1979 Sep 11;22:945−953.

A123. Albert ED, Baur MP, Mayr WR, editors. Histocompatibility Testing 1984. New York: Springer-Verlag, 1984.

A124. Alberti-Flor JJ. Chlorpromazine-induced lupus-like illness. Am Fam Physician 1983; 27:151−152.

A125. Alcala H, Alarcon-Segovia D. Ulceration and perforation of the nasal septum in systemic lupus erythematosus. N Engl J Med 1969 Sep 25;281:711−723.

A126. Alcocer-Varela J, Alarcon-Segovia D. Decreased production of and response to interleukin-2 by cultured lymphocytes from patients with systemic lupus erythematosus. J Clin Invest 1982 Jun;69:1388−1392.

A127. Alcocer-Varela J, Iglesias A, Llorente L, Alarcon-Segovia D. Effects of L-canavanine on T cells may explain the induction of systemic lupus erythematosus by alfalfa. Arthritis Rheum 1985 Jan;28(1):52−57.

A128. Alcocer-Varela J, Laffon A, Alarcon-Segovia D. Defective monocyte production of, and T lymphocyte response to, interleukin-1 in the peripheral blood of patients with systemic lupus erythematosus. Clin Exp Immunol 1983 Jan;55(1):125−132.

A129. Omitted.

A130. Alegre VA, Gastineau DA, Winklemann RK. Skin lesions associated with circulating lupus anticoagulant. Br J Dermatol 1989 Mar;120(3):419−429.

A131. Alegre VA, Winklemann RK, Gastineau DA. Cutaneous thrombosis, cerebrovascular thrombosis and the lupus anticoagulant—the Sneddon syndrome. Report of 10 cases. Int J Dermatol 1990 Jan−Feb;29(1):45−49.

A132. Alexander DR, Cantrell DA. Kinases and phophatases in T-cell activation. Immunol Today 1989;10(6):200−205.

A133. Alexander EL, Arnett FC, Provost TT, Stevens MB. Sjogren's syndrome-association of anti-Ro (SSA) antibodies with vasculitis, hematologic abnormalities, and serologic hyperreactivity. Ann Intern Med 1983 Feb;98:155−159.

A134. Alexander EL, Buyon JP, Lane J, Lafond-Walker A, Provost TT, Guarnieri T. Anti-SSA/Ro SSB/La antibodies bind to neonatal rabbit cardiac cells and preferentially inhibit in vitro cardiac repolarization. J Autoimmunol 1989;2:463−469.

A135. Alexander EL, Hirsh TJ, Arnett FC, Provost TT, Stevens MB. Ro(SSA) and La(SSB) antibodies in the clinical spectrum of Sjogren's syndrome. J Rheumatol 1982;9:239−246.

A136. Alexander EL, McNicholl J, Watson RM, Bias W, Reichlin M, Provost TT. The immunogenetic relationship between anti-Ro(SS-A)/La(SS-B) antibody positive Sjogren's/lupus erythematosus overlap syndrome and the neonatal lupus syndrome. J Invest Dermatol 1989 Dec;93(6):751−756.

A137. Alexander EL, Provost TT. Ro (SSA) and La (SSB) antibodies. Springer Semin Immunopathol 1981;4(3):253−273.

A138. Alexander NJ, Smythe NL, Jokinen MP. The type of dietary fat affects the severity of autoimmune disease in NZB/NZW mice. Am J Pathol 1987;127:106−121.

A138a. Alexander S. Lupus erythematosus in 2 patients after griseofulvin treatment of trichophyton rubrum infection. Br J Dermatol 1962;574:72.

A139. Alger M, Alarcon-Segovia D, Rivero SJ. Hemolytic anemia and thrombocytopenic purpura: two related subsets of systemic lupus erythematosus. J Rheumatol 1977 Winter;4: 351−357.

A140. Al-Hadithy H, Isenberg DA, Addison IE, Goldstone AH, Snaith ML. Neurophil function in systemic lupus erythematosus and other collagen diseases. Ann Rheumatol 1982;41: 33−38.

A141. Al-Husaini A, Jamal GA. Myelopathy as the main presenting feature of systemic lupus erythematosus. Eur Neurol 1985 Mar−Apr;24:94−105.

A142. Ali HM. Reduced ampicillin bioavailability following oral coadministration with chloroquine. J Antimicrob Chemother 1985 Jun;15(6):781−784.

A143. Al-Jitawi SA, Hakooz BA, Kazimi SM. False positive Monospot test in systemic lupus erythematosus. Br J Rheumatol 1987;26:71.

A144. Allan J, Mitchell T, Harborne N, Bohm L, Crane-Robinson C. Roles of H1 domains in determining higher order chromatin structure and H1 location. J Mol Biol 1986;187:591−601.

A145. Allard SA, Charles PJ, Herrick AL, McColl KE, Scott JT. Antinuclear antibodies and the diagnosis of systemic lupus erythematosus in patients with acute intermittent porphyria. Ann Rheum Dis 1990 Apr;49(4):246−248.

A146. Allegue F, Alonso ML, Rocamora A, Ledo A. Chilblain lupus erythematosus and antiphospholipid antibody syndrome. J Am Acad Dermatol 1988 Nov;19(5 Pt 1):908−910.

A147. Allen IV, Millar JHD, Kirk J, Shillington RK. Systemic lupus erythematosus clinically resembling multiple sclerosis and with unusual pathological and ultrastructural features. J Neuro Neurosurg Psychiatry 1979 May;42(5):392−401.

A148. Allen JB, Blatter D, Calandrea GB, Wilder RL. Sex hormonal effects on the severity of streptococcal cell wall induced polyarthritis in the rat. Arthritis Rheum 1983;26: 560−565.

A149. Allen JB, Wong HL, Guyre PM, Simon GL, Wahl SM. Association of circulating receptor FcRIII-positive monocytes in AIDS patients with elevated levels of transforming growth factor-β. J Clin Invest 1991;87:1773−1779.

A150. Allen JM, Seed B. Nucleotide sequence of three cDNAs for the human high affinity Fc receptor (FcRI). Nucl Acids Res 1988;16:118−124.

A151. Allen JM, Seed B. Isolation and expression of functional high affinity Fc receptor cDNAs. Science 1989;243:378−380.

A152. Allen TW, Glicksman M. Psychologic involvement in systemic lupus erythematosus: a psychometric approach. Clin Rheumatol Pract 1986;4:64−70.

A152a. Allison JH, Bettley FR. Rheumatoid arthritis with chronic leg ulceration. Lancet 1957;1:288−290.

A153. Almroth G, Westberg NG, Sandstrom BM. Normal zinc and selenium levels in patients with systemic lupus erythematosus. J Rheumatol 1985;12:633−634.

A154. Alonso JF, Ramos M, Castilla J, Silva A, Wichmann I, Torres M, Mateos J. Renal amyloidosis and systemic lupus erythematosus without renal involvement. Nefrologia 1986:113−116.

A155. Alonso-Ruiz A, Zea-Mendoza AC, Salazar-Vallinas JM, Rocamora-Ripoli A, Beltran-Gutierrez J. Toxic Oil Syndrome: A syndrome with features overlapping those of various forms of scleroderma. Semin Arthritis Rheum 1986;15:200−212.

A156. Alper CA, Rosen FS. Studies of the in vivo behavior of human C3 in normal subjects and patients. J Clin Invest 1967; 46:2021−2034.

A157. Alperin N, Babu S, Weinstein A. Acute adrenal insufficiency and the antiphospholipid syndrome [letter]. Ann Intern Med 1989 Dec;111(12):950.

A158. Alpert LI. Thrombotic thrombocytopenic purpura and systemic lupus erythematosus. Report of a case with immunofluorescence investigation of vascular lesions. J Mt Sinai Hosp NY 1968 Mar−Apr;35:165−173.

A159. Alpert MA, Goldberg SH, Singsen BH, Durham JB, Sharp GC, Ahmad M, Madigan NP, Hurst DP, Sullivan WD. Cardiovascular manifestations of mixed connective tissue disease in adults. Circulation 1983 Dec;68(6):1182–1193.

A160. Al-Rasheed SA, Al-Fawaz IM. Cryptococcal meningitis in a child with systemic lupus erythematosus. Ann Trop Paediatr 1990;10:323–326.

A161. Alsinet E, Ingl's-Esteve J, Vilella R, Lozano F, Mila J, Rojo I, Martorell J, Vives J, Gaya A. Differential effects of anti-CD45 monoclonal antibody on human B cell proliferation: A monoclonal antibody recognizing a neuraminidase-sensitive epitope of the T200 molecule enhances anti-immunoglobulin-induced proliferation. Eur J Immunol 1990;20:2801–2804.

A162. Alspaugh M, Maddison PJ. Resolution of the identity of certain antigen-antibody systems in systemic lupus erythematosus and Sjogren's syndrome. Arthritis Rheum 1979;22: 796–798.

A163. Alspaugh MA, Tan EM. Antibodies to cellular antigens in Sjogren's syndrome. J Clin Invest 1975 May;55:1067–1073.

A164. Alter BP. Systemic lupus erythematosus and ethosuccimide [letter]. J Pediatr 1970; 77:1093–1095.

A165. Altman A, Theofilopoulos AN, Weiner R, Katz DH, Dixon FJ. Analysis of T cell function in autoimmune murine strains. Defects in production of and responsiveness to interleukin 2. J Exp Med 1981 Sep 1;154(3):791–808.

A166. Altman R, Asch E, Bloch D, Bole G, Borenstein k, Brandt K, Christy W, Cooke TD, Greenwald M, Hochberg M, Howell D, Kaplan D, Koopman W, Longley S, Mankin H, McShane DJ, Medsger T, Meenan R, Mikkelsen W, Moskowitz R, Murphy W, Rothschild R, Segal M, Sokoloff L, Wolfe F. Development of criteria for the classification and reporting for osteoarthritis — classification of osteoarthritis of the knee. Arthritis Rheum 1986;29:1030–1049.

A167. Altomonte LA, Zoli A, Sommella L, Palumbo P, Greco AV, Magaro M. Concentration of serum bile acids as an index of hepatic damage in systemic lupus erythematosus. Clin Rheumatol 1984 Jun;3(2):209–212.

A168. Alund M, Olson L. Release of (14C) quinacrine from peripheral and central nerves. J Auton Nerv Syst 1980 Oct;2(3): 281–294.

A169. Alvarellos A, Ahearn JM, Provost TT, Dorsch CA, Stevens MB, Bias WB, Arnett FC. Relationships of HLA-DR and MT antigens to autoantibody expression in SLE. Arthritis Rheum 1983;26:1533–1535.

A170. Alvarez I, Vazquez JJ, Fontan G, Gil A, Barbado J, Ojeda JA. Neutrophil chemotaxis and serum chemotactic in systemic lupus erythematosus. Scand J Rheum 1978;7(1):69–74.

A171. Alverson DC, Chase HP. Systemic lupus erythematosus in childhood presenting as hyperlipoproteinemia. J Pediatr 1977;91:72–75.

A172. Alving AS, Eichelberger L, Craige B Jr, Whorton CM, Pullman TN. Studies on the chronic toxicity of chloroquine. J Clin Invest 1948;27:60–65.

A173. Alving BM, Baldwin PE, Richards RL, Jackson BJ. The dilute phospholipid APTT: a sensitive assay for verification of lupus anticoagulants. Thromb Hamostat 1985;54:709–712.

A174. Alving BM, Barr CF, Tang DB. Correlation between lupus anticoagulants and anticardiolipin antibodies in patients with prolonged activated partial thromboplastin times. Am J Med 1990;88:112.

A175. Amadio P Jr, Cummings DM, Dashow L. Procainamide, quinidine and lupus erythematosus [letter]. Ann Intern Med 1985 Mar;102:419–420.

A176. Amadori G, Fiore D. Diagnostic problems in hydantoin immunopathy. Review of literature and description of 3 cases. Minerva Med 1984; 75:2503–2509.

A177. Amano K, Azizuki M, Homma M. A case of systemic lupus erythematosus with urticarial vasculitis. Ryumachi 1989;29: 192–199.

A178. Amarenco P, Amarenco G, Malbec D, Bletry O, Roullet E, Marteau R. Vesical neuropathy in acute disseminated lupus erythematosus, 2 cases. Presse Med 1988 Jul 2;17(26):1367.

A179. Ambrosio G, Bigazzi MC, Tritto I, Focaccio A, Brigante F, Migliaccio C, Chiariello M. Limitation of the area of necrosis induced by quinacrine after coronary occlusion in the dog [English abstract]. G Ital Cardiol 1985 Dec;15(12): 1139–1146.

A180. Amend WJ Jr, Vincenti F, Feduska NJ, Salvatierra O Jr, Johnston WH, Jackson J, Tilney N, Garovoy M, Burwell EL. Recurrent systemic lupus erythematosus involving renal allografts. Ann Intern Med 1981 Apr;94(4 Pt 1):444–448.

A181. Amerding D, Katz DH. Activation of T and B lymphocytes in vitro. J Exp Med 1976;139:24–31.

A182. Amerian ML, Ahmad AR. Pemphigus erythematosus. Presenting of four cases and review of literature. J Am Acad Dermatol 1984 Feb;10(2):215–222.

A183. Ames D. Asherson RA, Ayers B, Cassar J, Hughes GR. Bilateral adrenal infarction, hypoadrenalism and splinter haemorrhages in 'primary' antiphospholipid syndrome. Br J Rheumatol 1992;31:117–120.

A184. Amino N, Miyai K, Kuro R, Tanizawa O, Azukizawa M, Takai S, Tanaka F, Nishi K, Kawashima M, Kumahara Y. Transient postpartum hypothyroidism: fourteen cases with autoimmune thyroiditis. Ann Intern Med 1977;87:155–159.

A185. Amit AG, Mariziuzza RA, Phillips SEV, Poljak RJ. Three-dimensional structure of an antigen-antibody complex at 2.8A resolution. Science 1986;233:747.

A186. Amor B, Kahan A, Pompidou A, Delbarre F. Efficacy of immunosuppressants in SLE. Comparison of a series of 13 treated cases and 12 controls [original in French]. Nouv Presse Med 1972;1:1699–1702

A187. Amorosi E, Ultmann J. Thrombotic thrombocytopenic purpura: report of 16 cases and review of the literature. Medicine 1966 Mar;45:139–159.

A188. Amrhein JA, Kenny FM, Ross D. Granulocytopenia, lupus-like syndrome and other complications of propylthiouracil therapy. J Pediatr 1970 Jan;76:54–63.

A189. Ananth JV, Minn K. Chlorpromazine-induced systemic lupus erythematosus [letter]. Can Med Assoc J 1973 Mar;108: 680–683.

A190. Andersen FG, Guckian JC. Systemic lupus erythematosus associated with fatal pulmonary coccidioidomycosis. Tex Rep Biol Med 1968;16:93–99.

A190a. Anderson J, Zieve G. Assembly and intracellular transport of snRNP particles. Bio Essays 1991 Feb;13:1–8.

A191. Andersen J, Feeney RJ, Zieve GW. Identification and characterization of the small nuclear ribonucleoprotein particle D' core protein. Mol Cell Biol 1990;10:4480–4485.

A192. Andersen P, Mosekilder L. Immunoglobulin levels and autoantibodies in epileptics in long-term anticonvulsant therapy. Acta Med Scand 1977;201(1–2):69–74.

A193. Anderson B, Rucker M, Entwisle R, Schmid FR, Wood GW. Plasma fibronectin is a component of cryoglobulins from patients with connective tissue and other diseases. Ann Rheum Dis 1981 Feb;40:50–54.

A194. Anderson B, Stillman MT. False positive FTA-ABS in hydralazine-induced lupus. JAMA 1978;139:1392–1393.

A195. Anderson CL. Isolation of the receptor for IgG from a human monocyte cell line (U937) and from human peripheral blood monocytes. J Exp Med 1982;156:1794–1806.

A196. Anderson CL, Abraham N. Characterization of the Fc receptor for IgG on a human macrophage cell line. U937. J Immunol 1980;125:2735–2741.

A197. Anderson CL, Looney RJ, Culp DJ, Ryan DH, Fleit HB, Utell MJ, Frampton MW, Manganiello P, Guyre PM. Human alveolar and peritoneal macrophages bear three distinct classes of Fc receptors for IgG. J Immunol 1990;145:196–201.

A198. Anderson CL, Shen L, Eicher DM, Wewers MD, Gill JK. Phagocytes mediated by three distinct Fcγ receptor classes on human leukocytes. J Exp Med 1990;171:1333–1345.

A199. Anderson CL, Stillman WS. Raji cell assay for immune complexes. Evidence for detection of Raji-directed immunoglobulin G antibody in sera from patients with systemic lupus erythematosus. J Clin Invest 1980 Aug;66:353–360.

A200. Anderson D, Bell D, Lodge R, Grant E. Recurrent cerebral ischemia and mitral valve vegetation in a patient with phospholipid antibodies. J Rheumatol 1987;14:839–841.

A201. Anderson FP, Wanerka GR. Drug-induced systemic lupus erythematosus due to quinidine. Conn Med 1972 Feb;36:84–85.

A202. Anderson GG, Rotchell Y, Kaiser DG. Placental transfer of methylprednisolone following maternal intravenous administration. Am J Obstet Gynecol 1981;140:699–701.

A203. Omitted.

A204. Anderson JM. Transplantation: Nature's success. Lancet 1971;2:1077–1082.

A205. See A206.

A206. Anderson JR, Gray KG, Beck JS, Buchanan WW, McElhinney AJ. Precipitating autoantibodies in the connective tissue diseases. Ann Rheum Dis 1962;21:360–369.

A207. Anderson MJ, Peebles CL, McMillar R, Curd JG. Fluorescent antinuclear antibodies and anti-SSA/Ro in patients with immune thrombocytopenia developing systemic lupus erythematosus. Ann Intern Med 1985;103:548–551.

A208. Anderson NE, Ali MR. The lupus anticoagulant, pulmonary thromboembolism and fatal pulmonary hypertension. Ann Rheum Dis 1984 Oct;43(5):760–763.

A209. Anderson P, Caligiuri M, O'Brien C, Manley T, Ritz J, Schlossman SF. Fcγ receptor type III (CD16) is included in the NK receptor complex expressed by human natural killer cells. Proc Natl Acad Sci USA 1990;87:2274–2278.

A210. Anderson P, Caligiuri M, Ritz J, Schlossman SF. CD3-negative natural killer cells express TCR as a part of a novel molecular complex. Nature 1989;341:159–162.

A211. Anderson PA, Harmon CE, Sjogren R. Anti-nuclear antibodies in chronic active hepatitis [abstract]. Arthritis Rheum 1982 Apr;25(4) Suppl:S109.

A212. Anderson PO. Drugs and breast feeding-A review. Drug Intelligence Clin Pharmacol 1977;11:208.

A213. Anderson WA, Torre D. Griseofulvin and lupus erythematosus. J Med Soc N J 1982 May;63:161–162.

A214. Andersson M, Hanson A, Englund G, Dohlback B. Inhibition of complement components C3 and C4 by cadralazine and its active metabolite. Eur J Clin Pharmacol 1991; 40:261–265.

A215. Ando DG, Sercarz EE, Hahn BH. Mechanisms of T and B cell collaboration in the in vitro production of anti-DNA antibodies in the NZB/NZW F1 murine SLE model. J Immunol 1987;138:3185–3190.

A216. Andonopoulos AP, Constantopoulos SH, Galanopoulou V, Drosos AA, Acritidis NC, Moutsopoulos HM. Pulmonary function of nonsmoking patients with systemic lupus erythematosus. Chest 1988;94:312–315.

A217. Andonopoulos AP, Skopouli FN, Dimou GS, Drosos AA, Moutsopoulos HM. Sjogren's syndrome in systemic lupus erythematosus. J Rheumatol 1990 Feb;17(2):201–204.

A218. Andreani T, Poupon R, Darnis F. Ascites disclosing systemic lupus erythematosus [abstract]. Gastroenterol Clin Biol 1986;10:845–847.

A219. Andreasen JO. Oral manifestation in discoid and systemic lupus erythematosus. I. Clinical Investigation. Acta Odontol Scand 1964 Aug;22:295–310.

A220. Andreason JO, Poulsen HE. Oral manifestations in discoid and systemic lupus erythematosus. II. Histological investigation. Acta Odontol Scand 1964 Oct;22:389–400.

A221. Andres BC, Accinni L, Beiser SM, Christian CL, Cinotti GA, Erlanger BF, Hsu KC, Seegal BC. Localization of fluorescein-labeled antinucleoside antibodies in glomeruli of patients with active systemic lupus erythematosus nephritis. J Clin Invest 1970 Nov;49:2106–2118.

A222. Andrew WF. Psychiatric illness associated with systemic lupus erythematosus. So Med J 1975 Oct;68:1207.

A223. Andre-Schwartz J, Datta SK, Shoenfeld Y, Isenberg DA, Stoller BD, Schwartz RS. Binding of cytoskeletal proteins by monoclonal anti-DNA lupus autoantibodies. Clin Immunol Immunopathol 1984 May;31(2):261–271.

A224. Andrews BS, Arora NS, Shadforth MF, Goldberg SK, Davis JS 4th. The role of immune complexes in the pathogenesis of pleural effusions. Am Rev Respir Dis 1981;124:152–161.

A225. Andrews BS, Eisenberg RA, Theofilopoulos AN, Izui SN, Wilson CB, McConahey PS, Murphy ED, Roths JB, Dixon FJ. Spontaneous murine lupus-like syndromes. Clinical and immunopathological manifestations in several strains. J Exp Med 1978 Nov 1;148(5):1198–1215.

A226. Andrews BS, Schenk A, Barr R, Friou G, Mirick G, Ross P. Immunopathology of cutaneous human lupus erythematosus defined by murine monoclonal antibodies. J Am Acad Dermatol 1986 Sep;15(3):474–481.

A227. Andrews DW, Capra JD. Complete amino acid sequence of variable domains from two monoclonal human anti-gamma globulins of the Wa cross-idiotypic group: suggestion that the J segments are involved in the structural correlate of the idiotype. Proc Natl Acad Sci USA 1981;78:3799.

A228. Andrews J, Hang L, Theofilopoulos AN, Dixon FJ. Lack of relationship between serum gp70 levels and the severity of systemic lupus erythematosus in MRL/l mice. J Exp Med 1986; 163:458–462.

A229. Andrews JM, Cancilla PA, Kunin J. Progressive spinal cord signs in a patient with disseminated lupus erythematosus. Bull Los Angeles Neurol Soc 1970 Apr;35:78–85.

A229a. Andrews RC. The side effects of antimalarial drugs indicates a polyamine involvement in both schizophrenia and depression. Medical Hypotheses 1985;18:11–18.

A230. Andrzejewski C Jr, Rauch J, Lafer F, Stollar BD, Schwartz RS. Antigen-binding diversity and idiotypic cross-reaction, among hybridoma autoantibodies to DNA. J Immunol 1981; 126:226–231.

A231. Anegon I, Cuturi MC, Trinchieri G, Perussia B. Interaction of Fc receptor (CD16) ligands induces transcription of interleukin 2 receptor (CD25) and lymphokine genes and expression of their products in human natural killer cells. J Exp Med 1988;167:452–472.

A232. Angello V, Pariser J, Gell J, Gelfand J, Turksoy RN. Preliminary observation on danazol therapy of systemic lupus erythematosus. J Rheumatol 1983;10:682–687.

A233. Angles-Cano E, Sultan Y, Clauvel JP. Predisposing factors to thrombosis in systemic lupus erythematosus: possible relationship to endothelial cell damage. J Lab Clin Med 1979 Aug; 94:312–323.

A233a. Editorial. Malaria in pregnancy. Lancet 1983;2:84–85.

A234. Anonymous. Clobetasol—A potent new topical corticosteroid. Med Lett 1986;28:57–59

A235. Anonymous. Drugs that cause photosensitivity. Med Lett 1986;28:50–51.

A236. Anonymous. Depression, stress and immunity [editorial]. Lancet 1987 Jun 27;1(8548):1467–1468.

A237. Anonymous. Editorial. J Rheumatol 1988;15:959–964.

A237a. Anonymous. Eosinophilia-myalgia syndrome and L-tryptophan containing products in New Mexico, Minnesota, Oregon and New York: MWWR 1989;38:785–788.

A238. Anonymous. HCV and autoimmune liver disease [editorial]. Lancet 1990 Dec 8;336(8728):1414–1415.

A239. Anonymous. A subdermal progestin implant for long-term contraception. Arthritis Rheum 1991;33:17–18.

A240. Anonymous. Sunscreens. Consumer Reports, 1991 Jun: 400–406.

A240a. Anonymous. Editorial. The antiphospholipid antibody story. World Neurol 1991:8.

A240b. Anonymous. Progestin-only pills. History, mechanism of action and effectiveness. Contraceptive Technology 1990–92: 314–322.

A240c. Anonymous. Package insert, ACE-inhibitors. 1992 Mar.

A241. Ansar Ahmed S, Aufdermoret TB, Chen JR, Montoya AI, Olive D, Talal N. Estrogen induces the development of antibodies and promotes salivary gland lymphoid infiltrates in normal mice. In Sjogren's Syndrome: Talal N, editor. Britain: Academic Press, 1989:235–244.

A242. Ansar Ahmed S, Dauphinee MJ, Montoya AI, Talal N. Estrogen induces normal murine CD$^+$B cells to produce autoantibodies. J Immunol 1989;142:2647–2653.

A243. Ansar Ahmed S, Dauphinee MJ, Talal N. Effects of short term administration of sex hormones on normal and autoimmune mice. J Immunol 1985;134:204–210.

A244. Ansar Ahmed S, Fischbach M, Talal N. Sex hormonal effects on ornithine decarboxylase activity in stimulated lymphocytes [in preparation]. 1990.

A245. Ansar Ahmed S, Penhale WJ. The influence of testosterone on the development of autoimmune thyroiditis in thymectomized and irradiated rats. Clin Exp Immunol 1982;48: 367–374.

A246. Ansar Ahmed S, Penhale WJ, Talal N. Sex hormones, immune responses and autoimmune diseases: mechanism of sex hormone action. Am J Pathol 1985;121:583–551.

A247. Ansar Ahmed S, Talal N. Sex hormones and the immune system—Part 2 Animal Data. Bailliere's Clinical Rheumatology 1980;4:13–31.

A248. Ansar Ahmed S, Talal N. The survival value of non-clonic target sites for sex hormone action in the immune and central nervous system. Clin Immunol Newslett 1985;6:97–99.

A249. Ansar Ahmed S, Talal N. Sex steroids, sex steroid receptors and autoimmune diseases. In: Sheridan PS, Blum K, Trachtenberg MC, editors. Steroid Receptors and Disease: Cancer, Autoimmune, Bone and Circulatory Disorders. New York, Basel: Marcel Dekker, 1988:289–316.

A250. Ansar Ahmed S, Talal N. Immune-endocrine interactions and autoimmune diseases. In: Kammuler ME, Bloksma N, Seinen W, editors. Autoimmunity and Toxicology. Holland: Elsevier, 1989:415–428.

A251. Ansar Ahmed S, Talal N, Christadoss P. Genetic regulation of testosterone-induced immune suppression. Cell Immunol 1987;104:91–98.

A252. Ansar Ahmed S, Young PR, Penhale WJ. The effects of female sex steroids on the development of autoimmune thyroiditis in thymectomized and irradiated rats. Clin Exp Immunol 1983;54:351–358.

A253. Ansar Ahmed S, Young PR, Penhale WJ. Beneficial effects of testosterone in the treatment of chronic autoimmune thyroiditis in rats. J Immunol 1986;136:143–147.

A254. Ansari A, Larson PH, Bates HD. Vascular manifestations of systemic lupus erythematosus. Angiology 1986 Jun;37(6): 423–432.

A255. Ansdell VE, Common JD. Corneal changes induced by mepacrine. J Trop Med Hyg 1979 Sep–Oct;82(9–10): 206–207.

A256. Ansel JC, Mountz J, Steinberg AD, DeFabo E, Green I.

Effects of UV radiation on autoimmune strains of mice: Increased mortality and accelerated autoimmunity in BXSB male mice. J Invest Dermatol 1985;85:181–186.

A257. Ansell BM, Lawrence JS. A family study in lupus erythematosus [abstract]. Arthritis Rheum 1963;5:260.

A258. Anselmino LM, Perussia B, Thomas LL. Human basophils selectively express the FcγRII (CDw32) subtype of IgG receptor. J Allergy Clin Immunol 1989;84:907–914.

A259. Antes U, Heniz H-P, Loos M. Evidence for the presence of autoantibodies to the collagen-like portion of Clq in SLE. Arthritis Rheum 1988;31:457–464.

A260. Antiplatelet Trialist' Collaboration. Secondary prevention of vascular disease by prolonged antiplatelet treatment. BMJ 1988;296:320–331.

A261. Antoine B, Ward PD. Histuria and fibrinuria in cases of systemic lupus erythematosus. Clin Exp Immunol 1970 Jan;6: 153–159.

A262. Aoki A, Ishigatsubo Y, Hagiwara E, Shirai A, Narita M, Matsunaga K, Tani K, Okubo T, Otani M, Miyagi Y, Aoki I, Misugi K, Okuda K. Comparison of serum antibody level and spleen antibody producing cell number in murine chronic graft-versus-host disease. Proc Jpn Soc Immunol 1989;19: 463–470.

A263. Aotsuka S, Nakamura K, Nakano T, Kawakami M, Goto M, Okawa-Takatsuji M, Kinoshita M, Yokohari R. Production of intracellular and extracellular interleukin-1 alpha and interleukin-1 beta by peripheral blood monocytes from patients with connective tissue diseases. Ann Rheum Dis 1991;50: 27–31.

A264. Apice AJ, Reti LL, Pepperell RJ, Fairley KF, Kincaid-Smith P. Treatment of severe preeclampsia by plasma exchange. Aust N Z J Obstet Gynecol 1990;20:231–235.

A265. Appel AE, Sablay LB, Golden RA, Barland P, Grayzel AI, Bank N. The effect of normalization of serum complement and anti-DNA antibody on the course of lupus nephritis: a two-year prospective study. Am J Med 1978 Feb;64(2):274–283.

A266. Appel GB, Cohen DJ, Pirani CL, Meltzer JI, Estes D. Long-term follow up of patients with lupus nephritis. A study based on the classification of the World Health Organization. Am J Med 1987;83:877–885.

A267. Appel GB, D'Agati V, Estes D. Intravenous pulse cytoxan (IVPC) treatment of lupus nephritis (LN). Kidney Int 1988; 33:179.

A268. Appel GB, Pirani CL, D'Agati VD. Renal vascular complications of systemic lupus erythematosus. In: Balow JE, editor. Lupus Nephritis. 1992. In press.

A269. Appel GB, Silva FG, Pirani CL, Meltzer JI, Estes D. Renal involvement in systemic lupus erythematosus: A study of 56 patients emphasizing histologic classification: Medicine 1978 Sep;57:371–410.

A270. Appel GB, Williams GX, Meltzer JI, Pirani CL. Renal vein thrombosis, nephrotic syndrome and systemic lupus erythematosus. Ann Intern Med 1976 Sep;85:310–317.

A271. Appelby P, Webber DG, Bowen JG. Murine chronic graft-versus-host disease as a model of systemic lupus erythematosus: effect of immunosuppressive drugs on disease development Clin Exp Immunol 78:449–453, 1989.

A272. Aptekar RG, Atkinson JP, Decker JL, Wolff SM, Chu EW. Bladder toxicity with chronic oral cyclophosphamide therapy in non-malignant disease. Arthritis Rheum 1973;16:461–467.

A273. Aptekar RG, Decker JL, Steinberg AD. Exacerbation of SLE nephritis after cyclophosphamide withdrawal. N Engl J Med 1972 May 25;286:1159–1160.

A274. Aragay AM, Diaz P, Daban JR. Association of nucleosome core particle DNA with different histone oligomers: Transfer of histones between DNA-(H2A,H2B) and DNA-(H3,H4) complexes. J Mol Biol 1988;204:141–154.

A275. Aragon Diez A, Garcia-Consuegra Sanchez-Camacho G, Hernandez Rodriguez I, Morillas Lopez L. Bleparoptosis and systemic lupus erythematosus. Rev Clin Exp 1987;181:173.

A276. Arai S, Yamamoto H, Itoh K, Kumagai K. Suppressive effect of human natural killer cells on pokeweed mitogen-induced B cell differentiation. J Immunol 1983;131:651.

A277. Aranegui P, Giner P, Lopez-Gomez M, el Amrani A, Jimenez-Alonso J. Danazol for Evan's syndrome due to SLE [letter]. DICP 1990 Jun;24(6):641–642.

A278. Aranow C, Enoch L, Barland P. Lipoprotein profiles and corticosteroid treatment in systemic lupus erythematosus [abstract]. Arthritis Rheum 1990;33 Suppl:S12.

A279. Arant SE, Griffin JA, Koopman EJ. V_H gene expression is restricted in anti-IgG antibodies from MRL autoimmune mice. J Exp Med 1986;164:1284–1300.

A280. Archer JD. The FDA does not approve uses of drugs [editorial]. JAMA 1984 Aug 24–31;250(8):1054–1055.

A281. Archer RL, Cunningham AC, Moore PF, Potter JA, Bliven ML, Otterness IG. Effects of dazmegrel, piroxicam and cyclophosphamide on the NZB/W model of SLE. Agents Actions 27:369–374, 1989.

A282. Areilla RA, Thilenius OG, Ranniger K. Congestive heart failure from suspected ductal closure in utero. J Pediatr 1969;75:74.

A283. Arend WP, Emmerich TE, Sturge JC, Starkebaum GA. Monocyte-reactive antibodies in patients with systemic lupus erythematosus. Arthritis Rheum 1977;20:1049–1057.

A284. Arend WP, Joslin FG, Massoni RJ. Effects of immune complexes on production by human monocytes of interleukin 1 or an interleukin 1 inhibitor. J Immunol 1985 Jun;134:3868–3875.

A285. Arend WP, Mannik M. Studies on antigen antibody complexes. II. Quantitation of tissue uptake of soluble complexes in normal and complement-depleted rabbits. J Immunol 1971;107:63–75.

A286. Ariga H, Edwards J, Sullivan DA. Androgen control of autoimmune expression in lacrimal gland of MRL-MP/lpr-lpr mice. Clin Immunol Immunopathol 1989;53:499–508.

A287. Arisaka O, Obinata K, Sasaki H, Arisaka M, Kaneko K. Chorea as an initial manifestation of systemic lupus erythematosus. Clin Pediatr 1984;23:298.

A288. Arita C, Kaibara N, Jingushi S, Takagishi K, Hotokebuchi T, Arai K. Suppression of collagen arthritis in rats by heterologous anti-idiotypic antisera against anticollagen antibodies. Clin Immunol Immunopathol 1987;43:374.

A289. Arman-Cruz R, Harnecker J, Ducach G, Jalil J, Gonzalez F. Clinical diagnosis of systemic lupus erythematosus. Am J Med 1958 Sep;25(3):409–419.

A290. Arnaiz-Villena A, Vasquez-Rodriguez JJ, Vicario JL, Lavilla P, Pascual D, Moreno F, Martinez-Laso J. Congenital heart block immunogenetics. Evidence for an additional role of HLA Class II antigens and independence of Ro antibodies. Arthritis Rheum 1989;32:1421–1426.

A291. Arnason BG, Richman DP. Effect of oral contraceptives on experimental demyelinating disease. Arch Neurol 1969;21:103–106.

A292. Arnett FC, Bias WB, Reveille JD. Genetic studies in Sjogren's syndrome and systemic lupus erythematosus. J Autoimmunity 1989;2:403–413.

A293. Arnett FC, Bias WB, Shulman LE. Studies in familial systemic lupus erythematosus [abstract]. Arthritis Rheum 1972;15:102.

A294. Arnett FC, Edworthy SM, Bloch DA, McShane DJ, Fries JF, Cooper NS, Healey LA, Kaplan SR, Liang HM, Luthra HS, Medsger TA, Mitchell DM, Neustadt DH, Pinals RS, Schaller JG, Sharp JT, Wilder RL, Hunder GG. The American Rheumatism Association 1987 revised criteria for the classification of rheumatoid arthritis. Arthritis Rheum 1988;31:315–324.

A295. Arnett FC, Goldstein R, Duvic M, Reveille JD. Major histocompatibility complex genes in systemic lupus erythematosus, Sjogren's syndrome and polymyositis. Am J Med 1988 Dec 23;85 Suppl 6A:38–41.

A296. Arnett FC, Hamilton RG, Reveille JD, Bias WB, Harley JB, Reichlin M. Genetic studies of Ro (SS-A) and La (SS-B) autoantibodies in families with systemic lupus erythematosus and primary Sjogren's syndrome. Arthritis Rheum 1989;32:413–419.

A297. Arnett FC, Hamilton RG, Roebber MG, Harley JB, Reichlin M. Increased frequencies of Sm and nRNP autoantibodies in American blacks compared to whites with systemic lupus erythematosus. J Rheumatol 1988;15:1773–1776.

A298. Arnett FC, Moulds JM. HLA class III molecules and autoimmune rheumatic diseases. Clin Exper Rheumatol 1991;9:289–296.

A299. Arnett FC, Olsen ML, Anderson KL, Reveille JD. Molecular analysis of major histocompatibility complex alleles associated with the lupus anticoagulant. J Clin Invest 1991;87:1490–1495.

A300. Arnett FC, Reveille JD, Wilson RW, Provost TT, Bias WB. Systemic lupus erythematosus current state of the genetic hypothesis. Semin Arthritis Rheum 1984 Aug;14:24–35.

A301. Arnett FC, Shulman LE. Studies in familial systemic lupus erythematosus. Medicine 1976 Jul;55:313–322.

A302. Arnold CM, Hochberg MC. Development and implementation of an immunization program for patients with rheumatoid arthritis. Arthritis Care Res 1990;2:162.

A303. Aronson AJ, Ordonez NG, Diddie KR, Ernest JT. Immune complex deposition in the eye in systemic lupus erythematosus. Arch Intern Med 1979 Nov;139(11):1312–1313.

A304. Aronson AJ, Soltani K, Aronson IK, Ong RT. Systemic lupus erythematosus and dermatitis herpeteformis: concurrence with Marfan's syndrome. Arch Dermatol 1979 Jan;115(1):68–70.

A305. Arroyaue CM, Taylor DG, Gallup P, Nakamura RM. Screening test for complement activation by counterimmunoelectrophoresis. Am J Clin Pathol 1978;69:440–445.

A306. Arterberry JD, Drexler E, Dubois EI. Significance of hematoxylin bodies in lupus erythematosus cell preparations. JAMA 1964 Feb 8;187:389–395.

A307. Arterberry JD, Durham WF, Elliott JW, Wolfe HR. Exposure to parathion. Measurement by blood cholinesterase level and urinary p-nitrophenol excretion. Arch Environ Health 1961 Oct;3:476–485.

A308. Arthur RP, Mason D. T cells that help B cells responses to soluble antigen are distinguishable from those producing interleukin 2 on mitogenic or allogeneic stimulation. J Exp Med 1986;163:774–786.

A309. Asano T, Furie BC, Furie B. Platelet binding properties of monoclonal lupus autoantibodies produced by human hybridomas. Blood 1985;66:1254–1260.

A310. Ascer K, Walker JA, Lief PD, Barland P, Bank N. Triad of glomerulonephritis, antinuclear antibodies, and positive skin immunofluorescence. Variant of systemic lupus erythematosus. Am J Med 1983 Jan;74(1):83–89.

A311. Ascheim JH. The adolescent and systemic lupus erythematosus: a developmental and educational approach. Issues-Compr-Pediatr-Nurs 1981 Sep–Dec;5(5–6):293–307.

A312. Asher RAJ. The dangers of going to bed. BMJ 1947 Dec 13;2:967–968.

A313. Asherson GL, Colizzi V, Zembala M. An overview of T-suppressor cell circuits. Annu Rev Immunol 1986;4:37–68.

A314. Asherson R. Antibodies to phospholipid and "the antiphospholipid syndrome." In: Immunology Update. N Williams Inc. 1989;1:1–8.

A314a. Asherson RA. Personal communication. 1992.

A315. Asherson RA. The catastrophic coagulation syndrome. J Rheumatol 1992 In Press.

A316. Asherson RA. A 'primary' antiphospholipid syndrome? J Rheumatol 1988;15:1742–1746.

A317. Asherson RA, Angus H, Matthews J, Meyers O, Hughes GR. The progressive systemic sclerosis/systemic lupus overlap: an unusual clinical progression [case report]. Ann Rheum Dis 1991 May;50(5):323–327.

A318. Asherson RA, Block S, Houssiau FA, Hughes GR. Systemic lupus erythematosus and lymphoma: Association with an antiphospholipid syndrome. J Rheumatol 1991;18:277–279.

A318a. Asherson RA, Cervera R. The antiphospholipid syndrome: a syndrome in evolution. Ann Rheum Dis 1991;51: 147–150.

A319. Asherson RA, Cruz DD, Stephens CJM, McKee PH, Hughes GRV. Urticarial vasculitis in a connective tissue disease clinic: Patterns, presentations, and treatment. Sem Arthritis Rheum 1991 April;20(5):285–296.

A320. Asherson RA, Derksen RH, Harris EN, Bingley PJ, Hoffbrand BI, Gharavi AE, Kater L, Hughes GR. Large vessel occlusion and gangrene in systemic lupus erythematosus and "lupus-like" disease. A report of six cases. J Rheumatol 1986 Aug; 13(4):740–747.

A321. Asherson RA, Derksen RH, Harris EN, Bouma BN, Gharavi AE, Kater L, Hughes GR. Chorea in systemic lupus erythematosus and "lupus-like" disease: association with antiphospholipid antibodies. Semin Arthritis Rheum 1987 May;16(4):253–259.

A322. Asherson RA, Gibson DG, Evans DW, Baguley E, Hughes GR. Diagnostic and therapeutic problems in two patients with antiphospholipid antibodies, heart valve lesions and transient ischemic attacks. Ann Rheum Dis 1988 Nov;47(11):947–953.

A323. Asherson RA, Harris EN. Anticardiolipin antibodies: clinical associations. Postgrad Med J 1986;62:1081–1087.

A324. Asherson RA, Harris EN, Ghavari AE, Hughes GR. Systemic lupus erythematosus, antiphospholipid antibodies, chorea, and oral contraceptives [letter]. Arthritis Rheum 1986 Dec; 29(12):1535–1536.

A325. Asherson RA, Harris EN, Hughes GR, Farquharson RG. Complications of oral contraceptives and antiphospholipid antibodies [letter]. Arthritis Rheum 1988 Apr;34(4):575–576.

A326. Asherson RA, Higenbottom TW, Dihn Xuan AT, Khamashta MA, Hughes GR. Pulmonary hypertension in a lupus clinic: experience with twenty-four patients. J Rheumatol 1990 Oct;17(10):1292–1298.

A327. Asherson RA, Hughes GR. Vocal cord paralysis in systemic lupus erythematosus complicated by pulmonary hypertension [letter]. J Rheumatol 1985 Oct;12(5):1029–1030.

A328. Asherson RA, Hughes GR. Antiphospholipid antibodies and chorea [letter]. J Rheumatol 1988 Feb;15(2):377–379.

A329. Asherson RA, Hughes GR. Recurrent deep vein thrombosis and Addison's disease in 'primary' antiphospholipid syndrome. J Rheumatol 1989 Mar;16(3):378–380.

A330. Asherson RA, Hughes GR. Hypoadrenalism, Addison's disease and antiphospholipid antibodies [editorial]. J Rheumatol 1991 Jan;18(1):1–4.

A331. Asherson RA, Jacobelli S, Rosenberg H, McKee P, Hughes GR. Skin nodules and macules resembling vasculitis in the antiphospholipid syndrome. Clin Exp Dermatol 1992 In press.

A332. Asherson RA, Junghers P, Liote F, Hughes GR. Ischemic necrosis of bone associated with the "lupus anticoagulant" and antibodies to cardiolipin. Proceedings of the XVIth International Congress of Rheumatology; Sydney, Australia, 1983: 373.

A333. Asherson RA, Khamashta MA, Baguley E, Oakley CM, Rowell NR, Hughes GR. Myocardial infarction and antiphospholipid antibodies in SLE and related disorders. Q J Med 1989 Dec;73(272):1103–1115.

A334. Asherson RA, Khamashta MA, Gil A, Vazquez JJ, Chan O, Baguley E, Hughes GR. Cerebrovascular disease and antiphospholipid antibodies in systemic lupus erythematosus, lupus-like disease, and the primary antiphospholipid syndrome. Am J Med 1989 Apr;86(4):391–399.

A335. Asherson RA, Khamashta MA, Hughes GR. Hepatic complications of the antiphospholipid syndrome. Clin Exp Rheumatol 1992;9:341–344.

A336. Asherson RA, Khamashta MA, Ordi-Ros J, Derksen RH, Machin SJ, Barquinero J, Outt HH, Harris EN, Vilardell-Torres M, Hughes GR. The 'primary' antiphospholipid syndrome: major clinical and serological features. Medicine 1989 Nov; 68(6):366–374.

A337. Asherson RA, Lanham JG, Hull RG, Boey ML, Gharavi AE, Hughes GR. Renal vein thrombosis in systemic lupus erythematosus: association with the 'lupus anticoagulant'. Clin Exp Rheumatol 1989;2:75–79.

A338. Asherson RA, Lubbe WF. Cerebral and valve lesions in SLE: association with antiphospholipid antibodies. J Rheumatol 1988 Apr;15(4):539–543.

A338a. Asherson RA, Mackworth-Young CG, Boey ML, Hill RG, Saunders A, Gharavi AG, Hughes GRV. Pulmonary hypertension in systemic lupus erythematosus. BMJ 1983;287: 1024–1025.

A338b. Asherson RA, Mayou SC, Merry P, Black MM, Hughes GRV. The spectrum of livedo reticularis and anticardiolipin antibodies. Br J Rheumatol 1989;120:215–221.

A339. Asherson RA, Mercey D, Phillips G, Sheehan N, Gharavi AE, Harris EN, Hughes GR. Recurrent stroke and multiinfarct dementia in systemic lupus erythematosus. Association with antiphospholipid antibodies. Ann Rheum Dis 1987 Aug;46(6): 605–611.

A340. Asherson RA, Merry P, Acheson JF, Harris EN, Hughes GR. Antiphospholipid antibodies: a risk factor occlusive Ocular vascular disease in systemic lupus erythematosus and the 'primary' antiphospholipid syndrome. Ann Rheum Dis 1989 May; 48(5):358–361.

A341. Asherson RA, Morgan SH, Harris EN, Gharavi AE, Krausz T, Hughes GR. Arterial occlusion causing large bowel infarction—a reflection of clotting diathesis in SLE. Clin Rheumatol 1986 Jan;5(1):102–106.

A342. Asherson RA, Oakley CM. Pulmonary hypertension and systemic lupus erythematosus. J Rheumatol 1986;13:1.

A343. Asherson RA, Tikly M, Staub H, Wilmshurst PT, Coltart DJ, Khamashta MA, Hughes GR. Infective endocarditis, rheumatoid factor, and anticardiolipin antibodies. Ann Rheum Dis 1990 Feb;49(2):107–108.

A344. Asherson RA, Zulman J, Hughes GRV. Pulmonary thromboembolism associated with procainamide induced lupus syndrome and anticardiolipin antibodies. Ann Rheum Dis 1989; 48:232–235.

A345. Ashinoff R, Werth VP, Franks AG Jr. Resistant discoid lupus erythematosus of palms and soles. Successful treatment with azathioprine. J Am Acad Dermatol 1988;19:961–965.

A346. Ashman RF, White RH, Wiesenhutter C, Cantor Y, Lasarow E, Liebling M, Talal N. Panhypogammaglobulinemia in systemic lupus erythematosus: In vitro demonstration of multiple cellular defects. J Allergy Clin Immunol 1982 Dec;70: 465–473.

A347. Askari A, Vignos PJ Jr, Moskowitz RW. Steroid myopathy in connective tissue disease. Am J Med 1976 Oct;61:485–492.

A348. Askari AD. Pericardial tamponade with hemorrhagic fluid in systemic lupus erythematosus. JAMA 1978;33:111–116.

A349. Atkins C, Rueffel L, Roddy J, Platts M, Robinson H, Ward

R. Rheumatic disease in the Nuu-Chah-Nulth Native Indians of the Pacific Northwest. J Rheumatol 1988;15:684–690.

A350. Atkinson JP. Complement deficiency. Predisposing factor in autoimmune syndromes. Am J Med 1988 Dec 23;85 Suppl 6A:45–57.

A351. Atkinson JP, Frank MM. Complement-independent clearance of IgG-sensitized erythrocytes: inhibition of cortisone. Blood 1974;44:629–637.

A352. Atkinson JP, Gorman JC, Curd J, Hyla JF, Deegan MJ, Keren DF, Abdou NI, Walker SE. Cold dependent activation of complement in discrepancy between clinical and laboratory parameters. Arthritis Rheum 1981;24:592–601.

A353. Atkinson JP, Schrieber AD, Frank MM. Effects of glucocorticoids and splenectomy on the immune clearance and destruction of erythrocytes. J Clin Invest 1973;52:1509–1517.

A354. Atkinson JR, Frank MM. Interaction of IgM antibody and complement in the immune clearance and destruction of erythrocytes in man. J Clin Invest 1975;54:339–348.

A355. Atkinson RA, Appenzeller O. Headache in small vessel disease of the brain: A study of patients with systemic lupus erythematosus. Headache 1978 Jan–Feb;15:198–204.

A356. Aucoin DP, Rubin RL, Peterson ME, Reidenberg MM, Drayer DE, Hurvitz AI, Lahita RG. Dose-dependent induction of anti-native DNA antibodies in cats by propylthiouracil. Arthritis Rheum 1988;31:688–692.

A357. Ausiello CM, Barbieri P, Spagnoli GC, Ciompi ML, Casciani CU. In vivo effects of chloroquine treatment on spontaneous and interferon-induced natural killer activities of rheumatoid arthritis patients. Clin Exp Rheumatol 1986 Jul–Sep;4(3):255–259.

A358. Ausio J, Dong F, Van Holde KE. Use of selectively trypsinized nucleosome core particles to analyze the role of the histone "tails" in the stabilization of the nucleosome. J Mol Biol 1989; 206:451–463.

A359. Ausio J, Van Holde KE. Histone hyperacetylation: Its effects on nucleosome conformation and stability. Biochemistry 1986;25:1421–1428.

A360. Austin HA 3d, Klippel JH, Balow JE, le Riche NG, Steinberg AD, Plotz PH, Decker JL. Therapy of lupus nephritis. Controlled trial of prednisone and cytotoxic drugs. N Engl J Med 1986 Mar 6;314(10):614–619.

A361. Austin HA 3d, Muenz LR, Joyce KM, Antonovych TA, Balow JE. Diffuse proliferative lupus nephritis: identification of specific pathologic features affecting renal outcome. Kidney Int 1984 Apr;25:689–695.

A362. Austin HA 3d, Muenz LR, Joyce KM, Antonovych TA, Kullich ME, Klippel JH, Decker JL, Balow JE. Prognostic factors in lupus nephritis: Contribution of renal histologic data. Am J Med 1983 Sep;75:382–391.

A363. Authi KS, Traynor JR. Stimulation of polymorphonuclear leucocyte phospholipase A2 activity by chloroquine and mepacrine. J Pharm Pharmacol 1982 Nov;34(11):736–738.

A364. Averbuch M, Levo Y. Longstanding intractable ascites as the initial and predominant manifestation of systemic lupus erythematosus. J Rheumatol 1986 Apr;13(2):442–443.

A365. Averill LE, Stein RL, Kammer GM. Control of human T-lymphocyte interleukin-2 production by a cAMP-dependent pathway. Cell Immunol 1988;115:88–99.

A366. Avinoach I, Amitel-Teplizki H, Kuperman O, Isenberg DA, Shoenfeld Y. Characteristics of antineuronal antibodies in systemic lupus erythematosus patients with and without central nervous system involvement: the role of mycobacterial cross-reacting antigens. Israel J Med Sci 1990;26:367.

A367. Avrameas S. Natural autoreactive B cells and autoantibodies: The "know thyself" of the immune system. Ann Inst Pasteur/Immunol 1986;137D:150–156.

A368. Avrameas S. Natural autoantibodies: from "horror autotoxicus" to "gnothi seauton." Immunol Today 1991;12:154–159.

A369. Awada HH, Mamo HL, Luft AG, Ponsin JC, Kahn MF. Cerebral blood flow in systemic lupus erythematosus with and without central nervous system involvement. J Neurol Neurosurg Psychiatry 1987 Dec;50(12):1597–1601.

A370. Awdeh JL, Raum D, Yunis EJ, Alper CA. Extended HLA/complement allele haplotypes evidence for T/t-like complex in man. Proc Natl Acad Sci USA 1983;80:259–263.

A371. Awdeh ZL, Raum DD, Glass D, Agnello V, Schur PH, Johnson RB Jr, Gelfand EW, Bollon M, Yunis E, Alper CA. Complement-HLA haplotypes in C2 deficiency. J Clin Invest 1981 67:581–583.

A372. Axelrod L. Glucocorticoid therapy. Medicine 1976 Jan;55:39–65.

A373. Axelrod L. Steroids. In: Kelley WF, editor. Textbook of Rheumatology. Philadelphia: Saunders, 1981.

A374. Axelson JA, LoBuglio AF. Immune hemolytic anemia. Med Clin North Am 1980 Jul;64:597–606.

A375. Aylward RD. Congenital heart block. Br Med J 1928;1:943.

A376. Ayoub WT, Torretti D, Harrington TN. Central nervous system manifestations after pulse therapy for systemic lupus erythematosus. Arthritis Rheum 1983 Jun;26:809–810.

A377. Ayres S Jr. Discoid lupus erythematosus: Thalidomide or Vitamin E? [letter] Int J Dermatol 1985 Nov;24(9):616.

A378. Ayvazian LF, Badger TL. Disseminated lupus erythematosus occurring among student nurses. N Engl J Med 1948 Oct 14;239:565–570.

A379. Azais-Noblinski B, Liscia G, Tubiana JM, Marsot-Dupuch K. Acute systemic lupus erythematosus associated with protein-losing enteropathy [English abstract]. Ann Radiol (Paris) 1988; 31(3):183–187.

A380. Azoury FJ, Jones HE, Derbes VJ, Gum OB. Intradermal tests and antinuclear factors in systemic lupus erythematosus. A comparative study. Ann Intern Med 1966 Dec;65(6):1221–1228.

B

B1. Baart de La Faille-Kuype EH. Lupus erythematosus-An immunohistochemical and clinical study of 485 patients. Thesis, 113 pages. Grafisch Bedriff Schotamus & Jens. Utrecht NV. 1969.

B2. Baart de la Faille-Kuype EH, Cormane RH. The occurrence of certain serum factors in the dermal-epidermal junction and vessel walls of the skin in lupus erythematosus and other (skin) diseases. Acta Dermatovener (Stockh) 1968;48:578–588.

B3. Babcock SK, Appel VB, Schiff M, Palmer E, Kotzin BL. Genetic analysis of the imperfect association of H-2 haplotype with lupus-like autoimmune disease. Proc Natl Acad Sci USA 1989 Oct;86(19):7552–7555.

B4. Babini SM, Arturi A, Marcos JC, Babini JC, Iniguez AM, Morteo OG. Laxity and rupture of the patellar tendon in systemic lupus erythematosus. Association with secondary hyperparathyroidism. J Rheumatol 1988 Jul;15(7):1162–1165.

B5. Babini SM, Cocco JA, Babini JC, de la Sota M, Arturi A, Marcos JC. Atlantoaxial subluxation in systemic lupus erythematosus: further evidence of tendinous alterations. J Rheumatol 1990 Feb;17(2):173–177.

B6. Babini SM, Cocco JA, de la Sota M, Babini JC, Arturi A, Marcos JC, Morteo OG. Tendinous laxity and Jaccoud's syndrome in patients with systemic lupus erythematosus. Possible role of secondary hyperparathyroidism. J Rheumatol 1989 Apr;16(4):494–498.

B7. Baccala R, Quang TV, Gilbert M, Ternynck T, Avrameas S.

Two murine natural polyreactive autoantibodies are encoded by non-mutated germ-line genes. Proc Natl Acad Sci USA 1989; 86:4624–4628.

B8. Bach JF. Transplantation immunity and cytotoxicity phenomena. In : Bach JF, Schwartz RS, editors. Immunology, 2nd ed. New York: Wiley, 1982:399.

B9. Bach M, Luhrmann R. Protein-RNA interactions in 20S U5 snRNPs. Biochim Biophy Acta 1991;1088:139–143.

B10. Bach M, Winkelmann G, Lurhmann R. 20S small nuclear ribonucleoprotein U5 shows a surprisingly complex protein composition. Proc Natl Acad Sci USA 1989;86:6038–6042.

B11. Bach MK. Reduction in the frequency of mutation to resistance to cytarabine in L1210 murine leukemic cells by treatment with quinacrine hydrochloride. Cancer Res 1969 Oct; 29:1881–1885.

B12. Bachmann M, Falke D, Schroder HC, Muller WEG. Intracellular distribution of the La antigen in Cv-1 cells after herpes simplex virus type 1 infection compared with the localization of U small nuclear ribonucleoprotein particles. J Gen Virol 1989;70:881–891.

B13. Bachmann M, Mayet WJ, Schroder HC, Pfeifer K, Meyer Zum Buschenfelde K-H, Muller WEG. Association of La and Ro antigens with intracellular structures of HEp-2 carcinoma cells. Pro Nat Acad Sci 1986;83:7770.

B14. Bachmann M, Pfiefer K, Schroder HC, Muller WEG. The La antigen shuttles between the nucleus and cytoplasm in CV-1 cells. Mol Cell Biochem 1989;85:103–114.

B15. Bachmann M, Pfiefer K, Schroder HC, Muller WEG. Characterization of the autoantigen La as a nucleic acid-dependent ATPase/dATPase with melting properties. Cell 1990;60: 85–93.

B16. Bacon PA, Myles AB, Beardwell CG, Daly JR, Savage O. Corticosteroid withdrawal in rheumatoid arthritis. Lancet 1966 Oct 29;2935–2937.

B17. Badui E, Garcia-Rubi D, Robles E, Jimenez J, Juan L, Deleze M, Diaz A, Mintz G. Cardiovascular manifestations in systemic erythematosus. Prospective study of 100 patients. Angiology 1985;431–440.

B18. Baehr G, Klemperer P, Schifrin A. Diffuse disease of the peripheral circulation usually associated with lupus erythematosus and endocarditis. Trans Assoc Am Physicians 1935;50: 139–155.

B19. Baer AN, Woosley RL, Pincus T. Further evidence for the lack of association between acetylator phenotype and systemic lupus erythematosus. Arthritis Rheum 1986;29: 508–514.

B20. Baer PA, Shore A, Ikeman RL. Transient fall in serum salicylate levels following intraarticular injection of steroid in patients with rheumatoid arthritis. Arthritis Rheum 1987 Mar; 30(3):345–347.

B21. Baethge BA, King JW, Husain F, Embree LJ. Herpes zoster myelitis occurring during treatment for systemic lupus erythematosus. Am J Med Sci 1989 Oct;298(4):264–266.

B22. Baethge BA, Lidsky MD. Intractable hiccups associated with high dose intravenous methylprednisolone therapy. Ann Intern Med 1986;104:58–59.

B23. Bafverstedt B. Lymphadenosis benign cutis (LABC), its nature, course and prognosis. Acta Dermatovener (Stockh) 1960;40:10–18.

B24. Baganz HM, Bailey WL. Systemic lupus erythematosus complicated by avascular necrosis of the hip. Medical and surgical management. Del Med J 1961 Feb;33:34–37.

B25. Baggenstoss AH. Symposium on systemic lupus erythematosus; visceral lesions in disseminated lupus erythematosus. Proc Mayo Clin 1952 Oct 22;27:412–419.

B25a. Bagley CM Jr, Bostick FW, DeVita VT Jr. Clinical pharma-

cology of cyclophosphamide. Cancer Res 1973 Feb;33: 226–233.

B26. Bahmanyar S, Morean-Dubois M-C, Brown P, Cathala F, Gajdusek DC. Serum antibodies to neurofilament antigens in patients with neurological and other diseases and in healthy controls. J Neuroimmunol 1983;5:190–196.

B27. Bahmanyar S, Srinvasappa J, Casali P, Fujinami RS, Oldstone MBA, Notkins AL. Antigenic mimicry between measles virus and human T lymphocytes J Infect Dis 1987;156:526–527.

B28. Bailey AA, Sayre GP, Clark EC. Neuritis associated with systemic lupus erythematosus; report of 5 cases with necropsy in 2. Arch Neurol & Psychiat 1956 March;75:251–259.

B28a. Bailey FA, Lilly M, Bertoli LF, Ball GV. An antibody that inhibits in vitro bone marrow proliferation in a patient systemic lupus erythematosus and aplastic anemia. Arthritis Rheum 1989;32:901–906.

B29. Bailey NC, Fidanza V, Mayer R, Mazza G, Fougereau M, Bona C. Activation of clones producing self-reactive antibodies by foreign antigen and anti-idiotype antibody carrying the internal image of the antigen. J Clin Invest 1989;84(3):744–756.

B30. Bain GO. The pathology of Mikulicz-Sjogren disease in relation to disseminated lupus erythematosus. A review of the autopsy findings and presentation of a case. Can Med Assoc J 1960 Jan 16;82:143–148.

B31. Bajaj SP, Bajaj MS, Joist JH, Gutmann T. Evidence that the anti-phospholipid antibodies are distinct from he anti-phospholipid antibodies in the lupus anticoagulant-hypoprothrombinemia syndrome [abstract]. Blood 1989;74 Suppl:136a.

B31a. See F139.

B32. Bajaj SP, Rapaport SI, Fierer DS, Herbst KD, Schwartz DB. A mechanism for the hypoprothrombinemia-lupus anticoagulant syndrome. Blood 1983 Apr;61:684–692.

B33. Baker DJ, Trist DG, Weatherall M. Proceedings: Inhibition of phagocytosis by mepacrine. Br J Pharmacol 1976 Mar; 56(3):346P-347P.

B34. Baker M. Psychopathology in systemic lupus erythematosus. I. Psychiatric observations. Semin Arthritis Rheum 1973; 3(2):95–110.

B35. Baker M, Hadler NM, Whitaker JN, Dunner DL, Gerwin RD, Decker JL. Psychopathology in systemic lupus erythematosus. II. Relation to clinical observations, corticosteroid administration, and cerebrospinal fluid C4. Semin Arthritis Rheum 1973; 2:111–126.

B36. Baker SB, Rovira JR, Campion EW, Mills JA. Late onset lupus erythematosus. Am J Med 1979 May;66(5):727–732.

B37. Bakir AA, Lopez-Majano V, Hyrhorczuk DO, Rhee HL, Dunea G. Appraisal of lupus nephritis by renal imaging with Gallium-67. Am J Med 1985;79:175–182.

B38. Bakir F, Saaed B. Systemic lupus erythematosus and periodic peritonitis (FMF) [letter]. Br J Rheumatol 1989 Feb; 28(1):81–82.

B39. Bakke AC, Gray JD, Abo W, Quismorio FP, Lash A, Cooper SM, Horwitz DA. Studies on human blood lymphocytes with iC3b (type 3) complement receptors. I. Granular, Fc-IgG receptor positive and negative subsets in healthy subjects and patients with systemic lupus erythematosus. J Immunol 1986; 136:1253–1259.

B40. Bakke AC, Kirkland PA, Kitridou RC, Quismorio FP, Rea T, Ehresmann GR, Horwitz DA. T lymphocyte subsets in systemic lupus erythematosus. Arthritis Rheum 1983 Jun;26:745–750.

B41. BAL Cooperative Steering Committee. Bronchoalveolar lavage constituents in healthy individuals, idiopathic pulmonary fibrosis and selected comparison group. Am Rev Respir Dis 1990;141:S169-S202.

B42. Balasch J, Font J, Lopez-Soto A, Cervera R, Jovi J, Casals FJ, Vanrell JA. Antiphospholipid antibodies in unselected patients with repeated abortion. Human Reprod 1990 Jan;5(1):43–46.

B43. Baldassare A, Weiss T, Tsai C, Auclair R, Zuckner J. Immune complexes in the skin of patients with rheumatoid arthritis (RA)[abstract]. Arthritis Rheum 1976;19:788.

B44. Balderas RS, Josimovic-Alasevic O, Diamantstein T, Dixon FJ, Theofilopoulos AN. Elevated titers of cell-free interleukin 2 receptor in serum of lupus mice. J Immunol 1987;139: 1496–1500.

B45. Baldi E, Emancipator SN, Hassan MO, Dunn MJ. Platelet activating factor receptor blockade ameliorates murine systemic lupus erythematosus. Kidney Int 1990;38:1030–1038.

B46. Baldini MG. Idiopathic thrombocytopenic purpura and the ITP syndrome. Med Clin North Am 1972 Jan;56:47–64.

B47. Baldwin DS. Chronic glomerulonephritis: nonimmunologic mechanisms of progressive glomerular damage. Kidney Int 1982;21:109.

B48. Baldwin DS. Clinical usefulness of the morphological classification of lupus nephritis. Am J Kidney Dis 1987 Jul;2 Suppl 1:142–149.

B49. Baldwin DS, Gluck ML, Lowenstein J, Gallo GR. Lupus nephritis: clinical course of related to morphologic forms and their transitions. Am J Med 1977 Jan;62:12–30.

B50. Baldwin DS, Lowenstein J, Rothfield NF, Gallo G, McCluskey RT. The clinical course of the proliferative and membranous forms of lupus nephritis. Ann Intern Med 1970 Dec;73:929–942.

B51. Baldwin DS, McLean PG, Chasis H, Goldring W. Effect of nitrogen mustard on clinical course of glomerulonephritis. Arch Intern Med 1953 Aug;92:162–167.

B52. Baldwin GB. Acute disseminated lupus erythematosus with report of a fatal case. Med J Aust 1945 Jul 7;2:11–15.

B53. Ballard DW, Voss EW Jr. Base specificity and idiotypy of anti-DNA antibodies reactive with synthetic nucleic acids. J Immunol 1985 Nov;135(5):3372–3380.

B54. Ballard PL, Grandberg P, Ballard RA. Glucocorticoid levels in maternal and cord serum after prenatal betamethasone therapy to prevent respiratory distress syndrome. J Clin Invest 1975;56:1548–1554.

B55. Ballas SK. Sideroblastic refractory anemia in a patient with systemic lupus erythematosus [case report]. Am J Med Sci 1973 Mar;265:225–231.

B56. Ballas ZK, Donta ST. Sulindac-induced aseptic meningitis. Arch Intern Med 1982 Jan;142(1):165–166.

B57. Ballico I. The cure of lupus erythematosus by means of ultraviolet rays [original in Italian]. Raggi Ultraviol 1930 Nov–Dec;6:182–187.

B58. Ballou SP, Khan MA, Kushner I. Clinical features of systemic lupus erythematosus: differences related to race and age of onset. Arthritis Rheum 1982 Jan;25(1):55–60.

B59. Ballou SP, Khan MA, Kushner I. Intravenous pulse methylprednisolone followed by alternate day corticosteroid therapy in lupus erythematosus: a prospective evaluation. J Rheumatol 1985;12:944–948.

B60. Ballou SP, Kushner I. Lupus patients who lack detectable anti-DNA. Clinical features and survival. Arthritis Rheum 1982 Sep;25:1126–1129.

B61. Ballow M, Parke A. The uses of intravenous immune globulin in collagen vascular disease. J Allergy Clin Immunol 1989 Oct;84(4 Pt 2):608–612.

B62. Balow JE. Therapeutic trials in lupus nephritis. Nephron 1981;27:171–176.

B63. Balow JE. Lupus as a renal disease. Hosp Pract (Off) 1988 Oct;23(10):129–146.

B64. Balow JE, Austin HA 3d, Muenz LR, Joyce KM, Antonovych TA, Klippel JH, Steinberg AD, Plotz PH, Decker JL. Effect of treatment on the evolution of renal abnormalities in lupus nephritis. N Engl J Med 1984 Aug 23;311(8):491–495.

B65. Balow JE, Austin HA 3d, Tsokos GC, Antonovych TA, Steinberg AD, Klippel JH. NIH conference: Lupus nephritis. Ann Intern Med 1987 Jan;106(1):79–94.

B66. Balow JE, Tsokos GC. T and B lymphocyte function in patients with lupus nephritis: correlation with renal pathology. Clin Nephrol 1984;21:93–101.

B67. Bambauer R, Jutzler GA, Pees H, Daus H, Schoenenberger HJ, Biro G, Keller HE. Ciclosporin (CyA) and therapeutic plasma exchange in steroid resistant SLE. In: Schindler R, editor. Ciclosporin in Autoimmune Diseases. Berlin: Springer-Verlag, 1985:346–355.

B68. Bambauer R, Pees H, Daus H, Biro G, Keller HE. Three year's experiences with ciclosporin A and therapeutic plasma exchange in severe cases of systemic lupus erythematosus. Clin Exp Rheumatol 1987;5 Suppl 2:124.

B69. Bambauer R, Weber U, Berberich R. Nephrotoxicity of cyclosporin A in the treatment of systemic lupus erythematosus. Nephropharmakologie 1990; ;452–454.

B70. Bamberg P, Malhotra S, Kaun U, Chadda R, Deodhar SD: Anorexia nervosa in a patient with systemic lupus erythematosus. Rheumatol Int. 1987;7(4):177–9.

B71. Bandziulis RJ, Swanson MS, Dreyfuss G. RNA binding proteins as developmental regulators. Genes Dev 1989;3: 431–437.

B72. Banerjee S, Haggi TM, Luthra HS, Stuart JM, David CS. Possible role of V beta T-cell receptor genes in susceptibility to collagen-induced arthritis in mice. J Exp Med 1988;167: 832–839.

B73. Banfi G, Mazzucco G, DiBelgiojoso GB, Bosiso MB, Stratta P, Confalonieri R, Ferrario F, Imbascati E, Monga G. Morphological patterns in lupus nephritis: their relevance for classification for relationship with clinical and histological findings and outcome. Q J Med 1985;55:153–168.

B74. Bang FDC, Wantzin GL, Christensen JD. Raynaud's phenomenon with oral manifestation in systemic lupus erythematosus. Dermatologica 1985;170:263–264.

B75. Bang NU. Frentizole in systemic lupus erythematosus: Current status. Arthritis Rheum 1982;23:1388–1390.

B76. Bangert J, Freeman R, Sontheimer RD, Gilliam JN. Subacute cutaneous lupus erythematosus and discoid lupus erythematosus. Comparative histopathologic findings. Arch Dermatol 1984;120:332–337.

B77. Bankhurst AD, Carlow TJ, Reidy RW. Exophthalmos in systemic lupus erythematosus. Ann Ophthalmol 1984 Jul;16(7): 669–671.

B78. Bankhurst AD, Witemeyer S. Williams RC. A population of human cord blood mononuclear cells with surface alpha fetoprotein. Immunol Commun 1978;7:187–208.

B79. Banks CN. Melanin: blackguard or red herring? Another look at chloroquine retinopathy. Aust NZ J Ophthalmol 1987 Nov;15(4):365–370.

B80. Banks PM, Witrak GA, Conn DL. Lymphoid neoplasia following connective tissue disease. Mayo Clin Proc 1979 Feb; 54:104–108.

B81. Bar El Y, Shimoni Z, Flatau E. Quinidine-induced lupus erythematosus. Am Heart J 1986; 111:1209–1210.

B82. Barada FA Jr, Andrews BS, Davis JS IV, Taylor RP. Antibodies to Sm in patients with systemic lupus erythematosus. Arthritis Rheum 1981;24:1236–1244.

B83. Barba Rubio J, Franco Martinez E. Discoid LE (Treatment with thalidomide) [original in Spanish]. Med Cut Iber Lat Am 1977;3:279–286.

B84. Barba Rubio J, Gonzalez FF. Discoid LE and thalidomide. Preliminary results [original in Spanish]. Dermatol Rev Mex 1975;19:131–139.

B85. Barber KA, Jackson R. Neonatal lupus erythematosus: five new cases with HLA typing. Can Med Assoc J 1983;129:139.

B86. Barbier F. The L.E. cell. Is it specific for systemic lupus erythematosus? [original in French] Acta Med Scand 1953;147: 325–330.

B87. Barbui T, Cortelazzo S, Galli M, Parazzini F, Radici E, Rossi E, Finazzi G. Antiphospholipid antibodies in early repeated abortions: a case-controlled study. Fertil Steril 1988 Oct; 50(4):589–592.

B88. Barcelli U, Rademacher R, Ooi YM, Ooi BS. Modification of glomerular immune complexes deposition in mice by activation of the reticuloendothelial system. J Clin Invest 1981;67: 20–27.

B89. Barcelo R, Pollak VE. A preliminary immunologic study of urinary proteins: The questionable value of protein clearances in kidney disease. Can Med Assoc J 1966 Feb 5;94:269–275.

B90. Barclay CS, French MA, Ross LD, Sokol RJ. Successful pregnancy following steroid therapy and plasma exchange in a woman with anti-Ro(SSA) antibodies. Case report. Br J Obstet Gynaecol 1987;94:369–371.

B91. Bardana EJ, Harbeck RJ, Hoffman AA, Pirofsky B, Carr RI. The prognostic and therapeutic implications of DNA. anti-DNA immune complexes in systemic lupus erythematosus. Am J Med 1975;59:515–522.

B92. Bardana EJ Jr, Manilow MR, Houghton DC, McNulty WP, Wuepper KD, Parker F, Pirofsky B. Diet-induced systemic lupus erythematosus (SLE) in primates. Am J Kidney Dis 1982; 1:345–352.

B93. Barden RP. Collagen disease and cancer. Radiology 1969 Apr;92:972–974.

B94. Barker GH. Cytotoxic drugs in pregnancy. In: Lewis P, editor. Clinical Pharmacology in Obstetrics. Bristol Wright DSG, 1983:144–155.

B95. Barnes SS, Moffatt TW, Lane CW, Weiss RS. Studies on the L.E. phenomenon. Arch Dermat & Syph 1950 Dec;62:771-785.

B96. Barnett EV, Bluestone R, Cracchiolo A 3d, Goldberg LS, Kantor GL, McIntosh RM. Cryoglobulinemia and disease. Ann Intern Med 1970 Jul;73:95–107.

B97. Barnett EV, Kantor G, Bickel YB, Forsen R, Gonick HC. Systemic lupus erythematosus. CA Med 1969 Dec;111: 467–481.

B98. Barnett EV, Leddy JP, Condemi JJ, Vaughan JH. Antinuclear factors in rheumatoid arthritis. Ann NY Acad Sci 1965 Jun 30; 124:896–903.

B99. Barnhill RL, McDougall AC. Thalidomide: use and possible mode of action in reactional lepromatous leprosy and in various other conditions. J Am Acad Dermatol 1982 Sep;7(3): 317–323.

B100. Baron M, Brisson ML. Pancreatitis in systemic lupus erythematosus. Arthritis Rheum 1982 Aug;25(8):1006–1009.

B101. Barr DP, Reader GG, Wheeler CH. Cryoglobulinemia: Report of two cases with discussion of clinical manifestations, incidence and significance. Ann Intern Med 1950 Jan;32:6–29.

B102. Barr WG, Hubbell EA, Robinson JA. Plasmapheresis and pulse cyclophosphamide in systemic lupus erythematosus [letter]. Ann Intern Med 1988 Jan;108(1):152–153.

B103. Barranco VP. Dapsone—other indications. Int J Dermatol 1982 Nov;21(9):513–514.

B104. Barrett C, Neylon N, Snaith ML. Oestrogen-induced systemic lupus erythematosus. Br J Rheumatol 1986 Aug;25(3): 300–301.

B105. Barrier J, Grolleau JY, Choimet P. Lupus induced by quinidine, detected by thrombocytopenic purpura [letter]. Nouvou Presse Med 1981;10:2991–2992.

B106. Barron KS, Person DA, Brewer EJ, Beale MG, Robson AM. Pulse methylprednisolone therapy in diffuse proliferative lupus nephritis. J Peds 1982 Jul;101:137–141.

B107. Barry JN. Lipstick and lupus erythematosus. N Engl J Med 1969; 281:620–621.

B108. Bartholomew BA. Antinuclear antibody tests as a clinically

selected screening procedure. Am J Clin Pathol 1974 Apr;61: 495–499.

B109. Bartholomew LE, Rynes RI. Use of antimalarial drugs in rheumatoid arthritis: Guidelines for ocular safety. Intern Med 1982;3:66–70.

B110. Barton DD, Fine JD, Gammon WR, Sams WM Jr. Bullous systemic lupus erythematosus: an unusual clinical course and detectable circulating autoantibodies to the epidermolysis bullosa acquisita antigen. J Am Acad Dermatol 1986 Aug;15(2 Pt 2):369–373.

B111. Barton LL, Johnson CR. Discoid lupus erythematosus and X-linked chronic granulomatous disease. Pediatr Dermatol 1986;3:376–379.

B112. Baserga SJ, Yang XW, Steitz JA. An intact Box C sequence in the U3 snRNA is required for binding of fibrillarin, the protein common to the major family of nucleolar snRNPs. Embo J 1991;20:2645–2651.

B113. Baskin L, Mee S, Matthay M, Carroll PR. Ureteral obstruction caused by vasculitis. J Urol 1989 Apr;141(4):933–935.

B114. Bass SW, Ramirez MA, Avaido DM. Cardiopulmonary effects of antimalarial drugs. VI. Adenosine, quinacrine and primaquine. Toxicol Appl Pharmacol 1972 Apr;21:464–481.

B115. Batchelor JR. Hormonal control of antibody formation. In: Cinader B, editor. Regulation of the antibody response. Springfield: Charles C Thomas, 1968:276–293.

B116. Batchelor JR, Fielder AHL, Walport MJ, David J, Lord DK, Davey N, Dodi IA, Malasit P, Wanachiwanawin W, Berstein R, Mackworth-Young C, Isenberg D. Family study of the major histocompatibility complex in HLA-DR3 negative patients with systemic lupus erythematosus. Clin Exp Immunol 1989; 70:364–371.

B117. Batchelor JR, Lombardi G, Lechler RI. Speculations on the specificity of suppression. Immunology Today 1989;10: 37–40.

B118. Batchelor JR, Welsh KL, Mansilla R, Tinoco R, Dollery CT, Hughes GRV, Bernstein R, Ryan P, Naish PF, Maber G, Bing RF, Russel GI. Hydralazine-induced systemic lupus erythematosus: influence of HLA-DR and sex on susceptibility. Lancet 1980 May 24;1:1107–1109.

B119. Bateman A, Singh A, Kral T, Solomon S. The immune-hypothalamic-pituitary-adrenal axis. Endocrin Rev 1989;10: 92–112.

B120. Bateman DE. Carbamazepine induced systemic lupus erythematosus: Case report. Br Med J (Clin Res) 1985; 291: 632–633.

B121. Bateman T. A practical synopsis of cutaneous disease, according to the arrangement of Dr. Willan, exhibiting a concise view of the diagnostic symptoms and the method of treatment, 2d ed. London: London, Longman, Hurst, Rees, Orme, and Brown, 1813 (also 2d Am ed. Philadelphia: Crissy J, 1824).

B122. Batsford SR, Takamiya H, Bogt A. A model of in situ formation of immune complex glomerulonephritis in the rat employing cationized ferritin. Clin Nephrol 1980;14:211.

B123. Bauer KA, Rosenberg RD. The pathophysiology of the prethrombotic state in humans. Insights gained from studies using markers of hemostatic system activation. Blood 1987; 70:343–350.

B124. Baum CG, Chiorazzi N, Frankel S, Shepherd GM. Conversion of systemic lupus erythematosus to common variable hypogammaglobulinemia. Am J Med 1989;87:449–456.

B125. Baum J. Epidemiology of juvenile rheumatoid arthritis. Arthritis Rheum 1977;20:158.

B126. Baum J, Stastny P, Ziff M. Effect of rheumatoid factor and antigen-antibody complexes on the vessels of the rat mesentery. J Immunol 1964 Dec;93:985–995.

B127. Baum J, Ziff M. Decreased 19S antibody response to bacterial antigens in systemic lupus erythematosus. J Clin Invest 1969 Apr;48:758–767.

B128. Baum WL. The Practical Medicine Year Books. Chicago: The Year Book Publishers. 1904;(10):8–9.

B129. Baur MP, Danilovs JA. Population analysis of HLA-A,B,C,DR and other genetic markers. In: Terasaki P, editor. Histocompatibility Testing 1980. Los Angeles: UCLA Tissue Typing Laboratory, 1981:955–975.

B130. Baur MP, Neugebauer M, Deppe H, Sigmund M, Luton T, Mayr WR, Albert ED. Population analysis on the basis of deducted haplotypes from random families, Histocompatibility Testing 1984. Albert ED, Bauer MP, Mayr WR, editors. New York: Springer Verlag, 1984.

B131. Bavykin SG, Usachenko SI, Zalensky AO, Mirzabekov AD. Structure of nucleosomes and organization of internucleosomal DNA in chromatin. J Mol Biol 1990;212:495–511.

B132. Baxevanis AD, Godfrey JE, Moudrianakis EN. Effect of aggregation of histone octamers in high-salt solutions on circular dichroism spectra. Biochemistry 1990;29:973–976.

B133. Baxevanis CN, Reclos GJ, Papamichail M, Tsokos GC. Prothymosin alpha restores the depressed autologous and allogeneic mixed lymphocyte responses in patients with systemic lupus erythematosus. Immunopharm Immunotoxicol 1987; 9(4):429–440.

B134. Bayliss C, Handa RK, Sorkin M. Glucocorticosteroids and control of glomerular filtration rate. Sem Nephrol 1990;10: 320–329.

B135. Bazinet P, Marin GA. Malabsorption in systemic lupus erythematosus. Am J Dig Dis 1971 May;16:460–466.

B136. Beall SS, Concannon P, Charmley P, McFarland HF, Gatti RA, Hood LE, McFarlin DE, Biddison WE. The germline repertoire of T-cell receptor beta-chain genes in patients with chronic progressive multiple sclerosis. J Neuroimmunol 1989; 21:59–66.

B137. Bean RB, Bean WB. Sir William Osler: Aphorisms from His Bedside Teachings and Writings, collected by R.B. Bean and edited by W.B. Bean. New York: Henry Schuman, 1950.

B138. Bean SF, Lynch FW. Senear-Usher syndrome (pemphigus erythematosus): immunofluorescent studies in a patient. Arch Dermatol 1970 Jun;101:642–645.

B139. Bean WB, editor. Aphorisms from Latham. Iowa City: The Prairie Press:1962.

B140. Bear R. Pregnancy and lupus nephropathy. Obstet Gynecol 1976;47:715–718.

B141. Beaucher WN, Garman RH, Condemi JJ. Familial lupus erythematosus: antibodies to DNA in household dogs. N Engl J Med 1977 Apr 28;296:982–984.

B142. Beaufils M, Donsimoni R, Uzan S, Colau JC. Prevention of pre-eclampsia by early antiplatelet therapy. Lancet 1985;1: 840–842.

B143. Beaulieu A, Quismorio FP Jr, Friou GJ, Vayuvegula B, Mirick G. IgG antibodies to double-stranded DNA in systemic lupus erythematosus sera. Arthritis Rheum 1979;22:565–570.

B144. Beaulieu A, Quismorio FP Jr, Kitridou RC, Friou GJ. Complement fixing antibodies to ds-DNA in SLE: A study using the immunofluorescent crithidia luciliae method. J Rheumatol 1979;6:389–396.

B145. Beaulieu AD, Valet JP, Strevey J. The influence of fibronectin on cryoprecipitate formation in rheumatoid arthritis and systemic lupus erythematosus. Arthritis Rheum 1981 Nov;24: 1383–1388.

B146. Beaumont V, Gioud-Paquet M, Kahn MF, Beaumont JL. Antiestrogen antibodies, oral contraception and systemic lupus erythematosus. Clin Physiol Biochem 1989;7(5): 263–268.

B147. Bechet PE. Lupus erythematosus hypertrophicus et profundus. Arch Dermatol 1942 Jan;45:33–39.

B148. Bechet PE. Aurotherapy in lupus erythematosus; study based on further experience of 14 years. N Y State J Med 1942 Apr 1;42:609–614.

B149. Beck DW, Strauss RG, Zisker T, Henricksen RA. An intrinsic coagulation pathway inhibitor in a 3-year-old child. Am J Clin Pathol 1979 Apr;71:470–472.

B150. Beck JS. Variations in the morphological patterns of autoimmune fluorescence. Lancet 1961;1:1203–1205.

B151. Beck JS, Oakley CL and Rowell NR. Transplacental passage of antinuclear antibody. Arch Dermatol 1966;93:656–662.

B152. Beck JS, Rowell NR. Discoid lupus erythematosus. A study of the clinical features and biochemical and serological abnormalities in 120 patients with observations on the relationship of this disease to systemic lupus erythematosus. Q J Med 1966 Jan;35:119–136.

B153. Becker EL, Henson PM. In vitro studies of immunologically induced secretion of mediators from cells and related phenomena. Adv Immunol 1973;17:94–193.

B154. Becker GJ, Waldburger M, Hughes GR, Pepys MB. Value of serum c-reactive protein measurement in the investigation of fever in systemic lupus erythematosus. Ann Rheum Dis 1980 Feb;39:50–52.

B155. Becker JC, Kolanus W, Lonnemann C, Schmidt RE. Human natural killer clones enhance in vitro antibody production by tumor necrosis factor alpha and gamma interferon. Scand J Immunol 1990;32:153–162.

B156. Becker NJ, Borek D, Abdou NI. Angioimmunoblastic lymphadenopathy presenting as SLE with GI protein loss [letter]. J Rheumatol 1988 Sep;15(9):1452–1454.

B157. Becker NJ, Crockett RS, Valenzeno DP, Abdou NI. Effect of in vitro ultraviolet radiation on the binding capacity of anti DNA and DNA in systemic lupus erythematosus. J Rheumatol 1989 Jun;16(6):773–776.

B158. Becker S, Daniel EG. Antagonistic and additive effects of IL-4 and interferon-gamma on human monocytes and macrophages: effects on Fc receptors, HLA-D antigens, and superoxide production. Cell Immunol 1990;129:351–362.

B159. Becker TM, Lizzio EF, Merchant B. Increased multiclonal antibody-forming cell activity in the peripheral blood of patients with SLE. Int Arch Allergy Appl Immunol 1981;66: 293–299.

B160. Beckett AG, Lewis JG. Familial lupus erythematosus. A report of two cases. Br J Dermatol 1959;71:360.

B161. Bedell SE, Bush BT. Erythrocyte sedimentation rate: From folklore to facts. Am J Med 1985 Jun;78:1001–1009.

B162. Beebe WE, Abbott RL, Fung WE. Hydroxychloroquine crystals in the tear film of a patient with rheumatoid arthritis. Am J Ophthalmol 1986 Mar 15;101(3):377–378.

B163. Beecham JE, Abd-Elrazak M. Concomitant herpes-monilial esophagitis in a patient with systemic lupus erythematosus: Successful systemic antiviral treatment. Saudi Med J 1987;8: 419–422.

B164. Been M, Thompson BJ, Smith MA, Ridgway JP, Douglas RHB, Berst JJK, Muir AL. Myocardial involvement in systemic lupus erythematosus detected by magnetic resonance imaging. Eur Heart J 1988;9:1250–1256.

B165. Beer AE, Billingham RE. Host response to intrauterine tissue of cellular and fetal allografts. J Reprod Fert 1974; 21(suppl):59–88.

B166. Beer AE, Sio JO. Placenta as in immunological barrier. Biol Reprod 1982;26:15–27.

B167. Behan PO, Behan WMH, Zacharias FJ, Nicholls JT. Immunological abnormalities in patients who had the oculmucocutaneous syndrome associated with practolol therapy. Lancet 1976 Nov 6;2:984–987.

B168. Behar SM, Corbet S, Diamond B, Scharff MD. The molecular origin of anti-DNA antibodies. Intern Rev Immunol 1989; 5:23–42.

B169. Behar SM, Scharff MD. Somatic diversification of the S107(T15) VH11 germ-line gene that encodes the heavy-chain variable region of antibodies to double-stranded DNA in (NZB × NZW)F1 mice. Proc Natl Acad Sci USA 1988 Jan; 85(11):3970–3974.

B170. Beigelman PM. Variants of the platelet thrombosis syndrome and their relationship to disseminated lupus. Arch Pathol 1951 Feb;51:213–223.

B171. Beilstein DP, Hawkins ES. Pedal manifestations of systemic lupus erythematosus. Clin Podiatr Med Surg 1988 Jan;5(1): 37–56.

B172. Beirne GJ, Brennan JT. Glomerulonephritis associated with hydrocarbon solvents. Arch Environ Health 1972;25: 365–369.

B173. Beitings IZ, Bayard F, Ances IG, Koworski A, Migeon CJ. The transplacental passage of prednisone and prednisolone in pregnancy near term. J Pediatr 1972;81:936–945.

B174. Beitings IZ, Bayard F, Ances IG, Kowarski A, Migeon CJ. The metabolic clearance rate, blood production, interconversion and transplacental passage of cortisol and cortisone in pregnancy near term. Pediatr Res 1973;7:509–519.

B175. Belch JF, Ansell D, Madhok R, O'Dowd A, Sturrock RD. Effects of altering dietary essential fatty acids on requirements for non-steroidal anti-inflammatory drugs in patients with rheumatoid arthritis: a double-blind placebo controlled study. Ann Rheum Dis 1988;47:96.

B176. Bell AL, Fleck B, Mitchell D, Thompson B, Hurst NP, Nuki G. Visual contrast sensitivity (VCS) testing for chloroquine retinopathy. Br J Rheumatol 1984 May;23:131.

B177. Bell CL. Hydroxychloroquine sulfate in rheumatoid arthritis: long-term response rate and predictive parameters. Am J Med 1983 Jul 18;75 Suppl 1A:46–51.

B178. Bell CL, Boh LE. The risk of retinopathy associated with hydroxychloroquine (HCQ) use in patients with rheumatoid arthritis (RA) [abstract]. Arthritis Rheum 1989 Jan;32(1) Suppl:R32.

B179. Bell CL, Partington C, Robbins M, Graziano F, Turski P, Kornguth S. Magnetic resonance imaging of central nervous system lesions in patients with lupus erythematosus: Correlation with clinical remission and antineurofilament and anticardiolipin antibody titers. Arthritis Rheum 1991 Apr;34(4): 432–441.

B180. Bell DA. Cell-mediated immunity in systemic lupus erythematosus: observations on in vitro cell-mediated immune responses in relationship to number of potentially reactive T cells, disease activity, and treatment. 1978 Mar;9:301–317.

B181. Bell DA. SLE in the elderly—is it really SLE or systemic Sjogren's syndrome? [editorial]. J Rheumatol 1988;15(5): 723–724.

B182. Bell DA, Cairns E, Cikalo K, Ly V, Block J, Pruzanski W. Anti-nucleic acid autoantibody responses of normal human origin: antigen specificity and idiotypic characteristics compared to patients with systemic lupus erythematosus and patients with monoclonal IgM. J Rheumatol 1987;14:127–131.

B183. Bell DA, Komar R, Chordiker WB, Block J, Girns E. A comparison of serologic reactivity among SLE patients with or without anti Ro(SSA) antibodies. J Rheumatol 1984;11: 315–317.

B184. Bell DA, Maddison PJ. Serologic subsets in systemic lupus erythematosus: An examination of autoantibodies in relationship to clinical features of disease and HLA antigens. Arthritis Rheum 1980 Nov;23:1268–1273.

B185. Bell DA, Morrison B. The spontaneous apoptotic cell death of normal human lymphocytes in vitro: the release of,

and immunoproliferative response to, nucleosomes in vitro. Clin Immunol Immunopathol 1991;60:13–26.

B186. Bell DA, Morrison B, Vanden Bygaart P. Immunogenic DNA-related factors. Nucleosomes spontaneously released from normal murine lymphoid cells stimulate proliferation and immunoglobulin synthesis of normal mouse lymphocytes. J Clin Invest 1990;85:1487–1496.

B187. Bell DA, Rigsby R, Stiller CR, Clark WF, Harth M, Ebers G. HLA Antigens in systemic lupus erythematosus: Relationship to disease severity, age at onset, sex. J Rheumatol 1984 Aug; 11:475–479.

B188. Bell EB. Thymus-derived and non-thymus-derived T-like cells: the origin and function of cells bearing gamma delta receptors. Thymus 1989;14:3–17.

B189. Bell EB, Sparshott SM. Interconversion of CD45R subsets of CD4 T cells in vivo. Nature 1990;348:163–166.

B190. Bell R, Lawrence DS. Chronic pleurisy in systemic lupus erythematosus. Br J Dis Chest 1976 Jul;73:324–326.

B191. Bell WR, Boss GR, Wolfson JS. Circulating anticoagulant in the procainamide-induced lupus syndrome. Arch Intern Med 1977 Oct;137:1471–1473.

B192. Belmont HM, Hopkins P, Edelson HS, Kaplan HB, Ludewig R, Weissmann G, Abramson S. Complement activation during systemic lupus erythematosus. C3a and C5a anaphylatoxins circulate during exacerbations of disease. Arthritis Rheum 1986;29:1085–1089.

B193. Belongia EA, Hedberg CW, Gleich GJ, White KE, Mayeno AN, Loegering DA, Dunnette SL, Pirie PL, McDonald KL, Osterholm MT. An investigation of the cause of the eosinophilia-myalgia syndrome associated with tryptophan use. N Engl J Med 1990;323:357–365.

B194. Belote GH. Lupus erythematosus disseminates: Its present status. Arch Dermat & Syph 1939 May:39:793–806.

B195. Beltran J, Herman LJ, Burk JM, Zuelzer WA, Clark RN, Lucas JG, Weiss LD, Yang A. Femoral head avascular necrosis MR imaging with clinical pathologic and radionuclide correlation. Radiology 1988 Jan;166(1 Pt 1):215–220.

B196. Ben-Asher S. Recurrent acute lupus erythematosus disseminatus: report of case which has survived 23 years after onset of systemic manifestations. Ann Intern Med 1951 Jan; 34:243–248.

B197. Ben-Chetrit E, Chan EKL, Sullivan KF, Tan EM. A 52-kD protein is a novel component of the SS-A/Ro antigenic particle. J Exp Med 1988;167:1560–1571.

B198. Ben-Chetrit E, Gandy BJ, Tan EM, Sullivan KF. Isolation and characterization of a cDNA clone encoding the 60-kD component of the human SS-A/Ro ribonucleoprotein autoantigen. J Clin Invest 1989;83:1284–1292.

B199. Ben-Chetrit E, Gross DJ, Braverman A, Weshler Z, Fuks Z, Slavin S, Eliakim M. Total lymphoid irradiation in refractory systemic lupus erythematosus. Ann Intern Med 1986 Jul; 105(1):58–60.

B200. Ben-Chetrit E, Pollack A, Flussaer D, Rubinow A. Coexistence of systemic lupus erythematosus and myasthenia gravis: two distinct populations of anti-DAN and anti-acetylcholine receptor antibodies. Clin Exp Rheumatol 1990;8:71–74.

B201. Benacerraf B. Immune response genes. Scand J Immunol 1974;3:381–386.

B202. Benacerraf B, Sebestyen MM, Schlossman S. A quantitative study of the kinetics of blood clearance of P^{32}-labelled Escherichia coli and Staphylococci by the reticuloendothelial system. J Exp Med 1959;10:27–46.

B203. Bencze G. Relationship of systemic lupus erythematosus (SLE) to rheumatoid arthritis (RA), discoid lupus erythematosus (DLE) Sjogren's syndrome, A clinical study. Acta Rheumatol Scand 1970;16:191–196.

B204. Bencze G, Tiboldi T, Lakatos L. Experiments on pathogenetic role of L.E. factor in dogs and guinea pigs. Acta Rheum Scand 1963;9:209.

B205. Bender A, Kabelitz D. CD4-CD8- human T cells: phenotypic heterogeneity and activation requirements of freshly isolated "double negative" T cells. Cell Immunol 1988;128: 542–554.

B206. Benenson EV, Mirrakhimova EM. Clinical effectiveness of prospidin in systemic lupus erythematosus: Results of a 6 month follow-up. Ter Arkh 1989;61:21–26.

B207. Bennaham DA, Messner RP, Shoop JD. The brain scan as a measure of activity in lupus cerebritis. [abstract]. Arthritis Rheum 1973 Jul–Aug;16:534.

B208. Benner EJ, Gourley RT, Cooper RA, Benson JA Jr. Chronic active hepatitis with lupus nephritis. Ann Intern Med 1968 Feb;68(2):405–413.

B209. Benner KG, Montanaro A. Protein-losing enteropathy in systemic lupus erythematosus. Diagnosis and monitoring immunosuppressive therapy by alpha-1-antitrypsin clearance in stool. Dig Dis Sci 1989 Jan;34(1):132–135.

B210. Bennet R, Hughes GRV, Bywaters EG, Holt PVL. Neuropsychiatric problems in systemic lupus erythematosus. BMJ 1972 Nov 11;4:342.

B211. Bennett JC, Holley HL. Intradermal hypersensitivity in systemic lupus erythematosus. Arthritis Rheum 1961 Feb;4: 64–73.

B212. Bennett RM. Scleroderma overlap syndromes. Rheum Dis Clin North Am 1990 Feb;16(1):185–198.

B213. Bennett RM, Bong DM, Spargo BH. Neuropsychiatric problems in mixed connective tissue disease. Am J Med 1978 Dec;65(6):955–962.

B214. Bennett RM, Davis J, Campbell S, Portnoff S. Lactoferrin binds to cell membrane DNA: Association of surface DNA with an enriched population of B cells and monocytes. J Clin Invest 1983;71:611–618.

B215. Bennett RM, Davis J, Merritt M. Anti-DNA antibodies react with DNA expressed on the surface of monocytes and B lymphocytes. J Rheumatol 1986;13:679–685.

B216. Bennett RM, Gabor GT, Merritt MM. DNA binding to human leukocytes: evidence for receptor-mediated association, internalization and degradation of DNA. J Clin Invest 1985;76:2182–2190.

B217. Bennett RM, Kotzin B, Merritt MJ. DNA receptor dysfunction in systemic lupus erythematosus and kindred disorders. Induction by anti-DNA antibodies, antihistone antibodies, and antireceptor antibodies. J Exp Med 1987 Oct 1;166(4): 850–863.

B218. Bennett RM, O'Connell DJ. Mixed connective tissue disease: a clinicopathologic study of 20 cases. Semin Arthritis Rheum 1980 Aug;10(1):25–51.

B219. Bennett RM, Spargo BH. Immune complex nephropathy in mixed connective tissue disease. Am J Med 1977 Oct;63(4): 534–541.

B220. Bennett WM, Bardana EJ, Houghton DC, Pirofsky B, Striker GD. Silent renal involvement in systemic lupus erythematosus. Int Arch All Appl Immunol 1977;55(4):420–428.

B221. Bennion SD, Ferris C, Lieu TS, Reimer CB, Lee LA. IgG subclasses in the serum and skin in subacute cutaneous lupus erythematosus and neonatal lupus erythematosus. J Invest Dermatol 1990;95:643–646.

B222. Benotti JR, Sataline CR, Sloss LJ, Conn LH. Aortic and mitral insufficiency complicating fulminant systemic lupus erythematosus. Chest 1984 Jul;86:141–143.

B223. Bensaid J, Aldigier JC, Gualde N. Systemic lupus erythematosus syndrome induced by pindolol. Br Med J 1979 Jun 16; 1:1603–1604.

B224. Benson MD, Cohen AS. Serum amyloid: A protein in amy-

loidosis, rheumatic and neoplastic diseases. Arthritis Rheum 1979 Jan;22(1):36–42.

B225. Bentley DL. Most kappa immunoglobulin mRNA in human lymphocytes is homologous to a small family of germ-line V genes. Nature 1984;307:77.

B226. Bently R, Keene J. Recognition of U1 and U2 small nuclear RNAs can be altered by a 5-amino acid segment in the U2 small nuclear ribonucleoprotein particle (snRNP) B″ protein and through interactions with U2 snRNP-A′ protein. Mol Cell Biol 1991;11:1829–1839.

B227. Bentson J, Reza M, Winter J, Wilson G. Steroids and apparent cerebral atrophy on computed tomography scans. J Comput Assist Tomogr 1978;2:16–23.

B228. Berbir N, Allen J, Dubois E. The risk of pericardiocentesis in SLE: Case report and literature review [original in French]. Rev du Rheumatisme 1976 Jun 15;44:359–362.

B229. Berbis P, Vernay-Vaisse C, Privot Y. Lupus cutane subaigu observe au cours d'un traitement par diuretiques thiazidiques. Ann Dermatol Venereol 1986;113:1245–1248.

B230. Berchtold P, Harris JP, Tani P, Piro L, McMillan R. Autoantibodies to platelet glycoproteins in patients with disease-related immune thrombocytopenia. Br J Haematol 1989;73: 365–368.

B231. Berczi I. The effects of growth hormone and related hormones on the immune system. In: Berczi I, editor. Pituitary function and immunity. Boca Raton: CRC Press, 1986: 133–160.

B232. Berden JH, Faaber P, Assmann KJ, Rijke TP. Effects of cyclosporin A on autoimmune disease in MRL/l and BXSB mice. Scand J Immunol 1986;24:405–411.

B233. Bereikene IP, Matulis AA, Shevchenko OP, Venalis AI. Levels of C4 component of the complement, lactoferrin and leukocytic thermostable alpha glycoprotein during the treatment of patients with systemic rheumatic diseases. Revmatologiia (Moskva) 1989;2:41–45.

B234. Berek C, Milstein C. Mutational drift and repertoire shift in the maturation of the immune response. Immunol Rev 1987;96:23–42.

B235. Bergemer AM, Fouquet B, Goupille P, Valat JP. Peripheral neuropathy as the initial manifestation of systemic lupus erythematosus. Report of a case. Sem Hop Paris 1987;63: 1979–1982.

B236. Bergen SS. Pericardial effusion. A manifestation of systemic lupus erythematosus. Circulating 1960 Jul;22:144–150.

B237. Omitted.

B238. Berglund S, Gottfries CG, Gottfries I, Stormby K. Chlorpromazine-induced antinuclear factors. Acta Med Scand 1970 Jan–Feb;187:67–74.

B239. Bergmeister R. Concerning primary and miliary tuberculosis of the retina [original in German]. Wien Med Wschr 1929 Aug 24;79:1116–1119.

B240. Bergroth V, Konttinen YT, Johansson E. Langerhans cells in SLE skin. A role in lymphocyte migration and activation in situ. Scand J Rheumatol 1985;14(4):411–416.

B241. Bergstein J, Wiens C, Fish AJ, Vernier RL, Michael A. Avascular necrosis of bone in systemic lupus erythematosus. J Pediatr 1974;85:31–35.

B242. Berinstein N, Campbell MJ, Lam K, Carswell C, Levy S, Levy R. Idiotypic variation in a human B lymphoma cell line. J Immunol 1990;144:752.

B243. Beris PH, Burger A, Favre L, Riodnel A, Miescher PA. Adrenocortical responsiveness after discontinuous corticosteroid therapy. Klin Wochenschr 1986 64:70–75.

B244. Berk MA, Sloan JB, Fretzin DF. Lupus erythematosus in a patient with long-standing multiple sclerosis. J Am Acad Dermatol 1988 Nov;19(5 Pt 2):969–972.

B245. Berkman EM, Orlin J, Wolfsdorf J. An antineutrophil antibody associated with propylthiouracil (PTU) induced lupus-like syndrome. Transfusion 1983;23:135–138.

B246. Berlin CM, Pascuzzi MJ, Yaffe SJ. Excretion of salicylate in human milk. Clin Pharmacol Ther 1980;27:245.

B247. Berliner RW, Earle DP, Taggert JV, Zubrod CG, Welch WJ, Conan NJ, Bauman E, Scudder ST, Shannon JA. Studies on the chemotherapy of the human malarials, the physiological disposition, antimalarial activity and toxicity of several derivations of 4-amino-quinidine. J Clin Invest 1948;27:98–107.

B248. Berlyne GM, Short IA, Vickers CFH. Placental transmission of the LE factor. Report of two cases. Lancet 1957;273:15–16.

B249. Berman J, Mellis S, Pollack R, Smith C, Suh HY, Kowal C, Surti U, Chess L, Cantor C, Alt F. Content and organization of the human Ig V_H locus: definition of this new V_H families and linkage to the Ig C_H locus. EMBO J 1988;7:727–738.

B250. Berman L, Axelrod AR, Goodman HL, McClaughry RI. So-called "lupus erythematosus inclusion phenomenon" of bone marrow and blood; morphologic and serologic studies. Am J Clin Pathol 1950 May;20:403–418.

B251. Bernabeu C, Carrera AC, De Landazuri MO, Sanchez Madrid F. Interaction between the CD45 antigen and phytohemagglutinin inhibitory effect on the lectin-induced T cell proliferation by anti-CD45 monoclonal antibody. Eur J Immunol 1987; 17:1461–1466.

B252. Bernal AL, Craft IL. Corticosteroid metabolism in vitro by human placenta, fetal membranes and decidua in early and late gestation. Placenta 1981;2:279–286.

B253. Bernard P, Barbeau C, Cardinaud F, Lasfargeas JP, Catanzano G, Bonnetblanc JM. Facial edema associated with a malar rash in systemic lupus erythematosus. Ann Dermatol Venereol 1986;113(12):1249–1250.

B254. Bernhard GC, Garancis JC, Piering WF. Prolonged cyclophosphamide or azathioprine therapy of lupus nephritis [abstract]. 1973 Jan–Feb;14(1):130.

B255. Bernhard GC, Lange RL, Hensley GT. Aortic disease with valvular insufficiency as the principal manifestation of systemic lupus erythematosus. Ann Intern Med 1969 Jul;71: 81–87.

B256. Bernstein BH, Stobie D, Singsen BH, Koster-King K, Kornreich HK, Hanson V. Growth retardation in juvenile rheumatoid arthritis. Arthritis Rheum 1977;20 Suppl:212–216.

B257. Bernstein NH. Chloroquine ocular toxicity. Survey Ophthal 1967 Oct;12:415–447.

B258. Bernstein HN. Ophthalmologic considerations and testing in patients receiving long-term antimalarial therapy. Am J Med 1983 Jul 18;75 Suppl 1A:25–34.

B259. Bernstein HN, Mills DW, Becker B. Steroid-induced elevation of intraocular pressure. Arch Ophthalmol 1963 Jul;70: 15–18.

B260. Bernstein JE, Soltani K, Cristancho N, Aronson AJ. Prognostic implications of cutaneous immunoglobulin deposits in systemic lupus erythematosus. Int J Dermatol 1983 Jan–Feb: 22(1):29–34.

B261. Bernstein ML, Salusinsky-Sternbach M, Bellefleur M, Esseltine DW. Thrombotic and hemorrhagic complications in children with the lupus anticoagulant. Am J Dis Child 1984 Dec; 138:1132–1135.

B262. Bernstein RM, Bunn CC, Hughes GRV, Francoeur AM, Mathews MB. Cellular protein and RNA antigens in autoimmune disease. Mol Biol Med 1984;2:105–120.

B263. Bernstein RM, Hobbs RN, Lee DJ, Ward DJ, Hughes GRV. Patterns of antihistone antibody specificity in systemic rheumatic disease. I. systemic lupus erythematosus, mixed connective tissue disease, primary sicca syndrome, and rheumatoid arthritis with vasculitis. Arthritis Rheum 1985;28:285–293.

B264. Berry CZ, Goldberg IC, Shepard WL. Systemic lupus ery-

thematosus complicated by coccidioidomycosis. JAMA 1968; 206:1083–1085.

B265. Bertouch JV, Roberts-Thompson PJ, Feng PH, Bradley J. C-reactive protein and serologic indices of disease activity in systemic lupus erythematosus. Ann Rheum Dis 1983;Feb;42: 655–568.

B266. Bertrand E, Cloitre B, Ticolat R, Bile RK, Gautier C, Abiyou GO, Bohui BY. Antiaggregation action of chloroquine [English abstract]. Med Trop (Mars) 1990 Jan–Mar;50(1):143–146.

B267. Berube S, Lister G, Towes WH, Creasy RK, Heymann MA. Congenital heart block and maternal systemic lupus erythematosus. Am J Obstet Gynecol 1978;130:595–596.

B268. Besana C, Lassarin A, Capsoni F, Caredda F, Moroni M. Phagocyte function in systemic lupus erythematosus. Lancet 1975;2:918.

B269. Bessler H, Sirota L, Dulitzky F, Djaldetti, M. Cord serum inhibits allogeneic mixed lymphocyte reactivity and stimulates lymphokine production. Reprod Immunol 1986;9(2): 103–110.

B270. Bessler H, Sirota L, Dulitzky F, Djaldetti, M. Production of interleukin 1 by mononuclear cells of newborns and their mothers. Clin Exp Immunol 1987;68(3):655–661.

B271. Best MM, Duncan CH. A lupus-like syndrome following propylthiouracil administration. J Ky Med Assoc 1964 Jan;62: 47–49.

B272. Best WR, Darling DR. A critical look at the splenectomy-SLE controversy. Med Clin N Am 1962 Jan;46:19–47.

B273. Bestagno M, Cerino A, Riva S, Ricotti GCBA. Improvements of Western blotting to detect monoclonal antibodies. Biochem Biophys Res Commun 1987;146:1509–1514.

B274. Bettley FR, Page F. Effect of mepacrine on light sensitivity in lupus. Br J Dermatol 1954 Aug–Sep; 66:287–293.

B275. Bettman JW Jr, Daroff RB, Sanders MD, Hoyt WF. Papilledema and asymptomatic intracranial hypertension in systemic lupus erythematosus. A fluorescein angiographic study of resolving papilledema. Arch Ophthalmol 1968 Aug;80: 189–193.

B276. Beurey J, Weber M, Delrous JL, Foos C. Acute lupus erythematosus perhaps induced by tegretol (carbamazepine) [original in French]. Bull Soc Fr Dermatol Syphilgr 1972;79: 186.

B277. Beutner EH, Chorzelski TP, Bean SF, editors. Immunopathology of the Skin, 2nd ed. New York: Wiley, 1979.

B278. Beutner EH, Krasny S, Kumar V, Taylor R, Chorzelski TP. Prospects and problems in the definition and standardization of immunofluorescence. I. Present levels of reproducibility and disease specificity of antinuclear antibody tests. Ann NY Acad Sci 1983 Dec 30;420:28–54.

B279. Beverley P. Immunological memory in T cells. Curr Opin Immunol 1991;3:355–360.

B280. Bevers EM. Anticardiolipin antibody cofactor. Lancet 1991;337:550.

B281. Bevers EM, Galli M. Beta 2—glycoprotein I for binding of anticardiolipin antibodies to cardiolipin. Lancet 1990;336: 952–953.

B282. Beynen AC. Could chloroquine be of value in the treatment of hypercholesterolemia? Artery 1986;13(6):340–351.

B283. Bharati S, De La Fuents D, Kallen RJ, Freij Y, Lev M. Conduction system in systemic lupus erythematous with atrioventricular block. Am J Cardiol 1975;35:299–304.

B284. Bharati S, Swerdlow MA, Vitullo D, Chiemmongoltip P, Lev M. Neonatal lupus with congenital atrioventricular block and myocarditis. PACE 1987;10:1058.

B285. Bhardwaj N, Santhanam V, Lau LL, Tatter SB, Ghrayeb J, Rivelis M, Steinman RM, Sehgal PB, May LT. IL-6/IFN-B2 in synovial effusions of patients with Rheumatoid Arthritis and other arthritides. J Immunol 1989;143:2153–2159.

B286. Bhathena DB, Sobel BJ, Migdal SD. Noninflammatory renal microangiopathy of systemic lupus erythematosus ("lupus vasculitis"). Am J Nephrol 1981 Oct;144–159.

B287. Bhattacharya-Chatterjee M, Chatterjee SK, Vasile S, Seon BK, Kohler H. Idiotype vaccines against human T cell leukemia. II. Generation and characterization of a monoclonal idiotype cascade (Ab1, Ab2, Ab3). J Immunol 1988;141:1398.

B288. Bhattacharya-Chatterjee M, Pride MW, Seon BK, Kohler H. Idiotype vaccines against human T cell acute lymphoblastic leukemia. I. Generation and characterization of biologically active monoclonal anti-idiotypes. J Immunol 1987;139:1354.

B289. Bhuyan UN, Malaviya AN, Dash SG, Malhotra KK. Prognostic significance of renal angiitis in systemic lupus erythematosus. Clin Nephrol 1983;20:109–113.

B290. Bhuyan UN, Malaviya AN, Kumar R, Malhotra KK, Tandin HD. Frequency and severity of renal lesions in systemic lupus erythematosus in north India. Indian J Med Res 1977 Dec;66:965–973.

B291. Bias WB, Reveille JD, Beaty TLH, Meyers DA, Arnett FC. Evidence that autoimmunity in man is a mendelian-dominant trait. Am J Hum Genet 198 6;39:584–602.

B292. Bich-Yhuy LT, Samarut C, Brochier J, Revillard JP. Suppression of the late stages of mitogen-induced human B-cell differentiation by Fcγ receptors released from polymorphonuclear neutrophils J Immunol 1981;127:1299–1403.

B293. Bickers JN, Buechner HA, Hood BJ, Alvarez-Chiesa G. Hypersensitivity reaction to antituberculosis drugs with hepatitis, lupus phenomenon, and myocardial infarction. N Engl J Med 1961 Jul 20;265:131–132.

B294. Bidani AK, Roberts JL, Schwartz MM, Lewis EJ. Immunopathology of cardiac lesions in fatal systemic lupus erythematosus. Am J Med 1980 Dec;69:849–858.

B295. Bielsa I, Herrero C, Ercilla G, Collado A, Font J, Ingelmo M, Mascaro JM. Immunogenetic findings in cutaneous lupus erythematosus. J Am Acad Dermatol 1991;25:251–257.

B296. Bielsa I, Herrero C, Font J, Masearo JM. Lupus erythematosus and toxic epidermal neurolysis. J Am Acad Dermatol 1987;16:1265–1267.

B297. Bielschowsky M, D'Ath EF. The kidneys of NZB-Bl, NZO-B1, NZC-B1 and NZY-B1 mice. J Pathol 1971 Feb;103:97–105.

B298. Bielschowsky M, Helyer BJ, Howie JB. Spontaneous haemolytic anaemia in mice of the NZB/Bl strain. Proc Univ Otago Med School (New Zealand) 1959 Jul;37:9–11.

B299. Biesecker G, Katz S, Koffler D. Renal localization of the membrane attack complex in systemic lupus erythematosus nephritis. J Exp Med 1981 Dec 1;154:1779–1791.

B300. Biesecker G, Lavin L, Ziskind M, Koffler D. Cutaneous localization of the membrane attack complex in discoid and systemic lupus erythematosus. N Engl J Med 1982 Feb 4;306:264–270.

B301. Biett T. Quoted in Arege Pratique des Maladies de la Peau, d'apres des Auteurs, les Plus Estimes, et Surtout d'apres les Documens Puises Dans les Lecons Cliniques de M. le Docteur Biett. Cazenave PLA, Schedel HE, editors. Paris, 1828:386.

B302. Bigby M, Stern R. Cutaneous reactions to non-steroidal anti-inflammatory drugs. A review. J Am Acad Dermatol 1985 May;12(5 Pt 1):866–876.

B303. Biggs R, Denson KWE. The mode of action of a coagulation inhibitor in the blood of 2 patients with disseminated erythematosus (DLE). Br J Haematol 1964 Apr;10:198–216.

B304. Biggs R, Douglas AS. The measurement of prothrombin in plasma. A case of prothrombin deficiency. J Clin Pathol 1953 Feb;6:15–22.

B305. Bignon YJ, Janin-Mercier A, Dubos Ult JJ, Ristori JM, Fonck Y, Alphonse JC, Sauvezie BJ. Angioimmunoblastic lymphadenopathy with dysproteinemia (AILD) and sicca syndrome. Ann Rheum Dis 1986 Jun;45(6):519–522.

B306. Bigot MC, Trenque T, Moulin M. Acebutolol and a lupus syndrome. Apropos of a case. Therapie 1984;39:571–575.

B307. Bilazarian SC, Baughman KL, Hutchins GM, Hellmann DB. Systemic lupus erythematosus presenting as acute severe mitral regurgitation. Am J Med 1990;88:60N-63N.

B308. Biller H, Schachtschabel DO, Leising HB, Pfab R, Hess F. Influence of x-rays and quinacrine (atebrine) for chloroquine (resochine)—alone or in combination—on growth and melanin formation of Harding-Passey melanoma cells in monolayer culture. Strahlentherapie 1982 Jul;158(7):450–456.

B308a. Billingsley LM, Yannakakis GD, Stevens MB. Evoked potentials (EPs) in central nervous system (CNS) systemic lupus erythematosus (SLE). Arthritis Rheum 1984 Apr;27 Suppl:S61.

B309. Billingsley LM, Yannakakis GD, Stevens MB. Evoked potentials (EPs): A sensitive test for CNS-SLE [abstract]. Arthritis Rheum 1985 Apr;28(4) Suppl:S22.

B310. Binstadt DH, L'Heureux PR. Pneumatosis cystoides intestinalis in childhood systemic lupus erythematosus. MN Med 1977;408.

B311. Binz H, Wigzell H. Shared idiotypic determinants on B and T lymphocytes reactive against the same antigenic determinant. I. Demonstration of similar or identical idiotypes on IgG molecules and T-cell receptors with specificity for the same alloantigen. J Exp Med 1975;142:197.

B312. Biriukov AV, Stenina MA, Anan'eva LP, Skripnik AIu, Cheredeev AN. Clinical effectiveness of the treatment of systemic lupus erythematosus with preparations of the methylxanthine group and T-activin. Klin Med (Mosk) 1987 Jan;65(1):107–111.

B313. Birmingham DJ, Hebert LA, Cosio FG, Van Aman M. Immune complex/erythrocyte complement receptor interactions in vivo during induction of glomerulonephritis in nonhuman primates. J Lab Clin Med 1990;116:242–252.

B314. Biron CA, Byron KS, Sullivan JL. Susceptibility to viral infections in an individual with a complete lack of natural killer cells. Nat Immun Cell Growth Regul 1988;7:47.

B315. Bishara SA, Matamoros N. Evaluation of several tests in screening for chloroquine maculopathy. Eye 1989;3(Pt 6):777–782.

B316. Bitran J, McShane D, Ellman MH. Arthritsi Rounds: Ascites as the major manifestation of systemic lupus erythematosus. Arthritis Rheum 1976 Jul–Aug;19(4):782–785.

B317. Bitter EQ, Parra CA, Ledesma de Prieto G, Briggs E, Ortiz Baeza O. Congenital ischemic onychodystrophy (Iso-Kikuchi syndrome) and chronic lupus erythematosus. Hautarzt (Ger) 1988;39:750–752.

B318. Bitter T, Bitter F, Silberschmidt R, Dubois EL. In-vivo and in-vitro study of cell-mediated immunity (CMI) during the onset of systemic lupus erythematosus (SLE) [abstract]. Arthritis Rheum 1971;14:152–153.

B319. Bitter T, Siegenthaler P, DePreux T, Martin E. Excretion in the urine of aminoacridine precipitable polyuronides (acid mucopolysaccharides) in patients with rheumatoid arthritis. Ann Rheum Dis 1970 Jul;29:427–433.

B320. Bizar-Scheebaum A, O'Dell JR, Kotzin BL. Anti-histone antibody production by peripheral blood cells in SLE. Arthritis Rheum. 1987;30:511.

B321. Bizzarro A, Valentini G, DiMartino G, Daponte A, DeBellis A, Iacono G. J Clin Endo Metabol 1987;64:32–36.

B322. Bjellerup M, Bruze M, Forsgren A, Krook G, Ljunggren B. Antinuclear antibodies during PUVA therapy. Acta Derm Venereol Stockh 1979;59:73–75.

B323. Bjorkman PJ, Saper MA, Samraoui B, Bennett WS, Strominger JL, Wiley DC. Structure of the human class I histocompatibility antigen, HLA-A2. Nature 1987;329:506–511.

B324. Bjorkman PJ, Saper MA, Samraoui B, Bennett WS, Strominger JL, Wiley DC. The foreign antigen binding site and T cell recognition regions of class I histocompatibility antigens. Nature 1987;329:512–518.

B325. Black AK, Greaves MW, Hensby CN, Plummer CA. Increased prostaglandins E2 and F2 in human skin at 6 and 24 hours after UV-B radiation. Br J Clin Pharmacol 1978;5: 431–436.

B326. Black CM, Maddison PJ, Welsh KI, Bernstein R, Woodrow JC, Pereira RS. HLA and immunoglobulin allotypes in mixed connective tissue disease. Arthritis Rheum 1988;31:131–134.

B327. Black CM, Perira S, McWhirter A, Welsh K, Laurent R. Genetic susceptibility to scleroderma-like syndrome in symptomatic and asymptomatic workers exposed to vinyl chloride. J Rheumatol 1986;13:1059–1062.

B328. Black RL, Oglesby RB, Von Sallmann L, Bunim JJ. Posterior subcapsular cataracts induced by corticosteroids in patients with rheumatoid arthritis. JAMA 1960;174:166–171.

B329. Blackman M, Kappler J, Marrack P. The role of the T cell receptor in positive and negative selection of developing T cells. Science 1990;248:1335–1341.

B330. Blaese RM, Grayson J, Steinberg AD. Elevated immunoglobulin secreting cells in the blood of patients with active systemic lupus erythematosus: Correlation of laboratory and clinical assessment of disease activity. Am J Med 1980;69: 345–350.

B331. Blair PB. Immunologic consequences of early exposure of experimental rodents to diethylstilbestrol and steroid hormones. In: Herbst AL, Bern HA, editor. Developmental effects of diethylstilbestrol in pregnancy. New York: Thieme-Stratton, 1981:167–178.

B332. Blake DR, Lunec J, Ahern M, Ring EF, Bradfield J, Gutteridge JM. Effect of intravenous iron dextran on rheumatoid synovitis. Ann Rheum Dis 1985 Mar;44(3):183–188.

B333. Blalock JE, Georgiades JA, Langford MP, Johnson HM. Purified human immune interferon has some potent anticellular activity than fibroblast or leukocyte interferon. Cell Immunol 1980 Feb;49:390–394.

B334. Blalock JE, Harbour-McMenamin D, Smith EM. Peptide hormones shared by the neuroendocrine and immunologic system. J Immunol 1985;135 Suppl:858S-861S.

B335. Blanc D, Kienzler JL. Lupus erythematosus gyratus repens. Report of a case associated with lung carcinoma. Clin Exp Dermatol 1982;7:129–134.

B336. Bland JH. Clinical recognition and management of disturbances of body fluids. 2nd ed. Philadelphia: Saunders, 1956: 101.

B337. Blaney DJ. On the etiology of lupus erythematosus. South Med J 1962;55:242–245.

B338. Blanford AT, Murphy BEP. In vitro metabolism of prednisolone, dexamethasone, betamethasone and cortisol by the human placenta. Am J Obstet Gynecol 1977;127:264–267.

B339. Blank M, Cohen J, Toder V, Shoenfeld Y. Induction of anti-phospholipid syndrome in naive mice with mouse lupus monoclonal and human polyclonal anti-cardiolipin antibodies. Proc Natl Acad Sci USA 1991;88:3069–3073.

B340. Blank M, Mendlovic S, Fricke H, Mozes E, Talal N, Shoenfeld Y. Sex Hormone involvement in the induction of experimental systemic lupus erythematosus by a pathogenic anti-DNA idiotype in native mice. J Rheumatol 1990;17:311–317.

B341. Blaszczyk M, Magaewski S, Wasik M, Chorzelski T, Jablonska S. Natural killer cell activity of peripheral blood mononuclear cells from patients with various forms of lupus erythematosus. Br J Dermatol 1987;117:709–714.

B342. Bleifeld CJ, Inglis AE. The hand in systemic lupus erythematosus. J Bone Joint Surg (Am) 1974 Sep;56–A(6): 1207–1215.

B343. Bleyer WA, Breckenridge RI. Adverse drug reactions in the newborn. II. Prenatal aspirin and newborn hemostasis. JAMA 1970;213:2049.

B344. Bloch KJ, Wohl MJ, Ship II, Oglesby RB, Bunim JJ. Sjogren's syndrome 1. Serologic reactions in patients with Sjogren's syndrome with and without rheumatoid arthritis. Arthritis Rheum 1960;3:287–297.

B345. Block SR, Gibbs CB, Stevens MB, Schulman LB. Delayed hypersensitivity in systemic lupus erythematosus. Ann Rheum Dis 1968;27:311–318.

B346. Block SR, Lockshin MD, Winfield JB, Weksler ME, Imamura M, Winchester RJ, Mellors RC, Christian CL. Immunologic observations on 9 sets of twins either concordant or discordant for SLE. Arthritis Rheum 1976;19:545–554.

B347. Block SR, Winfield JB, Lockshin MD, D'Angelo WA, Christian CL. Studies of twins with systemic lupus erythematosus. A review of the literature and presentation of 12 additional sets. Am J Med 1975 Oct;59:533–552.

B348. Blomback B, Blomback M, Edman P, Hessel B. Amino-acid sequence and occurrence of phosphorus in human fibrinopeptides. Nature 1962;193:883–884.

B349. Blomgren SE, Condemi JJ, Bignall MC. Antinuclear antibody induced by procainamide. A prospective study. N Engl J Med 1969 Jul 10;281:64–66.

B350. Blomgren SE, Condemi JJ, Vaughan JH. Procainamide-induced lupus erythematosus. Clinical and laboratory observations. Am J Med 1972 Mar;52:338–348.

B351. Bloom D. In: Discussion of H.O. Curth. Detection of genetic carriers of inherited disease. Arch Dermatol 1958;77: 342.

B352. Bloom EJ, Abrams DI, Rodgers G. Lupus anticoagulant in acquired immunodeficiency syndrome. JAMA 1986;256:491.

B353. Bloxham CA, Carr S, Ryan DW, Kesteven PJ, Bexton RS, Griffiths ID, Richards J. Disseminated zygomycosis and systemic lupus erythematosus [clinical conference]. Intensive Care Med 1990;16(3):201–207.

B354. Bluestein HG. Neurocytotoxic antibodies in serum of patients with system lupus erythematosus. Proc Natl Acad Sci USA 1978 Aug;75:3965–3969.

B355. Bluestein HG. Heterogeneous neurocytotoxic antibodies in systemic lupus erythematosus. Clin Exp Immunol 1979 Feb; 35:210–217.

B356. Bluestein HG. Neuropsychiatric disease systemic lupus erythematosus. In: Lahita RG, editor. Systemic lupus erythematosus. New York: John Wiley, 1987:593–614.

B357. Bluestein HG, Klippel JH, Zvaifler NJ. Antibodies to neuronal cells in antisera to SLE cryoproteins. Arthritis Rheum 1978;21:546.

B358. Bluestein HG, Weisman MH, Zvaifler NJ, Shapiro RF. Lymphocyte alteration by procainamide: relation to drug-induced lupus erythematosus syndrome. Lancet 1979; 2:816–819.

B359. Bluestein HG, Williams GW, Steinberg AD. Cerebrospinal fluid antibodies to neuronal cells: association with neuropsychiatric manifestations of systemic lupus erythematosus. Am J Med 1981 Feb;70(2):240–246.

B360. Bluestein HG, Zvaifler NJ. Brain-reactive lymphocytotoxic antibodies in the serum of patients with systemic lupus erythematosus. J Clin Invest 1976;57:509–516.

B361. Bluestein HG, Zvaifler HG. Antibodies reactive with central nervous system antigens. Human Pathol 1983 May;14: 424–428.

B362. Bluestone R, Goldberg LS, Cracchiolo A, Barnett EV. Detection and characterization of DNA in mixed IgG-IgM cryoglobulins. Int Arch Appl Allergy Immunol 1970;39(1):16–26.

B363. Bluestone HG, Redelman D, Zvaifler NJ. Procainamide-lymphocyte reactions. A possible explanation for drug-induced autoimmunity. Arthritis Rheum 1981;24:1019–1023.

B364. Blum A, Rubinow A, Galun E. Prominence of renal involvement in male patients with systemic lupus erythematosus [letter]. Clin Exp Rheumatol 1991;9:206–207.

B365. Blumenfeld HB, Kaplan SB, Mills DM, Clark GM. Disseminated lupus erythematosus in identical twins. JAMA 1963;185: 667–669.

B366. Blumenfield M. Psychological aspects of systemic lupus erythematosus. Primary Care 1978 Mar;5(1):159–171.

B367. Blunt RJ, Porter JM. Raynaud syndrome. Semin Arthritis Rheum 1981 May 10;10(4):282–308.

B368. Boardman PL, Hart FD. Clinical measurement of the antiinflammatory effects of salicylates in rheumatoid arthritis. BMJ 1967 Nov 4;4:264–268.

B369. Boardman PL, Robinson KC, Hart FD. Guanoxan and systemic lupus erythematosus. BMJ 1967 Jan 14;1:111.

B370. Boas NF, Soffer LJ. Hexosamine level in lupus erythematosus. Nutrition Rev 1951;9:219.

B371. Bobrie G, Liote F, Houllier P, Grunfeld JP, Jungers P. Pregnancy in lupus nephritis and related disorders. Am J Kidney Dis 1987;9:339–343.

B372. Bobrove AM, Miller P. Depressed in vitro B lymphocyte differentiation in SLE. Arthritis Rheum 1977;27:1326–1332.

B373. Bocanegra TS, Castaneda MO, Espinoza LR, Vasey FB, Germain BF. Sudden death after methylprednisolone pulse therapy. Ann Intern Med 1981 Jul;95:122.

B374. Bocckino SB, Blackmore PF, Wilson PB, Exton JH. Phosphatidate accumulation in hormone-treated hepatocytes via a phospholipase D mechanism. J Biol Chem 1987;262: 15309–15315.

B375. Bodmer JG, Marsh SGE, Parham P, Erlich HA, Albert E, Bodmer WF, Mach B, Mayr WR, Sasazuki T, Schreuder GM, Strominger JL, Svejgaard A, Terasaki PI. Nomenclature for factors of the HLA system, 1989. Human Immunol 1990;28: 326–342.

B376. Boeck C. Discussion on the etiology of lupus erythematosus. Br J Dermatol 1898;10:371–376.

B377. Boelens W, Scherly D, Beijer RP, Jansen EJ, Dathan NA, Mattaj IW, Van Venrooij WJ. A weak interaction between the U2A' protein and U2 snRNA helps to stabilize their complex with the U2B" protein. Nucleic Acids Res 1990;19:455–460.

B378. Boesken WH, Hsaio L, Stierle HE. Diagnostic relevance of quantitative and qualitative urinary protein analyses in SLE. Nieren- und Hochdruckkrankheiten Jahrgang 1987;16: 210–212.

B379. Boey ML, Colaco CB, Gharavi AE, Elkon KB, Loizou S, Hughes GR. Thrombosis in systemic lupus erythematosus: striking association with the presence of circulating lupus anticoagulant. Br Med J [Clin Res]. 1983;287:1021–1023.

B380. Boey ML, Peebles CL, Tsay G, Feng PH, Tan EM. Clinical and autoantibody correlations in Orientals with systemic lupus erythematosus. Ann Rheum Dis 1988;47:918–923.

B381. Boghossian SH, Isenberg DA, Wright G, Snaith ML, Segal AW. Effect of high-dose methylprednisolone therapy of phagocyte function in systemic lupus erythematosus. Ann Rheum Dis 1984 Aug;43:541–559.

B382. Boh E, Roberts LJ, Lieu TS, Gammon WR, Sontheimer RD. Epidermolysis bullosa acquisita preceding the development of systemic lupus erythematosus. J Am Acad Dermatol 1990; 22:587–593.

B383. Bohan A. Seronegative systemic lupus erythematosus. J Rheumatol 1979 Sep–Oct;6(5):534–540.

B384. Bohm L, Briand G, Sautiere P, Crane-Robinson C. Proteolytic digestion studies of chromatin core-histone structure: Identification of limit peptides from histone H2B. Eur J Biochem 1982;123:299–303.

B385. Boire G, Craft J. Human Ro ribonucleoprotein particles: characterization of native structure and stable association with the La polypeptide. J Clin Invest 1990;85:1182–1190.

B386. Boire G, Menard HA. Clinical significance of anti-Ro (SSA) antibody in rheumatoid arthritis. J Rheumatol 1988;15: 391–394.

B387. Boissier MC, Carlioz A, Fournier C. Experimental autoimmune arthritis in mice. Clin Immunol Immunopathol 1987; 48:225–237.

B388. Bojamini EM, Velez CA. Lupus erythematosus in identical twins. Antioguia Medica 1967;17(2):177.

B389. Bokemeyer B, Theile KG. Cluster analysis of 109 patients with systemic lupus erythematosus. Klin Wochenschrift 1984 Jan;63:79–83.

B390. Bole GG Jr, Friedlaender MH, Smith CK. Rheumatic symptoms and serological abnormalities induced by oral contraceptives. Lancet 1969 Feb 15;1:323–326.

B391. Bolgert M, Le Sourd M, Habib G. Subacute lupus erythematosus; Exanthematous onset with bullous lesions; Treatment with aureomycin [original in French]. Bull Soc Franc Dermat et Syph 1949 Nov–Dec;56:433–436.

B392. Boll TJ. The Halstead-Reitan neuropsychology battery. In: Filskov SB, Boll TJ, editors. Handbook of clinical neuropsychology. New York:Wiley 1981:577.

B393. Bolte J, Demuynck C, Lhomme J. Synthetic models deoxyribonucleic acid complexes with antimalarial compounds. I. Interaction of aminoquinoline with adenine and thymine. J Am Chem Soc 1976 Jan 21;98(2):613–615.

B394. Bolton WK, Schrock JH, Davis JS. Rheumatoid factor inhibition of in vitro binding of IgG complexes in the human glomerulus. Arthritis Rheum 1982 Mar;25:297–303.

B395. Bomalski JS, Talano JV, Perlman S. The value of echocardiography in patients with systemic lupus erythematosus [abstract]. Clin Res 1983;31:689A.

B396. Bombardier C, Gladman DD, Urowitz MB, Karon O, Chang CH, Committee on Prognosis Studies in SLE. Development and validation of the SLEDAI: a disease activity index for lupus patients. Submitted.

B397. Bona CA. V genes encoding autoantibodies: molecular and phenotypic characteristics. Annu Rev Immunol 1988;6: 327–358.

B398. Bonacossa IA, Chalmers IM, Rayner HL, Hunter T. Platelet bound IgG levels in patients with systemic lupus erythematosus. J Rheumatol 1985 Feb;12:78–80.

B399. Bonafede RP, van Staden M, Klemp P. Hepatitis B virus infection and liver function in patients with systemic lupus erythematosus. J Rheumatol 1986 Dec;13(6):1050–1052.

B400. Bonagura VR, Wedgwood JF, Agostino N, Hatam L, Mendez L, Jaffe I, Pernis B. Seronegative rheumatoid arthritis, rheumatoid factor cross reactive idiotype expression, hidden rheumatoid factors. Ann Rheum Dis 1989;48:488.

B401. Bonfa E, Elkon KB. Clinical and serologic associations of the antiribosomal P protein antibody. Arthritis Rheum 1986 Aug;29(8):981–985.

B402. Bonfa E, Golombek SJ, Kaufman LD, Skelly S, Weissbach H, Brot N, Elkon KB. Association between lupus psychosis and anti-ribosomal P protein antibodies. N Engl J Med 1987 Jul 30; 317(5):265–271.

B403. Bonfa E, Llovet R, Scheinberg M, de Souza JM, Elkon KB. Comparison between autoantibodies in malaria and leprosy with lupus. Clin Exp Immunol 1987 Dec;70(3):529–537.

B404. Bonfiglio TA, Botti RE, Hagstrom JWC. Coronary arteritis, occlusion, and myocardial infarction due to lupus erythematosus. Am Heart J 1972 Feb;83:153–158.

B405. Bongiovanni AM, McPadden AJ. Steroids during pregnancy and possible fetal consequences. Fertil Steril 1960;11: 181–186.

B406. Bonneau M, Latour M, Revillard JP, Robert M, Traeger J. Blocking antibodies eluted from human placenta. Transplant Proc 1973;5:589–592.

B407. Bonnin A, Besancenot JF, Caillot D, Auplat P, Cortet P. Perihepatitis and lupus erythematosus. Rev Med Interne 1985 Jun;6(3):301–302.

B408. Bonnin JA, Cohen AK, Hicks ND. Coagulation defects in a case of systemic lupus erythematosus with thrombocytopenia. Br J Haematol 1956 Apr;2:168–179.

B409. Boonpucknavig V, Boonpucknavig S, Vutvirojan O, Yaemboonruang C. Immunofluorescence skin test for lupus erythematosus. A correlation between frequency and patterns of skin test results, glomerular pathologic abnormalities, and immunologic findings. Arch Pathol Lab Med 1977;101:350–353.

B410. Boorman GA, Luster MI, Dean JH, Wilson RE. The effect of adult exposure of diethylstilbestrol in the mouse on macrophage function and numbers. J Reticuloendothel Soc 1980;28:547–559.

B411. Boot JHA, Geerts MEJ, Aarden LA. Functional polymorphisms of Fc receptors in human monocyte-mediated cytotoxicity toward erythrocytes induced by murine isotype switch variants. J Immunol 1989;142:1217–1223.

B412. Booth RJ, Wilson JD, Bullock JY. Beta adrenergic receptor blockers and antinuclear antibodies in hypertension. Clin Pharmacol Ther 1982 May;31:555–558.

B413. Bor I. Myocardial infarction and ischemic heart disease in infants and children. Arch Dis Child 1969;44:268–281.

B414. Border WA, Ward HJ, Kamil ES, Cohen AH. Induction of membranous nephropathy in rabbits by administration of an exogenous cationic antigen. J Clin Invest 1982 Feb;69:451–461.

B415. Borel Y, Borel H. Oligonucleotide linked to human gammaglobulin specifically diminishes anti-DNA antibody formation in cultured lymphoid cells from patients with SLE. J Clin Invest 1988;82:1901–1907.

B416. Borel Y, Lewis RM, Andre-Schwartz J, Stollar BD, Deinek E. Treatment of lupus nephritis in adult (NZB × NZW) F_1 mice by cortisone-facilitated tolerance to nucleic acid antigens. J Clin Invest 1978 Feb;61(2):276–286.

B417. Borel Y, Lewis RM, Stollar BD. Prevention of murine lupus nephritis by carrier-dependent induction of immunologic tolerance to denatured DNA. Science 1973;182:76–77.

B418. Borenstein DG, Fye WB, Arnett FC, Stevens MB. The myocarditis of systemic lupus erythematosus. Ann Intern Med 1978 Nov;89:619–624.

B419. Borsos T. Immunoglobulin classes and complement fixation. In: Amos B, editor. Progress in Immunology. New York: Academic Press, New York, 1971:841.

B420. Bose R, Mahadevan MM. Immunosuppressive activity in human embryo growth media is associated with successful pregnancy: effect of gonadotropin releasing hormone agonist (GnRHa) treatment of patients undergoing in vitro fertilization and embryo transfer (IVF-ET) J Clin Immunol 1990;10(3):175–181.

B421. Boston Collaborative Drug Surveillance Program. Acute adverse reactions to prednisone in relation to dosage. Clin Pharmacol Ther 1972;13:694–698.

B422. Boswell JM, Yui MA, Burt DW, Kelley VE. Increased tumor necrosis factor and IL-1 beta gene expression in the kidneys of mice with lupus nephritis. J Immunol 1988;141:3050–3054.

B423. Boswell JM, Yui MA, Endres S, Burt DW, Kelley VE. Novel and enhanced IL-1 gene expression in autoimmune mice with lupus. J Immunol 1988;141:118–124.

B424. Bottazzo GF, Dujol-Borell R, Hanafusa T, Feldman M. Role of aberrant HLA-DR expression and antigen presentation in induction of endocrine autoimmunity. Lancet 1983;11:1115–1119.

B425. Bottger BA, Sjolund M, Thyberg J. Chloroquine and monensin inhibit induction of DNA synthesis in rat arterial smooth muscle cells stimulated with platelet-derived growth factor. Cell Tissue Res 1988 May;252(2):275–285.

B426. Bottomly K. All idiotypes are equal, but some are more equal than others. Immunol Rev 1984;79:45–61.

B427. Bottomly K. A functional dichotomy of CD4+ T lymphocytes. Immunol Today 1988;9:268–274.

B428. Bottomly K, Luqman M, Greenbaum L, Carding S, West J, Pasqualini T, Murphy DB. A monoclonal antibody to murine CD45R distinguishes CD4 T cell populations that produce different cytokines Eur J Immunol 1989;19:617–623.

B429. Boulikas T, Bastin B, Boulikas P, Dupuis G. Increase in histone poly(ADP-Ribosylation) in mitogen-activated lymphoid cells. Exp Cell Res 1990;187:77–84.

B430. Boulter M, Brink A, Mathias C, Peart S, Stevens J, Stewart G, Unwin R. Unusual cranial and abdominal computed tomographic (CT) scan appearances in a case of systemic lupus erythematosus (SLE). Ann Rheum Dis 1987 Feb;46(2):162–165.

B431. Boulware DW, Hedgpeth MT. Lupus pneumonitis and Anti-SSA(Ro) antibodies. J Rheumatol 1989;16:479–481.

B432. Boulware DW, Makkena R, Karsh J. Monthly cyclophosphamide in lupus pneumonitis and myositis [letter]. J Rheumatol 1991 Jan;18(1):153.

B433. Boumpas DT, Barez S, Klippel JH, Balow JE. Intermittent cyclophosphamide for the treatment of autoimmune thrombocytopenia in systemic lupus erythematosus. Ann Intern Med 1990 May 1;112(9):674–677.

B434. Boumpas DT, Patronas NJ, Dalakas MC, Hakim CA, Klippel JH, Balow JE. Acute transverse myelitis in systemic lupus erythematosus: magnetic resonance imaging and review of the literature. J Rheumatol 1990 Jan;17(1):89–92.

B435. Boumpas DT, Popovic M, Mann DL, Balow JE, Isokos GC. Type C retroviruses of the human T cell leukemia family are not evident in patients with systemic lupus erythematous. Arthritis Rheum 1986;29:185.

B436. Boumpas DT, Yamada H, Patronas NJ, Scott D, Klippel JH, Balow JE. Intermittent pulse cyclophosphamide for the treatment of severe neuropsychiatric lupus [abstract]. Arthritis Rheum 1990 Sep;33(9) Suppl:S103.

B437. Bourke BE, de M Rudolf N. The value of electroencephalogram in cerebral systemic lupus erythematosus. XVI Int Congress Rheumatol, May 1985, Sydney, Australia, [abstract] F69.

B438. Bouterfa H, Doenecke D, Loffler M. Increased level of histone H1o messenger RNA in hypoxic ehrlich ascites tumor cells. Exp Cell Res 1990;188:160–163.

B439. Bouvier M, Colson F, Tebib JG, Noel E, Schott AM. Clinical analysis of neuropsychiatric disorders in systemic lupus erythematosus. Report of fourteen personal cases. Sem Hop Paris 1990;66:7–11.

B440. Bovin G, Jorstad S, Schrader H. Subdural hematoma presenting as headache in systemic lupus erythematosus. Cephalalgia 1990 Feb;10(1):25–29.

B441. Bovin G, Virstad S, Schrader H. Subdural hematoma presenting in systemic lupus erythematosus. Cephalgia 1990 (Feb);10(1):25–29.

B442. Bowie EJ, Thompson JH Jr, Pascuzzi CA, Owen CA Jr. Thrombosis in systemic lupus despite circulating anticoagulants. J Lab Clin Med 1963 Sep;62:416.

B443. Bowie PCW, Beaini AY. Normalization of dexamethasone suppression test: a correlate with clinical improvement in primary depressives. Psychiatry 1985;147:30–35.

B444. Bowman CA, Linthicum FH Jr, Nelson RA, Mikami K, Quismorio F. Sensorineural hearing loss associated with systemic lupus erythematosus. Otolaryngol Head Neck Surg 1986 Feb;94(2):197–204.

B445. Bowyer SL, Ragsdale CG, Sullivan DB. Factor VIII related antigen and childhood rheumatic diseases. J Rheumatol 1989; 16:1093–1097.

B446. Boxer M, Ellman L, Carvalho A. The lupus anticoagulant. Arthritis Rheum 1982 Nov–Dec;19:1244.

B447. Boyd AS. An overview of the retinoids. Am J Med 1989 May;86(5):568–574.

B448. Boye E, Morse M, Huttner I, Erlanger BF, MacKinnon KJ, Klassen J. Immune complex-mediated interstitial cystitis as a major manifestation of systemic lupus erythematosus. Clin Immunol Immunopath 1979 May;13(1):67–76.

B449. Boyer MH. Hyperposmolar anacidotic coma in association with glucocorticoid therapy. JAMA 1967 Dec 11;202:95.

B450. Boylan JJ, Owen DS, Chew JB. Phenytoin interference with dexamethasone. JAMA 1976 Feb 23;235:803–804.

B451. Boyle P, Craswell P, Hawley C, Searle J. Renal and myocardial infarcts associated with SLE and the lupus inhibitor. Kidney Int 1988;33:132–133.

B452. Bradley WG, Jacobs RP, Trew PA, Biava CG, Hopper J. Renal vein thrombosis; occurrence in membranous glomerulonephropathy and lupus nephritis. Radiology 1981 Jun;139: 571–576.

B453. Braester A, Varkel Y, Horn Y. Malabsorption and systemic lupus erythematosus [letter]. Arch Intern Med 1989 Aug; 149(8):1901.

B454. Branch DW, Andres R, Digre KB, Rote NS, Scott JR. The association of antiphospholipid antibodies with severe preeclampsia. Obstet Gynecol 1989;73:541–545.

B455. Branch DW, Rote NS, Scott JR. The demonstration of lupus anticoagulant by an enzyme-lined immunoadsorbent assay. Clin Immunol Immunopath 1986;39:298.

B456. Branch DW, Scott J, Kochenour N, Hershgold E. Obstetric complications associated with the lupus anticoagulant. N Engl J Med 1985;313:1322–1326.

B457. Brand C, Davidson A, Littlejohn G, Ryan P. Hydralazine-induced lupus: No association with HLA-DR4 [letter]. Lancet 1984 Feb 25;1:462.

B458. Brandslund I, Ibsen HHW, Klitgaard NA, Svehag SE, Simonsen E, Diederichsen H. Plasma concentrations of complement split product C3d and immune complexes after procainamide induced production of antinuclear antibodies. Acta Med Scand 1986;220:431–435.

B459. Brandt KD, Lessel S. Migranous phenomenon in systemic lupus erythematosus. Arthritis Rheum 1978 Jan–Feb;21(1): 7–16.

B460. Brandt L, Hedberg H. Impaired phagocytosis by peripheral blood granulocytes in systemic lupus erythematosus. Scand J Haematol 1969;6(5):348–353.

B461. Branson-Geokas B, Epstein MJ, Quismorio FP, Friou GJ. Sjogren's syndrome: Clinical and laboratory studies [abstract]. Arthritis Rheum 1971;14:152.

B462. Braude IA, Hochberg MC, Arnett FC, Waldman TA. In vitro suppression of anti-DNA antibody and immunoglobulin synthesis in systemic lupus erythematosus patients by human gamma interferon. J Rheumatol 1988;15:438–444.

B463. Braunstein EM, Weisman BN, Sosman JJ, Schur PH. Radiologic findings in late-onset systemic lupus erythematosus. AJR 1983 Mar;140(3):587–589.

B464. Bravo MG, Alarcon-Segovia D. C reactive protein in the differential diagnosis between infection and disease reactivation in SLE. J Rheumatol 1981 Mar–Apr;8:291–294.

B465. Bravo R, Celis JE. A search for differential polypeptide synthesis throughout the cell cycle of HeLa cells. J Cell Biol 1980;84:795–803.

B466. Bray KR, Gershwin ME, Ahmed A, Castles JJ. Tissue localization and biochemical characteristics of a new thymic antigen recognized by a monoclonal thymocytotoxic autoanti-

body from New Zealand black mice. J Immunol 1985 Jun; 134(6):4001–4008.

B467. Bray KR, Gershwin ME, Chused T, Ahmed A. Characteristics of a spontaneous monoclonal thymocytotoxic antibody from New Zealand Black mice: recognition of a specific NTA determinant. J Immunol 1984 Sep;133(3):1318–1324.

B468. Breathnach SM, Kofler H, Sepp N, Ashworth J, Woodrow D, Pepys MB, Hintner H. Serum amyloid P component binds to cell nuclei in vitro and to in vivo deposits of extracellular chromatin in systemic lupus erythematosus. J Exp Med 1989 Oct;170(4):1433–1438.

B469. Breckenridge RT, Moore RD, Ratnoff OD. A study of thrombocytopenia. New histologic criteria for the differentiation of idiopathic thrombocytopenia and thrombocytopenia associated with disseminated lupus erythematosus. Blood 1967 Jul;30:39–53.

B470. Breit S, Clark P, Penny R. Alpha-1 protease inhibitor (1-antitrypsin) phenotypes in rheumatic diseases. Aust NZ J Med 1980 Apr;10:272.

B471. Bremers HH, Golitz LE, Weston WL, Hays WG. Neonatal lupus erythematosus. Cutis 1979;24:287.

B472. Brendel W. The clinical use of ALG. Transplant Proc 1971 Mar;3:280–286.

B473. Brennan DC, Yui MA, Wuthrich RP, Kelley VE. Tumor necrosis factor and IL-1 in New Zealand Black/White mice. Enhanced gene expression and acceleration of renal injury. J Immunol 1989;143:3470–3475.

B473a. Brenner B, Blumenfeld Z, Markiewicz W, Reisner SA. Cardiac involvement in patients with primary antiphospholipid syndrome. JACC 1991;18:931–936.

B474. Brenner MB, McLean J, Dialynas DP, Strominger JL, Smith JA, Owen FL, Seidman JG, Ip S, Rosen F, Krangel MS. Identification of a putative second T-cell receptor. Nature 1986;322: 145–149.

B475. Brenner MK, Vyakarnam A, Reittie JE, Wimperis JZ, Grob JP, Hoffbrand AV, Prentice HG. Human large granular lymphocytes induce immunoglobulin synthesis after bone marrow transplantation. Eur J Immunol 1987;17:43.

B476. Brentjens JR, O'Connell DW, Paulowski IB, Hsu KC, Andres GA. Experimental immune complex disease of the lung. J Exp Med 1974;140:150–152.

B477. Brentjens JR, Sepulveda M, Baliah T, Bentzel C, Erlanger BF, Elwood C, Montes M, Hsu KC, Andres GA. Interstitial immune complex nephritis in patients with systemic lupus erythematosus. Kidney Int 1975 Jan;7:342–350.

B478. Bresnihan B, Grigor RR, Oliver M, Lewkonia RM, Hughes GRV, Lovins RE, Faulk WP. Immunological mechanism for spontaneous abortion in systemic lupus erythematosus. Lancet 1977;2:1205–1207.

B479. Bresnihan B, Hale GM, Bunn CC, Hughes GR. Immunoglobulin classes in skin basement membrane in systemic lupus erythematosus: clinical significance and comparison with classes of serum anti-DNA antibodies. Ann Rheum Dis 1979 Aug;38(4):351–355.

B480. Bresnihan B, Jasin HE. Suppressor function of peripheral blood mononuclear cells in normal individuals and in patients with systemic lupus erythematosus. J Clin Invest 1977 Jan;59: 106–116.

B481. Bresnihan B, Jenkins W, Chadwick YS, Hughes GR. Chronic active hepatitis in a patient presenting with clinical and serological evidence of SLE. J Rheumatol 1979 Jan–Feb; 6(1):38–42.

B482. Bresnihan B, Oliver M, Grigor R, Hughes GRV. Brain-reactivity of lymphocytotoxic antibodies in systemic lupus erythematosus with and without cerebral involvement. Clin Exp Immunol 1977;30:333.

B483. Bresnihan B, Oliver M, Williams B, Hughes GRV. An antineuronal antibody cross-reacting with erythrocytes and lymphocytes in systemic lupus erythematosus. Arthritis Rheum 1979 Apr;22:313–320.

B484. Bresser P, Toben FM, van Son WJ, Anema J, Beukhof JR. Current developments in the diagnosis and therapy of cytomegalovirus infections [English abstract]. Ned Tijdschr Geneeskd 1989 Mar;133(9):455–457.

B485. Bretscher P, Cohn M. A theory of self-nonself discriminations. Science 1970;163:1042–1049.

B486. Brick JE, Ong SH, Bathon JM, Walker SE, O'Sullivan FX, DeBartolomeo AG. Anti-histone antibodies in the serum of autoimmune MRL and NZB/NZW F1 mice. Clin Immunol Immunopathol 1990;54:372–381.

B487. Brick JE, Wilson DA, Walker SE. Hormonal modulation of responses to thymic independent and thymic-dependent antigens in autoimmune NZB/Q mice. J Immunol 1985;136:3693–3698.

B488. Bridge RG, Foley FE. Placental transmission of the lupus erythematosus factor. Am J Med Sci 1954;227:1–8.

B489. Brieva JA, Targan S, Stevens RH. NK and T cell subsets regulate antibody production by human in vivo antigen-induced lymphoblastoid B cells. J Immunol 1983;132:611.

B490. Brigden W, Bywaters EG, Lessof MH, Ross IP. The heart in systemic lupus erythematosus. Br Heart J 1960 Jan;22:1–16.

B491. Briggs DC, Senaldi G, Isenberg DA, Welsh KI, Vergani D. Influence of C4 null alleles on C4 activation in systemic lupus erythematosus. Ann Rheum Dis 1991;50:251–254.

B492. Briggs GG, Bodendorfer TW, Freeman RK, Yaffe SJ. Drugs in pregnancy and lactation: A reference guide to fetal and neonatal risk. Baltimore: Williams & Wilkins, 1983;65–66.

B493. Briley DP, Coull BM, Goodnight SH Jr. Neurological diseases associated with antiphospholipid antibodies. Ann Neurol 1989 Mar; 25(3):221–227.

B494. Brinet A, Fournel C, Faure JR, Venet C, Monier JC. Anti-histone antibodies (ELISA and immunoblot) in canine lupus erythematosus. Clin Exp Immunol 1988;74:105–109.

B495. Bringmann P, Luhrmann R. Purification of the individual snRNPs U1, U2, U5 and U4/U6 from HeLa cells and characterization of their protein constituents. Embo J 1986;5:3509–3516.

B496. Brinkman K, Termaat R, Berden JH, Smeenk RJ. Anti-DNA antibodies and lupus nephritis: the complexity of crossreactivity. Immunol Today 1990 Jul;11(7):232–234.

B497. Brissaud P, Laroche L, Krulik M, Prier AM, Saraux H, Canuel C, Debray J. Retinal vascularities and lupic disease [English abstract]. Rev Med Intern 1985 Jan;6(1):36–40.

B498. Brock W, Cullen SI. Triamcinolone acetonide in flexible collodion for dermatologic therapy. Arch Dermatol 1967 Aug; 96(2):193–194.

B499. Broder S, Cassidy JT, Goldberg CB, Whitehouse F Jr. F(ab')2-like immunoglobulin fragments in urine from patients with systemic lupus erythematosus. J Lab Clin Med 1972 Oct; 80:514–522.

B500. Brodeur GM, O'Neill PJ, Williams JA. Acquired inhibitors of coagulation in nonhemophiliac children. J Pediatr 1980;96:439.

B501. Brodman R, Gilfillan G, Glass D, Schur PH. Influenzal vaccine response in systemic lupus erythematosus. Ann Intern Med 1978 Jun;88(6):735–740.

B502. Brody S. Psychological factors associated with disseminated lupus erythematosus and effects of cortisone and ACTH. Psych Quart 1956;30:44.

B503. Brogadir SP, Myers AR. Chronic leg ulceration in systemic lupus erythematosus. J Rheumatol 1979 Mar–Apr;6(2):204–209.

B504. Bronshvag MM, Prystowsky SD, Traviesa DC. Vascular

headaches in mixed connective tissue disease. Headache 1978 Jul;18(3):154–160.

B505. Brook I, Controni G, Kassan SS, Moutsopoulos HM. Lactic acid levels in cerebrospinal fluid from patients with systemic lupus erythematosus. J Rheumatol 1979 Nov–Dec;6(6):691–693.

B506. Brook MS, Aldo-Benson M. Defects in antigen-specific immune tolerance in continuous B cell lines from autoimmune mice. J Clin Invest 1986;78:784–789.

B507. Brooker AE, Wiens AN, Wiens DA: Impaired brain functions due to diazepam and meprobamate abuse in a 53-year-old-male. J Nerv Ment Dis 1984 Aug;172(8):498–501.

B508. Brooks BJ Jr, Borxmeyer HE, Bryan CF, Leech SH. Serum inhibitor in systemic lupus erythematosus associated with aplastic anemia. Arch Intern Med 1984;144:1474–1477.

B509. Brooks DG, Qiu WQ, Luster AD, Ravetch JV. Structure and expression of a human IgG FcRII (CD32): Functional heterogeneity is encoded by the alternatively spliced products of multiple genes. J Exp Med 1989;170:1369–1386.

B510. Brooks MS, Aldo-Benson M. Defects in antigen-specific immune tolerance in continuous B cell lines from autoimmune mice. J Clin Invest 1986;78:784–789.

B511. Brooks PM, Day RO. Nonsteroidal anti-inflammatory drugs—differences and similarities. N Engl J Med 1991;324:1716–1725.

B512. Brooks PM, Needs CJ. The use of antirheumatic medication during pregnancy and in the puerperium. Rheum Dis Clin North Am 1989;15:789–806.

B513. Brouet JC, Clauvel JP, Danon F, Klein M, Seligmann M. Biologic and clinical significance of cryoglobulins: a report of 86 cases. Am J Med 1976 Nov;57:775.

B514. Brown C, Lieu TS, Sontheimer RD. The correlation between dermal interstitial immunoglobulin G and hypergammaglobulinemia. J Invest Dermatol 1991:373–377.

B515. Brown CD, Rao TKS, Maxey RW, Butt KMH, Friedman EA. Regression of clinical and immunological expression of systemic lupus erythematosus (SLE) consequent to development of uremia. Kidney Int 1979;16:884.

B516. Brown CH, Scanlon PJ, Haserick JR. Mesenteric arteritis with perforation of the jejunum in a patient with systemic lupus erythematosus. Cleve Clin Quart 1964 Jul;31:169–178.

B517. Brown CH, Shirey EK, Haserick JR. Gastrointestinal manifestations of systemic lupus erythematosus. Gastroenterology 1956;31:649–666.

B518. Brown J, Lewis V, Brown M, Horn G, Bowes JB. A comparison between transient amnesias induced by two drugs (diazepam or lorazepam) and amnesia of organic origin. Neuropsychologia 1982;20(1):55–70.

B519. Brown J, Winkelmann RK. Acanthosis nigricans: A study of 90 cases. Medicine 1968;47:33–51.

B520. Brown JH, Doherty CC, Allen DC, Morton P. Fatal cardiac failure due to myocardial microthrombi in systemic lupus erythematosus. BMJ (Clin Res) 1988 May 28; 296(6635):1505.

B521. Brown JH, Jardetzky T, Saper MA, Samraoui B, Bjorkman PJ, Wiley DC. A hypothetical model of the foreign antigen binding site of Class II histocompatibility molecules. Nature 1988;332:845–850.

B522. Brown MM, Yount WJ. Skin immunopathology in systemic lupus erythematosus. JAMA 1980;243:38–42.

B523. Brown RC, Cooke J, Losowsky MS. SLE syndrome, probably induced by labetalol [case report]. Postgrad Med 1981 Mar;57:189–190.

B524. Brown SL, Miller RA, Horning SJ, Czerwinski D, Hart SM, McElderry R, Basham T, Wanke RA, Merigan TC, Levy R. Treatment of B cell lymphoma with anti-idiotype antibodies alone and in combination with alpha interferon. Blood 1989;73:651.

B525. Brown SL, Miller RA, Levy R. Antiidiotype antibody therapy of B-cell lymphoma. Sem Oncol 1989;16:199.

B526. Brown WR, Williams AF. Lymphocyte cell surface glycoproteins which bind to soybean and peanut lectins. Immunology 1982;46:713.

B527. Browning CA, Bishop RL, Heilpern RJ, Singh JB, Spodick DH. Accelerated constrictive pericarditis in procainamide-induced systemic lupus erythematosus. Am J Cardiol 1984 Jan 15;53:376−377.

B528. Brozek CM, Hoffman CL, Savage SM, Searles RP. Systemic lupus erythematosus sera inhibit antigen presentation by macrophages to T cells. Clin Immunol Immunopathol 1988; 46:299−313.

B529. Bruce J, Sircus W. Disseminated lupus erythematosus of the alimentary tract. Lancet 1959 Apr 18;1(7077):795−798.

B530. Bruce-Chawat LJ. Malaria and pregnancy. Br Med J 1983; 286:1457−1458.

B531. Bruck C, Co MS, Slaoui M, Gaulton GN, Smith T, Fields BN, Mullins JI, Greene MI. Nucleic acid sequence of an internal image bearing monoclonal anti-idiotype and its comparison to the sequence of the external antigen. Proc Natl Acad Sci USA 1986;83:6578.

B532. Bruijn JA, VanElven EH, Hogendoorn PCW. Murine chronic graft-versus-host disease as a model of lupus nephritis. Am J Pathol 1988;130:639−641.

B533. Bruley-Rosset M, Dardenne M, Schuurs A. Functional and quantitative changes of immune cells of aging NZB mice treatment nandrolone deconate. Clin Exp Immunol 1985;62: 630−638.

B534. Brunda MJ, Tarnowski D, Davatelis V. Interaction of recombinant interferons with recombinant interleukin-2: Differential effects on natural killer cell activity and interleukin-2-activated killer cells. Int J Cancer 1986;37:787.

B535. Bruneau C, Benveniste J. Circulating DNA: anti-DNA complexes in systemic lupus erythematosus. Detection and characterization by ultracentrifugation. J Clin Invest 1979 Jul; 64(1):191−198.

B536. Bruneau C, Intrator L, Sobel A, Beaumont V, Billecocq A. Antibodies to cardiolipin and vascular complications in women taking oral contraceptives [letter]. Arthritis Rheum 1986 Oct;29(10):1294.

B537. Brunet C, Craft J, Nakamura M, Pachman L, Athreya B, Hardin J. Identification of nuclear antigens bound by sera from patients with juvenile rheumatoid arthritis (JRA) [abstract]. Arthritis Rheum 1986;29 Suppl:S67.

B538. Brunjes S, Ziked K, Julian R. Familial systemic lupus erythematosus. A review of the literature, with a report of ten additional cases in four families. Am J Med 1961;30:529−536.

B539. Brunner CM, Horwitz DA, Davis JS. Identical twins discordant for systemic lupus erythematosus An experiment in nature. Arthritis Rheum 1971;14:373.

B540. Brunner F, Wing AJ, Dykes SR, Brymger OA, Fassbinder W, Selwood NH. International review of renal replacement therapy: strategies and results. In: Maher JF, editor. Replacement of Renal Functional by Dialysis. Dordrecht: Kluwer Academic. 1989:697−719.

B541. Brunsting LA. Symposium on diseases of skin acute disseminated lupus erythematosus. Med Clin N Am 1951;35:399.

B542. Brunsting LA, Slocumb CH, Didcoct JW. Effects of cortisone on acute disseminated lupus erythematosus. Arch Dermatol 1951 Jan;63:39−48.

B543. Brunsting R, Sillevis Smitt JH, van der Meer JW, Weening RS. Discoid lupus erythematosus and other clinical manifestation in female carriers of chronic granulomatous disease [English abstract]. Ned Tijdschr Geneeskd 1988 Jan 2;132(1): 18−21.

B544. Brus I, Lewis SM. The haptoglobin content of serum in haemolytic anaemia. Br J Haematol 1959 Oct;5:348−355.

B545. Brustein D, Rodriguez JM, Murkin, Rabhun N. Familial lupus erythematosus. JAMA 1977;238:2294−2296.

B546. Bruyn GW, Padberg G. Chorea and lupus erythematosus. A critical review. Eur Neurol 1984 Nov−Dec;23(6):435−448.

B547. Bruze M, Forsgren A, Ljunggren B. Antinuclear antibodies in mice induced by long wave ultraviolet radiation (UVA). Acta Derm Venereal (Stockh) 1985;65:25−33.

B548. Bucala R, Lahita RG, Fishman J, Cerami A. Anti-oestrogen antibodies in users of oral contraceptives and in patients with systemic lupus erythematosus. Clin Exp Immunol 1987 Jan; 67(1):167−175.

B549. Buchanan IS, Humpston DJ. Nail-fold capillaries in connective-tissue disorders. Lancet 1968;1:845−847.

B550. Buchanan NMM, Morton KE, Khamashta MA, Hughes GRV. Management of the high risk lupus pregnancy. A prospective study of 87 pregnancies [abstract]. Arthritis Rheum 1991;34 Suppl:S95.

B551. Buchbinder R, Hall S, Littlejohn GO, Ryan PFJ. Neuropsychiatric manifestations of systemic lupus erythematosus. Aust NZ J Med 1988;18:679−684.

B552. Buckman KJ, Moore SK, Ebbin AJ, Cox MB, Dubois EL. Familial systemic lupus erythematosus. Arch Intern Med 1978 Nov;138(11):1674−1676.

B553. Budd RC Schumacher JH, Winslow G, Mosmann TR. Elevated production of interferon-gamma and interleukin 4 by mature T cells from autoimmune lpr mice correlates with Pgp-1 (CD44) expression. Eur J Immunol 1991;21:1081−1084.

B554. Budin JA, Feldman F. Soft tissue calcifications in systemic lupus erythematosus. AJR 1975;124:350−364.

B555. Budinsky RA, Roberts SM, Coates EA, Adams L, Hess EV. The formation of hydroxylamine by rat and human liver microsomes. Drug Metab Disp 1987;15:37−43.

B556. Budman D, Steinberg AD. Bone marrow in lupus erythematosus. Ann Intern Med 1977 Jun;86:831−832.

B557. Budman DR, Merchant EB, Steinberg AD, Doft B, Gershwin ME, Lizzio E, Reeves JP. Increased spontaneous activity of antibody-forming cells in the peripheral blood of patients with active SLE. Arthritis Rheum 1977 Apr;20:829−833.

B558. Budman DR, Steinberg AD. Hypertension and renal disease in systemic lupus erythematosus. Ann Intern Med 1976; 136:1003−1007.

B559. Budman DR, Steinberg AD. Hematologic aspects of systemic lupus erythematosus. Current concepts. Ann Intern Med 1977 Feb;86:220−226.

B560. Bukowski JF, Woda BA, Habu S, Olumura K, Welshe RM. Natural killer cell depletion enhances virus synthesis and virus-induced hepatitis in vivo. J Immunol 1983;131: 1531−1535.

B561. Bulgrin JG, Dubois EL, Jacobson G. Chest roentgenographic changes in systemic lupus erythematosus. Radiology 1960 Jan;74:42−49.

B562. Bulgrin JG, Dubois EL, Jacobson G. Peptic ulcer associated with corticosteroid therapy: Serial roentgenographic studies. Radiology 1960 Nov;75:712−721.

B563. Bulkley BH, Roberts WC. How steroid therapy has changed the heart of systemic lupus erythematosus (SLE) [abstract]. Am J Cardiol 1973 Jan;31:124.

B564. Bulkley BH, Roberts WC. The heart in systemic lupus erythematosus and the changes induced in it by corticosteroid therapy. A study of 36 necropsy patients. Am J Med 1975 Feb; 58:243−264.

B565. Bull HA, Machin SJ. The haemostatic function of the vascular endothelial cell. Blut 1987;55:71−80.

B566. Bulpitt KJ, Brahn E. Systemic lupus erythematosus and concurrent cytomegalic vasculitis: diagnosis by antemortem skin biopsy. J Rheumatol 1989 May;16(5):677–680.

B567. Bumgardner GL, Mauer SM, Ascher NL, Payne WD, Dunn DL, Fryd DS, Sutherland DE, Simmons RL, Najarian JS. Long-term outcome of renal transplantation in patients with systemic lupus erythematosus. Transplant Proc 1989 Feb;21(1 Pt 2):2031–2032.

B568. Bunim JJ. A broader spectrum of Sjogren's syndrome and its pathogenetic implications. Ann Rheum Dis 1961 Mar;20: 1–10.

B569. Bunker CB, Dowd PH. Giant cell arteritis and systemic lupus erythematosus. Br J Dermatol 1988 Jul;119(1): 115–120.

B570. Bunn CC, Bernstein RM, Mathews MB. Autoantibodies against alanyl tRNA synthetase coexist and are associated with myositis. J Exp Med 1986;163:1281–1291.

B571. Buntain WL, Wood JB, Woolley MM. Pancreatitis in childhood. J Pediatr Surg 1978;12:143–149.

B572. Bunting WL, Kiely JM, Campbell DC. Idiopathic thrombocytopenic purpura. Treatment in adults. Arch Intern Med 1961 Nov;108:733–738.

B573. Burge SM, Dawber RP. Stevens-Johnson syndrome and toxic epidermal neurolysis in a patient with systemic lupus erythematosus [letter]. J Am Acad Dermatol 1985 Oct;13(4): 665–666.

B574. Burge SM, Frith PA, Juniper RP, Wojnarowska F. Mucosal involvement in systemic and chronic cutaneous lupus erythematosus. Br J Dermatol 1989 Dec;121(6):727–741.

B575. Burger T, Brascgh G, Keszthelyi B. Iron metabolism and anemia in systemic lupus erythematosus and rheumatoid arthritis. Acta Med Acad Sci Hung 1967;23:95–104.

B576. Burgess ED, Render KC. Hypopharyngeal obstruction in lupus erythematosus [letter]. Ann Intern Med 1984 Feb; 100(2):319.

B577. Burkett G. Lupus nephropathy and pregnancy. Clin Obstet Gynecol 1985;28:310–323.

B578. Burkhardt R. The bone marrow in systemic lupus erythematosus. Seminars in Hematology. Grune and Stratton 1965 Jan;2:29–46.

B579. Burkly L, Lo D, Kanagawa O, Brinster RL, Flavell RA. T cell tolerance by clonal anergy in transgenic mice with non-lymphoid expression of MHC class III-E. Nature 1989;342: 564–566.

B580. Burkly LC, Lo D, Flavell RA. Tolerance in transgenic mice expressing major histocompatibility molecules extrathymically on pancreatic cells. Science 1990;248:1364–1368.

B581. Burlingame RW, Lowe WE, Wang B-C. Crystallographic structure of the octameric histone core of the nucleosome at a resolution of 3.3 A. Science 1985;228:546–553.

B582. Burlingame RW, Rubin RL. Subnucleosome structures as substrates in enzyme-linked immunosorbent assays. J Immunol Meth 1990; 134:187.

B583. Burlingame RW, Rubin RL. Drug-induced anti-histone antibodies display two patterns of reactivity with substructures of chromatin. J Clin Invest 1991;88:680–690.

B583a. Burlingame RW, Rubin RL. Drug-induced autoimmunity: A disorder at the interface between metabolism and immunity. Biochem Soc Trans 1991;19:153–159.

B584. Burman D, Oliver RAM. Placental transfer of the lupus erythematosus factor. J Clin Pathol 1958;11:43–44.

B584a. Burnet FM. Autoimmune disease, II. Pathology of the immune response. BMJ 1959 Oct 17;2:720–725.

B585. Burnet FM, Holmes MC. The natural history of the NZB/NZW F1 hybrid mouse: a laboratory model of systemic lupus erythematosus. Aust Ann Med 1965 Aug;14:185–191.

B586. Burnham TK. Immunofluorescent test for lupus erythema-

tosus: relation to renal disease [letter]. JAMA 1973 Feb 12; 223:798–799.

B587. Burnham TK, Fine G. The immunofluorescence "band" test for lupus erythematosus. I. Morphologic variations of localized immunoglobulins at the dermal-epidermal junction in lupus erythematosus. Arch Dermatol 1969;99:413–420.

B588. Burnham TK, Fine G. The immunofluorescent band test for LE: III. Employing clinically normal skin. Arch Dermatol 1971;103:24–32.

B589. Burnham TK, Neblett TR, Fine G. Application of fluorescent antibody technic to the investigation of lupus erythematosus and various dermatoses. J Invest Dermatol 1963 Dec;41: 451–456.

B590. Burns RP. Delayed onset of chloroquine retinopathy. N Engl J Med 1966;275:693–696.

B591. Burry JN. Lipstick and lupus erythematosus. N Engl J Med 1969;281:620–621.

B592. Bursztyn M, Many A, Rosenthal T. Nifedipine in the treatment of hypertension in systemic lupus erythematosus. Angiology 1987;359–362.

B593. Buskila D, Gladman DD. Stress fractures of the legs and swelling of the ankles in a patient with lupus: a diagnostic dilemma. Ann Rheum Dis 1990 Oct;49(10):783–784.

B594. Bustin M, Reisch J, Einck L, Klippel JH. Autoantibodies to nucleosomal proteins: antibodies to HMG-17 in autoimmune diseases. Science 1982 Mar 2;215:1245–1247.

B595. Butikofer P, Lin ZW, Kuypers FA, Scott MD, Xu C, Wagner GM, Chiu DTY, Lubin B. Chlorpromazine inhibits vesiculation, alters phosphoinositide turnover and changes deformability of ATP-depleted RBC's. Blood 1989;73:1699–1704.

B596. Butler PJG. The folding of chromatin. CRC Crit Rev Biochem 1983;15:57–91.

B597. Butler RC, Thomas SM, Thompson JM, Deat ACS. Anaplastic myeloma in systemic lupus erythematosus. Ann Rheum Dis 1984 Aug;43:653–655.

B598. Butler WT, Sharp JT, Rossen RD, Lidsky MD, Mittal KK, Gard DA. Relationship of the clinical course of systemic lupus erythematosus to the presence of circulating lymphocytotoxic antibodies. Arthritis Rheum 1972 May–Jun;15:231–238.

B599. Butterworth MB, McClellan B, Alansmith M. Influence of sex an immunoglobulin levels. Nature 1967;214:1224–1225.

B600. Buyon J, Roubey R, Swersky S, Pompeo L, Parke A, Baxi L, Winchester R. Compete congenial heart block: risk of occurrence and therapeutic approach to prevention. J Rheumatol 1988;15:1104–1108.

B601. Buyon JP. Complete heart block and antibodies to the SSA/Ro-SSB/La antigen systems. Clinical Aspects Autoimmunity 1990;48–17.

B602. Buyon JP, Ben-Chetrit E, Karp S, Roubey RA, Pompeo L, Reeves WH, Tan EM, Winchester R. Acquired congenital heart block. Pattern of maternal antibody response to biochemically defined antigens of the SSA/Ro-SSB/La system in neonatal lupus. J Clin Invest 1989;84:627–634.

B603. Buyon JP, Cronstein BN, Morris M, Tanner M, Weissman G. Serum complement values (C3 and C4) do differentiate between systemic lupus activity and preeclampsia. Am J Med 1986;81:194–200.

B604. See B600.

B605. Buyon JP, Swersky SH, Fox HE, Bierman FZ, Winchester RJ. Intrauterine therapy for presumptive fetal myocarditis with acquired heart block due to systemic lupus erythematosus. Arthritis Rheum 1987;30:44–49.

B606. Buyon JP, Winchester R. Congenital complete heart block: A human model of passively acquired autoimmune injury. Arthritis Rheum 1990;33:609–614.

B607. Bygbjerg IC, Flachs H. Effect of chloroquine on human lymphocyte proliferation. Trans R Soc Trop Med Hyg 1986; 80(2):231–235.

B608. Bygbjerg IC, Svenson M, Theander TG, Bendtzen K. Effect of antimalarial drugs of stimulation and interleukin 2 production of human lymphocytes. Int J Immunopharmacol 1987; 9(4):513–519.

B609. Byrd RB, Trunk G. Systemic lupus erythematosus presenting as pulmonary hemosiderosis. Chest 1973 Jul;64:128.

B610. Byrne JA, Butler JL, Cooper MD. Differential activation requirements for virgin and memory T cells. J Immunol 1988; 141:3249–3257.

B611. Byron MA, Allington MJ, Chapel HM, Mowat AG, Cederholm-Williams SA. Indications of vascular endothelial cell dysfunction in systemic lupus erythematosus Ann Rheum Dis 1987 Oct;46(10):741–745.

B612. Byron MA, Mowat AG. Thyroid disorders in systemic lupus erythematosus [letter]. Ann Rheum Dis 1987 Feb;46(2): 174–175.

B613. Bywaters EGL. Family studies of rheumatoid arthritis and lupus erythematosus in Great Britain. In: Kellgren JH, editor. The Epidemiology of Chronic Rheumatism, Philadelphia: Davis, 1961:255–257.

B614. Bywaters EGL. Classification criteria for systemic lupus erythematosus, with particular reference in lupus-like syndromes. Proc Roy Soc Med 1967;60:463–464.

B615. Bywaters EGL. Anatomic changes in Jaccoud's syndrome [abstract]. Arthritis Rheum 1971;14:153.

B616. Byyny RL. Withdrawal from glucocorticoid therapy. N Engl J Med 1976;295:30–32.

C

C1. Cade R, Spooner G, Schlein E, Pickering M, DeQuesada A, Holcomb A, Juncos L, Richard G, Shires D, Levin D, Hackett R, Free J, Hunt R, Fregly M. Comparison of azathioprine, prednisone and heparin alone or combined in treating lupus nephritis. Nephron 1973;10(1):37–56.

C2. Caeiro F, Michielson FMC, Bernstein R, Hughes GR, Ansell BM. Systemic lupus erythematosus in childhood. Ann Rheum Dis 1981 Aug;40:325–331.

C3. Caggiano V, Fernando LP, Schneider JM, Haesslein HC, Watson-Williams EJ. Thrombotic thrombocytopenic purpura. Report of fourteen cases-occurrence during pregnancy and response to plasma exchange. J Clin Apheresis 1983;1:71–85.

C4. Cagnoli L, Viglietta G, Madia G, Gattiani A, Orsi C, Rigotti A, Zucchelli A. Acute bilateral renal vein thrombosis superimposed on calcified thrombus of the inferior vena cava in a patient with membranous lupus nephritis. Nephrol Dial Transplant 1990;Supp 1:71–74.

C5. Cahn MM, Levy EJ, Schaffer B, Beerman H. Lupus erythematosus and polymorphous light eruptions; experimental study on their possible relationship. J Invest Dermatol 1953 Dec;21: 375–396.

C6. Caille B, Harpey P-J, Lejeune C, Sudre Y, Turpin R. Lupoid syndrome due to D-penicillamine associated with Wilson's disease. Clinical study of a case. Ann Med Interne (Paris) 1971; 122:255–260.

C7. Cairns E, Block J, Bell DA. Anti-DNA antibody producing hybridomas of normal lymphoid cell origin. J Clin Invest 1984; 74:880–887.

C8. Cairns E, Kwong PC, Misener V, Ip P, Bell DA, Siminovitch KA. Analysis of variable region genes encoding a human anti-DNA antibody of normal origin. Implications for the molecular basis of human autoimmune responses. J Immunol 1989 Jul 15;143(2):685–691.

C9. Cairns E, Massicotte H, Bell DA. Expression in systemic lupus erythematosus of an idiotype common to DNA-binding and

nonbinding monoclonal antibodies produced by normal human lymphoid cells. J Clin Invest 1989;83:1002–1009.

C10. Cairns E, St Germain J, Bell DA. The in vitro production of anti-DNA antibody by cultured peripheral blood or tonsillar lymphoid cells from normal donors and SLE patients. J Immunol 1985 Dec;135(6):3839–3844.

C11. Cairns SA, Acheson EJ, Corbett CL, Dosa S, Mallick NP, Lawler W, Williams G. The delayed appearance of an antinuclear factor and the diagnosis of systemic lupus erythematosus in glomerulonephritis. Postgrad Med J 1979 Oct;55(648): 723–727.

C12. Cairns SA, London A, Mallick NP. The value of three immune commplex assays in the management of systemic lupus erythematosus; an assessment of immune complex levels, size and immunochemical properties in relation to disease activity and manifestations. Clin Exp Immunol 1980 May;40:273–282.

C13. Calabrese JR, Kling MA, Gold PW. Alterations in immunocompetence during stress, bereavement and depression: focus on neuroendocrine regulation. Am J Psychiatry 1987 Sep; 144(9):1123–1134.

C14. Calabrese LH. The rheumatic manifestations of infection with the human immunodeficiency virus. Semin Arthritis Rheum 1989 May;18(4):225–239.

C15. Calaco CB, Eklin KB. The lupus anticoagulant. Arthritis Rheum 1985 Jan;28:67–74.

C16. Caldarelli DD, Rejowski JE, Corey JP. Sensorineural hearing loss in lupus erythematosus. Am J Otology 1986 May;7(3): 210–213.

C17. Calkins LL. Corneal epithelial changes occurring during chloroquine (aralen) therapy. Arch Ophthalmol 1958 Dec; 60(6):981–988.

C18. Callard RE, Smith SH, Scott KE. The role of interleukin 4 in specific antibody responses by human B cells. Int Immunol 1991; 3:157–163.

C19. Callen JP. Chronic cutaneous lupus erythematosus. Clinical, laboratory, therapeutic and prognostic examination of 62 patients. Arch Dermatol 1982 Jun;118(6):412–416.

C20. Callen JP. The effectiveness of colchicine for cutaneous vasculitis in lupus erythematosus. Clin Rheum in Practice 1984;2:176–179.

C20a. Callen JP. Systemic lupus erythematosus in patients with chronic cutaneous (discoid) lupus erythematosus. J Am Acad Dermatol 1985;12:278–288.

C21. Callen JP. Intralesional triamcinolone is effective for discoid lupus erythematosus of the palms and soles [letter]. J Rheumatol 1985 Jun;12(3):630–633.

C22. Callen JP, Fowler JF, Kulick KB. Serologic and clinical features of patients with discoid lupus erythematosus: relationship of antibodies to single-stranded deoxyribonucleic acid and of other antinuclear antibody subsets to clinical manifestations. J Am Acad Dermatol 1985 Nov;13(5 Pt 1):748–755.

C23. Callen JP, Fowler JF, Kulick KB, Stelzer G, Smith SZ. Neonatal lupus erythematosus occurring in one fraternal twin. Serologic and immunogenetic studies. Arthritis Rheum 1985; 28:271.

C24. Callen JP, Klein J. Subacute cutaneous lupus erythematosus. Clinical, serologic, immunogenetic and therapeutic considerations in seventy-two patients. Arthritis Rheum 1988 Aug; 31(8):1007–1013.

C25. Callen JP, Kulick KB, Stelzer G, Fowler JF. Subacute cutaneous lupus erythematosus. Clinical, serologic, and immunogenetic studies of 49 patients seen in a non-referral setting. J Am Acad Dermatol 1986;15:1227–1337.

C26. Callen JP, Ross L. Subacute cutaneous lupus erythematosus and porphyria cutanea tarda. Report of a case. J Am Acad Dermatol 1981;5:269–273.

C27. Callen JP, Spencer LV, Burruss JB, Holtman J. Azathioprine:

An effective, corticosteroid-sparing therapy for patients with recalcitrant cutaneous lupus erythematosus or with recalcitrant cutaneous leukocytoclastic vasculitis. Arch Dermatol 1991;127:515–522.

C28. Callender S, Race RR, Paykoc ZV. Hypersensitivity to transfused blood. Br Med J 1945 Jul 21;2:83–84.

C29. Callender ST, Race RR. Serological and genetical study of multiple antibodies formed in response to blood transfusion by a patient with lupus erythematosus diffusus. Ann Eugenics 1946 Aug;13:102–117.

C30. Calmes BA, Bartholomew BA. SSA-A(Ro) antibody in random mother-infant pairs. J Clin Pathol 1985 Jan;38:73–75.

C31. Calnan LD. Lymphocyte infiltration of the skin Jessner. Br J Derm 1957;69:169–173.

C32. Calzolari A. Recherches experimentales sur un rapport probable entra la function du thymus et celle des testiculus. Arch Ital Biol 1898;30:71–89.

C33. Cambiaggi A. Unusual ocular lesions in a case of systemic lupus erythematosus. Arch Ophthal 1957 Mar;57(3):451–453.

C34. Cameron B, Minota S, Stein L, Shaw M, Wilson J, Lemon S, Smiley L, Winfield JB. Autoantibody interrelationships in acute viral disease and childhood systemic lupus erythematosus [abstract]. Arthritis Rheum 1988 Apr;31(4) Suppl:S20.

C35. Cameron HA, Ramsay LE. The lupus syndrome induced by hydralazine: A common complication with low dose treatment. Br Med J 1984 Aug 18;289:410–412.

C36. Cameron JS. Immunosuppressant agents in the treatment of glomerulonephritis: 2. Cytotoxic drugs. J R Coll Physicians Lond 1971 Jul;5:301–322.

C37. Cameron JS, Boulton-Jones M, Robinson R, Ogg C. Treatment of lupus nephritis and cyclophosphamide. Lancet 1970; 2:846–849.

C38. Cameron JS, Lessof MH, Ogg CS, Williams BD, Williams DG. Disease activity in the nephritis of systemic lupus erythematosus in relation to serum complement concentrations. DNA-binding capacity and precipitating anti-DNA antibody. Clin Exp Immunol 1976;25:418–427.

C39. Cameron JS, Turner DR, Ogg CS, Williams DG, Lessof MH, Chantler C, Leibowitz S. Systemic lupus with nephritis: A long-term study. Q J Med 1979 Jan;48:1–24.

C40. Cameron R, Waterfield JD. Delineation of two defects responsible for T-cell hyporesponsiveness to concanavalin A in MRL congenic mice. Immunology 1986;59:187–193.

C41. Camisa C. Lichen planus and related conditions. Adv Dermatol 1987;2:47–69.

C42. Camisa C. Vesiculobullous systemic lupus erythematosus. A report of four cases. J Am Acad Dermatol 1988 Jan;18(1 Pt 1):93–100.

C43. Camisa C, Grinwood RE. Indirect immunofluorescence in vesiculobullous eruption of systemic lupus erythematosus [letter]. J Invest Dermatol 1986 May;86(5):606.

C44. Camisa C, Sharma HM. Vesiculobullous systemic lupus erythematosus. Report of two cases and a review of the literature. J Am Acad Dermatol 1983 Dec;9(6):924–933.

C45. Campbell CH. Skin pigmentation with camoquin as a malarial suppressive. Trans Roy Soc Trop Med Hyg 1959;53: 215–216.

C46. Campbell CH. Pigmentation of the nail-beds, palate, and skin occurring during malarial suppressive therapy with "camoquin." Med J Aust 1960 Jun 18;47(1):956–959.

C47. Campbell IL, Kay TWH, Oxbrow L, Harrison LC. Essential role for interferon-γ and interleukin-6 in autoimmune insulin-dependent diabetes in NOD/Wehi mice. J Clin Invest 1991; 87:739–742.

C48. Campbell MJ, Carroll W, Kon S, Thielemans K, Rothbard JB, Levy S, Levy R. Idiotype vaccination against murine B cell lymphoma: Humoral and cellular responses elicited by tumor-derived IgM and its molecular subunits. J Immunol 1987;139: 2825.

C49. Campbell MJ, Esserman L, Levy R. Immunotherapy of established murine B cell lymphoma. Combination of idiotype immunization and cyclophosphamide. J Immunol 1988;141: 3227.

C50. Campbell RD, Carroll MC, Porter RR. The molecular genetics of components of complement. Adv Immunol 1986;38: 203.

C51. Campbell RD, Law SKA, Reid KBM, Sim RB. Structure, organization and regulation of the complement genes. Ann Rev Immunol 1988;6:161–195.

C52. Campen DH, Horwitz DA, Quismorio FP Jr, Ehresmann GR, Martin WJ. Serum levels of interleukin-2 receptor and activity of rheumatic disease characterized by immune system activation. Arthritis Rheum 1988;31:1358–1364.

C53. Campion G, Maddison PJ, Goulding N, James I, Ahern MJ, Watt I, Sansom D. The Felty syndrome: a case-matched study of clinical manifestations and outcome, serologic features, and immunogenetic associations. Medicine 1990; 69:69–80.

C54. Camussi G, Tetta C, Coda R, Benveniste J. Release of platelet-activating factor in human pathology: evidence of the occurrence of basophil degranulation and release of platelet activating factor in systemic lupus erythematosus. Lab Invest 1981;44:241–251.

C55. Camussi G, Tetta C, Segolinia G, Coda R, Vercellone A. Localization of neutrophil cationic proteins and loss of anionic charges in glomeruli of patients with systemic lupus erythematosus glomerulonephritis. Clin Immunol Immunopathol 1982; 24:299–314.

C56. Canadian Hydroxychloroquine Study Group. A randomized study of the effect of withdrawing hydroxychloroquine sulfate in systemic lupus erythematosus. N Engl J Med 1991;324(3): 150–154.

C57. Cannat A, Seligmann M. Possible induction of antinuclear antibodies by isoniazid. Lancet 1966 Jan 22;1:185–187.

C58. Cannon AB, Orstein GG. Lupus erythematosus: Treatment with tuberculin. Arch Dermatol 1927;16:8–11.

C59. Cannon EF, Curtis AC. A survey of lupus erythematosus in the University of Michigan Hospital since 1948. Arch Dermatol 1958 Aug;78(2):196–199.

C60. Cano PO, Jerry LM, Sladowski JP, Osterland CK. Circulating immune complexes in systemic lupus erythematosus. Clin Exp Immunol 1977 Aug;29:197–204.

C61. Canoso JJ, Cohen AS. A review of the use, evaluations, and criticisms of the preliminary criteria for the classification of systemic lupus erythematosus. Arthritis Rheum 1979 Aug;22: 917–921.

C62. Canoso RT, deOliveira RM. Characterization and antigenic specificity of chlorpromazine-induced antinuclear antibodies. J Lab Clin Med 1986;108:213–216.

C63. Canoso RT, deOliveira RM. Chlorpromazine-induced anticardiolipin antibodies and lupus anticoagulant: absence of thrombosis. Am J Hematol 1988;27:272–275.

C64. Canoso RT, Lewis ME, Yunis EJ. Association of HLA-Bw44 with chlorpromazine-induced autoantibodies. Clin Immunol Immunopathol 1982;97:659–663.

C65. Canoso RT, Sise HS. Chlorpromazine-induced lupus anticoagulant and associated immunologic abnormalities. Am J Hematol 1982;13(2):121–129.

C66. Canoso RT, Zon LT, Groopman JE. Anticardiolipin antibodies associated with HTLV-III infection. Br J Haematol 1987;65: 495.

C67. Cantarovich M, Hiesse C, Lantz O, Charpentier B, Fries D. Renal transplantation and active lupus erythematosus [letter]. Ann Intern Med 1988 Aug 1;109(3):254–255.

C68. Canter JW, Shorb PE. Acute perforation of colonic diverticula associated with prolonged adrenocorticosteroid therapy. Am J Surg 1971 Jan;121:46–57.

C69. Cantor B, Tyler T, Nelson RM. Oligohydramnios and transient neonatal anuria. A possible association with the maternal use of prostaglandin synthetase inhibitors. J Reprod Med 1980; 24:220.

C70. Cantor H, McVay-Boudreau L, Hugenberger J, Naidorf D, Shen FW, Gershon RK. Immunoregulatory circuits among T cells. II. Physiological role of feedback inhibition in vivo: absence in NZB mice. J Exp Med 1978;147:1116–1122.

C71. Capel PJA, Preijers WMB, Allebes WA, Haanen C. Treatment of chronic lymphocytic leukemia with monoclonal anti-idiotype antibody. Neth J Med 1985;28:112.

C72. Caperton EM Jr, Bean SF, Dick FR. Immunofluorescent skin test in systemic lupus erythematosus. Lack of relationship with renal disease. JAMA 1972 Nov 20;222:935–937.

C73. Capra JD, Kehoe JM, Winchester RJ, Kunkel HG. Structure-function relationship among anti-gamma globulin antibodies Ann N Y Acad Sci 1971;190:371–381.

C74. Capra JD, Slaughter C, Milner ECB, Estess P, Tucker PW. The cross-reactive idiotype of A-strain mice: serological and structural analysis. Immunol Today 1982;3:332.

C75. Carbotte RM, Denburg SD, Denburg JA. Prevalence of cognitive impairment in systemic lupus erythematosus. J Nerv Ment Dis 1986 Jun;174(6):357–364.

C76. Carbotte RM, Denburg SD, Garnett S, Nahmias C, Firnau G, Denburg JA. Positron emission tomography (PET) of the brain and neurocognitive function in systemic lupus erythematosus (SLE): serial observations [abstract]. Arthritis Rheum 1988 Apr;31(4) Suppl:S56.

C77. Cardella CJ, Davies P, Allison AC. Immune complexes induce selective release of lysosomal hydrolyses from macrophages. Nature 1974;247:46–48.

C78. Carel RS, Shapiro MS, Shoham D, Gutman A. Lupus erythematosus cells in pleural effusion: initial manifestation of procainamide induced lupus erythematosus. Chest 1977 Nov;72: 670–672.

C79. Carette S, Jobin F. Acute adrenal insufficiency as a manifestation of the cardiolipin syndrome? Ann Rheum Dis 1989 May; 48(5):430–431.

C80. Carette S, Klippel JH, Decker JL, Austin HA, Plotz PH, Steinberg AD, Balow JE. Controlled studies of oral immunosuppressive drugs in lupus nephritis. A long term follow-up. Ann Intern Med 1983 Jul;99(1):1–8.

C81. Carette S, Macher AM, Nussbaum A, Plotz PH. Severe, acute pulmonary disease in patients with systemic lupus erythematosus: ten years of experience of the National Institutes of Health. Semin Arthritis Rheum 1985 Aug;14:52–59.

C82. Carette S, Urowitz MB. Systemic lupus erythematosus and diffuse soft tissue calcifications. Int J Dermatol 1983 Sep; 22(7):416–418.

C83. Carette S, Urowitz MB, Grosman H, St. Louis EL. Cranial computerized tomography in systemic lupus erythematosus. J Rheumatol 1982 Nov–Dec;9(6):855–859.

C84. Carey RA, Harvey AM, Howard JE. Effect of adrenocorticotropic hormone (ACTH) and cortisone on course of disseminated lupus erythematosus and periarteritis nodosa. Bull Johns Hopkins Hosp 1950 Nov;87:425–460.

C85. Cario JR, Rothfield NF, Ruddy S. Demonstration of B1H globulin together with C3 in the dermal-epidermal junction of patients with systemic lupus erythematosus. Arthritis Rheum 1979;2:13.

C86. Cariou R, Tobelem G, Belluci S, Soria J, Maclouf J, Soria C, Caen J. Effect of lupus anticoagulant on antithrombogenic properties of endothelial cells: inhibition of thrombomodulin-dependent protein C activation. Thromb Haemostas 1988;60: 54–58.

C87. Cariou R, Tobelem G, Soria C, Caen J. Inhibition of protein C activation by endothelial cells in the presence of lupus anticoagulant [letter]. N Engl J Med 1986 May 1;314(18): 1193–1194.

C88. Carlisle EJ, Leslie W. Primary hypoadrenalism in a patient with the lupus anticoagulant. J Rheumatol 1990 Oct;17(10): 1405–1407.

C89. Carlson JA, Hodder SR, Ucci AA, Madaio MP. Glomerular localization of circulating single-stranded DNA in mice. Dependence on the molecular weight of DNA. J. Autoimmunity. 1988;1:231–241.

C90. Carlston H, Tarkowski A. Expression of heterozygous lpr gene in MRL mice. I. Defective T-cell reactivity and polyclonal B-cell activation. Scand J Immunol 1989;30:457–462.

C91. Carmo-Fonseca M, Tollervey D, Pepperkok R, Barabino SML, Merdes A, Brunner C, Zamore PD, Green MR, Hurt E, Lamond A. Mammalian nuclei contain foci which are highly enriched in components of the pre-mRNA splicing machinery Embo J 1991;10:195–206.

C92. Caro XJ. Immunofluorescent detection of IgG at the dermal-epidermal junction in patients with apparent fibrositis syndrome. Arthritis Rheum 1984 Oct;27(10):1174–1179.

C93. Carol JR, Rothfeild NF, Ruddy S. Demonstration of B1H globulin together with C3 in the dermal epidermal junction of patients with systemic lupus erythematosus. Arthritis Rheum 1979;22:13–18.

C94. Carp HJA, Toder V, Gazit E, Orgad S, Mashiach S, Nebel L, Serr DM. Immunization by paternal leukocytes for prevention of primary habitual abortion: Results of a controlled matched trial. Gynecol Obstet Invest 1990;29:16–21.

C95. Carpenter JR, McDuffie FC, Sheps SG, Spiekerman RE, Brumfield H, King R. Prospective study of immune response to hydralazine and development of antideoxyribonucleoprotein in patients receiving hydralazine. Am J Med 1980 Sep;69: 395–400.

C96. Carpenter RR, Sturgill BC. The course of systemic lupus erythematosus. J Chronic Dis 1966 Feb;19:117–131.

C97. Carpentier N, Fontannaz J, Jeannet M, Nissen C, Speck B. Characteristics and clinical relevance of autolymphocytotoxins in patients with aplastic anemia. Transplantation 1986;42: 159–161.

C98. Carr R. Prolonged pharmacotherapy and the eye. A symposium. Chloroquine and organic changes in the eye. Dis Nerv Syst 1968;29 Suppl 3:36–39.

C99. Carr R, Forsyth S, Sadi D. Abnormal responses to ingested substances in murine systemic lupus erythematosus: apparent effect of a casein-free diet on the development of systemic lupus erythematosus in NZB/W mice. J Rheumatol 1987;14 Suppl 13:158–165.

C100. Carr RE, Henkind P, Rothfield N, Siege IM. Ocular toxicity of antimalarial drugs: Long-term follow-up. Am J Ophthal 1968;66:738–744.

C101. Carr RI, Wold RT, Farr RS. Antibodies to bovine gamma globulin (BGG) and occurrence of a BGG-like substance in systemic lupus erythematosus sera. J Allergy Clin Immunol 1972 Jul;50:18–30.

C102. Carratala J, Moreno R, Cabellos C, Miquel Nolla J, Pac V, Moga I. Neisseria meningitis monarthritis revealing systemic lupus erythematosus [letter]. J Rheumatol 1988 Mar;15(3): 532–533.

C103. Carreras LO, Perez G, Vega HR, Casavilla F. Lupus anticoagulant and recurrent fetal loss: successful treatment with gammaglobulin [letter]. Lancet 1988 Aug 13;2(8607): 393–394.

C104. Carreras LO, Defrey NG, Machin SJ, Vermylen J, Deman

R, Spitz B, Van Assche A. Arterial thrombosis, intrauterine death and "lupus" anticoagulant: Detection of immunoglobulin interfering with prostacyclin formation. Lancet 1981;1: 244–246.

C105. Carreras LO, Vermylen JG. 'Lupus' anticoagulant and thrombosis—possible role of inhibition of prostacyclin formation. Thromb Haemost 1982 Aug 24;48(1):38–40.

C106. Carr-Locke DL. Sulfasalazine-induced lupus syndrome in a patient with Crohn's disease. Am J Gastroenterol 1982 Sep; 77:614–616.

C107. Carroll GJ, Withers K, Bayliss CE. The prevalence of Raynaud's syndrome in rheumatoid arthritis. Ann Rheum Dis 1981 Dec 6;40(6):567–570.

C108. Carroll MC, Belt T, Palsdottir A, Yu Y. Molecular genetics of the fourth component of human complement and steroid 21-hydroxylase. Immunol Rev 1985;87:39–60.

C109. Carroll MC, Campbell RD, Porter RR. Mapping of component C4 genes in HLA, the major histocompatibility complex in man. Proc Natl Acad Sci USA 1985;82:521–525.

C110. Carroll MC, Katzman P, Alicot EM, Koller BH, Geraghty DE, Orr HT, Strominger JL, Spies T. Linkage map of the human histocompatibility complex including the tumor necrosis factor genes. Proc Nat Acad Sci USA 1987;84:8535–8539.

C111. Carroll MC, Palsdottir A, Belt KT, Porter RR. Deletion of complement C4 and 21-hydroxylase genes in the HLA class III region. EMBO J 1985;4:2547–2552.

C112. Carroll N, Barrett JA. Systemic lupus erythematosus presenting with cardiac tamponade. Br Heart J 1984 Apr;51: 452–453.

C113. Carroll P, Stafford D, Schwartz RS, Stollar BD. Murine monoclonal anti-DNA autoantibodies bind to endogenous bacteria. J Immunol 1985 Aug;135(2):1086–1090.

C114. Carroll WL, Lowder JN, Streifer R, Warnke R, Levy S, Levy R. Idiotype variant cell populations in patients with B cell lymphoma. J Exp Med 1986;164:1566.

C115. Carson DA, Chen PP, Kipps TJ. New roles for rheumatoid factor. J Clin Invest 1991;87:379–383.

C116. Carson DA, Chen PP, Kipps TJ, Radoux V, Jirik FR, Goldfien RD, Fox RI, Silverman GJ, Fong S. Idiotypic and genetic studies of human rheumatoid factors. Arthritis Rheum 1987; 30:1321.

C117. Carstens PH, Ogden LL Jr, Peak WP. Renal amyloidosis associated with systemic lupus erythematosus. Am J Clin Pathol 1980 Dec;74(6):835–838.

C118. Carter AE, Eban R, Perrett RD. Prevention of post-operative deep venous thrombosis and pulmonary embolism. BMJ 1971 Feb 6;1:312–314.

C119. Carter JB, Blieden LC, Edwards JE. Congenital heart block: anatomic correlations and review of the literature. Arch Pathol 1974;97:51.

C120. Carter ME, James VHT. Effect of alternate-day, single-dose, corticosteroid therapy on pituitary-adrenal function. Ann Rheum Dis 1972 Sep;31:379–383.

C121. Carter NG, Whitworth JA, Mackay IR. Impaired urinary acidification—its incidence in diseases with autoimmune features. Aust NZ J Med 1971 Feb;1:39–43.

C122. Carteron NL, Schimenti CL, Wofsy D. Treatment of murine lupus with F(ab')2 fragments of monoclonal antibody to L3T4. Suppression of autoimmunity does not depend on T helper cell depletion. J Immunol 1989;142:1470–1475.

C123. Carteron NL, Wofsy D, Schimenti C, Ermak TH. F(ab')2 anti-CD4+ and intact anti-CD4 monoclonal antibodies inhibit the accumulation of CD4+ T cells, CD8+ T cells, and B cells in the kidneys of lupus-prone NZB/NZW mice. Clin Immunol Immunopathol 1990;56:373–383.

C124. Caruana RJ, Barish CF, Buckalew VM Jr. Complete distal renal tubular acidosis in systemic lupus: clinical and laboratory findings. Am J Kidney Dis 1985 Jul;6(1):59–63.

C125. Casali P, Burastero SE, Nakamura M, Inghirami G, Notkins AL. Human lymphocytes making rheumatoid-factor and antibody to ssDNA belong to Leu-1 B cell subset. Science 1987; 236:77–81.

C126. Casali P, Notkins AL. CD5+ B lymphocytes, polyreactive antibodies and the human B cell repertoire. Immunol Today 1989;10:364–368.

C127. Casals SP, Friou GJ, Teague PO. Specific nuclear reaction pattern of antibody to DNA in lupus erythematosus sera. J Lab Clin Med 1963 Oct;62:625–631.

C128. Case DB, Atlas SA, Laragh J, Sealey JE. Clinical experience with blockade of the renin-angiotensin-aldosterone system by an oral converting enzyme inhibitor (SQ14,225,captopril) in hypertensive patients. Prog Cardiovasc Dis 1978;21:195–206.

C129. Case records of the Massachusetts General Hospital. Weekly clinicopathological exercises. Case 46–1973. N Engl J Med 1973 Apr 5;288:729–733.

C130. Case records of the Massachusetts General Hospital. Weekly clinicopathological exercises. Case 29–1976. N Engl J Med 1976;295:156–163.

C131. Case records of the Massachusetts General Hospital. Weekly clinicopathological exercises. Case 17–1976. N Engl J Med 1978;294:100.

C132. Case records of the Massachusetts General Hospital. Weekly clinicopathological exercises. Case 25–1978. N Engl J Med 1978 Jun 29;298(26);1463–1470.

C133. Case records of the Massachusetts General Hospital. Weekly clinicopathological exercises. Case 42–1979. N Engl J Med 1979 Oct 18;301:881–887.

C134. Case records of the Massachusetts General Hospital. Weekly clinicopathological exercises. Case 2–1985. N Engl J Med 1985;312:1–3-112.

C135. Case records of the Massachusetts General Hospital. Weekly clinicopathological exercises. Case 46–1986. Presentation Case. A 26-year old woman was admitted to the hospital because of secondary amenorrhea. N Engl J Med 1986;315: 1336.

C136. Case records of the Massachusetts General Hospital. Weekly clinicopathological exercises. Case 11–1990. N Engl J Med 1990;322:754–769.

C137. Casey TP. Systemic lupus erythematosus in NZB × NZW hybrid mice treated with the corticosteroid drug betamethazone. J Lab Clin Med 1968;71:390.

C138. Casey TP. Azathioprine (Imuran) administration and the development of malignant lymphomas in NZB mice. Clin Exp Immunol 1968;3:305.

C139. Casey TP. Immunosuppression by cyclophosphamide in NZB × NZW mice with lupus nephritis. Blood 1968;32:436.

C140. Casey TP, Howie JB. Autoimmune haemolytic anaemia in NZB/Bl mice treated with the corticosteroid drug betamethasone. Blood 1965;25:423.

C141. Caspary L, Schmees C, Schoetensak I, Hartung K, Stannat S, Deicher H, Creutzig A, Alexander K. Alterations of the nailfold capillary morphology associated with Raynaud phenomenon in patients with systemic lupus erythematosus. J Rheumatol 1991;18(4):559–566.

C142. Cass RM, Mongan ES, Jacox RF, Vaughan JH. Immunoglobulins G, A, and M in systemic lupus erythematosus. Relationship to serum complement titer, latex titer, antinuclear antibody, and manifestations of clinical disease. Ann Intern Med 1968 Oct;69:749–756.

C143. Cassidy JT. Clinical assessment of immune-complex disease in children with systemic lupus erythematosus. J Peds 1976 Sep;89:523–526.

C144. Cassidy JT, Burt A, Petty R, Sullivan D. Selective IgA deficiency in connective tissue diseases. N Engl J Med 1969;280: 275.

C145. Cassidy JT, Levinson JE, Bass JC, Baum J, Brewer EJ Jr, Fink CW, Hanson V, Jacobs JC, Masi AT, Schaller JG, Fries JF, McShane D, Young D. A study of classification criteria for a diagnosis of juvenile rheumatoid arthritis. Arthritis Rheum 1986 Feb;29(2):274–281.

C146. Cassidy JT, Petty RE. Textbook of Pediatric Rheumatology. 2nd Ed. New York: Churchill Livingston, 1990.

C147. Cassidy JT, Sullivan DB, Petty RE, Ragsdale C. Lupus nephritis and encephalopathy. Proceedings of the conference of rheumatic diseases in childhood. Arthritis Rheum 1977 Mar; 20 Suppl 2:315–322.

C148. Castaneda S, Herrero-Beaumont G, Valenzuela A, Vidal J, Molpenhauer F, Renedo G, Fernandez-Vallado P. Massive pulmonary hemorrhage: Fatal complication of systemic lupus erythematosus. J Rheumatol 1985 Feb;12:185–187.

C149. Casteneda S, Maldenhauen F, Herrero-Beaumont G, Yanez R. Protein losing enteropathy as the initial manifestation of systemic lupus erythematosus [letter]. J Rheumatol 1985 Dec; 12(6):1210–1212.

C150. Castro JE. Orchidectomy and the immune response. II. Response of orchidectomized mice to antigens. Proc R Soc Lond (Biol) 1974;185:437–451.

C151. Castrucci G, Alimandi L, Fichera A, Altomonte L, Zoli A. Changes in esophageal motility in patients with systemic lupus erythematosus: an esophago-manometric study [English abstract]. Minerva Dietol Gastroenterol 1990 Jan–Mar;36(1): 3–7.

C152. Catalano MA, Hoffmeier M. Frequency of systemic lupus erythematosus (SLE) among the ethnic groups of Hawaii. Arthritis Rheum 1989;32 Suppl 4:S30.

C153. Catania A, Mangone I, Motta P, Zanussi C. Administration of gonadotrophin-releasing hormone analog as adjunctive therapy in women with systemic lupus erythematosus [letter]. Arthritis Rheum 1989 Sep;32(9):1186–1188.

C154. Cathcart ES. Current concepts in the management of lupus nephritis. Hospital Practice 1977;12:59.

C155. Cathcart ES, O'Sullivan JB, Lincoln G. Standardization of the sheep cell agglutination test. The use of pooled reference sera and hemagglutination trays. Arthritis Rheum 1965 Aug;8: 530–537.

C156. Cathcart ES, Scheinberg MA. Systemic lupus erythematosus in a patient with amyloidosis. Discussion. Arthritis Rheum 1976 Mar–Apr;19(2):254–255.

C157. Cathcart ES, Scheinberg MA, Idelson BA, Couser WG. Beneficial effects of methylprednisolone "pulse" therapy in diffuse proliferative lupus nephritis. Lancet 1976 Jan 24;1:163.

C158. Catoggio LJ, Skinner RP, Smith G, Maddison PJ. Systemic lupus erythematosus in the elderly: clinical and serological characteristics. J Rheumatol 1984;11:175–181.

C159. Cats s, Terasaki PI, Perdue S, Mickey MR. Increased vulnerability of the donor organ in related kidney transplants for certain diseases. Transplantation 1984 Jun;37(6):575–579.

C160. Catterall RD. Biological false positive reactions and systemic disease. In: G. Walker, editor. Ninth Symposium on Advanced Medicine. Pitman Medical, London; 1973:97–111.

C161. Cattogio LJ, Skinner RP, Smith G, Maddison PJ. Systemic lupus erythematosus in the elderly: clinical and serological characteristics. J Rheumatol 1984 Apr;11:175–181.

C162. Caturla A, Colome JA, Bustos A, Chamorro MJ, Figueredo MA, Subiza JL, de la Concha EG. Occurrence of antibodies to protease-treated histones in a patient with vasculitis. Clin Immunol Immunopathol 1991;60:65–71.

C163. Cavalcant J, Shadduck RK, Winkelstein A, Zeiger Z, Mendelow H. Red cell hypoplasia and increased bone marrow reticulin in systemic lupus erythematosus: reversal with corticosteroid therapy. Am J Haematol 1978;5:253–263.

C164. Cavallo T, Cameron WR, Lapenas D. Immunopathology of early and clinically silent lupus nephropathy. Am J Pathol 1977 Apr;87:1–15.

C165. Cavallo T, Granholm NA. Bacterial lipopolysaccharide transforms mesangial into proliferative lupus nephritis without interfering with processing of pathogenic immune complexes in NZB/W mice. Am J Pathol 1990;137:971–978.

C166. Cavallo T, Granholm NA. Lipopolysaccharide from gram-negative bacteria enhances polyclonal B cell activation and exacerbates nephritis in MRL/lpr mice. Clin Exp Immunol 1990;82:515–521.

C167. Cavallo T, Graves K, Granholm NA. Murine lupus nephritis: effects of glucocorticoid on glomerular permeability. Lab Invest 1984;50:378–383.

C168. Cazenave A, Schedel HE. Abrege Pratique des Maladies de la Peau d'Apres les Auteurs les Plus Estimes, et Surtout d'apres des Documens Puises Dans les Lecons Cliniques de M. le Docteur Biett. Paris: Bechet, 1828 Jun.

C169. Cazenave A, Schedel HE. Abrege Pratique des Maladies de la Peau d'Apres le Auteurs les Plus Estimes, et Surtout d'apres des Documens Puises Dans les Lecons Clinique de M. le Docteur Biett, 2d ed. Paris: Bechet, 1833 Jun.

C170. Cazenave A, Schedel HE. Abrege Pratique des Maladies de la Peau d'Apres les Auteurs les Plus Estimes, et Surtout d'apres des Documens Puises Dans les Lecons Clinque de M. le Docteur Biett, 3d ed. Paris: Bechet, 1838 Jun.

C171. Cazenave PLA. Lupus erythemateux (Erytheme Centrifuge). Ann Malad Peau Syph 1850–1851;3:297–299.

C172. Cazenave PLA, Chausit M. Du lupus [Frey H, translation]. Ann Malad Peau Syph 1852;4:113–117.

C173. Cazenave PLA, Chausit M. Du lupus [Frey H, translation]. Ann Malad Peau Syph 1852;4:225–228.

C174. Cecchi E, Ferraris E. Desludging action of hydroxychloroquine in rheumatoid arthritis. Acta Rheum Scand 1962;8: 214–221.

C175. Cecere FA, Persellin RH. The interaction of pregnancy and the Rheumatic diseases. Clin Rheum Dis 1981;7:747–768.

C176. Cecere FA, Yoshinoya S, Pope RM. Fatal thrombotic thrombocytopenic purpura with systemic lupus erythematosus: circulating comune complexes. Arthritis Rheum 1981 Mar;24:550–553.

C177. Celada A, Barras C, Benzonana G, Jeannet M. Increased frequency of HLA-DRw3 in systemic lupus erythematosus. Tissue Antigens 1980;15:283–288.

C178. Celermajer DS, Thorner PS, Baumal R, Arbus GS. Sex differences in childhood lupus nephritis. Am J Dis Child 1984 Jun;138:586–588.

C179. Cellingsworth M, Scott DG. Acute systemic lupus erythematosus with fatal pneumonitis and disseminated intravascular coagulation. Ann Rheum Dis 1985 Jan;44:67.

C180. Center SA, Smith CA, Wilkinson E, Erb HN, Lewis RM. Clinicopathologic, renal immunofluorescent, and light microscopic features of glomerulonephritis in the dog: 41 cases (1975–1985). J Am Vet Med Assoc 1987;190:81–90.

C181. Ceppellini R, Polli E, Celada F. A DNA-reacting factor in serum of a patient with lupus erythematosus diffusus. Proc Soc Exp Biol Med 1957 Dec;96(3):572–574.

C182. Cerny J, Smith JS, Webb C, Tucker PW. Properties of anti-idiotypic T cell lines propagated with syngeneic B lymphocytes. I. T cells bind intact idiotypes and discriminate between the somatic idiotypic variants in a manner similar to the anti-idiotypic antibodies. J Immunol 1988;141:3718.

C182a. Cervera R, Font J, Khamashta MA, Hughes GRV. Antiphospholipid antibodies: which and when? Postgrad Med J 1990;66:889–891.

C183. Cervera R, Font J, Lopez-Soto A, Casals F, Pallares L, Bove A, Ingelmo M, Urbano-Marquez A. Isotype distribution of anticardiolipin antibodies in systemic lupus erythematosus: prospective analysis of a series of 100 patients. Ann Rheum Dis 1990 Feb;49(2):109–113.

C184. Cervera R, Font J, Pare C, Azqueta M, Perez-Villa F, Lopez-Soto A, Ingelmo M. Cardiac involvement in systemic lupus erythematosus. Prospective study of 70 patient patients. Ann Rheum Dis 1992;51:156–159.

C185. Cervera R, Khamashta MA, Font J, Lopez-Soto A, Ramirez G, D'Cruz D, Montalban J, Tripathi P, Ingelmo M, Hughes GRV. Antiendothelial cell antibodies in systemic lupus erythematosus patients with the antiphospholipid syndrome. I European Conference on Systemic Lupus Erythematosus. Amsterdam, The Netherlands; 1990; Nov 15–17.

C185a. Cervera R, Khamashta MA, Font J, Ramirez G, D'Cruz D, Montalban J, Lopez-Soto A, Asherson RA, Ingelmo M, Hughes GRV. Antiendothelial cell antibodies in patients with the antiphospholipid syndrome. Autoimmunity 1991;11:1–6.

C185b. Cervera R, Khamashta MA, Font J, Reyes PA, Vianna JL, Lopez-Soto A, Amigo MC, Asherson RA, Azqeta M, Pare C, Vargas J, Romero A, Ingelmo M, Hughes GRV. High prevalence of significant heart valve lesions in patients with the "primary" antiphospholipid syndrome. Lupus 1991;1:43–47.

C186. Ceuppens JL, Baroja ML, Van Vaeck F, Anderson CL. A defect in the membrane expression of high affinity 72 kD Fc receptors on phagocytic cells in four healthy subjects. J Clin Invest 1988;82:571–578.

C187. Ceuppens JL, Rodriguez MA, Goodwin JS. Non-steroidal anti-inflammatory agents inhibit the synthesis of IgM rheumatoid factor in vitro. Lancet 1982;528–530.

C188. Chagnac A, Kiberd BA, Farinas MC, Strober S, Sibley RK, Hoppe R, Myers BD. Outcome of the acute glomerular injury in proliferative lupus nephritis. J Clin Invest 1989 Sep;84(3):922–930.

C189. Chagnon A, Peres C, Camilleri G. Lupic syndrome induced by quinidine with thrombophlebitis alternans and circulating anti-factor IX anticoagulant [letter]. Nouvou Presse Med 1982;11:2020–2021.

C190. Chaiamnuay P, Johnston C, Maier J, Russell AS. Technique-related variation in results of FANA tests. Ann Rheum Dis 1984 Oct;43(5):755–757.

C191. Chalmers A, Thompson D, Stein HE, Reid G, Patterson AC. Systemic lupus erythematosus during penicillamine therapy for rheumatoid arthritis. Ann Intern Med 1982;97:659–663.

C192. Chamberlain WP Jr, Boles DJ. Edema of cornea precipitated by quinacrine (atabrine). Arch Ophthalmol 1946 Feb;35:120–134.

C193. Chambers JC, Denan D, Martin BJ, Keene JD. Genomic structure and amino acid sequence domains of the human La autoantigen. 1988;34:18043–18051.

C194. Chambers JC, Keene JD. Isolation and analysis of cDNA clones expressing human lupus antigen. Proc Natl Acad Sci USA 1985 Apr;82:2115–2119.

C195. Chambon P, Elgin S, Felsenfeld G, Guthrie C, Weintraub H, Yamamoto K. The Cell Nucleus. In: Alberts B, Bray D, Lewis J, Raff M, Roberts K, Watson JD, eds. Molecular Biology of the Cell. 2nd ed. New York: Garland, 1989:481–549.

C196. Chameides L, Truex RC, Vetter V, Rashkind WJ, Galioto FM, Noonan JA. Association of maternal systemic lupus erythematosus with congenital complete heart block. N Engl J Med 1977;297:1204–1207.

C197. Chan AC, Sack K. Danazol therapy for autoimmune hemolytic anemia associated with systemic lupus erythematosus [case report]. J Rheumatol 1991 Feb;18(2):280–282.

C198. Chan CN, Li E, Lai FM, Pang JA. An unusual case of systemic lupus erythematosus with isolated hypoglossal nerve palsy, fulminant acute pneumonitis and pulmonary amyloidosis. Ann Rheum Dis 1989 Mar;48(3):236–239.

C199. Chan EKL, Francoeur AM, Tan EM. Epitopes, structural domains, and asymmetry of amino acid residues in SS-B/La nuclear protein. J Immunol 1986;136:3744–3749.

C200. Chan EKL, Hamel JC, Buyon JP, Tan EM. Molecular definition and sequence motifs of the 52-kD component of human SS-A/Ro autoantigen. J Clin Invest 1991;87:68–76.

C201. Chan EKL, Sullivan KF, Tan EM. Ribonucleoprotein SS-B/La belongs to a protein family with consensus sequences for RNA-binding. Nucleic Acids Res 1989;17:2233–2244.

C202. Chan SH, Feng PH, Srinivasan N, Wee GB, Chan HC. HLA and systemic lupus erythematosus in Chinese. Hum Immunol 1981;3:345–350.

C203. Chandora DB. Delayed diazepam withdrawal syndrome: a case of auditory and visual hallucinations and seizures. J Med Assoc GA 1980 Sep;69(9):769–770.

C204. Chang R, Quismorio FP Jr. Transverse myelopathy in systemic lupus erythematosus (SLE). Arthritis Rheum 1990 Sep; 33 Suppl 9:S102.

C205. Chapel TA, Burns RE. Oral contraceptives and exacerbations of lupus erythematosus. Am J Obstet Gynecol 1971;110:366–369.

C206. Chaplin H, Avioli LV. Autoimmune hemolytic anemia. Arch Intern Med 1977 Mar;137:346.

C207. Chapman J, Bachar O, Korzyn AD, Wertman E, Michaelson DM. Alzheimers disease antibodies bind specifically to a neurofilament protein in torpedo cholinergic neurons. J Neurosci 1989;9:2710–2717.

C208. Charles GA, Schittecatte M, Rush AJ, Panzer M, Wilmotte J. Persistent cortisol non-suppression after clinical recovery predicts symptomatic relapse in unipolar depression. J Affective Disord 1989;17:271–278.

C209. Charlesworth A, Peake PW, Golding J, Mackie JD, Pussell BA, Timmermans K, Wakefield D. Hypercatabolism of C3 and C4 in active and inactive systemic lupus erythematosus. Ann Rheum Dis 1989;48:153–159.

C210. Charley MR, Bangert JL, Hamilton BL, Gilliam JN, Sontheimer RD. Murine graft vs. host disease: A chronologic and quantitative analysis of two histologic patterns. J Invest Dermatol 1983;81:412–417.

C211. Charley MR, Sontheimer RD. Clearing of subacute cutaneous LE around Molluscum contagiosum lesions. J Am Acad Dermatol 1982;6:529–533.

C212. Charmley P, Concannon T, Gatti RA. T-cell receptor β-chain DNA polymorphism frequencies in healthy HLA-DR homozygotes. Tissue Antigens 1990;35:157–164.

C213. Charpentier B, Carnoud C, Bach JF. Selective depression of the xenogeneic cell-mediated lympholysis in systemic lupus erythematosus. J Clin Invest 1979 Aug 64:351–360.

C214. Chartash EK, Lans DM, Paget SA, Qamar T, Lockshin MD. Aortic insufficiency and mitral regurgitation in patients with systemic lupus erythematosus and antiphospholipid syndrome. Am J Med 1989;86:407–412.

C215. Chase GJ, O'Shea PA, Collins E, Brem AS. Protein-losing enteropathy in systemic lupus erythematosus. Human Pathol 1981;3:1053–1055.

C216. Chasis H, Goldring W, Baldwin DS. Effect of febrile plasma, typhoid vaccine and nitrogen mustard on renal manifestations of human glomerulonephritis. Proc Soc Exp Biol & Med 1949 Aug;71:565–567.

C217. Chatenoud L, Bach MA. Abnormalities of T-cell subsets in glomerulonephritis and systemic lupus erythematosus. Kidney Int 1981 Aug;20:267–274.

C218. Chaudhuri KR, Taylor IK, Niven RM, Abbott RJ. A case of systemic lupus erythematosus presenting as Guillain-Barre syndrome. Br J Rheumatol 1989 Oct;28(5):440–442.

C219. Chavez-Legaspi M, Gomez-Vazquez A, Garcia-De La Torre I. Study of rheumatic manifestations and serologic abnormalities in patients with lepromatous leprosy. J Rheumatol 1985 Aug;12:738–741.

C220. Cheatum DE, Hurd ER, Strunk SW, Ziff M. Renal histology and clinical course of SLE: a prospective study. Arthritis Rheum 1973 Sep–Oct;16:670–676.

C221. Cheigh JS, Kim H, Stenzel KH, Tapia L, Sullivan JF, Stubenbord W, Riggio RR, Rubin AL. Systemic lupus erythematosus in patients with end-stage renal disease; long-term follow-up on the prognosis of patients and the evolution of lupus activity. Am J Kidney Dis 1990 Sep;16(3):189–195.

C222. Cheigh JS, Stenzel KH, Rubin AL, Chami J, Sullivan JF. Systemic lupus erythematosus in patients with chronic renal failure. Am J Med 1983 Oct;75(4):602–606.

C223. Chen PP, Albrandt K, Radoux V, Chen EW, Schrantz R, Liu F, Carson DA. Genetic basis for the cross-reactive idiotypes on the light chains of human IgM anti-IgG autoantibodies. Proc Natl Acad Sci USA 1986;83:8318.

C224. Chen PP, Liu ME, Sinha S, Carson DA. A 16/6 idiotype-positive anti-DNA antibody is encoded by a conserved VH gene with no somatic mutation. Arthritis Rheum 1988 Nov; 31(11):1429–1431.

C225. Chen PP, Liu MG, Glass CA, Sinha S, Kipps TJ, Carson DA. Characterization of two immunoglobulin V_H genes that are homologous to human rheumatoid factors. Arthritis Rheum 1989;32:72.

C226. Chen YS, Hu XE. Auricula-acupuncture in 15 cases of discoid lupus erythematosus. J Tradit Chin Med 1983;5: 261–262.

C227. Chen ZY, Dobson RL, Ainsworth SK, Silver RM, Rust RF, Maricq HR. Immunofluorescence in skin specimens from three different biopsy sites in patients with scleroderma. Clin Exp Rheumatol 1985 Jan–Mar;3(1):11–16.

C228. Cheng HM, Sam CK. Bacterial immunity and immunogenesis of normal human salivary IgA and serum IgG_2 antiphospholipid autoantibody: a link? Immunol Lett 1990 Oct;26(1): 7–10.

C229. Chetlin SM, Medsger TA, Caritas SN, di Bartolomeo AG. Serum complement values during pregnancy in systemic lupus erythematosus. Arthritis Rheum 1977;20:111.

C230. Chevalier J, Kazatchkine MD. Distribution in clusters of complement receptor type one (CR1) on human erythrocytes. J Immunol 1989;142:2031–2036.

C231. Chevalier X, Bourgeois P, Kahn MF. 3 cases of rheumatoid arthritis resulting in systemic lupus 15 years after the onset of polyarthritis. Rev Rhuem Mal Osteoartic 1990 Apr 25;57(4): 323–326.

C232. Chia BL, Mah EPK, Feng PH. Cardiovascular abnormalities in systemic lupus erythematosus. J Clin Ultrasound 1981 Jun; 9:237–243.

C233. Chiang B-L, Bearer E, Ansari A, Dorschkind K, Gershwin ME. The BM12 mutation and autoantibodies to dsDNA in NZB.H-2^{bm12}mice. J Immunol 1990;145:94–101.

C234. Chiarello M, Ambrosio G, Capelli-Bigazzi A, Capelli-Bigazzi M, Nevola E, Perrone-Filardi P, Marone G, Condorelli M. Inhibition of ischemia-induced phospholipase activation by quinacrine protects jeopardized myocardium in rats with coronary artery occlusion. J Pharmacol Exp Ther 1987 May; 241(2):560–568.

C235. Chiariello M, Ambrosio G, Capelli-Bigazzi M, Perrone-Filardi P, Tritto I, Nevola E, Golino P. Reduction in infarct size by the phospholipase inhibitor quinacrine in dogs with coronary artery occlusion. Am Heart J 1990 Oct;120(4):801–807.

C236. Chick TW, de Horatius RJ, Skipper BE, Messner RP. Pulmonary dysfunction in systemic lupus erythematosus without pulmonary symptoms. J Rheumatol 1976 Sep;3:262–268.

C237. Child S, Feizi T. Cross idiotypic specificity among heavy chains of macroglobulins with blood group I and i specificities. Nature 1975;255:562.

C238. Childs RA, Dalchau R, Scudder P, Hounsell EF, Fabre JW, Feizi T. Evidence for the occurrence of O-glucosidically linked oligosaccharides of poly-N-acetyllactosamine type on the human leukocyte common antigen. Biochem Biophys Res Commun 1983;110:424–431.

C239. Chin GL, Kong NCT, Lee BC, Rose IM. Penicillamine induced lupus-like syndrome in a patient with classical rheumatoid arthritis. J Rheumatol 1991; 947–948.

C240. Chiodi H. The relationship between the thymus and the sexual organs. Endocrinology 1940;89:211–215.

C241. Chirawong P, Nimmannit S, Vanichayakornkul S, Nilwarangkur S. Clinical course of lupus nephritis in Siriraj Hospital. J Med Assoc Thailand 1978 Jan;61 Suppl 1:177–183.

C242. Chiu D, Lubin B, Roelofsen B, Van Deenan LLM. Sickled erythrocytes accelerate clotting in vitro: an effect of abnormal membrane lipid asymmetry. Blood 1981;58:398–401.

C243. Chokron R, Robert A, Rozensztajn L. Procainamide-induced lupus with circulating anticoagulant [letter]. Nouv Presse Med 1982; 11:2568.

C244. Chong WK, Dewhurst AG, Dathan JR. Acute laryngeal stridor with respiratory arrest in drug induced systemic lupus erythematosus. BMJ 1988 Sep 10;297(6649):660–661.

C245. Chopra IJ, Tulchnisky D. Status of estrogen-androgen balance in hyperthyroid men with Graves' disease. J Clin Endocrinol Metabol 1974;38:269–277.

C246. Chorazak T. Cryoglobulins in chronic lupus erythematosus. Acta Dermatovener (Stockh) 1958;38:322–328.

C247. Chorzelski T, Blaszczyk M, Langner A. Effect of resochin on the formation of cells in vitro. Pol Med J 1966;5:201–205.

C248. Chorzelski T, Jablonska S. Coexistence of lupus erythematosus and scleroderma in light of immunopathological investigations. Acta Dermatvener (Stockh) 1970;50:81–85.

C249. Chorzelski T, Jablonska S, Blaszczyk M. Immunopathological investigations in the senear-usher syndrome (Coexistence of pemphigus and lupus erythematosus). Br J Dermatol 1968; 80:211–217.

C250. Chou CT, Lee FT, Schumacher HR. Modification of a screening technique to evaluate systemic lupus erythematosus in a Chinese population in Taiwan. J Rheumatol 1986;13: 806.

C251. Chou JY. Production of pregnancy-specific beta$_1$-glycoprotein by human placental cells and human fibroblasts. Oncodev Biol Med 1983;4:319–326.

C252. Choudhry V, Madan N, Sood SK, Ghai OP. Chloroquine-induced haemolysis and acute renal failure in subjects with G-6-PD deficiency. Trop Geogr Med 1978 Sep;30(3):331–335.

C253. Choukroun G, Quint L, Amoura Z, Boudes P, Guillevin L. Salmonella typhi murium spondylodiscitis in systemic lupus erythematosus. Ann Med Interne (Paris) 1988;139(6): 446–447.

C254. Christenson-Bravo B, Rodriguez JE, Vazquez G, Ramirez-Ronda Ch. Pseudomonas pseudomallei (meloidosis): acute septicemia and meningitis in patient with systemic lupus erythematosus. Bol Assoc Med PR 1986;78.347–349.

C255. Christian CL, Hatfield WB, Chase PH. Systemic lupus erythematosus, cryoprecipitation of sera. J Clin Invest 1963 Jun 48:823–829.

C256. Christmas TJ, Le Page S, Maddison PJ, Isenberg DA. Antinuclear antibodies in interstitial cystitis (IC) [abstract]. Br J Rheumatol 1989;28 Suppl 2:37.

C257. Christy NP. HPA failure and glucocorticoid therapy. Hosp Pract 1984; :77–89.

C258. Chu JL, Elkon KB. The small nuclear ribonucleoproteins,

Sm B and B′, are products of a single gene. Gene 1991;97: 311–312.

C259. Chuchana P, Blancher A, Brockly F, Alexandra D, Lefranc G, Lefranc M. Definition of the human immunoglobulin variable lambda (IGLV) gene subgroup. Eur J Immunol 1990; 20(6):1317–1325.

C260. Chudwin DS, Ammann AJ, Cowan MJ, Wara DW. Significance of a positive antinuclear antibody test in a pediatric population. Am J Dis Child 1983 Nov;137(11):1103–1106.

C261. Chung CS, Marianthopoulos NC. Racial and prenatal factors in major congenital malformations. Am J Human Gen 1968;20:44.

C262. Churchill PC, Churchill MC, McDonald FD. Quinacrine antagonizes the effects of Na, K-ATPase inhibitors on renal prostaglandin E2 release but not their effects on renin secretion. Life Sci 1985 Jan 21;36(3):277–282.

C263. Churg A, Franklin W, Chan KL, Kopp E, Carrington CB. Pulmonary hemorrhage and immune complex deposition in the lung: complications in a patient with systemic lupus erythematosus. Arch Pathol Lab Med 1980 Jul;104:388–391.

C264. Churg J, Sobin JH. Lupus nephritis. In: editors. Classification and Atlas of Glomerular Diseases. Tokyo: Igaku-Shoin, 1982;127–149.

C265. Chused TM, Kassan SS, Pelz GO, Moutsopoulos HM, Terasaki PI. Sjogren's syndrome associated with HLA-Dw3. N Engl J Med 1977;296:895–897.

C266. Chwalinska-Sadowski H, Milewski B, Maldyk H. Diagnostic troubles connected with differentiation of systemic lupus erythematosus against chronic hepatitis. Mater Medica Polona 1977;9:60–64.

C267. Ciabottoni G, Cinotti GA, Pierucci A, Simonetti BM, Manzi M, Pugilese F, Barsotti P, Pecci G, Taggi F, Patrono C. Effects of sulindac and ibuprofen in patients with chronic glomerular disease. Evidence for the dependence of renal function on prostacyclin. N Engl J Med 1984 Feb 2;310(5):279–283.

C268. Ciaccio M, Parodi A, Regora A. Myasthenia gravis and lupus erythematosus. Int J Dermatol 1989;28:317–321.

C269. Ciak J, Hahn FE. Chloroquine: mode of action. Science 1966 Jan 21;151:347–349.

C270. Cines DB. Antibodies reactive with surface membranes of cellular elements in the blood. Human Pathol 1983 May;14: 429–441.

C271. Cines DB, Lyss AP, Reeber M, Bina M, DeHoratius RJ. Presence of complement-fixing anti-endothelial cell antibodies in systemic lupus erythematosus. J Clin Invest 1984 Mar; 73:611–625.

C272. Cirino G, Peers SH, Flower RJ, Browning JL, Pepinsky RB. Human recombinant lipocortin 1 has acute local anti-inflammatory properties in the rat paw edema test. Proc Natl Acad Sci USA 1989;86:3428–3432.

C272a. Claman HN. Glucocorticoids. I. Anti-inflammatory mechanisms. 1983;18:123–134.

C273. Clark DJ, Hill CS, Martin SR, Thomas JO. Alpha-Helix in the carboxy-terminal domains of histones H1 and H5. EMBO J 1988;7:69–75.

C274. Clark DJ, Thomas JO. Differences in the binding of H1 variants to DNA: Cooperativity and linker-length related distribution. Eur J Biochem 1988;178:225–233.

C275. Clark EA, Ledbetter JA. Leukocyte cell surface enzymology: CD45 (LACA,T200) is a protein tyrosine phosphatase. Immunol Today 1989;10(7):225–228.

C276. Clark EC, Bailey AA. Neurological and psychiatric signs associated with systemic lupus erythematosus. JAMA 1956 Feb 11;160:455–457.

C277. Clark G, Reichlin M, Tomasi TB. Characterization of a soluble cytoplasmic antigen reactive with sera from patients with systemic lupus erythematosus. J Immunol 1969;102: 117–120.

C278. Clark JH, Hardin JW, Upchurch S, Ericksson H. Heterogeneity of estrogen binding sites in the cytosol of the rat uterus. J Biol Chem 1978;253:7630–7634.

C279. Clark M, Fountain RB. Oesophageal motility in connective tissue disease. Br J Dermatol 1967;79:449–452.

C280. Clark M, Sack K. Deforming arthropathy complicating primary biliary cirrhosis. J Rheumatol 1991;18:619–621.

C281. Clark MR, Lui L, Clarkson SB, Ory PA, Goldstein IM. An abnormality of the gene that encodes neutrophil Fc receptor III in a patient with systemic lupus erythematosus. J Clin Invest 1990;86:341–346.

C282. Clark RA, Kimball HR, Decker JL. Neutrophil chemotaxis in systemic lupus erythematosus. Ann Rheum Dis 1974 Mar; 33:167–172.

C283. Clark WF, Dau PC, Euler HH, Guillevin L, Hasford J, Heer AH, Jones JV, Kashgarian M, Knatterud G, Lockwood CM, Pusey CD, Rifle G, Robinson JA, Schroeder JO, Tan EM, Wallace DJ, Weiner SR. Plasmapheresis and subsequent pulse cyclophosphamide versus pulse cyclophosphamide alone in severe lupus: design of the LPSG trial. Lupus Plasmapheresis Study Group (LPSG). J Clin Apheresis 1991;6(1):40–47.

C284. Clark WF, Lewis ML, Cameron JS, Parsons V. Intrarenal platelet consumption in the diffuse proliferative nephritis of systemic lupus erythematosus. Clin Sci Mol Med 1975;49: 247–252.

C285. Clark WF, Lindsay RM, Cattran DC, Chodirker WB, Barnes CC, Linton AL. Monthly plasmapheresis for systemic lupus erythematosus with diffuse proliferative glomerulonephritis: a pilot study. Can Med Assoc J 1981 Jul 15;125(2):171–174.

C286. Clark WF, Lindsay RM, Ulan RA, Cordy PE, Linton AL. Chronic plasma exchange in SLE nephritis. Clin Nephrol 1981 Jul;16(1):20–23.

C287. Clark WF, Linton AL, Cordy PE, Keown PE, Lohmann RC, Lindsay RM. Immunologic findings, thrombocytopenia and disease activity in lupus nephritis. Can Med J 1978;118: 1191–1195.

C288. Clark WF, Parbtani A, Huff MW, Reid B, Holub BJ, Falardeau P. Omega-3 fatty acid dietary supplementation in systemic lupus erythematosus. Kidney Int 1989;36:653–660.

C289. Clark WF, Tevaarwerk GJM, Reid BD. Human platelet-immune complex interaction in plasma. J Lab Clin Med 1982 Dec;100:917–931.

C290. Clarke SH, Huppi K, Ruezinsky D, Staudt L, Gearhard W, Weigert M. Inter-and intraclonal diversity in the antibody response to influenza hemagglutinin. J Exp Med 1985;161: 687–704.

C291. Clarke SH, Rudikoff S. Evidence for gene conversion among immunoglobulin heavy chain variable region genes. J Exp Med 1984;159:773–782.

C292. Clarkson SB, Bussel JB, Kimberly RP, Valinsky JE, Nachman RL, Unkeless JC. Treatment of refractory immune thrombocytopenic purpura with an anti-Fc gamma receptor antibody. N Engl J Med 1986;314:1236–1239.

C293. Clarkson SB, Kimberly RP, Valinsky JE, Witmer MD, Bussel JB, Nachman RL, Unkeless JC. Blockade of clearance of immune complexes by an anti-Fc gamma receptor monoclonal antibody J Exp Med 1986;164:473–489.

C294. Clarkson SB, Ory PA. CD16: developmentally regulated IgG Fc receptors on cultured monocytes. J Exp Med 1988; 167:408–420.

C295. Cleigh JS, Reidenberg MM. Cyclophosphamide dose in renal failure [letter]. Am J Med 1978;64:725–726.

C296. Cleland LG, Bell DA, Williams M, Saurino BC. Familial lupus Family studies of HLA and serologic findings. Arthritis Rheum 1978;21:183–191.

C297. Cleland LG, French JK, Betts WH, Murphy GA, Elliott MJ. Clinical and biochemical effects of dietary fish oil supplements in rheumatoid arthritis. J Rheumatol 1988;15:1471–1475.

C298. Clemens LE, Siiteri PK, Stites, DP. Mechanisms of immuno-suppression of progesterone on lymphocyte activation during pregnancy. J immunol 1970;122:1978–1985.

C299. Clement LT, Yamashita N, Martin AM. The functionally distinct subpopulations of Human CD4+ helper/inducer T lymphocytes defined by anti-CD45R antibodies derive sequentially from a differentiation pathway that is regulated by activation-dependent post-thymic differentiation. J Immunol 1988;141:1464–1470.

C300. Clements PJ, Davis J. Cytotoxic drugs: their clinical application to the rheumatic diseases. Semin Arthritis Rheum 1986 May;15(4):231–254.

C301. Clemmensen O, Thomsen K. Porphyria cutanea tarda and systemic lupus erythematosus. Arch Dermatol 1982 Mar; 118(3):160–162.

C302. Clevinger B, Schilling J, Hood L, Davie JM. Structural correlates of crossreactive and individual idiotypic determinants on murine antibodies to a(1–3)dextran. J Exp Med 1980;151:1059.

C303. Clifford GO, McClure J, Conway M, Kahn R, Wolf P, Pearson B. Renal lesions in dogs produced by plasma from patients with systemic lupus erythematosus. J Lab Clin Med 1961;58:807.

C304. Clifton F, Greer CH. Ocular changes in acute systemic lupus erythematosus. Br J Ophthalmol 1955 Jan;39:1–10.

C305. Clive DM, Stoff JS. Renal syndromes associated with non-steroidal antiinflammatory drugs. N Engl J Med 1984 Mar;310:363–570.

C306. Closson RG. Liquid dosage form of chloroquine [letter]. Drug Intell Clin Pharm 1988 Apr;22(4):347.

C307. Clotet B, Guardia J, Pigrau C, Lience E, Murcia C, Pujol R, Bacardi R. Incidence and clinical significance of anti-ENA antibodies in systemic lupus erythematosus. Estimation by counter-immunoelectrophoresis. Scand J Rheumatol 1984; 13(1):15–20.

C308. Clough JD, Couri J, Youssofian H, Gephardt GN, Tubbs R. Antibodies against nuclear antigens: Association with lupus nephritis. Cleve Clin Q 1986;53:259–265.

C309. Clough JD, Lewis EJ, Lachin JM. Treatment protocols of the lupus nephritis collaborative study of plasmapheresis in severe lupus nephritis. The Lupus Nephritis Collaborative Study Group. Prog Clin Biol Res 1990;337:301–307.

C310. Clough JD, Valenzuela R. Relationship of renal histopathology in SLE nephritis to immunologic class of anti-DAN. Am J Med 1980 Jan;68:80.

C311. Coade SB, van Haaren E, Loizou S, Walport MJ, Denman AM, Pearson JD. Endothelial prostacyclin release in systemic lupus erythematosus. Thromb Haemost 1989;61:97–100.

C312. Cobb S. The frequency of the rheumatic diseases. Cambridge, Harvard University Press, 1971.

C313. Cobb S. The frequency of the rheumatic diseases. Cambridge, Harvard University Press, 1971:99.

C314. Coburn AF, Moore DH. The plasma proteins in disseminated lupus erythematosus. Bull Johns Hopkins Hosp 1943 Sep;73:196–221.

C315. Coburn PR, Shuster S. Dapsone and discoid lupus erythematosus. Br J Dermatol 1982 Jan;106(1):105–106.

C316. Cochran M, Nordin BE. Panhypopituitarism, testicular atrophy, alactasia, corticosteroid-induced osteoporosis and systemic lupus erythematosus induced by methion. Proc Roy Soc Med 1968 Jul;61:656.

C317. Cochrane CG, Koffler D. Immune complex disease in experimental animals and man. Adv Immunol 1973;16:185–253.

C318. Codding C, Targoff IN, McCarty GA. Aseptic meningitis in association with diclofenac treatment in a patient with systemic lupus erythematosus. Arthritis Rheum 1991;34:1340–1341.

C319. Cody RJ, Calabrese LH, Clough JD, Tarazi RC, Bravo EL. Development of antinuclear antibodies during acebutolol therapy. Clin Pharmacol Ther 1979 Jun;25:800–805.

C320. Coe MD, Hamer DH, Levy CS, Milner MR, Nam MH, Barth WF. Gonococcal pericarditis with tamponade in a patient with systemic lupus erythematosus. Arthritis Rheum 1990 Sep; 33(9):1438–1441.

C321. Cogen MS, Kline LB, Duvall ER. Bilateral internuclear ophthalmoplegia in systemic lupus erythematosus. J Clin Neuro Opthalmol 1987 Jun;7(2):69–73.

C322. Coggins CH. Overview of treatment of lupus nephropathy. Am J Kidney Dis 1982 Jul;2 Suppl 1:197–200.

C323. Cohen AJ, Philips TM, Kessler CM. Circulating coagulation inhibitors in the acquired immunodeficiency syndrome. Ann Intern Med 1986 Feb;104(2):175–180.

C324. Cohen AS, Canoso JJ. Criteria for the classification of systemic lupus erythematosus—Status 1972 [editorial]. Arthritis Rheum 1972 Sep–Oct;15:540–543.

C325. Cohen AS, Reynolds WE, Franklin EC, Kulka JP, Ropes MW, Shulman LE, Wallace SL. Preliminary criteria for the classification of systemic lupus erythematosus. Bull Rheum Dis 1971 May;21:643–648.

C326. Cohen IR, Cooke A. Natural autoantibodies might prevent autoimmune disease. Immunol Today 1986;7:363–364.

C327. Cohen J, Pinching AJ, Rees AJ, Peters DK. Infection and immunosuppression. A study of the infective complications of 75 patients with immunologically mediated disease. Q J Med 1982 Winter;51:1–15.

C328. Cohen JHM, Daniel L, Cordier G, Saez S, Revillard JP. Sex steroid receptors in peripheral T cells; absence of androgen receptors and restrictions of estrogen receptors to OKT-8 positive cells. J Immunol 1983;131;2767–2771.

C329. Cohen MG, Kevat S, Prowse MV, Ahern MJ. Two distinct quinidine-induced rheumatic syndromes. Ann Intern Med 1988; 108:369–371.

C330. Cohen MG, Webb J. Concurrence of rheumatoid arthritis and systemic lupus erythematosus: report of 11 cases. Ann Rheum Dis 1987 Nov;46(11):853–858.

C331. Cohen MG, Webb J. Antihistone antibodies in rheumatoid arthritis and Felty's syndrome. Arthritis Rheum 1989; 32:1319–1324.

C332. Cohen MN. Update on quinidine and procainamide. Angiology 1982; 33:454–463.

C333. Cohen P, Gardner FH, Barnett GO. Reclassification of the thrombocytopenias by the Cr 51 labeling method for measuring platelet life span. N Engl J Med 1961 Jun 22;264:1294–1295.

C334. Cohen PL, Litvin DA, Winfield JB. Association between endogenously activated T cells and immunoglobulin-secreting B cells in patients with active systemic lupus erythematosus. Arthritis Rheum 1982 Feb;25:168–173.

C335. Cohen PL, Rapoport R, Eisenberg RA. Characterization of functional T-cell lines derived from MRL mice. Clin Immunol Immunopathol 1986;40:485–496.

C336. Cohen S, Stastny P, Sontheimer RD. Concurrence of subacute cutaneous lupus erythematosus and rheumatoid arthritis. Arthritis Rheum 1986 Mar;29(3):421–425.

C337. Colaco CB, Elkon KB. The lupus anticoagulant. A disease marker in antinuclear antibody negative lupus that is cross-reactive with autoantibodies to double-stranded DNA. Arthritis Rheum 1985;28:67–74.

C338. Colaco CB, Male DK. Anti-phospholipid antibodies in syphilis and a thrombotic subset of SLE: distinct profiles of epitope specificity. Clin Exp Immunol 1985 Feb:449–456.

C339. Colardyn F, Van Hove W. Meningitis with LE-like cells in the cerebrospinal fluid. Acta Clin Belg 1975;30(6):504–510.

C340. Colburn KK, Gusewitch GA, Statian Pooprasert BS, Weisbart RH. Apheresis enhances the selective removal of antinuclear antibodies in systemic lupus erythematosus. Clin Rheumatol 1990;9:475–482.

C341. Cole EH, Schulman J, Urowitz M, Keystone E, Williams C, Levy GA. Monocyte procoagulant activity in glomerulonephritis associated with systemic lupus erythematosus. J Clin Invest 1985 Mar;75:861–868.

C342. Cole EH, Sweet J, Levy GA. Expression of macrophage procoagulant activity in murine systemic lupus erythematosus. J Clin Invest 1986;78:887–893.

C343. Cole FS, Whitehead AS, Auerbach HS, Lint T, Zeitz MJ, Kilbridge P, Colten HR. The molecular basis for genetic deficiency of the second component of human complement. N Engl J Med 1985;313:11–16.

C344. Cole RD. Microheterogeneity in H1 histones and its consequences. Int J Peptide Protein Res 1987;30:433–449.

C345. Cole RK, Kite JH, Witebsky W. Hereditary autoimmune thyroiditis in the fowl. Science 1968;160:1357–1358.

C346. Coleman WP 3d, Coleman WP, Derbes VI, Jolly HW, Nosbitt LT. Collagen disease in children. A review of 71 cases. JAMA 1977 March 14;237:1095–1100.

C347. Coles LS, Robins AJ, Madley LK, Wells JRE. Characterization of the chicken histone H1 gene complement: Generation of a complete set of vertebrate H1 protein sequences. J Biol Chem 1987;262:9656–9663.

C348. Coller BS, Owen J, Jesty J, Horowitz D, Reitman MJ, Spear J, Yeh T, Comp PC. Deficiency of plasma protein S, protein C, or antithrombin III and arterial thrombosis. Arteriosclerosis 1987;7:456–462.

C349. Collins DN, Oppenheim IA, Edwards MR. Cryptococcoses associated with systemic lupus erythematosus. Light and electron microscopic observations on a morphologic variant. Arch Pathol 1971 Jan;91:78–88.

C350. Collins E, Turner G. Maternal effects of regular salicylate ingestion in pregnancy. Lancet 1975;2:335–337.

C351. Collins JV, Tong D, Bucknall RG, Warin AP. Cryptococcal meningitis as a complication of systemic lupus erythematosus treated with systemic corticosteroids. Postgrad Med J 1972; 48:52–55.

C352. Collins RL, Turner RA, Nomeir AM, Hunt R, Johnson AM, McLean RL, Watts LE. Cardiopulmonary manifestations of systemic lupus erythematosus. J Rheumatol 1978 Fall;5: 299–305.

C353. Colten HR. Biosynthesis of complement. Adv Immunol 1976;22:67–118.

C354. Colten HR. Molecular genetics of the major histocompatibility linked complement genes. Springer Semin Immunopathol 1983;6:149.

C355. Comaish S. A case of hypersensitivity to corticosteroids. Br J Dermatol 1969 Dec;81:919–925.

C356. Comens P. Experimental hydralazine disease. Circulation 1955 Oct;12:688.

C357. Comens SM, Alpert MA, Sharp GC, Pressly TA, Kelly DL, Hazelwood SE, Mukerji V. Frequency of mitral valve prolapse in systemic lupus erythematosus, progressive systemic sclerosis and mixed connective tissue disease. Am J Cardiol 1989; 63:369–370.

C358. Comfurious P, Seden JMG, Tilly RHJ, Schroit AJ, Bevers EM, Zwarl RFA. Loss of membrane phospholipid asymmetry in platelets and red cells may be associated with calcium-induced shedding of plasma membrane and inhibition of ami-

nophospholipid translocase. Biochim Biophys Acta 1990; 1026:153–160.

C359. Committee on Prognosis Studies in SLE. Prognosis studies in SLE: an activity index [abstract]. Arthritis Rheum 1986;29 Suppl:S93.

C360. Comp PC, de Bault LE, Esmon NL, Esomon CT. Human thrombomodulin is inhibited by IgG from two patients with nonspecific anticoagulants [abstract]. Blood 1983;62:299a.

C361. Compton LJ, Steinberg AD, Sano H. Nuclear DNA degradation in lymphocytes of patients with systemic lupus erythematosus. J Immunol 1984;133:213–216.

C362. Conaway DC, DeFilipp G, Berney SN, Tourtellotte CD. Abnormal findings in magnetic resonance imaging in patients with active central nervous system lupus erythematosus [abstract]. Arthritis Rheum 1985 Apr;28(4) Suppl:S63.

C363. Condemi JJ, Grossman J, Callerame ML. Immunofluorescent studies on skin biopsies from patients with systemic lupus erythematosus and other antinuclear antibody positive diseases [abstract]. Arthritis Rheum 1972;15:433.

C364. Condemi JJ, Moore-Jones D, Vaughan JH. Antinuclear antibodies following hydralazine toxicity. N Engl J Med 1967 Mar 2:276:486–491.

C365. Conger J, Farrell T, Douglas S. Lupus nephritis complicated by fatal disseminated coccidioidomycosis. Calif Med 1973 Feb;118:60–65.

C366. Conger JD, Pike BL, Nossal GJ. Clonal analysis of the anti-DNA repertoire of murine B lymphocytes. Proc Natl Acad Sci USA 1987 May;84(9):2931–2935.

C367. Conklin KA, Chou SC. Antimalarials: effects on in vivo and in vitro protein synthesis. Science 1970 Dec 11;170: 1213–1214.

C367a. Conley CL, Rathbun HK, Morse WI 2d, Robinson JE Jr. Circulating anticoagulant as a cause of hemorrhagic diathesis in man. Bull Johns Hopkins Hosp 1948 Oct;83:288–296.

C368. Conley ME, Coopman WJ. Serum IgA1 and IgA2 in normal adults and patients with systemic lupus erythematosus and hepatic disease. Arthritis Rheum 1983 Mar;26:390–397.

C369. Conlon KC, Urba WJ, Smith JW, Steis RG, Longo DL, Clark JW. Exacerbation of symptoms of autoimmune disease in patients receiving alpha-interferon therapy. Cancer 1990;65: 2237–2242.

C370. Conn DL, Banks PM, Witrak GA. Influence of cytotoxic agents on the development of lymphoid neoplasms in connective tissue disease. Arthritis Rheum 1979 Aug;22;938–939.

C371. Conn HD, Blitzer BL. Nonassociation of adrenocorticosteroid therapy and peptic ulcer. N Engl J Med 1976 Feb 26;294: 473–475.

C372. Connolly KM, Stecher VJ, Snyder BW, Bohnet E, Potts GO. The effects of danazol in the MRL/lpr mouse model of autoimmune diseases. Agents Actions 1988;25:164–170.

C373. Omitted.

C374. Contractor SF, Davies H. Effect of human somatotropin and HCG on phytohemagglutinin-induced lymphocyte transformation. Nature 1973;243:284–286.

C375. Cook CD, Wedgwood RJP, Craig JM, Hartmann JR, Janeway CA. Systemic lupus erythematosus. Description of 37 cases in children and a discussion of endocrine therapy in 32 of the cases. Pediatrics 1960 Oct;26:570–585.

C376. Cook GC, Mulligan R, Sherlock S. Controlled prospective trial of corticosteroid therapy in active chronic hepatitis. QJ Med 1971 Apr;40:159–185.

C377. Cooke CA, Heck MMS, Earnshaw WC. The inner centromere protein (INCENP) antigens: movement from inner centromere to midbody during mitosis. J Cell Biol 1987;105: 2053–2067.

C378. Cooke CL, Lurie HI. Case report: fatal gastrointestinal hemorrhage in mixed connective tissue disease. Arthritis Rheum 1977 Sep−Oct;20(7):1421−1427.

C379. Coon WW. Splenectomy for cytopenias associated with systemic lupus erythematosus. Am J Surg 1988;155:301−394.

C380. Coons AH. Symposium on labelled antigens and antibodies; Fluorescent antibodies as histochemical tools. Fed Proc 1951 Jun;10:558−559.

C381. Cooper A, Bluestone R. Free immunoglobulin light chains in connective tissue diseases. Ann Rheum Dis 1968 Nov;27: 537−543.

C382. Cooper EL. Stress, Immunity and Aging. New York: Dekker, 1984.

C383. Cooper NR. The role of the complement system in host defense against virus disease. In: Notkins AL, Oldstone MBA, editors. Concepts in viral pathogenesis. New York: Spring Verlag, 1984:20.

C384. Coplon NS, Diskin CJ, Peterson J, Swenson RS. The long-term clinical course of systemic lupus erythematosus in end-stage renal disease. N Engl J Med 1983 Jan 27;308(4): 186−190.

C385. Coppeto J, Lessell S. Retinopathy in systemic lupus erythematosus. Arch Ophthalmol 1977 May;95:794−797.

C385a. Corke CE. Rheumatoid factor and renal disease in systemic lupus erythematosus. Rheumatol Rehab 1987 May;17: 76−78.

C386. Corman LC. The role of diet in animal models of systemic lupus erythematosus: possible implications of human lupus. Semin Arthritis Rheum 1985 Aug;15(1):61−69.

C387. Cormane RH. Band globulin in the skin of patients with chronic discoid lupus erythematosus and systemic lupus erythematosus. Lancet 1964;1:534−535.

C388. Cornacchia E, Golbus J, Maybaum J, Strahler J, Hanash S, Richardson B. Hydralazine and procainamide inhibit T cell DNA methylation and induce autoreactivity. J Immunol 1988; 140:2197−2200.

C389. Cornacoff JB, Hebert LA, Smead WL, VanAman ME, Birmingham DJ, Kimberly RP, Salmon JE, Edberg JC, Gibofsky A. The role of Fcγ receptors in mononuclear phagocyte system function. Clin Exp Rheum 1989;7 Suppl:130−138.

C390. Cornacoff JB, Hebert LA, Smead WL, VanAman ME, Birmingham DJ, Waxman FJ. Primate erythrocyte-immune complex-clearing mechanism. J Clin Invest 1983 Feb;71:236−247.

C391. Cornbleet T. Discoid lupus erythematosus treatment with plaquenil. Arch Dermatol 1956;73:572−575.

C392. Cornwell CJ, Schmitt MH. Perceived health status, self-esteem and body image in women with rheumatoid arthritis or systemic lupus erythematosus. Res Nurs Health 1990 Apr; 14(2):99−107.

C393. Correia P, Cameron JS, Lian JD, Hicks J, Ogg CS, Williams DG, Chantler C, Haycock DG. Why do patients with lupus nephritis die? BMJ 1985 Jan 12;290:126−131.

C394. Correia P, Cameron JS, Ogg CS, Williams DG, Bewick M, Hicks JA. End-stage renal failure in systemic lupus erythematosus with nephritis. Clin Nephrol 1984 Dec;22(6):293−302.

C395. Corrigan JJ Jr, Patterson JH, May NE. Incoaguability of the blood in systemic lupus erythematosus. A case due to hypoprothrombinemia and a circulating anticoagulant. Am J Dis Child 1970 Apr;119:365−369.

C396. Corvetta A, Della Bitta R, Gabrielli A, Spaeth PJ, Danieli G. Use of high dose intravenous immunoglobulin in systemic lupus erythematosus: report of three cases. Clin Exp Rheumatol 1989 May−Jun;7(3):295−299.

C397. Cosgriff TM, Martin AB. Low functional and high antigenic antithrombin III level in a patient with the lupus anticoagulant and recurrent thrombosis. Arthritis Rheum 1981;24:94.

C398. Cosio FG, Hebert LA, Birmingham DL, Dorval BL, Bakaletz AP, Kujala GA, Edberg JC, Taylor RP. Clearance of human anti-body/DNA immune complexes and free DNA from the circulation of nonhuman primate. Clin Immunol Immunopathol 1987;42:1−9.

C399. Cosio FG, Shen XP, Hebert LA. Immune complexes bind preferentially to specific subpopulations of human erythrocytes. Clin Immunol Immunopathol 1990;55:337−354.

C400. Costa JP, Bajador IP, Alonso EP, de la Serna AR. Prevalencia de lupus eritematoso generalizado en una poblacin psiquitrica. Med Clin (Barc) 1986;87:785−786.

C401. Costa O, Fournel C, Lotchouang E, Monier JC, Fontaine M. Specificities of antinuclear antibodies detected in dogs with systemic lupus erythematosus. Vet Immunol Immunopathol 1984;7:369−382.

C402. Costa O, Monier JC. Antihistone antibodies detected by ELISA and immunoblotting in systemic lupus erythematosus and rheumatoid arthritis. J Rheumatol 1986;13:722−725.

C403. Costa O, Tchouatcha-Tchouassom JC, Roux B, Monier JC. Anti-H1 histone antibodies in systemic lupus erythematosus: epitope localization after immunoblotting of chymotrypsin-digested H1. Clin Exp Immunol 1986;63:608−613.

C404. Costallat LTL, de Oliveira RM, Santiago MB, Cossermelli W, Samara AM. Neuropsychiatric manifestations of systemic lupus erythematosus: the value of anticardiolipin, antigangliosides and antigalactocerebrosides antibodies. Clin Rheumatol 1990;9:489−497.

C405. Costello C, Abdelaal M, Coomes EN. Pernicious anemia and systemic lupus erythematosus in a young woman. J Rheumatol 1985;12:798−799.

C406. Costello KB, Green FA. Patterns of in vitro aspirin hydrolysis rates in rheumatoid arthritis and systemic lupus erythematosus. J Rheumatol 1986;13:882−886.

C407. Cote CJ, Meuwissen HJ, Pickering RJ. Effects on the neonate of prednisone and azathioprine administered to the mother during pregnancy. J Pediatr 1974;85:324−328.

C408. Cotter PB, Weiter JT. Retinopathy in a patient with systemic lupus erythematosus. Ann Ophth 1978;14:470−473.

C409. Coulam CB, Silverfield JC, Kazmar RE, Fathman CG. T lymphocyte subsets during pregnancy and the menstrual cycle. Am J reprod Immunol 1983;4:88.

C410. Coull BM, Bourdette DN, Goodnight SH Jr, Briley DP, Hart R. Multiple cerebral infarctions and dementia associated with anticardiolipin antibodies. Stroke 1987 Nov−Dec;18(6): 1107−1112.

C411. Coulson IH, Mardsen RA. Lupus erythematosus cheilitis. Clin Exp Dermatol 1986 May;11(3):309−313.

C412. Courvalin JC, Lassoved K, Bartuil E, Blobel G, Wozniak RW. The 210 kD nuclear envelope polypeptide recognized by human autoantibodies in primary biliary cirrhosis is the major glycoprotein of the nuclear pore. J Clin Invest 1990;86: 297−285.

C413. Couser WG. Mechanisms of glomerular injury in immune-complex disease. Kidney Int 1985;28:569−583.

C414. Couser WG. Mediation of immune glomerular injury. J Am Soc Nephrol 1990;1:13−29.

C415. Couser WG, Salant DJ. In situ immune complex formation and glomerular injury. Kidney Int 1980;17:1−13.

C416. Couser WG, Salant DJ, Madaio MP, Adler S, Groggel GC. Factors influencing glomerular and tubulointerstitial patterns of injury in systemic lupus erythematosus. Am J Kidney Dis 1982 Jul;2 Suppl 1:126−134.

C417. Couser WG, Steinmuller DR, Stilmant MM, Salant DJ, Lowenstein LM. Experimental glomerulonephritis in the isolated perfused rat kidney. J Clin Invest 1978;62:1275−1287.

C418. Cowchock S, Fort J, Munoz S, Norberg R, Maddrey W. False positive ELISA tests for anticardiolipin antibodies in sera from patients with repeated abortion, rheumatologic disorders and primary biliary cirrhosis; correlation with elevated polyclonal IgM and implications for patients with repeated abortion. Clin Exp Immunol 1988 Aug;73(2):289–294.

C418a. Cowchock S, Rocco EA, Balaban D, Branch DW, Plouffe L. Repeated fetal losses associated with antiphospholipid antibodies: a collaborative randomized trial comparing prednisone to low dose heparin treatment. Am J Obstet Gynecol 1992 In press.

C419. Cowchock S, Smith JB, Gocial B. Antibodies in phospholipids and nuclear antigens in patients with repeated abortions. Am J Obstet Gynecol 1986;155:1002.

C420. Cowdery JS, Jacobi SM, Pitts AK, Tyler TL. Defective B cell clonal regulation and autoantibody production in NZB mice. J Immunol 1987;138:760–764.

C421. Cowdery JS, Pitts AK. Role of T cells in regulating expression of the B cell repertoire. J Immunol 1988;140:1380–1384.

C422. Crabtree GR, Munck A, Smith KA. Glucocorticoids inhibit expression of Fc receptors of the human granulocyte cell line HL-60. Nature 1979;279:338–339.

C422a. Craft J. Antibodies to snRNPs in systemic lupus erythematosus. Rheum Dis Clin 1992 In press.

C423. Craft J, Griffith A, Brunet C. Murine and Drosophila B proteins of Sm snRNPs. Mol Biol Rep 1991;15:159.

C424. Craft J, Hardin JA. Immunoprecipitation assays for the detection of soluble nuclear and cytoplasmic nucleoproteins. In: Rose N, Friedman H, Fahey J, editors. Manual of clinical laboratory immunology. 4th ed. Washington DC: American Society of Microbiology. 1991. In press.

C425. Craft J, Mimori T, Olsen TL, Hardin JA. The U2 small nuclear ribonucleoprotein particle as an autoantigen: Analysis with sera form patients with overlap syndrome. J Clin Invest 1988;8:1716–1724.

C426. Craft JE, Hardin JA. Linked sets of antinuclear antibodies: What do they mean? J Rheumatol 1987;14 Suppl:106–109.

C427. Craft JE, Radding JA, Harding MW, Bernstein RM, Hardin JA. Autoantigenic histone epitopes: a comparison between procainamide- and hydralazine-induced lupus. Arthritis Rheum 1987;30:689–694.

C428. Cranston WI, Hellon RF, Mitchell D, Townsend Y. Intraventricular injections of drugs which inhibit phospholipase A2 suppress fever in rabbits. J Physiol (Lond) 1983 Jun;339:97–105.

C429. Cras P, Franckx C, Martin JJ. Primary lymphoma in systemic lupus erythematosus treated with immunosuppressives. Clin Neuropathol 1989 Jul–Aug;8(4):200–205.

C430. Creagh MD, Malia RG, Cooper SM, Smith AR, Duncan SLB, Greaves M. Screening for lupus anticoagulant and anticardiolipin antibodies in women with fetal loss. J Clin Pathol 1991;44:45–47.

C431. Crews S, Griffin J, Huang H, Calame K, Hood L. A single V$_H$ gene segment encodes the immune responses to phosphorylcholine: Somatic mutation is correlated with the class of antibody. Cell 1981;25:59–66.

C432. Crews SJ. Posterior subcapsular lens opacities in patients on long-term corticosteroid therapy. Br Med J 1963 Jun 22;1:1644–1647.

C433. Crickx B, Crickx L, Vissuzaine C, Grossin M, Belaich S. Lupus erythematosus with lesions of polymorphic erythema. Ann Dermatol Venereol 1985;112(9):705–706.

C434. Cripps DJ, Rankin J. Action spectra of lupus erythematosus and experimental immunofluorescence. Arch Dermatol 1973 Apr;107:563–567.

C435. Crissey JT, Murray PF. Comparison of chloroquine and gold in the treatment of lupus erythematosus. Arch Dermatol 1956 Jul;74:69–72.

C436. Crockett-Torabi E, Fantoni JC. Soluble and insoluble immune complexes activate human neutrophil NADPH oxidase by distinct Fcγ receptor-specific mechanisms. J Immunol 1990;145:3026–3032.

C437. Croft SM, Schiffman G, Snyder E, Herrmann K, James K, Jarrett MP. Specific antibody response after in vivo antigenic stimulation in systemic lupus erythematosus. J Rheumatol 1984 Apr;11(2):141–146.

C438. Cronin ME, Balow JE, Tsokos GC. Immunoglobulin deficiency in patients with systemic lupus erythematosus. Clin Exp Rheumatol 1989;7:359–364.

C439. Cronin ME, Biswas RM, Van der Straeton C, Fleisher TA, Klippel JH. IgG and IgM anticardiolipin antibodies in patients with lupus with anticardiolipin antibody associated clinical syndromes. J Rheumatol 1988;15(5):795–798.

C440. Cronin ME, Leair DW, Jaronski S, Lightfoot RW Jr. Simultaneous use of multiple serologic tests in assessing clinical activity in systemic lupus erythematosus. Clin Immunol Immunopathol 1989;51:99–109.

C441. Cronlund M, Hardin J, Burton J, Lee L, Haber E, Bloch KJ. Fibrinopeptide A in plasma of normal subjects and patients with disseminated intravascular and systemic lupus erythematosus. J Clin Invest 1976 Jul;58:142–151.

C442. Crossland RD. Effect of chlorpromazine and quinacrine on the lethality in mice of the venoms and neurotoxins from several snakes. Toxicon 1989;27:655–663.

C443. Crouch MF, Roberts ML, Tennes KA. Mepacrine inhibition of bradykinin-induced contractions of the rabbit ear vein. Agents Actions 1981 Jul;11(4):330–334.

C444. Crovato F, Levi L. Clofazimine in the treatment of annular lupus erythematosus [letter]. Arch Dermatol 1981 May;117(5):249–250.

C445. Crozier IG, Li E, Milne MJ, Nicholls M. Cardiac involvement in systemic lupus erythematosus detected by echocardiography. Am J Cardiol 1990;65:1145–1148.

C446. Cruess AF, Schachat AP, Nicholl J, Augsburger JJ. Chloroquine retinopathy. Is fluorescein angiography necessary? Ophthalmology 1985 Aug;92(8):1127–1129.

C447. Cruickshank B. Lesions of joints and tendon sheaths in systemic lupus erythematosus. Ann Rheum Dis 1959 Jun;18:111–119.

C448. Cruz O, Sessums LR, Romanski R, Venkatachalam KK, Lewin NW. Mechlorethamine (NH2) therapy for severe SLE. Kidney Int 1982;21:148.

C449. Cruz PD, Bergstresser PR. Antigen processing and presentation by epidermal langerhans cells. Dermatol Clin 1990;8:633–647.

C450. Cruz PD, Coldiron BM, Sontheimer RD. Concurrent features of cutaneous lupus erythematosus and pemphigus erythematosus following myasthenia gravis and thymoma. J Am Acad Dermatol 1987;16:472–476.

C451. Csuka ME, Mc Carty DJ. Transient hypothermia after corticosteroid treatment of subcutaneous lupus erythematosus [letter]. J Rheumatol 1984 Feb;11(1):112–113.

C452. Cuenca R, Simeon CP, Montablan J, Bosch JA, Vilardell M. Facial nerve palsy due to angioedema in systemic lupus erythematosus. Clin Exp Rheumatol 1991;9:89–97.

C453. Cullen AP, Choalsy due to angioedema in systemic lupus erythematosus. Clin Exp Rheumatol 1991;9:89–97.

C453. Cullen AP, Chou BR. Keratopathy with low dose chloroquine therapy. J Am Optom Assoc 1986 May;57(5):368–372.

C454. Cunningham AJ. Active suppressor mechanism maintaining tolerance to some self components. Nature 1975;254:143–144.

C455. Cunningham E, Provost T, Brentjens J, Reichlin M, Venuto RC. Acute renal failure secondary to interstitial lupus nephritis. Arch Intern Med 1976 Oct;138:1560–1562.

C456. Cunningham PH, Andrews BS, Davis JS 4th. Immune complexes in progressive systemic sclerosis and mixed connective tissue disease. J Rheumatol 1980 May–Jun;7:301–308.

C457. Cunningham-Rundles S, Michelis MA, Masur H. Serum suppression of lymphocyte activation in vitro in acquired immunodeficiency disease. J Clin Immunol 1983;3:156–165.

C458. Curley JW, Byron MA, Bates GJ. Crico-arytenoid joint involvement in acute systemic lupus erythematosus. J Laryngol Otol 1986 Jun;100(6):727–732.

C459. Cush JJ, Lightfoot E, Duby AD, Lipsky PE. Cerebrospinal fluid (CSF) T cell clones from patients with active lupus cerebritis [abstract]. Arthritis Rheum 1989 Apr;32 Suppl 4:S120.

C460. Cush JJ, Lipsky PE, Postlethwaite AE, Schrohenloher RE, Saway A, Koopman WJ. Correlation of serologic indicators of inflammation with effectiveness of nonsteroidal anti-inflammatory drug therapy in rheumatoid arthritis. Arthritis Rheum 1990;33:19–28.

C461. Custer RP. Aplastic anemia in soldiers treated with atabrine (quinacrine). Am J Med Sci 1946 Aug;212:211–224.

C462. Cutolo M, Balleari E, Accardo S, Samanta E, Cimmino MA, Guist M, Monachesi M, Lomeo A. Preliminary results of serum androgen level testing in men with rheumatoid arthritis [letter]. Arthritis Rheum 1984;27:958–959.

C463. Cutolo M, Balleari E, Guisti M, Intra E, Accardo S. Androgen replacement therapy in male patients with rheumatoid arthritis. Arthritis Rheum 1991;34:1–5.

C464. Czop J, Nussenzweig V. Studies on the mechanism of solubilization of immune precipitates by serum. J Exp Med 1976; 143:615–630.

D

D1. Dabbous IA, Idriss HM. Occurrence of systemic lupus erythematosus in association with ethosuccimide therapy. [case report]. J Pediatr 1970 Apr;76:617–620.

D2. Dabski K, Winklemann RK. Histopathology of erythema nodosum in patients with coexisting lupus erythematosus [letter]. J Am Acad Dermatol 1988 Jul;19(1 Pt 1):131–132.

D3. Dacie JV. Autoimmune haemolytic anaemias. BMJ 1970 May 16;1:381–386.

D4. Dacie JV. Autoimmune hemolytic anemia. Arch Intern Med 1975 Oct:135:1293–1308.

D5. Daffus P, Parbtani A, Frampton C, Cameron JS. Intraglomerular localization of platelet related antigens platelet factor 4 and -thromboglobulin in glomerulonephritis. Clin Nephrol 1982 Jun;17:288–297.

D6. D'Agati V, Kunis C, Williams G, Appel GB. Anti- cardiolipin antibody and renal disease: a report of three cases. J Am Soc Nephrol 1990;1:777–784.

D7. D'Agati V, Seigle R. Coexistence of AIDS and lupus nephritis: a case report. Am J Nephrol 1990;10(3):243–247.

D8. D'Agati VD, Appel GB, Estes D, Knowles DM, Pirani CL. Monoclonal antibody identification of infiltrating leukocytes in lupus nephritis. Kidney Int 1986;30:573–581.

D9. Dagenais A, Bibor-Hardy V, Senecal JL. A novel autoantibody causing a peripheral fluorescent antinuclear antibody pattern is specific for nuclear pore complexes. Arthritis Rheum 1988; 31:1322–1327.

D10. Dahl MV. Usefulness of direct immunofluorescence in patients with lupus erythematosus. Arch Dermatol 1983;119: 1010–1017.

D11. Dahl MV. Lupus erythematosus and systemic sclerosis. Chapter 17. In: Dahl VM, editor. Clinical Immunodermatology 2d ed. Boca Raton: Yearbook Medical Publishers, 1988.

D12. Dahl MV, Gilliam JN. Direct immunofluorescence in lupus erythematosus. Ch. 30. In: Beutner EH, Chorzelski TP, Kumar V, editors. Immunopathology of the Skin, 3rd ed. New York: John Wiley 1987.

D13. Dahlback K, Lofberg H, Dahlback B. Vitronectin colocalizes with Ig deposits and C9 neoantigen in discoid lupus erythematosus and dermatitis herpetiformis, but not in bullous pemphigoid. Br J Dermatol 1989 Jun;120(6):725- 733.

D14. Dainiak N, Hardin J, Floyd V, Callahan M, Hoffman R. Humeral suppression of erythropoiesis in systemic lupus erythematosus (SLE) and rheumatoid arthritis. Am J Med 1980 Oct; 69:537–544.

D15. Dajee H, Hurley EJ, Szarnicki RJ. Cardiac valve replacement in systemic lupus erythematosus. J Thoracic Cardiovasc Surg 1983 May;85:718–726.

D16. Dale DC, Fauci AS, Guerry D IV, Wolff SM. Comparison of agents producing a neutrophilic leukocytosis in man: hydrocortisone, prednisone, endotoxin and etiocholanolone. J Clin Invest 1975;56:808–813.

D17. Dale DC, Fauci AS, Wolff SM. Alternate-day prednisone: Leukocyte kinetics and susceptibility to infection. N Engl J Med 1974 Nov 28;291:1154–1158.

D18. Dalqvist SR, Beckman G, Beckman L. Serum protein markers in systemic lupus erythematosus. Human Heredity 1988; 38:44–47.

D19. Daly D. Central nervous system in acute disseminated lupus erythematosus. J Nerv Ment Dis 1945 Nov;102:461- 465.

D20. Dalzier K, Going S, Cartwright PH, Marks R, Beveridge GW, Rowell NR. Treatment of chronic discoid lupus erythematosus with an oral gold preparation. Br J Dermatol 1985;113 Suppl: 25–26.

D21. Dalziel K, Going G, Cartwright PH, Marks R, Beveridge GW, Rowell NR. Treatment of chronic discoid lupus erythematosus with an oral gold compound (Auranofin). Br J Dermatol 1986; 115:211–216.

D22. D'Ambrosio R, Riggins R, Stadalnick R, Denado G. 99m Tc Diphosphonate scintigraphy validated with tetracycline labelling. Clin Ortho 1976;121:143–145.

D23. D'Amelio R, Bilotta P, Pachi A, Aiuti F. Circulating immune complexes in normal pregnant women and in some conditions complicating pregnancy. Clin Exp Immunol 1979;37:33–37.

D24. Dameshek W. Systemic lupus erythematosus: A complex autoimmune disorder? Ann Intern Med 1958 Mar;48: 707–730.

D25. Dameshek W, Reeves WH. Exacerbation of lupus erythematosus following splenectomy in "idiopathic" thrombocytopenic purpura and autoimmune hemolytic anemia. Am J Med 1956 Oct;21:560–566.

D26. Dameshek W, Schwartz R. Treatment of certain "autoimmune" diseases with antimetabolites; a preliminary report. Trans Assoc Am Physicians 1960;73:113–127.

D27. Damle NK, Childs AL, Doyle LV. Immunoregulatory T lymphocytes in man. Soluble antigen-specific suppressor- inducer T lymphocytes are derived from the CD4+ CD45R- p80+ subpopulation. J Immunol 1987;139:1501–1508.

D28. Damle NK, Linsley PS, Ledbetter JA. Direct helper T cell-induced B cell differentiation involves interaction between T cell antigen CD28 and B cell activation antigen B7. Eur J Immunol 1991;21:1277–1282.

D29. Damm J, Soonichsen N. Clinical examinations of chronic lupus erythematosus. [original in German] Derm Wschr 1964 Sep 12;150:268–278.

D30. Dammert K. Lupus erythematosus hypertrophicus et profundus. Acta Dermatovener (Stockh) 1971;51:315–320.

D31. Danao T, Reghetti G, Yen-Lieberman B, Starkey C, Wakasugi K, McLean-Johnson W, Clough J. Antibodies to the human T lymphocytotropic type I in systemic lupus erythematosus. Clin Exp Rheum 1991;9:55–58.

D32. Dang CV, Tan EM, Traugh JA. Myositis autoantibody reactivity and catalytic function of threonyl-tRNA synthetase. FASEB J 1988;2:2376–2379.

D33. Dang H, Harbeck RJ. The in vivo and in vitro glomerular deposition of isolated anti-double-stranded DNA antibodies in NZB/W mice. Clin Immunol Immunopathol 1984 Feb;31(2): 265–278.

D34. Dang H, Takei M, Isenberg D, Shoenfeld Y, Backimer R, Rauch J, Talal N. Expression of an interspecies idiotype in sera of SLE patients and their first-degree relatives. Clin Exp Immunol 1988;71:445.

D35. Dang H, Talal N. T-cell antigen receptor studies in mice expressing the lpr genetic defect. Cell Immunol 1988;115: 393–402.

D36. Daniel L, Sovweine G, Monier JC, Saez S. Specific estrogen binding sites in human lymphoid cells and thymic cells. J Steroid Biochem 1983;18:559–562.

D37. Daniel V, Schimpf K, Opelz G. Lymphocyte autoantibodies and alloantibodies in HIV-positive haemophilia patients. Clin Exp Immunol 1989;75:178–183.

D38. Daniel V, Weimer R, Schimpf K, Opelz G. Autoantibodies against CD4- and CD8 positive T lymphocytes in HIV- infected hemophilia patients. Vox Sang 1989;57:172–176.

D39. Daniels TE. Labial salivary gland biopsy in Sjogren's syndrome. Assessment as a diagnostic criterion in 362 suspected cases. Arthritis Rheum 1984 Feb;27(2):147–156.

D40. Danielson L, Christensen HE, Wanstrup J. Cutaneous amyloidosis: Classification, pathogenesis and relation to "collagen disease." Acta path Microbiol Scand Sect A 1970;78(3): 335–344.

D40a. Dannenberg AM Jr. Anti-inflammatory effects of glucocorticoids. Inflamm 1979;3:329–343.

D40b. Danneskiold-Samsoe B, Grimbly G. The influence of prednisone on the muscle morphology and muscle enzymes in patients with rheumatoid arthritis. CB Sci 1986;71:693- 701.

D41. Dano P. Connective tissue disease following anti- epileptic therapy. Epilepsia (Amst) 1969 Dec;10:481–486.

D42. Danon YL, Garty BZ. Autoantibodies to neuroblastoma cell surface antigens in neuropsychiatric lupus. Neuropediatrics 1986;17:23.

D43. Darby PL, Schmidt PJ. Psychiatric consultations in rheumatology: a review of 100 cases. Can J Psychiatry 1988 May; 33(4):290–293.

D44. Dardenne M, Savino W, Nabarra B, Bach JF. Male BXSB mice develop a thymic hormonal dysfunction with presence of intraepithelial crystalline inclusions. Clin Immunol Immunopathol 1989;52:392–405.

D45. Darken M, McBurney EI. Subacute cutaneous lupus erythematosus-like drug eruption due to combination diuretic hydrochlorothiazide and triamterene. J Am Acad Dermatol 1988; 18:38–42.

D46. Datta B, Weiner A. Genetic evidence for base pairing between U2 and U6 snRNA in mammalian mRNA splicing. Nature 1991;352:821–824.

D47. Datta SK, Manny N, Andrzejewski C, Andre-Schwartz J, Schwartz RS. Genetic studies of autoimmunity and retrovirus expression in crosses of New Zealand Black mice. I. Xenotropic virus. J Exp Med 1978 Mar 1;147(3):854–871.

D48. Datta SK, McConahey PJ, Manny N, Theofilopoulos AN, Dixon FJ, Schwartz RS. Genetic studies of autoimmunity and retrovirus expression in crosses of New Zealand Black mice. II. The viral envelope glycoprotein gp70. J Exp Med 1978; 147:872.

D49. Datta SK, Naparstek Y, Schwartz RS. In vitro production of an anti-DNA idiotype by lymphocytes of normal subjects and patients with systemic lupus erythematosus. Clin Immunol Immunopathol 1986;38:302.

D50. Datta SK, Owen FL, Womack JE, Riblet RJ. Analysis of recombinant inbred lines derived from 'autoimmune' (NZB) and 'high leukemia' (C58) strains: independent multigenic

D51. Datta SK, Patel H, Berry D. Induction of cationic shift in IgG anti-DNA autoantibodies. Role of T helper cells with classical and novel phenotype in three models of lupus nephritis. J Exp Med 1987 May 1;165(5):1252–1268.

D52. Datta SK, Stollar BD, Schwartz RS. Normal mice express idiotypes related to autoantibody idiotypes of lupus mice. Proc Natl Acad Sci USA 1983;80:2723.

D53. Dau PC, Callahan J, Parker R, Golbus J. Immunologic effects of plasmapheresis synchronized with pulse cyclophosphamide in systemic lupus erythematosus [case report]. J Rheumatol 1991 Feb;18(2):270–276.

D54. Daud AB, Nuruddin RN. Solitary paraventricular calcification in cerebral lupus erythematosus: a report of two cases. Neuroradiology 1988;30(1):84–85.

D55. Dauphinee MJ, Talal N. Characteristics of peritoneal lymphocytes form New Zealand black and normal mice autoreactive for mouse erythrocytes. J Clin Lab Immunol 1979;1: 355–360.

D56. Dausset J, Colombani J, Colombani M. Study of leucopenias and thrombocytopenias by the direct antiglobulin consumption test on leucocytes and/or platelets. Blood 1961 Dec;18: 672–690.

D57. Davatchi F, Akbarian M, Chams C, Shahram F. Evaluation of the 1988 classification tree [letter]. J Rheumatol 1990;17: 268–269.

D58. Davatchi F, Chams C, Akbarian M. Evaluation of the 1982 American Rheumatism Association revised criteria for the classification of SLE [letter]. Arthritis Rheum 1985 Jun;28:715.

D58a. Davey ME, Bleasdale K, Isenberg DA. Antibody affinity and IgG subclass of responses to tetanus toxoid in patients with rheumatoid arthritis and systemic lupus erythematosus. Clin Exp Immunol 1987;68:562–569.

D59. David CS, Banerjee S. T cell receptor genes and disease susceptibility. Arthritis Rheum 1989;32:105–107.

D60. David J. Hyperglucagonaemia and treatment with danazol for systemic lupus erythematosus. BMJ (Clin Res) 1985 Oct 26;291(6503):1170–1171.

D61. David KM, Thornton JC, Davis B, Sontheimer RD, Gilliam JN. Morbidity and mortality in patients with subacute cutaneous lupus erythematosus (abstract). J Invest Dermatol 1984;82:408.

D62. Davidson A, Halpern R, Diamond B. Speculation on the role of somatic mutation in the generation of anti-DNA antibodies. Ann N Y Acad Sci 1986;475:174–180.

D63. Davidson A, Manheimer-Lory A, Aranow C, Peterson R, Hannigan N, Diamond B. Molecular characterization of a somatically mutated anti-DNA antibody bearing two systemic lupus erythematosus-related idiotypes. J Clin Invest 1990 May; 85(5):1401–1409.

D64. Davidson A, Preud'homme JL, Solomon A, Chang MD, Beede S, Diamond B. Idiotypic analysis of myeloma proteins: anti- DNA activity of monoclonal immunoglobulins bearing an SLE idiotype is more common in IgG than IgM antibodies. J Immunol 1987;138:1515–1518.

D65. Davidson A, Shefner R, Livneh A, Diamond B. The role of somatic mutation of immunoglobulin genes in autoimmunity. Ann Rev Immunol 1987;5:85–108.

D66. Davidson A, Smith A, Katz J, Preud'homme JL, Solomon A, Diamond B. A cross-reactive idiotype on anti-DNA antibodies defines a heavy chain determinant present almost exclusively on IgG antibodies. J Immunol 1989;143:174–180.

D67. Davidson AG, Fox L, Gold JJ. Appearance of miliary tuberculosis following therapy with ACTH and cortisone in case of acute disseminated lupus erythematosus. Ann Intern Med 1953 April;38:852–862.

D68. Davidson AM, Birt AR. Quinine bisulfate as a desensitizing agent in the treatment of lupus erythematosus. Arch Dermat & Syph 1938 Feb;37:247–253.

D69. Davidson BL, Gilliam JN, Lipsky PE. Cimetidine-associated exacerbation of cutaneous lupus erythematosus. Arch Intern Med 1982 Jan;142:166.

D70. Davidson FF, Dennis EA, Powell M, Glenney JR. Inhibition of phospholipase A2 by "Lipocortins" and calpactins. J Biol Chem 1987;262:1698–1705.

D71. Davidson JR, Graziano FM, Rothenberg RJ. Methotrexate therapy for severe systemic lupus erythematosus [letter]. Arthritis Rheum 1987 Oct;30(10):1195–1196.

D72. Davies BM. Disseminated lupus erythematosus, with renal involvement, treated with nitrogen mustard. BMJ 1956 Mar 24;1:670.

D73. Davies KA, Hird V, Stewart S, Sivolapenko GB, Jose P, Epenetos AA, Walport MJ. A study of *in vivo* immune complex formation and clearance in man. J Immunol 1990;144: 4613–4620.

D74. Davies M, Coles GA, Huges KT. Glomerular basement membrane injury by neutrophil and monocyte neutral proteinases. Renal Physiol 1980;3(1–6):106–111.

D75. Davies MG, Marks R, Waddington E. Simultaneous systemic lupus erythematosus and dermatitis herpeteformis. Arch Dermatol 1976 Sep;112(9):1292–1294.

D76. Davignon JL, Cohen PL, Eisenberg RA. Rapid T cell receptor modulation accompanies lack of in vitro mitogenic responsiveness of double negative T cells to anti-CD3 monoclonal antibody in MRL/Mp-lpr mice. J Immunol 1988;141: 1848–1854.

D77. Davis AE, Harrison RA, Lachmann PJ. Physiologic inactivation of fluid phase C3b: Isolation and structural analysis of C3c, C3dg, and C3g. J Immunol 1984;132:1960-1966.

D78. Davis BM, Gilliam JN. Prognostic significance of subepidermal immune deposits in uninvolved skin of patients with systemic lupus erythematosus: a 10 year longitudinal study. J Inv Dermatol 1984 Oct;83(4):242-247.

D79. Davis GL, Davis JS. Detection of circulating DNA by counterimmunoelectrophoresis (CIE). Arthritis Rheum 1973 Jan–Feb;16:52–58.

D80. Davis JA, Cohen AH, Weisbart R, Paulus HE. Glomerulonephritis in rheumatoid arthritis. Arthritis Rheum 1979 Sep; 22(9):1018–1023.

D81. Davis JA, Weisman MH, Dail DH. Vascular disease in infective endocarditis: report of immune-mediated events in skin and brain. Arch Intern Med 1978 Mar;138(3):480-483.

D82. Davis JS, Bollet AJ. Protection of a complement-sensitive enzyme system by rheumatoid factor. J Immunol 1964;92: 139-144.

D83. Davis JS, Bollet AJ. Complement levels, rheumatoid factor and renal disease in SLE [abstract]. Arthritis Rheum 1966 Jun; 9:499–500.

D84. Davis JS, Godfrey SM, Winfield JB. Direct evidence for circulating DNA/anti-DNA complexes in systemic lupus erythematosus. Arthritis Rheum 1978 Jan–Feb;21:17–22.

D85. Davis M, Williams R, Chakraborty J, English J, Marks V, Ideo G, Tempini S. Prednisone or prednisolone for the treatment of chronic active hepatitis? A comparison of plasma availability. Br J Pharmacol 1978;5:502–505.

D86. Davis MM. Molecular genetics of the T-cell receptor beta chain. Annu Rev Immunol 1985;3:537–560.

D87. Davis MM, Bjorkman PJ. T-cell antigen receptor genes and T-cell recognition. Nature 1988;334:395–402.

D88. Davis MM, Kim SK, Hood LE. DNA sequences mediating class switching in immunoglobulins. Science 1980;209: 1360–1365.

D89. Davis MW, Gutridge GH. Disseminated lupus erythemato-

sus in identical twin sisters associated with diabetes mellitus in one case. J MO Med Assn 1951;48:446–450.

D90. Davis P, Atkins B, Hughes GR. Antibodies to native DNA in discoid lupus erythematosus. Br J Dermatol 1974;91:175-181.

D91. Davis P, Atkins B, Josse RG, Hughes GRV. Criteria for classification of SLE. Br Med J 1973;3:90–91.

D92. Davis P, Cumming RH, Verrier-Jones J. Relationship between Anti-DNA antibodies, complement consumption and circulating immune complexes in systemic lupus erythematosus. Clin Exp Immunol 1977 May;28:226–232.

D93. Davis P, Percy JS, Russell AS. Correlation between levels of DNA antibodies and clinical disease activity in SLE. Retrospective evaluation. Ann Rheum Dis 1977 Apr;36:157-159.

D94. Davis P, Stein M. Evaluation of criteria for the classification of SLE in Zimbabwean patients [letter]. Br J Rheumatol 1989; 28:546–556.

D95. Davis S, Furie BC, Griffin JH, Furie B, Willey R. Circulating inhibitors of blood coagulation associated with procainamide-induced lupus erythematosus. Am J Hematol 1978;4(4): 401–407.

D96. Davis TL, Lyde CB, Davis BM, Sontheimer RD. Perturbation of experimental ultraviolet light-induced erythema by passive transfer of serum from subacute cutaneous lupus erythematosus patients. Soc Invest Derm 1989;92:573–577.

D97. Davison JM, Lindheimer MD. Pregnancy in renal transplant recipients. J Reprod Med 1982;27:613–621.

D98. Dawkins RL, Christiansen FT, Kay PH, Garlepp M, McClusky J, Hollingsworth PM, Zuko PJ. Disease associations with complotypes, supratypes, and haplotypes. Immunol Rev 1983;70:5–22.

D99. Dawkins RL, Witt C, Richmond J, Sagenschneider K, Zilko PJ. Lymphocytotoxic antibodies in disease. Aust NZ J Med 1978;8 Suppl 1:81–86.

D100. Day NK, Winfield JB, Gee T, Winchester RJ, Teshima H, Kunkel HG. Evidence for immune complexes involving antilymphocyte antibodies associated with hypocomplementaemia in chronic lymphocyte leukemia (CLL). Clin Exp Immunol 1976;26:189–195.

D101. D'Cruz DD, Houssiau FA, Ramirez G, Baguley E, Mc Cutcheson J, Vianna J, Haga HJ, Swana GT, Khamashita MA, Taylor JC, Davies DR, Hughes GRV. Antibodies to endothelial cells in systemic lupus erythematosus: a potential marker for nephritis and vasculitis. Clin Exp Immunol 1991;85:254-261.

D102. Dean JH, Laver LD, Murray MJ, Lester MI, Neptun D, Adams DO. Functions of mononuclear phagocytes in mice exposed to diethylstilbestrol; A model of aberrant macrophage development. Cell Immunol 1986;102:315–322.

D103. Deapen DM, Weinrib L, Langholz B, Horwitz DA, Mack TM. A revised estimate of twin concordance in SLE a survey of 138 pairs [abstract]. Arthritis Rheum 1986;29 Suppl:S26.

D104. Deaton JG, Levin WC. Systemic lupus erythematosus and acute myeloblastic leukemia. Report of their coexistence and a survey of possible associating features. Arch Intern Med 1967 Sep;120:345–348.

D105. Deberkt R, van Hooren J, Biesbronck M, Amery W. Antinuclear factor positive mental depression: A single disease entity. Biol Psychiatry 1976;11(1):69–74.

D106. Debets JMH, van de Winkel JGJ, Ceuppens JL, Dieteren IEM, Buurman WA. Cross-linking of both FcγRI and FcγRII induces secretion of tumor necrosis factor by human monocytes, requiring high affinity Fc-FcγR interactions. J Immunol 1990;144:1304–1310.

D107. Debeyre N, Kahn MF, de Seze S. Lupoid syndrome after absorption of isoniazid. Study of 6 cases [original in French]. Sem Hop Paris 1967 Nov 26;43:3063–3071.

D108. De Boccardo G, Drayer D, Rubin AL, Novogrodsky A, Reidenberg MM, Stenzel KH. Inhibition of pokeweek mitogen-induced B cell differentiation by compounds containing primary amine or hydrazine groups. Clin Exp Immunol 1985;59: 69–76.

D109. de Boer PC, Moskowitz RW, Michel B. Skin basement membrane immunofluorescence in rheumatoid arthritis; lack of diagnostic correlation. Arthritis Rheum 1977;20:653- 658.

D110. de Castro P, Jorizzo JL, Solomon AR, Lisse JR, Daniels JC. Coexistent systemic lupus erythematosus and tophaceous gout. J Am Acad Dermatol 1985 Oct;13(4):650–654.

D111. Decaux G, Unger J, Marneffe C. Psychosis, central hyperventilation and inappropriate secretion of antidiuretic hormone in systemic lupus erythematosus. Postgrad Med J 1981 Nov;57(673):719–720.

D112. Decker JL. Cytotoxic agents in the management of systemic lupus erythematosus. Clin Rheum Dis 1975;1:665–677.

D113. Decker JL, Klippel JH, Plotz PH, Steinberg AD. Cyclophosphamide or azathioprine in lupus glomerulonephritis. A controlled trial: results at 28 months. Ann Intern Med 1975 Nov; 83(5):606–615.

D114. Decker JL, Steinberg AD, Reinersten JL, Plotz PH, Balow JE, Klippel JH. NIH Conference. Systemic lupus erythematosus: evolving concepts. Ann Intern Med 1979 Oct;91(4): 587–604.

D115. de Clerck LS, Couttenye MM, de Broe ME, Stevens WJ. Acquired immunodeficiency mimicking Sjogren's syndrome and systemic lupus erythematosus. Arthritis Rheum 1988 Feb; 31(2):272–275.

D116. de Clerck LS, Meijers KA, Cats A. Is MCTD a distinct entity? Comparison of clinical and laboratory findings in MCTD, SLE, PSS and RA patients. Clin Rheumatol 1989 Mar; 8(1):29–36.

D117. Decrop E, Ponette E, Baert AL, Verberckmoes R, Kerremans R, Geboes K. Pre-operative radiological diagnosis of acute necrotizing enteritis in systemic lupus erythematodes. J Belge Radkiol 1990 Jan;73(1):31–35.

D118. De Giorgio CM, Rabinowics AL, Olivas RD. Carbamazepine-induced antinuclear antibodies and systemic lupus erythematosus-like syndrome. Epilepsia 1991;32:128–129.

D119. Degos R, Garnier G, Darnis F, Vissian L. Subacute lupus erythematosus with signs of subactue dermatomyositis (electromyographic abnormalities) [original in French]. Bull Soc Franc Dermat et Syph 1949 Mar–Apr;56:114–116.

D120. DeHeer DH, Edgington TS. Clonal heterogeneity of the anti- erythrocyte defect underlying the anti-X autoantibody responses of NZB mice. J Immunol 1974 Oct;113(4):1184-1189.

D121. DeHeer DH, Edgington TS. Cellular events associated with the immunogenesis of anti-erythrocyte autoantibody response of NZB mice. Transplant Rev 1976;31:116–155.

D122. DeHeer DH, Edgington TS. Evidence for a B lymphocyte defect underlying the anti-X anti-erythrocyte autoantibody response of NZB mice. J Immunol 1977 May;118(5): 1858–1863.

D123. DeHoratius RJ. Lymphocytotoxic antibodies. Prog Clin Immunol 1980;4:151–174.

D124. DeHoratius RJ, Meissner RP. Lymphocytotoxic antibodies in family members of patients with SLE. J Clin Invest 1975; 550:1254–1258.

D125. DeHoratius RJ, Pillarisetty R, Messner RP, Talal N. Antinucleic acid antibodies in systemic lupus erythematosus patients and their families. Incidence and correlation with lymphocytotoxic antibodies. J Clin Invest 1975;56: 1149–1154.

D126. DeHoratius RJ, Tunk KSK, Pincus T. Reduced T-lymphocyte subsets in systemic lupus erythematosus: effects of immune complexes and lymphocytotoxic antibodies. Clin Immunol Immunopathol 1980 Oct;17:235–256.

D127. DeJongste JC, Neijens HJ, Duiverman EJ, Bogaard JM, Kerrebijn KF. Respiratory tract disease in systemic lupus erythematosus. Arch Dis Child 1986;61:478–483.

D128. Dekker A, O'Brien ME, Cammarata RJ. The association of thrombotic thrombocytopenic purpura with systemic lupus erythematosus: a report of two cases with successful treatment of one. Am J Med Sci 1974;267:243–249.

D129. DeLange RJ, Fambrough DM, Smith EL, Bonner J. Calf and pea histone IV. III. Complete amino acid sequence of pea seedling histone IV; comparison with the homologous calf thymus histone. J Biol Chem 1969;244:5669–5679.

D130. DeLange RJ, Smith EL, Fambrough DM, Bonner J. Amino acid sequence of histone IV: Presence of epsilon-N-acetylysine. Proc Natl Acad Sci USA 1968;61:1145–1146.

D131. de la Serna AR, Alarcon-Segovia D. Chronic interstitial cystitis as an initial major manifestation of systemic lupus erythematosus. J Rheumatol 1981;8:808–810.

D132. de la Sota M, Garcio-Morteo O, Maldonado-Cocco JA. Jaccoud's arthropathy of the knees in systemic lupus erythematosus. Arthritis Rheum 1985 Jul; 28(7):825–827.

D133. de la Sota M, Maldonado Cocco JA. Jaccoud's arthropathy in knees in systemic lupus erythematosus. Clin Rheumatol 1989;8:416–417.

D134. del Castillo M, Toblli JE, Rueda HJ, Trigo M, Hernaiz MA, Adara F. Infection and systemic lupus erythematosus. La Presna Medica Argentina 1988;75:49–60.

D135. Delektorskaya L, Janushkevich T, Okunev D. The significance of the assays of urinary enzymes activity in patients with systemic lupus erythematosus. Z Med Lab Diagn 1990; 31:375–379.

D136. Delepine N, Desbois JC, Taillard F, Allaneau C, Renoux G. Sodium diethyldithiocarbamate inducing long-lasting remission in case of juvenile systemic lupus erythematosus [letter]. Lancet 1985 Nov 30;2(8466):1246.

D137. Delespesse G, Gausset PH, Sarfati M, Dubi-Rucquoy M, Debisschop MJ, Van Haelst L. Circulating immune complexes in old people and in diabetics: correlation with autoantibodies. Clin Exp Immunol 1980;40:96–102.

D138. Deleze M, Alarcon-Segovia D, Oria CV, Sanchez-Guerrero J, Fernandez-Dominguez L, Gomez-Pacheco L, Ponce de Leon S. Hemocytopenia in systemic lupus erythematosus. Relationship to antiphospholipid antibodies. J Rheumatol 1989 Jul; 16(7):926–930.

D139. Deleze M, Oria CV, Alarcon-Segovia D. Occurrence of both hemolytic anemia and thrombocytopenic purpura (Evans' syndrome) in systemic lupus erythematosus. Relationship to antiphospholipid antibodies. J Rheumatol 1988 Apr; 15(4):611–615.

D140. Delfraissy JF, Second P, Galanaud P, Wallon C, Massias P, Dormont J. Depressed primary in vitro antibody response in untreated systemic lupus erythematosus. J Clin Invest 1980 Jul;11 141–142.

D141. Delgado EA, Malleson PN, Pirie GE, Petty RE. Pulmonary manifestations of childhood onset systemic lupus erythematosus. Semin Arthritis Rheum 1990;29:285–293.

D142. Del Guidice G, Elkon KB, Crow MK. Evidence for TGFβ-mediated suppression of T cell proliferative response in patients with systemic lupus erythematosus [abstract]. Arthritis Rheum 1991;34 Suppl:S137.

D143. Del Guidice GC, Scher CA, Athreya BH, Diamond GR. Pseudotumor cerebri and childhood systemic lupus erythematosus. J Rheumatol 1986;13:748–752.

D144. Delorme P, Giroux J-M. Solar urticaria as the presenting manifestation of systemic lupus erythematosus. Can Med Assoc J 1966;95:539–542.

D145. del Rio A, Vazquez JJ, Sorbrino JA, Gil A, Barbado J, Mate I, Ortiz-Vazquez J. Myocardial involvement in systemic lupus erythematosus: A noninvasive study of left ventricular function. Chest 1978 Oct;74:414–417.

D146. de Luis A, Pigrau C, Pahissa A, Fernandez F, Martinez-Vazquez JM. Infections in 96 cases of systemic lupus erythematosus. Med Clin (Barc) 1990 Apr 28;94(16):607-610.

D147. Demaine A, Welsh KI, Hawe BS, Farid NR. Polymorphism of the T cell receptor beta chain in Grave's disease. J Clin Invest 1987;65:643–646.

D148. Demaine AG, Vaughan RW, Taube DH, Welsh KI. Association of membranous nephropathy with T-cell receptor constant beta chain and immunoglobulin heavy chain switch region polymorphism. Immunogenetics 1988;27:19–23.

D149. Demis DJ, Brown CS, Crosby WH. Thioguanine in the treatment of certain autoimmune, immunologic, and related diseases. Am J Med 1964 Aug;37:195–205.

D150. Denburg JA. Clinical and subclinical involvement of the central nervous system in systemic lupus erythematosus. Res Publ Assoc Res Nerv Ment Dis 1990;68:171–178.

D151. Denburg JA, Behmann SA, Long AA, Carbotte RM, Denburg SD. Clinical associations of lymphocyte/neuronal autoantibodies in SLE [abstract]. Arthritis Rheum 1990 Sep;33(9) Suppl:S124.

D152. Denburg JA, Carbotte RM, Denburg SD. Neuronal antibodies and cognitive function in systemic lupus erythematosus. Neurology 1987 Mar;37(3):464–467.

D153. Denburg SD, Carbotte RM, Denburg JA. Cognitive impairment in systemic lupus erythematosus: a neuropsychological study of individual and group deficits. J Clin Exper Neuropsychol 1987 Aug;9(4):323–339.

D154. Denburg SD, Carbotte RM, Long AA, Denburg JA. Neuropsycho logical correlates of serum lymphocytotoxic antibodies in systemic lupus erythematosus. Brain Behav Immun 1988 Sep;2(3):222–234.

D155. Deng JS, Bair LW, Shen-Schwarz S, Ramsey-Goldman R, Medsger T. Localization of Ro(SS-A) antigen in the cardiac conduction system. Arthritis Rheum 1987;301:1232-1238.

D156. Deng JS, Sontheimer RD, Gilliam JN. Molecular characteristics of SS-B/La and SS-A/Ro cellular antigens. J Invest Dermatol 1985;84:86–90.

D157. Denko CW, Gabriel P. Serum proteins-transferrin, ceruloplasmin, albumin, alpha-1 glycoprotein, alpha-1 antitrypsin-in rheumatic diseases. J Rheumatol 1979 Nov–Dec;6:664–672.

D158. Denko CW, Zumpft CW. Chronic arthritis with splenomegaly and leukopenia. Arthritis Rheum 1962 Oct;5:478–491.

D159. Denman AM, Denman EJ. Proliferative activity in the lymphatic tissue of germ-free New Zealand black mice. Int J Cancer 1970 Jul 15;6:108–122.

D160. Denman AM, Russell AS, Denman EJ. Renal diseases in (NZB × NZW)F1 hybrid mice treated with antilymphocytic antibody. Clin Exp Immunol 1970;6:325.

D161. Denman AM, Russell AS, Loewi G, Denman EJ. Immunopathology of New Zealand black mice treated with antilymphocytic globulin. Immunology 1971;20:973.

D162. Dennis EJ, McFarland KF, Hester LL. The preeclampsia-eclampsia syndrome. In: Danforth DN, Editor. Obstetrics and Gynecology, 4th ed. Philadelphia: Harper & Rowe, 1982:455–474.

D163. Dennis GJ, West SG, Anderson PA. Identification of clinical subsets by serologic markers in systemic lupus erythematosus [abstract]. Arthritis Rheum 1983;26 Suppl:S13.

D164. Denzer BS, Blumenthal S. Acute lupus erythematosus disseminatus. 1937;53:525–540.

D165. Derksen OS. Pneumatosis intestinalis in a female patient with systemic lupus erythematosus. Radiol Clin (Basel) 1978 47(5):334–339.

D166. Derksen RH, Hasselaar P, Blokzijl L, de Groot PG. Lack of efficacy of plasma-exchange in removing antiphospholipid antibodies [letter]. Lancet 1987 Jul 25;2(8552):222.

D167. Derksen RH, Overbeek BP, Poeschmann PH. Serious bacterial cellulitis of the periorbital area in two patients with systemic lupus erythematosus. J Rheumatol 1988;15(5):840-844.

D168. Derksen RH, van Dam AP, Gmelig Meyling FHJ, Bijlsma JWJ, Smeenk RJT. A prospective study on antiribosomal P proteins in two cases of familial lupus and recurrent psychosis. Ann Rheum Dis 1990 Oct;49(10):779–782.

D169. Derksen RHWM, Beisma D, Bouma BN, Gmelig Meyling FHJ, Kater L. Discordant effects of prednisone on anti- cardiolipin antibodies and the lupus anticoagulant. Arthritis Rheum 1986;29:1295–1296.

D170. Derksen RHMW, Bouma BN, Kater L. The prevalence and clinical associations of the lupus anticoagulant in systemic lupus erythematosus. Scand J Rheumatol 1987;16:185.

D171. Derksen RHMW, Kater L. Lupus anticoagulant: revival of an old phenomenon. Clin Exp Rheumatol 1991;3:349–357.

D172. de Rooij DJ, Habets WJ, Van de Putte LB, Hoet MH, Verboek AL, Van Venrooij WJ. Use of recombinant RNP peptides 70K and A in an ELISA for measurement of antibodies in mixed connective tissue disease: a longitudinal follow up of 18 patients. Ann Rheum Dis 1990;49:391–395.

D173. Dersimonian H, McAdam PWJ, Mackworth-Young C, Stollar BD. The recurrent expression of variable region segments in human IgM anti-DNA autoantibodies. J Immunol 1989;142:4027.

D174. Dersimonian H, Schwartz RS, Barrett KJ, Stollar BD. Relationship of human variable region heavy chain germ- line genes to genes encoding anti-DNA autoantibodies. J Immunol 1987 Oct 1;139(7):2496–2501.

D175. Derue G, Englert H, Harris EN, Hughes GRV. Fetal loss in systemic lupus: association with anticardiolipin antibodies. J Obstet Gynaecol Neonatal Nurs 1985;2:207- 209.

D176. Desiderio S. Insertion of N regions into heavy chain genes is correlated with expression of terminal deoxytransferance in B cells. Nature 1984;311:752–755.

D177. de Silva JA, Elkon KB, Hughes GR, Dyck RF, Pepys MB. C- reactive protein levels in systemic lupus erythematosus: A classification criterion. Arthritis Rheum 1980 Jun;23:770–771.

D178. de Smet AA, Mahmood T, Robinson RG, Lindsley HB. Elevated sacroiliac joint uptake ratios in systemic lupus erythematosus. AJR 1984 Aug;143(2):351–354.

D179. Desnoyers MR, Bernstein S, Cooper AG, Kopelman RI. Pulmonary hemorrhage in lupus erythematosus without evidence of an immunologic cause. Arch Intern Med 1984 Jul 144:1398.

D180. DeSpain J, Clark DP. Subacute cutaneous lupus erythematosus presenting as erythroderma. J Am Acad Dermatol 1988; 19:388–392.

D181. Desrosiers R, Tanguay RM. The modifications in the methylation patterns of H2B and H3 after heat shock can be correlated with the inactivation of normal gene expression. Biochem Biophys Res Commun 1985;133:823–829.

D182. Dessein PH, Gledhill RF, Asherson RA. Anticardiolipin antibody negative occlusive vascular retinopathy in systemic lupus erythematosus [letter]. Ann Rheum Dis 1990 Feb;49(2):133–134.

D182a. Dessein PH, Lamperelli RD, Phillips SA, Rubechik IA, Zwi S. Severe immune thrombocytopenia and the development of skin infarctions in a patient with an overlap syndrome. J Rheumatol 1989;16:1494–1496.

D183. Desser KB, Sartiano GP, Cooper JL. Lupus livedo and cutaneous infarction. Angiology 1969 May;20:261.

D184. De Takats G, Fowler EF. Raynaud's phenomenon. JAMA 179;1:1962.

D185. Deutscher SL, Harley JB, Keene JD. Molecular analysis of the 60 kK human Ro ribonucleoprotein. Proc Natl Acad Sci USA 1988;85:9479–9483.

D186. DeVere R, Bradley WG. Polymyositis: Its presentation, morbidity and mortality. Brain 1975 Dec;98(4):637–666.

D187. Devey ME, Bleasdale K, Isenberg DA. Antibody affinity and IgG subclass of responses to tetanus toxoid in patients with rheumatoid arthritis and systemic lupus erythematosus. Clin Exp Immunol 1987;68:562–569.

D188. Devinsky O, Petito CK, Alonso DR. Clinical and neuropathological findings in systemic lupus erythematosus: the role of vasculitis, heart emboli, and thrombotic thrombocytopenic purpura. Ann Neurol 1988 Apr;23(4):380–384.

D189. Devoe LD, Loy GL. Serum complement levels and perinatal outcome in pregnancies complicated by systemic lupus erythematosus. Obstet Gynecol 1984;63:796–800.

D190. Devoe LD, Loy GL, Spargo BH. Renal histology and pregnancy performance in systemic lupus erythematosus. Clin Exper Hyper 1983;B2(2):325–340.

D191. Devoe LD, Taylor RL. Systemic lupus erythematosus in pregnancy. Am J Obstet Gynecol 1979;135:473–479.

D192. Devos P, Destee A, Prin L, Warot P. Multiple sclerosis and lupus [English abstract]. Rev Neurol (Paris) 1984;140(8-9):513–515.

D193. De Vries MJ, Hijmans W. Pathological changes of the thymic epithelial cells and autoimmune disease in NZB, NZW and (NZB × NZW) F1 mice. Immunology 1967 Feb;12:179–196.

D194. De Wolf F, Carreras LO, Moerman P, Vermylen J, Van Assche A, Renaer M. Decidual vasculopathy and extensive placental infarction in a patient with repeated thromboembolic accidents, recurrent fetal loss, and a lupus anticoagulant. Am J Obstet Gynecol 1982;142:829-834.

D195. Dhand AK, LaBrecque DR, Metzger J. Sulindac (Clinoril) hepatitis. Gastroenterology 1980 Mar;80(3):585–586.

D196. Dhillon VB, Davies MC, Hall ML, Round JM, Ell PJ, Jacobs HS, Snaith ML, Isenberg DA. Assessment of the effect of oral corticosteroids on bone mineral density in systemic lupus erythematosus: a preliminary study with dual energy x-ray absorptiometry. Ann Rheum Dis 1990 Aug;49(8):624-626.

D197. Diamond B, Scharff MD. Somatic mutation of the T15 heavy chain gives rise to an antibody with autoantibody specificity. Proc Natl Acad Sci USA 1984;81:5841–5844.

D198. Diaz-Jouanen E, Abud-Mendoza C, Inglesias-Gamarra A, Gonsalez-Amaro R. Ischemic necrosis of bone in systemic lupus erythematosus. Orthopedic Review 1985 May;14:303-309.

D199. Diaz-Jouanen E, Bankhurst AD, Messner RP, Williams RC Jr. Serum and synovial fluid inhibitors of antibody-mediated lymphocytotoxicity in rheumatoid arthritis and systemic lupus erythematosus. Arthritis Rheum 1976;19:142–149.

D200. Diaz-Jouanen E, Bankhurst AD, Williams RC. Antibody-mediated lymphocytotoxicity in rheumatoid arthritis and systemic lupus erythematosus. Arthritis Rheum 1976 Mar–Apr;19:133–141.

D201. Diaz-Jouanen E, de la Fuente JR, Llorente L, Rivero SJ, Alarcon-Segovia D. Does the thymus play opposite roles in SLE and myasthenia gravis? Arthritis Rheum 1978 May;21:492–493.

D202. Dicke B. Development of cancer in lupus erythematosus [original in German]. Derm Wschr 1925 May 25;44:24–40.

D203. Diddie KR, Aronson AJ, Ernest JT. Chorioretinopathy in a case of systemic lupus erythematosus. Trans Am Ophthalmol Soc 1977;75:122–131.

D204. Diedericksen H, Pyndt IC. Antibodies against neurons in a patient with systemic lupus erythematosus, cerebral palsy, and epilepsy. Brain 1970;93:407.

D205. Dietschi R, Panizzon R. Lupus-erythematosus-like Tinea faciei [English abstract]. Schweiz Rundsch Med Prax 1988 Oct 25;77(43):1171–1174.

D206. Dietze HJ, Voegele GE. Neuropsychiatric manifestations associated with systemic lupus erythematosus in children. Psychiatr Q 1966;40:59–70.

D207. Difino SM, Lachant NA, Krishner JJH, Gootlieb AJ. Adult idiopathic thrombocytopenic purpura. Am J Med 1980;69:430–442.

D208. Digeon M, Lauer M, Riza J, Back JF. Detection of circulating immune complexes in human sera by simplified assays with polyethylene glycol. J Immunol Meth 1977;16:165–183.

D209. Dighiero G, Lymberi P, Holmberg D, Lindquist I, Coutinho A, Avrameas S. High frequency of natural autoantibodies in normal newborn mice. J Immunol 1985;134:765–771.

D210. DiGiovanna JJ, Helfgott RK, Gerber LH, Peck GL. Extraspinal tendon and ligament calcification associated with long-term therapy with etretinate. N Engl J Med 1986;315:1177–1182.

D211. Dijkmans BA, de Vries E, de Vreede TM. Synergistic and additive effects of disease modifying anti-rheumatic drugs combined with chloroquine on the mitogen-driven stimulation of mononuclear cells. Clin Exp Rheumatol 1990 Sep–Oct;8(5):455–459.

D212. Dijkmans BA, de Vries E, de Vreede TM, Cats A. Effects of anti-rheumatic drugs on in vitro mitogenic stimulation of peripheral blood mononuclear cells. Transplant Proc 1988 Apr;20 Suppl 2:253–258.

D213. Dildrop R, Bruggermann M, Radbruch A, Rajewsky K, Beyreuther K. Immunoglobulin V region variants in hybridoma cells II. Recombination between V genes. EMBO J 1981;1:635.

D214. Dillard MG, Dujovne I, Pollak VE, Pirani CL. The effect of treatment with prednisone and nitrogen mustard on the renal lesions and life span of patients with lupus glomerulonephritis. Nephron 1973;10:273–291.

D215. Dillard MG, Tillman RL, Simpson GC. Lupus nephritis: correlation between the clinical course and presence of electron dense deposits. Lab Invest 1976 Mar;32:261–269.

D216. Dillon AM, Stein HB, Kassen BO, Ibbott JW. Hyposplenia in a patient with systemic lupus erythematosus. J Rheumatol 1980 Mar–Apr;7:196–198.

D217. Dillon CF, Jones JV, Reichlin M. Antibody to Ro in a population of patients with systemic lupus erythematosus: distribution, clinical and serological associations. J Rheumatol 1983;10:380.

D218. Dimant J, Ginzler EM, Diamond HS, Schlesinger M, Marino CT, Weiner M, Kaplan D. Computer analysis of factors influencing the appearance of aseptic necrosis in patients with SLE. J Rheumatol 1978 Summer;5(2):136–141.

D219. Dimant J, Ginzler EM, Schlesinger M, Diamond HS, Kaplan D. Systemic lupus erythematosus in the older age group: computer analysis. J Am Geriatr Soc 1979 Feb;27(2):58–61.

D220. Dimant J, Ginzler E, Schlesinger M, Sterba G, Diamond H, Kaplan D, Weiner M. The clinical significance of Raynaud's phenomenon in systemic lupus erythematosus. Arthritis Rheum 1979 Aug;22(8):815–819.

D221. Dinant HJ, Decker JL, Klippel JH, Balow JE, Plots PH, Steinberg AD. Alternative modes of cyclophosphamide and azathioprine therapy in lupus nephritis. Ann Intern Med 1982;96(6 Pt 1):728–736.

D222. Dinarello CA. Interleukin-1 and its biologically related cytokines. Adv Immunol 1989;44:153–205.

D223. Dinerman H, Goldenberg DL, Felson DT. A prospective evaluation of 118 patients with the fibromyalgia syndrome:

prevalence of Raynaud's, phenomenon, sicca symptoms, ANA, low complement, and Ig deposition at the dermal-epidermal junction. J Rheumatol 1986 Apr;13(2):368–373.

D224. Dionigi R, Zonta A, Albertario F, Galeazzi R, Bellinzona G. Cyclic variation in the response of lymphocytes to phytohemagglutinin in healthy individuals. Transplantation 1973;16:550.

D225. Di Paolo S, Lattanzi V, Guastamacchia E, Vincenti C, Balice AM, Montanaro N, Nardelli GM, Giorgino R. Extreme insulin resistance due to anti-insulin receptor antibodies: a direct demonstration of autoantibody secretion by peripheral lymphocytes. Diabetes Res Clin Pract 1990 Apr;9(1):65–73.

D226. Dise CA, Burch JW, Goodman DB. Direct interaction of mepacrine with erythrocyte and platelet membrane phospholipid. J Biol Chem 1982 May 10;257(9):4701–4704.

D227. Disney TF, Sullivan SN, Haddad RC, Lowe D, Goldbach MM. Budd-Chiari syndrome with inferior vena cava obstruction associated with systemic lupus erythematosus. J Clin Gastroenterol 1984 Jan;6(3):253–256.

D228. Distelmeier MR, Hayne ST, Rada DC. Neonatal lupus: a case report. Cutis 1984;33:191.

D229. Diumenjo MS, Lisanti M, Valles R, Rivero I. Allergic manifestations of systemic lupus erythematosus [English abstract]. Allergol Immunopathol (Madrid). 1985 Jul– Aug;13(4): 323–326.

D230. DiVittorio G, Wees S, Coopman WJ, Ball GV. Pancreatitis in systemic lupus erythematosus [abstract]. Arthritis Rheum 1982 Apr;25(4) Suppl:S6.

D231. Dixit R, Krieg AM, Atkinson JP. Thrombotic thrombocytopenic purpura developing during pregnancy in a C2-deficient patient with a history of systemic lupus erythematosus. Arthritis Rheum 1985;28:341–344.

D232. Dixon FJ. The role of antigen-antibody complexes in disease. Harvey Lectures 1962;58:21–51.

D233. Dixon FJ, Andrews BS, Eisenberg RA, McConahey PM, Theofilopoulos AN, Wilson CB. Etiology and pathogenesis of a spontaneous lupus-like syndrome in mice [abstract]. Arthritis Rheum 1978;21 Suppl:S64.

D234. Dixon FJ, Feldman JD, Vazquez JJ. Experimental glomerulonephritis. J Exp Med 1961;113:899–919.

D235. Dixon FJ, Oldstone MB, Tonietti G. Pathogenesis of immune complex glomerulonephritis of New Zealand mice. J Exp Med 1971 Sep 1;134 Suppl:65S-71S.

D236. Dixon FJ, Wilson CB. Immunological renal injury produced by formation and deposition of immune complexes. In: Wilson C, editor. Contemporary Issues in Nephrology. New York: Churchill, 1979:1–34.

D237. Dixon GH, Candido EPM, Honda BM. The biological roles of post-synthetic modifications of basic nuclear proteins. In: Bradbury EM, editor. The structure and function of chromatin. New York: American Elsevier, 1975:229.

D238. Dixon R, Rosse W, Ebbert L. Quantitative determination of antibody in idiopathic thrombocytopenic purpura. Correlation of serum and platelet-bound antibody with clinical response. N Engl J Med 1975 Jan 30;292:230–236.

D239. Dixon RB, Christy NP. On the various forms of corticosteroid withdrawal syndrome. Am J Med 1980;68:224- 229.

D240. Dixon RH, Rosse WF. Platelet antibody in auto-immune thrombocytopenia. Br J Haematol 1975 Oct;31:129–134.

D241. Doan CA, Bouroncle BA, Wiseman BK. Idiopathic and secondary thrombocytopenic purpura: clinical study and evaluation of 381 cases over a period of 28 years. Ann Intern Med 1960 Nov;53:861–876.

D242. Dobashi KS, Ono S, Murakami S, Takahama Y, Katoh Y, Hamaoka T. Polyclonal B cell activation by a B cell differentiation factor,B151-TRF-2. III B151-TRF-2 as a B cell differentia-

tion factor closely associated with autoimmune disease. J Immunol 1987;138:780–787.

D243. Dobos GJ, Meske S, Keller E, Riegel W, Vaith P, Peter HH, Schollmeyer P. Successful therapy of meningococcal sepsis in acute disseminated lupus erythematosus with plasmapheresis, immunosuppression, and antibiotics. Klin Wochenschr 1990 Oct 3;68(19):976–980.

D244. Dodson MG, Kerman RH, Lange CF, Stefani SS, O'Leary JA. T and B cells in pregnancy. Obstet Gynecol 1979;49:299–302.

D245. Dodson VN, Dinman BD, Whitehouse WM, Nasr ANM, Magnuson HJ. Occupational acroosteolysis. Arch Environ Health 1971;22:83–91.

D246. Doenecke D, Karlson P. Albrecht Kossel and the discovery of histones. Trends Bioc 1984;404–405.

D247. Doglia S, Graslund A, Ehrenberg A. Specific interactions between quinacrine and self-complementary deoxynucleotides. Anticancer Res 19 ;6:1363–1368.

D248. Doherty M, Maddison PJ, Grey RH. Hydralazine induced lupus syndrome with eye disease. BMJ (Clin Res) 1985 Mar 2;290(6469):675.

D248a. Doherty NE, Feldman G, Mauer G, Siegel RJ. Echocardiographic findings in systemic lupus erythematosus. Am J Cardiol 1988;61:1144–1145.

D249. Doherty NE, Siegel RJ. Cardiovascular manifestations of systemic lupus erythematosus. Am Heart J 1985;110:1257-1265.

D250. Dohi Y, Nisonoff A. Suppression of idiotype and generation of suppressor T cells with idiotype-conjugated thymocytes. J Exp Med 1979;150:909.

D251. Dohi Y, Yamada K, Ohno N, Aoki M, Takagaki Y, Nisonoff A, Shinka S. Naturally occurring cytotoxic T lymphocyte precursors with specificity for an Ig idiotype. J Immunol 1988; 141:3804.

D252. Domingo-Pedrol P, De la Serna A, Mancebo-Cortes J, Sanchez-Segura JM. Adult respiratory distress syndrome caused by systemic lupus erythematosus. Eur J Resp Dis 1985;67: 141–144.

D253. Domoto DT, Kashgarian M, Hayslett JP, Adler M, Siegel NJ. The significance of electron dense deposits in mild lupus nephritis. Yale J Biol Med 1980 Jul–Aug;53:314–324.

D254. Domz CA, McNamara DH, Holzapfel HF. Tetracycline provocation in lupus erythematosus. Ann Intern Med 1959 May 50:1217–1226.

D255. Domzig W, Stadler BM, Herberman RB. Interleukin 2 dependence on human natural killer cell activity. J Immunol 1983 Apr;130:1970–1973.

D256. Donadio JV, Burgess JG, Holley KE. Membranous lupus nephropathy: a clinicopathologic study. Medicine 1977 Nov; 56:527–536.

D257. Donadio JV, Holley KE, Ferguson RH, Ilstrup DM. Progressive lupus glomerulonephritis: Treatment with prednisone and combined prednisone and cyclophosphamide. Mayo Clin Proc 1976;51:484–494.

D258. Donadio JV, Holley KE, Wagoner RD, Ferguson RH, McDuffie FC. Treatment of patients with lupus nephritis with prednisone and combined prednisone-azathioprine. Ann Intern Med 1972 Dec;77(6):829–835.

D259. Donadio JV Jr, Holley KE, Ferguson RH, Ilstrup DM. Treatment of diffuse proliferative lupus nephritis with prednisone and combined prednisone and cyclophosphamide. N Engl J Med 1978 Nov 23;299(21):1151–1155.

D260. Donadio JV Jr, Holley KE, Ilstrup DM. Cytotoxic drug treatment of lupus nephritis. Am J Kidney 1982;2 Suppl 1: 178–181.

D261. Donaldson I, Mac G, Espiner EA. Disseminated lupus erythematosus presenting as chorea gravidarum. Arch Neurol 1971 Sep;24:240–244.

D262. Donaldson LB, de Alvarez RR. Further observations on lupus erythematosus associated with pregnancy. Am J Obstet Gynecol 1962;83:1461–1473.

D263. Donaldson PT, Hussain MJ, Mieli-Vergani G, Mowat AP, Vergani D. Anti-lymphocyte antibodies in autoimmune chronic active hepatitis starting in childhood. Clin Exp Immunol 1989;75:41–46.

D264. Doniach D, Roitt IM. Autoimmune thyroid disease. In: Miescher PA, Muller-Eberhard HJ, editors. Textbook of Immunopathology. Vol II. New York: Grune & Stratton, 1976: 715–736.

D265. Dore N, Synkowski D, Provost TT. Antinuclear antibody determinations in Ro(SSA)-positive, antinuclear antibody-negative lupus and Sjogren's syndrome patients. J Am Acad Dermatol 1983 May;8(5):611–615.

D266. Dore-Duffy P, Donaldson JO, Rothman BL, Zurier RB. Antinuclear antibodies in multiple sclerosis. Arch Neurol 1982 Aug;39(8):504–506.

D267. Dorf ME, Benacerraf B. Suppressor cells and immunoregulation. Annu Rev Immunol 1984;2:127–157.

D268. Dorfman DF. Histiocytic necrotizing lymphadenitis of Kirkuchi and Fujimoto. Arch Pathol Lab Med 1987;111:1026-1029.

D269. Dorfmann H, Kahn MF, de Seze S. Possible iatrogenic lupus induced by pheneturide (original in French). Ann Med Intern 1972 Apr;123:331–336.

D270. Doria A, Bonavina L, Anselmino M, Ruffatti A, Favaretto M, Gambari P, Peracchia A, Todesco S. Esophageal involvement in mixed connective tissue disease. J Rheumatol 1991;18: 685–690.

D271. Dorlon RE, Smith JM, Cook EH, Lobel DH, Mealing HG, Bailey JP. Staphylococcal pericardial effusion with tamponade in a patient with systemic lupus erythematosus. J Rheumatol 1982 Oct;9:813–814.

D272. Dorsch C, Meyerhoff J. Elevated plasma beta- thromboglobulin levels in systemic lupus erythematosus. Thrombosis Research 1980;20(5–6):617–622.

D273. Dorsch CA, Meyerhoff J. Mechanisms of abnormal platelet aggregation in systemic lupus erythematosus. Arthritis Rheum 1982 Aug;25:966–973.

D274. Dorsett B, Cronin W, Chuma V, Iochim HL. Anti-lymphocyte antibodies in patients with the acquired immune deficiency syndrome. Am J Med 1985;78:621–626.

D275. Dosa S, Mallick NP, Lawler W, Cairns SA, Slotki IN. The treatment of lupus nephritis by methylprednisolone pulse therapy. Postgrad Med J 1978 Sep;54:628–632.

D276. Doshi N, Smith B, Klionsky B. Congenital pericarditis due to maternal lupus erythematosus. J Pediatr 1980;96:699- 701.

D277. Dossetor JB. Creatininemia versus uremia. The relative significance of blood urea nitrogen and serum creatinine concentrations in azotemia. Ann Intern Med 1966 Dec;65: 1287–1299.

D278. Dotson AD, Raimer SS, Pursley TV, Tschen J. Systemic lupus erythematosus occurring in a patient with epidermolysis bullosa acquisita. Arch Dermatol 1981 Jul;117(7): 422–426.

D279. Dougados M, Job-Deslandre C, Amor B, Menkes CJ. Danazol therapy in systemic lupus erythematosus. A one-year prospective controlled trial on 40 female patients. Clin Trials J 1987;24:191–200.

D280. Dougherty TF, Brown HE, Berliner DL. Metabolism of hydrocortisone during inflammation. Endocrinology 1958 Apr;62:455–462.

D281. Douglass M, Lamberg SI, Lorincz AL, Good RA, Day NK. Lupus erythematosus-like syndrome with a familial deficiency of C2. Arch Dermatol 1976;112:671–674.

D282. Doutre MS, Beylot C, Bioulac P, Busquet M, Conte M. Skin lesion resembling malignant atrophic papulosis in lupus erythematosus. Dermatologica 1987;175(1):45–46.

D283. Douvas AS, Achten M, Tan EM. Identification of a nuclear protein (Sc1–70) as a unique target of human antinuclear antibodies in scleroderma. J Biol Chem 1979;254:10514-10522.

D284. Dowdy MJ, Nigra TP, Barth WF. Subacute cutaneous lupus erythematosus during PUVA therapy for psoriasis: case report and review of the literature. Arthritis Rheum 1989 Mar;32(3): 343–346.

D285. Downing JG, Messina SJ. Acute disseminated lupus erythematosus associated with finger lesions resembling lupus pernio. N Engl J Med 1942;227:408–409.

D286. Draznin TH, Esterly NB, Furey NL, DeBofsky H. Neonatal lupus erythematosus. J Am Acad Dermatol 1979;1:437–442.

D287. Drenkard C, Sanchez-Guerrero J, Alarcon-Segovia D. Fall in antiphospholipid antibody at time of thromboocclusive episodes in systemic lupus erythematosus. J Rheumatol 1989;16: 614.

D288. Dresser DW. Specific inhibition of antibody production. I. Protein-over-loading paralysis. Immunology 1962;5:161–168.

D289. Drew SI, Terasaki PI. Autoimmune cytotoxic granulocyte antibodies in normal persons and various diseases. Blood 1978;52:941–952.

D290. Dreyfus JN, Schnitzer TJ. Pathogenesis and differential diagnosis of the swan-neck deformity. Semin Arthritis Rheum 1983 Nov;13(2):200–211.

D291. Drinkard JP, Stanley TM, Dornfeld L, Austin RC, Barnett EV, Pearson CM, Vernier RL, Adams DA, Latta H, Gonick HC. Azathioprine and prednisone in the treatment of adults with lupus nephritis. Clinical, histological, and immunological changes with therapy. Medicine 1970 Sep;49(5):411–432.

D292. Drosos AA, Dimou GS, Siamopoulou-Mavridou A, Pennec YL, Youinou P, Moutsopoulos HM. The neonatal lupus erythematosus syndrome in Greece and France, a prospective study. Hungarian Rheumatology Abstracts of the XIIth European Congress of Rheumatology, 1991;XXXII:50 (SW14- 105).

D293. Drosos AA, Petris CA, Petroutsos GM, Moutsopoulos HM. Unusual eye manifestations in systemic lupus erythematosus patients. Clin Rheumatol 1989 Mar;8(1):49–53.

D294. Drosos AA, Constantopoulos SH, Moutsopoulos HM. Tuberculo sis spondylitis: a cause for paraplegia in lupus. Rheumatol Int 1985;5:185–186.

D295. Drouhin F, Fischer D, Vadrot J, Denis J, Johanet C, Abuaf N, Feldmann G, Labayle D. Idiopathic portal hypertension associated with connective tissue disease similar to systemic lupus erythematosus [English abstract]. Gastroenterol Clin Biol 1989 Oct;13(10):829–833.

D296. Druet P, Bernard A, Hirsch F, Weening JJ, Gengoux P, Mahieu P, Birkenland S. Immunologically mediated glomerulonephritis induced by heavy metals. Arch Toxicol 1982;50: 187–194.

D297. Druzin ML, Fox A, Kogut E, Carlson C. The relationship of the nonstress test to gestational age. Am J Obstet Gynecol 1985;153:386–389.

D298. Druzin ML, Gratacos J, Keegan KA, Paul RH. Antepartum fetal heart rate testing: The significance of fetal bradycardia. Am J Obstet Gynecol 1981;139:194–198.

D299. Druzin ML, Lockshin M, Edersheim TG, Hutson JM, Krauss AL, Kogut E. Second trimester fetal monitoring and preterm delivery in pregnancies with systemic lupus erythematosus and/or circulating anticoagulant. Am J Obstet Gynecol 1987; 157:1503–1510.

D300. Du LTH, Wechsler B, Lefebvre G, Piette JC, Darbois Y, Godeau P. Systemic lupus erythematosus and ovarian seminoma. Rev Med Interne 1988;9:133–135.

D301. Dubin HV, Courter MH, Harrell ER. Toxoplasmosis. A complication of corticosteroid and cyclophosphamide-treated lupus erythematosus. Arch Dermatol 1971 Nov;104: 547–550.

D302. Dubnow MH, McPherson JR, Bowie EJ. Lupus erythematosus presenting as an acute abdomen. Minn Med 1966 Apr;49: 577- 579.

D303. Dubois EL. Systemic lupus erythematosus: Recent advances in its diagnosis and treatment. Ann Intern Med 1951 Aug;45:163.

D304. Dubois EL. Symposium on recent advances in medicine; systemic lupus erythematosus. Med Clin North Am 1952 Jul; 36:1111–1125.

D305. Dubois EL. Acquired hemolytic anemia as presenting syndrome of lupus erythematosus disseminatus. Am J Med 1952 Feb;22:197–204.

D306. Dubois EL. Effect of LE cell test on clinical picture of systemic lupus erythematosus. Ann Intern Med 1953 Jun;38: 1265–1294.

D307. Dubois EL. Nitrogen mustard in treatment of systemic lupus erythematosus. Arch Intern Med 1954 May;93: 667–672.

D308. Dubois EL. Effect of quinacrine (atabrine) upon lupus erythematosus phenomenon. Arch Dermatol 1955 May;71: 570- 574.

D309. Dubois EL. Prednisone and prednisolone in the treatment of systemic lupus erythematosus. JAMA 1956 Jun 2;161:427-433.

D310. Dubois EL. Systemic lupus erythematosus: recent advances in its diagnosis and treatment. Ann Intern Med 1956 Aug;45:163–184.

D311. Dubois EL. Triamcinolone in the treatment of systemic lupus erythematosus. JAMA 1958 Jul 26;1590–1599.

D312. Dubois EL. Evaluation of steroids in systemic lupus erythematosus. Metabolism 1958 Jul;7:509–525.

D313. Dubois EL. Systemic lupus erythematosus: results of treatment with triamcinolone. CA Med 1958 Sep;89:195–203.

D314. Dubois EL. Methylprednisolone (Medrol) in the treatment of systemic lupus erythematosus. JAMA 1959 Jul 25;170: 1537–1542.

D315. Dubois EL. Current therapy of systemic lupus erythematosus. JAMA 1960 Aug 13;173:1633–1640.

D316. Dubois EL. Paramethasone in the treatment of systemic lupus erythematosus. Analysis of results in 51 cases with emphasis on single daily dose oral administration. JAMA 1963 May 11;184:463–469.

D317. Dubois EL. Management of systemic lupus erythematosus. Mod Treat 1966;3:1245–1279.

D318. Dubois EL. The relationship between discoid and systemic lupus erythematosus. Ch. 10 In: Dubois EL, editor. Lupus Erythematosus, 1st ed. New York: McGraw Hill, 1966.

D319. Dubois EL. Procainamide induction of a systemic lupus erythematosus-like syndrome. Presentation of six cases, review of the literature, and analysis and follow-up of reported cases. Medicine 1969;48:217–228.

D320. Dubois EL. Management and prognosis of systemic lupus erythematosus. Bull Rheum Dis 1968 Nov;18:477–482.

D321. Dubois E. Clinical Picture of Systemic Lupus Erythematosus [Ch 9]. In: Dubois E, editor. Lupus Erythematosus. Los Angeles: USC Press, 1974:232–379.

D322. Dubois EL. Ibuprofen for systemic lupus erythematosus [letter]. N Engl J Med 1975 Oct 9;293(15):779.

D323. Dubois EL, editor. Lupus Erythematosus. A Review of the Current Status of Discoid and Systemic Lupus Erythematosus and Their Variants, 2nd ed revised. Los Angeles: USC Press, 1976.

D324. Dubois EL, editor. Lupus Erythematosus. A Review of the Current Status of Discoid and Systemic Lupus Erythematosus and Their Variants, 2nd ed revised. Los Angeles: USC Press, 1976;232–242.

D325. Dubois EL. Antimalarials in the management of discoid and systemic lupus erythematosus. Semin Arthritis Rheum 1978 Aug;8(1):33–51.

D325a. Dubois EL, Adler DC. Single daily dose oral administration of corticosteroids in rheumatic disorders: An analysis of its advantages, efficacy, and side effects. Curr Ther Res 1963 Feb;5:43–56. [abstract] Arthritis Rheum 1962 Jun 5:293.

D326. Dubois EL, Bulgrin JG, Jacobson G. The corticosteroid-induced peptic ulcer; a serial roentgenological survey of patients receiving high dosages. Am J Gastroenterol 1960 Apr; 33:435–453.

D327. Dubois EL, Bulgrin JG, Jacobson G. The corticosteroid-induced peptic ulcer: A serial roentgenological survey of patients receiving high dosages. In: Mills LC, Moyer JH, editors. Inflammation and Diseases of Connective Tissue. A Hahnemann Symposium. Philadelphia: Saunders, 1961:648- 660.

D328. Dubois EL, Chandor S, Friou GJ, Bischel M. Progressive systemic sclerosis (PSS) and localized scleroderma (morphea) with positive LE cell test and unusual systemic manifestations compatible with systemic lupus erythematosus (SLE): presentation of 14 cases including one set of identical twins, one with scleroderma and the other with SLE. Review of the literature. Medicine 1971 May;50:199–222.

D329. Dubois EL, Commons RR, Starr P, Stein CS Jr, Morrison R. Corticotropin and cortisone treatment for systemic lupus erythematosus. JAMA 1952 Jul 12;149(11):995–1002.

D330. Dubois EL, Cozen L. Avascular (aseptic) bone necrosis associated with systemic lupus erythematosus. JAMA 1960 Oct 20;174:966–971.

D331. Dubois EL, Friou GJ, Chandor S. Rheumatoid nodules and rheumatoid granuloma in systemic lupus erythematosus. JAMA 1972 Apr 24;220:515–518.

D332. Dubois EL, Horowitz RE, Demopoulos HB, Teplitz R. NZB/ MZW mice as a model of systemic lupus erythematosus. JAMA 1966;195:285.

D333. Dubois EL, Katz YJ, Freeman V, Garbak F. Chronic toxicity studies of hydralazine in dogs. J Lab Clin Med 1957;50:119.

D334. Dubois EL, Martel S. Discoid lupus erythematosus; Analysis of its systemic manifestations. Ann Intern Med 1956 Mar; 44:482–496.

D335. Dubois EL, Patterson C. Ineffectiveness of beta-carotene in lupus erythematosus [letter]. JAMA 1976 Jul;236(2):138-139.

D336. Dubois EL, Ross GN, Quismorio FP, Siemsen JK. Brain scans in systemic lupus erythematosus (SLE) [abstract]. Clin Res 1976 Feb;24:149A.

D337. Dubois EL, Strain L. Effect of diet on survival and nephropathy of NZB-NZW hybrid mice. Biochem Med 1973;7: 336–342.

D338. Dubois EL, Strain L, Ehn M, Bernstein G, Friou GJ. LE cells after oral contraceptives [letter]. Lancet 1968;2:679.

D339. Dubois EL, Tallman E, Wonka RA. Chlorpromazine (Thorazine) induced systemic lupus erythematosus (SLE). Case report and review of the literature. JAMA 1972 Aug 7;221: 595–596.

D340. Dubois EL, Tuffanelli DL. Clinical manifestations of systemic lupus erythematosus. Computer analysis of 520 cases. JAMA 1964 Oct 12;190:104–111.

D341. Dubois EL, Wallace DJ. Clinical and laboratory manifestations of systemic lupus erythematosus. Ch. 18. In: Wallace DJ, Dubois EL, editors. Dubois' Lupus Erythematosus, 3rd ed. Philadelphia: Lea & Febiger, 1987.

D342. Dubois EL, Wierzchowiecki M, Cox MB, Weiner JM. Duration and death in systemic lupus erythematosus. An analysis of 249 cases. JAMA 1974 Mar 25;227:1399–1402.

D343. Dubois RW, Weiner JM, Dubois EL. Dermatoglyphic study of systemic lupus erythematosus. Arthritis Rheum 1976 Jan–Feb;19(1):83–87.

D344. Dubowitz LMS, Dubowitz V, Goldberg C. Clinical assessment of gestational age in the newborn infants. J Pediatr 1970; 77:1–4.

D345. Dubroff LM, Reid RI. Hydralazine-pyrimidine interactions may explain hydralazine-induced lupus erythematosus. Science 1980 Apr;208:404–406.

D346. Dubroff LM, Reid RI, Papalian M. Molecular models for hydralazine-related systemic lupus erythematosus. Arthritis Rheum 1981;24:1082–1085.

D347. Duchosal MA, Kofler R, Balderas RS, Aguado MT, Dixon FJ, Theofilopoulos AN. Genetic diversity of murine rheumatoid factors. J Immunol 1989;142:1737–1742.

D348. Du Clos TW, Marnell L, Zlock LR, Burlingame RW. Analysis of the binding of C-reactive protein to chromatin subunits. J Immunol 1991; 146:1220–1225.

D349. Duffus P, Parbtani A, Frampton G, Cameron JS. Intraglomerular localization of platelet related antigens, platelet factor 4 and beta thromboglobulin in glomerulonephritis. Clin Nephrol 1981;17:288–297.

D350. Dujovne I, Pollak VE, Pirani CL, Dillard M. The distribution and character of glomerular deposits in systemic lupus erythematosus. Kidney Int 1972 Jul;2:33-50.

D351. Dumas R. Lupus nephritis. Arch Dis Child 1985;60:126–128.

D352. Dumont F, Monier JC. Sex dependent lupus erythematosus like syndrome in (NZB × SJL/J) mice. Clin Immunol Immunopathol 1983;29:306–317.

D353. Dumont FJ, Habbersett RC. Alterations of the T-cell population in BXSB mice: early imbalance of 9F3-defined Ly-2 + subsets occurs in the males with rapid onset lupic syndrome. Cell Immunol 1986;101:39–50.

D354. Dunckley H, Gatenby PA, Hawkins B, Naito S, Serjeantson SW. Deficiency of C4A is a genetic determinant of systemic lupus erythematosus in three ethnic groups. J Immunogenet 1987;14:209–218.

D355. Dunckley H, Gatenby PA, Serjeantson SW. DNA typing of HLA-DR antigens in systemic lupus erythematosus. Immunogenet 1986;24:158–162.

D356. Dunckley H, Gatenby PA, Serjeantson SW. T-cell receptor and HLA class II RFLP's in systemic lupus erythematosus. Immunogenet 1988;27:392–395.

D357. Dunkel L, Taino VM, Savilahti E, Eskola J. Effect of endogenous androgens on lymphocyte subpopulations. Lancet 1985:440–441.

D358. Dunn EB, Bottomly K. T15-specific helper T cells: analysis of idiotype specificity by competitive inhibition analysis. Eur J Immunol 1985;15:728.

D359. Dunne JV, Carson DA, Spiegelberg HL, Alspaugh MA, Vaughan JH. IgA rheumatoid factor in the sera and saliva of patients with rheumatoid arthritis and Sjogren's syndrome. Ann Rheum Dis 1979 Apr;38:161–165.

D360. Dunoha CR, Pascual E, Abruzzo JL, Smukler NM. Quinidine-induced lupus erythematosus. Arthritis Rheum 1974;17:322.

D361. Dupont A, Six R. Lupus-like syndrome induced by methyldopa. Br Med J 1982 Sep 11;285:693–694.

D362. Dupont B, editor. In: Immunobiology of HLA, Vol I and II. New York: Springer-Verlag, 1989.

D363. Durback MA, Freeman J, Shumacher VR Jr. Recurrent ibuprofen induced aseptic meningitis: third episode after 200 mg of generic ibuprofen [letter]. Arthritis Rheum 1988 Jun;31(6):813–815.

D364. Dustan HP, Corcoran AC, Haserick JR. Urinary sediment in acute diffuse lupus erythematosus: Nature and response to treatment. National Meeting of the American Federation for Clinical Research; May 1951; NJ: Atlantic City.

D365. Dustan HP, Taylor RD, Corcoran AC, Page IH. Rheumatic and febrile syndromes during prolonged hydralazine therapy. JAMA 1954 Jan 2;154:23–29.

D366. Dustin ML, Springer TA. Role of lymphocyte adhesion receptors in transient interactions and cell locomotion. Ann Rev Immunol 1991;9:27.

D367. Dutt AK, Shaw T. Isonicotinic acid hydrazine (INH) induced syndrome of lupus erythematosus. Indian J Chest Dis Allied Sci 1976;18(3):146–151.

D368. Dutta P, Raiczyk GB, Pinto J. Inhibition of riboflavin metabolism in cardiac and skeletal muscles of rats by quinacrine and tetracycline. J Clin Biochem Nutr 1988;4:203–208.

D369. Duvic M, Jegasothy BV. Acquired ichthyosis with systemic lupus erythematosus. Arch Dermatol 1980 Aug;116(8):952-954.

D370. Duvic M, Steinberg AD, Klassen LW. Effect of the antiestrogen, Nafoxidine, on NZB/W autoimmune disease. Arthritis Rheum 1978 May;21(4):414–417.

D371. Dyadyk AI, Sinyachenko VV, Vasilenko IV, Sinyachenko OV, Chernykh OS, Kobets VG. Lupoid glomerulonephritis in males. 1988;3:5–7.

D372. Dyer HR, Zweiman B. In vivo LE cells. Arthritis Rheum 1969;12:64.

D373. Dykman TR, Cole JL, Iida K, Atkinson J. Polymorphism of the human erythrocyte C3b/C4b receptor. Proc Natl Acad Sci USA 1983;80:1698–1702.

D374. Dykman TR, Gluck OS, Murphy WA, Hahn TJ, Hahn BH. Evaluation of factors associated with glucocorticoid- induced osteopenia in patients with rheumatic diseases. Arthritis Rheum 1985 Apr;28(4):361–368.

D375. Dykman TR, Haralson KM, Gluck OS, Murphy WA, Teitelbaum SL, Hahn TJ, Hahn BH. Effects of oral 1.25-dihydroxy vitamin D and calcium on glucocorticoid-induced osteopenia in patients with rheumatic diseases. Arthritis Rheum 1984 Dec;27(1):1336–1343.

D376. Dykman TR, Hatch JA, Aqua MS, Atkinson J. Polymorphism of the human C3b/C4b receptor: Identification of a rare variant. J Immunol 1985;134:1787–1789.

D377. Dykman TR, Hatch JA, Atkinson JP. Polymorphism of the human C3b/C4b receptors: identification of third allele and analysis of receptor phenotypes in families and patients with systemic lupus. J Exp Med 1989;159:691–703.

D378. Dyrberg T. Molecular mimicry and diabetes. Curr Top Microbiol Immunol 1989; 145:117–126.

D379. Dyrberg T, Petersen JS, Oldstone MBA. Immunological cross-reactivity between mimicking epitopes on a virus protein and a human autoantigen depends on a single amino acid residue. Clin Immunol Immunopathol 1990;54:290–297.

D380. Dyson PJ, Knight AM, Fairchild S, Simpson E, Tomonari K. Genes encoding ligands for deletion of V beta 11 T cells cosegregate with mammary tumor vorus genomes. Nature 1991;349:531–532.

D381. Dzau VJ, Schur PH, Weinstein L. Vibrio fetus endocarditis in a patient with systemic lupus erythematosus. Am J Med Sci 1976 Nov–Dec;272(3):331–334.

D382. Dziubinski EH, Winkelmann RK, Wilson RB. Systemic lupus erythematosus and pregnancy. Am J Obstet Gynecol

E

E1. Eagen JW, Memoli VA, Roberts JL, Matthew GR, Schwartz MM, Lewis EJ. Pulmonary hemorrhage in systemic lupus erythematosus. Medicine 1978 Nov;57(6):545–560.

E2. Eaker EY, Toskes PP. Case report: Systemic lupus erythematosus presenting initially with acute pancreatitis and a review of the literature. Am J Med Sci 1989 Jan;297(1):38–41.

E3. Early P, Huang H, Davis M, Calame K, Hood L. An immunoglobulin heavy chain variable region is generated from three segments of DNA: V_H, D, and J_H. Cell 1980;19:981–992.

E4. Earnshaw WC. Mitotic chromosome structure. BioEssays 1988; 9:147–150.

E5. Earnshaw WC, Rothfield NF. Identification of a family of human centromere proteins using autoimmune sera from patients with scleroderma. Chromosoma 1985; 91:313–321.

E6. East WR, Lumpkin CR. Systemic lupus erythematosus in the newborn. Minn Med 1969;53:477.

E7. Eastcott JW, Schwartz RS, Datta SK. Genetic analysis of the inheritance of B cell hyperactivity in relation to the development of autoantibodies and glomerulonephritis in NZB × SWR crosses. J Immunol 1983 Nov;131(5):2232–2239.

E8. Easterbrook M. The use of Amsler grids in early chloroquine retinopathy. Ophthalmology 1984 Nov;91(11):1368–1372.

E9. Easterbrook M. Dose relationships in patients with early chloroquine retinopathy. J Rheumatol 1987 Jun;14(3):472-475.

E10. Easterbrook M. Ocular effects and safety of antimalarial agents. Am J Med 1988 Oct 14;85 Suppl 4A:23–29.

E11. Easterbrook M. Useful and diagnostic tests in the detection of early chloroquine retinopathy [abstract]. Arthritis Rheum 1989 Jan;32(1) Suppl:R8.

E12. Easterbrook M. Is corneal deposition of antimalarial any indication of retinal toxicity? Can J Ophthalmol 1991 Aug; 25(5):249–251.

E13. Eberhard A, Shore A, Silverman E, Laxer R. Bowel perforation and interstitial cystitis in childhood systemic lupus erythematosus [case report]. J Rheumatol 1991; :746.

E14. Eberhard BA, Silverman ED, Eddy A, Laxer RM. Occurrence of thyroid abnormalities in childhood systemic lupus erythematosus, [abstract]. Arthritis Rheum 1990 Sep;33(9) Supp: S144.

E15. Ebling FM, Ando DG, Panosian-Sahakian N, Kalunian KC, Hahn BH. Idiotypic spreading promotes the production of pathogenic autoantibodies. J Autoimmunity 1988;1:47–61.

E16. Ebling FM, Hahn BH. Restricted subpopulations of DNA antibodies in kidneys of mice with systemic lupus. Comparison of antibodies in serum and renal eluates. Arthritis Rheum 1980;23(4):392–403.

E17. Ebling FM, Hahn BH. Pathogenic subsets of antibodies to DNA. Intern Rev Immunol 1989;5:79–95.

E18. Ebling FM, Kalunian KC, Fronek Z, Panosian-Sahakian N, Louie JS, McDevitt HO, Hahn BH. Idiotypic characteristics of immunoglobulins associated with human systemic lupus erythematosus. Association of high serum levels of IdGN2 with nephritis but not with HLA Class II genes predisposing to nephritis. Arthritis Rheum 1990;33:978–984.

E19. Edberg JC, Barinsky M, Redecha PB, Salmon JE, Kimberly RP. FcγRIII expressed on cultured monocytes is a N-glycosylated transmembrane protein distinct from FcγRIII expressed on natural killer cells. J Immunol 1990;144:4729–4734.

E20. Edberg JC, Kujala GA, Taylor RP. Rapid immune adherence reactivity of nascent, soluble antibody/DNA immune complexes in the circulation. J Immunol 1987;139:1240–1244.

E21. Edberg JC, Kujala GA, Taylor RP. Clearance kinetics and immunochemistry in rabbits of soluble antibody/DNA immune complexes. J Immunol 1987;139:180–187.

E22. Edberg JC, Salmon JE, Kimberly RP. The functional capacity of Fcγ receptor III (CD16) on human neutrophils. Pathobiology 1992 In press.

E23. Edberg JC, Salmon JE, Whitlow M, Kimberly RP. Preferential expression of human Fcγ $RIII_{PMN}$ (CD16) in paroxysmal nocturnal hemoglobinuria. J Clin Invest 1991;87:58–67.

E24. Edberg JC, Taylor PR. Quantitative aspects of lupus anti-DNA autoantibody specificity. J Immunol 1986;136: 4581–4587.

E25. Edberg JC, Tosic CL, Taylor RP. Immune adherence and the processing of soluble complement-fixing antibody/DNA immune complexes in mice. Clin Immunol Immunopathol 1989;51:118–132.

E26. Edberg JC, Tosic CL, Wright E, Sutherland W, Taylor RP. Quantitative analysis of the relationship between C3 consumption, C3b capture, and immune adherence of complement fixing antibody/DNA complexes. J Immunol 1988;141: 4258–4265.

E27. Edberg JC, Wright E, Taylor RP. Quantitative analyses of the binding of soluble complement-fixing antibody/dsDNA immune complexes to CR1 on human red blood cells. J Immunol 1987;139:3739–3747.

E28. Edelen JS, Lockshin MD, LeRoy EC. Gonococcal arthritis in two patients with active lupus erythematosus. A diagnostic problem. Arthritis Rheum 1971 Sep– Oct;14:557–559.

E29. Edelstein PH. Legionnaires' disease [letter]. Arthritis Rheum 1978 Jul;22(7):806.

E30. Edison M, Philen RM, Sewell CM, Voorhess R, Kilbourne EM. L-tryptophan and eosinophilic-myalgia syndrome in New Mexico. Lancet 1990;335:645–648.

E31. Omitted.

E32. Edmunds SE, Ganju V, Beveridge BR, French MA, Quinlan MF. Protein-losing enteropathy in systemic lupus erythematosus. Aust N Z J Med 1988 Dec;18(7):868–871.

E33. Edon JR, Vogt JM, Hasegawa DR. Abnormal prothrombin crossed-immunoelectrophoresis in patients with lupus inhibitors. Blood 1984;64:807.

E34. Edwards JCW, Snaith ML, Isenberg DA. A double blind controlled trail of methylprednisolone infusions in systemic lupus erythematosus using individualized outcome assessment. Ann Rheum Dis 1987;46:773–776.

E35. Edwards JM, Moulds JJ, Judd WJ. Chloroquine dissociation of antigen-antibody complexes. A new technique for typing red blood cells with a positive direct antiglobulin test. Transfusion 1982 Jan– Feb;22(1):59–61.

E36. Edwards RL, Rick ME, Wakem CJ. Studies on a circulating anticoagulant in procainamide-induced lupus erythematosus. Arch Intern Med 1981 Nov;141:1688–1690.

E37. Edworthy SM, Albridge K, Farinas C, Bloch DA, Strober S. Renal outcome and survival of lupus patients treated with total lymphoid irradiation (TLI) compared with two control groups: Biologically matched pairs and intention to treat patients [abstract]. Arthritis Rheum 1989 Jan;32(1) Suppl:R20.

E38. Edworthy SM, Bloch DA, Mc Shane DJ, Segal MR, Fries JF. A "state model" of renal function in systemic lupus erythematosus: Its value in the prediction of outcome in 292 patients. J Rheumatol 1989;16:29–35.

E39. Edworthy SM, Fritzler MJ, Kelly JK, McHattie JD, Shaffer EA. Protein-losing enteropathy in systemic lupus erythematosus associated with intestinal lymphangiectasia. Am J Gastroenterol 1990 Oct;85(10):1398–1402.

E40. Edworthy SM, Zatarain E, McShane DJ, Bloch DA. Analysis of the 1982 ARA lupus criteria data set by recursive partitioning methodology: new insights to the relative merit of individual criteria. J Rheumatol 1988;15:1493- 1498.

E41. Egido J, Crespo MS, Lahoz C, Garcia R, Lopez-Trascasea M, Hernando L. Evidence of an immediate hypersensitivity mechanism in systemic lupus erythematosus. Ann Rheum Dis 1980 Aug;39:321–327.

E42. Ehlers S, Smith KA. Differentiation of T cell lymphokine gene expression: The in vitro acquisition of T cell memory. J Exp Med 1991;173:25–36.

E43. Ehrenfeld M, Nesher R, Merin S. Delayed-onset chloroquine retinopathy. Br J Ophthalmol 1986 Apr;70(4):281–283.

E44. Ehrfeld H, Renz M, Seelig HP, Hartung K, Delcher H, Coldewey R. Antibodies to recombinant U1–70K and U1-A protein in systemic lupus erythematosus (SLE). Mol Biol Reports 1991;15:190.

E45. Eichacker PQ, Pinsker K, Epstein A, Schiffenbauer J, Graysez A. Serial Pulmonary function testing in patients with systemic lupus erythematosus. Chest 1988;94:129–132.

E46. Eichmann K, Rajewsky K. Production of T and B cell immunity by anti-idiotypic antibodies. Eur J Immunol 1975;5:661.

E47. Eichner HL, Schambelan M, Biglieri EG. Systemic lupus erythematosus with adrenal insufficiency. Am J Med 1973 Nov;55:700–705.

E48. Eidinger D, Garrett TJ. Studies of the regulatory effects of sex hormones on antibody formation and stem cell differentiation. J Exp Med 1972;136:1098–1162.

E49. Eilat D. Cross-reactions of anti-DNA antibodies and the central dogma of lupus nephritis. Immunol Today 1985;6:123-127.

E50. Eilat D, Hochberg M, Tron F, Jacob L, Bach JF. The Vh gene sequences of anti-DNA antibodies in two different strains of lupus-prone mice are highly related. Eur J Immunol 1989;19:1241–1246.

E51. Eilat D, Rischel R, Zlotnick A. A central anti-DNA idiotype in human and murine systemic lupus erythematosus. Eur J Immunol 1985;15:187–193.

E52. Eilat D, Webster DM, Rees AR. V region sequences of anti-DNA and anti-RNA autoantibodies from NZB/NZW F1 mice. J Immunol 1988 Sep 1;141(5):1745–1753.

E53. Eilat DR, Rischel R, Zlotnick A. A central anti-DNA idiotype in human and murine systemic lupus erythematosus. Eur J Immunol 1985;15:368.

E54. Einck L, Dibble R, Frado LLY, Woodcock CLF. Nucleosomes as antigens: Characterization of determinants and cross-reactivity. Exp Cell Res 1982; 139:101–110.

E55. Einhorn S, Horowitz Y, Einhorn M. Ischemic colitis in systemic lupus erythematosus. Treatment with corticosteroids. Rev Rheum Mal Osteoartic 1986 Nov;53(11):669.

E56. Eisen B, Demis DJ, Crosby WH. Thioguanine therapy. Systemic lupus erythematosus, atopic dermatitis, and other non-malignant disorders. JAMA 1982:789–791.

E57. Eisenberg H, Dubois EL, Sherwin RP, Balcum OJ. Diffuse interstitial lung disease in systemic lupus erythematosus. Ann Intern Med 1973;79:37–45.

E58. Eisenberg RA, Cohen PL. Mechanisms of autoantibody production in systemic lupus erythematosus. Clin Aspects Autoimmunity 1988;2:8–17.

E59. Eisenberg RA, Craven SY, Cohen PL. The stochastic control of anti-Sm autoantibodies in MRL/Mp-lpr/lpr mice. J Clin Invest 1987;80:691–697.

E60. Eisenberg RA, Craven SY, Cohen PL. Isotype progression and clonality of anti-Sm autoantibodies in MRL/Mp-lpr/lpr mice. J Immunol 1987;139:728–733.

E61. Eisenberg RA, Craven SY, Fisher CL, Morris SC, Rapoport R, Pisetsky DS, Cohen PL. The genetics of autoantibody production in MRL/lpr lupus mice. Clin Exp Rheumatol 1989;7 Suppl 3:S35-S40.

E62. Eisenberg RA, Dixon FJ. Effect of castration of male- determined acceleration of autoimmune disease in BXSB mice. J Immunol 1980;125:1959–1963.

E63. Eisenberg RA, Dyer K, Craven SY, Fuller CR, Yount WJ. Subclass restriction and polyclonality of the systemic erythematosus marker antibody anti-Sm. J Clin Invest 1985;75:1270–1277.

E64. Eisenberg RA, Izui S, McConahey PJ, Hang L, Peters CJ, Theofilopoulos AN, Dixon FJ. Male determined accelerated autoimmune disease in BXSB mice transfer by bone marrow and spleen cells. J Immunol 1980;125:1032.

E65. Eisenberg RA, Pisetsky DS, Craven SY, Grudier JP, O'Donnell MA, Cohen PL. Regulation of the anti-Sm autoantibody response in SLE mice by non-anti-Sm antibodies. J Clin Invest 1990;85:86–92.

E66. Eisenberg RA, Theofilopoulos AN, Dixon FJ. Use of bovine conglutinin for the assay of immune complexes. J Immunol 1977;118:1428–1434.

E67. Eisenberg RA, Winfield JB, Cohen PL. Subclass restriction of anti-Sm antibody in MRL mice. J Immunol 1982;129:2146–2149.

E68. Eiser AR, Katz SM, Swartz C. Clinically occult diffuse proliferative lupus nephritis: An age related phenomenon. Arch Int Med 1979 sep;139:1022–1025.

E69. Ekelund M, Ahren B, Hakanson R, Lindquist T, Sundler F. Quinacrine accumulates in certain peptide hormone-producing cells. Histochemistry 1980;66(1):1–9.

E70. Elder MG, de Swiet M, Robertson A, Elder MA, Floyd E, Hawkins DF. Low-dose aspirin in pregnancy [letter]. Lancet 1988 Feb 20;1(8582):410.

E71. Eldredge NT, Robertson WVB, Miller JJ. The interaction of lupus-inducing drugs with deoxyribonucleic acid. Clin Immunol Immunopathol 1974;3:263–271.

E72. El Ghobarey A, Grennan D, Hadidi T, El-Bodawy S. Aortic incompetence in systemic lupus erythematosus. Br Med J 1976 Oct 16;2:915–916.

E73. el-Habib R, Laville M, Traeger J. Specific adsorption of circulating antibodies by extracorporeal plasma perfusions over antigen coated collagen flat-membranes: Application to systemic lupus erythematosus. J Clin Lab Immunol 1984;15:111–117.

E74. Elias M, Eldor A. Thromboembolism in patients with the 'lupus'-type circulating anticoagulant. Arch Intern Med 1984 Mar;144(3):510–515.

E75. Elkayam U, Weiss S, Laniado S. Pericardial effusion and mitral valve involvement in systemic lupus erythematosus: echocardiographic study. Ann Rheum Dis 1977 Aug;36:349–353.

E76. Elkinton JR, Hunt AD Jr, Godrey L, McCrory WW, Rogerson AG, Stokes J Jr. Effects of pituitary adrenocorticotropic hormone (ACTH) therapy. JAMA 1949 Dec 31;141:1273–1279.

E77. Elkon KB, Bonfa E, Llovet R, Eisenberg RA. Association between anti-Sm and anti-ribosomal P protein autoantibodies in human systemic lupus erythematosus and MRL/lpr mice. J Immunol 1989;143:1549–1554.

E78. Elkon KB, Hines JJ, Chu JL, Parnassa A. Epitope mapping of recombinant HeLa Sm B and B' peptides obtained by the polymerase chain reaction. J Immunol 1990;145:636–643.

E79. Elkon KB, Parnassa AP, Foster CL. Lupus antibodies target ribosomal P proteins. J Exp Med 1985;162;459- 471.

E80. Elkon KB, Sewell JR, Ryan PF, Hughes GRV. Splenic function in non-renal systemic lupus erythematosus. Am J Med 1980; 69:80–82.

E81. Elkon KB, Skelly S, Parnassa AP, Moller W, Danko W, Weissbach H, Brot N. Identification and chemical synthesis of a ribosomal protein antigenic determinant in systemic lupus erythematosus. Proc Natl Acad Sci USA 1986;83:7419.

E82. Elkon KB, Walport MJ, Rynes RI, Black CM, Batchelor JR, Hughes GRV. Circulating c1q binding immune complexes in relatives of patients with systemic lupus erythematosus. Arthritis Rheum 1983;26:921–924.

E83. Elling P. On the incidence of antinuclear factors in rheumatoid arthritis. Acta Rheumatol Scand 1967;13:102- 112.

E84. Ellis FA, Bereston ES. Lupus erythematosus associated with pregnancy and menopause. Arch Dermatol Syph 1952;65:170–176.

E85. Ellis SG, Verity MA. Central nervous system involvement in systemic lupus erythematosus: a review of neuropathologic findings in 57 cases. 1955–1977. Semin Arthritis Rheum 1979 Feb;8(3):212–221.

E86. Ellman MH, Pachman L, Medof ME. Raynaud's phenomenon and initially seronegative mixed connective tissue disease. J Rheumatol 1981 Jul–Aug;8(4):632–634.

E87. Ellrodt AG, Murata GH, Riedinger MS, Stewart ME, Mochizuki C, Gray R. Severe neutropenia associated with sustained-release procainamide. Ann Intern Med 1984;100:197–201.

E88. Elman A, Gullberg R, Nilsson E, Rendahl E, Wachtmeister L. Chloroquine retinopathy in patients with rheumatoid arthritis. Scand J Rheumatol 1976;5:161–166.

E89. Elmasry MN, Fox EJ, Rich RR. Sequential effects of prostaglandins and interferon-γ on differentiation of CD8+ suppressor cells. J Immunol 1987;139:688–694.

E90. El Mouzan MI, Ahmad MAM, Saleh ALF, Al Sohaiban MO. Myelofibrosis and pancytopenia in systemic lupus erythematosus. Acta Haematol 1988;80:219–222.

E91. Elner VM, Schaffner T, Taylor K, Glagov S. Immunophagocytic properties of retinal pigment epithelium cells. Science 1981 Jan 2;211(4477):74–76.

E92. El-Roeiy A, Sela O, Isenberg DA, Feldman R, Colaco CB, Kennedy RC, Shoenfeld Y. The sera of patients with Klebsiella infections contain a common anti-DNA idiotype (16/6) Id and anti-polynucleotide activity. Clin Exp Immunol 1987;67:507–515.

E93. el Tahir KE. Influence of niridazole and chloroquine on arterial and myometrial prostacyclin synthesis. Br J Pharmacol 1987;92:567–572.

E94. Emancipator SN, Iida K, Nustenzweig V, Gallow GR. Monoclonal antibodies to human complement receptor (CR1). Clin Immunol Immunopathol 1983 May;27:170–175.

E95. Emberger J-M, Navarro M, Oules C, Vallat G, Brunel M. Presence of Sternberg type cells in a case of lupus adenopathy [original in French]. Nouv Presse Med 1976 Sep 25;5:1994.

E96. Emilie D, Wechsler B, Belmatoug N, Etienne P, Godeau P. Perihepatitis and lupus. Rev Med Interne 1985 Oct;6(4):462–463.

E97. Emlen W, Ansari R, Burdick G. DNA-anti-DNA immune complexes. Antibody protection of a discrete DNA fragment from DNase digestion in vitro. J Clin Invest 1984 Jul;74(1):185–190.

E98. Emlen W, Burdick G. Clearance and organ localization of small DNA anti-DNA immune complexes in mice. J Immunol 1988;140:1816–1822.

E99. Emlen W, Burdick G, Carl V, Lachmann PJ. Binding of immune complexes to erythrocyte CR1 facilitates immune complex uptake by macrophages. J Immunol 1989;142:4366–4371.

E100. Emlen W, Mannik M. Effect of DNA size and strandedness on the in vivo clearance and organ localization of DNA. Clin Exp Immunol 1984 Apr;56(1):185–192.

E101. Emlen W, Pisetsky DS, Taylor RP. Antibodies to DNA. A perspective. Arthritis Rheum 1986 Dec;29(12):1417–1426.

E102. Emlen W, Rifai A, Magilavy D, Mannik M. Hepatic binding of DNA is mediated by a receptor on non-parenchymal cells. Am J Pathol 1988;133:40–47.

E103. Emody L, Molnar L, Kellermayer M, Paal M, Wadstrom T. Urinary Escherichia coli infection presenting with jaundice. Scand J Infect Dis 1989;21(5):579–582.

E104. Endo L, Croman LC, Panush RS: Clinical utility of assays for circulating immune complexes. Med Clin NA 1985;69:623-636.

E105. Endre N, Klara V, Istvan J. Verrucous lupus erythematosus. Borgy Venereol Szemie 1989;65:175–178.

E106. Engel GL, Romano J, Ferris EB. Effect of quinacrine (atabrine) on the central nervous system; clinical and electroencephalographic studies. Arch Neurol & Psychiat 1947 Sep;58:337–350.

E107. Engelfriet CA, Van Loghem JJ. Studies on leucocyte iso- and auto-antibodies. Br J Haematol 1961 apr;7:223–238.

E108. Engle EW, Callahan CF, Pincus T, Hochberg MC. Learn helplessness in systemic lupus erythematosus: analysis the rheumatology attitudes index. Arthritis Rheum 1990 Feb;33(2):281.

E109. Englert HJ, Derue GM, Loizou S, Hawkins DF, Elder MG, de Swiet M, Walport MJ, Hughes GRV. Pregnancy and lupus: prognostic indicators and response to treatment. Q J Med 1988;66:125–136.

E110. Englert HJ, Loizou S, Derue GG, Walport MJ, Hughes GR. Clinical and immunologic features of livedo reticularis in lupus: A case-controlled study. Am J Med 1989 Oct;87(4):408–410.

E111. Englund JA, Lucas RV. Cardiac complications in children with systemic lupus erythematosus. Pediatrics 1983;72:724–730.

E112. Enomoto K, Kaji Y, Maymi T, Tsuda Y, Kanaya S, Nagasawa K, Kujino T, Niho Y. Frequency of valvular regurgitation by color doppler echocardiography in systemic lupus erythematosus. Am J Cardiol 1991;67:209–211.

E113. Enriquez JL, Rajaraman S, Kalla A, Brouhard BH, Travis LB. Isolated antinuclear antibody-negative lupus nephropathy in young children. Child Nephrol Urol 1988- 89;9:340–346.

E114. Enzenauer RJ, McKoy J, Vincent D, Gates R. Disseminated cutaneous and synovial Mycobacterium marinum infection in a patient with systemic lupus erythematosus. South Med J 1990 Apr;83(4):471–474.

E115. Enzenauer RJ, West SG, Rubin RL. D-penicillamine-induced lupus erythematosus. Arthritis Rheum 1990;33:1582–1585.

E116. See A237a.

E117. Epstein A, Barland P. The diagnostic value of antihistone antibodies in drug-induced lupus erythematosus. Arthritis Rheum 1985 Feb;28:158–162.

E118. Epstein A, Greenberg M, Halbert S, Kramer L, Barland P. The clinical application of an ELISA technique for the detection of antihistone antibodies. J Rheumatol 1986;13:304–307.

E119. Epstein HC, Litt JZ. Discoid lupus erythematosus in a newborn infant. N Engl J Med 1961;265:1106.

E120. Epstein RJ, Ogler RF, Gatenby PA. Lupus erythematosus and panhypogammaglobulinemia. Ann Intern Med 1984 Jan;100:162–163.

E121. Epstein W, Grausz H. Favorable outcome in diffuse proliferative glomerulonephritis of systemic lupus erythematosus (SLE) [abstract]. Arthritis Rheum 1972;15:437.

E122. Epstein WV. Immunologic events preceding clinical exacerbation of systemic lupus erythematosus. Am J Med 1973 May;54:631–636.

E123. Epstein WV, Tan M. Increased of L-chain proteins in the sera of patients with systemic lupus erythematosus and the synovial fluids of patients with peripheral rheumatoid arthritis. Arthritis Rheum 1966;9:713–719.

E124. Epstein WV, Tan M. Effect of adrenocorticosteroid therapy on L-Chain abnormalities of patients with systemic lupus erythematosus [abstract]. Arthritis Rheum 1967 Jun;10:277.

E125. Erasmus LD. Scleroderma in gold-miners on the Witwatersrand with particular reference to pulmonary manifestations. S Afr J Clin Lab 1957;3:209–231.

E126. Erbe DV, Collins JE, Shen L, Graziano RF, Fanger MW. The effects of cytokines on the expression and function of Fc receptors for IgG on human myeloid cells. Mol Immunol 1990;25:57–67.

E127. Erbsloh F, Baedeker WD. Lupus myopathy. A clinical, electromyographic and bioptic histological study [original in German]. Deutsch Med Wschr 1962 Nov 30;87:2464–2470.

E128. Erhardt CC, Mumford P, Maini RN. Differences in immunochemical characteristics of cryoglobulins in rheumatoid arthritis and systemic lupus erythematosus and their complement-binding properties. Ann Rheum Dis 1984 Jun;43: 451–455.

E129. Erice A, Jordan MC, Chace BA, Fletcher C, Chinnock BJ, Balfour HH Jr. Ganciclovir treatment of cytomegalovirus disease in transplant recipients and other immunocompromised hosts. JAMA 1987 Jun 12;257(22):3082–3087.

E130. Erikson J, personal communication.

E131. Erikson J, Radic MZ, Camper SA, Hardy RR, Carmack C, Weigert M. Expression of anti-DNA immunoglobulin transgenes in non-autoimmune mice. Nature 1991;349: 331–334.

E132. Ermakava TM, Isaeva LA, Curbanov VP. Systemic lupous erythematosus in two uniovular adolescent twins. Vopr. Revmatizma (Russian) 1973;3:32.

E133. Erman A, Azuri R, Raz A. Prostaglandin biosynthesis in rabbit kidney: mepacrine inhibits renomedullary cyclooxygenase. Biochem Pharmacol 1984 Jan 1;33(1):79-82.

E134. Errington SL, Cox KO. Limiting dilution analysis of age and gender-related differences in autoantibody production against bromelain-modified RBC. Int Arch Allergy Appl Immunol 1986;79:276–281.

E135. Ertl HCJ, Skinner MA, Finberg RW. Induction of anti-viral immunity by an anti-idiotypic antibody directed to a Sendai virus specific T helper cell clone. Intern Rev Immunol 1986; 1:41.

E136. Ervin PE, Strom T. Beta-2 microglobulin and its binding activity in serum from patients with SLE. Ann Rheum Dis 1984 Apr;43:267–274.

E137. Esaguy N, Aquas AP, Van Emboden JDA, Silva MT. Mycobacteria and human autoimmune disease. Infect Immun 1991; 59:1117–1125.

E138. Escolar G, Font J, Reverter JC, Lopez-Soto A, Garrido M, Cervera R, Ingelmo M, Castillo R, Ordinas A. Plasma from systemic lupus erythematosus patient with antiphospholipid antibodies promotes platelet aggregation: studies in a perfusion system. Arteriosclerosis 1992;12:196–200.

E139. Esdaile JM, Danoff D, Rosenthall L, Gutkowski A. Deforming arthritis in systemic lupus erythematosus. Ann Rheum Dis 1981 Apr;40(2):124–126.

E140. Esdaile JM, Levinton C, Federgreen W, Hayslett JP, Kashgarian M. The clinical and renal biopsy predictors of long-term outcome in lupus nephritis: A study of 87 patients and review of the literature. Q J Med 1989;72:779–833.

E141. Esdaile JM, Sampalis JS, Lacaille D, Danoff D. The relationship of socioeconomic status to subsequent health status in systemic lupus erythematosus [abstract]. Arthritis Rheum 1988;31:423–427.

E142. Eshhar Z, Benacerraf B, Katz DH. Induction of tolerance to nucleic acid determinants by administration of a complex of nucleoside d-glutamic acid and d-lysine (D-GL). J Immunol 1975;114:872–876.

E143. Eskreis BD, Eng AM, Furey NL. Surgical excision of trauma-induced verrucous lupus erythematosus. J Dermatol Surg Oncol 1988 Nov;14(11):1296–1299.

E144. Espana A, Gutierrez JM, Soria C, Gila L, Ledo A. Recurrent laryngeal palsy in systemic lupus erythematosus. Neurology 1990 Jul;40(7):1143–1144.

E145. Espinoza LR, Jara LJ, Silveira LH. Anticardiolipin antibodies in polymyalgia rheumatica-giant cell arteritis: association with severe vascular complications. Am J Med 1991;90:474–478.

E146. Esscher E, Scott JS. Congenital heart block and maternal systemic lupus erythematosus. Br Med J 1979;1:1235–1238.

E147. Estes D, Christian CL. The natural history of systemic lupus erythematosus by prospective analysis. Medicine 1971 Mar;50:85–95.

E148. Estes D, Larson DL. Systemic lupus erythematosus and pregnancy. Clin Obstet Gynecol 1965;8:307–321.

E149. Estes ML, Ewing-Wilson D, Chou SM, Mitsumoto H, Hanson M, Shirey E, Ratliff NB. Chloroquine neuromyotoxicity. Clinical and pathologic perspective. Am J Med 1987;82(3): 447–455.

E150. Eto H, Arai H, Nishiyama S. Cluster analysis of systemic lupus erythematosus. J Inv Derm 1980 Jun;74:448.

E151. Ette EI, Essien EE, Ogonor JI, Brown-Awala EA. Chloroquine in human milk. J Clin Pharmacol 1987 Jul;27(7): 499–502.

E152. Ette EI, Essien EE, Thomas WO, Brown-Awala EA. Pharmacokinetics of chloroquine and some of its metabolites in healthy volunteers: a single dose study. J Clin Pharmacol 1989 May;29(5):457–462.

E153. Ettinger WH, Bender WL, Goldberg AP, Hazzard WR. Dyslipoproteinemia in systemic lupus erythematosus: effect of corticosteroids. Am J Med 1987;83:503–508.

E154. Ettinger WH, Goldberg AP, Appelbaum-Bowden D, Hazzard WR. Dyslipoproteinemia in systemic lupus erythematosus. Effects of corticosteroids. Am J Med 1987;83:503–508.

E155. Ettinger WH, Hazzard WR. Elevated apolipoprotein-B levels in corticosteroid-treated patients with systemic lupus erythematosus. J Clin Endocrinol Metab 1988;67:425–428.

E156. Euler HH, Gutschmidt HJ, Schmuecking M, Schroeder JO, Loffler H. Induction of remission in severe SLE after plasma exchange synchronized with subsequent pulse cyclophosphamide. Prog Clin Biol Res 1990;337:319–320.

E157. Evans DAP, Bullen MF, Houston J, Hopkins CA, Vetters JM. Antinuclear factor in rapid and slow acetylator patients with isoniazid. J Med Genet 1972 Nar;9:53–56.

E158. Evans J, Reuben A, Craft J. PBC 95 K, a 95-kilodalton nuclear autoantigen in primary biliary cirrhosis. Arthritis Rheum 1991;34:731–736.

E159. Evans JA, Hastings DE, Urowitz MB. The fixed lupus hand deformity and its surgical correction. J Rheumatol 1977;4: 170–175.

E160. Evans OB, Lexow SS. Painful ophthalmoplegia in systemic lupus erythematosus. Ann Neurol 1978 Dec;4(6):584–585.

E161. Evans PM, Lanham DF. Effects of inhibitors of arachidonic acid metabolism on intercellular adhesion of SV40–3T3 cells. Cell Biol Int Rep 1986 Sep;10(9):693–698.

E162. Evans RL, Khalid S, Kinney JL. Antimalarial psychosis revisited. Arch Dermatol 1984 Jun;120(6):765–767.

E163. Evanson S, Passo MH, Aldo-Benson MA, Benson MD. Methylprednisolone pulse therapy for non-renal lupus erythematosus. Ann Rheum Dis 1980;39:399–380.

E164. Everett MA, Coffey CM. Intradermal administration of chloroquine for discoid lupus erythematosus and lichen sclerosus et atrophicus. Arch Dermatol 1961 Jun;83:977–979.

E165. Evertson LR, Gauthier RJ, Shrifin BS. Antepartum fetal heart rate testing: I. Evolution of the non-stress test. Am J Obstet Gynecol 1979;133:29.

E166. Ewald SJ, Refling PH. Analysis of structural differences between Ly-5 molecules of T- and B-cells. Mol Immunol 1985; 22:581–588.

E167. Exner T. Similar mechanisms of lupus anticoagulants. Thromb Haemost 1985 Feb 18;53:15.

E168. Exner T. Comparison of two simple tests for the lupus anticoagulant. Am J Clin Pathol 1985 Feb;83(2):215-218.

E169. Exner T, Koutts J. Autoimmune cardiolipin-binding antibodies in oral anticoagulant patients. Aust N Z J Med 1988 Aug;18(5):669–673.

E170. Exner T, Rickard KA, Kronenberg BH. A sensitive test demonstrating lupus anticoagulant and its behavioral patterns. Br J Haematol 1978 Sep 40:143–151.

E171. Exner T, Rickard KA, Kronenberg H. Studies on phospholipids in the action of a lupus coagulation inhibitor. Pathology 1975 Oct;7(4):319–328.

E172. Exner T, Triplett DA, Taberner DA. Comparison of test methods for the lupus anticoagulant; international survey on lupus anticoagulants -I (ISLA-1). Thromb Haemost 1990;64: 478–484.

E173. Exner T, Triplett DA, Taberner D, Machin SJ. Guidelines for testing and revised criteria for lupus anticoagulants. Thromb Haemost 1991;65:320–322.

E174. Eyanson S, Greist MC, Brandt KD, Skinner B. Systemic lupus erythematosus: association with psoralen- ultraviolet-A treatment of psoriasis. Arch Dermatol 1979 Jan;115(1): 54–56.

E175. Eyanson S, Passo MH, Aldo-Benson MA, Benson MD. Methylprednisolone pulse therapy for nonrenal lupus erythematosus. Ann Rheum Dis 1980 Aug;39:377.

E176. Eyster ME, Jenkins DE Jr. Erythrocyte coating substances in patients with positive direct antiglobulin reactions. Am J Med 1969 Mar;46:360–371.

F

F1. Faaber P, Capel PJ, Rijke GP, Vierwinden G, van de Putte LB, Koene RA. Cross-reactivity of anti-DNA antibodies with proteoglycans. Clin Exp Immunol 1984 Mar;55(3):502–508.

F2. Faaber P, Rijke TP, van de Putte LB, Capel PJ, Berden JH. Cross-reactivity of human and murine anti-DNA antibodies with heparin sulfate. The major glycosaminoglycan in glomerular basement membranes. J Clin Invest 1986 Jun;77(6): 1824–1830.

F3. Fabian RH. Uptake of antineural IgM by CNS neurons: comparison with antineuronal IgG. Neurology 1990;40:419.

F4. Fabré VC, Hodge SJ, Callen JP. Twenty percent of biopsies from sun exposed skin of normal young adults demonstrate positive immunofluorescence [abstract]. Arthritis Rheum 1990 Sep;33(9) Suppl:S129.

F5. Fabré VC, Lear S, Reichlin M, Hodge SJ, Callen JP. Twenty percent of biopsy specimens from sun-exposed skin of normal young adults demonstrates positive immunofluorescence. Arch Dermatol 1991;127:1006–1011.

F6. Fahey JL, Sarna G, Gale RP, Seeger R. Immune interventions in disease. [published erratum appears in Ann Intern Med 1987 May;106(5):783]. Ann Intern Med 1987 Feb;106(2): 257–274.

F7. Fahey PH, Utell MJ, Condemi JJ, Green R, Hyde RW. Raynaud's phenomenon of the lung. Am J Med 1984 Feb;76: 263–269.

F8. Faig D, Karpatkin S. Cumulative experience with a simplified solid-phase radioimmunoassay for the detection of bound anti-platelet IgG, serum auto-allo-, and drug-dependent antibodies. Blood 1982 Oct;60:807–813.

F9. Fairfax MJ, Osborn TG, Williams GA, Tsai CC, Moore TL. Endomyocardial biopsy in patients with systemic lupus erythematosus. J Rheumatol 1988;15:593–596.

F10. Falherty MJ, Winer MH. Antibodies to thrombin in postsurgical patients. Blood 1989;73:1386.

F11. Falk RJ, Dalmasso AP, Kim Y, Lam S, Michael A. Radioimmunoassay of the attack complex of complement in serum from patients with systemic lupus erythematosus. N Engl J Med 1985;315:1584–1589.

F12. Fallett GH, Lospalluto J, Ziff M. Chromatographic and electrophoretic studies of the LE factor. Arthritis Rheum 1958;1: 419–425.

F13. Faludi G, Mills LC, Chayes ZW. Effect of steroids on muscle. Acta Endocrinol (Kobenhavn) 1964;45:68–78.

F14. Falus A, Merety G, Glickman G, Svehag SE, Fabian F, Bozsoky S. Beta-2 microglobulin containing IgG complexes in sera and synovial fluids of rheumatoid arthritis and systemic lupus erythematosus. Scand J Immunol 1980;13(11):25–34.

F15. Fan JL, Himeno K, Tsuru S, Nomoto K. Treatment of autoimmune MRL/Mp-lpr/lpr mice with cholera toxin. Clin Exp Immunol 1987;94–101.

F16. Fan PT, Clements PJ, Eisman J, Yu DT, Fowlston S, Bluestone R. Effects of corticosteroids on the human immune response: Comparison of 1 and 3 daily 1 G intravenous pulses of methylprednisolone. J Lab Clin Med 1978 Apr;91:625–634.

F17. Fanger MW, Shen L, Graziano RF, Guyre PM. Cytotoxicity mediated by human Fc receptors for IgG. Immunol Today 1989;10:92–99.

F18. Farid N, Anderson J. S.L.E.-like reaction after phenylbutazone therapy. Lancet 1971 May 15;1:1022–1023.

F19. Farid NR, Bear JC. Two major genes, linked to HLA and Gm control susceptibility to Graves' disease. Nature 1982;295: 629.

F20. Farid NR, Newton RM, Noel EP, Marshall WH. Gm phenotypes in autoimmune thyroid disease. J Immunogenet 1977;4: 429.

F21. Farnam J, Lavastida MT, Grant JA, Reddi RC, Daniels JC. Antinuclear antibodies in the serum of normal pregnant women: A prospective study. J Allergy Clin Immunol 1984; 73:596–599.

F22. Fassler R, Dietrich H, Kroemer G, Bock G, Brezinschek H, Panel G, Wick G. The role of testosterone in spontaneous autoimmune thyroiditis of obese strain chickens. J Autoimmun 1988;1:97–108.

F23. Fasy TM, Inoue A, Johnson EM, Allfrey VG. Phosphorylation of H1 and H5 histones by cyclic AMP-dependent protein kinase reduces DNA binding. Biochim Biophys Acta 1979;564: 322–334.

F24. Fauci AS, Dale DC, Balow JE. Glucocorticosteroid therapy: mechanisms of action and clinical considerations. Ann Intern Med 1976 Mar;84:304–315.

F25. Fauci AS, Moutsopoulos HM. Polyclonally triggered B cells in the peripheral blood and bone marrow of normal individuals and in patients with systemic lupus erythematosus and Sjogren's syndrome. Arthritis Rheum 1981 Apr;24:577–583.

F26. Fauci AS, Steinberg AD, Haynes BF, Whalen G. Immunoregulatory aberrations in systemic lupus erythematosus. J Immunol 1978;121:1473.

F27. Faulhaber G, Lechner W. Urticarial-Vasculitis with bullous eruptions in systemic lupus erythematosus. Z Hautkr 1987 Jun 1;62(11):839–844.

F28. Faulk WP, Galbraith GM. Transferrin and transferrin-receptors of human trophoblast. In: Hemmings WA, editor. Protein transmissions through living membranes: Proceedings, 2nd Brambell Symposium. Amsterdam: Elsevier/North-Holland, 1979:55–61.

F29. Faulk WP, Jeannet M, Creighton WD, Carbonara A. Immunological studies of the human placenta: characterization of immunoglobulins on trophoblastic basement membranes. J Clin Invest 1974;54:1011–1019.

F30. Faulk WP, Temple A, Lovins RE, Smith N. Antigens of human trophoblast: a working hypothesis for their role in normal and abnormal pregnancies. Proc Nat Acad Sci 1978;75: 1947–1951.

F31. Fava GA, Sonino N. Hypothalamic-pituitary-adrenal axis disturbances in depression. IRCS Med Sci 1986; 14:1058–1061.

F32. Favre H, Chatelanat F, Miescher PA. Autoimmune hematologic diseases associated with infraclinical systemic lupus erythematosus in four patients: a human equivalent of the NZB mice. Am J Med 1979 Jan;66:91–95.

F33. Favre H, Miescher PA, Huang YP, Chatelanat F, Mihatsch MJ. Ciclosporin in the treatment of lupus nephritis. Am J Nephrol 1989;9 Suppl 1:57–60.

F34. Fayemi AO. The lung in systemic lupus erythematosus: a clinico-pathologic study of 20 cases. Mt Sinai J Med N Y 1975 Mar–Apr;142:110–118.

F35. Fazekas T, Szekeres L. Effect of chloroquine in experimental myocardial ischemia. Acta Physiol Hung 1988;72(2): 191–199.

F36. Fearon DT. Identification of the membrane glycoprotein that is the C3b receptor of the human erythrocyte, polymorphonuclear leucocyte, B lymphocyte, and monocyte. J Exp Med 1980;152:20–30.

F37. Fearon DT. Complement as a mediator of inflammation. Clin Immunol Allergy 1981;1:225–242.

F38. Fearon DT. Cellular receptors for fragments of the third component of complement. Immunol Today 1984;5: 105–110.

F39. Fearon DT, Wong WW. Complement ligand-receptor interactions that mediate biological responses. Ann Rev Immunol 1983;1:243–271.

F40. Federlin K, Becker H. Borrelia infection and systemic lupus erythematosus [English abstract]. Immun Infekt 1989 Dec; 17(6):195–198.

F41. Fedorko M. Effect of chloroquine on morphology of cytoplasmic granules in maturing human leukocytes-an ultrastructural study. J Clin Invest 1967 Dec;46:1932–1942.

F42. Fedrick JA, Pandey JP, Chen Z, Fudenberg HH, Ainsworth SK, Dobson RL. Gm allotypes in blacks with systemic lupus erythematosus. Arthritis Rheum 1985;28:828–830.

F43. Feeney AJ. Lack of N regions in fetal and neonatal mouse immunoglobulin V-D-J junctional sequences. J Exp Med 1990; 172:1377–1390.

F44. Feinberg BB, Gonik B. General precepts of the immunology of pregnancy. Clin Obstet Gynecol 1991;34:3–16.

F45. Feinfield RE, Hesse RJ, Rosenberg SA. Orbital inflammatory disease associated with systemic lupus erythematosus. S Med J, S Med Assoc 1991 Jan;84(1):98–99.

F46. Feinglass EJ, Arnett FC, Dorsch CA, Zizic TM, Stevens MB. Neuropsychiatric manifestations of systemic lupus erythematosus; diagnosis, clinical spectrum, and relationship to other feature so the disease. Medicine 1976 Jul;55(4):323–339.

F47. Feinstein D, Rapaport SI. Lupus anticoagulant and other hemostatic problems. In: Wallace DJ, Dubois EL, editors. Lupus erythematosus. Philadelphia: Lea & Febiger, 1987:271.

F48. Feinstein DE, Rapaport SI. Acquired inhibitors of blood coagulation. Prog Hemost Thromb 1968;1:75.

F49. Feinstein DI. Lupus anticoagulant, thrombosis, and fetal loss. N Engl J Med 1985;33:1348.

F50. Feld S, Landau Z, Gefel D, Green L, Resnitzky P. Pernicious anemia, Hashimoto's thyroiditis and Sjogren's in a woman with SLE and autoimmune hemolytic anemia (letter). J Rheumatol 1989 Feb;16(2):258–259.

F51. Feldaker M, Brunsting LA, McKenzie BF. Paper electrophoresis of serum proteins in selected dermatoses. J Invest Dermatol 1956 Apr;26:293–310.

F52. Feldman D, Feldman D, Ginzler E, Kaplan D. Rheumatoid factor in patients with systemic lupus erythematosus. J Rheumatol 1989 May;16(5):618–622.

F53. Feldman MD, Huston DP, Karsh J, Balow JE, Klima E, Steinberg AD. Correlation of serum IgG, IgM and anti-native DNA antibodies with renal and clinical indexes of activity in systemic lupus erythematosus. J Rheumatol 1982 Jan–Feb;9: 52–58.

F54. Feldmann J, Becker MJ, Moutsopoulos H, Fye K, Blackman

M, Epstein WV, Talal N. Antibody dependent cell-mediated cytotoxicity in selected autoimmune diseases. J Clin Invest 1976;58:173.

F55. Fellows G, Gittoes N, Scott DGI, Coppock JS, Wainwright A, Goodall M, Turner BM. Individual variation in the isotype profile of anti-histone autoantibodies in systemic lupus erythematosus. Clin Exp Immunol 1988;72:440–445.

F56. Felson DT, Anderson JA. Treatment of lupus nephritis. N Engl J Med 1986;315:458.

F57. Felson DT, Anderson JJ. Across-study evaluation of association between steroid dose and bolus steroids and avascular necrosis of bone. Lance L 1987 Apr 18;1(8538):902–906.

F58. Feng CS. Atypical lupus erythematosus cells in pleural fluid. Pathology 1989;19:317–319.

F59. Feng PH, Oon CJ, Yo SL, Lan YK. Levamisole in the treatment of systemic lupus erythematosus—preliminary results. Singapore Med J 1978 Sep;19(3):120–124.

F60. Feng PH, Tan TH. Tuberculosis in patients with systemic lupus erythematosus. Ann Rheum Dis 1982 Feb;41(1):11–14.

F61. Fenton DA, Black MM. Low-dose dapsone in the treatment of subacute cutaneous lupus erythematosus. Clin Exp Dermatol 1986 Jan;11(1):102–103.

F62. Fernandes G, Alonso DR, Tanaka T, Taler HT, Yunis EJ, Good RA. Influence of diet on vascular lesions in autoimmune-prone B/W mice. Proc Natl Acad Sci USA 1983;80:874–877.

F63. Fernandes G, Friend P, Yunis EJ, Good RA. Influence of dietary restriction on immunologic function and renal disease in (NZB × NZW) F1 mice. Proc Natl Acad Sci USA 1978;75: 1500–1504.

F64. Fernandes G, Venkatraman J, Khare A, Horback GJ, Friendrichs W. Modulation of gene expression in autoimmune disease and aging by food restriction and dietary lipids. Proc Soc Exp Biol Med 1990;193:16–22.

F65. Fernandes G, Yunis EJ, Good RA. Influence of diet on survival of mice. Proc Natl Acad Sci USA 1976 Apr;73(4): 1279–1283.

F66. Fernandes G, Yunis EJ, Jose DG, Good RA. Dietary influence on antinuclear antibodies and cell-mediated immunity in NZB mice. Int Arch Allergy 1973;44:770–782.

F67. Fernandes G, Yunis EJ, Smith J, Good RA. Dietary influence on breeding behavior, hemolytic anemia and longevity in NZB mice. Proc Soc Exp Biol Med 1972;139:1189–1196.

F68. Fernandez-Botran R, Sanders VM, Mossman TR, Vitetta ES. Lymphokine-mediated regulation of the proliferative response of T helper 1 and T helper 2 cells. J Exp Med 1988;168: 543–558.

F69. Ferrante A, Rowan-Kelly B, Seow WK, Thong YH. Depression of human polymorphonuclear leucocyte function by antimalarial drugs. Immunology 1986 May;58(1):125–130.

F70. Ferreira SJ, Vane JR. New aspects of the mode of action of nonsteroid anti-inflammatory drugs. Ann Rev Pharmacol 1974;14:57.

F71. Ferreiro JE, Reiter WM, Saldana MJ. Systemic lupus erythematosus presenting as an chronic serositis with no demonstrable antinuclear antibodies. Am J Med 1984 Jun;76(6): 1100–1105.

F72. Ferrick DA, Ohashi PS, Wallace V, Schilham M, Mak TW. Thymic ontogeny and selection of γδ and αβ T cells. Immunology Today 1989;10:403–407.

F73. Ferrick DA, Ohashi PS, Wallace VA, Schilham M, Mak TW. Transgenic mice as an in vivo model for self-reactivity. Immunol Rev 1990;118:257–283.

F74. Fessel WJ. Systemic lupus erythematosus in the community. Incidence, prevalence, outcome, and first symptoms; the high prevalence in black women. Arch Intern Med 1974 Dec;134: 1027–1035.

F75. Fessel WJ. Mixed connective tissue diseases [letter]. N Engl J Med 1977 Feb 24;296(8):450.

F76. Fessel WJ. ANA-negative systemic lupus erythematosus. Am J Med 1978 Jan;64(1):80–86.

F77. Fessel WJ. Megadose corticosteroid therapy in systemic lupus erythematosus. J Rheumatol 1980 Jul–Aug;7:486–500.

F78. Fessel WJ. Epidemiology of systemic lupus erythematosus. Rheum Dis Clin North Am 1988;14:15.

F79. Fessel WJ, Solomon GF. Psychosis and systemic lupus erythematosus: Review of the literature and case report. CA Med 1960;92:266–270.

F80. Feutren G, Querin S, Tron F, Noel LH, Chatenoud L, Lesavre P, Bach JF. The effects of cyclosporine in patients with systemic lupus. Transplantation Proceedings 1986;18:643–644.

F81. Ficat RP, Arlet J. Ischemia and necrosis of bone. DS Hungerford editor. Baltimore: Williams & Wilkins, 1980:171–182.

F82. Fiedler AHL, Walport MJ, Batchelor JR, Rynes RI, Black CM, Dodi IA, Hughes GRV. Family study of the major histocompatibility complex in patients with systemic lupus erythematosus: Importance of null alleles of C4A and C4B in determining disease susceptibility. Br Med J [Clin Res] 1983;286:425–428.

F83. Field M, Brennan FM, Melson RD, McCarthy D, Mumford P, Maini RN. MRL mice show an age-related impairment of IgG aggregate removal from the circulation. Clin Exp Immunol 1985;61:195–202.

F84. Field M, Williams DG, Charles P, Maini RN. Specificity of anti-Sm antibodies by ELISA for systemic lupus erythematosus: increase sensitivity of detection using purified peptide antigens. Ann Rheum Dis 1988;47:820–825.

F85. Fielder AH, Walport MJ, Batchelor JR, Rynes RI, Black CM, Dodi IA, Hughes GR. Family study of the major histocompatibility complex in patients with systemic lupus erythematosus: importance of null alleles of C4A and C4B in determining disease susceptibility. Br Med J [Clin Res] 1983;286(6363):425–428.

F86. Fields RA, Sibbitt WL, Toubbeh H, Bankhurst AD. Neuropsychiatric lupus erythematosus, cerebral infarctions, and anticardiolipin antibodies. Ann Rheum Dis 1990 Feb;49(2):114–117.

F87. Fields RA, Toubbeh H, Searles RP, Bankhurst AD. The prevalence of anticardiolipin antibodies in a healthy elderly population and its associations with antinuclear antibodies. J Rheumatol 1989 May;16(5):623–625.

F88. Filippov A, Skatova G, Porotikov V, Kobrinsky E, Saxon M. Ca2 + -antagonistic properties of phospholipase A2 inhibitors, mepacrine and chloroquine. Gen Physiol Biophys 1989 Apr; 8(2):113–118.

F88a. Finazzi G, Cortelazzo S, Viero P, Galli M, Barbui T. Maternal lupus anticoagulant and fatal neonatal thrombosis. Thromb Haemost 1987;58:238.

F89. Finbloom DS, Plotz PH. Studies of reticuloendothelial function in the mouse with model immune complexes. II. Serum clearance, tissue uptake, and reticuloendothelial saturation in NZB/W mice. J Immunol 1979;123:1600–1603.

F90. Finbloom DS, Silver K, Newsome DA, Gunkel R. Antimalarial use and the development of toxic maculopathy [abstract]. Arthritis Rheum 1981;24 Suppl:S82.

F91. Finbloom DS, Silver K, Newsome DA, Gunkel R. Comparison of hydroxychloroquine and chloroquine use and the development of retinal toxicity. J Rheumatol 1985 Aug;12(4): 692–694.

F92. Finch SC, Ross JF, Ebaugh FC Jr. Immunologic mechanisms of leukocyte abnormalities. J Lab Clin Med 1953 Oct;42: 555–569.

F93. Findlay JW, DeAngelis RL, Kearney MF Welch RM, Findlay JM. Analgesic drugs in breast milk and plasma. Clin Pharmacol Ther 1981;29:625–633.

F94. Findlay RF, Odom RB. Toxic shock syndrome in a patient with systemic lupus erythematosus. Int J Dermatol 1982 Apr; 21(3):140–141.

F95. Fine LG, Barnett EV, Danovitch GM, Nissenson AR, Conolly ME, Lieb SM, Barrett CT. Systemic lupus erythematosus in pregnancy Ann Intern Med 1981;94:667–677.

F96. Fine RM. Subacute cutaneous lupus erythematosus associated with hydrochlorothiazide therapy. Int J Dermatol 1989; 28:375–376.

F97. Fingerote RJ, Seigel S, Atkinson MH, Lewkonia RM. Disseminated zygomycosis associated with systemic lupus erythematosus [case report]. J Rheumatol 1990;17(12):1692–1694.

F98. Finkbiner RB, Decker JP. Ulceration and perforation of the intestine due to necrotizing arteriolitis. New Engl J Med 1963 Jan 3;268:14–18.

F99. Finkel HE, Brauer MJ, Taub RN, Dameshek W. Immunologic aberrations in the Di Guglielmo syndrome. Blood 1966 Nov; 28:634–369.

F100. Finn P, Rudolf N, Ade M. The electroencephalogram in systemic lupus erythematosus. Lancet 1978 Jun 10;1:1255.

F101. Finol HJ, Montagnani S, Marquez A, Montes de Oca I, Muller B. Ultrastructural pathology of skeletal muscle in systemic lupus erythematosus. J Rheumatol 1990 Feb;17(2): 210–219.

F102. Firkin BG, Buchanan RRC, Pfueller S, Ryan P. Lupoid thrombocytopenia. Aust N Z J Med 1987;17:295–300.

F103. Firkin BG, Howard MA, Radford N. Possible relationship between lupus inhibitor and recurrent abortion in young women [letter]. Lancet 1980 Aug;2:366.

F104. Fischman AS, Abeles M, Zanetti M, Weinstein A, Rothfield NF. The coexistence of rheumatoid arthritis and systemic lupus erythematosus: A case report and review of the literature. J Rheumatol 1981 May–Jun;8(3):405–415.

F105. Fish AJ, Blau EB, Westberg NG, Burke BA, Vernier RL, Michael AF. Systemic lupus erythematosus within the first two decades of life. Am J Med 1977 Jan;62:99–117.

F106. Fish F, Ziff M. The in vitro and in vivo induction of antidouble-stranded DNA antibodies in normal and autoimmune mice. J Immunol 1982(1);128:409–414.

F107. Fishbein E, Alarcon-Segovia D, Vega JM. Antibodies to histones in systemic lupus erythematosus. Clin Exp Immunol 1979;36:145–150.

F108. Fishbein E, Ramon-Niembro F, Alacon-Segovia D. Free serum ribonucleoprotein in mixed connective tissue disease and other connective tissue diseases. J Rheumatol 1978 Winter;5(4):384–390.

F109. Fisher C, Gibb WRG, Cohen SL, Collins R, Potter A, Isenberg DA. Lupus-like nephritis heralding the definitive manifestation of systemic lupus erythematosus. Br J Rheumatol 1984; 24:256–262.

F110. Fisher CL, Eisenberg RA, Cohen PL. Quantitation and IgG subclass distribution of antichromatin autoantibodies in SLE mice. Clin Immunol Immunopathol 1988 Feb;46(2): 205–213.

F111. Fisher CL, Shores EW, Eisenberg RA, Cohen PL. Cellular interactions for the in vitro production of antichromatin autoantibodies in MRL/Mp-lpr/lpr mice. Clin Immunol Immunopathol 1989;50:231–240.

F112. Fisher DA, Epstein JH, Kay DN, Tuffanelli DL. Polymorphous light eruption and lupus erythematosus. Differential diagnosis by fluorescent microscopy. Arch Dermatol 1970 Apr; 101:458–461.

F113. Fisher DE, Bickel WH. Corticosteroid-induced avascular necrosis. A clinical study of 77 patients. J Bone Joint Surg (Am) 1971 Jul;53A:859–873.

F114. Fisher DE, Bickel WH, Holley KE. Histologic demonstration of fat emboli in aseptic necrosis associated with hypercortisonism. Mayo Clin Proc 1969 Apr;44:252–259.

F115. Fisher DE, Reeves WH, Wisniewolski R, Lahita RG, Chiorazzi N. Temporal shifts from Sm to ribonucleoprotein reactivity in systemic lupus erythematosus. Arthritis Rheum 1985;28:1348–1356.

F116. Fisher KA, Luger A, Spargo BH, Lindheimer MD. Hypertension in pregnancy: clinical-pathological correlations and remote prognosis. Medicine 1981;60:267–76.

F117. Fishl B, Caspi D, Eventov I, Avrahami E, Yaron M. Multiple osteonecrotic lesions in systemic lupus erythematosus. J Rheumatol 1987;14:601–604.

F118. Fishman A, Kinsman JM. Hypoplastic anemia due to atabrine. Blood 1949 Aug;4:970–976.

F119. Fishman J, Martucci C. Biological properties of 16 alpha-hydroxystrone Implications in estrogen physiology and pathophysiology. J Clin Endo Metab 1980;51:611.

F120. Fitchen JJ, Cline MJ, Saxon A, Golde DW. Serum inhibitors of hematopoiesis in a patient with aplastic anemia and systemic lupus erythematosus: recovery after plasmapheresis. Am J Med 1979 Mar;66:537–542.

F121. Fitzgerald A, Russell AS. Identical twins discordant for SLE. Clin Exp Rheumatol 1983;1:73.

F122. Fitzgerald OM, Barnes L, Woods R, McHugh L, Barry C, O'Laughlin S. Direct immunofluorescence of normal skin in rheumatoid arthritis. Br J Rheumatol 1985 Nov;24(4):340–345.

F123. Fitzpatrick EP, Chesen N, Rahn EK. The lupus anticoagulant and retinal vaso-occlusive disease. Ann Ophthalmol 1990 Apr;22(4):148–152.

F124. Fitzsimmons JS, Crawford MJ, Reeves WG. Congenital discoid lupus in the newborn. J Med Genet 1977;14:283–286.

F125. Flaegstad T, Fredriksen K, Dahl B, Traavik T, Rekvig OP. Inoculation with BK virus may break immunological tolerance to histone and DNA antigens. Proc Natl Acad Sci USA 1988;85:8171–8175.

F125a. Flaherty MJ, Winer MH. Antibodies to thrombin in postsurgical patients [letter]. Blood 1987;73:1386.

F126. Flanigan RC, McDougal WS, Griffen WO. Abdominal complications of collagen vascular disease. Am Surg 1983 May;49(5):241–244.

F127. Fleck BW, Bell AL, Mitchell JD, Thomson BJ, Hurst NP, Nuki G. Screening for antimalarial maculopathy in rheumatology clinics. BMJ (Clin Res) 1985 Sep 21;291(6498):782–785.

F128. Fleck RA, Rapaport SI, Rao VM. Antiprothrombin antibodies and the lupus anticoagulant. Blood 1988;Blood 72:512.

F129. Fleming HG, Bergfeld WF, Tomecki KJ, Tuthill RJ, Norris M, Benedetto EA, Weber LA. Bullous systemic lupus erythematosus. Int J Dermatol 1989;28:321–326.

F130. Fletcher JE, Kistler P, Rosenberg H, Michaux K. Dantrolene and mepacrine antagonize the hemolysis human red blood cells by halothane and bee venom phospholipase A2. Toxicol Appl Pharmacol 1987 Sep 30;90(3):410–419.

F131. Flores RH, Stevens MB, Arnett FC. Familial occurrence of progressive systemic sclerosis and systemic lupus erythematosus. J Rheumatol 1984;11:321–323.

F132. Floyd M, Tesar JT. The role of IgM rheumatoid factor in experimental immune vasculitis. Clin Exp Immunol 1979 Apr;36:165–174.

F133. Flynn A. Expression of Ia and the production of interleukin-1 by peritoneal exudate macrophages activated in vivo by steroids. Life Sciences 1986;38:2455–2460.

F134. Flynn JT. Inhibition of complement-mediated hepatic thromboxane production by mepacrine, a phospholipase inhibitor. Prostaglandins 1987 Feb;33(2):287–299.

F135. Foad B, Litwin A, Zimmer H, Hess EV. Acetylator pheno-

type in systemic lupus erythematosus. Arthritis Rheum 1977;20:815.

F136. Folb PI, Trounce JR. Immunological aspects of candida infection complicating steroid and immunosuppressive drug therapy. Lancet 1970 Nov 28;2:1112–1114.

F137. Foldes J. Acute systemic lupus erythematosus. Am J Clin Pathol 1948 Mar;16:160–173.

F138. Foley J. Systemic lupus erythematosus presenting as polymyalgia rheumatica [letter]. Ann Rheum Dis 1987 Apr;46(4):351.

F139. Follea G, Coiffier B, Viale JP, Dechavanne M. Antiprothrombinase and factor ii deficiency in a non-SLE patient [letter]. Thromb Haemost 1981 Oct;46:670.

F140. Folomeev M, Alekberova Z. Impotence in systemic lupus erythematosus [Reply]. J Rheumatol 1990;17(1):117–118.

F141. Folomeev M, Alekberova Z. Survival pattern of 120 males with systemic lupus erythematosus. J Rheumatol 1990;17:856–858.

F142. Folomeev MIu. Use of androgens in the complex treatment of men with systemic lupus erythematosus. Ter Arkh 1986;58:57–59.

F143. Folomeev MIu, Folomeev IuV. Use of androgens in the complex treatment of men with systemic lupus erythematosus. Revmatologiia (Moskva) 1986;Oct–Dec (4):24–26.

F144. Folomeeva DO, Nassonova VA, Alekberova AS, Talal N, Williams RD Jr. Comparative studies of antilymphocyte, antipolynucleotide, and antiviral antibodies among families of patients with systemic lupus erythematosus. Arthritis Rheum 1978;21:23–27.

F145. Fong HJ, Cohen AH. Ibuprofen-induced acute renal failure with acute tubular necrosis, Am J Nephrol 1982;2(1):28–31.

F146. Fong KY, Poh WT, Ng HS. Cryptococcoses of the liver in a systemic lupus erythematosus patient. Singapore Med J 1988 Jun;29(3):309–310.

F147. Fong PH, Chan HL. Systemic lupus erythematosus and pemphigus vulgaris [letter]. Arch Dermatol 1985 Jan;121(1):26–27.

F148. Fonkalsrud EW, Henney P, Riemenschneider TA, Barker WF. Management of pancreatitis in infants and children. Am J Surg 1968;116:198–203.

F149. Font J, Bosch X, Ferrer J, Perez-Villa F, Ingelmo M. Systemic lupus erythematosus and ulcerative colitis [letter]. Lancet 1988 Apr;1(8588):770.

F150. Font J, Bosch X, Ingelmo M, Herrero C, Bielsa I, Mascaro JM. Acquired ichthyosis in a patient with systemic lupus erythematosus [letter]. Arch Dermatol 1990 Jun;126(6):829.

F151. Font J, Cervera R, Lopez-Soto A Pallares L, Bosch X, Ampurdanes S, Casals FJ, Ingelmo M. Anticardiolipin antibodies in patients with autoimmune diseases: isotype distribution and clinical associations. Clin Rheumatol 1989 Dec;8(4):475–483.

F152. Font J, Cervera R, Pallares L, Lopez-Soto A, Ingelmo M. Systemic lupus erythematosus and monoclonal gammopathy. Br J Rheumatol 1988;27:412–413.

F153. Font J, Coca A, Molina R, Ballesta A, Cardellach F, Ingelmo M, Balague A, Balcells A. Serum beta-2 microglobulin as a marker of activity in systemic lupus erythematosus. Scand J Rheumatol 1986;15:201–205.

F154. Font J, Herrero C, Bosch X, Cervera R, Ingelmo M, Mascaro JM. Systemic lupus erythematosus in a patient with partial lipodystrophy. J Am Acad Dermatol 1990 Feb;22(2 Pt 2):337–340.

F155. Font J, Lopez-Soto A, Cervera R, Balasch J, Pallares L, Navarro M, Bosch X, Ingelmo M. The 'primary' antiphospholipids syndrome: Antiphospholipid antibody pattern and clinical features of a series of 23 patients. Autoimmunol 1991;9:69–75.

F156. Font J, Pallares L, Cervera R, Lopez-Soto M, Navarro M,

Bosch X, Ingelmo M. Systemic lupus erythematosus in the elderly. Clinical and serological characteristics. Ann Rheum Dis 1991;50:702−705.

F157. Font J, Torras A, Cevera R, Darnell A, Revert L, Ingelmo M. Silent renal disease in systemic lupus erythematosus. Clin Nephrol 1987;27:283−288.

F158. Fontagne J, Roch-Arveiller M, Giroud JP, Lechat P. Effects of some antimalarial drugs on rat inflammatory polymorphonuclear leukocyte function. Biomed Pharmacother 1989; 43(1):43−51.

F159. Foote RA, Kimbrough SM, Stevens JC. Lupus myositis. Muscle Nerve 1982 Jan;5(1):65−68.

F160. Ford PM. The effect of manipulation of reticuloendothelial system activity on glomerular deposition of aggregated protein and immune complexes in two different strains of mice. Br J Exp Pathol 1975;56:523−529.

F161. Ford PM. Glomerular localization of aggregated protein in mice:effect of strain differences in relationship to systemic macrophage function. Br J Exp Pathol 1976;56:307−313.

F162. Ford PM. Interaction of rheumatoid factor with immune complexes in experimental glomerulonephritis-possible role of antiglobulins in chronicity. J Rheumatol 1983 Dec;Suppl 11:81−84.

F163. Ford PM, Ford SE, Lillicrap DP. Association of lupus anticoagulant with severe valvular heart disease in systemic lupus erythematosus. J Rheumatol 1989;15:597−600.

F164. Ford PM, Kosatka I. The effect of human IgM rheumatoid factor on renal glomerular immune complex deposition in passive serum sickness in the mouse. Immunol 1982 Aug;46: 761−768.

F165. Ford PM, Kosatka I. In situ immune complex formation in the mouse glomerulus: reactivity with human IgM rheumatoid factor and the effect on subsequent immune complex deposition. Clin Exp Immunol 1983 Feb;51:285−291.

F165a. Fordyce J. Lupus erythematosus in a tuberculosis subject: Autopsy report. J Cutaneous Genito-Urin Dis 1899;17: 113−116.

F166. Formica N, Shornick J, Parke A. Resistant cutaneous lupus responds to isoretinoin (Accutane) [abstract]. Arthritis Rheum 1989 Apr;32(4) Suppl:S75.

F167. Fornasieri A, Sinico R, Fiorini G, Goldaniga D, Colasanti G, Bendemia F, Gibelli A, D'Amic G. T-lymphocyte subsets in primary and secondary glomerulonephritis. Proc Eur Dial Transplant Assoc 1983;19:635−641.

F168. Forrister J, Globus J, Brede D, Hudson J, Richardson B. B cell activation in patients with active procainamide induced lupus. J Rheumatol 1988;15:1384−1388.

F169. Forsdyke DR. Evidence for a relationship between chloroquine and complement from studies with lymphocyte mitogens: Possible implications for the mechanism of action of chloroquine in disease. Can J Microbiol 1975 Oct;21(10): 1581−1586.

F170. Fort JG, Cowchock FS, Abruzzo JL, Smith JB. Anticardiolipin antibodies in patients with rheumatic diseases. Arthritis Rheum 1987 Jul;30(7):752−760.

F171. Fortenberry JD, Shew ML. Fatal pneumocystis carinii in an adolescent with systemic lupus erythematosus. J Adolesc Health Care 1989 Nov;10(6):570−572.

F172. Fossaluzza V, Dal Mas P. Proptosis and systemic lupus erythematosus (letter). Clin Exp Rheumatol 1987 Apr−Jun; 5(2):192−193.

F173. Fournie GJ. Circulating DNA and lupus nephritis [editorial review]. Kidney Intern 1988;33(2):487−497.

F174. Fournie GJ, Dueymes JM, Gayral-Taminh H. Pourrat JP, Mignon-Coute MA, Conte JJ. Anti-DNA antibody idiotypes in SLE. Lancet. 1984;2:821−844.

F175. Fournie GJ, Gayral-Taminh M, Bouche JP, Conte JJ. Recovery of nanogram quantities of DNA from plasma and quantitative measurement using labelling by Nick Translation. Anal Biochem 1986;158:250−256.

F176. Fournie GJ, Lambert PH, Miescher PA. Release of DNA in circulating blood and induction of anti-DNA antibodies after injection of bacterial lipopolysaccharides. J Exp Med 1974; 140:1189−1206.

F177. Fowler JF Jr, Callen JP. Cutaneous mucinosis associated with lupus erythematosus. J Rheumatol 1984 Jun;11(3): 380−383.

F178. Fox D, Millard JA, Treisman J, Zeldes W, Bergman A, Depper J, Dunne R, McCune WJ. Defective CD2 pathway T cell activation in systemic lupus erythematosus. Arthritis Rheum 1991;34:561−571.

F179. Fox DA, Faix JD, Coblyn J, Fraser J, Smith B, Weinblatt ME. Thrombotic thrombocytopenic purpura and systemic lupus erythematosus. Ann Rheum Dis 1986;45:319−322.

F180. Fox H. Pathology of the Placenta. Major problems in Pathology. Vol VII. Toronto, 1978.

F181. Fox IS, Spence AM, Wheelis RF, Healey LA. Cerebral embolism in Libman-Sacks endocarditis. Neurology 1980 May;30: 487−491.

F182. Fox R, Hawkins DF. Fetal-pericardial effusion in association with congenital heart block and maternal systemic lupus erythematosus. Case report. Br J Obstet Gynecol 1990;97: 638−640.

F183. Fox R, Lumb MR, Hawkins DF. Persistent fetal sinus bradycardia associated with maternal anti-Ro antibodies. Case report. Br J Obstet Gynecol 1990;7:1151−1153.

F184. Fox RA, Rosahn PD. Lymph nodes in disseminated lupus erythematosus. Am J Pathol 1943 Jan;19:73−99.

F185. Fox RI, Pearson G, Vaughan JH. Detection of Epstein-Barr virus-associated antigens and DNA in salivary gland biopsies from patients with Sjögren's syndrome. J Immunol 1986;137: 3162−3168.

F186. Fox RJ Jr, McCuiston CH, Schoch EP Jr. Systemic lupus erythematosus association with previous neonatal lupus erythematosus. Arch Dermatol 1979;115:340.

F187. Fradis M, Podoshin L, Ben-David J, Statter P, Pratt H, Nahir M. Brainstem auditory evoked potentials with increased stimulus rate in patients suffering from systemic lupus erythematosus. Laryngoscope 1989 Mar;99(3):325−329.

F188. Fraga A, Armendares S, Mintz G, Mora J, Cortes R. Dermatoglyphic patterns in systemic lupus erythematosus (SLE) and their changes in patients with increased fetal wastage. J Rheumatol 1974;1 Suppl:35.

F189. Fraga A, Mintz G. Splinter hemorrhage in SLE. Arthritis Rheum 1966;9:648−649.

F190. Fraga A, Mintz G, Orozco J, Orozco JH. Sterility and fertility rates, fetal wastage and maternal morbidity in systemic lupus erythematosus. J Rheumatol 1974;1:293−298.

F191. Frampton G, Cameron JS. purified antiphospholipid antibodies form lupus nephritis patients enhance thromboxane (TXB2) production by activated platelets [abstract]. Clin Exp Rheumatol 1988;6:203.

F192. Frampton G, Cameron JS, Thom M, Jones S, Raftery M. Successful removal of antiphospholipid antibody during pregnancy using plasma exchange and low-dose prednisone. Lancet 1987;2:1023−1024.

F192a. Frampton G, Hicks J, Cameron JS. Significance of antiphospholipid antibodies in patients with lupus nephritis. Kidney Intern 1991;39:1225−1231.

F193. Frampton G, Perl S, Bennett A, Cameron JS. Platelet associated DNA and anti-DNA antibody in systemic lupus erythematosus. Clin Exp Immunol 1986;63:621−628.

F194. Frampton G, Winer JP, Cameron JS, Hughes RA. Severe Guillain-Barre syndrome: an association with IgA anticardiolipin antibody in a series of 92 patients. J Neuroimmunol 1988 Aug;19(1–2):133–139.

F195. Frances C, Boisnic S, Lefebvre C, Bletry O, Agulhon F, Chomette G, Godeau P. Rare cutaneous manifestations in the course of lupus: Cutaneous skin necrosis. Ann Dermatol Venereol 1986;113:976–977.

F196. Frances C, Tribout B, Boisnic S, Drouet L, Piette AM, Piette JC, Bletry O, Wechsler B, Godeau P. Cutaneous necrosis associated with the lupus anticoagulant. Dermatologica 1989; 178(4):194–201.

F197. Franceschini F, Bertoli MT, Martinelli M, Tincani A, Malagoli A, Faden D, Tarantini M, Balestrieri G, Cattaneo R. The neonatal lupus erythematosus associated with isolated La(SSB) antibodies. J Rheumatol 1990;17:415–416.

F198. Francis DA. Pure red-cell aplasia: association with systemic lupus erythematosus with primary autoimmune hypothyroidism. BMJ (Clin Res) 1982 Jan 9;284(6309):85.

F199. Francis RB Jr. Antiphospholipid antibodies in sickle cell anemia. Blood 1989;74 Suppl 1:308a.

F200. Francis RB Jr. Elevated fibrin-D-dimer fragment in sickle cell anemia: evidence for activation of coagulation during the steady state as well as in painful crisis. Haemostasis 1989;19: 105–111.

F201. Francis RB Jr, McGehee WG, Feinstein DI. Endothelial-dependent fibrinolysis in subjects with the lupus anticoagulant and thrombosis. Thromb Haemost 1988;59:412–414.

F202. Francis RB Jr, Neely S. Effect of the lupus anticoagulant on endothelial fibrinolytic activity in vitro. Thromb Haemost 1989;61:314–317.

F203. Franco AE, Schur PH. Hypocomplementemic rheumatoid arthritis (RA) [abstract]. Arthritis Rheum 1971 Jan–Feb;14: 162.

F204. Franco HL, Weston WL, Peebles C, Forstot SL, Phanuphak P. Autoantibodies directed against sicca syndromes antigens in neonatal lupus syndrome. J Am Acad Dermatol 1981 Jan;4: 67–72.

F205. Francoeur AM. Anti-histones. Scand J Rheumatol [Suppl] 1985; 56:46–48.

F206. Francoeur AM, Peebles CL, Gompper P, Tan EM. Identification of Ki (Ku p70/p80) autoantigens and analysis of anti-Ki autoantibody reactivity. J Immunol 1986;136:1648–1653.

F207. Francotte M, Urbain J. Induction of anti-tobacco mosaic virus antibodies in mice by rabbit anti-idiotypic antibodies. J Exp Med 1984;160:1485.

F208. Francotte M, Urbain J. Enhancement of antibody response by mouse dendritic cells pulsed with tobacco mosaic virus or with rabbit anti-idiotypic antibodies raised against a private rabbit idiotype. Proc Natl Acad Sci USA 1985;82:8149.

F209. Frank AO. Apparent predisposition to systemic lupus erythematosus in Chinese patients in West Malaysia. Ann Rheum Dis 1980 Jun;39(2):266–169.

F210. Frank MB, McArthur R, Harley JB, Fujisaku A. Anti-Ro (SSA) autoantibodies are associated with T cell receptor β genes in systemic lupus erythematosus patients. J Clin Invest 1990;85:33–39.

F211. Frank MM. Complement in the pathophysiology of human disease. N Engl J Med 1987;316:1525–1530.

F212. Frank MM, Atkinson JP. complement in clinical medicine. DM 1975 Jan:1–54.

F213. Frank MM, Hamburger MI, Lawley TJ, Kimberly RP, Plot PH. Defective reticuloendothelial system Fc-receptor function in systemic lupus erythematosus. N Engl J Med 1979 Mar 8; 300(10):518–523.

F214. Frank MM, Lawley TJ, Hamburger MI, Brown E. Immunoglobulin G Fc receptor-mediated clearance in autoimmune disease. Ann Intern Med 1983;98:206–218.

F215. Frank MM, Schreiber AD, Atkinson JP, Jaffe CJ. Pathophysi-

ology of immune hemolytic anemia. Ann Intern Med 1977 Aug;87:210–222.

F216. Frankel WN, Rudy C, Coffin JM, Huber BT. Linkage of Mls genes to endogenous mammary tumor viruses of inbred mice. Nature 1991;349:526–528.

F217. Franklin CM, Torretti D. Systemic lupus erythematosus and Down's syndrome [letter]. Arthritis Rheum 1985 May; 28(5):598–599.

F218. Franklin EC, Kunkel HG. Comparative levels of high molecular (19S) gamma globulin in maternal and umbilical cord sera. J Lab Clin Med 1958:724.

F219. Franzen P, Friman C, Pettersson T, Fyhrquist F, Ruutu T. Combined pure red cell aplasia and primary autoimmune hypothyroidism in systemic lupus erythematosus. Arthritis Rheum 1987 Jul;30(7):837–840.

F220. Fraser FC, Fainstat TD. Production of congenital defects in the offspring of pregnant mice treated with cortisone. Pediatrics 1951;8:527.

F221. Frayha RA, Jizi I, Saadeh G. Salmonella typhimurium bacteriuria. An increased infection rate in systemic lupus erythematosus. Arch Intern Med 1985 Apr;145(4):645–647.

F222. Frazer IH, Mackay IR. T lymphocyte subpopulations defined by two sets of monoclonal antibodies in chronic active hepatitis and systemic lupus erythematosus. Clin Exp Immunol 1982 Oct;50:107–114.

F223. Freddo L, Hays AP, Nickerson KG, Spatz L, McGinnis S, Lieberson R, Vedeler CA, Shy ME, Autilio-Gambetti L, Grauss FC, Petito F, Chess L, Laov N. Monoclonal anti-DNA IgM kappa in neuropathy binds to myelin and to a conformational epitope formed by phosphatidic acid and gangliosides. J Immunol 1986 Dec;137(12):3821–3825.

F223a. Fredriksen K, Traavik T, Flaegstad T, Rekvig OP. BK virus terminates tolerance to dsDNA and histone antigens in vivo. Immunol Invest 1990;19:133–151.

F224. Freedman AS, Freeman G, Whitman J, Segil J, Daley J, Levine H, Nadler LM. Expression and regulation of CD5 on in vitro activated human B cells. Eur J Immunol 1989;19: 849–855.

F225. Freedman P, Markowitz AS. Gamma globulin and complement in the diseased kidney. J Clin Invest 1962 Feb;41: 328–334.

F226. Freeman RG, Knox J, Owens DW. Cutaneous lesions of lupus erythematosus induced by monochromatic light. Arch Dermatol 1969 Dec;100:677–682.

F227. Freeman RW, Uetrecht JP, Woosley RL, Oates JA, Harrison RD. Covalent binding of procainamide in vitro and in vivo to hepatic protein in mice. Drug Metab Dispos 1981;9:188–192.

F228. Freeman RW, Woosley RL, Oates JA, Harrison RD. Evidence for biotransformation of procainamide to a reactive metabolite. Toxicol Appl Pharmacol 1979;50:9–16.

F229. Freemont AJ, Denton J, Chuck A, Holt PJL, Davies M. Diagnostic value of synovial fluid microscopy : a reassessment and rationalization. Ann Rheum Dis 1991 Feb;50(2):101–107.

F230. Same as F223a.

F231. Freigang DM, Fritzler MJ. Proliferative responses of lymphocytes to chromatin components. Clin Invest Med. In press.

F232. Freitas AA, Guilbert B, Holmberg D, Wennerstron G, Coutinho A, Avrameas S. Analysis of autoantibody reactivities in hybridoma collections derived from normal adult BALB/C mice. Ann Inst Pasteur Immunol 1986;137D:33–45.

F233. French JK, Hurst NP, O'Donnell ML, Betts WH. Uptake of chloroquine and hydroxychloroquine by human blood leukocytes in vitro: relation to cellular concentrations during antirheumatic therapy. Ann Rheum Dis 1987 Jan;46(1):42–45.

F234. French DL, Laskov R, Scharff MD. The role of somatic hypermutation in the generation of antibody diversity. Science 1989;244:1152–1157.

F235. Freni-Titulaer LWJ, Kelley DB, Grow AG, McKinley TW, Arnett FC, Hochberg MC. Connective tissue disease in southeastern Georgia: A case control study of etiologic factors. Am J Epidemiology 1989;130:404–409.

F236. Frenkel JK. Role of corticosteroids as predisposing factors in fungal diseases. Lab Invest 1962 Nov;11:1192–1208.

F237. Frenkel M. Safety of hydroxychloroquine [letter]. Arch Ophthalmol 1982 May;100(5):841.

F238. Fresco LD, Harper DS, Keene JD. Leucine periodicity of U2 small nuclear ribonucleoprotein particle (snRNP) A′ protein is implicated in snRNP assembly via protein-protein interactions. Mol Cell Biol 1991;11:1578–1589.

F239. Fresco R. Virus-like particles in systemic lupus erythematosus. N Engl J Med 1970;283:1231–1233.

F240. Fretwell MD, Altman LC. Exacerbation of a lupus-erythematosus-like syndrome drug treatment of a non-C_1-esterase-inhibitor-dependent angioedema with danazol. J Allergy Clin Immunol 1982;69:306–310.

F241. Fretwell MD, Altman LC, Van Arsdel PP. Angioedema associated with a lupus-erythematosus syndrome in a 70-year old man. J Allergy Clin Immunol 1979;63:187.

F242. Freundlich B, Makover D, Maul GG. A novel antinuclear antibody associated with a lupus-like paraneoplastic syndrome. Ann Intern Med 1988 Aug 15;109(4):295–297.

F243. Freyer DR, Morganroth ML, Rogers CE, Arnaout MA, Todd RF 3d. Modulation of surface CD11/CD18 glycoproteins (Mo1,LFA-1,P150,95) by human mononuclear phagocytes. Clin Immunol Immunopathol 1988;46:272–283.

F244. Fricchione GL, Kaufman LD, Gruber BL, Fink M. Electroconvulsive therapy and cyclophosphamide in combination for severe neuropsychiatric lupus with catatonia. Am J Med 1990 Apr;88(4):442–443.

F245. Frick PG. Acquired circulating anticoagulants in systemic "collagen disease"; autoimmune thromboplastin deficiency. Blood 1955 Jul;10:691–706.

F246. Friedberg CK, Gross L, Wallach K. Nonbacterial thrombotic endocarditis associated with prolonged fever, arthritis, inflammation of serous membranes and wide-spread vascular lesions. Arch Intern Med 1936 Oct;58:662–684.

F247. Friederich HC. Skin transplantation and skin grafts in chronic discoid LE [original in German]. Hautarzt 1969 Mar; 20:119–122.

F248. Friederich HC. Results of autotransplantation in chronic discoid lupus erythematosus [original in German]. Arch Klin Exp Derm 1970;237:71–75.

F249. Friedman D, Nettl F, Schreiber AD. Effect of estradiol and steroid analogues on the clearance of immunoglobulin G-coated erythrocytes. J Clin Invest 1985;75:162–167.

F250. Friedman DM, Lazarus HM, Fierman AH: Acute myocardial infarction in pediatric systemic lupus erythematosus. J Pediatr 1990;117:263–266.

F251. Friedman EA, Rutherford JW. Pregnancy and lupus erythematosus. Obstet Gynecol 1956;8:601–610.

F251a. Friedman IA, Sickley JF, Poske RM, Black A, Bronsky D, Hartz WH Jr, Feldhake C, Reeder PS, Katz EM. The L.E. phenomenon in rheumatoid arthritis. Ann Intern Med 1957 Jun; 46:113–1136.

F252. Friedman SJ. Leukonychia striata associated with systemic lupus erythematosus. J Am Acad Dermatol 1986;15:536–538.

F253. Friedman SM, Posnett DN, Tumang JR, Cole BC, Crow MK. A potential role for microbial superantigens in the pathogenesis of systemic autoimmune disease. Arthritis Rheum 1991;34: 468–480.

F254. Friedman WF, Hirschklau MJ, Printz MP, Pitlick PT, Kirkpatrick SF. Pharmacologic closure of the patent ductus arteriosus in the premature infant. N Engl J Med 1976;295:526–529.

F255. Friend PS, Kim Y, Michael AF, Donadio JV. Pathogenesis of membranous nephropathy in systemic lupus erythematosus; possible role of non-precipitating DNA antibody. BJM 1977;1: 25

F256. Fries J, Holman H. Systemic Lupus Erythematosus: A Clinical Analysis. Philadelphia: Saunders, 1975.

F257. Fries JF. The clinical aspects of systemic lupus erythematosus. Med Clin North Am 1977 Mar;61:229–240.

F258. Fries JF. Immunosuppressive drugs plus prednisone versus prednisone alone in lupus nephritis. N Engl J Med 1985;312; 921–922.

F259. Fries JF. Methodology of validation of criteria for systemic lupus erythematosus. Scand J Rheumatol 1987;65 Suppl: 25–30.

F260. Fries JF. The epidemiology of systemic lupus erythematosus, 1950–1990. Conceptual advances and the ARAMIS data banks. Clin Rheumatol 1990;9:5–9.

F261. Fries JF, Hunder GG, Block DA, Michel BA, Arend WP, Calabrese LH, Fauci AS, Leavitt RY, Lie JT, Lightfoot RW, Masi AT, McShane DJ, Mills JA, Stevens MB, Wallace SL, Zvaifler NJ. The American College of Rheumatology 1990 criteria for the classification of vasculitis: summary. Arthritits Rheum 1990; 33:1135–1136.

F262. Fries JF, Porta J, Liang MH. Marginal benefit of renal biopsy in systemic lupus erythematosus. Arch Intern Med 1978 Sep; 138:1386–1389.

F263. Fries JF, Sharp GC, McDevitt HO, Holman HR. Cyclophosphamide therapy in systemic lupus erythematosus and polymyositis. Arthritis Rheum 1973 Mar–Apr;16(2):154–162.

F264. Fries JF, Siegel RC. Testing the "preliminary criteria for classification of SLE." Ann Rheum Dis 1973 Mar;32:171–177.

F265. Fries JF, Singh G, Lenert L, Furst DE. Aspirin, hydroxychloroquine, and hepatic enzyme abnormalities with methotrexate in rheumatoid arthritis. Arthritis Rheum 1990 Nov;33(11): 1611–1619.

F266. Fries LF, Brickman CM, Frank MM. Monocyte receptors for the Fc portion of IgG increases in number in autoimmune hemolytic anemic and other hemolytic states and are decreased by glucocorticoid therapy. J Immunol 1983;131: 1240–1245.

F267. Fries LF, Hall RP, Lawley TJ, Crabtree GR, Frank MM. Monocyte receptors for the Fc portion of IgG studied with monomeric human IgG1: Normal *in vitro* expression of Fcγ receptors in HLA-B8/DRw3 subjects with defective Fcγ-mediated *in vivo* clearance. J Immunol 1982;129:1041–149.

F268. Fries LF, Mullin WW, Cho KR, Plotz PH, Frank MM. Monocyte receptors for the Fc portion of IgG are increased in systemic lupus erythematosus. J Immunol 1984;132:695–700.

F269. Friman C, Nordstrom D, Eronen I. Plasma glycosaminoglycans in systemic lupus erythematosus. J Rheumatol 1987;14: 1132–1134.

F270. Friou GJ. Clinical application of lupus serum: Nucleoprotein reaction using fluorescent antibody technique [abstract]. J Clin Invest 1957;36:890.

F271. Friou GJ. The significance of the lupus globulin-nucleoprotein reaction. Ann Intern Med 1958 Oct;49:866–874.

F272. Friou GJ. Identification of the nuclear component of the interaction of lupus erythematosus globulin and nuclei. J Immunol 1958;80:476–481.

F273. Friou GJ, Finch SC, Detre KD. Interaction of nuclei and globulin from lupus erythematosus serum demonstrated with fluorescent antibody. J Immunol 1958 Apr;80:324–329.

F274. Frith P, Burge SM, Millard PR, Wojnarowska F. External ocular findings in lupus erythematosus: a clinical and immunopathological study. Br J Ophthalmol 1990 Mar;74(3): 163–167.

F275. Fritz A, Parisot R, Newmeyer D, De Robertis EM. Small nuclear U-ribonucleoproteins in Xenopus laevis development.

Uncoupled accumulation of the protein and RNA components. J Mol Biol 1984;178:273–285.

F276. Fritzler MJ. Immunofluorescent antinuclear antibody tests. In: Rose NR, Friedman H, Fahey JL, editors. Manual of Clinical Laboratory Immunology. 3rd ed. Washington, DC: American Society for Microbiology, 1986:733–739.

F277. Fritzler MJ, Pauls JD, Kinsella TD, Bowent J. Antinuclear, anticytoplasmic and anti-Sjogren's syndrome antigen A (SS-A/Ro) antibodies in female blood donors. Clin Immunol Immunopathol 1985;36:120–128.

F278. Fritzler MJ, Ryan JP, Kinsella TD. Clinical features of SLE patients with antihistone antibodies. J Rheumatol 1982 Jan;9: 46–51.

F279. Fritzler MJ, Salazar M. Diversity and origin of rheumatologic autoantibodies. Clin Microbiol Rev 1991;4:256–269.

F280. Fritzler MJ, Tan EM. Antibodies to histone in drug-induced and idiopathic lupus erythematosus. J Clin Invest 1978 Sep; 62:560–567.

F281. Fritzler MJ, Tan EM. Antinuclear antibodies and the connective tissue diseases. In: Cohen AS, editor. Laboratory Diagnostic Procedures in the Rheumatic Diseases. 3rd ed. Toronto: Grune & Stratton, 1985:207–247.

F282. Fritzler MJ, Valencia DW, McCarty GA. Speckled pattern antinuclear antibodies resembling anticentromere antibodies. Arthritis Rheum 1984;27:92–96.

F283. Frocht A, Leek JC, Robbins DL. Gout and hyperuricemia in systemic lupus erythematosus. Br J Rheumatol 1987 Aug; 26(4):303–306.

F284. Froelich CJ, Goodwin JS, Bankhurst AD, Williams RC. Pregnancy, a temporary fetal graft of suppressor cells in autoimmune disease? Am J Med 1980;69:329–331.

F285. Froelich CJ, Guiffaut S, Sosenko M, Muth K. Deficient interleukin-2-activated killer cell cytotoxicity in patients with systemic lupus erythematosus. Clin Immunol Immunopathol 1989;50:132–145.

F286. Froham M, Francfort JW, Carving C. T-dependent destruction of thyroid isografts exposed to IFN-Gamma. J Immunol 1991;2227–2234.

F287. Fromer JL. Use of testosterone in chronic lupus erythematosus: Preliminary report. Lahey Clin Bull 1950 Jul;7:13–17.

F288. Fronek Z, Lentz D, Berliner N, Duby AD, Klein KA, Seidman JG, Schur PH. Systemic lupus erythematosus is not genetically linked to the beta chain of the T cell receptor. Arthritis Rheum 1986;29:1023–1025.

F289. Fronek Z, Timmerman LA, Alper CA, Hahn BH, Kalunian KC, Peterlin BM, McDevitt HO. Major histocompatibility complex genes and susceptibility to systemic lupus erythematosus. Arthritis Rheum 1990 Oct;33(10):1542–1553.

F290. Frost BF, Park KS, Tuck M, Disa S, Kim S, Paik WK. Site-specificity of histone H1 methylation by two H1-specific protein-Lysine N-methyltransferases from Euglena gracilis. Int J Biochem 1989;21:1061–1070.

F291. Fruchter L, Gauthier B, Marino F. The use of plasmapheresis in a patient with systemic lupus erythematosus and necrotizing cutaneous ulcers [letter]. J Rheumatol 1983 Apr;10(2): 341–343.

F292. Frutos MA, Rivilla A, Garcia I, Burgos D, Valera A, Martin-Reyes G, Cabello M, Lopez de Novales E. Intravenous pulse cyclophosphamide therapy in severe lupus nephritis. Nefrologia 1990;10 Suppl 5:88–93.

F293. Fu J-Y, Masferrer JL, Seibert K, Raz A, Neddleman P. The induction and suppression of prostaglandin H2 synthase (cyclooxygenase) in human monocytes. J Biol Chem 1990; 265:16737–16740.

F294. Fu XD, Maniatis T. Factor required for mammalian spliceosome assembly is localized to discrete regions in the nucleus. Nature 1990;343:437–441.

F295. Fuetren G, Querin S, Noel LH, Chatenoud L, Beaurain G, Tron F, Lesavre P, Bach JF. Effects of cyclosporine in severe systemic lupus erythematosus. J Pediatr 1987;111: 1063–1068.

F296. Fugger L, Morling N, Ryder LP, Georgsen J, Jakobsen BK, Svejgard A, Andersen V, Oxholm P, Pedersen FK, Friis J, Halberg P. NcoI restriction fragment length polymorphism (RFLP) of the tumor necrosis factor (TNFα) region in four autoimmune diseases. Tissue Antigens 1989;34:17–22.

F297. Fugger L, Morling N, Ryder LP, Jakobsen BK, Andersen V, Oxholm P, Dalhoff K, Heilmann C, Pedersen FK, Fries J, Halberg P, Spies T, Strominger JL, Svejgard A. Restriction fragment length polymorphism of two HLA-B-associated transcript genes in five autoimmune diseases. Hum Immunol 1991;30: 27–31.

F298. Fujii Y, Kobayashi Y, Fujii H, Higaki T, Hara H, Usui T. Systemic lupus erythematosus in a boy, with a review of the Japanese literature. Eur J Pediat 1977;125(1):15–20.

F299. Fujinami RS, Oldstone MB. Molecular mimicry as a mechanism for virus-induced autoimmunity. Immunol Res 1989;8: 3–15.

F300. Fujisaku A, Frank MB, Neas B, Reichlin M, Harley JB. HLA-DQ gene complementation and other histocompatibility relationships in man with the Ro/SSA autoantibody response of systemic lupus erythematosus. J Clin Invest 1990;86: 606–611.

F301. Fujiwara M, Cinader B. Cellular aspects of tolerance. IV Strains variations of tolerance inducibility. Cell Immunol 1974;12:11–29.

F302. Fukasawa T, Arai T, Naruse T, Maekawa T. Hyperviscosity syndrome in a patient with systemic lupus erythematosus. Am J Med Sci 1977 May–Jun;273:329–334.

F303. Fuks Z, Smith KC. Effect of quinacrine on x-ray sensitivity and the repair of damaged DNA in Escherichia coli K-12. Radiat Res 1971 Oct;48:63–73.

F304. Fukumoto S, Tusmagari T, Kinjo M, Tanaka K. Acta Pathol Jpn 1987;37:1–9.

F305. Fukushima T, Kobayashi K, Kasama T, Kasahara K, Tabata M. Inhibition of interleukin-2 by serum in healthy individuals and in patients with autoimmune disease. Int Arch Allergy Applied Immunol 1987;84:135–141.

F306. Fulcher D, Stewart G, Exner T, Trudinger B, Jeremy R. Plasma exchange and the cardiolipin syndrome in pregnancy. Lancet 1989;2:171.

F307. Fulford KWM, Catterall RD, Delhanty JJ, Doniach D, Kremer M. A collagen disorder of the nervous system presenting as multiple sclerosis. Brain (Part II) 1972;95:373–386.

F308. Fulkerson JP, Ladenbauer-Bellis IM, Chrisman OD. In vitro hexosamine depletion of intact articular cartilage by E-prostaglandins: prevention by chloroquine. Arthritis Rheum 1979 Oct;22(10):1117–1121.

F309. Fullcher D, Stewart G, Exner T, Trudinger B, Jeremy R. Plasma exchange and the anticardiolipin syndrome in pregnancy [letter]. Lancet 1989 Jul 15;2(8655):171.

F310. Fultz PN, Siegel RL, Brodie A, Mawle AC, Stricker RB, Swenson RB, Anderson DC, McCluve HM. Prolonged CD4+ lymphocytopenia and thrombocytopenia in a chimpanzee persistently infected with human immunodeficiency virus type 1. J Infect Dis 1991;163:441–447.

F311. Funata N. Cerebral vascular changes in systemic lupus erythematosus. Bull Tokyo Med Dent Univ 1979 Jun;26(2): 91–112.

F312. Funauchi M, Sugishima H, Minoda M, Horiuchi A. Effect of interferon-gamma on B lymphocytes of patients with systemic lupus erythematosus. J Rheumatol 1991;18:368–372.

F313. Fundenberg HH, Strelkauskas AJ, Goust J-M, Osborne D, Fort D, Vasily D. "Discoid" lupus erythematosus: Dramatic clinical and immunological response to dialyzable leukocyte extract (Transfer factor). Trans Assoc Am Phys 1981;94:279–281.

F314. Funkhouser JD, Peevy KJ, Mockridge PB Hughes ER. Distribution of dexamethasone between mother and fetus after maternal administration Pediatr Res 1978;12:1053.

F315. Furie R, Kaell A, Petrucci R, Farber B, Kaplan M. Systemic lupus erythematosus complicated by infection with human immunodeficiency virus (HIV) [abstract]. Arthritis Rheum 1988 Apr;31(4) Suppl:S56.

F316. Furie RA, Chartash EK. Tendon rupture in systemic lupus erythematosus. Semin Arthritis Rheum 1988 Nov;18(2):127–133.

F317. Furner BB. Treatment of Subacute cutaneous lupus erythematosus. Int J Dermatol 1990;29:542–547.

F318. Furst C, Smiley WK, Ansell BM. Steroid cataract. Ann Rheum Dis 1966 Jul;25:364–368.

F319. Furszyfer J, Kurland LT, Woolner LB, Elveback LR, McConahey WM. Hashimoto's thyroiditis in Olmsted County, Minnesota, 1935 through 1967. Mayo Clin Proc 1970;45:586–596.

F320. Furukawa F, Kashihara-Sawami M, Lyons MB, Norris DA. Binding of antibodies to the extractable nuclear antigens SS-A/Ro and SS-B/La is induced on the surface of human keratinocytes by ultraviolet light (UVL): Implications for the pathogenesis of photosensitive cutaneous lupus. J Invest Dermatol 1990;94:77–85.

F321. Furukawa F, Lyons MB, Lee L, Coulter SN, Norris DA. Estradiol enhances binding to cultured human keratinocytes of antibodies specific for SS-A/Ro and SS-B/La. Another possible mechanism for estradiol influence of lupus erythematosus. J Immunol 1988;141:1480–1488.

F322. Futcher PH. Enlargement and round cell infiltration of the salivary glands associated with systemic disease. Bull Johns Hopkins Hosp 1959 Sep;105:97–107.

F323. Futran J, Shore A, Urowitz MB, Grossman H. Subdural hematoma in systemic lupus erythematosus: report and review of the literature [case report]. J Rheumatol 1987 Apr;14(2):378–381.

F324. Futrell N, Millikan C. Frequency, etiology and prevention of stroke in patients with systemic lupus erythematosus. Stroke 1989 May;20(5):583–591.

F325. Fye KH, Terasaki PI, Michalski JP, Daniels TE, Pelz GO, Talal N. Relationship of HLA-Dw3 and HLA-B8 to Sjogren's syndrome. Arthritis Rheum 1978;21:337–342.

G

G1. Gaal JC, Pearson CK. Eukaryotic nuclear ADP-ribosylation reactions. Biochem J 1985;230:1–18.

G2. Gaal JC, Smith KR, Pearson CK. Cellular euthanasia mediated by a nuclear enzyme: a central role for nuclear ADP-ribosylation in cellular metabolism. Trends Bioc 1987;12:129–130.

G3. Gabbe SG. Drug therapy in autoimmune diseases. Clin Obstet Gynecol 1983;26:635–641.

G4. Gabriel A, Agnello V. Detection of immune complexes. The use of radioimmunoassays with C1q and monoclonal rheumatoid factor. J Clin Invest 1977;59:990–1001.

G5. Gabrielli A, Corvetta A, Montroni M, Rupoli S, Danieli G. Immune deposits in normal skin of patients with systemic lupus erythematosus: relationship to the serum capacity to solubilize immune complexes. Clin Immunopath Immunopathol 1985 Sep;36(3):266–274.

G6. Gaedicke G, Teller WM, Kohne E, Dopfer R, Niethammer D. IgG therapy in systemic lupus erythematosus—two case reports. Blut 1984 Jun;48(6):387–390.

G7. Gahring L, Baltz M, Pepys MB, Daynes R. Ro − SS-A: Effect of

ultraviolet radiation on the production of ETAF/IL-1 inn vivo and in vitro. Proc Natl Acad Sci USA 1984;81:1198–1202.

G8. Gaither KK, Bias WB, Harley JB. The frequency of SLE autoantibodies in normal sera and correlations with Class II HLA antigens [abstract]. Arthritis Rheum 1987;30 Suppl 4:S22.

G9. Gaither KK, Fox OF, Yamagata H, Mamula MJ, Reichlin M, Harley JB. Implications of anti-Ro/Sjogren's syndrome A antigen autoantibody in normal sera for autoimmunity. J Clin Invest 1987;79:841–846.

G10. Galeazzi M, Sebastiani GD, Passiu G, Angelina G, Delfino L, Asherson RA, Khamashta MA, Hughes GRV. HLA-DP genotyping in patients with systemic lupus erythematosus: correlation with autoantibody subsets. J Rheumatol 1991;19:42–46.

G11. Galeazzi M, Tuzi T, De Pita O, Ruffelli M, Sarti P. Repeat skin biopsies of nonlesional skin in patients with systemic lupus erythematosus [letter]. Arthritis Rheum 1983 Oct;26(10):1294–1295.

G12. Gall JG. Spliceosomes and snurposomes. Science 1991;252:1499–1500.

G13. Gallagher RB, Cambier JC. Signal transmission pathways and lymphocyte function [news]. Immunol Today 1990;11:187–189.

G14. Gallant C, Kenny P. Oral glucocorticoids and their complications. J Am Acad Dermatol 1986;14:161–177.

G15. Galli M, Comfurius P, Maassen C, Hemker HC, de Baets MH, van Breda-Vriesman PJ, Barbui T, Zwaal RF, Bevers EM. Anticardiolipin antibodies (ACA) directed not to cardiolipin but to a plasma protein cofactor. Lancet 1990 Jun 30;335(8705):1544–1547.

G16. Galli R, Beguin S, Lindout T, Hemker CH. Inhibition of phospholipid and platelet-dependent prothrombinase activity in the plasma of patients with lupus anticoagulants. Br J Haematol 1989;72:549–555.

G17. Galliano D, Cardesi E, Gandolfo S, Gatto V. Keratotic lesions of the oral cavity. Notes on histopathologic differential diagnosis in leukoplakia, lichen planus, lupus erythematosus [English abstract]. Minerva Stomatol 1989 Apr;38(4):481–487.

G18. Gallien M, Schnetzler J-P, Morin J. Antinuclear antibodies and lupus induced by phenothiazines in 600 hospitalized patients [original in French]. Ann Med Psychol (Paris) 1975 Feb;1:237–248.

G19. Gallo GR, Caulin-Glaser T, Lamm ME. Charge of circulating immune complexes as a factor in glomerular basement membrane localization in mice. J Clin Invest 1981 May;67(5):1305–1313.

G20. Gallo R, Graves TK, Granholm MA, Izui S. Association of glycoprotein gp70 with progression or attenuation of murine lupus nephritis. J Clin Lab Immunol 1985;18:63.

G21. Galofre J, Bielsa I, Casademont J, Herrero C, Cardellach F. Papulonodular mucinosis and late-onset SLE associated with Hashimoto's thyroiditis and Sjogren's syndrome [letter]. Rev Clin Esp 1989 May;184(8):446–447.

G22. Same as G75.

G23. Galve E, Candell-Riera J, Pigrau C, Permanyer-Miralda G, Gardia-Del-Castillo H, Soler-Soler J. Prevalence, morphologic types, and evolution of cardiac valvular disease in systemic lupus erythematosus. N Engl J Med 1988;319:817–823.

G24. Galve E, Ordi J, Candell-Riera J, Permanyer-Miralda G, Vilardell M, Soler-Soler J. Valvular heart disease in systemic lupus erythematosus [letter]. N Engl J Med 1989;320:740–741.

G25. Gammon WR, Briggaman RA, Inaman AO 3d, Merritt CC, Wheeler CE Jr. Evidence supporting a role for immune complex mediated inflammation in the pathogenesis of bullous lesions of systemic lupus erythematosus. J Invest Dermatol 1983 Oct;81(4):320–325.

G26. Gammon WR, Heise ER, Burke WA, Fine JD, Woodley DT, Briggaman RA. Increased frequency of HLA-DR2 in patients with autoantibodies to epidermolysis bullosa acquisita antigen evidence that the expression of autoimmunity to type VII collagen is HLA class II allele associated. J Invest Dermatol 1988; 91:228–232.

G27. Gammon WR, Woodley DT, Dole KC, Briggaman RA. Evidence that anti-basement membrane zone antibodies in bullous eruption of systemic lupus erythematosus recognize epidermolysis bullosa acquisita autoantigen. J Invest Dermatol 1985 Jun;84(6):472–476.

G28. Gamsu B, Webb WR. Pulmonary hemorrhage in systemic lupus erythematosus. J Can Assoc Radiol 1978 Mar;29:66–68.

G29. Ganczarczyk L, Urowitz MB, Gladman DD. "Latent lupus." J Rheumatol 1989 Apr;16(4):475–478.

G30. Ganczarczyk ML, Lee P, Fornasier VL. Early diagnosis of osteonecrosis in systemic lupus erythematosus with magnetic resonance imaging. Failure of core decompression. J Rheumatol 1986 Aug;13(4):814–817.

G31. Gange KW, Levene GM. A distinctive eruption in patients receiving oxprenolol. Clin Exp Dermatol 1979;4:87–97.

G32. Ganor S, Sagagen F. Systemic lupus erythematosus changing to the chronic discoid type. Dermatologica 1962;125:81–92.

G33. Gant NF. Lupus erythematosus, the lupus anticoagulant and the anticardiolipin antibody. Williams Obstetrics 1986 May/Jun;Suppl 6:1–11.

G34. Ganz VH, Gurland BJ, Beming WE, Fisher B. The study of psychiatric symptoms of systemic lupus erythematosus. Psychosomat Med 1972 May–Jun;34:207.

G35. Gao X, Ball EJ, Dombrausky L, Olsen NJ, Pincus T, Khan MA, Wolfe F, Stastny P. Class II human leukocyte antigen genes and T cell receptor polymorphisms in patients with rheumatoid arthritis. Am J Med 1988;85:14–16.

G36. Garancis JC, Komorowski RA, Bernhard GC, Straumfjiord JV. Significance of cytoplasmic microtubules in lupus nephritis. Am J Pathol 1971 Jul;64:1–12.

G37. Garancis JC, Piering WF. Prolonged cyclophosphamide or azathioprine therapy of lupus nephritis [abstract]. Clin Pharmacol Ther 1973;14:130.

G38. Garb J. Nevus verrucous unilateris cured with podophyllin ointment. Ointment applied as occlusive dressing; report of a Case. Arch Dermatol 1960 Apr;81:606–609.

G39. Garber EK, Fan PT, Bluestone R. Realistic guidelines of corticosteroid therapy in rheumatoid diseases. Semin Arthritis Rheum 1981 Nov;11:231–256.

G40. Garcia-de la Torre I, Hernandez-Vazquez L, Angulo-Vazquez J, Romero-Ornelas A. Prevalence of antinuclear antibodies in patients with habitual abortion and in normal and toxemic pregnancies. Rheumatol Int 1984;4:87–89.

G41. Garcia-de la Torre I, Sanchez-Guerrero A, Salmon-de la Torre G, Hernandez-Vazquez L. Prevalence of anti-SSA(Ro) antibodies in a Mexican population of patients with various systemic rheumatic diseases. J Rheumatol 1987;14:479–481.

G42. Garcia-Morteo O, Maldonado-Cocco JA. Lupus-like syndrome during treatment with nomifensine [letter]. Arthritis Rheum 1983;26:936.

G43. Garcia-Morteo O, Nitsche A, Maldonado-Cocco JA, Barcelo HA. Eosinophilic fascitis and retroperitoneal fibrosis in a patient with systemic lupus erythematosus [letter]. Arthritis Rheum 1987 Nov;30(11):1314–1315.

G44. Garcia-Penarrubia P, Koster FT, Kelley RO, McDowell TD, Bankhurst AD. Antibacterial activity of human natural killer cells. J Exp Med 1989;169:99–113.

G45. Garcia Ruiz PJ, Guerrero Sola A, Garcia Urra D. Sensory neuralgia of the trigeminal nerve and systemic lupus erythematosus. Neurologia 1988;3:248.

G46. Gare A, Fasth A, Anderson J, Berglund G, Ekstrom H, Eriksson M, Hammeren L, Holmquist L, Ronge E, Thilen A. Incidence and prevalence of juvenile chronic arthritis. Ann Rheum Dis 1987;46:277–281.

G47. Gargour G, MacGaffey K, Locke S, Stein MD. Anterior radiculopathy and lupus erythematosus cells: report of a case. Br Med J 1964 Sep 26;5412:799–801.

G48. Garin E, Shulman ST, Donnelly WH, Richard GA. Systemic lupus erythematosus glomerulonephritis in children. Pediatr 1981 Jan;10:351–367.

G49. Garin EH, Donnelly WH, Fenell RS, Richard GA. Nephritis in systemic lupus erythematosus in children. J Pediatr 1976; 89:366–371.

G50. Garin EH, Donnelly WH, Shulman ST, Fernandez R, Finton C, Williams RL, Richard GA. The significance of serial measurements of serum complement C3 and C4 components and DNA binding capacity in patients with lupus nephritis. Clin Nephrol 1979 Oct;12:148–155.

G51. Garland LH, Sisson MA. Roentgen findings in "collagen" disease. AJR 1954 Apr;71:581–598.

G52. Garlepp MJ, Hart DA, Fritzler MJ. Regulation of plasma complement C4 and factor b levels in murine systemic lupus erythematosus. J Clin Lab Immunol 1989;28:137–141.

G53. Garlund B. The lupus inhibitor in thromboembolic disease and intrauterine death in the absence of systemic lupus. Acta Med Scand 1984;215(4):293–298.

G54. Garner BF, Burns P, Bunning RD, Laureno R. Acute blood pressure elevation can mimic arteriographic appearance of cerebral vasculitis (a postpartum case with relative hypertension). J Rheumatol 1990 Jan;17(1):93–97.

G55. Garnier JL, Merino R, Kimoto M, Izui S. Resistance to tolerance induction to human gamma globulin (HGG) in autoimmune BXSB/MpJ mice: functional analysis of antigen-presenting cells and HGG-specific T helper cells. Clin Exp Immunol 1988;73:283–288.

G56. Garovich M, Agudelo C, Pisko E. Oral contraceptives and systemic lupus erythematosus. Arthritis Rheum 1980 Dec;23: 1396–1398.

G57. Garrett R, Paulus H. Complications of intravenous methylprednisolone pulse therapy [abstract]. Arthritis Rheum 1980 Jun;28:677.

G58. Garsenstein M, Pollak VE, Kark RM. Systemic lupus erythematosus and pregnancy. N Engl J Med 1962;267:165–169.

G59. Garty BZ, Stark H, Yaniv I, Varsano I, Danon YL. Pulmonary nocardiosis in a child with systemic lupus erythematosus. Pediatr Infect Dis 1985;4:66–68.

G60. Garwryl MA, Chudwin DS, Longlois PF, Lint TF. The terminal complement complex, C5b-9, a marker of disease activity in patients with systemic lupus erythematosus. Arthritis Rheum 1988;31:188–195.

G61. Gaskill HS, Fitz-Hugh T Jr. Toxic psychosis following atabrine. Bull US Army M Dept 1945 Mar;86:63–69.

G62. Gastineau DA, Kazmier FJ, Nichols WL, Bowie EJ. Lupus anticoagulant: an analysis of the clinical and laboratory features of 219 cases. Am J Haematol 1985;19:265–275.

G63. Gatenby PA. Systemic lupus erythematosus and pregnancy. Aust NZ J Med 1989;19:261–278.

G64. Gatenby PA, Cameron K, Shearman RP. Pregnancy loss with antiphospholipid antibodies: improved outcome with aspirin containing treatment. Aust N Z J Obstet Gynaecol 1989 Aug; 29 (Part 2):294–298.

G65. Gatenby PA, Smith H, Krwan P, Lauer CS. Systemic lupus erythematosus and thrombotic thrombocytopenic purpura. A case report and review of the relationship. J Rheumatol 1981 May–Jun;8:504–508.

G66. Gatrill AJ, Munk ME, Kaufmann SH. Gamma/delta T cells and bacteria. Res Immunol 1990;141:641–644.

G67. Gaulton GN, Greene MI. Anti-idiotypic antibodies of reovirus as biochemical and immunological mimics. Intern Rev Immun 1986;1:79.

G68. Gause WC, Jackson JV, Dietert RR, Marsch JA. Autoantithyroglobulin production in obese chickens: Influence of age and sex as a measure of ELISA. Develop Comp Immunol 1985;9: 107–118.

G69. Gause WC, Marsh JA. Effect of testosterone treatments for varying periods on autoimmune thyroiditis. Clin Immunol Immunopathol 1986;20:240–245.

G70. Gauthier VJ, Mannik M. A small proportion of cationic antibodies in immune complexes is sufficient to mediate their deposition in glomeruli. J Immunol 1990 Nov 15;145(10): 3348–3352.

G71. Gauthier VJ, Mannik M, Striker GE. Effect of cationized antibodies in preformed immune complexes on deposition and persistence in renal glomeruli. J Exp Med 1982 Sep 1;156: 766–777.

G72. Gauthier VJ, Striker GE, Mannik M. Glomerular localization of preformed immune complexes prepared with anionic antibodies or with cationic antigens. Lab Invest 1984;50: 636–644.

G73. Gavalchin J, Datta SK. The NZB × SWR model of lupus nephritis. II. Autoantibodies deposited in renal lesions show a distinctive and restricted idiotypic diversity. J Immunol 1987 Jan 1;138(1):138–148.

G74. Gavalchin J, Nicklas JA, Eastcott JW, Madaio MP, Stollar BD, Schwartz RS, Datta SK. Lupus prone (SWR × NZB)F1 mice produce potentially nephritogenic autoantibodies inherited from the normal SWR parent. J Immunol 1985 Feb;134(2): 885–894.

G75. Gavalchin J, Seder RA, Datta SK. The NZB × SWR model of lupus nephritis. I. Cross-reactive idiotypes of monoclonal anti-DNA antibodies in relation to antigenic specificity, charge and allotype. Identification of inter-connected idiotype families inherited from the normal SWR and the autoimmune NZB parents. J Immunol 1986 Jan 1;138(1):128–137.

G76. Gawkrodger DJ, Beveridge GW. Neonatal lupus erythematosus in four successive siblings born to a mother with discoid lupus erythematosus. Br J Dermatol 1984;111:683.

G77. Gaylis NG, Altman RD, Ostrov S, Quencer R. The selective value of computed tomography of the brain in cerebritis due to system lupus erythematosus. J Rheumatol 1982 Nov– Dec; 9(6):850–854.

G78. Gearhart P, Johnson MD, Douglas R, Hood L. IgG antibodies to phosphorylcholine exhibit more diversity than their IgM counterparts. Nature 1981;291:28–34.

G79. Geggel RL, Tucker L, Szer I. Postnatal progression from second- to third-degree heart block in neonatal lupus syndrome. J Pediatr 1988;113:1049–1052.

G80. Gehrz RC, Christianson WR, Linner KM, Conroy MM, McCue SA, Balfour HH. A longitudinal analysis of lymphocyte proliferative responses to mitogens and antigens during normal pregnancy. Am J Obstet Gynecol 1981;40:665.

G81. Gelbracht D, Shapiro L. Temporomandibular joint erosions in patients with systemic lupus erythematosus [letter]. Arthritis Rheum 1982 May;25(5):597.

G82. Gelfand EW, Cheung RK, Grinstein S, Mills GB. Characterization of the role for calcium influx in mitogen-induced triggering of human T cells. Identification of calcium-dependent and calcium-independent signals. Eur J Immunol 1986;16: 907–912.

G83. Gelfand EW, Cheung RK, Mills GB, Grinstein S. Uptake of extracellular Ca^{2+} and not recruitment from internal stores is essential for T lymphocyte proliferation. Eur J Immunol 1988;18:917–992.

G84. Gelfand J, Truong L, Stern L, Pirani C, Appel GB. Thrombotic thrombocytopenic purpura in systemic lupus erythematosus. Treatment with plasma infusion. Am J Kidney Dis 1985; 6:154–160.

G85. Gelfand MC, Steinberg AD. Therapeutic studies in NZB/W mice. II. Relative efficacy of azathioprine, cyclophosphamide and methylprednisolone. Arthritis Rheum 1972 May–Jun;15: 247–252.

G86. Gelmers HJ. Exacerbation of systemic lupus erythematosus, aseptic meningitis and acute mental symptoms, following metrizamide lumbar myelography. Neuroradiology 1984; 26(1):65–66.

G87. Gembruch U, Hansmann M, Redel DA, Bald R, Knoepfle G. Fetal complete heart block: antenatal diagnosis, significance and management. Eur J Obstet Gynecol Reprod Biol 1989;31: 9–22.

G88. Genez BM, Wilson MR, Houk RW, Weiland FL, Unger HR Jr, Shields NN, Rugh KS. Early osteonecrosis of the femoral head: detection in high-risk patients with MR imaging. Radiology 1988 Aug;168(2):521–524.

G88a. Gennerich W. The present state of the lupus erythematosus question [original in German]. Arch Derm u Syph 1922; 138:403–410.

G89. Genth E, Zarnowski H, Mierau R, Wohltmann D, Hartl OW. HLA-DR4 and Gm (1,3;5,21) are associated with U1-nRNP antibody positive connective tissue disease. Ann Rheum Dis 1987;46:189–196.

G90. George JN, Snaith SJ. Clinical importance of acquired abnormalities of platelet function. N Engl J Med 1991;324: 27–39.

G91. Geppert TD, Davis LS, Gur H, Wacholtz MC, Lipsky PE. Accessory cell signals involved in T-cell activation. Immunol Rev 1990;117:5–66.

G92. Gerard JM, Stoupel N, Collier A, Flament-Durand J. Morphologic study of neuromyopathy caused by prolong chloroquine treatment. Eur Neurol 1973;9(6):363–379.

G93. Gerber DA. Effect of chloroquine on the sulfhydryl group and the denaturation of bovine serum albumin. Arthritis Rheum 1964;7(3):193–200.

G94. Gerbracht DD, Steen VD, Ziegler GL, Medsger TA Jr, Rodnan GP. Evolution of primary Raynaud's phenomenon (Raynaud's disease) to connective tissue disease. Arthritis Rheum 1985 Jan;28(1):87–92.

G95. Gergely P. Treatment of systemic lupus erythematosus (SLE) with piroxicam (Hotemin-Egis). Ther Hung 1989; 37(2):83–85.

G96. Gerding DN, Staples PJ, Gordon RS, Decker JL. Bacterial and mycotic infections in systemic lupus erythematosus [abstract]. Arthritis Rheum 1970 May–Jun;13(3):317–318.

G97. Germuth FG, Rodriguez E. Immunopathology of the renal glomerulus 1. Boston: Brown, 1973.

G98. Germuth FG Jr, Rodriguez E, Lorelle CA, Trump E, Milano L, Wise O. Passive immune complex glomerulonephritis in mice: models for various lesions found in human disease: II Low avidity complexes and diffuse proliferative glomerulonephritis with subepithelial deposits. Lab Invest 1979 Oct;41: 366–377.

G99. Gershon RK, Kondo K. Infectious immunological tolerance. Immunology 1971;21:903–914.

G100. Gershoni JM, Palade GE. Protein blotting: Principles and applications. Anal Biochem 1983;131:1–15.

G101. Gershwin ME, Castles JJ, Saito W, Ahmed A. Studies of congenitally immunologically mutant New Zealand mice. VII: TSP the ontogeny of thymic abnormalities and reconstitution of nude NZB/W mice. J Immunol 1982 Nov;129(5): 2150–2155.

G102. Gershwin ME, Ikeda RM, Kruse WL, Wilson F, Shifrine M, Spangler W. Age-dependent loss in New Zealand mice of morphological and functional characteristics of thymic epithelial cells. J Immunol 1978 Mar;120(3):971–979.

G103. Gershwin ME, Steinberg AD. Qualitative characteristics of anti-DNA antibodies in lupus nephritis. Arthritis Rheum 1974 Nov–Dec;17(6):947–954.

G104. Geschickter CF, Athanasiadou PA, O'Malley WE. The role of mucinolysis in collagen disease. Am J Clin Pathol 1958;30:93–111.

G105. Geschwind NBP. Left-handedness: association with immune disease, migraine, and developmental learning disorder. Proc Natl Acad Sci USA. 1982;79:5097–5100.

G106. Geschwind NBPO. Laterality, hormones, and immunity, cerebral dominance. In: Geschwind AM, Galaburda AM, editors. The Biological Foundations. Cambridge: Harvard University Press, 1984:211–224.

G107. Geschwind NGAM. Cerebral lateralization: biological mechanisms, associations, and pathology: a hypothesis and a program for research: Part I. Arch Neurol 1985;42:428–459.

G108. Geschwind NGAM. Cerebral lateralization: biological mechanisms, associations, and pathology: a hypothesis and a program for research: Part II. Arch Neurol 1985;42:529–552.

G109. Geschwind NGAM. Cerebral lateralization: biological mechanisms, associations, and pathology: hypothesis and a program for research: Part III. Arch Neurol 1985;42:634–654.

G110. Gewanter HL, Baum J. The frequency of juvenile arthritis. J Rheumatol 1989;16:556.

G111. Gewurz A, Lint TF, Robert JL, Zeitz H, Gewurz H. Homozygous C2 deficiency with fulminant lupus erythematosus. Arthritis Rheum 1978;21:28–36.

G112. Gewurz H, Page AR, Pickering RJ, Good RA. Complement activity and inflammatory neutrophil exudation in man. Int Arch Allergy 1967;32:64–90.

G113. Gharavi AE, Chu JL, Elkon KB. Autoantibodies to intracellular proteins in humans SLE are not due to random polyclonal B cell activation. Arthritis Rheum 1988;31:1337–1345.

G114. Gharavi AE, Harris EN, Asherson RA, Hughes GR. Anticardiolipin antibodies: isotype distribution and phospholipid specificity. Ann Rheum Dis 1987 Jan;46(1):1–6.

G115. Gharavi AE, Harris EN, Lockshin MD, Hughes GR, Elkon KB. IgG subclass and light chain distribution of anticardiolipin and anti-DNA antibodies in systemic lupus erythematosus. Ann Rheum Dis 1988 Apr;47(4):286–290.

G116. Gharavi AE, Mellors RC, Elkon KB. IgG anticardiolipin antibodies in murine lupus. Clin Exp Immunol 1989;78:233–238.

G117. Ghatak S, Sainis K, Owens FL, Datta SK. T-cell-receptor beta and I-A-chain genes of normal SWR mice are linked with the development of lupus nephritis in NZB × SWR crosses. Proc Natl Acad Sci USA 1987 Oct;84(19):6850–6853.

G118. Ghose K, Coppen A, Hurdle AD, McIllroy I. Antinuclear antibodies, affective disorders and lithium therapy. Pharmakopsychiatry & Neuropsychopharmakology 1977 Jul;10:243–245.

G119. Giampietri A, Fioretti MC, Goldin A, Bonmasser E. Drug-mediated antigenic changes in murine leukemia cells: Antagonistic effects of quinacrine, an antimutagenic compound. JNCI 1980;64(2):297–301.

G120. Gibbons RB, Westerman E. Acute nonlymphocytic leukemia following short-term, intermittent, intravenous cyclophosphamide treatment of lupus nephritis. Arthritis Rheum 1988 Dec;31(12):1552–1554.

G121. Gibofsky AM, Winchester RJ, Patarroyo M, Fotino M, Kunkel HG. Disease association of the Ia-like human alloantigens Contrasting patterns in rheumatoid arthritis and systemic lupus erythematosus. J Exp Med 1978;148:1728–1732.

G122. Gibson AL, Herron JN, Ballard DW, Voss EW Jr, He XM, Patrick VA, Edmundson AB. Crystallographic characterization of the Fab fragment of a monoclonal anti-ss-DNA antibody. Mol Immunol 1985 Apr;22(4):499–502.

G123. Gibson GJ, Edmonds JP, Hughes GRV. Diaphragm function and lung involvement in systemic lupus erythematosus. Am J Med 1977 Dec;63:926–932.

G124. Gibson T, Myers AR. Nervous system involvement in systemic lupus erythematosus. Ann Rheum Dis 1975 Oct;35(5):398–406.

G125. Gibson T, Myers AR. Subclinical liver disease in systemic lupus erythematosus. J Rheumatol 1981 Sep;8(5):752–759.

G126. Gibson TP, Dibona GF. Use of the American Rheumatism Association's preliminary criteria for the classification of systemic lupus erythematosus. Ann Intern Med 1972 Nov;77:754–756.

G127. Gilbert CW, Zaroukian MH, Esselman WJ. Poly-N-acetyllactosamine structures on murine cell surface T200 glycoprotein participate in natural killer cell binding to YAC-1 targets. J Immunol 1988;140:2821–2828.

G128. Gilchrest BA, Soter NA, Stoff JS, Mimh MC. The human sunburn reaction: Histologic and biochemical studies. J Am Acad Dermatol 1981;5:411–422.

G129. Gilchrist DM, Friedman JM. Teratogenesis and IV cyclophosphamide [letter]. J Rheumatol 1989 Jul;16(7):1008–1009.

G130. Giles RC, DeMars R, Chang CC, Capra JD. Allelic polymorphism and transassociation of molecules encoded by the HLA-DQ subregion. Proc. Natl Acad Sci USA 1985;82:1776–1780.

G131. Giles RC, Capra JD. Biochemistry of MHC class II molecules. Tissue Antigens 1985;25:57–58.

G132. Gilgor RS, Tindall JP, Elson M. Lupus-erythematosus-like tinea of the face (tinea faciale). JAMA 1971 Mar 29;215:2091–2094.

G133. Gilkeson GS, Grudier JP, Karounos DG, Pisetsky DS. Induction of anti-double stranded DNA antibodies in normal mice by immunization with bacterial DNA. J Immunol 1989;142:1482–1486.

G134. Gill D. Rheumatic complaints of women using anti-ovulatory drugs. An evaluation. J Chronic Dis 1968 Oct;21:435–444.

G135. Gill KS, Hayne OA, Zayed E. Another case of procainamide-induced pancytopenia [letter]. Am J Hematol 1989;31:298.

G136. Gill TJ 3d. Immunological and genetic factors influencing pregnancy. In: Knobil E, Neill JD, editors. The physiology of reproduction. New York: Raven Press, 1988:2023.

G137. Gilleece MH, Evans CC, Bucknall RC. Steroid resistant pleural effusion in the systemic lupus erythematosus treated with tetracycline pleurodesis. Ann Rheum Dis 1988;47:1031–1032.

G138. Gillespie JP, Lindsley CB, Linshaw MA, Richardson WP. Childhood systemic lupus erythematosus with negative antinuclear antibody test. J Pediatr 1981 Apr;98(4):578–581.

G139. Gilliam J. Immunopathology and pathogenesis of cutaneous lupus erythematosus. In: Safai RA, Good RA, editors. Comparative immunology: Immunodermatology. New York: Plenum, 1980;21:323–332.

G140. Gilliam JN. The cutaneous signs of lupus erythematosus. Continuing Education for the Family Physician 1977;6:34–40.

G141. Gilliam JN, Cheatum DE, Hurd ER, Stastny P, Ziff M. Immunoglobulin in clinically uninvolved skin in systemic lupus erythematosus: Association with renal disease. J Clin Invest 1974;43:1434–1440.

G142. Gilliam JN, Cheatum DE, Hurd ER, Ziff M. The prognostic significance of the LE fluorescent band test [abstract]. Arthritis Rheum 1973;16:545–546.

G143. Gilliam JN, Prystowsky SD. Conversion of discoid lupus erythematosus to mixed connective tissue disease. J Rheumatol 1977 Summer;4(2):165–169.

G144. Gilliam JN, Sontheimer RD. Distinctive cutaneous subsets in the spectrum of lupus erythematosus. J Am Acad Dermatol 1981;4:471–475.

G145. Gilliam JN, Sontheimer RD. Skin manifestations of systemic lupus erythematosus. Clin Rheum Dis 1982;8:207–218.

G146. Gilliland BC, Leddy JP, Vaughan JH. The detection of cell-bound antibody on complement-coated human red cells. J Clin Invest 1970 May;49:898–906.

G147. Gilliland BC, Turner E. Mechanism of complement binding by the red cell in rheumatoid arthritis. Arthritis Rheum 1969 Oct;12:498–503.

G148. Gilman AG. G proteins: transducers of receptor-generated signals. Ann Rev Biochem 1987;56:615–649.

G149. Gimmi CD, Freeman GJ, Gribben JG, Sugita K, Freedman AS, Morimoto C, Nadler LM. B-cell surface antigen B7 provides a costimulatory signal that induces T cells to proliferate and secrete interleukin 2. Proc Natl Acad Sci USA 1991;88:6575–6579.

G150. Gimovsky ML, Brenner P, Montoro M, Platt LD, Berne T, Paul RH. Successful pregnancy in a patient with systemic lupus erythematosus, renal transplantation and chronic renal failure: a case report. J Reprod Med 1983;28:677–680.

G151. Gimovsky ML, Montoro M, Paul RH. Pregnancy outcome in women with systemic lupus erythematosus. Obstet Gynecol 1984;63:686–692.

G152. Ginsberg HM, O'Malley M. Serum factors releasing serotonin from normal platelets: relation to the manifestation of systemic lupus erythematosus. Ann Intern Med 1977;87:564–569.

G153. Ginsburg K, Alpert M, Larson M, Wright E, Fossel H, Rogers M, Schur P, Liang M. Prevalence of neurocognitive symptoms and dysfunction in unselected patients with systemic lupus erythematosus and rheumatoid arthritis [abstract]. Arthritis Rheum 1990 Sep;33(9) Suppl:S29.

G154. Ginsburg WW, Conn DL, Bunch TW, McDuffie FC. Comparison of clinical and serologic markers in systemic lupus erythematosus and overlap syndrome: a review of 247 patients. J Rheumatol 1983 Apr;10(2):235–241.

G155. Ginsburg WW, Finkelman FD, Lipsky PE. Circulating and pokeweed mitogen-induced immunoglobulin-secreting cells in systemic lupus erythematosus. Clin Exp Immunol 1979 Jan;35:76–88.

G156. Ginzler AM, Fox TT. Disseminated lupus erythematosus: cutaneous manifestations of systemic disease (Libman-Sacks) [case report]. Arch Intern Med 1940 Jan;65:26–50.

G157. Ginzler E, Berg A. Mortality in systemic lupus erythematosus. J Rheumatol 1987;14 Suppl 13:218.

G158. Ginzler E, Diamond H, Guttadauria M, Kaplan D. Prednisone and azathioprine compared to prednisone plus low dose azathioprine and cyclophosphamide plus low dose azathioprine and cyclophosphamide in the treatment of diffuse lupus nephritis. Arthritis Rheum 1976;19:693–699.

G159. Ginzler E, Diamond H, Kaplan D, Weiner M, Schlesinger M, Seleznick M. Computer analysis of factors influencing frequency of infection in systemic lupus erythematosus. Arthritis Rheum 1978 Jan–Feb;21(1):37–44.

G160. Ginzler E, Feldman D, Giovaniello G, Fruchter R, Schorn K, Singer J. The association of cervical neoplasia (CN) and SLE [abstract]. Arthritis Rheum 1989 Apr;32(4) Suppl:S30.

G161. Ginzler EM, Bollet AJ, Friedman EA. The natural history and response to therapy of lupus nephritis. Ann Rev Med 1980;31:462–487.

G162. Ginzler EM, Diamond HS, Weiner M, Schlesinger M, Fries JF, Wasner C, Medsger TA Jr, Zieger G, Klippel JH, Hadler NM, Albert DA, Hess EV, Spencer-Green G, Grayzel A, Worth D, Hahn BH, Barnett EV. A multicenter study of outcome of systemic lupus erythematosus. I. Entry variables as predictors of progress. Arthritis Rheum 1982 Jun;25(6):601–611.

G163. Ginzler EM, Nicastri AD, Chen CK, Friedman EA, Diamond HS, Kaplan D. Progression of mesangial and focal to diffuse nephritis. N Engl J Med 1974 Oct 3;291:693–696.

G164. Giordano M, Gallo M, Chianese U, Maniera A, Tirri G. Acute pancreatitis as the initial manifestation of systemic lupus erythematosus. Z Rheumatol 1986 Mar–Apr;45(2):60–63.

G165. Gioud M, Ait Kaci M, Monier JC. Histone antibodies in systemic lupus erythematosus. Arthritis Rheum 1982 Apr;25:407–413.

G166. Girand MT, Hjaltadottir S, Fejes-Toth AN, Guyre PM. Glucocorticoids enhance the gamma-interferon augmentation of human monocyte immunoglobulin G Fc receptor expression. J Immunol 1987;138:3235–3241.

G167. Girard TJ, McCourt D, Novotny WF, McPhail LA, Likert KM, Broze GJ. The lipoprotein-associated coagulation inhibitor is phosphorylated at serine-2 [abstract]. Blood 1989;74 Suppl 1:95a.

G168. Girgis FL, Popple AW, Bruckner FE. Jaccoud's arthropathy. A case report and necropsy study. Ann Rheum Dis 1978 Dec;37(6):561–565.

G169. Gitlow S, Goldmark C. Generalized capillary and arteriolar thrombosis: report of two cases with a discussion of the literature. Ann Intern Med 1939 Dec;13:1046–1047.

G170. Gladman D, Urowitz M, Tozman E. Glynn M. Hemostatic abnormalities in systemic lupus erythematosus. Q J Med 1983 Summer;52:424–433.

G171. Gladman DD, Chalmers A, Urowitz MB. Systemic lupus erythematosus with negative LE cells and antinuclear factor. J Rheumatol 1978 Summer;5:142–147.

G172. Gladman DD, Goldsmith CH, Urowitz MB, Bombardier C, Isenberg D, Kalunian K, Liang MH, Maddison P, Nived O, Richter M, Snaith M, Symmonds D, Zoma A. Cross-cultural validation and reliability of three disease activity indices in systemic lupus erythematosus. J Rheumatol 1992;19:608–611.

G173. Gladman DD, Ross T, Richardson B, Kulkarni S. Bowel involvement in systemic lupus erythematosus: Crohn's disease or lupus vasculitis. Arthritis Rheum 1985 Apr;28(4):466–470.

G174. Gladman DD, Sternberg L. Pulmonary hypertension in systemic lupus erythematosus. J Rheumatol 1985 Apr;12:365–367.

G175. Gladman DD, Terasaki PI, Park MS, Iwaki Y, Louie S, Quismorio FP, Barnett EV, Liebling MR. Increased frequency of HLA-DRw2 in SLE. Lancet 1972;2:902–905.

G176. Gladman DD, Urowitz MB. Venous syndromes and pulmonary embolism in systemic lupus erythematous. Ann Rheum Dis 1980 Aug;39:340–343.

G177. Gladman DD, Urowitz MB. Morbidity in systemic lupus erythematosus. J Rheumatol 1987;14 Suppl 13:223.

G178. Gladman DD, Urowitz MB, Cole E, Ritchie S, Chang CH, Churg J. Kidney biopsy in SLE. I. A clinical-morphologic evaluation. Q J Med 1989;73:1125–1133.

G179. Gladman DD, Urowitz MB, Keystone EC. Serologically active clinically quiescent systemic lupus erythematosus: a discordance between clinical and serological features. Am J Med 1979 Feb;66(2):210–215.

G180. Glagov S, Gechman E. Familial occurrence of disseminated lupus erythematosus. N Engl J Med 1956;255:936–940.

G181. Glas-Greenwalt P, Kant KS, Allen C, Pollak VE. Fibrinolysis n health and disease: severe abnormalities in systemic lupus erythematosus. J Lab Clin Med 1984 Dec;104:962–976.

G182. Glass D, Fearon DT, Austen KF. Inherited abnormalities of the complement system. In: Stanbury JB, Wyngaarden JB, editors. Metabolic basis of inherited disease, 5th ed. New York: McGraw-Hill, 1983:1934–1955.

G183. Glass D, Raum D, Gibson D, Stillman JS, Schur PH. Inherited deficiency of the second component of complement. Rheumatic disease associations. J Clin Invest 1976;58: 853–861.

G184. Glass D, Schur PH. Autoimmunity and systemic lupus erythematosus. In: Talal N, editor. Autoimmunity: genetic, immunologic, virologic and clinical aspects. New York: Academic, 1977:532–560.

G185. Glassman AB, Bennett CE, Christopher JB, Self S. Immunity during pregnancy: lymphocyte subpopulations and mitogen responsiveness. Ann Clin Lab Sci 1985;15:357.

G186. Glassock RJ, Goldstein DA. Recurrent acute renal failure in a patient with mixed connective tissue disease. Am J Nephrol 1982;2(5)282–290.

G187. Glavinskaia TA, Pavlova LT, Dorofeichuk VG. Lysozyme in the combined therapy of erythematosus [English abstract]. Vestn Dermatol Venereol 1990;(3):21–25.

G188. Glazer GH. Lesions of the central nervous system in disseminated systemic lupus erythematosus. Arch Neurol 1952 Jun;67:745.

G189. Gledhill RF, Dessein PH. Autonomic neuropathy in systemic lupus erythematosus [letter]. J Neurol Neurosurg Psychiatry 1988 Sep;51(9):1238–1240.

G190. Gleichman H. SLE triggered by diphenylhydantoin [letter]. Arthritis Rheum 1982;25:1377–1378.

G191. Gleichman H. Systemic lupus erythematosus triggered by diphenylhydantoin [letter]. Arthritis Rheum 1982 Nov;25: 1387–1388.

G192. Gleichmann E, Pals ST, Rolink AG, Radaskiewicz T, Gleichmann H. Graft-versus-host reactions: clues to the etiopathology of a spectrum of immunological diseases. Immunol Today 1984;5:324–332.

G193. Gleichmann E, Van Elven EH, Van der Veen JP. A systemic lupus erythematosus (SLE)-like disease in mice induced by abnormal T-B cell cooperation. Preferential formation of autoantibodies characteristic of SLE. Eur J Immunol 1982;182:129.

G194. Gleichmann E, Van Elven F, Gleichman H. Immunoblastic, lymphadenopathy, systemic lupus erythematosus, and related disorders. Possible pathologenetic pathways. Am J Clin Pathol 1979 Oct;72 Suppl 4:708–723.

G195. Gleichmann H, Gleichmann E, Andre-Schwartz J, Schwartz RS. Chronic allogeneic disease. III. Genetic requirements for the induction of glomerulonephritis. J Exp Med 1972;135:516–532.

G196. Glickstein M, Neustadter L, Dalinka M, Kricun M. Periosteal reaction in systemic lupus erythematosus. Skeletal Radiol 1986;15(8):610–612.

G197. Glidden RS, Mantzouranis EC, Borel Y. Systemic lupus erythematosus in childhood: clinical manifestations and improved survival in fifty-five patients. Clin Immunol Immunopathol 1983 Nov;29(2):196–210.

G198. Glinski W, Gershwin ME, Budman DR, Steinberg AD. Study of peripheral blood lymphocyte subpopulations in normal humans and patients with systemic lupus erythematosus by fractionation of peripheral blood lymphocytes on a discontinuous Ficoll gradient. Clin Exp Immunol 1976 Nov;26: 228–238.

G199. Glinski W, Gershwin ME, Steinberg AD. Fractionation of cells on a discontinuous Ficoll gradient. Study of subpopulations of human T cells using anti-T cell antibodies from patients with systemic lupus erythematosus. J Clin Invest 1976 Mar;57:604–614.

G200. Glovsky MM, Louie JS, Pitts WH Jr, Alenty A. Reduction of pleural fluid complement activity in patients with systemic lupus erythematosus and rheumatoid arthritis. Clin Immunol Immunopathol 1976 Jul;6:31–41.

G201. Gluch OS, Murphy WA, Hahn TJ, Hahn BH. Bone loss in adults receiving alternate day glucocorticoid therapy: a comparison with daily therapy. Arthritis Rheum 1981;24: 892–898.

G202. Glueck CJ, Levy RI, Glueck HI, Gralnick HR, Greten H, Fredrickson DS. Acquired type 1 hyperlipoproteinemia with systemic lupus erythematosus, dysglobulinemia and heparin resistance. Am J Med 1969 Aug;47(2):318–324.

G203. Glueck HI, Kant KS, Weiss MA, Pollak VE, Miller MA, Coots M. Thrombosis in systemic lupus erythematosus: relation to the presence of circulating anticoagulants. Arch Intern Med 1985 Aut;145:1389–1395.

G204. Go T, Lockshin M. Latex-negative ANA-positive erosive arthritis. Prognosis more like SLE than RA [abstract]. Arthritis Rheum 1975 Jul–Aug;18:401.

G205. Gocken NE, Thompson JS. Conditions affecting the immunosuppressive properties of human AFP. J Immunol 1977;119: 139–146.

G206. Godeau P, Aukert M, Imbert JD, Herreman G. SLE and active isoniazid levels in 47 cases [original in French]. Ann Med Intern 1973 Mar;124:181–186.

G207. Godeau P, Guillevin L, Fechner J, Bletry O, Herreman G. Conduction abnormalities in the hearts of lupus patients: frequency in 112 patients [original in French]. Ann Med Interne 1981;132(4):234–242.

G208. Godeau P, Piette C, Balafrej M. A study of blood chloroquine concentration in patients with retinotoxicity and neuromyopathies [English abstract]. Sem Hosp Paris 1979 May 18–25;55(19–20:955–957.

G209. Godfrey DG, Stimson WH, Watson J, Belch JF, Sturrock RD. Effects of dietary supplementation on autoimmunity in the MRL/lpr mouse: a preliminary investigation. Ann Rheum Dis 1986;45:1019–1024.

G210. Godfrey DG, Stimson WH, Watson J, Belch JF, Sturrock RD. The modulation of auto-immunity in the MRL-mp-lpr/lpr mouse by dietary fatty-acid supplementation. Prog Lipid Res 1986;25:288.

G211. Godfrey JE, Baxevanis AD, Moudrianakis EN. Spectropolarimetric analysis of the core histone octamer and its subunits. Biochemistry 1990;29:965–972.

G212. Godman GC, Deitch AD. A cytochemical study of the L.E. bodies of systemic lupus erythematosus. I. Nucleic acids. J Exp Med 1957 Sep;106:575. II. Proteins, ibid 1957;Sep:593–616.

G213. Goeckerman WH. Lupus erythematosus as a systemic disease. JAMA 1923;80:542–547.

G214. Goegel KM, Gassel WD, Goebel FD. Evaluation of azathioprine in autoimmune thrombocytopenia and lupus erythematosus. Scand J Haematol 1973;10:28–34.

G215. Goette DK. Sweet's syndrome in subacute cutaneous lupus erythematosus. Arch Dermatol 1985;121:789–791.

G216. Goggans FC, Weisberg LJ, Koran LM. Lithium prophylaxis of prednisone psychosis: a case report. J Clin Psychiatry 1983; 44:3–4.

G217. Goh KL, Wang F. Thyroid disorders in systemic lupus erythematosus. Ann Rheum Dis 1986 Jul;45(7):579–583.

G218. Gohill J, Cary PD, Couppez M. Antibodies from patients with drug-induced and idiopathic lupus erythematosus react with epitopes restricted to the amino and carboxyl termini of histone. J Immunol 1985;135:3116–3121.

G219. Gohill J, Fritzler MJ. Antibodies in procainamide-induced and systemic lupus erythematosus bind the C-terminus of histone 1 (H1). Mol Immunol 1987;24:275–285.

G220. Gohill J, Pauls JD, Fritzler MJ. Purification of histone H1 polypeptides by high-performance cation-exchange chromatography. J Chromatogr 1990; 502:47–57.

G221. Golan DT. Exposure to UV light in the pathogenesis of systemic lupus erythematosus (SLE). Isr J Med Sci 1988 Jul; 24(7):360–362.

G222. Golan DT, Borel Y. Increased photosensitivity to near-ultraviolet light in murine SLE. J Immunol 1984;132:705–710.

G223. Golan DT, Borel Y. Spontaneous increase of DNA turnover in murine systemic lupus erythematosus. Eur J Immunol 1983 May;13(5):430–433.

G224. Golan TD, Foltyn V, Roueff A. Increased susceptibility to in vitro ultraviolet B radiation in fibroblasts and lymphocytes cultured from systemic lupus erythematosus patients. Clin Immunol Immunopathol 1991 Feb;58(2):289–304.

G225. Golbus J, Salata M, Greenwood J, Hudson J, Richardson BC. Increased immunoglobulin response to gamma-interferon by lymphocytes from patients with systemic lupus erythematosus. Clin Immunol Immunopathol 1988;46:129–140.

G226. Gold AP, Yahr MD. Childhood lupus erythematosus. Trans Am Neurol Assoc 1960;85:96–102.

G227. Gold DH, Morris DA, Henkind P. Ocular findings in systemic lupus erythematosus. Br J Ophthalmol 1972 Nov;56:800–804.

G228. Gold EF, Ben-Efraim S, Faivisewitz A, Steiner Z, Klajman A. Experimental studies on the mechanism of induction of antinuclear antibodies by procainamide. Clin Immunol Immunopathol 1977; 7:176–186.

G229. Gold MS, Sweeney DR. Perphenazine-induced systemic lupus erythematosus-like syndrome. J Nerv Ment Dis 1978; 166:442–445.

G230. Gold S. Role of sulphonamides and penicillin in the pathogenesis of systemic lupus erythematosus. Lancet 1951;1: 268–272.

G231. Gold SC, Gowing NFC. Systemic lupus erythematosus. A clinical and pathological study. Q J Med 1953 Oct;22: 457–481.

G232. Gold W, Jennings D. Pulmonary function in systemic lupus erythematosus. Clin Res 1964 Apr;12:291.

G233. Gold WM, Jennings DB. Pulmonary function in patients with systemic lupus erythematosus. Am Rev Resp Dis 1966 Apr;93:556–567.

G234. Goldberg HI, Dodds WJ. Cobblestone esophagus due to Monilial infection. AJR 1968 Nov;104:608–612.

G235. Goldberg IM, McCord R, Schwartz AA. Right lower quadrant pain and systemic lupus erythematosus. Am Surg 1979 Jan;45(1):52–53.

G236. Goldberg J, Dlesk A. Successful treatment of Raynaud's phenomenon with pentoxifylline [letter]. Arthritis Rheum 1986 Aug;29(8):1055-1056.

G237. Goldberg J, Pinals RS. Felty syndrome. Semin Arthritis Rheum 1980 Aug;10(1):52–65.

G238. Goldberg JW, Lidsky MD. Pulse methylprednisolone therapy for persistent subacute cutaneous lupus. Arthritis Rheum 1984 Jul 27:837–838.

G239. Goldberg LC. Lupus erythematosus; treatment with oxophenarsine hydrochloride. Arch Dermat & Syph 1945 Aug;52: 89–90.

G240. Goldberg LC, Diamond A. Presumptive congenital lupus erythematosus in the newborn. Cutis 1973;11:143.

G241. Goldberg M, Chitanondh H. Polyneuritis with albuminocytologic dissociation in the spinal fluid in systemic lupus erythematosus; report of a case, with review of pertinent literature. Am J Med 1959 Aug;27:342–350.

G242. Goldberg MA, Arnett FC, Bias WB, Shulman LE. Histocompatibility antigens in systemic lupus erythematosus. Arthritis Rheum 1976;19:129–132.

G243. Goldblatt S. Treatment of lupus erythematosus with vitamin B12; preliminary report of 4 cases. J Invest Dermatol 1951 Dec;17:303–304.

G244. Goldblatt S. Cyanocobalamin (vitamin B12) therapy of lupus erythematosus; further observations. Acta Dermatovener (Stockh) 1953;33:216–235.

G245. Golden CJ, Moses JA, Fishburn FJ, Engum E, Lewis GP, Wisniewski AM, Conley FK, Berg RA, Graber B. Cross-validation of the Luria-Nebraska neuropsychological battery for the presence, lateralization, and localization of brain damage. J Consul Clinical Psychol 1981;49:491–507.

G246. Golden HE, McDuffie FC. Role of lupus erythematosus factor and accessory serum factors in production of extracellular nuclear material. Ann Intern Med 1967 Oct;67:780–790.

G247. Golden RL. Livedo reticularis in systemic lupus erythematosus. Arch Dermatol 1963 Mar;87:299–301.

G248. Goldenberg DL, Cohen AS. Synovial membrane histopathology in the differential diagnosis of rheumatoid arthritis, gout, pseudogout, systemic lupus erythematosus, infectious arthritis and degenerative joint disease. Medicine 1978 May; 57(3):239–252.

G249. Goldenberg DL, Leff G, Grayzel AI. Pericardial tamponade in systemic lupus erythematosus. N Y State Med J 1975;75: 910–914.

G250. Goldenberg GJ, Paraskevas F, Israels LG. Lymphocyte and plasma cell neoplasms associated with autoimmune diseases. Semin Arthritis Rheum 1971 Aug;1:174–193.

G251. Goldenstein-Schainberg C, Rodrigues Pereira RM, Cossermelli W. Linear scleroderma and systemic lupus erythematosus [letter]. J Rheumatol 1990;17:1427–1428.

G252. Golding PL, Smith M, Williams R. Multisystem involvement in chronic liver disease. Studies on the incidence and pathogenesis. Am J Med 1973 Dec;55:772–782.

G253. Goldings EA. Defective B-cell tolerance in New Zealand Black mice Fc receptor-independence of resistance to low-epitope-density tolerogens. Cell Immunol 1988;113: 183–191.

G254. Goldings EA. Defective B cell tolerance induction in New Zealand Black mice. I Macrophage independence and comparison with other autoimmune strains. J Immunol 1983;131: 2630–2634.

G255. Goldings EA, Cohen PL, McFadden SF, Ziff M, Vitetta ES. Defective B cell tolerance in adult (NZBxNZW) F1 mice. J Exp Med 1980;152:730–735.

G256. Goldman DD, Ross T, Richardson B, Kulkarni S. Bowel involvement in systemic lupus erythematosus: Crohn's disease or lupus vasculitis. Arthritis Rheum 1985;28:466–470.

G257. Goldman JA, Chiapella J, Casey H, Bass N, Graham J, McClatchey W, Dronavalli RV, Brown R, Bennett WJ, Miller SB, Wilson CH, Pearson B, Haun C, Persinski L, Huey H, Muckerheide M. Laser therapy of rheumatoid arthritis. Laser Surg Med 1980;1(1):93–101.

G258. Goldman JA, Litwin A, Adams LE, Krueger RC, Hess EV. Cellular immunity to nuclear antigens in systemic lupus erythematosus. J Clin Invest 1972 Oct;51:2669–2677.

G259. Goldman JA, Klimek GA, Ali R. Allergy in systemic lupus erythematosus, IgE levels and reaginic phenomenon. Arthritis Rheum 1976 Jul–Aug;19:669–676.

G260. Goldman JA, Litwin A, Adams LE, Krueger RC, Hess EV. Cellular immunity to nuclear antigens in systemic lupus erythematosus. J Clin Invest 1972;51:2669–2677.

G261. Goldman L, Cole DP, Preston RH. Chloroquine diphosphate in treatment of discoid lupus erythematosus. JAMA 1953 Aug 8;152:1428–1429.

G262. Goldman M, Druet P, Gleichmann E. T_H2 cells in systemic autoimmunity: insights from allogeneic diseases and chemically-induced autoimmunity. Immunology Today 1991;12: 223–271.

G263. Goldsmith DP. Neonatal rheumatic disorders. View of the pediatrician. Rheum Dis Clin North Am 1989;15:287–305.

G264. Goldsmith MA, Weiss A. Early signal transduction by the antigen receptor without commitment to T cell activation. Science 1988;240:1029–1031.

G265. Goldstein AL, Zatz MM, Low TL, Jacobs R. Potential role of thymosin in the treatment of autoimmune diseases. Ann NY Acad Sci 1981;377:486–495.

G266. Goldstein G, MacKay I. The thymus in SLE: a quantitative, histopathological analysis and comparison with stress involution. Br M J 1967;2:475–478.

G267. Goldstein JL, Brown MS. The LDL pathway in human fibroblasts. A receptor-mediated mechanism for the regulation of cholesterol metabolism. Curr Top Cell Regul 1976;11: 147–181.

G268. Goldstein JL, Brunschede GY, Brown MS. Inhibition of the proteolytic degradation of low density lipoprotein in human fibroblasts by chloroquine, concanavalin A and Triton WR 1339. J Biol Chem 1975 Oct 10;250(19):7854–7862.

G269. Goldstein R, Arnett FC, McLean RH, Bias WB, Duvic M. Molecular heterogeneity of complement component C4-null and 21-hydroxylase genes in systemic lupus erythematosus. Arthritis Rheum 1988;31:736–744.

G270. Goldstein R, Izaguirre C, Smith CD, Mierins E, Karsh J. Systemic lupus erythematosus and common absence of circulating B cells. Arthritis Rheum 1985 Jan;28:100–103.

G271. Goldstein R, Krupen KI, Crawford YM, Bias WB, Duvic M, Arnett FC. Interaction of the T cell receptor beta chain gene and HLA-DR in systemic lupus erythematosus [abstract]. Arthritis Rheum 1987 Suppl;30(4):S22.

G272. Goldstein R, Sengar DPS. Comparative study of HLA associations and C4A gene deletion in French-Canadian and non-French-Canadian Caucasians with systemic lupus erythematosus (SLE), Fifteenth Annual Meeting of the American Society for Histocompatibility and Immunogenetics, Toronto, Sep 12–21, 1989.

G273. Goldstein R, Smith CD, Sengar DPS. MHC class II studies of primary antiphospholipid antibody (APLA) syndrome and of serum antiphospholipid antibodies in systemic lupus erythematosus (SLE) [abstract]. Arthritis Rheum 1990;33 Suppl: S125.

G274. Goldstein R, Thompson FE, McKendry RJ. Diagnostic and predictive value of the lupus band test in undifferentiated connective tissue disease. A follow-up study. J Rheumatol 1985 Dec;12(6):1093–1096.

G275. Goldsteyn EJ, Fritzler MJ. The role of the thymus-hypothalamus-pituitary-gonadal axis in normal immune processes and autoimmunity. J Rheumatol 1987;14(5):982–990.

G276. Golombek SJ, Graus F, Elkon KB. Autoantibodies in the cerebrospinal fluid of patients with systemic lupus erythematosus. Arthritis Rheum 1986 Sep;29(9):1090–1097.

G277. Golombek SJ, Magid SK. Cerebrospinal fluid beta 2-microglobulin in central nervous system lupus erythematosus [abstract]. Arthritis Rheum 1985 Apr;28(4) Suppl:S23.

G278. Gomez F, Chien P, King M, McDermott P, Levinson AI, Rossman MD, Schreiber AD. Monocyte Fcγ receptor recognition of cell-bound and aggregated IgG. Blood 1989;74: 1058–1065.

G279. Gompertz NR, Isenberg DA, Turner BM. Correlation between clinical features of systemic lupus erythematosus and levels of antihistone antibodies of the IgG, IgA, and IgM isotypes. Ann Rheum Dis 1990;49:524–527.

G280. Goni F, Chen PP, Pons-Estel B, Carson DA, Frangione B. Sequence similarities and cross-idiotypic specificity of L chains among human monoclonal IgM$_k$ with anti-gammaglobulin activity. J Immunol 1985;135:4073.

G281. Gonnerman WA, Mortensen RF, Tebo JM, Conte J, Leslie CA, Cathcart ES. Dietary fish oil modulates macrophage fatty acids and decreases arthritis susceptibility in mice. J Exp Med 1988;162:1336–1349.

G281a. Gonnerman WA, Mortensen RF, Tebo JM, Conte JM, Leslie CA, Cathcart ES. Dietary fish oil modulation of macro-

phage amyloid P component responses in mice. J Immunol 1988;140:796–799.

G282. Gonyea L, Herdman R, Bridges RA. The coagulation abnormalities in systemic lupus erythematosus. Thromb Diath Haemorrh 1968 Dec;20:457–464.

G283. Gonzalez T, Gantes M, Bustabad S, Diaz-Flores L. Formation of rheumatoid nodules in systemic lupus erythematosus [English abstract]. Med Clin (Barc) 1985 Nov 23;85(17): 711–714.

G284. Gonzalez-Dattoni H, Tron F. Membranous glomerulopathy in systemic lupus erythematosus. In: Grunfeld JP, Maxwell MH, editors. Advances in Nephrology. Chicago: Year Book, 1985:347–364.

G285. Gonzalez-Scarano F, Lisak RP, Bilaniuk LT, Zimmerman RA, Atkins PC, Zweiman B. Cranial computed tomography in the diagnosis of systemic lupus erythematosus. Ann Neurol 1979;5:158–165.

G286. Good JT, King TE, Antony VD, Sahn SA. Lupus pleuritis. Clinical features and pleural fluid characteristics with special reference to pleural fluid antinuclear antibodies. Chest 1983 Dec;84:714–718.

G287. Good RA, Venters H, Page AR, Good TA. Diffuse connective tissues in children: With a special comment on connective tissue diseases with agamma-globulinemia. Lancet 1961 May; 81:192–204.

G288. Goodman HC, Fahey JL, Malmgren RA. Serum factors in lupus erythematosus and other diseases reacting with cell nuclei and nucleoprotein extracts: electrophoretic, ultracentrifugal and chromatographic studies. J Clin Invest 1960;36: 1595–1603.

G289. Goodman LS, Gilman A. The Pharmacological Basis of Therapeutics (2nd ed). New York: Macmillan, 1954: 1167–1173.

G290. Goodman LS, Goodman A. The Pharmacologic Basis of Therapeutics. (5th ed). New York: Macmillan, 1975: 1045–1069.

G291. Goodnow CC, Adelstein S, Basten A. The need for central and peripheral tolerance in the B cell repertoire. Science 1990;248:1373–1379.

G292. Goodnow CC, Crosbie J, Adelstein S, Lavoie TB, Smith-Gill SJ, Brink RA, Pritchard-Briscoe H, Wotherspoon JS, Loblay RH, Raphael K, Trent RJ, Basten A. Altered immunoglobulin expression and functional silencing of self-reactive B lymphocytes in transgenic mice. Nature 1988;334:676–682.

G293. Goodnow CC, Crosbie J, Jorgensen H, Brink RA, Basten A. Induction of self-tolerance in mature peripheral B lymphocytes. Nature 1989;342:385–391.

G294. Goodwin GH, Johns EW. Isolation and characterization of two calf-thymus chromatin non-histone proteins with high contents of acidic and basic amino acids. Eur J Biochem 1973; 40:215–219.

G295. Goodwin J, Goodwin J, Kellner R. Psychiatric symptoms in disliked medical patients. JAMA 1979 Mar 16;241:1117.

G296. Goodwin JS, Geuppens J. Regulation of the immune response by prostaglandins. J Clin Immunol 1983;3:295–310.

G297. Goodwin JS, Goodwin JM. Cerebritis in lupus erythematosus [letter]. Ann Intern Med 1979 Mar;90(3):437–438.

G298. Gordan MF, Stolley PD, Schinnar R. Trends in recent systemic lupus erythematosus mortality rate. Arthritis Rheum 1981 Jun;24:762–769.

G299. Gordon BL 2d, Keenan JP. The treatment of systemic lupus erythematosus (SLE) with the T-cell immunostimulant drug levamisole: A case report. Ann Allergy 1975 Dec;35(6): 343–355.

G300. Gordon BL 2d, Yanagihara R. Treatment of systemic lupus erythematosus with T-cell immunopotentiator levamisole: a follow-up report of 16 patients under treatment for a minimum period of four months. Ann Allergy 1977 Oct;39(4): 227–236.

G301. Gordon C, Ranges GE, Greenspan JS, Wofsy D. Chronic therapy with recombinant tumor necrosis factor-alpha in autoimmune NZB/NZW F1 mice. Clin Immunol Immunopathol 1989;52:421–434.

G302. Gordon C, Wofsy D. Effects of recombinant murine tumor necrosis factor-alpha on immune function. J Immunol 1990; 144:1753–1758.

G303. Gordon T, Dunn EC. Systemic lupus erythematosus and right recurrent laryngeal nerve palsy. Br J Rheumatol 1990 Aug;29(4):308–309.

G304. Gordon T, Isenberg D. The endocrinologic associations of the autoimmune rheumatic diseases. Semin Arthritis Rheum 1987 Aug;17(1):58–70.

G305. Gorevic PD, Katler EI, Agus B. Pulmonary nocardiosis. Occurrence in men with systemic lupus erythematosus. Arch Intern Med 1980 Mar;140(3):361–363.

G306. Gorla R, Airo P, Franceschini F, Stefani E, Braga S, Tincani A, Cattaneo R. Decreased number of peripheral blood Cd4 + CD29 + lymphocytes and increased spontaneous production of anti-DNA antibodies in patients with active systemic lupus erythematosus. J Rheumatol 1990;17:1048–1053.

G307. Gorst DW, Rawlinson VI, Merry RH, Stratton F. Positive direct antiglobulin test in normal individuals. Vos Sang 1989; 398:99–105.

G308. Goshen E, Livneh A, Nagy J, Sarov I, Shoenfeld Y. Antinuclear autoantibodies in sera of patients with IgA nephropathy. Nephron 1990; 55:33–36.

G309. Gossar DM, Walls RS. Systemic lupus erythematosus in later life. M J 1982 Apr 3;1(7):297–299.

G310. Gosset D, Foucher C, Lecouffe P, Savinel P. Asymptomatic sacroiliitis in systemic lupus erythematosus [letter]. J Rheumatol 1988 Jan;15(1):152–153.

G311. Goter Robinson CJ, Abraham AA, Balazs T. Induction of antinuclear antibodies by mercuric chloride in mice. Clin Exp Immunol 1984;58:300–306.

G312. Goter Robinson CJ, Balazs T, Egorov IK. Mercuric chloride-, gold sodium thiomalate-and D-Penicillamine-induced antinuclear antibodies in mice. Toxicol Appl Pharmacol 1986; 86:159–169.

G313. Goto M, Tanimoto K, Horiuchi Y. Natural cell mediated cytotoxicity in systemic lupus erythematosus. Suppression by anti-lymphocyte antibody. Arthritis Rheum 1980 Nov;23: 1274–1281.

G314. Gotoff SP, Isaacs EW, Muehrcke RC, Smith RD. Serum beta *IC* globulin in glomerulonephritis and systemic lupus erythematosus. Ann Intern Med 1969 Aug;71:327–333.

G315. Gottlieb AB, Lahita RG, Chiorazzi N, Kunkel HG. Immune function in systemic lupus erythematosus. Impairment of in vitro T-cell proliferation and in vivo antibody response to exogenous antigen. J Clin Invest 1979 May;63:885–892.

G316. Gottlieb E, Steitz JA. The RNA binding protein La influences both the accuracy and the efficiency of RNA polymerase III transcription in vitro. Embo J 1989;8:841–850.

G317. Gottlieb E, Steitz JA. Function of the mammalian La protein: evidence for this action in transcription termination by RNA polymerase III. Embo J 1989;8:851–861.

G318. Gotze O, Muller-Eberhard HJ. The C3-activator system: an alternative pathway of complement activation. J Exp Med 1971; 134:905–1085.

G319. Gouet D, Marchaud R, Aucouturier P. Atenolol induced systemic lupus erythematosus syndrome. J Rheumatol 1986; 13:11–32.

G320. Gougerot A, Stopopa-Lyonnet D, Poirer JC, Schmid M, Busson M, Marcelli A. HLA markers and complotypes: risk factors in SLE. Ann Dermatol Venerol 1987;113:329–334.

G321. Gougerot H, Carteaud A, Desvignes P. Acute eruption in facial lupus erythematosus. Kaposi-Besnier-Libman-Sacks syndrome apparently healed by streptomycin [original in French]. Bull Soc Franc Dermat et Syph 1949 Jan– Feb;56:41.

G322. Gough W, Lightfoot RW, Christian CL. Cryoglobulins and complement in immune complex disease [abstract]. Arthritis Rheum 1974;17:497.

G323. Gould DB, Soriano RZ. Acute alveolar hemorrhage in lupus erythematosus. Ann Intern Med 1975 Dec;83:836–837.

G324. Gould DM, Daves ML. Roentgenologic findings in systemic lupus erythematosus. Analysis of 100 cases. J Chron Dis 1955 Aug;2:136–145.

G325. Gould ES, Taylor S, Naidich JB, Furie R, Lane L. MR appearance of bilateral spontaneous patellar tendon rupture in systemic lupus erythematosus. J Comp Assist Tomogr 1987 Nov–Dec;11(6):1096–1097.

G326. Grabowska A, Carter N, Loke YW. Human trophoblast cells in culture express an unusual major histocompatibility complex class I-like antigen. Am J Reprod Immunol 1990;23: 10–18.

G327. Grace AW, Combes FC. Remission of disseminated lupus erythematosus induced by adrenocorticotropin. Proc Soc Exp Biol Med 1949 Dec;72:563–565.

G328. Graciansky P de. Two forms of dermatomyositis [original in French]. Sem Hop Paris 1949 May 2;25(33):1406–1413.

G329. Graciansky P de. Remarks concerning six cases of dermatomyositis [original in French]. Sem Hop Paris 1953 May 20; 29(33):1621–1633.

G330. Graff RJ, Lappe MA, Snell CD. The influence of gonads and adrenal glands on the immune response to skin grafts. Transplantation 1969;7:105–111.

G331. Graham DY, Agrawal N, Roth SH. Prevention of NSAID induced gastric ulcer with misoprostol: multicentre, double-blind, placebo-controlled trial. Lancet 1988;2:1277–1280.

G332. Graham IL, Gresham H, Brown EJ. An immobile subset of plasma membrane CD11b/CD18 (Mac-1) is involved in phagocytosis of targets recognized by multiple receptors. J Immunol 1989;142:235–2358.

G333. Graham S, Wilner H, Goodman D, Fichman M. Hyperkalemia in lupus nephritis associated with hyporeninemic hypoaldosteronism, [abstract]. Clin Res 1980;28:62A.

G334. Gral T, Schroth P, Sellers A, Fichman M, Maxwell M, DePalma J. Terminal lupus nephropathy (TLN) treated with chronic hemodialysis (CHD)[abstract]. Clin Res 1970;18:150.

G335. Granados J, Oliveras I, Melin H, Andrade F, Alarcon-Segovia D. Further evidence of the role of complement genotypes in susceptibility to systemic lupus erythematosus (SLE) obtained from Mexican family studies [abstract]. Arthritis Rheum 1987;30 Suppl:S21.

G336. Granier F, Vayssairat M, Priollet P, Housset E. Nailfold capillary microscopy in mixed connective tissue diseases. Comparison with systemic sclerosis and systemic lupus erythematosus. Arthritis Rheum 1986 Feb;29(2):189–195.

G337. Grant JM. Annular vesicular lupus erythematosus. Cutis 1981;28:90–92.

G338. Grant KD, Adams LE, Hess EV. Mixed connective tissue disease-a subset with sequential clinical and laboratory features. J Rheumatol 1981 Jul–Aug;8(4):587–598.

G339. Grant KD, Kant KS, Pollak VE, Weiss MA, Hess EV. Thrombosis in the lupus kidney. Arthritis Rheum 1982 Jan;25:117.

G340. Grausz H, Earley LE, Stephens BG, Lee JC, Hopper J Jr. Diagnostic import of virus-like particles in the glomerular endothelium of patients with systemic lupus erythematosus. N Engl J Med 1970;283:506–511.

G341. Gray JD, Horwitz DA. Lymphocytes expressing type 3 complement receptors proliferate in response to interleukin

2 and are the precursors of lymphokine-activated killer cells. J Clin Invest 1988;81:1247.

G342. Gray JD, Lash A, Baake AC, Horwitz DA. Studies on human blood lymphocytes with iC3b (type 3) complement receptors: III. Abnormalities in patients with active systemic lupus erythematosus. Clin Exp Immunol 1987;67:556–564.

G343. Graybill JR, Alford RH. Variability of sequential studies of lymphocyte blastogenesis in normal adults. Clin Exp Immunol 1976;25:28.

G344. Grayzel A, Solomon A, Aranow C, Diamond B. Antibodies elicited by pneumococcal antigens bear an anti-DNA associated idiotype. J Clin Invest 1991;87:842–846.

G345. Greaves MW, Sondergaard J. Pharmacologic agents released in ultraviolet light inflammation studied by continuous skin perfusion. J Invest Dermatol 1970 May;54:365–367.

G346. Grebenau MD. Personal communication.

G347. Green BJ, Wyse DG, Duff HJ, Mitchell LB, Matheson DS. Procainamide in vivo modulates suppressor T cell activity. Clin Invest Med 1988;11:425–429.

G348. Green DR, Flood PM, Gershon RK. Immunoregulatory T-cell pathways. Annu Rev Immunol 1983;1:439–464.

G349. Green JA, Dawson AA, Walker W. SLE and lymphoma. Lancet 1978 Oct 7;2:753–756.

G350. Green JE, Hinrichs SH, Vogel J, Jay G. Exocrinopathy resembling Sjögren's syndrome in HTLV-1 tax transgenic mice. Nature 1989;341(6237):72–74.

G351. Green SG, Piette WW. Successful treatment of hypertrophic lupus erythematosus with isotretinoin. J Am Acad Dermatol 1987 Aug;17(2 Pt 2):364–368.

G352. Greenberg JH, Lutcher CL. Drug-induced systemic lupus erythematosus. A case with life-threatening pericardial tamponade. JAMA 1972 Oct 1;222:191–193.

G353. Greenberg RA, Eaglstein WH, Turnier H, Hondek PV. Orally given indomethacin in blood flow response to UVL. Arch Dermatol 1975 Mar;111:328–330.

G354. Greenfield DI, Fong JS, Barth WF. Systemic lupus erythematosus and gout. Semin Arthritis Rheum 1985 Feb;14(3):176–179.

G355. Greenfield DI, Trinh P, Fulenwider A, Barth WF. Kaposi's sarcoma in a patient with SLE. J Rheumatol 1986;13:637–640.

G356. Greenspan EM. Survey of clinical significance of serum mucoprotein level. Arch Intern Med 1954 Jun;93:863–874.

G357. Greer JM, Panush RS. Incomplete lupus erythematosus. Arch Intern Med 19889;149:2473.

G358. Greger WP, Choy SH, Rantz LA. Experimental determination of the hypersensitive diathesis in man. J Immunol 1985;66:445–450.

G359. Gregersen PK. Biology of disease. HLA class II polymorphism implications for genetic susceptibility to autoimmune disease. Lab Invest 1989;615:19.

G360. Gregersen PK, Kao H, Nunez-Roldan A, Hurley CK, Karr RW, Silver J. Recombination sites in the HLA class II region are haplotype dependent. J Immunol 1988;141:1365–1368.

G361. Gregersen PK, Silver J, Winchester RJ. The shared epitope hypothesis. An approach to understanding the molecular genetics of susceptibility to rheumatoid arthritis. Arthritis Rheum 1987;30:1205–1213.

G362. Gregory CD, Shah LP, Lee H, Scott IV, Golding PR. Cytotoxic reactivity of natural killer (NK) cells during normal pregnancy: a longitudinal study. J Clin Lab Immunol 1985;18:175.

G363. Greiner AC, Berry K. Skin pigmentation and corneal and lens opacity with prolonged chlorpromazine therapy. Can Med Assoc J 1964 Mar 14;90:663–665.

G364. Greisman SG, Redecha PB, Kimberly RP, Christian CL. Differences among immune complexes: association of C1q in systemic lupus erythematosus immune complexes with renal diseases. J Immunol 1987;138:739.

G365. Greisman SG, Thayaparan LS, Godwin TA, Lockshin MD. Occlusive vasculopathy in systemic lupus erythematosus. Association with anticardiolipin antibody. Arch Intern Med 1991 Feb;151(2):389–392.

G366. Grennan DM, Ferguson M, Ghobarey AE, Williamson J, Dick WC, Buchanan WW. Sjogren's syndrome in SLE: Part 2. An examination of the clinical significance of Sjogren's syndrome by comparison of its frequency in typical and atypical forms of SLE, overlap syndromes and scleroderma. N Z Med J 1977 Oct 26;86(598):376–379.

G367. Grennan DM, Ferguson M, Williamson J, Mavrikakis M, Dick WC, Buchanan WW. Sjogren's syndrome in SLE: Part 1. The frequency of the clinical and subclinical feature of Sjogren's syndrome in patients with SLE. N Z Med J 1977 Oct 26; 86(598):374–376.

G368. Grennan DM, McCormick JN, Wojtacha D, Carty M, Behan W. Immunological studies of the placenta in systemic lupus erythematosus. Ann Rheum Dis 1978;37:129–134.

G369. Grennan DM, Moseley A, Sloane D, Pumphrey R, Dick WC, Buchanan WW. The significance of serial measurement of serum antinative DNA antibodies and complement C3 and C4 components in the management of systemic lupus erythematosus. Aust N Z J Med 1977 Dec;7:625–629.

G370. Gresham HD, Ray CJ, O'Sullivan FX. Defective neutrophil function in the autoimmune mouse strain MRL/lpr. J Immunol 1991;146:3911–3921.

G371. Grey RE, Jenkins EA, Hall MA, Kanski JJ, Ansell BM. Recurrent acute proptosis in atypical systemic lupus erythematosus. Clin Rheumatol 1989;8:785–786.

G372. Gribetz D, Henley WL. Systemic lupus erythematosus in childhood. J Mount Sinai Hosp 1959;26:289–296.

G373. Griffey RH, Brown MS, Bankhurst AD, Sibbitt RR, Sibbitt WL Jr. Depletion of high-energy phosphates in the central nervous system of patients with systemic lupus erythematosus, as determined by phosphorus-31 nuclear magnetic resonance spectroscopy. Arthritis Rheum 1990 Jun;33(6):827–833.

G374. Griffin JD, Hercend T, Beveridge R, Schlossman SF. Characterization of an antigen expressed by human natural killer cells. J Immunol 1983;130:2947–2951.

G375. Griffin SW, Ulloa A, Holley HL. The familial occurrence of systemic lupus erythematosus: a case report. Arthritis Rheum 1958;1:544–547.

G376. Griffing WL, Moore SB, Luthra HS, McKenna CH, Fathman CG. Associations of antibodies to native DNA with HLA-DRw3 A possible major histocompatibility linked human immune response gene. J Exp Med 1980;152:3195–3205.

G377. Griffith AJ, Schumauss C, Craft J. The Sm protein is highly conserved between species and its murine gene contains a nonfunctional splice junction. 1992 In press.

G378. Griffith GC, Vural IL. Acute and subacute disseminated lupus erythematosus: correlation of clinical and postmortem findings in eighteen cases. Circulation 1951 Apr;3:492–500.

G379. Griffith HW, McEvers J, Becker R, Editors. Instructions for obstetric and gynecologic patients. Philadelphia: Saunders, 1984:113.

G380. Griffiths GM, Berek C, Kaartinen M, Milstein C. Somatic mutation and the maturation of immune response to 2-phenyl oxazolone. Nature 1984;312:271–275.

G381. Griffiths I, Kane S. Sulfasalazine-induced lupus syndrome in ulcerative colitis. BMJ 1977 Nov 5; 2:1188–1189.

G382. Griffiths ID, Richardson J. Lupus-like illness associated with labetalol. BMJ 1979 Aug 25;2:496–497.

G383. Griffiths HJ. Etiology, pathogenesis and early diagnosis of ischemic necrosis of the hip. JAMA 1981 Dec 4;246(22): 2615–2617.

G384. Griffits ME, DeWitt CW. Modulation of collagen-induced arthritis in rats by non-RTl-linked genes. J Immunol 1984;133: 3043–3046.

G385. Grigor R, Edmonds J, Lewkonia R, Bresnihan B, Hughes GR. Systemic lupus erythematosus. A prospective analysis. Ann Rheum Dis 1978 Apr;37(2):121–128.

G386. Grigor REJ, Lewkonia R, Bresnihan B, Hughes GRV. Systemic lupus erythematosus: A prospective analysis. Ann Rheum Dis 1978 Apr;37:127.

G387. Grigor RR, Shervington PC, Hughes GRV, Hawkins DF. Outcome of pregnancy in systemic lupus erythematosus. Proc Roy Soc Med 1977;70:99–100.

G388. Grimes DA, LeBolt SA, Grimes KR, Wingo PA. Systemic lupus erythematosus and reproductive function: a case-control study. Am J Obstet Gynecol 1985;153–179–186.

G389. Grimley PM, Decker JL, Michelitch HJ, Frantz MM. Abnormal structures in circulating lymphocytes from patients with systemic lupus erythematosus and related diseases. Arthritis Rheum 1978;16:313–323.

G390. Grimley PM, Kang YH, Silverman RH, Davis G, Hoofnagle JH. Blood lymphocyte inclusions associated with alpha-interferon [abstract]. Lab Invest 1983 Jan;48:30A.

G391. Grimm EA, Mazumder A, Zhang HZ, Rosenberg SA. Lymphokine-activated killer cells phenomenon. Lysis of natural killer-resistant fresh solid tumor cells by interleukin 2-activated autologous human peripheral blood lymphocytes. J Exp Med 1982;155:1823.

G392. Griner PF, Hoyer LW. Megakaryocytic thrombocytopenia in systemic lupus erythematosus Arch Intern Med 1970;125: 328–332.

G393. Grinlinton FM, Vuletic JC, Gow PJ. Rapidly progressive calcific periarthritis occurring in a patient with lupus nephritis receiving chronic ambulatory peritoneal dialysis. J Rheumatol 1990;17(8):1100–1103.

G394. Gripenberg M, Helve T, Kurki P. Profiles of Antibodies to Histones, DNA and IgG in Patients with Systemic Rheumatic Diseases Determined by ELISA. J Rheumatol 1985; 12: 934–939.

G395. Grishman E, Churg J. Ultrastructure of dermal lesions in systemic lupus erythematosus. Lab Invest 1970 Mar;22: 189–197.

G396. Grishman E, Porush JC, Rosen SM, Churg J. Lupus nephritis with organized deposits in the kidneys. Arch Pathol Lab Med 1967;103:573.

G397. Grishman E, Venkataseshan VS. Vascular lesions in lupus nephritis. Modern Pathol 1988;1:235–241.

G398. Griso D, Macri A, Biolcati G, Topi G. Does an association exist between PCT and SLE? Results of a study on autoantibodies in 158 patients affected with PCT. Arch Dermatol Res 1989;281(4):291–292.

G399. Gristanti MAA, Vergara EF, Cartier RL, Guzman BL. Central nervous system involvement in systemic lupus erythematosus. Rev Med Chile 1985;113:1194–1202.

G400. Gritzmacher C. Molecular aspects of heavy-chain class switching. Critical Reviews in Immunology. 1989;9:173–200.

G401. Grob JJ, Collet-Villette AM, Andrac L, Bonerandi JJ. Fibrosing lupus erythematosus panniculitis in a pregnant woman with anti-Ro/SSA antibodies in mother and child. Ann Dermatol Venereol 1987;114(8):973–977.

G402. Grob PJ, Muller-Schoop JW, Hacki MA, Joller-Jemelka HI. Drug-induced pseudolupus. Lancet 1975 Jul 26;2:144–148.

G403. Groothuis JR, Groothuis DR, Mukhopadhyay D, Grossman BJ, Altemeier WA. Lupus-associated chorea in childhood. Am J Dis Child 1977 Oct;131(10):1131–1134.

G404. Gross DS, Garrard WT. Poising chromatin for transcription. Trends Bioc 1987; 12:293–297.

G405. Gross L. The heart in atypical verrucous endocarditis (Libman-Sacks). In: Contributions to the Medical Sciences in Honor of Dr. Emanuel Libman by His Pupils, Friends, and Colleagues. New York: The International Press 1932;2:527–550.

G406. Gross L. Cardiac lesions in Libman-Sacks disease with consideration of its relationship to acute diffuse lupus erythematosus. Am J Pathol 1940 Jul;16:375–408.

G407. Gross L. Influence of sex on the evolution of a transplant mouse sarcoma. Proc Soc Exp Biol Med 1941;47:273–276.

G408. Gross M, Esterly JR, Earle RH. Pulmonary alterations in systemic lupus erythematosus. Am Rev Resp Dis 1972 Apr; 105:572–577.

G409. Grosse-Wilde H, Genth E, Grevesmuhl A, Vogeler U, Zarnowski H, Mierau R, Doxiadis G, Doxiadis I, Maas D. HLA-DR4 and Gm 121 haplotypes are associated with pseudolupus induced by Venopyrum dragees. Arthritis Rheum 1987;30: 878–883.

G410. Grossman CB, Bragg DG, Armstrong D. Roentgen manifestations of pulmonary nocardiosis. Radiology 1970 Aug;96: 325–330.

G411. Grossman CJ. Regulation of the immune system by sex steroids. Endocrin Reve 1984;5:435–454.

G412. Grossman J, Schwartz RH, Callerame ML, Codemi JJ. Systemic lupus erythematosus in a 1-year-old child. Am J Dis Child 1975 Jan;129:123–125.

G413. Grossman L, Barland P. Histone reactivity of drug-induced antinuclear antibodies. Arthritis Rheum 1981;24:927–931.

G414. Grottolo A, Ferrari V, Mariano M, Zambruni A, Tincani A, Del Bono R. Primary adrenal insufficiency, circulating lupus anticoagulant and anticardiolipin antibodies in a patient with multiple abortions and recurrent thrombotic episodes. Haematologica (Pavia) 1988 Nov–Dec;73(6):517–519.

G415. Gruber MF, Bjorndahl JM, Nakamura S, Fu SM. Anti-CD45 inhibition of human B cell proliferation depends on the nature of activation signals and the state of B cell activation. A study with anti-IgM and anti-CDw40 antibodies. J Immunol 1989; 142:4144–4152.

G416. Grumet FC, Coukell A, Bodmer JG, Bodmer WF, McDevitt HO. Histocompatibility (HL-A) antigens associated with systemic lupus erythematosus. A possible genetic predisposition to disease. N Engl J Med 1971;285:193–196.

G417. Grundmann M, Bayer A. Effects of chloroquine on adrenocortical function. H. Histological, histochemical and biochemical changes in suprarenal gland of rats on long-term administration of chloroquine. Arzneim Forsch 1976;26:2029–2035.

G418. Grundy HO, Peltz G, Moore KW, Golbus MS, Jackson LG, Lebo RV. The polymorphic Fcγ receptor II gene maps to human chromosome 1q. Immunogenetics 1989;29:331–339.

G419. Grupper C, Marcel GA. Lupus erythematosus and psychotropic drugs [original in French]. Bull Soc Fr Dermatol Syphilgr (Paris) 1965 Oct; 72:714–721.

G420. Guardia J, Richart C, Martinez-Vazquez JM, Martin C. Pseudo-lupus induced by a vasculotropic drug [English abstract]. Nouv Press Med 1977 Oct 1;6(32):2873–2875.

G421. Guckian JC, Byers EH, Perry JE. Arizona infection of man. Report of a case and review of the literature. Arch Intern Med 1967 Feb;119(2):170–175.

G422. Guery JC, Druet E, Glotz D, Hirsch F, Mandet C, DeHeer E, Druet P. Specificity and cross reactive idiotypes of antiglomerular basement membrane autoantibodies in HgCl2-induced autoimmune glomerulonephritis. Eur J Immunol 1990; 20:93–100.

G423. Guilbert B, Dighiero G, Avrameas S. Naturally occurring antibodies against nine common antigens in human sera: I.

detection, isolation, and characterization. J Immunol 1982; 128:2779–2787.

G424. Guillet G, Sassolas B, Plantin P, Cledes J, Youinou P, Masse R. Anti-Ro-positive lupus and hereditary angioneurotic edema. A 7-year follow-up with worsening of lupus under danazol treatment. Dermatologica 1988;177(6):370–375.

G425. Guilly MN, Damon F, Bovet JC, Borners M, Courvalin JC. Autoantibodies to nuclear lamin B in a patient with thrombopenia. Eur J Cell Biol 1987;43:266–272.

G426. Guisti AM, Chien NC, Zack DJ, Shin S-U, Scharff MD. Somatic diversification of S107 from an anti-phosphocholine to an anti-DNA autoantibody is due to a single base change in its heavy chain variable region. Proc Natl Acad Sci USA 1987;84: 2926–2930.

G427. Guldner HH, Szostecki C, Vosberg HP, Lakonilk HJ, Penner E, Bautz FA. Scl70 autoantibodies from scleroderma patients recognize a 95 kDa protein identified as DNA topoisomerase I. Chromosome 1986;94:132–138.

G428. Gupta RC, Kohler PF. Identification of HBsAg determinants in immune complexes from hepatitis B virus-associated vasculitis. J Immunol 1984;132:1223–1228.

G429. Gupta S, Funkhouser JW. Treatment of thrombotic thrombocytopenic purpura with plasma exchange: Five cases. J Clin Apheresis 1984;2:195–199.

G430. Gurian LE, Rogoff TM, Ware AJ, Jordan RE, Combes B, Gilliam JN: The immunologic diagnosis of chronic active "autoimmune" hepatitis: distinction from systemic lupus erythematosus. Hepatology 1985 May–Jun;5(3):397–402.

G431. Gusterson BA, Fitzharris BM. Angio-immunoblastic lymphadenopathy with lupus erythematosus cells. Br J Haematol 1979 Sep;43(1):149–150.

G432. Guthaner DF, Stathers GM. Salmonella typhimurium and septicaemia complicating disseminated lupus erythematosus. Med J Aust 1969;2:1156.

G433. Gutierrez G, Dagnino R, Mintz G. Polymyositis/dermatomyositis and pregnancy. Arthritis Rheum 1984;27:291–294.

G434. Gutierrez F, Valenzuela JE, Ehresmann GR, Quismorio FP, Kitridou RC. Esophageal dysfunction in patients with mixed connective tissue diseases and systemic lupus erythematosus. Digestive Dis and Sciences 1982;27:592–597.

G435. Gutierrez-Ramos JC, Andreu JL, de Alboran IM, Rodriguez J, Leonardo E, Kroemer G, Marcos MAR, Martinez A C. Insights into autoimmunity: From classical models to current perspectives. Immunol Rev 1990;118:73–101.

G436. Gutierrez-Rodriguez O, Starusta-Bacal P, Gutierrez-Montes O. Treatment of refractory rheumatoid arthritis—The thalidomide experience. J Rheumatol 1989 Feb;16(2):158–163.

G437. Guttman M, Lang AE, Garnett ES, Nahmias C, Firnau G, Tyndel FJ, Gordon AS. Regional cerebral glucose metabolism in SLE chorea: further evidence that striational hypometabolism is not a correlated of chorea. Mov Disord 1987;2: 201–210.

G438. Guyre PM, Campbell AS, Kniffin W, Fanger MW. Monocytes and polymorphonuclear neutrophils of patients with streptococcal pharyngitis express increased numbers of type I IgG Fc receptors. J Clin Invest 1990;86:1892–1896.

G439. Guyre PM, Morganelli PM, Miller R. Recombinant immune interferon increases immunoglobulin G Fc receptors on cultured human mononuclear phagocytes. J Clin Invest 1983;72: 393–397.

G440. Guze SB. The occurrence of psychiatric illness in systemic lupus erythematosus. Am J Psychiatry 1967 Jun;123: 1562–1540.

G441. Guzman L, Avalos E, Ortiz R, Gurrola R, Lopez E, Herrera R. Placental abnormalities in systemic lupus erythematosus: In situ deposition of antinuclear antibodies. J Rheumatol 1987; 14:924–929.

G442. Gyorkey F, Min K-W, Sincovics JG, Gyorkey P. Systemic lupus erythematosus and myxovirus. N Engl J Med 1969;280:

H

H1. Haakenstad AO, Case JB, Mannik M. Effect of cortisone on the disappearance kinetics and tissue localization of soluble immune complexes. J Immunol 1975;114:1153–1160.

H2. Haakenstad AO, Mannik M. Saturation of the reticuloendothelial system with soluble immune complexes. J Immunol 1974;112:1939–1948.

H3. Haakenstad AO, Mannik M. The disappearance kinetics of soluble immune complexes prepared with reduced and alkylated antibodies and with intact antibodies in mice. Lab Invest 1976;35:283–292.

H4. Haakenstad AO, Striker GE, Mannik M. The glomerular deposition of soluble immune complexes prepared with reduced and alkylated antibodies and with intact antibodies in mice. Lab Invest 1976;35:293–301.

H5. Haas M, Meshorer A. Reticulum cell neoplasms induced in C57B1/6 mice by cultured virus grown in stromal hematopoietic cell lines. J Natl Cancer Inst 1979;63:427.

H6. Habara Y, Williams JA, Hootman SR. Antimuscarinic effects of chloroquine in rat pancreatitic acini. Biochem Biophys Res Commun 1986 Jun 13;137(2):664–669.

H7. Habets WJ, de Rooij DJ, Salden MH, Verhagen AP, Van Eekelen CAG, Van de Putte LB, Van Venrooij WJ. Antibodies against distinct nuclear matrix proteins are characteristic for mixed connective tissue disease. Clin Exp Immunol 1983;54: 265–276.

H8. Habets WJ, Hoet M, Bringmann P, Luhrmann R, Van Venrooij W. Autoantibodies to ribonucleoprotein particles containing U2 small nuclear RNA. Embo J 1985;4:1545–1550.

H9. Habets WJ, Sillekens PTG, Hoet MH, McAllister MR, Lerner MR, Van Venrooij WJ. Small nuclear RNA-associated proteins are immunologically related as revealed by mapping of autoimmune reactive B cell epitopes. Proc Natl Acad Sci USA 1989; 86:4674–4678.

H10. Habets WJ, Sillekens PTG, Hoet MH, Schalken JA, Roebrook AJM, Leunissen JAM, Van de Ven WJM, Van Venrooij WJ. Analysis of a cDNA clone expressing a human autoimmune antigen: Full-length sequence of the U2 small nuclear RNA-associated B″ antigen. Proc Natl Acad Sci USA 1987;84: 2421–2425.

H11. Hackett ER, Martinez RP, Larson PF, Paddison RM. Optic neuritis in SLE. Arch Neurol 1974;31:9–11.

H12. Hadidi T, Decker JL, El-Nagdy L, Samy M. Ineffectiveness of levamisole in systemic lupus erythematosus: a controlled trial. Arthritis Rheum 1981 Jan;24(1):60–63.

H13. Hadler NM, Gerwin RD, Frank MM, Whitaker JN, Baker M, Decker JL. The fourth component of complement in the cerebrospinal fluid in SLE. Arthritis Rheum 1973 Jul–Aug;16: 507–521.

H14. Hadley AG, Byron MA, Chapel HM, Bunch C, Holburn AM. Anti-granulocyte opsonic activity in sera from patients with systemic lupus erythematosus. Br J Haematol 1987;65:61–65.

H15. Hadron PY, Bouchez B, Wattel A, Arnott G, Devulder B. Chorea, systemic lupus erythematosus, circulating anticoagulant. J Rheumatol 1986;13:991–993.

H16. Haeger-Aronsen B, Krook G, Abdulla M. Oral carotenoids for photosensitivity in patients with erythrohepatic protoporphyria, polymorphous light eruption and lupus erythematodes discoides. Int J Dermatol 1979 Jan–Feb;18(1): 73–82.

H17. Haga HJ, Christopoulos C, Machin S, Khamashta MA, Hughes GR. Lack of specific binding of anticardiolipin antibodies to platelet demonstration by a flow-cytometric method. J Rheumatol. In press.

H18. Hagberg B, Leonhardt T, Skogh M. Familial occurrence of collagen diseases. 1. Progressive systemic sclerosis and systemic lupus erythematosus. Acta Med Scand 1961;169:727.

H19. Hagihara M, Nagatsu T, Ohashi M, Miura T. Concentrations of neopterin and biopterin in serum from patients with rheumatoid arthritis or systemic lupus erythematosus and in synovial fluids from patients with rheumatoid or osteoarthritis. Clin Chemistry 1990;36:705.

H20. Hagiwara M, Katayose K, Kan R, Takahashi Y, Yashima Y, Kumashiro H. The feature of epileptic seizures in systemic lupus erythematosus. Jap J Psych Neurol 1987;41:533–534.

H21. Hahn BH. Characteristics of pathogenic subpopulations of antibodies to DNA. Arthritis Rheum 1982;24:747–752.

H22. Hahn BH. Current concepts of the pathogenesis and treatment of autoimmune diseases. Ann Roy Coll Phy Surg Canada 1990;23:253–264.

H23. Hahn BH. Lupus nephritis: therapeutic decisions. Hosp Practice (Office) 1990;Mar 30;25(3A):89–104.

H24. Hahn BH, Ando DG, Dunn K, Ebling FM, Sercarz E. Idiotype regulatory networks promote autoantibody formation. J Rheumatol 1987;14 Suppl 13:143.

H25. Hahn BH, Bagby MK, Hamilton TR, Osterland CK. Comparison of therapeutic and immunosuppressive effects of azathioprine, prednisone, and combined therapy in NZB/NZW mice. Arthritis Rheum 1973;16:163.

H26. Hahn BH, Bagby MK, Osterland CK. Abnormalities of delayed hypersensitivity in systemic lupus erythematosus. Am J Med 1973 Jul;55:25–31.

H27. Hahn BH, Ebling FM. A public idiotypic determinant is present on spontaneous cationic IgG antibodies to DNA from mice of unrelated lupus-prone strains. J Immunol 1984;133:3015–3019.

H28. Hahn BH, Ebling FM. Suppression of NZB/NZW murine nephritis by administration of a syngeneic monoclonal antibody to DNA. Possible role of anti-idiotypic antibodies. J Clin Invest 1983;71:1728.

H29. Hahn BH, Ebling FM. Suppression of murine lupus nephritis by administration of an anti-idiotypic antibody to anti-DNA. J Immunol 1984 Jan;132:187–190.

H30. Hahn BH, Ebling FM. Idiotypic restriction in murine lupus: high frequency of three public idiotypes on serum IgG in nephritic NZB/NZW F1 mice. J Immunol 1987 Apr;138(7):2110–2118.

H31. Hahn BH, Ebling FM, Freeman S, Clevinger B, Davie J. Production of monoclonal murine antibodies to DNA by somatic cell hybrids. Arthritis Rheum 1980 Aug;23(8):942–945.

H32. Hahn BH, Ebling FM, Panosian-Sahakian N, Klotz J, Kronenberg M, Tsao B, Kalunian KC, Ando D. Idiotype selection is an immunoregulatory mechanism which contributes to the pathogenesis of systemic lupus erythematosus. J Autoimmunity 1989;1:673.

H33. Hahn BH, Kantor OS, Osterland CK. Azathioprine plus prednisone compared with prednisone alone in the treatment of systemic lupus erythematosus. Report of a prospective controlled trial in 24 patients. Ann Intern Med 1975 Nov;83(3):597–605.

H34. Hahn BH, Kalunian KC, Fronek Z, Panosian-Sahakian N, Louie JS, McDevitt HO, Ebling FM. Idiotypic characteristics of immunoglobulins associated with human systemic lupus erythematosus. Arthritis Rheum 1990;33:978–984.

H35. Hahn BH, Knotts L, Hamilton TR. Influence of cyclophosphamide on neoplasia in NZB/NZW mice. Arthritis Rheum 1975 Mar–Apr;18:145–152.

H36. Hahn BH, Knotts L, Mehta JM. The effect of altered lymphocyte function on the immunologic disorders of NZB/NZW mice. II. Response to anti-thymocyte globulin. Clin Immunol Immnopathol 1977;8:225.

H37. Hahn BH, Pletcher LS, Muniain M, Mac-Dermott RP. Suppression of the normal autologous mixed lymphocyte reaction by sera from patients with systemic lupus erythematosus. Arthritis Rheum 1982 Apr;25:381–389.

H38. Hahn BH, Sharp GC, Irvin WS, Kantor OS, Gardner CA, Bagby MK, Perry HM, Osterland CK. Immune response to hydralazine and nuclear antigens in hydralazine-induced lupus erythematosus. Ann Intern Med 1972;76:365–374.

H39. Hahn BH, Shulman LE. Autoantibodies and nephritis in the white strain (NZW) of New Zealand mice. Arthritis Rheum 1969 Aug;12:355–364.

H40. Hahn TJ, Hahn BH. Osteopenia in patients with rheumatic disease: Principles of diagnosis and therapy. Semin Arthritis Rheum 1976 Nov;6:165–188.

H41. Hahn TJ, Halstead LR, Teitelbaum SL, Hahn BH. Altered mineral metabolism in glucocorticoid-induced osteopenia. Effect of 25-hydroxyvitamin D administration. J Clin Invest 1979 Aug;64(2):655–665.

H42. Haider YS, Roberts WC. Coronary arterial disease in systemic lupus erythematosus: quantification of degrees of narrowing in 22 necropsy patients (21 women) aged 16–37 years. Am J Med 1981 Apr;70:775–781.

H43. Haidushka I, Zlatev S. Isoprinosine in patient with systemic lupus erythematosus [letter]. Lancet 1987 Jul 18;2(8551):153.

H44. Haim S, Shafrir A. The nature of discoid lupus erythematosus. Acta Dermatovener (Stockh) 1970;50(2):86–88.

H45. Hajiroussou VJ. Hypoparathyroidism associated with systemic lupus erythematosus. Postgrad Med J 1981 Sep;57(671):597–598.

H46. Halberg P, Alsbjorn B, Tolle Balslov J, Gerstoft J, Lorenzen I, Ullman S, Wiik A. Systemic lupus erythematosus: Follow-up study of 148 patients, I: Classification, clinical and laboratory findings, course and outcome. Clin Rheumatol 1987;6:13–21.

H47. Halberg P, Alsbjorn B, Tolle Balslev J, Lorenzen I, Gerstoft J, Ullman S, Wiik A. Systemic lupus erythematosus: Follow-up study of 148 patients, II: Predictive factors of importance for course and outcome. Clin Rheumatol 1987;6:22–26.

H48. Halberg P, Ullman S, Jorgensen F. The lupus band test as a measure of disease activity in systemic lupus erythematosus. Arch Dermatol 1982 Aug;118(8):572–576.

H49. Hale GM, Highton J, Kalmakoff J, Palmer DG. Changes in anti-DNA antibody affinity during exacerbations of systemic lupus erythematosus. Scand J Rheumatol 1986;15:243–250.

H50. Halevy S, Ben-Bassat M, Joshua H, Hazaz B, Feuerman E. Immunofluorescent and electron-microscope findings in the uninvolved skin of patients with systemic lupus erythematosus. Acta Dermatovener (Stockh) 1979;59(5):427–433.

H51. Same as H53a.

H52. Hall ND, Goulding NJ, Snaith ML, Davies J, Maddison PJ. Antimalarial drugs and the immune system. Br J Clin Prac 1987;41 Suppl 52:60–63.

H53. Hall RCW. Psychiatric presentations of medical illness: Somatopsychic disorders. New York: Septrum, 1980.

H53a. Hall RCW. Psychiatric adverse drug reactions: Steroid psychosis. Clinical Advances in Psychiatric Disorders. 1991 Apr–May;5(2).

H54. Hall RCW, Beresford TP. Psychiatric manifestations of physical illness. In: Michels R, Cavenar JO, Brodie HKH, et al, editors. Psychiatry. Philadelphia: Lippincott, 1989;2:9.

H55. Hall RCW, Popkin MK, Kirkpatrick B. Tricyclic exacerbation of steroid psychosis. J Nerv Ment Dis 1978; 166(10):738–742.

H56. Hall RCW, Popkin MK, Stickney SK, Gardner ER. Presentation of the steroid psychoses. J Nerv Ment Dis 1979;167:229–236.

H57. Hall RN, Goldstein AL. In: Fenichel RL, Chirigos MA, editors. Endocrine regulation of host immunity on immunomodulation agents and their mechanisms. New York: Mercel-Dekker, 1984:533–563.

H58. Hall RP, Lawley TJ, Smith HR, Katz SI. Bullous eruption of systemic lupus erythematosus. Dramatic response to dapsone therapy. Ann Intern Med 1982 Aug;97(2):165–170.

H59. Hall S, Buettner H, Luthra HS. Occlusive retinal vascular disease in systemic lupus erythematosus. J Rheumatol 1984; 11:846–850.

H60. Hall S, Czaja AJ, Ginsburg WW. How lupoid is lupoid hepatitis? [abstract]. Arthritis Rheum 1984 Apr;27(4) Suppl:S62.

H61. Hall S, Czaja AJ, Kaufman DK, Markowitz H, Ginsburg WW. How lupoid is lupoid hepatitis? J Rheumatol 1986 Feb;13(1): 95–98.

H62. Halla JT, Hardin JG. Clinical features of the arthritis of mixed connective tissue disease. Arthritis Rheum 1978 Jun; 219(4):497–503.

H63. Halla JT, Schrohenloher RE, Volanakis JE. Immune complexes and other laboratory features of pleural effusions: A comparison of rheumatoid arthritis, systemic lupus erythematosus and other diseases. Ann Intern Med 1980 Jun;92: 748–752.

H64. Halla JT, Volanakis JE, Schrohenloher RE. Circulating immune complexes in mixed connective disease. Arthritis Rheum 1979 May;22(5):484–489.

H65. Hallaq H, Sellmayer A, Smith TW, Leaf A. Protective effect of eicosapentaenoic acid on ouabain toxicity in neonatal rat cardiac myocytes. Proc Natl Acad Sci USA 1990;87: 7834–7838.

H66. Hallgren R, Hakansson L, Venge P. Kinetic studies of phagocytosis. I. The serum independent particle uptake by PMN from patients with rheumatoid arthritis and systemic lupus erythematosus. Arthritis Rheum 1978 Jan–Feb;21:107–113.

H67. Halliwell RE. Autoimmune diseases in domestic animals. J Am Vet Med Assoc. 1982;181:1088–1096.

H68. Halloran PF, Cole EH, Bookman AA, Urowitz MB, Clarke WTW. Possible beneficial effect of ciclosporin in some cases of severe systemic lupus erythematosus. In: Schindler R, editor. Ciclosporin in Autoimmune Diseases. Berlin: Springer-Verlag, 1985:357–361.

H69. Halloran PF, Urmson J, Rammassar V, Laskin C, Autenried P. Increased class I and class II MHC products and mRNA in kidneys of MRL-lpr/lpr mice during autoimmune nephritis and inhibition by cyclosporine. J Immunol 1988;141:2303–2312.

H70. Halma C, Breedveld FC, Daha MR, Blok D, Evers-Schouten JH, Hermans J, Pauwels EK, van Es LA. Elimination of soluble ^{123}I-labeled aggregates of IgG in patients with systemic lupus erythematosus. Effect of serum IgG and number of erythrocyte complement receptor type 1. Arthritis Rheum 1991;34: 442–452.

H71. Halma C, Daha MR, van Furth R, Camps JAJ, Evers-Schouten JH, Pauwels EK, Lobatto S, van Es LA. Elimination of soluble ^{123}I-labeled aggregates of IgG in humans: the effects of splenectomy. Clin Exp Immunol 1989;77:62–66.

H72. Halmay O, Ludwig K. Bilateral band-shaped deep keratitis and iridocyclitis in systemic lupus erythematosus. Br J Opthalmol 1964;44:558–562.

H73. Halpern AA, Horwitz BG, Nagel DA. Tendon ruptures associated with corticosteroid therapy. West J Med 1977 Nov; 127(5):378–382.

H74. Halpern R, Davidson A, Lazo A, Solomon G, Lahita R, Diamond B. Familial systemic lupus erythematosus. Presence of a cross-reactive idiotype in healthy family members. J Clin Invest 1985;76:731–736.

H75. Hamberg M. Inhibition of prostaglandin synthesis in man. Biochem Biophys Res Comm 1972;49:720–726.

H76. Hamblin TJ, Mufti GJ, Bracewell A. Severe deafness in systemic lupus erythematosus: its immediate relief by plasma exchange. BMJ (Clin Res) 1982 May 8;284(6326):1374.

H77. Hamburger M, Hodes S, Barland P. The incidence and clinical significance of antibodies to extractable nuclear antigens. Am J Med Sci 1977 Jan–Feb;273(1):21–28.

H78. Hamburger MI. A long-term study of plasmapheresis (PEX) and cyclophosphamide (C) in systemic lupus erythematosus (SLE). J Clin Apheresis 1984;2(1):143.

H79. Hamburger MI, Gerardi EN, Fields TR, Bennett RS. Reticuloendothelial system Fc receptor function and plasmapheresis in systemic lupus erythematosus. Artif Organs 1981 Aug;5(3): 264–268.

H80. Hamburger MI, Lawley TJ, Kimberly RP, Plotz PH, Frank MM. A serial study of splenic reticuloendothelial system Fc receptor functional activity in systemic lupus erythematosus. Arthritis Rheum 1982;25;48–54.

H81. Hamburger MI, Moutsopoulus HM, Lawley TJ, Sharp GC, Frank MM. Reticuloendothelial system Fc receptor function in mixed connective tissue disease [abstract]. Arthritis Rheum Jun;22:618–619.

H82. Hamburger RN. Induction of the lupus erythematosus ("L.E.") cell in vitro in peripheral blood. Yale J Biol 1950;22: 407–410.

H83. Hamed I, Lindeman RD, Czerwinski AW. Acute pancreatitis following corticosteroid and azathioprine therapy [case report]. Am J Med Sci 1978 Sep–Oct;276(2):211–219.

H84. Hamilton CR, Tumulty PA. Thrombosis of renal veins and inferior vena cava complicating lupus nephritis. JAMA 1968 Dec 2;206:2315–2316.

H85. Hamilton M, Normansell DE, Garrett MA, Davis JS 4th. Mitogen stimulation of human lymphocytes. II. Effect of exogenous DNA on lymphocyte function in systemic lupus erythematosus. Clin Immunol Immunopathol 1982 Feb;22:238–246.

H86. Hamilton ME, Winfield JB. T gamma cells in systemic lupus erythematosus. Arthritis Rheum 1979 Jan;22:1–6.

H87. Hamilton RG, Harley JB, Bias WB, Roebber M, Reichlin M, Hochberg MC, Arnett FC. Two Ro (SS-A) autoantibody responses in systemic lupus erythematosus correlation of HLA-DR/DQ specificities with quantitative expression of Ro (SS-A) autoantibody. Arthritis Rheum 1988;31:496–505.

H88. Hammar JA. Uber Gewicht Involution und Persistenz der tavmus im Post-fetal-leben des Menschen. Arch F Anta U Physiol Anat Abt Supple Bd 1906:91.

H89. Hammer O, Saltissi D. Response of acute cerebral lupus in childhood to pulse methylprednisolone in reduced dosage. Ann Rheum Dis 1986;45:606–607.

H90. Hammond A, Rudge AC, Loizou S, Bowook SJ, Walport MJ. Reduced numbers of complement receptors type 1 on erythrocytes are associated with increased levels of anticardiolipin antibodies. Findings in patients with systemic lupus erythematosus and the antiphospholipid syndrome. Arthritis Rheum 1989;32:259–264.

H91. Hamsten A, Norbert R, Bjorkholm M, de Faire U, Holm G. Antibodies to cardiolipin in young survivors of myocardial infarctions: An association with recurrent cardiovascular events. Lancet 1986;1:113–115.

H92. Hamza M, Elleuch M, Meddeb S, Moalla M. Arthritis and osteomyelitis caused by Salmonella typhimurium. In a case of disseminated lupus erythematosus. Rev Rheum Mal Osteoartic 1990 Oct;57(9):670.

H93. Hanada T, Saito K, Nagasawa T, Kabashima T, Nakahara S, Okuyama A, Takita H. Intravenous gammaglobulin therapy for thromboneutropenic neonates of mothers with systemic lupus erythematosus. Eur J Haematol 1987 May;38(5): 400–404.

H94. Hanauer LB, Christian CL. Studies of cryoproteins in SLE. J Clin Invest 1967 Mar;46:400–408.

H95. Hancock WK, Barnett EV. Demonstration of anti-idiotypic antibodies directed against IgM rheumatoid factor in the serum of rheumatoid arthritis patients. Clin Exp Immunol 1989;75:25.

H96. Handley AJ. Thrombocytopenia and LE cells after oxyphenbutazone. Lancet 1971 Jan 30;1:245–246.

H97. Hang L, Aguado MT, Dixon FJ, Theofilopolous AN. Induction of severe autoimmune disease in normal mice by simultaneous action of multiple immunostimulators. J Exp Med 1985;161:423–434.

H98. Hang L, Izui S, Slack JH, Dixon FJ. The cellular basis for resistance to induction of tolerance in BXSB SLE male mice. J Immunol 1982;129:787–789.

H99. Hang L, Theofilopoulous AN, Dixon FJ. A spontaneous rheumatoid arthritis-like disease in MRL/l mice. J Exp Med 1982;155:1690–1701.

H100. Hanly JG, Behmann S, Denburg SD, Carbotte RM, Denburg JA. The association between sequential changes in serum antineuronal antibodies and neuropsychiatric systemic lupus erythematosus. Postgrad Med J 1989;65:622–627.

H101. Hanly JG, Gladman DD, Rose TH, Laskin CA, Urowitz MB. Lupus pregnancy: a prospective study of placental changes. Arthritis Rheum 1988;31:358–66.

H102. Hanly JG, Sherwood G, Jones E, Jones JV, Eastwood B, Fisk JD. Cognitive impairment in unselected patients with systemic lupus erythematosus (SLE) [abstract]. Arthritis Rheum 1991 May;34(5) May:R37.

H103. Hanna N, Nelken D. A two-stage agglutination test for the detection of antithrombocyte antibodies. Vox Sang 1970 Apr; 18:342–348.

H104. Hannestad K. Certain rheumatoid factors react with both IgG and an antigen associated with cell nuclei. Scand J Immunol 1978;7(2):127–136.

H105. Hannestad K, Johannessen A. Polyclonal human antibodies to IgG (rheumatoid factors) which cross-react with cell nuclei. Scand J Immunol 1976;5(5):541–547.

H106. Hannestad K, Rekvig OP, Husebekk A. Cross-reacting rheumatoid factors and lupus erythematosus (LE) actors. Springer Semin Immunopathol 1981; 4:133–160.

H107. Hannestad K, Stollar BD. Certain rheumatoid factors react with nucleosomes. Nature (Lond) 1978;275:671–673.

H108. Hanrahan GE. Three cases of disseminated lupus erythematosus with psychosis. Can Med Assoc J 1954 Oct;71:374.

H109. Hansen JA, Martin PJ, Nowinski RC. Monoclonal antibodies identifying a novel T cell antigen and Ia antigens of human lymphocytes. Immunogenetics 1980;10:247.

H110. Hansen JR, McCray PB, Bale JF, Corbett AJ, Flanders DJ. Reye syndrome associated with aspirin therapy for systemic lupus erythematosus. Pediatrics 1985;76:202–205.

H111. Hansen OP, Hansen TM, Jans H, Hippe E. Red blood cell membrane-bound IgG: demonstration of antibodies in patients with autoimmune hemolytic anemia and immune complexes in patients with rheumatic diseases. Clin Lab Haemat 1984;6:341–349.

H112. Hansen TH, Koprak SL, Wormstall EM, Olson BJ, Jackson RD. Long-term passive enhancement of allogeneic skin grafts with monoclonal antibodies. J Immunogenet 1985;12:167.

H113. Hanson V, Drexler E, Kornreich H. DNA antibodies in childhood scleroderma. Arthritis Rheum 1970 Nov–Dec;17: 798–801.

H114. Hanssen AD, Cabanela ME, Michet CJ. Hip arthroplasty in patients with systemic lupus erythematosus, J Bone Joint Surg (Am) 1987 Jul;69(6):807–814.

H115. Hara K, Suzuki T, Tanaka M, Ohno S, Matuo H. A case of pseudohypoparathyroidism type I with systemic lupus erythematosus. Ryumachi 1989;29:200–206.

H116. Harata N, Sasaki T, Osaki H, Saito T, Shibata S, Muryoi T, Takai O, Yoshinaga K. Therapeutic treatment of New Zealand mouse disease by a limited number of anti-idiotypic antibodies conjugated with neocarzinostatin. J Clin Invest 1990;86: 769–786.

H117. Harata N, Sasaki T, Shibata S, Kameoka J, Hirabayashi Y, Osaki H, Tamate E, Yoshinaga K. Selective absorption of anti-DNA antibodies and their idiotype positive cells in vitro using an anti-idiotype antibody-affinity column: Possible application to plasma exchange. J Clin Apheresis 1991;6:34–39.

H118. Harbeck RJ, Hoffman AA, Hoffman SA, Shucard DW, Carr RI. A naturally occurring antibody in New Zealand mice cytotoxic to dissociated cerebellar cells. Clin Exp Immunol 1978 Feb;31(2):313–320.

H119. Hardie RJ, Isenberg DA. Tetraplegia as a presenting feature of systemic lupus erythematosus complicated by pulmonary hypertension. Ann Rheum Dis 1985 Jul;44(7):491–493.

H120. Hardin JA. The lupus autoantigens and the pathogenesis of systemic lupus erythematosus. Arthritis Rheum 1986 Apr; 29(4):457–460.

H121. Hardin JA, Thomas JO. Antibodies to histones in systemic lupus erythematosus: localization of prominent autoantigens on histone H1 and H2B. Proc Natl Acad Sci USA 1983;80: 7410–7414.

H122. Hardy BG, Lemieux C, Walker SE, Bartle WR. Interindividual and intraindividual variability in acetylation: characterization with caffeine. Clin Pharmacol Ther 1988;44:152–157.

H123. Hardy DA, Bell JI, Long EO, Lindsten T, McDevitt HO. Mapping of the class II region of the human major histocompatibility complex by pulsed-field gel electrophoresis. Nature 1986;323:453–455.

H124. Hardy JD, Solomon S, Banwell GS, Beach R, Wright V, Howard FM. Congenital complete heart block in the newborn associated with maternal systemic lupus erythematosus and other connective tissue disorders. Arch Dis Child 1979;54: 7–13.

H125. Hardy RR, Hayakawa K. Development and physiology of Ly-1 B and its human homolog, Leu-1 B. Immunol Rev 1986; 93:53–79.

H126. Hardy RR, Hayakawa K, Shimizu M, Yuamasaki K, Kishimoto T. Rheumatoid-factor secretion from human Leu-1 B cells. Science 1987;236:81–83.

H127. Hare WSC, Mackay IR. Radiological assessment of thymic size in myasthenia gravis and systemic lupus erythematosus. Lancet 1963 Apr 6;1:746–478.

H128. Hargraves MM. Discovery of the LE cell and its morphology. Mayo Clin Proc 1969 Sep;44:579–599.

H129. Hargraves MM, Richmond H, Morton R. Presentation of 2 bone marrow elements; "tart" cell and "L.E." cell. Proc Staff Meet Mayo Clin 1948 Jan 21;23:25–28.

H130. Hariharan S, Pollak VE, Kant KS, Weiss MA, Wadhwa NK. Diffuse proliferative lupus nephritis: long-term observations in patients treated with ancrod. Clin Nephrol 1990;34:61–69.

H131. Harisdangkul V, Benson CH, Myers A. Renal cell carcinoma presenting as necrotizing vasculitis with digital gangrene. Intern Med 1984 Feb;5:108–117.

H132. Harisdangkul V, Nilganuwonge S, Rockhold L. Cause of death in systemic lupus erythematosus: A pattern based on age at onset, Southern Med J 1987;80:1249–1253.

H133. Harkiss GD, Hendrie F, Nuki G. Cross-reactive idiotypes in anti-DNA antibodies of systemic lupus erythematosus patients. Clin Immunol Immunopathol 1986;39:421–430.

H134. Harley JB, Alexander EL, Arnett FC, Bias WB, Fox OF, Reichlin M, Yamagata H. Anti-Ro/SSA and anti-La/SSB in patients with Sjogren's syndrome. Arthritis Rheum 1986;29: 196−206.

H135. Harley JB, Kaine JL, Fox OF, Reichlin M, Gruber B. Ro (SS-A) antibody and antigen in a patient with congenital complete heart block. Arthritis Rheum 1985;28:1321−1325.

H136. Harley JB, McArthur R, Fujisaku A, Neas B, Frank MB. HLA-DQ gene complementation is synergistic with T cell receptor polymorphisms in the anti-Ro response of systemic lupus erythematosus [abstract]. Clin Res 1990;38:238A.

H137. Harley JB, Reichlin M, Arnett FC, Alexander EL, Bias WB, Provost TT. Gene interaction at the HLA-DQ locus enhances autoantibody production in primary Sjogren's syndrome. Science 1986;232:1145−1147.

H138. Harley JB, Sestak AL, Willis LG, Fu SM, Hansen JA, Reichlin M. A model for disease heterogeneity in systemic lupus erythematosus. Relationships between histocompatibility antigens, autoantibodies, and lymphopenia or renal disease. Arthritis Rheum 1989 Jul;32(7):826−836.

H139. Harley JB, Yamagata H, Reichlin M. Anti-La/SSB antibody is present in some normal sera and is coincident with anti-Ro/SSA precipitins in systemic lupus erythematosus. J Rheumatol 1984;11:309−314.

H140. Harmon CE, Deng JS, Peebles CL, Tan EM. The importance of tissue substrate in the SSA/Ro antigen-antibody system. Arthritis Rheum 1984;27:116−173.

H141. Harmon CE, Lee LA, Huff JC, Norris DA, Weston WL. The frequency of antibodies to the SS-A/Ro antigen in pregnancy sera. Arthritis Rheum 1974;27 Suppl 4:S20.

H142. Same as M280.

H143. Harrington WJ, Minnich V, Arimura C. The auto-immune thrombocytopenias. Prog Hematol 1956;1:166−192.

H144. Harrington WJ, Sprague CC, Minnich V, Moore CV, Aulvin RC, Dubach R. Immunologic mechanisms in idiopathic and neonatal thrombocytopenic purpura. Ann Intern Med 1953 Mar;38:433−469.

H145. Harris ED Jr. Retinoid therapy for rheumatoid arthritis. Ann Intern Med 1984 Jan;100(1):146−147.

H146. Harris EN. Antiphospholipid antibodies. Br J Haematol 1990 Jan;74(1):1−9.

H147. Harris EN, Asherson RA, Gharaval AE, Morgan SH, Derue E, Hughes GR. Thrombocytopenia in SLE and related autoimmune disorders: Association with anticardiolipin antibody. Br J Haematol 1985 Feb;59(2):227−230.

H148. Harris EN, Asherson RA, Hughes GRV. Antiphospholipid antibodies—autoantibodies with a difference. Ann Rev Med 1988;39:261.

H149. Harris EN, Baguley E, Asherson RA, Hughes GR. Clinical and serological features of the antiphospholipid syndrome (APS) [abstract]. Br J Rheumatol 1987;26:19.

H149a. Harris EN, Bos K. An acute disseminated coagulopathy-vasculopathy associated with the antiphospholipid syndrome. Arch Intern Med 1991;15:231−233.

H150. Harris EN, Chan JK, Asherson RA, Aber VR, Gharavi AE, Hughes GR. Thrombosis, recurrent fetal loss, and thrombocytopenia. Predictive value of the anticardiolipin antibody test. Arch Intern Med 1986 Nov;146(11):2153−2156.

H151. Harris EN, Gharavi AE, Asherson RA, Boey ML, Hughes GR. Cerebral infarction in systemic lupus: association with anticardiolipin antibodies. Clin Exp Rheumatol 1984 Jan−Mar; 2(1):47−51.

H152. Harris EN, Gharavi AE, Boey ML, Patel BM, Mackworth-Young CG, Loizou S, Hughes GR. Anticardiolipin antibodies: detection by radioimmunoassay and association with thrombosis in systemic lupus erythematosus. Lancet 1983 Nov 26; 2(8361):1211−1214.

H153. Harris EN, Gharavi AE, Hedge U, Derue G, Morgan SH, Englert H, Chan JK, Asherson RA, Hughes GR. Anticardiolipin

antibodies in autoimmune thrombocytopenic purpura. Br J Haematol 1985;59:231−234.

H154. Harris EN, Gharavi AE, Hughes GR. Anti-phospholipid antibodies. Clin Rheum Dis 1985 Dec;11(3):591−609.

H155. Harris EN, Gharavi AE, Loizou S, Derue G, CHan JK, Patel BM, Mackworth-Young CG, Bunn CC, Hughes GRV. Cross-reactivity of antiphospholipid antibodies. J Clin Lab Immunol 1985;16:1−6.

H156. Harris EN, Gharavi AE, Mackworth-Young CG, Patel BM, Derue G, Hughes GR. Lupoid sclerosis: a possible pathogenetic role for antiphospholipid antibodies. Ann Rheum Dis 1985 Apr;44(4):281−283.

H157. Harris EN, Gharavi AE, Patel SP, Hughes GR. Evaluation of the anti-cardiolipin antibody test: report of an international workshop held 4 April 1986. Clin Exp Immunol 1987 Apr; 68(1):215−222.

H158. Harris EN, Gharavi AE, Tincani A, Chan JK, Engler TH, Mantelli P, Allegro F, Ballestrieri G, Hughes GR. Affinity purified anti-cardiolipin and anti-DNA antibodies. J Clin Lab Immunol 1985 Aug;17(4):155−162.

H159. Harris EN, Gharavi AE, Wasley GD, Hughes GR. Use of an enzyme-linked immunosorbent assay and of inhibition studies to distinguish between antibodies to cardiolipin from patients with syphilis or autoimmune disorders. J Infect Dis 1988 Jan; 157(1):23−31.

H160. Harris EN, Phil M, editors. The second international anti-cardiolipin standardization workshop/The Kingston Antiphospholipid Antibody Study (KAPS) Group [Special Report]. Am J Clin Pathol 1990 Oct;94(4):474−484.

H161. Harris EN, Phil M, Bos K. An acute disseminated coagulopathy-vasculopathy associated with the antiphospholipid syndrome [editorial]. Arch Intern Med 1991 Feb;15(2):231−233.

H161a. Harris EN, Spinnato JA. Should anticardiolipin tests be performed in otherwise healthy pregnant women? Am J Obstet Gynecol 1991;165;1272−1277.

H162. Harris EN, Williams E, Shah DJ, De Ceulaer K. Mortality of Jamaican patients with systemic lupus erythematosus. Br J Rheumatol 1989;28:113−117.

H163. Harris L, Downar E, Shaikh NA, Chen T. Antiarrhythmic potential of chloroquine: new use for an old drug. Can J Cardiol 1988 Sep;4(6):295−300.

H164. Harris RB, Winkelmann RK. Lupus mastitis. Arch Dermatol 1978;114:410−412.

H165. Harris-Jones JN, Pein NK. Disseminated lupus erythematosus complicated by miliary tuberculosis during cortisone therapy. Lancet 1952 Jul 19;2:115−117.

H166. Harrison DJ, Thomson D, McDonald MK. Membranous glomerulonephritis. J Clin Pathol 1986;39:167−171.

H167. Harrison GN, Lipham M, Elguindi AS, Loebl DH. Acute sarcoidosis occurring in the course of systemic lupus erythematosus. South Med J 1979 Nov;72(11):1387−1388.

H168. Harrison LC, Kahn CR. Autoantibodies to the insulin receptor. Clinical significance and experimental applications. Prog Clin Immunol 1980;4:107−125.

H169. Harrist TJ, Mihm MC Jr. The specificity and clinical usefulness of the lupus band test. Arthritis Rheum 1980 Apr;23(4): 479−490.

H170. Hart CW, Naunton RF. The ototoxicity of chloroquine phosphate. Arch Otolaryngol 1964;80:407−412.

H171. Hart FD, Golding JR. Rheumatoid neuropathy. Br Med J 1960 May 28;5186:1594−1600.

H172. Hart HH, Grigor RR, Caughey DE. Ethnic difference in the prevalence of systemic lupus erythematosus. Ann Rheum Dis 1983 Oct;42:529−532.

H173. Hart RG, Miller VT, Coull BM, Bril V. Cerebral infarction association with lupus anticoagulants; preliminary report. Stroke 1984;15(4):293−298.

H174. Harter JG, Reddy WJ, Thorn GW. Studies on an intermittent corticosteroid dosage regimen. N Engl J Med 1963 Sep 19;169:591–596.

H175. Harth M. LE cells and positive direct Coombs' test induced by methyldopa. Can Med Assoc J 1968 Aug 10;99:277–280.

H176. Hartikainen-Sorri AL, Kaila J. Systemic lupus erythematosus and habitual abortion. Case report. Br J Obstet Gynaecol 1980 Aug;87(8):729–731.

H176a. Hartzband PI, Van Herle AJ, Sorger L, Cope D. Assessment of hypothalamic-pituitary-adrenal (HPA) axis dysfunction: comparison of ACTH stimulation, insulin-hypoglycemia and metyrapone. J Endocrinol Invest 1988;11:769–776.

H177. Harvey AM, Howard JE, Winkenwerder WL, Bordley JE, Carey RA, Kattus A. Observations on effect of adrenocorticotropic hormone (ACTH) on disseminated lupus erythematosus, drug hypersensitivity reactions; and chronic bronchial asthma. Trans Am Clin Climat Assoc 1950;61:221–228.

H178. Harvey JP Jr, Corcos J. Large cysts in lower leg originating in the knee, occurring in patients with rheumatoid arthritis. Arthritis Rheum 1960 Jun;3:218–228.

H179. Haserick JR. Unpublished data.

H180. Haserick JR. Modern concepts of systemic lupus erythematosus: review of 126 cases. J Chronic Dis 1955 Mar;1:317–334.

H181. Haserick JR, Corcoran AC, Dustan HP. ACTH and cortisone in acute crisis of systemic lupus erythematous. JAMA 1951 Jun 16;146:643–645.

H182. Haserick JR, Lewis LA, Bortz DW. Blood factor in acute disseminated lupus erythematosus; determination of gamma globulin as specific plasma fraction. Am J Med Sci 1950 Jun;219:660–663.

H183. Haserick JR, Long R. Systemic lupus erythematosus preceded by false-positive serological tests for syphilis: presentation of five cases. Ann Intern Med 1952 Sep;37:559–565.

H184. Hashimoto C. Studies on synthesis of interleukin-6 and gammaglobulin in peripheral blood mononuclear cells of patients with systemic lupus erythematosus. Tohoku J Exp Med 1990;162:323–335.

H185. Hashimoto H, Shiokawa Y. Changing patterns in the clinical features and prognosis of systemic lupus erythematosus—A Japanese experience. J Rheumatol 1982 May–Jun;9:386–389.

H186. Hashimoto H, Shiokawa Y 3d. Lupus erythematosus: Supplementary treatment and prognosis of lupus nephritis. Jpn J Med 1980 Jul;19:250–251.

H187. Hashimoto H, Tsuda H, Kanai Y, Kobayashi S, Hirose S, Shinoura H, Yokohari R, Kinoshita M, Aotsuka S, Yamada H, Takahashi K, Yoshinoya S, Miyamoto T. Selective removal of anti-DNA and anticardiolipin antibodies by adsorbent plasmapheresis using dextran sulfate columns in patients with systemic lupus erythematosus. J Rheumatol 1990;18:545–551.

H188. Hashimoto H, Tsuda H, Matsumoto T, Nasu H, Takasaki Y, Shiokawa Y, Hirose S, Terasaki PI, Iwaki Y. HLA antigens associated with systemic lupus erythematosus in Japan. J Rheumatol 1985;12:919–923.

H189. Hashimoto H, Tsuda H, Takasaki Y, Fujimaki N, Suzuki M, Shiokawa Y. Digital ulcers/gangrene and immunoglobulin classes/complement fixation of anti-ds-DNA in systemic lupus erythematosus patients. J Rheumatol 1983 Oct;10(5):727–732.

H190. Hashimoto H, Utagawa Y, Yamagata J, Okada T, Shiokawa Y, Suzuki S, Tomiyama T. The relationship of renal histopathological lesions to immunoglobulin classes and complement fixation of anti-native DNA antibodies in systemic lupus erythematosus. Scand J Rheumatol 1983;12(3)209–214.

H191. Hashimoto K, Thompson DF. Discoid lupus erythematosus. Electron microscopic studies of paramyxovirus-like structures. Arch Dermatol 1970 May;101:565–567.

H192. Hashimoto N, Handa H, Taki W. Ruptured cerebral aneurysms in patients with systemic lupus erythematosus. Surg Neurol 1986 Nov;26(5):512–516.

H193. Hashimoto S, Michalsky JP, Berman MA, McCombs C. Mechanism of a lymphocyte abnormality associates with HLA-B8/DR3: Role of interleukin-1. Clin Exp Immunol 1990;79:227–232.

H194. Hashimoto Y, Ziff M, Hurd ER. Increased endothelial cell adherence aggregation and superoxide generation by neutrophils incubated in systemic lupus erythematosus and Felty's syndrome sera. Arthritis Rheum 1982;25:1409–1418.

H195. Hasler P, Schultz LA, Kammer GM. Defective cAMP-dependent phosphorylation of intact T lymphocytes in active systemic lupus erythematosus. Proc Natl Acad Sci USA 1990;87:1978–1982.

H196. Hasper MF. Chronic cutaneous lupus erythematosus. Thalidomide treatment of 11 patients. Arch Dermatol 1983 Oct;119(10):812–815.

H197. Hasper MF, Klokke AH. Thalidomide in the treatment of chronic discoid lupus erythematosus. Acta Dermatovener (Stockh) 1982;62:321–324.

H198. Hasselaar P, Derksen RH, Blokzijl L, de Groot PG. Thrombosis associated with antiphospholipid antibodies cannot be explained by effects on endothelial and platelet prostanoid synthesis. Thromb Haemost 1988 Feb 25;59(1):80–85.

H199. Hasselaar P, Derksen RHWM, Blokzijl L, de Groot PG. Cross-reactivity of antibodies directed against cardiolipin, DNA, endothelial cells and blood platelets. Thromb Haemost 1990;63:169–173.

H200. Hasselaar P, Derksen RHWM, Blokzijl L, Hessing M, Nieuwenhuis HR, Bouma BN, De Groot P. Risk factors of thrombosis in lupus patients. Ann Rheum Dis 1989;48:933–940.

H201. Hasselaar P, Triplett DA, LaRue A, Derkson RH, Blokzijl L, de Groot PG, Wagenknecht DR, McIntyre JA. Heat treatment of serum plasma induces false positive results in the antiphospholipid antibody ELISA. J Rheumatol 1990 Feb;17(2):186–191.

H202. Hasselbacher P. Immunoelectrophoretic assay for synovial fluid C3 with correction for synovial fluid globulin. Arthritis Rheum 1979 Mar;22(3):243–250.

H203. Hasselbacher P, LeRoy EC. Serum DNA binding activity in healthy subjects and in rheumatic disease. Arthritis Rheum 1974 Jan–Feb;17:63–71.

H204. Hasselbacher P, Myers AR, Passero FC. Serum amylase and macroamylase in patients with systemic lupus erythematosus. Br J Rheumatol 1988 Jun;27(3):198–201.

H205. Hatakeyama M, Sumiya M, Gonda N, Kano S, Takaku F. Clinical study of systemic lupus erythematosus and pregnancy. Ryumachi 1983;23:93–99.

H206. Hauck L. The positive reaction of the Wassermann-Neisser-Bruck test in acute lupus erythematosus [original in German]. Muchen Med Wschr 1910 Jan 4;57:17.

H207. Haupt HM, Moore GW, Hutchins GM. The lung in systemic lupus erythematosus. Analysis of the pathologic changes in 120 patients. Am J Med 1981 Nov;71:791–798.

H208. Hauser GJ, Lidoe A, Zakuth V, Rosenberg H, Bino T, David MP, Spirer Z. Immunocompetence in pregnancy; production of IL2 by peripheral blood lymphocytes. Cancer Detection Prevention 1987;1 Suppl:39–42.

H209. Havran WL, Digiusto DL, Cambier JC. mIgM:mIgD ratios on B cells. Mean IgD expression exceeds mIgM by 10 fold on most splenic B cells. J Immunol 1984;132:1712–1716.

H210. Havre DC. Cataracts in children on long-term corticosteroid therapy. Arch Ophthalmol 1965 Jun;73:818.

H211. Same as H217.

H212. Same as H223a.

H213. Same as H224.

H214. Hawker G, Laskin CA, Bombardier C, Raboud J, Shewchuck AB, Mandel F, Ritchie K, Hannah M, Soloninka C, Spitzer K. Autoantibodies in healthy women and in women with a history of unexplained recurrent fetal loss [abstract]. Arthritis Rheum 1991;34 Suppl:S95.

H215. Hawkins BR, Wong KL, Wong RW, Chan KH, Dunckley H, Serjeantson SW. Strong associations between the major histocompatibility complex and systemic lupus erythematosus in southern Chinese. J Rheumatol 1987;14:1128–1131.

H216. Haxthausen H. Treatment of lupus erythematosus by intravenous injections of gold chloride. Arch Dermat & Syph 1930 Jul;22:77–90.

H217. Hay FC, Niveham LJ, Roitt IM. Routine assay for the detection of known immunoglobulin class using solid phase C1q. Clin Exp Immunol 1976;24:396–400.

H218. Hayakawa K, Hardy RR. Normal, autoimmune, and malignant CD5+ B cells: The Ly-1 B lineage? Ann Rev Immunol 1988;6:197–218.

H219. Hayakawa K, Hardy RR, Herzenberg LA. Peritoneal Ly-1 B cells: genetic control, autoantibody production, increased lambda light chain expression. Eur J Immunol 1986 Apr; 16(14):450–456.

H220. Hayakawa K, Hardy RR, Honda M, Herzenberg LA, Steinberg AD. Ly-1 B cells: Functionally distinct lymphocytes that secrete IgM autoantibodies. Proc Natl Acad Sci USA 1984 Apr;81:2494–2498.

H221. Hayakawa K, Hardy RR, Parks DR, Herzenberg LA. The 'Ly-1 B' cell subpopulation in normal, immunodefective, and autoimmune mice. J Exp Med 1983 Jan 1;157(1):202–218.

H222. Hayes JJ, Clark DJ, Wolffe AP. Histone contributions to the structure of DNA in the nucleosome. Proc Natl Acad Sci USA 1991; 88:6829–6833.

H223. Haynes DC, Gershwin ME, Robbins DL, Miller JJ 3d, Cosca D. Autoantibody profiles in juvenile arthritis. J Rheumatol 1986; 13:358–363.

H223a. Hayslett JP, Kashgarian M, Cook CD, Spargo BH. The effect of azathioprine on lupus glomerulonephritis. Medicine 1972 Sep;51:393.

H224. Hayslett JP, Lynn RI. Effect of pregnancy in patients with lupus nephropathy. Kidney Int 1980;18:207–220.

H225. Hazeltine M, Rauch J, Danoff D, Esdaile JM, Tannenbaum H. Antiphospholipid antibodies in systemic lupus erythematosus: evidence of an association with positive Coombs' and hypocomplementemia. J Rheumatol 1988;15:80–86.

H226. Hazelton RA, Lowe GD, Forbes CD, Sturrock RD. Increased blood and plasma viscosity in systemic lupus erythematosus. J Rheumatol 1985;616–617.

H227. Hazelton RA, McCruden AB, Sturrock RD, Stimson WH. Hormonal manipulation of the immune response in systemic lupus erythematosus: a drug trial of an anabolic steroid, 19-nortestosterone. Ann Rheum Dis 1983 Apr;42(2):155–157.

H228. Same as A238.

H229. Heaton JM. Sjogren's syndrome and systemic lupus erythematosus. BMJ 1959 Feb 21;5120:466–469.

H230. Hebbes TR, Thorne AW, Crane-Robinson C. A direct link between core histone acetylation and transcriptionally active chromatin. EMBO J 1988;7:1395–1402.

H231. Hebert L. The clearance of immune complexes from the circulation of man and other primates. Am J Kidney Dis 1991; 17:352–361.

H232. Hebert L, Nielsen E, Pohl M, Lachin J, Hunsicker L, Lewis E. Clinical course of severe lupus nephritis during the controlled trial of plasmapheresis therapy. Kidney Int 1987;31: 201.

H233. Hebert LA, Cosio FG. The erythrocyte-immune complex-

glomerulonephritis connection in man. Kidney Int 1987;31: 877–885.

H234. Hebert LA, Cosio FG, Birmingham DJ, Van Man ME. Experimental immune complex-mediated glomerulonephritis in the nonhuman primate. Kidney Int 1991;39:44–56.

H235. Hebra F. Hebra's Hautkrankheiten, Wien. 1845; B. 3, Theil 1.

H236. Hebra F. Report on accomplishments in dermatology. [original in German]. Jahresbericht uber die Fortschritte der Gesammten Medicin in Allen Landern im Jahre 1945. Drs. Canstatt and Eisenmann, editors. Erlangen, Ferdinand Enke, 1948:(3).

H237. Hebra F, Kaposi M. On diseases of the skin, including the exanthemata. Tay W translator, Fagge C Hilton, editor. London: The New Sydenham Society 1866–1880, 1874;(4).

H238. Hecaen H. Les Gaushers. Paris, Presses Universitaires de France, 1984.

H239. Hecht B, Siegel N, Adler M, Kashgarian M, Hayslett JP. Prognostic indices in lupus nephritis. Medicine 1976 Mar;55: 163–181.

H240. Heck LW, Alarcon GS, Ball GV, Phillips RL, Kline LB, Moreno H, Hirschowitz BI, Baer AN, Dessypris EN. Pure red cell aplasia and protein-losing enteropathy in a patient with systemic lupus erythematosus. Arthritis Rheum 1985 Sep;28(9): 1059–1061.

H241. Hedge UM, Gordon-Smith EC, Worlledge S. Platelet antibodies in thrombocytopenic patients. Br J Haematol 1977 Jan; 35:113–182.

H242. Hedgpeth, MT, Boulware DW. Interstitial pneumonitis in antinuclear antibody-negative systemic lupus erythematosus: a new clinical manifestation and possible association with anti-Ro (SS-A) antibodies. Arthritis Rheum 1988;31:545–548.

H243. Heibel RH, O'Toole JD, Curtiss EJ, Medsger TA, Reddy SP, Shaver JA. Coronary arteritis in systemic lupus erythematosus. Chest 1976 May;69:700–703.

H244. Heiberg E, Wolverson MK, Sundaram M, Shields JB. Body computed tomography findings in systemic lupus erythematosus, CT. J Comput Tomogr 1988 Jan;12(1):68–74.

H245. Heine BE. Psychiatric aspects of systemic lupus erythematosus. Acta Psychiatry Scand 1969;45(4):307.

H246. Heiter P, Korsmeyer SJ, Waldmann TA, Leder P. Human immunoglobulin kappa light chain genes are deleted or rearranged in lambda producing B cells. Nature 1981;290: 368–372

H247. Hejtmanicik MR, Wright JC, Quint R, Jennings FL. Cardiovascular manifestations of systemic lupus erythematosus. Am Heart J 1964 Jul;68:119–230.

H248. Hekman A, Sluyser M. Antigenic Determinants on Lysine-Rich Histones. Biochim Biophys Acta 1973; 295:613–620.

H249. Helin H, Korpela M, Mustonen J, Pasternack A. Rheumatoid factor in rheumatoid arthritis associated renal disease in lupus nephritis. Ann Rheum Dis 1986;45:508–511.

H250. Heller CA, Schur PH. Serological and clinical remission in systemic lupus erythematosus. J Rheumatol 1985;12: 916–918.

H251. Heller M, Owens JO, Mushinski JF, Rudikoff S. Amino acids at the site of V_K—J_K recombination not encoded by germline sequences. J Exp Med 166:637–646 (1987).

H252. Helliwell M, Crisp AJ, Grahame R. Co-existent tophaceous gout and systemic lupus erythematosus. Rheumatol Rehab 1982 Aug;21(3):161–163.

H253. Helliwell TR, Flook D, Whitworth J, Day DW. Arteritis and venulitis in systemic lupus erythematosus resulting in massive lower intestinal haemorrhage. Histopathology 1985 Oct; 9(10):1103–1113.

H254. Hellmann DB, Petri M, Whiting-O'Keefe Q. Fatal infections in systemic lupus erythematosus: the role of opportunistic organisms. Medicine 1987 Sep;66(5):341–348.

H255. Helm KF, Peters MS. Immunodermatology update: the immunologically mediated vesiculobullous diseases. Mayo Clin Proc 1991 Feb;66(2):187–202.

H256. Helmke K, Otten A, Maser E, Wolf H, Federlin K. Islet cell antibodies, circulating immune complexes and antinuclear antibodies in diabetes mellitus. Horm Metab Res 1987 Jul;19(7): 312–315.

H257. Helve T. Prevalence and mortality rates of systemic lupus erythematosus and causes of death in SLE patients in Finland. Scand J Rheumatol 1985;14(1):43–46.

H258. Helyer BJ, Howie JB. Positive lupus erythematosus tests in a cross-bred strain of mice NZB/Bl-NZY/Bl. Proc Univ Otago (New Zealand) Med School 1961 Jul;39:3–4.

H259. Helyer BJ, Howie JB. The thymus and autoimmune disease. Lancet 1963 Nov 16;2:1026–1029.

H260. Hench PA. The potential reversibility of rheumatoid arthritis. Mayo Clin Proc 1949;24:167–178.

H261. Hench PS, Kendall EC, Slocumb CH, Polley HF. Effect of hormone of adrenal cortex (17-Hydroxy-11-Dehydrocorticosterone: compound E) and of pituitary adrenocorticotropic hormone on rheumatoid arthritis; Preliminary report. Proc Mayo Clin 1949 Apr 13;24:181–197.

H262. Hench PS, Kendall EC, Slocumb CH, Polley HF. Effects of cortisone acetate and pituitary ACTH on rheumatoid arthritis, rheumatic fever and certain other conditions; Study in clinical physiology. Arch Intern Med 1950 Apr;85:545–666.

H263. Henderson DL, Odom JC. Laser treatment of discoid lupus [case report]. Lasers Surg Med 1986;6(1):12–15.

H264. Henke CJ, Yelin EH, Ingbar ML, Epstein WV. The university rheumatic disease clinic: Provider and patient perceptions of cost. Arthritis Rheum 1977 Mar;20:751–758.

H265. Henkind P, Rothfield NF. Ocular abnormalities in patients treated with antimalarial drugs. New Engl J Med 1963 Aug 29; 269:433–439.

H266. Henningsen NC, Cederberg A, Hanson A, Johansson BW. Effects of longterm treatment with procainamide. Acta Med Scand 1975; 198:475–482.

H267. Henry AK, Brunner CM. Relapse of lupus transverse myelitis mimicked by vertebral fractures and spinal cord compression. Arthritis Rheum 1985 Nov;28(11):1307–1311.

H268. Henry R, Williams AV, McFadden NR, Pilia PA, Histopathologic evaluation of lupus patients with transient renal failure, Am J Kidney Dis 1986 Dec;8(6):417–421.

H269. Henry RE, Goldberg LS, Sturgeon P, Ansel RD. Serological abnormalities associated with L-dopa therapy. Vox Sang 1971 Apr; 20:306–316.

H270. Hera A, Marcos MAR, Toribio ML, Marquez C, Gaspar ML, Martinez-a C. Development of Ly-1 B cells in immunodeficient CBA/n mice. J Exp Med 1987;166:804–809.

H271. Herberman RB, Holder HT. Natural cell-mediated immunity. Adv Cancer Res 1978;27:305–370.

H272. Hercend T, Griffin Bensussan A, Schmidt RE, Edson MA, Brennan A, Murray C, Daley JF, Schlossman SF, Ritz J. Generation of monoconal antibodies to a human natural killer clone. Characterization of two natural killer-associated antigens, NKH1A and NKH2, expressed on a subset of large granular lymphocytes. J Clin Invest 1985;75:932.

H273. Hercend T, Schmidt RE. Characteristics and uses of natural killer cells. Immunol Today 1988;9:291–293.

H274. Herd JK, Medhi M, Uzendoski DM, Saldivar VA. Chorea associated with systemic lupus erythematosus. Pediatrics 1978;61:308–315.

H275. Herman JH, Khosla RC. Nd: YAG laser modulation of synovial tissue metabolism. Clin Exp Rheumatol 1989 Sep–Oct; 7(5):505–512.

H276. Hermann G. Intussusception secondary to mesenteric arteritis. Complication of systemic lupus erythematosus in a 5-year-old child. JAMA 1967;200:180–181.

H277. Herreman G, Broquie G, Metzger JP, Godeau P. Treatment of SLE and other collagenoses with anti-lymphocyte globulin. A propos of 10 cases [original in French]. Nouv Presse Med 1972;1:2035–2039.

H278. Herreman G, Ferme I, Morel S, Batisse J, Unon NP, Meyer O. Fetal death caused by myocarditis and isolated congenital complete heart block. Presse Med 1985;14:1547–1550.

H279. Herrera-Acosta J, Reyes PA, Lopez Manay G, Padilla L, Cerdas Calderon M, Ruiz A, Perez Grovas H. Inhibition of prostaglandin synthesis results in suppression of renal functional reserve in lupus nephritis [English abstract]. La Rev Invest Clin (Spa) 1987 Apr–Jun;39(2):107–114.

H280. Herrero C, Bielsa I, Font J, Lozano F, Ercilla G, Lecha M, Ingelman M, Masearo JM. Subacute cutaneous lupus erythematosus: Clinical pathologic findings in 13 cases. J Am Acad Dermatol 1988;19:1057–1062.

H281. Herrman WP, Koch H, Hoft G. Catamnestic studies on the course of chronic erythematosus. Hautarzt (Ger) 1962 Jul;13: 309–315.

H282. Herron A, Dettleff G, Hixon B, Brandwin I, Ortbals D, Hornick R, Hahn B. Influenza vaccination in patients with rheumatic diseases: Safety and Efficacy. JAMA 1979 Jul 6; 242(1):53–56.

H283. Herron LR, Coffman RL, Bond MW, Kotzin BL. Increased autoantibody production by NZB/NZW B cells in response to IL-5. J Immunol 1988;141:842–848.

H284. Herron LR, Coffman RL, Kotzin BL. Enhanced response of autoantibody-secreting B cells from young NZB/NZW mice to T cell-derived differentiation signals. Clin Immunol Immunopathol 1988;46:314.

H285. Hershko A. Ubiquitin-mediated protein degradation. J Biol Chem 1988;263:15237–15240.

H286. Herson D, Krivitzky A, Douche C, Jeantils A, Lemaitre MD, Delzant G. Familial lupus and Adie's tonic pupil. Ann Med Interne (Paris) 1989;140(1):56–57.

H287. Hertzman PA, Falk H, Kilbourne EM, Page S, Shulman LE. The eosinophilia-myalgia syndrome: The Los Alamos Conference. J Rheumatol 1991;18:867–873.

H288. Heslop HE, Gottlieb DJ, Bianchi ACM, Meager A, Prentice HG, Mehta AB, Hoffbrand AV, Brenner MK. In vivo induction of gamma interferon and tumor necrosis factor by interleukin-2 infusion following intensive chemotherapy or autologous marrow transplantation. Blood 1989;74:1374–1380.

H289. Hess E. Drug-related lupus. N Engl J Med 1988;318:1460.

H290. Hess EV. Drug-related lupus: The same or different? Systemic Lupus Erythematosus. Wiley Medical:New York 1987: 869–880.

H291. Hess EV. Introduction to drug-related lupus. Arthritis Rheum 1981; 24:6–9.

H292. Hess EV, Baum J. Antinuclear factor and LE cells in pregnant women. Lancet 1971;2:877.

H293. Hess EV, Litwin A. Drug-related rheumatic diseases. Basic Mechanisms. Immunol Rheum Dis 1985:651–668.

H294. Hetherington GW, Jetton RL, Knox JM. The association of lupus erythematosus and porphyria. Br J Dermatol 1970 Feb;82:118–124.

H295. Heymann W, Grupe WE. Increase in proteinuria due to steroid medication in chronic renal disease. J Pediatr 1969 mar;74:346–363.

H296. Hibbs ML, Selvaraj P, Carpen O, Springer TA, Kuster H, Jouvin MH, Kinet JP. Mechanisms for regulating expression of membrane isoforms of FcγRIII (CD16). Science 1989;246: 1608–1611.

H297. Hicklin JA. Chloroquine neuromyopathy. Ann Phys Med 1968 Feb;9:189–192.

H298. Hicks JD, Burnet FM. Renal lesions in the "autoimmune" mouse strains NZB and F1 NZB × NZW. J Pathol 1966 Apr; 91:467–477.

H299. Hicks JT, Aulakh GS, McGrath PP, Washington GC, Kim E, Alepa FP. Search for Epstein-Barr and type C oncornaviruses in systemic lupus erythematosus. Arthritis Rheum 1979;22: 845–857.

H300. Higgs GA, Salmon JA, Henderson B, Vane JR. Pharmacokinetics of aspirin and salicylate in relation to inhibition of arachidonate cyclooxygenase and antiinflammatory activity. Proc Natl Acad Sci USA 1987;84:1417–1420.

H301. Hijmans W, Doniach D, Roitt IM, Holborow EJ. Serological overlap between lupus erythematosus, rheumatoid arthritis, and thyroid auto-immune disease. BMJ 1961 Oct 7;5257: 909–914.

H302. Hill AGS. C-reactive protein in the chronic rheumatic diseases. Lancet 1951 Nov 3;261:807–811.

H303. Hill CS, Thomas JO. Core histone-DNA interactions in sea urchin sperm chromatin: The N-terminal tail of H2B interacts with linker DNA. Eur J Biochem 1990;187:145–153.

H304. Hill G. Systemic lupus erythematosus and mixed connective tissue disease. In: Heptinstall RH, editor. Pathology of the kidney. Boston: Little Brown, 1983:839–906.

H305. Hill GS, Hinglais N, Tron F, Bach JF. Systemic lupus erythematosus. Morphologic correlations with immunologic and clinical data at the time of biopsy. Am J Med 1978 Jan;64: 61–79.

H306. Hill HM, Kirshbaum JD. Miliary tuberculosis developing during prolonged cortisone therapy of systemic lupus erythematosus. Ann Intern Med 1956 April;44:781–790.

H307. Hiller RI. A study of quinacrine dihydrochloride in the human breast in vitro and in vivo. Am J Surg 1970 Mar;119: 317–321.

H308. Hillson JL, Perlmutter RM. Autoantibodies and the fetal antibody repertoire. Int Rev Immunol 1990;5:215–229.

H309. Hillyer CD, Berkman EM, Schwartz RS. Autoimmune hemolytic anemia and cold agglutinin disease; autoantibodies, mechanisms and therapy. Clin Aspects Autoimmunity 1990;5: 22–32.

H310. Himeno K, Good RA. Marrow transplantation from tolerant donors to treat and prevent autoimmune diseases in BXSB mice. Proc Natl Acad Sci USA 1988;85:2235–2239

H311. Hind CRK, Ng SC, Feng PH, Papys MB. Serum C-reactive protein measurement in the detection of intercurrent infection in Oriental patients with systemic lupus erythematosus. Ann Rheum Dis 1985 Apr;44:260–261.

H312. Hinkle SC, Merkatz IR, Gyves MT, Michel B, Moskowitz RW. Antinuclear factor and anti-DNA in sera of pregnant women. Arthritis Rheum 1979;22(2):201–202.

H313. Hinrichs JV, Mewaldt SP, Ghoneim MM, Berie JL. Diazepam and Leading: assessment of acquisition deficits. Pharmacol Biochem Behav 1982 Jul;17(1):165–170.

H314. Hinrichsen H, Barth J, Ferstl R, Kirch W. Changes of immunoregulatory cells induced by acoustic stress in patients with systemic lupus erythematosus, sarcoidosis, and in healthy controls. Eur J Clin Invest 1989 Aug;19(4):372–377.

H315. Hinterberger M, Pettersson I, Steitz JA. Isolation of small nuclear ribonucleoproteins containing U1, U2, U4, U5, and U6 RNAs. J Biol Chem 1983;258:2604–2613.

H316. Hirahara F, Gorai I, Tanaka K, Matsuzaki Y, Sumiyoshi Y, Shiojima Y. Cellular immunity in pregnancy: subpopulations of T lymphocytes bearing Fc receptors for IgG and IgM in pregnant women. Clin Exp Immunol 1980;41:353–357.

H317. Hirano T, Taga T, Yasukawa K, Nakajima K, Nakano N, Takatsuki F, Shimizo M, Murashima A, Tsunasawa S, Sakiyama F, Kishimoto T. Human B cell differentiation factor defined by an antipeptide antibody and its possible role in autoantibody production. Proc Natl Acad Sci 1987;84:228–231.

H318. Hirata Y, Omori Y, Takei M, Nakazawa M. Autoimmunity in diabetes mellitus. Gunma Symp Endocrinol 1980;17:81.

H319. Hirawa M, Nonaka C, Abe T, Lio M. Positron emission tomography in systemic lupus erythematosus: Relation to cerebral vasculitis to PET findings. Am J N Rad 1983 May–Jun;4: 541–543.

H320. Hirohata S, Hirose S, Miyamoto T. Cerebrospinal fluid IgM, IgA, and IgG indexes in systemic lupus erythematosus. Their use as estimates of central nervous system disease activity. Arch Intern Med 1985 Oct;145(10):1843–1846.

H321. Hirohata S, Iwamoto S, Miyamoto T, Sugiyama H, Nakano K, Inokuma S. A patient with systemic lupus erythematosus presenting both central nervous system lupus and steroid induced psychosis. J Rheumatol 1988 Apr;15(4):706–710.

H322. Hirohata S, Lipsky PE. T cell regulation of human B cell proliferation and differentiation. Regulatory influences of CD45+ and CD45R⁻ T4 cell subsets. J Immunol 1989;142: 2597–2607.

H323. Hirohata S, Miyamoto T. Increased intrathecal immunoglobulin synthesis of both kappa and lambda types in patients with systemic lupus erythematosus and central nervous involvement. J Rheumatol 1986 Apr;13(4):715–721.

H324. Hirohata S, Miyamoto T. Elevated levels of interleukin-6 in cerebrospinal fluid from patients with systemic lupus erythematosus and central nervous system involvement. Arthritis Rheum 1990 May;33(5):644–649.

H325. Hirohata S, Taketani T. A serial study of changes in intrathecal immunoglobulin synthesis in a patient with central nervous system systemic lupus erythematosus. J Rheumatol 1987 Oct;14(5):1055–1057.

H326. Hirose S, Kinoshita K, Nozawa S, Nishimura H, Shirai T. Effects of major histocompatibility complex on autoimmune disease of H-2-congenic New Zealand mice. Intern Immunol 1991;2:1091–1095.

H327. Hirose S, Ogawa S, Nishimura H, Hashimoto H, Shirai T. Association of HLA-DR2/DR4 heterozygosity with systemic lupus erythematosus in Japanese patients. J Rheumatol 1988; 15:1489–1492.

H328. Hirose T. Spontaneous production of interleukin-1 and B cell stimulating factors by B cells from patients with systemic lupus erythematosus. Ryumachi 1989;29:277–283.

H329. Hishikawa T, Tokano Y, Sekigawa I, Ando S, Takasaki Y, Hashimoto H, Hirose S, Okumura K, Abe M, Shirai T. HLA-DP + T cells and deficient interleukin-2 production in patients with systemic lupus erythematosus. Clin Immunol Immunopathol 1990;55:285–296.

H330. Hissung A, Dertinger H, Heinrich G. The action of ionizing radiation on DNA in the presence os quinacrine. I. UV absorption and fluorescence measurements. Radiat Environ Biophys 1975 Jun 13;12(1):5–12.

H331. Hjortjoer Petersen H, Nielsen H, Hansen M, Stensgaard-Hansen F, Helin P. High- dose immunoglobulin therapy in pericarditis caused by SLE [letter]. Scand J Rheumatol 1990; 19(1):91–93.

H332. Ho MS, Teh LB, Goh HS. Ischaemic colitis in systemic lupus erythematosus—report of case and review of the literature. Ann Acad Med Singapore 1987 Jul;16(3):501–503.

H333. Ho C-H, Chiang Y-M, Chong L-L, Lin H-Y. Development of chronic lymphocytic leukemia in a case of Sjogren's syndrome with systemic lupus erythematosus. Scand J Haematol 1985; 35:246–248.

H334. Hobart MJ, Lachman PJ. Allotypes of complement components in man. Transplant Rev 1976;32:26–42.

H335. Hobbs HE, Eadie SP, Somerville F. Ocular lesions after treatment with chloroquine. Br J Ophthal 1961;45:284–297.

H336. Hobbs RN, Clayton AL, Bernstein RM. Antibodies to the five histones and poly(adenosine diphosphate-ribose) in drug-induced lupus: implications for pathogenesis. Ann Rheum Dis 1987; 46:408–416.

H337. Hobbs RN, Lea DJ, Phua KK, Johnson PM. Binding of isolated rheumatoid factors to histone proteins and basic polycations. Ann Rheum Dis 1983 Dec;42:435–438.

H338. Hoch S, Schur PH, Schwaber J. Frequency of anti-DNA antibody producing cells from normal and patient with systemic lupus erythematosus. Clin Immunol Immunopathol 1983 Apr;27(1):28–37.

H339. Hoch S, Schwaber J. Identification and sequence of the V_H gene elements encoding a human anti-DNA antibody. J Immunol 1987;139:1689–1693.

H340. Hochberg MC. The incidence of systemic lupus erythematosus in Baltimore, Maryland, 1970–1977. Arthritis Rheum 1985 Jan;28:80–86.

H341. Hochberg MC. Prevalence of systemic lupus erythematosus in England and Wales, 1981–1982. Ann Rheum Dis 1987; 46:664.

H342. Hochberg MC. Mortality from systemic lupus erythematosus in England and Wales, 1974–1983. Br J Rheumatol 1987; 26:437–441.

H343. Hochberg MC. The application of genetic epidemiology to systemic lupus erythematosus. J Rheumatol 1987;14: 867–869.

H344. Hochberg MC. Genetic epidemiology of systemic lupus erythematosus. In Proceedings of the Second International Conference on Systemic Lupus Erythematosus, Tokyo, 1989: 9.

H345. Hochberg MC. Racial differences in the descriptive and clinical epidemiology of systemic lupus erythematosus in the United States. In Proceedings of the Second International Conference on Systemic Lupus Erythematosus, Tokyo, 1989:32.

H346. Hochberg MC. Systemic lupus erythematosus. Rheum Dis Clin North Am 1990;16:671.

H347. Hochberg MC, Boyd RE, Ahearn JM, Arnett FC, Bias WB, Provost TT, Stevens MB. Systemic lupus erythematosus: A review of clinico-laboratory features and immunogenetic markers in 150 patients with emphasis on demographic subsets. Medicine 1985 Sep;64(5):285–295.

H348. Hochberg MC, Dorsch CA, Feinglass EJ, Stevens MB. Survivorship in systemic lupus erythematosus; effect of antibody to extractable nuclear antigen. Arthritis Rheum 1981 Jan;24: 54–59.

H349. Hochberg MC, Engle EW. Physical disability and psychosocial dysfunction in systemic lupus erythematosus: comparison with rheumatoid arthritis. Arthritis Rheum 1989;32 Suppl 4:S88.

H350. Hochberg MC, Engle EW, Pruitt A, Petri M. Correlation of disease activity with physical disability in systemic lupus erythematosus. Arthritis Rheum 1990;33 Suppl 5:R22.

H351. Hochberg MC, Florsheim P, Scott J, Arnett FC. Familial aggregation of systemic lupus erythematosus [abstract]. Arthritis Rheum 1985;28:523.

H352. Hochberg MC, Florsheim F, Scott J, Arnett F. Familial aggregation of systemic lupus erythematosus. Am J Epidemiol 1985;122:526–527.

H353. Hochberg MC, Kaslow RA. Risk factors for the development of systemic lupus erythematosus: A case-control study. Clin Res 1983;31:732A.

H354. Hochberg MC, Sutton JD. Physical disability and psychosocial dysfunction in systemic lupus erythematosus. J Rheumatology. 1988;15:959–964.

H355. Hochberg MC, Sutton JD, Engle EW. Longitudinal course of physical disability and psychosocial dysfunction in systemic lupus erythematosus [abstract]. Arthritis Rheum 1988;31 Suppl 4:S94.

H356. Hodge JV, Casey TP. Methyldopa and the direct antiglobulin (Coombs') test. N Z Med J 1968 Oct;68:240–246.

H357. Hodgman JE, Elhassani S, Dubois EL. Growth and development of children born to steroid treated mothers. Lupus, Pregnancy and Neonatal Lupus, Ch. 23 In: Wallace DJ, Dubois EL, editors. Dubois' Lupus Erythematosus, 3rd ed. Philadelphia: Lea & Febiger, 1987:572.

H358. Hodgson SF. Corticosteroid-induced osteoporosis. Endocrinol Metabol Clin North Am 1990;19:95–111.

H359. Hodus HN, Quismorio FP, Wickham E, Blankenhorn DH. The lipid-lowering effects of hydroxychloroquine in humans: A case control study [abstract]. Arteriosclerosis 1990;10:753a.

H360. Hoffbrand BI, Beck ER. "Unexplained" dyspnoea and shrinking lungs in systemic lupus erythematosus. Br Med J 1965 May 15;1:1273–1277.

H361. Hoffman BI, Katz WA. The gastrointestinal manifestations of systemic lupus erythematosus: a review of the literature. Semin Arthritis Rheum 1980 May;9(4):237–247.

H362. Hoffman BJ. Sensitivity of sulfadiazine resembling acute disseminated lupus erythematosus. Arch Dermatol Syph 1945; 51:190–192.

H363. Hoffman RW, Rettenmaier LJ, Takeda Y, Hewett JE, Pettersson I, Nyman U, Luger AM, Sharp GC. Human autoantibodies against the 70-kd polypeptide of U1 small nuclear RNP are associated with HLA-DR4 among connective tissue disease patients. Arthritis Rheum 1990;33:666–673.

H364. Hoffman RW, Sharp GC, Irvin WS, Anderson SK, Hewett JE, Pandey JP. Association of immunoglobulin Km and Gm allotypes with specific antinuclear antibodies and disease susceptibility among connective tissue disease patients. Arthritis Rheum 1991;34:453–458.

H365. Hoffman RW, Yang HK, Waggie KS, Durham JB, Burge JB, Walker SE. Band keratopathy in MRL/l and MRL/n mice. Arthritis Rheum 1983;26:645.

H366. Hoffman SA, Arbogast DN, Ford PM, Shucard DW, Harbeck RJ. Brain-reactive autoantibody levels in the sera of ageing autoimmune mice. Clin Exp Immunol 1987;70:74–83.

H367. Hoffman SL, Prescott SM, Majerus PW. The effects of mepacrine and p-bromophenlacyl bromide on arachidonic acid release in human platelets. Arch Biochem Biophys 1982 Apr 15;215(1):237–244.

H368. Hoffman T. Natural killer function in systemic lupus erythematosus. Arthritis Rheum 1980 Jan;23:30–35.

H369. Hoffsten PE, Swerdlin A, Bartell M, Hill CL, Venverloh J, Brotherson K, Klahr S. Reticuloendothelial and mesangial function in murine immune complex glomerulonephritis. Kidney Int 1979;15:144–159.

H370. Hogan MJ, Brunet DG, Ford PM, Lillicrap D. Lupus anticoagulant, antiphospholipid antibodies and migraine. Can J Neurol Sci 1988 Nov;15(4):420–425.

H371. Hogg N. The structure and function of Fcγ receptors. Immunol Today 1988;9:185–187.

H372. Hogg GR. Congenital, acute lupus erythematosus associated with subendocardial fibroelastosis. Report of a case. Am J Clin Path 1954;28:648.

H373. Hoh YK, Lim EH, Ooi SO, Kon OL. Fatty acid modulation of antiestrogen action and antiestrogen-binding protein in cultured lymphoid cells. Experentia 1991;46:1032–1037.

H374. Holborow EJ, Barnes RD, Tuffrey M. A new red-cell autoantibody in NZB mice. Nature (London) 1965 Aug 7;207: 601–604.

H375. Holborow EJ, Weir DM. Histone: An essential component for the lupus erythematosus antinuclear reaction. Lancet 1959;1:809–810.

H376. Holborow J, Johnson GD. Antinuclear factor in systemic lupus erythematosus. A consideration of immunofluorescent method of detecting antinuclear antibodies with results obtained in a family study. Arthritis Rheum 1964;7:119.

H377. Holborow J, Weir DM, Johnson GD. A serum factor in lupus erythematosus with affinity for tissue nuclei. BMJ 1957; 2:732–734.

H378. Holden M. Massive pulmonary fibrosis due to systemic lupus erythematosus. N Y State J Med 1973 Feb 1;73:462–465.

H379. Holers VM, Seya T, Brown E, O'Shea JJ, Atkinson JP. Structural and functional studies on the human C3b/C4b receptor (CR1) purified by affinity chromatography using a monoclonal antibody. Complement 1986;3:63–78.

H380. Holgate ST, Glass DN, Haslam P, Maini RN, Turner-Warwick M. Respiratory involvement in systemic lupus erythematosus: a clinical and immunologic study. Clin Exp Immunol 1976 Jun;24:385–395.

H381. Hollander JL, Jessar RA, McCarty DJ. Synovianalysis: an aid in arthritis diagnosis. Bull Rheum Dis 1961;12:263–264.

H382. Hollcraft RM, Dubois EL, Lundberg GD, Chandor SB, Gilbert SB, Quismorio FP, Barbour BH, Friou GJ. Renal damage in systemic lupus erythematosus with normal renal function. J Rheumatol 1976 Sep;3:251–261.

H383. Hollenhorst RW, Henderson JW. Ocular manifestations of diffuse collagen diseases. Am J Med Sci 1951 Feb;221: 211–222.

H384. Hollinger FB, Sharp JT, Lidsky MD, Rawls WE. Antibodies to viral antigens in systemic lupus erythematosus. Arthritis Rheum 1971;14:1–11.

H385. Hollingworth P, de Vere R, Tyndall ADV, Ansell BM, Platts-Mills I, Gumpel JM, Mertin J, Smith DS, Denman AM. Intensive immunosuppression versus prednisolone in the treatment of connective tissue diseases. Ann Rheum Dis 1982 Dec;41(6): 557–562.

H386. Holman HR. Partial purification and characterization of an extractable nuclear antigen which reacts with SLE sera. Ann N Y Acad Sci 1965 Jun 30;124:800–806.

H387. Holman HR, Deicher HR. The reaction of the L.E. cell factor with deoxyribonucleoprotein of the cell nucleus. J Clin Invest 1959 Nov;38:2059–2072.

H388. Holman HR, Deicher HR. The appearance of hypergammaglobulinemia, positive serological reactions for rheumatoid arthritis and complement fixation reactions with tissue constituents in the sera of relatives with systemic lupus erythematosus [abstract]. Arthritis Rheum 1960:3244.

H389. Holman HR, Deicher HR, Kunkel HG. The L.E. cell and the L.E. serum factors. Bull N Y Acad Med 1959 Jul;35:409–418.

H390. Holman HR, Kunkel HG. Affinity between the lupus erythematosus serum factor and cell nuclei and nucleoprotein. Science 1957 Jul 19;126(3264):162–163.

H391. Holman WR, Dineen P. The role of splenectomy in the treatment of thrombocytopenic purpura due to systemic lupus erythematosus. Ann Surg 1978 Jan;187:52–56.

H392. Holmberg D, Forsgren S, Forni L, Ivars F, Coutinho A. Idiotype determinant of natural IgM antibodies that resemble self Ia antigens. Proc Natl Acad Sci USA 1984;81:3175.

H393. Holme E, Fyfe A, Zoma A, Veitch J, Hunter J, Whaley K. Decreased C3b receptors (CR1) on erythrocytes from patients with systemic lupus erythematosus. Clin Exp Immunol 1986;63:41–48.

H394. Holmes E, Sibbitt WL Jr, Bankhurst AD. Serum factors which suppress natural cytotoxicity in cancer patients. Int Arch Allergy Appl Immunol 1986;80:39–43.

H395. Holmes FF, Stubbs DW, Larsen WE. Systemic lupus erythematosus and multiple sclerosis in identical twins. Arch Intern Med 1967;119:302–304.

H396. Holmes MC, Burnet FM. The natural history of autoimmune disease in NZB mice. A comparison with the pattern of human autoimmune manifestations. Ann Intern Med 1963 Sep; 59:265–276.

H397. Holsboer F, Liebl R, Hofschuster E. Repeated dexamethasone suppression test during depressive illness. J Affective Disord 1982;4:93–101.

H398. Holsboer F, Steiger A, Maier W. Four cases of reversion to abnormal dexamethasone suppression test response as indicator of clinical relapse. Biol Psychiatry 1983;18:911–916.

H399. Holsti MA, Raulet DH. IL-6 and IL-1 synergize to stimulate IL-2 production and proliferation of peripheral T cells. Center for Cancer Research, Massachusetts Institute of Technology, Cambridge 02139. J Immunol 1989;143:2514–2519.

H400. Holtman JH, Neustadt DH, Klein J, Callen JP. Dapsone is an effective therapy for the skin lesions of subacute cutaneous lupus erythematosus and urticarial vasculitis in a patient with C2 deficiency [case report]. J Rheumatol 1990 Sep;17(9): 1222–1225.

H401. Homcy CJ, Liberthson RR, Fallon JT, Gross S, Miller LM. Ischemic heart disease in systemic lupus erythematosus in the young patient: Report of 6 cases. Am J Cardiol 1982 Feb;49: 478–484.

H402. Homma M, Mimori T, Takeda Y, Akama H, Yoshida T, Ogasawara T, Akizuki M. Autoantibodies to the Sm antigen: immunological approach to clinical aspects of systemic lupus erythematosus. J Rheumatol 1987;14 Suppl 13:188–193.

H403. Homsy J, Morrow WJ, Levy JA. Nutrition and autoimmunity: a review. Clin Exp Immunol 1986 Sep;65(3):473–488.

H404. Honda BM, Candido EPM, Dixon GH. Histone methylation: its occurrence in different cell types and relation to histone H4 metabolism in developing trout testis. J Biol Chem 1975; 250:8686–8689.

H405. Honig S, Gorevic P, Weissmann G. C-reactive protein in systemic lupus erythematosus. Arthritis Rheum 1977 Jun;20: 1065–1070.

H406. Honjo T, Habu S. Origin of immune diversity: genetic variation and selection. Ann Rev Biochem 1985;54:803.

H407. Hontani N, Horino K, Fukui J. Lupus erythematosus observed in a newborn infant. A case report and review of the literature. Acta Pediatr Japan 1971;75:171.

H408. Hood AF, Jerden MS, Moore W, Callen JP. Histopathologic comparison of the subsets of lupus erythematosus. Arch Dermatol 1990;126:52–55.

H409. Hook JJ, Moutsopoulos HM, Geis SA, Stahl NI, Decker JL, Notkins AL. Immune interferons in the circulation of patients with autoimmune disease. N Engl J Med 1979;310:5–8.

H410. Hooper JE, Sequeira W, Martellotto JN, Siegel MB, Skosey JS. Clinical relapse in systemic lupus erythematosus: Correlation with antecedent elevation of urinary free light chain immunoglobulin. J Clin Immunol. in press.

H411. Hoover ML, Angelini G, Ball E, Stastny P, Marks J, Rosenstock J, Raskin P, Ferrara GB, Tosi R, Capra JD. HLA-DQ and T-cell receptor genes in insulin-dependent diabetes mellitus. Cold Spring Harbor Symp Quant Biol 1986;51:803–809.

H412. Hoover R, Fraumeni JF Jr. Risk of cancer in renal-transplant recipients. Lancet 1973 July 14;2:55–57.

H413. Hope RR, Bates LA. The frequency of procainamide-induced systemic lupus erythematosus. Med J Aust 1972 Aug 5; 2:298–303.

H414. Hopkins P, Belmont HM, Buyon J, Philips M, Weissmann G, Abramson SB. Increased levels of plasma anaphylatoxins in systemic lupus erythematosus predict flares of the disease and may elicit vascular injury in lupus cerebritis. Arthritis Rheum 1988 May;31(5):632–641.

H415. Hopper JE, Sequeira W, Martllotto J, Papagiannes E, Perna L, Skosey JL. Clinical relapse in systemic lupus erythematosus:

Correlation with antecedent elevation of urinary free light-chain immunoglobulin. J Clin Immunol 1989;9:338–350.

H416. Horak ID, Gress RE, Lucas PJ, Horak EM, Waldmann TA, Bolen JB. T-lymphocyte interleukin 2-dependent tyrosine protein kinase signal transduction involves the activation of p56^{lck}. Proc Natl Acad Sci USA 1991;88:1996–2000.

H417. Horgan C, Burge J, Crawford L, Taylor RP. The kinetics of [3H]dsDNA/anti-DNA immune complex formation, binding by red blood cells, and release into serum: Effect of DNA m.w. and conditions of antibody excess. J Immunol 1984;133:2079–2084.

H418. Horgan C, Johnson RJ, Gauthier J, Mannik M, Emlen W. Binding of double-stranded DNA to glomeruli of rats in vivo. Arthritis Rheum 1989 Mar;32(3):298–305.

H419. Horgan C, Taylor RP. Studies on the kinetics of binding of complement-fixing dsdna/anti-DNA immune complexes to the red blood cells of normal individuals and patients with systemic lupus erythematosus. Arthritis Rheum 1984;27:320–329.

H420. Horigome I, Seino J, Sudo K, Kinoshita Y, Saito T, Yoshinaga K. Terminal complement complex in plasma from patients with systemic lupus erythematosus and other glomerular disease. Clin Exp Immunol 1987;70:417–424.

H420a. Horiguchi Y, Furukawa F, Hamashima Y, Imamura S. Ultrastructural lupus band test in the skin of RML mice. Arch Dermatol Res 1986;278:474–480.

H421. Horkay I, Nagy E, Varga L, Krajczar J, Alfoldi G. Effect of chloroquine on DNA synthesis in the skin of DLE patients. Acta Dermatovener (Stockh) 1979;59(5):435–439.

H422. Horn JR, Kapur JJ, Walter SE. Mixed connective tissue disease in siblings. Arthritis Rheum 1978 Jul–Aug;21(6):709–714.

H423. Horowitz MD, Rosenbluth D, Kohtz DS, Puszkin S, Speira H. Evidence for the presence of a brain-specific antigen recognized by antibodies in the serum of patients with CNS-SLE [abstract]. Arthritis Rheum 1989 Jan;32(1) Suppl:R5.

H424. Horowitz RE, Dubois EL, Weiner PH, Strain L. Cyclophosphamide treatment of mouse systemic lupus erythematosus. Lab Invest 1969;21:199.

H425. Horrobin DF, Manku MS, Karmazyn M, Asly AL, Morgan RD, Karmali RA. Quinacrine is a prostaglandin antagonist. Biochemical Biophysical Comm 1977;76:1188–1193.

H426. Horsfall AC, Venabler PJW, Mumford PA, Maini RN. Interpretation of the Raji cell assay in sera containing anti-nuclear antibodies and immune complexes. Clin Exp Immunol 1981;44:405–415.

H427. Horton RC, Sheppard MC, Emery P. Propylthiouracil-induced systemic lupus erythematosus [letter]. Lancet 1989 Sep;2(8662):568.

H428. Horwitz DA. Impaired delayed hypersensitivity in systemic lupus erythematosus. Arthritis Rheum 1972 Jul–Aug;15:353–359.

H429. Horwitz DA. Selective depletion of B lymphocytes with cyclophosphamide in patients with rheumatoid arthritis and systemic lupus erythematosus: guidelines for dosage. Arthritis Rheum 1974 Jul–Aug;17:363–374.

H430. Horwitz DA. Mechanisms producing decreased mitogenic reactivity in patients with systemic lupus erythematosus and other rheumatic diseases in mitogens. In: Oppenheim JJ, Rosenstreich DL, editors. Mitogens and immunobiology. New York: Academic Press, 1976.

H431. Horwitz DA, Basin K, Gray JD. Evidence for a post-thymic T-cell developmental defect in SLE [abstract]. Clin Res 1991;39:249A.

H432. Horwitz DA, Cousar JB. A relationship between impaired cellular immunity, humoral suppression of lymphocytes func-

tion and severity of systemic lupus erythematosus. Am J Med 1975 Jun;58:829–835.

H433. Horwitz DA, Garrett MA. Lymphocyte reactivity to mitogens in subjects with systemic lupus erythematosus, rheumatoid arthritis and scleroderma. Clin Exp Immunol 1977 Jan;27:92–99.

H434. Horwitz DA, Garrett MA, Criag AH. Serum effects on mitogenic reactivity in subjects with systemic lupus erythematosus, rheumatoid arthritis and scleroderma. Clin Exp Immunol 1977 Jan;27:100–110.

H435. Horwitz DA, Juul-Nielsen K. Human blood I, lymphocytes in patients with active systemic lupus erythematosus, rheumatoid arthritis, and scleroderma. Clin Exp Immunol 1977 Dec;30:370–378.

H436. Horwitz DA, Linker-Israeli M, Gray JD, Lemoine C. Functional properties of CD8 positive lymphocyte subsets in systemic lupus erythematosus. J Rheumatol 1987;14:49–52.

H437. Horwitz DA, Stastny P, Ziff M. Circulating deoxyribonucleic acid-synthesizing mononuclear leukocytes. I. Increased numbers of proliferating mononuclear leukocytes in inflammatory disease. J Lab Clin Med 1970;76:391–402.

H438. Hosea SW, Brown EJ, Hamburger MI, Frank MM. Opsonic requirements for intravascular clearance after splenectomy. N Engl J Med 1981;304:245–250.

H439. Hosie J, Ghafoor S. Ocular, systemic, and antinuclear antibody changes with acebutolol. J Roy Coll Gen Prac 1983 Dec;33:779–782.

H440. Hossiau FA, D'Cruz D, Vianna J, Hughes GRV. Lupus nephritis: The significance of serological tests at the time of biopsy. Clin Exp Rheumatol 1991;9:345–349.

H441. Hostetter TH, Olson JL, Rennke HG, Brenner BM. Hyperfiltration in remnant nephrons: a potentially adverse response to renal ablation. Am J Physiol 1985;241:F85.

H442. Hospital Practice, April 15, 1990

H443. Hou S. Pregnancy in women with chronic renal disease. N Engl J Med 1985;312:836–839.

H444. Hou SH, Grossman SD, Madias NE. Pregnancy in women with renal disease and moderate renal insufficiency. Am J Med 1985;78:185–194.

H445. Hough W. Discoid lupus erythematosus. A study of sex and age at onset. Acta Dermatol Verereol 1966;46:240–241.

H446. Houghton AN, Mintzer D, Cordon D, Cardo C, Welt S, Fliegel B, Vadhan S, Carswell E, Melamed MR. Oettgen HF, Old IJ. Mouse monoclonal IgG3 antibody detecting GD3 ganglioside: a phase I trial in patients with malignant melanoma. Proc Natl Acad Sci USA 1985;82:1242.

H447. Hourdebaigt-Larrusse P, Ziza JM, Grivaux M. A new case of lupus induced by acebutolol. Ann Cardiol Angiol 1985;34:421–423.

H448. Houser MT, Fish AJ, Tagatz GE, Williams PP, Michael AF. Pregnancy and systemic lupus erythematosus. Am J Obstet Gynecol 1980;138:409–413.

H449. Houssiau FA, Haga HJ, D'Cruz DP, Hughes GR. Initial treatment of lupus nephritis by low does intravenous (IV) cyclophosphamide (CPM): An alternative to high doses of steroids [abstract]. Arthritis Rheum 1990 Sep;33(9) Suppl:S129.

H450. Houssiau FA, D'Cruz D, Vianna J, Hughes GRV. Lupus nephritis: the significance of serologic tests at the time of biopsy. Clin Exp Rheumatol 1991;9:345–349.

H451. Houssiau FA, Lebacq EG. Neonatal lupus erythematosus with congenital heart block associated with maternal systemic lupus erythematosus. Clin Rheumatol 1986;5:505.

H452. Houtman PM, Kallenberg CG, Limburg PC, van Leeuwen MA, van Rijswijk MH, The TH. Fluctuations in anti-NRNP levels in patients with mixed connective tissue disease are related to disease activity as part of a polyclonal B cell response. Ann Rheum Dis 1986 Oct;45(10):800–808.

H453. How A, Den PD, Liao SK, Denburg JD. Antineuronal antibodies in neuropsychiatric systemic lupus erythematosus. Arthritis Rheum 1985 Jul;28(7):789–795.

H454. Howard MA, Firkin BG. Investigations of the lupus-like inhibitor bypassing activity of platelets. Thromb Haemost 1983 Dec 30;50:775.

H455. Howard PF, Hochberg MC, Bias WB, Arnett FC Jr, McLean RH. Relationship between C4 null genes, HLA-D region antigens and genetic susceptibility to systemic lupus erythematosus in Caucasians and black Americans. Am J Med 1986;81:187–193.

H456. Howard RF, Maier WP, Gordon DS, Miller SB. Clinical and immunological investigation of intravenous human immunoglobulin (IVIG) therapy in SLE-associated thrombocytopenia [abstract]. Arthritis Rheum 1989 Apr;32(4) Suppl:S75.

H457. Howard RL, Beck LK, Schneebaum A. Systemic lupus erythematosus presenting as hypoglycemia with insulin receptor antibodies. West J Med 1989 Sep;151(3):324–325.

H458. Howard TW, Iannini MJ, Burge JJ, Davis JS. Rheumatoid factor, cryoglobulinemia, anti-DNA, and renal disease in patients with systemic lupus erythematosus. J Rheumatol 1991;18:826–830.

H459. Howe SE, Lynch DM. Platelet antibody binding in systemic lupus erythematosus. J Rheumatol 1987;14:482–486.

H460. Howie JB, Helyer BJ. The immunology and pathology of NZB mice. Adv Immunol 1968;9:215–266.

H461. Howqua J, Mackay IR. L.E. cells in lymphoma. Blood 1963 Aug;22:191–198.

H462. Hoyle C, Ewing DJ, Parker AC. Acute autonomic neuropathy in association with systemic lupus erythematosus. Ann Rheum Dis 1985 Jun;44(6):420–424.

H463. Hoyoux C, Foidart J, Rigo P, Mahieu P, Geubelle F. Effects of methylprednisolone on Fcγ receptor function of human reticuloendothelial system *in vivo*. Eur J Clin Invest 1984;14:60–66.

H464. Huang CT, Hennigar GR, Lyons HA. Pulmonary dysfunction in systemic lupus erythematosus. N Engl J Med 1965 Feb 11;272:288.

H465. Huang CT, Lyons HA. Comparison of pulmonary function in patients with systemic lupus erythematosus, scleroderma, and rheumatoid arthritis. Am Rev Resp Dis 1966 Jun;93:865–875.

H466. Huang S-W, Kao K-J. Plasma thrombospondin measurement in clinical practice. Intern Med 1990;11:52–70.

H467. Huang YP, Miescher PA, Zubler RH. The interleukin 2 secretion defect in vitro in systemic lupus erythematosus is reversible in rested cultured T cells. J Immunol 1986;137:3515–3520.

H468. Huang YP, Perrin LH, Miescher PA, Zubler RH. Correlation of T and B cell activities in vitro and serum IL-2 levels in systemic lupus erythematosus. J Immunol 1988;141:827–833.

H469. Hubbard HC, Portnoy B. Systemic lupus erythematosus in pregnancy treated with plasmapheresis. Br J Dermatol 1979 Jul;101(1):87–90.

H470. Huber C, Pfister R, Stingl G. Complement-dependent lymphocytotoxic antibodies (CLA) in systemic lupus erythematosus preferentially inhibit the generation of allo-reactive cytotoxic T cells in secondary CML. Clin Exp Immunol 1982;50:525–533.

H471. Huber SA, Job PL, Auld JK, Woodruff JF. Sex related differences in the rapid production of cytotoxic spleen cells against uninfected myofibers during coxsackievirus-B infection. J Immunol 1981;126:1336–1340.

H472. Hubscher O, Elsner B. Nodular transformation of the liver in a patient with systemic lupus erythematosus [letter]. J Rheumatol 1989 Mar;16(3):410–412.

H473. Hughes ER, Ely RS, Kelley VC. Plasma adrenocortical hormones in connective tissue diseases. Am J Dis Child 1962 Dec;104:610–613.

H474. Hughes GR. Thrombosis, abortion, cerebral disease and the lupus anticoagulant [editorial]. BMJ (Clin Res) 1983 Oct;287(6399):1088–1089.

H475. Hughes GR. Antimalarials in SLE. Br J Clin Prac 1987;41 Suppl 52:10–12.

H476. Hughes GR, Harris EN, Gharavi AE. The anticardiolipin syndrome. J Rheumatol 1986 Jun;13(3):486–489.

H477. Hughes GR, Mackworth-Young C, Harris EN, Gharavi AE. Veno-occlusive disease in systemic lupus erythematosus: possible association with anti-cardiolipin antibodies? [letter]. Arthritis Rheum 1984 Sep;27(9):1071.

H478. Hughes GRV. The treatment of SLE. Clin Rheum Dis 1982;8:299–313.

H479. Hughes GRV, Asherson RA. A typical lupus with special reference to ANA negative lupus and lupus subsets. In: Grunfeld JP, Maxwell MH, editors. Advances in neprology. Chicago: Year Book, 1985:333–346.

H480. Hughes GRV, Cohen SA, Lightfoot RW, Meltzer JJ, Christian CL. The release of DNA into serum and synovial fluid. Arthritis Rheum 1971 Mar–Apr;14:259–266.

H481. Hughes JT, Esiri M, Oxbury JM, Whitty CWM. Chloroquine myopathy. QJ Med 1971;40:85–93.

H482. Hughes RA, Cameron JS, Hall SM, Heaton J, Payan J, Tech R. Multiple mononeuropathy as the initial presentation of systemic lupus erythematosus-nerve biopsy and response to plasma exchange. J Neurol 1982;228(4):239–247.

H483. Hughes-Jones NC, Ghosh S. Anti-D coated Rh-positive red cells will bind the first component of the complement pathway, C1q. Febs Lett 1981;128:318–320.

H484. Hugli TE, Muller-Eberhard HJ. Anaphylatoxins: C3a and C5a. Adv Immunol 1978;26:1–55.

H485. Huizinga TWJ, De Haas M, Kleijer M, Nuijens JH, Roos D, Von dem Borne AEG Kr. Soluble Fcγ receptor III in human plasma originates from release by neutrophils. J Clin Invest 1990;86:416–423.

H486. Huizinga TWJ, Dolman KM, Van der Linden NJM, Kleijer M, Nuijens JH, Von dem Borne AEG, Roos D. Phosphatidylinositol-linked FcRIII mediates exocytosis of neutrophil granule proteins, but does not mediate initiation of the respiratory burst. J Immunol 1990;144:1432–1437.

H487. Huizinga TWJ, Kleijer M, Roos D, Von dem Borne AEG Kr. Differences between FcRIII of human neutrophils and human K/NK lymphocytes in relation to the NA antigen system. In: Knapp W, et al editors. Leucocyte Typing IV. Oxford: Oxford University Press, 1989:582.

H488. Huizinga TWJ, Kleijer M, Tetteroo PAT, Roos D, von dem Borne AEGKr. Biallelic neutrophil NA-antigen system is associated with a polymorphism on the phosphoinositol-linked Fcγ receptor III (CD16). Blood 1990;75:213–217.

H489. Huizinga TWJ, Kuijpers RWAM, Kleijer M, Schulpen TWJ, Cuypers TM, Roos D, von dem Borne AEG Kr. Maternal genomic neutrophil FcRIII deficiency leading to neonatal isoimmune neutropenia. Blood 1990;76:1927–1932.

H490. Huizinga TWJ, Van der Schoot CE, Jost C, Klaassen R, Kleijer M, Von dem Borne AEG Kr, Roos D, Tetteroo PAT. The PI-linked receptor FcRIII is released on stimulation of neutrophils. Nature 1988;333:667–669.

H491. Huizinga TWJ, Van der Schoot CE, Roos D, Weening RS. Induction of neutrophil Fcγ receptor I expression can be used as a marker for biological activity of recombinant interferon-γ *in vivo*. Blood 1991;77:2088–2090.

H492. Huletsky A, De Murcia G, Muller S, Hengartner M, Menard L, Lamarre D, Poirier GG. The effect of poly(ADP-ribosyl)ation on native and H1-depleted Ccromatin. a role of poly(ADP-ribosyl)ation on core nucleosome structure. J Biol Chem 1989;264:8878–8886.

H493. Hull B, editor. Summary from questionnaires: history of diseases in members' families. Lupus Lifeline, 1975.

H494. Hull D, Binns BAO, Joyce D. Congenital heart block and widespread fibrosis due to maternal lupus erythematosus. Arch Dis Child 1966;41:688–690.

H495. Hull RG, Harris EN, Morgan SH, Hughes GRV. Anti-Ro antibodies and abortions in women with SLE. Lancet 1983;2: 1138.

H496. Hultman P, Enestrom S, Pollard KM, Tan EM. Anti-fibrillarin autoantibodies in mercury-treated mice. Clin Exp Immunol 1989;78:470–472.

H497. Humphreys EM. Cardiac lesions of acute disseminated lupus erythematosus. Ann Intern Med 1948 Jan;28:12–14.

H498. Hunder GG, McDuffie FC. Hypocomplementemia in rheumatoid arthritis. Am J Med 1973 Apr;54:461–472.

H499. Hunder GG, McDuffie FC, Huston KA, Elveback LR, Hepper NG. Pleural fluid complement, complement conversion and immune complexes immunologic and nonimmunologic diseases. J Lab Clin Med 1977 Dec;90:971–980.

H500. Hunder GG, Mullen BJ, McDuffie FC. Complement in pericardial fluid lupus erythematosus. Ann Intern Med 1974; 80:453–458.

H501. Hunder GG, Pierre RV. In vivo LE cell formation in synovial fluid. Arthritis Rheum 1970 Jul–Aug;13:448–454.

H502. Hungerford DS, Zizic TM. II. The early diagnosis of ischemic necrosis of bone. Medicine 1980 Mar;59(2):143–148.

H503. Hunkapiller T, Hood L. The growing immunoglobulin gene superfamily. Nature 1986;323:15–16.

H504. Hunter T. Protein-tyrosine phosphatase: The other side of the coin. Cell 1989;58:1013–1016.

H505. Hunter T, Arnott JE, McCarthy DS. Feature of systemic lupus erythematosus and sarcoidosis occurring together. Arthritis Rheum 1980 Mar;23:364.

H506. Hunter T, Plummer FA. Infectious arthritis complicating systemic lupus erythematosus. Can Med Assoc J 1980 Apr; 122(7):791–793.

H507. Huntley AC, Fletcher MP, Ikeda RM, Gershwin ME. Shared antigenic determinants between rabbit antihuman brain and rabbit antihuman thymocyte sera: Relationship to the lymphocytotoxic antibodies of systemic lupus erythematosus. Clin Immunol Immunopathol 1977 March;7:269–280.

H508. Hurd ER, Jasin JE, Gilliam JN. Correlation of disease activity and C1-binding immune complexes with the neutrophil inclusions which form in the presence of SLE sera. Clin Exp Immunol 1980;40:283–291.

H509. Hurd ER, Johnston JM, Okita JR, MacDonald PC, Ziff M, Gilliam JN. Prevention of glomerulonephritis and prolonged survival in New Zealand black/New Zealand white F1 hybrid mice fed an essential fatty-acid deficient diet. J Clin Invest 1981;67:476.

H510. Hurley CK, Gregersen P, Steiner N, Bell J, Hartzman R, Nepom G, Silver J, Johnson AH. Polymorphism of the HLA-D region in American blacks. A DR3 haplotype generated by recombination. J Immunol 1988;140:885–892.

H511. Hurley CK, Gregersen PK, Gorski J, Steiner N, Robbins FM, Hartzman R, Johnson AH, Silver J. The DR3 (w18), DQw4 haplotype differs from DR3(w17), DQw2 haplotypes at multiple class II loci. Hum Immunol 1989;25:37–50.

H512. Hurst NP, French JK, Bell AL, Nuki G, O'Donnell ML, Betts WH, Cleland LG. Differential effects of mepacrine, chloroquine and hydroxychloroquine on superoxide anion generation, phospholipid methylation and arachidonic acid release by human blood monocytes. Biochem Pharmacol 1986 Sep 15;35(18):3083–3089.

H513. Hurst NP, French JK, Gorjatschko L, Betts WH. Studies on the mechanism of inhibition of chemotactic tripeptide stimulated human neutrophil polymorphonuclear leucocyte superoxide production by chloroquine and hydroxychloroquine. Ann Rheum Dis 1987 Oct;46(10):750–756.

H514. Hurst NP, French JK, Gorjatschko L, Betts WH. Chloroquine and hydroxychloroquine inhibit multiple sites in metabolic pathways leading to neutrophil superoxide release. J Rheumatol 1988 Jan;15(1):23–27.

H515. Hurst NP, Nuki G, Wallington T. Evidence for intrinsic cellular defects of 'complement' receptor-mediated monocyte phagocytosis in patients with systemic lupus erythematosus (SLE). Clin Exp Immunol 1984;55:303–312.

H516. Hurvitz D, Hirschhorn K. Suppression of in vitro lymphocyte responses by chloroquine. N Engl J Med 1965 Jul 1;273: 23–26.

H517. Huston KA, Gupta RC, Donadio JV, McDuffie FC, Ilstrup DM. Circulating immune complexes in systemic lupus erythemato sus. Association with other immunologic abnormalities but not with changes in renal function. J Rheumatol 1978;5: 423–432.

H518. Hutchins GM, Harvey AM. The thymus in systemic lupus erythematosus. Bull Johns Hopkins Hosp 1964 Nov;115: 355–378.

H519. Hutchinson J. Harvelian lectures on lupus: Lecture 1, Common lupus-The head of a family and not a solitary disease. BMJ 1888 Jan 7;1:6–10. Lecture II, Varieties of common lupus. Ibid. 1888;Jan 14;58–63. Lecture III, On the various forms of lupus vulgaris and erythematosus. Ibid 1888 Jan 21;113–118.

H520. Hutchinson J. Lupus erythematosus. Med Times Gazette 1879 Jan 4;1:1.

H521. Hutchinson J. On lupus and its treatment. Br Med J 1880 May 1;1:650.

H522. Hutchinson M, Bresnihan B. Neurological lupus erythematosus with tonic seizures simulating multiple sclerosis [letter]. J Neurol Neurosurg Psychiatry 1983 Jun;46(6):583–585.

H523. Hymes K, Schur PH, Karpatkin S. Heavy-chain subclass of bound antiplatelet IgG autoimmune hemolytic anemia. Blood 1980 Jul;56:84–87.

H524. Hymes SR, Russell TJ, Jordon RE. The anti-Ro antibody system. Int J Dermatol 1986;25:1–7.

I

I1. Iacobelli D, Bianchi L, Hashimoto K. Passive transfer of photosensitivity by intradermal injection of vesiculobullous lupus erythematosus serum and ultraviolet light irradiation in the guinea pig. Photodermatol 1987 Dec;4(6):288–295.

I2. Ibels LS, Alfrey AC, Haut L, Huffer WE. Preservation of function in experimental renal disease by dietary restriction of phosphate. N Engl J Med 1978 Jan 19;298(3):122–126.

I3. Igarashi T, Nagaoka S, Matsunaga K, Katoh K, Ishigatsubo Y, Tani K, Okubo T, Lie JT. Aortitis syndrome (Takayasu's arteritis) associated with systemic lupus erythematosus. J Rheumatol 1989 Dec;16(12):1579–1583.

I4. Ihle BU, Whitworth JA, Dowling JP, Kincaid-Smith P. Hydralazine and lupus nephritis. Clin Nephrol 1984;22:230–238.

I5. Iida K, Mornaghi R, Nussenzweig V. Complement receptor (CR1) deficiency in erythrocytes from patients with systemic lupus erythematosus. J Exp Med 1982;155:1427–1438.

I6. Ikehara S, Nakamura T, Sekita K, Muso E, Hasumizu R, Ohtsuki H, Hamashima Y, Good R. Treatment of systemic and organ-specific autoimmune disease in mice by allogeneic bone marrow transplantation. Prog Clin Biol Res 1987;229:131–146.

I7. Iliffe GD, Naidoo S, Hunter T. Primary biliary cirrhosis associated with systemic lupus erythematosus. Dig Dis Sci 1982 Mar; 27(3):274–278.

I8. Ilowite NT, Samuel P, Ginzler E, Jacobson MS. Dyslipoproteinemia in pediatric systemic lupus erythematosus. Arthritis Rheum 1988;31:859–863.

I9. Ilowite NT, Wedgwood JF, Bonagura VR. Expression of the major rheumatoid factor cross-reactive idiotype in juvenile rheumatoid arthritis. Arthritis Rheum 1989;32:265.

I10. Imaoka K, Kanai Y, Yoshikawa Y, Yamanouchi K. Temporary breakdown of immunological tolerance to dsdna and nucleohistone antigens in rabbits infected with rinderpest virus. Clin Exp Immunol 1990;82:522–526.

I11. Imbasciati E, Surian M, Bottino S, Cosci P, Colussi G, Ambroso GC, Massa E, Minetti L, Pardi G, Ponticelli C. Lupus nephropathy and pregnancy. Nephron 1984;36:46–51.

I12. Inaba M, Marauyama E. Reversal of resistance to vincristine in P388 leukemia by various polycyclic clinical drugs, with a special emphasis on quinacrine. Cancer Res 1988 Apr;48(8): 2064–2067.

I13. Inada Y, Kamiyama M, Kanemitsu T, Ikegami H, Watanabe K, Clark WS, Asai Y. In vivo binding of circulating immune complexes by C3b receptors (CR1) of transfused erythrocytes. Ann Rheum Dis 1989;48:287–294.

I14. Inai S, Akagaki Y, Moriyama T, Fukumori Y, Yoshimura K, Ohnoki S, Yamaguhi HTI. Inherited deficiencies of the late-acting complement components other than C9 found among healthy blood donors. Int Arch Allergy Appl Immunol 1989; 90:274–279.

I15. Inam S, Sidki K, Al-Marshedy AR, Judzewitsch R. Addison's disease, hypertension, renal and hepatic microthrombosis in 'primary' antiphospholipid syndrome. Postgrad Med J 1991; 67:385–388.

I16. Inghirami G, Simon J, Balow JE, Tsokos GC. Activated T lymphocytes in the peripheral blood of patients with systemic lupus erythematosus induce B cells to produce immunoglobulin. Clin Exp Rheumatol 1988:269–276.

I17. Ingle DJ, Baker BL. Physiological and therapeutic effects of corticotropin (ACTH) and cortisone. Springfield, IL:Charles C. Thomas, 1953.

I18. Inman RD. Immune complexes in SLE. Clin Rheum Dis 1982:8:49–62.

I19. Inman RD, Day NK. Immunologic and clinical aspects of immune complex disease. Am J Med 1981;70:1097–1106.

I20. Inman RD, Fong JKK, Pussell BA, Ryan PJ, Hughes GRV. The C1q binding assay in SLE: discordance with disease activity. Arthritis Rheum 1980 Nov;23:1282–1286.

I21. Inman RD, Jovanovic L, Markenson JA, Longcope C, Dawood MY, Lockshin MD. Systemic lupus erythematosus in men. Genetic and endocrine features. Arch Intern Med 1982 Oct; 142(10):1813–1815.

I22. Inman RD, McDougal JS, Redecha PB, Lockshin MD, Stevens CE, Christian CL. Isolation and characterization of circulating immune complexes in patients with hepatitis systemic vasculitis. Clin Immunol Immunopathol 1981;21:364–374.

I23. Innes A, Cunningham C, Power DA, Catto AR. Fetus as an allograft: non-cytotoxic maternal antibodies to HLA-linked paternal antigens. Am J Reprod Immunol 1989;19(4):146–150.

I24. Inoue K, Nishioka J, Hukuda S. Altered lymphocyte proliferation by low dosage laser irradiation. Clin Exp Rheumatol 1989 Sep–Oct;7(5):521–523.

I25. Inoue T, Kanayama Y, Kato N, Ohe A, Amatsu K, Okamura M, Horiguchi T. Significance of C-reactive protein elevation in the pretreatment stage of systemic lupus erythematosus. Scand J Rheum 1981;10(3):222–224.

I25a. Inoue T, Kanayama Y, Ohe A, Kato N, Horiguchi T, Ishii M, Shiota K. Immunopathologic studies of pneumonitis in systemic lupus erythematosus. Ann Intern Med 1979 Jul;91: 30–34.

I26. Inoue T, Takeda T, Koda S, Negoro N, Okamura M, Amatsu K, Kohno M, Horiguchi T, Kanayama Y. Differential diagnosis of fever in systemic lupus erythematosus using discriminant analysis. Rheumatol Int 1986;6(2):69–77.

I27. Irgang S. Lupus erythematosus profundus. Arch Dermatol Syphiligr 1940;42:97–108.

I28. Irons EM, Ayer JP, Brown RG, Armstrong SH Jr. ACTH and cortisone in diffuse collagen disease and chronic dermatoses; Differential therapeutic effects. JAMA 1951 Mar 24;145: 861–865.

I29. Irving BA, Weiss A. The cytoplasmic domain of the T cell receptor zeta chain is sufficient to couple to receptor-associated signal transduction pathways. Cell 1991;64:891–901.

I30. Isaacs A, Richardson P, Hibbert D, Oram S, Cooper P, Ferguson R, Toghill P, Walker M. Aortic incompetence in systemic lupus erythematosus. BMJ 1976 Nov 20;2:1260–1261.

I31. Isenberg DA, Colaco CB, Dudeney C, Todd-Pokropek A, Snaith ML. The relationship of anti-DNA antibody idiotypes and anticardiolipin antibodies to disease activity in systemic lupus erythematosus. Medicine 1986;65:46–55.

I32. Isenberg DA, Dudeney C, Williams W, Todd-Pokropek A, Stollar BD. Disease activity in systemic lupus erythematosus related to a range of antibodies binding DNA and synthetic polynucleotides. Ann Rheum Dis 1988;47:717–724.

I33. Isenberg DA, Madaio MP, Reichlin M, Schoenfeld Y, Rauch J, Stollar BD, Schwartz RS. Anti-DNA antibody idiotypes in systemic lupus. Lancet 1984 Aug 25;2:419–422.

I34. Isenberg DA, Meyrick-Thomas D, Snaith ML, McKeran RO, Royston JP. A study of migraine in systemic lupus erythematosus. Ann Rheum Dis 1982 Feb;41(1):30–32.

I34a. Isenberg DA, Morrow WJ, Snaith ML. Methyl prednisolone pulse therapy in the treatment of systemic lupus erythematosus. Ann Rheum Dis 1982 Aug;41:347–351.

I35. Isenberg DA, Shoenfeld Y, Madaio MP, Rauch J, Reichlin M, Stollar BD, Schwartz RS. Anti-DNA antibody idiotypes in systemic lupus erythematosus. Lancet Aug 25; 2(8400): 417–422.

I36. Isenberg DA, Shoenfeld Y, Schwartz RS. Multiple serologic reactions and their relationship to clinical activity in systemic lupus erythematosus. Arthritis Rheum 1984 Feb;27(2): 132–138.

I37. Isenberg DA, Shoenfeld Y, Walport M, Mackworth-Young C, Dudeney C, Todd-Pokropek A, Brill S, Weinberger A, Pinkhas J. Detection of cross-reactive anti-DNA antibody idiotypes in the serum of systemic lupus erythematosus patients and of their relatives. Arthritis Rheum 1985;28:999–1007.

I38. Isenberg DA, Snaith ML. Muscle disease in systemic lupus erythematosus: a study of its nature, frequency and cause. J Rheumatol 1981 Nov–Dec;8(6):917–924.

I39. Isenberg DA, Snaith ML, Morrow WJ, Al-Khader AA, Cohen SL, Fisher C, Moubray J. Cyclosporin A for the treatment of systemic lupus erythematosus. Int J Immunopharmacol 1981; 3(2):163–169.

I40. Isenberg DA, Williams W, Axford J, Bell D, Diamond B, Ebling F, Hahn B, Harkiss G. Mackworth-Young C, Rauch J, Ravirajan CT, Schwartz R, Staines N, Todd-Pokropek A, Tucker L, Zouali M. Comparison of 17 DNA antibody idiotypes in patients with autoimmune diseases, healthy relatives and spouses and normal controls—Results of an international study from 10 laboratories. J Autoimmunity 1990;3:393–414.

I41. Isenberg I. Histones. Ann Rev Biochem 1979; 48:159–191.

I42. Ishibashi Y, Watanabe R, Hommura S, Koyama A, Ishikawa T, Mikami Y. Endogenous Nocardia asteroides endophthalmitis in a patient with systemic lupus erythematosus. Br J Ophthalmol 1990 Jul;74(7):433–436.

I43. Ishida H, Kumagai S, Unehara H, Sano H, Tagaya Y, Yodoi J, Imura H. Impaired expression of high affinity interleukin 2 receptor on activated lymphocytes from patients with systemic lupus erythematosus. J Immunol 1987;139:1070–1074.

I44. Ishigatsubo Y, Sakamoto H, Hagiwara E, Aoki A, Shirai A, Tani K, Okubo T, Klinman DM. Quantitation of autoantibody-secreting B cells in Systemic Lupus Erythematosus. Autoimmunity 1990;5:71–80.

I45. Ishiguro N, Tomino Y, Fujito K, Nakayama S, Koide H. A case of massive ascites due to lupus peritonitis with a dramatic response to steroid pulse therapy. Jap J Medicine 1989 Sep–Oct;28(5):608–611.

I46. Ishii Y, Nagasawa K, Mayumi T, Niho Y. Clinical importance of persistence of anticardiolipin antibodies in systemic lupus erythematosus. Ann Rheum Dis 1990 Jun;49(6):387–390.

I47. Ishikawa S, Segar WE, Gilbert EF, Burkholder PM, Levy JM, Visekul C. Myocardial infarction in a child with systemic lupus erythematosus. Am J Dis Child 1978 Jul;132:696–699.

I48. Iskander MK, Khan MA. Chorea as the initial presentation of oral contraceptive related systemic lupus erythematosus [letter]. J Rheumatol 1989 Jun;16(6):850–851.

I49. Isobe T, Tanaka K, Yamauchi Y, Matsumoto J, Horimatsu T. Intradermal tests in SLE versus in other connective tissue disease. Jpn J Med 1978;17:212–216.

I50. Israel E, Dermarkarian R, Rosenberg M, Sperling R, Taylor G, Rubin P, Drazen JM. The effects of a 5-lipoxygenase inhibitor on asthma induced by cold, dry air. N Engl J Med 1990; 323:1740–1744.

I51. Israel HL. Pulmonary manifestations of disseminated lupus erythematosus. Am J Med Sci 1953 Oct;226:387–392.

I52. Itabashi HH, Kokmen E. Chloroquine neuromyopathy, a reversible granulovacuolar myopathy. Arch Pathol 1972 Mar; 93:209–218.

I53. Ito H, Harada R, Uchida Y, Odashiro K, Uozumi K, Yawumoto Y, Ohashi T, Yamashita W, Uematsu T, Hanada S, Arima T, Tanoue Y. Lupus nephritis and adult T cell leukemia. Nephron 1990;55:325–328.

I54. Ito M, Kagiyama Y, Moura I, Hiramatsu Y, Jurata E, Kanaya S, Ito S, Fujino T, Kusaba T, Kimi S. Cardiovascular manifestations in systemic lupus erythematosus. Jpn Circ J 1979 Nov; 43:985–994.

I55. Ito S, Ueno M, Arakawa M, Saito T, Aoyagi T, Fujiwara M. Therapeutic effect of 15-deoxyspergualin on the progression of lupus nephritis in MRL mice. I. Immunopathological analyses. Clin Exp Immunol 1990;81:446–453.

I56. Itoh Y, Rader MD, Reichlin M. Heterogeneity of the Ro/SSA antigen and autoanti-Ro/SSA response: evidence of the four antigenically distinct forms. Clin Exp Immunol 1990;81: 45–51.

I57. Itoh K, Itoh Y, Frank MB. Protein heterogeneity of the human ribonucleoprotein: the 52 and 60 kD Ro/SSA autoantigens are encoded by separate genes. J Clin Invest 1991;87: 177–186.

I58. Itoh Y, Reichlin M. Ro/SS-A antigen in human platelets: different distributions of the isoforms of Ro/Ss-A protein and the Ro/SS-A binding RNA. Arthritis Rheum 1991;34:888–893.

I59. Itoh Y, Sekine H, Hosono O, Takeuchi T, Koide J, Takano M, Abe T. Thrombotic thrombocytopenic purpura in two patients with systemic lupus erythematosus: clinical significance of antiplatelet antibodies. Clin Immunol Immunopathol 1990; 57:125–136.

I60. Ivanova MM, Nassonova VA, Soloviev SK, Akhnazarova VD, Speranski AI. Controlled trial of cyclophosphamide, azathioprine and chlorambucil in lupus nephritis (a double-blind trial). Vopr Revum 1981 Apr–Jun;(2):11–18.

I61. Ivanova MM, Nassonova VA, Soloviev SK, Speransky AI, Akhanzarova VD, Decker JL, Steinberg AD. Cyclophosphamide azathioprine or chlorambucil for systemic lupus erythematosus nephritis. Arthritis Rheum 1979;22:624–625.

I62. Ivey KJ, DenBesten L. Pseudotumor cerebri associated with corticosteroid therapy in an adult. JAMA 1969 Jun 2;28: 1698–1700.

I63. Ivey KJ, Hwang YF, Sheets RF. Scleroderma associated with thrombocytopenia and Coombs-positive hemolytic anemia. Am J Med 1971 Dec;51:815–817.

I63a. Iwahara Y, Niiya K, Yamato K, Myoshi I. Thrombocytopenic purpura in a patient with lupus anticoagulant: Requirement of both immunosuppressive and antithrombotic therapies. Am J Haematol 1990;33:75–77.

I64. Izui S, Kelley VE, Masudak K, Yoshida H, Roths JB, Murphy ED. Induction of various autoantibodies by mutant gene lpr in several strains of mice. J Immunol 1984;133:227.

I65. Izui S, Higaki M, Morrow D, Merino R. The Y chromosome from autoimmune BXSB/MpJ induces a lupus-like syndrome in (NZW × C57Bl/6) F1 male mice, but not in C57Bl/6J male mice. Eur J Immunol 1988;18:911–915.

I66. Izui S, Lambert PH, Fournie GJ, Turler H, Miescher PA. Features of systemic lupus erythematosus in mice injected with bacterial lipopolysaccharides: identification of circulating DNA and renal localization of DNA-anti-DNA complexes. J Exp Med 1977 May 1;145(5):1115–1130.

I67. Izui S, Lambert PH, Miescher PA. In vitro demonstration of a particular affinity of glomerular basement membrane and collagen for DNA. A possible basis for a local formation of DNA-anti-DNA complexes in systemic lupus erythematosus. J Exp Med 1976 Aug 1;144(2):428–443.

I68. Izui S, Lambert PH, Miescher PA. Failure to detect circulating DNA-anti-DNA complexes by four radio-immunological methods in patients with systemic lupus erythematosus. Clin Exp Immunol 1977 Dec;30:384–392.

I69. Izui S, Masuda K. Resistance to tolerance induction is not prerequisite to development of murine SLE. J Immunol 1984; 133:3010–3014.

I70. Izui S, McConahey PJ, Theofilopoulos AN, Dixon FJ. Association of circulating retroviral gp70-anti-gp70 immune complexes with murine systemic lupus erythematosus. J Exp Med 1979;149:1099–1107.

I71. Izui SP, McConahey PJ, Dixon FJ. Increased spontaneous polyclonal activation of B lymphocytes in mice with spontaneous autoimmune disease. J Immunol 1978;121:2213–2219.

I72. Izumi AK, Takiguchi P. Lupus erythematosus panniculitis. Arch Dermatol 1983 Jan;119:61–64.

J

J1. Jablonska S, Chorzelski T, Blaszczyk M, Maciejewski W. Pathogenesis of pemphigus erythematosus. Arch Dermatol Res 1977;258:135–140.

J2. Jabs DA, Arnett FC, Bias WB, Beale MG. Familial abnormalities of lymphocyte function in a large Sjogren's syndrome kindred. J Rheumatol 1985;13:320–326.

J3. Jabs DA, Enger C, Prendergast RA. Murine models of Sjogren's syndrome. Evolution of the lacrimal gland inflammatory lesions. Invest Ophthalmol Vis Sci 1991;32:371.

J4. Jabs DA, Fine SL, Hochberg MC, Newman SA, Heiner GG, Stevens MB. Severe retinal vaso-occlusive disease in systemic lupus erythematosus. Arch Ophthalmol 1986 Apr;104(4): 558–563.

J5. Jabs DA, Heiner GG, Stevens MB. Severe ocular disease in systemic lupus erythematosus: Ocular and systemic manifestations [abstract]. Arthritis Rheum 1985 Apr;28(4) Suppl:S22.

J6. Jabs DA, Henneken AM, Schachat AP, Fine SL. Choroidopathy in systemic lupus erythematosus. Arch Ophthalmol 1988 Feb; 106(2):230–234.

J7. Jabs DA, Miller NR, Newman SA, Johnson MA, Stevens MB. Optic neuropathy in systemic lupus erythematosus. Arch Ophthalmol 1986 Apr;104(4):564–568.

J8. Jackson G, Miller M, Littlejohn G, Helme R, King R. Bilateral internuclear ophthalmoplegia in systemic lupus erythematosus. J Rheumatol 1986 Dec;13(6):1161–1162.

J9. Jackson R. Discoid lupus in a newborn infant of a mother with lupus erythematosus. Pediatrics 1964;33:425–430.

J10. Jackson R, Gulliver M. Neonatal lupus erythematosus progressing into systemic lupus erythematosus a 15 year follow-up. Br J Dermatol 1979;101:81–86.

J11. Jackson V. Deposition of newly synthesized histones: new histones H2A and H2B do not deposit in the same nucleosome with new histones H3 and H4. Biochemistry 1987;26:2315–2325.

J12. Jackson V. Deposition of newly synthesized histones: misinterpretations due to cross-linking density-labeled proteins with Lomant's reagent. Biochemistry 1987;26:2325–2334.

J13. Jackson V. Deposition of newly synthesized histones: hybrid nucleosomes are not tandemly arranged on daughter DNA strands. Biochemistry 1988;27:2109–2120.

J14. Jacob CO, Aiso S, Michie SA, McDevitt HO, Acha-Orbea H. Prevention of diabetes in nonobese diabetic mice by tumor necrosis factor (TNF): similarities between TNF-α and interleukin 1. Proc Natl Acad Sci USA 1990;87:968–972.

J15. Jacob CO, Fronek Z, Lewis GD, Koo M, Hansen JA, McDevitt HO. Heritable major histocompatibility complex class II- associated differences in production of tumor necrosis factor alpha: relevance to genetic predisposition to systemic lupus erythematosus. Proc Natl Acad Sci USA 1990;87:1233–1237.

J16. Jacob CO, McDevitt HO. Tumour necrosis factor-alpha in murine autoimmune 'lupus' nephritis. Nature 1988;331:356-358.

J17. Jacob HS. Pulse steroids in hematologic disease. Hosp Pract 1985 Aug 15;5:87–94.

J18. Jacob JR, Weisman MH, Rosenblatt SI. Bookstein. Chronic pernio. A historical perspective of cold-induced vascular disease. Arch Intern Med 1986 Aug;146(8):1589–1592.

J19. Jacob L, Lety MA, Bach JF, Louvard D. Human systemic lupus erythematosus sera contain antibodies against cell- surface protein(s) that share(s) epitope(s) with DNA. Proc Natl Acad Sci USA 1986;83:6970–6974.

J20. Jacob L, Lety MA, Louvard D, Bach JF. Binding of a monoclonal anti-DNA autoantibody to identical protein(s) present at the surface of several human cell types involved in lupus pathogenesis. J Clin Invest 1985 Jan;75(1):315–317.

J21. Jacob L, Tron F, Bach JF, Louvard D. A monoclonal anti-DNA antibody also binds cell surface proteins. Proc Natl Acad Sci USA 1984;81:3843–3845.

J22. Jacob L, Viard JP, Allenet B, Anin MF, Slama FBH, Vandekerckhove J, Primo J, Markovitz J, Jacob F, Bach JF, Le Pecq JB, Louvard D. A monoclonal anti-double-stranded DNA autoantibody binds to a 94-kDa cell-surface protein on various cell types via nucleosomes or a DNA-histone complex. Proc Natl Acad Sci USA 1989;86:4669–4673.

J23. Jacob L, Viard JP, Louvard D, Bach JF. Recent advances in the pathogenesis of systemic lupus erythematosus [review]. Adv Nephrol 1990;19:237–255.

J24. Jacobs HJ. Acute disseminated lupus erythematosus with hemolytic anemia in a 10-year-old child. J Pediatr 1953;42:728–730.

J25. Jacobs J, Bernhard M, Delgado A, Strain J. Screening for organic mental syndromes in the mentally ill. Ann Intern Med 1977;86:40.

J26. Jacobs JC. Systemic lupus erythematosus in childhood. Report of 35 cases with discussion of seven apparently induced by anticonvulsant medication, and of prognosis and treatment. Pediatr 1963 Aug;32:257–264.

J27. Jacobs JC. Childhood-onset systemic lupus erythematosus.

Modern management and improved prognosis. NY State J Med 1977 Dec;77:2231.

J28. Jacobs JC. Fever on drug-free day of alternate-day steroid therapy [letter]. Am J Med 1984;76:A91-A92.

J29. Jacobs JR, Waters RC, Toomey JM. Head and neck manifestations of SLE. Am Fam Physician 1979;20(6):97–99.

J30. Jacobs L, Kinkel PR, Costello PB, Alukal MK, Kinkel WR, Green FA. Central nervous system lupus erythematosus: the value of magnetic resonance imaging. J Rheumatol 1988 Apr; 15(4):601–606.

J31. Jacobs P, Wood L, Dent DM. Splenectomy and the thrombocytopenia of systemic lupus erythematosus. Ann Intern Med 1986;105:971–972.

J32. Jacobson EJ, Reza MJ. Constrictive pericarditis in systemic lupus erythematosus. Arthritis Rheum 1978 Nov– Dec;21:972–974.

J33. Jacox RF, Stuard ID. Legionnaires' disease in a patient with systemic lupus erythematosus. Arthritis Rheum 1978 Nov–Dec;21(8):975–977.

J33a. Jadassohn J. Handbuch der Hautkrankheiten. Quoted by Harvey AM et al. Berlin: F. Mraech 1940;(3):298–424.

J34. Jaeger A, Sauder J, Kopferschmitt FF, Flesch F. Hypokalemia as evidence of chloroquine toxicity. Presse Med 1987 Oct 10; 16(33):1658–1659.

J35. Jaenichen HR, Pech M, Lindenmaier W, Weldgruber N, Zachau HG. Composite human V_K genes and a model of their evolution. Nuc Acids Res 1984;12:5249–5263.

J36. Jaffe CJ, Vierling JM, Jones EA, Lacoley T, Frank MM. Receptor-specific clearance by the reticuloendothelial system in chronic liver diseases. Demonstration of defective C3b-specific clearance in primary biliary cirrhosis. J Clin Invest 1978; 62:1069–1077.

J37. Jakes JT, Dubois EL, Quismorio FP Jr. Antileprosy drugs and lupus erythematosus [letter]. Ann Intern Med 1982 Nov; 97(5):788.

J38. James TN, Rupe CE, Monto RW. Pathology of the cardiac conduction system in systemic lupus erythematosus. Ann Intern Med 1965 Sep 16:402–410.

J39. James AP. Intradermal triamcinolone acetonide in localized lesions. J Invest Dermatol 1960 Mar;34:175–176.

J40. James DG. Sarcoidosis of the skin. Ch. 161. In: Fitzpatrick TB, Eisen AZ, Wolff K, Freedberg IM, Austen KF. Dermatology and General Medicine, 3d ed. New York: McGraw Hill, 1987.

J41. Jandl RC, George JL, Silberstein DS, Eaton RB, Schur PH. The effect of adherent cell-derived factors on immunoglobulin and anti-DNA synthesis in systemic lupus erythematosus. Clin Immunol Immunopathol 1987;42:344–359.

J42. Janeway C. Mls: makes little sense. Nature 1991;349:459–461.

J43. Janeway CA. Natural killer cells—A primitive immune system. Nature 1989;341:108.

J44. Janin A. Histopathologic aspects of the minor salivary glands in lupus erythematosus [English abstract]. Ann Med Interne (Paris) 1990;141(3):247–249.

J45. Jankovic J, Patten BM. Blepharospasm and autoimmune diseases. Movement Disorders 1987;2:159–163.

J46. Jans H, Dybkjaer E, Halberg P. Circulating immune complexes in healthy persons. Scand J Rheumatol 1982;11:194–198.

J47. Jansen GT, Dillaha CJ, Honeycutt WM. Discoid lupus erythematosus. Is systemic treatment necessary? Arch Dermatol 1965 Sep;92:283–285.

J48. Jansen HM, Schutte AJH, Elema JD, Giessen MVD, Reig RP, Leeuwen MAV, Sluiter HF, The TH. Local immune complexes and inflammatory response in patients with chronic interstitial pulmonary disorders associated with collagen vascular diseases. Clin Exp Immunol 1984;56:311–320.

J49. Jansson L, Mattsson A, Mattsson R, Holmdahl R. Estrogen induced suppression of collagen arthritis. V: Physiological level of estrogen in DBA/1 mice is therapeutic on established arthritis, suppresses anti-type II collagen T-cell dependent immunity and stimulates polyclonal B-cell activity. J Autoimmun 1990;3:257–270.

J50. Jara LJ, Capin NR, Lavalle C. Hyperviscosity syndrome as the initial manifestation of systemic lupus erythematosus. J Rheumatol 1989 Feb;16(2):225–230.

J51. Jara LJ, Gomez-Sanchez C, Silveira L, Seleznick MJ, Martinez-Osuna P, Espinoza LR. Hyperprolactinemia in systemic lupus erythematosus [abstract]. Arthritis Rheum 1991 May;34 Suppl 5:R24.

J52. Jara LJ, Gomez-Sanchez C, Silveira LH, Martinez-Osuna P, Seleznick M, Vasey F, Espinoza LR. Hyperprolactinemia in systemic lupus erythematosus (SLE). Association with immunological and clinical activity [abstract]. Arthritis Rheum 1991; 34:S163.

J53. Jara LJ, Lavalle C, Fraga A, Gomez-Sanchez C, Silveira LH, Martinez-Osuna P, Germain BF, Espinoza LR. Prolactin, immunoregulation, and autoimmune diseases. Semin Arthritis Rheum 1991;20:273–284.

J54. Jara-Quesada L, Graef A, Lavalle C. Prolactin and gonadal hormones during pregnancy in systemic lupus erythematosus. J Rheumatol 1991;18:349–353.

J55. Jarcho S. Notes on the early modern history of lupus erythematosus. J Mt Sinai Hosp (NY) 1957 Nov–Dec;24:939- 944.

J56. Jarrett MP, Sablay LB, Walter L, Barland P, Grayzel AL. The effect of continuous normalization of serum hemolytic complement on the course of lupus nephritis. A five year prospect study. Am J Med 1981;70:1067–1072.

J57. Jarrett MP, Santhanam S, Del Greco F. The clinical course of end-stage renal disease in systemic lupus erythematosus. Arch Intern Med 1983 Jul;143(7):1353–1356.

J58. Jarrett MP, Schiffman G, Barland P, Grayzel AL. Impaired response to pneumococcal vaccine in systemic lupus erythematosus. Arthritis Rheum 1980 Nov;23(11):1287–1293.

J59. Jawad AS, Scott DG. Immunization triggering rheumatoid arthritis? [letter] Ann Rheum Dis 1989 Feb;48(2):174.

J60. Jeanette JC, Kskandar SS, Dalldorf FG. Pathologic differentiation between lupus and non-lupus membranous glomerulopathy. Kidney Int 1985 Sep;24:377–385.

J61. Jeffrey PJ, Asherson RA, Rees PJ. Recurrent deep vein thrombosis in thromboembolic pulmonary hypertension in the 'primary' antiphospholipid syndrome. Clin Exp Rheumatol 1989 Sep–Oct;7(5):567–569.

J62. Jeffries R. Structure/function relationships of IgG subclasses: *In*: Shakib F, editor. The Human IgG Subclasses: Molecular Analysis of Structure, Function, and Regulation. Oxford: Pergamon Press, 1990:93–108.

J63. Jelinek DF, Lipsky PE. Enhancement of human B cell proliferation and differentiation by tumor necrosis factor-α and interleukin 1. J Immunol 1987;139:2970–2976.

J64. Jendryczko A, Drozdz M. DNA damage in liver and kidney of rats after treatment with hydralazine in vitro. Exp Pathol 1989; 36:53–57.

J65. Jendryczko A, Drozdz M, Magner K. Carbamazepine induced systemic lupus erythematosus [letter]. Br Med J 1985;291: 1198–1200.

J66. Jenkins D. Pharmacology of prednisone, prednisolone, 6 methylprednisolone, and triamcinolone. In: Mills LC, Moyer JC, editors. Inflammation and diseases of connective tissue. A Hahnemann Symposium. Philadelphia: Saunders, 1961: 328–335.

J67. Jenkins MK, Pardoll DM, Mizuguchi J, Quill H, Schwartz RH. T-cell unresponsiveness in vivo and in vitro: fine specificity of

induction and molecular characterization of the unresponsive state. Immunol Rev 1987;95:113–135.

J68. Jennett JC, Falk RJ. Antineurophil cytoplasmic autoantibodies and associated diseases. A review. Am J Kidney Dis 1990; 15:517–529.

J69. Jensen S, Glud TK, Bacher T, Ersgaard H. Ibuprofen-induced meningitis in a male with systemic lupus erythematosus, Acta Med Scand 1987;221(5):509–511.

J70. Jeong HD, Teale JM. V$_H$ gene family repertoire of resting B cells: Preferential use of D-proximal families early in development may be due to distinct B cell subsets. J Immunol 1989; 143:2752–2760.

J71. Jerdan MS, Hood AF, Moore GW, Callen JP. Histopathologic comparison of the subsets of lupus erythematosus. Arch Dermatol 1990 Jan;126(1):52–55.

J72. Jerne NK. Towards a network theory of the immune system. Ann Immunol (Paris) 1974;125:373–389.

J73. Jerne NK. The generative grammar of the immune system. Science 1985;229:1057.

J74. Jerne NK, Roland J, Cazenave P-A. Recurrent idiotypes and internal images. EMBO J 1982;1:243.

J75. Jessar RA, Lamont-Havers RW, Ragan C. Natural history of lupus erythematosus disseminatus. Ann Intern Med 1953; 38(4):717–731.

J76. Jick H, Holmes LB, Hunter JR, Madsen S, Stergachis A. First trimester drug use and congenital disorders. JAMA 1981:246: 343–346.

J77. Jimenez RA, Haakenstad AO, Mannik M. Hepatic uptake of small-latticed immune complexes does not alter mononuclear phagocyte system function. Immunology 1983;48:205–210.

J78. Jindal BK, Martin MF, Gayner A. Gangrene developing after minor surgery in a patient with undiagnosed systemic lupus erythematosus and lupus anticoagulant. Ann Rheum Dis 1983 Jun;42(3):347–349.

J79. Jira M, Strejcek J, Zavadil Z, Antosova E, Rejholec V. Interleukin-2 activated cells from peripheral blood of patients with systemic lupus erythematosus. Z Rheumatol 1990;49: 30–33.

J80. Job-Deslandre C, Delrieu F, Delbarre F, Carlioz A. Relapsing polychondritis and systemic lupus erythematosus [letter]. J Rheumatol 1983 Aug;10(4):666–668.

J81. Joffe RT, Denicoff KD, Rubinow DR, Tsokos G, Balow JE, Pillemer SE. Mood effects of alternate-day corticosteroid therapy in patients with systemic lupus erythematosus. Gen Hosp Psychiatry 1988 Jan;10(1):56–60.

J82. Joffe RT, Wolkowitz OM, Rubinow DR, Denicoff K, Tsokos G, Pillemer S. Alternate-day corticosteroid treatment, mood and plasma HVA in patients with systemic lupus erythematosus. Neuropsychobiology 1988;19(1):17–19.

J83. Johansson E, Kanerva L, Niemi KM, Valimaki MM. Diffuse soft tissue calcifications (calcinosis cutis) in a patient with discoid lupus erythematosus. Clin Exp Dermatol 1988 May; 13(3):193–196.

J84. Johansson E, Niemi KM, Halme H. The ribonucleic acid (RNA) skin test in systemic lupus erythematosus and other connective tissue disorders. Br J Dermatol 1979 Feb;100(2): 127–130.

J84a. Johansson E, Niemi KM, Mustakallio KK. A peripheral vascular syndrome overlapping with systemic lupus erythematosus. Dermatologica 1977;15(5):257–267.

J85. Johansson E, Pyrhonen S, Rostila T. Wart and wart virus antibodies in patients with systemic lupus erythematosus [abstract]. BMJ 1977;1:74–75.

J86. Johansson-Stephansson E, Koskimes S, Partanen J, Kariniemi AL. Subacute cutaneous lupus erythematosus: Genetic markers and clinical and immunological findings in patients. Arch Dermatol 1989;125:791–796.

J87. Johns DG, Rutherford LD, Leighton PG, Vogel CL. Secretion of methotrexate into human milk. Am J Obstet Gynecol 1972; 112:978–980.

J88. Johnson BC, Gajjar A, Kubo C, Good RA. Calories versus protein in onset of renal disease in NZB × NZW mice. Proc Natl Acad Sci USA 1986;83:5659–5662.

J89. Johnson CA, Densen P, Hurford R, Colten HR, Wetsel RA. Deficiency of human complement C2 type 1: A 28 bp gene deletion leads to a splicing defect [abstract]. Clin Res 1991: 39:304A.

J90. Johnson DA, Diehl AM, Finkleman FD, Cattau EL Jr. Crohn's disease and systemic lupus erythematosus. Am J Gastroenterology 1985 Nov;80(11):869–870.

J91. Johnson GD, Holborow EJ, Glynn LE. Antibody to liver in lupoid hepatitis. Lancet 1966 Aug 20;2:416–418.

J92. Johnson HM. Effect of splenectomy in acute systemic lupus erythematosus. Arch Dermat & Syph 1953 Dec;68:699–713.

J93. Johnson JG, Jemmerson R. Relative frequencies of secondary B cells activated by cognate vs other mechanisms. Eur J Immunol 1991;21:951–958.

J94. Johnson PM. IgM rheumatoid factors cross-reactive with IgG and a cell nuclear antigen: Apparent "masking" in original serum. Scand J Immunol 1979;9(5):461–466.

J95. Johnson RT. Neurologic and neuropathologic observations in lupus erythematosus. N Engl J Med 1962 Apr 26;266:895.

J96. Johnson RT, Richardson EP. The neurological manifestations of systemic lupus erythematosus. A clinical-pathological study of 24 cases and review of the literature. Medicine 1968 Jul;47:337–369.

J97. Johnson SAM, Meyer O, Brown JW, Rasmussen AF Jr. Failure of chloranpenicol (chloromycetin) in treatment of 3 cases of lupus erythematosus disseminatus. J Invest Dermatol 1950 May;14:305–307.

J98. Joint Report of Armored Medical Research Laboratory, Fort Knox, KY, and Commission on Tropical Diseases, Army Epidemiological Board, Preventive Medicine Service, Office of the Surgeon General, United States Army. Plasma quinacrine concentration as a function of dosage and environment. Arch Intern Med 1946;78:64–107.

J99. Jokinen EJ, Alfthan OS, Oravisto KJ. Antitissue antibodies in interstitial cystitis. Clin Exp Immunol 1972 Jul;11:333–339.

J100. Jokinen EJ, Jankala EO. Antitissue antibodies in monozygotic twins with systemic lupus erythematosus. Ann Rheum Dis 1970;29:677–680.

J101. Jokinen EJ, Lassus A, Salo OP, Alfthan O. Discoid lupus erythematosus and interstitial cystitis. The presence of bound immunoglobulins in the bladder mucosa. Ann Clin Res 1972 Feb;4:23–25.

J102. Jonas J, Kolble K, Volcker HE, Kalden JR. Central retinal artery occlusion in Sneddon's disease associated with antiphospholipid antibodies. Am J Ophthalmol 1986 Jul 15; 102(1):37–40.

J103. Jondal M, Pross H. Surface markers on human B and T lymphocytes. VI. Cytotoxicity against cell lines as a functional marker for lymphocyte subpopulations. Int J Cancer 1975;15: 596.

J104. Jones BR. Lacrimal and salivary precipitating antibodies in Sjogren's syndrome. Lancet 1958;11:773–776.

J105. Jones CJ, Salisbury RS, Jayson MI. The presence of abnormal lysosomes in lymphocytes and neutrophils during chloroquine therapy: a quantitative ultrastructural study. Ann Rheum Dis 1984 Oct;43(5):710–715.

J106. Jones DH, Looney RJ, Anderson CL. Two distinct classes of IgG Fc receptors on a human monocyte line (U937) defined by differences in binding of murine IgG subclasses at low ionic strength. J Immunol 1985;135:33–48.

J107. Jones FJ Jr, Spivey CG Jr. Spread of pulmonary coccidioido-

mycosis associated with steroid therapy: Report of a case with a lupus-like reaction to anti-tuberculosis chemotherapy. J Lancet 1966 May;86:226–230.

J107a. Jones HW, Tocantins LM. Purpura hemorrhagica: further notes on treatment. Trans Assoc Am Physicians 1936;51:59–68.

J108. Jones JF, Ray CG, Minnich LL, Hicks MJ, Kibler R, Lucas DO. Evidence for active Epstein-Barr virus infection in patients with persistent, unexplained illnesses: elevated anti-early antigen antibodies. Ann Intern Med 1985 Jan;102(1): 1–7.

J109. Jones JP, Engleman EP, Steinbach HL, Murray WR, Rambo ON. Fat embolization as a possible mechanism producing avascular necrosis [abstract]. Arthritis Rheum 1965;8:448.

J110. Jones JV. Plasmapheresis in SLE. Clin Rheum Dis 1982 Apr; 8(1):243–260.

J111. Jones JV. The Application of Plasmapheresis in Systemic Lupus Erythematosus: Therapeutic Apheresis and Plasma Perfusion. New York: Liss, 1982:81–89.

J112. Jones JV, Cumming RH, Bacon PA, Evers J, Fraser ID, Bothamley J, Tribe CR, Davis A, Hughes GR. Evidence for a therapeutic effect of plasmapheresis on patients with systemic lupus erythematosus? Q J Med 1979 Oct;48(192):555–576.

J113. Jones JV, Cumming RH, Bucknall RC, Asplin CM, Fraser ID, Bothamley J, Davis P, Hamblin TJ. Plasmapheresis in the management of acute systemic lupus erythematosus? Lancet 1976;1:709–711.

J114. Jones JV, Jones E, Forsyth SJ, Skanes VM, Reichlin M, MacSween JM, Eastwood S, Carr RI. Familial systemic lupus erythematosus evidence for separate loci controlling C4 deficiency and formation of antibodies to DNA, nRNP, Ro and La. J Rheumatol 1987;14:263–267.

J115. Jones JV, Robinson MF, Parciany RK, Layfer LF, McLeod B. Therapeutic plasmapheresis in systemic lupus erythematosus. Effect on immune complexes and antibodies to DNA. Arthritis Rheum 1981 Sep;24(9):1113–1120.

J116. Jones MB, Osterholm RK, Wilson RB, Martin FH, Commers JR, Bachmayer JD. Fatal pulmonary hypertension and resolving immune-complex glomerulonephritis in mixed connective tissue disease. A case report and review of the literature. Am J Med 1978 Nov;65(5):855–863.

J117. Jones PE, Rawchiffe P, White N, Segal AW. Painless ascites in systemic lupus erythematosus. BMJ 1977;1:1513.

J118. Jongen PJH, Boerbooms AM Th, Lamers KJB, Raes BC, Vierwin den G. Diffuse CNS involvement in systemic lupus erythematosus: Intrathecal synthesis of the 4th component of complement. Neurology 1990;40(10):1593–1596.

J119. Jonsson H, Nived O, Sturfelt G. The effect of age on clinical and serological manifestations in unselected patients with systemic lupus erythematosus. J Rheumatol 1988 Mar;15(3): 505–509.

J120. Jonsson H, Nived O, Sturfelt G. Thyroid disorders are related to secondary Sjogren's syndrome in unselected systemic lupus erythematosus patients [letter]. Arthritis Rheum 1988 Aug;31(8):1079–1080.

J121. Jonsson H, Nived O, Sturfelt G. Outcome in systemic lupus erythematosus: a prospective study of patients from a defined population. Medicine 1989;68:141–150.

J122. Jonsson J, Norberg R. Symptomatology and diagnosis in connective tissue disease. II. Evaluations and follow-up examinations in consequence of a speckled antinuclear immunofluorescence pattern. Scand J Rheumatol 1978;7(4):229–236.

J123. Jonsson R, Heyden G, Westberg NG, Nyberg G. Oral mucosal lesions in systemic lupus erythematosus: A clinical, histopathological and immunopathological study. J Rheumatol 1884;11:38–42.

J124. Jonsson R, Lindvall AM, Nyberg G. Temporomandibular joint involvement in systemic lupus erythematosus. Arthritis Rheum 1983 Dec;26(12):1506–1510.

J125. Jonsson R, Nyberg G, Kristensson-Aas A, Westberg NG. Lupus band test in uninvolved oral mucosa in systemic lupus erythematosus. Acta Med Scand 1983;213(4):269–273.

J126. Jordan E, Burnstein SL, Calabro JJ, Henderson ES. Multiple myeloma complicating the course of seronegative systemic lupus erythematosus. Arthritis Rheum 1978 Mar;21:260–265.

J127. Jordan JM, Valenstein P, Kredich DW. Systemic lupus erythematosus with Libman-Sacks endocarditis in a 9-month- old infant with neonatal lupus erythematosus and congenital heart block. Pediatrics 1989;84:574–577.

J128. Jordon RE, Muller SA, Hale WL, Beutner EH. Bullous pemphigoid associated with systemic lupus erythematosus. Arch Dermatol 1969 Jan;99(1):17–25.

J129. Jordan SC, Ho W, Ettenger R, Salusky IB, Fine RN. Plasma exchange improves the glomerulonephritis of systemic lupus erythematosus in selected pediatric patients. Pediatr Nephrol 1987;1:276–280.

J130. Joselow SA, Gown A, Mannik M. Cutaneous deposition of immune complexes in chronic serum sickness of mice induced with cationized or unaltered antigen. J Invest Dermatol 1985;85:559–563.

J131. Joseph RR, Tourtellotte CD, Barry WE, Smalley RV, Durant JR. Prolonged immunological disorder terminating in hematological malignancy. A human analogue of animal disease. Ann Intern Med 1970 May;72:699–703.

J132. Joseph RR, Zarafonetis CJD. Fatal systemic lupus erythematosus in identical twins: case reports and review of the literature. Am J Med Sci 1965;249:190–199.

J133. Joshi BC, Dwivedi C, Powell A, Holscher M. Immune complex nephritis in rats induced by long-term oral exposure to cadmium. J Comp Pathol 1981;91:11–15.

J134. Joske RA, King WE. "L.E.-Cell" phenomenon in active chronic viral hepatitis. Lancet 1955 Sep 3;2:477–480.

J135. Jothy S, Samka RJ. Presence of monocytes in systemic lupus erythematosus—associated glomerulonephritis. Marker studies and significance. Arch Pathol Lab Med 1981 Nov;105: 590–593.

J136. Jouhikainen T, Keomaki R, Leirisalo-Repo M, Backland T, Myllyla G. Platelet autoantibodies detected by immunoblotting in systemic lupus erythematous; association with the lupus anticoagulant, and with history of thrombosis and thrombocytopenia. Eur J Haematol 1990;44:234–239.

J137. Jouvin MH, Wilson JG, Bourgeois P, Fearon DT, Kazatchkine MD. Decreased expression of C3b receptor (CR1) on erythrocytes of patients with SLE contrasts with its normal expression in other systemic diseases and does not correlated with the occurrence or severity of SLE nephritis. Complement 1986;3:88–96.

J138. Joyce K, Berkebile C, Hastings C, Yarboro C, Yocum D. Heath status and disease activity in SLE. Arthritis Care Res (June) 1989;2(2):65–69.

J139. Juan H. Inhibition of the algesic effect of bradykinin and acetylcholine by mepacrine. Naunyn Schmiedebergs Arch Pharmacol 1977 Dec;301(1):23–27.

J140. Juhl RP, Daugherty VM, Kroboth PD. Incidence of next-day anterograde amnesia caused by fluorazepam hydrochloride and triazolam. Clin Pharm 1984 Nov–Dec;3(6):622–625.

J141. Jungers P, Dougados M, Pelissier C, Kuttenn F, Tron F, Lesavre P, Bach JF. Influence of oral contraceptive therapy on the activity of systemic lupus erythematosus. Arthritis Rheum 1982;25:618–623.

J142. Jungers P, Dougados M, Pelissier C, Kuttenn F, Tron F, Lesavre P, Bach JF. Lupus nephropathy and pregnancy. Arch Intern Med 1982;142:771–776.

J143. Jungers P, Kuttenn F, Liote F, Pelissier C, Athea N, Laurent MC, Viriot J, Dougados M, Bach JF. Hormonal modulation in systemic lupus erythematosus. Preliminary clinical and hormonal results with cyproterone acetate. Arthritis Rheum 1985 Nov;28(11):1243–1250.

J144. Jungers P, Liote F, Pelissier C, Viriot J, Laurent MC, Athea N, Dougados M, Lesavre P, Kuttenn F, Bach JF. The hormonomodulation in systemic lupus erythematosus: preliminary results with Danazol (D) and cyproterone- acetate (CA) [English abstract]. Ann Med Interne (Paris) 1986;137(4):313–319.

J145. Jungers P, Nahoui K, Pelissier C, Dougados M, Tron F, Bach JF. Low plasma androgens in women with active or quiescent lupus erythematosus. Arthritis Rheum 1982 Apr;25:454–457.

J146. Jurjus A, Wheeler DA, Gallo RC, Witz IP. Placenta-bound immunoglobulins. Arthritis Rheum 1979;22:1308–1313.

J147. Jyonouchi A, Kimmel MD, Lee G, Kincade PW, Good RA. Humoral Factors in very young NZB mice that enhance the maturation of normal B cell precursors: partial purification and characterization. J Immunol 1985;135:1891–1899.

K

K1. Kabat EA, Wu TT. Attempts to locate complementarily determining residues in the variable positions of light and heavy chains. Ann NY Acad Sci 1971;190:382–393.

K2. Kabat EA, Nickerson KG, Liao J, Grossbard L, Osserman EF, Glickman E, Chess L, Robbins TB, Schneerson R, Yang Y. A human monoclonal macroglobulin with specificity for alpha C-28 linked poly-N-acetyl neuraminic acid, the capsular polysaccharide of group B meningococci and Escherichia coli K1, which cross reacts with polynucleotides and denatured DNA. J Exp Med 1986;164:642–654.

K3. Kabbash L, Esdaile J, Shenker S, Danoss D, Fuks A, Shuster J. Reticuloendothelial system Fc receptor function in systemic lupus erythematosus. J Rheumatol 1982;9:374–379.

K3a. Kabir DI, Malkinson FD. Lupus erythematosus and calcinosis cutis. Arch Dermatol 1969;100:17–22.

K4. Kachru RB, Sequeira W, Mittal KK, Siegel ME, Telischi M. A significant increase of HLA-DR3 and DR2 in systemic lupus erythematosus among blacks. J Rheumatol 1984;11:471–474.

K5. Kadin M, Dubois EL. Keratoconjunctivitis sicca, corneal and lens changes associated with lupus erythematosus and its treatment [unpublished observations].

K6. Kaelin WG Jr, Spivak JL. Systemic lupus erythematosus and myelofibrosis. Am J Med 1986;81:935–940.

K7. Kaell AT, Shetty M, Lee BC, Lockshin MD. The diversity of neurologic events in systemic lupus erythematosus. Prospective clinical and computed tomographic classification of 82 events in 71 patients. Arch Neurol 1986 Mar;43(3):273–276.

K8. Kagami M, Koike T, Takabayashi K, Tomioka H, Yoshida S. Antibody to activated lymphocytes in patients with systemic lupus erythematosus. J Rheumatol 1987;14:907–912.

K9. Kagen LJ. Myoglobinemia in inflammatory myopathies. JAMA 1977;237-2448–2452.

K10. Kahl LE, Al-Sabbagh R, Greenberg A, Medsger TA. Comparison of hemodialysis (HD) and peritoneal dialysis (PD) in systemic lupus erythematosus (SLE) patients with end stage renal failure (ESRF) [abstract]. Arthritis Rheum 1986 Apr; 29(4) Suppl:S97.

K11. Kahl LE, Sheetz KE. Similarity of SLE in multicase families vs sporadic cases. Arthritis Rheum 1990 Sep;33(9) Suppl:S130.

K12. Kahn G, Davis BP. In vitro studies on longwave ultraviolet light-dependent reactions of the skin photosensitizer chlorpromazine with nucleic acids purines, and pyrimidines. J Invest Dermatol 1970 Jul;55:47–52.

K13. Kahn MF. Jaccoud's syndrome in a rheumatology unit. Clin Rheum in Practice 1986;(Winter):153–155.

K14. Kahn MF, Peltier AP, Degraeve B, Mery JP, Morel-Maroger L, de Seze S. Successive connective tissue diseases: Scleroderma, then lupus. Clinical and biological study of 4 cases [original in French]. Ann Med Interne 1977 Jan;128:1–8.

K15. Kahn MF, Solnica J, Bourgeois P. Disappearance of clinical and biological evidence of SLE after removal of an ovarian seminoma: 21 years' follow-up. J Rheumatol 1986;13:834.

K16. Kaine JL. Refractory massive pleural effusion in systemic lupus erythematosus treated with talc poudrage. Ann Rheum Dis 1985 Jan;44:61–64.

K17. Kaiser IH. Specificity of periarterial fibrosis of the spleen in disseminated lupus erythematosus. Bull Johns Hopkins Hosp 1942 Jul;71:31.

K18. Kaiser W, Biesenbach G, Stuby U, Grafinger P, Zazgornik J. Human adjuvant disease: Remission of silicone induced autoimmune disease after explanation of breast augmentation. Ann Rheum Dis 1990;49:937–938.

K19. Kajdaosy-Balla A, Doe EM, Bagasra O. Activation of factor B of the alternative pathway of complement. Assessment by rocket immunoelectrophoresis. Am J Clin Pathol 1987;88: 66–73.

K20. Kakkanaiah VN, Nagarkatti M, Nagarkatti PS. Evidence for the existence of distinct heterogeneity among the peripheral CD4-CD8- T cells from MRL-lpr/lpr mice based on the expression of the J11d marker, activation requirements, and functional properties. Cell Immunol 1990;127:442–457.

K21. Kakkanaiah VN, Ptle RH, Nagarkatti M, Nagarkatti PS. Evidence for major alterations in the thymocyte subpopulations in murine models of autoimmune diseases. J Autoimmun 1990;3:271–288.

K22. Kalabay L, Jakab L, Cseh K, Pozsonyi T, Jakab LA. Correlations between serum alpha 2-HA-glycoprotein and conventional laboratory parameters in systemic lupus erythematosus. Acta Medica Hungarica 1990;47:53–64.

K23. Kalb RE, Grossman ME. Chronic perianal herpes simplex in immunocompromised hosts. Am J Med 1986 Mar;80(3): 486–490.

K24. Kalina P, Prochazkova L, Hauftova D. A syndrome similar to systemic lupus erythematosus caused by penicillamine in patients with Wilson's disease. Bratisl Lek Listy 1985; 84: 336–340.

K25. Kalla AA, Learmonth ID, Klemp P. Early treatment of avascular necrosis in systemic lupus erythematosus. Ann Rheum Dis 1986 Aug;45(8):649–652.

K26. Kalland T. Decreased and disproportionate T cell population in the adult male after neonatal exposure to diethylstilbestrol. Cell Immunol 1980;51:55–63.

K27. Kalland T. Reduced natural killer activity in female mice after neonatal exposure to diethylstilbestrol. J Immunol 1980; 124:1297–1300.

K28. Kalland T. Alterations of antibody response in female mice after neonatal exposure to diethylstilbestrol. J Immunol 1980; 24:194–198.

K29. Kalland T, Forsberg JC. Natural killer cell activity and tumor susceptibility in female mice treated neonatally with diethylstilbestrol. Cancer Res 1981;41:5134–5140.

K30. Kallen PS, Nies KM, Louie JS, Fritchen JH. Serum inhibition of erythropoiesis in systemic lupus erythematosus [abstract]. Arthritis Rheum 1981 Apr;24 Suppl:S108.

K31. Kallenback J, Zwi S, Goldman HI. Airway obstruction in a case of disseminated lupus erythematosus. Thorax 1978;33: 814–815.

K32. Kallenberg CG, de Jong MC, Walstra TM, Kardaun S, The TH. In vivo antinuclear antibodies (ANA) in biopsies of normal skin: diagnostic significance and relation to serum ANA. J Rheumatol 1983 Oct;10(5):733–740.

K33. Kallenberg CG, Limburg PC, Van Slochteren C. The T helper B cell activity in SLE: Depressed in vivo humoral immune response to a primary antigen (haemocyanin) and de-

creased in vitro spontaneous Ig synthesis. Clin Exp Immunol 1983;53:371–378.

K34. Kallenberg CG, Wouda AA, Hoet MH, Van Venrooij WJ. Development of connective tissue disease in patients with Raynaud's phenomenon: a six year follow up with emphasis on the predictive value of antinuclear antibodies as detected by immunoblotting. Ann Rheum Dis 1988 Aug;47(8): 634–641.

K35. Kallenberg CG, Wouda AA, The TH. Systemic involvement and immunologic findings in patients presenting with Raynaud's phenomenon. Am J Med 1980 Nov;69(5):675–680.

K36. Kallenberg CGM, ter Borg EJ, Horst G, Hummel E, Limburg PC. Predictive value of anti-double stranded DNA antibody levels in SLE: A long term prospective study. Clin Rheumatol 1989;8:49–50.

K37. Kallenberg CGM, ter Borg EJ, Jaarsma D, Limburg PC. Detection of autoantibodies to ribonucleoproteins by counterimmunoelectrophoresis, immunoblotting and RNA-immunoprecipitation: comparison of results. Clin Exp Rheumatol 1990 Jan–Feb;8(1):35–40.

K38. Kalter H, Warkany J. Experimental production of congenital abnormalities in mammals by metabolic procedure. Physiol Rev 1959;39:69.

K39. Kalunian KC, Gladman DD, Bacon PA, Bombardier C, Chang C, Goldsmith C, Hahn B, Isenberg D, Liang M, Maddison P, Nived O, Richter M, Snaith M, Symmons D, Urowitz M, Zoma A. Development and assessment of a computerized index of clinical disease activity in systemic lupus erythematosus. Submitted.

K40. Kalunian KC, Hahn BH, Bassett L. Magnetic resonance imaging identifies early femoral head ischemic necrosis in patients receiving glucocorticoid therapy. J Rheumatol 1989 Jul; 16(7):959–963.

K41. Kalunian KC, Panosian-Sahakian N, Ebling FM, Cohen AH, Louie JS, Kaine J, Hahn BH. Idiotypic characteristics of immunoglobulins associated with human systemic lupus erythematosus. Studies of antibodies deposited in glomeruli of humans. Arthritis Rheum 1989 May;32(5);513–522.

K42. Kalunian KC, Peter JB, Middlekauff HR, Sayre J, Ando DG, Mangotich M, Hahn BH. Clinical significance of a simple test for anti-cardiolipin antibodies in patients with systemic lupus erythematosus. Am J Med 1988 Nov;85(5):602–608.

K43. Kambic H, Hyslop L, Nose Y. Topics in plasmapheresis: A bibliography of therapeutic applications and new techniques. Cleveland:ISAO Press, 1985.

K44. Kameda S, Aito SN, Tanaka K, Kajiyama K, Kunihiro K, Nishigouri S, Jimi S, Yanese T. HLA antigens of patients with systemic lupus erythematosus. Tissue Antigens 1981;20: 221–222.

K45. Kammer GM. Impaired T cell capping and receptor regeneration in active systemic lupus erythematosus. Evidence for a disorder intrinsic to the T lymphocyte. J Clin Invest 1983; 72:1686–1697.

K46. Kammer GM, Mitchell E. Impaired mobility of human T lymphocyte surface molecules during inactive systemic lupus erythematosus. Relationship to a defective CAMP pathway. Arthritis Rheum 1988;31:88–98.

K47. Kanai H, Tshuchida A, Yano S, Naruse T. Intraplatelet and urinary serotonin concentrations in systemic lupus erythematosus with reference to its clinical manifestations. J Med 1989; 20:371–377.

K48. Kanauchi H, Furukawa F, Imamura S. Evaluation of ATPase-positive Langerhans' cells in skin lesions of lupus erythematosus and experimentally induced inflammations. Arch Dermatol Res 1989;281(5):327–332.

K49. Kanayama Y, Kim T, Inariba H, Negoro N, Okamura M, Takeda T, Inoue T. Possible involvement of interferon alpha in the pathogenesis of fever in systemic lupus erythematosus. Ann Rheum Dis 1989 Oct;48(10):861–863.

K50. Kanayama Y, Peebles C, Tan EM, Curd JG. Complement-activating abilities of defined antinuclear antibodies. Arthritis Rheum 1986; 29:748–754.

K51. Kanayama Y, Shiota K, Horiguchi T, Kato N, Oha A, Inoue T. Correlation between steroid myopathy and serum lactid denyorogenase in systemic lupus erythematosus. Arch Intern Med 1981 Aug;141:1176–1179.

K52. Kanof ME, Strober W, Kwan WC, O'Connell NA, James SP. CD4+ Leu-8 + T cell supernatant activity that inhibits Ig production. J Immunol 1991;147:155–161.

K53. Kant KS, Pollak VE, Dosekun A, Glas-Greenwalt P, Weiss MA, Glueck HI. Lupus nephritis with thrombosis and abnormal fibrinolysis: effect of ancrod. J Lab Clin Med 1985 Jan;105:77–88.

K54. Kant KS, Pollak VE, Weiss MA, Glueck HI, Miller AN, Hess EV. Glomerular thrombosis in systemic lupus erythematosus: prevalence and significance. Medicine 1981 Mar;60(2):71–86.

K55. Kantor GL, Bickel YB, Barnett EV. Coexistence of systemic lupus erythematosus and rheumatoid arthritis. Report of a case and review of the literature, and clinical, pathologic and serologic observations. Am J Med 1969 Sep;47:433–444.

K56. Kanyerezi BR, Lwanga SK, Bloch KJ. Fibrinogen degradation products in serum and urine of patients with systemic lupus erythematosus. Relation in renal disease and pathogenic mechanism. Arthritis Rheum 1971 Mar–Apr 1;14:267–275.

K57. Kaplan AP, Curl FD, Decker JL. Central hyperventilation and inappropriate antidiuretic hormone secretion in systemic lupus erythematosus. Am J Med 1970 May;48:661–667.

K58. Kaplan C, Champeix P, Blanchar D, Muller JY, Cartron JP. Platelet antibodies in systemic lupus erythematosus. Br J Haematol 1990;67:89–93.

K59. Kaplan D. The onset of disease in twins and siblings with systemic lupus erythematosus. J Rheumatol 1984:648–652.

K60. Kaplan D, Ginzler EM, Feldman J. Arthritis and nephritis in patients with systemic lupus erythematosus. J Rheumatol 1991;18:223–229.

K61. Kaplan E. A process approach to neuropsychology. In: Ball T, Briant K, editors. Clinical Neuropsychology and BF; Research Measurement and Practice. Washington DC, American Psychological Association, 1988.

K62. Kaplan PE, Betts HB. Lupoid sclerosis: evaluation and treatment. Arch Phys Med Rehabil 1977 Jan;58(1):24–28.

K63. Kaplan RE, Springate JE, Feld LG, Cohen ME. Pseudotumor cerebri associated with cerebral venous sinus thrombosis, internal jugular vein thrombosis, and systemic lupus erythematosus. J Pediatr 1985 Aug;107(2):266–268.

K64. Kaplan RP, Callen JP. Pemphigus associated diseases and induced pemphigus. Clin Dermatol 1983;1:42–71.

K65. Kaposi M. New reports on knowledge of lupus erythematosus [original in German]. Arch Dermat u Syph 1872;4:36–78.

K66. Kappas A, Jones HE, Roitt IM. Effects of steroid sex hormones on immunological phenomenon. Nature 1963;198:902.

K67. Kappes J, Schoepflin G, Bardana E, Bennett R. Lupoid sacroarthropathy-A previously undescribed association. Arthritis Rheum 1980 Jun;23:699–700.

K68. Kappler JW, Roehm N, Marrack P. T cell tolerance by clonal elimination in the thymus. Cell 1987;49:273–280.

K69. Kappler JW, Staerz V, White J, Marrack PC. Self-tolerance eliminates T cells specific for Mls-modified products of the major histocompatibility complex. Nature 1988;332:35–40.

K70. Karas SP, Rosse WF, Kurlander RJ. Characterization of IgG-FC receptor on human platelets. Blood 1982 Dec;60:1277–1282.

K71. Karen E, Reichlin MW, Koscec M, Fugate RD, Reichlin M. Autoantibodies to the ribosomal P protein react with a plasma membrane related target on human cells. Arthritis Rheum 1991;34:S75.

K72. Karjalainen TK, Tomich CE. A histopathologic study of oral mucosal lupus erythematosus. Oral Surg Oral Med Oral Pathol 1989 May;67(5):547–554.

K73. Kark RM, Pollak VE, Soothill JF, Pirani CL, Muehrcke RC. Simple test of renal function in health and disease. I. A reappraisal of their value in the light of serial renal biopsies. Arch Intern Med 1957 Feb;99:176–189.

K74. Karoleva NI, Kaladze NN, Kirichenko A, Ya A. Collage disease in twins. Vopt Revmatizma (Russian) 1973:2:32.

K75. Karpatkin S. Autoimmune thrombocytopenic purpura. Blood 1980 Sep;56:329–343.

K76. Karpatkin S. Autoimmune thrombocytopenic purpura. Sem Hematol 1985;22:260–288.

K77. Karpatkin S, Schur PH, Strick N, Siskind GW. Heavy chain subclass of human anti-platelet antibodies. Clin Immunol Immunopath 1973 Nov;2:1–8.

K78. Karpatkin S, Siskind GW. In vitro detection of platelet antibody in patients with idiopathic thrombocytopenic purpura and SLE. Blood 1969 Jun;33:795–812.

K79. Karpatkin S, Strick N, Karpatkin M, Siskind GW. Cumulative experience in the detection of antiplatelet antibody in 234 patients with idiopathic thrombocytopenic purpura, systemic lupus erythematosus and other clinical disorders. Am J Med 1972 Jun;52:776–785.

K80. Karpatkin SI, Lackner HL. Association of antiplatelet antibody with functional platelet disorders, autoimmune thrombocytopenic purpura, systemic lupus erythematosus and thrombopathy. Am J Med 1975 Nov;59:599–604.

K81. Karpiak SE, Graf L, Rappaport MM. Antiserum to brain gangliosides produces recurrent epileptiform activity. Science 1976;194:735.

K82. Karpik AG, Schwartz MM, Dickey LE, Streeten BW, Roberts JL. Ocular immune reactants in patients dying with systemic lupus erythematosus. Clin Immunol Immunpathol 1985 Jun;35(3):295–312.

K83. Karpus WJ, Swanborg RH. CD4+ suppressor cells inhibit the function of effector cells of experimental autoimmune encephalomyelitis through a mechanism involving transforming growth factor-beta. J Immunol 1991;146:1163–1168.

K84. Karsh J, Dorval G, Osterland CK. Natural cytotoxicity in rheumatoid arthritis and systemic lupus erythematosus. Clin Immunol Immuopathol 1981 Jun;19:437–446.

K85. Karsh J, Kimberly RA, Stahl NI, Plotz PH, Decker JL. Comparative effects of aspirin and ibuprofen in the management of systemic lupus erythematosus. Arthritis Rheum 1980 Dec;23(12):1401–1404.

K86. Karsh J, Klippel JH, Balow JE, Decker JL. Mortality in lupus nephritis. Arthritis Rheum 1979 Jul;22:764–769.

K87. Karsh J, Vergalla J, Jones EA. Alpha-1 antitrypsin phenotypes in rheumatoid arthritis and systemic lupus erythematosus. Arthritis Rheum 1979 Feb;22:111–113.

K88. Karthikeyan G, Wallace SL, Blum L. Systemic lupus erythematosus and sickle cell disease. Arthritis Rheum 1978 Sep–Oct 21:862–863.

K89. Kasai N, Parbtani A, Cameron JS, Yewdall V, Shepherd P, Verroust P. Platelet aggregating immune complexes and intraplatelet serotonin in idiopathic glomerulonephritis and systemic lupus. Clin Exp Immunol 1981 Jan;43:64–72.

K90. Kasid A, Director EP, Rosenberg SA. Induction of endogenous cytokine-MRNA in circulating peripheral blood mononuclear cells by IL-2 administration to cancer patients. J Immunol 1989;143:736–739.

K91. Kasinath BS, Katz AI. Delayed maternal lupus after delivery of offspring with congenital heartblock. Arch Intern Med 1982;142:2317.

K92. Kaslow RA. High rate of death caused by systemic lupus erythematosus among US residents of Asian descent. Arthritis Rheum 1982 Apr;25:414–416.

K93. Kaslow RA, Masi AT. Age, sex, and race effects on mortality from systemic lupus erythematosus in the United States. Arthritis Rheum 1978 May;32:493–497.

K94. Kass GH. Hypothermia following cortisone administration. Am J Med 1955 Jan;18:146–149.

K95. Kass S, Tyc K, Steitz JA, Sollner-Webb B. The U3 small nucleolar ribonucleoprotein functions in the first step of preribosomal RNA processing. Cell 1990;60:897–908.

K96. Kassan SS, Akizuki M, Steinberg AD, Reddick RL, Chused TM. Antibody to a soluble acidic nuclear antigen in Sjogren's syndrome. Am J Med 1977 Sep;63(3):328–335.

K97. Kassan SS, Gardy M. Sjogren's syndrome: an update and overview. Am J Med 1978 Jun;64(6):1037–1046.

K98. Kassan SS, Kagen LJ. Elevated levels of cerebrospinal fluid guanosine 3',5'-cyclic monophosphate (C-GMP) in systemic lupus erythematosus. Am J Med 1978 May;64(5):732–741.

K99. Kassan SS, Kagen LJ. Central nervous system lupus erythematosus: measurement of cerebrospinal fluid cyclic GMP and other clinical markers of disease activity. Arthritis Rheum 1979 May;22(5):449–457.

K100. Kastner DL, McIntire TM, Mallett CP, Hartman AD, Steinberg AD. Direct quantitative in situ hybridization studies of IgVh gene utilization. A comparison between unstimulated B cells from autoimmune and normal mice. J Immunol 1989; 143:2761–2767.

K101. Kasukawa R, Sharp GC, editors. Mixed Connective Tissue Diseases and Antinuclear Antibodies. Amsterdam: Elsevier, 1987.

K102. Kasukawa R, Tojo T, Miyawaki S. Preliminary diagnostic criteria for classification of mixed connective tissue disease. In: Kasukawa R, Sharp GC, editors. Mixed Connective Tissue Diseases and Anti-nuclear antibodies. Amsterdam: Elsevier, 1987:41–47.

K103. Katagiri K, Katagiri T, Eisenberg RA, Ting J, Cohen PL. Interleukin 2 responses of lpr and normal L3T4-/Lyt2- T cells induced by TPA plus A23187. J Immunol 1987;138:149–156.

K104. Katagiri T, Cohen PL, Eisenberg RA. The lpr gene causes an intrinsic T cell abnormality that is required for hyperproliferation. J Exp Med 1988;167:741–751.

K105. Katayama I, Kondo S, Kawana S, Nishioka K, Nishiyama S. Neonatal lupus erythematosus with a high anticardiolipin antibody titer. J Am Acad Dermatol 1989;21:490–492.

K106. Katayama S, Chia D, Knutson S, Burnett EV. Decreased FcR avidity and degradative function of monocytes from patients with systemic lupus erythematosus. J Immunol 1983; 131:217–222.

K107. Kato N, Hiro OH, Fumio H. Nucleotide sequence of 45S RNA (C8 or hY5) from HeLa cells. Biochem Biophys Res Commun 1982;108:363–370.

K108. Kato M, Noma K, Takeuchi Y, Nagano M. A case of idiopathic portal hypertension supervening on SLE (systemic lupus erythematosus)—a study of the possible role of SLE in the pathogenesis of IPH. Nippon Naiki Gakkai Zasshi 1986 Dec;75(12):1836–1840.

K109. Katsanis E, Hsu E, Luke KH, McKee JA. Systemic lupus erythematosus and sickle hemoglobinopathies: a report of two cases and review of the literature. Am J Hematol 1987;25: 211–214.

K110. Kattwinkel N, Cook L, Agnello V. Overwhelming fatal infection in a young woman after intravenous cyclophosphamide therapy for lupus nephritis [case report]. J Rheumatol 1991;18(1):79–81.

K111. Katz AI, Davison JM, Hayslett JP, Singson E, Lindheimer MD. Pregnancy in women with kidney disease. Kidney Int 1980;18:192–206.

K112. Katz FH, Duncan DR. Entry of prednisolone into human milk. N Engl J Med 1975;293:1154.

K113. Katz P, Mitchell SR, Cupps TR, Evans M, Whalen G. Suppression of B cell responses by natural killer cells is mediated through direct effects on T cells. Cell Immunol 1989; 119:130–142.

K114. Katz P, Zaytoun AM, Lee JH Jr, Panush RS, Longley S. Abnormal natural killer cell activity in systemic lupus erythematosus: an intrinsic defect in the lytic event. J Immunol 1982 Nov;129:1966–1971.

K115. Katz VL, Thorp JM Jr, Watson WJ, Fowler L, Heine RP. Humlan immunoglobulin therapy for preeclampsia associated with lupus anticoagulant and anticardiolipin antibody. Obstet Gynecol 1990;76(2 Pt 2):986–988.

K116. Katz WA, Ehrlich GE. Acute salivary gland inflammation associated with systemic lupus erythematosus (SLE). Ann Rheum Dis 1972 Sep;31:384–387.

K117. Katz WA, Ehrlich GE, Gupta VP, Shapiro B. Salivary gland dysfunction in systemic lupus erythematosus and rheumatoid arthritis diagnostic importance. Arch Intern Med 1980 Jul; 140(7):949–951.

K118. Kaudewitz P, Ruzicka T, Meurer M, Rieber P, Braun-Falco O. Epidermal synthesis and expression of HLA-DR on keratinocytes in lupus erythematosus. Arch Dermatol Res 1985; 277(6):444–447.

K119. Kaufman JL, Bancilla E, Slade J. Lupus vasculitis with tibial artery thrombosis and gangrene [letter]. Arthritis Rheum 1986 Oct;29(10):1291–1292.

K120. Kaufman LD, Gomez-Reino JJ, Heinicke MH, Gorevic PD. Male lupus: Retrospective analysis of the clinical and laboratory features of 52 patients, with a review of the literature. Semin Arthritis Rheum 1989;18:189–197.

K121. Kaufman LD, Heinicke MH, Hamburger M, Gorevic PD. Male lupus: prevalence of IgA deficiency, 7S IgM and abnormalities of Fc-receptor function. Clin Exp Rheumatol 1991;9: 265–269.

K122. Kaufman RL, Kitrodou RC. Pregnancy in mixed connective tissue disease: comparison with systemic lupus erythematosus. J Rheumatol 1982 Jul–Aug;9:549–555.

K123. Kavai M, Lukacs K, Sonkloly I, Paloczi K, Szegedi G. Circulating immune complexes and monocyte Fc receptor function in autoimmune diseases. Ann Rheum Dis 1979;38:79–83.

K124. Kavai M, Zsindely A, Sonkloly I, Major M, Demjan I, Szegedi G. Signals of monocyte activation in patients with SLE. Clin Exp Immunol 1983;51:255–260.

K125. Kawahara DJ, Miller A, Sercarz EE. The induction of helper and suppressor cells with secondary anti-hen egg-white lysozyme B hybridoma cells in the absence of antigen. Eur J Immunol 1987;17:1101.

K126. Kawai T, Katoh K, Narita M, Tani K, Okubo T. Deficiency of the 9th component of complement (C9) in a patient with systemic lupus erythematosus. J Rheumatol 1989;16: 542–543.

K127. Kawai T, Katoh K, Tani K, Okuda K, Okubo T. HLA antigens in Japanese patients with central nervous system lupus. Tissue Antigens 1990 Jan;35(1):45–46

K128. Kawanishi K, Ueda H, Nagase M, Ofuji T. Decreased plasma post heparin lipolytic activity in systemic lupus erythematosus. Acta Med Okayama 1977 Oct;31(5):319–324.

K129. Kawashima I, Sakabe K, Seiki K, Fuki-Hanamoto H. Effect of sex steroids on T-cell differentiation in the thymus of castrated C57BL/6NJcl mice. Med Sci Res 1990;18:261–262.

K130. Kay DR, Bole GG Jr, Ledger WJ. Antinuclear antibodies, rheumatoid factor, and C-reactive protein in serum of normal women using oral contraceptives. Arthritis Rheum 1971 Mar–Apr;14:239–248.

K131. Kay DR, Valentine TV, Walker SE, Valentine MH, Bole GG. Frentizole therapy of active systemic lupus erythematosus. Arthritis Rheum 1980 Dec;23(12):1381–1387.

K132. Kay HD, Horwitz DA. Evidence by reactivity with hybridoma antibodies for a probable myeloid origin of peripheral blood cells active in natural cytotoxicity and antibody-dependent cell-mediated cytotoxicity. J Clin Invest 1980;66:847.

K133. Kay RA, Wood KJ, Bernstein RM, Holt PJL, Pumphrey RS. An IgG subclass imbalance in connective tissue disease. Ann Rheum Dis 1988;47:536–541.

K134. Kaye BR. Rheumatic manifestations of infection with human immunodeficiency virus (HIV). Ann Intern Med 1989 Jul;111(2):158–167.

K135. Kaye EM, Butler IJ. Myelopathy in neonatal and infantile lupus erythematosus. Ann Neurol 1985;18:392.

K136. Kaye EM, Butler IJ, Conley S. Myelopathy in neonatal and infantile lupus erythematosus. J Neurol Neurosurg Psychiatry 1987;50:923.

K137. Kazatchkine MD, Fearon DT, Appay MD, Maudet C, Bariety J. Immunohistochemical study of human glomerular C3b receptor in normal kidney and in seventy-five cases of renal diseases. Loss of C3b receptor antigen in focal hyalinosis and in proliferative nephritis of systemic lupus erythematosus. J Clin Invest 1982 Apr;69:900–912.

K138. Keane WF, Kasiske BL. Hyperlipidemia in the nephrotic syndrome. New Engl J Med 1990;323:603–604.

K139. Keats TE. The collagen diseases: a demonstration of the nonspecificity of their extrapulmonary manifestations. AJR 1961 Nov;86:938–943.

K140. Keefer EB, Felty AR. Acute disseminated lupus erythematosus. Bull Johns Hopkins Hosp 1924 Sep;35:294–304.

K141. Keene JD, Query CC. Nuclear RNA binding proteins. In: Moldave K, Cohn W, editors. Progress in Nucleic Acid Research and Molecular Biology 41. Orlando: Academic 1991: 179–202.

K142. Kehrl JH, Wakefield LM, Roberts AB, Anderson PM, Roberts AB, Jakowiew S, Alvarez-Mon M, Derynck R, Sporn MB, Fauci AS. Production of transforming growth factor β by human T lymphocytes and its potential role in the regulation of T cell growth. J Exp Med 1986;163:1037.

K143. Keil H. Relationship between lupus erythematosus and tuberculosis: critical review based on observations at necropsy. Arch Dermatol 1933 Dec;28:765–779.

K144. Keil H. Conception of lupus erythematosus and its morphologic variants with particular reference to "systemic" lupus erythematosus. Arch Dermat & Syph 1937 Oct;36: 729–757.

K145. Keil H. Dermatomyositis and systemic lupus erythematosus; I. Clinical report of "transitional" cases, with consideration of lead as possible etiologic factor. Arch Intern Med 1940 Jul;66:109–139.

K146. Keil H. Dermatomyositis and systemic lupus erythematosus; II. Comparative study of essential clinicopathologic features. Arch Intern Med 1940 Aug;66:339–383.

K147. Keith NM, Rowntree LG. Study of renal complications of disseminated lupus erythematosus: report of four cases. Trans Assoc Am Physicians 1922;37:487–502.

K148. Kellett HA, Collier A, Taylor R, Sawers JS, Benton C, Doig A, Baird D, Clarke BF. Hyperandrogenism, insulin resistance, acanthosis nigracans and systemic lupus erythematosus associated with insulin receptor antibodies. Metabolism 1988 Jul; 37(7):656–659.

K148a. Kelley RE, Berger JR. Ischemic stroke in a girl with lupus anticoagulant. Pediatr Neurol 1987;3:58–61.

K149. Kelley RE, Stokes N, Reyes P, Harik SI. Cerebral transmural

angiitis and ruptured aneurysm: a complication of systemic lupus erythematosus. Arch Neurol 1980 Aug;37(8)::526–527.

K150. Kelley S, McGarry P, Hutson Y. A typical cells in pleural fluid characteristic of systemic lupus erythematosus. Acta Cytol 1971 Jul–Aug;15:357–362.

K151. Kelley VE, Ferreti A, Izui S, Strom TB. A fish oil diet rich in eicosapentaenoic acid reduces cyclooxygenase metabolites, and suppresses lupus in MRL/lpr mice. J Immunol 1985; 134:1914–1919.

K152. Kelley VE, Izui S, Halushka PV. Effect of ibuprofen, a fatty acid cyclooxygenase inhibitor, on murine lupus. Clin Immunol Immunopathol 1982;25:223–231.

K153. Kelley VE, Sneve S, Musinski S. Increased renal thromboxane production in murine lupus nephritis. J Clin Invest 1986; 77:252–259.

K153a. Kelley VE, Winkelstein A. Age-and sex-related glomerulonephritis in New Zealand White mice. Clin Immunol Immunopathol 1980;16:142.

K154. Kellum RE, Haserick JR. Mechlorethamine therapy for systemic lupus nephropathy. Analysis and review of ten years' experience and a clinical study of 211 cases including 81 patients treated with mechlorethamine. Arch Dermatol 1963 Mar;87:289–298.

K155. Kellum RE, Haserick JR. Systemic lupus erythematosus. A statistical evaluation of mortality based on a consecutive series of 299 patients. Arch Intern Med 1964 Feb;113:200–207.

K156. Kelly MC, Denburg JA. Cerebrospinal fluid immunoglobulins and neuronal antibodies in neuropsychiatric systemic lupus erythematosus and related conditions. J Rheumatol 1987 Aug;14(4):740–744.

K157. Kelly RH, Vertosick FT Jr. Systemic lupus erythematosus: a role for anti-receptor antibodies? Medical Hypotheses 1986 May;20(1):95–101.

K158. Kelly TA. Cardiac tamponade in systemic lupus erythematosus. An unusual initial manifestation. South Med J 1987;80: 514–515.

K159. Kelsey PR, Stevenson KJ, Poller L. The diagnosis of lupus anticoagulant by the activated partial thromboplastin time—the central role of phophatidly serine. Thromb Haemost 1984;52:172.

K160. Kelton JG. The measurement of platelet-bound immunoglobulins: an overview of the methods and the biological relevance of platelet-associated IgG. Prog Hematol 1983;13: 183–199.

K161. Kelton JG, Gibbons S. Autoimmune platelet destruction. Idiopathic thrombocytopenic purpura. Semin Throm Hemostasis 1982;Apr;8(Pt 1):8:83–104.

K162. Kelton JG, Giles AR, Neame PB, Powers P, Hageman N, Hirsh J. Comparison of two direct assays for platelet-associated IgG (PAIgG) in assessment of immune and nonimmune thrombocytopenia. Blood 1980 Mar;55:424–429.

K163. Kelton JG, Keystone J, Moore J, Denomme G, Tozman E, Glynn M, Neame PL, Gauldie J. Immune mediated thrombocytopenia of malaria. J Clin Invest 1983 Apr;71:832–836.

K164. Kelton JG, Powers PJ, Carter C. A prospective study of the usefulness of the measurement of platelet-associated IgG for the diagnosis of idiopathic thrombocytopenic purpura. Blood 1982 Oct;60:1050–1063.

K165. Kelton JG, Singer J, Rodger C, Gauldie J, Horsewood P, Dent P. The concentration of IgG in the serum is a major determinant of Fc-dependent reticuloendothelial function. Blood 1985;66:490–495.

K166. Kemp ME, Atkinson JP, Skanes VM, Levine RP, Chaplin DD. Deletion of C4A genes in patients with systemic lupus erythematosus. Arthritis Rheum 1987;30:1015–1022.

K167. Kenik JA, Krohn K, Kelly RB, Bierman M, Hammeke MD, Hurley JA. Transverse myelitis and optic neuritis in systemic lupus erythematosus: a case report with magnetic resonance imaging findings. Arthritis Rheum 1987 Aug;30(8):947–950.

K168. Kenik JG, Maricq HR, Bole GG. Blind evaluation of the diagnostic specificity of nailfold capillary microscopy in the connective tissue diseases. Arthritis Rheum 1981 Jul;24(7): 885–891.

K169. Kennedy RC, Adler-Stortz C, Burns JW, Henkel RD, Dreesman GR. Anti-idiotype modulation of herpes simplex virus infection leading to increased pathogenicity. J Virol 1984;50: 951.

K170. Kennedy RC, Dreesman GR. Anti-idiotypic antibodies as idiotope vaccines that induce immunity against infectious agents. Intern Rev Immunol 1986;1:67.

K171. Kennedy RC, Eichberg JW, Dreesman GR. Lack of genetic restriction by a potential anti-idiotype vaccine for type B viral hepatitis. Virology 1986;148:369.

K172. Kennedy RC, Melnick JL, Dreesman GR. Antibody to hepatitis B virus induced by injecting antibodies to the idiotype. Science 1984;223:930.

K173. Kephart DC, Hood AF, Provost TT. Neonatal lupus erythematosus: new serological findings. J Invest Dermatol 1981 Sep; 77:331–333.

K174. Kern AB, Schiff BL. Discoid lupus erythematosus following trauma; report of cases and analysis of a questionnaire. Arch Dermatol 1957 Apr 5;75(4):685–688.

K175. Kern JA, Lamb RJ, Reed JC, Daniele RP, Nowell PC. Dexamethasone inhibition of interleukin-1 beta production by human monocytes. Posttranscriptional mechanisms. J Clin Invest 1988;81:237–244.

K176. Kerr LD, Adelsberg BR, Schulman P, Spiera H. Factor B activation products in patients with systemic lupus erythematosus. A marker of severe disease activity. Arthritis Rheum 1989;32:1406–1413.

K177. Kerr LD, Adelsberg BR, Spiera H. Complement activation in systemic lupus erythematosus: a marker of inflammation. J Rheumatol 1986;13:313–319.

K178. Kersley GD, Palin AG. Amodiaquine and hydroxychloroquine in rheumatoid arthritis. Lancet 1959 Nov 21;2: 886–888.

K179. Keshgegian AA. Lupus erythematosus cells in pleural fluid. Am J Clin Path 1978 May;69:570–571.

K180. Kessler HS. A laboratory model for Sjogren's syndrome. Am J pathol 1968;42:671–685.

K181. Kettler AH, Bean SF, Duffy JO, Gammon WR. Systemic lupus erythematosus presenting as a bullous eruption in a child. Arch Dermatol 1988 Jul;124(7):1083–1087.

K182. Kettler AH, Stone MS, Bruce S, Tschen JA. Annular eruptions of infancy and neonatal lupus erythematosus. Arch Dermatol 1987;123:298–199.

K183. Kewalramani LS, Saleem S, Bertrand D. Myelopathy associated with systemic lupus erythematosus (erythema nodosum). Paraplegia 1978–1979 Nov;16(3):282–294.

K184. Khamashta MA, Asherson RA, Hughes GR. Possible mechanisms of action of the antiphospholipid binding antibodies. Clin Exp Rheumatol 1989 Sep–Oct;7 Suppl 3:S85–89.

K185. Khamashta MA, Cervera R, Asherson RA, Font J, Gil A, Caltart DJ, Vazquez JJ, Pare C, Ingelmo M, Oliver J, Hughes GR. Association of antibodies against phospholipids with heart valve disease in systemic lupus erythematosus. Lancet 1990 Jun 30;335(8705):1541–1544.

K186. Khamashita MA, Gil A, Anciones B, Lavilla P, Valencia ME, Pintado V, Vazquez JJ. Chorea in systemic lupus erythematosus: association with antiphospholipid antibodies. Ann Rheum Dis 1988 Aug;47(8):681–683.

K187. Khamashita MA, Harris EN, Gharavi AE, Derue G, Gil A, Vazquez JJ, Hughes GR. Immune mediated mechanism for

thrombosis: antiphospholipid antibody binding to platelet membranes. Ann Rheum Dis 1988 Oct;47(10):849–854.

K188. Khan MA, Ballou SP. Tendon rupture in systemic lupus erythematosus. J Rheumatol 1981 Mar–Apr;8(2):308–310.

K189. Khan MA, Sbar S. Cryptococcal meningitis in steroid-treated systemic lupus erythematosus. Postgrad Med J 1975 Sep;51(599):660–662.

K190. Khanduja S, Arnett FC, Reveille JD. HLA-DQ beta genes encode an epitope for lupus specific DNA antibodies [abstract]. Clin Res 1991;38:975A.

K191. Khansari N, Whittier HD, Fudenberg HH. Phencyclidine-induce immunodepression. Science 1986;225:76–78.

K192. Kharazmi A. Antimalarial drugs and human neutrophil oxidative metabolism. Trans R Soc Trop Med Hygiene 1986; 80(1):94–97.

K193. Khoury MI. Ulcerative proctitis in juvenile systemic lupus erythematosus after ibuprofen treatment. J Rheumatol 1989 Feb;16(2):217–218.

K194. Kieber-Emmons R, Kohler H. Toward a unified theory of immunoglobulin structure-function relations. Immunol Rev 1986;90:29.

K195. Kieber-Emmons T, Ward RE, Raychaudhuri S, Rein R, Kohler H. Rational design and application of idiotope vaccines. Intern Rev Immunol 1986;1:1.

K196. Kiel H. Conception of lupus erythematosus and its morphologic variants. With particular references to systemic lupus erythematosus. Arch Dermatol 1937;36:729–757.

K197. Kiener PA, Mittler RS. CD45-protein tyrosine phosphatase cross-linking inhibits T cell receptor CD3-mediated activation in human T cells. J Immunol 1989;143:23–28.

K198. Kievits JH, Goslings J, Schuit HRE, Hijmans W. Rheumatoid arthritis and the positive L.E.-cell phenomenon. Ann Rheum Dis 1956 Sep;15:211–216.

K199. Kilbourne EM, Swygert LA, Philen RM, Sun RK, Auerbach SB, Miller L, Nelson DE, Falk H. Interim guidance on the eosinophilia-myalgia syndrome. Ann Intern Med 1990;112:85–86.

K200. Killian PJ, Hoffman GS. Coexistence of systemic lupus erythematosus and myasthenia gravis. South Med J 1980;73: 244–246.

K201. Kilpatrick DC, Weston WL. Immune complex assays and their limitations. Med Lab Sci 1985;42:178–185.

K202. Kim KE, Onesti G, Ramirez O, Brest AN, Swartz C. Creatinine clearance in renal disease. A reappraisal. Br Med J 1969 Oct 4;5674:11–14.

K203. Kim S, Davis M, Sinn E, Pattern P, Hood L. Antibody diversity: Somatic hypermutation of rearranged V_H genes. Cell 1981;27:573–581.

K204. Kim S, Wadhwa NK, Kant KS, Pollak VE, Glas-Greenwalt P, Weiss MA, Hong CD. Fibrinolysis in glomerulonephritis treated with ancrod: renal functional, immunologic and histopathologic effects. Q J Med 1988;69:795–815.

K205. Kim T, Kanayama Y, Okamura M, Takeda T, Inoue T. Serum levels of interferons in patients with systemic lupus erythematosus. Clin Exp Immunol 1987;70:562–569.

K206. Kimata H, Saxon A. Subset of natural killer cells is induced by immune complexes to display Fc receptor for IgE and IgA and demonstrates isotype regulatory function. J Clin Invest 1988;82:160.

K207. Kimata H, Shanahan F, Brogan M, Targan S, Saxon A. Modulation of ongoing human immunoglobulin synthesis by natural killer cells. Cell Immunol 1987;107:74–88.

K208. Kimata H, Sherr EH, Saxon A. Human natural killer (NK) cells produce a late-acting B-cell differentiation activity. J Clin Immunol 1988:8.

K209. Kimball HR, Wolff SM, Talal N, Plotz PH, Decker JL. Marrow granulocyte reserves in the rheumatic diseases. Arthritis Rheum 1973 May–Jun;16:345–352.

K210. Kimberly RP. Immune complexes in rheumatic diseases. *In*: Pisetsky DS, Snyderman R, editors. Immunology of the rheumatic diseases. Rheum Dis Clin North Am 1987;13: 583–596.

K211. Kimberly RP, Bowden RE, Keiser HR, Plotz PH. Reduction of renal function by newer nonsteroidal anti-inflammatory drugs. Am J Med 1978;64:804–807.

K212. Kimberly RP, Edberg JC, Merriam LT, Clarkson SB, Unkeless JC, Taylor R. *In vivo* handling of soluble complement fixing Ab/dsDNA immune complexes in chimpanzees. J Clin Invest 1989;84:962–970.

K213. Kimberly RP, Gibofsky A, Salmon JE, Fotino M. Impaired Fc-mediated mononuclear phagocyte system clearance in HLA-DR2 and MT1-positive healthy young adults. J Exp Med 1983;157:1698–1703.

K214. Kimberly RP, Gill JR, Bowden RE, Keiser HR, Plotz PH. Elevated urinary prostaglandins and the effects of aspirin on renal function in lupus erythematosus. Ann Intern Med 1978 Sep;89(3):336–341.

K215. Kimberly RP, Lockshin MD, Sherman RL, Beary JF, Mouradian J, Cheigh JS. "End-stage" lupus nephritis. Medicine 1981; 60:277–287.

K216. Kimberly RP, Lockshin MD, Sherman RL, McDougal JS, Inman RD, Christian CL. High-dose intravenous methylprednisolone pulse therapy in systemic lupus erythematosus. Am J Med 1981 Apr;70;817–824.

K217. Kimberly RP, Lockshin MD, Sherman RL, Mouradian J, Saal S. Reversible 'end stage' lupus nephritis. analysis of patients able to discontinue dialysis. Am J Med 1983 Mar;74(3): 361–368.

K218. Kimberly RP, Meryhew NL, Runquist OA. Mononuclear phagocyte function in SLE I. Bipartite Fc- and complement-dependent dysfunction. J Immunol 1986;137:91–96.

K219. Kimberly RP, Parris TM, Inman RD, McDougal JS. Dynamics of mononuclear phagocyte system Fc receptor function in systemic lupus erythematosus. Relation to disease activity and circulating immune complexes. Clin Exp Immunol 1983 Feb; 51:261–268.

K220. Kimberly RP, Plotz PH. Aspirin-induced depression of renal function. N Engl J Med 1977;Feb 24;296(8):418–424.

K221. Kimberly RP, Salmon JE, Bussel JB, Crow MK, Hilgartner MW. Modulation of mononuclear phagocyte function by intravenous γ-globulin. J Immunol 1984;132:745–750.

K222. Kimberly RP, Salmon JE, Edberg JC, Gibofsky A. The role of Fcγ receptors in mononuclear phagocyte system function. Clin Exp Rheum 1989;7 Suppl:S130-S138.

K223. Kimberly RP, Salmon JE, Edberg JC, Shen L, Barinsky M, Brogel N, Triscari C. HLA class II-associated differences in FcγR-mediated phagocytosis are mediated by FcγRI. Arthritis Rheum 1990;33:S108.

K224. Kimberly RP, Sherman RL, Mouradian J, Lockshin MD. Apparent acute renal failure associated with therapeutic aspirin and ibuprofen administration. Arthritis Rheum 1979 Mar; 22(3):281–285.

K225. Kimmel CA, Wilson JG, Schumacher HJ. Studies on metabolism and identification of the causative agent in aspirin teratogenicity in rats. Teratology 1971;4:15–24.

K226. Kimura K, Hatakeyama M, Miyagi J, Takeda A, Sumiya M, Kano S, Takaku F, Yamamoto K. A case of systemic lupus erythematosus with cryptococcal meningitis successfully treated with amphotericin B and 5-FC. Nippon Naika Gakkai Zasshi 1986 Mar;75(3):406–413.

K227. Kimura M, Van Rappard-Van Der Veen FM, Gleichmann E. Requirement of H-2 subregion differences for graft-versus-host autoimmunity in mice: superiority of the differences at class II H-2 antigens (I-A/I-E). Clin Immunol Immunopathol 1986;65:542.

K228. Kimura T, Satoh S. Inhibitory effect of quinacrine on myocardial reactive hyperthermia in the dog. J Pharmacol Exp Ther 1985 Jan;232(1):269–274.

K229. Kincaid-Smith P, Fairley KF, Kloss M. Lupus anticoagulant associated with renal thrombotic microangiopathy and pregnancy-related renal failure. Q J Med 1988;68:795–815.

K230. Kind P, Goerz G. Clinical and differential diagnosis of cutaneous lupus erythematosus. Z Hautkr 1987 Sep 15; 62(18):1337–1347.

K231. Kind P, Lipsky P, Sontheimer RD. Circulating T and B cell abnormalities in cutaneous lupus erythematosus. J Invest Dermatol 1986;86:235–239.

K232. King KK, Kornreich HK, Bernstein BH, Singsen BH, Hanson V. The clinical spectrum of systemic lupus erythematosus in childhood. Proceedings of the conference on rheumatic diseases of childhood. Arthritis Rheum 1977 Mar; 20 Suppl: 287–294.

K233. King RW Jr, Falls WF Jr. Renal amyloidosis: development in a case of systemic lupus erythematosus [letter]. Clin Nephrol 1976 Nov;6(5):497–499.

K234. King-Smith D. External irritation as a factor in the causation of lupus erythematosus discoides. Arch Dermatol 1926 Nov;14:547–549.

K235. Kinlaw CS, Dusing-Swartz SK, Berget SM. Human U1 and U2 small nuclear ribonucleoproteins contain common and unique polypeptides. Mol Cell Biol 1982;2:1159–1166.

K236. Kinlaw CS, Robberson BL, Berget SM. Fractionation and characterization of human small nuclear ribonucleoproteins containing U1 and U2 RNAs. J Biol Chem 1983;258: 7181–7189.

K237. Kinlough-Rathbone RL. Platelets, drugs and thrombosis. the effects of some other drugs in platelet formation. Basel: Karger, 1975:124–131.

K238. Kinney EJ, Wynn J, Ward S, Babb JD, Wine-Schaffer C, Zelis R. Ruptured chordae tendinea: Its association with systemic lupus erythematosus. Arch Pathol Lab Med 1980 Nov; 104:595–596.

K239. Kinney WW, Angelillo VA. Bronchiolitis in systemic lupus erythematosus. Chest 1982;82:646–648.

K240. Kinoshita M, Aotsuka S, Funahashi T, Tani N, Yokohari R. Selective removal of anti-double-stranded DNA antibodies by immunoadsorption with dextran sulphate in a patient with systemic lupus erythematosus. Ann Rheum Dis 1989 Oct; 48(11):856–860.

K241. Kinoshita M, Aotsuka S, Yokohari R. Cross-reactive rheumatoid factors in rheumatoid arthritis with extra-articular disease. Clin Exp Immunol 1990;79:72–77.

K242. Kinsella TD, Fritzler MJ. CRP: An immunoregulatory protein. J Rheumatol 1980 May–Jun;7:272.

K243. Kintz P, Ritter-Lohner S, Lamant JM, Tracqui A, Mangin P, Lugnier AA, Chaumont AJ. Fatal chloroquine self-poisoning. Hum Toxicol 1988;7(6):541–543.

K244. Kipps TJ. The CD5 B cell. Adv Immunol 1989;47: 117–185.

K245. Kipps TJ, Fong S, Tomhave E, Chen PP, Goldfein RD, Carson DA. High frequency expression of a conserved kappa variable region gene in chronic lymphocytic leukemia. Proc Natl Acad Sci USA 1987;84:2916.

K246. Kirby JD, Dieppe PA, Huskisson EC, Smith B. D-penicillamine and immune complex deposition. Ann Rheum Dis 1979 Aug;38:344–346.

K247. Kirkpatrick RA. Witchcraft and lupus erythematosus. JAMA 1981 May 15;245(19):1937.

K248. Kirshon B, Wasserstrum N, Willis R, Herman GE, McCabe ER. Teratogenic effects of first-trimester cyclophosphamide therapy. Obset Gynecol 1988 Sep;72(3 Pt 2):462–464.

K249. Kirsner AB, Diller JG, Sheon RP. Systemic lupus erythematosus with cutaneous ulceration. Correlation of immunologic factors with therapy and clinical activity. JAMA 1971 Aug 9; 271:821–823.

K250. Kishimoto T. Factors affecting B cell growth and differentiation. Ann Rev Immunol 1985;3:133.

K251. Kisielow P, Bluthmann H, Staerz U, Steinmetz M, von Boehmer H. Tolerance in T cell receptor transgenic mice involves deletion of nonmature CD4+CD8+ thymocytes. Nature 1988;333:742–746.

K252. Kisielow P, The HS, Bluthmann H, von Boehmer H. Positive selection of antigen-specific T cells in thymus by restricting MHC molecules. Nature 1988;335:730–733.

K253. Kistin MG, Kaplan MM, Harrington JT. Diffuse ischemic colitis associated with systemic lupus erythematosus— response to subtotal colectomy. Gastroenterology. 1978 Dec; 75(6):1147–1151.

K254. Kitagawa H, Iho S, Yokochi T, Hoshino T. Detection of antibodies to the Epstein-Barr virus nuclear antigens in the sera from patients with systemic lupus erythematosus. Immunol Lett 1988 Mar;17(3):249–252.

K255. Kitagawa Y, Gotoh F, Koto A, Okayasu H. Stroke in systemic lupus erythematosus. Stroke 1990;21(11):1533–1539.

K256. Kitajima I, Yamamoto K, Sato K, Nakajima Y, Nakajima T, Maruyama I, Osame M, Nishioka K. Detection of human T cell lymphotropic virus type I proviral DNA and its Gene expression in Synovial cells in Chronic inflammatory arthropathy. J Clin Invest 1991;88:1315–1322.

K257. Kitamura H, Kitamura H, Ito T, Kanisawa M, Kato K. Systemic lupus erythematosus with multiple calcified fibrous nodules of the spleen. Acta Pathol Japan 1985;35(1):213–226.

K258. Kitani A, Hara M, Hirose T, Norioka K, Harigai M, Hirose W, Suzuki K, Kawakami M, Kawagoe M, Nakamura H. Heterogeneity of B cell responsiveness to interleukin 4, interleukin 6 and low molecular weight B cell growth factor in discrete stages of B cell activation in patients with systemic lupus erythematosus. Clin Exp Immunol 1989;77:31–36.

K259. Kitridou RC. Leprosy: The great imitator of rheumatic diseases [abstract]. XVI International Congress of Rheumatology, Sydney, Australia, 1985:P247.

K260. Kitridou RC. Pregnancy in mixed connective tissue disease, poly/dermatomyositis and scleroderma. Clin Exper Rheumatol 1988;6:173–178.

K261. Kitridou RC, Akmal M, Ehresman GR, Quismorio FP, Massry S. Nephropathy in mixed connective tissue disease. Arthritis Rheum 1980 Jun;23:704.

K262. Kitridou RC, Akmal M, Turkel SB, Ehresmann GR, Quismorio FP Jr, Massry SG. Renal involvement in mixed connective tissue disease: a longitudinal clinicopathologic study. Semin Arthritis Rheum 1986 Nov;16(2):135–145.

K263. Kitridou RC, Wittmann AL, Quismorio FP Jr. Chondritis in systemic lupus erythematosus: clinical and immunopathologic studies. Clin Exp Rheumatol 1987 Oct–Dec;5(4):349–353.

K264. Kitzmiller JL, Benirschke K. Immunofluorescent study of placental blood vessels in preeclampsia of pregnancy. Am J Obstet Gynecol 1973;115:248–251.

K265. Klajman A, Camin-Belsky N, Kimchi A, Ben-Efraim S. Occurrence, immunoglobulin pattern and specificity of antinuclear antibodies in sera of procainamide treated patients. Clin Exp Immunol 1970 Nov;7:641–649.

K266. Klajman A, Farkas R, Gold E, Ben-Efraim S. Procainamide-induced antibodies to nucleoprotein, denatured and native DNA in human subjects. Clin Immunol Immunopathol 1975; 3(4):525–530.

K267. Klajman A, Kafri B, Shohat T, Drucker I, Moalem T, Jaretzky A. The prevalence of antibodies to histones induced by procainamide in old people, in cancer patients, and in rheumatoid-like disease. Clin Immunol Immunopathol 1983;27:1–8.

K268. Klareskog K, Forusum V, Paterson PA. Hormonal regulation of the expression of Ia antigens on mammary gland epithelium. Eur J Immunol 1980;10:958–963.

K269. Klashman DJ, Martin RA, Martinez-Maza O, Stevens RH. In vitro regulation of B cell differentiation by interleukin-6 and soluble CD23 in systemic lupus erythematosus B cell subpopulations and antigen-induced normal B cells. Arthritis Rheum 1991;34:276–286.

K270. Klausner RD, Samelson LE. T cell antigen receptor activation pathways: The tyrosine kinase connection. Cell 1991;64: 875–878.

K271. Klavis G, Drommer W. Goodpasture's syndrome and effect of benzene. Arch Toxik 1970;26:40–50.

K272. Klein AM, Buskila D, Gladman D, Bruser B, Malkin A. Cortisol catabolism by lymphocytes of patients with systemic lupus erythematosus and rheumatoid arthritis. J Rheumatol 1990;17(1):30–33.

K273. Klein B, Kalden JR. Toxoplasmic encephalitis with fatal outcome as an opportunistic infection in systemic lupus erythematosus. Akt Rheumatol 1989;14:62–66.

K274. Klein MB, Pereira FA, Kantor I. Kaposi's sarcoma complicating systemic lupus erythematosus treated with immunosuppression. Arch Dermatol 1974 Oct;110:602–604.

K275. Kleiner RC, Najarian LV, Schatten S, Jabs DA, Patz A, Kaplan HJ. Vaso-occlusive retinopathy associated with antiphospholipid antibodies (lupus anticoagulant retinopathy). Ophthalmology 1989 Jun;96(6):896–904.

K276. Kleinfield R, Hardy RR, Tarlinton D, Danyl J, Herzenberg LA, Weigert M. Recombination between an expressed immunoglobulin heavy-chain gene and a germline variable gene segment in a Lyl$^+$ B cell lymphoma. Nature 1986;322: 843–846.

K277. Kleinman P, Meyers MA, Abbott G, Kazan E. Necrotizing enterocolitis with pneumatosis intestinalis in systemic lupus erythematosus and polyarteritis. Radiology 1976;121: 595–598.

K278. Kleinman S, Nelson R, Smith L. Positive direct antiglobin tests and immune hemolytic anemia in patients receiving procainamide. N Engl J Med 1984 Sep 27;311:809–812.

K279. Klemp P, Majoos FL, Chalton D. Articular mobility in systemic lupus erythematosus (SLE). Clin Rheumatol 1987 Jan; 6(2):202–207.

K280. Klemp P, Meyers OL, Keyzer C. Atlanto-axial subluxation in systemic lupus erythematosus: a case report. S Afr Med J 1977 Aug 13;52(8):531–532.

K281. Klemp P, Timme AH, Sayers GM. Systemic lupus erythematosus and nodular regenerative hyperplasia of the liver. Ann Rheum Dis 1986 Feb;45(2):167–170.

K282. Klemperer P. Concept of collagen diseases. Am J Pathol 1950 Jul;26:505–519.

K283. Klemperer P, Gueft B, Lee SL, Leuchtenberger C, Pollister AW. Cytochemical changes of acute lupus erythematosus. Arch Pathol 1950 May;49:503–516.

K284. Klemperer P, Pollack AD, Baehr G. Pathology of disseminated lupus erythematosus. Arch Pathol 1941 Oct;32: 569–631.

K285. Klemperer P, Pollack AD, Baehr G. Diffuse collagen disease: Acute disseminated lupus erythematosus and diffuse scleroderma. JAMA 1942 May 23;119:331–332.

K286. Kletzel M, Melloni L, Terrez A, Rosenthal J. Systemic lupus erythematosus proceeding acute lymphoblastic leukemia. J Arkansas Med Soc 1986;82:563–565.

K287. Klickstein LB, Wong WW, Smith JA, Weiss JH, Wilson JG, Fearon DT. Human C3b/C4b receptor: Demonstration of long homologous repeating domains that are composed of the short consensus repeats characteristic of C3/C4 binding proteins. J Exp Med 1987;165:1095–1112.

K288. Klinefelter HF, Windenwerder WL, Bledsoe T. Single day prednisone therapy. JAMA 1979 Jun 22;241:2721–2723.

K289. Klinenberg JR, Miller F. Effect of corticosteroids on blood salicylate concentration. JAMA 1965 Nov 8;194:601–604.

K290. Klinkoff AV, Thompson CR, Reid GD, Tomlison CW. M-mode and two dimensional echocardiography abnormalities in systemic lupus erythematosus. JAMA 1985;253;3273–3277.

K291. Klinman DM. B cells and autoimmune disease. ISI Atlas of Science: Immunology 1988;1:185–271.

K292. Klinman DM. Current Advances in Murine Lupus. Curr Opin Immunol 1989;1:740–746.

K293. Klinman DM. IgG1 and IgG2a production by autoimmune B cells treated in vitro with IL-4 and IFN-gamma. J Immunol 1990;144:2529–2534.

K294. Klinman DM. Polyclonal B cell activation in lupus-prone mice precedes and predicts the development of autoimmune disease. J Clin Invest 1990;86:1249–1254.

K295. Klinman DM, Banks S, Hartman A, Steinberg AD. Natural murine autoantibodies and conventional antibodies exhibit similar degrees of antigenic cross-reactivity. J Clin Invest 1988;82:652–657.

K296. Klinman DM, Eisenberg RA, Steinberg AD. Development of the autoimmune B cell repertoire in MRL-lpr/lpr mice. J Immunol 1990;1440:506–512.

K297. Klinman DM, Holmes KL. Differences in the repertoires expressed by peritoneal and splenic Ly-1 (CD5) B cells. J Immunol 1990;144:4520–4526.

K298. Klinman DM, Ishigatsubo Y, Steinberg AD. Acquisition and maturation of expressed B cell repertoires in normal and autoimmune mice. J Immunol 1988;141:801–806.

K299. Klinman DM, Ishigatsubo Y, Steinberg AD. Pathogenesis of generalized autoimmunity: In vivo studies of the interaction between B cells and their internal milieu. Cell Immunol 1988;17:360–368.

K300. Klinman DM, Shirai A, Ishigatsubo Y, Conover J, Steinberg AD. Quantitation of IgG and IgM secreting B cells in the peripheral blood of patients with systemic lupus erythematosus. Arthritis Rheum. In press.

K301. Klinman DM, Steinberg AD. Proliferation of anti-DNA producing NZB B cells in a non-autoimmune environment. J Immunol 1986;137:69–75.

K302. Klinman DM, Steinberg AD. Similar in vivo expansion of B cells from normal DBA/2 and autoimmune NZB mice in xid recipients. J Immunol 1987;139:2284–2289.

K303. Klinman DM, Steinberg AD. Systemic autoimmune disease arises from polyclonal B cell activation. J Exp Med 1987;165:1755–1760.

K304. Klinman NR. The mechanism of antigenic stimulation of primary and secondary clonal precursor cells. J Exp Med 1972;136:241–260.

K305. Klinman NR, Riley RL, Stone MR, Wylie D, Zharhary D. The specificity repertoire of prereceptor and mature B cells. Ann NY Acad Sci 1986;179:130–138.

K305a. Klippel JH. Personal communication.

K306. Klippel JH. Morbidity and mortality, pp. 89–92, In: Balow JE, moderator, Austin HA 3d, Tsokos GC, Antonovych TT, Steinberg AD, Klippel JH. Lupus nephritis. Ann Intern Med 1987;106:79–94.

K307. Klippel JH. How to alter the course of lupus nephritis. J Musculoskeletal Dis 1988;5:29–43.

K308. Klippel JH, Austin HA 3d, Balow JE, leRiche NG, Steinberg AD, Plotz PH, Decker JL. Studies of immunosuppressive drugs in the treatment of lupus nephritis. Rheum Dis Clin North Am 1987 Apr;13(1):47–56.

K309. Klippel JH, Bluestein HG, Zvaifler NJ. Lymphocyte reactivity of antisera to cryoproteins in systemic lupus erythematosus. Clin Immunol Immunopathol 1979 Jan;12:52–61.

K310. Klippel JH, Gerberg LH, Pollak L, Decker JL. Avascular necrosis in systemic lupus erythematosus: Silent symmetric osteonecrosis. Am J Med 1979 Jul;67(1):83–87.

K311. Klippel JH, Karsh J, Stahl NI, Decker JL, Steinberg AD, Schiffman G. A controlled study of pneumococcal polysaccharide vaccine in systemic lupus erythematosus. Arthritis Rheum 1979 Dec;22(12):1321–1325.

K312. Klippel JH, Zvaifler NJ. Neuropsychiatric abnormalities in systemic lupus erythematosus. Clin Rheum Dis 1975 Dec;1:621–638.

K313. Klipper AR, Stevens MB, Zizic TM, Hungerford DS. Ischemic necrosis of bone in systemic lupus erythematosus. Medicine 1976;55:251–157.

K314. Omitted.

K315. Klobeck HG, Meindl A, Combriato G, Solomon A, Zachau HG. Human immunoglobulin kappa light chain genes of subgroups II and III. Nuc Acids Res 1985;13:6499–6514.

K316. Klobeck HG, Bornkamm GW, Cabriato G, Mocikat R, Pohlenz HD, Zachau HG. Subgroup IV of human immunoglobulin K light chains is encoded by a single germline gene. Nuc Acids Res 1985;13:6515–6530.

K317. Kloster BE, Tomar RH, Spira TJ. Lymphocytotoxic antibodies in the acquired immune deficiency syndrome (AIDS). Clin Immunol Immunopathol 1984;30:330–335.

K318. Knapp HR. Reduced allergen-induced nasal congestion and leukotriene synthesis with an orally active 5-lipoxygenase inhibitor. N Engl J Med 1990;323:1745–1748.

K319. Knecht A, Rosenthal T, Many A, Stern N, Militeanu J. Terminal ileitis in a patient with systemic lupus erythematosus. Israel J Med Sci 1985;21:67–68.

K320. Knight JG, Adams DD. Genes determining autoimmune disease in New Zealand mice. J Clin Lab Immunol 1981 May;5(5):165–170.

K321. Knight KL, Becker RS. Molecular basis of the allelic inheritance of rabbit immunoglobulin V_H allotypes: implications for the generation of antibody diversity. Cell 1990;60:963–710.

K322. Knodell RG, Manders SJ. Staphylococcal pericarditis in a patient with systemic lupus erythematosus. Chest 1974 Jan;65:103–105.

K323. Knop J, Bonsmann G, Happle R, Ludolph A, Matz DR, Mifsud EJ, Macher E. Thalidomide in the treatment of sixty cases of chronic discoid lupus erythematosus. Br J Dermatol 1983 Apr;108(4):461–466.

K324. Knop J, Happle R, Bonsmann G, Vakilzadeh F, Macher E. Treatment of chronic discoid lupus erythematosus with thalidomide. Arch Dermatol Res 1981;271:165–170.

K325. Ko LW, Sheu KF, Young O, Thaler H, Blass JP. Expression in cultured human neuroblastoma cells of epitopes associated with affected neurons in Alzheimer's disease. Am J Pathol 1990;146:867.

K326. Kobayashi K, Asakura H, Shinozawa T, Yoshida S, Ichikawa Y, Tsuchiya M, Brown WR. Protein-losing enteropathy in systemic lupus erythematosus. Observations by magnifying endoscopy. Dig Dis Sci 1989 Dec;34(12):1924–1928.

K327. Kobayasi T, Asboe-Hansen G. Virus particles in lupus erythematosus. Acta Dermatol Venerol (Stockh) 1972;52:425–437.

K328. Kobiler D, Fuchs S, Samuel D. The effect of antisynaptosomal plasma membrane antibodies on memory. Brain Res 1976;115:129.

K329. Kobori JA, Strauss E, Minard K, Hood L. Molecular analysis of the hotspot of recombination in the murine major histocompatibility complex. Science 1986;234:173–179.

K330. Kobzik L, Brown MC, Cooper AG. Demonstration of an idiotypic antigen on a monoclonal cold agglutinin and on its isolated heavy and light chains. Proc Natl Acad Sci USA 1976; 73:1702.

K331. Kochchiyama A, Oka D, Ueki H. T cell subsets in lesions of systemic and discoid lupus erythematosus. J Cutaneous Pathol 1985;12:493–499.

K332. Kocks C, Rajewsky K. Stepwise intraclonal maturation of antibody affinity through somatic mutation. Proc Natl Acad Sci USA 1988;85:8206–8210.

K333. Kocks C, Rajewsky K. Stable expression and somatic hypermutation of antibody V regions in B-cell developmental pathways. Ann Rev Immunol 1989;537–559.

K334. Kodaira, M, Kinashi T, Umemura I, Matsuda F, Noma T, Ono Y, Honjo T. Organization and evolution of variable region genes of the human immunoglobulin heavy chain. J Mol Biol 1986;190:529–541.

K335. Koffler D. Immunopathogenesis of systemic lupus erythematosus. Annu Rev Med 1974;25:149–164

K336. Koffler D, Agnello V, Carr RI, Kunkel HG. Variable patterns of immunoglobulin and complement deposition in the kidneys of patients with systemic lupus erythematosus. Am J Pathol 1969 Sep;56:305–316.

K337. Koffler D, Agnello V, Thoburn R, Kunkel HG. Systemic lupus erythematosus:prototype of immune complex nephritis in man. J Exp Med 1971;134:1695–1795.

K338. Koffler D, Bieseker G. Immunopathogenesis of tissue injury. In: Schur PH, editor. The clinical management of systemic lupus erythematosus. New York: Grune & Stratton, 1983:29–47.

K339. Koffler D, Carr R, Agnello V, Thoburn R, Kunkel HG. Antibodies to human polynucleotides in human sera: Antigenic specificity and relation to disease. J Exp Med 1971;134: 294–312.

K340. Koffler D, Kunkel HG. Mechanisms of renal injury in systemic lupus erythematosus. Am J Med 1968;45:165–169.

K341. Koffler D, Schur PH, Kunkel HG. Immunological studies concerning the nephritis of systemic lupus erythematosus. J Exp Med 1967 Oct;126:607–623.

K342. Koffler S. The role of neuropsychological testing in systemic lupus erythematosus. In Lahita RG, editor. Systemic lupus erythematosus. New York: Wiley, 1987:847–853.

K343. Kofler R, Dixon FJ, Theofilopoulos AN. The genetic origin of autoantibodies [review]. Immunol Today 1987;80: 375–380.

K344. Kofler R, Noonan DJ, Levy DE, Wilson MC, Moller NA, Dixon FJ, Theofilopoulos AN. Genetic elements used for a murine lupus anti-DNA autoantibody are closely related to those for antibodies to exogenous antigens. J Exp Med 1985 Apr 1;161(4):805–815.

K344a. Kofler R, Noonan DJ, Strohal R, Balderas RS, Moller NPH, Dixon FJ, Theofilopoulos AN. Molecular analysis of the murine lupus-associated anti-self response: involvement of a large number of heavy and light chain variable region genes. Eur J Immunol 1987;17:91–95.

K345. Koga T, Pearson CM, Narita T, Kotani S. Polyarthritis induced in the rat with cell walls from several bacteria and two streptomyces species. Proc Soc Exp Biol Med 1973;143: 824–827.

K346. Kohda S, Kanayama Y, Okamura M, Amatsu K, Negoro N, Takeda T, Inoue T. Clinical significance of antibodies to histones in systemic lupus erythematosus. J Rheumatol 1989;16: 24–28.

K347. Kohl LE, Atkinson JP. Autoimmune aspects of complement deficiency. Clin Aspects Autoimmunity 1988;2:8–20.

K348. Kohler H, Kieber-Emmons T, Srinivasan S, Kaveri S, Morrow WJ, Muller S, Kang DY, Raychaudhuri S. Revised immune network concepts. Clin Immunol Immunopathol 1989;52: 104.

K349. Kohler PE, Percy J, Smyth CJ, Campion WW. Hereditary angioedema and "familial" lupus erythematosus in identical twin boys. Am J Med 1974;56:406–411.

K350. Kohler PF, Ten Bensel R. Serial complement component alteration in acute glomerulonephritis and SLE. Clin Exp Immunol 1969;4:191–199.

K351. Kohno Y, Naito N, Saito K, Hoshioka A, Niimi H, Nakajima H, Hosoya T. Anti-thyroid peroxidase antibody activity in sera of patients with systemic lupus erythematosus. Clin Exp Immunol 1989 Feb;75(2):217–221.

K352. Kohsaka H, Yamamoto K, Fujii H, Miura H, Miyasaka N, Nishioka K, Miyamoto T. Fine epitope mapping of the human Ss-B/La protein. Identification of a distinct autoepitope homologous to a viral gag polyprotein. J Clin Invest 1990;85: 1566–1574.

K353. Koike T, Ichikawa K, Suzuki T, Ishihara S, Tomioka H, Yoshida S. Specificity of monoclonal hybridoma antibodies to cardiolipin from SLE-prone mice [abstract]. Clin Exp Rheumatol 1990;8 Suppl 2:207.

K354. Koike T, Kagami M, Takabayshi K, Maruyama N, Tomioka H, Yoshida H. Antibodies to human T cell leukemia virus are absent in patients with systemic lupus erythematosus. Arthritis Rheum 1985;28:481–484.

K355. Koike T, Kobayashi S, Yoshiki T, Itoh T, Shirai T. Differential sensitivity of functional subsets of T cells to the cytotoxicity of natural T-lymphocytotoxic autoantibody of systemic lupus erythematosus. Arthritis Rheum 1979 Feb;22:123–129.

K356. Koike T, Sueishi M, Funaki H, Tomioka H, Yoshida S. Antiphospholipid antibodies and biological false positive serological test for syphilis in patients with systemic lupus erythematosus. Clin Exp Immunol 1984 Apr;56(1):193–199.

K357. Koike T, Tomioka H, Kumagai A. Antibodies cross-reactive with DNA and cardiolipin in patients with systemic lupus erythematosus. Clin Exp Immunol 1982 Nov;50(2):298–302.

K358. Koivisto O, Sotaniemi E, Vesikari T. Recurrent virus infections in identical twins with systemic lupus erythematosus. Acta Rheumatol Scand 1971;17:304–311.

K359. Koller SR, Johnson CL, Moncure CW, Waller MV. Lupus erythematosus cell preparation-Antinuclear factor incongruity. A review of diagnostic tests for systemic lupus erythematosus. Am J Clin Path 1976 Sep;66:495–505.

K360. Koller BH, Geraghty DE, DeMars R, Duvick L, Rich SS, Orr HT. Chromosomal organization of the human major histocompatibility complex class I gene family. J Exp Med 1989;169: 469–480.

K361. Kolstee HJ. A patient with disseminated lupus erythematosus caused by the use of carbamazepine (Tegretol). Ned Tijdschr-Geneeskd 1983 Aug;127:1588–1590.

K362. Komisar JL, Yeung KY, Crawley RC, Talal N, Teale JM. IgVH gene family repertoire of plasma cells derived from lupus-prone MRL/lpr and MRL/ + + mice. J Immunol 1989;143: 340–347.

K363. Komori S, Siegel RM, Yui K, Katsumata M, Greene MI. T-cell receptor and autoimmune disease. Immunol Res 1990;9: 245–264.

K364. Konenkov VI, Prokofiev VF, Yu I, Glazycheva VS, Kozhevnikov VS, Yu N, Naumov N, Petova ED, Voronova IA, Petrova EM, Lozovoi VP. Changes in the level of soluble HLA antigens and their light chains (Beta-2 microglobulin) in rheumatoid arthritis and systemic lupus erythematosus. Terapt Ark 1986; 7:57–59.

K365. Kong NCT, Cheong IKS, Phang KS. Low dose intravenous cyclophosphamide (IV-CY) in diffuse proliferative lupus nephritis [abstract]. 2nd International Conference on SLE, Singapore, 1989:92.

K366. Kong TQ, Kellum RE, Haserick JR. Clinical diagnosis of cardiac involvement in systemic lupus erythematosus. A correlation of clinical and autopsy findings in thirty patients. Circulation 1962 Jul;26:7–11.

K367. Konikoff F, Isenberg DA, Barrison I, Theodor E, Schoenfeld Y. Antinuclear autoantibodies in chronic liver diseases. Hepatogastroenterology 1989 Oct;36(5):341–345.

K368. Konikoff F, Swissa M, Shoenfeld Y. Autoantibodies to histones and their subfractions in chronic liver diseases. Clin Immunol Immunopathol 1989;51:77–82.

K369. Kono DH, Klashman DJ, Gilbert RC. Successful IV pulse cyclophosphamide in refractory PM in 3 patients with SLE [letter]. J Rheumatol 1990 Jul;17(5):982–983.

K370. Kono I, Sakurai T, Kabashima T, Yamane K, Kashiwagi H. Fibronectin binds to Clq: possible mechanisms for their coprecipitation in cryoglobulins from patients with systemic lupus erythematosus. Clin Exp Immunol 1983 May;52:305–310.

K371. Konstantinov K, Russanova V, Russeva V. Antibodies to histones and disease activity in systemic lupus erythematosus: A comparative study with an enzyme-linked immunosorbent assay and immunoblotting. Arch Dermatol Res 1986;278:410–415.

K372. Konttinen YT, Tolvanen E, Johansson E, Reitamo S, Wegelius O. Skin response to intradermal DNA and RNA in systemic lupus erythematosus. Arthritis Rheum 1982 Nov;25(11):1284–1290.

K373. Koo AP, Segal AM, Smith JW, Smith DS, Krakauer RS. Continuous flow cryofiltration in the treatment of systemic vasculitis [abstract]. Arthritis Rheum 1983 Apr;26(4) Suppl:S67.

K374. Koolwijk P, Spierenburg GT, Frasa H, Boot JHA, van de Winkel JGJ, Bast BJEG. Interaction between hybrid monoclonal antibodies and the human high affinity IgG FcR, huFc-γRI, on U937: Involvement of only one of the mIgG heavy chains in receptor binding. J Immunol 1989;143:1656–1662.

K375. Kopelman RG, Zolla-Panzer S. Association of human immunodeficiency virus infection and autoimmune phenomena. Am J Med 1988 Jan;84(1):82–88.

K376. Koransky JS, Esterly NB. Lupus panniculitis (profundus). J Pediatr 1981 Feb;98(2):241–244.

K377. Same as K384a.

K378. Same as K384b.

K379. Korbet SM, Block LJ, Lewis EJ. Laryngeal complications in a patient with inactive systemic lupus erythematosus. Arch Intern Med 1984 Sep;144(9):1867–1868.

K380. Korbet SM, Corwin JL. Pernicious anemia in a patient with systemic lupus erythematosus in a young women. J Rheumatol 1986;12:193–194.

K381. Korbet SM, Corwin HL, Patel SK, Schwartz MM. Intraperitoneal hemorrhage associated with systemic lupus erythematosus [letter]. J Rheumatol 1987 Apr;14(2):398–400.

K382. Korbet SM, Schwartz MM, Lewis EJ. Immune complex deposition and coronary vasculitis in systemic lupus erythematosus. Report of 2 cases. Am J Med 1984 Jul;77:141–146.

K383. Korn S, Barbieri EJ, de Horatius RJ. Cerebrospinal fluid (CSF) substance P (SP) in neuropsychiatric systemic lupus erythematosus (NP-SLE) [abstract]. Arthritis Rheum 1989 Jan;32(1) Suppl:R34.

K384. Korn S, Huppert A, Spitzer S, de Horatius RJ. Systemic lupus erythematosus presenting with lingual infarction. J Rheumatol 1988 Aug;15(8):1281–1283.

K384a. Kornberg RD. Structure of chromatin. Ann Rev Biochem 1977; 46:931–954.

K384b. Kornberg RD, Klug A. The nucleosome. Sci Am 1981; 244:52–64.

K385. Korsmeyer SJ. A hierarchy of immunoglobulin gene rearrangements in human leukemic pre B-cells. Proc Natl Acad Sci USA 1981;78:7096–7100.

K386. Koskela P, Vaarala O, Makitalo R, Palosuo T, Aho K. Significance of false positive syphilis reactions and anticardiolipin antibodies in a nationwide series of pregnant women. J Rheumatol 1988;15:70–73.

K387. Kosmetatos N, Blackman MS, Elrad H, Aubry RH. Congenital complete heart block in the infant of a woman with collagen vascular disease. A case report. J Reprod Med 1979;22:213–216.

K388. Kosowsky BD, Taylor J, Lown B, Ritchie RF. Long-term use of procainamide following acute myocardial infarction. Circulation 1973 Jun;47:1204–1210.

K389. Kossard S, Doherty E, McColl I, Ryman W. Autofluorescence of clofazimine in discoid lupus erythematosus. J Am Acad Dermatol 1987 Nov;17(5 Pt 2):867–871.

K390. Kotzin BL, Arndt R, Okada S, Ward R, Thach AB, Strober S. Treatment of NZB/NZW mice with total lymphoid irradiation: long-lasting suppression of disease without generalized immune suppression. J Immunol 1986;136:3259–3265.

K391. Kotzin BL, Babcock SK, Herron LR. Deletion of potentially self-reactive T cell receptor specificities in L3T4-, Lyt-2- T cells of lpr mice. J Exp Med 1989;169:2221–2229.

K392. Kotzin BL, Barr VL, Palmer E. A large deletion within the T cell receptor beta-chain gene complex in New Zealand White mice. Science 1985;229:167–171.

K393. Kotzin BL, Herron LR, Babcock SK, Portanova JP, Palmer E. Self-reactive T cells in murine lupus: analysis of genetic contributions and development of self-tolerance. Clin Immunol Immunopathol 1989 Nov;53(2 Pt 2):S35–46.

K394. Kotzin BL, Kappler JW, Marrack PC, Herron LR. T cell tolerance to self antigens in New Zealand hybrid mice with lupus-like disease. J Immunol 1989;143:89–94.

K395. Kotzin BL, Palmer E. The contribution of NZW genes to lupus-like disease in (NZB × NZW) F1 mice. J Exp Med 1987 May 1;165(5):1237–1251.

K396. Kotzin BL, Palmer E. Genetic contributions to lupus-like disease in NZB/NZW mice. Am J Med 1988;85(6A):29–31.

K397. Kotzin BL, Strober S. Reversal of NZB/NZW disease with total lymphoid irradiation. J Exp Med 1979;150:371.

K398. Kountz DS, Kolander SA, Rozovsky A. False positive urinary pregnancy test in the nephrotic syndrome. N Engl J Med 1989;321:1416.

K399. Kovarsky J. Clinical pharmacology and toxicology of cyclophosphamide: emphasis on use in rheumatoid disease. Semin Arthritis Rheum 1983 May;12(4):359–372.

K400. Kovarsky J. Otorhinolaryngologic complications of rheumatic disease. Semin Arthritis Rheum 1984 Nov;14(2):141–150.

K401. Kozeny GA, Barr W, Bansal VK, Vertuno LL, Fresco R, Robinson J, Hano JE. Occurrence of renal tubular dysfunction in lupus nephritis. Arch Intern Med 1987;147:891–895.

K402. Kozeny GA, Hurley RM, Fresco R, Vertuno LL, Bansal VK, Hano JE. Systemic lupus erythematosus presenting with hyporeninemic hypoaldosteronism in a 10 year old girl. Am J Nephrol 1986;6(4):321–324.

K403. Kozlowski CL, Johnson MJ, Gorst DW, Willey RF. Lung cancer, immune thrombocytopenia and the lupus inhibitor. Postgrad Med J 1987 Sep;63(743):793–795.

K404. Kozlowski RD, Steinbrunner JV, MacKenzie AH, Clough JD, Wilke WS, Segal AM. Outcome of first-trimester exposure to low-dose methotrexate in eight patients with rheumatic disease. Am J Med 1990;88:589–592.

K405. Kozower M, Veatch L, Kaplan MM. Decreased clearance of prednisolone, a factor in the development of corticosteroid side effects. J Clin Endocrinol Metabol 1974;38:407–417.

K406. Krainin MJ, Clark JI. Quinidine-induced lupus erythematosus [letter]. Arch Intern Med 1985;145:1740–1741.

K407. Kramer LS, Ruderman JE, Dubois EL, Friou GJ. Deforming, nonerosive arthritis of the hands in chronic systemic lupus erythematosus (SLE) [abstract]. Arthritis Rheum 1970;13:329–330.

K408. Krantz SB, Moore WH, Zaentz SD. Studies of red cell aplasia. J Clin Invest 1973;52:324–336.

K409. Kraus A. Erythromelalgia in a patient with systemic lupus erythematosus treated with clonazepam. J Rheumatol 1990 Jan;17(1):120.

K410. Kraus A, Cervantes G, Barojas E, Alarcon-Segovia D. Retinal vasculitis in mixed connective tissue disease. A fluoroangiographic study. J Rheumatol 1985 Dec;12(6):1122–1124.

K411. Kraus A, Guerra-Bautista G, Chavarria P. Paragonimiasis: an infrequent but treatable cause of hemoptysis in systemic lupus erythematosus [case report]. J Rheumatol 1990;17(2):244–246.

K412. Krause I, Cohen I, Blank M, Bakimer R, Cartman A, Hohmann A, Velesini G, Asherson RA, Khamashta MA, Hughes GRV, Shoenfeld P. Distribution of two cross-reactive idiotypes of anti-cardiolipin antibodies in sera of patients with primary anti-phospholipid syndrome, systemic lupus erythematosus and monoclonal gammopathies. Lupus 1992;1:91–96.

K413. Krawinkel U, Zoebelin G, Bruggemann M, Radbruch A, Rajewsky K. Recombination between antibody heavy chain variable region genes: evidence for gene conversion. Proc Natl Acad Sci USA 1983;80:4997–5001.

K414. Kremer JM, Bigauoette J, Michalek AV, Timchalk MA, Lininger L, Rynes RI, Huyck C, Zieminski J, Bartholomew LE. Effects of manipulation of dietary fatty acids on clinical manifestations of rheumatoid arthritis. Lancet 1985;1:184–187.

K415. Kremer JM, Jubiz W, Michalek A, Rynes RI, Bartholomew LE, Bigaouette J, Timchalk M, Beeler D, Lininger L. Fish-oil fatty acid supplementation in active rheumatoid arthritis. Ann Intern Med 1987;106:497–502.

K416. Kremer JM, Lawrence DA, Jubiz W, DiGiacomo R, Rynes R, Bartholomew LE, Sherman M. Dietary fish oil and olive oil supplementation in patients with rheumatoid arthritis. Arthritis Rheum 1990;33:810–820.

K417. Kremer JM, Michalek AV, Linninger L, Huyck C, Biggouette J, Timchalk MA, Rynes RI, Zieminski J, Bartholomew LE. Effects of manipulation of dietary fatty acids on clinical manifestations of rheumatoid arthritis. Lancet 1985;1:184–187.

K418. Kremer JM, Rynes RI, Bartholomew LE, Rodichok LD, Pelson EW, Block EA, Tassinari RB, Silver RJ. Non-organic non-psychotic psychopathology (NONPP) in patients with systemic lupus erythematosus. Semin Arthritis Rheum 1981;11:182–189.

K419. Krensky AM, Weiss A, Crabtree G, Davis MM, Parham P. T-lymphocyte-antigen interactions in transplant rejection. N Engl J Med 1990;322:510.

K420. Krieg AM. Environmental and infectious factors, pp 553–555. In: Steinberg AD, moderator. Systemic Lupus Erythematosus. Ann Intern Med 1991;115:548–559.

K421. Krieg AM, Khan AS, Steinberg AD. Expression of an endogenous retroviral transcript is associated with murine lupus. Arthritis Rheum 1989;32:322–329.

K422. Krill AE, Potts AM, Johanson CE. Chloroquine retinopathy. Investigation of discrepancy between dark adaptation and electroretinographic findings in advance stages. Am J Ophthal 1971 Feb;71:530–543.

K423. Krippner H, Springer B, Merle B, Pirlet K. Antibodies to histones of the IgG and IgM class in systemic lupus erythematosus. 1984;58:49–56.

K424. Kris M, White DA. Treatment of eclampsia by plasma exchange. Plasma Ther 1981;2:143–147.

K425. Krishman C, Kaplan MH. Immunopathologic studies of systemic lupus erythematosus. II. Antinuclear reaction of gamma-globulin eluted from homogenates and isolated glomeruli of kidneys from patients with lupus nephritis. J Clin Invest 1967;46:569–572.

K426. Krishnan G, Thacker L, Angstadt JD, Capelli JP. Multicenter analysis of renal allograft survival in lupus patients. Transplant Proc 1991 April;23(2):1755–1756.

K427. Krivanek J, Paver WK, Kossard S, Cains G. Clofazimine (Lamprene) in the treatment of discoid lupus erythematosus. Australasian J Dermatol 1976;17:108–110.

K428. Krivanek JF, Paver WK. Further study of the use of clofazimine in discoid lupus erythematosus [letter]. Australasian J Dermatol 1980 Dec;21(3):169.

K429. Kroemer G, Martinez AC. Cytokines and autoimmune disease. Clin Immunol Immunopathol 1991;61:275–295.

K430. Kroemer G, Wick G. The role of interleukin 2 in autoimmunity. Immunol Today 1989;10(7):246–251.

K431. Kromman N, Green A. Epidemiologic studies in the Upernavik district, Greenland. Acta Med Scand 1980;208:401–406.

K432. Kronenberg M, Siu G, Hood LE, Shastri N. The molecular genetics of the T-cell antigen receptor and T-cell antigen recognition. Annu Rev Immunol 1986;4:529–591.

K433. Kronful Z, Schlesser M, Tsuang MT. Catatonia and systemic lupus erythematosus. Dis Nerv Sys 1977 Sep;38:729.

K434. Krulik M, Aylberait D, Vittecoq D, Audebert AA, Debray J. Primary biliary cirrhosis associated with systemic lupus erythematosus: Case report [original in French]. La Nouvelle Presse Medicale 1980 Jan 5;8:31–34.

K435. Krupp LB, LaRocca NG, Muir J, Steinberg AD. A study of fatigue in systemic lupus erythematosus. J Rheumatol 1990;17(11):1450–1452.

K436. Krupp LB, LaRocca NG, Muir-Nash J, Steinberg AD. The fatigue severity scale. Application to patients with multiple sclerosis and systemic lupus erythematosus. Arch Neurol 1989 Oct;46(10):1121–1123.

K437. Krutmann J, Kirnbauer R, Kock A, Schwartz T, Schopf E, May LT, Sehgal PB, Luger TA. Cross-linking Fc receptors on monocytes triggers IL-6 production. J Immunol 1990;145:1337–1342.

K438. Kruyswijk MR, Keuning JJ. Cutaneous cryptococcoses in a patient receiving immunosuppressive drugs for systemic lupus erythematosus. Dermatologica 1980;161(4):280–284.

K439. Krzych U, Strausser HR, Bressler JP, Goldstein AL. Effects of sex hormones of some T and B cell functions. Am J Reprodu Immunol 1981;1:73–85.

K440. Kubba R, Steck WD, Clough JD. Antinuclear antibodies and PUVA photochemotherapy. Arch Dermatol 1981;117:474–477.

K441. Kubo T, Hirose S, Aoki S, Kaji T, Kitagawa M. Canada-Cronkhite syndrome associated with systemic lupus erythematosus. Arch Intern Med 1986 May;146 (5):995–996.

K442. Kucharz EJ, Sierakowski S, Goodwin JS. Decreased activity of interleukin-2 inhibitor in plasma of patients with systemic lupus erythematosus. Clin Rheumatol 1988;7:87–90.

K443. Kuehn MW, Oellinger R, Kustin G, Merkel KH. Primary testicular manifestation of systemic lupus erythematosus. Eur Urol 1989;16(1):72–73.

K444. Kugler SL, Costakos DT, Aron AA, Speira H. Hypothermia and systemic lupus erythematosus [case report]. J Rheumatol 1990;17(5):680–681.

K445. Kuharz EJ, Goodwin JS. Hydralazine causes nonspecific binding of antibodies to human lymphocytes in vitro. Immunopharmacol 1990;19:1–4.

K446. Kuhn A, Kaufmann I. Subakuter kutaner lupus erythematodes als paraneoplastisches syndrom. Z. Hautkr 1986;61: 581–583.

K447. Kuhn H, Sprecher H, Brash AR. On singular or dual positional specificity of lipoxygenases. The number of choral products varies with alignment of methylene groups at the active site of the enzyme. J Biol Chem 1990;265:16300–16305.

K448. Kuhns WJ, Bauerlein TC. Exchange transfusion in hemolytic anemia complicating disseminated lupus erythematosus; report of case of acquired hemolytic disease associated with rare blood group antibodies following whole blood transfusions. Arch Intern Med 1953 Aug;92:284–292.

K449. Kulesha D, Moldofsky H, Urowitz M, Zeman R. Brain scan lateralization and psychiatric symptoms in systemic lupus erythematosus. Biol Psychiatry 1981 Apr;16(4):407–412.

K450. Kulick KB, Mogavero H Jr, Provost TT, Reichlin M. Serologic studies in patients with lupus erythematosus and psoriasis. J Am Acad Dermatol 1983 May;8(5):631–634.

K451. Kulick KB, Provost TT, Reichlin M. Antibodies to single-stranded DNA in patients with discoid lupus erythematosus. Arthritis Rheum 1982 Jan;25(6):639–646.

K452. Kumagai S, Sredni B, House S, Steinberg AD, Green I. Defective regulation of B lymphocyte colony formation in patients with systemic lupus erythematosus. J Immunol 1982 Jan;128:258–262.

K453. Kumagai S, Steinberg AD, Green I. Antibodies to T cells in patients with systemic lupus erythematosus can induce antibody-dependent cell-mediated cytotoxicity against human T cells. J Clin Invest 1981 Mar;67:605–614.

K454. Kumagai S, Steinberg AD, Green I. Immune responses to hapten-modified self and their regulation in normal individuals and patients with systemic lupus erythematosus. J Immunol 1981 Oct;127:1643–1658.

K455. Kumagai Y, Shiokawa Y, Medsger TA Jr, Rodnan GP. Clinical spectrum of connective tissue disease after cosmetic surgery. Arthritis Rheum 1984;27:1–12.

K456. Kumano K, Sakai T, Mashimo S, Endo T, Koshiba K, Elises JS, Iitaka K. A case of recurrent lupus nephritis after renal transplantation. Clin Nephrol 1987 Feb;27(2):94–98.

K457. Kumar A, Kumar P, Schur PH. DR3 and non-DR3 associated complement component C4A deficiency in systemic lupus erythematosus. Clin Immunol Immunopathol 1991;60: 55–64.

K458. Kumar V, Kono DH, Urban JL, Hood L. The T-cell receptor repertoire and autoimmune diseases. Annu Rev Immunol 1989;7:657–682.

K459. Kunci RW, Duncan G, Watson D, Alderson K, Rogawski MA, Peper M. Colchicine myopathy and neuropathy. N Engl J Med 1987;316:1562–1568.

K460. Kunimi K, Nagano K, Misaki T, Hisazumi H. A case of lupus cystitis [English abstract]. Hinyokika Kiyo 1989 Apr;35(4): 685–688.

K461. Kunin CM, Schwartz R, Yaffe S, Napp J, Janeway CA, Findland M. Antibody response to influenza virus in children with nephrosis: Effects of cortisone. Pediatrics 1959;23:54–62.

K462. Kunkel HG, Agnello V, Joslin FG, Winchester RJ, Capra JD. Cross-idiotypic specificity among monoclonal IgM proteins with anti-gammaglobulin activity. J Exp Med 1973;137: 331.

K463. Kunkel HG, Holman HR, Deicher HR. Multiple autoantibodies to cell constituents in systemic lupus erythematosus. Ciba Foundation Symposium Cellular Aspects of Immunology, London. Boston: Little Brown, 1960:429–437.

K464. Kunkel HG, Mannik M, Williams RC. Individual antigenic specificity of isolated antibodies. Science 1963;140:1218.

K465. Kunkel HG, Winchester RJ, Joslin FG. Similarities in the light chains of anti-gamma-globulins showing close idiotypic specificities. J Exp Med 1974;139:120.

K466. Kuno M, Gardner P. Ion channels activated by inositol 1,4,5-trisphosphate in plasma membrane of human T-lymphocytes. Nature 1987;326:301–304.

K467. Kuntz MM, Innes JB, Weksler ME. Lymphocyte transformation induced by autologous cells. IV. Human T-lymphocyte proliferation induced by autologous or allogeneic non-T lymphocytes. J Exp Med 1976 May;143:1042–1054.

K468. Kuntz MM, Innes JB, Weksler ME. The cellular basis of the impaired autologous mixed lymphocyte reaction in patients with systemic lupus erythematosus. J Clin Invest 1979 Jan;63:151–153.

K469. Kupper TS, Chau AO, Flood P, McGuire J, Gubler U. Interleukin-1 gene expression in cultured human keratinocytes is augmented by ultraviolet light exposure irradiation. J Clin Invest 1987;80:430–436.

K470. Kurilla MG, Keene JD. The leader RNA of vesicular stomatitis virus is bound by a cellular protein reactive with anti-La lupus antibodies. Cell 1983;34:837–845.

K471. Kurita Y, Tsuboi R, Numata K, Ogawa H. A case of multiple urate deposition, without gouty attacks, in a patient with systemic lupus erythematosus. Cutis 1989 Mar;43(3):273–275.

K472. Kurki P, Helve T, Dahl D, Virtanen I. Neurofilament antibodies in systemic lupus erythematosus. J Rheumatol 1986; 13:69.

K473. Kurland LT, Hauser WA, Ferguson RH, Holley KE. Epidemiologic features of diffuse connective tissue disorders in Rochester, Minn., 1951 through 1967, with special reference to systemic lupus erythematosus. Mayo Clin Proc 1969 Sep; 44:649–663.

K474. Kurlander DJ, Kirsner JB. The association of chronic "nonspecific" inflammatory bowel disease with lupus erythematosus. Ann Intern Med 1964 May;60:799–813.

K475. Kurnick NB. Rational therapy of systemic lupus erythematosus. Arch Intern Med 1956 May;97:562–575.

K476. Kurokawa Y, Ueno T, Obara T, Gotohda T, Fukatsu R, Yamashita I. Hyperkinetic mutism within the scope of consciousness disorder in a case of systemic lupus erythematosus. Jap J Psychiatry Neurol 1989;43(1).

K477. Kurosaki T, Ravetch JV. A single amino acid in the glycosyl phosphatidylinositol attachment domain determines the membrane topology of FcγRIII. Nature 1989;342:805.

K478. Kurosawa Y, Tonegawa S. Organization, structure and assembly of immunoglobulin heavy chain diversity DNA segments. J Exp Med 1982;155:201–218.

K479. Kurwa AR, Evans AJ. Discoid lupus erythematosus treated by dermabrasion. Br J Dermatol 1979;101 Suppl:53–54.

K480. Kurz O. Eye changes in lupus erythematosus [original in German]. Ztschr f Augenh 1938 Sep;95:315–322.

K481. Kushimoto K, Nagasawa K, Ueda A, Mayumi T, Ishii Y, Yamauchi Y, Tada Y, Tsukamoto H, Kusaba T, Niho Y. Liver abnormalities and liver membrane autoantibodies in systemic lupus erythematosus. Ann Rheum Dis 1989 Nov;48(11): 946–952.

K482. Kushner MJ, Chawluk J, Fazekas F, Mandell B, Burke A, Jaggi J, Rosen M, Reivich M. Cerebral blood flow in systemic lupus erythematosus with or without cerebral complications. Neurology 1987 Oct;37(10):1596–1598.

K483. Kushner MJ, Tobin M, Fazekas F, Chawluk J, Jamieson D, Freundlich B, Grenell S, Freemen L, Reivich M. Cerebral blood flow variations in CNS lupus. Neurology 1990 Jan;40(1): 99–102.

K484. Kustimur S, Gulmezoglu E. Selective IgA deficiency in patients with systemic lupus erythematosus and rheumatoid arthritis. Mikrobiyol Bul 1985;19:190–199.

K485. Kutner KC, Busch HM, Mahmood T, Racis SP, Krey PR. Neuropsychological dysfunction in systemic lupus erythematosus (SLE) [abstract]. Arthritis Rheum 1988 Jan;31(1) Suppl: R4.

K486. Kutti J, Safai-Kutti S, Good RA. The platelet Factor 3 assay and circulating immune complexes as studied on non-thrombocytopenic patients with systemic lupus erythematosus. Scand J Haematol 1982;29(1):31−35.

K487. Kutti-Sarolainen ER, Kivirikko KI, Laitinen O. Serum immunoreactive propyl hydroxylase in inflammatory rheumatic diseases. Ann Rheum Dis 1980 Jun;39−217−221.

K488. Kuwano KK, Arai S, Munakata T, Tomita Y, Yoshitake Y, Kumagai K. Suppressive effect of human natural killer cells on Epstein-Barr virus-induced immunoglobulin synthesis. J Immunol 1986;137:1462.

K489. Kuzel TM, Springer E, Roenigk HH Jr, Rosen ST. Mycosis fungoides: time to define the best therapy. J Natl Cancer Inst 1990 Feb 7;82(3):183−185.

K490. Kwakye-Berko F, Meshnick S. Sequence preference of chloroquine binding to DNA and prevention of Z-DNA formation. Molecular Biochem Parasitol 1990 Mar;39(2):275−278.

K491. Kwan KC, Breault GO, Davis RL, Lei BW, Czerwinski AW, Besselaar GH, Duggan DE. Effects of concomitant aspirin administration in the pharmacokinetics of indomethacin in man. J Pharmacokinet Biopharm 1978 Dec;6(6):451−476.

K492. Kwok WW, Thurtle P, Nepom GT. A genetically controlled pairing anomaly between HLA-DQα and HLA-DQβ chains. J Immunol 1989;143:3598−3601.

K493. Kwong YL, Wong KL, Kung IT, Chan PC, Lam WK. Concomitant alveolar haemorrhage and cytomegalovirus infection in a patient with systemic lupus erythematosus. Postgrad Med J 1988 Jan;64(747):56−59.

K494. Kyle RA, Bartholomew LG. Variations in pigmentation from quinacrine. Report of case mimicking chronic hepatic

L

L1. Laasonen L, Gripenberg M, Leskinen R, Skrifvars B, Edgren J. A subset of systemic lupus erythematosus with progressive cystic bone lesions. Ann Rheum Dis 1990 Feb;49(2):118−120.

L2. Laborde H, Rodrigue S, Catoggio PM. Mycobacterium fortuitum in systemic lupus erythematosus. Clin Exp Rheumatol 1989 May−Jun;7(3):291−293.

L3. Labowitz R, Schumacher HR Jr. Articular manifestations of systemic lupus erythematosus. Ann Intern Med 1971 Jun;74: 911−921.

L4. Labro MT, Babin-Chevaye CB. Effects of amodiaquine, chloroquine and mefloquine on human polymorphonuclear neutrophil function in vitro. Antimicrob Agents Chemother 1988 Aug;32(8):1124−1130.

L4a. Lacasa JTM, Palacin AV, Ferranz VP, Sampere IM, Cerezales MS, Fernandez-Nogues F. Systemic lupus erythematosus presenting as Lahita RG, *salmonella enteriditis* bacteremia. J Rheumatol 1991;18:785.

L5. Lachmann PJ. An attempt to characterize the lupus erythematosus cell antigen. Immunology 1961 Apr;4:153−163.

L6. Lachmann PJ, Muller-Eberhard HJ, Kunkel HG, Paronetto F. The localization of in vivo bound complement in tissue sections. J Exp Med 1962 Jan;15:63−82.

L7. Lacks S, White P. Morbidity associated with childhood systemic lupus erythematosus. J Rheumatol 1990;17:941−945.

L8. Lacour JP, Juhlin L, el Baze P, Duplay H, Ortonne JP. Hyperpigmented acral papular mucinosis, systemic lupus erythematosus and universal alopecia. Acta Derm Venereol (Stockh) 1989;69(3):212−216.

L9. Ladd AT. Procainamide-induced lupus erythematosus. N Engl J Med 1962;267:1357−1358.

L10. Lafer EM, Rauch J, Andrzejewski C Jr, Mudd D, Furie B, Schwartz RS, Stollar DB. Polyspecific monoclonal lupus auto-

antibodies reactive with both polynucleotides and phospholipids. J Exp Med 1981 Apr;153(4):897−909.

L11. Lafeuillade A, Aubert L, Quilichini R. Systemic lupus and chorea. Two personal cases with a review of the literature. Sem Hop Paris 1988;64:3109−3116.

L12. Lafont H, Chanussot F, Dupuy C, Lechene P, Lairon D, Charbonnier-Augiere M, Chalbert C, Portugal H, Pauli AM, Hauton JC. Influence of acute injection of chloroquine on the biliary secretion of lipids and lysosomal enzyme in rats. Lipids 1984 Mar;19(3):195−201.

L13. Lagana FJ, McCarthy DJ. Podiatric implications of lupus erythematosus. J Am Podiatr Med Assoc 1988 Nov;78(11): 577−583.

L14. Lahita R, Kluger J, Drayer DE, Koffler D, Reidenberg MM. Antibodies to nuclear antigens in patients treated with procainamide or acetylprocainamide. N Engl J Med 1979 Dec 20; 301:1382−1385.

L15. Lahita RG. Sex and age in systemic lupus erythematosus. In: Lahita RG, editor. Systemic lupus erythematosus. New York: Wiley, 1984:523−539.

L16. Lahita RG. Current comment Sex steroids and the rheumatic diseases. Arthritis Rheum 1985;28:121−126.

L17. Lahita RC, Bradlow HL, Fishman J, Kunkel HG. Abnormal estrogen and androgen metabolism in the human with systemic lupus erythematosus. Am J Kid Dis 1983;2 Suppl 1: 206−211.

L18. Lahita RG, Bradlow HL, Kunkel HG, Fishman J. Alterations of estrogen metabolism in systemic lupus erythematosus. Arthritis Rheum 1979;22:1195−1198.

L19. Lahita RG, Bradlow HL, Kunkel HG, Fishman J. Increased 16 alpha-hydroxylation of estradiol in systemic lupus erythematosus. J Clin Endocrinol Metab 1981 Jul;53(1):174−178.

L20. Lahita RG, Bradlow L, Fishman J, Kunkel HG. Estrogen metabolism in systemic lupus erythematosus: patients and family members. Arthritis Rheum 1982 Jul;25:843−846.

L21. Lahita RG, Bradlow L, Ginzler E, Pang S, New M. Low androgen levels in females with active systemic lupus erythematosus. Arthritis Rheum 1984;30(3):241−248.

L22. Lahita RG, Bradlow L, Ginzler E, Pang S, New M. Low androgen levels in females with active systemic lupus erythematosus [abstract]. Arthritis Rheum 1984 Apr

L23. Suppl;27:539.

L24. Lahita RG, Chiorazzi N, Gibofsky A, Winchester RJ, Kunkel HG. Familial systemic lupus erythematosus in males. Arthritis Rheum 1983;26:39−44.

L25. Lahita RG, Geschwind N. Evidence for right cerebral laterality in patients with systemic lupus erythematosus and their male relatives. Arthritis Rheum 1985 Apr;28 Suppl:S62.

L26. Lahita RG, Kunkel HG. Treatment of systemic lupus erythematosus (SLE) with the androgen 19-nor testosterone (Nandrolone) [abstract]. Arthritis Rheum 1984 Apr;27(4) Suppl: S65.

L27. Lahita RG, Kunkel HG, Bradlow HL. Increased oxidation of testosterone in systemic lupus erythematosus. Arthritis Rheum 1983 Dec;26:1517−1521.

L28. Lai FM, Lai KN, Lee JC, Hom BL. Hepatitis B virus-related glomerulopathy in patients with systemic lupus erythematosus. Am J Clin Path 1987;88(4):412−420.

L29. Lai KN, Lai FM, Lo S, Leung A. Is there a pathogenetic role of hepatitis B virus in lupus nephritis? Arch Pathol Lab Med 1987 Feb;111(2):185−188.

L30. Laing TJ. Gastrointestinal vasculitis and pneumatosis intestinalis due to systemic lupus erythematosus: successful treatment with pulse intravenous cyclophosphamide. Am J Med 1988 Oct;85(4):555−558.

L31. Laitman RS, Glicklich D, Sablay LB, Grayzel AI. Effect of long-term normalization of serum complement levels on the course of lupus nephritis. Am J Med 1989;87:132–138.

L32. Lamarre D, Talbot B, De Murcia G, Laplante C, Leduck Y, Mazel A, Poirier GG. Structural and functional analysis of poly(ADP ribose) polymerase: an immunological study. Biochim Biophys Acta 1988;950:147–160.

L33. Lamas-Robles C, Gonzalez-Mendoza A, Perez-Suarez G, Mejia-Arreguin S. Use of human skin to demonstrate antinuclear antibodies in lepromatous leprosy patients. Int J Leprosy Other Mycobact Dis 1985 Sep;53(3):373–377.

L34. Lamb JH, Lain ES, Keaty C, Hellbaum A. Steroid hormones; metabolic studies in dermatomyositis, lupus erythematosus, and polymorphic light-sensitivity eruptions. Arch Dermat & Syph 1948 May;57:785–801.

L35. Lambert D, Beer F, Godard W, Dalac S, Chavanet P, Portier H. Bullous systemic lupus erythematosus. Immunoelectronic study [English abstract]. Ann Dermatol Venereol 1986;113(8): 665–669.

L36. Lambert PH, Dixon FJ. Pathogenesis of the glomerulonephritis of NZB/W mice. J Exp Med 1968 Mar 1;127:507–522.

L37. Lambert PH, Dixon FJ. Genesis of antinuclear antibody in NZB-W mice: role of genetic factors and of viral infections. Clin Exp Immunol 1970 Jun;6:829–839.

L38. Lambert PH, Dixon FJ, Xubler RH, Agnello V, Cambiaso C, Casali P, Clarke J, Cowdery JS, McDuffie FC, Hay FC, MacLennon ICM, Masson P, Muller-Eperhard HJ, Penttinen K, Smith M, Tappeiner G, Theofilopoulos AN, Verroust P. A WHO collaborative study for the evaluation of eighteen methods for detecting immune complexes in serum. J Clin Lab Immunol 1978;1:1–15.

L39. Lambie P, Kaufman R, Beardmore T. Septic ischial bursitis in systemic lupus erythematosus presenting as a perirectal mass. J Rheumatol 1989 Nov;16(11):1497–1499.

L40. Lamy P, Valla D, Bourgeois P, Rueff B, Benhamou JP. Primary sclerosing cholangitis and systemic lupus erythematosus. Gastroenterol Clin Biol 1988 Dec;12(12):962–964.

L41. Lance NJ, Blaszak W, Swartz TJ. Bullous skin lesions in systemic lupus erythematosus. Semin Arthritis Rheum 1991 Jun;20(6):396–404.

L42. Lancman ME, Mesropian H, Granillo RJ. Chronic aseptic meningitis in a patient with systemic lupus erythematosus. Can J Neurol Sci 1989 Aug;16(3):354–356.

L43. Landau NR, Shatz DG, Rosa M, Baltimore D. Increased frequency of N-region insertion in a murine pre-B-cell line infected with a terminal deoxynucleotidyl transferase retroviral expression vector. Mol Cell Biol 1987;7:3237–3243.

L44. Landi G, Calloni MV, Sabbadini MG. Recurrent ischemic attacks in young adults with the lupus anticoagulant. Stroke 1983;14:377.

L45. Landry M. Phagocyte function and cell-mediated immunity in systemic lupus erythematosus. Arch Dermatol 1977 Feb; 113:147–154.

L46. Lane AT, Watson RM. Neonatal lupus erythematosus. Am J Dis Child 1984 Jul;138:663–666.

L47. Lane JR, Newmann DA, Lafond-Walker A, Herskowitz A, Rose NR. LPS promotes CB3-induced myocarditis in resistant B10.A mice. Submitted.

L48. Lane PJL, Ledbetter JA, McConnel FM, Draves K, Deans J, Schieven GL, Clark EA. The role of tyrosine phosphorylation in signal transduction through surface Ig in human B cells: Inhibition of tyrosine phosphorylation prevents intracellular calcium release. J Immunol 1991;146:715–722.

L49. Lange K, Ores R, Strauss W, Wachstein M. Steroid therapy of systemic lupus erythematosus based on immunologic considerations. Arthritis Rheum 1965 Apr;8:244–259.

L50. Langevitz P, Buskila D, Lee P, Urowitz MB. Treatment of refractory ischemic skin ulcers in patients with Raynaud's phe-

nomenon with PGE1 infusions. J Rheumatol 1989 Nov; 16(11):1433–1435.

L51. Langhof H. Target therapy of the vascular injuries with subacute lupus erythematosus with Igrapyrin [original in German]. Derm Wschr 1953;128:877–884.

L52. Langhoff E, Landeforged J. Relative immunosuppressive potency of various corticosteroids measured in vitro. Eur J Clin Pharmacol 1983;25:459–462.

L53. Langley FA. Disseminated ectopic calcification in a newborn infant. Arch Dis Child 1971;46:884.

L54. Langlo L. The efficiency of local application of chloroquine and mepacrine in preventing the effects of ultraviolet rays on human skin. Acta Dermatovener (Stockh) 1975;37:85–87.

L55. Lanham JG, Brown MM, Hughes GRV. Cerebral systemic lupus erythematosus presenting with catatonia. Postgraduate Med J 1985 Apr;61:329.

L56. Lanham JG, Hughes GRV. Antimalarial therapy in SLE. Clin Rheum Dis 1982;8:279–299.

L57. Lanham JG, Walport MJ, Hughes GRV. Congenital heart block and familial connective tissue disease. J Rheumatol 1983;10:823–825.

L58. Lanier LL, Benike CJ, Phillips JH, Engleman EG. Recombinant interleukin 2 enhanced natural killer cell-mediated cytotoxicity in human lymphocyte populations expressing Leu 7 and Leu 11 antigens. J Immunol 1985 Feb;134:794–801.

L59. Lanier LL, Cwirla S, Phillips JH. Human natural killer cells isolated from peripheral blood do not rearrange T cell antigen receptor chain genes. J Exp Med 1986;163:209.

L60. Lanier LL, Cwirla S, Yu G, Testi R, Phillips JH. Membrane anchoring of a human IgG Fc receptor (CD16) determined by a single amino acid. Science 1989;246:1611–1613.

L61. Lanier LL, Le AM, Civin CI, Loken MR, Phillips JH. The relationship of CD16 (Leu-11) and Leu-19 (NKH-1) antigen expression on human peripheral blood NK cells and cytotoxic T lymphocytes. J Immunol 1986;136:4480.

L62. Lanier LL, Phillips JM, Hackett J, Tutt M, Kumar V. Natural killer cells: definition of a cell type rather than a function. J Immunol 1986;137:2735.

L63. Lanier LL, Testi R, Bindl J, Phillips JH. Identity of Leu19 (CD56) leucocyte differentiation antigen and neural cell adhesion molecule. J Exp Med 1990;169:2233.

L64. Lanier LL, Weiss A. Presence of Ti (WT31) negative T lymphocytes in normal blood and thymus. Nature 1987;324: 268–270.

L65. Lanier LL, Yu G, Philips JH. Co-associations of CD3 with a receptor (CD16) for IgG Fc on human natural killer cells. Nature 1989;342:803–805.

L66. Lapeyre B, Bourbon H, Amalric F. Nucleolin, the major nucleolar protein of growing eukaryotic cells: An unusual protein structure revealed by the nucleotide sequence. Proc Natl Acad Sci USA 1987;84:1472–1476.

L67. Larbre JP, Perret P, Collet P, Llorca G. Antinuclear antibodies during pyrithioxine treatment. Br J Rheumatol 1901;29: 496–497.

L68. Larocca LM, Piantelli M, Leone G, Sica S, Teofili L, Panici PB, Scambia G, Mancuso S, Capelli A, Ranelletti FO. Type II oestrogen binding sites in acute lymphoid and myeloid leukaemias: growth inhibitory effect of oestrogen and flavonoids. Br J Haematol 1990;75:489–495.

L69. Laroche CM, Mulvey DA, Hawkins PN, Walport MJ, Strickland B, Moxham J, Green M. Diaphragm strength in the shrinking lung syndrome of systemic lupus erythematosus. Q J Med 1990;265:429–439.

L70. LaRochelle G, Lacks S, Borenstein D. IV cyclophosphamide therapy of steroid resistant neuropsychiatric SLE (NPSLE) [abstract]. Arthritis Rheum 1990 May;33 Suppl 5:R21.

L71. Larsen RA. Family studies in systemic lupus erythematosus.

I. A proband material from central eastern Norway. Acta Med Scand Suppl 1972;543:11–19.

L72. Larsen RA. Family studies in systemic lupus erythematosus. 3. Presence of LE factor in relatives and spouses. Acta Med Scand Suppl 1972;543:31–41.

L73. Larsen RA. Family studies in systemic lupus erythematosus (SLE). VI. Presence of rheumatoid factors in relatives and spouses. J Chronic Dis 1972;25:191–203.

L74. Larsen RA, Gotal T. Family studies in systemic lupus erythematosus (SLE) IX. Thyroid diseases and antibodies. J Chronic Dis 1972;25:225- .

L75. Larsen RA, Solheim BG. Family studies in systemic lupus erythematosus. V. Presence of antinuclear factors (ANTFs) in relatives and spouses of selected SLE probands. Acta Med Scand 1972;543 Suppl:55–64.

L76. Larson DL. Systemic Lupus Erythematosus. Boston: Little Brown, 1961.

L77. Larson P, Holmdahl R. Estrogen-induced suppression of collagen arthritis. II. Treatment of rats suppresses development of arthritis but does not affect the anti-type II collagen humoral response. Scand J Immunol 1987;27:579–583.

L78. Larsson KS, Bostrom H, Ericson B. Salicylate- induced malformations in mouse embryos. Acta Paediatr (Stockh) 1963 Jan;52:36–40.

L79. Larsson O. Thymoma and systemic lupus erythematosus in the same patient. Lancet 1963 Sep 28;2:665–666.

L80. Larsson O, Leonhardt T. Hereditary hypergammaglobulinemia and systemic lupus erythematosus. I. Clinical and electrophoretic studies. Acta Med Scand 1959;165:371.

L81. Laser U, Kierat L, Grob PJ, Hitzig WH, Frater-Schroder M. Transcobalamin II, a serum protein reflecting autoimmune disease activity, the plasma dynamics and the relationship to establish serum parameters in systemic lupus erythematosus. Clin Immunol Immunopathol 1985;36:345–357.

L82. Lash AD, Wittman AL, Quismorio FP Jr. Myocarditis in mixed connective tissue disease: clinical and pathologic study of three cases and review of literature. Semin Arthritis Rheum 1986;15:288–296.

L83. Lasisz B, Zdrojewicz Z, Dul W, Markiewicz A, Strychalski J. Possibility of using TFX (Thymus factor X) in the treatment of systemic lupus erythematosus [English abstract]. Pol Tyg Lek 1989 Jul;44(30–31):724–725.

L84. Laskin CA, Smathers PA, Reeves JP, Steinberg AD. Studies of defective tolerance induction in NZB mice. Evidence for a marrow pre-T cell defect. J Exp Med 1982;155:1025–1036.

L85. Laskin CA, Taurog JD, Smathers PA, Steinberg AD. Studies of defective tolerance in murine lupus. J Immunol 1981;127:1743–1747.

L86. Laskin CA, Vidins E, Blendis LM, Soloninka CA. Autoantibodies in alcoholic liver disease [comments]. Am J Med 1990 Aug;89(2):127–128.

L87. Lassoved K, Guilly MN, Audre C, Paintraud M, Dhumeaux D, Danon F, Brouet AC, Courvalin JC. Autoantibodies to 200 kD polypeptide(s) is of the nuclear envelope: a new serological nuclear of primary biliary cirrhosis. Clin Exp Immunol 1988;74:283–288.

L88. Laszlo MH, Alvarez A, Feldman F. Association of thrombotic thrombocytopenic purpura and disseminated lupus erythematosus [case report]. Ann Intern Med 1955 Jun;42:1308–1320.

L89. Lau KS, White JC. Myelosclerosis associated with systemic lupus erythematosus in patients in West Malaysia. J Clin Pathol 1969;22:43–438.

L90. Laudenslager ML, Ryan SM, Drugan RC, Hyson RL, Maier SF. Coping and immunosuppression: Inescapable but not escapable shock suppresses lymphocyte proliferation. Science 1983 Aug 5;221:568–570.

L91. Laurell AB, Malmquist J. Hypergammaglobulinemia, circulating anticoagulant, and biologic false positive Wassermann reactions; a study of two cases. J Lab Clin Med 1957 May;49:694–707.

L92. Laut J, Barland P, Glicklich D, Senitzer D. Soluble interleukin-2 receptors in lupus nephritis. Arthritis Rheum 1990;33 Suppl:S129.

L93. Lauter SA, Espinoza LR, Osterland CK. The relationship between C-reactive protein and systemic lupus erythematosus. Arthritis Rheum 1979 Dec;22:1421.

L94. Laux B, Korting GW. Simultaneous occurrence of lupus erythematosus and hepatic porphyria—coincidence or chance association [English abstract]. Z Hautkr 1985 Nov 1;60(21):1714–1724.

L95. Lavalle C, Gonzales-Barcenas D, Graef A, Fraga A. Gonadotropins pituitary secretion in systemic lupus erythematosus. Clin Exp Rheumatol 1984;2:163–166.

L96. Lavalle C, Layo E, Paniague R, Bermudez JA, Graef A, Herrera J, Navarete R, Gonzalez-Barcena D, Fraga A. Correlation study between prolactin and androgens in male patients with systemic lupus erythematosus. J Rheumatol 1987;14:268–272.

L97. Lavalle C, Pizarro S, Drenkard C, Sanchez-Guerrero J, Alarcon-Segovia D. Transverse myelitis: manifestation of systemic lupus erythematosus strongly associated with antiphospholipid antibodies. J Rheumatol 1990 Jan;17(1):34–37.

L98. Lavastida MT, Goldstein AL, Daniels JS. Thymosin administration in autoimmune disorders. Thymus 1981;2(4–5):287–295.

L99. Laver WG, Gillian MA, Webster RG, Smith-Gill SJ. Epitopes on protein antigens: misconceptions and realities. Cell 1990;61:553–556.

L100. Lavie CH, Biundo J, Quinet BJ, Waxman J. Systemic lupus erythematosus (SLE) induced by quinidine. Arch Intern Med 1985 Mar;145:700–702.

L101. Lawley TJ. Immune complexes and reticuloendothelial system function in human disease. J Invest Dermatol 1980;74:339–343.

L102. Lawley TJ, Hall RP, Fauci AS, Katz SI, Hamburger MI, Frank MM. Defective Fc-receptor functions associated with HLA-B8/DRw3 haplotype. Studies in patients with dermatitis herpetiformis and normal subjects. N Engl J Med 1981;304:185–192.

L103. Lawrence JS, Martins CL, Drake GL. A family survey of lupus erythematosus. 1. Heritability. J Rheumatol 1987;14:913–921.

L104. Lawrence N, Bligard CA, Storer J, Courrege ML. Neonatal lupus in twins. South Med J 1989;82:657–660.

L105. Lawrence RA. Breastfeeding: A guide for the Medical Profession. 3rd ed. St. Louis: Mosby, 1989:256–284, 571.

L106. Lawrence RC, Hochberg MC, Kelsey JL, McDuffie FC, Medsger TA, Felts WR, Shulman LE. Estimates of prevalence of selected arthritis and musculoskeletal diseases in the United States. J Rheumatol 1989;16:427–441.

L107. Lawson JP. The joint manifestations of the connective tissue diseases. Semin Roentgen 1982 Jan;17(1):25–38.

L108. Laxer RM, Cameron BJ, Silverman ED. Occurrence of Kawasaki disease and systemic lupus erythematosus in a single patient. J Rheumatol 1988 Mar;15(3):515–516.

L109. Laxer RM, Roberts EA, Gross KR, Britton JR, Cutz E, Dimmick J, Petty RE, Silverman ED. Liver disease and neonatal lupus erythematosus. J Pediatr 1990 Feb;116(2):238–242.

L110. Layer P, Englehard M. Tuberculostatics-induced systemic lupus erythematosus. Dtsch Med Wochenschr 1986;11:1603–1605.

L111. Lazaro MA, Maldonado-Cocco JA, Catoggio LJ, Babini SM, Messina OD, Garcio Morteo O. Clinical and serologic characteristics of patients with overlap syndrome: is mixed connective disease a distinct clinical entity. Medicine 1989 Jan;68(1): 58–65.

L112. Lazarte RA, Goldson E. Perinatal diagnosis of complete congenital heart block: four cases. VA Med 1984;111:223.

L113. Leaf A, Weber PC. Cardiovascular effects of n-3 fatty acids. N Engl J Med 1988;318;549–557.

L114. Leak AM, Ansell BM, Burman SJ. Antinuclear antibody studies in juvenile chronic arthritis. Arch Dis Child 1986 Feb; 61(2):168–172.

L115. Leaker B, MacGregor AJ, Isenberg DA, Neil G. Insidious loss of renal function in patients with anticardiolipin antibodies (ACLA) and absence of overt nephritis [abstract]. Br J Rheumatol 1990;19 Suppl 2:108.

L116. Leaker BR, Becker GJ, Dowling JP, Kincaid-Smith PS. Rapid improvement in severe lupus glomerular lesions following intensive plasma exchange associated with immunosuppression. Clin Nephrol 1986;25(5):236–244.

L117. LeBihan G, Birembaut JC, Bourreille J. Primary biliary cirrhosis and lupus: Role of D-penicillamine? [letter]. Gastroenterol Clin Biol 1982;6:405–406.

L118. Lecha V, Herrera C, Bordas X, Lecha M, Mascaro JM, Gelpi C, Rodriguez JL. Lupus erythemateux neonatal. Ann Dermatol Venereol 1982;109:779–780.

L119. Lechner K, Pabinger-Fasching I. Lupus anticoagulant and thrombosis. A study of 25 cases and review of the literature. Hemostasis 1985;15:254.

L120. Ledbetter JA, Rose LM, Spooner CE, Beatty PG, Martin PJ, Clark EA. Antibodies to common leukocyte antigen p220 influence human T cell proliferation by modifying IL 2 receptor expression. J Immunol 1985;135:1819–1825.

L121. Ledbetter JA, Schieven GL, Uckun FM, Imboden JB. CD45 cross-linking regulates phospholipase C activation and tyrosine phosphorylation of specific substrates in CD3-Ti stimulated T cells J Immunol 1991;146:1577–1583.

L122. Ledbetter JA, Tonks NK, Fischer EH, Clark EA. CD45 regulates signal transduction and lymphocyte activation by specific association with receptor molecules on T or B cells. Proc Natl Acad Sci USA 1988;85:8628–8632.

L123. Leddy JP, Peterson P, Yeaw MA, Bakemeier RF. Patterns of serologic specificity of human Gamma G erythrocyte autoantibodies. Correlation of antibody specificity with complement-fixing behavior. J Immunol 1970 Sep;105:677–686.

L124. Leden I. Digoxin-hydroxychloroquine interaction? Acta Med Scand 1982;211(5):411–412.

L125. Leden I. Antimalarial drugs 350 years. Scand J Rheumatol 1981;10(4):307–312.

L126. LeDuc G, Marion P, Davignon A. Le bloc articulo-ventriculaire complet congenital. Union Med du Canada 1968;97: 1029.

L127. Lee AK, Mackay IR, Rowley MJ, Yap CY. Measurement of antibody-producing capacity to flagellin in man. IV. Studies in autoimmune disease, allergy and after azathioprine treatment. Clin Exp Immunol 1971;9:507–518.

L128. Lee BW, Yap HK, Low PS, Saw AH, Tay JSH, Wong HB. A 10 year review of systemic lupus erythematosus in Singapore children. Aust Paediatr J 1987;23:163–165.

L129. Lee CK, Hansen HT, Weiss AB. The "silent hip" of idiopathic ischemic necrosis of the femoral head in adults. J Bone Joint Surg 1981;62A:795–800.

L130. Lee FO, Quismorio FP Jr, Troum OM, Anderson PW, Do YS, Hsueh WA. Mechanisms of hyperkalemia in systemic lupus erythematosus. Arch Intern Med 1988 Feb;148(2):397–401.

L131. Lee HM, Rich S. Co-stimulation of T cell proliferation by transforming growth factor-beta 1. J Immunol 1991;147: 1127–1133.

L132. Lee HS, Spargo BH. A renal biopsy study of lupus nephrop-

athy in the United States and Korea. Am J Kidney Dis 1985;5: 242–250.

L133. Lee LA, Bias WB, Arnett FC, Huff JC, Norris DA, Harmon C, Provost TT, Weston WL. Immunogenetics of neonatal lupus syndrome. Ann Intern Med 1983;99:592–596.

L134. Lee LA, Coulter S, Erner S, Chu H. Cardiac immunoglobulin deposition in congenital heart block associated with maternal anti-Ro autoantibodies. Am J Med 1987;83:793–796.

L135. Lee LA, David KM. Cutaneous lupus erythematosus. Curr Prob Dermatol 1989;1:161–200.

L136. Lee LA, Gaither KK, Coulter SN, Norris DA, Harley JB. The pattern of cutaneous immunoglobulin G deposition in subacute cutaneous lupus erythematosus is reproduced by infusing purified anti-Ro (SSA) autoantibodies into human skin-grafted mice. J Clin Invest 1989;83:1556–1562.

L137. Lee LA, Harmon CE, Huff JC, Norris DA, Weston WL. Demonstration of SSA/Ro antigen in human fetal tissues and in neonatal and adult skin. J Invest Dermatol 1985;85:143–146.

L138. Lee LA, Lillis PJ, Fritz KA, Huff JC, Norris DA, Weston WL. Neonatal lupus in successive pregnancies. J Am Acad Dermatol 1983;9:401–406.

L139. Lee LA, Weston WL. New findings in neonatal lupus syndrome. Am J Dis Child 1984;138:233–236.

L140. Lee LA, Weston WL, Krueger GG, Emam M, Reichlin M, Stevens JO, Surbrugg SK, Vasil A, Norris DA. An animal model of antibody binding in cutaneous lupus. Arthritis Rheum 1986; 29:782–788.

L141. Lee P, Urowitz MB, Bookman AA, Koehler BE, Smythe HA, Gordon DA, Ogryzlo MA. Systemic lupus erythematosus: A review of 110 cases with reference to nephritis, the nervous system, infections, aseptic necrosis and prognosis. Q J Med 1977 Jan;46(181):1–32.

L140a. Lee SI. Four novel U RNAs are encoded by a herpesvirus. Ph.D. Thesis, Yale University, 1990.

L142. Lee SI, Murthy SCS, Trimble JJ, Desrosiers RC, Steitz JA. Four novel U RNAs are encoded by a herpesvirus. Cell 1988; 54:599–607.

L143. Lee SL, Meiselas LE, Zingale SB, Richman R. Antibody production in systemic lupus erythematosus (SLE) and rheumatoid arthritis (RA) [abstract]. J Clin Invest 1960 Jun;39(6): 1005.

L144. Lee SL, Meiselas LE, Zingale SB, Richman SM. Effect of 6-mercaptopurine administration on antibody production and clinical course in systemic lupus erythematosus. Report of a case. Arthritis Rheum 1961 Feb;4:56–63.

L145. Lee SL, Michael SR, Vural IL. The L.E. (lupus erythematosus) cell; clinical and chemical studies. Am J Med 1951 Apr; 10:446–451.

L146. Lee SL, Rivero I. Cryoglobulins in SLE as circulating immune complexes [abstract] Arthritis Rheum 1964;7:321.

L147. Lee SL, Rivero I, Siegel M. Activation of systemic lupus erythematosus by drugs. Arch Intern Med 1966 May;117: 620–626.

L148. Lee T, Hoover RL, Williams JD, Sperling RI, Ravalese J 3d, Spur BW, Robinson DR, Corey EJ, Lewis RA, Austen KF. Effect of dietary enrichment with eicosapentaenoic and docosahexaenoic acids on in vitro neutrophil and monocyte leukotriene generation and neutrophil function. N Engl J Med 1985 May; 312:1217–1224.

L149. Lee TD, Lee A, Shi WX. HLA-A,B,DR and DQ antigens in black North Americans. Tissue Antigens 1991;37:79–83.

L150. Lee TD, Lee G, Zhao TM. HLA-DR, DQ antigens in North American Caucasians. Tissue Antigens 1990;37:79–83.

L151. Lee TH, Israel E, Drazen JM, Leitch AG, Ravalese J 3d, Corey EJ, Robinson DR, Lewis RA, Austen KF. Enhancement of plasma levels of biologically active leukotriene B compounds during anaphylaxis in guinea pigs pretreated by indomethacin or by a fish oil-enriched diet. J Immunol 1986;136: 2575–2582.

L152. Leechawengwong M, Berger H, Sukumaran M. Diagnostic significance of antinuclear antibodies in pleural effusion. Mt Sinai J Med 1979 Mar–Apr 46:137–139.

L153. Leehey DJ, Katz AI, Azaran AH, Aranson AJ, Spargo BH. Silent diffuse lupus nephritis: Long term follow-up. Am J Kidney Dis 1982 Jul;2 Suppl 1:188–196.

L154. Leeper RW, Allende MF. Antimalarials in treatment of discoid lupus erythematosus; special reference to amodiaquin (camoquin). Arch Dermatol 1956 Jan;73:50–57.

L155. LeFeber WP, Norris DA, Ryan SR, Huff JC, Lee LA, Kubo M, Boyce ST, Kotzin BL, Weston WL. Ultraviolet light induces binding of antibodies to selected nuclear antigens of cultured human keratinocytes. J Clin Invest 1984;74:1545–1551.

L156. Lefford F, Edwards JC. Nailfold capillary microscopy in connective tissue disease: a quantitative morphological analysis. Ann Rheum Dis 1986 Sep;45(9):741–749.

L157. Lefkert AK. Anti-acetylcholine receptor antibody related idiotypes in myasthenia gravis. J Autoimmunol 1988;1:63.

L158. Lefkert AK. The start of an autoimmune disease: idiotypic network during early progression of myasthenia gravis. Ann Inst Pasteur Immunol 1988;139:633.

L159. Lefrancois L, Bevan MJ. Functional modifications of cytotoxic T-lymphocyte T200 glycoprotein by monoclonal antibodies. Nature 1985;315:449–452.

L160. Lefrancois L, Puddington L, Machamer CE, Bevan MJ. Acquisition of cytotoxic T lymphocyte-specific carbohydrate differentiation antigens. J Exp Med 1985;162:1275–1293.

L161. Leger JM, Puifoulloux H, Dancea S, Hauw JJ, Bouche P, Rougemont D, Laplane D. Chloroquine neuromyopathies: 4 cases during antimalarial prevention [English abstract]. Rev Neurol (Paris) 1986;142(10):746–752.

L162. Leggett B, Collins R, Prentice R, Powell LW. CAH or SLE? [letter]. Hepatology 1986 Mar–Apr;6(2):341–342.

L163. Legros J, Rosner I, Berger C. Influence of the ambient light level on the ocular modifications induced by hydroxychloroquine in the rat. Arch Ophthalmol (Paris) 1973 May;33: 417–424.

L164. Lehman DH, Wilson CB, Dixon FJ. Extra glomerular immune deposits in human nephritis. Am J Med 1975;58: 765–786.

L165. Lehman P, Holzle E, Kind P, Goerz G, Plewig G. Experimental reproduction of skin lesions in lupus erythematosus by UVA and UVB radiation. J Am Acad Dermatol 1990;22: 181–187.

L166. Lehman TJ, Bernstein B, Hanson V, Kornreich H, King K. Meningococcal infection complicating systemic lupus erythematosus. J Pediatr 1981 Jul;99(1):94–96.

L167. Lehman TJ, Sherry DD, Wagner-Weiner L, McCurdy DK, Emery HM, Magilavy DB, Kovalesky A. Intermittent intravenous cyclophosphamide therapy for lupus nephritis. J Pediatr 1989 Jun;114(6):1055–1060.

L168. Lehman TJA. Current concepts in immunosupressives drug therapy of systemic lupus erythematosus. J Rheumatol. In press.

L169. Lehman TJA. Long term outcome of systemic lupus erythematosus in childhood. Rheum Dis Clin N Am. In press.

L170. Lehman TJA, Curd JG, Zvaifer NJ, Hanson V. The association of antinuclear antibodies, antilymphocyte antibodies, and C4 activation among the relatives of children with systemic lupus erythematosus: preferential activation of complement in sisters. Arthritis Rheum 1982;25:556–561.

L171. Lehman TJA, Hanson V, Singsen BH, Kornreich HK, Bernstein B, King K. The role of antibodies directed against double-stranded DNA in the manifestations of sytemic lupus erythematosus in childhood. J Pediatr 1980;96:657–661.

L172. Lehman TJA, Hanson V, Zvaifler N, Sharp G, Alspaugh M. Antibodies to nonhistone nuclear antigens and antilymphocyte antibodies among children and adults with systemic lupus erythematosus and their relatives. J Rheumatol 984;11: 644–647.

L173. Lehman TJA, McCurdy D, Spencer C, Silverman E, Harley J. Prognostic value of antibodies to Ro/SSA, SSB/La, and RNP in children with systemic lupus erythematosus. Arthritis Rheum 1990;33 Suppl:S154.

L174. Lehman TJA, McCurdy DK, Bernstein BH, King KK, Hanson V. Systemic lupus erythematosus in the first decade of life. Pediatrics 1989;83:235–239.

L175. Lehman TJA, Palmeri ST, Hastings C, Klippel JH, Plotz PH. Bacterial endocarditis complicating systemic lupus erythematosus. J Rheumatol 1983 Aug;10:655–658.

L176. Lehman TJA, Reichlin M, Harley JB. Familial concordance for antibodies to Ro/SSA among female relatives of children with systemic lupus erythematosus. Evidence for the 'supergene' hypothesis? [abstract]. Arthritis Rheum 1990;33 Suppl: S125.

L177. Lehman TJA, Reichlin M, Santner TJ, Silverman E, Petty RE, Spencer CH, Harley JB. Maternal antibodies to Ro (SS-A) are associated with both early onset of disease and male sex among children with systemic lupus erythematosus. Arthritis Rheum 1989;32:1414–1420.

L178. Lehman TJA, Sherry DD, Wagner-Weiner L, McCurdy DK, Emery HM, Magilavy DB, Kovalesky A. Intermittent intravenous cyclophosphamide therapy for lupus nephritis. J Pediatr 1989;114:1055–1060.

L179. Lehmann P, Holzle E, Kind P, Goerz G, Plewig G. Experimental reproduction of skin lesions in lupus erythematosus by UVA and UVB radiation. J Am Acad Dermatol 1990 Feb; 22(2 Pt 1):181–187.

L180. Lehmeier T, Foulaki K, Luhrmann R. Evidence for three distinct D proteins, which react differentially with anti-Sm autoantibodies, in the cores of the major snRNPs U1, U2, U4/U6 and U5. Nucleic Acids Res 1990;18:6475–6484.

L181. Lehuen A, Carnaud C. Characterization of two molecules at 30,33 kDa as major target antigens of natural thymocytotoxic autoantibodies. Cell Immunol 1988 Apr;112(2): 381–390.

L182. Leibowitch M, Droz D, Noel LH, Avril MF, Leibowitch J. Clq deposits at the dermoepidermal junction: a marker discriminating for discoid and systemic lupus erythematosus. J Clin Immunol 1981 Apr;1(2):119–124.

L183. Leikola J, Perkins HA. Enzyme-linked antiglobulin test: An accurate and simple method to quantify red cell antibodies. Transfusion 1980 Mar–Apr;20:138–144.

L184. Leitch AG, Lee TH, Ringel EW, Prickett JD, Robinson DR, Pyne SG, Corey EJ, Drazen JM, Austen KF, Lewis RA. Immunologically induced generation of tetraene and pentane leukotrienes in the peritoneal cavities of menhaden-fed rats. J Immunol 1984;132:2559–2565.

L185. Lemmer JP, Curry NH, Mallory JH, Waller MV. Clinical characteristics and course in patients with high titer anti-RNP antibodies. J Rheumatol 1982 Jul–Aug;9(4):536–542.

L186. Leng JJ, Mbanzulu PN, Akbaraly JP, Albin H, Guibert S, Gravier J, Demotes-Mainard F. Transplacental passage of chloroquine sulphate: in vitro study [English abstract]. Path Biol (Paris) 1987 Sep;35(7):1051–1054.

L187. Lennek R, Baldwin AS Jr, Waller SJ, Morley KW, Taylor RP. Studies of the physical biochemistry and complement-fixing properties of DNA/anti-DNA immune complexes. J Immunol 1981 Aug;127(2):602–608.

L188. Lentz RD, Michael AF, Fried PS. Membranous transformation of lupus nephritis. Clin Immunol Immunopathol 1981 Apr;19:131–138.

L189. Leohirun L, Thuvasethakul P, Sumethkul V, Phoicharoen T, Boonpucknavig V. Urinary neopterin in patients with systemic lupus erythematosus. Clin Chem 1991;37:47–50.

L190. Leonhardt ETG. Family studies in systemic lupus erythematosus. Clin Exp Immunol 1967;2:743–759.

L191. Leonhardt T. Familial hypergammaglobulinemia and systemic lupus erythematosus. Lancet 1957;273:1200–1203.

L192. Leonhardt T. Family studies in systemic lupus erythematosus. Acta Med Scand 1964;176 Suppl:416.

L191a. Leonhardt T. Long-term prognosis of systemic lupus erythematosus. Acta Med Scand 1966;445 Suppl:440–443.

L193. Le Page SH, Williams W, Parkhouse D, Cambridge G, Mackenzie L, Lyndyard PM, Isenberg DA. Relation between lymphocytotoxic antibodies, anti-DNA antibodies and a common anti-DNA antibody idiotype PR4 in patients with systemic lupus erythematosus, their relatives and spouses. Clin Exp Immunol 1989;77:314–318.

L194. Lerer RJ. Cardiac tamponade as an initial finding in systemic lupus erythematosus. Am J Dis Child 1972 Sep;124:436–437.

L195. Lerner A, Barnum C, Watson J. Studies on cryoglobulins: II. The spontaneous precipitation of protein from serum at 50 degree C in various disease states. Am J Med Sci 1947 Oct;214:15–21.

L196. Lerner MR, Boyle JA, Mount SN, Wolin SL, Steitz JA. Are snRNPs involved in splicing? Nature 1980;283:220–224.

L197. Lerner MR, Steitz JA. Antibodies to small nuclear RNAs complexes with proteins are produced by patients with systemic lupus erythematosus. Proc Natl Acad Sci USA 1979 Nov; 76:5495–5499.

L198. LeRoy EC, Maricq HR, Kahaleh MB. Undifferentiated connective tissue syndromes. Arthritis Rheum 1980 Mar;23(3): 341–343.

L199. Leslie CA, Gonnerman WA, Ullman MD, Hayes KC, Franzblau C, Cathcart ES. Dietary fish oil modulates macrophage fatty acids and decreases arthritis susceptibility in mice. J Exp Med 1985;162:1336–1349.

L200. Leskinen RH, Skrifvars BV, Laasonen LS, Edgren KJ. Bone lesions in systemic lupus erythematosus. Radiology 1984 Nov; 153(2):349–352.

L201. Lesperance B, David M, Rauch J, Infante-Rivard C, Rivard GE. Relative sensitivity of different tests in the detection of low titer lupus anticoagulants. Thromb Haemost 1988;60: 217–218.

L202. Lesser RS, Metzger DS, deHoratius RJ. Hypothyroidism in an outpatient SLE population [abstract]. Arthritis Rheum 1988 Jan;31(1) Suppl:R4.

L203. Lester RS, Burnham TK, Fine G, Murray K. Immunologic concepts of light reactions in lupus erythematosus and polymorphous light eruptions. I. The mechanism of action of hydroxychloroquine. [clinical studies] Arch Dermatol 1967 Jul; 96(1):1–10.

L204. Leung DYM, Burns JC, Newburger JW. Reversal of lymphocyte activation in vivo in the Kawasaki syndrome by intravenous gammaglobulin. J Clin Invest 1987;79:468–475.

L205. Leung W, Lau C, Wong C, Leung C. Fatal cardiac tamponade in systemic lupus erythematosus—a hazard of anticoagulation. Am Heart J 1990;119:422–423.

L206. Leung WH, Wong K-L, Lau C-P, Wong C-K, Liu H-W. Association between antiphospholipid antibodies and cardiac abnormalities in patients with systemic lupus erythematosus. Am J Med 1990 Oct;89(4):411–419.

L207. Leung WH, Wong KL, Lau CP, Wong CK, Cheng CH, Tai YT. Doppler echocardiographic evaluation of left ventricular diastolic function in patients with systemic lupus erythematosus. Am Heart J 1990;120:82–87.

L208. Levene NA, Buskila D, Dvilansky A, Horowitz Y, Sukenik S. Pernicious anemia in a patient with systemic lupus erythematosus. Irs Med Sci 1987;23:846–847.

L209. Levene NA, Berrebi A. Systemic lupus erythematosus associated with refractory anemia with excess of blast. Eur J Haematol 1990;44:79–80.

L210. Levenson AI, Zweiman B, Lisak RP. Immunopathogenesis and treatment of myasthenia gravis. J Clin Immunol 1987;7: 187–197.

L211. Leventhal LJ, Kobrin S, Callegari PE. Systemic lupus erythematosus and the syndrome inappropriate secretion of antidiuretic hormone. J Rheumatol 1991;18(4):613–616.

L212. Leveque E, Dreno B, Planchon B, Bureau B, Litoux P, Barriere H. The etiology of skin immunofluorescence in patients with antinuclear antibodies [English abstract]. Ann Dermatol Venereol 1986;113(8):655–664.

L213. Levi-Strauss M, Carroll MC, Steinmetz M, Meo T. A previously undetected MHC gene with an unusual periodic structure. Science 1988;240:201–204.

L214. Levin AS, Fudenberg HH, Petz LD, Sharp GC. IgG levels in cerebrospinal fluid of patients with central nervous system manifestations of systemic lupus erythematosus. Clin Immunol Immunopathol 1972 Oct;1:1–5.

L215. Levin DC. Proper interpretation of pulmonary roentgen changes in systemic lupus erythematosus. Am J Roentgenol Radum Ther Nucl Med 1971 Mar;11:510–517.

L216. Levin DL, Fixler DE, Moriss FC, Tyson J. Morphologic analysis of the pulmonary vascular bed in infants exposed in utero to prostaglandin synthetase inhibitors. J Pediatr 1987; 92:478–484.

L217. Levin DL, Roenigk HH, Caro WA, Lyons M. Histologic, immunofluorescent, and antinuclear antibody findings in PUVA-treated patients. J Am Acad Dermatol 1982;6:328–333.

L218. Levin RE, Weinstein A, Peterson M, Testa MA, Rothfield NF. A comparison of the sensitivity of the 1971 and 1982 American Rheumatism Association criteria for the classification of systemic lupus erythematosus. Arthritis Rheum 1984 May;27:530–538.

L219. Levine RP, Dodds AW. The thioester bond of C3. Curr Top Microbiol Immunol 1989;153:73–82.

L220. Levine S, Shearn MA. Thrombotic thrombocytopenic purpura and systemic lupus erythematosus. Arch Intern Med 1964 Jun;113:826–836.

L221. Levine SR, Crofts JW, Lesser GR, Floberg J, Welch KM. Visual symptoms associated with the presence of a lupus anticoagulant. Ophthalmology 1988 May;95(5):686–692.

L222. Levine SR, Deegan MJ, Futrell N, Welch KM. Cerebrovascular and neurologic disease associated with antiphospholipid antibodies: 48 cases. Neurology 1990 Aug;40(8):1181–1189.

L223. Levine SR, Joseph R, D'Andrea G, Welch KM. Migraine and the lupus anticoagulant: Case reports and review of the literature. Cehalalgia 1987 Jun;7(2):93–99.

L224. Levine SR, Langer SL, Albers JW, Welch KM. Sneddon's syndrome: an antiphospholipid antibody syndrome? Neurology 1988 May;38(5):798–800.

L225. Levine SR, Welch KM. Cerebrovascular ischemia associated with lupus anticoagulant. Stroke 1987 Jan–Feb;18(1): 257–263.

L226. Levinsky RJ, Cameron JS, Soothill JF. Serum immune complexes and disease activity in lupus nephritis. Lancet 1977 Mar 12;1:564–567.

L227. Levinson AI, Dziarski A, Pincus T, DeHoratius RJ, Zweiman B. Heterogeneity of polyclonal B cell activity in SLE. J Clin Lab Immunol 1981;5:17–24.

L228. Levitt JI. Deterioration of renal function after discontinuation of long-term prednisone-azathioprine therapy in primary renal disease. N Engl J Med 1970 May 14;282:1125–1127.

L229. Levy AB. Delirium and seizures due to abrupt alprazolam withdrawal: case report. J Clin Psychiatry 1984 Jan;45(1): 38–39.

L230. Levy EN, Ramsey-Goldman R, Kahl LE. Adrenal insufficiency in two women with anticardiolipin antibodies: Cause and effect? Arthritis Rheum 1990 Dec;33(12):1842–1846.

L231. Levy G. Clinical pharmacokinetics of aspirin. Pediatrics 1978;62:867.

L232. Levy J, Barnett EV, MacDonald NS, Klinenberg JR. Altered immunoglobulin metabolism in systemic lupus erythematosus and rheumatoid arthritis. J Clin Invest 1970 Apr;49:708–715.

L233. Levy JA, Pincus T. Demonstration of biological activity of a murine leukemia virus of New Zealand Black mice. Science 1970;170:326–327.

L234. Levy M, Buskila D, Gladman DD, Urowitz MB, Koren G. Pregnancy outcome following first trimester exposure to chloroquine. Am J Perinatal 1991;8:174–178.

L235. Levy M, Eldor A, Lotanc SZ, Mayder SD, Yatziv S. Circulating anticoagulant and recurrent deep vein thrombosis in a 12-year-old girl. Eur J Pediatr 1983;140(4):343–345.

L236. Levy NA. A case of chronic factitious illness. Int J Psych Med 1976;7(3):257–267.

L237. Levy R, Levy S. Cleary ML Carroll W, Schinchiro K, Bind J, Sklan J. Somatic mutations in human B cell tumors. Immunol Rev 1987;96:43.

L238. Levy S, Mendel E. Kon S, Avner Z, Levy R. Mutational hot spots in Ig V region genes of human follicular lymphomas. J Exp Med 1988;168:475.

L239. Levy SB, Goldsmith LA, Morohashi M, Hashimoto K. Tubuloreticular inclusions in neonatal lupus erythematosus. JAMA 1976;235:2743–2744.

L240. Lewis BI, Sinton BW, Knott JR. Central nervous system involvement in disorders of collagen. Arch Intern Med 1954 Mar;93:315–327.

L241. Lewis CD, Laemmli UK. Higher order metaphase chromosome structure: evidence for metalloprotein interactions. Cell 1982;17:849–858.

L242. Lewis DA, Smith RE. Steroid-induced psychiatric syndromes. A report of 14 cases and a review of the literature. J Affective Disord 1983 Nov;5(4):319–332.

L243. Lewis E, Lachin J. Primary outcomes in the controlled trial of plasmapheresis therapy in severe lupus nephritis. Kidney Int 1987;31:208.

L244. Lewis EJ, Carpenter CB, Schur PH. Serum complement components levels in human glomerulonephritis. Ann Intern Med 1971;75:555–560.

L245. Lewis GP, Jusko WJ, Burke CW, Graves L. Prednisone side effects and serum protein levels: a collaborative study. Lancet 1971;2:778–781.

L246. Lewis HM, Frumess GM. Plaquenil in the treatment of discoid lupus erythematosus; preliminary report. Arch Dermatol 1956 Jun;73:576–581.

L247. Lewis KS. Living with chromic illness. Postgrad Med. 1983 (Sept) 74(3):179–183.

L246a. Lewis R, Laversen NH, Birnbaum S. Malaria associated with pregnancy. Obstet Gynecol 1973 42:696–700.

L248. Lewis RA, Austen KF, Soberman RJ. Leukotrienes and other products of the 5-lipoxygenase pathway. Biochemistry and relation to pathobiology in human diseases. N Engl J Med 1990;323:645–655.

L249. Lewis RB, Castor CW, Knisley RE, Bole GG. Frequency of neoplasia in systemic lupus erythematosus and rheumatoid arthritis. Arthritis Rheum 1976 Nov–Dec;19:1244–1248.

L250. Lewis RB, Schulman JD. Influence of acetylsalicylic acid, an inhibitor of prostaglandin synthesis on the duration of human gestation and labor. Lancet 1973;2:1159–1161.

L251. Lewis RM, Andre-Schwartz J, Hirsch MC, Black P, Schwartz

RS. The transmissibility of canine systemic lupus erythematosus (SLE) [abstract]. J Clin Invest 51:57a.

L252. Lewis RM, Schwartz RS. Canine systemic lupus erythematosus. Genetic analysis of an established breeding colony. J Exp Med 1971;134:417.

L253. Lewis RM, Schwartz RS, Gilmore CE. Autoimmune diseases in domestic animals. Part l. Ann NY Acad Sci 1965;124: 178–200.

L254. Lewis VM, Twomey JJ, Steinberg AD, Goldstein G. Serum thymic hormone activity and systemic lupus erythematosus. Clin Immunol Immunopathol 1981 Jan 18:61–67.

L255. Ley AB, Reader GG, Sorensen CW, Overman RS. Idiopathic hypothrombinemia associated with hemorrhagic diathesis and the effect of vitamin K. Blood 1951 Aug;6:740–755.

L256. Leyh F, Wendt V, Scherer R. Systemic lupus erythematosus and hyperimmunoglobulinemia E syndrome in a 13 year old girl. Z Hautkr 1985;61:611–614.

L257. Li EK, Chan MSY. Is pseudotumor cerebri in systemic lupus erythematosus a thrombotic event [letter]. J Rheumatol 1990 Jul;17(5):983–984.

L258. Li EK, Ho PC. Pseudotumor cerebri in systemic lupus erythematosus. J Rheumatol 1989 Jan;16(1):113–116.

L259. Li JZ, Steinman CR. Plasma DNA in systemic lupus erythematosus. Arthritis Rheum 1989;32:726–733.

L260. Li-Zhen P, Dauphinee MJ, Ansar Ahmed S, Talal N. Alteral natural killer and natural cellular activities in lpr mice. Scand J Immunol 1986;23:415–423.

L261. Liang M, Rogers M, Swafford J, Schur PH. The psychological impact systemic lupus erythematosus rheumatoid arthritis. Arthritis Rheum 1984 Jan;27:13.

L262. Liang MH, Meenan RE, Cathcart ES, Schur PH. A screening strategy for population studies in systemic lupus erythematosus. Series design. Arthritis Rheum 1980 Feb;23:153–157.

L263. Liang MH, Socher SA, Larson MG, Schur PH. Reliability and validity of six systems for the clinical assessment of disease activity in systemic lupus erythematosus. Arthritis Rheum 1989 Sep;32(9):1107–1118.

L264. Liang MH, Socher SA, Roberts WN, Esdaile JM. Measurement of systemic lupus erythematosus activity in clinical research. Arthritis Rheum 1988;31:817–825.

L265. Liang TJ. Gastrointestinal vasculitis and pneumatosis intestinalis due to systemic lupus erythematosus: successful treatment with pulse intravenous cyclophosphamide [case report]. Am J Med 1988 Oct;85:555–558.

L266. Liano F, Mampaso F, Garcia Martin F, Pardo A, Orte L, Teruel JL, Quereda C, Ortuno J. Allograft membranous glomerulonephritis and renal-vein thrombosis in a patient with a lupus anticoagulant factor. Nephrol Dial Transplant 1988;3: 684–689.

L267. Liao CD, Lin CY, Chen WP, Hwang BT, Tasi ST. Neonatal lupus erythematosus: report of one case. Acta Paediatrica Sinica 1989;30:191–195.

L268. Liautard JP, Sri-Wadada J, Brunel C, Jeanteur P. Structural organization of ribonucleoproteins containing small nuclear RNAs from HeLa cells. J Mol Biol 1982;162:623–643.

L269. Libertini LJ, Ausio J, Van Holde KE, Small EW. Histone hyperacetylation: its effects on nucleosome core particle transitions. Biophys J 1988;53:477–487.

L270. Libman E, Sacks B. A hitherto undescribed form of valvular and mural endocarditis. Arch Intern Med 1924 Jun;33: 701–737.

L271. Lichon FS, Sequeira W, Pilloff A, Skosey JL. Retroperitoneal fibrosis associated with systemic lupus erythematosus: a case report and brief review. J Rheumatol 1984 Jun;11(3): 373–374.

L272. Lider O, Reshef T, Beraud E, Bun-Nun A, Cohen IR. Anti-idiotypic network induced by T cell vaccination against experimental autoimmune encephalomyelitis. Science 1988;239: 181.

L273. Lidz T, Kahn RL. Toxicity of quinacrine (atabrine) for the central nervous system; experimental study on human subjects. Arch Neurol & Psychiat 1946 Sep;56:284−299.

L274. Lie JT. Medical complications of cocaine and other illicit drug abuse simulating rheumatic disease. J Rheumatol 1990; 17:736−737.

L275. Lie TH, Rothfield NF. An evaluation of the preliminary criteria for the diagnosis of systemic lupus erythematosus. Arthritis Rheum 1972 Sep−Oct;15:532−534.

L276. Lieberman E, Heuser E, Hanson V, Kornreich H, Donnell GN, Landing BH. Identical 3-year old twins with disseminated lupus erythematosus: one with nephrosis and one with nephritis. Arthritis Rheum 1968;11:22−32.

L277. Lieberman JD, Schatten S. Treatment. Disease-modifying therapies. Rheum Dis Clin N Am 1988 Apr;14(11):223−243.

L278. Lieberman R, Vrana M, Humphrey W, Chien C, Potter M. Idiotypes of inulin binding myeloma proteins localized to variable region light and heavy chains: genetic implications. J Exp Med 1977;146:1294.

L279. Liebling MR, Gold RH. Erosions of the temporomandibular joint in systemic lupus erythematosus. Arthritis Rheum 1981 Jul 24;29(7):948−950.

L280. Liebling MR, McLaughlin K, Boonsue S, Raskin J, Barnett EV. Monthly pulses of methylprednisolone in SLE nephritis. J Rheumatol 1982 Jul−Aug;9:543−548.

L281. Liebling MR, Wong C, Radosevich J, Louie JS. Specific suppression of anti-DNA production in vitro. J Clin Immunol 1988;8:362−371.

L282. Lief PD, Barland P, Bank N. Diagnosis of lupus nephritis by skin immunofluorescence, in the absence of extrarenal manifestations of systemic lupus erythematosus. Am J Med 1977 Sep;63(3):441−448.

L283. Liegler DG, Henderson ES, Hahn MA, Oliverio VT. The effect of organic acids on renal clearance of methotrexate in man. Clin Pharmacol Ther 1969;10:849−857.

L284. Lies RB, Messner RP, Williams RC Jr. Relative T-cell specificity of lymphocytotoxins from patients with systemic lupus erythematosus. Arthritis Rheum 1973 May−Jun;16:369−375.

L285. Liew CT, Kanel GC. Lupoid hepatitis and hepatocellular carcinoma (HCC). Hepatology 1985;5:1051.

L286. Lightfoot RW Jr, Hughes GRV. Significance of persisting serologic abnormalities in SLE. Arthritis Rheum 1976 Sep−Oct;19:837.

L287. Lightfoot RW Jr, Lotke PA. Osteonecrosis of metacarpal heads in systemic lupus erythematosus. Value of radiostrontium scintimetry in differential diagnosis. Arthritis Rheum 1972 Sep−Oct;15:486−492.

L288. Lillard S, Harmon C, Sharp G, Hurst D. Pulmonary manifestations in an active systemic connective tissue syndrome [abstract]. Clin Res 1977 Oct;25:590A.

L289. Lillicrap DP, Pinto M, Benford K, Ford PM, Ford S. Heterogeneity of laboratory test results for antiphospholipid antibodies in patients treated with chlorpromazine and other phenothiazines. Am J Clin Pharm 1990;6:771−775.

L290. Lillquist KB, Dyerberg J, Krogh-Jensen M. The absence of factor II in a child with systemic lupus erythematosus. Acta Pediatr Scand 1978 Jul;67:533.

L291. Lim L, Ron MA, Ormerod ID, David J, Miller DH, Logsdail SJ, Walport MJ, Hardin AE. Psychiatric and neurological manifestations in systemic lupus erythematosus. QJ Med 1988 Jan; 66(249):27−38.

L292. Lim TK, Fong KY. Hyperkalemic distal renal tubular acidosis with hyporeninemic hypoaldersteronism in a patient with systemic lupus erythematosus—a case report. Singapore Med J 1987 Dec;28(6):560−561.

L293. Lim VS, DeGowin RL, Zavala D, Kirchner PT, Abels R, Perry P, Fangman J. Recombinant human erythropoetinic treatment in pre-dialysis patients. Ann Intern Med 1989;110: 108−114.

L294. Lin CY. Improvement in steroid and immunosuppressive drug resistant lupus nephritis by intravenous prostaglandin E1 therapy. Nephron 1990;55(3):258−264.

L295. Lin CY, Hsu HC, Chang H. Improvement of histological and immunological change in steroid and immunosuppressive drug-resistant lupus nephritis by high-dose intravenous gamma globulin. Nephron 1989;53(4):303−310.

L296. Lin R, Leone JW, Cook RG, Allis CD. Antibodies specific to acetylated histones document the existence of deposition- and transcription-related histone acetylation in Tetrahymena. J Cell Biol 1989;108:1577−1588.

L297. Lin RY, Cohen-Addad N, Krey PR, Schwartz RA, de Cotis A, Lambert WC. Neonatal lupus erythematosus, multiple thromboses, and monoarthritis in a family with Ro antibody. J Am Acad Dermatol 1985;12:1022−1025.

L298. Lin RY, Landsman L, Krey PR, Lambert WC. Multiple dermatofibromas and systemic lupus erythematosus. Cutis 1986 Jan;37(1):45−49.

L299. Linares LF, Roces A, Padrino JM, Zubieta J, Castillo A. Avascular necrosis in systemic lupus erythematosus [English abstract]. Rev Clin Esp 1987 Feb;180(2):71−73.

L300. Lindahl G, Hedfors E. Lymphocytic infiltrates and epithelial HLA-DR expression in lip salivary glands in connective tissue disease patients lacking sicca: a prospective study. Br J Rheumatol 1989 Aug;28(4):293−298.

L301. Lindeman RD, Pederson JA, Matter BJ, Laughlin LD, Mandal AK. Long term azathioprine-corticosteroid therapy in lupus nephritis and idiopathic nephrotic syndrome. J Chronic Dis 1976;29(3):189−204.

L302. Lindenmayer JP, Vargas P. Toxic psychosis following use of quinacrine. J Clin Psychiat 1981;42:162−164.

L303. Linder E, Edgington TS. Antigenic specificity of antierythrocyte autoantibody responses by NZB mice: Identification and partial characterization of erythrocyte surface autoantigen. J Immunol 1972 Jun;108:1615−1623.

L304. Lindner H, Wesierska-Gadek J, Helliger W, Puschendorf B, Sauermann G. Identification of ADP-ribosylated histones by the combined use of high-performance liquid chromatography and electrophoresis. J Chromatogr 1989;472:243−249.

L305. Lindqvist KJ, Makene WJ, Shaba JD, Nantulya V. Immunofluorescence and electron microscopic studies of kidney biopsies from patients with nephrotic syndrome, possibly induced by skin lightening creams containing mercury. E Afr Med J 1974;51:168−169.

L306. Lindqvist T. Lupus erythematosus disseminatus after administration of mesantoin. Report of two cases. Acta Med Scand 1957 Aug 13;158:131−138.

L307. Lindsey GG, Orgeig S, Thompson P, Davies N, Maeder DL. Extended C-terminal tail of wheat histone H2A interacts with DNA of the "linker" region. J Mol Biol 1991;218:805−813.

L308. Lindskov R, Reymann F. Dapsone in the treatment of cutaneous lupus erythematosus. Dermatologica 1986;172(4): 214−217.

L309. Lindstedt G, Lundberg PA, Westberg G, Kaijser B. SLE nephritis and positive tests for antibodies against native DNA but negative tests for antinuclear antibodies. Lancet 1977 Jul 16;2:135.

L310. Ling BN, Bourke E, Campbell WG Jr, Delaney VB. Naproxen-induced nephropathy in systemic lupus erythematosus. Nephron 1990;54(3):249−255.

L311. Ling MHM, Perry PJ, Tsuang MT. Side effects of corticosteroid therapy. Arch Gen Psychiatry 1981;38:471−477.

L312. Linker-Israeli M, Bakke AC, Kitridou RC, Gendler S, Gillis

S, Horwitz DA. Defective production of interleukin 1 and interleukin 2 in patients with systemic lupus erythematosus (SLE). J Immunol 1983 Jun;130:2651–2655.

L313. Linker-Israeli M, Baake AC, Quismorio FP Jr, Horwitz DA. Correlation of interleukin-2 production in patients with systemic lupus erythematosus by removal of spontaneously activated suppressor cells. J Clin Invest 1985 Feb;75:762–768.

L314. Linker-Israeli M, Casteel N. Partial purification of systemic lupus erythematosus-derived factors that suppress production of interleukin-2. J Rheumatol 1988;15:952–958.

L315. Linker-Israeli M, Deans RJ, Wallace DJ, Prehn J, Ozeri-Chen T, Klinenberg JR. Elevated levels of endogenous IL-6 in systemic lupus erythematosus. A putative role in pathogenesis. J Immunol 1991;147:117–123.

L316. Linker-Israeli M, Gray JD, Quismorio FP Jr, Horwitz DA. Characterization of lymphocytes that suppress IL-2 production in systemic lupus erythematosus. Clin Exp Immunol 1988;73:236–241.

L317. Linker-Israeli M, Quismorio FP Jr, Horwitz DA. Further characterization of interleukin-2 production by lymphocytes of patients with sytemic lupus erythematosus. J Rheumatol 1988;15:1216–1222.

L318. Linker-Israeli M, Quismorio FP Jr, Horwitz DA. CD8+ lymphocytes from patients with systemic lupus erythematosus sustain, rather than suppress, spontaneous polyclonal IgG production and synergies with CD4+ cells to support autoantibody synthesis. Arthritis Rheum 1990;33:1216–1225.

L319. Linn JE, Hardin JG, Halla JT. A controlled study of ANA+RF- arthritis. Arthritis Rheum 1978 Jul–Aug;21(6):645–651.

L320. Linssenn WH, Fiselier TJ, Gabreels FJ, Wevers RA, Cuppen MP, Rotteveel JJ. Acute transverse myelopathy as the initial manifestation of probable systemic lupus erythematosus in a child. Neuropediatrics 1988;19:212–215.

L321. Linton P-J, Decker DJ, Klinman NR. Primary antibody forming cells and secondary B cells are generated from separate precursor cell subpopulations. Cell 1989;59:1049–1059.

L322. Linton PL, Rudie A, Klinman NR. Tolerance susceptibility of newly generated memory B cells. J Immunol 1991;146:4099–4104.

L323. Lipnick RN, Karsh J, Stahl NI, Blackwelder WC, Schiffman G, Klippel JH. Pneumococcal immunization in patients with systemic lupus erythematosus treated with immunosuppressives. J Rheumatol 1985 Dec;12(6):1118–1121.

L324. Lipnick RN, Tsokos GC. Immune abnormalities in the pathogenesis of juvenile rheumatoid arthritis. Clin Exp Rheumatol 1990;8:177–186.

L325. Lippman SM, Arnett FC, Conley CL, Ness PM, Myers DA, Bias WB. Genetic factors predisposing to autoimmune diseases. Autoimmune hemolytic anemia, chronic thrombocytopenic purpura, and systemic lupus erythematosus. Am J Med 1982;73:827–840.

L326. Lipsey A, Mahnovsky V. Septicemia with allescheria boydii in a patient with systemic lupus erythematosus. Lab Invest 1978;38:390.

L327. Lipsmeyer EA. Development of malignant cerebral lymphoma in a patient with systemic lupus erythematosus treated with immunosuppression. Arthritis Rheum 1972 Mar–Apr;15:183–188.

L328. Lischwe MA, Oochs RL, Reddy R, Cook RG, Yeoman LC, Tan EM, Reichlin M, Busch H. Purification and partial characterization of a nucleolar scleroderma antigen (Mr = 34,000 + 8.5) rich in Ng dimethylarginine. J Biol Chem 1985;260:14304–14310.

L329. Lishner M, Ravid M. Methyl-prednisolone pulse therapy of recurrent peritonitis and cerebritis in systemic lupus ery-

thematosus [English abstract]. Harefuah 1986 Dec;111(12):424–425.

L330. List AF, Doll DC. Thrombosis associated with procainamide-induced lupus anticoagulant. Acta Hematol 1989;82:50–52.

L331. Lister RG, File SE. The nature of lorazepam-induced amnesia. Psychopharmacology (Berlin) 1984;83(2):183–187.

L332. Liston TE, Roberts LJ. Metabolic fate of radiolabeled prostaglandin D2 in a normal human male volunteer. J Biol Chem 1985;260:13172–13180.

L333. Litsey SE, Noonan JA, O'Connor WN, Cottrill CM, Mitchell B. Maternal connective tissue disease and congenital heart block. Demonstration of immunoglobulin in cardiac tissue. N Engl J Med 1985;312:98–100.

L332a. Litvin DA, Cohen PL, Winfield JB. Characterization of warm-reactive IgG anti-lymphocyte antibodies in systemic lupus erythematosus. Relative specificity for mitogen-activated T cells and their soluble products. J Immunol 1983 Jan;130:181–186.

L334. Litwin A, Adams LE, Zimmer H. Prospective study of immunologic effects of hydralazine in hypertensive patients. Clin Pharmacol Ther 1981;29:447–456.

L335. Litwin A, Adams LE, Zimmer H, Hess EV. Immunologic effects of hydralazine in hypertensive patients. Arthritis Rheum 1981 Aug;24:1074–1078. Same as L332a.

L336. Liu S, Miller N, Waye JD. Retrograde amnesia effects of intravenous diazepam in endoscopy patients. Gastrointest Endosc 1984 Dec;30(6):340–342.

L337. Livneh A, Coman EA, Cho S, Lipstein-Kresch E. Strongyloides stercoralis hyperinfection mimicking systemic lupus erythematosus flare [letter]. Arthritis Rheum 1988 Jul;31(7):930–931.

L338. Livneh A, Halpern A, Perkins D, Lazo A, Halpern R, Diamond B. A monoclonal antibody to a cross-reactive idiotype on cationic human anti-DNA antibodies expressing lambda light chains: A new reagent to identify a potentially differential pathogenic subset. J Immunol 1987;138:123.

L339. Llach F, Koffler A, Kinck E, Massry SG. On the incidence of renal vein thrombosis in nephrotic syndrome. Arch Intern Med 1977 Mar;137:333–336.

L340. Lloyd LA, Hiltz JW. Ocular complications of chloroquine therapy. Can Med Assoc J 1965 Mar 6;92:508–513.

L341. Lloyd W, Schur PH. Immune complexes, complement, and anti-DNA in exacerbations of systemic lupus erythematosus (SLE). Medicine 1981 May;60:208–217.

L342. Lluberas-Acosta G. "Pseudolupus" [letter]. South Med J 1989 Dec;82(12):1587.

L343. Lo JS, Berg RE, Tomecki KJ. Treatment of discoid lupus erythematosus. Int J Dermatol 1989 Oct;28(8):497–507.

L344. Lobatto S, Daha MR, Breedveld FC, Pauwels EK, Evers-Schouten JH, Voetman AA, Cats A, Van Es LA. Abnormal clearance of soluble aggregates of human immunoglobulin G in patients with systemic lupus erythematosus. Clin Exp Immunol 1988;72:55–59.

L345. Lobatto S, Daha MR, Voetman AA, Evers-Schouten JH, van Es AA, Pauwels EK, van Es LA. Clearance of soluble aggregates of human immunoglobulin G in healthy volunteers and chimpanzees. Clin Exp Immunol 1987;69:133–141.

L346. Lockshin MD. Lupus pregnancy. Clin Rheum Dis 1985;11:611–632.

L347. Lockshin MD. Anti-cardiolipin antibody. Arthritis Rheum 1987;30:471.

L348. Lockshin MD. Pregnancy does not cause systemic lupus erythematosus to worsen. Arthritis Rheum 1989;32:665–670.

L349. Lockshin MD, Bonfa E, Elkon K, Druzin ML. Neonatal lupus risk to newborns of mothers with systemic lupus erythematosus. Arthritis Rheum 1988;31:697–701.

L350. Lockshin MD, Druzin ML, Goei S, Qamar T, Magid MS, Jovanovic L, Ferenc M. Antibody to cardiolipin as a predictor of fetal distress or death in pregnant patients with systemic lupus erythematosus. N Engl J Med 1985 Jul 18;313(3): 152–156.

L351. Lockshin MD, Druzin ML, Qamar T. Prednisone does not prevent recurrent fetal death in women with antiphospholipid antibody. Am J Obstet Gynecol 1989;160:439–443.

L352. Lockshin MD, Gibofsky A, Peebles CC, Gigli I, Fotino M, Hurwitz S. Neonatal lupus erythematosus with heart block: family study of a patient with anti-SS-A and SS-B antibodies. Arthritis Rheum 1983 Feb;26:210–213.

L353. Lockshin MD, Harpel PC, Druzin ML, Becker CG, Klein RF, Watson RM, Elkon KB, Reinitz E. Lupus pregnancy. II. Unusual pattern of hypocomplementemia and thrombocytopenia in the pregnant patient. Arthritis Rheum 1985;28:58–66.

L354. Lockshin MD, Qamar T, Druzin ML, Goei S. Antibody to cardiolipin, lupus anticoagulant, and fetal death. J Rheumatol 1987 Apr;14(2):259–262.

L355. Lockshin MD, Qamar T, Levy RA, Best MP. IgG but not IgM anti-phospholipid antibody binding is temperature dependent. J Clin Immunol 1988 May;8(3):188–192.

L356. Lockshin MD, Reinitz E, Druzin ML, Murrman M, Estes D. Lupus pregnancy. Case-control prospective study demonstrating absence of lupus exacerbation during or after pregnancy. Am J Med 1984;77:893–898.

L357. Lockshin ME, Eisenhauer AC, Kohn R, Weksler M, Block S, Mushlin DS. Cell-mediated immunity in rheumatic diseases. II. Mitogen responses in RA, SLE and other illnesses: Correlation with T and B lymphocyte populations. Arthritis Rheum 1975 May–Jun 18:245–250.

L358. Lockwood CJ, Romero RD, Feinberg RF, Clyne LP, Coster B, Hobbins JC. The prevalence and biologic significance of lupus anticoagulant in a general obstetric population. Am J Obstet Gynecol 1989;161:369–373.

L359. Lockwood CM, Pussell B, Wilson CB, Peters DK. Plasma exchange in nephritis. Adv Nephrol 1979;8:383–418.

L360. Lodin H. Discoid lupus erythematosus and trauma. Acta Dermatovener (Stockh) 1963;43:142–148.

L361. Loeliger A. Prothrombin as co-factor of the circulating anticoagulant in systemic lupus erythematosus? Thromb Diath Haemorrh 1959;3(2/3):237.

L362. Logar D, Kveder T, Rozman B, Dobovisek J. Possible association between anti-Ro antibodies and myocarditis or cardiac conduction defects in adults with systemic lupus erythematosus. Ann Rheum Dis 1990;49:627–629.

L363. Logue GL, Shimm DS. Autoimmune granulocytopenia. Ann Rev Med 1980;31:191–200.

L364. Loizou S, McCrea JD, Rudge AC, Reynolds A, Boyle CC, Harris EN. Measurement of anti-cardiolipin antibodies by an enzyme-linked immunosorbent assay (ELISA): standardization and quantitation of results. Clin Exp Immunol 1985 Dec; 62(3):738–745.

L365. Loizou S, Mackworth-Young CG, Cofiner C, Walport MJ. Heterogeneity of binding reactivity to different phospholipids of antibodies from patients with systemic lupus erythematosus (SLE) and with syphilis. Clin Exp Immunol 1990 May;80(2): 171–176.

L366. Loke YW, King A. Immunology of pregnancy: quo vadis? Human Reprod 1989;4:613–615.

L367. Loke YW, King A, Grabowska A. Antigenic expression by migrating trophoblast and its relevance to implantation. In: Denker HW, Aplin JD, editors. Trophoblast Invasion and Endometrial Receptivity. Novel Aspects of the Cell Biology of Embryo Implantation. New York: Plenum. Trophoblast Res 1990; 4:191–207.

L368. Lom-Orta H, Alarcon-Segovia D, Diaz-Jouanen E. Systemic lupus erythematosus. Differences between patients who do, and who do not fulfill classification criteria at the time of diagnosis. J Rheumatol 1980 Nov–Dec;7:831–837.

L369. Lom-Orta H, Diaz-Jouanen E, Alarcon-Segovia D. Lymphocytotoxic antibodies and pregnancy in systemic lupus erythematosus. Lancet 1979;1:1034–1035.

L370. Lom-Orta H, Diaz-Jouanen E, Alarcon-Segovia D. Protein-caloric malnutrition and systemic lupus erythematosus. J Rheumatol 1980 Mar–Apr;7:178–182.

L371. Long AA, Denburg DS, Carbotte RM, Singal DP, Denburg JA. Serum lymphocytotoxic antibodies and neurocognitive function in systemic lupus erythematosus. Ann Rheum Dis 1990 Apr;49(4):249–253.

L372. Looney RJ, Abraham GN, Anderson CL. Human monocytes and U937 cells bear two distinct Fc receptors for IgG. J Immunol 1986;136:1641–1647.

L373. Looney RJ, Anderson CL, Ryan DH, Rosenfeld SI. Structural polymorphism of the human platelet Fcγ receptor. J Immunol 1988;141:2680–2683.

L374. Looney RJ, Ryan DH, Takahashi K, Fleit HB, Cohen HJ, Abraham GN, Anderson CL. Identification of a second class if IgG Fc receptors on human neutrophils: A 40 kD molecule also found on eosinophils. J Exp Med 1986;163:826–836.

L375. Loor F, Forni L, Pernis B. The dynamic state of the lymphocyte membrane. Factors affecting the distribution and turnover of surface immunoglobulins. Eur J Immunol 1972;2: 203–212.

L376. Lopes Cardozo P. Treatment of lupus erythematosus by means of a splenectomy: a familial case. Nederl T Geneesk 1955;99:3271.

L377. Lopez-Acuna D, Hochberg MC, Gittelsohn AM. Do persons of Spanish-heritage have an increased mortality from systemic lupus erythematosus compared to other Caucasians? Arthritis Rheum 1982;25 Suppl:S67.

L378. Lopez-Acuna D, Hochberg MC, Gittelsohn AM. Mortality from discoid and systemic lupus erythematosus in the United States, 1968–1978. Arthritis Rheum 1982;25 Suppl:S80.

L379. Lopez-Soto A, Casals FJ, Font J, Cervera R, Ingelmo M. Detection of antiphospholipid antibodies by ELISA-method with bovine thromboplastin as antigen. Thromb Res 1989 Mar 15;53(6):623–628.

L380. Lorber A, Bovy RA, Chang CC. Sulfhydryl deficiency in connective tissue disorders: Correlation with disease activity and protein alterations. Metabolism 1971 May;20:446–455.

L381. Lorcerie B, Marchal G, Borsotti JP, Guard O, Giroud M, Dumas R, Martin F. Multiple sclerosis with biologic features of systemic lupus erythematosus: case report and anatomic study. Rev Med Intern 1989;10:471–474.

L382. Lorig K, Lonkol L, Gonzalez V. Arthritis patient education: a review of the literature. Patient Educ Counsel 1987;10: 207–252.

L383. Lortholary A, Varache N, Bouachour G, Szapiro N, Bourrier P, Alquier P. Generalized status epilepticus following ingestion of ibuprofen (Brufen) disclosing a systemic lupus erythematosus. La Revue de Medecine Interne 1990;11:243–244.

L384. Lorz HM, Frumin AM. Spontaneous remission in chronic idiopathic thrombocytopenic purpura during pregnancy. Obstet Gynecol 1961;17:362–363.

L385. Lospalluto J, Dorward B, Miller W Jr, Ziff M. Cryoglobulinemia based on interaction between a gamma macroglobulin and 79 gamma globulin. Am J Med 1962 Jan;32:142–147.

L386. Lot TY. The in vitro pharmacology of chloroquine and quinacrine. Med Biol 1986;64(4):207–213.

L387. Lot TY, Bennett T. Comparison of the effects of chloroquine, quinacrine and quinidine on autonomic neuroeffector mechanisms. Med Biol 1982 Dec;60(6):307–315.

L388. Lotke PA, Steinberg ME. Osteonecrosis of the hip and knee. Bull Rheum Dis 1985;35(2):1–8.

L389. Louderback AL, Shanbrom E. Hepatoglobulin electrophoresis. JAMA 1968 Oct 7;206:362–363.

L390. Loudon JR. Hydroxychloroquine and postoperative thromboembolism after total hip replacement. Am J Med 1988 Oct 14;85 Suppl 4A:57–61.

L391. Louie JS, Liebling MR, Nies KM. In vitro anti-DNA production by SLE following KLH immunization [abstract]. Arthritis Rheum 1984 Apr;27(4) Suppl:S39.

L392. Love PE, Santoro SA. Antiphospholipid antibodies: anticardiolipin and the lupus anticoagulant in systemic lupus erythematosus (SLE) and in non-SLE disorders. Prevalence and clinical significance. Ann Intern Med 1990 May 1;112(9):682–698.

L393. Lovy MR, Ryan PF, Hughes GR. Concurrent systemic lupus erythematosus and salmonellosis. J Rheumatol 1981;8(4):605–612.

L394. Low A, Hotze A, Krapf F, Schranz W, Manger BJ, Mahlstedt J, Wolf F, Kalden JR. The nonspecific clearance function of the reticuloendothelial system in patients with immune complex mediated diseases before and after therapeutic plasmapheresis. Rheumatol Int 1985;5(2):69–72.

L395. Lowe NJ. Photoprotection. Semin Dermatol 1990;9:78–83.

L396. Lowenstein MB, Rothfield NF. Family study of systemic lupus erythematosus: analysis of the clinical history, skin immunofluorescence, and serologic parameters. Arthritis Rheum 1977;20:1293–1303.

L397. Lozier JR, Friedlaender MH. Complications of antimalarial therapy. Int Ophthalmol Clin 1989 Fall;29(3):172–178.

L398. Luban NLC, Boeck RL, Barr O. Sickle cell anemia and systemic lupus erythematosus. J Peds 1980 Jun;96:1120.

L399. Lubbe WF. Low-dose aspirin in prevention of toxemia of pregnancy. Does it have a place? Drugs 1987;34:515–518.

L400. Lubbe WF, Butler WS, Palmer SJ, Liggins GC. Fetal survival after prednisone suppression of maternal lupus anticoagulant. Lancet 1983;1:1361–1366.

L401. Lubbe WF, Butler WS, Palmer SJ, Liggins GC. Lupus anticoagulant in pregnancy. Br J Obstet Gynaecol 1984;91:357–363.

L402. Lubbe WF, Liggins GC. Lupus anticoagulant and pregnancy. Am J Obstet Gynecol 1985 Oct 1;153(3):322–327.

L403. Lubbe WF, Palmer SJ, Butler WS, Liggins GC. Fetal survival after prednisone suppression of maternal lupus anticoagulant. Lancet 1983 Jun 18;1:1361–1363.

L404. Lubbe WF, Pattison N, Liggins G. Antiphospholipid antibodies and pregnancy. N Engl J Med 1985;313:1351.

L405. Lucas GF. A survey of platelet serology in UK laboratories (1987): an assessment of the efficacy of using chloroquine-treated platelets to distinguish between platelet-specific and anti-HLA antibodies. The UK Platelet and Granulocyte Serology Workshop Group. Clin Lab Haematol 1990;12(2):185–200.

L406. Lucas JA, Ansar Ahmed S, Casey ML, MacDonald PC. The prevention of autoantibody formation and prolonged survival in NZB/NZW F1 mice fed dehydroisoandrosterone. J Clin Invest 1985;75:2091–2093.

L407. Luce EB, Montgomery MT, Redding SW. The prevalence of cardiac valvular pathosis in patients with systemic lupus erythematosus. Oral Surg Oral Med Oral Pathol 1990 Nov;705(5):590–592.

L408. Ludmerer KM, Kissane JM. Headache, mental status changes, and death in a 36-year-old woman with lupus. Am J Med 1989;86:94–102.

L409. Ludolph A, Matz DR. Electrophysiologic changes in thalidomide neuropathy under treatment for discoid LE [English abstract] [original in German] EEG EMG 1982 Dec;13(4):167–170.

L410. Luedke CE, Cerami A. Interferon-gamma overcomes glucocorticoid suppression of cacectin/tumor necrosis factor biosynthesis by murine macrophages. J Clin Invest 1990;86:1234–1240.

L411. Luetje CM. Theoretical and practical implications for plasmapheresis in autoimmune inner ear disease. Laryngoscope 1989 Nov;99(11):1137–1146.

L412. Luger TA, Smolen JS, Chused TM, Steinberg AD, Oppenheim JJ. Human lymphocytes with either OKT4 or OKT8 phenotype produce interleukin 2 in culture. J Clin Invest 1982;70:470–473.

L413. Luhrmann R. snRNP proteins. In: Birnstiel ML. Structure and function of major and minor small nuclear ribonuclear ribonucleoprotein particles. Heidelberg, FRG: Springer Verlag, 1988:71–99.

L414. Luhrmann R. Formation of the U snRNPs. Mol Biol Reports 1990;14:183–192.

L415. Luhrmann R, Kastner B, Bach M. Structure of splicesomal snRNPs and their role in pre-mRNA splicing. Biochim Biophy Acta 1990;1087:265–292.

L415a. Lukert BP, Raisz LG. Glucocorticoid-induced osteoporosis: Pathogenesis and management. Ann Intern Med 1990;112:352–364.

L416. Lumpkin LR, Hall J, Hogan JD, Tucker SB, Jordan RE. Neonatal lupus erythematosus. A report of three cases associated with anti-Ro/ssa antibodies. Arch Dermatol 1985;121:377–381.

L417. Lunardi C, Marguerie C, Bowness P, Walport MJ. Reduction in Tγδ cell numbers and alteration in subset distribution in systemic lupus erythematosus. Arthritis Rheum 1991;34 Suppl:S162.

L418. Lund T, O'Reilly L, Hutchings P, Kanagawa O, Simpson E, Gravely R, Chandler P, Dyson J, Picard JK, Edwards A, Kioussis D, Cooke A. Prevention of insulin-dependent diabetes mellitus in non-obese diabetic mice by transgenes encoding modified I-A beta-chain or normal I-E alpha-chain. Nature 1990;345:727–729.

L419. Lundberg I, Hedfors E. Clinical course of patients with anti-RNP antibodies. J Rheumatol 1991;18:1511–1519.

L420. Lundberg PO, Werner I. Trigeminal sensory neuropathy in systemic lupus erythematosus. Acta Neurol Scand 1972;48(3):330–340.

L421. Lundquist I, Ahren B, Hakanson R, Sundler F. Quinacrine accumulation in pancreatic islet cells of rat and mouse: relationship to functional activity and effects on basal and stimulated insulin secretion. Diabetologia 1985 Mar;28(3):161–166.

L422. Luo SF, Huang CC, Wang JW. Neonatal lupus erythematosus: report of a case. Taiwan I Hsueh Hui Tsa Chih-J Formosan Med Assoc 1989;88:832–835.

L423. Luqman M, Johnson P, Trowbridge I, Bottomly K. Differential expression of the alternatively spliced exons of murine CD45 in T_h1 and T_h2 cell clones. Eur J Immunol 1991;21:17–22.

L424. Lurie DP, Kanaleh MR. Pulse corticosteroid therapy for refractory thrombocytopenia in systemic lupus erythematosus. J Rheumatol 1982 Mar–Apr;9:311–314.

L425. Luster MI, Boorman G, Dean JH, Luebke RW, Lawson LD. Effects of in utero exposure to diethylstilbestrol on the immune response in mice. Toxicol Appl Pharmacol 1979;47:287–293.

L426. Luster MI, Boorman GA, Dean JH, Luebke RW, Lawson LD. The effects of adult exposure to diethylstilbestrol in the mouse: Alterations in immunological functions. J Reticuloendothel Soc 1980;28:561.

L427. Lutz-Freyermuth C, Keene JD. The U1 RNA-binding site of the U1 small nuclear ribonucleoprotein (snRNP)-associated A protein suggests a similarity with U2 snRNPs. Mol Cell Biol 1989;9:2975–2982.

L428. Lutz-Freyermuth C, Query CC, Keene JD. Quantitative determination that one of the two potential RNA-binding domains of the A protein component of the U1 small nuclear ribonucleoprotein complex binds with high affinity to stem-loop II of U1 RNA. Proc Natl Acad Sci USA 1990;87:6393–6397.

L429. Lutzker LG, Alavi A. Bone and marrow imaging in sickle cell disease: diagnosis of infarction. Semin Nucl Med 1976 Jan;6(1):83–93.

L430. Lutzker S, Rothman P, Pollack R, Coffman R, Alt FW. Mitogen-and IL-4-regulated expression of germ-line Ig 2b transcripts: Evidence for directed heavy chain class switching. Cell 53:177–184 (1988).

L431. Lydyard PM, Isenberg D, De Sousa B, Mackenzie L, Cooke A. A cross-reactive idiotype on anti-DNA and lymphocytotoxic antibodies. Clin Exp Immunol 1987;67:500–506.

L432. Lynch A, Marlar R, Murphy J, Davila G, Emlen W. Prospective study of the value of antiphospholipid antibodies in predicting pregnancy outcome [abstract]. Arthritis Rheum 1991;34:S95.

L433. Lynch RG. Immunoglobulin-specific suppressor T cells. Adv Immunol 1987;40:135–151.

L434. Lyon JM. Acute lupus erythematosus. Am J Dis Child 1993 Mar;45:572–583.

L435. See L341.

M

M1. Ma AS, Soltani K, Bristol LA, Bernstein JE, Sorensen LB. Cutaneous immunofluorescence studies in adult rheumatoid arthritis in sun-exposed and non-sun-exposed areas. Int J Dermatol 1984 May;23(4):269–272.

M2. Maas D, Schubothe H. Lupus erythematosus-like syndrome with antimitochondrial antibodies [original in German]. Dtsch Med Wochenschr 1973 Jan 26;98:131–139.

M3. Macchia D, Parronchi P, Piccinni MP, Simonelli C, Mazzetti M, Ravina A, Milo D, Maggi E, Romagnani S. In vitro infection with HIV enables human CD4⁺ T cell clones to induce noncognate contact-dependent polyclonal B cell activation. J Immunol 1991;146:3413–3418.

M4. MacDonald HR, Schneider R, Lees RK, Howe RC, Acha-Orbea H, Festenstein H, Zinkernagel RM, Hengartner H. T-cell receptor V beta use predicts reactivity and tolerance to Mlsa-encoded antigens. Nature 1988;322:40–45.

M5. Mac DS, Kumar R, Goodwin DW. Anterograde amnesia with oral lorazepam. J Clin Psychiatry 1985 Apr;46(4):137–138.

M6. MacGregor RR, Sheagren JN, Lipsett MB, Wolff SM. Alternate-day prednisone therapy. Evaluation of delayed hypersensitivity responses, control of disease and steroid side effects. N Engl J Med 1969 Jun 26;280:1427–1431.

M7. Mach PS, Auscher C, Le Go A, Pasquier C, Delbarre F. Study of alpha 2 macroglobulin, alpha 1 antitrypsin and their antitryptic activity in the serum in rheumatic disease and collagen diseases [original in French]. Eur Etud Clin Biol 1972 May;17:462–470.

M8. Machold KP, Smolen JS. Interferon-gamma induced exacerbation of systemic lupus erythematosus. J Rheumatol 1990 Jun;17(6):831–832.

M9. Mackay IR. Lupoid hepatitis and primary biliary cirrhosis. Autoimmune diseases of the liver? Bull Rheum Dis 1968;18:487–494.

M10. Mackay IR. The effects in active chronic (lupoid) hepatitis of three long-term "suppressive" treatment regimes. Gastroenterology 1971;60:693.

M11. Mackay IR. Autoimmunity and the liver. Clinical Aspects of Autoimmunity 1988;2:8–17.

M12. Mackay IR, Cowling DC, Hurley TH. Drug induced autoimmune disease: Hemolytic anemia and lupus cells after treatment with methyldopa. Med J Aust 1968 Dec 7;2:1047–1050.

M13. Mackay IR, DeGail P. Thymic "germinal centres" and plasma cells in systemic lupus erythematosus. Lancet 1963 Sep 28;3:667.

M14. Mackay IR, Goldstein G, McConchie IH. Thymectomy in systemic lupus erythematosus. BMJ 1963 Sep 28;5360:792–793.

M15. Mackay IR, Perry BT. Autoimmunity in human thyroid disease. Aust Ann Med 1960 May;9:84–92.

M16. Mackay IR, Smalley M. Results of the thymectomy in SLE: observations on clinical course and serological reactions. Clin Exp Immunol 1966;1:129–138.

M17. Mackay IR, Taft LI, Cowling DC. Lupoid hepatitis and the hepatic lesions of systemic lupus erythematosus. Lancet 1959 Jan 10;1(7063):65–69.

M18. Mackay IR Weiden S, Ungar B. Treatment of active chronic hepatitis and lupoid hepatitis with 6-mercaptopurine and azathioprine. Lancet 1964;1:899–902.

M19. Mackay IR, Wood IJ. Lupoid hepatitis: comparison of 22 cases with other types of chronic liver disease. Q J Med 1962 Oct;31:485–507.

M20. Mackay IR, Wood IJ. The course and treatment of lupoid hepatitis. Gastroenterology 1963 Jul;45:4–13.

M21. Mackenzie AH. Pharmacologic actions of 4-aminoquinoline compounds. Am J Med 1983 Jul 18;75 Suppl 1A:5–10.

M22. Mackenzie AH. Dose refinements in long-term therapy of rheumatoid arthritis with antimalarials. Am J Med 1983 Jul;75 Suppl 1A:40–45.

M23. Mackenzie AH, Parker W, Gonzalez L. New sialographic criteria for Sjogren's syndrome [abstract]. Arthritis Rheum 1969;12:679.

M24. Mackenzie AH, Szilagyi PJ. Light may provide energy for retinal damage during chloroquine treatment. Arthritis Rheum 1968;11:496–497.

M25. MacKenzie MR, Creevy CC. Hemolytic anemia with cold detectable IgG antibodies. Blood 1970 Nov;36:549.

M26. Mackey JP, Barnes T. Clofazimine in the treatment of discoid lupus erythematosus. Br J Dermatol 1974 Jul;92:93–96.

M27. Mackiewicz A, Marcinkowska-Pieta R, Ballou S, Mackiewicz S, Kushner I. Microheterogeneity of alpha 1-acid glycoprotein in the detection of intercurrent infection in systemic lupus erythematosus. Arthritis Rheum 1987 May;30(5):513–518.

M27a. Mackworth-Young C. Antiphospholipid antibodies: more than just a disease marker? Immunol Today 1990;11:60–65.

M28. Mackworth-Young CG, Chan JKH, Bunn CC, Hughes GRV, Gharavi AE. Complement fixation by anti-dsdna antibodies in SLE: Measurement by radioimmunoassay and relationship with disease activity. Ann Rheum Dis 1986;45:314–318.

M29. Mackworth-Young CG, David J, Morgan SH, Hughes GRV. A double blind, placebo controlled trial of intravenous methylprednisolone in systemic lupus erythematosus. Ann Rheum Dis 1988;47:496–502.

M30. Mackworth-Young CG, Harris EN, Steere AC, Rizvi R, Malawista SE, Hughes GR, Gharavi AE. Anticardiolipin antibodies in Lyme disease. Arthritis Rheum 1988 Aug;31(8):1052–1056.

M31. Mackworth-Young CG, Loizou S, Walport MJ. Primary antiphospholipid syndrome: features of patients with raised anticardiolipin antibodies and no other disorder. Ann Rheum Dis 1989;48(5):362–367.

M32. Mackworth-Young CG, Morgan SH, Hughes GRV. Intravenous methylprednisolone in the treatment of systemic lupus erythematosus. Scand J Rheum 1983 Sep 16;54 Suppl:16–18.

M33. Mackworth-Young CG, Parke AL, Morley KD, Folherby K, Hughes GRV. Sex hormones in male patients with systemic lupus erythematosus. Eur J Rheum Inflam 1983;6:228–232.

M34. Mackworth-Young CG, Sabbaga J, Schwartz RS. Idiotypic markers of polyclonal B cell activation: Public idiotypes shared by monoclonal antibodies derived from patients with systemic lupus erythematosus and leprosy. J Clin Invest 1987; 79:572–581.

M35. Mackworth-Young CG, Walport MJ, Hughes GRV. Thrombocytopenia in a case of systemic lupus erythematosus: repeated administration of "pulse" methylprednisolone. Br J Rheumatol 1984;23:298–300.

M36. MacLean K, Robinson HS. Sjogren's Syndrome. Can Med Assoc J 1954 Dec;71:597–599.

M37. MacNeill A, Grennan DM, Ward D, Dick W. Psychiatric problems in SLE. Br J Psychiatry 1976 Mar;128:442–445.

M38. MacSween RNM, Dalakos TG, Jasani MK, Boyle JA, Buchanan WW, Goudie RB. A clinicoimmunological study of serum and synovial fluid antinuclear factors in rheumatoid arthritis and other arthritides. Clin Exp Immunol 1968;3: 17–24.

M39. MacSween RNM, Dalakos TK, Jasani MK, Wilson ME, Buchanan WW, Goudie RB. Antinuclear factors in synovial fluids. Lancet 1967;1:312–314.

M40. Madaio MP, Carlson J, Cataldo J, Ucci A, Migliorini P, Pankewycs O. Murine monoclonal anti-DNA antibodies bind directly to glomerular antigens and form immune deposits. J Immunol 1987;138:2883–2893.

M41. Madden JF. Comparison of muscle biopsies and bone marrow examinations in dermatomyositis and lupus erythematosus. Arch Dermat & Syph 1950 Aug;62:192–205.

M42. Maddison PJ. Overlap syndromes, mixed connective tissue disease and eosinophilic fascitis. Curr Opin Rheumatol 1989; 1:523–528.

M43. Maddison PJ. Anti-Ro antibodies and neonatal lupus. Clin Rheumatol 1990;9:116–122.

M44. Maddison PJ, Bell DA. HLA antigens in relationship to serologic subsets of systemic lupus erythematosus. Arthritis Rheum 1980;23:714–715.

M45. Maddison PJ, Isenberg DA, Goulding NJ, Leddy J, Skinner RP. Anti La(SSB) identifies a distinctive subgroup of systemic lupus erythematosus. Br J Rheumatol 1988;27:27–31.

M46. Maddison PJ, Mogavero H, Provost TT, Reichlin M. The clinical significance of autoantibodies to a soluble cytoplasmic antigen in systemic lupus erythematosusand other connective tissue diseases. J Rheumatol 1979;6:189–195.

M47. Maddison PJ, Mogavero H, Reichlin M. Antibodies to nuclear ribonucleoprotein. J Rheumatol 1978 Winter;5: 407–411.

M48. Maddison PJ, Provost TT, Reichlin M. Serological findings in patients with 'ANA-Negative' systemic lupus erythematosus. Medicine 1981 Mar;60(2):87–94.

M49. Maddison PJ, Reichlin M. Quantitation of precipitating antibodies to certain soluble nuclear antigens in systemic lupus erythematosus. Their contribution to hyperglobulinemia. Arthritis Rheum 1977;20:819–824.

M50. Maddison PJ, Reichlin M. Deposition of antibodies to a soluble cytoplasmic antigen in the kidneys of patients with systemic lupus erythematosus. Arthritis Rheum 1979 Aug; 22(8):858–863.

M51. Maddisson PJ, Skinner RP, Vlahoyeannopoulos P, Brennand DM, Dough D. Antibodies to nRNP, Sm, Ro (SSA), and La (SSB) detected by ELISA: Their specificity and interrelationship in connective tissue disease sera. Clin Exp Immunol 1985;62: 337–345.

M52. Maddison JP, Sukhum P, Williamson DP, Campion BC. Echocardiography and fetal heart sounds in the diagnosis of fetal heart block. Am Heart J 1979;98:505–509.

M53. Madhok R, Zoma R, Capell H. Fatal exacerbation of systemic lupus erythematosus after treatment with griseofulvin. Br Med J 1985;291:249–250.

M54. Madi N, Paccaud JP, Steiger G, Schifferli JA. Immune complex binding efficiency of erythrocyte complement receptor 1 (CR1). Clin Exp Immunol 1991;84:9–15.

M55. Madi N, Steiger G, Estreicher J, Schifferli JA. Defective immune adherence and elimination of hepatitis B surface antigen/antibody complexes in patients with mixed essential cryoglobulinemia type II. J Immunol 1991;147:495–502.

M56. Madow BP. Use of hydroxychloroquine in the treatment of hyperlipidemia, hypercholesterolemia, and (sic) sludging of blood [abstract]. Arteriosclerosis 1990;10:754a.

M57. Madsen JR, Anderson BV. Lupus erythematosus and pregnancy. Obstet Gynecol 19691;8:492–494.

M58. Maegawa H, Kobayashi M, Watanabe N, Ishibashi O, Takata T, Shigeta Y. Inhibition of down regulation by chloroquine in cultured lymphocytes (RPMI-1788 line). Diabetes Res Clin Pract 1985 Oct;1(3):145–153.

M59. Magalhaes MM, Magalhaes MC. Effects of ovariectomy and estradiol administration on the adrenal macrophage systemic of the rat. Cell Tissue Res 1984;138:559–564.

M60. Magil AB, Putterman ML, Ballon HS, Chan V, Lirenman DS, Rae A, Sutton RAL. Prognostic factors in diffuse proliferative lupus glomerulonephritis. Kidney Int 1988;34:511–517.

M61. Magil AB, Tyler M. Tubulo-interstitial disease in lupus nephritis: a morphometric study. Histopathol 1984 Jan;8:81–87.

M62. Magilavy DB, Rothstein JL. Spontaneous production of tumor necrosis factor alpha by Kupffer cells of MRL/lpr mice. J Exp Med 1988;168:789–794.

M63. Maguire A. Amodiaquine hydrochloride in the treatment of chronic discoid lupus erythematosus. Lancet 1962 Mar 31; 1:665–667.

M64. Mahajan SK, Ordonez NG, Feitelson PJ, Lim VS, Spargo BH, Katz AI. Lupus nephritis without clinical renal involvement. Medicine 1977 Nov;56:493–501.

M65. Mahana W, Guilbert B, Avrameas S. Suppression of anti-DNA antibody production in MRL mice by treatment with anti-idiotypic antibodies. Clin Exp Immunol 1987;70: 538–545.

M66. Mahowald ML, Dalmasso AP. Lymphocyte destruction by antibody-dependent cellular cytotoxicity mediated in vitro by antibodies in serum from patients with systemic lupus erythematosus. Ann Rheum Dis 1982;41:593–598.

M67. Mahowald ML, Weir EK, Ridley DJ, Messner RP. Pulmonary hypertension in systemic lupus erythematosus: effect of vasodilators on pulmonary hemodynamics. J Rheumatol 1985;12: 773–777.

M68. Maier WP, Gordon DS, Howard RF, Saleh MN, Miller SB, Lieberman JD, Woodlee PM. Intravenous immunoglobulin therapy in systemic lupus erythematosus-associated thrombocytopenia. Arthritis Rheum 1990 Aug;33(8):1233–1239.

M69. Majer RV, Hyde RD. High dose intravenous immunoglobulin in the treatment of autoimmune hemolytic anemia. Clin Lab Haemat 1988;10:391–395.

M70. Makila U-M, Viinikka L, Ylikorkala O. Increased thromboxane A2 production but normal prostacyclin by the placenta in hypertensive pregnancies. Prostaglandins 1984;27:87–95.

M71. Makin M, Fumiwara M, Watanabe H. Studies on the mechanisms of the development of lupus nephritis in BXSB mice. I. Analyses of immunological abnormalities at the onset period. J Clin Lab Immunol 1987;22:127–131.

M72. Makino M, Fujiwara M, Aoyagi T, Umezawa H. Immunosuppressive activities of deoxyspergualin. I. Effect of the longterm administration of the drug on the development of murine lupus. Immunopharmacology 1987;14:107–113.

M73. Makoul GT, Robinson DR, Bhalla AK, Glimcher LH. Prostaglandin E$_2$ inhibits the activation of cloned T cell hybridomas. J Immunol 1985;134:2645–2650.

M74. Makover D, Freundlich B, Zurier RB. Relapse of systemic lupus erythematosus in a patient receiving cyclosporin A. J Rheumatol 1988 Jan;15(1):117–119.

M75. Maksymowych W, Russell AS. Antimalarials in rheumatology: efficacy and safety. Semin Arthritis Rheum 1987 Feb; 16(3):206–221.

M76. Malas D, Weiss S. Progressive multifocal leukoencephalopathy and cryptococcal meningitis with systemic lupus erythematosus and thymoma. Ann Neurol 1977 Feb;1:188–191.

M77. Malave I, Cuadra C. Impaired function of peripheral lymphocytes in systemic lupus erythematosus. Intern Arch Allergy Appl Immunol (NY) 1977;55:412–419.

M78. Malave I, Searles RP, Montano J, Williams RC Jr. Production of tumor necrosis factor/cachectin by peripheral blood mononuclear cells in patients with systemic lupus erythematosus. Int Arch Allergy Appl Immunol 1989;89:355–361.

M79. Malia RG, Kitchen S, Greaves M, Preston FE. Inhibition of activated protein C and its cofactor protein S by antiphospholipid antibodies. Br J Haematol 1990;76:101–107.

M80. Malinow MR, Bardana EJ Jr, Pirofsky B, Craig S, McLaughlin P. Systemic lupus erythematosus-like syndrome in monkeys fed alfalfa sprouts: Role of a nonprotein amino acid. Science 1982 Apr 23;216(4544):415–417.

M81. Malinow MR, McLaughlin P, Bardana EJ Jr, Craig S. Elimination of toxicity from diets containing alfalfa seeds. Food Chem Toxicol 1984;22:583–587.

M82. Malipiero UV, Levy NS, Gearhart PJ. Somatic mutation in anti-phosphorylcholine antibodies. Immunol Rev 1987;96: 59–74.

M83. Malleson P, Petty RE, Fung M, Candido PM. Reactivity of antinuclear antibodies with histones and other antigens in juvenile rheumatoid arthritis. Arthritis Rheum 1989;32: 919–923.

M84. Malleson P, Petty RE, Nadel H, Dimmick JE. Functional asplenia in childhood onset systemic lupus erythematosus. J Rheumatol 1988;15:1648–1652.

M85. Malleson PN. The role of renal biopsy in childhood onset systemic lupus erythematosus: a viewpoint. Clin Exp Rheumatol 1989;7:563–566.

M86. Mamula MJ, O'Brien CA, Harley JB, Hardin JA. The Ro ribonucleoprotein particle: induction of autoantibodies and the detection of Ro RNAs among species. Clin Immunol Immunopathol 1989;52:435–446.

M87. Manchester D, Margolis HS, Sheldon RE. Possible association between maternal indomethacin therapy and primary pulmonary hypertension of the newborn. Am J Obstet Gynecol 1976;126:467–469.

M88. Mandel MJ, Carr R, Weston WL, Sams WM Jr, Harbeck RJ, Krueger GG. Anti-native DNA antibodies in discoid lupus erythematosus. Arch Dermatol 1972 Nov;106(5):668–670.

M89. Mandell BF, Raps EC. Severe systemic hypersensitivity reaction to ibuprofen occurring after prolonged therapy. Am J Med 1987 Apr;82(4):817–820.

M90. Mandler R, Birch RE, Polmar SH, Kammer GM, Rudolph SA. Abnormal adenosine-induced immunosuppression and CAMP metabolism in T lymphocytes of patients with systemic lupus erythematosus. Proc Natl Acad Sci USA 1982;79:7542–7546.

M91. Manilow MR, Bardana EJ Jr, Goodnight SH. Pancytopenia during ingestion of alfalfa seeds. Lancet 1981;1:615.

M92. Manilow MR, Bardana EJ Jr, Piroksky B, Craig S, McLaughlin P. Systemic lupus erythematosus-like syndrome in monkeys

fed alfalfa sprouts: Role of a nonprotein amino acid. Science 1982;216:415–416.

M93. Manku MS, Horrobin DF. Chloroquine, quinine, procaine, quinidine, tricyclic antidepressants, and methylxanthines as prostaglandin agonists and antagonists. Lancet 1976 Nov 20; 2(7995):1115–1117.

M94. Manly SW, Knight A, Adams DD. The thyrotropin receptor. Springer Semin Immunopathol 1982;5:413–431.

M95. Mannik M. Pathophysiology of circulating immune complexes. Arthritis Rheum 1982;25:783–787.

M96. Mannik M. Mechanisms of tissue deposition of immune complexes [review]. J Rheumatol 1987 Jun;14 Suppl 13: 35–42.

M97. Mannik M. Immune complexes. In: Lahita RG, editor. Systemic lupus erythematosus. New York: Wiley, 1987:333–351.

M98. Mannik M, Arend WP. Fate of preformed immune complexes in rabbits and rhesus monkeys. J Exp Med 1971;134 Suppl:19S-31S.

M99. Mannik M, Arend WP, Hall AP, Gilliland BC. Studies on antigen-antibody complexes. I. Elimination of soluble complexes from rabbit circulation. J Exp Med 1971;133:713–739.

M100. Mannik M, Striker GE. Deposition and removal of glomerular immune complexes. Relationships to the mononuclear phagocyte system. In: Cummings S, Michael AF, Wilson CB, editors. Immune Mechanisms of Renal Disease. New York: Plenum 1982:151–165.

M101. Manning PJ, Watson RM, Margolskee DJ, Williams VC, Schwartz JI, O'Byrne PM. Inhibition of exercise-induced bronchoconstriction by MK-571, a potent leukotriene D4-receptor antagonist. N Engl J Med 1990;323:1736–1739.

M102. Mannucci PM, Canciani MT, Mari D, Meucci P. The varied sensitivity of partial thromboplastin and prothrombin time reagents in the demonstration of the lupus-like anticoagulant. Scand J Haematol 1979;22(5):423–432.

M103. Manny N, Datta SK, Schwartz RS. Synthesis of IgM by cells of NZB and SWR mice and their crosses. J Immunol 1979 Apr; 122(4):1220–1227.

M104. Manohar V, Brown E, Leiserson WM, Chused TM. Expression of Lyt-1 by a subset of B lymphocytes. J Immunol 1982 Aug;129(2):532–538.

M105. Manoharan A, Gibson L, Rush B, Feery BJ. Recurrent venous thrombosis with a "lupus" coagulation inhibitor in the absence of systemic lupus. Aust N Z J Med 1977 Aug;7: 422–426.

M106. Manoharan A, Gottlieb P. Bleeding in patients with lupus anticoagulant. Lancet 1984 Jul 21;2:171.

M107. Manoharan A, Williams NT, Sparrow R. Acquired megakaryocytic thrombocytopenia: report of a case and review of literature. Q J Med 1989;70:234–252.

M108. Manoussakis MN, Papadopoulos GK, Drosos AA, Moutsopoulos HM. Soluble interleukin 2 receptor molecules in the serum of patients with autoimmune diseases. Clin Immunol Immunopathol 1989;50:321–332.

M109. Manoussakis MN, Tzioufas AG, Silis MP, Pange PJ, Goudevenos J, Moutsoupoulos HM. High prevalence of anticardiolipin and other autoantibodies in a health elderly population. Clin Exp Immunol 1987 Sep;69(3):557–565.

M110. Manser T, Gefter ML. The molecular evolution of the immune response: idiotype specific suppression indicates that B cells express germ-line-encoded V genes prior to antigenic stimulation. Eur J Immunol 1986;16:1439–1444.

M111. Manser T, Wysocki LJ, Margolies MN, Gefter ML. Evolution of antibody variable region structure during the immune response. Immunol Rev 1987;96:141–162.

M112. Mansilla-Tinoco R, Harland SJ, Ryan PJ, Bernstein RM, Dollery CT, Hughes GRV, Bulpitt CJ, Morgan A, Jones JM. Hydralazine, antinuclear antibodies, and the lupus syndrome. Br Med J 1982 Mar 27;284:936–939.

M113. Manthei U, Nickells MW, Barnes SH, Ballard LL, Cui WY, Atkinson JP. Identification of a C3b/iC3b binding protein of rabbit platelets and leukocytes. A CR1-like candidate for the immune adherence receptor. J Immunol 1988;140: 1228–1235.

M114. Manthorpe R, Andersen V, Jensen OA, Oxholm P, Prause JU, Schiodt M. Editorial comments to the four sets of criteria for Sjogren's syndrome. Scand J Rheumatol 1986;61 Suppl: 31–35.

M115. Manthorpe R, Bendixen G, Schioler H, Viderbaek A. Jaccoud's syndrome: A nosographic entity associated with systemic lupus erythematosus. J Rheumatol 1980 Mar–Apr;7(2): 169–177.

M116. Manthorpe R, Ellig H, van der Meulen JJ, Sorensen SF. Two fatal cases of mixed connective tissue disease: description of case histories terminating as progressive systemic sclerosis. Scand J Rheumatol 1980;9(1):7–10.

M117. Manthorpe R, Morling N, Platz P, Ryder LP, Svejgard A, Thomsen M. HLA-D antigen frequencies in Sjogren's syndrome: differences between primary and secondary forms. Scand J Rheumatol 1981;10:124–128.

M118. Manthorpe R, Teppo AM, Bendixen G, Wegelius O. Antibodies to SS-B in chronic inflammatory connective tissue diseases. Relationship with HLA-Dw2 and HLA-Dw3 antigens in primary Sjogren's syndrome. Arthritis Rheum 1982 Jun;25(6): 662–667.

M119. Manzi S, Urbach AH, McCune AB, Altman HA, Kaplan SS, Medsger TA Jr, Ramsey-Goldman R. Systemic lupus erythematosus in a boy with chronic granulomatous disease: Case report and review of the literature [brief report]. Arthritis Rheum 1991 Jan;34(1):101–105.

M120. Marabani M, Zoma A, Hadley D, Sturrock RD. Transverse myelitis occurring during pregnancy in a patient with systemic lupus erythematosus. Ann Rheum Dis 1989 Feb;48(2): 160–162.

M121. Maragou M, Siotsiou F, Sfondouris H, Nicolia Z, Vayopoulos G, Dantis P. Late-onset systemic lupus erythematosus presenting as polymyalgia rheumatica. Clin Rheumatol 1989 Mar;8(1):91–97.

M122. Marchesi SL, Aptekar RG, Steinberg AD, Gralnick HR, Decker JL. Urinary fibrin split products in lupus nephritis: correlation with other parameters of renal disease. Arthritis Rheum 1974 Mar–Apr;17:158–164.

M123. Marciniak E, Romond EH. Impaired catalytic function of activated protein C: a new in vitro manifestation of lupus anticoagulant. Blood 1989;74:2426.

M124. Marcus RM, Grayzel AI. A lupus antibody syndrome associated with hypernephroma. Arthritis Rheum 1979 Dec; 22(12):1396–1398.

M125. Marcus ZH, Hess EV. Antisperm antibodies in patients with systemic lupus erythematosus [letter]. Arthritis Rheum 1980 Mar;24(3):569–570.

M126. Marcus-Bagley D, Alper CA. Personal communication.

M127. Marghescu S. Rosacea like dermatitis—Lupus variant. Hautarzt (Ger) 1988;392:382–383.

M128. Margolies MN, Wysocki LJ, Sato VL. Immunoglobulin idiotype and anti-anti-idiotype utilize the same variable region genes irrespective of antigen specificity. J Immunol 1983;130: 515–517.

M129. Margolius A Jr, Jackson DP, Ratnoff OD. Circulating anticoagulants: A study of 40 cases and review of literature. Medicine (Balt) 1961 May;40:145–202.

M130. Maricq HR, LeRoy EC. Patterns of finger capillary abnormalities in connective tissue disease by "wide-field" microscopy. Arthritis Rheum 1973 Sep–Oct;16:619–628.

M131. Mariette X, Gozlan J, Clerc D, Bisson M, Morinet F. Detection of Epstein-Barr virus DNA by in situ hybridization and polymerase chain reaction in salivary gland biopsy specimens from patients with Sjögren's syndrome. Am J Med 1991;90: 286–294.

M132. Marino C, Cook P. Danazol for lupus thrombocytopenia. Arch Intern Med 1985 Dec;145(12):2251–2252.

M133. Marino CT, Pertschuk LP. Pulmonary hemorrhage in systemic lupus erythematosus. Arch Intern Med 1981 Feb;141: 201–203.

M134. Marion C, Cook P. Danazol for lupus thrombocytopenia. Arch Intern Med 1988;108:703–706.

M135. Marion TN, Bothwell AL, Briles DE, Janeway CA Jr. IgG anti-DNA autoantibodies within an individual autoimmune mouse are the products of clonal selection. J Immunol 1989 Jun 15;142(12):4269–4274.

M136. Marion TN, Lawton AR, Kearney JF, Briles DE. Anti-DNA autoantibody in (NZB/NZW) F1 mice are clonally heterogeneous but the majority share a common idiotype. J Immunol 1982;128:668.

M137. Marion TN, Tillman DM, Jou N. Interclonal and intraclonal diversity among anti-DNA antibodies from an (NZBXNZW) F_1 mouse. J Immunol 1990;145:2322–2332.

M138. Markenson JA, Lockshin MD, Fuzesi L, Warburg M, Joachim C, Morgan JW. Suppressor monocytes in patients with systemic lupus erythematosus. Evidence of suppressor activity associated with a cell-free soluble product of monocytes. J Lab Clin Med 1980 Jan;95:40–48.

M139. Markowitz SS, McDonald CJ, Fethiere W, Kerzner MS. Occupational acroosteolysis. Arch Dermatol 1971;106: 219–233.

M140. Marks JS. Chloroquine retinopathy: is there a safe daily dose? Ann Rheum Dis 1982 Feb;41(1):52–58.

M141. Marks JS, Power BJ. Is chloroquine obsolete in treatment of rheumatoid disease? Lancet 1979 Feb 17;1(8112): 371–373.

M142. Markusse HM, Haan J, Tan WD, Breedveld FC. Anterior spinal artery syndrome in systemic lupus erythematosus. Br J Rheumatol 1989 Aug;28(4):344–346.

M143. Markusse HM, Vecht JC. Is neurologic disease with positive lupus serology sufficient for a diagnosis of systemic lupus erythematosus? Br J Rheumatol 1986 Aug;25(3):302–305.

M144. Marlow AA, Peabody HD Jr, Nickel WR. Familial occurrence of systemic lupus erythematosus. JAMA 1960;173: 1641–1643.

M145. Marmont A, Damasio E. The place of indomethacin in the treatment of SLE. In: Atti del Simposio Internationazionale su Recenti Acquisizioni nella Terapia Antireumatica nonsteroidea. Turin: Minerva Medica, 1965:219–258.

M146. Marmont AM, Rossi F, Damasio E. Indomethacin in the treatment of rheumatic lupus erythematosus. In: Proceedings of an International Symposium on Non-Steroidal Anti-Inflammatory Drugs. (Milan) Series No. 82, Excerpta Medica International Congress, New York: Excerpta Medica Foundation, 1964:364–372.

M147. Marmont AM. Systemic Lupus Erythematosus [original in Italian]. Rome: L Pozzi, 1980.

M148. Marrack PC, Kushnir E, Kappler J. A maternally inherited superantigen encoded by a mammary tumor virus. Nature 1991;349:524–526.

M149. Marschalko M, Dobozy E, Daroczy J, Gyimesi E, Horvath A. Subacute cutaneous lupus erythematosus: a study of 15 cases. Orvosi Hetilap 1989;130:2623–2628.

M150. Marsh FP, Vince FP, Pollock DJ, Blandy JP. Cyclophosphamide necrosis of bladder causing calcification, contracture and reflux; Treated by colocystoplasty. Br J Urol 1971;43: 324–332.

M151. Marshall AJ, McGraw ME, Barritt DW. Positive antinuclear factor tests with prazocin. BMJ 1979 Jan 20;1:165–166.

M152. Marshall JB, Kretschmar JM, Gerhardt DC, Winship DH, Winn D, Treadwell EL, Sharp GC. Gastrointestinal manifestations of mixed connective tissue disease. Gastroenterology 1990 May;98(5 Pt 1):1232–1238.

M153. Marshall PJ, Kulmacz RJ, Lands WEM. Constraints on prostaglandin biosynthesis in tissues. J Biol Chem 1987;262:3510–3517.

M154. Marten RH, Blackburn EK. Lupus erythematosus; Clinical hematological studies in seventy-seven cases. Arch Dermatol 1956;73:1–14.

M155. Marten RH, Blackburn EK. Lupus erythematosus: A five year follow-up of 77 cases. Arch Dermatol 1961 Mar;83:430–436.

M156. Martens H, Zamber R, Rubin RL, Starkebaum GA. Drug-induced lupus (DLE) caused by ophthalmic timolol. Arthritis Rheum 1991;34 Suppl:R20.

M157. Martens J, Demedts M, Vanmeenen MT, Dequeker J. Respiratory muscle dysfunction in systemic lupus erythematous. Chest 1983 Aug;83:170–175.

M158. Martenstein H. Subacute lupus erythematosus and tubercular cervical adenopathy. Treatment with plasmochin [original in German]. Zbl Haut Geschlechtskr 1928;27:248–249.

M159. Martin JN, Files JC, Blake PG, Norman PH, Martin RW, Hess LW, Morrison JC, Wiser WL. Plasma exchange for preeclampsia. I. Postpartum use for severe preeclampsia-eclampsia with HELLP syndrome. Am J Obstet Gynecol 1990;162:126–137.

M160. Martin L, Chalmers IM. Photosensitivity to fluorescent light in a patient with systemic lupus erythematosus. J Rheumatol 1983 Oct;10(5):811–812.

M161. Martin LJ, Bergan RL, Dobrow HR. Delayed onset chloroquine retinopathy: case report. Ann Ophthalmol 1978 Jun;10(6):723–726.

M162. Martin LM, Pauls JD, Ryan JP, Fritzler MJ. Antibodies to both histone and centromere define a subset of patients with severe scleroderma [abstract]. Clin Invest Med 1990;13:798.

M163. Martin RW, Duffy J, Engel AG, Lie JT, Bowles CA, Moyer TP, Gleich GJ. The clinical spectrum of the eosinophilia-myalgia syndrome associated with L-tryptophan ingestion. Clinical features in 20 patients and aspects of pathophysiology. Ann Intern Med 1990;113:124–134.

M164. Martin T, Knapp AM, Muller S, Pasquali JL. Polyclonal human rheumatoid factors cross-reacting with histone H3: characterization of an idiotope on the H3 binding site. J Clin Immunol 1990;10:211–219.

M165. Martinez-Cairo Cueto S, Ramirez-Lacayo ML, Veladiz-Saint-Martin P, Lopez-Roman M. Deterioration of intracellular destruction capacity of S. aureus in children with systemic lupus erythematosus. Arch Invest Med (Mex) 1986 Jan–Mar;17(1):25–36.

M166. Martinez-Cordero E, Lopez Zepeda J, Andrade-Ortega L, Selman M. Mutilans arthropathy in systemic lupus erythematosus. Clin Exp Rheumatol 1989 Jul–Aug;7(4):427–429.

M167. Martinez Lacasa JT, Palacin AV, Pac Ferranz V, Moga Sampere I, Santin Cerezales M, Fernandez-Nogues F. Systemic lupus erythematosus presenting as Salmonella Enteritidis bacteremia [letter]. J Rheumatol 1990:18():785.

M168. Martinez-Lavin M, Vaughan JH, Tan EM. Autoantibodies and the spectrum of Sjogren's syndrome. Ann Intern Med 1979 Aug;91(2):185–190.

M169. Martini A, Ravelli A, Viola S, Burgio RG. Systemic lupus erythematosus with Jaccoud's arthropathy mimicking juvenile rheumatoid arthritis. Arthritis Rheum 1987 Sep;30(9):1062–1064.

M170. Martins CR, Squiquera HL, Diaz LA. Pemphigus vulgaris and pemphigus foliaceus. Current Problems Dermatol 1989;1(2):31–61.

M171. Martorell J, Vilella R, Borche L, Rojo I, Vives J. A second signal for T cell mitogenesis provided by monoclonal antibodies CD45 (T200). Eur J Immunol 1987;17:1447–1451.

M172. Maruyama N, Furukawa F, Nakai Y, Saski Y, Ohta K, Ozaki S, Hirose S, Shirai T. Genetic studies of autoimmunity in New Zealand mice. IV.Contribution of NZB and NZW genes to the spontaneous occurrence of retroviral gp70 immune complexes in (NZB × NZW)F1 hybrid and the correlation to renal disease. J Immunol 1983 Feb;130(2):740–746.

M173. Masi AT. Family, twin, and genetic studies: a general review illustrated by systemic lupus erythematosus. Population studies of the Rheumatic Diseases. Bennet PH, Wood PHN, editors. Proceedings of the Third International Symposium, New York. International Congress series No 148. Amsterdam, Excerpta Medica Foundation 1968:267–286.

M174. Masi AT. Clinical epidemiologic perspective of systemic lupus erythematosus. In: Lawrence RC, Shulman LE, editors. Epidemiology of the rheumatic diseases. New York: Gower Medical Publishing Ltd, 1984:145.

M175. Masi AT, D'Angelo WA, Shulman LE. Comparative mortality of the diffuse connective tissue diseases (systemic lupus erythematosus, polyarteritis, systemic sclerosis, and dermatomyositis): An epidemiologic survey [abstract]. Arthritis Rheum 1966 Jun;9:523.

M176. Masi AT, Hartmann WH, Hahn BH, Abbey H, Shulman LE. Hashimoto's disease. A clinicopathological study with matched controls. Lack of significant associations with other "autoimmune" disorders. Lancet 1965 Jan 16;1:123–126.

M177. Masi AT, Kaslow RA. Sex effects in systemic lupus erythematosus. A clue to pathogenesis. Arthritis Rheum 1978 May;21:480–484.

M178. Mason JC, Venables PJW, Smith PR, Maini RN. Characterization of non-histone nuclear proteins cross reactive with purified rheumatoid factors. Ann Rheum Dis 1985 May;44:287–293.

M179. Mass D, Schubothe H, Sennekamp J, Genth E, Maerker-Alzer G, Droeser M, Hartl PW, Schumacher K. On the question of drug-induced pseudo-LE syndrome: Preliminary results in 58 cases [original in German]. Dtsch Med Wochenschr 1975 Jul;100:155–1557.

M180. Masson PL, Deline M, Cambiaso CL. Circulating immune complexes in normal human pregnancy. Nature 1977;266:542.

M181. Mastaglia FL, Papadimitrion JM, Dawkins RL, Beveridge B. Vacuolar myopathy associated with chloroquine, lupus erythematosus and thymoma. J Neurol Sci 1977 Dec;34:315–328.

M182. Masys DR, Bajaj SP, Rapaport SI. Activation of human factor VII by activated factors and IX and X. Blood 1982 Nov;60:1143–1150.

M183. Matei I, Ghyka G, Savi I, Tudor A. Correlation of serum interferon with some clinical and humoral signs of systemic lupus erythematosus. Med Interne 1990;28:289–294.

M184. Mathews MB, Francoeur AM. La antigen recognizes and binds to the 3'-oligouridylate tail of a small RNA. Mol Cell Biol 1984;4:1134–1140.

M185. Mathews MB, Reichlin M, Hughes GRV, Bernstein RM. Anti-theonyl tRNA synthetase, a second myositis related autoantibody. J Exp Med 1984;160:420–434.

M186. Mathieu DDP, Mura CV, Frado LLY, Woodcock CLF, Stollar BD. Differing accessibility in chromatin of the antigenic sites of regions 1–58 and 63–125 of histone H2B. J Cell Biol 1981; 91:135–141.

M187. Mathur AK, Gatter RA. Chorea as the initial presentation of oral contraceptive induced systemic lupus erythematosus [letter]. J Rheumatol 1988 Jun;15(6):1042–1043.

M188. Matis LA, Fry AM, Cron RQ, Cotterman MM, Dick RF, Bluestone JA. Structure and specificity of a class II MHC alloreactive T cell receptor heterodimer. Science 1989;245: 746–749.

M189. Matsanuga A, Miller BC, Cottam GL. Dehydroisoandrosterone prevention of autoimmune disease in NZB/W F1 mice: lack of an effect on associated immunological abnormalities. Biochim Biophys Acta 1989;992:265–271.

M190. Matsiota P, Druet P, Dosquet P, Guilbert B, Avrameas S. Natural autoantibodies in systemic lupus erythematosus. Clin Exp Immunol 1987;69:79–88.

M191. Matsumaga A, Miller BC, Cottam CL. Dehydroepiandrosterone prevention of autoimmune disease in NZB/NZW F1 mice: Lack of an effect on associated immunological abnormalities. Biochem Biophys Acta 1989;15:265–271.

M192. Matsumoto N, Ishihara T, Fujii H, Makamura H, Uchino F, Miwa S. Fine structure of the spleen in autoimmune hemolytic anemia associated with systemic lupus erythematosus. Tohoku J Exp Med 1978 Mar;124:223–232.

M193. Matsumura O, Kawashima Y, Kato S, Sanaka T, Teraoka S, Kawai T, Honda H, Fichinoue S, Takahashi K, Toma K, Ota K, Sugino N. Therapeutic effect of cyclosporin in thrombocytopenia associated with autoimmune disease. Transplant Proceed 1988 20 Suppl;4:317–322.

M194. Matsuoka C, Liouris J, Andrianakos A, Papademetriou C, Karvountizis G. Systemic lupus erythematosus and myelofibrosis. Clin Rheumatol 1989;8:402–407.

M195. Matsuoka I, Suzuki T. Mapacrine-induced elevation of cyclic GMP levels and acceleration of reversal of ADP-induced aggregation in washed rabbit platelets. J Cyclic Nucleotide Protein Phosphor Res 1983;9(4–5):341–353.

M196. Matsuoka LY, Wortsman J, Pepper JJ. Acute arthritis during isotretinoin treatment for acne. Arch Intern Med 1984 Sep;144(9):1870–1871.

M197. Matsuoka M, Yoshida K, Maeda T, Usuda S, Sakano H. Switch Circular DNA formed in cytokine-treated mouse splenocytes: Evidence for intramolecular DNA deletion in immunoglobulin class switching. Cell 1990;62:135–142.

M198. Matsuura E, Igarashi Y, Fujimoto M. Anticardiolipin cofactor(s) and differential diagnosis of autoimmune disease. Lancet 1990;336:177–178.

M199. Matsuyama T, Anderson P, Daley JF, Schlossman S, Morimoto C. CD4+CD45R+ cells are preferentially activated through the CD2 pathway. Eur J Immunol 1988;18: 1473–1476.

M200. Matsuzawa Y, Hostetler KY. Studies on drug-induced lipidosis: subcellular localization of phospholipid and cholesterol in the liver of rats treated with chloroquine or 4,4'bis (diethylaminoethoxy)alpha, beta-diethyldiphenylethane. J Lipid Res 1980 Feb;21(2):202–214.

M201. Matsuzawa Y, Hostetler KY. Inhibition of lysosomal phospholipase A and phospholipase C by chloroquine and 4, 4' bis(diethylaminoethoxy) alpha, beta-diethylidphenylethane. J Biol Chem 1980 Jun 10;255(11):5190–5194.

M202. Mattaj IW. Cap trimethylation of U snRNA is cytoplasmic and dependent on U snRNP protein binding. Cell 1986;46: 905–911.

M203. Mattaj IW. Functions of the abundant U snRNPs. In: Birnstiel ML, editor. Structure and function of major and minor small nuclear ribonuclear ribonucleoprotein particles. Heidelberg FRG: Springer Verlag, 1988:100–114.

M204. Matter L, Wilhelm JA, Nyffenegger T, Parisot RF, De Robertis EM. Molecular characterization of ribonucleoprotein antigens bound by antinuclear antibodies; a diagnostic evaluation. Arthritis Rheum 1982;25:1278–1283.

M205. Matthay RA, Schwartz MI, Petty TL, Stanford RE, Gupta RS, Salus SA, Steigerwald JC. Pulmonary manifestations of systemic lupus erythematosus: Review of twelve cases of acute lupus pneumonitis. Medicine 1975 Sep;54:397–409.

M206. Matthews CNA, Saihan EM, Warin RP. Urticaria-like lesions associated with systemic lupus erythematosus: response to dapsone. Br J Dermatol 1978 Oct;99(4):455–457.

M207. Matthews JB, Potts AJ, Hamburger J, Scott DG, Struthers G. An immunohistochemical study of lymphocyte subsets and expression of glandular HLA-DR in labial salivary glands from patients with symptomatic xerostomia, rheumatoid arthritis and systemic lupus erythematosus. Scand J Rheumatol 1986; 61 Suppl:56–60.

M208. Matthews JB, Potts AJ, Hamburger J, Struthers G, Scott DG. Immunoglobulin producing cells in labial salivary glands of patients with rheumatoid arthritis and systemic lupus erythematosus. J Oral Path 1986 Nov;15(10):520–523.

M209. Mattioli M, Reichlin M. Characterization of a soluble nuclear ribonucleoprotein antigen reactive with SLE sera. J Immunol 1971;107:1281–1290.

M210. Mattioli M, Reichlin M. Physical association of two nuclear antigens and mutual occurrence of their antibodies: the relationship of the Sm and RNA protein (Mo) systems in SLE sera. J Immunol 1973;110:1318–1324.

M211. Mattioli M, Reichlin M. Heterogeneity of RNA protein antigens reactive with sera of patients with systemic lupus erythematosus. Description of a cytoplasmic nonribosomal antigen. Arthritis Rheum 1974 Jul–Aug;17:421–429.

M212. Matveikov GP, Titova IP, Kaliia ES, Dosin IuM. Immunopathological manifestations of systemic lupus erythematosus and their correction during long-term dispensary observation. Ter Arkh 1987;59:27–31.

M213. Mauff G, Alper CA, Dawkins R, Doxiadis G, Giles CM, Hauptmann G, Rittner C, Schneider PM. C4 nomenclature statement (1190). Complement & Inflammation 1990;7: 261–268.

M214. Maul GG, French BT, van Veurooij WJ, Jiminez SA. Topoisomerase I identified by scleroderma 70 antisera: enrichment of topoisomerase I at the centromere in mouse mitotic cells before anaphase. Proc Natl Acad Sci USA 1986;83:5145–5149.

M215. Maumenee AE. Retinal lesions in lupus erythematosus. Am J Ophthal 1940 Sep;23:971.

M216. Maury CP, Teppo AM. Tumor necrosis factor in the serum of patients with systemic lupus erythematosus. Arthritis Rheum 1989;32:146–150.

M217. Maury CP, Teppo AM. Cachectin/tumor necrosis factor-alpha in the circulation of patients with rheumatic disease. Int J Tissue Reactions 1989;11:189–193.

M218. Maury CP, Teppo AM, Wegelius O. Relationship between urinary sialylated saccharides, serum amyloid A protein and C-reactive protein in rheumatoid arthritis and systemic lupus erythematosus. Ann Rheum Dis 1982 Jun;41:268–271.

M219. Mayer JW, Antoine JE, deHoratius RJ, Messner RP. Aseptic necrosis in systemic lupus erythematosus: Early detection by radionuclide scan. Report of case. Rocky Mt Med J 1977 Nov–Dec:74(6):324–326.

M220. Mayer MM. Complement, past and present. Harvey Lett 1978;72:139–193.

M221. Mayou SC, Wojnarowska F, Lovell CR, Asherson RA, Leigh IM. Anticardiolipin and antinuclear antibodies in discoid lupus erythematosus—their clinical significance. Clin Exp Dermatol 1988 Nov;13(6):389–392.

M222. Mazza G, Ollier P, Comme G, Moinier D, Rocca-Serra J, Van Rietschoten J, Theze J, Fougereau M. A structural basis for the internal image in the idiotypic network; antibodies against synthetic Ab2-D regions cross-react with the original antigen. Ann Immunol 1985;136D:259.

M223. McAllister G, Amara SG, Lerner MR. Tissue-specific expression and cDNA cloning of N: a novel snRNP-associated polypeptide. Proc Natl Acad Sci USA 1988;85:5296–5300.

M224. McAllister G, Roby-Shemkovitz A, Amara SG, Lerner MR. cDNA sequence of the rat U snRNP-associated protein N: description of a potential Sm epitope. Embo J 1989;8: 1177–1181.

M225. McAllister HA, Ferrans VJ, Hall RJ, Strickman NE, Bossart MI. Chloroquine-induced cardiomyopathy. Arch Pathol Lab Med 1987 Oct;111(10):953–956.

M226. McCain GA, Bell DA, Chodirker WB, Komar RR. Antibody to extractable nuclear antigen in the rheumatic diseases. J Rheumatol 1978 Winter;5(4):399–406.

M227. McCarty GA, Lister KA, Kendrick DG, Bias WB, Petri MA, Reveille JD, Arnett FC. Autoantibodies to cardiolipin (aCL) and to phosphatidyl serine (aPS) and HLA-DQ associations in Mexican-American and Black patients with systemic lupus erythematosus (SLE). Arthritis Rheum [abstract]. In press.

M228. McCarty GA, Rice JR, Bembe ML, Pisetsky DS. Independent expression of autoantibodies in SLE. J Rheumatol 1982; 9:691–695.

M229. McCauliffe DP, Zappi E, Lieu TS, Michalak M, Sontheimer RD, Capra JD. A human Ro/SS-A autoantigen is the homologue of calreticulin and is highly homologous with onchocercal RAL-1 antigen and an aplasia "memory molecule." J Clin Invest 1990;86:332–335.

M230. McChesney EW, Nachod FC, Tainter ML. Rationale for treatment of lupus erythematosus with antimalarials. J Invest Derm 1957 Aug;29(2):97–104.

M231. McClary AR, Meyer E, Weitzman EL. Observations on the role of depression in some patients with disseminated lupus erythematosus. Psychosomat Med 1955 Jul–Aug;17(4): 311–321.

M232. McCluskey RT. Lupus nephritis. In: Sommers SC, editor. Kidney Pathology Decennial 1966–1975. New York: Appleton-Century-Crofts 1975:435–670.

M233. McCluskey RT. Evidence for an immune complex disorder in systemic lupus erythematosus (SLE). Am J Kidney Dis 1982 Jul;2 Suppl 1:119–125.

M234. McCluskey RT. The value of the renal biopsy in lupus nephritis. Arthritis Rheum 1982 Jul;25:867–876.

M235. McCluskey RT, Bhan AK. Cell-mediated mechanisms in renal diseases. Kidney Int 1982 May;21 Suppl;S6-S12.

M236. McCluskey RT, Feinberg R. Vasculitis in primary vasculitides, granulomatoses and connective tissue diseases. Human Pathol 1983 Apr;14:305–315.

M237. McCollum CN, Sloan ME, Davidson AM, Giles GR. Ruptured hepatic aneurysm in systemic lupus erythematosus. Ann Rheum Dis 1979 Aug;38(4):396–398.

M238. Mc Combe PA, Chalk JB, Pender MP. Familial occurrence of multiple sclerosis with thyroid disease and systemic lupus erythematosus. J Neurol Sci 1990 Jul;97(2–3):163–171.

M239. McCombe PA, McLeod JG, Pollard JD, Guo YP, Ingall TJ. Peripheral sensorimotor and autonomic neuropathy associated with systemic lupus erythematosus. Clinical, pathological and immunological features. Brain 1987 Apr;110(Pt 2): 533–549.

M240. McConkey DJ, Orrenius S, Jondal M. Cellular signalling in programmed cell death (apoptosis). Immunol Today 1990; 11:120–121.

M241. McCoombs RP, Patterson JF. Factors influencing the course and prognosis of systemic lupus erythematosus. N Engl J Med 1959 Jun 11;260:1195–1204.

M242. McCormack GD, Barth WF. Quinidine induced lupus syndrome. Semin Arthritis Rheum 1985; 15:73–79.

M243. McCormack GD, Barth WF. Congenital complete heart block with maternal primary Sjogren's syndrome. South Med J 1985;78:471.

M244. McCormack LS, Elgart ML, Turner ML. Annular subacute cutaneous lupus erythematosus responsive to dapsone. J Am Acad Dermatol 1984;11:397–401.

M245. McCormick DL. Anticarcinogenic activity of quinacrine in the rat mammary gland. Carcinogenesis 1988;9:175–178.

M246. McCormick JN, Day J. The association of rheumatoid factor with antinuclear factor activity. Lancet 1963 Sep 14;2: 554–557.

M247. McCormick JN, Faulk WP, Fox H, Fudenberg HH. Immunohistological and elution studies of the human placenta. J Exp Med 1971;133:1–18.

M248. McCoubrey-Hoyer A, Okarma TB, Holman HR. Partial purification and characterization of plasma DNA and its relation to disease activity in SLE. Am J Med 1984;77:23–34.

M249. McCoy KL, Kendrick L, Chused TM. Tolerance defects in New Zealand Black and New Zealand Black × New Zealand White F1 mice. J Immunol 1986;136:1217–1222.

M250. McCracken M, Benson EA, Hickling P. Systemic lupus erythematosus induced by aminoglutethimide. BMJ 1980 Nov 8;281:1254.

M251. McCrea JM, Robinson P, Gerrard JM. Mepacrine (quinacrine) inhibition of thrombin-induced platelet responses can be overcome by lysophosphatidic acid. Biochim Biophys Acta 1985 Oct 17;842(2–3):189–194.

M252. McCue CM, Mantakas ME, Tingelstad JB, Ruddy S. Congenital heart block in newborns of mothers with connective tissue disease. Circulation 1977;56:82–90.

M253. McCuiston CF, Moser KM. Studies in pericarditis. I. Differentiation of the acute idiopathic form from that occurring in disseminated lupus. Am J Cardiol 1959 Jul;4:42–55.

M254. McCuiston CH, Schoch EP Jr. Possible discoid lupus erythematosus in newborn infant. Report of case with subsequent development of acute systemic lupus erythematosus in mother. Arch Dermatol 1954;70:782–785.

M255. McCune AB, Weston WL, Lee LA. Maternal and fetal outcome in neonatal lupus erythematosus. Ann Intern Med 1987; 106:518–523.

M256. McCune WJ, Dunne RB, Millard J, Gilson BK, Fox DA. Two year follow-up of patients with severe systemic lupus (SLE) treated with pulse cyclophosphamide [abstract]. Arthritis Rheum 1990 Sep;33(9) Suppl:S103.

M257. McCune WJ, Fox D. Intravenous cyclophosphamide therapy of severe SLE. Rheum Dis Clin North Am 1989 Aug;15(3): 455–477.

M258. McCune WJ, Golbus J, Zeldes W, Bohlke P, Dunne R, Fox DA. Clinical and immunologic effects of monthly administration of intravenous cyclophosphamide in severe systemic lupus erythematosus. N Engl J Med 1988 Jun 2;318(22): 1423–1431.

M259. McCune WJ, MacGuire A, Aisen A, Gebarski S. Identification of brain lesions in neuropsychiatric systemic lupus erythematosus by magnetic resonance scanning. Arthritis Rheum 1988 Feb;31(2):159–166.

M260. McCune WJ, MacGuire AM, Aisen AM. Improved identification of focal brain lesions in cerebral lupus by magnetic resonance imaging [abstract]. Arthritis Rheum 1985 Apr; 28(4) Suppl:S23.

M261. McCurdy D, Kovalesky A, Katz AR, Turner M, Bernstein B. Intravenous pulse cyclophosphamide therapy (IVCY) for childhood lupus nephritis (LN) [abstract]. Arthritis Rheum 1989 Jan;32(1) Suppl:R20.

M262. McCurdy D, Lehman TJA, Hanson V, Sherry D, King K, Bernstein B. Lupus nephritis in childhood: A retrospective study of renal outcome in childhood SLE [abstract]. Arthritis Rheum 1984 Apr;27 Suppl:S17.

M263. McCurdy DK, Lehman TJA, Bernstein B, Hanson V, King

KK, Nadorra R, Landing BH. Lupus nephritis: Prognostic factors in children. Pediatrics. In press.

M264. McDonald E, Jarrett MP, Schiffman G, Grayzel AI. Persistence of pneumococcal antibodies after immunization in patients with systemic lupus erythematosus. J Rheumatol 184; 11:306–308.

M265. McDonald EM, Mann AH, Thomas HC. Interferons as mediators of psychiatric morbidity. An investigation in a trial of recombinant alpha-interferon in hepatitis B carriers. Lancet 1987 Nov 21;2(8569):1175–1178.

M266. McDonald J, Fam A, Paton T, Senn J. Allopurinol hypersensitivity in a patient with coexistent systemic lupus erythematosus and tophaceous gout. J Rheumatol 1988;15(5): 865–868.

M267. McDonald K, Hutchinson M, Bresnihan B. The frequent occurrence of neurological disease in patients with late-onset systemic lupus erythematosus. Br J Rheumatol 1984 Aug; 23(3):186–189.

M268. McDougal JS, Hubbard M, Strobel PL, McDuffie FC. Comparison of five assays for immune complexes in the rheumatic diseases. Performance characteristics of the assays. J Lab Clin Med 1982;100:705–719.

M269. McDougal JS, Kennedy MS, Kalyanaraman VS, McDuffie F. Failure to demonstrate (cross reacting) antibodies to human T lymphotropic viruses in patients with rheumatic diseases. Arthritis Rheum 1985;28:1170–1174.

M270. McDougal JS, McDuffie FC. Immune complexes in man: detection and clinical significance. Adv Clin Chem 1985;24: 1–60.

M271. McDougall AC, Horsfall WR, Hede JE, Chaplin AJ. Splenic infarction and tissue accumulation of crystals associated with the use of clofazamine (Lamprene B663) in the treatment of pyoderma gangrenosum. Br J Dermatol 1980;102:227–230.

M272. McDuffie FC. Bone marrow depression after drug therapy in patients with systemic lupus erythematosus. Ann Rheum Dis 1965 May;24:289.

M273. McDuffie FC. Relationship between immune response to hydralazine and to deoxyribonucleoprotein in patients receiving hydralazine. Arthritis Rheum 1981;24:1079–1081.

M274. McDuffie FC, Blondin C, Golden HE. Immunologic factors in lupus erythematosus cell formation. May Clin Proc 2969; 44:620–629.

M275. McFadden N. PUVA-induced lupus erythematosus in a patient with polymorphous light eruption. Photodermatol 1984;1:148–150.

M276. McFarland HI, Bigley NJ. Sex-dependent, early cytokine production by NK-like spleen cells following infection with the D variant of encephalomyocarditis virus. Viral Immunol 1989;2:205–214.

M277. McGalliard J, Bell AL. Acquired Brown's syndrome in systemic lupus erythematosus: another ocular manifestation [case report]. Clin Rheumatol 1990;9(3):399–400.

M278. McGee CD, Makowski EL. Systemic lupus erythematosus in pregnancy. Am J Obstet Gynecol 1970;107:1008–1012.

M278a. McGehee WG, Patch MJ, Klotz T, Feinstein DI. Thrombosis and the LE anticoagulant: resistance to the effect of PGE1 in patients with recent thrombosis [abstract]. Blood 1982;60 Suppl 1:217a.

M279. McGehee WG, Patch MJ, Lingao JU, Feinstein DI. Detection of the lupus anticoagulant: A comparison of the kaolin clotting time (KCT) with the tissue thromboplastin inhibition (TTI) test [abstract]. Blood 1983 Nov;62(5) Suppl:276a.

M280. McGehee Harvey A, Shulman LE, Tumulty AP, Lockard Conley C, Schoenrich EH. Systemic lupus erythematosus: Review of the literature and clinical analysis of 138 cases. Medicine 1954 Dec;33(4):291–437.

M281. McGhee JD. The structure of interphase chromatin. In:

Risley MS, ed. Chromosome Structure and Function. New York: Van Nostrand Reinhold Company, 1986:1–38.

M282. McGhee JD, Felsenfeld G. Nucleosome structure. Ann Rev Biochem 1980; 49:1115–1156.

M283. McGhee JD, Nickol JM, Felsenfeld G, Rau DC. Histone hyperacetylation has little effect on the higher order folding of chromatin. Nucleic Acids Res 1983; 11:4065–4075.

M284. McGill NW, Gow PJ. Nailfold capillaroscopy: a blinded study of its discriminatory value in scleroderma, systemic lupus erythematosus and rheumatoid arthritis. Aust NZ J Med 1986 Aug;16(4):457–460.

M285. McGrath H Jr, Bak E, Michalski JP. Ultraviolet-A light prolongs survival and improves immune function in (New Zealand Black × New Zealand White) F₁ hybrid mice. Arthritis Rheum 1987;30:557–561.

M286. McGrath H Jr, Biundo JJ Jr. A longitudinal study of high and los avidity antibodies to double stranded DNA in systemic lupus erythematosus. Arthritis Rheum 1985;28:425–430.

M287. McGrath H Jr, Scopelitis E, Nesbitt LT Jr. Subacute cutaneous lupus erythematosus during psoralen ultraviolet A therapy [letter]. Arthritis Rheum 1990 Feb;33(2):302–303.

M288. McHugh N, James I, Maddison P. Clinical significance of antibodies to a 68kDa U1RNP polypeptide in connective tissue disease. J Rheumatol 1990 Oct;17(10):1320–1328.

M289. McHugh NJ, Campbell GJ, Landreth JJ, Laurent MR. Polyarthritis and angioimmunoblastic lymphadenopathy. Ann Rheum Dis 1987 Jul;46(7):555–558.

M290. McHugh NJ, Maddison PJ. HLA-DR antigens and anticardiolipin antibodies in patients with systemic lupus erythematosus [letter]. Arthritis Rheum 1989 Dec;32(12):1623–1624.

M291. McHugh NJ, Maddison PJ, MacCleod TIF, Dean SG, James IE, Goulding NJ, Tan RSH. Papular lesions and cutaneous lupus erythematosus: A comparative clinical and histological study using monoclonal antibodies. J Rheumatol 1988;15: 1097–1103.

M292. McHugh NJ, Maymo J, Skinner RP, James I, Maddison PJ. Anticardiolipin antibodies, livedo reticularis, and major cerebrovascular and renal disease in systemic lupus erythematosus. Ann Rheum Dis 1988 Feb;47(2):110–115.

M293. McHugh NJ, Reilly PA, McHugh LA. Pregnancy outcome and autoantibodies in connective tissue disease. J Rheumatol 1989;16:42–46.

M294. McIlvanie DK, Dittman WA. Chlorambucil in treatment of SLE. Med Tribune 1962 Oct 8;2.

M295. McInerney MF, Clough JD, Senitzer D, Cathcart MK. Two distinct subsets of patients with systemic lupus erythematosus. Clin Immunol Immunopathol 1988;49:116–132.

M296. McIntosh RM, Kulvinskas C, Kaufman DB. Cryoglobulins II. The biological and chemical properties of cryoproteins in acute post streptococcal glomerulonephritis. Int Arch Allergy Appl Immunol 1971;41(5):700–715.

M297. McIntyre JA. In search of trophoblast-lymphocyte cross-reactive (TLX) antigens. Am J Reprod Immunol Microbiol 1988;17:100–110.

M298. McIntyre JA, Faulk WP. Allotypic trophoblast-lymphocyte cross reactive (TLX) cell surface antigens. Hum Immunol 1982;4:27.

M299. McKay DG. Hematologic evidence of disseminated intravascular coagulation in eclampsia. Obstet Gynecol Surv 1972; 27:399.

M300. McKeever U, Mordes JP, Greiner DL, Appel MC, Rozing J, Handler ES, Rossini AA. Adoptive transfer of autoimmune diabetes and thyroiditis to thymic rats. Proc Natl Acad Sci USA 1990;87:7618–7622.

M301. McKenna CH, Schroeter AL, Kierland RR, Stilwell GG, Pien FD. The fluorescent treponemal antibody absorbed (FTA-

ABS) test beading phenomenon in connective tissue diseases. Mayo Clin Proc 1973;48:545–548.

M302. McKenna CH, Wieman KC, Shulman LE. Oral contraceptives, rheumatic disease, and autoantibodies [abstract]. Arthritis Rheum 1969;12:313–314.

M303. McKenzie AW, Stoughton RB. Method for comparing percutaneous absorption of steroids. Arch Dermatol 1962 Nov; 86:606–610.

M304. McKenzie SA, Selley JA, Agnew JE. Secretion of prednisolone into breast milk. Arch Dis Child 1975;50:894–896.

M305. McLaughlin J, Gladman DD, Urowitz MB, Bombardieri C, Farewell VT, Cole E. Kidney biopsy in systemic lupus erythematous: II. Survival, analysis according to biopsy results. Arthritis Rheum 1991;34:1268–1273.

M306. McLean RH, Winkelstein JA. Genetically determined variation in the complement system: Relationship to disease. J Pediatr 1984;105:179–188.

M307. McLelland J, Jack W. Phenytoin/dexamethasone interaction a clinical problem. Lancet 1978 May 20;1:1096.

M308. McLeod B, Lewis E, Schnitzer T, Katz R, Korbet S, Neighbour A, Wong W. Therapeutic immunoadsorption of anti-native DNA antibodies in SLE: Clinical studies with a device utilizing monoclonal anti-idiotypic antibody [abstract]. Arthritis Rheum 1988 Apr;31(4) Suppl:S15.

M309. McMillan R. Chronic idiopathic thrombocytopenic purpura. N Engl J Med 1981 May 7;304:1135–1147.

M310. McNamara MK, Ward RE, Kohler H. Monoclonal idiotope vaccine against Streptococcus pneumonia infection. Science 1984;226:1325.

M311. McNeil HP, Chesterman CN, Krilis SA. Anticardiolipin antibodies and lupus anticoagulants comprise separate antibody subgroups with different phospholipid binding characteristics. Br J Haemost 1989;73:506.

M312. McNeil HP, Chesterman CN, Krilis SA. Immunology and clinical importance of antiphospholipid antibodies. Adv Immunol 1991;49:193–280.

M313. McNeil HP, Gavaghan TP, Krilis SA, Geczy AP, Chesterman CN. HLA-DR antigens and anticardiolipin antibodies [letter]. Clin Exp Rheumatol 1990 Jul–Aug;8(4):425–426.

M314. McNeil HP, Hunt JE, Krilis SA. New aspects of anticardiolipin antibodies [editorial]. Clin Exp Rheumatol 1990 Nov–Dec;8(6):525–527.

M315. McNeil HP, Simpson RJ, Chesterman CN, Krilis SA. Antiphospholipid antibodies are directed against a complex antigen that includes a lipid-binding inhibitor of coagulation: beta 2-glycoprotein I (apolipoprotein H). Proc Natl Acad Sci USA 1990 Jun;87(11):4120–4124.

M316. McNeilage LJ, Whittingham S, Jaack I, Mackay IR. Molecular analysis of the RNA and protein components recognized by anti-La(SS-B) autoantibodies. Clin Exp Immunol 1985;62: 685–695.

M317. McNevin S, MacKay M. Chlorprothixene-induced systemic lupus erythematosus. J Clin Psychopharmacol 1982 Dec;2:411–412.

M318. McPhaul JJ Jr. Cryoimmunoglobulinemia in patients with primary renal disease and systemic lupus erythematous. I. IgG and DNA binding assessed by co-precipitation. Clin Exp Immunol 1978 Jan;31:131–140.

M319. McPhaul JJ Jr, Montgomery WR. Cryoimmunoglobulinemia in patients with renal disease. II. Attempts to demonstrate that cryoprecipitates contain autoantibodies and/or antigen. Clin Exp Immunol 1981 Jun;44:560–566.

M320. McShane DJ, Porta J, Fries JF. Comparison of therapy in severe systemic lupus erythematosus employing stratification techniques. J Rheumatol 1978 Spring;5(1):51–58.

M321. Medal LS, Lisker R. Circulating anticoagulants in disseminated lupus erythematosus. Br J Haemost 1959 Jul;5:284–293.

M322. Meddings J, Grennan DM. The prevalence of systemic lupus erythematosus (SLE) in Dunedin. N Z Med J 1980;91: 205.

M323. Medeiros LJ, Kaynor B, Harris NL. Lupus lymphadenitis: Report of a case with immunohistologic studies on frozen section. Human Pathol 1989; 20:295–299.

M324. Medicus RG, Melamed J, Arnaout MA. Role of human factor I and C3b receptor in the clearance of surface-bound C3bi molecules. Eur J Immunol 1983;13:465–470.

M325. Medina F, Fraga A, Lavalle C. Salmonella septic arthritis in systemic lupus erythematosus. The importance of chronic carrier state. J Rheumatol 1989 Feb;16(2):203–208.

M326. Medof ME. Complement-dependent maintenance of immune complex solubility. In: Rother K, Till GO, editors. The Complement System. Berlin: Springer Verlag, 1988:418.

M327. Medof ME, Iida K, Mold C, Nussenzweig V. Unique role of the complement receptor CR1 in the degradation of C3b associated with immune complexes. J Exp Med 1982;156: 1739–1754.

M328. Medof ME, Lam T, Prince GM, Mold C. Requirement for human red cells in inactivation of C3b in immune complexes and enhancement of binding to spleen cells. J Immunol 1983; 130:1336–1340.

M329. Medof ME, Prince GM. Immune complex alterations occur in the human red blood cell membrane. Immunology 1983;50:11–18.

M330. Medof ME, Prince GM, Mold C. Release of soluble immune complexes from immune adherence receptors on human erythrocytes is mediated by C3b inactivator independently of B1H and is accompanied by generation of C3c. Proc Natl Acad Sci USA 1982;79:5047–5051.

M331. Medof ME, Prince GM, Oger JJF. Kinetics of interaction of immune complexes with complement receptors on human red blood cells: Modification of complexes during interaction with red cells. Clin Exp Immunol 1982;48:715.

M332. Medof ME, Scarborough D, Miller G. Ability of complement to release systemic lupus erythematosus complexes from cell receptors. Clin Exp Immunol 1981;44:416.

M333. Medsger TA Jr. Raynaud's, carpal tunnel associated but distinct [questions and answers]. J Musculoskeletal Med 1991 June;15–16.

M334. Meehan RT, Dorsey JK. Pregnancy among patients with systemic lupus erythematosus receiving immunosuppressive therapy. J Rheumatol 1987;14:252–258.

M335. Meek K, Jeske D, Slaoui M, Leo O, Urbain J, Capra J. Complete amino acid sequence of heavy chain variable region derived from two monoclonal anti-p-azophenyl arsenate antibodies of BALB/c mice expressing the major cross-reactive idiotype of the A/J strain. J Exp Med 1984;160:1070.

M336. Meek KD, Hasemann CA, Capra JD. Novel rearrangements at the immunoglobulin D locus. Inversions and fusions add to IgH somatic diversity. J Exp Med 1989;170(1):39–57.

M337. Meeker TC, Lowder J, Maloney DG, Miller RA, Thielmans K, Warnke R, Levy R. A clinical trial of anti-idiotype therapy for B cell malignancy. Blood 1985;65:1349.

M338. Meilof JF, Bantjes I, De Jong J, Van Dam AP, Smeenk RJ. The detection of anti-Ro/SSA and anti-La/SSB antibodies: A comparison of counterimmunoelectrophoresis with immunoblot, ELISA, and RNA precipitation assays. J Immunol Methods 1990;133:215–226.

M339. Meindl A, Klobeck HG, Ohnheiser R, Zachau HA. The V kappa gene repertoire in the human germ line. Eur J Immunol 1990;20(8):1855–1863.

M340. Meiselas LE, Zingale SB, Lee SL, Richman S, Siegel M. Antibody production in rheumatic diseases. The effect of brucella antigen. J Clin Invest 1961 Oct;40:1872–1881.

M341. Meislin AG, Rothfield N. Systemic lupus erythematosus

in childhood. Analysis of 42 cases, with comparative data on 200 adult cases followed concurrently. Pediatrics 1968 Jul; 42:37–49.

M342. Meisner DJ, Carlson RJ, Gottlieb AJ. Thrombocytopenia following sustained-release procainamide. Arch Intern Med 1985;145:446–448.

M343. Meissner WA, Diamdopoulos GTH. Neoplasia. In: Anderson WA, Kissane JM, editors. St Louis: Mosby, 1977:674–683.

M344. Mejia G, Zimmerman SW, Glass NR, Miller DT, Sollinger HW, Belzer FO. Renal transplantation in patients with systemic lupus erythematosus. Arch Intern Med 1983 Nov;143(11): 2089–2092.

M345. Mekori VA, Schneider M, Yaretzkty A, Klajman A. Pancreatitis in systemic lupus erythematosus-A case report and review of the literature. Postgrad Med J 1980;56:145–147.

M346. Melkild A, Gaarder PI. Does prazocin induce formation of antinuclear factor? [letter]. BMJ 1979 Mar 3;1:620–621.

M347. Mellman IS, Plutner H, Steinman RM, Unkeless JC, Cohn ZA. Internalization and degradation of macrophage Fc receptors during receptor-mediated phagocytosis. J Cell Biol 1983; 96:887–895.

M348. Mellors RC, Aoki T, Huebner FJ. Further implications of murine leukemia-like virus in the disorders of NZB mice. J Exp Med 1969;129:1045–1061.

M349. Mellors RC, Mellors JW. Antigen related to mammalian type C RNA viral p30 proteins is located in renal glomeruli in human systemic lupus erythematosus. Proc Natl Acad Sci USA 1976;73:233–237.

M350. Mellors RC, Ortega LC, Holman HR. Role of gamma globulins in pathogenesis of renal lesions in systemic lupus erythematosus and chronic membranous glomerulonephritis, with an observation on lupus erythematosus cell reaction. J Exp Med 1957 Aug 1;106:191–202.

M351. Melnick JL. Virus vaccines: principles and prospects. Bull World Health Organ 1989;67:105.

M352. Menard HA, Boire G, Lopez-Longo FJ, Masson C, Lapointe S. Rhupus: An RA subset predicted and defined by the presence of anti-native Ro antibody [abstract]. Arthritis Rheum 1989 Apr;32(4) Suppl:S16.

M352a. Mendelson E, Bustin M. Monoclonal antibodies against distinct determinants of histone H5 bind to chromatin. Biochemistry 1984;23:3459–3466.

M352b. Mendelson E, Smith BJ, Bustin M. Mapping the binding of monoclonal antibodies to histone H5. Biochemistry 1984; 23:3466–3471.

M353. Mendlovic S, Brocke S, Shoenfeld Y, Ben-Bassat M, Meshorer A, Bakimer R, Mozes E. Induction of a systemic lupus erythematosus-like disease in mice by a common human anti-DNA idiotype. Proc Natl Acad Sci USA 1988 Apr;85(7): 2260–2264.

M354. Mendlovic S, Fricke H, Shoenfeld Y, Mozes E. The role of anti-idiotypic antibodies in the induction of experimental systemic lupus erythematosus in mice. Eur J Immunol 1989; 19:729–734.

M355. Merino R, Shibata T, DeKossodo S, Izui S. Differential effect of the autoimmune Yaa and lpr genes on the acceleration of lupus-like syndrome in MRL/MpJ mice. Eur J Immunol 1989;19:2131–2137.

M356. Merkenschlager M, Beverley PC. Evidence for differential expression of CD45 isoforms for memory dependent and independent cytotoxic responses: Human CD8 memory CTL precursors selectively express CD45RO (UCHL1). Int Immunol 1989;1:450–457.

M357. Merkenschlager M, Terry L, Edwards R, Beverley PC. Limiting dilution analysis of proliferative responses in human lymphocyte populations defined by the monoclonal antibody

UCHL1: implications for differential CD45 expression in T cell memory formation. Eur J Immunol 1988;18:1653–1661.

M358. Meroni P, Harris EN, Brucato A, Tincani A, Barcellini W, Vismara A, Balestrieri G, Hughes GR, Zanussi C. Anti-mitochondrial type M5 and anti-cardiolipin antibodies in autoimmune disorders: studies on their association and cross-reactivity. Clin Exp Immunol 1987 Mar;67(3):484–491.

M359. Merrell M, Shulman LE. Determination of prognosis in chronic disease, illustrated by systemic lupus erythematosus. J Chron Dis 1955 Jan;1:12–32.

M360. Merrill JA. Cortisone in disseminated lupus erythematosus during pregnancy. Report of a case and review of the literature. Obstet Gynecol 1955;6:637.

M361. Merwin CF, Winkelmann RK. Dermatologic clinics. 2. Antimalarial drugs in the therapy of lupus erythematosus. Proc Mayo Clin 1962 Apr 25;37:253–268.

M362. Mery J-P, Morel-Maroger L, Boelaert J, Richet G. Clinical and anatomical evaluation of diffuse and focal glomerulonephritis in the course of systemic lupus erythematosus. J Urol Neprol (Paris) 1973 Apr–May;79:321–332.

M363. Meryhew N, Runquist OA. A kinetic analysis of immune-mediated clearance of erythrocytes. J Immunol 1981;126: 2443–2449.

M364. Meryhew NL, Handwerger BS, Messner RP. Monoclonal antibody-induced murine hemolytic anemia. J Lab Clin Med 1984 Oct;104(4):591–601.

M365. Meryhew NL, Kimberly RP, Messner RP, Runquist OA. Mononuclear phagocyte system in SLE II. A kinetic model of immune complex handling in systemic lupus erythematosus. J Immunol 1986;137:97–102.

M366. Meryhew NL, Messner RP, Wasiluk KR, Runquist OA. Assessment of mononuclear phagocyte system function by clearance of anti-D sensitized erythrocytes: The role of complement. J Lab Clin Med 1985;105:277–281.

M367. Meryhew NL, Shaver C, Messner RP, Runquist OA. Mononuclear phagocyte system dysfunction in murine SLE: Abnormal clearance kinetics precedes clinical disease. J Lab Clin Med 1991;117:181–193.

M368. Meryhew NL, Zoschke DC, Messner RP. Anti beta-2 microglobulin antibodies in systemic lupus erythematosus and ankylosing spondylitis: Effects on in vitro lymphocyte function. J Rheumatol 1986;13:83–89.

M369. Messenger AG, Church RE. Subacute cutaneous lupus erythematosus and malabsorption. Br J Dermatol 1986;115 Suppl 30:56–57.

M370. Messer J, Reitman D, Sacks HS, Smith H Jr, Chalmers TC. Association of adrenocorticosteroid therapy and peptic-ulcer disease. N Engl J Med 1983 Jul 7;309:212–224.

M371. Messner RP, De Horatius RJ, Ferrone S. Lymphocytotoxic antibodies in systemic lupus erythematosus patients and their relatives. Reactivity with the HLA antigenic molecular complex. Arthritis Rheum 1980 Mar;23:265–272.

M372. Messner RP, Kennedy MS, Kelinek JG. Antilymphocyte antibodies in systemic lupus erythematosus. Effect on lymphocyte surface characteristics. Arthritis Rheum 1975 May–Jun; 18:201–206.

M373. Messner RP, Kindstrom FD, Williams JR Jr. Peripheral blood lymphocyte cell surface markers during the course of systemic lupus erythematosus. J Clin Invest 1973;52: 3046–3056.

M374. Metzger AL, Coyne M, Lee S, Kramer LS. In vivo LE formation in peritonitis due to systemic lupus erythematosus. J Rheumatol 1974;1:130–133.

M375. Meuer SC, Hussey RE, Penta AC, Fitzgerald KA, Stadler BM, Schlossman SF, Reinherz EL. Cellular origin of interleukin 2 (IL 2) in man: evidence for stimulus-restricted IL 2 production by T4+ and T8+ T lymphocytes. J Immunol 1982;129: 1076–1079.

M376. Meuer SC, Roux MM, Schraven B. The alternative pathway of T cell activation: biology, pathophysiology, and perspectives for immunopharmacology. Clin Immunol Immunopathol 1989;50:S133-S139.

M377. Meuleman J, Katz P. The immunologic effects, kinetics and use of glucocorticoids. Med Clin North Am 1985;69: 805–816.

M378. Meyer GJ, Schober O, Stoppe G, Wildhagen K, Seidel JW, Hundeshagen H. Cerebral involvement in systemic lupus erythematosus (SLE): comparison of positron emission tomography (PET) with other imaging methods. Psychiatry Res 1989 Sep;29(3):367–368.

M379. Meyer O, Cyna L, Haim T. IgG-type anti-histone antibodies. Diagnostic value in rheumatoid polyarthritis, scleroderma, spontaneous and drug-induced lupus. Rev Rheum Mal Osteoartic 1984;51:303–310.

M380. Meyer O, Hauptmann G, Tappeiner G. Genetic deficiency of C4, C2 or C1q and lupus syndromes. Association with anti-Ro(SS-A) antibodies. Clin Exp Immunol 1985;62:678–684.

M381. Meyer O, Hauptmann G, Tappeiner G, Ochs HD, Mascart-Lemone F. Genetic deficiency of C4, C2 or C1q and lupus syndromes. Association with anti-Ro (SSA) antibodies. Clin Exp Immunol 1985;62:678–684.

M382. Meyer O, Piette JC, Bourgeois P, Fallas P, Bletry O, Jungers P, Kahn MF, Godeau P, Ryckewaert A. Antiphospholipid antibodies: a disease marker in 25 patients with antinuclear antibody negative systemic lupus erythematosus (SLE): comparison with a group of 91 patients with antinuclear antibody positive SLE. J Rheumatol 1987 Jun;14(3):502–506.

M383. Meyer RA, Hooley JR. Systemic lupus erythematosus with circulating anticoagulant discovered after post-extraction hemorrhage. Oral Surg 1967;24:22–26.

M384. Meyer RJ, Hoffman R, Zanjani ED. Autoimmune hemolytic anemia and periodic pure red cell aplasia in systemic lupus erythematosus: recovery after plasmapheresis. Am J Med 1978 Aug;65:342–345.

M385. Meyerhoff J, Dorsch CA. Decreased platelet serotonin levels in systemic lupus erythematosus. Arthritis Rheum 1981; 24:1495–1500.

M386. Meyers MC. Results of treatment in 71 patients with idiopathic thrombocytopenic purpura. Am J Med Sci 1961 Sep; 242:295–302.

M387. Michael SR, Vural IL, Bassen FA, Schaefer L. The hematologic aspects of disseminated (systemic) lupus erythematosus. Blood 1951 Nov;6:1059–1072.

M388. Michaelson M, Engle MA. Congenital complete heart block: an international study of the natural history. In: Cardiovasc Clin N A. Philadelphia: FA Davis. 1972;4(3):85–101.

M389. Michaiski JP, Snyder SM, McLeod RL, Talal N. Monozygotic tissues with Klinefelter's Syndrome discordant for systemic lupus erythematosus and symptomatic Myasthenia Gravis. Arthritis Rheum 1978;21:306–309.

M390. Michalevicz R, Many A. Predominance of T cells in pleural fluid of a patient with systemic lupus erythematosus. N Engl J Med 1977 Jan 6;196:51–52.

M391. Michet CJ Jr, McKenna CH, Elveback LR, Kaslow RA, Kurland LT. Epidemiology of systemic lupus erythematosus and other connective tissue disease in Rochester, Minnesota, 1950 through 1979. Mayo Clin Proc 1985 Feb;60:105–113.

M392. Michiels JJ. Erythromelalgia in SLE [letter]. J Rheumatol 1991;18(3):481–482.

M393. Michl J, Unkeless JC, Pieczonka MM, Silverstein SC. Modulation of Fc receptors of mononuclear phagocytes by immobilized antigen-antibody complexes. J Exp Med 1983;157: 1746–1757.

M394. Middlekoop E, Lubin BH, Bevers EM, Op den Kamp JAF, Comfurius P, Chiu DTY, Zwaal RFA, Van Deenen LLM, Roelofsen B. Studies on sickle erythrocytes provide evidence that the asymmetric distribution of phosphatidylserine in the red cell membrane is maintained by both ATP-dependent translocation and interaction with membrane skeletal proteins. Biochem Biophys Acta 1988;937:281–288.

M395. Mier A, Weir W. Ascites in systemic lupus erythematosus. Ann Rheum Dis 1985 Nov;44(11):778–779.

M396. Miescher P, Fauconnet M. L'absorption du facteur "L.E." par des noyaux cellulaires isol's. Experientia 1954; 10:252.

M397. Miescher P, Strassle R. New serological methods for the detection of LE factor. Vox Sang 1975;2:283.

M398. Miescher PA. Autoantibodies against thrombocytes and leukocytes. In: Miescher PA, Muller-Eberhard HJ, editors. Textbook of Immunopathology, Volume II. New York: Grune & Stratton 1969:500–506.

M399. Miescher PA, Favre H, Chatelanat F, Mihatsch MJ. Combined steroid-cyclosporin treatment of chronic autoimmune diseases. Clinical results and assessment of nephrotoxicity by renal biopsy. Klin Wochenschr 1987 Aug;65(15):727–736.

M400. Miescher PA, Miescher A. Combined ciclosporin-steroid treatment of systemic lupus erythematosus. In: Schindler R, editor. Ciclosporin in Autoimmune Diseases. Berlin: Springer-Verlag, 1985:338–345.

M401. Miescher PA, Riethmuller D. Diagnosis and treatment of systemic lupus erythematosus. Seminars in Hematology: Grune & Stratton 1965;2:1–28.

M402. Migliaresi S, Di Iorio G, Picillo U, Tedeschi G, Santanelli P, Di Constanzo A, Della Cloppa G, Fasolino M, Diano A, Bonavita V. Neurological manifestations of systemic lupus erythematosus. Study of 53 cases. Ann Ital Med Int 1989;4:10–5.

M403. Mihalakis N, Miller OJ, Erlanger BF. Antibodies to histones and histone-histone complexes: immunochemical evidence for secondary structure in histone 1. Science 1976;192: 469–471.

M404. Mihara M, Ohsugi Y, Saito K, Miyai T, Togashi M, Ono S, Muakami S, Dobashi K, Hirayama F, Hamaoka T. Immunologic abnormality in NZB/NZW F1 mice. Thymus-independent occurrence of B cell abnormality and requirement for T cells in the development of autoimmune disease, as evidenced by an analysis of the athymic nude individuals. J Immunol 1988;141: 85–90.

M405. Mijer F, Olsen RM. Transplacental passage of the lupus erythematosus factor. J Pediatr 1958;52:690–693.

M406. Mikecz K, Sonkoly I, Meszaros C, Szegedi G. Serum IgE level in systemic lupus erythematosus. Acta Med Hung 1985; 42:59–65.

M407. Mikhail MH, Heine MJ, Pengo V, Shapiro SS. The interaction of lupus anticoagulants with human platelets [abstract]. Circulation 1988;78 Suppl II:514.

M408. Mikhalev ID, Kurennaia NN, Morozov VN. A case of systemic lupus erythematosus associated with cancer of the lung. Revmatologiia (Moskva) 1989;1:68–70.

M409. Milch RA. Blood supply and the localization of tetracycline fluorescence in arthritic femoral heads. Arthritis Rheum 1963 Aug;6:377–380.

M410. Milich DR, Gershwin ME. The pathogenesis of autoimmunity in New Zealand mice. Semin Arthritis Rheum 1980 Nov; 10:111–147.

M411. Milich DR, Gershwin ME. Murine autoimmune hemolytic anemia via xenogeneic erythrocyte immunization: III. Difference of sec. Clin Immunol Immunopathol 1981;18:1–11.

M412. Millard LG, Rowell NR. Chilblain lupus erythematosus (Hutchison). A clinical and laboratory study of 17 patients. Br J Dermatol 1978 May;98(5):497–506.

M413. Millard LG, Rowell NR. Abnormal laboratory tests results and their relationship to prognosis in discoid lupus erythematosus. A long-term follow-up study of 92 patients. Arch Dermatol 1979 Sep;115(9):1055–1058.

M414. Miller BJ, Pauls JD, Fritzler MJ. Human monoclonal antibodies demonstrate polyspecificity for histones and the cytoskeleton. J Autoimmun In press.

M415. Miller D, Fiechtner J. Hydroxychloroquine overdosage [letter]. J Rheumatol 1989 Jan;16(1):142–143.

M416. Miller DG. The association of immune disease and malignant lymphoma. Ann Intern Med 1967 Mar;66:507–521.

M417. Miller DR, Fiechtner JJ, Carpenter JR, Brown RR, Stroshane RM, Stecher VJ. Plasma hydroxychloroquine concentrations and efficacy in rheumatoid arthritis. Arthritis Rheum 1987 May;30(5):567–571.

M418. Miller FW, Love LA. Prevention of predictable Raynaud's phenomenon by sublingual nifedipine [letter]. N Engl J Med 1987 Dec 3;317(23):1476.

M419. Miller FW, Moore GF, Weintraub BD, Steinberg AD. Prevalence of thyroid disease and abnormal thyroid function test results in patients with systemic lupus erythematosus. Arthritis Rheum 1987 Oct; 30(10):1124–1131.

M420. Miller FW, Santoro TJ, Papadopoulos NM. Idiopathic anasarca associated with oligoclonal gammopathy in systemic lupus erythematosus. J Rheumatol 1987 Aug;14(4):842–843.

M421. Miller FW, Waite KA, Biswas T, Plotz PH. The role of an autoantigen, histidyl-tRNA synthetase in the induction and maintenance of autoimmunity. Proc Natl Acad Sci USA 1990; 87:9933–9937.

M422. Miller IW, Morman WH. Learned helplessness in humans: a review and attribution theory model. Psychol Bull 1979;86: 93–118.

M423. Miller JF, Dawnham TF, Chapel TA. Co-existent bullous pemphigoid and systemic lupus erythematosus. Cutis 1978; 21:368–373.

M424. Miller KB, Salem D. Immune regulatory abnormalities produced by procainamide in vitro suppressor cell function of IgG secretion. Am J Med 1982 Apr;73:487–492.

M425. Miller KB, Schwartz RS. Familial abnormalities of suppressor-cell function in systemic lupus erythematosus. N Engl J Med 1979;301:803–809.

M426. Miller LG. Cigarettes and drug therapy: pharmacokinetic and pharmacodynamic considerations. Clin Pharmacol 1990; 9:125–135.

M427. Miller MH. Pulmonary hypertension, systemic lupus erythematosus, and the contraceptive pill: another report [case report]. Ann Rheum Dis 1987 Feb;46(2):159–161.

M428. Miller MH. Impotence in systemic lupus erythematosus [comment]. J Rheumatol 1990;17(1):118.

M429. See M435a.

M430. Miller MH, Urowitz MB, Gladman DD. Significance of thrombocytopenia in systemic lupus erythematosus. Arthritis Rheum 1983;26;1181–1186.

M431. Miller MH, Urowitz MB, Gladman DD, Blendis LM. The liver in systemic lupus erythematosus. Q J Med 1984 Summer; 53(211):401–409.

M432. Miller MH, Urowitz MB, Gladman DD, Killinger DW. Systemic lupus erythematosus in males. Medicine 1983;62: 327–334.

M433. Miller MH, Urowitz MB, Gladman DD, Tozman ECS. Chronic adhesive lupus serositis as a complication of systemic lupus erythematosus. Refractory chest pain and small bowel obstruction. Arch Intern Med 1984 Sep;144:1863–1864.

M434. Miller ML, Chacko JA. Autoimmune CD4 + T cells interfere with immune tolerance to a thymic-independent antigen. J Immunol 1988;140:4108–4114.

M435. Miller ML, Raveche ES, Laskin CA, Klinman DM, Steinberg AD. Genetic studies in NZB mice. VI. Association of autoimmune traits in recombinant inbred lines. J Immunol 1984 Sep; 133(3):1325–1331.

M435a. Miller MN, Baumal R, Poucell S, Steele BT. Incidence and prognostic importance of glomerular crescents in renal diseases of childhood. Am J Nephrol 1984;4:244–247.

M436. Miller RA, Wener MH, Harnisch JP, Gilliland BC. The limited spectrum of antinuclear antibodies in leprosy. J Rheumatol 1987 Feb;14(1):108–110.

M437. Miller RW, Salcedo JR, Fink RJ, Murphy TM, Magilavy DB. Pulmonary hemorrhage in pediatric patients with systemic lupus erythematosus. J Pediat 1986;108:576–579.

M438. Millet VG, Usera G, de la Ossa JMA, Ruilope LM, Ortuno MT, Rodicio JL. Renal vein thrombosis, nephrotic syndrome and focal lupus glomerulonephritis. Br Med J 1978 Jan 7;1: 24–25.

M439. Millette TJ, Subramony SH, Wee AS, Harisdangkul V. Systemic lupus erythematosus presenting with recurrent acute demyelinating polyneuropathy. Eur Neurol 1986;25(6): 397–402.

M440. Millman RP, Cohen TB, Levinson AI, Kelley MA, Sachs ML. Systemic lupus erythematosus complicated by acute pulmonary hemorrhage: recovery following plasmapheresis and cytotoxic therapy. J Rheumatol 1981 Nov–Dec;8:1021–1022.

M441. Mills PV, Beck M, Power BJ. Assessment of the retinal toxicity of hydroxychloroquine. Trans Ophthal Soc UK 1981; 101:109–113.

M442. Millus JL, Muller SA. The coexistence of psoriasis and lupus erythematosus: An analysis of 27 cases. Arch Dermatol 1980 Jun;116:658–663.

M443. Millwad BA, Welsh KI, Leslie RDG, Pyke DA, Demaine AG. T-cell receptor beta chain polymorphisms are associated with insulin-dependent diabetes. Clin Exp Immuno 1987;70: 152–157.

M444. Milne JA, Anderson JR, McSween RN, Fraser K, Short I, Stevens J, Shaw GB, Tankel HI. Thymectomy in acute SLE and rheumatoid arthritis. BMJ 1967;1:461–464.

M445. Milner GR, Holt PJ, Bottomley J, Maciver JE. Practolol therapy associated with a systemic lupus-like syndrome and an inhibitor to Factor XIII. J Clin Pathol 1977 Aug;30:770–773.

M446. Mimori T, Akizuki M, Yamagata H, Inada S, Yoshida S, Homma M. Characterization of a high molecular weight acidic protein recognized by autoantibodies in sera from patients with polymyositis-scleroderma overlap. J Clin Invest 1981;68: 611–620.

M447. Omitted.

M448. Omitted.

M449. Mimori T, Fujii T, Hama N, Suwa A, Akizuki M, Tojo T, Homma H. Newly identified autoantibodies to U4/U6 small nuclear ribonucleoprotein particle in a patient with primary Sjogren's syndrome. Arthritis Rheum 1991;34 Suppl:S46.

M450. Mimori T, Hardin J, Steitz JA. Characterization of the DNA binding protein antigen Ku recognized by autoantibodies from patients with rheumatic disorders. J Biol Chem 1986; 261:2274–2278.

M451. Mimori T, Hardin JA. Mechanisms of interaction between Ku protein and DNA. J Biol Chem 1986;261:10375–10379.

M452. Mimori T, Hinterberger M, Pettersson I, Steitz JA. Autoantibodies to the U2 small nuclear ribonucleoprotein in a patient with scleroderma-polymyositis overlap syndrome. J Biol Chem 1984;259:560–565.

M453. Mimura T, Fernsten P, Jarjour W, Winfield JB. Autoantibodies specific for different isoforms of CD45 in systemic lupus erythematosus. J Exp Med 1990;172:653–656.

M453a. Mimura T, Fernstein P, Shaw M, Jarjour W, Winfield JB. Glycoprotein specificity of cold-reactive IgM anti-lymphocyte autoantibodies in systemic lupus erythematosus. Arthritis Rheum 1990;33:1226–1232.

M454. Minakuchi R, Wacholtz MC, Davis LS, Lipsky PE. Delineation of the mechanisms of inhibition of human T cell activation by PEG2. J Immunol 1990;145:2616–2625.

M455. Minetti L, Bardiano di Belgiojoso G, Taratino A, Rovati C, Civati G, Imbascati E. Segni immunoistologici di attiuita della nefrite lupica. Minerva Nefrologica 1973 May–Jun;20: 136–147.

M456. Miniter MF, Stollar BD, Agnello V. Reassessment of the clinical significance of native DNA antibodies in systemic lupus erythematosus. Arthritis Rheum 1979 Sep 22:959–968.

M457. Minker E, Blazso G, Kadar T. Inhibitory effect on gastric motility of chloroquine and mepacrine. Acta Physiol Acad Sci Hung 1978;52(4):455–458.

M458. Minker E, Kadar T, Matejka Z. Effect of chloroquine and mepacrine on the spontaneous and evoked movements of the rat portal vein. Acta Physiol Acad Sci Hung 1980;55(1):71–80.

M459. Minkin W, Rabhan NB. Office nailfold capillary microscopy using the ophthalmoscope. J Am Acad Derm 1982;7: 190–193.

M460. Minnigerode B, Leitner C. Transient, directional changing spontaneous and provoked nystagmus in the course of lupus erythematodes visceralis [English abstract]. Klin Wochenschr 1985 Mar 1;63(5):230–232.

M461. Minoda M, Horiuchi A. The function of thymic reticuloepithelial cells in New Zealand mice. Thymus 1983 Sep;5(5–6): 363–374.

M462. Minoda M, Horiuchi A. The effects of macrophages on interleukin 2 production in thymocytes of New Zealand black mice. J Clin Lab Immunol 1987 Jan;22(1):29–34.

M463. Minoda M, Senda S, Horiuchi A. The relationship between the defect in the syngeneic mixed lymphocyte reaction and thymic abnormality in New Zealand mice. J Clin Lab Immunol 1987 Jun;23(2):101–108.

M464. Minota S, Cameron B, Welch WJ, Winfield JB. Autoantibodies to the constitutive 73-kD member of the hsp 70 family of heat shock proteins in systemic lupus erythematosus. J Exp Med 1988;168:1475–1480.

M465. Minota S, Jarjour WN, Suzuki N, Notima Y, Roubey RAS, Mimura T, Akira Y, Hosoya T, Takaku F, Winfeld JB. Autoantibodies to nucleolin in systemic lupus erythematosus and other diseases. J Immunol 1991;146:2249–2252.

M466. Minota S, Koyasu S, Yahara I, Winfield J. Autoantibodies to the heat shock protein hsp 90 in systemic lupus erythematosus. J Clin Invest 1988;81:106–109.

M467. Minota S, Terai C, Nojima Y, Takano K, Takai E, Miyakawa Y, Takaku F. Low C3b receptor reactivity on erythrocytes from patients with systemic lupus erythematosus detected by immune adherence hemagglutination and radioimmunoassays with monoclonal antibody. Arthritis Rheum 1984;27: 1329–1335.

M468. Minota S, Winfield JB. Nature of IgG anti-lymphocyte autoantibody-reactive molecules shed from activated T cells in systemic lupus erythematosus. Rheumatol Int 1988;8: 165–170.

M469. Mintz G, Acevedo-Vazquez E, Gutierrez-Espinosa G, Avelar-Garnica F. Renal vein thrombosis and inferior vena cava thrombosis in systemic lupus erythematosus: Frequency and risk factor. Arthritis Rheum 1984 May;27(5):539–544.

M470. Mintz G, Galindo LF, Fernandez-Diez J, Jimenez FJ, Robles-Saaverda E, Enrique-Casillas RD. Acute massive pulmonary hemorrhage in systemic lupus erythematosus. J Rheumatol 1978 Spring;5:39–50.

M471. Mintz G, Gutierrez G, Deleze M, Rodriguez E. Contraception with progestagens in systemic lupus erythematosus. Contraception 1984 Jul;30(1):29–38.

M472. Mintz G, Niz J, Gutierrez G, Garcia-Alonso A, Karchmer S. Prospective study of pregnancy in systemic lupus erythema-

tosus. Results of a multidisciplinary approach. J Rheumatol 1986;13:732–739.

M473. Mintz G, Rodriquez-Alvarez E. Systemic lupus erythematosus. Rheum Dis Clin N A 1989;15:255–278.

M474. Mirzabekov AD, Pruss DV, Ebralidse KK. Chromatin superstructure-dependent crosslinking with DNA of the histone H5 residues Thr1, His25 and His62. J Mol Biol 1989;211: 479–491.

M475. Misra R, Venables PJW, Zyberk CP, Watkins PF, Maini RN. Anti-cardiolipin antibodies in infectious mononucleosis react with the membrane of activated lymphocytes. Clin Exp Immunol 1989;75:35–40.

M476. Misteli M, Conen D. Acute transverse myelitis in systemic lupus erythematosus treated with cyclophosphamide and prednisone. Schweiz Med Wschr 1991;121:77–80.

M477. Mistilis SP. Active Chronic Hepatitis. In: Schiff L editor. Diseases of the Liver, 3rd edition. Philadelphia: Lippincott, 1969:645–671.

M478. Mistilis SP, Blackburn CRB. The treatment of active chronic hepatitis with 6-mercaptopurine and azathioprine. Aust Ann Med 1967 Nov;305–311.

M479. Mitchell AJ, Rusin LJ, Diaz LA. Circumscribed scleroderma with immunologic evidence of systemic lupus erythematosus. A report of a case and review of the literature. Arch Dermatol 1980 Jan;116(1):69–73.

M480. Mitchell DG. Using MR imaging to probe the pathophysiology of osteonecrosis. Radiology 1989 Apr;171(1):25–26.

M481. Mitchell DG, Steinberg MC, Dalinka MK, Rao VM, Fallon M, Kressel HY. Magnetic resonance imaging of the ischemic hip. Alterations within the osteonecrotic, viable and reactive zone. Clin Orthop 1989 Jul;(244):60–72.

M482. Mitchell DM, Fitzharris P, Knight RA, Schild GC, Snaith ML. Kinetics of specific anti-influenza antibody production by cultured lymphocytes from patients with systemic lupus erythematosus following influenza immunization. Clin Exp Immunol 1982 Aug;49(2):290–296.

M483. Mitchell DR, Lyles KW. Glucocorticoid-induced osteoporosis: mechanisms for bone loss; evaluation of strategies for prevention. J Gerontol: Med Sci 1990 Sep;45(5): M153–158.

M484. Mitchell HW. Pharmacological studies into cyclo-oxygenase, lipoxygenase and phospholipase in smooth muscle contraction in the isolated trachea. Br J Pharmacol 1984 Jul; 82(3):549–555.

M485. Mitchell JA, Batchelor JR, Chapel H, Spiers CN, Sim E. Erythrocyte complement receptor type 1 (CR1) expression and circulating immune complex (CIC) levels in hydralazine-induced SLE. Clin Exp Immunol 1987;68:446–456.

M486. Mitchell JA, Sim RB, Sim E. CR1 polymorphism in hydralazine-induced systemic lupus erythematosus. Clin Exp Immunol 1989;78:354–358.

M487. Mitchell SR, Nguyen PQ, Katz P. Risk of Neisserial infections in systemic lupus erythematosus (SLE) [abstract]. Arthritis Rheum 1990 May;33(5) Suppl:R22.

M488. Mitchell SR, Nguyen PQ, Katz P. Increased risk of neisserial infections in systemic lupus erythematosus. Semin Arthritis Rheum 1990;20:174–184.

M489. Mitchell WD, Thompson TL. Psychiatric distress in systemic lupus erythematosus outpatient. Psychosomatics 1990 Summer, 31(3):293–300.

M490. Mittal KK, Rossen RD, Sharp JT, Lidsky MD, Butler WT. Lymphocyte cytotoxic antibodies in SLE. Nature 1970 Mar 28; 225:1255–1256.

M491. Mittler RS, Greenfield RS, Schacter BZ, Richard NF, Hoffmann MK. Antibodies to the common leukocyte antigen (T200) inhibit an early phase in the activation of resting human B cells. J Immunol 1987;138:3159–3166.

M492. Mitzutani W, Quismorio FP. Lupus foot: Deforming arthropathy of the feet in systemic lupus erythematosus. J Rheumatol 1984;11:80–82.

M493. Miyachi K, Fritzler MJ, Tan EM. Autoantibody to a nuclear antigen in proliferating cells. J Immunol 1978;121: 2228–2234.

M494. Miyachi Y. A possible action of thalidomide on rheumatoid arthritis [letter]. Arthritis Rheum 1985 Jul;28(7):836.

M495. Miyachi Y, Yoshioka A, Imamura S, Niwa Y. Antioxidant action of antimalarials. Ann Rheum Dis 1986 Mar;45(3): 244–248.

M496. Miyagi J, Minato N, Sumiya M, Kasahara T, Kano S. Two types of antibodies inhibiting interleukin-2 production by normal lymphocytes in patients with systemic lupus erythematosus. Arthritis Rheum 1989;32:1356–1364.

M497. Miyagawa S, Dohi K, Yoshioka A, Shirai T. Female predominance of immune response to SSA/Ro antigens and risk of neonatal lupus erythematosus. Br J Dermatol 1990;123: 223–227.

M498. Miyagawa S, Kitamura W, Yoshioka J, Sakamoto K. Placental transfer of anticytoplasmic antibodies in annular erythema of newborns. Arch Dermatol 1981;117:569–572.

M499. Miyagawa S, Okuchi T, Shiomi Y, Sakamoto K. Subacute cutaneous lupus erythematosus lesions precipitated by griseofulvin. J Am Acad Dermatol 1989;21:343–346.

M500. Miyagi J, Minato N, Sumiya M, Kasahara T, Kano S. Two types of antibodies inhibiting interleukin-2 production by normal lymphocytes in patients with systemic lupus erythematosus. Arthritis Rheum 1989;32:1356–1364.

M501. Miyakawa M, Sato K, Sato Y. Presentation of a case of Graves' disease with neutropenia and splenomegaly: Propylthiouracil-induced autoimmune neutropenia and review of the literature on the drug-induced lupus-like syndrome. Nippon Naika Gakkai Zasshi 1984;73:538–545.

M502. Miyakawa Y, Yamada A, Kosaka K, Tsuda F, Kosugi E, Mayumi M. Defective immune adherence (C3b) receptor on erythrocytes from patients with systemic lupus erythematosus. Lancet 1981;2:493–497.

M503. Miyasaka N, Nakamura T, Russell IJ, Talal N. Interleukin-2 deficiencies in rheumatoid arthritis and systemic lupus erythematosus. Clin Immunol Immunopathol 1984 Apr;31: 109–117.

M504. Miyazaki M, Endoh M, Suga T, Yabno N, Kuramoto T, Matsumoto Y, Eguchi K, Ygame M, Miura M, Nomoto Y, Sakai H. Rheumatoid factors and glomerulonephritis. Clin Exp Immunol 1990;81:250–255.

M505. Miyazaki T, Uno M, Uehira M, Kikutani H, Kishimoto T, Kimoto M, Nishimoto H, Miyazaki J, Yamamura K. Direct evidence for the contribution of the unique I-A to the development of insulitis in non-obese mice. Nature 1990;345: 722–742.

M506. Miyoshi K, Miyamura T, Kobayashi Y, Hakwra T, Nishijo K, Higashibara M, Shiragami H, Ohno F. Hypergammaglobulinemia by prolonged adjuvanticity in man. Disorders developed after augmentation mammoplasty. Jpn Med J 1964;2122: 9–14.

M507. Mizushima Y, Shoji Y, Hoshi K, Kiyokawa S. Detection and clinical significance of IgE rheumatoid factors. J Rheumatol 1984 Feb;11:22–26.

M508. Mizutani WT, Hutchinson M, Quismorio FP Jr. Association of migraine headache (MH) and Raynaud's phenomenon (RP) in systemic lupus erythematosus (SLE) [abstract]. Arthritis Rheum 1985 Apr;28(4) Suppl;S63.

M509. Moalla M, Elleuch M, Bergaoui N, Hamza M, Chaffai M, Ben Osmane A, Dallagi K, Ben Ayed H. Association of ankylosing spondylitis, discoid lupus and a dermatofibrosarcoma. Sem Hop Paris 1987;63:1457–1461.

M510. Modena V, Marengo C, Amoroso A, Rosina F, Constantini

P, Bellando P, Coppo R, Rizzetto M. Primary biliary cirrhosis and rheumatic diseases: a clinical, immunological and immunogenetical study. Clin Exp Rheumatol 1986 Apr–Jun;4(2): 129–134.

M511. Modore SJ, Wieben ED, Pederson T. Eukaryotic mall ribonucleoproteins: anti-La human autoantibodies react with U1 RNA-protein complexes. J Biol Chem 1984;259:1929–1933.

M512. Mody CK, Miller BL, McIntyre HB, Cobb SK, Goldberg MA. Neurologic complications of cocaine abuse. Neurology 1988;38:1189–1193.

M513. Moeller E, Boehme J, Vargerdi MA, Ridderstad A, Olerup O. Speculation on mechanisms of HLA associations with autoimmune diseases and the specificity of autoreactive T lymphocytes. Immunol Rev 1990;118:5–19.

M514. Moens PB, Pearlman RE. Chromatin organization at meiosis. Bio Essays 1988;9:151–153.

M515. Moersch HJ, Purnell DC, Good CA. Pulmonary changes occurring in disseminated lupus erythematosus. Dis Chest 1956 Feb;29:166–173.

M516. Moffat MP, Tsushima RG. Functional and electrophysiological effects of quinacrine on the response of ventricular tissues to hypoxia and reoxygenation. Can J Physiol Pharmacol 1989 Aug;67(8):929–935.

M517. Mogadem M, Dobbins WO, Korelitz RI, Ahmed SW. Pregnancy in inflammatory bowel disease: Effect of sulfasalazine and corticosteroids on fetal outcome. Gastroenterol 1981;80: 72–76.

M518. Mohacsi G, Julesz J, Berger Z, Ormos J. Bilateral renal malacoplakia in systemic lupus erythematosus and andrenogenital syndrome. Int Urol Nephrol 1989;21(1):31–38.

M519. Mohagheghpour N, Damle NK, Takada S, Engleman EG. Generation of antigen receptor-specific suppressor T cell clones in man. J Exp Med 1986;164:950.

M520. Mohammad SF, Martin BA, Hershgold KJ. The importance of reagents in the laboratory detection of lupus anticoagulants. Thromb Haemost 1985 Jul;54:82.

M521. Moidel RA, Good AE. Coexistent gout and systemic lupus erythematosus. Arthritis Rheum 1981 Jul;24(7):969–971.

M522. Molad Y, Rachmilewitz B, Sidi Y, Pinkhas J, Weinberger A. Serum cobalamin and transcobalamin levels in systemic lupus erythematosus. Am J Med 1990;88:141–144.

M523. Molad Y, Weinberger A, David M, Garty B, Wysenbeek AJ, Pinkas J. Clinical manifestations and laboratory data of subacute cutaneous lupus erythematosus. Isr J Med Sci 1987;23: 278–280.

M524. Molden DP, Klipple GL, Peebles CL, Rubin RL, Nakamura RM, Tan EM. IgM anti-histone H-3 antibody associated with undifferentiated rheumatic disease syndromes. Arthritis Rheum 1986;29:39–46.

M525. Moldenhauer F, David J, Felder AHL, Lachmann PJ, Walport MJ. Inherited deficiency of erythrocyte complement receptor type 1 does not cause susceptibility to systemic lupus erythematosus. Arthritis Rheum 1988;30:961–966.

M526. Molina J, Dubois EL, Bilitch M, Bland SL, Friou GJ. Procainamide-induced serologic changes in asymptomatic patients. Arthritis Rheum 1969;12:608–614.

M527. Molina Boix M, Ortega Gonzalez G, Perez Garcia B, Perez Gracia A. Perforation of the colon in systemic lupus erythematosus. Rev Esp Enferm Apar Dig 1988 Aug;74(2):187–188.

M528. Moller DE, Ratner RE, Borenstein DG, Taylor SI. Antibodies to the insulin receptor as a cause of autoimmune hypoglycemia in systemic lupus erythematosus. Am J Med 1988 Feb; 84(2):334–338.

M529. Mollison PL, Crome P, Hughes-Jones NC, Rocha E. Rate of removal from the circulation of red cells sensitized with different amounts of antibody. Br J Haematol 1965;11: 461–470.

M530. Monash S. Oral lesions of lupus erythematosus. Dental Cosmos 1931;73:511–513.

M531. Moncayo-Naveda H, Moncayo R, Benz R, Wolf A, Lauritzen C. Organ-specific antibodies against ovary in patients with systemic lupus erythematosus. Am J Obstet Gynecol 1989 May;160(5 Pt 1):1227–1229.

M532. Mond CB, Peterson MG, Rothfield NF. Correlation of anti-Ro antibody with photosensitivity rash in systemic lupus erythematosus patients. Arthritis Rheum 1986;29:421–425.

M533. Mond CB, Peterson MG, Rothfield NF. Correlation of anti-Ro antibody with photosensitivity rash in systemic lupus erythematosus patients. Arthritis Rheum 1989 Feb;32(2): 202–204.

M534. Mond CB, Rothfield NF. Anti-Ro antibody correlates with photosensitive rash in SLE patients [abstract]. Arthritis Rheum 1988;31 Suppl:S55.

M535. Monestier M. Variable region genes of anti-histone autoantibodies from a MRL/Mp- lpr/lpr mouse. Eur J Immunol 1991; 21:1725–1731.

M536. Monestier M, Bonin B, Migliorini P, Dang H, Datta S, Kuppers R, Rose N, Maurer P, Talal N, Bona C. Autoantibodies of various specificities encoded by genes from the $V_H J558$ family bind to foreign antigens and share idiotypes of antibodies specific for self and foreign antigens. J Exp Med 1987;166: 1109–1124.

M537. Monestier M, Fasy TM. Specificities and variable region genes of murine anti-histone autoantibodies. FASEB J 1991;5: 1087.

M538. Monestier M, Fasy TM, Debbas ME, Bohm L. Specificities of IgM and IgG anti-histone H1 autoantibodies in autoimmune mice. Clin Exp Immunol 1990;81:39–44.

M539. Monestier M, Losman JA, Fasy TM, Babbas ME, Massa M, Albani S, Bohm L, Martini A. Antihistone antibodies in antinuclear antibody-positive juvenile arthritis. Arthritis Rheum 1990;33:1836–1841.

M540. Monestier M, Manheimer-Lory A, Bellon B, Painter C, Dang H, Talal N, Zanetti M, Schwartz R, Pisetsky D, Kuppers R, Rose N, Brochier J, Klareskog L, Holmdahl R, Erlanger B, Alt F, Bona C. Shared idiotypes and restricted immunoglobulin variable region heavy chain genes characterize murine autoantibodies of various specificities. J Clin Invest 1986;78: 753–759.

M541. Monga G, Mazzucco G, di Belgiojoso B, Busnach G. The presence and possible role of monocyte infiltration in human chronic proliferation glomerulonephritis. Am J Pathol 1979 Feb;94:271–284.

M542. Mongan ES, Leddy JP, Atwater EC, Barnett EV. Direct antiglobulin (Coombs) reactions in patients with connective tissue diseases. Arthritis Rheum 1967 Dec;10:502–508.

M543. Mongey A, Hess EV. Antinuclear antibodies and disease specificity. Adv Intern Med 1991;36:151–169.

M544. Mongey AB, Glynn D, Hutchinson M, Bresnihan B. Clinical neurophysiology in the assessment of neurological symptoms in systemic lupus erythematosus. Rheumatol Int 1987; 7(2):49–52.

M545. Mongey AB, Hess EV. Drug-related lupus. Curr Science 1989;353–359.

M546. Monier JC, Fournel C, Lapras M, Dardenne M, Randle T, Fontaine CM. Systemic lupus erythematous in a colony of dogs. Am J Vet Res 1988;49:46–51.

M547. Monplaisir N, Valette I, Pierre-Louis S, Yoyo M, Sobesky G, Verpre FC, Quist D, Arfi S, Gervaise G, Gabriel JM, Artax H, Raffoux C. Study of HLA antigens in systemic lupus erythematosus in the French West Indies. Tissue Antigens 1988;31: 238–242.

M548. Montanaro A, Bardana EJ. Dietary amino acid-induced systemic lupus erythematosus. Rheum Dis Clin N Am 1991; 17:323–332.

M549. Montgomery H. Pathology of lupus erythematosus. J Invest Dermatol 1939 Dec;2:343–359.

M550. Montgomery H, McCreight WG. Disseminated lupus erythematosus. Arch Dermat & Syph 1949;60:356–372.

M551. Montgomery WW, Lofgren RH. Usual and unusual causes of laryngeal arthritis. Arch Otolaryngology 1963 Jan;77: 29–33.

M552. Monto RW, Rizek RA, Rupe CE, Rebuck JW. The L.E. cell. Significance and relation to collagen disease. In: Mills LC, Moyer JH, editors. Inflammation and diseases of connective tissue. A Hahnemann Symposium. Philadelphia: Saunders 1961:200–205.

M553. Montzka K, Steitz JA. Additional low-abundance human small nuclear ribonucleoproteins: U11, U12, etc. Proc Natl Acad Sci USA 1988;85:8885–8889.

M554. Mook WH, Weiss RS, Bromberg LK. Lupus erythematosus disseminatus. Arch Dermatol 1931 Nov;786–829.

M555. Mooney E, Wade TR. Subacute cutaneous lupus erythematosus in Iceland. Int J Dermatol 1989;28:104–106.

M556. Moore CP, Willkens RF. The subcutaneous nodule: Its significance in the diagnosis of rheumatic disease. Semin Arthritis Rheum 1977 Aug;7(1):63–79.

M557. Moore GF, Yarboro C, Sebring NG, Robinson DR, Steinberg AD. Eicosapentanoic acid (EPA) in the treatment of systemic lupus erythematosus (SLE). Arthritis Rheum 1987; 30 Suppl:S33.

M558. Moore JE, Lutz WB. Natural history of systemic lupus erythematosus: approach to its study through chronic biologic false positive reactors. J Chronic Dis 1955 Mar;1:297–316.

M559. Moore JE, Mohr CF. Biologically false positive serologic tests for syphilis; type, incidence, and cause. JAMA 1952 Oct 4;150:467–473.

M560. Moore JS, Hoover RG. Defective isotype-specific regulation of IgA anti-erythrocyte autoantibody-forming cells in NZB mice. J Immunol 1989;142:4282–4288.

M561. Moore PJ. Maternal systemic lupus erythematosus associated with fetal congenital heart block. A case report. S A Med J 1981;60:285–286.

M562. Moore TL, Osborn TG, Dorner RW. Cross-reactive antiidiotypic antibodies against human rheumatoid factors from patients with juvenile rheumatoid arthritis. Arthritis Rheum 1989;32:699.

M563. Moore TL, Osborn TG, Weiss TD, Sheridan PW, Eisenwinter RK, Miller AV, Dorner RW, Zuckner J. Autoantibodies in juvenile arthritis. Semin Arthritis Rheum 1984 May;13(4): 329–336.

M564. Moorthy AV, Zimmerman S, Mejia G, Sollinger HW, Belzer FO. Recurrence of lupus nephritis after renal transplantation. Kidney Int 1987;31:464.

M565. Mor F, Beigel Y, Inbal A, Goren M, Wysenbeek AJ. Hepatic infarction in a patient with a lupus anticoagulant. Arthritis Rheum 1989 Apr;32(4):491–495.

M566. Morahan G, Allison J, Miller JF. Tolerance of class I histocompatibility antigens expressed extrathymically. Nature 1989;339:622–624.

M567. Morel P, Marinho E, Bruneau C, Civatte J, Puissant A. Deep skin lesions of lupus erythematosus [English abstract]. Ann Med Interne (Paris) 1986;137(4):320–323.

M568. Morel-Maroger L, Mery JP, Droz E, Godin M, Verroust P, Kourilsky O, Richet GA. The course of lupus nephritis: contribution in serial renal biopsies. In: Hamburger J, Crosnier J, Maxwell MH. Chicago: Year Book, 1976:79–118.

M569. Moretta LM, Mingari MC, Webb SR, Pearl ER, Lydyard PM, Grossi CE, Lawton AR, Cooper MD. Imbalances in T cell subpopulations associated with immunodeficiency and autoimmune syndromes. Eur J Immunol 1984;7(10):696–700.

M570. Morgan AG, Steward MW. Macrophage clearance function and immune complex disease in New Zealand Black/White F₁ hybrid mice. Clin Exp Immunol 1976;26:133–136.

M571. Morgan MC, Matteson E, Dunne R, Brown M, Fox DA, McCune WJ. Complications of intravenous cyclophosphamide: Association of infections with high daily doses of prednisone in lupus patients [abstract] Arthritis Rheum 1990 May;28(5) Suppl:R27.

M572. Morgan SH, Kennett RP, Dudley C, Mackworth-Young C, Hull R, Hughes GR. Acute polyradiculoneuropathy complicating systemic lupus erythematosus. Postgrad Med J 1986 Apr; 62(726):291–294.

M573. Morgan WS. Probable systemic nature of Mikulicz's disease and its relation to Sjogren's syndrome. N Engl J Med 1954 Jul 1;251:5–10.

M574. Mori T, Takai Y, Minakuchi R, Yu B, Nishizuka Y. Inhibitory action of chlorpromazine, dibucaine and other phospholipid-interacting drugs on calcium-activated phospholipid dependent protein kinase. J Biol Chem 1980;255:8378–8387

M575. Morimoto C, Abe T, Toguchi T, Kiyotaki H, Homma M. Studies of anti-lymphocyte antibody in patients with active SLE. Scand J Immunol 1979 Sep;10:213–221.

M576. Morimoto C, Abe T, Toguchi T, Kiyotaki H, Homma M. Studies of anti-lymphocyte antibody in patients with active SLE. II. Effect of anti-lymphocyte antibody on autoreactive cell clones. Scand J Immunol 1980 May;11:479–488.

M577. Morimoto C, Letvin NL, Boyd AW, Hagan M, Brown HM, Kornacki MM, Schlossman SF. The isolation and characterization of the human helper inducer subset. J Immunol 1985; 134:3762–3769.

M578. Morimoto C, Letvin NL, Distaso JA, Aldrich WR, Schlossman SF. The isolation and characterization of the human suppressor inducer T cell subset. J Immunol 1985 Mar; 134:1508–1515.

M579. Morimoto C, Reinherz EL, Abe T. Characteristics of anti-T cell antibodies in systemic lupus erythematosus. Evidence for selective reactivity with normal suppressor cells defined by monoclonal antibodies. Clin Immunol Immunopathol 1980 Aug;16:474–484.

M580. Morimoto C, Reinherz EL, Distaso JA, Steinberg AD, Schlossman SF. Relationship between systemic lupus erythematosus T cell subsets, anti-T cell antibodies and T cell functions. J Clin Invest 1984 Mar;73;689–700.

M581. Morimoto C, Reinherz EL, Schlossman SF, Schur PH, Mills JA, Steinberg AD. Alteration in T cell subsets in active systemic lupus erythematosus. J Clin Invest 1980 Nov;66:1171–1174.

M582. Morimoto C, Sano H, Abe T, Homma M, Steinberg AD. Correlation between clinical activity of systemic lupus erythematosus and the amounts of DNA in DNA/anti-DNA antibody immune complexes. J Immunol 1982;139:1960–1965.

M583. Morimoto C, Schlossman SF. Antilymphocyte antibodies and systemic lupus erythematosus. Arthritis Rheum 1987;30: 225–228.

M584. Morimoto C, Steinberg AD, Letvin NL, Hagan M, Takeuchi T, Daley J, Levine H, Schlossman SF. A defect of immunoregulatory T cell subsets in systemic lupus erythematosus patients demonstrated with anti-2H4 antibody. J Clin Invest 1987;79: 762–768.

M585. Morimoto I, Shiozawa S, Tanaka Y, Fujita T. L-canavanine acts on suppressor-inducer T cells to regulate antibody synthesis: Lymphocytes of systemic lupus erythematosus are specifically unresponsive to L-canavanine. Clin Immunol Immunopathol 1990;55:97–108.

M586. Morishima Y, Ogata S, Collins NH, DuPont B, Lloyd KO. Carbohydrate differences in human high molecular weight antigens of B- and T-cell lines. Immunogenetics 1982;15: 529–535.

M587. Moriuchi J, Ichikawa Y, Takaya M, Shimizu H, Tokunaga M, Eguchi T, Izumi M, Ohta W, Katsuoka Y, Nakajima I, Tsutsumi Y, Arimori S. Lupus cystitis and perforation of the small bowel in a patient with systemic lupus erythematosus and overlapping syndrome. Clin Exp Rheumatol 1989;7:533–536.

M588. Moriwaka F, Tashiro K, Fukazawa T, Akino M, Yasuda I, Sagawa A, Hida K. A case of systemic lupus erythematosus—its clinical and MRI resemblance to multiple sclerosis. Jap J Psychiatry Neurol 1990 Sep;44(3):601–605.

M589. Morland C, Michael J, Adu D, Kizaki T, Howie AJ, Morgan A, Staines NA. Anti-idiotype and immunosuppressant treatment of murine lupus. Clin Exp Immunol 1991;83:126–132.

M590. Morley KD, Bernstein RM, Bunn CC, Gharavi AE, Fortin MT, Chipping PM, Hughes GRV. Thrombocytopenia and anti-Ro. Lancet 1981;11:940.

M591. Morley KD, Leung A, Rynes RI. Lupus foot. BMJ (Clin Res) 1982 Feb 20;284(6315):557–558.

M592. Morley KD, Parke A, Hughes GR. Systemic lupus erythematosus' two patients treated with danazol. BMJ (Clin Res) 1982 May 15;284(6327):1431–1432.

M593. Moroi Y, Peebles C, Fritzler MJ, Steigerwald J, Tan EM. Autoantibody to centromere (Kinetochore) in scleroderma sera. Proc Natl Acad Sci 1980 Mar;77:1627–1631.

M594. Morquio L. Sur une maladie enfantile et familiale caracterisee par des modifications des pouls, des attaques syncopales et epileptiformes et la mort subite. Arch Med Enfants 1901;4:467.

M595. Morris JL, Zizic TM, Stevens MB. Proteus polyarthritis complicating systemic lupus erythematosus. Johns Hopkins Med J 1973 Nov;133:262–269.

M596. Morris MC, Cameron JS, Chantler C, Turner DR. Systemic lupus erythematosus with nephritis. Arch Dis Child 1981 Oct; 56:779–783.

M597. Morris MH. Acute lupus erythematosus disseminate treated with penicillin. N Y State J Med 1946 Apr 15;46: 917–918.

M598. Morris RC Jr. Renal tubular acidosis. Mechanisms, classification and implications. N Engl J Med 1969 Dec 18;281: 1405–1413.

M599. Morris RJ, Freed CR, Kohler PF. Drug acetylation phenotype unrelated to development of spontaneous systemic lupus erythematosus. Arthritis Rheum 1979 Jul;22:777–780.

M600. Morris RJ, Guggenheim SJ, McIntosh RM, Rubin RI, Kohler PF. Simultaneous immunologic studies of skin and kidney in systemic lupus erythematosus: Clinicopathologic correlations. Arthritis Rheum 1979 Aug;22(8):864–870.

M601. Morris SC, Cheek RL, Cohen PL, Eisenberg RA. Autoantibodies in chronic graft versus host result from cognate T-B interactions. J Exp Med 1990;171:503–517.

M602. Morris SC, Cheek RL, Cohen PL, Eisenberg RA. Allotype-specific immunoregulation of autoantibody production by host B cells in chronic graft-versus-host disease. J Immunol 1990;144:916–922.

M603. Morrow JD, Schroeder HA, Perry HM Jr. Studies on the control of hypertension by Hyphex. II. Toxic reactions and side effects. Circulation 1953;8:829–839.

M604. Morrow M, Hager C, Berger D, Djordjevic B. Chloroquine as a hyperthermia potentiator. J Surg Res 1989 Jun;46(6): 637–639.

M605. Morrow WJ, Ohashi Y, Hall J, Pribnow J, Hirose S, Shirai T, Levy JA. Dietary fat and immune function. I. Antibody responses, lymphocyte and accessory cell function in (NZB × NZW)F1 mice. J Immunol 1985;135:3857–3863.

M606. Morrow WJW, Isenberg DA, Parry HF, Shen L, Okolie EE, Farzaneh F, Shall S, Snaith ML. Studies on autoantibodies to poly (adenosine diphosphate-ribose) in SLE and other autoimmune disease. Ann Rheum Dis 1982 Aug;41:396–402.

M607. Morrow WJW, Isenberg DA, Parry HF, Snaith ML. C-reactive protein in sera from patients with systemic lupus erythematosus. J Rheumatol 1981 May–Jun;8:599–604.

M608. Morrow WJW, Isenberg DA, Todd-Pokropek A, Parry HF, Snaith ML. Useful laboratory measurements in the management of systemic lupus erythematosus. Q J Med 1982 Spring; 51:125–138.

M609. Morrow MJW, Williams DJP, Ferec C, Casburn-Budd R, Isenberg DA, Paice E, Snaith ML, Youinou P, LeGoff P. The use of C3d as a means of monitoring clinical activity in systemic lupus erythematosus and rheumatoid arthritis. Ann Rheum Dis 1983 Dec;42(6):668–671.

M610. Morse HC 3d, Davidson WF, Yetter RA, Murphy ED, Roths JB, Coffman RL. Abnormalities induced by the mutant gene lpr: expansion of a unique lymphocyte subset. J Immunol 1982 Dec;129(6):2612–2615.

M611. Morse JH, Stearns G, Arden J. The effects of crude and purified human gonadotropin on in vitro stimulated human lymphocyte cultures. Cell Immunol 1976;5:178.

M612. Morse PF, Horrobin DF, Manku MS, Stewart JCM, Allen R, Littlewood S, Wright S, Burton J, Gould DJ, Holt PJ, Jansen CT, Mattila L, Meigel W, Dettke TH, Wexler D, Guenther L, Bordon A, Patrizi A. Meta-analysis of placebo-controlled studies of the efficacy of Epogam in the treatment of altopic eczema: relationship between plasma essential fatty acid changes and clinical response. Br J Dermatol 1989;121:75–90.

M613. Morsman CD, Livesey SJ, Richards IM, Jessop JD, Mills PV. Screening for hydroxychloroquine retinal toxicity: is it necessary? Eye 1990;4(Pt 4):572–576.

M614. Morteo OG, Franklin EC, McEwen C, Phythyon J, Tanner M. Clinical and laboratory studies of relatives with systemic lupus erythematosus. Arthritis Rheum 1961;4:356–361.

M615. Mortley KP, Parke A, Hughes GRV. SLE: Two patients treated with Danazol. BMJ 1982;284:1431–1432.

M616. Morton H, Kolfe B, Clunie GJA, Anderson MJ, Morrison J. An early pregnancy factor detected in human serum by the rosette inhibition test. Lancet 1977;1:394–397.

M617. Morton JI, Siegel BV. Transplantation of autoimmune potential. I. Development of antinuclear antibodies in H-2 histocompatible recipients of bone marrow from New Zealand black mice. Proc Natl Acad Sci USA 1974 Jun;71:2162–2165.

M618. Morton JI, Siegel BV, Moore RD. Transplantation of autoimmune potential. II. Glomerulonephritis in lethally irradiated DBA/2 recipients of NZB bone marrow cells. Transplantation 1975 Jun;19(6):464–469.

M619. Morton RE, Miller AI, Kaplan R. Systemic lupus erythematosus: unusual presentation with gastric polyps and vasculitis. South Med J 1976 Apr;69(4):507–509.

M620. Morton RO, Gershwin ME, Brady C, Steinberg AD. The incidence of systemic lupus erythematosus in North American Indians. J Rheumatol 1976 Jun;3:186–190.

M621. Moscovitch M, Rosenmann E, Neeman Z, Slavin S. Successful treatment of autoimmune manifestations in MRL/l and MRL/n mice using total lymphoid irradiation (TLI). Exp Mol Pathol 1983;38:33–47.

M622. Moses RE, McCormick A, Nickey W. Fatal arrhythmia after pulse methylprednisolone. Ann Intern Med 1981 Dec;95: 781–782.

M623. Moskowitz R, Strober S, Trentham D. Total lymphoid irradiation: A viable therapeutic approach for connective tissue disease? Point/Counterpoint 1990;7:3–12.

M624. Moskowitz RW, Katz D. Chondrocalcinosis coincidental to other rheumatic disease. Arch Intern Med 1965 Jun;115: 680–683.

M625. Moss C, Hamilton PJ. Thrombocytopenia in systemic lupus erythematosus responsive to dapsone. BMJ (Clin Res) 1988 Jul 23;297(6643):266.

M626. Mossard JM, Walter P, Brechenmacher C, Voegtlin R. Cardiac injury in the course of SLE [original in French]. Arch des Malades de Coeur 1977 Nov;70:1203–1208.

M627. Motoo Y, Wakatsuki T, Tanaka N, Hinoue Y, Kobayashi K, Hattori N, Matsui O, Izumi R, Nakanuma Y, Ohta H. Resected case of hepatocellular carcinoma associated with lupoid hepatitis. J Gastroenterol Hepatol 1989;4:295–298.

M628. Mottironi VD, Terasaki PI. Lymphocytotoxins in disease. I. Infectious mononucleosis, rubella, and measles. In: Terasaki PI, editor. Histocompatibility Testing. 1970:301.

M629. Moudgil A, Kishore K, Srivastava RN. Neonatal lupus erythematosus, late onset hypocalcemia, and recurrent seizures. Arch Dis Child 1987;62:736.

M630. Mountz JD, Gause WC, Finkelman FD, Steinberg AD. Prevention of lymphadenopathy in MRL-lpr/lpr mice by blocking peripheral lymph node homing with Mel-14 in vivo. J Immunol 1988;140:2943–2949.

M631. Mountz JD, Mushinski JF, Mark GE, Steinberg AD. Oncogene expression in autoimmune mice. J Mol Cell Immunol 1985;2:121–131.

M632. Mountz JD, Smith HR, Wilder RL, Reeves JP, Steinberg AD. Cs-A therapy in MRL-lpr/lpr mice: Amelioration of immunopathology despite autoantibody production. J Immunol 1987;138:157–163.

M633. Mountz JD, Smith TM, Toth KS. Altered expression of self-reactive T cell receptor V beta regions in autoimmune mice. J Immunol 1990 Mar;144(6):2159–2166.

M634. Moutsopoulos HM, Boehm-Truitt M, Kassan SS, Chused TM. Demonstration of activation of B lymphocytes in New Zealand black mice at birth by an immunoradiometric assay for murine IgM. J Immunol 1977 Nov;119(5):1639–1644.

M635. Moutsopoulos HM, Gallagher JD, Decker JL, Steinberg AD. Herpes zoster in patients with systemic lupus erythematosus. Arthritis Rheum 1978 Sep–Oct;21(7):798–802.

M636. Moutsopoulos HM, Klippel JH, Pavlidis N, Wolf RO, Sweet JB, Steinberg AD, Chu FC, Tarpley TM. Corrective histologic and serologic findings of sicca syndrome in patients with systemic lupus erythematosus. Arthritis Rheum 1980 Jan;23(1): 36–40.

M637. Moutsopoulos HM, Mann DL, Johnson AH, Chused TM. Genetic differences between primary and secondary sicca syndrome. N Engl J Med 1979;301:761–763.

M638. Mowry KL, Steitz JA. Identification of the human U7 snRNP as one of the several factors involved in the 3' end maturation of histone premessenger RNAs. Science 1987;238: 1682–1687.

M639. Moxey-Mims MM, Preston K, Fivush B, McCurdy F. Heptavax-B in pediatric dialysis patients: effect of systemic lupus erythematosus. Chesapeake Pediatric Nephrology Study Group. Pediatr Nephrol 1990 Mar;4(2):171–173.

M640. Mubagwa K, Adler J. Muscarinic antagonist action of clinical doses of chloroquine in healthy volunteers. J Auton Nerv Syst 1988 Sep;24(1–2):147–155.

M641. Mueh JR, Herbst KD, Rapaport SI. Thrombosis in patients with the lupus anticoagulant. Ann Intern Med 1980 Feb;92: 156–159.

M642. Muehrcke RC, Kark RM, Pirani CL, Pollak VE. Lupus nephritis: A clinical and pathologic study based on renal biopsies. Medicine 1957 Feb;36:1–145.

M643. Mukherjee P, Mastro AM, Hymer WC. Prolactin induction of interleukin-2 receptors on rat splenic lymphocytes. Endoimmunology 1990;120:88–94.

M644. Mukwayan G. Immunosuppressive effects and infections associated with corticosteroid therapy. Pediatr Infect Dis J 1988;7:499–504.

M645. Mulhern LM, Masi AT, Shulman LE. Hashimoto's disease. A search for associated disorders in 170 clinically detected cases. Lancet 1966;2:508–512.

M646. Muller S, Barakat S, Watts R, Joubaud P, Isenberg D. Longitudinal analysis of antibodies to histones, Sm-D peptides and ubiquitin in the serum of patients with systemic lupus erythematosus, rheumatoid arthritis and tuberculosis. Clin Exp Rheumatol 1990;8:445–453.

M647. Muller S, Bonnier D, Thiry M, Van Regenmortel MHV. Reactivity of Autoantibodies in Systemic Lupus Erythematosus with Synthetic Core Histone Peptides. Int Arch Allergy Appl Immunol 1989;89:288–296.

M648. Muller S, Briand JP, Van Regenmortel MHV. Presence of antibodies to ubiquitin during the autoimmune response associated with systemic lupus erythematosus. Proc Natl Acad Sci USA 1988; 85:8176–8180.

M649. Muller S, Chaix ML, Briand JP, Van Regenmortel MHV. Immunogenicity of free histones and of histones complexed with RNA. Mol Immunol 1991;28:763–772.

M650. Muller S, Rother U, Westerhausen M. Complement activation by cryoglobulin. Clin Exp Immunol 1976 Feb;23: 233–241.

M651. Muller S, Van Regenmortel MHV. Specificity of anti-histone autoantibodies in systemic rheumatic disease. Int J Immunopathol Pharmacol 1988;1:139–148.

M652. Muller-Eberhard HJ. The complement system and nephritis. Adv Nephrol 1974;4:3–14.

M653. Muller-Eberhard HJ. The membrane attack complex of complement. Ann Rev Immunol 1986;4:503–528.

M654. Mullins JF, Watts FL, Wilson CJ. Plaquenil in the treatment of lupus erythematosus. JAMA 1956 Jun 30;161:879–881.

M655. Mullins WW Jr, Plotz PH, Schriebner L. Soluble immune complexes in lupus mice: clearance from blood and estimation of formation rates. Clin Immunol Immunopathol 1987; 42:375–385.

M656. Mulshine J, Lucas FV, Clough JD. Platelet-bound IgG in systemic lupus erythematosus with and without thrombocytopenia. J Immunol Methods 1981;275(3):275.

M657. Mund A, Simson J, Rothfield NF. Effect of pregnancy on course of systemic lupus erythematosus. JAMA 1963;183: 917–922.

M658. Muniain M, Spilberg I. Opera-glass deformity and tendon rupture in a patient with systemic lupus erythematosus. Clin Rheumatol 1985 Sep;4(3):335–339.

M659. Munns TW, Liszewski MK, Hahn BH. Antibody-nucleic acid complexes. Conformational and base specificities associated with spontaneously occurring poly- and monoclonal anti-DNA from autoimmune mice. Biochemistry Jun 19;23(13): 2964–2970.

M660. Munves EF, Schur PH. Antibodies to Sm and RNP. Prognosticators of disease involvement. Arthritis Rheum 1983 Jul; 26(7):848–853.

M661. Murai K, Oku H, Takeuchi K, Kanayama Y, Inoue T, Takeda T. Alterations in myocardial systolic diastolic function in patients with active lupus erythematosus. Am Heart J 1987; 11:966–971.

M662. Murakawa Y, Sakane T. Deficient phytohemagglutinin-induced interleukin-2 activity in patients with inactive systemic lupus erythematosus is correctable by the addition of phorbol myristate acetate. Arthritis Rheum 1988;31:826–833.

M663. Murakawa Y, Takada S, Ueda Y, Suzuki N, Hoshino T, Sakane T. Characterization of T lymphocyte subpopulations responsible for deficient interleukin 2 activity in patients with systemic lupus erythematosus. J Immunol 1985 Jan;134: 187–195.

M664. Murashima A, Takasaki Y, Ohgaki M, Hashimoto H, Shirai T, Hirose S. Activated peripheral blood mononuclear cells de-tected by murine monoclonal antibodies to proliferating cell nuclear antigen in active lupus patients. J Clin Immunol 1990; 10:28–37.

M665. Murphy ED, Roths JB. A single gene for massive lymphoproliferation with immune complex disease in a new mouse strain MRL. In: Proceedings of the 16th International Congress in Hematology. Amsterdam: Excerpta Medica, 1976:69.

M666. Murphy ED, Roths JB. New Inbred strains. Mouse News Letter 1978;58:51.

M667. Murphy ED, Roths JB. A Y chromosome associated factor in strain BXSB producing accelerated autoimmunity and lymphoproliferation. Arthritis Rheum 1979;22:1188–1194.

M668. Murphy EL Jr, DeCeulaer K, Williams W, Clark JW, Saxinger C, Gibbs SWn, Blattner WA. Lack of relation between human T-lymphotropic virus Type I infection and systemic lupus erythematosus in Jamaica, West Indies. JAIDS 1988;1: 18–22.

M669. Murphy JJ, Leach IH. Findings at necropsy at the heart of a patient with anticardiolipin syndrome. Br Heart J 1989 Jul; 62(1):61–64.

M670. Murphy RC, Falck JR, Lumin S, Yadagiri P, Zirrolli JA, Balazy M, Masferrer JL, Abraham NG, Schwartzman ML. 12(4)-hydroxy eicosatrienoic acid: a vasodilator cytochrome P-450-dependent arachidonate metabolite from the bovine corneal epithelium. J Biol Chem 1988;263:17197–17202.

M671. Murphy S, LoBuglio AF. Drug therapy of autoimmune hemolytic anemia. Sem Haematol 1976;13:323–337.

M672. Murray FA. Lupus erythematosus in pregnancy. J Obstet Gynecol Pr Emp 1956;65:401.

M673. Murray FT, Fuleihan DS, Cornwall CS, Pinals RS. Acute mitral regurgitation from ruptured chordae tendinae in systemic lupus erythematosus. J Rheumatol 1975;2:454–459.

M674. Murray-Lyon IM, Stern RB, Williams R. Controlled trial of prednisone and azathioprine in active chronic hepatitis. Lancet 1973 Apr 7;1:735–737.

M675. Muryoi T, Sasaki T, Hatakeyama A, Shibata S, Suzuki M, Seino J, Yoshinaga K. Clonotypes of anti-DNA antibodies expressing specific idiotypes in immune complexes of patients with active lupus nephritis. J Immunol 1990 May;144(10): 3856–3861.

M676. Muryoi T, Sasaki T, Sekiguchi Y, Tamate E, Takai O, Yoshinaga K. Impaired accessory cell function of monocytes in systemic lupus erythematosus. J Clin Lab Immunol 1989;28: 123–128.

M677. Muschel LH. Systemic lupus erythematosus and normal antibodies. Proc Soc Exp Biol Med 1961 Mar;106;622–625.

M678. Musher DR. Systemic lupus erythematosus. A cause of "medical peritonitis." Am J Surg 1972 Sep;124:368–372.

M678a. Mustafa MH, Mispireta LA, Pierce LE. Occult pulmonary embolism presenting with thrombocytopenia and elevated fibrin split products. Am J Med 1989;86:490–491.

M679. Mustakallio KK, Lassus A, Putkonen T, Wager O. Cryoglobulins and rheumatoid factor in systemic lupus erythematosus. Acta Dermatovener (Stockh) 1967;47(4):241–248.

M680. Muzellec Y, Le Goff P, Jouquan J, Fauquert P, Muller S, Youinou P. Antibodies to histones in rheumatoid arthritis. Diag Clin Immunol 1988;5:326–331.

M681. Muzes G, Vien CV, Gonzalez-Cabello R, Feher J, Gergely P. Defective production of interleukin-1 and tumor necrosis factor alpha by stimulated monocytes from patients with systemic lupus erythematosus. Acta Medica Hungarica 1989;46: 245–252.

M682. Myers JL, Katzenstein AA. Microangitis in lupus-induced pulmonary hemorrhage. Am J Clin Path 1986;85:552–556.

M683. Mylvaganam R, Ahn YS, Harrington W, Kim CI. Immune modulation by danazol in autoimmune thrombocytopenia. Clin Immunol Immunopathol 1987;42:281–287.

N

N1. Naafs B, Bakkers EJM, Flinterman J, Faber WR. Thalidomide treatment of subacute cutaneous lupus erythematosus. Br J Dermatol 1982;107:83–86.

N2. Naama JK, Holme E, Hamilton E, Whaley K. Prevention of immune precipitation by purified components of the alternative pathway. Clin Exp Immunol 1984;60:169–177.

N3. Nadorra RL, Landing BH. Pulmonary lesions in childhood onset systemic lupus erythematosus. Pediatr Path 1987;7:1–18.

N4. Nadorra RL, Nakazato Y, Landing BH. Pathologic features of gastrointestinal tract lesions in childhood-onset systemic lupus erythematosus: study of 26 patients, with review of the literature. Pediatr Pathol 1987;7(3):245–259.

N5. Nagasawa K, Ishii Y, Mayumi T, Tada Y, Ueda A, Yamauchi Y, Kusaba T, Niho Y. Avascular necrosis of bone in systemic lupus erythematosus: possible role of haemostatic abnormalities. Ann Rheum Dis 1989 Aug;48(8):672–676.

N6. Nagasawa K, Yamauchi Y, Tada Y, Kusaba T, Niho Y, Yoshikawa H. High incidence of herpes zoster in patients with systemic lupus erythematosus: an immunological analysis. Ann Rheum Dis 1990 Aug;49(8):630–633.

N7. Nagasawa T, Sakurai T, Kashiwagi H, Abe T. Cell mediated megakaryocytic thrombocytopenia associated with systemic lupus erythematosus. Blood 1986;67:479–483.

N8. Nagata M, Ogawa Y, Hisana S, Ueda K. Crohn disease in systemic lupus erythematosus: a case report. Eur J Pediatr 1989 Apr;148(6):525–526.

N9. Nagayama Y, Fukase M. Suppression of 3H-thymidine incorporation into PHA-stimulated lymphocytes ty testosterone. Acta Haematol Jpn 1978;41:11–16.

N10. Nagayama Y, Kazuyama Y. Serum anti-herpes virus antibody titre in patients with active systemic lupus erythematosus. Int J Immunotherapy 1987;3:59–64.

N11. Nagayama Y, Kusudo K, Imura H. A case of central nervous system lupus associated with ruptured cerebral berry aneurysm. Jpn J Med 1989 Jul–Aug;28(4):530–533.

N12. Nagayama Y, Namura Y, Tamura T, Muso R. Beneficial effect of prostaglandin E1 in three cases of lupus nephritis with nephrotic syndrome. Ann Allergy 1988 Oct;61(4):289–295.

N13. Nagler-Anderson C, van-Vollenhove RF, Gurish MF, Bober LA, Siskind GW, Thorbecke GJ. A cross-reactive idiotype on anti-collagen antibodies in collagen-induced arthritis: identification and relevance to disease. Cell Immunol 1988;113:447.

N14. Nagy E, Balogh E. Bullous form of chronic discoid lupus erythematodes accompanied by L.E. cell symptoms. Dermatologica (Basel) 1961 Jan;122:6–10.

N15. Nagy E, Kocsar L. Experiments on the antihistaminic action of Atabrine. Derm Wschr 1956;133:265–269.

N16. Nahm MH, Clevinger BL, Davie JM. Monoclonal antibodies to streptococcal group A carbohydrate. I. A dominant idiotypic determinant is located on V_k. J Immunol 1982;129:1513.

N17. Naides SJ. Suppression of antigen-specific interleukin 2 production in the MRL/MpJ-lpr/lpr mouse. J Immunol 1986;136:4113–4121.

N18. Naimiuchi S, Kumagai S, Imura H, Suginoshita T, Hattori T, Hirata F. Quinacrine inhibits the primary but not secondary proliferative response of human cytotoxic T cells to allogeneic non-T cell antigens. J Immunol 1984 Mar;132(3):1456–1461.

N19. Nai-Zheng C. Rheumatic diseases in China. J Rheumatol 1983 Nov;10 Suppl 10:41–44.

N20. Nai-Zheng Z. Epidemiology of systemic lupus erythematosus (SLE) in China. In: Proceedings of the Second International Conference on Systemic Lupus Erythematosus. Tokyo. 1989:29.

N21. Nakae K, Furusawa F, Kasukawa R, et al. A nationwide epidemiological survey on diffuse collagen diseases: estimation of prevalence rate in Japan. In: Kasukawa R, Missouri GC, editors. Mixed connective tissue disease and anti-nuclear antibodies. Amsterdam: Elsevier, 1987:9.

N22. Nakai Y, Yoshida H, Maruyama N, Shirai T, Hamashima Y. Association between circulating immune complexes and renal disease in New Zealand mice. Clin Exp Immunol 1981;43:240–245.

N23. Nakamura H, Uehara H, Okada T, Kambe H, Kimura Y, Ito H, Hayashi E, Yamamoto H, Kishimoto S. Occlusion of small hepatic veins associated with systemic lupus erythematosus with the lupus anticoagulant and anti-cardiolipin antibody. Hepatogastroenterology 1989 Oct;36(5):393–397.

N24. Nakano I, Mannen T, Mizutani T, Yokohari R. Peripheral white matter lesions of the spinal cord with changes in small arachnoid arteries in systemic lupus erythematosus. Clin Neuropathol 1989 Mar–Apr;8(2):102–108.

N25. Nakao Y, Miyazaki T, Ota K, Matsumoto H, Nishitani H, Fusita T, Tsuji K. Gm allotypes in myasthenia gravis. Lancet 1980 Mar 29;1:677–680.

N26. Nakao Y, Matsumoto H, Miyazaki T, Nishitani H, Takatsuki K, Kasukawa R, Nakayama S, Izumi S, Fujita T, Tsuji K. IgG heavy chain allotypes (Gm) in autoimmune diseases. Clin Exp Immunol 1980;42:20–26.

N27. Nakazato Y, Hirato J, Ishida Y, Hoshi S, Haseqawa M, Fukuda T. Swollen cortical neurons in Creutzfeldt-Jakob disease contain a phosphorylated neurofilament epitope. J Neuropathol Exp Neurol 1990;49:197.

N28. Naparstek Y, Andre-Schwartz J, Manser T, Wysocki L, Breitman L, Stollar BD, Schwartz RS. A single V_H germline gene segment of normal A/J mice encodes autoantibodies characteristic of systemic lupus erythematosus. J Exp Med 1986;164:614–626.

N29. Naparstek Y, Ben-Yehuda A, Madaio MP, Bar-Tana R, Schuger L, Pizov G, Neeman Z, Cohan IR. Binding of anti-DNA antibodies and inhibition of glomerulonephritis in MRL-lpr/lpr mice by heparin. Arthritis Rheum 1990;33:1554–1559.

N30. Naparstek Y, Duggan D, Schattner A, Madaio MP, Goni F, Frangione G, Stollar BD, Kabat EA, Schwartz RS. Immunochemical similarities between monoclonal anti-bacterial Waldenstrom's macroglobulins and monclonal anti-DNA lupus autoantibodies. J Exp Med 1985;161:1525–1538.

N31. Naparstek Y, Kupolovic J, Tur-Kaspa R, Rubinger D. Focal glomerulonephritis in the course of hydralazine-induced lupus syndrome. Arthritis Rheum 1984 Jul;27:822–825.

N32. Narula AA, Powell RJ, Davis A. Frequency solving ability in systemic lupus erythematosus. Br J Audiol 1989;23:69–72.

N33. Nashel D, Ulmer C. Systemic lupus erythematosus, Important considerations in the adolescent. J Adol Health Care 1982;2:273.

N34. Nashel DJ, Leonard A, Mann DL, Guccion JG, Katz AL, Sliwinski AJ. Ankylosing spondylitis and systemic lupus erythematosus. A rare HLA combination. Arch Intern Med 1982 Jun;142(6):1227–1228.

N35. Nassberger L, Johansson AC, Bjorck S, Sjoholm AG. Antibodies to neutrophil granulocyte myeloperoxidase and elastase: autoimmune responses in glomerulonephritis and due to hydralazine treatment. J Intern Med 1991;229:261–265.

N36. Nassberger L, Sjoholm AG, Johnson H, Sturfelt G, Akesson A. Autoantibodies against neutrophil cytoplasm components in systemic lupus erythematosus and in hydralazine-induced lupus. Clin Exp Immunol 1990;81:380–383.

N37. Nassonova VA, Alekberova ZS, Folomeyev MY, Mylov NM. Sacroiilitis in male systemic lupus erythematosus. Scand J Rheumatol 1984;53 Suppl:23–29.

N38. Nastasi G, Crema F, Attardo-Parrinello G, Spaghi A, Pezzali M, Mazzone A, Rizzo SC. Intrahepatic cholestasis due to azathioprine during treatment of systemic lupus erythematosus. A case report. Medicina-Riv EMI 1987;7:69−70.

N39. Natali PG, DeMartino C, Marcellini M, Quaranta V, Ferrona S. Expression of Ia-like antigens on the vasculature of the human kidney. Clin Immunol Immunopathol 1981 Jan;20: 11−20.

N40. Natali PG, Mottoles N, Noctra NR. Immune complex formation in NB/W mice after ultraviolet light radiation. Clin Immunol Immunopathol 1978;10:414−419.

N41. Natali PG, Tan EM. Experimental renal disease induced by DNA anti-DNA immune complexes. J Clin Invest 1972;51: 345−355.

N42. Natali PG, Tan EM. Experimental skin lesions in mice resembling systemic lupus erythematosus. Arthritis Rheum 1973;16:579−589.

N43. Natelson KA, Cyprus GS, Hettig RA. Absent factor II in systemic lupus erythematosus. Immunologic studies and response to corticosteroid therapy. Arthritis Rheum 1976 Jan−Feb;19:79−82.

N44. Nathan DJ, Snapper I. Simultaneous placental transfer of factors responsible for L.E. cell formation and thrombocytopenia. Am J Med 1958 Oct;25:647−653.

N45. Nation RL, Hacket LP, Dusci LJ, Ilett KF. Excretion of hydroxychloroquine in human milk. Br J Clin Pharmacol 1984; 17:368−369.

N46. Natour J, Montezzo LC, Moura LA, Atra E. A study of synovial membrane of patients with systemic lupus erythematosus (SLE). Clin Exp Rheumatol 1991;9:221−225.

N47. Neary BA, Mura CV, Stollar BD. Serological homologies between H1 degrees and H5 include the carboxyl terminus domain. J Biol Chem 1985;260:15850−15855.

N48. Neary BA, Stollar BD. The carboxyl-terminal domain of murine H1o: Immunochemical and partial amino acid sequence comparisons with other H1o/H1/H5 histones. Eur J Biochem 1987;168:161−167.

N49. Needleman P, Turk J, Jakschik BA, Morrison AR, Lefkowith JB. Aracidonic acid metabolism. Ann Rev Biocem 1986;55: 69−102.

N50. Needleman SW, Silber RA, Von Brecht JH, Goeken JA. Systemic lupus erythematosus complicated by disseminated sarcoidosis. Report of a case associated with circulating immune complexes. Am J Clin Pathol 1982 Jul;78(1):105−107.

N51. Needs CJ, Brooks PM. Antirheumatic medication during lactation. Br J Rheumatol 1985;24:291−297.

N52. Negoro N, Kanayama Y, Takeda T, Amatsu K, Koda S, Inoue Y, Kim T, Okamura M, Inoue T. Clinical significance of U1-RNP immune complexes in mixed connective tissue disease and systemic lupus erythematosus. Rheumatol Int 1987;7(1): 7−11.

N53. Negoro N, Okamura M, Takeda T, Koda S, Amatsu K, Inoue T, Curd JG, Kanayama Y. The clinical significance of iC3b neoantigen expression in plasma from patients with systemic lupus erythematosus. Arthritis Rheum 1989;32:1233−1242.

N54. Neilan BA, Barney SN. Hyposplenism in systemic lupus erythematosus. J Rheumatol 1983 Apr;10:332−334.

N55. Neill WA, Panayi GS, Duthie JJR, Prescott RJ. Action of chloroquine phosphate in rheumatoid arthritis. II. Chromosome damaging effect. Ann Rheum Dis 1973;32:547−550.

N56. Neiman RA, Fye KH. Methotrexate induced false photosensitivity reaction. J Rheumatol 1985 Apr;12(2);354−355.

N57. Nel AE, Bouic P, Lattanze GR, Stevenson HC, Miller P, Dirienzo W, Stefanini GF, Galbraith MR. Reaction of T lymphocytes with anti-T3 induces translocation of C-kinase activity to the membrane and specific substrate phosphorylation. J Immunol 1987;138:3519−3524.

N58. Nelissen RLH, Heinrichs V, Habets WJ, Simons F, Luhrmann R, van Venrooij WJ. Zinc-finger like structure in U1-specific protein C is essential for specific binding to U1 snRNP. Nucleic Acids Res 1991;19:449−454.

N59. Nelson A, Fogel B. Faust D. Bedside cognitive screening instruments. J Nerv Mental Dis 1986;174:73−83.

N60. Nelson AA, Fitzhugh OG. Chloroquine; pathologic changes observed in rats which have been fed various proportions for 2 years. Arch Pathol 1948 Apr;45:454−462.

N61. Nelson AM, Conn DL. Glucocorticoids in rheumatic disease. Mayo Clin Proc 1980 Dec;55:758−769.

N62. Nelson DS. Immune adherence. Adv Immunol 1963;3: 131−180.

N63. Nelson RA. The immune adherence phenomenon: an immunologically specific reaction between micro-organisms and erythrocytes leading to enhanced phagocytosis. Science 1953; 118:733−737.

N64. Nelson RA Jr, Mayer NM. Immobilization of treponema pallidum in vitro by antibody produced in syphilitic infection. J Exp Med 1949 Apr;89:369−393.

N65. Nemazee DA, Burki K. Clonal deletion of B lymphocytes in a transgenic mice bearing anti-MHC class I antibody genes. Nature 1989;337:562−566.

N66. Nepom BS, Schaller JG. Childhood systemic lupus erythematosus. Prog Clin Rheumatol 1984;1:33−69.

N67. Nesbitt LT Jr. Cutaneous immunofluorescence in dermatomyositis. Int J Dermatol 1980 Jun;19(5):270−278.

N68. Neu HC, Silva M, Hazen E, Rosenheim SH. Necrotizing nocardial pneumonitis [case report]. Ann Intern Med 1967 Feb;66(2):274−284.

N69. Neumann R, Schmidt JB, Niebauer G. Subacute lupus erythematosus-like gyrate erythema. Report of a case associated with a breast cancer. Dermatologica 1986;173:146−149.

N70. Newbold KM, Allum WH, Downing R, Symmons DP, Oates GD. Vasculitis of the gall bladder in rheumatoid arthritis and systemic lupus erythematosus. Clin Rheumatol 1987 Jun;6(2): 287−289.

N71. Newbold PC. Beta-carotene in the treatment of discoid lupus erythematosus. Br J Dermatol 1976 Jul;95(1):100−101.

N72. Newkirk MM, Mageed RA, Jefferis R, Chen PP, Capra JD. Complete amino acid sequences of variable regions of two human IgM rheumatoid factors, BOR and KAS of the Wa idiotypic family, reveal restricted use of heavy and light chain variable and joining region gene segments. J Exp Med 1987;166: 550.

N73. Newland AC. Annotation: The use and mechanism of action of intravenous immunoglobulin, an update. Br J Haematol 1989;72:301−305.

N74. Newman DM, Walter JB. Multiple dermatofibromas in patients with systemic lupus erythematosus on immunosuppressive therapy. N Engl J Med 1973 Oct 18;289:842−843.

N75. Newman W, Fast LD, Rose LM. Blockade of NK cell lysis is a property of monoclonal antibodies that bind to distinct regions of T-200. J Immunol 1983;131:1742−1747.

N76. Newport JW, Forbes DJ. The nucleus: structure, function, and dynamics. Ann Rev Biochem 1987; 56:535−565.

N77. Newton P, Aldridge RD, Lessels AM, Best PV. Progressive multifocal leukoencephalopathy complicating systemic lupus erythematosus. Arthritis Rheum 1986 Mar;29(3):337−343.

N78. Newton RC, Jorizzo JL, Solomon AR, Sanchez RL, Daniels JC, Bell JD, Cavallo T. Mechanism-oriented assessment of isotretinoin in chronic or subacute cutaneous lupus erythematosus. Arch Dermatol 1986 Feb;122(2):170−176.

N79. Ng HS, Ng HW, Sinniah R, Feng PH. A case of systemic lupus erythematosus with sideroblastic anemia terminating in erythroleukemia. Ann Rheum Dis 1981 Aug;40:422−426.

N80. Ng MHL, Li EK, Feng CS. Gelatinous transformation of the bone marrow in systemic lupus erythematosus. J Rheumatol 1989;16:989−992.

N81. Ng RCK, Craddock PR. End-stage renal disease in systemic lupus erythematosus. N Engl J Med 1983;308:1357.

N82. Ng YC, Schifferli JA, Walport MJ. Immune complexes and erythrocyte CR1 (complement receptor type I): Effect of CR1 numbers on binding and release reactions. Clin Exp Immunol 1988;71:481–485.

N83. Ngo AW, Straka C, Fretzin D. Pemphigus erythematosus: A unique association with systemic lupus erythematosus. Cutis 1986 Sep;38(3):160–163.

N84. Nice CM Jr. Congenital disseminated lupus erythematosus. AJR 1962;86:585–587.

N85. Nichols CJ, Mieler WF. Severe retinal vaso-occlusive disease secondary to procainamide-induced lupus. Ophthalmology 1989 Oct;96(10):1535–1540.

N86. Nickel BE, Allis CD, Davie JR. Ubiquitinated histone H2B is preferentially located in transcriptionally active chromatin. Biochemistry 1989;28:958–963.

N87. Nickel BE, Davie JR. Structure of polyubiquitinated histone H2A. Biochemistry 1989;28:964–968.

N88. Nickerson KG, Berman J, Glickman E, Chess L, Alt FW. Early human IgH gene assembly in Epstein-Barr virus-transformed fetal B cell lines: Preferential utilization of the most J_H-proximal D segment (DQ52) and two unusual V_H-related rearrangements. J Exp Med 1989;169:1391–1403.

N89. Nicolas JF, Thivolet J, Kanitakis J, Lyonnet S. Response of discoid and subacute cutaneous lupus erythematosus to recombinant interferon alpha 2a. J Invest Dermatol 1990;95 Suppl 6:142S-145S.

N90. Nieboer C, Tak-Diamand Z, Van Leeuwen-Wallau AG. Dust-like particles: A specific direct immunofluorescence pattern in subacute cutaneous lupus erythematosus. Br J Dermatol 1988;118:725–734.

N91. Niebyl JR, editor. Drug Use in Pregnancy. Philadelphia: Lea & Febiger, 1982.

N92. Niebyl JR, Blake DA, White RD, Kumor KM, Dubin NH, Robinson JC, Egner PG. The inhibition of premature labor with indomethacin. Am J Obstet Gynecol 1980;136:1014–1019.

N93. Nies K, Boyer R, Stevens R, Louie J. Anti-tetanus toxoid antibody synthesis after booster immunization in systemic lupus erythematosus: Comparison of the in vitro and in vivo responses. Arthritis Rheum 1980 Dec;23(12):1343–1350.

N94. Nies KM, Brown JC, Dubois EL, Quismorio FP, Friou GJ, Terasaki PI. Histocompatibility (HLA) antigens and lymphocytotoxic antibodies in systemic lupus erythematosus (SLE). Arthritis Rheum 1974 Jul–Aug;17(4):397–402.

N95. Nies KM, Stevens RH, Louie JS. Normal T cell regulation of IgG synthesis in systemic lupus erythematosus. J Clin Lab Immunol 1980 Sep;4:69–75.

N96. Nievoer C. Lupus erythematosus/lichen planus (LE/LP) overlap syndrome. J Am Acad Dermatol 1985;13:297.

N97. Nigg EA, Baeuerie PA, Luhrmann R. Nuclear import-export; in search of signals and mechanisms. Cell 1991;66:15–22.

N98. Nihoyannopoulos P, Gomez PM, Joshi J, Loizou S, Walport MJ, Oakley CM. Cardiac abnormalities in systemic lupus erythematosus. Association with raised anticardiolipin antibodies [comments]. Circulation 1990 Aug;82(2):369–375; 636–638.

N99. Nilsen KH. Systemic lupus erythematosus and avascular bone necrosis. N Z Med J 1977 Jun 8;85(589):472–475.

N100. Nilsson IM, Astedt B, Hedner U, Berezin D. Intrauterine death and circulating anticoagulant, "antithromboplastin." Acta Med Scand 1975;197:153–159.

N101. Nimelstein SH, Brody S, McShane D, Holman HR. Mixed connective tissue disease: subsequent evaluation of the 25 original patients. Medicine 1980 Jul;59(4):239–248.

N102. Nishikai M, Okano Y, Mukohda Y, Sato A, Ito M. Serial estimation of anti-RNP antibody titers in systemic lupus ery-

thematosus, mixed connective tissue disease and rheumatoid arthritis. J Clin Lab Immunol 1984;13:15–19.

N103. Nishikai M, Sekiguchi S. Relationship of autoantibody expression and HLA phenotype in Japanese patients with connective tissue diseases. Arthritis Rheum 1985;28:579–581.

N104. Nishiya K, Kawabata F, Ota Z. Elevated urinary ferritin in lupus nephritis. J Rheumatol 1989;16:1513–1514.

N105. Nishizuka Y. The role of protein kinase C in cell surface signal transduction and tumor promotion. Nature 1984;308:693–698.

N106. Nisonoff A, Lamoyi E. Implications of the presence of an internal image of the antigen in anti-idiotypic antibodies: Possible application to vaccine production. Clin Immunol Immunopathol 1989;21:397.

N107. Nissenson AR, Port FK. Outcome of ESRD in patients with rare causes of renal failure: III Systemic/vascular disorders. Q J Med 1990;74:63–74.

N108. Nitta Y, Ohashi M. Neonatal lupus syndrome and microtubular structure. J Dermatol 1989;16:54–58.

N109. Nived D, Linder C, Odeberg H, Svensson B. Reduced opsonisation of protein A containing Staphylococcus aureus in sera with cryoglobulins from patients with active systemic lupus erythematosus. Ann Rheum Dis 1985 Apr;44:252–259.

N110. Nived O, Sturfelt G. Epidemiology of systemic lupus erythematosus. Monogr Allergy 1987;21:197.

N111. Nived O, Sturfelt G, Wollheim F. Systemic lupus erythematosus in an adult population in Southern Sweden: incidence, prevalence and validity of ARA revised classification criteria. Br J Rheumatol 1985;24:147.

N112. Nived O, Sturfelt G, Wollheim F. Systemic lupus erythematosus and infection: a controlled and prospective study including an epidemiological group. Q J Med 1985 Jun;55(218):271–287.

N113. Niwa Y, Kanoh T. Immune deficiency states and immune imbalance in systemic lupus erythematosus and other autoimmune diseases. Clin Immunol Immunopathol 1979 Mar;12(3):289–300.

N114. Noel LH, Dorz D, Rothfield NF. Clinical and serologic significance of cutaneous deposits of immunoglobulins, C3, C1g in SLE patients with nephritis. Clin Immunol Immunopathol 1978 Aug;10(4):381–388.

N115. Nolan RJ, Shulman ST, Victorica BE. Congenital complete heart block associated with maternal mixed connective tissue disease. J Pediatrics 1979;95:420–422.

N116. Nolle B, Specks U, Ludemann J, Rohrback MS, DeRemee RA, Gross WL. Anticytoplasmic autoantibodies; their immunodiagnostic value in Wegener granulomatosis. Ann Int Med 1989;111:28–40.

N117. Nollet D, Herreman G, Piette JC, Herson S, Cabane J, Godeau P. Psychic disorders in systemic lupus erythematosus. Prospective study of 35 cases. Pressee Med 1985 Feb 16;14(7):401–404.

N118. Nolten WE, Rueckert PA. Elevated free cortisol index in pregnancy: Possible regulatory mechanisms. Am J Obstet Gynecol 1981;139:492–498.

N119. Nomura M, Okada N, Okada M, Yoshikawa K. Large subcutaneous calcification in systemic lupus erythematosus. Arch Dermatol 1990 Aug;126(8):1057–1059.

N120. Nomura S, Kumagai N, Kanoh T, Uchino H, Kurihara J. Pulmonary amyloidosis associated with systemic lupus erythematosus [brief report]. Arthritis Rheum 1986 May;29(5):680–682.

N121. Noonan CD, Odone DT, Englemann EP, Splitter SD. Roentgenographic manifestations of joint disease in systemic lupus erythematosus. Radiology 1963 May;80:837–843.

N122. Noonan DJ, Kofler R, Singer PA, Cardenas G, Dixon FJ, Theofilopoulos AN. Delineation of a defect in T cell receptor beta genes of NZW mice predisposed to autoimmunity. J Exp Med 1986 Mar;163(3):644–653.

N123. Norberg R, Nived O, Sturfelt G, Unander M, Arfors L. Anticardiolipin and complement activation: relation to clinical symptoms. J Rheumatol 1987;18:149–153.

N124. Nordstrom DM, West SG, Andersen PA. Basal ganglia calcifications central nervous system lupus erythematosus. Arthritis Rheum 1985 Dec;28(12):1412–1416.

N125. Nordstrom DM, West SG, Rubin RL. Methyldopa-induced systemic lupus erythematosus. Arthritis Rheum 1989;32:205–208.

N126. Nordstrom RE. Hair transplantation. The use of hair bearing compound grafts for correction of alopecia due to chronic discoid lupus erythematosus, traumatic alopecia, and male pattern baldness. Scand J Plast Reconstr Surg 1976;14 Suppl: 1–37.

N127. Noriko T, Katayama I, Arai, H, Eto H, Kamimura K, Uetsuka M, Kondo S, Nishioka K, Nishiyama S. Annular erythema: A possible association with primary Sjogren's syndrome. J Am Acad Dermatol 1989;20:596–601.

N128. Norins LC, Loan LC, Lantz MA. Apparent false-positive reactions in a serologic test for syphilis and presence of antinuclear factor in hybrids of NZB and A-J mice. J Immunol 1970 Nov;105:1108–1110.

N129. Norman DA, Fleischman RM. Gastrointestinal systemic sclerosis in serologic mixed connective tissue disease. Arthritis Rheum 1978 Sep–Oct;21(7):811–819.

N130. Norris DA, Ryan SR, Fritz KA, Kubo M, Tan EM, Deng JS, Weston WL. The role of RNP, Sm and SSA/Ro specific antisera from patients with lupus erythematosus in inducing antibody-dependent cellular cytotoxicity of targets coated with non-histone antigens. Clin Immunol Immunopathol 1984 Jun;31: 311–320.

N131. Norris DG, Colon AR, Stickler GB. Systemic lupus erythematosus in children: the complex problems of diagnosis and treatment encountered in 101 such patients at the Mayo Clinic. Clin Pediatr (Phila) 1977 Sep;16(4):774–778.

N132. Northway JD, Tan EM. Differentiation of antinuclear antibodies giving speckled staining patterns in immunofluorescence. Clin Immunol Immunopathol 1972;1:140–154.

N133. Norton SD, Hovinen DE, Jenkins MK. IL-2 secretion and T cell clonal anergy are induced by distinct biochemical pathways. J Immunol 1991;146:1125–1129.

N134. Norton WL. Comparison of the microangiopathy of systemic lupus erythematosus, dermatomyositis, scleroderma, and diabetes mellitus. Lab Invest 1970 Apr;22:301–308.

N135. Norton WL, Hurd ER, Lewis DC, Ziff M. Evidence of microvascular injury in scleroderma and systemic lupus erythematosus: Quantitative study of the microvascular bed. J Lab Clin Med 1968;71:919–933.

N136. Nosal R, Ericsson O, Sjoqvist F, Durisova M. Distribution of chloroquine in human blood fractions. Methods Find Exp Clin Pharmacol 1988 Sep;10(9):581–587.

N137. Nosanchuk JS, Kim CW. Lupus erythematosus cells in CSF. JAMA 1976 Dec 20;236(25):2883–2884.

N138. Noseworthy JH, Fields BN, Dichter MA, Sobotka C, Pizer E, Perry LL, Nepom JT, Greene MI. Cell receptors for mammalian reovirus. I. Syngeneic monoclonal anti-idiotypic antibody identified a cell surface receptor for reovirus. J Immunol 1983; 131:2533.

N139. Nossal GJV. Cellular mechanisms of immunological tolerance. Annu Rev Immunol 1983;1:33–62.

N140. Nossal GJV. Bone marrow pre B cells and the clonal anergy theory of immunologic tolerance. Intern Rev Immunol 1987;217:321–338.

N141. Nossal GJV. Immunologic tolerance: Collaboration between antigen and lymphokines. Science 1989;245:147–153.

N142. Nossent HC, Henzen-Logmans SC, Vroom TM, Berden JHM, Swaak TJG. Contribution of renal biopsy data in predicting outcome in lupus nephritis: analysis of 116 patients. Arthritis Rheum 1990;33:970.

N143. Nossent HC, Swaak TJ, Berden JH. Systemic lupus erythematosus: analysis of disease activity in 55 patients with end-stage renal failure treated with hemodialysis or continuous ambulatory peritoneal dialysis. Dutch Working Party on SLE. Am J Med 1990 Aug;89(2):169–174.

N144. Nossent HC, Swaak TJG. Systemic lupus erythematosus. VI. Analysis of the interrelationship with pregnancy. J Rheumatol 1990;17:771–776.

N145. Nossent HC, Swaak TJG, Berden JHM, The Dutch Working Party on SLE. Systemic lupus erythematosus after renal transplantation: Patient and graft survival and disease activity. Ann Intern Med 1991 Feb 1;114(3):183–188.

N146. Nossent JC, Bronsveld W, Swaak AJ. Systemic lupus erythematosus. III. Observations on clinical renal involvement and follow up of renal function: Dutch experience with 110 patients studied prospectively. Ann Rheum Dis 1989 Oct; 48(10):810–816.

N147. Nossent JC, Henzen-Logmans SC, Vroom TM, Huysen V, Berden JHM, Swaak AJG. Relation between serological data at the time of biopsy and renal histology in lupus nephritis. Rheumatol Int 1991;11:77–82.

N148. Nossent JC, Swaak AJ. Pancytopenia in systemic lupus erythematosus related to azathioprine. J Intern Med 1990 Jan; 227(1):69–72.

N149. Notman DD, Kurata N, Tan EM. Profiles of antinuclear antibodies in systemic rheumatic diseases. Ann Intern Med 1975;83:464–469.

N150. Novotny EA, Raveche ES, Sharrow S, Ottinger M, Steinberg AD. Analysis of thymocyte subpopulations following treatment with sex hormone. Clin Immunol Immunopathol 1983; 28:205–217.

N151. Nowak D, Piasecka G, Hrabec E. Chemotactic activity of histones for human polymorphonuclear leukocytes. Exp Pathol 1990;40:111–116.

N152. Nyberg G, Eriksson O, Westberg NG. Increased incidence of cervical atypia in women with systemic lupus erythematosus treated with chemotherapy. Arthritis Rheum 1981 May; 24(5):648–650.

N153. Nydegger UE, Kazatchkine MD. Modulation by complement of immune complex processing in health and disease in man. Prog Allergy 1986;39:361–392.

N154. Nydegger UE, Lambert PH, Gerber H, Miescher PA. Circulating immune complexes in the serum in systemic lupus erythematosus and in carriers of hepatitis B antigen. Quantitation by binding to radiolabelled C1q. J Clin Invest 1974;54: 297–309.

N155. Nyman KE, Bangert R, Machleder H, Paulus HE. Thoracic duct drainage in SLE with cutaneous vasculitis. Arthritis Rheum 1979;20:1129–1134.

O

O1. Oberg KE. Development of an SLE syndrome in a patient with malignant carcinoid tumor after treatment with alpha interferon. Interferon & Cytokines 1989;12:30–32.

O2. Obraski TP, Stoller JK, Weinstein C, Hayden S. Splenic infarction. Cleve Clin J Med 1989;56:174–176.

O3. O'Brien CA, Harley JB. A subset of Y RNAs are associated with erythrocyte Ro ribonucleoproteins. Embo J 1990;9: 3683–3689.

O4. O'Brien RM, Cram DS, Coppel RL, Harrison LC. T-cell epitopes on the 70-kDa protein of the (U1) RNP complex in autoimmune disorders. J Autoimmunity 1990;3:747–757.

O5. O'Brien RL, Olnenick JG, Hahn FE. Reactions of quinine, chloroquine, and quinacrine with DNA and their effects on the DNA and RNA polymerase reactions. Proc Natl Acad Sci USA 1966;55:1511–1517.

O6. O'Brien WM, Bagby GF. Carprofen: a new nonsteroidal anti-inflammatory drug. Pharmacology, clinical efficacy and adverse effects. Pharmacotherapy 1987 Jan–Feb;7(1):16–24.

O7. Ochi T, Goldings EA, Lipsky PE, Ziff M. Immunomodulatory effect of procainamide in man. J Clin Invest 1983;71:36–45.

O8. Ochs HD, Rosenfeld SI, Thomas ED, Giblett ER, Alper CA, Dupont B, Schaller JG, Gilliland BC, Hansen JA, Wedgwood RJ. Linkage between the gene (or genes) controlling synthesis of the fourth component of complement and the major histocompatibility complex. N Engl J Med 1977;296:470–475.

O9. Ochs HD, Wedgwood RJ, Heller SR, Beatty PG. Complement, membrane glycoproteins, and complement receptors: their role in regulation of the immune response. Clin Immunol Immunopathol 1986;40:94–104.

O10. O'Connor JF. Psychoses associated with systemic lupus erythematosus. Ann Intern Med 1959 Sep;51:526.

O11. O'Connor JF, Musher DM. Central nervous system involvement in systemic lupus erythematosus. A study of 150 cases. Arch Neurol 1966 Feb;14:157–164.

O12. O'Dell JR, Hays RC, Guggenheim SJ, Steigerwald JC. Systemic lupus erythematosus without clinical renal abnormalities: renal biopsy findings and clinical course. Ann Rheum Dis 1985;44:415–419.

O13. O'Duffy JD, Colgan JP, Phyliky RL, Ferguson RH. Frentizone therapy of thrombocytopenia in systemic lupus erythematosus and refractory idiopathic thrombocytopenic purpura. Mayo Clin Proc 1980;55(10):601–605.

O14. Oen K, Petty RE, Schroeder ML, Briggsa EJN, Bishop AH. Thrombotic thrombocytopenic purpura in a girl with systemic lupus erythematosus. J Rheumatol 1980;7:727–729.

O15. Office of the Surgeon General: Circular letter no. 153; The drug treatment of malaria, suppressive and clinical. JAMA 1943;123:205–208.

O16. Offner H, Konat G, Legg NJ, Raun NE, Winterberg H, Clausen J. Antigenic stimulation of active E-rosette-forming lymphocytes in multiple sclerosis, systemic lupus erythematosus, and rheumatoid arthritis. Clin Immunol Immunopathol 1980 Jul;16:367–373.

O17. Ogata K, Ogata Y, Takasaki Y, Tan EM. Epitopes on proliferating cell nuclear antigen recognized by human lupus autoantibody and murine monoclonal antibody. J Immunol 1987;139(9):2942–2946.

O18. Ogawa K, Sano T, Hisano G, Tsubura E. Levamisole in systemic lupus erythematosus. Ann Allergy 1979 Sep;43(3):187–189.

O19. Ogawa M, Hirakawa T, Saida Y, Fujisawa R, Ito S, Sugisaki T. Clinical signification of localization of S protein and late components in the skin from lupus patients [English abstract]. Nippon Hifuka Gakkai Zasshi 1989 Apr;99(4):435–441.

O20. Ogawa S, Kurumatani N, Shibaike N, Yamazoe S. Progression of retinopathy long after cessation of chloroquine therapy [letter]. Lancet 1979 Jun 30;1(8131):1408.

O21. O'Grady JH, Looney RJ, Anderson CL. The valence for ligand of the human mononuclear phagocyte 72 kD high affinity IgG Fc receptor is one. J Immunol 1986;137:2307–2310.

O22. Ogryzlo MA. The LE (lupus erythematosus) cell reaction. Can Med Assoc J 1956;75:980.

O23. Ogryzlo MA. Systemic lupus erythematosus in rheumatic disease. Duthie JJR, Alexander WRM, editors. Baltimore 1968:189–203.

O24. Ogryzlo MA, Maclachlan M, Dauphinee JA, Fletcher AA. The serum proteins in health and disease, filter paper electrophoresis. Am J Med 1959 Oct;27:596–616; Med Serv J Canada 1960 Mar;16:208–238.

O25. Ohe Y, Hayashi H, Iwai K. Human spleen histone H1. isolation and amino acid sequences of three minor variants, H1a, H1c, and H1d. J Biochem 1989;106:844–857.

O26. Ohgaki M, Ueda G, Shiota J, Nishimura H, Hirose S, Sato H, Sirai T. Two distinct monoclonal natural thymocytotoxic autoantibodies from New Zealand black mouse. Clin Immunol Immunopathol 1989 Dec;53(3):475–487.

O27. Ohkawa S, Ozaki M, Izumi S. Lepromatous leprosy complicated with systemic lupus erythematosus. Dermatologica 1985 Feb;170:80–83.

O28. Ohmoto A, Taneichi K, Chimoto T, Konno T, Shibaki H. The coexistence of systemic lupus erythematosus and psoriatic arthritis [English abstract]. Ryumachi 1986 Aug;26(4):278–283.

O29. Ohnishi K, Mitchell B, Ebling FM, Tsao B, Hahn BH. Comparison of pathogenic and non-pathogenic monoclonal antibodies to DNA: Ability of pathogens to bind heparin sulfate via antibody/DNA/histone complexes. Clin Res. In press.

O30. Ohno S. Many peptide fragments of alien antigens are homologous with host proteins, thus canalizing T-cell responses. Proc Natl Acad Sci USA 1991; 88:3065–3068.

O31. Ohosona Y, Akizuki M, Hirakata M, Satoh M, Yamagata H, Homma M. In vitro production of autoantibodies to U1 ribonucleoproteins by peripheral blood mononuclear cells from patients with connective tissue diseases. Arthritis Rheum 1986;29:1343–1350.

O32. Ohosone Y, Mimori T, Griffith A, Akizuki M, Homma M, Craft J, Hardin JA. Molecular cloning of cDNA encoding Sm autoantigen: derivation of a cDNA for a B polypeptide of the U series of small nuclear ribonucleoprotein particles [published erratum appears in Proc Natl Acad Sci USA 1989;86:8982]. Proc Natl Acad Sci USA 1989;86:4249–4253.

O33. Ohsawa M, Takahashi K, Otsuka F. Induction of anti-nuclear antibodies in mice orally exposed to cadmium at low concentrations. Clin Exp Immunol 1988;73:98–102.

O34. Ohsugi Y, Gershwin MC, Ahmed A, Skelly RR, Milich DR. Studies of congenitally immunologic mutant New Zealand mice. VI. Spontaneous and induced autoantibodies to red cells and DNA occur in New Zealand X-linked immunodeficient (Xid) mice without phenotypic alterations of the Xid gene or generalized polyclonal B cell activation. J Immunol 1982 May; 128(5):2220–2227.

O35. Ohtaki N, Miyamoto C, Orita M, Koya M, Matsuo M. Concurrent multiple morphea and neonatal lupus erythematosus in an infant boy born to a mother with SLE. Br J Dermatol 1986 July;115(1):85–90.

O36. Oite T, Batsford SR, Mihatsch MJ, Takamiya H, Vogt A. Quantitative studies of In Situ immune complex glomerulonephritis in the rat induced by planted, cationized antigen. J Exp Med 1982;155:460–474.

O37. Oka M, Vainio V. Effect of pregnancy on the prognosis and serology of rheumatoid arthritis. Acta Rheum Scand 1966;12:47–52.

O38. Okada M. Methylprednisolone pulse therapy: a histopathological evaluation. Kidney and Dialysis 1980;8:535.

O39. Okano Y, Medsger T. Newly identified U4/U6 snRNP-binding proteins by serum autoantibodies from a patient with systemic sclerosis. J Immunol 1991;146:535–542.

O40. Okano Y, Medsger T. Novel serum autoantibodies reactive with U5 small nuclear ribonucleoprotein particle (snRNP) specific proteins obtained from a patient with systemic sclerosis-polymyositis overlap. Arthritis Rheum 1991;34 Suppl: S103.

O41. Okayasu I, Kong YM, Rose NR. Effect of castration and sex hormones on experimental autoimmune thyroiditis. Clin Immunol Immunopathol 1981;20:240–245.

O42. O'Keefe TL, Bandyopadhyay S, Datta SK, Imanishi-Kari T. V region sequences of an idiotypically connected family of pathogenic anti-DNA autoantibodies. J Immunol 1990 Jun 1; 144(11):4275–4283.

O43. Okhawa S, Ozaki M, Izumi S. Lepromatous leprosy complicated with systemic lupus erythematosus. Dermatologica 1985;170:80–83.

O44. Okor RS, Nwankwo MU. Chloroquine absorption in children from polyethylene glycol base suppositories. J Clin Pharm Ther 1988 Jun;13(3):219–223.

O45. Oksenberg JR, Gaiser CN, Cavali-Sforza LL, Steinman L. Polymorphic markers of human T cell-receptor alpha and beta genes. Family studies and comparison of frequencies in healthy individuals and patients with multiple sclerosis and myasthenia gravis. Hum Immunol 1988;22:111–121.

O46. Okudaira K, Nakai H, Hayakawa T, Kashiwado T, Tanimoto K, Horiuchi Y, Juji T. Detection of anti-lymphocyte antibody with two-color method in systemic lupus erythematosus and its heterogeneous specificities against human T-cell subsets. J Clin Invest 1979;64:1213–1220.

O47. Okudaira K, Searles RP, Ceuppens JL, Goodwin JS, Williams RC Jr. Anti-Ia reactivity in sera from patients with systemic lupus erythematosus. J Clin Invest 1982 Jan;69:17–24.

O48. Omitted.

O49. Okudaira K, Searles RP, Goodwin JS, Williams RC Jr. Antibodies in the sera of patients with systemic lupus erythematosus that block the binding of monoclonal anti-Ia to Ia-positive targets also inhibit the autologous mixed lymphocyte response. J Immunol 1982 Aug;129:582–586.

O50. Okudaira K, Tanimoto K, Horiuchi Y. Effect of anti-lymphocyte antibody in systemic lupus erythematosus on in vitro Ig synthesis. Clin Immunol Immunopathol 1981 Nov;21: 162–171.

O51. Okun E, Gouras P, Bernstein H, von Sallmann L. Chloroquine retinopathy. A report of eight cases with ERG and dark-adaption findings. Arch Ophthal 1963;69:59.

O52. Olansky AJ, Briggaman RA, Gammon WR, Kelly TF, Sams WM Jr. Bullous systemic lupus erythematosus. J Am Acad Dermatol 1982 Oct;7(4):511–520.

O53. Oldham RK, Foon KA, Morgan AC, Woodhouse CS, Schroff RW, Abrams PG, Fer M, Schoenberger CS, Farrell M, Kimbell E, Sherwin SA. Monoclonal antibody therapy of malignant melanoma: in vivo localization in cutaneous metastasis after intravenous administration. J Clin Oncol 1984;2:1235.

O54. Olding LB, Oldstone MBA. Lymphocytes from human newborns abrogate mitoses of their mother's lymphocytes. Nature 1974;249:161–163.

O55. Oldstone MBA. Molecular mimicry and autoimmune disease. Cell 1987;50:819–820.

O56. Oldstone MBA. Molecular Mimicry as a Mechanism for the Cause and as a Probe Uncovering Etiologic Agent(s) of Autoimmune Disease. Curr Top Microbiol Immunol 1989; 145:127–135.

O57. Oldstone MBA. Virus-induced autoimmunity: molecular mimicry as a route to autoimmune disease. J Autoimmun 1989;2 Suppl:187–194.

O58. Oldstone MBA, Notkins AL. Molecular Mimicry. In: Notkins AL, Oldstone MBA, editors. Concepts in Viral Pathogenesis II. 2nd ed. New York: Springer-Verlag, 1986:195–202.

O59. O'Leary PA. Disseminated lupus erythematosus. Minnesota Med 1934 Nov;17:637–644.

O60. O'Leary PA, Brunsting LA, Kierland RR. Quinacrine (atabrine) hydrochloride in treatment of discoid lupus erythematosus. Arch Dermatol 1953;67:633–634.

O61. O'Leary PA, Lambert EH, Sayre GP. Muscle studies in cutaneous disease. J Invest Dermatol 1955 Mar;24:301–310.

O62. O'Leary TJ, Jones G, Yip A, Lohnes D, Cohanim M, Yendt ER. The effects of chloroquine on serum 1,25-dihydroxyvitamin D and calcium metabolism in sarcoidosis. N Engl J Med 1986 Sep 18;315(12):727–730.

O63. Olee T, Yang P-M, Siminovitch KA, Olsen NJ, Hillson J, Wu J, Kozin F, Carson DA, Chen PP. Molecular basis of an autoantibody-associated restriction fragment length polymorphism that confers susceptibility to autoimmune diseases. J Clin Invest 1991;88:193–203.

O64. Oleinick A. Leukemia or lymphoma occurring subsequent to an autoimmune disease. Blood 1967 Jan;29:144–153.

O65. Oleinick A. Family studies in systemic lupus erythematosus. I. Prenatal factors. Arthritis Rheum 1969;12:10–16.

O66. Oleinick A, Mantel N. Family studies in systemic lupus erythematosus. II. Mortality among siblings and offspring of index cases with a statistical appendix concerning life table analysis. J Chron Dis 1970;22:617.

O67. Olenginski TP, Harrington TM, Carlson JP. Transverse myelitis secondary to sulfasalazine [letter]. J Rheumatol 1991;18: 304.

O68. Olivieri I, Gemignani G, Balagi M, Pasquariello A, Gremignai G, Pasero G. Concomitant systemic lupus erythematosus and ankylosing spondylitis. Ann Rheum Dis 1990 May;49(5): 323–324.

O69. Olivotto IA, Fairey RN, Gillies JH, Stein H. Fatal outcome of pelvic radiotherapy for carcinoma of the cervix in a patient with systemic lupus erythematosis <sic>. Clin Radiol 1989; 40:83–84.

O70. O'Loughlin S, Schroeter AL, Jordon RE. Chronic urticaria-like lesions in systemic lupus erythematosus. Arch Dermatol 1978 Jun;114(6):879–883.

O71. O'Loughlin S, Schroeter AL, Jordon RE. A study of lupus erythematosus with particular reference to generalized discoid lupus. Br J Dermatol 1978 Jul;99(1):1–11.

O72. Olsen EGJ, Lever JV. Pulmonary changes in systemic lupus erythematosus. Br J Dis Chest 1972;66:71–77.

O73. Olsen ML, Arnett FC, Reveille JD. Anti-Sm and anti-RNP antibodies are associated with distinct and different HLA-DQα and β chain genes [abstract]. Arthritis Rheum 1990;33 Suppl: S100.

O74. Olsen ML, Dimou GS, Papasteriades C, Moutsopoulos HM, Arnett FC. MHC class II and III genes in Greek patients with systemic lupus erythematosus (SLE) [abstract]. Arthritis Rheum 1992 In press.

O75. Olsen ML, Goldstein R, Arnett FC, Duvic M, Pollack M, Reveille JD. C4A gene deletion and HLA associations in black Americans with systemic lupus erythematosus. Immunogenet 1989;30:27–33.

O76. Olson NY, Lindsley CB, Peter JB. Immunoglobulin G subclasses in childhood systemic lupus erythematosus and systemic onset juvenile rheumatoid arthritis [abstract]. Arthritis Rheum 1988;31 Suppl:R28.

O77. Olszynski WP, Sibley JT, De Coteau WE, Sundaram WBM. Central nervous system (CNS) involvement in systemic lupus erythematosus (SLE) [abstract]. Arthritis Rheum 1989 Jan; 32(1) Suppl:R8.

O78. Omdal R, Dickstein K, Von Brandis C. Cardiac tamponade in systemic lupus erythematosus. J Rheumatol 1988;17: 55–57.

O79. Omdal R, Mellgren SI, Husby G. Clinical neuropsychiatric and neuromuscular manifestations in systemic lupus erythematosus. Scand J Rheumatol 1988;17(2):113–117.

O80. Omdal R, Selseth B, Klow NE, Husby G, Mellgren SI. Clinical neurological, electrophysiological, and cerebral CT scan findings in systemic lupus erythematosus. Scand J Rheumatol 1989;18(5):283–289.

O81. O'Neil S, Thomson J, Strong AMM, Lang W. Systemic lupus erythematosus presenting as a recurrent sore throat and oral ulceration. Br J Dermatol 1977;96:211–213.

O82. O'Neill GJ, Yang SY, Dupont B. Two HLA-linked loci controlling the fourth component of human complement. Proc Natl Acad Sci USA 1978;75:5165–5169.

O83. Ooi BS, Ooi YM, Pesce AJ, Pollak V. Antibodies to Beta 2 microglobulin in the sera of patients with systemic lupus erythematosus. Immunology 1977 Oct;33:535–541.

O84. Ooi BS, Orlina AR, Pesce AJ, Mendoza N, Masaitis L, Pollak VE. Lymphocytotoxic antibodies in patients with systemic lupus erythematosus. Clin Exp Immunol 1974 Jun;17: 237–243.

O85. Ooi YM, Ooi BS, Pollack VE. Relationship of circulating immune complexes to histologic patterns of nephritis: a comparative study of membranous glomerulonephropathy and diffuse proliferative glomerulonephritis. J Lab Clin Med 1977 Nov;90:891–900.

O86. Oosterhuis HJGH, de Haas WHD. Rheumatic diseases in patients with myasthenia gravis. Acta Neurol Scand 1968; 44(2):22–219.

O87. Op den Kamp JAF. Lipid asymmetry in membranes. Ann Rev Biochem 1979;48:47–71.

O88. Oppenheimer EH. Lesions of the adrenals of an infant following maternal corticosteroid therapy. Bull Johns Hopkins Hosp 1964;114:146–51.

O89. Oppenheimer EH, Boitnott JK. Pancreatitis in children following adrenal cortico-steroid therapy. Bull Johns Hopkins Hosp 1960 Dec;107:297–306.

O90. Oppenheimer S, Hoffbrand BI. Optic neuritis and myelopathy in systemic lupus erythematosus. Can J Neurol Sci 1986 May;13(2):129–132.

O91. O'Quinn S, Cole J, Many H. Problems of disability in patients with chronic skin diseases. Arch Dermatol 1972 Jan; 105:35–41.

O92. Ordi J, Barquinero J, Vilardell M, Jordana R, Tolosa A, Selva A, Genover E. Fetal loss treatment in patients with antiphospholipid antibodies. Ann Rheum Dis 1989 Oct;48(10): 798–802.

O93. Ordi J, Vargas V, Vilardell M, Barquinero J, Guardia J. Lupus anticoagulant and portal hypertension [letter]. Am J Med 1988 Mar;84(3 Pt 1):566–568.

O94. Ordi J, Vilardell M, Oristrell J, Veldes M, Knobel A, Alijotas J, Monasterio Y, Flores P. Bleeding in patients with lupus anticoagulant. Lancet 1984 Oct 13;2:868–869.

O95. O'Regan S. The clearance of preformed immune complexes in rats with Heymann's nephritis. Clin Exp Immunol 1979;37: 432–435.

O96. Orenstein JM, Schulof RS, Simon GL. Ultrastructural markers in acquired immunodeficiency syndrome [letter]. Arch Pathol Lab Med 1984;108:857–859.

O97. Ores RO, Lange K. Skin test for the diagnosis of systemic lupus erythematosus. Am J Med Sci 1964 Nov;248:562–566.

O98. Orozco JH, Jasin HE, Ziff M. Defective phagocytosis in patients with systemic lupus erythematosus (SLE) [abstract]. Arthritis Rheum 1970 May–Jun;13:342.

O99. Orser B. Thrombocytopenia and cocaine abuse. Anesthesiology 1991;74:195–196.

O100. Ory PA, Clark MR, Kwoh EE, Clarkson SB, Goldstein IM. Sequences of complementary DNAs that encode the NA1 and NA2 forms of Fc receptor III on human neutrophils. J Clin Invest 1989;84:1688–1691.

O101. Ory PA, Goldstein IM, Kwoh EE, Clarkson SB. Characterization of polymorphic forms of FcRIII on human neutrophils. J Clin Invest 1989;83:1676–1681.

O102. Osa SR, Weksler ME. Demonstration of significant differences in the proliferative capacity of lymphocytes from normal human subjects. Cell Immunol 1977;32:391.

O103. Osathanondh A, Tulchinsky D, Kamali H, de M Fenci M, Taeusch HW. Dexamethasone levels in treated pregnant women and newborn infants. J Pediatr 1977;90:617–620.

O104. Osborn TG, Patel NJ, Moore TI, Zuckner J. Use of the HEp-2 cell substrate in the detection of antinuclear antibodies in juvenile rheumatoid arthritis. Arthritis Rheum 1984 Nov; 27(11):1286–1289.

O105. Osborne ED, Jordon JW, Hoak FC, Pschierer FJ. Nitrogen mustard therapy in cutaneous blastomatous disease. JAMA 1947 Dec 27;135:1123–1128.

O106. Oshimi K, Sumiya M, Gonda N, Kano S, Takaku F. Natural killer cell activity in untreated systemic lupus erythematosus. Ann Rheum Dis 1982 Aug;41:417–420.

O107. Osler W. On the visceral complications of erythema exudativum multiforme. Am J Med Sci 1895;110:629–646.

O108. Osler W. The visceral lesions of the erythema group. Br J Dermatol 1900;12:227–245.

O109. Osler W. On the visceral manifestations of the erythema group of skin diseases. Trans Assoc Am Physicians 1903;18: 599–624.

O110. Osler W. On the visceral manifestations of the erythema group of skin diseases. Am J Med Sci 1904;127:1–23.

O111. Omitted.

O112. Ost L, Wettrel G, Bjorkhem I, Rane A. Prednisolone excretion in human milk. J Pediatr 1985;106:1008–1011.

O113. Ostensen M, Fredriksen K, Kass E, Rekvig OP. Identification of antihistone antibodies in subsets of juvenile chronic arthritis. Ann Rheum Dis 1989;48:114–117.

O114. Osterland CK. Immune complexes in systemic lupus erythematosus. In: Espinoza LR, Osterland CK, editors. Circulating Immune Complexes. Futura 1983:63–86

O115. Ostrer M, Stamberg J, Perinchief P. Two chromosome aberrations in the child of a woman with systemic lupus erythematosus treated with azathioprine and prednisone. Am J Med Genetics 1984;17:627–632.

O116. Ostuni PA, Lazzarin P, Pengo V, Ruffatti A, Schiavon F, Gambari P. Renal artery thrombosis and hypertension in a 13 year old girl with antiphospholipid syndrome. Ann Rheum Dis 1990 Mar;49(3):184–187.

O117. O'Sullivan FX, Fassbender HG, Gay S, Koopman WJ. Etiopathogenesis of the rheumatoid arthritis-like disease in MRL/l mice. I. The histomorphologic basis of joint destruction. Arthritis Rheum 1985 May;28(5):529–536.

O118. Ota T, Uemura A, Eto S, Suzuki H. Clinical significance of serum sialic acid in rheumatoid arthritis and systemic lupus erythematosus. Sangyo Ika Daigaku Zasshi 1985;7:401–407.

O119. Otani A. Lupus erythematosus hypertrophicus et profundus. Br J Dermatol 1977;96:75–78.

O120. Otani H, Engleman RM, Breyer RH, Rousou JA, Lemeshow S, Das DK. Mepacrine, a phospholipase inhibitor. A potential tool for modifying myocardial reperfusion injury. J Thorac Cardiovasc Surg 1986 Aug;92(2):247–254.

O121. Otto R, Mackay IR. Psycho-social and emotional disturbances to systemic lupus erythematosus. Med J Aust 1967 Sep 9;2:488–493.

O122. Ottolenghi-Lodigiani F. Local intradermal application of acridine preparations for treatment of chronic lupus erythematosus. Hautarzt 1955 Jan;6:24–27.

O123. Oudin J, Cazenave PA. Similar idiotypic specificities in immunoglobulin fractions with different antibody functions or even without detectable antibody function. Proc Natl Acad Sci USA 1971;68:2616–2620.

O124. Oudin J, Michel M. Une nouvelle forme d'allotypic des globulines du serum de lapin apparemment liee a la fonction et a la specificite anticorps. CR Hebd Seance Acad Sci Ser D, Sci Natur Paris 1963;257:805.

O125. Out HJ, De Groot PG, Hasselaar P, Van Vliet M, Derksen RHWM. Fluctuations of anticardiolipin antibody levels in patients with systemic lupus erythematosus: a prospective study. Ann Rheum Dis 1989 Dec;48(12):1023

O126. Out HJ, De Groot PG, Van Vliet M, De Gast GC, Niuwenhuis HK, Derksen RHWM. Antibodies to platelets in patients with antiphospholipid antibodies. Blood 1991;77:2655–2659.

O127. Out HJ, Derksen RHWM, Christiaens GCML. Systemic lupus erythematosus and pregnancy. Obstet Gynecol Survey 1989;44:585–591.

O128. Owen JA, De Gruchy GC, Smith H. Serum haptoglobins in haemolytic states. J Clin Pathol 1960 Nov;13:478–482.

O129. Owen RD. Immunogenetic consequences of vascular anastomoses between bovine twins. Science 1945;102: 400–401.

O130. Owens T. A role for adhesion molecules in contact-dependent T help for B cells. Eur J Immunol 1991;21:979–983.

O131. Owhashi M, Heber-Katz E. Protection from experimental allergic encephalomyelitis conferred by a monoclonal antibody directed against a shared idiotype on rat T cell receptors specific for myelin basic protein. J Exp Med 1988;168: 2153–2164.

O132. Oxenhandler R, Hart M, Corman L, Sharp G, Adelstein E. Pathology of skeletal muscle in mixed connective tissue disease. Arthritis Rheum 1977 May;20:985–988.

O133. Oxenhandler R, Hart MN, Bickel J, Scearce D, Durham J, Irvin W. Pathologic features of muscle in systemic lupus erythematosus: a biopsy series with comparative clinical and immunopathologic observations. Hum Pathol 1982 Aug; 13(8):745–757.

O134. Oxholm P, Oxholm A, Manthorpe R. Epidermal IgG deposits in patients with chronic inflammatory connective tissue diseases: diagnostic value and correlation to clinical and immunological parameters in patients with primary Sjogren's syndrome. Clin Exp Rheumatol 1987 Jan–Mar;5(1):5–9.

O135. Ozturk GE, Kohler PF, Horsburgh CR Jr, Kirkpatrick CH. The significance of antilymphocyte antibodies in patients with acquired immune deficiency syndrome (AIDS) and their sexual partners. J Clin Immunol 1987;7:130–139.

O136. Ozturk GE, Terasaki PI. Non-HLA lymphocyte cytotoxins in various diseases. Tissue Antigens 1979;14:52–58.

P

P1. Paavonen T, Anderson LC, Adlercreutz H. Sex hormone regulation of in vitro immune responses. J Exp Med 1981;154: 1935–1945.

P2. Paccaud J-P, Carpentier J-L, Schifferli JA. Direct evidence for the clustered nature of complement receptors type I on the erythrocyte membrane. J Immunol 1988;141:3889–3894.

P3. Paccaud J-P, Carpentier J-L, Schifferli JA. Difference in the clustering of complement receptor type 1 (CR1) on polymorphonuclear leukocytes and erythrocytes: effect on immune adherence. Eur J Immunol 1990;20:283–289.

P4. Paccaud JP, Steiger G, Sjoholm AG, Spaeth PJ, Schifferli JA. Tetanus toxoid-anti-tetanus toxoid complexes: A model to study the human complement transport system for immune complexes. Clin Exp Immunol 1987;69:468–476.

P5. Pacifici R, Paris L, DiCarlo S, Pichini S, Zuccarao P. Immunologic aspects of carbamazepine treatment in epileptic patients. Epilepsia 1991;32:122–127.

P6. Packer SH, Logue GL. Quantitation of warm reactive IgG antilymphocyte autoantibodies in systemic lupus erythematosus. Clin Immunol Immunopathol 1980 Dec;17:515–529.

P7. Page AR, Condie RM, Good RA. Suppression of plasma cell hepatitis with 6-mercaptopurine. Am J Med 1964 Feb;36: 200–213.

P8. Page F. Treatment of lupus erythematosus with mepacrine. Lancet 1951 Oct 27;2:755–758.

P9. Pagel W, Treip CS. Viscero-cutaneous collagenosis; study of intermediate forms of dermatomyositis, scleroderma and disseminated lupus erythematosus. J Clin Path 1955 Feb;8: 1–18.

P10. Pahl MV, Vaziri ND, Saiki JK, Upham T, Ness R. Chronic hemodialysis in end-stage lupus nephritis: changes of clinical and serological activities. Artif Organs 1984 Nov;8(4): 423–428.

P11. Painter CJ, Monestier M, Chew A, Bona-Dimitriu A, Kasturi K, Bailey C, Scott VE, Sidman CL, Bona CA. Specificities and V genes encoding monoclonal autoantibodies from viable motheaten mice. J Exp Med 1988;167:1137–1153.

P12. Pal B, Gibson C, Passmore J, Griffiths ID, Dick WC. A study of headaches and migraine in Sjogren's syndrome and other rheumatic disorders. Ann Rheum Dis 1989 Apr;48(4): 312–316.

P13. Paladini G, Tonazzi C, Maring L. Pulmonary eosinophilia and lupus-like syndrome secondary to carbazepine. J Clin Pharm Res 1982;2 Suppl:43–45.

P14. Palfi Z, Bach M, Solymosy F, Luhrmann R. Purification of the major U snRNPs from broad bean nuclear extracts and characterization of their protein constituents. Nucleic Acids Res 1989;17:1445–1458.

P15. Palit J, Holt PJL, Still PE, Mawer EB. Effect of chloroquine on serum vitamin D in rheumatoid arthritis. Br J Rheumatol 1988;27 Suppl:131–132.

P16. Palmer A, Gjorstrup G, Severn A, Welsh K, Taube D. Treatment of systemic lupus erythematosus by extracorporeal immunoadsorption [letter]. Lancet 1988 Jul 30;2(8605):272.

P17. Palmer DG. Synovial cysts in rheumatoid disease. Ann Intern Med 1969 Jan;70:61–68.

P18. Palmer DG. Systemic lupus erythematosus with cerebral complications [letter]. N Z Med J 1988 Feb 24;101(840):91.

P19. Palmer DK, O'Day K, Trong HL, Charbonneau H, Margolis RL. Purification of the centromere-specific protein CENP-A and demonstration that it is a distinctive histone. Proc Natl Acad Sci USA 1991;88:3734–3738.

P20. Palmer RG, Dore CJ, Denman AM. Cyclophosphamide induces more chromosome damage than chlorambucil in patients with connective tissue diseases. Q J Med 1986 Apr; 59(228):395–400.

P21. Paloyan D, Levin B, Simonowitz D. Azathioprine-associated acute pancreatitis. Am J Dig Dis 1977 Sep;22(9):839–840.

P22. Palvio DH, Christensen KS. Systemic lupus erythematosus with rectal stenosis simulating tumor or diverticulosis [case report]. Acta Chir Scand 1987 Jan;153(1):63–65.

P23. Pancer LB, Milazzo MF, Morris VL, Singhal SK, Bell DA. Immunogenicity and characterization of supernatant DNA released by murine spleen cells. J Immunol 1981 Jul;127(1): 98–104.

P24. Pandy JP, Goust JM, Salier JP, Fudenberg HH. Immunoglobulin G heavy chain (Gm) allotypes in multiple sclerosis. J Clin Invest 1981;67:1797.

P25. Pandya MR, Agus B, Grady RF. In vivo LE phenomenon in pleural fluid. Arthritis Rheum 1976;19:962–966.

P26. Panem S, Ordonez NG, Kirsten WH, Katz AI, Spargo GH. Type-C virus expression in systemic lupus erythematosus. N Engl J Med 1976;295:470–475.

P27. Panfieue L, Magnard P. Degenerescence retinienne chez deux enfants consecutive a un traitement preventif antipaludeen chez la mere pendant la grossesse. Bull Soc Ophthal Fr 1969;69:466–467.

P28. Pangborn MC. A new serologically active phospholipid from beef heart. Proc Soc Exp Biol & Med 1941 Nov;48:484–486.

P29. Panja RK, Sengupta KP, Aikat BK. Seromucoid in lupus erythematosus scleroderma. J Clin Path 1964 Nov;17:658–659.

P30. Pankewycz OG, Migliorini P, Madaio MP. Polyreactive autoantibodies are nephritogenic in murine lupus nephritis. J Immunol 1987 Nov 15;139(10):3287–3294.

P31. Panosian-Sahakian N, Klotz JL, Ebling F, Kronenberg M, Hahn BH. Diversity of Ig V gene segments found in anti-DNA autoantibodies from a single (NZB × NZW)F1 mouse. J Immunol 1989 Jun 15;142(12):4500–4506.

P32. Panush RS, Edwards L, Longley S, Webster E. "Rhupus" syndrome. Arch Intern Med 1988 Jul;148(7):1633–1636.

P33. Panush RS, Stroud RM, Webster EM. Food-induced (allergic) arthritis. Arthritis Rheum 1986;29:220–226.

P34. Paolozzi FP, Goldberg J. Acute granulocytic leukemia following systemic lupus erythematosus. Am J Med Sci 1985;290:32–35.

P35. Papa MZ, Shiloni E, Vetto JT, Kastner DL, McDonald HD. Surgical morbidity in patients with systemic lupus erythematosus. Am J Surg 1989 Mar;157(3):295–298.

P36. Papero PH, Bluestein HG, White P, Lipnick RN. Neuropsychologic deficits and antineuronal antibodies in pediatric systemic lupus erythematosus. Clin Exp Rheumatol 1990 Jul–Aug;8(4):417–424.

P37. Papoian R, Pillarisetty R, Talal N. Immunological regulation of spontaneous antibodies to DNA and RNA. II. Sequential switch from IgM to IgG in NZB/NZW F1 mice. Immunology 1977 Jan;32(1):75–79.

P38. Pappas MG, Nussenzweig RS, Nussenzweig V, Shear HL. Complement-mediated defect in clearance and sequestration of sensitized, autologous erythrocytes in rodent malaria. J Exp Med 1981;67:183–192.

P39. Pappenfort RB, Lockwood JH. Amodiaquin (camoquin) in treatment of chronic discoid lupus erythematosus; preliminary report, with special reference to successful response of patients resistant to other antimalarial drugs. Arch Dermatol 1956 Oct;74:384–386.

P40. Parbtani A, Frampton G, Yewdall V, Kasai N, Cameron JS. Platelet and plasma serotonin in glomerulonephritis III. The nephritis of systemic lupus erythematosus. Clin Nephrol 1980 Oct;14:164–172.

P41. Paredes RA, Morgan H, Lachelin GC. Congenital heart block associated with maternal primary Sjogren's syndrome. Case report. Br J Obstet Gynaecol 1983;90:870.

P41a. Parillo JE, Fauci AS. Mechanism of glucocorticoid action on immune processes. Ann Rev Pharmacol Toxicol 1979;19:179–201.

P42. Park CL, Balderas RS, Fieser TM, Slack JH, Prud'Homme GJ, Dixon FJ, Theofilopoulos, AN. Isotypic profiles and other fine characteristics of immune responses to exogenous thymus-dependent and independent antigens by mice with lupus syndromes. J Immunol 1983 May;130(5):2161–2167.

P43. Park K, Fasman GD. The histone octamer, a conformationally flexible structure. Biochemistry 1987;26:8042–8045.

P44. Park MH, D'Agati VD, Appel GB, Pirani CL. Tubulo-interstitial disease in lupus nephritis: relationship to immune deposits, interstitial inflammation, glomerular changes, renal function, and prognosis. Nephron 1986;44:309–319.

P45. Park MS, Terasaki PI, Bernoco D. Autoantibodies against beta lymphocytes. Lancet 1977;2:465–467.

P46. Parke A, Maier D, Wilson D, Andreoli J, Ballow M. Intravenous gamma-globulin, antiphospholipid antibodies and pregnancy [letter]. Ann Intern Med 1989 Mar 15;110(6):495–496.

P47. Parke AL. Antimalarial drugs, SLE and pregnancy. J Rheumatol 1988;15:607–610.

P48. Parke AL. Antiphospholipid antibody syndromes. Rheum Dis Clin N A 1989;15:275–286.

P49. Parke AL, Maier D, Wilson D, Andreoli J, Ballow M. Intravenous gamma-globulin, antiphospholipid antibodies, and pregnancy. Ann Intern Med 1989;110:495–496.

P50. Parke AL, Rothfield NF. Congenital heart block, systemic lupus erythematosus, and anti-Ro antibodies. Arthritis Rheum 1985;28:1077.

P51. Parke AL, Wilson D, Maier D. The prevalence of antiphospholipid antibodies in women with recurrent spontaneous abortion, women with successful pregnancies, and women who have never been pregnant. Arthritis Rheum 1991;34:1231–1235.

P52. Parker LP, Hahn BH, Osterland CK. Modification of NZB/NZW F1 autoimmune disease by development of tolerance to DNA. J Immunol 1974 Jul;113:292–297.

P53. Parker RL, Schmid FR. Phagocytosis of particular complexes of gamma globulin and rheumatoid factor. J Immunol 1962 Apr;88:519.

P54. Parnass SM, Goodwin JA, Patel DV, Levinson DJ, Reinhard JD. Dural sinus thrombosis: a mechanism for pseudotumor cerebri in systemic lupus erythematosus [case report]. J Rheumatol 1987 Feb;14(1):152–155.

P55. Parris TM, Kimberly RP, Inman RD, McDougal JS, Gibofsky A, Christian CL. Defective Fc receptor-mediated function of the mononuclear phagocyte system in lupus nephritis. Ann Intern Med 1982;97:526–532.

P56. Parrish LC, Kennedy RJ, Hurley HJ. Palmar lesions in lupus erythematosus. Arch Dermatol 1967 Sep;96:273–276.

P57. Partanen J, Koskimies S, Johansson E. C_4 null phenotypes among lupus erythematosus patients are predominantly the result of deletions covering C_4 and closely linked C_{21}-hydroxylase A genes. J Med Genetics 1988;25:387–391.

P58. Pascher F, Sawicky HH, Silverberg MG, Emmet R. Therapeutic assays of New York Skin and Cancer Unit, Post-graduate Medical School, New York University-Bellevue Medical Center; Aurol sulfide (Hille). J Invest Dermatol 1949;13:151–155.

P59. Pascher F, Silverberg MG, Loewenstein LW, Sawicky HH. Therapeutic Assays of New York Skin and Cancer Unit, Post-Graduate Medical School, New York University-Bellevue Medical Center; aurol-sulfide (Hille). J Invest Dermat 1949 Sep;13:151–155.

P60. Pascual V, Capra JD. Human immunoglobulin heavy chain variable region genes: organization, polymorphism, and expression. Adv Immunol 1991;49:1–74.

P61. Pasquali JL, Azerad G, Martin T, Muller S. The double reactivity of a human monoclonal rheumatoid factor to IgG and histones is related to distinct binding sites. Eur J Immunol 1988; 18:1127–1130.

P62. Passaleva A, Massai G, Emmi L, Stenardi L, Valesini G. Plasma exchange in the treatment of acute systemic lupus erythematosus without circulating immune complexes. Clin Exp Rheumatol 1985 Jul–Sep;3(3):255–257.

P62a. Passas CM, Wond RL, Peterson M, Testa MA, Rothfield NF. A comparison of the specificity of the 1971 and 1982 American Rheumatism Association criteria for the classification of systemic lupus erythematosus. Arthritis Rheum 1985 Jun;28:620–623.

P63. Passlick B, Flieger D, Siegler-Heitbrock HWL. Identification and characterization of a novel monocyte subpopulation in human peripheral blood. Blood 1989;74:2527–2534.

P64. Patarroyo M. Leucocyte adhesion to cells. Molecular basis, physiological relevance, and abnormalities. Scand J Immunol 1989;30:129.

P65. Pathak MA, Fitzpatrick TB, Greither FJ, Kraus EW. Principles of photoprotection in sunburn and suntanning, and topical and systemic photoprotection in health and diseases. J Dermatol Surg Oncol 1985;11:575–579.

P66. Patri P, Nigro A, Rebora A. Lupus erythematosus-like eruption from captopril. Acta Derm Venereol 1985;65:447–448.

P67. Patrignani P, Filabozzi P, Patrono C. Selective cumulative inhibition of platelet thromboxane production by low-dose aspirin in healthy subjects. J Clin Invest 1982;69:1366–1372.

P68. Patrono C, Ciabattoni G, Remuzzi G, Gotti E, Bombardieri S, Di Munno O, Tartarelli G, Cinotti GA, Simonetti BM, Pierucci A. Functional significance of renal prostacyclin and thromboxane A2 production in patients with systemic lupus erythematosus. J Clin Invest 1985 Sep;76(3):1011–1018.

P69. Patrucco R, Rothfield NF, Hirschhorn K. The response of cultured lymphocytes from patients with systemic lupus erythematosus to DNA. Arthritis Rheum 1967 Feb;10:32–37.

P70. Paty JG Jr, Sienknecht CW, Townes AS, Hanissian AS, Miller JB, Masi AT. Impaired cell-mediated immunity in systemic lupus erythematosus (SLE). A controlled study of 23 untreated patients. Am J Med 1975 Dec;59:769–779.

P71. Pauciullo P, de Simone B, Rubba P, Mancini M. A case of association between Type I hyperlipoproteinemia and systemic lupus erythematosus (SLE). Effects of steroid treatment. J Endocrinol Invest 1986;9:517–520.

P72. Paul E, Manheimer-Lory A, Livneh A, Solomon A, Aranow C, Ghossein C, Shefner R, Offen D, Pillinger M, Diamond B. Pathogenic anti-DNA antibodies in SLE: Idiotypic families and genetic origins. Intern Rev Immunol 1990;5:295–313.

P73. Paulino-Netto A, Dreiling DA. Pancreatitis in disseminated lupus erythematosus. J Mount Sinai Hosp NY 1960;27:291–295.

P74. Paull AM. Occurrence of the "L.E." phenomenon in a patient with a severe penicillin reaction. N Engl J Med 1955 Jan 27;252:128–129.

P75. Pauls JD, Edworthy SM, Fritzler MJ. Epitope mapping of histone 5 (H5) with systemic lupus erythematosus, procainmide-induced lupus and hydralazine-induced lupus sera. J Immunol 1991 (submitted)

P76. Pauls JD, Gohill J, Fritzler MJ. Antibodies from patients with systemic lupus erythematosus and drug-induced lupus react with determinants on histone 5 (H5). Molec Immunol 1990;27:701–711.

P77. Pauls JD, Silverman E, Laxer RM, Fritzler MJ. Antibodies to histones H1 and H5 in sera of patients with juvenile rheumatoid arthritis. Arthritis Rheum 1989;32:877–883.

P78. Paulus HE, Okun R, Calabro JJ. Depression of bone marrow granulocyte reserves in systemic lupus erythematosus (SLE) [abstract]. Arthritis Rheum 1970 May–Jun;13:344.

P79. Paulus HE, Okun R, Calabro JJ. Immunosuppressive therapy: guidelines for drug dosage. Depression of bone marrow granulocyte reserves in systemic lupus erythematosus. Arthritis Rheum 1972 Jan–Feb;15:29–35.

P80. Pawlak L, Hart D, Nisonoff A. Requirements for prolonged suppression of an idiotypic specificity in adult mice. J Exp Med 1973;137:1442.

P81. Payne JF. A postgraduate lecture on lupus erythematosus. Clin J 1894;4:223–229.

P82. Payne TC, Leavitt F, Garron DC, Katz RS, Golden HE, Glickman PB, Vanderplate C. Fibrositis and psychologic disturbance. Arthritis Rheum 1982 Feb;25(2):213–217.

P83. Pazmino NH, Yuhas JM, Tennant RW. Inhibition of murine RNA tumor virus replication and oncogenesis of chloroquine. Int J Cancer 1974 Sep 15;14(3):379–385.

P84. Peake PW, Greenstein JD, Timmermans V, Gavrilovic L, Charlesworth JA. Lymphocytotoxic antibodies in systemic lupus erythematosus: studies of their temperature dependence, binding characteristics, and specificity in vitro. Ann Rheum Dis 1988;47:725–732.

P85. Pearson CM. Vacuolar myopathy in a patient with a positive LE cell preparation. Discussion. Arthritis Rheum 1967;10:147.

P86. Pearson CM. Development of arthritis, periarthritis, periostitis in rats given adjuvants. Proc Soc Exp Biol Med 1956;91:95–101.

P87. Pearson CM, Yamazaki JN. Vacuolar myopathy is systemic lupus erythematosus. Am J Clin Path 1958 May;29(5):455–463.

P88. Pearson L, Lightfoot RW Jr. Correlation of DNA-Anti-DNA association rates with clinical activity in systemic lupus erythematosus. J Immunol 1981;126:16–19.

P89. Peck B, Hoffman GS, Franck WA. Thrombophlebitis in systemic lupus erythematosus. JAMA 1978 Oct 13;240:1728–1730.

P89a. Pederson AK, Fizgerald GA. Dose-related kinetics of aspirin. Presystemic acetylation of platelet cyclooxygenase. N Engl J Med 1984;311:1206–1211.

P90. Pedersen BK, Beyer JM, Rasmussen A, Klarlund K, Pederson BN, Helin P. Methylprednisolone pulse therapy induced fall in natural killer cell activity in rheumatoid arthritis. Acta Path Microbiol Immunol Scand 1984;92:319–323.

P91. Pedersen BK, Bygbjerg IC, Theander TG, Andersen BJ. Effects of chloroquine, mefloquine and quinine on natural killer cell activity in vitro. An analysis of the inhibitory mechanism. Allergy 1986 Sep;41(7):537–542.

P92. Pedersen SE, Taylor RP, Morley KW, Wright E. Stability of DNA/anti-DNA complexes. IV. Complement fixation. J Immunol Methods 1980;38:269–280.

P93. Omitted.

P94. Pehrson M. Lupus erythematosus disseminatus treated with ACTH. Acta Paediatrica 1952;41:478–483.

P95. Pekin TJ Jr, Zvaifler NJ. Synovial fluid findings in systemic lupus erythematosus (SLE). Arthritis Rheum 1970 Nov–Dec;13:777–785.

P95a. Pelkonen P, Simell O, Rasi V, Vaarala O. Venous thrombosis associated with lupus anticoagulant and anticardiolipin antibodies. Acta Paediatr Scand 1988;77:767–772.

P96. Pelton BK, Speckmaier M, Hylton W, Farrant J, Denman AM. Cytokine-independent progression of immunoglobulin production in vitro by B lymphocytes from patients with systemic lupus erythematosus. Clin Exp Immunol 1991;83:274–279.

P97. Pelzig A, Witten VH, Sulzberger MB. Chloroquine for chronic discoid lupus erythematosus. Intralesional injections. Arch Dermatol 1961 Jan;83:146–148.

P98. Pena AS. Systemic lupus erythematosus, Sjogren's syndrome, and purpura in a patient with coeliac disease. Neth J Med 1987 Dec;31(5–6):305–307.

P99. Pender MP, Chalk JB. Connective tissue disease mimicking multiple sclerosis. Aust N Z J Med 1989 Oct;19(5):469–472.

P100. Pengo V, Thiagarajan P, Shapiro SS, Heine MJ. Immunological specificity and mechanism of action of IgG lupus anticoagulants. Blood 1987;70:69–77.

P101. Penhale WJ, Ansar Ahmed S. Autoimmune thyroiditis in rats induced by thymectomy and irradiation. Am J Pathol 1982;106:300–302.

P102. Penhale WJ, Farmer A, Urbanaik SJ, Irvine WY. Susceptibility of inbred rat strains to experimental thyroiditis: Quantitation of thyroglobulin binding cells and assessment of T cell function in susceptible and nonsusceptible strains. Clin Exp Immunol 1975;19:179–191.

P103. Penn AS, Rowan AJ. Myelopathy in systemic lupus erythematosus. Arch Neurol 1968 Apr;18:337–349.

P104. Penn J, Makowski E, Drogemueller N, Halgrimson C, Starzl TE. Parenthood and in renal homograft reactions. JAMA 1971 Jun 14;216:1755–1762.

P105. Pennebaker JB, Gilliam JN, Ziff M. Immunoglobulin classes of DNA binding activity in serum and skin in systemic lupus erythematosus. J Clin Invest 1977 Dec;60(6):1331–1338.

P106. Penner E, Muller S, Zimmermann D, Van Regenmortel MHV. High prevalence of antibodies to histones among patients with primary biliary cirrhosis. Clin Exp Immunol 1987; 70:47–52.

P107. Penner E, Reichlin M. Primary biliary cirrhosis associated with Sjogren's syndrome: evidence for circulating and tissue-deposited Ro/anti-Ro immune complexes. Arthritis Rheum 1982;25:1250–1253.

P108. Penneys NS, Wiley HE. Herpetiform blisters in systemic lupus erythematosus. Arch Dermatol 1979;115:1429–1428.

P109. Pentland AP, Mahoney M, Jacobs SC, Holtzman MJ. Enhanced prostaglandin synthesis after ultraviolet injury is mediated by endogenous histamine stimulation. A mechanism for irradiation erythema. J Clin Invest 1990;86:566–574.

P110. Penttinen K, Myllyla G, Makela O, Vaheri A. Soluble antigen-antibody complexes and platelet aggregation. Acta Pathol Microbiol Scand 1969;77:309–317.

P111. Peppercorn MA, Docken WP, Rosenberg S. Esophageal motor dysfunction in systemic lupus erythematosus. Two cases with unusual features. JAMA 1979 Oct;242(17): 1895–1896.

P112. Pepys MB, Lanham JG, deBeer FC. C-reactive protein in SLE. Clin Rheum Dis 1982 Apr;8:91–103.

P113. Perednia DA, Curosh NA. Lupus-associated protein-losing enteropathy. Arch Intern Med 1990 Sep;150(9):1806–1810.

P114. Pereyo N. Tartrazine and drug-induced lupus. Schock Lett 1980;30:1.

P115. Pereyo N. Hydrazine derivatives and induction of systemic lupus erythematosus [letter]. J Acad Dermatol 1986;14: 514–515.

P116. Pereyo N. Tartrazine, hydrazine, amino compounds and systemic lupus erythematosus. Science-Ciencia 1987;14: 31–35.

P117. Pereyo-Torrellas N. p-Aminobenzoic acid related compounds and systemic lupus. Arch Dermatol 1978 Jul;114: 1097.

P118. Perez HD, Andron RI, Goldstein IM. Infection in patients with systemic lupus erythematosus. Association with a serum inhibitor of complement-derived chemotactic activity. Arthritis Rheum 1979 Dec;22(12):1326–1333.

P119. Perez HD, Katler E, Embury S. Idiopathic thrombocytopenic purpura with high titer speckled pattern antinuclear antibodies: possible marker for systemic lupus erythematosus. Arthritis Rheum 1985 May;28(5):596–597.

P120. Perez HD, Kimberly RP, Kaplan HB, Edelson H, Inman RD, Goldstein IM. Effect of high dose methylprednisolone infusion on polymorphonuclear leukocyte function in patients with systemic lupus erythematosus. Arthritis Rheum 1981 May; 24(5):641–647.

P121. Perez HD, Kramer N. Pulmonary hypertension in systemic lupus erythematous: report of 4 cases and review of the literature. Semin Arthritis Rheum 1981 Aug;11:177–181.

P122. Perez MC, Wilson WA, Scopelitis E. Cyclophosphamide use in a young woman with antiphospholipid antibodies and recurrent cerebrovascular accident. South Med J 1989 Nov; 82(11):1421–1424.

P123. Perez-Gutthann S, Petri M, Hochberg MC. Risk factors for coronary heart disease in patients with systemic lupus erythematosus. Arthritis Rheum 1990 Sep;33 Suppl 9:S12.

P124. Perez-Gutthann S, Petri M, Hochberg MC. Comparison of different methods of classifying patients with systemic lupus erythematosus. J Rheumatol 1991. In press.

P124a. See P125.

P125. Perez-Ruiz F, Zea AC, Orte FJ. Antiphospholipid antibodies may play a role in the pathogenesis of nodular regenerative hyperplasma of the liver [abstract]. Br J Rheumatol 1990;29 Suppl 2:107.

P126. Perkins DL, Michaelson J, Glaser RM, Marshak-Rothstein A. Selective elimination of non-lpr lymphoid cells in mice undergoing lpr-mediated graft-vs-host disease. J Immunol 1987;139:1406–1413.

P127. Perkins HA, Acra DJ. The circulating anticoagulant in disseminated lupus erythematosus. Thromb Diath Haemorrh 1960 Dec;5:250–255.

P128. Perkins PS, Young RW. Comparisons of histones in retinal and brain nuclei from newborn and adult mice. Dev Brain R 1987; 33:161–168.

P129. Permin H, Juhl F, Wiik A, Balsv JT. Immunoglobulin deposit in the dermoepidermal junction zone in patients with systemic lupus erythematosus, rheumatoid arthritis and temporal arteritis compared by serologic testing including macroglobulin. Scand J Rheumatol 1977;6:105–110.

P130. Perri NA, Lipkowitz GS, Honig JH, Manis T, Friedman EA, Butt KMH. Cyclosporine markedly improves patient and graft survival in renal transplantation. Kidney Int 1987;31:466.

P131. Perry HM, Chaplin H, Carmody S. Immunologic findings in patients receiving methyldopa: A prospective study. J Lab Clin Med 1971; 78:905–917.

P132. Perry HM Jr. Late toxicity of hydralazine resembling systemic lupus erythematosus or rheumatoid arthritis. Am J Med 1973 Jan;54:58–72.

P133. Perry HM Jr, Schroeder HA. Syndrome simulating collagen disease caused by hydralazine (Apresoline). JAMA 1954 Feb 20;154:670–673.

P134. Perry HM Jr, Tan EM, Carmody S, Sakamoto A. Relationship of acetyl transferase activity to antinuclear antibodies and toxic symptoms in hypertensive patients treated with hydralazine. J Lab Clin Med 1970;76:114–125.

P135. Persellin RH. The effect of pregnancy on rheumatoid arthritis. Bull Rheum Dis 1977;27:922–927.

P136. Persellin RH, Takeuchi A. Antinuclear antibody-negative systemic lupus erythematosus: loss in body fluids. J Rheumatol 1980 Jul–Aug;7(4):547–550.

P137. Pertschuk LP, Moccia LF, Rosen Y, Lyons H, Marino CM, Rashford AA, Wollschlager CM. Acute pulmonary complications in systemic lupus erythematosus: Immunofluorescence and light microscopic study. Am J Clin Path 1977 Nov;68: 553–557.

P138. Perussia B, Acuto O, Terhorst C, Faust J, Lazarus R, Fanning V, Trinchieri G. Human natural killer cells analyzed by B73.1, a monoclonal antibody blocking FcR functions. II. Studies of B73.1 antibody-antigen interaction on the lymphocyte membrane. J Immunol 1983;130:2142–2148.

P139. Perussia B, Dayton ET, Lazarus R, Fanning V, Trinchieri G. Immune interferon induces the receptor for monomeric IgG1 on human monocytic and myeloid cells. Exp Med 1983;158: 1092–1113.

P140. Perussia B, Starr S, Abraham S, Fanning V, Trinchieri G. Human natural killer cells analyzed by B73.1, a monoclonal antibody blocking Fc receptor functions. I. Characterization of the lymphocyte subset reactive with B73.1. J Immunol 1983;130:2133.

P141. Peter JB, Spezialetti R, Bluestein HG. CNS-systemic lupus erythematosus (SLE: Clinical utility of immunological abnormalities) [abstract]. Arthritis Rheum 1990 Sep;33(9) Suppl: S102.

P142. Peter LD. Autoimmune hemolytic anemia. Hum Pathol 1983;14:251–255.

P143. Peters MS, Su WP. Lupus erythematosus panniculitis. Med Clin North Am 1989 Sep;73(5):1113–1126.

P144. Petersdorf RG, Beeson PB. Fever of unexplained origin: report on 100 cases. Medicine 1961 Feb;40:1–30.

P145. Petersen HH, Nielsen H, Hansen M, Stensgaard-Hansen F, Helin P. High dose immunoglobulin therapy in pericarditis caused by SLE. Scand J Rheumatol 1990;19:91–93.

P146. Peterson LL. Hydralazine-induced systemic lupus erythematosus presenting as pyoderma gangrenosum-like ulcers. J Am Acad Dermatol 1984;10:379–384.

P147. Peterson MW, Monick M, Hunninghake GW. Prognostic role of eosinophils in pulmonary fibrosis. Chest 1987;92:51–56.

P148. Peterson RD, Good RA. Interrelationships of the mesenchymal diseases with consideration of possible genetic mechanisms. Ann Rev Med 1963;14:1.

P149. Peterson RDA, Vernier RL, Good RA. Lupus erythematosus. Pediatr Clin North Am 1963;10:941–975.

P150. Peterson T, Klockars M, Hellstrom PE. Chemical and immunological features of pleural effusions: comparison between rheumatoid arthritis and other diseases. Thorax 1982;37:354–361.

P151. Petri M, Bockenstedt L, Colman J, Whiting-O'Keefe Q, Fitz G, Sebastian A, Hellmann D. Serial assessment of glomerular filtration rate in lupus nephropathy. Kidney Int 1988;34:832–839.

P152. Petri M, Genovese M, Engle E, Hochberg MC. Definition, incidence and clinical description of flare in systemic lupus erythematosus: a prospective cohort study. Arthritis Rheum 1991;34:937–944.

P153. Petri M, Hellmann DB, Hochberg MC. Validity and reliability of the lupus activity index (LAI): comparison with the Toronto activity index (SLEDAI) and systemic lupus activity measure (SLAM) [abstract]. Arthritis Rheum 1989 Apr;32 Suppl 4):S30.

P153a. Petri M, Howard D, Repke J. Frequency of lupus flare of pregnancy. The Johns Hopkins Lupus Pregnancy Center experience. Arthritis Rheum 1991;34:1538–1545.

P154. Petri M, Katzenstein P, Hellmann D. Laryngeal infection in lupus: Report of nocardiosis and review of laryngeal involvement in lupus. J Rheumatol 1985;15:1014–1015.

P155. Petri M, Perez-Guttham S, Longenecker C, Hochberg MC. The association of black race with morbidity in patients with systemic lupus erythematosus is explained by socioeconomic status and compliance [abstract]. Arthritis Rheum 1990;33 Suppl:S83.

P156. Petri M, Perez-Guttham S, Longenecker JC, Hochberg MC. Morbidity of Systemic Lupus Erythematosus: role of race and socioeconomic status. Am J Med 1991. In press.

P157. Petri M, Rheinschmidt M, Whiting-O'Keefe Q, Hellmann D, Corash L. The frequency of lupus anticoagulant in systemic lupus erythematosus. A study of sixty consecutive patients by activated partial thromboplastin time, Russel viper venom time, and anticardiolipin antibody level. Ann Intern Med 1987;106:524–531.

P158. Petri M, Watson R, Hochberg MC. Anti-Ro antibodies and neonatal lupus. Rheum Dis Clin N A 1989;15:335–360.

P159. Petrova TR, Akopova VL. Systemic lupus erythematosus in uniovular twins. Ter Arkh (Russian) 1972;44:111.

P160. Petrucco OM, Seamark RF, Holmes K, Forbes IJ, Symons RG. Changes in lymphocyte function during pregnancy. Br J Obstet Gynecol 1976;83:245.

P161. Pettersson I, Hinterberger M, Mimori T, Gottlieb E, Steitz A. The structure of mammalian small nuclear ribonucleoproteins. J Biol Chem 1984;259:5907–5914.

P162. Pettersson I, Wang G, Smith EI, Wigzell H, Hedfors E, Horn J, Sharp GC. The use of immunoblotting and immunoprecipitation of (U) small nuclear ribonucleoproteins in the analysis of sera of patients with mixed connective tissue disease and systemic lupus erythematosus. A cross-sectional, longitudinal study. Arthritis Rheum 1986 Aug;29(8):986–996.

P163. Pettersson T, Tornroth T, Totterman KJ, Fortelius P, Maury CP. AA amyloidosis in systemic lupus erythematosus. J Rheumatol 1987 Aug;14(4):835–838.

P164. Pettijohn DE. Histone-like proteins and bacterial chromosome structure. J Biol Chem 1988;263:12793–12796.

P165. Petty BG, Zahka KG, Bernstein MT. Aspirin hepatitis associated with encephalopathy. J Pediatr 1978 Nov;93(5):881–882.

P166. Petz LD. Autoimmune hemolytic anemia. Hum Pathol 1983;14:251–255.

P167. Petz LD, Sharp GC, Cooper NR, Irvin WS. Serum and cerebral spinal fluid complement and serum autoantibodies in systemic lupus erythematosus. Medicine 1971 Jul;50:259–275.

P168. Pfab R, Schachtschabel DO, Kern HF. Ultrastructural studies of the effect of x-rays and quinacrine (Atebrin) or chloroquine (Resochine)—alone or in combination —on Harding-Passey melanoma cells in monolayer culture. Strahlentherapie 1985 Nov;161(11):711–718.

P169. Pfeffer U, Ferrari N, Tosetti F, Vidali G. Histone acetylation in conjugating Tetrahymena thermophila. J Cell Biol 1989;109:1007–1014.

P170. Phadke K, Trachtman H, Nicastri A, Chen CK, Tejani A. Acute renal failure as the initial manifestation of systemic lupus erythematosus in children. J Pediatr 1984;105:38–41.

P171. Pham BN, Prin L, Gosset D, Hatron PY, Devulder B, Capron A, Dessaint JP. T lymphocyte activation in systemic lupus erythematosus analyzed by proliferative response to nucleoplasmic proteins on nitrocellulose immunoblots. Clin Exp Immunol 1989;77:168–174.

P172. Pheiffer CA. The impact of gender-role socialization on women coping with a rheumatic disease. Clin Rheumatol Pract 1986 Mar:75–80.

P173. Phi NC, Chien DK, Binh VV, Gergely P. Cathepsin D-like activity in serum of patients with systemic lupus erythematosus. J Lab Clin Immunol 1990;29:185–188.

P174. Phi NC, Takáts A, Binh VH, Vien CV, González-Cabello R, Gergely P. Cyclic AMP level of lymphocytes in patients with systemic lupus erythematosus and its relation to disease activity. Immunol Lett 1989;23:61–64.

P174a. Philips PE. The potential role of microbial agents in the pathogenesis of systemic lupus erythematosus. J Rheumatol 1981;8:344.

P174b. Philips PE, Christian CL. Myxovirus antibody increases in human connective tissue disease. Science 1970;168:982–984.

P175. Phillips JH, Gemlo BT, Myers WW, Rayner AA, Lanier LL. In vivo and in vitro activation of natural killer cells in advanced cancer patients undergoing combined recombinant interleukin-2 and LAK cell therapy. J Clin Oncol 1987;5:1933.

P176. Phillips JH, Lanier LL. Dissection of the lymphokine-activated killer phenomenon. Relative contribution of peripheral blood natural killer cells and T lymphocytes to cytolysis. J Exp Med 1986;164:814.

P177. See 174a.

P178. See 174b.

P179. Phipps RP, Spaulding M, Szakos J. DNA is a potent immunogen for spleen cells and for guanosine-binding B lymphocytes. Cell Immunol 1988;113:202–213.

P180. Pichler WJ, Schindler L, Staubli M, Stadler BM. Anti-amiodarone antibodies: detection and relationship to the development of side effects. Am J Med 1988; 85:197.

P181. Pickering G, Bywaters EGL, Damielli JF, Gell PG, Kellgren JH, Long DA, Neuberger A, Nicholson H, Prunty FTG, Robb-Smith AHT, Payling Wright G, Conybeare ET, Duthie JJR. Treatment of systemic lupus erythematosus with steroids. Report to the Medical Research Council by the Collagen Diseases and Hypersensitivity Panel. BMJ 1961 Oct 7;5257:915–920.

P182. Picking WL, Smith C, Petrucci R, Scheffel J, Levich JD,

Stetler DA. Anti-RNA polymerase I antibodies in the urine of patients with systemic lupus erythematosus. J Rheumatol 1990;1308–1313.

P183. Pierangeli S, Robinson E, Harris EN. Gold-labelled affinity-purified anti-cardiolipin antibodies specifically bind human-platelet membrane [abstract]. Arthritis Rheum 1989 Apr; 32(4) Suppl:S122.

P184. Pierce DA, Stern R, Jaffe R, Zulman J, Talal N. Immunoblastic sarcoma with features of Sjogren's syndrome and systemic lupus erythematosus in a patient with immunoblastic lymphadenopathy. Arthritis Rheum 1979 Aug;22(8):911–916.

P185. Pierucci A, Simonetti BM, Pecci G, Mavrikakis G. Improvement of renal function with selective thromboxane antagonism in lupus nephritis. N Engl J Med 1989 Feb 16;320(7): 421–425.

P186. Omitted.

P187. Piette JC, Bourgeois P, Herson S, Etienne S, Kahn MF, Godeau P. Acebutolol-induced lupus (AIL). Arthritis Rheum 1985 Apr;28 Suppl:S52.

P188. Pigott PV. Captopril and drug-induced lupus. Br Med J 1982 Jun 12;284:1786.

P189. Piliero P, Furie R. Functional asplenia in systemic lupus erythematosus. Semin Arthritis Rheum 1990;20:185–189.

P190. Pillemer SR, Austin HA, Tsokos GC, Balow JE. Lupus nephritis: Association between serology and renal biopsy measurements. J Rheumatol 1988;15:284–288.

P191. Pillsbury DM, Jacobson C. Treatment of chronic discoid lupus erythematosus with chloroquine (aralen). JAMA 1954 Apr 17;154:1330–1333.

P192. Pinching AJ, Travers RL, Hughes GR, Jones T, Moss S. Oxygen-15 brain scanning for detection of cerebral involvement in systemic lupus erythematosus. Lancet 1978 Apr 29; 1(8070):898–900.

P193. Pincus T. Studies regarding a possible function for viruses in the pathogenesis of systemic lupus erythematosus. Arthritis Rheum 1982 Jul;25:847–856.

P194. Pincus T, Hughes GRV, Pincus D, Tina LU, Bellanti JA. Antibodies to DNA in childhood systemic lupus erythematosus. J Pediatr 1971;78:981–984.

P195. Pincus T, Olsen NJ, Russel J, Wolfe F, Harris ER, Schnitzer TJ, Boccagno JA, Drantz S. Multicenter study of recombinant human erythropoietin in correction of anemia in rheumatoid arthritis. Am J Med 1990;89:161–166.

P196. Pincus T, Schur PH, Rose JA, Decker JL, Talal N. Measurement of serum anti-DNA binding activity in systemic lupus erythematosus. N Engl J Med 1970;281:701–705.

P197. Pincus T, Summey JA, Soraci SA, Wallston KA, Hummon NP. Assessment of patient satisfaction in activies of daily living using a modified Stanford Health Assessment Questionnaire. Arthritis Rheum 1983;26:1346–1353.

P198. Pingel JT, Thomas ML. Evidence that the leukocyte-common antigen is required for antigen-induced T lymphocyte proliferation. Cell 1989;58:1055–1065.

P199. Pinillos RM, Solle JMN, Roura XJ, Ferranz VP, Palacin AV, Sampere IM. Rheumatoid factor in patients with systemic lupus erythematosus. Ann Rheum Dis 1987;46:877–878.

P199a. Piper JM, Ray WA, Daugherty JR, Griffin MR. Corticosteroid use and peptic ulcer disease: Role of nonsteroidal anti-inflammatory drugs. Ann Intern Med 1991;114:735–740.

P200. Pipitone V, Carrozzo M. Modern views on the treatment with anabolics in the therapy of osteoporosis in the course of chronic arthropathy. In: Osteoporosis e Malattie Reumatiche. Bari 13–14. Febbraio, 1976:213–243.

P201. Pirani CL. Evaluation of kidney biopsy specimens. In: Brenner BM, editor. Renal Pathology. Philadelphia: Lippincott, 1989:11–42.

P202. Pirani CL, Olesnicky L. Role of electromicroscopy in the classification of lupus nephritis. Am J Kidney Dis 1982;2 Suppl 1:150–163.

P203. Pirani CL, Pollak VE. Systemic lupus erythematosus (SLE) Glomerulonephritis (lupus nephritis). In: McCluskey RT, Andres GA, editors. Immunologically mediated renal diseases. New York: Marcel Dekker 1978:11–69.

P204. Pirani CL, Silva FG. The kidney in systemic lupus erythematosus and other collagen diseases. In: Churg J, Spargo BH, Mostofi KF, Abell MR, editors. Baltimore: Williams, 1979: 98–139.

P205. Pirner K, Rosler W, Kalden JR, Manger B. Long-term remission after i.v. immunoglobulin therapy in acquired antihemophilic factor hemophilia with systemic lupus erythematosus. Z Rheumatol 1990 Nov–Dec;49(6):378–381.

P206. Pirofsky B. Hereditary aspects of autoimmune hemolytic anemia A retrospective analysis. Vox Sang 1968;14:334–347.

P207. Pirofsky B, Bardana EJ, Bayracki C, Porter GA. Antilymphocyte antisera in immunologically mediated renal disease. JAMA 1969;210:1059–1064.

P208. Pirofsky B, Shearn MA. The familial occurrence of disseminated lupus erythematosus. NY J Med 1953;53:3022–3024.

P209. Pischel KD, Bluestein HG, Woods VL Jr. Molecular characterization of lymphocyte cell surface proteins reactive with systemic lupus erythematosus (SLE) autoantibodies. Arthritis Rheum 1984;27:83.

P210. Pisetsky DS. Inhibition of in vitro NZB antibody responses by cyclosporine. Clin Exp Immunol 1988;71:155–158.

P211. Pisetsky DS, Grudier JP. Polyspecific binding of Escherichia coli beta-galactosidase by murine antibodies to DNA. J Immunol 1989 Dec 1;143(11):3609–3613.

P212. Pisetsky DS, Grudier JP, Gilkeson GS. A role for immunogenic DNA in the pathogenesis of systemic lupus erythematosus. Arthritis Rheum 1990;33:153–159.

P213. Pisetsky DS, Hoch SO, Klatt CL, O'Donnel MA, Keene JD. Specificity and idiotypic analysis of a monoclonal anti-Sm antibody with anti-DNA activity. J Immunol 1985 Dec;135(6): 4080–4085.

P213a. Pisetsky DS, Jelinek DF, McAnally LM, Reich CF, Lipsky PE. In vitro autoantibody production by normal adult and cord blood B cells. J Clin Invest 1990;85:899–903.

P214. Pisetsky DS, Semper KF, Eisenberg RA. Idiotypic analysis of a monoclonal anti-Sm antibody. II. Strain distribution of a common idiotypic determinant and its relationship to anti-Sm expression. J Immunol 1984;133:2085.

P215. Pishkin V, Lovallo WR, Fishkin SM, Shurley JT. Residual effects of temazepam and other hypnotic compounds on cognitive function. J Clin Psychiatry 1980 Oct;41(10):358–63.

P216. Pistiner M, Wallace DJ, Nessim S, Metzger AL, Klinenberg JR. Lupus erythematosus in the 1980s: A survey of 570 patients. Semin Arthritis Rheum 1991 Aug;21(1):55–64.

P217. Pizarro S, Medina F, Jara J, Fernandez M, Cevera H, Medina A. Efficacy of danazol therapy vs splenectomy in systemic lupus erythematosus patients with hematologic onset [abstract]. Arthritis Rheum 1990 Sep;33(9) Suppl:S165.

P218. Pizzi F, Cararra PM, Aldeghi A, Eridani S. Immunofluorescence of megakaryocytes in the thrombocytopenic purpuras. Blood 1966 Apr;27:521–526.

P219. Plant RK, Steven RA. Complete A-V block in a fetus. Case report. Am Heart J 1945;30:615–618.

P220. Plantey F. Antinuclear factor in affective disorders. Biol Psych 1978 Feb;13:149–150.

P221. Platt JL, Burke BA, Fish AJ, Kim Y, Michael AF. Systemic lupus erythematosus in the first two decades of life. Am J Kidney Dis 1982 Jul;2 Suppl 1:212–222.

P222. Platt LD, Manning FA, Gray C, Guttenburg M, Turkel SB. Antenatal detection of fetal A-V dissociation utilizing real-time B-mode ultrasound. Obstet Gynecol 1979;53 Suppl:59S-61S.

P223. Plotnick H, Burnham TK. Lichen planus and coexisting lupus erythematosus versus lichen planus-like lupus erythematosus. Clinical, histologic, and immunopathologic considerations. J Am Acad Dermatol 1986 May;14(5 Pt 2):931–938.

P223a. Plotz CM, Knowlton AI, Ragan C. Natural history of Cushing's syndrome. Am J Med 1952 Nov;13:597–614.

P224. Plotz PH. Autoantibodies are antiidiotype antibodies to antiviral antibodies. Lancet 1987;2:824–826.

P225. See P223a.

P226. Plotz PH, Dalakas M, Leff RL, Love LA, Miller FW, Cronin ME. Current concepts in the idiopathic inflammatory myopathies: polymyositis, dermatomyositis, and related disorders. Ann Intern Med 1989 Jul 15;111(2):143–157.

P227. Podolsky M. Hair "permanent wave" preparation allergy presenting as lupus erythematosus. Ann Allergy 1980 Jan;44; 49.

P228. Pohl MA, Lan S-P, Berl T, Lupus Nephritis Collaborative Study Group. Plasmapheresis does not increase the risk for infection in immunosuppressed patients with severe lupus nephritis. Ann Intern Med 1991 June 1;114(11):924–929.

P229. Pohle EL, Tuffanelli DL. Study of cutaneous lupus erythematosus by immunohistochemical methods. Arch Dermatol 1968;97:520–526.

P230. Pohlgeers AP, Eid MS, Schikler KN, Shearer LT. Systemic lupus erythematosus: Pulmonary presentation in childhood. South Med J 1990;83:712–714.

P231. Polano MK, Cats A, van Olden GAJ. Agranulocytosis following treatment with hydroxychloroquine sulphate. Lancet 1965;1:1275.

P232. Poldre PA. Splenic hypofunction in systemic lupus erythematosus response to pneumococcal vaccine. J Rheumatol 1989;16:1130–1131.

P233. Polednak AP. Connective tissue responses in Blacks in relation to disease: further observations. Am J Phys Anthropol 1974;41:49.

P234. Polishuck WZ, Beyth Y, Izak G. Antinuclear factor and LE cells in pregnant women. Lancet 1971;2:270.

P235. Poljak RJ, Anzel LM, Avey HP, Chen BL, Phizackerley P, Saul F. Three dimensional structure of the Fab' fragment of a human immunoglobulin at 2.8 A. Proc Natl Acad Sci USA 1973; 70:3305–3310.

P236. Pollak O, Ziskind JM. Death during sulfonamide treatment; finding of liver cells in brain. J Nerv Ment Dis 1943 Dec;98: 648–655.

P237. Pollak VE. Antinuclear antibodies in families of patients with systemic lupus erythematosus. N Engl J Med 1964 Jul 23; 271:165–171.

P238. Pollak VE, Dosekun AK. Evaluation of treatment in lupus nephritis: effects of prednisone. Am J Kidney Dis 1982;2 Suppl 1:170–177.

P239. Pollak VE, Kant KS. Nephritis in systemic lupus erythematosus. Ricera Clinica Laboratorio (Milano) 1981 Jan–Mar;11: 1–10.

P240. Pollak VE, Kant KS, Hariharan S. Diffuse and focal proliferative lupus nephritis: treatment approaches and results. Nephron 1991;59:177–193.

P241. Pollak VE, Mandema E, Doig AB, Moore M, Kark RM. Observations on electrophoresis of serum proteins from healthy North American caucasian and negro subjects and from patients with systemic lupus erythematosus. J lab Clin Med 1961 Sep;58:353–365.

P242. Pollak VE, Mandema E, Kark RM. Antinuclear factors in the serum of relatives of patients with systemic lupus erythematosus. Lancet 1960;2:1061–1063.

P243. Pollak VE, Pirani CL, Dujovne I, Dillard MG. The clinical course of lupus nephritis. In: Kincaid-Smith P, Mathew TH,

Becker EL, editors. Glomerulonephritis. New York: Wiley, 1973:1167–1181.

P244. Pollak VE, Pirani CL, Kark RM. Effect of large doses of prednisone on the renal lesions and life span of patients with lupus glomerulonephritis. J Lab Clin Med 1961 Apr;57: 495–511.

P245. Pollak VE, Pirani CL, Schwartz F. Natural history of the renal manifestations of systemic lupus erythematosus. J Lab Clin Med 1964 Apr;63:537–550.

P246. Pollak VE, Schwartz FD, Pirani CL. Systemic lupus erythematosus: the failure of urinalysis and simple renal function tests to predict reliably the underlying renal pathology. Presbyterian-St. Luke's Hospital Med Bull 1964 Jul;3:94–103.

P247. Omitted.

P248. Pollard KM, Furphy LJ, Webb J. Anti-Sm and anti-DNA antibodies in paired serum and synovial fluid samples from patients with SLE. Rheumatol Int 1988;8(5):197–204.

P248a. Pollard KM, Steele R, Hogg S, Webb J. Measurement of serum DNA binding in chronic active hepatitis and systemic lupus erythematosus using the Farr assay. Rheumatol Int 1986; 6(3):139–144.

P249. Pollock CA, Ibels LS. Dialysis and transplantation in patients with renal failure due to systemic lupus erythematosus. The Australian and New Zealand experience. Aust N Z J Med 1987 Jun;17(3):321–325.

P250. Pomeroy C, Knodell RG, Swaim WR, Arneson P, Mahowald ML. Budd-Chiari syndrome in a patient with the lupus anticoagulant. Gastroenterology 1984 Jan;86(1):158–161.

P251. Pompougnac E, Doutre MS, Beylot C, Beylot J, Lacoste D, Bioulac P. Chilblain lupus erythematosus: a peculiar form of lupus. A study of four patients. Sem Hop Paris 1986 Apr 17; 62(18):1233–1235.

P252. Pons M, Nolla JM, Bover J, Mateo L, Rozadilla A, Climent EM. Concurrence of rheumatoid arthritis and systemic lupus erythematosus. A case report with diffuse proliferative glomerulonephritis. Nefrologia 1991;9:80–83.

P253. Ponticelli C, Moroni G, Banfi G. Discontinuation of therapy in diffuse proliferative lupus nephritis. Am J Med 1988; 85:275–276.

P254. Ponticelli C, Zuchelli P, Banfi G, Cagnoli L, Scalia P, Pasquali S, Imasciati E. Treatment of diffuse proliferative lupus nephritis by intravenous high-dose methyl-prednisolone. Q J Med 1982 Winter;51:18–24.

P255. Ponticelli C, Zucchelli P, Moroni G, Cagnoli L, Banfi G, Pasquali S. Long-term prognosis of diffuse lupus nephritis. Clin Nephrol 1987;28:263–271.

P256. Pope JM, Canny CLB, Bell DA. Cerebral ischemic events assoc with endocarditis, retinal vascular disease, and lupus anticoagulant. Am J Med 1991;90:299–309.

P257. Pope RM, Keightley R, McDuffy S. Circulating autoantibodies to IgD in rheumatic diseases. J Immunol 1982;128: 1860–1863.

P258. Pope RM, McDuffy SJ. IgG rheumatoid factor. Arthritis Rheum 1979 Sep;22:968–998.

P259. Porac C, Coren S. Lateral preferences and human behavior. New York: Springer-Verlag, 1981.

P260. Porcel JM, Selva A, Tornos MP, Galve E, Soler-Soler J. Resolution of cardiac tamponade in systemic lupus erythematosus with indomethacin. Chest 1989 Nov;96(5):1193–1194.

P261. Porges AJ, Christian CL. Patients with systemic lupus erythematosus at high risk for pneumocystis carinii pneumonia [abstract]. Arthritis Rheum 1990 May;33 Suppl 5:R46.

P262. Portanova JP, Arndt RE, Tan EM. Anti-histone antibodies in idiopathic and drug-induced lupus recognized distinct intrahistone regions. J Immunol 1987;138:293–296.

P263. Portanova JP, Cherouis JC, Blodgett JK, Kotzin BL. Histone autoantigens in murine lupus. Definition of a major epitope within an accessible region of chromatin. J Immunol 1990; 144:4633–4639.

P264. Portanova JP, Ebling FM, Hammond WS, Hahn BH, Kotzin BL. Allogeneic MHC antigen requirements for lupus-like autoantibody production and nephritis in murine graft-vs-host disease. J Immunol 1988;141:3370–3376.

P265. Portanova JP, Rubin RL, Joslin FG. Reactivity of anti-histone antibodies induced by procainamide and hydralazine. Clin Immunol Immunopathol 1982;25:67–79.

P266. Porter JM, Bardana EJ, Baur GM, Wesche DH, Andrasch RH, Rosch J. The clinical significance of Raynaud's syndrome. Surgery 1976;80:756–764.

P267. Porter RR. Complement polymorphism, the major histocompatibility complex and associated disease: a speculation. Molec Biol Med 1983;1:161–167.

P268. Portnoy JZ, Callen JP. Ophthalmologic aspects of chloroquine and hydroxychloroquine therapy. Int J Dermatol 1983;22(5):273–278.

P269. Posey WC, Nelson HS, Pearlman DS. The effects of acute corticosteroid therapy for asthma on serum immunoglobulin levels. J Allergy Clin Immunol 1980;62:440–444.

P270. Posner DI, Guill MA 3d. Coexistent leprosy and lupus erythematosus. Cutis 1987 Feb;39(2):136–138.

P271. Posner MA, Gloster ES, Bonagura VR, Valacer DJ, Ilowite NT. Burkitt's lymphoma in a patient with systemic lupus erythematosus. J Rheumatol 1990 Mar;17(3):380–382.

P272. Posnett DN, Gottlieb A, Bussel JB, Friedman SM, Chiorazzi N, Li Y, Szabo P, Farid NR, Robinson MA. T cell antigen receptors in autoimmunity. J Immunol 1988;141:1963–1969.

P273. Posnick J. Systemic lupus erythematosus. The effect of corticotropin and adrenocorticoid therapy on survival rate. CA Med 1963 Jun;98:308–312.

P274. Potasman I, Bassan HM. Multiple tendon rupture in systemic lupus erythematosus: case report and review of the literature. Ann Rheum Dis 1984 Apr;43(2):348–347.

P275. Poulton TA, Gallagher G, Beck J. Suppression of the increase in free cytosilic calcium during the inhigition of T-cell activation by an autoantibody present in the serum of leprosy patients. Immunology 1989;68:353–358.

P276. Powell AL, Joshi B, Dwivedi C, Green LD. Immunopathological changes in cadmium treated rats. Veterinary Pathol 1979;16:116–118.

P277. Powell TJ Jr, Streilein JW. Neonatal tolerance induction by class II alloantigens activates IL-4-secreting, tolerogen-responsive T cells. J Immunol 1990;144:854–859.

P278. Prager D, Levitt LP. Chronic pericarditis with effusion due to lupus erythematosus. Harefuah 1978 Jun 15;90:568–569.

P279. Pratilas V, Pratila M. Anesthesia in the presence of complete fetal atrioventricular heart block: an anesthetics dilemma. Mt Sinai J Med 1990;57:157–159.

P280. Pratt EE. Analysis of Leanon Lupus Erythematosus Club Questionnaire. Unpublished data.

P281. Praz F, Halbwachs L, Lesavre P. Genetic aspects of complement and glomerulonephritis. In: Grunfeld JP, Maxwell MH, editors. Advances in nephrology. Chicago: Year Book, 1984: 271–296.

P282. Preble OT, Black RJ, Friedman RM, Klippel J, Vilcek J. Systemic lupus erythematosus: presence in human serum of the unusual acid labile leukocyte interferon. Science 1982 Apr 23;216:429–431.

P283. Preble OT, Rothko K, Klippel JH, Friedman RM, Johnston MI. Interferon-induced 2'-5' adenylate synthetase *in vivo* and interferon production by lymphocytes from systemic lupus erythematosus patients with and without circulating interferon. J Exp Med 1983;157:2140–2146.

P284. Prelich G, Tan CK, Kostura M, Mathews MB, So AG, Downey KM, Stillman B. Functional identity of proliferating cell nuclear antigens and a DNA polymerase delta auxiliary protein. Nature 1987;326:517–520.

P285. Prentice RL, Gatenby PA, Loblay RH, Shearman RP, Kronenberg H, Basten A. Lupus anticoagulant in pregnancy. Lancet 1984;2:464.

P286. Present PA, Comstock GW. Tuberculin sensitivity in pregnancy. Am Rev Respir Dis 1975;112:413.

P287. Presley AP, Kahn A, Williamson N. Antinuclear antibodies in patients on lithium carbonate. Br Med J 1976 Jul 31;2: 280–281.

P288. Presthus J, Skulstad A. Cortisone therapy in lupus erythematosus disseminatus with affection of the central nervous system. J Lancet 1957 Jan;77:11–13.

P289. Prete P. The mechanism of action of L-canavanine in inducing autoimmune phenomena. Arthritis Rheum 1985;28: 1198–2000.

P290. Prete PE. The mechanisms of action of L-canavanine in inducing autoimmune phenomena [letter]. Arch Intern Med 1985;145:1926–1927.

P291. Prete PE. The mechanism of action of L-canavanine in inducing autoimmune phenomenon [letter]. Arthritis Rheum 1985 Oct;28(10):1198–1200.

P292. Prete PE. Effects of L-canavanine on immune function in normal and autoimmune mice: disordered B-cell function by a dietary amino acid in the immunoregulation of autoimmune disease. Can J Physiol Pharmacol 1985;63:843–854.

P293. Price J, Klestov A, Beacham B, Roberts C. A case of cerebral systemic lupus erythematosus treated with methylprednisolone pulse therapy. Aust NZ J Psychiatry 1985 Jun;19(1): 184–188.

P294. Price JE, Rigler LG. Widening of the mediastinum resulting from fat accumulation. Radiology 1970 Sep;96:497–500.

P295. Prickett JD, Robinson DR, Steinberg AD. Dietary enrichment with the polyunsaturated fatty acid eicosapentaenoic acid prevents proteinuria and prolongs survival in NZB × NZW F1 mice. J Clin Invest 1981;68:556.

P296. Prickett JD, Robinson DR, Steinberg AD. Effects of dietary enrichment with eicosapentaenoic acid upon autoimmune nephritis in female NZB × NZW/F1 mice. Arthritis Rheum 1983; 26:133–139.

P297. Prickett JD, Trentham DE, Robinson DR. Dietary fish oil augments the induction of arthritis in rats immunized with type II collagen. J Immunol 1984;132:725–729.

P298. Priofsky B. Immune haemolytic disease: the autoimmune haemolytic anemias. Clin Haematol 1975;4:167–180.

P299. Priollet P, Vayssairat M, Housset E. How to classify Raynaud's phenomenon. Long-term follow-up study of 73 cases. Am J Med 1987 Sep;83(3):494–498.

P300. Pritchard CH, Berney S. Patellar tendon rupture in systemic lupus erythematosus. J Rheumatol 1989 Jun;16(6): 786–788.

P301. Pritchard MH, Jessop JD, Trenchard P, Whittaker JA. Systemic lupus erythematosus. Repeated abortions and thrombocytopenia. Ann Rheum Dis 1978;37:476.

P302. Pritzker MR, Ernst JD, Caudill C, Wilson CS, Weaver WF, Edwards JE. Acquired aortic stenosis in systemic lupus erythematosus. Ann Intern Med 1980 Sep;93:434–436.

P303. Procopio ADG, Allavena P, Ortaldo JR. Noncytotoxic functions of natural killer (NK) cells: large granular lymphocytes (LGL) produce a B cell growth factor (BCGF). J Immunol 1985:135.

P304. Prokoptchouk AJ. Treatment of lupus erythematosus with acridine. [abstract] [original in German]. Z Haut Geschlechtskr 1940;66:112.

P304a. Prokoptchouk AJ. Article translated into English. Arch Dermatol & Syph 1955;71:520.

P305. Propper DJ, Bucknall RC. Acute transverse myelopathy complicating systemic lupus erythematosus. Ann Rheum Dis 1989 Jun;48(6):512–515.

P306. Provost TT. The relationship between discoid lupus erythematosus and systemic lupus erythematosus: a hypothesis. Am J Dermatapathol 1979;1:181–186.

P307. Provost TT, Andres G, Maddison PJ, Reichlin M. Lupus band test in untreated SLE patients: correlation of immunoglobulin deposition in the skin of the extensor forearm with clinical renal disease and serologic abnormalities. J Invest Dermatol 1980 Jun;74(6):407–415.

P308. Provost TT, Arnett FC, Reichlin M. Homozygous C2 deficiency, lupus erythematosus and anti-Ro(SS-A) antibodies. Arthritis Rheum 1983 Oct;26:1279–1282.

P309. Provost TT, Levin LS, Watson RM, Mayo M, Ratrie H. Detection of anti Ro(SSA) antibodies by gel double diffusion and a sandwich ELISA in systemic and subacute cutaneous lupus erythematosus and Sjogren's syndrome. J Autoimmunity 1991; 4:87–96.

P310. Provost TT, Ratrie H. Autoantibodies and autoantigens in lupus erythematosus and Sjogren's syndrome. Current Prob Dermatol 1990;2:150–208.

P311. Provost TT, Reichlin M. Antinuclear antibody-negative lupus erythematosus. J Am Acad Dermatol 1981 Jan;4(1): 84–89.

P312. Provost TT, Talal N, Bias W, Harley JB, Reichlin M, Alexander EL. Ro (SS-A) positive Sjogren's/lupus erythematosus (SC/LE) overlap patients are associated with the HLA-DR3 and/or DRw6 phenotypes. J Invest Dermatol 1988 Oct;91(4): 369–371.

P313. Provost TT, Talal N, Harley JB, Reichlin M, Alexander E. The relationship between anti-Ro (SS-A) antibody-positive Sjogren's syndrome and anti-Ro (SS-A) antibody-positive lupus erythematosus. Arch Dermatol 1988 Jan;124(1):63–71.

P314. Provost TT, Tomasi TB Jr. Evidence for complement activation via the alternative pathway in skin diseases, herpes gestationis, systemic lupus erythematosus, and bullous pemphigoid. J Clin Invest 1973 Jul;52:1779–1787.

P315. Provost TT, Watson R, Gammon WR, Radowsky M, Harley JB, Reichlin M. The neonatal lupus syndrome associated with U1RNP (nRNP) antibodies. N Engl J Med 1987;315: 1135–1139.

P316. Provost TT, Watson R, Gammon WR, Radowsky M, Harley JB, Reichlin M, Yamagata H, Arnett FC. Anti-Ro/SSA and anti-La/SSB in Sjogren's syndrome. Arthritis Rheum 1986;29: 196–206.

P317. Provost TT, Zone JJ, Synkowski DR, Maddison PJ, Reichlin M. Unusual cutaneous manifestations of SLE: Urticaria-like lesions; correlation with clinical and serologic abnormalities. J Invest Dermatol 1980;75:495–499.

P318. Prud'homme GJ, Balderas RS, Dixon FJ, Theofilopoulos AN. B cell dependence on and response to accessory signals in murine lupus strains. J Exp Med 1983;157:1815–1827.

P319. Prud'homme GJ, Park CL, Fieser TM, Kofler R, Dixon FJ, Theofilopoulos AN. Identification of a B cell differentiation factor (s) spontaneously produced by proliferating T cells in murine lupus strains of the lpr/lpr genotype. J Exp Med 1983; 157:730–742.

P320. Pruitt RE, Tumminello VV, Reveille JD. Pneumatosis cystoides intestinalis and benign peritoneum in a patient with antinuclear antibody negative systemic lupus erythematosus. J Rheumatol 1988;15:1575–1577.

P321. Prupas HM, Patzakis M, Quismorio FP Jr. Total hip arthroplasty for avascular necrosis of the femur in systemic lupus erythematosus. Clin Ortho 1981 Nov–Dec;(161): 186–190.

P322. Pruzanski W, Sarraf D, Klein M, Lau KY, Richardson JE. Lymphocytotoxins in vasculitis. Correlation with clinical manifestations and laboratory variables. J Rheumatol 1986;13: 1066–1071.

P323. Prystowsky SD. Mixed connective tissue disease. West J Med 1980 Apr;132(4):288–293.

P324. Prystowsky SD, Gilliam JN. Discoid lupus erythematosus as part of a larger disease spectrum. Arch Dermatol 1975;111: 1448–1452.

P325. Prystowsky SD, Gilliam JN, Tuffanelli DL. Epidermal nucleolar IgG deposition in clinically normal skin: clinical and serologic features of eight patients. Arch Dermatol 1978 Apr; 114(8):536–538.

P326. Prystowsky SD, Herdon JH Jr, Gilliam JN. Chronic cutaneous lupus erythematosus (DLE)—a clinical and laboratory investigation of 80 patients. Medicine 1976 Mar;55(2): 183–191.

P327. Prystowsky SD, Tuffanelli DL. Speckled (particulate) epidermal nuclear IgG deposition in normal skin: Correlation of clinical features and laboratory findings in 46 patients with a subset of connective tissue disease characterized by antibody to extractable nuclear antigen. Arch Dermatol 1978 May; 114(5):705–710.

P328. Puccetti A, Migliorini P, Sabbaga J, Madaio MP. Human and murine anti-DNA antibodies induce the production of anti-idiotypic antibodies with autoantigen-binding properties (epibodies) through immune-network interactions. J Immunol 1990;145:4229–4237.

P329. Pugh S, Pelton B, Raferty EB, Denman AM. Abnormal lymphocyte function is secondary to drug-induced autoimmunity. Ann Rheum Dis 1976;35:344–348.

P330. Pulido R, Cebrian M, Acevedo A, De Landazuri MO, Sanchez-Madrid F. Comparative biochemical and tissue distribution study of four distinct CD45 antigen specificities. J Immunol 1988;140:3851–3857.

P331. Pulido R, Sanchez-Madrid F. Biochemical nature and topographic localization of epitopes defining four distinct CD45 antigen specificities conventional CD45, CD45R, 180KDa (UCHL1) and 220/205/190 kDa. J Immunol 1989;143(6): 1930–1936.

P332. Pulido R, Sanchez-Madrid F. Glycosylation of CD45: Carbohydrate composition and its role in acquisition of CD45R0 and CD45RB T cell maturation-relation antigen specificities during biosynthesis. Eur J Immunol 1990;20:2667–2671.

P333. Pullen AM, Marrack P, Kappler JW. The T-cell repertoire is heavily influenced by tolerance to polymorphic self-antigens. Nature 1988;335:796–801.

P334. Pung OJ, Tucker AN, Vore SH, Luster MI. Influence of estrogen on host resistance: Increased susceptibility of mice to Listeria monocytogenes correlates with depressed production of interleukin-2. Infect Immunol 1985;50:91–96.

P335. Puram V, Giuliani D, Morse BS. Circulating immune complexes and platelet IgG in various diseases. Clin Exp Immunol 1984 Dec;58:672–676.

P336. Purnell DC, Baggestoss AH, Olsen AM. Pulmonary lesions in disseminated lupus erythematosus. Ann Intern Med 1955 Mar;42:619–628.

Q

Q1. Qamar T, Levy RA, Sammaritano L, Gharavi AE, Lockshin MD. Characteristics of high-titer IgG antiphospholipid antibody in systemic lupus erythematosus patients with and without fetal death. Arthritis Rheum 1990;33:501–504.

Q2. Qi-Ling W, Jia-ning Y, Zhong-rong H. A case of fulminant systemic lupus erythematosus complicated by severe aspergillar septicemia confirmed by pathologic findings. Chinese Med J 1986;99:93–497.

Q3. Qiu WQ, de Bruin D, Brownstein BH, Pearse R, Ravetch JV.

Organization of the human and mouse low affinity Fc R genes: Evidence for duplication and recombination. Science 1990; 248:732–735.

Q4. Quatraro A, Consoli G, Magno M, Caretta F, Nardozza A, Ceriello A, Giugliano D. Hydroxychloroquine in decompensated, treatment-refractory noninsulin-dependent diabetes mellitus. A new job for an old drug? Ann Intern Med 1990 May 1;112(9):678–681.

Q5. Query CC, Bently RC, Keene JD. A common RNA recognition motif identified within a defined U1 RNA binding domain of the 70K U1 snRNP protein. Cell 1989;57:89–101.

Q6. Query CC, Bently RC, Keene JD. A specific 31-nucleotide domain of U1 RNA directly interacts with the 70K small nuclear ribonucleoprotein component. Mol Cell Biol 1989;9: 4872–4881.

Q7. Query CC, Keene JD. A human autoimmune protein associated with U1 RNA contains a region of homology that is cross reactive with retroviral p30 gag antigen. Cell 1987;51: 211–220.

Q7a. Quimby SR, Perry HO. Livedo reticularis and cerebrovascular accidents. J Am Acad Dermatol 1980;3:377–383.

Q8. Quin JW, Charlesworth JA, Lee CH, Macdonald GJ. Studies of lymphocytotoxins in infectious mononucleosis: reduced lymphocyte killing in the acute phase. Clin Exp Immunol 1980;39:588–592.

Q8a. Quinn JP, Weinstein RA. Eosinophilic meningitis and ibuprofen therapy. Neurology 1984;34:108–109.

Q9. Quismorio FP, Friou GJ. Serological factors in SLE and their pathogenetic significance. CRC Crit Rev Clin Lab Sci 1970;1: 639–715.

Q10. Quismorio FP, Stimmler MM. Serum antibodies to ribosome P protein in systemic lupus erythematosus (SLE) [abstract]. Arthritis Rheum 1990 Sep;33(9) Suppl:S12.

Q11. Quismorio FP, Tay A. Axillary vein thrombosis after nitrogen mustard therapy for SLE [letter]. J Rheumatol 1988 Nov; 15(11):1732–1733.

Q12. Quismorio FP Jr. Immune complexes in the pericardial fluid in systemic lupus erythematosus. Arch Intern Med 1980 Jan;140:112–114.

Q13. Quismorio FP Jr. Clinical and pathologic features of lung involvement in systemic lupus erythematosus. Semin Resp Dis 1988;9:297–304.

Q14. Quismorio FP Jr, Bjarnason DF, Dubois EL, Friou GJ. Chlorpromazine-induced antinuclear antibodies [abstract]. Arthritis Rheum 1972 Jul–Aug;15:451.

Q15. Quismorio FP Jr, Bjarnason DF, Kiely WF, Dubois EL, Friou GJ. Antinuclear antibodies in chronic psychotic patients treated with chlorpromazine [brief communication]. Am J Psychiatry 1975 Nov;132:1204–1206.

Q16. Quismorio FP Jr, Dubois EL. Septic arthritis in systemic lupus erythematosus. J Rheumatol 1975 Mar;2(1):73–82.

Q17. Quismorio FP Jr, Friou GJ. Antibodies reactive with neurons in SLE in patients with neuropsychiatric manifestations. Int Arch Allergy Appl Immunol 1972;43(5):740–748.

Q18. Quismorio FP Jr, Friou GJ. Serological factors in systemic lupus erythematosus and their pathogenetic significance. CRC Crit Rev Clin Lab Sci 1979 Dec;1:639–684.

Q19. Quismorio FP Jr, Johnson C. Serum autoantibodies in patients with sickle cell anemia. Am J Med Sci 1984;287:13–15.

Q20. Quismorio FP Jr, Kaufman RL, Hoefs JC. Immune complexes and cryoproteins in ascitic fluid of patient with alcoholic liver disease. Int Arch Allergy Appl Immunol 1981;64: 190–194.

Q21. Quismorio FP Jr, Sharma O, Koss M, Boylen T, Edmiston AW, Thornton PJ, Tatter D. Immunopathologic and clinical studies in pulmonary hypertension associated with systemic lupus erythematosus. Semin Arthritis Rheum 1984 May;13(4): 349–359.

R

R1. Rabhan NB. Pituitary-adrenal suppression and Cushing's syndrome after intermittent dexamethasone therapy. Ann Intern Med 1956 Dec;69:1141–1148.

R2. Rabinovich CE, Schanberg LE, Kredich DW. Intravenous immunoglobulin and bromocriptine in the treatment of refractory neuropsychiatric systemic lupus erythematosus. Arthritis Rheum 1990 May;33(5) Suppl:R22.

R3. Rabinovitch M, Manejias RE, Nussenzweig V. Selective phagocytic paralysis induced by immobilized immune complexes. J Exp Med 1975;142:827–838.

R4. Rabinowitz Y, Dameshek W. Systemic lupus erythematosus after "idiopathic: thrombocytopenic purpura: a review. A study of systemic lupus erythematosus occurring after 78 splenectomies for "idiopathic" thrombocytopenic purpura. Ann Intern Med 1960;52:28.

R5. Rabson A, Blank S, Lomnitzer R. Effect of levamisole on in vitro suppressor cell function in normal humans and patients with systemic lupus erythematosus. Immunopharmacology 1980 Apr;2(2):103–108.

R6. Radcliffe R, Nemerson Y. Activation and control of factor VII by activated factor X and thrombin. Isolation and characterization of a single chain form of factor VII. J Biol Chem 1975 Jan; 250(2):388.

R7. Rader MD, O'Brien CO, Harley JB, Liu Y, Reichlin M. Heterogeneity of the Ro/SSA antigen: different molecular forms in lymphocytes and red blood cells [abstract]. Arthritis Rheum 1987;30:S55.

R8. Rafferty P, Young AC, Haeney MR. Sulphasalazine-induced cerebral lupus erythematosus. Postgrad Med J 1982 Feb;58: 98–99.

R9. Raghoebar M, Peeters PA, van den Berg WB, van Ginneken CA. Mechanisms of cell association of chloroquine to leucocytes. J Pharmacol Exp Ther 1986 Jul;238(1):302- 306.

R10. Ragsdale CG, Petty RE, Cassidy JT, Sullivan DB. The clinical progression of apparent juvenile rheumatoid arthritis to systemic lupus erythematosus. J Rheumatol 1980 Jan–Feb;7(1): 50–55.

R11. Raij L, Sibley RK, Keane WF. Mononuclear phagocyte stimulation. Protective role from glomerular immune complex deposition. J Lab Clin Med 1981;98:558–567.

R12. Raijman I, Schrager M. Hemorrhagic acalculous cholecystitis in systemic lupus erythematosus [letter]. Am J Gastroenterol 1989 Apr;84(4):445–447.

R13. Raines MF, Bhargava SK, Rosen ES. The blood-retinal barrier in chloroquine retinopathy. Invest Opthalmol Vis Sci 1989 Aug;30(8):1726–1731.

R14. Rainsford KD. Effects of antimalarial drugs on interleukin-1-induced cartilage proteoglycan degradation in-vitro. J Pharm Pharmacol 1986 Nov;38(11):829–833.

R15. Raizman MB, Baum J. Discoid lupus keratitis. Arch Ophthalmol 1989 Apr;107(4):545–547.

R16. Rajagopalan N, Humphrey PR, Bucknall RC. Torticollis and blepharospasm in systemic lupus erythematosus. Move Disord 1989;4(4):345–348.

R17. Rajagopalan S, Zordan T, Tsokos GC, Datta SK. Pathogenic anti-DNA autoantibody-inducing T helper cell lines from patients with active lupus nephritis. Isolation of CD4–8–T helper cell lines that express the gamma delta T-cell antigen receptor. Proc Natl Acad Sci USA 1990;87:7020–7024.

R18. Rajani KB, Ashbacher LV, Kinney TR. Pulmonary hemorrhage and systemic lupus erythematosus. J Pediat 1978 Nov; 93:810–812.

R19. Rajewsky K, Takemori T. Genetics, expression and function of idiotypes. Ann Rev Immunol 1983;1:569–603.

R20. Rakov HL, Taylor JS. Acute disseminated lupus erythematosus without cutaneous manifestations and with heretofore undescribed pulmonary lesions. Arch Intern Med 1974 Jul;70:88–100.

R21. Rallison ML, Carlisle JW, Lee RE Jr, Vernier RL, Good RA. Lupus erythematosus and Steven's Johnson syndrome. Occurrence as reactions to anticonvulsant therapy. Am J Dis Child 1961 Jun;101:725–738.

R22. Raman SB, Abraham JP, Saeed SM, Sawdyk M. Azathioprine-induced reversible severe dyserythropoiesis as a cause of anemia. Henry Ford Hosp Med J 1986;34(3):202–206.

R23. Ramirez F, Williams RC, Sibbitt WL, Searles RP. Immunoglobulin from systemic lupus erythematosus serum induces interferon release by normal mononuclear cells. Arthritis Rheum 1986;29:326–336.

R24. Ramirez G, Khamashta MA, Hughes GRV. The ANCA test: its clinical relevance. Ann Rheum Dis 1990;49:741–744.

R25. Ramirez RE, Glasier C, Kirks D, Shackelford GD, Locey M. Pulmonary hemorrhage associated with systemic lupus erythematosus in children. Radiology 1984;152:409–412.

R26. Ramirez-Mata M, Reyes PA, Alarcon-Segovia D, Garva R. Esophageal motility in systemic lupus erythematosus. Am J Dig Dis 1974 Feb;19(2):132–136.

R27. Ramkissoon RA. Thrombotic thrombocytopenic purpura and systemic lupus erythematosus. CA Med 1966 Mar;104:212-214.

R28. Ramos-Niembro F, Alarcon-Segovia D. Familial aspects of mixed connective tissue disease (MCTD). I. Occurrence of systemic lupus erythematosus in another family member in two families and aggregation of MCTD in another family. J Rheumatol 1978 Winter;5(4):433–440.

R29. Ramos-Niembro F, Alarcon-Segovia D. Development of sicca symptoms in systemic lupus erythematosus with existing subclinical abnormalities of lacrimal and/or salivary glands. Arthritis Rheum 1979 Aug;22(8):935-936.

R30. Ramos-Niembro F, Alarcon-Segovia D, Hernandez-Ortiz J. Articular manifestations of mixed connective tissue disease. Arthritis Rheum 1979 Jan;22(1):43–51.

R31. Ramot B, Singer K. An unusual circulating anticoagulant in systemic lupus erythematosus. Acta Haemat (Basel) 1956 Aug;16:158.

R32. Ramsey-Goldman R. Pregnancy in systemic lupus erythematosus. Rheum Dis Clin N A 1988;14:169.

R33. Ramsey-Goldman R, Franz T, Solano FX, Medsger TA Jr. Hydralazine induced lupus and Sweet's syndrome. Report and review of the literature. J Rheumatol 1990;17:682–684.

R34. Ramsey-Goldman R, Hom D, Deng J-S, Ziegler GC, Kahl LE, Steen VD, LaPorte RE, Medsger TA. Anti-SS-A antibodies and fetal outcome in maternal systemic lupus erythematosus. Arthritis Rheum 1986;29:1269–1273.

R35. Ramsey-Goldman R, Mientus JM, Medsger TA. Toxicity of nonsteroidal anti-inflammatory drugs (NSAIDS) in patients with systemic lupus erythematosus (SLE) I. Patient reported side effects. [abstract]. Arthritis Rheum 1989 Apr;32(4) Suppl:S75.

R36. Ramsey-Goldman R, Mientus JM, Medsger TA. Pregnancy outcome in women with systemic lupus erythematosus (SLE) treated with immunosuppressive drugs [abstract]. Arthritis Rheum 1990;33 Suppl:S28.

R37. Randall T. Thalidomide's back in the news, but in more favorable circumstances [news]. JAMA 1990 Mar 16;263(11):1467–1468.

R38. Randen I, Thompson K, Forre O, Natviq JB. Evidence for in vivo affinity maturation of a somatically mutated human autoantibody. FASEB J 1991;50:1087.

R39. Randle HW, Millns JL, Schroeter AL, Winkelmann RK. Cutaneous immunofluorescence in primary biliary cirrhosis. JAMA 1981 Oct 9;246(15):1679–1681.

R40. Ranelletti FP, Carmigani M, Marchetti P, Natoli C, Jacobelli S. Estrogen binding by neoplastic human thymus cytosols. Eur J Cancer 1980;16:951–955.

R41. Rao BK, Coldiron BM, Freeman RF, Sontheimer RD. Subacute cutaneous lupus erythematosus lesions progressing to morphea. J Am Acad Dermatol 1990;23:1019–1022.

R42. Rao RH, Vagnucci AH, Amico JA. Bilateral massive adrenal haemorrhage: early recognition and treatment. Ann Intern Med 1989 Feb 1;110(3):227–235.

R43. Rapaport SI, Ames SB, Duvall BJ. A plasma coagulation defect in systemic lupus erythematosus arising form hypothrombinemia combined with antiprothrombinase activity. Blood 1960 Feb;15:212–227.

R44. Rapp F. Localization of antinuclear factors from lupus erythematosus sera in tissue culture. J Immunol 1962;88:732–740.

R45. Rappaport EF, Cassel DL, McKenzie SE, Meister RP, Surrey S, Schreiber AD, Schwartz E. An FcγRII-A transcript encoding a soluble receptor can arise by alternative splicing of the transmembrane exon. Blood 1992 In press.

R46. Rappaport RS, Dodge GR. Prostaglandin E inhibits the production of human interleukin 2. J Exp Med 1982;155:943–948.

R47. Rappersberger K, Tschachler E, Tani M, Wolff K. Bullous disease in systemic lupus erythematosus. J Am Acad Dermatol 1989 Oct;21(4 Pt 1):745–752.

R48. Raptis L, Menard HA. Quantitation and characterization of plasma DNA in normals and patients with systemic lupus erythematosus. J Clin Invest 1980;66:1391–1399.

R49. Rasheed FN, Locniskar M, McCloskey DJ, Hasan RS, Chiang TJ, Rose P, de Soldenhoff R, Festenstein H, McAdam PWJ. Serum lymphocytotoxic activity in leprosy. Clin Exp Immunol 1989;76:391–397.

R50. Rasheed KA, Whisenant EC, Ghai RD, Papaioannou VE, Bhatnagar YM. Biochemical and immunocytochemical analysis of a histone H1 variant from the mouse testis. J Cell Sci 1989;94:61–71.

R51. Rasmussen EK, Ullman S, Hoier-Madsen M, Sorensen SF, Halberg P. Clinical implications of ribonucleoprotein antibody. Arch Dermatol 1987 May;123(5):601–605.

R52. Rasmussen S, Petersen J, Nielsen IL, Christensen P, Hilden T. Effect of acetylsalicylic acid on renal function in systemic lupus erythematosus. Eur J Clin Pharmacol 1982;23(6):505–508.

R53. Rasponi L. Antibiotics in pemphigus vulgaris and in acute lupus erythematosus. Postgrad Med J 1982;58:98-99.

R54. Ratain JS, Petri M, Hochberg MC, Hellmann DB. Accuracy of creatinine clearance in measuring glomerular filtration rate in patients with systemic lupus erythematosus without clinical evidence of renal disease. Arthritis Rheum 1990;33:277–280.

R55. Ratliff NB, Estes ML, Myles JL, Shirey EK, Mc Mahon JT. Diagnosis of chloroquine cardiomyopathy by endomyocardial biopsy. N Engl J Med 1987;316:191–193.

R56. Ratner D, Skouge J. Discoid lupus erythematosus scarring and dermabrasion. A case report of discussion. J Am Acad Dermatol 1990;22:314–316.

R57. Rauch J, Massicotte H, Tannenbaum H. Specific and shared idiotypes found on hybridoma anti-DNA autoantibodies derived from rheumatoid arthritis and systemic lupus erythematosus patients. J Immunol 1985;135:2385–2392.

R58. Rauch J, Meng QH, Tannenbaum H. Interaction of human hybridoma lupus anticoagulant and antiphospholipid antibodies with platelets [abstract]. Clin Exp Rheumatol 1988;6:211.

R59. Rauch J, Murphy E, Roths JB, Stollar BD, Schwartz RS. A high frequency idiotype marker of anti-DNA autoantibodies in MRL-lpr/lpr mice. J Immunol 1982 Jul;129(1):236–241.

R60. Rauch J, Tannenbaum H, Stollar BD, Schwartz RS. Monoclonal anti-cardiolipin antibodies bind to DNA Eur J Immunol 1984;14:529–539.

R61. Rauch J, Tannenbaum H, Straaton K, Massicotte H, Wild J. Human-human hybridoma autoantibodies with both anti-DNA and rheumatoid factor activities. J Clin Invest 1986 Jan;77(1): 106–112.

R62. Raud J, Dahlen SE, Sydbom A, Lindbom L, Hedqvist P. Enhancement of acute allergic inflammation by indomethacin is reversed by prostaglandin E2: apparent correlation with in vivo modulation of mediator release. Proc Natl Acad Sci USA 1990;85:2315–2319.

R63. Rauh AJ, Hornig H, Luhrmann R. At least three distinct B cell epitopes reside in the C-terminal half of La protein, as determined by a recombinant DNA approach. Eur J Immunol 1988;18:2049–2057.

R64. Raulet DH. Antigens for γδT Cells. Nature 1989;339: 342–343.

R65. Raum D, Donaldson VH, Rosen FS, Alper CA. Genetics of complement. Current topics in hematology. Hematology 1980;3:111–174.

R66. Raveche ES, Chused TM, Steinberg AD, Laskin CA, Edison LJ, Tjio JH. Comparison of response to stem cell differentiation signals between normal and autoimmune mouse strains. J Immunol 1985;134:865–873.

R67. Raveche ES, Lalor P, Stall A, Conroy J. In vivo effects of hyperdiploid Ly-1+ B cells of NZB origin. J Immunol 1988 Dec 15;141(12):4133–4139.

R68. Raveche ES, Novotny EA, Hansen CT, Tijo JH, Steinberg AD. Genetic studies of NZB mice V. Recombinant inbred lines demonstrate that separate genes control autoimmune phenotype. J Exp Med 1981 May 1;153(5):1187–1197.

R69. Raveche ES, Tijo JH, Boegel W, Steinberg AD. Studies on the effects of sex hormones on autosomal and X-linked genetic control of induced and spontaneous antibody production. Arthritis Rheum 1979;22:1177–1187.

R70. Raveche ES, Tijo JH, Steinberg AD. Genetic studies in NZB mice: IV. The effect of sex hormones on spontaneous anti-T cell antibodies. Arthritis Rheum 1980;23:48–56.

R71. Ravelli A, Caporali C, Bianchi E, Viola S, Solmi M, Montecucco C, Martini A. Anticardiolipin syndrome in childhood: a report of two cases. Clin Exp Rheumatol 1990;8: 95–98.

R72. Ravetch JV, Anderson CL. FcγR Family: Proteins, Transcripts, and Genes. In: Metzer H, editor. Fc receptors and the action of antibodies. Washington DC: Am Soc Microbiol, 1990: 211–235.

R73. Ravetch JV, Kinet JP. Fc receptors. Ann Rev Immunol 1991; 9:457–492.

R74. Ravetch JV, Perussia B. Alternative membrane forms of FcγRIII (CD16) on human NK cells and neutrophils: Cell-type specific expression of two genes which differ in single nucleotide substitutions. J Exp Med 1989;170:481-497.

R75. Rawsthorne L, Ptacin M, Choi P, Olinger G, Bamrah V. Lupus valvulitis necessitating double valve replacement. Arthritis Rheum 1981 Mar;24:561–564.

R76. Ray P, Berman JD. Prevention of muscarinic acetylcholine receptor-down regulation by chloroquine: antilysosomal or antimuscarinic mechanisms. Neurochem Res 1989 Jun;14(6): 533–535.

R77. Raychaudhuri S, Kohler H, Saeki Y, Chen JJ. Potential role of anti-idiotype antibodies in active tumor immunotherapy. Crit Rev Oncol/Hematol 1989;9:109.

R78. Rayer PF. Theoretical and practical treatise on skin diseases; based upon new research in anatomy and pathology [original in French]. Paris, Vailliere, 1826:(1).

R79. Raz A. Mepacrine blockade of arachidonate-induced washed platelet aggregation: relationship to mecaprine inhibition of platelet cyclooxygenase. Thromb Haemost 1983 Dec; 50(4):784–786.

R80. See R81a.

R81. Raz A, Wyche A, Siegel N, Needleman P. Regulation of fibroblast cyclooxygenase synthesis by interleukin-1. J Biol Chem 1988;263:3022–3028.

R81a. Raz E, Brezis M, Rosenmann E, Eilat D. Anti-DNA antibodies bind directly to renal antigens and induce kidney dysfunction in the isolated perfused rat kidney. J Immunol 1989 May; 142(9):3076–3082.

R82. Razis DV, Diamond HD, Craver LF. Hodgkin's disease associated with other malignant tumors and certain neo- neoplastic diseases. Am J Med Sci 1959 Sep;128:327–335.

R83. Raziuddin S, Nur MA, Al Wabel AA. Increased circulating HLA-DR+ CD4+ T cells in systemic lupus erythematosus: alterations associated with prednisolone therapy. Scand J Immunol 1990;31:139–145.

R84. Raziuddin S, Nur MA, Al Wabel AA. Selective loss of the CD4+ inducers of suppressor T cell subsets (2H4+) in active systemic lupus erythematosus. J Rheumatol 1991;16: 1315–1319.

R85. Read NG, Trist DG. Mepacrine uptake by granulocytes [proceedings]. Br J Pharmacol 1978 Jun;63 Suppl 2:410P.

R86. Read NG, Trist DG. The uptake of mepacrine horse polymorphonuclear leucocytes in vitro. J Pharm Pharmacol 1982 Nov;34(11):711–714.

R87. Read WK, Bay WW. Basic cellular lesion in chloroquine toxicity. Lab Invest 1971;24:246–259.

R88. Reagan KJ, Wunner WH, Wiktor TJ, Koprowski H. Anti-idiotypic antibodies induce neutralizing antibodies to rabies virus glycoprotein. J Virol 1984;48:660.

R89. Rebhun J, Quismorio FP Jr, Dubois EL, Helner DC. Systemic lupus erythematosus activity and IgE. Ann Allergy 1983 Jan; 50:34–36.

R90. Reckart MD, Eisendrath SJ. Exogenous corticosteriod effects on mood and cognition: case presentations. Int J Psychosom 1990;37(1–4):58–61.

R91. Reda MG, Baigelman W. Pleural effusion in systemic lupus erythematosus. Acta Cytologica 1980 Nov– Dec;24:553–557.

R92. Reddy R, Busch H. Small nuclear RNAs: RNA sequences, structure, and modifications. In: Birnstiel ML, editor. Structure and function of major and minor small nuclear ribonuclear ribonucleoprotein particles. Heidelberg FRG: Springer-Verlag, 1988:1–37.

R93. Reddy R, Henning D, Busch H. Primary and secondary structure of U8 small nuclear RNA. J Biol Chem 1985;260: 10930–10935.

R94. Redisch W, Messina GH, McEwen C. Capillaroscopic observations in rheumatic diseases. Ann Rheum Dis 1970;29: 244–253.

R95. Reece EA, Gabrielli S, Cullen MT, Zheng XZ, Hobbins JC, Harris N. Recurrent adverse pregnancy outcome and antiphospholipid antibodies. Am J Obstet Gynecol 1990;163:162–169.

R96. Reed BR, Huff JC, Jones SK, Orton DW, Lee LA, Norris DA. Subacute cutaneous lupus erythematosus associated with hydrochlorothiazide therapy. Ann Intern Med 1985;103: 49–51.

R97. Reed BR, Lee LA, Harmon C, Wolfe R, Wiggins J, Peebles C, Weston WL. Autoantibodies to SS-A/Ro in infants with congenital heart block. J Pediatr 1983;103:889–891.

R98. Reed WB, May SB, Tuffanelli DL. Discoid lupus erythematosus in a newborn. Arch Dermatol 1967;96:64.

R99. Rees EG, Wilkinson M. Serum proteins in systemic lupus erythematosus. BMJ 1959 Oct 24;5155:795−798.

R100. Rees L, Chantler C. Growth and endocrine function in children receiving long-term steroid therapy for renal disease. Acta Paediat Scand 1990;366 Suppl:93−96.

R101. Reeves JA. Keratopathy associated with systemic lupus erythematosus. Arch Ophthalmol 1965 Aug;74:159−160.

R102. Reeves WH. Use of monoclonal antibodies for the characterization of novel DNA-binding proteins recognized by human autoimmune sera. J Exp Med 1985;161:18−39.

R103. Reeves WH, Chaadbury N, Salerno A, Blobel G. Lamin B autoantibodies in sera of certain patients with systemic lupus erythematosus. J Exp Med 1987;165:750−762.

R104. Reeves WH, Chiorazzi N. Interaction between anti-DNA and anti-DNA binding protein autoantibodies in cryoglobulins from sera of patients with systemic lupus erythematosus. J Exp Med 1986;164:1029−1042.

R105. Reeves WH, Fisher DE, Lahita RG, Kunkel HG. Autoimmune sera reactive with Sm antigen contain high levels of RNP-like antibodies. J Clin Invest 1985;75:580−587.

R106. Reeves WH, Fisher DE, Wisniewolski R, Gottlieb AB, Chiorazzi N. Psoriasis and Raynaud's phenomenon associated with autoantibodies to U1 and U2 small nuclear ribonucleoproteins. N Engl J Med 1986;315:105- 111.

R107. Reeves WH, Pierani A, Chou CH, Ng T, Nicastri C, Roeder RG, Sthoeger ZM. Epitopes of the p70 and p80 (Ku) lupus autoantigens. J Immunol 1991;146:2678−2686.

R108. Reeves WH, Sthoeger Z, Lahita R. Role of antigen selectivity in autoimmune responses to the Ku (p70/p80) antigen. J Clin Invest 1989;84:562−567.

R109. Regan M, Lackner H, Karpatkin S. Platelet function and coagulation profile in lupus erythematosus; studies in 50 patients. Ann Intern Med 1974;Oct;81:462−468.

R110. Regeste RT, Painter P. False-positive radioimmunoassay pregnancy test in nephrotic syndrome. JAMA 1981;246:1237−1238.

R111. Reiches AJ. The lupus erythematosus syndrome: the relationship of discoid (cutaneous) lupus erythematosus to systemic (disseminated) lupus erythematosus. Ann Intern Med 1957 Apr;46(4):678−684.

R112. Reichlin M. Progressive systemic sclerosis. In: Bigazi PE, Reichlin M, editors. Systemic autoimmunity. Marcell Decker, In Press.

R113. Reichlin M. Diagnostic criteria and serology. In: The Clinical Management of Systemic Lupus Erythematosus. Schur PH, editor. New York: Grune & Stratton 1983.

R114. Reichlin M. Antinuclear antibodies. In: Kelley W, Harris E, Ruddy S, Sledge C, editors. Textbook of Rheumatology, 3rd ed. Philadelphia: Saunders, 1989:208- 225.

R115. Reichlin M, Arnett FC. Multiplicity of antibodies in myositis. Arthritis Rheum 1984;27:1150−1156.

R116. Reichlin M, Friday K, Harley JB. Complete congenital heart block followed by the development of antibodies to Ro/SSA in adult life: Serological clinical and HLA studies in an informative family. Am J Med 1988;84:339- 344.

R117. Reichlin M, Haas GG Jr. Association of antisperm antibodies with lupus erythematosus [abstract]. Arthritis Rheum 1985 Apr;28(4) Suppl:S67.

R118. Reichlin M, Harley JB. Antibodies to Ro(SSA) and the heterogeneity of systemic lupus erythematosus. J Rheumatol 1987;14:112.

R119. Reichlin M, Mattioli M. Correlation of a precipitating reaction to an RNA protein antigen and a low prevalence of nephritis in patients with systemic lupus erythematosus. N Engl J Med 1972;286:908−911.

R120. Reichlin M, Mattioli M. Description of a serologic reaction characteristic of polymyositis. Clin Immunol Immunopathol 1976 Jan;5:12−20.

R121. Reichlin M, Rader M, Harley JB. Autoimmune responses to Ro/SSA is directed to the human antigen. Clin Exp Immunol 1989;76:373−377.

R122. Reichlin M, Reichlin MW. Autoantibodies to the ro/SSA particle react preferentially with the human antigen. J Autoimmun 1989;2:359−361.

R123. Reichlin M, van Venrooij WJ. Autoantibodies to the URNP particles: relationship to clinical diagnosis and nephritis. Clin Exp Immunol 1991;83:286−290.

R124. Reid JM, Coleman EN, Doig W. Complete congenital heart block. Report of 35 cases. Br Heart J 1982;48:236.

R125. Reidenberg MM. The chemical induction of systemic lupus erythematosus and lupus-like illnesses. Arthritis Rheum 1981;24:1004−1008.

R126. Reidenberg MM. Aromatic amines and the pathogenesis of lupus erythematosus. Am J Med 1983 Dec;75:1037−1042.

R127. Reidenberg MM, Case DB, Drayer DE, Reis S, Lorenzo B. Development of antinuclear antibody in patients treated with high doses of captopril. Arthritis Rheum 1984 May;27:579−581.

R128. Reidenberg MM, Durant PJ, Harris RA, De Boccardo G, Lahita R, Stenzel KH. Lupus erythematosus-like disease due to hydrazine. Am J Med 1983 Aug;75(2):365−370.

R129. Reidenberg MM, Levy M, Drayer DE. Acetylator phenotype in idiopathic systemic lupus erythematosus. Arthritis Rheum 1980;23:569−573.

R130. Reifenstein EC, Reifenstein EC Jr, Reifenstein GH. Variable symptom complex of undetermined etiology with fata termination, including conditions described as visceral erythema group (Osler), disseminated lupus erythematosus atypical verrucous endocarditis (Libman- Sacks), fever of unknown origin Christian) and diffuse peripheral vascular disease (Baehr and others). Arch Intern Med 1939 Mar;63:553−574.

R131. Reilly PA, Evison G, McHugh NJ, Maddison PJ. Arthropathy of hands and feet in systemic lupus erythematosus. J Rheumatol 1990;17:777−784.

R132. Reilly PA, Maddison PJ. Painful, swollen calf in a patient with SLE [letter]. Br J Rheumatol 1987 Aug;26(4):319−320.

R133. Reimer G, Steen VD, Penny CA, Medsger TA Jr, Tan EM. Correlates between autoantibodies to nucleolar antigens and clinical features in patients with systemic sclerosis (scleroderma). Arthritis Rheum 1988;31:525- 532.

R134. Rein CR, Fleischmajer R. The treatment of lupus erythematosus and infiltration of the skin with A.P.A. 5533. Br J Dermatol 1957 May;69(5):174−177.

R135. Rein CR, Kostant GH. Lupus erythematosus: serologic and chemical aspects. Arch Dermat & Syph 1950 Jun;61:898−903.

R136. Reinertsen JL, Kaslow RA, Klippel JH, Hurvitz AI, Lewis RM, Rothfield NF, Zvaifler NJ, Steinberg AD, Decker JL. An epidemiologic study of households exposed to canine systemic lupus erythematosus. Arthritis Rheum 1980;23:564−568.

R137. Reinertsen JL, Klippel JH, Johnson AH, Steinberg AD, Decker JL, Mann DL. B-lymphocyte alloantigens associated with systemic lupus erythematosus. N Engl J Med 1978;299−515.

R138. Reinertsen JL, Klippel JH, Johnson AH, Steinberg AD, Decker JL, Mann DL. Family studies of B lymphocyte alloantigens in systemic lupus erythematosus. J Rheumatol 1982;9:253−262.

R139. Reinhard J, Bennett R. Chloroquine inhibition of anti-DNA binding [abstract]. Clin Res 1980;28;77A.

R140. Reinhart A. Experiences with Wassermann-Neisser-Bruck's syphilis reaction [original in German]. Munchen Med Wschr 1990 Oct 12;56:2092−2097.

R141. Reinharz D, Tiercy JM, Mach B, Jeannet M. Absence of DRw15/3 and of DRw15/7 heterozygotes in Caucasian patients with systemic lupus erythematosus. Tissue Antigens 1991;37:10–15.

R142. Reinisch JM, Simon NG, Karow WG, Gandelman R. Prenatal exposure to prednisone in humans and animals retards intrauterine growth. Science 1978;202:436–438.

R143. Reinitz E, Barland P. Adverse reactions to dapsone. Lancet 1981 Jul;2:184–185.

R144. Reinitz E, Grayzel A, Barland P. Specificity of Sm antibody [letter]. Arthritis Rheum 1980;23:868.

R145. Reinitz E, Hubbard D, Grayzel AI. Central nervous system systemic lupus erythematosus versus central nervous infection: low cerebral spinal glucose and pleocytosis in a patient with a prolonged course. Arthritis Rheum 1982 May;25(5): 583–587.

R146. Reinitz E, Hubbard D, Zimmerman RD. Central nervous system disease in systemic lupus erythematosus: axial tomographic scan as an aid to differential diagnosis [letter]. J Rheumatol 1984 Apr;11(2):252–253.

R147. Reinter M, Cox J, Bernheim C, Vischer TL. Two cases of disseminated lupus erythematosus with terminal Moschowitz syndrome. Schweiz Med Wochenschr 1968 Oct 19;98: 1691–1692.

R148. Reisin LH, Reisin I, Darawshi A, Aviel E. Central retinal-artery occlusion in a patient with circulating lupus anticoagulant. Ann Ophthalmol 1989 Jul;21(7):269- 271.

R149. Reitan RM. Manual for administration of neuropsychological test batteries for adults and children. Indianapolis, privately printed, not dated.

R150. Rekant SI, Becker LE. Auto-immune annular erythema. A variant of lupus erythematosus? Arch Dermatol 1973 Mar;107: 424–426.

R151. Rekvig OP. Intrinsic cell membrane antigens recognized by antichromatin autoantibodies; The membrane antigens do not derive from the nucleus. Scand J Immunol 1989;29:7–13.

R152. Rekvig OP, Hannestad K. Certain polyclonal anti-nuclear antibodies cross-react with the surface membrane of human lymphocytes and granulocytes. Scand J Immunol 1977;6: 1041–1054.

R153. Rekvig OP, Hannestad K. The specificity of human autoantibodies that react with both cell nuclei and plasma membranes: the nuclear antigen is present on core mononucleosomes. J Immunol 1979;123:2673–2681.

R154. Rekvig OP, Hannestad K. Lupus erythematosus (LE) factors recognize both nucleosomes and viable human leukocytes. Scand J Immunol 1981;13:597–604.

R155. Rekvig OP, Muller S, Briand JP, Skogen B, Van Regenmortel MHV. Human antinuclear autoantibodies crossreacting with the plasma membrane and the N-Terminal region of histone H2B. Immunol Invest 1987;16:535–547.

R156. Rembecki RM, Kumar V, David CS, Bennett M. Polymorphism of Hh-1, the mouse hemopoietic histocompatibility locus. Immunogenetics 1988;28:158–170.

R157. Remington JS. The compromised host. Hosp Practice 1972;7:59–70.

R158. Remvig L, Thomsen BS, Baek L, Svenson M, Bendtzen K. Interleukin 1, but not interleukin 1 inhibitor, is released from human monocytes by immune complexes . Scand J Immunol 1990;32:255–261.

R159. Renauld JC, Vink A, Van Snick J. Accessory signals in murine cytolytic T cell responses. Dual requirement for IL-1 and IL-6. J Immunol 1989;143:1894–1898.

R160. Rendall JR, Wilkinson JD. Neonatal lupus erythematosus. Clin Exp Dermatol 1978;3:69.

R161. Rene RM, Pearson CM. The familial occurrence of systemic lupus erythematosus [abstract]. Arthritis Rheum 1960; 3:460.

R162. Repke JT, Kuhajda F, Hochberg MC, Johnson TRB, Winn K, Provost T. Fetal viral myocarditis and congenital complete heart block in a pregnancy complicated by systemic lupus erythematosus: a case report. J Reprod Med 1987;32: 217–220.

R163. Res PC, Bredveld FC, Van Embden JDA, De Vries RPR, Schaar CG, Van Eden W, Cohen IR. Synovial fluid T cell reactivity against 65 Kd heat shock protein of mycobacteria in early chronic infections. Lancet 1988;11:478–480.

R164. Reth M, Gehrmann P, Petrac E, Wiese P. A novel V_H to V_H DJ_H joining mechanism in heavy-chain-negative (null) pre-B cells results in heavy-chain production. Nature 1986;322: 840–842.

R165. Omitted.

R166. Reuter R, Luhrmann R. Immunization of mice with purified U1 small nuclear ribonucleoprotein (RNP) induces a pattern of antibody specificities characteristic of the anti-Sm and anti-RNP autoimmune response of patients with lupus erythematosus, as measured by monoclonal antibodies. Proc Natl Acad Sci USA 1986;83:8689–8693.

R167. Reuter R, Rothe S, Habets W, van Venrooij W, Luhrmann R. Autoantibody production against the U small nuclear ribonucleoprotein particle proteins E, F, and G in patients with connective tissue diseases. Eur J Immunol 1990;20:437–440.

R168. Reuter R, Tessaro G, Vohr HW, Gleichmann E, Luhrmann R. Mercuric chloride induces autoantibodies against U3 small nuclear ribonucleoprotein in susceptible mice. Proc Natl Acad Sci USA 1989;86:237–241.

R169. Reveille JD, Anderson KL, Schrohenloher RE, Acton RT, Barger BO. Restriction fragment length polymorphism analysis of HLA-DR, DQ, DP and C4 alleles in Caucasians with systemic lupus erythematosus. J Rheumatol 1991;18:14–18.

R170. Reveille JD, Arnett FC. The immunogenetics of Sjogren's syndrome. Rheum Dis Clin North Am. In press.

R171. Reveille JD, Arnett FC, Wilson RW, Bias WB, McLean RH. Null alleles of the fourth component of complement and HLA haplotypes in familial systemic lupus erythematosus. Immunogenetics 1985;21:299–311.

R172. Reveille JD, Bias WB, Winkelstein JA, Provost TT, Dorsch CA, Arnett FC. Familial systemic lupus erythematosus Immunogenetic studies in eight families. Medicine 1983;62:21–35.

R173. Reveille JD, Bartolucci A, Alarcon GS. Prognosis in systemic lupus erythematosus. Negative impact of increasing age at onset, Black race, and thrombocytopenia, as well as causes of death. Arthritis Rheum 1990;33:37–48.

R174. Reveille JD, MacLeod MJ, Whittington K, Arnett FC. Specific amino acid residues in the second hypervariable region of HLA-DQA1 and DQB1 chain genes promote the Ro (SS-A)/La (SS-B) autoantibody responses. J Immunol 1991;146: 3871–3876.

R175. Reveille JD, MacLeod MJ, Whittington K, Small D, Bias WB, Arnett FC. HLA-DR, DQ and DP genotypes in Mexican-Americans with systemic lupus erythematosus the importance of autoantibody subsets in HLA/disease associations [abstract]. Arthritis Rheum 1992 In press.

R176. Reveille JD, Schrohenloher RE, Acton RT, Barger BO. DNA analysis of HLA-DR and DQ genes in American Blacks with systemic lupus erythematosus. Arthritis Rheum 1989;32: 1243–1251.

R177. Reveille JD, Wilson RW, Provost TT, Bias WB, Arnett FC. Primary Sjogren's syndrome and other autoimmune diseases in families. Prevalence and immunogenetic studies in six kindreds. Ann Intern Med 1984;101:748–756.

R178. Revillard JP, Vincent C, Rivera S. Anti-Beta 2 microglobulin lymphocytotoxic autoantibodies in systemic lupus erythematosus. J Immunol 1979 Feb;122:614–618.

R179. Reyes-Lopez PA, Santos G, Forsbach GB. Absence of ANA in pregnancy. Arthritis Rheum 1980;23(3):378.

R180. Reynaud C, Anquez V, Dahan A, Weill J. A single rearrangement event generates most of the chicken immunoglobulin light chain diversity. Cell 1985;40:283- 291.

R181. Reynaud CA, Anquez V, Grimal H, Weill JC. A hyperconversion mechanism generates the chicken light chain preimmune repertoire. Cell 1987;48:379–388.

R182. Reynolds TB, Edmonson HA, Peters RL, Redeker A. Lupoid hepatitis. Ann Intern Med 1964 Oct;61(4):650–666.

R183. Reynolds TB, Peters RL, Yamada S. Chronic active and lupoid hepatitis caused by a laxative, oxyphenisatin. N Engl J Med 1971 Oct 7;285:813–820.

R184. Reza MJ, Dornfeld L, Goldberg LS. Hydralazine therapy in hypertensive patients with idiopathic systemic lupus erythematosus. Arthritis Rheum 1975 Jul–Aug;18:335–338.

R185. Reznikova MM, Trofimova IB. Exacerbation of lupus erythematosus during treatment by the reinfusion of UV- irradiated blood [English abstract]. Vestn Dermatol Venerol 1986; (7):51–52.

R186. Rheins LA, Karp RD. Effect of gender on the inducible humoral immune response to honeybee venom in American Cockroach (periplaneta America). Dev Comp Immunol 1985; 9:41–49.

R187. Rhodes K, Markham RL, Maxwell PM, Monk-Jones NE. Immunoglobulins and X-chromosomes. Br Med J 1969;3:439-441.

R188. Rhodus NL, Johnson DK. The prevalence of oral manifestations of systemic lupus erythematosus. Quintessence Int 1990; 21(6):461–465.

R189. Ribaute E, Weill B, Ing H, Badelon I, Menkes CJ. Occulomotor paralysis in disseminated lupus erythematosus [English abstract]. Ophthalmologie 1989 Apr–May;3(2):125–128.

R190. Rich S, Kieras K, Hart K, Groves BM, Stobo JD, Brundage BH. Antinuclear antibodies in primary pulmonary hypertension. J Am Coll Cardiol 1986 Dec;8(6):1307- 1311.

R191. Rich SA. Human lupus inclusion and interferon. Science 1981 Aug 14;213:772–775.

R192. Rich SA, Owens TR, Anzola C, Bartholomew LE. Induction of lupus inclusions by sera from patients with systemic lupus erythematosus. Arthritis Rheum 1986;29:501–507.

R193. Richards DS, Wagman AJ, Cabaniss ML. Ascites not due to congestive heart failure in a fetus with lupus-induced heart block. Obstet Gynecol 1990 Nov;76(5 Pt 2):957- 959.

R194. Richards RM, Fulkerson WJ. Constrictive pericarditis due to hydralazine-induced lupus erythematosus. Am J Med 1990; 88:56N-59N.

R195. Richardson B, Cornacchia E, Globus J, Maybaum J, Strahler J, Hanash S. N-acetylprocainamide is a less potent inducer of T cell autoreactivity than procainamide. Arthritis Rheum 1988;31:995–999.

R196. Richardson BC, Liebling MR, Hudson JL. CD4 + cells treated with DNA methylation inhibitors induce autologous B cell differentiation. Clin Immunol Immunopathol 1990;55: 368–381.

R197. See A229a.

R198. Richlin C, Chabot R, Roubey R, Dwyer E, Eberle M, Sulkowitz K, Buyon J, Belmont H, Abramson S. Quantitative EEG in patients with systemic lupus erythematosus (SLE) and neuropsychiatric dysfunction [abstract]. Arthritis Rheum 1989 Apr;32(4) Suppl:S48.

R199. Richmond DE. Thiamphenicol as an immunosuppressant in active systemic lupus erythematosus with nephritis. Aust NZ J Med 1979 Dec;9(6):670–675.

R200. Richmond TJ, Finch JT, Rushton B, Rhodes D, Klug A.

Structure of the nucleosome core particle at 7 A Resolution. Nature 1984;311:532–537.

R201. Richter MB, Woo P, Panayi GS, Trull A, Unger A, Sheperd P. The effects of intravenous pulse methylprednisolone on immunological and inflammatory processes in ankylosing spondylitis. Clin Exp Immunol 1983;53:51–59.

R202. Rider LG, Sherry DD, Glass ST. Neonatal lupus erythematosus simulating transient myasthenia gravis at presentation. J Pediatr 1991;118:417–419.

R203. Ridley MG, Maddison PJ, Tribe CR. Amyloidosis and systemic lupus erythematosus. Ann Rheum Dis 1984 Aug;43(4): 649–650.

R204. Ridolfi RL, Bell WR. Thrombotic thrombocytopenic purpura. Medicine 1981;60:413–428.

R205. Rieber M, Rieber MS. DNA on membrane receptors: a target for monoclonal anti-DNA antibody induced by a nucleoprotein shed in systemic lupus erythematosus. Biochem Biophys Res Commun 1989;159:1441–1447.

R206. Riedel N, Wolin S, Guthrie C. A subset of yeast snRNA's contains functional binding sites for the highly conserved Sm antigen. Science 1987;125:328–331.

R207. Riehm MR, Harrington RE. Histone-histone interaction mediates chromatin unfolding at physiological ionic strength. Biochemistry 1989;28:5787–5793.

R208. Riemenshneider TA, Wilson JF, Vernier RL. Glucocorticoid-induced pancreatitis in children. Pediatrics 1968 Feb;41: 428–437.

R209. Rifle G, Bielfeld P, Chalopin JM, Besancenot JF, Guiguet M, Mousson C, Tanter Y, Poirier D, Cortet P. Selective IgA deficiency and systemic lupus erythematosus. Ann Med Interne 1988;139:134–137.

R210. Rillema JA. Actions of quinacrine on RNA and casein syntheses in mouse mammary gland explants. Prostaglandins Med 1979 Feb;2(2):155–160.

R211. Rillema JA, Etindi RN, Cameron CM. Prolactin actions on casein and lipid biosynthesis in mouse and rabbit mammary gland explants are abolished by p-bromphenacyl bromide and quinacrine, phospholipase A2 inhibitors. Horm Metab Res 1986 Oct;18(10):672–674.

R212. Rimon R, Kronqvist K, Helve T. Overt Psychopathology in systemic lupus erythematosus. Scand J Rheumatol 1988; 27(2):143–146.

R213. Rinke J, Steitz JA. Precursor molecules of both human 5S ribosomal RNA and transfer RNAs are bound by a cellular protein reactive with anti-La lupus antibodies. Cell 1982;29: 149.

R214. Riou B, Barriot P, Riamailho A, Baud FJ. Treatment of severe chloroquine poisoning. N Engl J Med 1988 Jan 7; 318(1):1–6.

R215. Risdon RA, Sloper JC, de Wardener HE. Relationship between renal function and histologic changes found in renal biopsy specimens from patients with persistent glomerular nephritis. Lancet 1968 Aug 17;2:363–366.

R216. Riska H, Fyhrquist F, Selander RK, Hellstrom PE. Systemic erythematosus and DNA antibodies in pleural effusions. Scand J Rheumatol 1978 Jan;7:159–160.

R217. Ritchlin C, Dobro J, Senie R, Buyon J, Winchester R, Abramson S. Opportunistic infections in patients with systemic lupus erythematosus [abstract]. Arthritis Rheum 1989 Apr;32(4) Suppl:S115.

R218. Ritchlin CT, Dobro JS, Buyon JP, Abramson S. Opportunistic infections in patients with systemic lupus erythematosus [abstract]. Arthritis Rheum 1988 Jan;31(1) Suppl:R4.

R219. Rittner C, Bertrams J. On the significance of C2, C4, and Factor B polymorphism in disease. Hum Genet 1981;56: 235–247.

R220. Riuz P, Gomez F, King M, Lopez R, Darby C, Schreiber

AD. In vivo glucocorticoid modulation of guinea pig splenic macrophage Fcγ receptors. J Clin Invest 1991;88:149–157.

R221. Rivera E, Maldonado N, Velez-Garcia E, Grillo AJ, Malaret G. Hyperinfection syndrome with Strongyloides stercoralis. Ann Intern Med 1970;72:199–204.

R222. Rivera J, Escalante A, Stohl W, Horwitz DA. Unpublished observations.

R223. Rivera J, Horwitz DA. Regulatory effects of activated CD3+ double negative (CD4-CD8-) T cells and a novel triple negative (CD3-CD4-CD8-) subset on CD4+ helper cell activity [abstract]. Arthritis Rheum 1991;34 Suppl:S164.

R224. Rivera M, Marcen R, Pascual J, Naya MT, Orofina L, Ortuno J. Kidney transplantation in systemic erythematosus lupus nephritis: A one center experience. Nephron 1990;56:148–151.

R225. Rivero I, Morales J. Bisegmental neutrophils and lymphocytes in diagnosis of leukopenia associated with systemic lupus erythematosus (SLE) [original in Spanish]. Rev Med Chil 1972 May;100:526–528.

R226. Rivero SJ, Alger M, Alarcon-Segovia D. Splenectomy for hemocytopenia in systemic lupus erythematosus: a controlled reappraisal. Arch Intern Med 1979 Jul;139:773–776.

R227. Rivero SJ, Diaz-Jouanen E, Alarcon-Segovia D. Lymphopenia in systemic lupus erythematosus. Arthritis Rheum 1978 Apr;21:295–305.

R228. Rivero SJ, Llorente L, Diaz-Jouanen E, Alarcon-Segovia D. T-lymphocyte subpopulation in untreated systemic lupus erythematosus. Variations with disease activity. Arthritis Rheum 1977 Jul–Aug;20:1169–1173.

R229. Robb-Nicholson LC, Daltroy L, Eaton H, Gall V, Wright E, Hartley LH, Schur PH, Liang MH. Effects of aerobic conditioning in lupus fatigue: a pilot study. Br J Rheumatol 1989 Dec; 28(6):500–505.

R230. Robberecht W, Bednarik J, Bourgeois P, van Hees J, Carton H. Myasthenic syndrome caused by direct effect of chloroquine on neuromuscular junction. Arch Neurol 1989 Apr; 46(4):464–468.

R231. Robbey SJ, Lewis EJ, Schur PJ, Colman RW. Circulating anticoagulants to factor VIII. Am J Med 1957 Dec;49:575–579.

R232. Omitted.

R233. Robbins ML, Kornguth SE, Cell CL, Kalinke T, England D, Turski P, Graziano FM. Antineurofilament antibody evaluation in neuropsychiatric systemic lupus erythematosus. Combination with anticardiolipin antibody assay and magnetic resonance imaging. Arthritis Rheum 1988 May;31(5):623–631.

R234. Robbins WC, Holman HR, Deicher H, Kunkel HG. Complement fixation with cell nuclei and DNA in lupus erythematosus. Proc Soc Exp Biol Med 1957 Dec;96(3):575–579.

R235. Roberts AB, Sporn MB. Transforming growth factor. Adv Cancer Res 1988;51:107–145.

R236. Roberts DL. Subacute cutaneous lupus erythematosus and gluten sensitive enteropathy. Br J Dermatol 1988;118: 731–732.

R237. Roberts JL. Diagnosis of systemic lupus erythematosus and lupus nephritis. Contrib Nephrol 1983;35:150–169.

R238. Roberts JL, Hayashi JA. Exacerbation of SLE associated with alfalfa ingestion [letter]. N Engl J Med 1983 Jun 2; 308(22):1361.

R239. Roberts JL, Lewis EJ. Identification of anti-native DNA antibodies to cryoglobulinemic states. Am J Med 1978 Sep;65: 437–445.

R240. Roberts JL, Lewis EJ. Immunochemical demonstration of cryoprecipitable anti-native DNA antibody and DNA in the serum of patients with glomerulonephritis. J Immunol 1980 Jan;124:127–133.

R241. Roberts JL, Robinson MF, Lewis EJ. Low molecular weight plasma cryoprecipitable anti-native DNA: Polynucleotide

complexes in lupus glomerulonephritis. Clin Immunol Immunopathol 1981 Apr;19:75–90.

R242. Roberts JL, Schwartz MM, Lewis EJ. Hereditary C2 deficiency and systemic lupus erythematosus associated with severe glomerulonephritis. Clin Exp Immunol 1978;31: 328–338.

R243. Roberts PJ, Isenberg DA, Segal AW. Defective degradation of bacterial DNA by phagocytes from patients with systemic and discoid lupus erythematosus. Clin Exp Immunol 1987 Jul; 69(1):68–78.

R244. Roberts SM, Adams LE, Donovan-Brand R, Budinsky R, Skoulis NP, Zimmer H, Hess EV. Procainamide hydroxylamine lymphocyte toxicity—I. Evidence for participation by hemoglobin. Int J Pharmacol 1989;11:419–427.

R245. Roberts WN, Hauptman HW, Ruddy S. Reversal of the vasospastic component of lupus vasculopathy by prostaglandin E1 infusion [abstract]. Arthritis Rheum 1989 Apr;32(4) Suppl:S74.

R246. Roberts-Thompson PJ, Shepherd K, Bradley J, Boey ML. Frequency and role of low molecular weight IgM in systemic lupus erythematosus. Study of patients from different ethnic origins. Rheumatol Int 1990;10:95–98.

R247. Robineaux R, Pinet J. The Hargraves cell. Description, significance, and research techniques. Rev Practicien 1965 Jul 1;15:2523.

R248. Robinson DR, Prickett JD, Makoul GT, Steinberg AD, Colvin RB. Dietary fish oil reduces progression of established renal disease in (NZB × NZW)F1 mice and delays renal disease in BXSB and MRL/l strains. Arthritis Rheum 1986 Apr; 29(4):539–546.

R249. Robinson DR, Prickett JD, Polisson R, Steinberg AD, Levine L. The protective effect of dietary fish oil on murine lupus. Prostaglandins 1985;30:51–75.

R250. Robinson DR, Skoskiewicz M, Bloch KJ, Castorena G, Hayes E, Lowenstein E, Melvin C, Michelassi F, Zapol WM. Cyclooxygenase blockade elevates leukotriene E4 production during acute anaphylaxis in sheep. J Immunol 1986;163: 1509–1517.

R251. Robinson DR, Zvaifler NJ, editors. Rheumatic Disease Clinics of North America, Vol 13. Pathogenesis of chronic inflammatory arthritis. New York: Saunders, 1987:385.

R252. Robinson HJ Jr, Hartleben PD, Lund G, Schreiman J. Evaluation of magnetic resonance imaging in the diagnosis of osteonecrosis of the femoral head. Accuracy compared with radiographs, core biopsy, and intraosseous pressure measurements. J Bone Joint Surg (Am) 1989 Jun;71(5): 650–663.

R253. Rock GA. Plasma exchange in treatment of Rhesus hemolytic disease: A review. Plasma Ther 1981;2:211.

R254. Rock GA, Shumak KH, Buskard NA, Blanchette VS, Kelton JG, Nair RC, Spasoff RA, Canadian Apheresis Study Group. Comparison of plasma exchange with plasma infusion in the treatment of thrombotic thrombocytopenic purpura. N Engl J Med 1991;325:393–397.

R255. Rocklin RE, Kitzmiller JL, Carpenter CB, Garovoy MR, David JR. Maternal-fetal relation: absence of an immunologic blocking factor from the serum of women with chronic abortions. N Engl J Med 1976;295:1209–1213.

R256. Rodby RA, Korbet SM, Lewis EJ. Persistent of clinical and serologic activity in patients with systemic lupus erythematosus undergoing peritoneal dialysis. Am J Med 1987 Oct;83(4): 613–618.

R256a. Roddy SM, Giang DW. Antiphospholipid antibodies and stroke in an infant. Pediatrics 1991;87:933–935.

R257. Roden DM, Riele SB, Higgins SB, Wilkinson GR, Smith RF, Oates JA, Woolsey RL. Antiarrhythmic efficacy, pharmacokinetics and safety of N-acetylprocainamide in human subjects:

Comparison with procainamide. Am J Cardiol 1980 Sep;46: 463–468.

R258. Rodkey LS. Autoregulation of immune responses via idiotype network interactions. Microbiol Rev 1980;44:631.

R259. Rodnan GP. Scleroderma, calcinosis and eosinophilic fascitis. In: McCarty DJ, editor. Arthritis and Allied Conditions, 9th ed. Philadelphia: Lea & Febiger, 1979:762–809.

R260. Rodnan GP, Benedek TG, Medsger TA Jr, Cammarta RJ. The association of progressive systemic sclerosis (scleroderma) with coal miners' pneumoconiosis and other forms of silicosis. Ann Intern Med 1967;66:323–334.

R261. Rodnan GP, Maclachlan MJ, Creighton AS. Study of serum proteins and serologic reactions in relatives of patients with SLE [abstract]. Clin Res 1960;8;197.

R262. Rodrigue S, Laborde H, Catoggio PM. Systemic lupus erythematosus and thyrotoxicosis: a hitherto little recognized association. Ann Rheum Dis 1989 May;48(5):424–427.

R263. Rodriquez MA, Paul H, Abadi I, Bravo JR, Armas P. Multiple microcrystal deposition in a patient with systemic lupus erythematosus. Ann Rheum Dis 1984 Jun;43(3):498–502.

R264. Rodriguez SU, Leikin SL, Hiller MC. Neonatal thrombocytopenia associated with anti-partum administration of thiazide drugs. N Engl J Med 1964;270:881–884.

R265. Rodriquez-Iturbe B, Garcia R, Rubio L, Serrano H. Immunohistologic findings in systemic lupus erythematosus. Arch Pathol Lab Med 1977 Jul;101:342- 344.

R266. Roehrig JT, Huna AR, Mathews JH. Equine encephalitis. In: The 1984 High Techology Route to Virus Vaccines. 1984: 32.

R267. Roehrs T, McLenaghan A, Koshorek G, Zorick F, Roth T. Amnesic effects of lormetazepam. Psychopharmacol 1984;9 Suppl 1:165–172.

R268. Roehrs T, Zoric FJ, Sicklesteel JM, Wittig RM, Harse KM, Roth T. Effects of hypnotics on memory. J Clin Psychopharmacol 1983 Oct;3(5):310–313.

R269. Roenigk HH Jr. Dermabrasion from miscellaneous cutaneous scars (exclusive of scarring from acne). J Dermatol Surg Oncol 1977;3:322–328.

R270. Roennblom LE, Alm GV, Oberg K. Autoimmune phenomena in patients with malignant carcinoid tumors during interferon-alpha treatment. Acta Oncol 1991;30:537–450.

R271. Rogers M. Psychiatric aspects. In: Schur P, editor. Clinical management of systemic lupus erythematosus. New York: Grune & Stratton, 1983:189–210.

R272. Rogers MA, Dubey D, Reich P. The influence of the psyche and the brain on immunity and disease susceptibility: A critical review. Psycho Med 1979;41(2):147.

R273. Rohn RJ, Bond WH. Some effects of nitrogen mustard and trimethylene melamine in acute disseminated lupus erythematosus. Am J Sci 1950;226:179–190.

R274. Roitt IM, Doniach D, Campbell PN, Hudson RV. Autoantibodies in Hashimoto's disease (lymphadenoid goiter); preliminary communications. Lancet 1956 Oct 20;2:820- 821.

R275. Rojas C, Jacobelli S, Massardo L, Rosenberg H, Rivero S. Disseminated lupus erythematosus without abnormalities in urinary sediment. Rev Med Chile 1987;115:120–125.

R276. Rokeach LA, Haselby JA, Hoch SA. Molecular cloning of a cDNA encoding the human Sm-D autoantigen. Proc Natl Acad Sci USA 1988;85:4832–4836.

R277. Rokeach LA, Jannatipour M, Haselby JA, Hoch SO. Primary structure of a human small nuclear ribonucleoprotein polypeptide as deduced by cDNA analysis. J Biol Chem 1989;264: 5024–5030.

R278. Rokeach LA, Jannatipour M, Hoch S. Heterologous expression and epitope mapping of a human small nuclear ribonucleoprotein-associated Sm-B'/B autoantigen. J Immunol 1990;144:1015–1022.

R279. Rolink AG, Gleichmann E. Allosuppressor and allohelper T cells in acute and chronic graft-versus-host (GVH) disease. III. Different Lyt subsets of T cells induce different pathological lesions. J Exp Med 1983;158:546.

R280. Rolink AG, Gleichmann H, Gleichmann E. Diseases caused by reactions of T lymphocytes to incompatible structures of the MHC. J Immunol 1983;130:209–215.

R281. Rolink AG, Pals ST, Gleichmann E. Allosuppressor and allohelper T cells in acute and chronic graft-vs-host disease. IIF1 recipients carrying mutations at H-2K and/or I-A. J Exp Med 1983; 157:755–771.

R282. Romac J, Bouley JP, Van Regenmortel MHV. Enzyme-linked immunosorbent assay in the study of histone antigens and nucleosome structure. Anal Biochem 1981 May 15;113: 366–371.

R283. Romano C, Pongiglione R, Ruffa G, Bezante T, Villa- Venzano G. Blocco atrioventricolare congenito di alto grado. Minerva Pediatrica 1976;27:1632–1649.

R284. Romero RW, Nesbitt LT Jr, Ichinose H. Mikulicz disease and subsequent lupus erythematosus development. JAMA 1977 Jun 6;237(23):2507–2510.

R285. Romero RW, Nesbitt LT Jr, Reed RJ. Unusual variant of lupus erythematosus on lichen planus. Clinical, histopathologic and immunofluorescence studies. Arch Dermatol 1977; 113:741–748.

R286. Rongioletti F, Parodi A, Rebora A. Papular and nodular mucinosis as a sign of lupus erythematosus. Dermatologica 1990;180(4):221–223.

R287. Rongioletti F, Rebora A. Papular and nodular mucinosis associated with systemic lupus erythematosus. Br J Dermatol 1986 Nov;115(5):631–636.

R288. Rook AH, Lane HC, Folks T, McCoy S, Alter H, Fauci AS. Sera from HTLV-III/LAV antibody-positive individuals mediate antibody-dependent cellular cytotoxicity against HTLV-III/LAV-infected T cells. J Immunol 1987;138:1064- 1067.

R289. Rook AH, Tsokos GC, Quinnan GV Jr, Balow JE, Ramsey KM, Stocks N, Phelan MA, Djeu JY. Cytotoxic antibodies to natural killer cells in systemic lupus erythematosus. Clin Immunol Immunopathol 1982 Aug;24:179–185.

R290. Rook GAW. Rheumatoid arthritis, mycobacterial antigens, and agalactosyl IgG. Scand J Immunol 1988;28:487–492.

R291. Rooney PJ, Decker JL, Steinberg AD. A controlled trial of cyclophosphamide and azathioprine in lupus glomerulonephritis. a report on the status at four years of follow up [abstract]. Arthritis Rheum 1978;19:819.

R292. Omitted.

R293. Ropes MW. Observations on the natural course of disseminated lupus erythematosus. Medicine 1964 May;43:387–391.

R294. Ropes MW. Systemic Lupus Erythematosus. Cambridge MA: Harvard University Press, 1976.

R295. Ropes MW. Systemic Lupus Erythematosus. Cambridge MA: Harvard University Press, 1976:19.

R296. Ropes MW, Bennett GA, Cobb S, Jacox R, Jessar RA. 1958 revision of diagnostic criteria for rheumatoid arthritis. Bull Rheum Dis 1958 Dec;9:175–176.

R297. Rosa MA, Gottlieb E, Lerner RM, Steitz JA. Striking similarities are exhibited by two small Epstein-Barr virus-encoded ribonucleic acids and the adenovirus- associated ribonucleic acids VAI and VAII. Mol Cell Biol 1981;1:785–796.

R298. Rosal EJ, Maricq HR. Comparison of digital artery pressure responses to local cooling in Raynaud phenomenon associated with systemic lupus erythematosus, systemic sclerosis and primary Raynaud's phenomenon [abstract]. Arthritis Rheum 1989 Jan;32(1) Suppl:R45.

R298a. Rose C, Goldsmith DP. Childhood adrenal insufficiency, chorea and antiphospholipid antibodies. Ann Rheum Dis 1990;49:421–422.

R299. Rose E, Pillsbury DM. Lupus erythematosus (erythematoides) and ovarian function: observations on possible relationship with report of 6 cases. Ann Intern Med 1944 Dec;21: 1022–1034.

R300. Rosemarin JI, Nigro EJ, Levere RD, Mascarenhas BR. Systemic lupus erythematosus and acute intermittent porphyria: coincidence or association. Arthritis Rheum 1982 Sep;25(9): 1134–1137.

R301. Rosen PJ, Cramer AD, Dubois EL, Lukes RJ. Systemic lupus erythematosus and myelofibrosis. A possible pathogenetic relationship [abstract]. Clin Res 1973 Apr;21:565.

R302. Rosenbaum J, Pottinger BE, Woo P, Block CM, Loizou S, Byron MA, Pearson JD. Measurement and characterization of circulating anti-endothelial cell IgG in connective tissue diseases. Clin Exp Immunol 1988 Jun;72(3):450- 456.

R303. Rosenberg AM. The clinical associations of antinuclear antibodies in juvenile rheumatoid arthritis. Clin Immunol Immunopathol 1988 Oct;49(1):19–27.

R304. Rosenberg AM, Petty RE, Cumming GR, Koehler BE. Pulmonary hypertension in a child with mixed connective tissue disease. J Rheumatol 1979 Nov–Dec;6(6):700–704.

R305. Rosenberg FJ, Phillips PG, Druzba PG. Platelets and thrombosis. Use of a rabbit extracorporeal shunt in the assay of antithrombotic and thrombotic drugs. Baltimore: University Park Press, 1974:233–234.

R306. Rosenberg RD, Bauer KA. Thrombosis in inherited deficiencies of antithrombin III, protein C, and protein S. Human Pathol 1987;18:253–262.

R307. Rosenberg S. Lymphokine-activated killer cells: A new approach to A immunotherapy of cancer. JNCI, J Natl Cancer Inst 1985:75:595.

R308. Rosenberg YJ, Steinberg AD, Santoro TJ. The basis of autoimmunity in MRL-lpr/lpr mice: a role for self Ia-reactive T cells. Immunol Today 1984;5:64–67.

R309. Rosenow EC 3d, Hurley BT. Disorders of the thymus. Arch Intern Med 1984;144:763–770.

R310. Rosenstein ED, Sobelman J, Kramer N. Isolated, pupil-sparing third nerve palsy as initial manifestation of systemic lupus erythematosus. J Clin Neuro Opthalmol 1989 Dec;9(4): 285–288.

R311. Rosenstein ED, Wieczorek R, Raphael BG, Agus B. Systemic lupus erythematosus and angioimmunoblastic lymphadenopathy: case report and review of the literature. Semin Arthritis Rheum 1986 Nov;16(2):146- 151.

R312. Rosenthal CJ, Franklin EC. Deficiency of cell mediated immunity (CMI) in active SLE: Changing patterns after steroid therapy [abstract]. Arthritis Rheum 1973;16:565.

R313. Rosenthal CJ, Franklin EC. Depression of cellular- mediate mediated immunity in systemic lupus erythematosus. Relation to disease activity. Arthritis Rheum 1975 May–Jun;18: 207–217.

R314. Rosenthal DS, Sack B. Autoimmune hemolytic anemia in scleroderma. JAMA 1971 Jun 21;216:2011–2012.

R315. Rosenthal M. Sharp syndrome (mixed connective tissue disease): Clinical and laboratory evaluation on 40 patients. Eur J Rheumatol 1979;2(2):237–242.

R316. Omitted.

R317. Omitted.

R318. Omitted.

R319. Rosling AE, Rhodes EL, Watson B. Removal of a blocking factor from the sera of patients with systemic lupus erythematosus with Levamisole. Clin Exp Dermatol 1978 Mar;3(1): 39–42.

R320. Rosner E, Pauzner R, Lusky A, Modan M, Mang A. Detection and quantitative evaluation of lupus circulating anticoagulant activity. Thromb Haemost 1987;57:144–147.

R321. Rosner S, Ginzler EM, Diamond HS, Weiner M, Schlesinger M, Fries JF, Wasner C, Medsger TA Jr, Ziegler G, Klippel JH, Hadler NM, Albert DA, Hess EV, Spencer-Green G, Grayzel A, Worth D, Hahn BH, Barnett EV. A multicenter study of outcome in systemic lupus erythematosus. II. Causes of death. Arthritis Rheum 1982 Jun;25:612–619.

R322. Rosoff PM, Savage N, Dinarello CA. Interleukin-1 stimulates diacylglycerol production in T lymphocytes by a novel mechanism. Cell 1988;54:73–81.

R322a. Rosove MH, Brewer PMC, Runge A, Hirji K. Simultaneous lupus anticoagulant and anticardiolipin assays and clinical detection of antiphospholipids. Am J Haemat 1989;32:148–149.

R322b. Rosove MH, Ismail M, Koziol BJ, Runge A, Kaspar CK. Lupus anticoagulants: improved diagnosis with kaolin clotting time using rabbit brain phospholipid in standard and high concentrations. Blood 1986;68:472- 478.

R322c. Rosove MH, Tabsh K, Wasserstrum N, Howard P, Hahn BH, Kalunian KC. Heparin therapy and prevention of pregnancy loss in women with lupus anticoagulant or anticardiolipin antibodies. Obstet Gynecol 1990;75:630- 634.

R322d. See R322c.

R323. Ross GD, Lambris JD, Cain JA, Newman SL. Generation of three different fragments of bound C3 with purified factor I or serum: Requirement of factor H vs CR1 cofactor activity. J Immunol 1982;129:2051–2060.

R324. Ross GD, Medof ME. Membrane complement receptors specific for bound fragments of C3. Adv Immunol 1985;37: 217–267.

R325. Ross GD, Walport MJ, Parker CJ, Lentine AF, Fuller CR, Yount WJ, Myones BL, Winfield JB, Lachmann PJ. Acquired loss of erythrocyte CR1 (C3b-receptor) in systemic lupus erythematosus and other diseases with autoantibodies and/or complement activation [abstract]. 1984;27 Suppl:S28.

R326. Ross GD, Yount WJ, Walport MJ, Winfield JB, Parker CJ, Fuller CR, Taylor RP, Myones BL, Lachmann PJ. Disease- associated loss of erythrocyte complement receptors (CR1, C3b receptors) in patients with systemic lupus erythematosus and other diseases involving autoantibodies and/or complement activation. J Immunol 1985;135:2005–2014.

R327. Ross SC, Densen P. Complement deficiency states and infection: Epidemiology, pathogenesis and consequences of Neisserial and other infections in an immune deficiency. Medicine 1984 Sep;63:243–273.

R328. Ross SW, Wells BB. Systemic lupus erythematosus; Review of the literature. Am J Clin Pathol 1953;23:139–160.

R329. Rosse WF. The antiglobulin test in autoimmune hemolytic anemia. Ann Rev Med 1975;26:331–337.

R330. Rosse WF. The mechanisms of destruction of antibody-altered cells. Clin Lab Med 1982 Mar;2:211–219.

R331. Rosse WF, Adams JP, Yount WJ. Subclasses of IgG antibodies in immune thrombocytopenic purpura (ITP). Br J Haematol 1980 Sep;46:109–114.

R332. Rossen RD, Reisberg MA, Sharp JT, Suki WD, Schloeder FX, Hill LL, Eknoyan G. Antiglobulins and glomerulonephritis. J Clin Invest 1975 Aug;56:427–437.

R333. Rossen RD, Rickaway RH, Reisberg MA, Singer DB, Schloeder FX, Suki WS, Hill LL, Eknoyan G. Renal localization of antiglobulins in glomerulonephritis and after renal transplantation. Arthritis Rheum 1977 May;20:947–961.

R334. Rote NS, Dostal-Johnson D, Ng AK, Ault K, Carmody M. Platelet and endothelial cell reactivity of monoclonal antibodies against phosphatidylserine and cardiolipin [abstract]. Clin Exp Rheumatol 1990;8 Suppl 2:210.

R335. See R336a.

R336. Roth D, Milgrom M, Esquenazi V, Strauss J, Zilleruelo G, Miller J. Renal transplantation in systemic lupus erythematosus: one center's experience. Am J Nephrol 1987;7(5): 367–374.

R336a. Roth M. Contribution to knowledge of varicose hypertrophy of nerve fibers [original in German]. Virchow Arch Path Anat 1872;55:197–217.

R337. Rothenberg RJ, Graziano FM, Grandone JT, Goldberg JW, Bjarnason DF, Finesilver AG. The use of methotrexate in steroid-resistant systemic lupus erythematosus. Arthritis Rheum 1988 May;31(5):612–615.

R338. Rother U, Rother K, Flad HD, Miescher PA. Bithermic complement activation in cryoglobulinemic serum. Eur J Clin Invest 1972 Jan;2:59–65.

R339. Rothfield N. Systemic lupus erythematosus. Clinical and laboratory aspects. In: McCarty D, editor. Arthritis and Allied Conditions. 9th ed. Philadelphia: Lea & Febiger, 1979: 691–715.

R340. Rothfield N. Clinical features of systemic lupus erythematosus. In: Kelly WN, Harris ED, Ruddy S, Sledge CB, editors. Textbook of Rheumatology. Philadelphia: Saunders, 1981: 1106–1132.

R341. Rothfield N. Cardiopathy manifestations. In: Schur P, editor. The clinical management of systemic lupus erythematosus. New York: Grune & Stratton, 1983:113–122.

R342. Rothfield N. Clinical features of systemic lupus erythematosus. In: McCarty DJ, editor. Arthritis and Allied Conditions. 10th ed. Philadelphia: Lea & Febiger, 1985:1091.

R343. Rothfield N. Efficacy of antimalarials in systemic lupus erythematosus. Am J Med 1988 Oct 14;85 Suppl 4A:53–56.

R344. Rothfield N, Marino C. Studies of repeat skin biopsies of nonlesional skin in patients with systemic lupus erythematosus. Arthritis Rheum 1982 Jun;25(6):624–630.

R345. Rothfield N, Ross HA, Minta JO, Lepow IH. Glomerular and dermal deposition of properdin in systemic lupus erythematosus. N Engl J Med 1972;287:681–685.

R346. Rothfield N, Weissman G. Bullae in systemic lupus erythematosus. Arch Intern Med 1961 Jun;107:908–914.

R347. Rothfield NF. General considerations in the treatment of systemic lupus erythematosus. Mayo Clin Proc 1969 Sep;44: 691–696.

R348. Rothfield NF. Nasal septum perforation in systemic lupus erythematosus. N Engl J Med 1974;291:51.

R349. Rothfield NF. Current approaches to SLE and its subsets. DM 1982 Oct;29(1):1–62.

R350. Rothfield NF, Bierer WF, Garfield WJ. Isoniazid induction of antinuclear antibodies. A prospective study. Ann Intern Med 1978 May:650–652.

R351. Rothfield NF, Evans AS, Niederman JC. Clinical and laboratory aspects of raised virus antibody titers in systemic lupus erythematosus. Ann Rheum Dis 1973;32:238–246.

R352. Rothfield NF, March C, Miescher P, McEwen C. Chronic discoid lupus erythematosus. A study of 65 patients and 65 controls. N Engl J Med 1963 Nov 28;269 (22):1155- 1161.

R353. Rothfield NF, McCluskey RT, Baldwin DS. Renal disease in systemic lupus erythematosus. N Engl J Med 1963 Sep;269: 537–544.

R354. Rothfield NF, Stollar BD. The relation of immunoglobulin class, pattern of anti-nuclear antibody, and complement-fixing antibodies to DNA in sera from patients with systemic lupus erythematosus. J Clin Invest 1967 Nov;46:1785–1794.

R355. Rothschild BM. Serine esterase inhibition and immune modulation. Semin Arthritis Rheum 1984 Feb;13:274–292.

R356. Rothschild BM, James KK, Jones JV, Thompson LD, Pifer DD, Chesney CM. Significance of elevated C-reactive protein in patients with SLE. Arthritis Rheum 1982 Apr;25 Suppl:S82.

R357. Rothschild BM, Jones JV, Chesney C, Pifer DD, Thompson LD, James KK, Badger H. Relationship of clinical findings in systemic lupus erythematosus to seroreactivity. Arthritis Rheum 1983 Jan;26(1):45–51.

R358. Rotman M, Dorfmann H, de Seze S, Kahn MF. Coexistence of systemic lupus erythematosus and seminoma of the ovary. Apparent rapid cure of the lupus after removal of the tumor. Seven years follow up [original in French]. La Nouvelle Presse Med 1972 March 25;1:853- 857.

R359. Roubenoff R, Drew H, Moyer M, Petri M, Whiting-O'Keefe Q, Hellmann DB. Oral cimetidine improves the accuracy and precision of creatinine clearance in lupus nephritis. Ann Intern Med 1990;113:501–506.

R360. Roubenoff R, Hochberg MC. Systemic lupus erythematosus. In: Bellamy N, editor. Prognosis in the Rheumatic Diseases. Lancaster: Kluwer Academic Publishers Ltd, 1991:193.

R361. Roubinian J, Papoian R, Talal N. Androgenic hormones modulate auto-antibody responses and improve survival in murine lupus. J Clin Invest 1977;59:1066.

R362. Roubinian J, Talal N, Siiteri PK, Sadakian JA. Sex hormone modulation of autoimmunity in NZB/NZW mice. Arthritis Rheum 1979 Nov;22(11):1162–1169.

R363. Roubinian JR, Talal N, Greenspan JS, Goodman JR, Nussenzweig V. Danazol's failure to suppress autoimmunity in NZB/ NZW F1 mice. Arthritis Rheum 1979;22:1399–1402.

R364. Roubinian JR, Talal N, Greenspan JS, Goodman JR, Siiteri PK. Delayed androgen treatment prolongs survival in murine lupus. J Clin Invest 1979 May;63(5):902–911.

R365. Roubinian JR, Talal N, Greenspan JS, Goodman JR, Siiteri PK. Effect of castration and sex hormone treatment on survival, anti-nucleic acid antibodies and glomerulonephritis in NZB/NZW F1 mice. J Exp Med 1983 Jun 1;147:1568–1583.

R366. Roudot-Thoraval F, Gouault-Heilmann M, Zafrani ES, Barge J, Dhumeaux D. Budd-Chiari syndrome and the lupus anticoagulant. Gastroenterology 1985;87:605.

R367. Roujeau JC, Andre C, Bertolus S, Lemann M, Touraine R. Lupus cutane subaigu: Etude critique. Ann Med Intern 1987; 138:592–594.

R368. Roumm AD, Greenberg A, Buckingham RB. The effects of ibuprofen in renal function in lupus nephritis [abstract]. Clin Res 1985;33:793A.

R369. Roundtree J, Weigand D, Burgdorf W. Lupus erythematosus with oral and preianal mucous membrane involvement. Arch Dermatol 1982 Jan;118(1):55–56.

R370. Roura M, Lopez-Gil F, Umbert P. Systemic lupus erythematosus exacerbated by piroxicam. Dermatologica 1991;182: 56–58.

R371. Rouzer CA, Scott WA, Hamill AL, Cohn ZA. Dynamics of leukotriene C production by macrophages. J Exp Med 1980; 152:1236–1247.

R372. Rouzer CA, Scott WA, Kempe J, Cohn ZA. Prostaglandin synthesis by macrophages requires a specific receptor- ligand interaction. Proc Natl Acad Sci USA 1980;77:4279- 4282.

R373. Rovensky J, Cebecauer L, Zitnan D, Lukac J, Ferencik M. Levamisole treatment of systemic lupus erythematosus [letter]. Arthritis Rheum 1982 Apr;25(4):470–471.

R374. Rovensky J, Lukac J, Zitnan D, Pekarek J, Cebecauer L. Results of immunomodulatory therapy in systemic lupus erythematosus. Int J Immunother 1986;2:193–198.

R375. Rowell NR. Treatment of chronic discoid lupus erythematosus with intralesional triamcinolone. Br J Dermatol 1962 Oct;74:354–357.

R376. Rowell NR. Laboratory abnormalities in the diagnosis and management of systemic lupus erythematosus. Br J Dermatol 1970 Mar;84:210–216.

R377. Rowell NR. The natural history of lupus erythematosus. Clin Exp Dermatol 1984 May;9(3):217–231.

R378. Rowell NR. Chilblain lupus erythematosus responding to etretinate. Br J Dermatol 1987;117 Suppl 32:100–101.

R379. Rowell NR. Discoid lupus erythematosus and systemic sclerosis. Br J Dermatol 1987;117 Suppl 32:106–107.

R380. Rowell NR, Beck JS, Anderson JR. Lupus erythematosus and erythema multiforme-like lesions. A syndrome with characteristic immunological abnormalities. Arch Dermatol 1963 Aug;88:176–180.

R381. Rowell NR, Tate GM. The lupus anticoagulant in systemic lupus erythematosus and systemic sclerosis. Br J Dermatol 1987;117 Suppl 32:13–14.

R382. Rowland LP, Clark C, Olarte M. Therapy for dermatomyositis and polymyositis. Adv Neurol 1977;17:63–97.

R383. Rubenstein DJ, Huntley AC. Keratotic lupus erythematosus: treatment with isotretinoin. J Am Acad Dermatol 1986 May;14(5 Pt 2):910–914.

R384. Rubin BR, DeHoratius RJ. Acute visual loss in lupus erythematosus. J Am Osteopath Assoc 1989 Jan;89(1):73- 77.

R384a. Rubin L, Urowitz MB, Pruzanski W. Systemic lupus erythematosus with paraproteinemia. Arthritis Rheum 1984 Jun; 27:638–644.

R385. Rubin LA, Urowitz MB. Shrinking lung syndrome in SLE—A clinical pathologic study. J Rheumatol 1983 Dec;10: 973–976.

R386. Rubin LA, Urowitz MB, Gladman DD. Mortality in systemic lupus erythematosus: the bimodal pattern revisited. Q J Med 1985;55:87–98.

R387. Rubin M, Bernstein HN, Zvaifler NJ. Studies on the pharmacology of chloroquine. Recommendations for the treatment of chloroquine retinopathy. Arch Ophthalmol 1963 Oct; 70:474–481.

R388. Rubin RL. Autoimmune reactions induced by procainamide and hydralazine. In: Kammuller ME, Bloksma N, Seinen W, editors. Autoimmunity and Toxicology. New York: Elsevier, 1989:119–150.

R389. Omitted.

R390. Rubin RL, Burlingame RW, Bell SA. Specific anti-histone antibody common to lupus induced by diverse drugs [abstract]. Arthritis Rheum 1991;34:S104.

R391. Rubin RL, Carr RI. Anti-DNA activity of IgG F(ab') from normal human serum. J Immunol 1979 Apr;122(4):1604-1607.

R391a. Rubin RL, Curnutte JT. Metabolism of procainamide to the cytotoxic hydroxylamine by neutrophils activated in vitro. J Clin Invest 1989;83:1336–1343.

R392. Rubin RL, Joslin FG, Tan EM. Specificity of antihistone antibodies in systemic lupus erythematosus. Arthritis Rheum 1982;25:779–782.

R393. Rubin RL, Joslin FG, Tan EM. A solid-phase radioimmunoassay for antihistone antibodies in human sera: comparison with an immunofluorescence assay. Scand J Immunol 1982; 15(1):63–70.

R394. Rubin RL, McNally EM, Nusinow SR, Robinson CA, Tan EM. IgG antibodies to the histone complex H2A-H2B characterize procainamide-induced lupus. Clin Immunol Immunopathol 1985;36:49–59.

R395. Rubin RL, Nusinow SR, Johnson AD, Rubenson AD, Curd JG, Tan EM. Serologic changes during induction of lupus-like disease by procainamide. Am J Med 1986;80:999–1002.

R396. Rubin RL, Nusinow SR, McNally EM, Curd JB, Tan EM. Specificity of anti-histone antibodies and relation to clinical symptoms in drug-induced lupus [abstract]. Arthritis Rheum 1984 Apr;27 Suppl:S44.

R397. Rubin RL, Reimer G, McNally EM, Nusinow SR, Searles RP, Tan EM. Procainamide elicits a selective autoantibody immune response. Clin Exp Immunol 1986;63:58–67.

R398. Rubin RL, Tang FL, Chan EKL, Pollard KM, Tsay G, Tan EM. IgG subclasses of autoantibodies in systemic lupus erythematosus, Sjogren's syndrome, and drug-induced autoimmunity. J Immunol 1986;137:2528–5334.

R399. Rubin RL, Tang FL, Lucas AH, Spiegelberg HL, Tan EM. IgG subclasses of anti-tetanus toxoid antibodies in adult and newborn normal subjects and in patients with systemic lupus erythematosus, Sjogren's syndrome, and drug-induced autoimmunity. J Immunol 1986 Oct 15;137(8):2522–2527.

R400. Rubin RL, Tang FL, Tsay G, Pollard KM. Pseudoautoimmunity in normal mice: Anti-histone antibodies elicited by immunization versus induction during graft-versus-host reaction. Clin Immunol Immunopathol 1990;54:320–332.

R401. Rubin RL, Theofilopoulos AN. Monoclonal autoantibodies reacting with multiple structurally related and unrelated macromolecules. Intern Rev Immunol 1988 Mar;3(1–2):71–95.

R402. Rubin RL, Uetrecht JP, Jones JE. Cytotoxicity of oxidative metabolites of procainamide. J Pharmacol Exp Ther 1987; 242:833–841.

R403. Rubin RL, Waga S. Antihistone antibodies in systemic lupus erythematosus. J Rheumatol 1987;14:118–126.

R404. Rudders RA, Jespersen DL, Zacks J, Sikorski A, DeDellis RA, Krontiris T. Clonal diversity in human B cell lymphoma. I. Idiotypic and genetic analysis of lymphoma heterohybrids. J Immunol 1990;144:396.

R405. Ruddy S. Complement, rheumatic diseases and the major histocompatibility complex. Clin Rheum Dis 1977;3:215.

R406. Ruddy S. Complement and its components. In: Cohen A, editor. Laboratory diagnostic procedures in the rheumatic diseases. 3d ed. Boston: Little, Brown, 1985:137.

R407. Ruddy S, Carpenter CB, Chin KW, Knostman JN, Soter NA, Gotze O, Muller-Eberhard H, Austen KF. Human complement metabolism: an analysis of 144 studies. Medicine 1975;54: 165–178.

R408. Ruderman M, McCarty DJ Jr. Arthritis rounds: (4). Aseptic necrosis in systemic lupus erythematosus. Report of a case involving six joints. Arthritis Rheum 1964 Dec;7;709–721.

R409. Ruderman M, Miller LM, Pinals RS. Clinical and serologic observations on 27 patients with Felty's syndrome. Arthritis Rheum 1968 Jun;11:377–384.

R410. Rudikoff S. Structural correlates of idiotypes expressed on galactan-binding antibodies. In: Greene MI, Nisonoff A, editors. The Biology of Idiotypes. New York: Plenum Press 1984: 15.

R411. Rudin DO. The choroid plexus and system disease in mental illness. I systemic lupus erythematosus: A combined transport dysfunction model for schizophrenia. Biol Psych 1981 Apr;16:373.

R412. Rudnicki RD, Gresham GE, Rothfield NF. The efficacy of antimalarials in systemic lupus erythematosus. J Rheumatol 1975 Sep;2(3):323–330.

R413. RuDusky DM. Recurrent Osler's nodes in systemic lupus erythematosus. Angiology 1969 Jan;20:33–37.

R414. Ruiz-Arguelles A, Presno-Bernal M. Demonstration of a cross-reactive idiotype (IdRQ) in rheumatoid factors from patients with rheumatoid arthritis but not in rheumatoid factors from healthy, aged subjects. Arthritis Rheum 1989;32:134.

R415. Ruiz-Arguelles A, Ruiz-Arguelles GJ, Presno-Bernal J, Deleze M, Ortiz-Lopez R, Vazques-Prado J. Protein C (PC) dysfunction in systemic lupus erythematosus (SLE) and in primary antiphospholipid syndrome (PAPS). Relationship to antiphospholipid antibodies (APLA) [abstract]. Arthritis Rheum 1988 Apr;31(4) Suppl:S67.

R416. Ruiz-Arguelles GJ, Ruiz-Arguelles A, Alarcon-Segovia D, Drenkard C, Villa A, Cabiedes J, Presno-Bernal M, Deleze M, Ortiz-Lopez R, Vazquez-Prado J. Natural anticoagulants in systemic lupus erythematosus. Deficiency of protein S bound to C4bp associates with recent history of venous thromboses, antiphospholipid antibodies, and the antiphospholipid syndrome. J Rheumatol 1991;18:552–558.

R417. Ruiz-Carrillo A, Affolter M, Renaud J. Genomic organization of the genes coding for the six main histones of the chicken: complete sequence of the H5 gene. J Mol Biol 1983; 170:843–859.

R418. Rummelt JD. Assessment of neuropsychological functioning in Systemic Lupus Erythematosus. Dissertation Abstracts International 1990.

R419. Rumore P, Steinman C. Nucleosome-like characteristics of circulating DNA in SLE [abstract]. Arthritis Rheum 1988;31: D32.

R420. Rumore PM, Steinman CR. Endogenous circulating DNA in systemic lupus erythematosus: Occurrence as multimeric complexes bound to histone. J Clin Invest 1990;86(1):69–74.

R421. Runge LA. Risk/benefit analysis of hydroxychloroquine sulfate treatment of rheumatoid arthritis. Am J Med 1983 Jul 18;75 Suppl 1A:52–56.

R422. Runyon BA, LaBrecque DR, Anuras S. The spectrum of liver disease in systemic lupus erythematosus: Report of 33 histologically-proved cases and review of the literature. Am J Med 1980 Aug;69(2):187–194.

R423. Rupin A, Gruel Y, Poumier-Gashard P, Chassaigne M, Leroy J, Bardos P. Thrombocytopenia in systemic lupus erythematosus: association with antiplatelet and anticardiolipin antibodies. Clin Immunol Immunopathol 1990;55:418–426.

R424. Ruppert GB, Barth WF. Tolmetin-induced aseptic meningitis. JAMA 1981 Jan 2;245(1):67–68.

R425. Rupprecht T, Wenzel D, Michalk D. Pancreatitis as the first symptom of lupus erythematodes in childhood [English abstract]. Monatsschr Kinderheilkd 1988 Mar;136(3): 143–145.

R426. Rush PJ, Baumal R, Shore A, Balfe JW, Schreiber M. Correlation of renal histology with outcome in children with lupus nephritis. Kidney Int 1986;29:1066–1071.

R427. Ruskin J, Remington JS. The compromised host and infection. I. Pneumocystis carinii pneumonia. JAMA 1967 Dec 18; 202:1070–1074.

R428. Ruskin J, Remington JS. Pneumocystis carinii pneumonia. JAMA 1968;203:162–163.

R429. Russell AS, Ziff M. Natural antibodies to procainamide. Clin Exp Immunol 1968 Nov;3:901–909.

R430. Russell GI, Bing RF, Jones JAG, Thurston H, Swales JD. Hydralazine sensitivity: clinical features, autoantibody changes and HLA-DR phenotype. Q J Med 1987;65:845–852.

R431. Russell ML, Hanna WM. Ultrastructural pathology of skeletal muscle in various rheumatic diseases. J Rheumatol 1988 Mar;15(3):445–453.

R432. Russell PJ, Hicks JD, Burnet RM. Cyclophosphamide treatment of kidney diseases in (NZB × NZW) F1 mice. Lancet 1966;1:1279.

R433. Russell PW, Haserick JR, Zuker EM. Epilepsy in systemic lupus erythematosus; effect of cortisone and ACTH. Arch Intern Med 1951 Jul;88:78–92.

R434. Russell RI, Allan JG, Patrick R. Active chronic hepatitis after chlorpromazine ingestion. BMJ 1973 Mar 17;1:655–656.

R435. Rustagi AK, Currie MS, Logue GL. Complement-activating antineutrophil antibody in systemic lupus erythematosus. Am J Med 1985;78:971–977.

R436. Rustagi AK, Peppercorn MA. Gluten-sensitive enteropathy and systemic lupus erythematosus. Arch Intern Med 1988 Jul; 148(7):1583–1584.

R437. Rustin MH, Bull HA, Machin SJ, Koro O, Dowd PM. Effects of the lupus anticoagulant in patients with systemic lupus erythematosus on endothelial cell prostacyclin release and procoagulant activity. J Invest Dermatol 1988 May;90(5): 744–748.

R438. Rutherford BD. Procainamide-induced systemic lupus erythematosus. N Z Med J 1968 Oct;68:235–240.

R439. Ruzicka T, Goerz G. Dapsone in the treatment of lupus erythematosus. Br J Dermatol 1981;104:53–56.

R440. Ruzicka T, Meurer M, Bieber T. Efficiency of acitretin in the treatment of cutaneous lupus erythematosus. Arch Dermatol 1988 Jun;124(6):897–902.

R441. Ruzicka T, Meurer M, Braun-Falco O. Treatment of cutaneous lupus erythematosus with etretinate. Acta Derm Venerol (Stockh) 1985;65:324–329.

R442. Ryan PFJ, Hughes GRV, Bernstein R, Mansilla R, Dollery CT. Lymphocytotoxic antibodies in hydralazine-induced lupus erythematosus. Lancet 1979;2:1248–1249.

R443. Ryan WE, Ellefson RD, Ward LE. Clinical conference: Lipid synovial effusion. Unique occurrence in systemic lupus erythematosus. Arthritis Rheum 1973 Nov– Dec;16:759–764.

R444. Rynes RI. Ophthalmologic safety of long-term hydroxychloroquine sulfate treatment. Am J Med 1983 Jul 18;75 Suppl 1A:35–39.

R445. Rynes RI. Side effects of antimalarial therapy. Br J Clin Prac 1987;41 Suppl 52:42–45.

R446. Rynes RI, Krohel G, Falbo A, Reinecke RD, Wolfe B, Bartholomew LE. Ophthalmologic safety of long-term hydroxychloroquine treatment. Arthritis Rheum 1979 Aug;22(8): 832–836.

S

S1. Saal JG, Daniel PT, Berg PA. Inbuprofen induced aplastic anemia in active connective tissue disease detected by drug-specific lymphocyte transformation. Klin Wochenschr 1986 May 15;64(10):481–485.

S2. Saarikoski S, Seppala M. Immunosuppression during pregnancy. Transmission of azathioprine and its metabolites from the mother to the fetus. Am J Obstet Gynecol 1973;115: 1100–1106.

S3. Sabbaga J, Line SR, Potocnjak P, Madaio MP. A murine nephritogenic monoclonal anti-DNA autoantibody binds directly to mouse laminin, the major non-collagenous protein component of the glomerular basement membrane. Eur J Immunol 1989 Jan;19(1):137–143.

S4. Sabban EL, Kuhn LJ, Sarmalkar M. Chloroquine and monensin alter the post translational processing and secretion of dopamine beta-hydroxylase and other proteins from PC 12 cells. Ann NY Acad Sci 1986;493:399–402.

S5. Sabbour MS, Osman LM. Comparison of chlorambucil, azathioprine or cyclophosphamide combined with corticosteroids in the treatment of lupus nephritis. Br J Dermatol 1979 Feb; 100(2):113–125.

S6. Sabharwal UK, Vaughan JH, Kaplan RA, Robinson CA, Curd JG. Frentizole therapy in systemic lupus erythematosus. Arthritis Rheum 1980 Dec;23(12):1376–1380.

S7. Sablitzky F, Wildner G, Rajewsky K. Somatic mutation and clonal expansion of B cells in an antigen-driven immune response. EMBO J 1985;4:345–350.

S8. Sabo I. The lanthanic or undifferentiated collagen disease. Hiroshima J Med Sci 1969 Dec;18:259–264.

S9. Sacco RL, Owen J, Mohr JP, Tatemichi T, Grossman BA. Free protein S deficiency: a possible association with cerebrovascular occlusion. Stroke 1989;20:1657–1661.

S10. Sachs DH. Anti-idiotype to MHC receptors—a possible route to specific transplantation tolerance? Intern Rev Immunol 1988;3:313.

S11. Sacks DL, Esser KM, Sher A. Immunization of mice against African trypanosomiasis using anti-idiotypic antibodies. J Exp Med 1982;155:1108.

S12. Sadeh M, Sarova-Pinhas I, Ohry A. Sensory ataxia as an initial symptom of systemic lupus erythematosus [letter]. J Rheumatol 1980 May–Jun;7(3):420–421.

S13. Sadiq SA, van den Berg LH, Kilidereas K, Harp AP, Latov N. Human monoclonal antineurofilament antibody cross-reacts with a neuronal surface protein. J Neurosci Res 1991;29:319.

S14. Saga Y, Tung J-S, Shen F-W, Boyse EA. Alternative use of 5' exons in the specification of Ly-5 isoforms distinguishing hemato-poietic cell lineages. Proc Natl Acad Sci USA 1987;84: 5364–5368.

S15. Sagawa A, Abdou NI. Suppressor-cell antibody in systemic lupus erythematosus. Possible mechanism for suppressor-cell dysfunction. J Clin Invest 1979 Mar;63:536–539.

S16. Saiki O, Saeki Y, Tanaka T, Doi S, Hara H, Negoro S, Igarashi T, Kishimoto S. Development of selective IgM deficiency in systemic lupus erythematosus patients with disease of long duration. Arthritis Rheum 1987;30:1289–1292.

S17. Saiki O, Tanaka T, Kishimoto S. Defective expression of p70/75 interleukin-2 receptor in T cells from patients with systemic lupus erythematosus: a possible defect in the process of increased intracellular calcium leading to p70/p75 expression. J Rheumatol 1990;17:1303–1307.

S18. Sainis K, Datta SK. CD4 T cell lines with selective patterns of autoreactivity as well as CD4,CD8 negative helper cell lines augment the production of idiotypes shared by pathogenic anti-DNA autoantibodies in the NZB x SWR model of lupus nephritis. J Immunol 1988;140:2215–2224.

S19. St. Clair EW, Kenan D, Burch JA Jr, Keene JD, Pisetsky DS. Anti-La antibody production by MRL-lpr/lpr mice. Analysis of fine specialty. J Immunol 1991:146:1885–1892.

S20. St. Clair EW, Pisetsky DS, Reich CG, Chambers J, Keene JD. Quantitative immunoassay of anti-La antibodies using purified recombinant La antigen. Arthritis Rheum 1988;31:506–514.

S21. St. Clair EW, Pisetsky DS, Reich CG, Keene JD. Analysis if the autoantibody binding to different regions of the human LA antigen expressed in recombinant proteins. J Immunol 1988;141:4173–4180.

S22. St. Clair EW, Query CC, Bentley R, Keene JD, Polisson RP, Allen NB, Caldwell DS, Rice JR, Cox C, Piesetsky DS. Expression of autoantibodies to recombinant (U1) RNP-associated 70K antigen in systemic lupus erythematosus. Clin Immunol Immunopathol 1990;54:266–280.

S23. St. Hill CA, Finn R, Denye V. Depression of cellular immunity in pregnancy due to a serum factor. BMJ 1973;3:513–514.

S24. Saissy JM, Gohard R, Diatta B, Kempf J, Raux O. The role of diazepam as monotherapy in the treatment of chloroquine intoxication. Presse Med 1989 Dec;18(41):2022–2023.

S25. Saito H. Tyrosine phosphatases: Cellular superstars in the offing. J NIH Res 1990;2:62–66.

S26. Saito I, Servenius B, Compton T, Fox RI. Detection of Epstein-Barr virus DNA by polymerase chain reaction in blood and tissue biopsies from patients with Sjögren's syndrome. J Exp Med 1989;169:2191–2198.

S26a. Sakaki T, Morimoto T, Utsumi S. Cerebral transmural angiitis and ruptures cerebral aneurysms in patients with systemic lupus erythematosus. Neurochirugia 1990 Jul;33(4): 132–135.

S27. Sakane T, Kotani H, Takada S, Murakawa Y, Ueda Y. A defect in the suppressor circuits among OKT4+ cell populations in patients with systemic lupus erythematosus occurs independently of a defect in the OKT8+ suppressor T cell function. J Immunol 1983 Aug;181:753–756.

S28. Sakane T, Murakawa Y, Nhoboru S, Ueda Y, Tsuchida T, Takada S, Yamauchi Y, Tsunematsu T. Familial occurrence of impaired interleukin-2 activity and increased peripheral blood B cells actively secreting immunoglobulins in systemic lupus erythematosus. Am J Med 1989;86:385–390.

S29. Sakane T, Steinberg AD, Arnett FC, Reinertsen JL, Green I. Studies of immune functions of patients with systemic lupus erythematosus. III. Characterization of lymphocyte subpopulations responsible for defective autologous mixed lymphocyte reactions. Arthritis Rheum 1979 Jul;22:770–776.

S30. Sakane T, Steinberg AD, Green I. Failure of autologous mixed lymphocyte reactions between T and non-T cells in patients with systemic lupus erythematosus. Proc Natl Acad Sci USA 1978 Aug;75:3464–3468.

S31. Sakane T, Steinberg AD, Reeves JP, Green I. Studies of immune functions of patients with systemic lupus erythematosus: Complement-dependent immunoglobulin-M anti-thymus derived cell antibodies preferentially inactive suppressor cells. J Clin Invest 1979 May;63:954–965.

S32. Sakane T, Steinberg AD, Reeves JP, Green I. Studies of immune functions of patients with systemic lupus erythematosus. 4. T-cell subsets and antibodies to T-cell subsets. J Clin Invest 1979 Nov;64:1260–1269.

S33. Sakane T, Suzuki N, Takada S, Ueda Y, Muarkawa Y, Tsuchida T, Yamauchi T, Kishimoto T. B cell hyperreactivity and its relation to distinct clinical features and the degree of disease activity in patients with SLE. Arthritis Rheum 1988;31:80–87.

S34. Sakano H, Maki R, Kurosawa Y, Roeder W, Tonegawa S. Two types of somatic recombination are necessary for the generation of complete immunoglobulin heavy-chain genes. Nature 1980;286:676–683.

S35. Sakata S, Nakamura S, Nagai K, Komaki T, Kawade M, Niwa T, Miura K. Two cases of systemic lupus erythematosus associated with hypothyroidism. Jpn J Med 1987 May;26(3): 373–376.

S36. Sakata S, Yamamoto M, Takuno H, Fuwa Y, Chimori K, Miura K. A case of systemic lupus erythematosus (SLE) associated with anti-thyrotropin (TSH) autoantibodies. Nippon Naika Gakkai Zasshi 1989 Apr;78(4):571–572.

S37. Sakemi T, Yamaguchi M, Fujimi S, Nagano Y, Uchida M. Effects of the methylprednisolone pulse therapy on renal function. Am J Nephrol 1991;11:48–53.

S38. Saki S, Tanaka K, Fujisawa M, Shiomi S, Saitoh S, Sakagami Y, Matsui T, Mizoguchi Y, Kuroki T, Harihara S. A patient with asymptomatic primary biliary cirrhosis in association with Sjogren syndrome developing features of systemic lupus erythematosus. Nippon Shokakibyo Gakkai Zasshi 1986;83: 2445–2449.

S39. Sakiya S, Iwasaki H, Takeda B, Takamizawa H. Endometrial carcinoma following chronic anovulation in a premenopausal woman with systemic lupus erythematosus. Acta Obstet Gynecol Scand 1988;67:553–536.

S40. Sakon SJ, Gershenson J, translators. Prokopchuk A 1A. Treatment of lupus erythematosus with acriquine [Clinical notes]. Introduction of Quinacrin in treatment of lupus erythematosus. Arch Dermatol Syph 1955;71:520.

S41. Saladino CF, Ben-Hur E. Quinacrine-enhanced killing response of cultured Chinese hamster cells by x-rays. Res Commun Chem Pathol Pharmacol 1978 Dec;22(3):629–632.

S42. Salazar-Paramo M, Garcia-de la Torre I, Hernandez-Vazquez L, Ortiz-Cadena A. Evidence of a new antigen-antibody system (anti-Mic-1) in patients with systemic lupus erythematosus and hyperthyroidism. J Rheumatol 1989 Feb;16(2):175–180.

S43. Salcedo JR, Spiegler BJ, Gibson E, Magilavy DB. The autoimmune disease systemic lupus erythematosus is not associated with left-handedness. Cortex 1985;21:645–647.

S44. Salmeron S, Lipsky PE. Immunosuppressive potential of antimalarials. Am J Med 1983;5:19–24.

S45. Salmon D, Verdier F, Malhotra K, Pussard E, Clavier F, Le Bras J, Vilde JL, Pocidalo JJ. Absence of effect of chloroquine in vivo on neutrophil oxidative metabolism in human subjects. J Antimocrob Chemother 1990 Mar;25(3):367–370.

S46. Salmon JE, Brogle NL, Edberg JE, Kimberly RP. Fcγ receptor III induces actin polymerization in human neutrophils and primes phagocytosis mediated by Fcγ receptor II. J Immunol 1991;146:997–1004.

S47. Salmon JE, Edberg JC, Brogle NL, Kimberly RP. Functional consequences of allelic variants of Fcγ receptors on human phagocytosis. Arthritis Rheum 1990;33:S108.

S48. Salmon JE, Edberg JC, Kimberly RP, Mensa E, Ryan R. Fcγ receptor III on human neutrophils: Allelic variants have functionally distinct capacities. J Clin Invest 1990;85:1287–1295.

S49. Salmon JE, Kapur S, Kimberly RP. Gammaglobulin for intravenous use induces an Fcγ receptor-specific decrement in phagocytosis by blood monocytes. Clin Immunol Immunopath 1987;43:23–33.

S50. Salmon JE, Kapur S, Kimberly RP. Opsonin-independent ligation of Fc gamma receptors. The 3G8-bearing receptors on neutrophils mediate the phagocytosis of concanavalin-A treated erythrocytes and non-opsonized Escherichia coli. J Exp Med 1987;166:1798–1813.

S51. Salmon JE, Kapur S, Meryhew NL, Runquist OA, Kimberly RP. High-dose, pulse intravenous methylprednisolone enhances Fcγ receptor-mediated mononuclear phagocyte function in systemic lupus erythematosus. Arthritis Rheum 1989; 32:717–725.

S52. Salmon JE, Kimberly RP. Phagocytosis of concanavalin A-treated erythrocytes is mediated by the Fcγ receptor. J Immunol 1986;137:456–462.

S53. Salmon JE, Kimberly RP, Gibofsky A, Fotino M. Defective mononuclear phagocyte function in systemic lupus erythematosus: Dissociation of Fc receptor-ligand binding and internalization. J Immunol 1984;133:2525–2531.

S54. Salmon JE, Kimberly RP, Gibofsky A, Fotino M. Altered phagocytosis by monocytes from HLA-DR2 and DR3-positive healthy adults is Fcγ receptor-specific. J Immunol 1986;136: 3625–3632.

S55. Salo OP, Tallberg T, Mustakallio KK. Demonstration of fibrin in skin diseases. I. Lichen rubor planus and lupus erythematosus. Acta Dermatovener (Stockh) 1972;52:291–294.

S56. Sambrook PN, Eisman JA, Champion GD, Pocock NA. Sex hormonal status and osteoporosis in postmenopausal women with rheumatoid arthritis. Arthritis Rheum 1988;31:973–978.

S57. Sammaritano LR, Gharavi AE, Lockshin MD. Antiphospholipid antibody syndrome: Immunologic and clinical aspects. Semin Arthritis Rheum 1990 Oct;20(2):81–96.

S58. Sammartino L, Webber LM, Hogarth PM, McKenzie IFC, Garson OM. Assignment of the gene coding for human FcRII (CD32) to bands q23q24 on chromosome 1. Immunogenetics 1988;28:380–381.

S59. Samsoen M, Grosshaus E, Basset A. Thalidomide in the treatment of chronic lupus erythematosus [English abstract]. Ann Dermatol Vernereol (Paris) 1980 Jun;107(6):515–523.

S60. Samtleben VW, Gurland HJ. Plasmapheresis in lupus nephritis: rational (sic) and clinical experiences. Nieren-und Hochdruckkrankheiten 1986;15:104–108.

S61. Samuels P, Pfeifer SM. Autoimmune disease in pregnancy. The obstetrician's view. Rheum Dis N A 1989;15:307–322.

S62. Samuelson CO, Williams HJ. Ibuprofen associated aseptic meningitis in systemic lupus erythematosus. West Med J 1979 Jul;131:57–59.

S63. Samuelsson B, Dahlen S-E, Lindgren JA, Rouzer CA, Serhan CA. Leukotrienes and lipoxins: structures, biosynthesis, and biological effects. Science 1987;237:1171–1176.

S64. Sanchez NP, Peters MS, Winkelmann RK. The histopathology of lupus erythematosus panniculitis. J Am Acad Dermatol 1981;5:673–680.

S65. Sanchez R, Jonsson R, Ahlfors E, Backman K, Czerkinsky C. Oral lesions of lupus erythematosus patients in relation to other chronic inflammatory oral diseases: an immunologic study. Scand J Dent Res 1988 Dec;96(6):569–578.

S66. Sanchez-Guerrero J, Alarcon-Segovia D. Salmonella pericarditis with tamponade in systemic lupus erythematosus. Br J Rheumatol 1990;29:69–71.

S67. Sanders ME, Alexander EL, Koski CL, Frank MM, Joiner KA. Detection of activated terminal complement (C5b-9) in cerebrospinal fluid from patients with central nervous system involvement of primary Sjogren's syndrome or systemic lupus erythematosus. J Immunol 1987;138(7):2095–2099.

S68. Sands ML, Ryczak M, Brown RB. Recurrent aseptic meningitis followed by transverse myelitis as a presentation of systemic lupus erythematosus. J Rheumatol 1988 May;15(5): 862–864.

S69. Sandyk R. Transient global amnesia induced by lorazepam. Clin-Neuropharmacol 1985;8(3):297–298.

S70. Sankoorikal A, Stimmler M, Quismorio FP Jr. Contrasting effects of IgM rheumatoid factor on clinical manifestations of SLE. Arthritis Rheum 1990;34:5129.

S71. Sano H, Imokawa M, Steinberg AD, Morimoto C. Accumulation of guanine-cytosine-enriched low M.W. DNA fragments in lymphocytes of patients with systemic lupus erythematosus. J Immunol 1983 Jan;130(1):187–190.

S72. Sano H, Kumagai S, Namiuchi S, Uchiyama T, Yodoi J, Maeda M, Takatsuki K, Suginoshita T, Imura H. Systemic lupus erythematosus sera antilymphocyte reactivity; detection of antibodies to Tac-antigen positive T cell lines. Clin Exp Immunol 1986;63:8–16.

S73. Santen RJ, Wright IS. Systemic lupus erythematosus associated with pulmonary nocardiosis. Arch Intern Med 1967 Feb; 119(2):202–205.

S74. Santiago A, Satriano J, DeCandido S, Holthofer H, Schreiber R, Unkeless J, Schlondorff D. Specific Fcγ receptor on cultured rat mesangial cells. J Immunol 1989;143:2575–2582.

S75. Santoro TJ, Portanova JP, Kotzin BL. The contribution of L3T4 + T cells to lymphoproliferation and autoantibody production in MRL-lpr/lpr mice. J Exp Med 1988;167:1713–1718.

S76. Sanz I, Capra JD. The genetic origin of human autoantibodies. J Immunol 1988;140:3283–3285.

S77. Sanz I, Casali P, Thomas JW, Notkins AL, Capra JD. Nucleotide sequences of eight human natural autoantibody V_H regions reveals apparent restricted use of V_H families. J Immunol 1989;142:4054–4061.

S78. Sanz I, Kelly P, Williams C, Scholl S, Tucker P, Capra JD. The smaller human V_H gene families display remarkably little polymorphism. EMBO J 1989;8:3741–3748.

S79. Sappington JT, Fiorito EM. Thermal feedback in Raynaud's phenomenon secondary to systemic lupus erythematosus: long term remission of target symptoms. Biofeedback Self Regul 1985 Dec;10(4):335–341.

S80. Sargent CA, Dunham I, Trowsdale J, Campbell RD. Human major histocompatibility complex contains genes for the major heat shock protein HSP70. Proc Nat Acad Sci USA 1989; 86:1968–1972.

S81. Sargent IL, Wilkins T, Redman CW. Maternal immune responses to the fetus in early pregnancy and recurrent miscarriage. Lancet 1988;2(8620):1099–1104.

S82. Sartoris DJ, Resnick D, Gershuni D, Bielecki D, Meyers M. Comuted tomography with multiplanar reformation and 3-dimensional image analysis in the preoperative evaluation of ischemic necrosis of the femoral head. J Rheumatol 1986 Feb; 13(1):153–163.

S83. Sarvetnick N, Fox RI. Interferon-gamma and sexual dimorphism of autoimmunity. Mol Biol Med 1990;7(4):323–331.

S84. Sasaki T, Muryoi T, Takai O, Tamate E, Ono Y, Koide Y, Ishida N, Yoshinaga K. Selective elimination of anti-DNA antibody-producing cells by antiidiotypic antibody conjugated with neocarzinostatin. J Clin Invest 1986;77:1382–1386.

S85. Sasaki T, Shibata S, Hirabayashi Y, Sekiguchi Y, Yoshinaga K. Accessory cell activity of monocytes in anti-DNA antibody production in systemic lupus erythematosus. Clin Exp Immunol 1989;77:37–42.

S86. Sasaki T, Tamate E, Muryoi T, Takai O, Yoshinaga K. In vitro manipulation of human anti-DNA antibody production by anti-idiotypic antibodies conjugated with neocarzinostatin. J Immunol 1989;142:1159–1165.

S87. See H116.

S88. Sasamura H, Nakamoto H, Ryuzaki M, Kamagai K, Abe S, Suzuki H, Hirakata M, Tojo T, Handa M, Yamamoto M. Repeated intestinal ulcerations in a patient with systemic lupus erythematosus and high serum antiphospholipid antibody levels. South Med J 1991 Apr;84(4):515–517.

S89. Sassani JW, Brucker AJ, Cobbs W, Campbell C. Progressive chloroquine retinopathy. Ann Ophthalmol 1983 Jan;15(1): 19–22.

S90. Sasson S, Mayer M. Effect of androgenic steroids on rat thymus thymocytes in suspension. J Steroid Biochem 1981; 14:509–512.

S91. Satake Y, Takada K, Ikeda K, Shiosaka T, Fujita S, Kobayashi Y. A case of primary liver cell cancer complicating lupoid hepatitis. Jap J Med 1988 Feb;27(1):83–86.

S92. Sato EH, Edwards JA, Soo C, Ariga H, Vendramini AC, Sullivan DA. ARVO. Res presentations on Sjogren's Syndrome, 1991.

S93. Sato K, Miyasaka N, Yamaoka K, Okuda M, Yata J, Nishioka K. Quantitative defect of CD4 + 2H4 + cells in systemic lupus. Arthritis Rheum 1987;30:1407–1411.

S94. Satz P, Soper HV. Left-handedness, dyslexia, and autoimmune disorder: A critique. J Clin Exp Neuropsychol. 1986;8: 453–458.

S95. Saulsbury FT. Antinuclear antibody specificity in juvenile rheumatoid arthritis [abstract]. Clin Res 1985; 33:512A.

S96. Saulsbury FT. Antibody to ribonucleoprotein in pauciarticular juvenile rheumatoid arthritis. J Rheumatol 1988 Feb;15(2): 295–297.

S97. Saulsbury FT, Kesler RW, Kennaugh JM, Barber JC, Chevalier RT. Overlap syndrome of juvenile rheumatoid arthritis and systemic lupus erythematosus. J Rheumatol 1982 Jul–Aug;9(4):610–612.

S98. Savi M, Ferraccioli GF, Neri TM, Zanelli P, Dall Aglio PP, Tincani A, Bales G, Cattaneo R. HLA-DR antigens and anticardiolipin antibodies in northern Italian systemic lupus erythematosus patients. Arthritis Rheum 1988 Dec;31(12):1568–1570.

S99. Savitz MH, Katz SS, Lestch SD, Boltin HN, Becker A. Mirror-image intracerebral hemorrhages in a patient with systemic lupus erythematosus. Mt Sinai J Med (NY) 1987 Sep;54(6): 522–524.

S100. Sawada S, Talal N. Characteristics of in vitro production of antibodies to DNA in normal and autoimmune mice. J Immunol 1979;122:2309–2315.

S101. Saxe PA, Altman RD, Igarashi T, Tani K, Lie JT. Aortitis syndrome (Takayasu's Arteritis) associated with SLE [letter]. J Rheumatol 1990;17:1251–1252.

S102. Sayers G. Adrenal cortex and homeostasis. Physiol Rev 1950 Jul;30:241–320.

S103. Scambia G, Ranelletti FO, Benedetti Panici P, Piantelli M, Rumi C, Battaglia F, Larocca LM, Capelli A, Mancuso S. Type II-estrogen binding sites in a lymphoblastoid cell line and growth inhibitory effects of estrogen, anti-estrogen bioflavonoiditis. Int J Cancer 1990;46:1112–1116.

S104. Scarpelli DG, McCoy FW, Scott JK. Acute lupus erythematosus with laryngeal involvement. N Engl J Med 1959 Oct 1; 261:691–694.

S105. Schaff Z, Barry DW, Grimley PM. Cytochemistry of tubuloreticular structures in lymphocytes from patients with systemic lupus erythematosus and in cultures human lymphoid cells: comparison to a paramyxovirus. Lab Invest 1973;29(6): 557–586.

S106. Schaison G, Najean Y, Seligmann M, Flandrin G, Jacquillat C, Weil M, Cannat A, Ripault J, Dreyfus B, Bernard J. Acute leukemia with prolonged course and lupus syndrome [original in French]. Nouv Rev Fr Hematol 1969 May–Jun;9:329–448.

S107. Schaller J. Illness resembling lupus erythematosus in mothers of boys with chronic granulomatous disease. Ann Intern Med 1972;76:747–750.

S108. Schaller J. Lupus in childhood. Clin Rheum Dis 1982 Apr; 8(1):219–228.

S109. Schalier JG, Gilliland BG, Ochs HD, Leddy JP, Agodoa LC, Rosenfeld SI. Severe systemic lupus erythematosus with nephritis in a boy with deficiency of the fourth component of complement. Arthritis Rheum 1977;20:1519–1525.

S110. Scharf M, Khosia N, Brocker N, Goff P. Differential amnestic properties of short and long-acting benzodiazepines. J Clin Psychiatry 1984 Feb;45(2):51–53.

S111. Scharf MB, Khosia N, Lysaght R, Brocker N, Moran J. Anterograde amnesia with oral lorazepam. J Clin Psychiatry 1983 Oct;44(10):362–364.

S112. Scharre D, Petri M, Engman E, DeArmond S. Large intracranial arteritis with giant cells in systemic lupus erythematosus. Ann Intern Med 1986 May;104(5):661–662.

S113. Schatten S, Howard RL, Judd RL. Treatment of severe lupus nephritis with combined monthly intravenous cyclophosphamide and methylprednisolone [abstract]. Arthritis Rheum 1989 Apr;32(4) Suppl:S75.

S114. Schattner A, Miller KB, Kaburaki Y, Schwartz RS. Suppressor cell function and anti-DNA antibody idiotypes in the serum of SLE patients and their first-degree relatives. Clin Immunol Immunopathol 1986;41:417–426.

S115. Schatz M, Patterson R, Zeitz S, O'Rourke J, Melam H. Corticosteroid therapy for the pregnant asthmatic patient. JAMA 1975;223:804.

S116. Schechner RS, Greenstein SM, Glicklich D, Mallis M, Quinn T, Sablay B, Veith FJ, Tellis VA. Renal transplantation in the black population with systemic lupus erythematosus: a single center experience. Transplant Proc 1989 Dec;21(6): 3937–3938.

S117. Scheib JS, Waxman J. Congenital heart block in successive pregnancies: A case report and evaluation of risk with therapeutic consideration. Obstet Gynecol 1989;73:481–484.

S118. Scheinbart LS, Johnson MA, Gross LA, Edelstein SR, Richardson BC. Procainamide inhibits DNA methyltransferase in a human T cell line. J Rheumatol 1991;18:530–534.

S119. Scheinberg L. Polyneuritis in systemic lupus erythematosus; review of literature and report of case. N Engl J Med 1956 Aug 30;255:416–421.

S120. Scheinberg MA, Cathcart ES. Antibody-dependent direct cytotoxicity of human lymphocytes. I. Studies on peripheral blood lymphocytes and sera of patients with systemic lupus erythematosus. Clin Exp Immunol 1976 May;24:317–322.

S121. Scheinberg MA, Cathcart ES, Goldstein AL. Thymosin-induced reduction of "null cells" in peripheral-blood lymphocytes of patients with systemic lupus erythematosus. Lancet 1975;1:424–446.

S122. Schenfeld L, Gray RG, Poppo MJ, Gaylis NB, Gottlieb NL. Bacterial monarthritis due to Neisseria meningitidis in systemic lupus erythematosus. J Rheumatol 1981 Jan–Feb;8(1): 145–148.

S123. Scherak O, Smolen JS, Mayr WR. Prevalence of HLA-DRw2 not increased in systemic lupus erythematosus. N Engl J Med 1979;301:612.

S124. Scherak O, Smolen JS, Mayr WR. HLA-DRw3 and systemic lupus erythematosus. Arthritis Rheum 1980;23:954–957.

S125. Scherak O, Smolen JS, Menzel EJ, Kojer M, Kolarz G. Effect of levamisole on immunological parameters in patients with systemic lupus erythematosus. Scand J Rheumatol 1980;9(2): 106–112.

S126. Scherly D, Boelens W, Dathan NA, van Venrooij WJ, Mattaj IW. Major determinants of the specificity of interaction between small nuclear ribonucleoproteins U1A and U2B″ and their cognate RNAs. Nature 1990;345:502–508.

S127. Scherly D, Boelens W, van Venrooij WJ, Dathan NA, Hamm J, Mattaj IW. Identification of the RNA binding segment of human U1 A protein and definition of its binding site on U1 snRNA. Embo J 1989;8:4163–4170.

S128. Scherly D, Dathan NA, Boelens W, van Vanrooij WJ, Mattaj IW. The U2B″ RNP motif as a site of protein interaction. Embo J 1990;9:3675–3681.

S129. Schewach-Millet M, Shapiro D, Ziv R, Trau H. Subacute cutaneous lupus erythematosus associated with breast carcinoma. J Am Acad Dermatol 1988;19:406–408.

S130. Schiff C, Milili M, Fougereau M. Functional and pseudogenes are similarly organized and may equally contribute to the extensive antibody diversity of the Ig V$_H$II family. EMBO J 1985;4:1225–1230.

S131. Schiff C, Milili M, Hue I, Rudikoff S, Fougereau M. Genetic basis for expression of the idiotypic network. One unique Ig V$_H$ germ line gene accounts for the major family of Ab1 and Ab3 (Ab1′) antibodies of the GAT system. J Exp Med 1986;163:573–587.

S132. Schiffenbauer J, McCarthy DM, Nygard NR, Woulfe SL, Didier DK, Schwartz BD. A unique sequence of the NZW I-E beta chain and its possible contribution to autoimmunity in the (NZB × NZW)F1 mouse. J Exp Med 1989 Sep;170(3):971–984.

S133. Schiffenbauer J, Wegrzyn L. Sequence of class II major histocompatibility complex genes from MRL mice: conserved amino acids in the I-E beta chains for autoimmune mice. Arthritis Rheum 1991;34:1411–1415.

S134. Schifferli JA. Hydralazine and isoniazid reduce the formation of soluble immune complexes by complement. Immunol Lett 1985;9:297–299.

S135. Schifferli JA, Bartolotti SR, Peters DK. Inhibition of immune precipitation by complement. Clin Exp Immunol 1980;1:387–394.

S136. Schifferli JA, Ng YC, Estreicher J, Walport MJ. The clearance of tetanus toxoid/anti-tetanus toxoid immune complexes from the circulation of humans. Complement-and erythrocyte complement receptor 1-dependent mechanisms. J Immunol 1988;140:899–904.

S137. Schifferli JA, Ng YC, Paccaud J-P, Walport MJ. The role of hypocomplementaemia and low erythrocyte complement receptor type 1 numbers in determining abnormal immune complex clearance in humans. Clin Exp Immunol 1989;75:329–335.

S138. Schifferli JA, Ng YC, Peters DK. The role of complement and its receptor in the elimination of immune complexes. N Engl J Med 1986;315:488–495.

S139. Schifferli JA, Steiger G, Hauptmann G, Spaeth PJ, Sjoholm AG. Formation of soluble immune complexes by complement in sera of patients with various hypocomplementemic states. Difference between inhibition of immune precipitation and solubilization. J Clin Invest 1985;74:2127–2133.

S140. Schifferli JA, Taylor RP. Physiological and pathological aspects of circulating immune complexes. Kidney Int 1989;35:993–1003.

S141. Schilling PJ, Kurzrock R, Kantarjian H, Gutterman JU, Talpaz M. Development of systemic lupus erythematosus after interferon therapy for chronic myelogenous leukemia. Cancer 1991;68:1536–1537.

S142. Schiodt M. Oral discoid lupus erythematosus. II. Skin lesions and systemic lupus erythematosus in sixty-six patients with 6-year follow-up. Oral Surg 1984 Feb;57(2):177–180.

S143. Schiodt M. Oral discoid lupus erythematosus . III. A histo-pathologic study of sixty-six patients. Oral Surg 1984 Mar;57:281–293.

S144. Schiodt M. Oral manifestations of lupus erythematosus. Int J Oral Surg 1984 Apr;13(2):101–147.

S145. Schleicher EM. LE cells after oral contraceptives. Lancet 1968 Apr 13;1:821–822.

S146. Schleider MA, Nachman RL, Jaffe EA, Coleman M. A clinical study of the lupus anticoagulant. Blood 1976 Oct;48:499–509.

S147. Schleissner LA, Sheehan WW, Orselli RC. Lupus erythematosus in a patient with amyloidosis, adrenal insufficiency, and subsequent immunoblastic sarcoma. Demonstration of the LE phenomenon in the lung. Arthritis Rheum 1976 Mar–Apr;19(2):249–255.

S148. Schmauss C, Lerner MR. The closely related small nuclear ribonucleoprotein polypeptides N and B′/B are distinguishable by antibodies as well as by differences in their mHNAs and gene structures. J Biol Chem 1990;265:10733–10739.

S149. Schmauss C, McAllister G, Ohosone Y, Hardin JA, Lerner MR. A comparison of snRNP associated autoantigens: human N, rat N, and human B/B′. Nucleic Acids Res 1989;17:1733–1743.

S150. Schmid I, Anasetti C, Petersen FB, Storb R. Marrow transplantation for severe aplastic anemia associated with exposure to quinacrine. Blut 1990 Aug–Sep;61(2–3):52–54.

S151. Schmiedeke TM, Stockl FW, Weber R, Sugisaki Y, Batsford SR, Vogt A. Histones have high affinity for the glomerular basement membrane. J Exp Med 1989 Jun 1;169(6):1879–1894.

S152. Schneebaum AB, Singleton JD, West SG, Blodgett JK, Allen LG, Cheronis JC, Kotzin BL. Association of psychiatric manifestations with antibodies to ribosomal P proteins in systemic lupus erythematosus. Am J Med 1991;90:54–62.

S153. Schneider J, Chin W, Friou GJ, Cooper SM, Harding B, Hill RL, Quismorio FP. Reduced antibody-dependent cell-mediated cytotoxicity in systemic lupus erythematosus. Clin Exp Immunol 1975 May;20:187–192.

S154. Schneider M, Berning T, Waldendorf M, Glaser J, Gerlach U. Immunoadsorbent plasma perfusion in patients with systemic lupus erythematosus. J Rheumatol 1990 Jul;17(7):900–907.

S155. Schneider M, Hengst K, Waldendorf M, Hogelmann B, Gerlach U. The value of serum laminin Pl in monitoring disease activity in patients with systemic lupus erythematosus. Scand J Rheumatol 1988;17:417–422.

S156. Schnitzer B. Reactive lymphoid hyperplasia in surgical pathology of the lymph nodes and related organs. In: Jaffe ES, editor. Major problems in pathology series. Philadelphia: Saunders, 1985;16:46.

S157. Schocket AL, Lain D, Kohler PF, Steigerwald J. Immune complex vasculitis as a cause of ascites and pleural effusions in systemic lupus erythematosus. J Rheumatol 1978 Spring;5(1):33–38.

S158. Schoenfeld Y, Liuni E, Shaklai M, Pinkhas J. Sensitization to ibuprofen in systemic lupus erythematosus. JAMA 1980 Aug 8;244:547–548.

S158a. Schoenfeld Y, El-Roeiy A, Ben-Yehuda O, Pick AI. Detection of anti-histone activity in sera of patients with monoclonal antibodies. Clin Immunol Immunopathol 1987;42:250–258.

S159. Schoenfeld Y, Pick AL, Danziger Y, Kalaczi I, Frolichman R, Pinkhas J. Immunoglobulin chantes in systemic lupus erythematosus. Ann Allergy 1977 Aug;39:99–111.

S159a. Shoenfeld Y, Segol G, Segol O, Neary B, Klajman A, Stollar BD, Isenberg DA. Detection of antibodies to total histones and their subfractions in systemic lupus erythematosus patients and their asymptomatic relatives. Arthritis Rheum 1987;30:169–175.

S159b. Schoenfeld Y, Segol O. Anti-histone antibodies in SLE and other autoimmune diseases. Clin Exp Rheumatol 1989; 7: 265–271.

S160. Schoenfeld Y, Vilner Y, Reshef T, Klajman A, Skibin A, Kooperman O, Kennedy RD. Increased presence of common systemic lupus erythematosus (SLE) anti-DNA idiotypes (16/6 ld, 32/15 ld) is induced by procainamide. J Clin Immunol 1987;7:410–419.

S161. Schofer K, Feldges A, Baelocher K, Parisot RF, Wilhelm JA, Matter L. Systemic lupus erythematosus in staphylococcus aureus hyperimmunoglobulinemia E syndrome. BMJ 1983 Aug 20;287:524–526.

S162. Scholtz JR. Topical therapy of psoriasis with fluocinolone acetonide. Arch Dermatol 1961 Dec;84:1029–1030.

S163. Scholz W, Isakov N, Mally MI, Theofilopoulos AN, Altman A. Lpr T cell hyporesponsiveness to mitogens linked to deficient receptor-stimulated phosphoinositide hydrolysis. J Biol Chem 1988;263:3626–3631.

S164. Schonhofer PS, Groticke J. Fatal necrotizing vasculitis associated with nomifensine. Lancet 1985;2:221.

S165. Schorer AE, Wickman NWR, Watson KV. Lupus anticoagulant induces a selective defect in thrombin-mediated endothelial prostacyclin release and platelet aggregation. Br J Haematol 1989;71:399.

S166. Schorlemmer HU, Davies P, Allison A. Ability of activated complement components to induce lysosomal enzyme release from macrophages. Nature 1976;261:48–52.

S167. Schot LPC, Verheul HAM, Schuurs AHWN. Effect of nandralone decanoate on Sjogren's Syndrome-like disorders in NZBW mice. Clin Exp Immunol 1984;57:571–574.

S168. Schousboe JT, Koch AE, Chang RW. Chronic lupus peritonitis with ascites; review of the literature with a case report. Sem Arthritis Rheum 1988 Nov;18(2):121–126.

S169. Schrager NA, Rothfield NF. Clinical significance of serum properdin levels and properdin deposition at the dermal epidermal junction in lupus erythematosus. J Clin Invest 1976; 57:212–216.

S170. Schraven B, Roux M, Hutmacher B, Meuer S. Alternative pathway activation of human T-lymphocytes involves the CD45 glycoproteins. In: Knapp W, Dorken B, Gilks WR, et al. Leucocyte Typing IV. Oxford: Oxford University Press, 1989: 640–643.

S171. Schraven B, Roux M, Hutmacher B, Meuer SC. Triggering of the alternative pathway of human T cell activation involves member of the T 200 family of glycoproteins. Eur J Immunol 1989;19:397–403.

S172. Schraven B, Samstag Y, Altevogt P, Meuer SC. Association of CD2 and CD45 on human T lymphocytes. Nature 1990; 345:71–74.

S173. Schreiber AD. Autoimmune hemolytic anemia. Ped Clin North Am 1980 May;27:253–267.

S174. Schreiber AD, Chien P, Tomaski A, Cines DB. Effects of danazol in immune thrombocytopenic purpura. N Engl J Med 1987;316:503–508.

S175. Schreiber AD, Frank MM. The role of antibody and complement in the immune clearance and destruction of erythrocytes. I. In vivo effects of IgG and IgM complement fixing sites. J Clin Invest 1972 Mar;51:575–582.

S176. Schreiber AD, Frank MM. The roles of antibody and complement in the immune clearance and destruction of erythrocytes. II. Molecular nature of IgG and IgM complement fixing sites and effects of their interaction with serum. J Clin Invest 1972 Mar;51:583–589.

S177. Schreiber AD, Nettl FM, Sanders MC, King M, Szabolcs P, Friedman D, Gomez F. Effect of endogenous and synthetic sex steroids on the clearance of antibody-coated cells. J Immunol 1988;141:2959–2966.

S177a. Schreiber AD, Parsons J, McDermott P, Cooper RA. Effect of glucocorticoids on the human monocyte IgG and complement receptors. J Clin Invest 1975;56:1189–1197.

S178. Schreiber JR, Patawaran M, Tosi M, Lennon J, Pier GB. Anti-idiotype-induced, lipopolysaccharide-specific antibody response to Pseudomona aeruginosa. J Immunol 1990;144: 1023.

S179. Schreiner GE. The nephrotic syndrome. In: Strauss MB, Welt LG, editors. Diseases of the Kidney. Boston: Little Brown 1963:335–444.

S180. Schreiner GF, Cotran RS, Pardo V, Unanue EM. A mononuclear cell component in experimental immunological glomerulonephritis. J Exp Med 1978 Feb;147:369–384.

S181. Omitted.

S182. Schroeder HW Jr, Hillson JL, Perlmutter RM. Early restriction of the human antibody repertoire. Science 1987;238: 791–793.

S183. Schroeder JL, Hahn BH, Beale MG, Pietscher LS. Genetic, hormonal, and immune studies in a pair of identical twin boys discordant for lupus. Arthritis Rheum 1983;26:1399–1404.

S184. Schroeder JO, Euler HE, Loffler H. Synchronization of plasmapheresis and pulse cyclophosphamide in severe systemic lupus erythematosus. Ann Intern Med 1987 Sep;107(3): 344–346.

S185. Schulz EJ, Menter MA. Treatment of discoid and subacute lupus erythematosus and cyclophosphamide. Br J Dermatol 1971;85 Suppl:60.

S186. Schulze P, Audring H, Sonnichsen N. Erythema elevatum diutinum—a rare variant of skin changes in systemic lupus erythematosus. Dermatol Monatsschr 1989;175(10): 628–634.

S187. Schumacher HJ. Electron microscopic study of synovial fluid cells in systemic lupus erythematosus [abstract]. Arthritis Rheum 1978 Jun;21(5):590.

S188. Schumacher HR Jr, Sieck MS, Rothfuss S, Clayburne GM, Baumgarten DF, Mochan BS, Kant JA. Reproducibility of synovial fluid analysis. A study among four laboratories. Arthritis Rheum 1986 Jan;29(6):770–774.

S189. Schumann D, Kubicka-Muranyi M, Mirtschewa J, Gunther J, Kind P. Adverse immune reactions to gold. I. Chronic treatment with an Au (I) drug sensitizes mouse T cells not to Au (I), but to Au (III) and induces autoantibody formation. J Immunol 1990;145:2132–2139.

S190. Schupbach CW, Wheeler CE, Briggaman, RA, Warner NA, Kanof EP. Cutaneous manifestations of disseminated cryptococcosis. Arch Dermatol 1976;112:1734–1740.

S191. Schur P, Monroe M, Rothfield N. The subclass of antinuclear and antinucleic acid antibodies. Arthritis Rheum 1972; 15:174–182.

S192. Schur PH. Human gamma G subclasses. Prog Clin Immunol 1972;1:71–104.

S193. Schur PH. Complement in lupus. Clin Rheum Dis 1975;1: 519–543.

S194. Schur PH. Genetics of complement testing in the diagnosis of immune and autoimmune disease. Am J Clin Pathol 1977; 68:647–659.

S195. Schur PH. Genetics of complement deficiencies associated with lupus-like syndromes. Arthritis Rheum 1978 Jun;21 Suppl:S153-S160.

S196. Schur PH. Complement and lupus erythematosus. Arthritis Rheum 1982 Jul;25:793–798.

S197. Schur PH, editor. The Clinical Management of Systemic Lupus Erythematosus. Orlando: Grune & Stratton. 1983

S198. Schur PH. Inherited complement component abnormalities. Ann Rev Med 1986;37:333–346.

S199. Schur PH. Handedness in systemic lupus erythematosus. Arthritis Rheum 1986;29:419–420.

S200. Schur PH. Complement and immune complexes in systemic lupus erythematosus. In: Wallace DJ, Dubois EL, editors. Dubois' Lupus Erythematosus, 3d ed. Philadelphia: Lea & Febiger, 1987.

S201. Schur PH. Caucasian ethnic variation and the evaluation of genetic, clinical and immunological factors in patients with SLE [abstract]. Clin Res 1988;36:537A.

S202. Schur PH. Fingerprint analysis of patients with systemic lupus erythematosus and their relatives. J Rheumatol 1990 Apr;17(4):482–484.

S203. Schur PH, Carpenter CB. Sharing of HLA haplotypes by parents of patients with systemic lupus erythematosus. Arthritis Rheum 1983;26:1104–1110.

S204. Schur PH, Marcus-Bagley D, Awdeh Z, Yunis EJ, Alper CA. The effect of ethnicity on major histocompatibility complex complement allotypes and extended haplotypes in patients with systemic lupus erythematosus. Arthritis Rheum 1990;33:985–992.

S205. Schur PH, Meyer I, Garovoy M, Carpenter CB. Associations between systemic lupus erythematosus and the major histocompatibility complex: clinical and immunological considerations. Clin Immunol Immunopathol 1982 Aug;24:263–275.

S206. Schur PH, Pandey JP, Fedrick JA. Gm allotypes in white patients with systemic lupus erythematosus. Arthritis Rheum 1985;28:828–830.

S207. Schur PH, Sandson J. Immunologic factors and clinical activity in systemic lupus erythematosus. N Engl J Med 1968 May 7;278:533–538.

S208. Schurmans S, Heusser CH, Qin HY, Merino J, Brighouse G, Lambert PH. In vivo effects of anti-IL-4 monoclonal antibody on neonatal induction of tolerance and on an associated autoimmune syndrome. J Immunol 1990;145:2465–2473.

S209. Schuurman HJ, Schemmann MH, de Weger RA, Aanstoot H, Hene R. Epstein-Barr virus in the sublabial salivary gland in Sjögren's syndrome. Am J Clin Pathol 1989;91:461–463.

S210. Schwartz IS, Grishman E. Rheumatoid nodules of the vocal cords as the initial manifestation of systemic lupus erythematosus. JAMA 1980 Dec 19;244(24):2751–2752.

S211. Schwartz MM, Fennell JS, Lewis EJ. Pathologic changes in the renal tubule in systemic lupus erythematosus. Human Pathol 1982 Jun;13:534–547.

S212. Schwartz MM, Kawala K, Roberts JL, Humes C, Lewis EJ. Clinical and pathological features of membranous glomerulonephritis of systemic lupus erythematosus. Am J Nephrol 1984 Sep–Oct;29:311.

S213. Schwartz R, Andre J. The chemical suppression of immunity. In: Grabar P, Miescher P, editors. International Symposium on Immunopathology 2d Brook Lodge, 1961. Mechanism of Cell and Tissue Damage Produced by Immune Reaction. New York: Grune & Stratton, 1962:385–409.

S214. Schwartz R, Dameshek W. The treatment of autoimmune hemolytic anemia with 6-mercaptopurine and thioguanine. Blood 1962 Apr;19:483–500.

S215. Schwartz RH. T-lymphocyte recognition of antigen in association with gene products of the major histocompatibility complex. Annu Rev Immunol 1985;3:237–261.

S216. Schwartz RH. A cell culture model for T lymphocyte clonal anergy. Science 1990;248:1349–1356.

S217. Schwartz RS. Immunologic and genetic aspects of systemic lupus erythematosus. Kidney Int 1981 Mar;29:474–484.

S218. Schwartz RS, Stollar BD. Origins of anti-DNA antibodies [review]. J Clin Invest 1985 Feb;75(2):321–327.

S219. Schwartzman ML. Modification of arachidonic acid metabolism via the cytochrome P450-related monooxygenase system. Adv Prostaglandin Thromboxand & Leukotriene Res 1990;20:241–249.

S220. See B443.

S221. Scofield RH, Harley JB. Autoantigenicity of Ro/SSA antigen is related to a nucleocapsid protein of vesicular stomatitis virus. Proc Natl Acad Sci USA 1991;88:3343–3347.

S222. Scolari F, Harms M, Gilardi S. Thalidomide in the treatment of LE [English abstract]. Dermatologica 1982 Oct;165(4):355–362.

S223. Scoles PV, Yoon YS, Makley JT, Kalamchi A. Nuclear magnetic resonance imaging in Legg-Calve-Perthes disease. J Bone Joint Surg (Am) 1984 Dec;66(9):1357–1363.

S224. See S227.

S225. Scopelitis E, Biundo JJ, Alspaugh MA. Anti-SSA antibody and other antinuclear antibodies in systemic lupus erythematosus. Arthritis Rheum 1980;23:287–293.

S226. Scott A, Rees EG. The relationship of systemic lupus erythematosus and discoid lupus erythematosus; a clinical and hematological study. Arch Dermatol 1959 Apr;79(4):422–435.

S227. Scott AA, Purohit DM. Neonatal renal failure: A complication of maternal antihypertensive therapy. Am J Obstet Gynecol 1989;160:1223–1224.

S228. Scott DE, Lindahl M, Gourley M, Balow J, Austin H, Plotz P, Wilder R, Blau C, Steinberg AD. Randomized trial of monthly methylprednisolone (IV-MP) versus cyclophosphamide (IV-CY) in lupus nephritis [abstract]. Arthritis Rheum 1990 Sep;33(9) Suppl:S12.

S229. Scott JR, Branch DW, Kochenour NK, Ward K. Intravenous immunoglobulin treatment of pregnant patients with recurrent pregnancy loss caused by antiphospholipid antibodies and Rh immunization. Am J Obstet Gynecol 1988;159:1055–1056.

S230. Scott JS, Maddison PJ, Taylor PJ, Escher E, Scott O, Skinner RP. Connective-tissue disease, antibodies to ribonucleoprotein, and congenital heart block. N Engl J Med 1983 Jul 28;39:209–212.

S231. Scott RAH. Anti-cardiolipin antibodies and preeclampsia. Br J Obstet Gynecol 1987;94:604–605.

S232. Scott TF, Goust JM, Strange CB, Brillman J. SLE, thrombocytopenia, and HTLV-1 [letter]. J Rheumatol 1990 Nov;17(11):1565–1566.

S233. Screpanti I, Morrone S, Meco D, Santoni A, Gulino A, Paolini R, Crisanti A, Mathieson BJ, Frati L. Steroid sensitivity of thymocytic subpopulations during intrathymic differentiation. Effects of 17 B estradiol and dexamethasone on subsets expressing T cell antigen receptor or IL-2 receptor. J Immunol 1989;142:3378–3383.

S234. Scribner C, Steinberg AD. The role of splenic colony-forming units in autoimmune disease. Clin Immunol Immunopathol 1988;49:133–142.

S235. Sculley DG, Sculley TB, Pope JH. Reactions of sera from patients with rheumatoid arthritis, systemic lupus erythematosus and infectious mononucleosis to Epstein-Barr virus-induced polypeptides. J Gen Virol 1986 Oct;67(Pt 10):2253–2258.

S236. Scully RE, Galdabini JJ, McNeely BU. Case records of the Massachusetts General Hospital. Weekly clinicopathological exercises. Case 17–1978. N Engl J Med 1978 May 4;198:1463–1470.

S237. Seaman AJ, Christerson JW. Demonstration of L.E. cells in pericardial fluid. Report of a case. JAMA 1952 May 10;149:145–147.

S238. Seaman WE, Blackman MA, Gindhart TD, Roubinian JR, Loeb JM, Talal N. B-estradiol reduced natural killer cells in mice. J Immunol 1978;121:2193–2198.

S239. Seaman WE, Ishak KG, Plotz PH. Aspirin-induced hepatotoxicity in patients with systemic lupus erythematosus. Ann Intern Med 1974 Jan;80:1–8.

S240. Seaman WE, Plotz PH. Effect of aspirin on liver tests in patients with RA or SLE and in normal volunteers. Arthritis Rheum 1976;19:155–160.

S241. Searles RP, Mladimich EK, Messner RP. Isolated trigeminal sensory neuropathy: early manifestation of mixed connective tissue disease. Neurology (Minneap) 1978 Dec;28(12): 1286–1289.

S242. Searles RP, Plymate SR, Troup GM. Familial thiomide-induced lupus syndrome in thyrotoxicosis. J Rheumatol 1981 May–June;8:498–500.

S243. Sears D, Osman N, Tate B, McKenzie IFC, Hogarth PM. Molecular cloning and expression of the mouse high affinity Fc receptor for IgG. J Immunol 1990;144:371–378.

S244. Sears HF, Atkinson B, Mattis J, Ernst C, Herlyn D, Steplewski Z, Hayry P, Koprowski H. Phase I clinical trial with monoclonal antibody treatment of gastrointestinal tumors. Lancet 1982;1:762.

S245. Sears HF, Herlyn D, Steplewski Z, Koprowski H. Phase II clinical trial of a murine monoclonal antibody cytotoxic for gastrointestinal adenocarcinoma. Cancer Res 1985;45:5910.

S246. Sebastiani GD, Lulli P, Passiu G, Trabace S, Bellucci M, Morellini M, Galaezzi M. Anticardiolipin antibodies: their relationship with HLA-DR antigens in systemic lupus erythematosus. Br J Rheumatol 1991;30:156–157.

S247. Sedgwick RP, Von Hagen KO. Neurological manifestations of lupus erythematosus and periarteritis nodosa; report of 10 cases. Bull Los Angeles Neurol Soc 1948 Sep;13:129–142.

S248. Segal AM, Calabrese LH, Ahmad M, Tubbs RR, White CS. The pulmonary manifestations of systemic lupus erythematosus. Semin Arthritis Rheum 1985 Feb;14:202–224.

S249. Segal-Eiras A, Segura GM, Babini JC, Arturi AS, Frapuela JM, Marcos JC. Effect of antimalarial treatment on circulating immune complexes in rheumatoid arthritis. J Rheumatol 1985 Feb;12(1):87–89.

S250. Sege K, Peterson PA. Use of anti-idiotypic antibodies as cell-surface receptor probes. Proc Natl Acad Sci USA 1978;75: 2443.

S251. Seguin J, Berta P, Saussine M, Chaptal PA. Mepacrine, a phospholipase inhibitor [letter]. J Thorac Cardiovasc Surg 1987 Aug;94(2):312–314.

S252. Sehgal VN, Rege VL, Vadiraj SN. An unusual cutaneous manifestation of systemic lupus erythematosus [letter]. Arch Dermatol 1971 Apr;103:463–464.

S253.

S254. Seibold JR, Buckingham RB, Medsger TA Jr, Kelly RH. Cerebrospinal fluid immune complexes in systemic lupus involving the central nervous system. Semin Arthritis Rheum 1982 Aug;12(1):68–76.

S255. Seibold JR, Knight PJ, Peter JB. Anticardiolipin antibodies in systemic sclerosis [letter]. Arthritis Rheum 1986 Aug;29(8): 1052–1053.

S256. Seibold JR, Medsger TA Jr, Buckingham RB, Kelly RH. Central nervous system (CNS) involvement in systemic lupus erythematosus (SLE). Clinical features and response to therapy [abstract]. Arthritis Rheum 1981 Apr;24 Suppl 4:S70.

S257. Seibold JR, Wechsler LE, Cammarata RJ. LE cells in intermittent hydrarthrosis. Arthritis Rheum 1980 Aug;28(8): 958–959.

S258. Seidman JG, Max EE, Leder P. A K-immunoglobulin gene is formed by site-specific recombination without further somatic mutation. Nature 1979;280:370–375.

S259. Seiger E, Roland S, Goldman S. Cutaneous lupus treated with topical Tretinoin: A case report. Cuts 1991 May;47: 351–355.

S260. Seigneurin JM, Guilbert B, Bourgeat MJ, Avrameas S. Polyspecific natural antibodies and autoantibodies secreted by human lymphocytes immortalized with Epstein-Barr virus. Blood 1988;71:581–585.

S261. Seip M. Systemic lupus erythematosus in pregnancy with haemolytic anaemia, leucopenia and thrombocytopenia in the mother and her newborn infant. Arch Dis Child 1960;35: 364–366.

S262. Sekigawa I, Groopmen J, Allan JD, Ikeuch K, Biberfield G, Takatsuki K, Byrn RA. Characterization of autoantibodies to CD4 molecule in human immunodeficiency virus infection. Clin Immunol Immunopathol 1991;58:145–153.

S263. Sekigawa I, Okada T, Noguchi K, Ueda G, Hirose S, Sato H, Shirai T. Class-specific regulation of anti-DNA antibody synthesis and the age-associated changes in (NZB × NZW)F1 hybrid mice. J Immunol 1987;138:2890–2895.

S264. Sekita K, Doi T, Muso E, Yoshida H, Kanatsu K, Hamashima Y. Correlation of C3d fixing circulating immune complexes with disease activity and clinical parameters in patients with systemic lupus erythematosus. Clin Exp Immunol 1984;55: 487–494.

S265. Seleznick MJ, Fries JF, Brown BW. Prognostic subgroups in systemic lupus erythematosus (SLE) by recursive partitioning analysis [abstract]. Arthritis Rheum 1984 Apr;27 Suppl:S55.

S266. Seligmann M. Demonstration in the blood of patients with disseminated lupus erythematosus a substance determining a precipitation reaction with desoxyribonucleic acid. C rend Acad Sc (Paris) 1957 Jun 24;244(26):243–245.

S267. Seligmann M. Immuno-electrophoretic study of the serum during the course of systemic lupus erythematosus. In: Grabar P, Burtin P, editors. Immuno-Electrophoretic Analyses. Applications to Human Biological Fluids. New York: Elsevier Publishing Co, 1964:209–214.

S268. Selling JA, Hogan DL, Aly A, Koss MA, Isenberg JI. Indomethacin inhibits duodenal mucosal bicarbonate secretion and endogenous prostaglandin E2 output in human subjects. Ann Intern Med 1987;106:368–371.

S269. Sellmayer A, Uedelhoven WM, Weber PC, Bonventre JV. Endogenous noncyclooxygenase metabolites of arachidonic acid modulate growth and mRNA levels of immediate-early response genes in rat mesangial cells. J Biol Chem 1991;266: 3800–3807.

S270. Selvaraj P, Carpen O, Hibbs ML, Springer TA. Natural killer cell and granulocyte Fcγ receptor III (CD16) differ in membrane anchor and signal transduction. J Immunol 1989;143: 3283–3288.

S271. Selvaraj P, Rosse WF, Silber R, Springer TA. The major Fc receptor in blood has a phosphatidylinositol anchor and is deficient in paroxysmal nocturnal haemoglobinuria. Nature 1988;333:565–567.

S272. Semenzato G, Bambara LM, Biasi D, Frigo A, Vinante F, Zuppini B, Trentin L, Feruglio C, Chilosi M, Pizzolo G. Increased serum levels of soluble interleukin-2 receptor in patients with systemic lupus erythematosus and rheumatoid arthritis. J Clin Immunol 1988;8:447–452.

S273. Semon HC, Wolff E. Acute lupus erythematosus with fundus lesions. Proc Roy Soc Med 1933 Dec;27:153–157.

S274. Semprini AE, Vucetich A, Garbo S, Agostoni G, Pardi G. Effect of prednisone and heparin treatment in 14 patients with poor reproductive efficiency related to lupus anticoagulant. Fetal Ther 1989;4:73–76.

S275. Senaldi G, Ireland R, Bellingham AJ, Vergani D, Veerapan K, Wang F. IgM reduction in systemic lupus erythematosus. Arthritis Rheum 1988;31:1213.

S276. Senaldi G, Makinde VA, Vergani D, Isenberg DA. Correlation of the activation of the fourth component of complement (C4) with disease activity in systemic lupus erythematosus. Ann Rheum Dis 1988;47:913–917.

S277. Sendagorta EM, Matarredona J, Brieva JA, Rodriguez ML, Ledo A. Systemic lupus erythematosus in association with smoldering multiple myeloma. J Am Acad Dermatol 1987;16: 135–136.

S278. Senear FE, Usher B. An unusual type of pemphigus combining features of lupus erythematosus. Arch Derm & Syph 1926; 13:761–781.

S279. Senecal JL, St. Antoine P, Beliveau C. Legionella pneumophilia lung abscess in a patient with systemic lupus erythematosus. Am J Med Sci 1987 May;293(5):309–314.

S280. Senecal JL, Rauch J. Hybridoma lupus autoantibodies can bind major cytoskeletal filaments in the absence of DNA-binding activity. Arthritis Rheum 1988;31:864–875.

S281. Senecal JL, Raymund Y. Autoantibodies to DNA, Lamins, and pore complex proteins produce distinct peripheral fluorescent antinuclear antibody patterns and Hep2 substrate. Arthritis Rheum 1991;34:249–251.

S282. Senyk G, Hadley WK, Attias MR, Talal N. Cellular immunity in systemic lupus erythematosus. Arthritis Rheum 1974 Sep–Oct;17:553–562.

S283. Sepp N, Hintner H, Shuler G, Wick G. Dust-and rod-like particles in cutaneous biopsies of patients with systemic lupus erythematosus [letter]. Br J Dermatol 1989 Jun;120(6): 851–853.

S284. Sequeira JH. Lupus erythematosus in two sisters. Br J Dermatol 1903;15:171.

S285. Sequeira JH, Balean H. Lupus erythematosus: A clinical study of seventy-one cases. Br J Dermatol 1902;14:367–379.

S286. Sequeira W, Polisky RB, Alrenga DP. Neutrophilic dermatosis (Sweet's syndrome). Association with a hydralazine-induced lupus syndrome. Am J Med 1986;81:558–560.

S287. Serdula MK, Rhoads GG. Frequency of systemic lupus erythematosus in different ethnic groups in Hawaii. Arthritis Rheum 1979 Apr;22(4):328–333.

S288. Sergent JS, Lockshin MD, Klempner MS, Lipsky BA. Central nervous system disease in systemic lupus erythematosus. Therapy and prognosis. Am J Med 1975 May;58(5):644–654.

S289. Sergent JS, Sherman RL, Al-Mondhiry H. Fibrinogen catabolism in systemic lupus erythematosus. Arthritis Rheum 1976 Mar–Apr;19:195–198.

S290. Sergott TJ, Limoli JP, Baldwin CM Jr, Laub DR. Human adjuvant disease, possible autoimmune disease after silicone implantation: A review of the literature case studies, and speculation for the future. Plast Reconstruct Surg 1986;78: 104–114.

S291. Serhan CN. Components of the arachidonic acid signalling cascade: a brief update and hypothesis. In: Advances in Rheuamtology and Inflammation. Cular Publishers, 1991:(1). In press.

S292. Serra A, Lauzurica R, Bonal J, Texido J, Bonet J, Boix J, Romero R, Caralps A. Lupus crisis versus cytomegalovirus infection. Role of digestive endoscopy for the differential diagnosis. Med Clin (Barc) 1987;88:25–27.

S293. Serrano G, Bonillo J, Aliaga A, Gargallo E, Pelufo C. UVA Piroxicam induced photosensitivity in vivo and in vitro studies of its photosensitizing potential. J Am Acad Dermatol 1984 Jul;11(1):113–120.

S294. Servitje O, Ribera M, Juanola X, Rodriguez-Moreno J. Acute neutrophilic dermatosis associated with hydralazine-induced lupus. Arch Dermatol 1987;123:1435–1436.

S295. Sessions S, Mehta K, Kovarsky J. Quantitation of proteinuria in systemic lupus erythematosus by random, spot urine collection. Arthritis Rheum 1983 Jul;26:918–920.

S296. Sessoms SL, Kovarsky J. Monthly intravenous cyclophosphamide in the treatment of severe systemic lupus erythematosus. Clin Exp Rheumatol 1984 Jul–Sep;2(3):247–251.

S297. Sewell KL, Livneh A, Aranow CB, Grayzel AI. Magnetic resonance imaging versus computed tomographic scanning in neuropsychiatric systemic lupus erythematosus. Am J Med 1989 May;86(5):625–626.

S298. Sewell RB, Barham SS, LaRusso NF. Effect of chloroquine on the form and function of hepatocyte lysosomes. Morphologic modifications and physiologic alterations related to the biliary excretion of lipids and proteins. Gastroenterology 1983 Nov;85(5):1146–1153.

S299. Sghirlanzoni A, Mantegazza R, Mora M, Pareyson D, Cornelio F. Chloroquine myopathy and myasthenia-like syndrome. Muscle Nerve 1988 Feb;11(2):114–119.

S300. Sha WC, Nelson CA, Newberry RD, Kranz DM, Russell JH, Loh D. Selective expression of an antigen receptor on CD8-bearing T lymphocytes in transgenic mice. Nature 1988;335: 271–274.

S301. Shader RI, Greenblatt DJ. Triazolam and anterograde amnesia: all is not well in the Z-zone editorial. J Clin Psychopharmacol 1983 Oct;3(5):273.

S302. Shafer RB, Gregory DH. Systemic lupus erythematosus presenting as regional ileitis. Minn Med 1970 Jul;53:789–792.

S303. Shaffer B, Cahn MM, Levy EJ. Absorption of antimalarial drugs in human skin; spectroscopic and chemical analysis in epidermis and Corium. J Invest Dermatol 1951;30:341–345.

S304. Shalit M, Gross DJ, Levo Y. Pneumococcal epiglottitis in systemic lupus erythematosus on high dose corticosteroids. Ann Rheum Dis 1982 Dec;41(1):615–616. Shames JL, Fast A. Gluteal abscess causing sciatica in a patient with systemic lupus erythematosus. Arch Phys Med Rehabil 1989 May;70(5): 410–411.

S305. Shamiss A, Thaler M, Nussinovitch N, Zissin R, Rosenthal T. Multiple Salmonella enteritidis leg abscesses in a patient with systemic lupus erythematosus. Postgrad Med J 1990;66: 486–488.

S306. Shan SA. The Pleura. Am Rev Respir Dis 1988;138: 184–234.

S307. Shanley KJ. Lupus erythematosus in small animals. Clin Dermatol 1985;3:131–138.

S308. Shanlian E, Shoenfield Y, Berliner S, Shaklai M, Pinkhas J. Surgery in patients with circulating lupus anticoagulants. Int Surg 1981;66:157–159.

S309. Shannon MF, Wells JRE. Characterization of the six chicken histone H1 proteins and alignment with their respective genes. J Biol Chem 1987;262:9664–9668.

S310. Shapeero LG, Myers A, Oberkircher PE, Miller WT. Acute reversible lupus vasculitis of the gastrointestinal tract. Radiology 1974;112:569–574.

S311. Shapira Y, Mor F, Friedler A, Wysenbeek AW, Weinberger A. Antiproteinuric effect of captopril in a patient with lupus nephritis and intractable nephrotic syndrome [case report]. Ann Rheum Dis 1990 Sep;49(9):723–727.

S312. Shapiro H. Personal correspondence, unpublished.

S313. Shapiro HS. Depression in lupus, Official Information Pamphlet issued by the National Lupus Foundation of America Office, Washington, D.C. [no date].

S314. Shapiro HS. Depression in lupus. Lupus News. 1987;7(3) Washington D.C.

S315. Shapiro HS. Personality traits that often interfere with the lupus patient's adjustment. Reprinted in Lupus/Scleroderma Bulletin, Australia (Publication SAW 2654) 1989 Apr.

S316. Shapiro HS. Psychopharmacological effects and considerations of the various medications used in the treatment of SLE, Fall-Winter proceeding of Lupus News, Washington, D.C. 1990;10(2).

S317. Shapiro HS. Psychiatric side effects and problems associated with drugs used in the treatment of SLE, Lupus. Ridgeway, Ontario, Canada 1990 Fall:9–12.

S318. Shapiro HS. The physicians' ordeal on becoming a patient, reprint Minn. News and Notes (LFA), 1983 Oct:40 from address before the National Lupus Foundation of America, Annual Meeting, 1983 Jul.

S319. Shapiro HS. Rap groups: aid to lupus management, the Newsletter of the British Columbia Association (Vancouver), The Lupus Lighthouse, 1986 Winter;7(4).

S320. Shapiro KS, Pinn VW, Harrington JT, Levey AS. Immune complex glomerulonephritis in hydralazine-induced SLE. Am J Kidney Dis 1984;3:270–274.

S321. Shapiro L, Cohen HJ. Tinea faciei simulating other dermatoses. JAMA 1971 Mar 29;215:2106–2107.

S322. Shapiro RF, Gamble CN, Wiesner KB, Castles J, Wolf AW, Hurley EJ, Salel AF. Immunopathogenesis of Libman Sachs endocarditis. Assessment by light and immunofluorescent microscopy in two cases. Ann Rheum Dis 1977 Dec;36:508–516.

S323. Shapiro SH, Wessely Z, Lipper S. Concentric membranous bodies in hepatocytes from a patient with systemic lupus erythematosus. Ultrastruct Pathol 1985;8(23):241–247.

S324. Shapiro SS, Thiagarajan P. Lupus anticoagulants. Prog Hemostat Thromb 1982;6:263.

S325. Sharfstein SS, Sack DS, Fauci AS. Relationship between alternate-day corticosteroid therapy and behavioral abnormalities. JAMA 1982 Dec 10;248:2987–2989.

S326. Sharon E, Jones J, Diamond H, Kaplan D. Pregnancy and azathioprine in systemic lupus erythematosus. Am J Obstet Gynecol 1974;118:25–28.

S327. Sharon E, Kaplan D, Diamond HS. Exacerbation of systemic lupus erythematosus after withdrawal of azathioprine therapy. N Engl J Med 1973 Jan 18;288:122–124.

S328. Sharon Z, Roberts JL, Fennell JS, Lewis EJ. Plasmapheresis in lupus nephritis. Plasma Therapy 1982;3:165–169.

S329. Sharp GC. Mixed connective tissue disease: Current concepts. Proceedings of the Conference Commemorating the 25th Anniversary, Research Fellowships Program. The Arthritis Foundation. Arthritis Rheum 1977 Jul–Aug;20 Suppl 6: S181.

S330. Sharp GC. Mixed connective tissue disease. In: McCarty D, editor. Arthritis and Allied Conditions. 9th ed. Philadelphia: Lea & Febiger 1979:737–741.

S331. Sharp GC. Diagnostic criteria for classification of MCTD. In: Kasukawa R, Sharp GC, editors. Mixed connective tissue diseases and antinuclear antibodies. Amsterdam: Elsevier, 1987:23–32.

S332. Sharp GC, Anderson PC. Current concepts in the classification of connective tissue diseases; Overlap syndromes and mixed connective tissue disease (MCTD). J Am Acad Dermatol 1980 Apr;2(4):269–279.

S333. Sharp GC, Irvin WS, LaRoque RL, Velez C, Daly V, Kaiser AD, Holman HR. Association of auto-antibodies to different nuclear antigens with clinical patterns to rheumatic disease and responsiveness to therapy. J Clin Invest 1971 Feb;50: 350–359.

S334. Sharp GC, Irvin WS, May CM, Holman HR, McDuffie FC, Hess EV, Schmid FR. Association of antibodies to ribonucleoprotein and Sm antigens with mixed connective-tissue disease, systemic lupus erythematosus and other rheumatic diseases. N Engl J Med 1976 Nov 18;295:1149–1154.

S335. Sharp GC, Irvin WS, Northway JD, Tan EM. Specificity of antibodies to extractable nuclear antigens (ENA) in mixed connective tissue disease (MCTD) and systemic lupus erythematosus (SLE) [abstract]. Arthritis Rheum 1972;15:125.

S336. Sharp GC, Irvin WS, Tan EM, Gould RG, Holman HR. Mixed connective tissue disease-an apparently distinct rheumatic disease syndrome associated with a specific antibody to an extractable nuclear antigen (ENA). Am J Med 1972 Feb;52: 148–159.

S337. Shay CE, Foster PG, Neelin JM. Immunological relationships among vertebrate lysine-rich histones. Comp Biochem Physiol [B] 1988; 91B:69–78.

S338. Shear HL, Wofsy D, Talal N. Effects of castration and sex hormones on immune clearance and autoimmune disease in MRL/Mp-lpr and MRL/MP— +/+ mice. Clin Immunol Immunopathol 1983;26:361–369.

S339. Shearn MA. The heart in systemic lupus erythematosus. Am Heart J 1959 Sep;58:452–466.

S340. Shearn MA. Sjogren's Syndrome. Philadelphia: Saunders, 1971:262.

S341. Shearn MA, Epstein WV, Engelman EP. Serum viscosity in rheumatic diseases and macroglobulinemia. Arch Intern Med 1963 Nov;112:684–687.

S342. Shearn MA, Hooper J, Biava CG. Membranous lupus nephropathy initially seen as idiopathic membranous nephropathy: possible diagnostic value of tubular reticular structures. Arch Intern Med 1980 Nov;140:1521–1523.

S343. Shearn MA, Pirofsky B. Disseminated lupus erythematosus; analysis of 34 cases. Arch Intern Med 1952 Dec;90:790–807.

S344. Sheehy JL. Doctor's discussion. Am J Otol 1981;2: 405–407.

S344a. Shefner R, Kleiner G, Turken A, Papazian L, Diamond B. A novel class of anti-DNA antibodies identified in BALB/c mice. J Exp Med 1991;173:287–296.

S345. Sheft DJ, Shrago G. Esophageal moniliasis. The spectrum of the disease. JAMA 1970 Sep 14;213:1859–1862.

S346. Shehade S. Successful treatment of generalized discoid skin lesions with azathioprine [letter]. Arch Dermatol 1986 Apr;122(4):376–377.

S347. Sheldon PJ, Williams WR. Procainamide-induced systemic lupus erythematosus. Ann Rheum Dis 1970 May;29:236–243.

S348. Shelley WB, Crissey JT. Alphee Cazenave. In: classics in clinical dermatology with biographical sketches. Springfield IL: Charles C. Thomas, 1953.

S349. Shen L, Guyre PM, Fanger MW. Polymorphonuclear leukocyte function triggered through the high affinity Fc receptor for monomeric IgG. J Immunol 1987;139:534–538.

S350. Shenker L, Reed KL, Anderson CF, Marx GR, Sobonya RE, Graham AR. Congenital heart block and cardiac anomalies in the absence of maternal connective tissue disease. Am J Obstet Gynecol 1987;157:248–253.

S351. Sherertz EF. Lichen planus following procainamide induced lupus erythematosus. Cutis 1988;42:51–53.

S352. Shergy WJ, Kredich DW, Pisetsky DS. The relationship of anticardiolipin antibodies to disease manifestations in pediatric systemic lupus erythematosus. J Rheumatol 1988;15: 1389–1394.

S352a. Sheridan-Pereira M, Porreco RP, Hays T, Burke MS. Neonatal aortic thrombosis associated with the lupus anticoagulant. Obstet Gynecol 1988;71:1016–1018.

S353. Sherlock S. The immunology of liver disease. Am J Med 1970 Nov;49:693–706.

S354. Sherlock S. Chronic active hepatitis. Definition, diagnosis and management. Postgrad Med 1971;50:206–211.

S354a. Sherman GF, Galaburda AM, Geschwind N. Cortical anomalies in brains of New Zealand mice: a neuropathologic model of dyslexia? Proc Natl Acad Sci USA 1985 Dec;82(23): 8072–8074.

S355. Sherman JD, Love DE, Harrington JF. Anemia, positive lupus and rheumatoid factors with methyldopa. A report of 3 cases. Arch Intern Med 1967 Sep;120:321–326.

S356. See S354a.

S357. Shero HJ, Bordwell B, Rothfield NF, Earnshaw WC. High titers of autoantibodies to topoisomerase I in sera from scleroderma patients. Science 1986;231:737–740.

S358. Shetlar MR, Payne RW, Padron J, Felton F, Kishmael W. Objective evaluation of patients with rheumatic diseases. I.

Comparison of serum glycoprotein, cold hemagglutination, C-reactive protein and other tests with clinical evaluation. J Lab Clin Med 1956 Aug;48:94–200.

S359. Shiba K, Stohl W, Gray JD, Horwitz DA. A novel role for accessory cells in T cell-dependent B cell differentiation. 1990;127:458–469.

S360. Shiel WC Jr, Jason M. The diagnostic associations of patients with antinuclear antibodies referred to a community rheumatologist. J Rheumatol 1989 Jun;16(6):782–785.

S361. Shields AF, Berenson JA. Procainamide-associated pancytopenia. Am J Hematol 1988;27:299–301.

S362. Shilling PJ, Kurzrock R, Kantarjian H, Gutterman JU, Talpaz M. Development of systemic lupus erythematosus after interferon therapy for chronic myelogenous leukemia. Cancer 1991;68:1536–1538.

S363. Shimizu T, Ino T, Nishimoto K, Iwahara M, Yamashiro Y, Yabuta K. Advanced atrioventricular block in a neonate with lupus erythematosus and anti-SSA antibodies. Ped Cardiol 1988;9:121–124.

S364. Shimomura C, Eguchi K, Kawakami A, Migita K, Nakao H, Otsubo T, Ueki Y, Tezuka H, Yamashita S, Matsunaga M, Nagataki S. Elevation of a tumor associated antigen CA 19–9 levels in patients with rheumatic diseases. J Rheumatol 1989;16:1410–1415.

S365. Shimuzu A, Honjo T. Immunoglobulin class switching. Cell 1984;36:801–803.

S366. Shiohara T, Moriya N, Tsuchiya K, Nagashima M, Narimatsu H. Lichenoid tissue reaction induced by local transfer of Ia-reactive T-cell clones. J Invest Dermatol 1986;87:33–38.

S367. Shiozawa S, Kuroki Y, Kim M, Hirohata S, Ogino T. Alpha-interferon in lupus psychosis [abstract]. Arthritis Rheum 1991;34 Suppl:S51.

S368. Shipton EA. Hunner's ulcer (chronic interstitial cystitis). A manifestation of collagen disease. Br J Urol 1965 Aug;37:443–449.

S369. Shirai T. The genetic basis of autoimmunity in murine lupus. Immunol Today 1982;3:187–194.

S370. Shirai T, Mellors RC. Natural thymocytotoxic autoantibody and reactive antigen in New Zealand black and other mice. Proc Natl Acad Sci USA 1971 Jul;68:1412–1415.

S371. Shirakawa F, Yamashita U, Suzuki H. Monocyte (macrophage)-specific antibodies in patients with systemic lupus erythematosus (SLE). J Clin Immunol 1987;7:121–129.

S372. Omitted.

S373. Shivakumar S, Tsokos GC, Datta SK. T cell receptor alpha/beta expressing double negative(CD4-/CD8-) and CD4+ T helper cells in human augment the production of pathogenic anti-DNA autoantibodies associated with lupus nephritis. J Immunol 1989;143:103–112.

S374. Shlomchik M, Mascelli M, Shan H, Radic MZ, Pisetsky D, Marshak-Rothstein A, Weigert M. Anti-DNA antibodies from autoimmune mice arise by clonal expansion and somatic mutation. J Exp Med 1990 Jan 1;171(1):265–292.

S375. Shlomchik MJ, Aucoin AH, Pisetsky DS, Weigert MG. Structure and function of anti-DNA autoantibodies derived from a single autoimmune mouse. Proc Natl Acad Sci USA 1987 Dec;84(24):9150–9154.

S376. Shlomchik MJ, Marshak-Rothstein A, Wolfowicz CB, Rothstein TL, Weigert MG. The role of clonal selection and somatic mutation in autoimmunity. Nature 1987;328:805–811.

S377. Shlomchik MJ, Nemazee D, van Snick J, Weigert M. Variable region sequences of murine IgM anti-IgG monoclonal autoantibodies (rheumatoid factors). II. Comparison of hybridomas derived by lipopolysaccharide stimulation and secondary protein immunization. J Exp Med 1987;165:970–987.

S378. Shlomchik MJ, Nemazee DA, Sato VL, van Snick J, Carson DA, Weigert MG. Variable region sequences of murine IgM anti-IgG monoclonal autoantibodies (rheumatoid factors). J Exp Med 1986;164:407–427.

S379. Shoenfeld H, Isenberg DA, Rauch J, Madaio MP, Stollar BD, Schwartz RS. Idiotypic cross-reactions of monoclonal human lupus autoantibodies. J Exp Med 1983;158:718.

S380. Shoenfeld R, Isenberg DA. DNA antibody idiotypes: a review of their genetic, clinical and immunopathological features [review]. Semin Arthritis Rheum 1987;16:215–252.

S381. Shoenfeld Y, Andre-Schwartz J, Stollar BD, Schwartz RS. Anti-DNA antibodies [review]. In: Lahita R, editor. Systemic Lupus Erythematosus. New York: Wiley, 1987:213–255.

S382. Omitted.

S383. Shoenfeld Y, Isenberg DA, Rauch J, Madaio MP, Stollar BD, Schwartz RS. Idiotypic cross-reactions of monoclonal human lupus autoantibodies. J Exp Med 1983;158:718–730.

S384. Shoenfeld Y, Mozes E. Pathogenic idiotypes in autoimmunity: lessons from new experimental models of SLE. FASEB J 1990;4:2646–2651.

S385. Shoenfeld Y, Rauch J, Masicotte H, Datta SK, Andre-Schwartz J, Stollar BD, Schwartz RS. Polyspecificity of monoclonal lupus autoantibodies produced by human-human hybridomas. N Engl J Med 1983 Feb 24;303(8):414–420.

S386. See S159a.

S387. See S159b.

S388. Shoenfeld Y, Vilner Y, Coates ARM, Rauch J, Lavie G, Shaul D, Pinkhas J. Monoclonal anti-tuberculosis antibodies react with DNA and monoclonal anti-DNA antibodies react with Mycobacterium tuberculosis. Clin Exp Immunol 1986;66:255–261.

S389. Shoenfeld Y, Zamir R, Joshua H, Lavie G, Pinkhas J. Human monoclonal anti-DNA antibodies react as lymphocytotoxic antibodies. Eur J Immunol 1985;15:1024–1028.

S390. Shohat B, Hirsh M, Tardena O, Henrig J, Levy I, Trainin N. Cellular immune aspects of the human fetal-maternal relationship. Am J Reprod Immunol Microbiol 1986;11(4):125–129.

S391. Shores EW, Eisenberg RA, Cohen PL. Role of the Sm antigen in the generation of anti-Sm antibodies in the SLE-prone MRL mouse. J Immunol 1987;136:3662–3667.

S392. Shores EW, Eisenberg RA, Cohen PL. T-B collaboration in the in vitro anti-Sm autoantibody response of MRL/Mp-lpr/lpr mice. J Immunol 1988;140:2977–2982.

S393. Shornick JK, Formica N, Parke AL. Isotretoin for refractory lupus erythematosus. J Am Acad Dermatol 1991 Jan;24(1):49–52.

S394. Short TS. Fatal case of acute lupus erythematosus. Br J Dermatol 1907 Aug;19:271–274.

S395. Shou L, Schwartz S, Good RA. Suppressor cell activity after concanavalin A treatment on lymphocytes from normal donors. J Exp Med 1978 May 1;143:1100–1110.

S396. Shou-yi S, Shu-fang F, Kang-huang L, Li F, Ke-fei K. Clinical study of 30 cases of subacute cutaneous lupus erythematosus. Chin Med J 1987;100:45–48.

S397. Shrank AB, Doniach D. Discoid lupus erythematosus. Correlation of clinical features with serum auto-antibody pattern. Arch Dermatol 1963 Jun;87:677–685.

S398. Shukla VR, Borison RL. Lithium and lupus-like syndrome [letter]. JAMA 1982 Aug 27;248:921–922.

S399. Shulman HJ, Christian CL. Aortic insufficiency in systemic lupus erythematosus. Arthritis Rheum 1969 Apr;12:138–145.

S400. Shulman IA, Branch DR, Nelson JM, Thompson JC, Saxena S, Petz LD. Autoimmune hemolytic anemia with both cold and warm autoantibodies. JAMA 1985;253;1746–1748.

S401. Shulman NR, Marder VJ, Weinrach RS. Similarities between known antiplatelet antibodies and the factor responsible for thrombocytopenia in idiopathic purpura, physiologic, serologic and isotopic studies. Ann N Y Acad Sci 1965 Jun 30;124; 499–542.

S402. Siame JL. Exophtalmie basedowienne isole, maladie lupique revelee par une neuropathie peripherique associee a une angiete necrosante. Presse Med 1988 Mar 5;17(8):391.

S403. Siamopoulou-Mavridou A, Manoussakis MN, Mavridias AK, Moutsoponlos HM. Outcome of pregnancy in patients with autoimmune rheumatic diseases before the disease onset. Ann Rheum Dis 1988;47:982–987.

S404. Sibbitt WL Jr, Gibbs DL, Kenny C, Bankhurst AD, Searles RP, Ley KD. Relationship between circulating interferon and anti-interferon antibodies and impaired natural killer cell activity in systemic lupus erythematosus. Arthritis Rheum 1985 Jun;28:624–629.

S405. Sibbitt WL Jr, Kenny C, Spellman CW, Ley KD, Bankhurst AD. Lympokines in autoimmunity: relationship between interleukin-2 and interferon-gamma production in systemic lupus erythematosus. Clin Immunol Immunopathol 1984 Aug; 32:166–173.

S406. Sibbitt WL Jr, Likar L, Spellman CW, Bankhurst AD. Impaired natural killer cell function in systemic lupus erythematosus. Relationship to interleukin-2 production. Arthritis Rheum 1983 Nov;26:1316–1320.

S407. Sibbitt WL Jr, Sibbitt RR, Griffey RH, Eckel C, Bankhurst AD. Magnetic resonance and computed tomographic imaging in the evaluation of acute neuropsychiatric disease in systemic lupus erythematosus. Ann Rheum Dis 1989 Dec;48(12): 1014–1022.

S408. Siddiqui FA, Lina EC-Y. Novel platelet-agglutinating protein form a thrombotic thrombocytopenic purpura plasma. J Clin Invest 1985;76:1330–1340.

S409. Sidiq M, Kirsner AB, Shoen RP. Carpal tunnel syndrome: First manifestation of systemic lupus erythematosus. JAMA 1972 Dec 11;222:1416–1417.

S410. Sidman CL, Shultz LD, Hardy RR, Hayakawa K, Herzenberg LA. Production of immunoglobulin isotypes by Ly-1 + B cells in viable motheaten and normal mice. Science 1986;232: 1423–1425.

S411. Sieber C, Grimm E, Follath F. Captopril and systemic lupus erythematosus syndrome. BMJ 1990;301:669.

S412. Siegel BM, Friedman IA, Kessler S, Schwartz SO. Thrombohemolytic thrombocytopenic purpura and lupus erythematosus. Ann Intern Med 1957 Nov;27:1022–1029.

S413. Siegel I, Liu TL, Gleichner N. The red cell immune system. Lancet 1981;2:556–559.

S414. Siegel M, Gwon N, Lee SL, Rivero I, Wong W. Survivorship in systemic lupus erythematosus: Relationship to race and pregnancy. Arthritis Rheum 1969 Apr;12:117–125.

S415. Siegel M, Holley H, Lee SL. Epidemiologic studies on systemic lupus erythematosus, comparative data for New York City and Jefferson County, AL. 1956–1965. Arthritis Rheum 1970 Nov–Dec;13:802–811.

S416. Siegel M, Lee SL. The epidemiology of systemic lupus erythematosus. Semin Arthritis Rheum 1973;3(1):1–54.

S417. Siegel M, Lee SL, Widelock D, Gwon NV, Kravitz H. A comparative family study of rheumatoid arthritis and systemic lupus erythematosus. N Engl J Med 1965;273:893–897.

S418. Siegel RM, Katsumata M, Komori S, Wadsworth S, Gill-Morse L, Jerrold-Jones S, Bhandoola A, Greene MI, Yui K. Mechanisms of autoimmunity in the context of T cell tolerance : Insights from natural and transgenic animal model systems. Immunol Rev 1990;118:165–192.

S419. Siegert C, Daha M, Westedt ML, van der Voort E, Breedveld F. IgG autoantibodies against C1q are corre lated with nephritis, hypocomplementemia, and dsDNA antibodies in systemic lupus erythematosus. J Rheumatol 1991;18:230–234.

S420. Siekevitz M, Kocks C, Rajewsky K, Dildrop R. Analysis of somatic mutation and class switching in naive and memory B cells generating adoptive primary and secondary responses. Cell 1987;48:757–770.

S421. Siemsen JK, Brook J, Meister L. Lupus erythematosus and avascular bone necrosis: a clinical study of three cases and review of the literature. Arthritis Rheum 1962 Oct;5: 492–501.

S422. Sierakowski S, Kucharz EJ, Lightfoot RW, Goodwin JS. Impaired T-cell activation in patients with systemic lupus erythematosus. J Clin Immunol 1989;9:469–476.

S423. Sierakowski S, Kucharz EJ, Lightfoot RW Jr, Goodwin JS. Interleukin-1 production by monocytes from patients with systemic lupus erythematosus. Clin Rheum 1987;6:403–407.

S423a. Sietsema WK. The absolute oral bioavailability of selected drugs. Int J Clin Pharmacol Ther Toxicol 1989;27:179–211.

S424. Sieving RR, Kauffman CA, Watanakunakorn C. Deep fungal infection in systemic lupus erythematosus—three cases reported, literature reviewed. J Rheumatol 1975 Mar;2(1): 61–72.

S425. Sigal LH. Chronic inflammatory polyneuropathy complicating SLE: successful treatment with monthly oral pulse cyclophosphamide [letter]. J Rheumatol 1989 Nov;16(11): 1518–1519.

S426. Siiteri PK, Febres F, Clemens LE, Chang RJ, Gondos B, Stites DP. Progesterone and the maintenance of pregnancy: is progesterone nature's immunosuppressant? Ann NY Acad Sci 1977;286:384–397.

S427. Sikder SK, Borden, P, Gruezo F, Akolkar PN, Bhattacharya SB, Morrison SL, Kabat EA. Amino acid substitutions in V_H CDR2 change the idiotype but not the antigen-binding of monoclonal antibodies to alpha(1—>6)dextrans. J Immunol 1989;142:888.

S428. Silber TJ, Chatoor I, White PH. Psychiatric manifestations of systemic lupus erythematosus in children and adolescents: a review. Clin Pediatr 1984 Jun;23(6):331–335.

S429. Silberberg DH, Laties AM. Increased intracranial pressure in disseminated lupus erythematosus. Arch Neurol 1973 Aug; 29:88–90.

S430. Silberstein SL, Barland P, Grayzel AI, Koerner SK. Pulmonary dysfunction in systemic lupus erythematosus: Prevalence, classification and correlation with other organ involvement. J Rheumatol 1980 Mar–Apr;7:187–195.

S431. Sillekens PTG, Habets WJ, Beijer RP, van Venrooij WJ. cDNA cloning of the human U1 snRNP associated A protein: extensive homology between U1 and U2 snRNP specific proteins. Embo J 1987;6:3841–3848.

S432. Sillekens PTG, Beijer RP, Habets WJ, van Venrooij WJ. Human U1 sn RNP specific C protein: complete cDNA and protein sequence and identification of a multigene family in mammals. Nucleic Acids Res 1988;16:8307–8321.

S433. Sillekens PTG, Beijer RP, Habets WJ, van Venrooij WJ. Molecular cloning of the cDNA for the human U2 snRNP-specific A′ protein. Nucleic Acids. Res. 1989;17:1893–1906.

S434. Sills EM. Systemic lupus erythematosus in a patient previously diagnosed as having Shulman disease [letter]. Arthritis Rheum 1988 May;31(5):694–695.

S435. Silva FG. The nephropathies of systemic lupus erythematosus. In: Rosen S, editor. Pathology of glomerular diseases. New York: Churchill Livingston, 1983:79–124.

S436. Silva H, Hall EW, Hill KR, Shaldon S, Sherlock S. Renal involvement in active "juvenile" cirrhosis. J Clin Pathol 1965; 18:157–163.

S437. Silveira LH, Hubble CL, Jara JL, Martinez-Osuna P, Seleznick MJ, Espinoza LR. Prevention of anticardiolipin antibodies-related pregnancy losses with prednisone and aspirin. Arthritis Rheum 1991;34 Suppl:S95.

S438. Silver M, Steinbrocker O. The musculoskeletal manifestations of systemic lupus erythematosus. JAMA 1961 Jun;176: 1001–1003.

S439. Silverberg DS, Kidd EG, Shnitka TK, Ulan RA. Gold nephropathy. A clinical and pathologic study. Arthritis Rheum 1970;13:812–825.

S440. Silverman E, Mamula M, Hardin JA, Laxer R. Importance of the immune response to the Ro/La particle in the development of congenital heart block and neonatal lupus erythematosus. J Rheumatol 1991;18:120–124.

S441. Silverman JA, Pascucci VL, Chatterji DC, Klippel JH. The pharmacokinetics of bolus oral cyclophosphamide in systemic lupus erythematosus [abstract]. Arthritis Rheum 1984 Apr; 27(4) Suppl:S64.

S442. Silverman SL, Cathcart ES. Natural killing in systemic lupus erythematosus: inhibitory effects of serum. Clin Immunol Immunopathol 1980 Oct;17:219–226.

S443. Silverstein AM. Essential hypocomplementemia; report of a case. Blood 1960;16:1338–1341.

S444. Silverstein MD, Albert DA, Hadler NM, Ropes MW. Prognosis in SLE: Comparison of Markov model to life table analysis. J Clin Epidemiol 1988;41:623–633.

S445. Silvestris F, Edwards BS, Sadeghi OM, Frassanito MA, Williams RC, Dammacco F. Isotype, distribution and target analysis of lymphocyte reactive antibodies in patients with human immunodeficiency virus infection. Clin Immunol Immunopathol 1989;53:329–340.

S446. Sim E. Drug-induced immune complex disease. Biochem Soc Trans 1991;19:164–170.

S447. Sim E, Gill EW, Sim RB. Drugs that induce systemic lupus erythematosus inhibit complement component C4. Lancet 1984 Aug 25;1:422–424.

S448. Sim E, Stanley L, Gill EW, Jones A. Metabolites of procainamide and practolol inhibit complement proteins C3 and C4. Biochem J 1988;251:323–326.

S449. Simel DL, St Clair EW, Adams J, Greenberg CS. Correction of hypoprothrombinemia by immunosuppressive treatment of the lupus anticoagulant-hypoprothrombinemia syndrome. Am J Med 1987 Sep;83(3):563–566.

S450. Simeon-Aznar CP, Cuenca-Luque R, Solans-Laque R, Fernandez-Cortijo J, Bosch-Gil JA, Vilardell-Tarres M. Fulminant soft tissue infection by Salmonella enteritidis in SLE [letter]. J Rheumatol 1990;17(11):1570–1571.

S451. Simeone JF, McCloud T, Putman CE, Marsh J. Thymoma and systemic lupus erythematosus. Thorax 1975;30:670–679.

S452. Siminovitch KA, Misener V, Kwong PC, Yang PM, Laskin CM, Cairns E, Bell D, Rubin CA, Chen PP. A human anticardiolipin autoantibody is encoded by developmentally restricted heavy and light chain variable region genes. Autoimmunity 1990;8:97–105.

S453. Simkin NJ, Jelinek DF, Lipsky PE. Inhibition of human B cell responsiveness by prostaglandin E$_2$. J Immunol 1987;138: 1074–1081.

S454. See S457.

S455. Simon J, Simon O. Effect of passive transfer of anti-brain antibodies to a normal recipient. Exp Neurol 1975;47:523.

S456. Simone JV, Cornet JA, Abildagaard CF. Acquired von Willebrand's syndrome in systemic lupus erythematosus. Blood 1968 Jun;31:803–812.

S457. Simons-Ling N, Schachner L, Pennys N, Gorman H, Zillereulo G, Strauss J. Childhood systemic lupus erythematosus: Association with pancreatitis, subcutaneous fat necrosis and calcinosis cutis. Arch Dermatol 1983 Jun;119:491–494.

S458. Simonson JS, Schiller NB, Petri M, Hellmann DB. Pulmonary hypertension in systemic lupus erythematosus. J Rheumatol 1989;16:918–925.

S459. Simopoulos AP, Kifer RR, Martin RE, editors. Health effects of polyunsaturated fatty acids in seafoods. New York: Academic Press, 1986.

S460. Simpson DG, Walker JH. Hypersensitivity to para-aminosalicylic acid. Am J Med 1960 Aug;29:297–306.

S461. Simpson JL, Mills JL. Methodologic problems in determining fetal loss rates: revelance to chorionic villi samplings. In: Fraccaro M, Simoni G, Brabati R, editors. First trimester fetal diagnosis. Berlin: Springer Verlag, 1985:321.

S462. Simpson RT. Nucleosome positioning in vivo and in vitro. Bio Essays 1986;4:172–176.

S463. Singer J, Denburg JA, Ad Hoc Neuropsychiatric Lupus Workshop Group. Diagnostic criteria for neuropsychiat ric systemic lupus erythematosus: The results of a consensus meeting [workshop report]. J Rheumatol 1990 Oct;17(10): 1397–1402.

S464. Singer JM. The latex fixation test in rheumatic diseases. Am J Med 1961 Nov;31:766–779.

S465. Singer JZ, Ginzler EM, Kaplan D. Solganol (Aurothioglucose) for treatment of arthritis of systemic lupus erythematosus (SLE) [abstract]. Arthritis Rheum 1987 Jan;30(1) Suppl: S14.

S466. Singer PA, Balderas RS, McEvilly RJ, Bobardt M, Theofilopoulos AN. Tolerance-related V beta clonal deletions in normal CD4−8-, TCR-alpha/beta + and abnormal lpr and gld cell populations. J Exp Med 1989 Dec;170(6):1869–1877.

S467. Singer PA, McEvilly RJ, Noonan DJ, Dixon FJ, Theofilopoulos AN. Clonal diversity and T-cell receptor beta-chain variable gene expression in enlarged lymph nodes of MRL-lpr/lpr lupus mice. Proc Natl Acad Sci USA 1986;83:7018–7022.

S468. Singer PA, Theofilopoulos AN. T-cell receptor V beta repertoire expression in murine models of SLE. Immunol Rev 1990;118:103–127.

S469. Singer PA, Theofilopoulos AN. Novel origin of lpr and gld cells and possible implications in autoimmunity. J Autoimmun 1990;3:123–135.

S470. Singh RR, Prasad K, Kumar A, Misra A, Padmakumar K, Malaviya AN. Cerebellar ataxia in systemic lupus erythematosus: three case reports. Ann Rheum Dis 1988 Nov;47(11): 954–956.

S471. Singh VK, Yamaki K, Donoso LA, Shinohara T. Sequence homology between yeast histone H3 and uveitopathogenic site of S-antigen: lymphocyte cross-reaction and adoptive transfer of the disease. Cell Immunol 1989;119:211–221.

S472. Singleton JD, Schneebaum AB, West SG, Cheronis J, Kotzin BL. Clinical associations of antibodies to ribosomal P proteins [abstract]. Arthritis Rheum 1989 Apr;32(4) Suppl:S48.

S473. Singsen BH. Epidemiology of Rheumatic Diseases: Rheumatic diseases of childhood. Rheum Dis Clin North Am 1990; 16:581–599.

S474. Singsen BH, Bernstein BH, King KK, Hanson V. Systemic lupus erythematosus in childhood: Correlations between changes in disease activity and serum complement levels. J Pediatr 1976;89:358–365.

S475. Singsen BH, Kornreich HK, Koster-King K, Brink SJ, Bernstein BH, Hanson V, Tan EM. Mixed connective tissue disease in children. Proceedings of the conference on rheumatic diseases in childhood. Arthritis Rheum 1976 Mar;20 Suppl: 355–360.

S476. Singsen BH, Nevon P, Wang G, Sharp GC. Anti-SSA and other antinuclear antibodies (ANA) in healthy pregnant women and in newborn cord bloods [abstract]. J Rheumatol 1986;13:984.

S477. Singsen BH, Platzker CG. Pulmonary involvement in the rheumatic disorders of childhood. Disorders of the Respiratory tract in children, 4th ed. Kendig EL, Chernick V, editors. Philadelphia: Saunders, 1983:846–872.

S478. Singsen BH, Swanson VL, Bernstein BH, Heuser ET, Hanson

V, Landing BH. A histologic evaluation of mixed connective tissue disease of childhood. Am J Med 1980 May;68(5): 710–717.

S479. Sinha AA, Lopez MT, McDevitt HO. Autoimmune diseases: The failure of self tolerance. Science 1990;248:1380–1387.

S480. Sinniah R, Feng PH. Lupus nephritis: correlation between light, electromicroscopic and immunofluorescent findings and renal function. Clin Nephrol 1976 Aug;6:340–351.

S481. Sipos A, Csortos C, Sipka S, Gergely P, Sonkoly I, Szegedi G. The antigen/receptor specificity of antigranulocyte antibodies in patient with SLE. Immunol Lett 1988;19:329–334.

S482. Sires RL, Adler SG, Louie JS, Cohen AH. Poor prognosis in end-stage lupus nephritis due to nonautologous vascular access site associated septicemia and lupus flares. Am J Nephrol 1989;9(4):279–284.

S483. Sitton NG, Dixon JS, Bird HA, Wright V. Serum biochemistry in rheumatoid arthritis, seronegative arthropathies, osteoarthritis, SLE and normal subjects. Br J Rheumatol 1987;26: 131–135.

S484. Siurala M, Julkunen H, Tolvonen S, Pelkonen R, Saxen E, Pitkanen E. Digestive tract in collagen disease. Acta Med Scan 1965;178:13–25.

S485. Skibin A, Quastel MR, Kuperman O, Segal S. Suppression of lymphocyte activation by a soluble factor released from the human placental chorionic membrane: chemical analysis and functional characterization. Am J Reprod Immunol 1989; 19(3):85–91.

S486. Skinner MD, Schwartz RS. Immunosuppressive therapy. 2. N Engl J Med 1972 Aug 10;287:281–286.

S487. Skinner RP, Maddison PJ. Analysis of polyethylene glycol precipitates from SLE sera antibody enrichment in association with disease activity. Clin Exp Rheumatol 1990;8:553–560.

S488. Skinnider LF, Laxdal V. Effect of progesterones, estrogens, and hydrocortisones on mitogenic response of lymphocytes to phytohaemagglutin in pregnant and non-pregnant women. Por J Obsetet Gynaecol 1981;88:110–117.

S489. Slattery RM, Kjer-Nielsen L, Allison J, Charlton B, Mandel TE, Miller JFAP. Prevention of diabetes in non-obese diabetic I-AK transgenic mice. Nature 1990;345:724–726.

S490. Slavin S. Successful treatment of autoimmune disease in (NZB × NZW) F1 female mice by using fractionated total lymphoid irradiation. Proc Natl Acad Sci USA 1979;76: 5274–5276.

S491. Sliwinski AJ, Zvaifler NJ. Decreased synthesis of the third component in hypo-complementemic systemic lupus erythematosus. Clin Exp Immunol 1972;11:21–29.

S492. Sloan JB, Berk MA, Gebel HM, Fretzin DF. Multiple sclerosis and systemic lupus erythematosus. Occurrence in two generations of the same family. Arch Intern Med 1987 Jul; 147(7):1317–1320.

S493. Slone D, Heinonen OP, Kaufman D, Siskind V, Monson RR, Shapiro S. Aspirin and congenital malformations. Lancet 1976; 1:1373–1375.

S494. Sluiter HE, Kallenberg CGM, VanSon WJ, Weening JJ, van der Meulen J, The TH, Van der Hem GK. When to perform a renal biopsy in systemic lupus erythematosus (SLE)? Neth J Med 1981;24(6):217–223.

S495. Small P, Frank H, Kreisman H, Wolkove N. An immunological evaluation of pleural effusions in systemic lupus erythematosus. Ann Allergy 1982 Aug 49:101–103.

S496. Small P, Frenkiel S. Relapsing polychondritis. A feature of systemic lupus erythematosus. Arthritis Rheum 1980 Mar; 23(3):361–363.

S497. Small P, Mass MF, Kohler PF, Harbeck RJ. Central nervous system involvement in SLE: Diagnosis profile and clinical features. Arthritis Rheum 1977 Apr;20:869–878.

S498. Smathers PA, Santoro TJ, Chused TM, Reeves JP, Steinberg AD. Studies of lymphoproliferation in MRL/lpr/lpr mice. J Immunol 1984;133:1955.

S499. Smeenk R, Brinkman K, van den Brink H, Termaat RM, Berden J, Nossent H, Swaak T. Antibodies to DNA in patients with systemic lupus erythematosus. Their role in the diagnosis, the follow-up and the pathogenesis of the disease [review]. Clin Rheumatol 1990 Mar;9(1) Suppl 1:100–110.

S500. Smeenk RJT, Lucassen WAM, Swaak TJG. Is anticardiolipin activity a cross-reaction of anti-DNA or a separate entity? Arthritis Rheum 1987;30:607–617.

S501. Smeeton WMI, Doak PB, Simpson IJ, Herdson PB. Lupus nephritis: clinicopathological correlations. N Z Med J 1983 Jan 26;96:39–42.

S502. Smith CD, Marino C, Rothfield NF. The clinical utility of the lupus band test. Arthritis Rheum 1984 Apr;27(4): 382–387.

S503. Smith ECI, Borgonovo L, Carlsson B, Hammarstrom L, Rabbitts TH. Molecular probing of disease susceptibility genes in myasthenia gravis patients : an analysis of T cell receptor and HLA class II genes using restriction fragment length polymorphism. Ann NY Acad Sci 1987;505:388–397.

S504. Smith FE, Sweet DE, Brunner CM, Davis JS 4th. Avascular necrosis in SLE. An apparent predilection for young patients. Ann Rheum Dis 1976 Jun;35(3):227–232.

S505. Smith GA, Ward PH, Berci G. Laryngeal lupus erythematosus. J Laryngol Otol 1978 Jan;92(1):67–73.

S506. Smith GD, Amos TA, Mahler R, Peters TJ. Effect of chloroquine on insulin and glucose homeostasis in normal subjects and patients with non-insulin dependent diabetes mellitus. BMJ 1987 Feb 21;294(6570):465–467.

S507. Smith GM, Leyland MJ. Plasma exchange for cerebral lupus erythematosus. Lancet 1987;1:103.

S508. Smith HR, Chused TM, Smathers PA, Steinberg AD. Evidence for thymic regulation of autoimmunity in BXSB mice: Acceleration of disease by neonatal thymectomy. J Immunol 1983;130:1200.

S509. Smith HR, Green DR, Raveche ES, Smathers PA, Gerson RK, Steinberg AD. Studies of the induction of anti-DNA antibodies in normal mice. J Immunol 1982;129;2332–2336.

S510. Smith HR, Hansen CL, Rose R, Canoso RT. Autoimmune MRL-lpr/lpr mice are an animal model for the secondary antiphospholipid syndrome. J Rheumatol 1990 Jul;17(7): 911–915.

S511. Smith HR, Steinberg AD. Autoimmunity— a perspective. Annu Rev Immunol 1983;1:175–210.

S512. Smith JA, Margolies MN. Complete amino acid sequences of the heavy and light chain variable regions from two A/J mouse antigen non-binding monoclonal antibodies bearing the predominant p-azophenylarsonate idiotype. Biochemistry 1987;26:604.

S513. Smith JF. Interlesional triamcinolone as an adjunct to antimalarial drugs in the treatment of chronic discoid lupus erythematosus. Br J Dermatol 1962 Oct;74:350–353.

S514. Smith JK, Caspary EA, Field EJ. Lymphocyte reactivity to antigen in pregnancy. Am J Obstet Gynecol 1972;113: 602–606.

S515. Smith RM, Rill RL. Mobile histone tails in nucleosomes. Assignments of mobile segments and investigations of their role in chromatin folding. J Biol Chem 1989;264: 10574–10581.

S516. Smith V, Barrell BG. Cloning of a yeast U1 snRNP 70K protein homologue: functional conservation of an RNA-binding domain between humans and yeast. Embo J 1991;10: 2627–2634.

S517. Smolen J, Scherak O, Menzel J, Kojer M, Kolarz G. Levamisole in systemic lupus erythematosus [letter]. Arthritis Rheum 1977 Nov–Dec;20(8):1558–1559.

S518. Smolen JS, Bettelheim P, Koller U, McDougal S, Graninger W, Luger TA, Knapp W, Lechner K. Deficiency of the autologous mixed lymphocyte reaction in patients with classic hemophilia treated with commercial factor VIII concentrate. Correlation with T cell subset distribution, antibodies to lymphadenopathy-associated or human T lymphotropic virus, and analysis of the cellular basis of the deficiency. J Clin Invest 1985;75:1828–1834.

S519. Smolen JS, Chused TM, Leiserson WM, Reeves JP, Alling D, Steinberg AD. Heterogeneity of immunoregulatory T-cell subsets in systemic lupus erythematosus. Am J Med 1982 May;72:783–790.

S520. Smolen JS, Klippel JH, Penner E, Reichlin M, Steinberg AD, Chused TM, Scherak O, Graninger W, Hartter E, Zielinski CC, Wolf A, Davey RJ, Mann DL, Mayr WR. HLA-DR antigens in systemic lupus erythematosus association with specificity of autoantibody responses to nuclear antigens. Ann Rheum Dis 1987;46:457–462.

S521. Smolen JS, Morimoto C, Steinberg AD, Wolf A, Schlossman SF, Steinberg RT, Penner E, Reinherz E, Reichlin M, Chused TM. Systemic lupus erythematosus: Delineation of subpopulations by clinical serologic and T cell subset analysis. Am J Med 1985;289:139–148.

S522. Smorodinsky NI, Ghendler Y, Bakimer R, Chaitchuk S, Keydar I, Shoenfeld Y. Towards an idiotype vaccine against mammary tumors. Induction of an immune response to breast cancer-associated antigens by anti-idiotypic antibodies. Eur J Immunol 1988;18:1713.

S523. Smythe H. Fibrositis and other diffuse musculoskeletal syndromes. In: McCarty DJ, editor. Arthritis and Allied Conditions, Philadelphia: Lea & Febiger, 1985:481–489.

S524. Smythe HA, editor. Prostaglandins and benoxaprofen [editorial]. Proceedings of international symposium on benoxaprofen. J Rheumatol 1980;6 Suppl 1:1–3, 143.

S525. Snaith MI, Holt JM, Oliver DO, Dunnill MS, Halley W, Stephenson AC. Treatment of patients with systemic lupus erythematosus including nephritis and chlorambucil. BMJ 1973;2:197–201.

S526. Snapp RH. Lupus vulgaris of forty years' duration with mitotic process in lupo. Arch Dermatol 1950 Jul;62:166–167.

S527. Snapper CM, Finkelman FD, Stefany D, Conrad DH, Paul WE. Il-4 induces co-expression of intrinsic membrane IgG1 and IgE by murine B cells stimulated with lipopolysaccharide. J Immunol 1988;141:489–498.

S527a. Sneddon IB. Cerebrovascular lesions and livedo reticularis. Br J Dermatol 1965;77:180–185.

S528. Snyder S. Cutaneous effects of topical indomethacin, an inhibitor of prostaglandin synthesis in UV damaged skin. J Invest Dermatol 1975;64:322–325.

S529. Snyers B, Lambert M, Hardy JP. Retinal and choroidal vaso-occlusive disease in systemic lupus erythematosus associated with antiphospholipid antibodies. Retina 1990;10(4):255–260.

S530. So AK, Fielder AH, Warner CA, Isenberg DA, Batchelor JR, Walport MJ. DNA polymorphism of major histocompatibility complex class II and class III genes in systemic lupus erythematosus. Tissue Antigens 1990;35:144–147.

S531. Soares R, Paulini E, Pereira JP. Concentration and elimination of chloroquin by the placental circulation and milk in patients receiving chloroquin salt. Bull Trop Dis 1959;56:412.

S532. Sobel ES, Katagiri T, Katagiri K, Morris SC, Cohen PL, Eisenberg RA. An intrinsic B cell defect is required for the production of autoantibodies in the lpr model of murine systemic autoimmunity. J Exp Med 1991;173:1441–1449.

S533. Sobhon P, Jirasattham C. Effects of sex hormones on the thymus and lymphoid tissue of ovariectomized rats. Acta Ana 1974;89:211–225.

S534. Sobota WL, Brickman CM, Doyle TH, Rummelt JK. Serial Neuropsychological Examination during fluctuating systemic lupus erythematosus disease activity. In: Lahita R, editor. Systemic Lupus Erythematosus. New York: Wiley & Sons, 1987:847–853.

S535. Soffer LJ, Bader R. Corticotropin and cortisone in acute disseminated lupus erythematosus: results of long-term use. JAMA 1952 Jul 12;149:1002–1008.

S536. Sokal JE, Lessman EM. Effects of cancer chemotherapeutic agents on the human fetus. JAMA 1966;172:1765–1771.

S537. Sokol RJ, Hewill S, Stamps BK. Autoimmune hemolysis: an 18 year study of 865 cases referred to a regional transfusion center. Br J Med 1981;282:2023–2027.

S538. Sola MA, Soto de Delas J, Vazquez Doval J, Quintanilla E. Molluscum contagiosum gigante en lupus eritematoso sistemico. Med Clin (Barc) 1990 Feb 24;94(7):276–277.

S539. Solary E, Caillot D, Guy H, Olsson NO, Tanter Y, Chalopin JM. Systemic lupus erythematosus occurring in a patient with multiple myeloma. Arthritis Rheum 1986;29:933–934.

S540. Solheim BG, Larsen RA. Family studies in systemic lupus erythematosus. IV. Presence of antinuclear factors (ANFs) in the total populations of relatives and spouses, and the correlation to rheumatic disease. Acta Med Scand Suppl 1972;543:43–53.

S541. Solinger AM. Drug-related lupus. Clinical and etiological considerations. Rheum Dis Clin North Am 1988;14:187–202.

S542. Solinger AM, Adams LE, Friedman-Kien AE, Hess EV. Acquired immune deficiency syndrome (AIDS) and autoimmunity-mutually exclusive entities? J Clin Immunol 1988;8:32–42.

S543. Sollazzo J, Hasemann CA, Meek KD, Glotz D, Capra JD, Zanetti M. Molecular characterization of the V_H region of murine autoantibodies from neonatal and adult BALB/c mice. Eur J Immunol 1989;19:453.

S544. Solomon G, Schiffenbauer J, Keiser HD, Diamond B. Use of monoclonal antibodies to identify shared idiotypes on human antibodies to native DNA from patient with systemic lupus erythematosus. Proc Natl Acad Sci USA 1983 Feb;80(3):850–854.

S545. Solomon GF, Amkraut AA Psychoneuroendocrinological effects of the immune response. Annual Rev Microbiol 1981;35:155–184.

S546. Solomon GF, Moos RH. Emotions, immunity and disease. Arch Gen Psych 1974;11:657.

S547. Soloninka CA, Anderson MJ, Laskin CA. Anti-DNA and anti-lymphocyte antibodies during acute infection with human parvovirus B19. J Rheumatol 1989 Jun;16(6):777–781.

S548. Solovera JJ, Farinas MC, Strober S. Changes in B lymphocyte function in rheumatoid arthritis and lupus nephritis after total lymphoid irradiation. Arthritis Rheum 1988 Dec;31(12):1481–1491.

S549. Soloway RD, Baggenstoss AH, Elveback LR, Schoenfield LJ, Stubbs BL, Summerskill WHJ. The treatment of chronic active liver disease (CALD) [abstract]. Gastroenterology 1971;60:167.

S550. Soloway RD, Summerskill WHJ, Baggenstoss AH, Schoenfield LJ. "Lupoid" hepatitis, a nonentity in the spectrum of chronic active liver disease. Gastroenterology 1972 Sep;63(3):458–465.

S551. Soltani K, Pacernick LJ, Lorincz AL. Lupus erythematosus-like lesions in newborn infants. Arch Dermatol 1974;110:435.

S552. Sones DA, McDuffie FC, Hunder GG. Clinical significance of the RA cell. Arthritis Rheum 1968 Jun;11:400–403.

S553. Sonies BC, Klippel JH, Gerber RB, Gerber LH. Cognitive performance in systemic lupus erythematosus [abstract]. Arthritis Rheum 1982 Apr;25(4) Suppl:S80.

S554. Sonnenblick M, Abraham AS. Ibuprofen hypersensitivity in systemic lupus erythematosus. Br Med J 1978 Mar 11;1: 619–620.

S555. Sonnhog C, Karlson E. Procainamide-induced lupus erythematosus-like syndrome in relation to acetylator phenotype and plasma levels of procainamide. Acta Med Scand 1979; 206(4):245–251.

S556. Sonpal GM, Abramovici B. Acute abdomen in systemic lupus erythematosus with spontaneous hemoperitoneum [letter]. J Rheumatol 1987 Jun;14(3):636–637.

S557. Sontheimer RD. Clinical significance of subacute cutaneous lupus erythematosus skin lesions. J Dermatol (Japan) 1985;12:205–212.

S558. Sontheimer RD. Subacute cutaneous lupus erythematosus. Ch. 6. In: Callen J, editor. Clinics in dermatology. Philadelphia: Lippincott 1985;3(3):58–68.

S559. Sontheimer RD. The anticardiolipin syndrome. A new way to slice an old pie or a new pie to slice? Arch Dermatol 1987; 123:590–595.

S560. Sontheimer RD. Lupus Erythematosus. In: Provost TT, Farmer ER, editors. Current Therapy in Dermatology-2. Philadelphia: BC Decker, 1988:123–128.

S561. Sontheimer RD. Subacute cutaneous lupus erythematosus: a decade's perspective. Med Clin North Am 1989 Sep;73(5): 1073–1090.

S562. Sontheimer RD, Gilliam JN. DNA antibody class, subclass, and complement fixation in systemic lupus erythematosus with and without nephritis. Clin Immunol Immunopathol 1978 Aug;10(4):459–467.

S563. Sontheimer RD, Gilliam JN. A reappraisal of the relationship between subepidermal immunoglobulin deposits and DNA antibodies in systemic lupus erythematosus: a study using the Crithidia luciliae immunofluorescence anti-DNA assay. J Invest Dermatol 1979 Jan;72(1):29–32.

S564. Sontheimer RD, Gilliam JN. Regional variation in the deposition of subepidermal immunoglobulin in NZB/WF1 mice: Association with epidermal DNA synthesis. J Invest Dermatol 1979;72:25–28.

S565. Sontheimer RD, Gilliam JN. Subacute cutaneous lupus erythematosus. Current Concepts in Skin Disorders 1983;4: 11–17.

S566. Sontheimer RD, Maddison PJ, Reichlin M, Jordon RE, Stastny P, Gilliam JN. Serologic and HLA associations in subacute cutaneous lupus erythematosus: a clinical subset of lupus erythematosus. Ann Intern Med 1982 Nov;97:664–671.

S567. Sontheimer RD, Stastny P, Gilliam JN. Human histocompatibility antigen associations in subacute cutaneous lupus erythematosus. J Clin Invest 1981;67:312–316.

S568. Sontheimer RD, Thomas JR, Gilliam JN. Subacute cutaneous lupus erythematosus—A cutaneous marker for a distinct lupus erythematosus subset. Arch Dermatol 1979;115: 1409–1415.

S569. Soppi E, Viander M, Meurman I, Ekfors T, Forsstrom J. Triad of nephrotic syndrome, antinuclear antibodies and positive lupus band test [letter]. Clin Exp Rheumatol 1984 Oct–Dec;2(4):355–357.

S570. Soto-Aguilar MC, Boulware DW. Sarcoidosis presenting as antinuclear antibody positive glomerulonephritis. Ann Rheum Dis 1988 Apr;47(4):337–339.

S571. Sotolongo JR Jr, Swerdlow F, Schiff HI, Schapira HE. Successful treatment of lupus erythematosus cystitis with DMSO. Urology 1984 Feb;23(2):125–127.

S572. Souadjian JV, Enriquez P, Silverstein MN, Pepin J. The spectrum of diseases associated with thymoma. Arch Intern Med 1974;134:374–379.

S573. Soulier JP, Boffa MC. Avortements a repetition, thrombose et anticoagulant circulant anti-thromboplastine. Nouv Presse Med 1980;9:859–864.

S574. Souroujon MC, Rubinstein DB, Schwartz RS, Barrett KJ. Polymorphisms in human H chain V region genes from the V_HIII gene family. J Immunol 1989;143:706–711.

S575. Soya LF, Saxena KM. Alternate day steroid therapy for nephrotic children. JAMA 1965;192:125–130.

S576. Spaeth GL. Corneal staining in systemic lupus erythematosus. N Engl J Med 1967;276:1168–1171.

S577. Spagnuolo C, Galli C, Omini C, Folco GC. Antipyretic action of mepacrine without blockade of prostaglandin (PG): the kinetics of quinacrine (mepacrine) block. J Physiol (Lond) 1980;306:262–281, 283–306.

S578. Spangelo BL, Ross PC, Judd AM, MacLeod RM. Thymic stromal elements contain an anterior pituitary hormone-stimulating activity. J Neuroimmunol 1989;25:37–46.

S579. Spann CR, Callen JP, Klein JB, Kulick KB. Clinical, serological and immunogenetic studies in patients with chronic cutaneous (discoid) lupus erythematosus who have verrucous and/or hypertrophic skin lesions. J Rheumatol 1988;15: 256–261.

S580. Sparshott SM, Bell EB, Sarawar SR. CD45R CD4 T cell subset-reconstituted nude rats: subset-dependent survival of recipients and bi-directional isoform switching. Eur J Immunol 1991;21:993–1000.

S581. Spears CJ, Batchelor JR. Drug-induced autoimmune disease. Adv Nephrol 1987;16:219–230.

S582. Speira H, Rothenberg RR. Myocardial infarction in four young patients with systemic lupus erythematosus. J Rheumatol 1983 Jun;10:464–466.

S583. Speirs C, Fielder AH, Chapel H, Davey NJ, Batchelor JR. Complement system protein C4 and susceptibility to hydralazine-induced systemic lupus erythematosus. Lancet 1989;1: 922–924.

S584. Speller DC, Fakunie F, Cairns SA, Stephens M. Cryptococcal meningitis complicating systemic lupus erythematosus: two patients treated with flucytosine and amphotericin B. J Clin Path 1977;30:254–261.

S585. Spencer RW, Andelman SY. Steroid cataracts. Posterior subcapsular cataract formation in rheumatoid arthritis patients on long term steroid therapy. Arch Ophthalmol 1965 Jul;74:38–40.

S586. Spencer RP, Sziklas JJ, Rosenberg RJ. Waxing and waning of abdominal organ 67Ga uptake in a male with lupus: a potential for organ-specific therapy [letter]. Int J Rad Appl Instrum [B] 1987;14(2):161–162.

S587. Spencer-Green G, Adams LE, Hurtubise P, Kravatz G, Hess E. Familial alterations of immunoregulation in systemic lupus erythematosus. J Rheumatol 1985;2:498–503.

S588. Sperling R, Wachtel EJ. The histones. Adv Protein Chem 1981;34:1–60.

S589. Sperling RI, Weinblatt M, Robin JL, Ravalese J 3d, Hoover RL, House F, Coblyn JS, Fraser PA, Spur BW, Robinson DR, Lewis RA, Auste KF. Effects of dietary supplementation with marine fish oil on leukocyte lipid mediator generation and function in rheumatoid arthritis. Arthritis Rheum 1987;30: 988–997.

S590. Spezialetti R, Peter JB, Bluestein HG. Clinical correlations between anti-ribosomal P and anti-neuronal cell antibodies in CNS-SLE [abstract]. Arthritis Rheum 1990 Sep;33(9) Suppl: S102.

S591. Spickett GP, Brandon MR, Mason DW, Williams AF, Woollett GR. MRC OX-22, a monoclonal antibody that labels a new subset of T lymphocytes and reacts with the high molecular weight form of the leukocyte-common antigen. J Exp Med 1983;158:795–810.

S592. Spiegelberg HL. Biological activities of immunoglobulins of different classes and subclasses. Adv Immunol 1974;19: 259–294.

S593. Spiegler BJ, Yeni-Koshian GH. Incidence of left handed writing in college population with reference to family patterns of hand preference. Neuropsychologia 1983;21:651–659.

S594. Spiera H, Rothenberg RR. Myocardial infarction in four young patients with systemic lupus erythematosus. J Rheumatol 1983;10:464.

S595. Spiers C, Fielder AHL, Chapel H, Davey NJ, Batchelor JR. Complement system protein C4 and susceptibility to hydralazine-induced systemic lupus erythematosus. Lancet 1989;1:922–924.

S596. Spies T, Blanck G, Bresnahan M, Sands J, Strominger JL. A new cluster of genes within the human major histocompatibility complex. Science 1989;243:214–217.

S597. Spies T, Morton CC, Nedospasov SA, Fiers W, Pious D, Stominger JL. Genes for the tumor necrosis factors α and β are linked to the human major histocompatibility complex. Proc Nat Acad Sci USA 1986;83:8699–8702.

S598. Spinozzi F, Capodicasa E, Gerli R, Bertotto A, Rambotti P, Grignani F. Systemic lupus erythematosus following total body irradiation for malignant lymphoma. Allergol Immunopathol (Madr) 1986;14:241–244.

S599. Spiva DA, Cecere FA. The use of combination plasmapheresis/leukocytapheresis in the treatment of refractory systemic lupus erythematosus. Plasma Ther Trans Tech 1983;4:151–164.

S600. Spriggs B, Epstein W. Clinical correlation of elevated urine L-chain concentrations in SLE [abstract]. Clin Res 1973 Feb;21:213.

S601. Spritz RA, Strunk K, Surowy CS, Hoch SO, Barton DE, Francka U. The human U1/UK protein: cDNA cloning, chromosomal localization, expression, alternative splicing and RNA-binding. Nucleic Acids Res 1987;15:10373–10391.

S602. Spurney RF, Ruiz P, Pisetsky DS, Coffman TM. Enhanced renal leukotriene production in murine lupus: role of lipoxygenase metabolites. Kidney Int 1991;39:95–102.

S603. Spurr C, in discussion of Osborne, ED, Jordon JW, Hoak FC, Pschierer FJ. Nitrogen mustard therapy in cutaneous blastomatous disease. JAMA 1947;135:1123–1128.

S604. Sreebny LM, Valdini A. Xerostomia: A neglected symptom. Arch Intern Med 1987 Jul;147(7):1333–1337.

S605. Stafford-Brady FJ, Gladman DD, Urowitz MB. Successful pregnancy in systemic lupus erythematosus with an untreated lupus anticoagulant. Arch Intern Med 1988;148:1647–1648.

S606. Stafford-Brady FJ, Urowitz MB, Gladman DD, Easterbrook M. Lupus retinopathy. Patterns, associations and prognosis. Arthritis Rheum 1988;31(9):1105–1110.

S607. Stage DE, Mannik M. 7S gamma M-globulin in rheumatoid arthritis. Evaluation of its clinical significance. Arthritis Rheum 1971 Jul–Aug;14:400–450.

S608. Stahl NI, Klippel JH, Decker JL. Fever in systemic lupus erythematosus. Am J Med 1979 Dec;67(6):935–940.

S609. Stamenkovic I, Favre H, Donath A, Assimacopoulos A, Chatelenat F. Renal biopsy in SLE irrespective of clinical findings: long-term follow-up. Clin Nephrol 1986;26:109–115.

S610. Standiford TJ, Strieter RM, Chensue SW, Westwick J, Kasahara K, Kunkel SL. IL-4 inhibits the expression of IL-8 from stimulated human monocytes. J Immunol 1990;145:1435–1439.

S611. Stanford DR, Kehl M, Perry CA, Holicky E, Harvey SE, Rohleder AM, Rehder K, Luhrmann R, Wieben ED. The complete primary structure of the human snRNP E protein. Nucleic Acids Res 1988;16:10593–10605.

S612. Staples PJ, Gerdin DN, Decker JL, Gordon RS. Incidence of infection in systemic lupus erythematosus. Arthritis Rheum 1974;17:1–10.

S613. Staples PJ, Steinberg AD, Talal N. Induction of immunologic tolerance in older New Zealand mice repopulated with young spleen, bone marrow or thymus. J Exp Med 1970;131:1223–1238.

S614. Staples PJ, Talal N. Relative inability to induce tolerance in adult NZB and NZB/NZW F1 mice. J Exp Med 1969;129:123–129.

S615. Staples PJ, Talal N. Rapid loss of tolerance induced in weanling NZB and B/W F1 mice. Science 1969;163:1215–1216.

S616. Starkebaum G, Arend WP. Neutrophil-binding immunoglobulin G in systemic erythematosus. J Clin Invest 1979;64:902–912.

S617. Starkebaum G, Price TH, Lee MY, Arend WP. Autoimmune neutropenia in systemic lupus erythematosus. Arthritis Rheum 1978 Jun;21:504–512.

S618. Stary A, Schwartz T, Duschet P, Gschnait F. Lichen ruber planus—lupus erythematosus/overlap syndrome [English abstract]. Z Hautkr 1987 Mar;62(5):381–394.

S619. Starzl TE, Porter KA, Andres G, Halgrimson CG, Hurwitz R, Giles G, Terasaki PI, Penn I, Schroter GT, Lilly J, Starkie SJ, Putman CW. Long-term survival after renal transplantation in humans: (with special reference to histocompatibility matching, thymectomy, homograft glomerulonephritis, heterologous ACG, and recipient malignancy). Ann Surg 1970 Sep;172(3):437–472.

S620. Stasny P. The distribution of HL-A antigens in black patients with systemic lupus erythematosus (SLE) [abstract]. Arthritis Rheum 1972;15:455.

S621. Stasny P. Association of the B-cell alloantigen DRw4 with rheumatoid arthritis. N Engl J Med 1978;298:869–871.

S622. Stasny P. HLA-D and Ia antigens in rheumatoid arthritis and systemic lupus erythematosus. Arthritis Rheum 1978;21:1728.

S623. Stastny P, Ziff M. Cold-insoluble complexes and complement levels in SLE. N Engl J Med 1969 Jun 19;280:1376–1381.

S624. Stastny P, Ziff M. Lymphocyte and platelet autoantibodies in SLE. Lancet 1971 Jun 12;1:1239–1249.

S625. Stastny P, Ziff M. Antibodies against cell membrane constituents in systemic lupus erythematosus and related diseases. I. Cytotoxic effect of serum from patients with systemic lupus erythematosus for allogeneic and for autologous lymphocytes. Clin Exp Immunol 1971 Apr;8:543–550.

S626. Staub HL, Harris EN, Khamashta MA, Savidge G, Chahade WH, Hughes GR. Antibody to phosphatidylethanolamine in a patient with lupus anticoagulant and thrombosis. Ann Rheum Dis 1989 Feb;48(2):166–169.

S627. Stecher VJ, Connolly KM, Speight PT. Fibronectin and macrophages as parameters of disease-modifying antirheumatic activity. Br J Clin Prac 1987;41 Suppl:64–71.

S628. Stedman E. Cell specificity of histones. Nature 1950; 166:780–781.

S629. Stedman E. Phil Trans R Soc Lond [Biol] 1951;235:565.

S630. Steele EJ, Cunningham AJ. High proportion of Ig-producing cells making autoantibody in normal mice. Nature 1978 Aug 3;274(5670):483–484.

S631. Steen VD, Ramsey-Goldman R. Phenothiazine-induced systemic lupus erythematosus with superior vena cava syndrome: case report and review of the literature. Arthritis Rheum 1988;31:923–926.

S632. Stein A, Winkelstein A, Agarwal A. Concurrent systemic lupus erythematous and common variable hypogammaglobulinemia. Arthritis Rheum 1985 Apr;28:462–465.

S633. Stein H, Walters K, Dillon A, Schulzer M. Systemic lupus erythematosus: a medical and social profile. J Rheumatol 1986;13:570–576.

S634. Stein KE, Soderstrom T. Neonatal administration of idiotype or antiidiotype primes for protection against Escherichia coli K13 infection in mice. J Exp Med 1984;160:1011.

S635. Steinberg AD. Studies of immune regulation in patients with systemic lupus erythematosus: Evolving concepts. Ann Intern Med 1979;91:101–587.

S636. Steinberg AD. The treatment of lupus nephritis [clinical conference]. Kidney Int 1986 Nov;30(5):769–787.

S637. Steinberg AD, Decker JL. Immunoregulatory drugs. In McCarty, editor. Arthritis and Allied Conditions, Philadelphia: Lea & Febiger 1979:375–390.

S638. Steinberg AD, Decker JL, Aptekar RG. Completed ten-week trial of cyclophosphamide or azathioprine or placebo in lupus nephritis [abstract]. Arthritis Rheum 1973;16:572.

S639. Steinberg AD, Gourley MF, Klinman DM, Tsokos GC, Scott DE, Krieg AM. Systemic Lupus Erythematosus. Am J Med. In Press.

S640. Steinberg AD, Gourley MF, Klinman DM, Tsokos GC, Scott DE, Kreig AM. NIH conference: Systemic lupus erythematosus. Ann Intern Med 1991;115:548–559.

S641. Steinberg AD, Huston DP, Taurog JD, Cowdery JS, Raveche ES. The cellular and genetic basis of murine lupus. Immunol Rev 1981;55:121–154.

S642. Steinberg AD, Klassen LW, Budman DR, Williams GW. Immunofluorescence studies of anti-T cell antibodies and T cells in systemic lupus erythematosus. Arthritis Rheum 1979 Feb;22:114–122.

S643. Steinberg AD, Klinman DM. Pathogenesis of systemic lupus erythematosus. Rheum Dis Clin North Am 1988;14: 25–41.

S644. Steinberg AD, Krieg AM, Gourley MF, Klinman DM. Theoretical and experimental approaches to generalized autoimmunity. Immunol Rev 1990;118:129–163.

S645. Steinberg AD, Law LW, Talal N. The role of the NZB/NZW F1 thymus in experimental tolerance and autoimmunity. Arthritis Rheum 1970;13:369–377.

S646. Steinberg AD, Melez KA, Raveche ES, Reeves JP, Boegel WA, Smathers PA, Taurog JD, Weinlein LM, Duvic M. Approach to the study of the role of sex hormones in autoimmunity. Arthritis Rheum 1979 Nov;22(11):1170–1176.

S647. Steinberg AD, Raveche ES, Laskin CA, Miller ML, Steinberg RT. Genetic environmental and cellular factors in the pathogenesis of systemic lupus erythematosus. Arthritis Rheum 1982;25:734–743.

S647a. Steinberg AD, Raveche ES, Laskin CA, Smith HR, Santoro T, Miller ML, Plotz PH. Systemic lupus erythematosus: Insights from animal models. Ann Intern Med 1984 May;100:714–727.

S648. Steinberg AD, Roths JB, Murphy ED, Steinberg RT, Raveche ES. Effects of thymectomy or androgen administration upon the autoimmune disease of MRL/Mp-lpr/lpr mice. J Immunol 1980;125:871–873.

S649. Steinberg AD, Smathers PA, Boegel WB. Effects of sex hormones on autoantibody production by NZB mice and modification by environmental factors. Clin Immunol Immunopathol 1980;17:562–572.

S650. Steinberg AD, Smith HR, Laskin CA, Steinberg BJ, Smolen JS. Studies of immune abnormalities in systemic lupus erythematosus. Am J Kidney Dis 1982 Jul;2 Suppl 1:101–110.

S651. Steinberg AD, Steinberg BJ. Lupus disease activity associated with menstrual cycle [letter]. J Rheumatol 1985 Aug; 12(4):816–817.

S652. Steinberg AD, Steinberg SC. Long-term preservation of renal function in patients with lupus nephritis receiving treatment that includes cyclophosphamide versus those treated with prednisone only. Arthritis Rheum 1991;34:945–950.

S653. Steinberg AD, Talal N. The coexistence of Sjogren's syndrome and systemic lupus erythematosus. Ann Intern Med 1971 Jan;74:55–61.

S654. Steinberg B, Smathers P, Frederiksen K, Steinberg A. Ability of the xid gene to prevent autoimmunity in (NZBxNZW)

F1 mice during the course of their natural history, after polyclonal stimulation, or following immunization with DNA. J Clin Invest 1982;70:587–597.

S655. Steinman CR. Circulating DNA in systemic lupus erythematosus. Association with central nervous system involvement and systemic vasculitis. Am J Med 1978 Sep;67(3): 429–435.

S655a. Steinman CR. Circulating DNA in systemic erythematosus. Isolation and characterization. J Clin Invest 1984;73: 832–841.

S656. Steinman CR, Ackad A. Appearance of circulating DNA during hemodialysis. Am J Med 1977;62:693–697.

S657. Steitz JA. Snurps. Sci Am 1988 Jun:56–63.

S658. Steitz JA, Black DL, Gerke V, Parker KA, Kramer A, Frendewey D, Keller W. Functions of the abundant U-snRNPs. In: Birnstiel ML, editor. Structure and function of major and minor small nuclear ribonuclear ribonucleoprotein particles. Heidelberg FRG: Springer Verlag, 1988:115–154.

S659. Stejskal J, Pirani CL, Okada M, Mandalenakis N, Pollak VE. Discontinuities (gaps) of the glomerular capillary wall and basement membrane in renal diseases. Lab Invest 1973 Feb; 28:149–169.

S660. Stekman IL, Blasini AM, Leon-Ponte M, Baroja ML, Abadi I, Rodriguez MA. Enhanced CD3-mediated T lymphocyte proliferation in patients with systemic lupus erythematosus. Arthritis Rheum 1991;34:459–467.

S661. Stenseth K, Thyberg J. Monensin and chloroquine inhibit transfer to lysosomes of endocytosed and macromolecules in cultured mouse peritoneal macrophages. Eur J Cell Biol 1989 Aug;49(2):326–333.

S662. Stenszky V, Kozma L, Szegedi G, Farid NR. Interplay of immunoglobulin G heavy chain markers (Gm) and HLA in predisposing to systemic lupus erythematosus. J Immunogenet 1986;13:11–17.

S663. Stephano JE. Purified lupus antigen La recognizes an oligo uridylate stretch common to the 3' termini of RNA polymerase III transcripts. Cell 1984;36:145–154.

S664. Stephens HAF, Fitzharris P, Knight RA, Snaith ML. Inhibition of proliferative and suppressor responses in the autologous mixed lymphocyte reaction by serum from patients with systemic lupus erythematosus. Ann Rheum Dis 1982 Oct;41: 495–501.

S665. Stephensen O, Cleland WP, Hallidie-Smith K. Congenital complete heart block and persistent ductus arteriosus associated with maternal systemic lupus erythematosus. Br Heart J 1981;46:104–106.

S666. Stern JL, Johnson TRB. Antineoplastic drugs and pregnancy. In: Niebyl JR, editor. Drug use in Pregnancy. Philadelphia: Lea & Febiger, 1982:67–90.

S667. Stern M, Robbins ES. Psychoses in systemic lupus erythematosus. Arch Gen Psychiatry 1960 Aug;3:205–212.

S668. Stern MP, Kolterman OG, McDevitt H, Reaven GM. Acquired type 3 hyperlipoproteinemia. Arch Intern Med 1972 Dec;130:817–821.

S669. Stern R, Fishman J, Brushman H, Kunkel HG. Systemic lupus erythematosus associated with Klinefelter's syndrome. Arthritis Rheum 1977;20:18–22.

S670. Stern R, Fu SM, Fotino M, Agnello V, Kunkel H. Hereditary C2-deficiency. Arthritis Rheum 1976;19:517–522.

S671. Stern RS. Phototoxic reactions to piroxicam and other nonsteroidal anti-inflammatory agents [letter]. N Engl J Med 1983 Jul 21;309(3):186–187.

S672. Stern RS, Docken W. An exacerbation of SLE after visiting a tanning salon. JAMA 1986;255:3120.

S673. Stern RS, Morison WL, Thibodeau LA, Kleinerman RA, Parish JA, Geer DE Jr. Antinuclear antibodies and oral methoxsalen photochemotherapy (PUVA) for psoriasis. Arch Dermatol 1979;115:1320–1324.

S674. Stern W, Macdonald VE. Factors affecting the sensitivity of APTT reagents to lupus inhibitors (LI). Thromb Haemost 1985 Jul;54:146.

S675. Stetler DA, Cavallo T. Anti-RNA polymerase I antibodies: potential role in the induction and progression of murine lupus nephritis. J Immunol 1987 Apr 1;138(7):2119–2123.

S676. Stetler DA, Sipes DE, Jacob ST. Anti-RNA polymerase I antibodies in sera of MRL lpr/lpr and MRL +/+ autoimmune mice. Correlation of antibody production with delayed onset of lupus-like disease in MRL +/+ mice. J Exp Med 1985;162:1760–1770.

S677. Stevanovic G, Cramer AD, Taylor CR, Lukes RJ. Immunoblastic scaroma in patients with systemic lupus erythematosus. Arch Pathol Lab Med 1983 Nov;107(11):589–592.

S678. Steven MM, Tanner AR, Holdstock GE, Cockrell R, Smith J, Smith DS, Hamblin TJ, Wright R. The effect of plasma exchange on the in vitro monocyte function of patients with immune complex diseases. Clin Exp Immunol 1981 Aug;45(2):240–245.

S679. Stevens MB. Systemic lupus erythematosus, Clinical issues. Springer Semin Immunopathol 1986;9(2–3):251–270.

S680. Stevens MB. Musculoskeletal manifestations. In: Schur PH, editor. The Clinical Management of Systemic Lupus Erythematosus. New York: Grune & Stratton, 1983, 63–84.

S681. Stevens MB, Hookman P, Siegel CI, Esterly JR, Hendrix TR, Shulman LE. The "slcerodermatosus" esophagus and Raynaud's phenomenon [abstract]. Arthritis Rheum 1963;6:301–302.

S682. Stevens MB, Knowles B. Significance of urinary gamma globulin in lupus nephritis. 1. Electrophoretic analysis. N Engl J Med 1962 Dec 6;267:1159–1166.

S683. Stevens MB, Zizic TM, Young N. Urinary fibrinogen fragments in lupus nephritis [abstract]. Arthritis Rheum 1970 May–Jun;13:352.

S684. Stevens WMR, Burdon JGW, Clemens LE, Webb J. The "Shrinking lung syndrome" an infrequently recognized feature of systemic lupus erythematosus. Aust N Z J Med 1990;20:67–70.

S685. Stevenson FK, Wrightham M, Glennie MJ, Jones DB, Cattan AR, Teizi T, Hamblin TJ, Stevenson GT. Antibodies to shared idiotypes as agents for analysis and therapy for human B cell tumors. Blood 1986;68:430.

S686. Stevenson GH, Pindar A, Slade CJ. A chimeric antibody with dual Fc regions (bisFabFc) prepared by manipulations at the IgG hinge. Anticancer Drug Des 1989;3:219.

S687. Steward MW, Hay FC. Changes in immunoglobulin class and subclass of anti-DNA antibodies with increasing age in NAB/NZW F1 hybrid mice. Clin Exp Immunopathol 1976 Nov;26(2):363–370.

S688. Stewart CC, Goeckerman WH. Lupus erythematosus disseminatus acutus in a juvenile. Am J Dis Child 1931;42:864–869.

S689. Stewart SJ, Prpic V, Powers FS, Bocckino SB, Isaacks RE, Exton JH. Perturbation of the human T-cell antigen receptor-T3 complex leads to the production of inositol tetrakisphosphate: evidence for conversion from inositol trisphosphate. Proc Natl Acad Sci USA 1986;83:6098–6102.

S690. Stiehm ER, Ashida E, Kim KS, Winston DJ, Haas A, Gale RP. Intravenous immunoglobulins as therapeutic agents [clinical conference]. Ann Intern Med 1987 Sep;107(3):367–382.

S691. Stimmler MM, Chen DCP, Quismorio FP Jr, Ma GQ, Colletti PM, Siegel ME. Single photon emission computed tomography (SPECT) and magnetic resonance imaging (MRI) of the brain in neuropsychiatric SLE [NP-SLE] [abstract]. Arthritis Rheum 1990 Sep;33(9) Suppl:S103.

S692. Stimmler MM, Colletti PM, Quismorio FP Jr. Magnetic resonance imaging in neuropsychiatric systemic lupus erythematosus (NP-SLE) [abstract]. Arthritis Rheum 1990 Sep;33(9) Suppl:S30.

S693. Stimmler MM, Quismorio FP Jr, McGehee WG, Boylen T, Sharma OP. Anticardiolipin antibodies in acquired immunodeficiency syndrome. Arch Intern Med 1989 Aug;149(8):1833–1835.

S694. Stimson WH. Ostrogen and human T lymphocytes: Presence of specific receptors in the T-suppressor/ cytotoxic/subset. Scand J Immunol 1988;28:345–350.

S695. Stimson WH, Hunter IC. Estrogen induced immunoregulation mediated through the thymus. J Clin Lab Immunol 1980;4:27–33.

S696. Stimson WH, Strachan AF, Shepherd A. Studies on the maternal immune response to placental antigens: absence of a blocking factor from the blood of abortion-prone women. Br J Obstet Gynecol 1979;86:41–45.

S697. Stites DP, Pavia CS, Clemens LE, Kuhn RW, Siiteri PK. Immunologic regulation in pregnancy. Arthritis Rheum 1979;22:1300–1307.

S698. Stohl W. Impaired generation of polyclonal T cell-mediated cytolytic activity despite normal polyclonal T cell proliferation in systemic lupus erythematosus. Clin Immunol Immunopathol 1992 In press.

S699. Stohl W, Crow MK, Kunkel HG. Systemic lupus erythematosus with deficiency of the T4 epitope on T helper/inducer cells. N Engl J Med 1985;312:1671–1678.

S700. Stohl W, Singer JZ. Correlation between systemic lupus erythematosus and T4 epitope phenotype. Arthritis Rheum 1987;30:1412–1415.

S701. Stokes-Turner L, Mones M, Addison I, Mansell M, Isenberg DA. Does rheumatoid factor protect lupus nephritis from the development of nephritis. Ann Rheum Dis 1989;48:14–16.

S702. Stoll DM, King LE Jr. Association of bullous pemphigoid with systemic lupus erythematosus. Arch Dermatol 1984 Mar;120(3):362–366.

S703. Stollar BD. Varying specificity of systemic lupus erythematosus sera for histone fractions and a periodate-sensitive antigen associated with histone. J Immunol 1969;103(4):804–808.

S704. Stollar BD. Reactions of systemic lupus erythematosus sera with histone fractions and histone-DNA complexes. Arthritis Rheum 1971 Jul–Aug;14:485–492.

S705. Stollar BD. The specificity and application of antibodies to helical nucleic acids. C R C Crit Rev Biochem 1975;3:45–69.

S706. Stollar BD. The antigenic potential and specificity of nucleic acids, nucleoproteins, and their modified derivatives. Arthritis Rheum 1981 Aug;24:1010–1018.

S707. Stollar D, Levine L. Antibodies to denatured deoxyribonucleic in lupus erythematosus serum. V. Mechanism of DNA—anti-DNA inhibition by chloroquine. Arch Biochem 1963 May;101:335–341.

S708. Stollar BD, Schwartz RS. Monoclonal anti-DNA antibodies: The targets and origins of SLE autoantibodies. Ann NY Acad Sci 1986;465:192–199.

S709. Stollar BD, Zon G, Pastor RW. A recognition site on synthetic helical oligonucleotide for monoclonal anti-native DNA autoantibody. Proc Natl Acad Sci USA 1986 Jan;83(12):4469–4473.

S710. Stolzenburg T, Binz H, Fontana A, Felder M, Wagenhaeuser FJ. Impaired mitogen-induced interferon-gamma production in rheumatoid arthritis and related diseases. Scand J Immunol 1988;27:73–81.

S711. Stoner GL, Best PV, Mazio M, Ryschkewitsch CF, Walker DL, de F Webster H. Progressive multifocal leukoencephalopathy complicating systemic lupus erythematosus: Distribution of JC virus in chronically demyelinated cerebellar lesions. J Neuropath Exp Neurol 1988;47:307.

S712. Stoppe G, Wildhagen K, Meyer GJ, Schober O. FDG-PET in the diagnosis of neuropsychiatric lupus erythematosus and comparison with computed tomography and magnetic resonance imaging [English abstract]. Nuklearmedizin 1989 Oct; 28(5):187–192.

S713. Stoppe G, Wildhagen K, Seidel JW, Meyer GJ, Schober O, Heintz P, Kunkel H, Deicher H, Hundeshagen H. Positron emission tomography in neuropsychiatric lupus erythematosus. Neurology 1990 Feb;40(2):304–308.

S714. Storck H, Berzups S. On lupus erythematosus, with special reference to transition from localized to generalized form [original in German]. Dermatologica (Basel) 1962.124: 142–154.

S715. Stott DI. Immunoblotting and dot blotting. J Immunol Methods 1989;119:153–187.

S716. Stoudemire A, Stork M, Simel D, Houpt JL. Neuro-ophthalmic systemic lupus erythematosus misdiagnosed as hysterical blindness [clinical and research reports]. Am J Psychiatry 1982;139:1194–1196.

S717. Stowers JH. Lupus erythematosus in a child. Br J Dermatol 1892;20:236; cited in Stewart CC, Goeckerman WH. Lupus erythematosus disseminatus acutus in a juvenile. Am J Dis Child 1931;42:864–869.

S718. Straaton KV, Chatham WW, Reveille JD, Koopman WJ, Smith SH. Clinically significant valvular heart disease in systemic lupus erythematosus. Am J Med 1988;85:645–650.

S719. Strack van Schijndel RJ, Bronsveld W, Boen-Tan TN. The patient with pseudotumor cerebri and disseminated lupus erythematosus [English abstract]. Ned Tijdschr Geneeskd 1986 Jan 18;130(3):123–126.

S720. Straka P, Grossman R, Makover D, Freundlich B. Disease quiescence following renal transplantation in patients with systemic lupus erythematosus [abstract]. Arthritis Rheum 1989 Apr;32(4) Suppl:S115.

S721. Strakosch EA. Acute lupus erythematosus disseminatus treated with penicillin; report of case. Arch Dermat & Syph 1946 Aug;54:197–199.

S722. Strate M, Brandrup F, Wang P. Discoid lupus erythematosus-like skin lesions in a patient with autosomal recessive chronic granulomatous disease. Clin Genetics 1986 Sep; 30(3):184–190.

S723. Stratton F, cited by Lachman PJ. Genetic deficiencies of the complement system. Boll 1st Sieroter Milan 1974;53 Suppl 1:195–207.

S724. Stratton MA. Drug-induced systemic lupus erythematosus. Clin Pharmacol 1985;4:657.

S725. Straub RL, Black FW. Mental status examination. In: Organic Brain Syndrome, 1990; Ch 3.

S726. Strauer BE, Brune I, Schenk H, Knoll D, Perings E. Lupus cardiomyopathy: Cardiac mechanics, hemodynamics and coronary blood flow in uncomplicated systemic lupus erythematosus. Am Heart J 1976 Dec;92:715–722.

S727. Strauss J, Abitbol C, Zilleruelo G, Scott G, Paredes A, Malaga S, Montane B, Mitchell C, Parks W, Pardo V. Renal disease in children with the acquired immunodeficiency syndrome. N Engl J Med 1989 Sep 7;321(10):625–630.

S728. Strejcek J. Lecba solemi zlata a systemovy erythematodes [English abstract]. Cas Lek Cesk 1983 Apr 15;122(15): 469–472.

S729. Streuli M, Hall LR, Saga Y, Schlossman SF, Saito H. Differential usage of three exons generates at least five different mRNA encoding human leukocyte common antigens. J Exp Med 1987;166:1548–1566.

S730. Stricker RB, Corash L. Antibodies to thrombin in postsurgical patients. Blood 1989;73:1386.

S731. Stricker RB, Lane PK, Lefferet JD, Rodgers GM, Shuman MA, Corash L. Development of antithrombin antibodies following surgery in patients with prosthetic cardiac valves. Blood 1988;72:1375–1380.

S732. Stricker RB, Shuman MA. Aplastic anemia complicating systemic lupus erythematosus: response to androgens in two patients. Am J Hematol 1984;17:193–201.

S733. Strickland RW, Limmani A, Wall JG, Krishnan J. Hairy cell leukemia presenting as a lupus-like illness. Arthritis Rheum 1988 Apr;31(4):566–568.

S734. Striker GE, Kelly MR, Quadracci LJ, Scribner BH. The course of lupus nephritis: a clinico-pathologic correlation of 50 patients. In: Kincaid-Smith P, Mathew TH, Becker EL, editors. Glomerulonephritis. New York: Wiley, 1973:1141–1166.

S735. Strober S, Farinas MC, Field EH, Solovera JJ, Kiberd BA, Myers BD, Hoppe RT. Lupus nephritis after total lymphoid irradiation: persistent improvement and reduction of steroid therapy. Ann Intern Med 1987 Nov;107(5):689–690.

S736. Strober S, Farinas MC, Field EH, Solovera JJ, Kiberd BA, Myers BD, Hoppe RT. Treatment of lupus nephritis with total lymphoid irradiation. Observations during a 12–79 month follow-up. Arthritis Rheum 1988 Jul;31(7):850–858.

S737. Strober S, Field E, Hoppe RT, Kotzin BL, Shemesh O, Engleman E, Ross JC, Myers BD. Treatment of intractable lupus nephritis with total lymphoid irradiation. Ann Intern Med 1985 Apr;102(4):450–458.

S738. Struyf NJ, Snoeck HW, Bridts CH, DeClerck LS, Stevens WJ. Natural killer cell activity in Sjogren's syndrome and systemic lupus erythematosus: stimulation with interferons and interleukin 2 and correlation with immune complexes. Ann Rheum Dis 1990;49:690.

S739. Stuart MJ, Gross SJ, Elrad H, Graber JE. Effects of acetylsalicylic acid ingestion on maternal and neonatal hemostasis. N Engl J Med 1982;307:909–913.

S740. Stuckey M, Dawkins R, Zilko P, Williamson J, Edelman J. MCTD in children: Development of SLE with CNS involvement. Aust NZ J Med 1982 Oct;12:576.

S741. Studenski S, Allen NB, Caldwell DS, Rice JR, Polisson RP. Survival in systemic lupus erythematosus. A multivariate analysis of demographic factors. Arthritis Rheum 1987;30: 1326–1332.

S742. Studenski SA, Bembe ML, Caldwell DS, Polisson RP, Rice JR. Late onset systemic lupus erythematosus—Race and sex factors [abstract]. Clin Res 1984;32–469A.

S743. Stulberg BN, Levine M, Bauer TW, Belhobek GH, Pflanze W, Feiglin DH, Roth AI. Multimodality approach to osteonecrosis of the femoral head. Clin Orthop 1989 Mar;(240): 181–193.

S744. Stumpf WE, Sar M. In: Pasqualini JF, editor. Receptor and mechanisms of action of steroid hormones. New York & Basel: Marcell Dekker, 1976:41–84.

S745. Sturfelt G, Johnson U, Sjoholm AG. Sequential studies of complement activation in systemic lupus erythematosus. Scand J Rheumatol 1985;14:184–196.

S746. Sturfelt G, Mousa F, Jonsson H, Nived O, Thysell H, Wollheim F. Recurrent cerebral infarction and the antiphospholipid syndrome: effect of intravenous gammaglobulin in a patient with systemic lupus erythematosus. Ann Rheum Dis 1990 Nov;49(11):939–941.

S747. Sturfelt G, Sjoholm AG. Complement components, complement activation and acute phase response in systemic lupus erythematosus. Int Arch All Appl Immunol 1984;75(1): 75–83.

S748. Sturfelt G, Truedsson L, Johansen P, Jonsson H, Nived O, Sjoholm AG. Homozygous C4A deficiency in SLE; analysis of patients from a defined population. Clin Genetics 1990;38: 427–433.

S749. Sturgess AD, Evans DT, Mackay IR, Riglar A. Effects of the oestrogen antagonist tamoxifen on disease indices in systemic lupus erythematosus. J Clin Lab Immunol 1984;13(1):11–14.

S750. Sturgess AD, Peterson MG, McNeilage LJ, Whittingham S, Coppel RL. Characteristics and epitope mapping of a cloned human autoantigen La. J Immunol 1988;140:3212–3218.

S751. Su TP, London ED, Jaffee JH. Steroid binding at o receptors suggests a link between endemic, venous and immune systems. Science 1988;240:219–221.

S752. Subiza JL, Caturla A, Pascual-Salcedo D, Chamorro MJ, Gazapo E, Fiqueredo MA, De La Concho EG. DNA-anti-DNA complexes account for part of the antihistone activity found in patients with systemic lupus erythematosus. Arthritis Rheum 1989;32:406–412.

S753. Suchman AL, Condemi JJ, Leddy JP. Seizure after pulse therapy with methylprednisolone. Arthritis Rheum 1983 Jan; 26:117–118.

S754. Suciu-Foca N, Buda JA, Thiem T, Reemtsa K. Impaired responsiveness of lymphocytes in patients with systemic lupus erythematosus. Clin Exp Immunol 1974 Nov;18:295–302.

S755. Sugasawa K, Ishimi Y, Yamada M, Hanaoka F, Ui M. Heterogeneous assembly of nascent core histones to form nucleosomal histone octamers in mouse FM3A cells. Eur J Biochem 1989;185:55–61.

S756. Sugimoto M, Sato Y, Kumagai Y, Suenaga M, Hashimoto H, Hiross S. A case of systemic lupus erythematosus with lupus nephritis occurring in Crohn's disease. Nippon Naika Gakkai Zasshi 1989 Apr;78(4):583–584.

S757. Sugimura K, Wada Y, Kimura T, Ohno T, Kobayashi S, Azuma I. Abnormal behavior of gamma-committed B lymphocytes probed by a lymphocytes blastogenesis inhibitory factor in autoimmune MRL mice. Eur J Immunol 1990;20: 1899–1904.

S758. Sugisaki T, Shiwachi S, Yonekura M, Kitazawa K, Yamamoto J, Uchida J, Saito K, Shibata T, Kawasum H, Takase T, Soeda K. High does intravenous gamma globulin for membranous nephropathy (MN), membranoproliferative glomerulonephritis (MPGN) and lupus nephritis (LN). Fed Proc 1982; 41(3):692.

S759. Sugiyama T, Kiwamoto H, Esa A, Park YC, Kaneko S, Kurita T. Neurogenic bladder in patients with SLE [English abstract]. Nippon Hinyokika Gakkai Zasshi 1987 Sep;78(9):1613–1617.

S760. Sullivan DA. Hormonal influence on the secretory immune systemic of the eye. In: Frier S, editor. The neuroendocrine-immune network. Bocka Rotan: CRC Press, 1990:200–237.

S761. Sulzberger MB, Witten VH. Thin pliable plastic films in topical dermatologic therapy. Arch Dermatol 1961 Dec;84: 1027–1028.

S762. Sulzberger MB, Wolf J, Witten VH, Kopf AW. Dermatology, Diagnosis and Treatment, 2d ed. Chicago: Year Book Medical Publishers, 1961.

S763. Sun D, Qin Y, Chluba J, Epplen JT, Wekerle H. Suppression of experimentally induced autoimmune encephalomyelitis by cytolytic T-T cell interactions. Nature 1988;332:843.

S764. Sundblad A, Hauser S, Holmberg D, Cazenave PA, Coutinho A. Suppression of antibody responses to the acetylcholine receptor by natural antibodies. Eur J Immunol 1989;19: 1425.

S765. Surowy CS, van Santen VL, Scheib-Wixted SM, Spritz RA. Direct, sequence-specific binding of the human U1 70K ribonucleoprotein antigen protein to loop 1 of U1 small nuclear RNA. Mol Cell Biol 1989;9:4179–4186.

S766. Surwit RS, Gilgor RS, Allen LM, Duvic M. A double-blind study of prazosin in the treatment of Raynaud's phenomenon in scleroderma. Arch Dermatol 1984 Mar;120(3):329–331.

S767. Sussman GL, Rivera VJ, Kohler PF. Transition form systemic lupus erythematosus to common variable hypogammaglobulinema. Ann Intern Med 1986 Jul;99:32–35.

S767a. Suster S, Rosai J. Histology of the normal thymus. Am J Surg Pathol 1990;14:284–303.

S768. Sutej PG, Gear AJ, Morrison RC, Tikly M, de Beer M, Dos Santos L, Sher R. Photosensitivity and anti-Ro (SSA) antibodies in black patients with systemic lupus erythematosus (SLE). Br J Dermatol 1989 Aug;28(4):321–324.

S769. Sutjita M, Hohmann A, Comacchio R, Boey ML, Bradley J. A common anti-cardiolipin antibody idiotype in autoimmune disease: identification using a mouse monoclonal antibody directed against a naturally-occurring anti-phospholipid antibody. Clin Exp Immunol 1989;75:211.

S770. Sutton JD, Griffin PE, Hochberg MC. Hospitalization in systemic lupus erythematosus [abstract]. Arthritis Rheum 1987;30 Suppl:S63.

S771. Suzuki K, Hara M, Nakajima S, Hirose T, Kitani A, Norioka K, Harigai M, Kawakami M, Tabata H, Kawagoe M. Analysis of systemic lupus erythematosus (SLE) involving the central nervous system by magnetic resonance imaging (MRI) [English abstract]. Ryumachi 1989 Apr;29(2):88–96.

S772. Suzuki K, Ishizuka T, Harigai M, Kawagoe M, Hara M, Hirose T, Kitani K, Nakamura H. Continuous anti-ds DNA antibody apheresis in systemic lupus erythematosus. Lancet 1990; 336:753–754.

S773. Suzuki N, Sakane T, Engleman EG. Anti-DNA antibody production by CD5+ and CD5- B cells of patients with systemic lupus erythematosus. J Clin Invest 1990;85:238–247.

S774. Suzuki Y, Kitagawa Y, Matsuoka Y, Fukuda J, Mizushima Y. Severe cerebral and systemic necrotizing vasculitis developing during pregnancy in a case of systemic lupus erythematosus [case report]. J Rheumatol 1990 Oct;17(10):1408–1411.

S775. Svec KH, Weisberger AS, Post RS, Naff GB. Immunosuppression by a chloramphenicol analogue in patients with lupus glomerulonephritis. J Lab Clin Med 1968;72:1023.

S776. Svedersky LP, Shepard HM, Spencer SA, Shalaby MR. Augmentation of human natural cell-mediated cytotoxicity by recombinant human interleukin 2. J Immunol 1984;133:714.

S777. Svensson B. Monocyte in vitro function in systemic lupus erythematosus (SLE). Scand J Rheumatol 1980;31 Suppl: 29–41.

S778. Svensson B. Occurrence of deficient monocyte yeast cell phagocytosis in presence of rheumatic sera. Scand J Rheumatol 1980;31 Suppl:21–28.

S779. Swaak AJ, Statius van Eps LW, Aarden LA, Feltkamp TE. Azathioprine in the treatment of systemic lupus erythematosus. A three-year prospective study. Clin Rheumatol 1984 Sep; 3(3):285–291.

S780. Swaak AJ, van Rooyen A, Aarden LA. Interleukin-6 (IL-6) and acute phase proteins in the disease course of patients with systemic lupus erythematosus. Rheumatol Int 1989;8: 263–268.

S781. Swaak AJG. Central nervous system involvement in systemic lupus erythematosus. Neth J Med 1986;29:221–228.

S782. Swaak AJG, Aarden LA, Statius van Eps LW, Feltkamp TEW. Anti-ds DNA and complement profiles as prognostic guides in systemic lupus erythematosus. Arthritis Rheum 1979 Mar;22: 226–235.

S783. Swaak AJG, Groenwold J, Aarden LA, Statius van Eps LW, Feltcamp TEW. Prognostic value of anti-ds DNA in SLE. Ann Rheum Dis 1982 Aug;41:388–395.

S784. Swaak AJG, Gorenwold J, Bronsveld W. Predictive value of complement profiles and anti-dsDNA in systemic lupus erythematosus. Ann Rheum Dis 1986;45:359–366.

S785. Swaak AJG, Nossent JC, Bronsveld W, van Rooyen A, Nieuenhuys EJ, Theuns L, Smeek RJT. Systemic lupus erythematosus. I: Outcome and survival: Dutch experience with 110 patients studied prospectively. Ann Rheum Dis 1989;48: 447–454.

S786. Swaak T, Smeenk R. Detection of anti-ds DNA as a diagnostic tool: A prospective study in 441 nonsystemic lupus erythematosus patients with anti-ds DNA antibody (anti-dsDNS). Ann Rheum Dis 1985 Apr;44:245–251.

S787. Swanepoel CR, Floyd A, Allison H, Learmouth GM, Cassidy MJD, Pascoe MD. Acute acalculous cholecystitis complicating systemic lupus erythematosus: case report and review. BMJ (Clin Res) 1983 Jan 22;286(6361):251–252.

S788. Swartz C. Lupus-like reaction to phenelzine. JAMA 1978 Jun 23;239:2693.

S789. Omitted.

S790. Sweeny P. Ultraviolet light denatured DNA/anti ultraviolet light denatured DNA immune complex nephritis in rabbits. J Lab Clin Med 1980;95:791–795.

S791. Sweet J, Bear RA, Lang AP. Amyloidosis and systemic lupus erythematosus. Hum Pathol 1981 Sep;12(9):853–856.

S792. Swezey RL, Bjarnason DM, Alexander SJ, Forrester DB. Resorptive arthropathy and the opera-glass hand syndrome. Semin Arthritis Rheum 1972–1973;2:191–244.

S793. Syed AA. Congenital heart block and hypothyroidism. Arch Dis Child 1978;53:256.

S794. Sylvester R, Daniels T, Claypool R, Tabbara K, Powell M, Greenspan J, Talal N. Outpatient study of Sjogren's syndrome (SS) utilizing newer diagnostic techniques [abstract]. Arthritis Rheum 1973;16:574–575.

S795. Sylvester RA, Attias M, Talal N, Tuffanelli DL. Antibodies to viral and synthetic double-stranded RNA in discoid lupus erythematosus. Arthritis Rheum 1973 May–Jun;16:383–387.

S796. Symmons DPM, Coopock JS, Bacon PA, Bresnihan B, Isenberg DA, Maddison P, McHugh N, Snaith ML, Zoma AS. Development and assessment of a computerized index of clinical disease activity in systemic lupus erythematosus. Q J Med 1988;68:927–937.

S797. Synkowski DR, Provost TT. Characterization of the inflammatory infiltrate in lupus erythematosus lesions using monoclonal antibodies. J Rheumatol 1983;10:920–924.

S798. Synkowski DR, Reichlin M, Provost TT. Serum autoantibodies in systemic lupus erythematosus and correlation with cutaneous features. J Rheumatol 1982;9:380.

S799. Syrop CH, Varner MW. Systemic lupus erythematosus. Obstet Gynecol 1983;26:547–582.

S800. Szer IS, Jacobs JC. Systemic lupus erythematosus in childhood. In: Lahita R, editor. Systemic Lupus Erythematosus. New York: Wiley & Sons, 1987:383–413.

S801. Szilagyi T, Kavai M. The effect of chloroquine on the antigen-antibody reaction. Acta Physiol Acad Sc Hung 1970;38: 411–417.

S802. Szostecki C, Goldner HH, Netter HJ, Will H. Isolation and characterization of cDNA encoding a human nuclear antigen predominantly recognized by autoantibodies from patients with primary biliary cirrhosis. J Immunol 1990;145: 4338–4347.

S803. Sztejnbok M, Stewart A, Diamond H, Kaplan D. Azathioprine in the treatment of systemic lupus erythematosus: A controlled study. Arthritis Rheum 1971;14:639–645.

T

T1. Tabata H, Hara M, Kitani A, Hirose T, Norioka K, Harigai M, Suzuki K, Kawakami M, Kawagoe M, Nakamura H. Expression of TLiSA1 on T cells from patients with rheumatoid arthritis and systemic lupus erythematosus. Clin Immunol Immunopathol 1989;52:366–375.

T2. Tabibzadeh SS, Santhanam V, Sehgal PB, May LT. Cytokine-induced production of IFN-B2/IL-6 by freshly explanted human endometrial stromal cells. J Immunol 1989;142: 3134–3139.

T3. Tabuenca JM. Toxic-allergic syndrome caused by ingestion of rapeseed oil denatured with aniline. Lancet 1981;2: 567–568.

T4. Tada T, Ohzeki S, Utsumi K, Takiuchi H, Muramatsu M, Li XF, Shimizu J, Fujiwara H, Hamaoka T. Transforming growth factor-beta-induced inhibition of T cell function. Susceptibility difference in T cells of various phenotypes and functions and its relevance to immunosuppression in the tumor-bearing state. J Immunol 1991;146:1077–1082.

T5. Tada Y, Nagasawa K, Yamauchi Y, Tsukamoto H, Niho Y. A defect in the protein kinase C system in T cells from patients with systemic lupus erythematosus. Clin Immunol Immunopathol 1991;60:220–231.

T6. Taieb A, Hehunstre JP, Goetz J, Bazeille JE, Fizet D, Hauptmann G, Maleville J. Lupus erythematosus panniculitis with partial genetic deficiency of C2 and C4 in a child. Arch Dermatol 1986 May;122(5):576–582.

T7. Taft LI, Mackay IR, Cowling DC. Autoclasia: a perpetuating mechanism in hepatitis. Gastroenterology 1960 Apr;38: 563–566.

T8. Taft LI, Mackay IR, Larkin L. Hepatitis complicated by manifestations of lupus erythematosus. J Path Bact (Lond) 1958 Apr;75(2):399–404.

T9. Takada S, Magira T, Yamamura M. Alteration of DNA primase activity by phosphorylation and de-phosphorylation of histone H1. Biochem Biophys Res Commun 1989;160:711–714.

T10. Takada S, Ueda Y, Suzuki N, Murakawa Y, Hosino T, Green L, Steinberg AD, Horwitz DA, Sakane T. Abnormalities in autologous mixed lymphocyte reaction-activated immunologic processes in systemic lupus erythematosus and their possible correction by interleukin 2. Eur J Immunol 1985 Mar;15: 262–267.

T11. Takahashi H, Terasaki PI, Iwaki Y, Nakata S. Identification of surface IgM as the target antigen of cold lymphocytotoxins. Tissue Antigens 1980;16:176–180.

T12. Takahashi T, Gray JD, Horwitz DA. Human CD8+ lymphocytes stimulated in the absence of CD4+ cells enhance IgG production by antibody-secreting B cells. Clin Immunol Immunopathol 1991;58:352–365.

T13. Takasugi M, Mickey MR, Terasaki PI. Reactivity of lymphocytes from normal persons on cultured tumor cells. Cancer Res 1973;33: 2898.

T14. Takeda Y, Wang GS, Wang RJ, Anderson SK, Pettersson I, Amaki S, Sharp GC. Enzyme-linked immunosorbent assay using isolated (U) small nuclear ribonucleoprotein polypeptides as antigens to investigate the clinical significance of autoantibodies to these polypeptides. Clin Immunol Immunopathol 1989; 50:213–230.

T15. Takehara K, Nojima Y, Kikuchi K, Igarashi A, Soma Y, Tsuchida T, Ishibashi Y. Systemic lupus erythematosus associated with antiribosomal P protein antibody. Arch Dermatol 1990 Sep;126:1184–1186.

T16. Takei M, Kang H, Tomura K, Amaki S, Hirata M, Karasaki M, Sawsda S, Amaki I. Aberration of monokine production and monocyte subset in patients with systemic lupus erythematosus. J Clin Lab Immunol 1987;22:169–173.

T17. Takeuchi F, Otsuka F, Enomoto T, Hanaoka F, Yamada MA, Kamatani N, Nakano K, Matsuta K, Tanimoto K, Morita T, Miyamoto T. Decrease in the reaction of DNA repair synthesis in response to nicotinamide or 3-aminobenzamide to ultraviolet irradiated systemic lupus erythematosus lymphocytes. J Rheumatol 1985;12:504–507.

T18. Takeuchi T, Abe T, Kiyotaki M, Toguchi T, Koide J, Morimoto C, Homma M. In vitro immune response of SLE lymphocytes. The mechanism involved in B-cell activation. Scand J Immunol 1982 Nov;16:369–377.

T19. Takeuchi T, Abe T, Koide J, Hosono O, Morimotos C, Homma M. Cellular mechanism of DNA-specific antibody synthesis by lymphocytes from systemic lupus erythematosus patients. Arthritis Rheum 1984 Jul;27:766–773.

T20. Takeuchi T, Rudd CE, Schlossman SF, Morimoto C. Induction of suppression following autologous mixed lymphocyte reaction; role of a novel 2H4 antigen. Eur J Immunol 1987;17:97–103.

T21. Takeuchi T, Rudd CE, Tanaka S, Rothstein DM, Schlossman SF, Morimoto C. Functional characterization of the CD45R (2H4) molecule on CD3 (T8) cells in the autologous mixed lymphocyte reaction system. Eur J Immunol 1989;19:474–755.

T22. Takeuchi T, Tanaka S, Steinberg AD, Matsuyama T, Daley J, Schlossman SF, Morimoto C. Defective expression of the 2H4 molecule after autologous mixed lymphocyte reaction activation in systemic lupus erythematosus patients. J Clin Invest 1988;82:1288–1294.

T23. Takuwa N, Kojima I, Ogata E. Lupus-like syndrome—a rare complication of thionamide treatment for Graves' disease. Endocrinol Jpn 1981 Oct;28(5):663–667.

T24. Talal N. Disordered immunologic regulation and autoimmunity. Transplant Rev 1976;31:240–263.

T25. Talal N. Autoimmunity and the immunologic network. Arthritis Rheum 1978 Sep–Oct;21:853–867.

T26. Talal N. Sjogren's syndrome and connective tissue disorders with other immunologic disorders. In: McCarty DJ, editor. Arthritis and Allied Conditions, 10th ed. Philadelphia: Lea & Febiger, 1985:1037–1046.

T27. Talal N, Dauphinee MJ, Ansar Ahmed S, Christadoss P. Sex factors in immunity and autoimmunity. In: Yamamura Y, Tada T, editors. Progress in Immunology V. Tokyo: Academic Press, 1983;1589–1600.

T28. Talal N, Dauphinee MJ, Dang H, Alexander SS, Hart DJ, Garry RF. Detection of serum antibodies to retroviral proteins in patients with primary Sjögren's syndrome (autoimmune exocrinopathy). Arthritis Rheum 1990;33:774–781.

T29. Talal N, Dauphinee MJ, Wofsy D. Interleukin-2 deficiency, genes, and systemic lupus erythematosus. Arthritis Rheum 1982;25:838–842.

T30. Talal N, Garry RF, Schur PH, Alexander S, Dauphinee MJ, Livas IH, Ballester A, Takei M, Dang H. A conserved idiotype and antibodies to retroviral proteins in systemic lupus erythematosus. J Clin Invest 1990;85:1866–1871.

T31. Talal N, Steinberg AD. The pathogenesis of autoimmunity in NZB mice. In: Arberg W, editor. Current Topics in Microbiology and Immunology. New York: Springer-Verlag, 1974:79–103.

T32. Talal N, Steinberg AD. The pathogenesis of autoimmunity in NZB mice. Curr Top Microbiol Immunol 1974;64:79–85.

T33. Talbott JH. Historical background of discoid and systemic lupus erythematosus. Ch. 1. In: Wallace DJ, Dubois EL, editors. Dubois' Lupus Erythematosus, 3d ed. Philadelphia: Lea & Febiger, 1987.

T34. Talbott JH, Ferrandis RM. Collagen Diseases, Including Systemic Lupus Erythematosus, Polyarteritis, Dermatomyositis, Systemic Scleroderma, Thrombotic Thrombocytopenic Purpura. New York: Grune & Stratton, 1956.

T35. Tamura G, Kaizuka H, Iwasaki T, Satodate R, Abe H, Ishida M, Mori S. A case report of angiosarcoma of the breast. Gan No Rinsho 1987;33:1085–1089.

T36. Tan C-K, Sullivan K, Li X, Tan EM, Downey KM, So AG. Autoantibody to the proliferating cell nuclear antigen neutralizes the activity of the auxiliary protein for DNA polymerase delta. Nucleic Acids Res 1987;15:9299–9308.

T37. Tan EM. Drug-induced autoimmune disease. Fed Proc 1974 Aug; 33:1894–1897.

T38. Tan EM. An immunologic precipitin system between soluble nucleoprotein and serum antibody in systemic lupus erythematosus. J Clin Invest 1967;46:735–745.

T39. Tan EM. Relationship of nuclear staining patterns with precipitating antibodies in systemic lupus erythematosus. J Lab Clin Med 1967;70:800–812.

T40. Tan EM. Drug-induced autoimmune disease. Fed Proc 1974; 33:1894–1897.

T41. Tan EM. Immunopathology and pathogenesis of cutaneous involvement in systemic lupus erythematosus. J Invest Dermatol 1976 Sep;67(3):360–365.

T42. Tan EM. Autoantibodies to nuclear antigens (ANA): their immunobiology and medicine. Adv Immunol 1982;33:167–240.

T43. Tan EM. Antinuclear antibodies: Diagnostic markers for autoimmune diseases and probes for cell biology. Adv Immunol 1989;44:93–151.

T44. Tan EM, Chan EKL, Sullivan KF, Rubin RL. Short analytical review: Diagnostically specific immune markers and clues toward the understanding of systemic autoimmunity. Clin Immunol Immunopathol 1988;47:121–141.

T45. Tan EM, Chaplin H JR. Antinuclear antibodies in Coombs-positive acquired hemolytic anemia. Vox Sang 1968;15(3):161–170.

T46. Tan EM, Cohen AS, Fries JF, Masi AT, McShane DJ, Rothfield NF, Schaller JG, Talal N, Winchester RJ. Special article: The 1982 revised criteria for the classification of systemic lupus erythematosus. Arthritis Rheum 1982 Nov;25(11):1271–1277.

T47. Tan EM, Kunkel HG. An immunofluorescent study of the skin lesions in systemic lupus erythematosus. Arthritis Rheum 1966 Feb;9:37–46.

T48. Tan EM, Kunkel HG. Characteristics of a soluble nuclear antigen precipitating with sera of patients with systemic lupus erythematosus. J Immunol 1966;96:464–471.

T49. Tan EM, Robinson J, Robitaille P. Studies on antibodies to histones by immunofluorescence. Scand J Immunol 1976; 5(6–7):811–818.

T50. Tan EM, Rubin RL. Autoallergic reactions induced by procainamide. J Allergy Clin Immunol 1984;74:631–634.

T51. Tan EM, Schur PH, Carr RI, Kunkel HG. Deoxyribonucleic acid (DNA) and antibodies to DNA in the serum of patients with systemic lupus erythematosus. J Clin Invest 1966;45:1732–1740.

T52. Tan P, Pang G, Wilson JD. Immunoglobulin production in vitro by peripheral blood lymphocytes in systemic lupus erythematosus: helper T cell defect and B cell hyperreactivity. Clin Exp Immunol 1981 Jun;44:548–554.

T53. Tan PLJ, Borman GB, Wigley RD. Testing clinical criteria for systemic lupus erythematosus in other connective tissue disorders. Rheumatol Int 1981;1(3):147–149.

T54. Tan PLJ, Pang GTM, Wilson JD, Cullinane G. Immunoglobulin secreting cells in SLE. Correlation with disease activity. J Rheumatol 1980;7:807–813.

T55. Tan RF, Gladman DD, Urowitz MB, Milne N. Brain scan diagnosis of central nervous system involvement in systemic lupus erythematosus. Ann Rheum Dis 1978 Aug;37(4):357–362.

T56. Tanaka S, Matsuyama T, Steinberg AD, Schlossman SF, Morimoto C. Antilymphocyte antibodies against CD4 + 2H4 + cell populations in patients with systemic lupus erythematosus. Arthritis Rheum 1989;32(4):398–405.

T56a. Tanaka T, Saiki O, Negoro S, Igarashi T, Kuritani T, Hara H, Suemura M, Kishimoto S. Decreased expression of interleukin-2 binding molecules (p70/75) in T cells from patients with systemic lupus erythematosus. Arthritis Rheum 1989;32:552–559.

T57. Tanaka Y, Saito K, Shirakawa F, Ota T, Suzuki H, Eto S, Yamashita U. Production of B cell-stimulating factors by B cells in patients with systemic lupus erythematosus. J Immunol 1988;141:3043–3049.

T58. See T56a.

T59. Tanaka Y, Saito K, Suzuki H, Eto H, Yamashita U. Inhibitory effect of anti-class II antibody on the spontaneous activation of B cells in patients with systemic lupus erythematosus. Analysis with IL-1 production and IL-1 receptor expression. J Immunol 1989;143:1584–1590.

T60. Tanigaki T, Kanda R, Sato K. Epidermodysplasia verruciformis (L-L, 1922) in a patient with systemic lupus erythematosus. Arch Dermatol Res 1986;278(3):247–248.

T61. Tannenbaum H, Schur PH. Development of reticulum cell sarcoma during cyclophosphamide therapy. Arthritis Rheum 1974 Jan–Feb;17:15–18.

T62. Tannenbaum SH, Finko R, Cines DB. Antibody and immune complexes induce tissue factor production by human endothelial cells. J Immunol 1986;137:1532–1537.

T63. Tanphaichitr K, Hahn BH. Studies of tolerance to DNA in NZ/NZW F1 mice. J Immunol 1977;119:330–336.

T64. Tanter Y, Rifle G, Chalopin JM, Mousson C, Besancenot JF. Plasma exchange in central nervous system involvement of systemic lupus erythematosus. Plasma Ther Transfus Technol 1987;8:161–168.

T65. Tao W, Bothwell AL. Development of B cell lineages during a primary anti-hapten immune response. J Immunol 1990;145:3216–3222.

T66. Tappeiner G, O'Loughlin S, Jordan RE. Clq binding activity in lupus erythematosus: correlation with the "lupus band test." J Invest Dermatol 1978 Apr;70:187–190.

T67. Tareyeva IE, Shilov EM, Gordovskaya NB. The effects of azathioprine and prednisolone on T- and B-lymphocytes in patients with lupus nephritis and chronic glomerulonephritis. Clin Nephrol 1980 Nov;14(5):233–237.

T68. Targoff IN, Arnett FC, Berman L, O'Brien CD, Reichlin M. Anti-KJ: a new antibody associated with the syndromes of polymyositis and intestinal lung disease. J Clin Invest 1989;84:162–172.

T69. Targoff IN, Reichlin M. Unmasking of cytoplasmic fluorescence of anti-Jo1 by purification of antibody [abstract]. Arthritis Rheum 1985;28:S74.

T70. Targoff IN, Johnson AE, Miller FW. Antibody to signal recognition particle in polymyositis. Arthritis Rheum 1990;33:1361–1370.

T71. Targum SD. Persistent neuroendocrine dysregulation in major depressive disorder: a marker for early relapse. Biol Psychiatry 1984;19:305–318.

T72. Tarkowski A, Westerberg G. Rheumatoid factor isotypes and renal disease in systemic lupus erythematosus. Scand J Rheumatol 1987;16:309–312.

T73. Tarzy BJ, Garcia C-R, Wallach EE, Zweiman B, Myers AR. Rheumatic disease, abnormal serology, and oral contraceptives. Lancet 1972 Sep 9;2(7776):501–503.

T74. Tatelman M, Keech MK. Esophageal motility in systemic lupus erythematosus, rheumatoid arthritis, and scleroderma. Radiology 1966 Jun;86:1041–1046.

T75. Tateno S, Kobayashi Y, Shigenmatsu H, Hiki Y. Study of lupus nephritis: its classification and the significance of subendothelial deposits. Q J Med 1983 Summer;52:311–331.

T76. Tauber AI, Simmons ER. Dissociation of human neutrophil membrane depolarization, respiratory burst stimulation and phospholipid metabolism by quinacrine. FEBS Lett 1983 May 30;156(1):161–164.

T77. Tauber U, Haack D, Nieuweboer B, Kloss G, Vecsei P,

Wendt H. The pharmacokinetics of fluocortolone and prednisolone after intravenous and oral administration. Int J Clin Pharmacol Ther Toxicol 1984;22:48–55.

T78. Taurog JD, Moutsopoulos HM, Rosenberg YJ, Chused TM, Steinberg AD. CBA/N X-linked B cell defect prevents NZB B-cell hyperactivity in F1 mice. J Exp Med 1979 Jul 1;150(1):31–43.

T79. Taurog JD, Raveche ES, Smathers PA, Glimcher LH, Huston DP, Hansen CT, Steinberg AD. The cell abnormalities in NZB mice occur independently of autoantibody production. J Exp Med 1981;153:221.

T80. Taurog JD, Sandberg GP, Mahowald ML. The cellular basis of adjuvant arthritis. I. Enhancement of cell-mediated passive transfer by concanavalin A and by immunosuppressive treatment of the recipient. Cell Immunol 1983;75:271.

T81. Taurog JD, Smathers PA, Lieberman R, Steinberg AD. Evidence for abnormalities in separate lymphocyte populations in NZB mice. J Immunol 1980;125:485–491.

T82. Taylor HG, Stein CM. Systemic lupus erythematosus in Zimbabwe. Ann Rheum Dis 1986;45:645–648.

T83. Taylor PV, Hancock KW. Antigenicity of trophoblast and possible antigen-masking effect during pregnancy. Immunol 1975;28:973.

T84. Taylor PV, Scott JS, Gerlis LM, Path FRC, Esscher E, Scott O. Maternal antibodies against fetal cardiac antigens in congenital complete heart block. N Engl J Med 1986;315:667–672.

T85. Taylor PV, Taylor KF, Norman A, Griffiths S, Scott JS. Prevalence of maternal Ro(SS-A) and La(SS-B) autoantibodies in relation to congenial heart block. Br J Rheumatol 1988;27:128–132.

T86. Taylor RP, Horgan C, Buschbacher R, Brunner CM, Hess CE, O'Brien WM, Wanebo HJ. Decreased complement mediated binding of antibody/3H-dsDNA immune complexes to the red blood cells of patients with systemic lupus erythematosus, rheumatoid arthritis, and hematologic malignancies. Arthritis Rheum 1983;26:736–744.

T87. Taylor RP, Kujala G, Wilson K, Wright E, Harbin A. In vivo and in vitro studies of the binding of antibody/dsDNA immune complexes to rabbit and guinea pig platelets. J Immunol 1985;134:2550–2558.

T88. Taylor RP, Weber D, Broccoli AV, Winfield JB. Stability of DNA/anti-DNA complexes. J Immunol 1979 Jan;122(1):115–120.

T89. Tchouatcha-Tchouassom JC, Julliard JH, Roux B. Isolation and characterization of five histone H1 subtypes from adult rat liver. Biochim Biophys Acta 1989;1009:121–128.

T90. Te Velde AA, Huijbens RJF, De Vries JE, Figdor CG. IL-4 decreases FcγR membrane expression and FcγR-mediated cytotoxic activity of human monocytes. J Immunol 1990;144:3046–3051.

T91. Tebbe B, Orfanos CE. Cutaneous lupus erythematosus. An analysis of 97 patients [English abstract]. Z Hautkr 1987 Nov 15;62(22):1563–1584.

T92. Tebib JG, Alcocer-Verela J, Alarcon-Segovia D, Schur PH. Association between a T cell receptor restriction fragment length polymorphism and systemic lupus erythematosus. J Clin Invest 1990;86:1961–1967.

T93. Tebib JG, Martinez C, Granados J, Alarcon-Segovia D, Schur PH. The frequency of complement receptor type 1 (CR1) gene polymorphisms in nine families with multiple cases of systemic lupus erythematosus. Arthritis Rheum 1989;32:1465–1468.

T94. Tedesco F, Silvani CM, Agelli M, Giovanetti AM, Bombardieri S. A lupus like syndrome in a patient with deficiency of the sixth component complement. Arthritis Rheum 1981;24:1438–1440.

T95. Tegner R, Tome FM, Godeau P, Lhermitte F, Fardeau M.

Morphological study of peripheral nerve changes induced by chloroquine treatment. Acta Neuropathol (Berl) 1988;75(3): 253–260.

T96. Teh LS, Amos N, Bedwell AE, Williams BD. Antiribosomal P-protein in systemic lupus erythematosus (SLE) [abstract]. Arthritis Rheum 1990 Sep;33(9) Suppl:S102.

T97. Teichner M, Krumbacher K, Doxiadis I, Doxiadis G, Fournel C, Rigal D, Monier JC, Grosse-Wilde H. Systemic lupus erythematosus in dogs: association to the major histocompatibility complex class I antigen DLA-A7. Clin Immunol Immunopathol 1990;55:255–262.

T98. Teitelbaum D, Rauch J, Stollar BD, Schwartz RS. In vivo effects of antibodies against a high frequency idiotype of anti-DNA antibodies in MRL mice. J Immunol 1984;132:1282.

T99. Teitsson I, Thorsteinsson J. Systemic lupus erythematosus in Iceland. Iceland Med J 1978;64 Suppl 3:116.

T100. Tejani A, Khawar M, Butt KMH. Drug therapy, dialysis and transplantation in children with diffuse proliferative lupus nephritis [abstract]. Pediatr Res 1987;21:485A.

T101. Tejani A, Nicastri AD, Chen C-K, Fikrig S, Gurumurthy K. Lupus nephritis in black and Hispanic children. Am J Dis Child 1983 May;137:481–483.

T102. Temesvari A, Denburg J, Denburg S, Carbotte R, Bensen W, Singal D. Serum lymphocytotoxic antibodies in neuropsychiatric lupus: a serial study. Clin Immunol Immunopathol 1983 Aug;28(2):243–251.

T103. Temple A, Loewi G. The effect sera from patients with connective tissue diseases on red cell binding and phagocytosis by monocytes. Immunology 1977;33:109–114.

T104. ter Borg E, Horst G, Limburg P, Van Venrooij W, Kallenberg CGM. Changes in levels of antibodies against 70 kDa and a polypeptides of the U1RNP complex in relation to exacerbations of systemic lupus erythematosus. J Rheumatol 1991;18: 363–367.

T105. ter Borg EJ, de Jong PE, Meijer S, Kallenberg CG. Renal effects of indomethacin in patients with systemic lupus erythematosus. Nephron 1989;53(3): 238–243.

T106. ter Borg EJ, de Jong PE, Meyer S, van Rijswijk MH, Kallenberg CGM. Indomethacin and ibuprofen induced reversible acute renal failure in a patient with systemic lupus erythematosus. Neth J Med 1987;31:181–187.

T107. ter Borg EJ, Groen H, Horst G, Limburg PC, Wouda AA, Kallenberg CGM. Clinical associations of antiribonucleo-protein antibodies in patients with systemic lupus erythematosus. Semin Arthritis Rheum 1990;20:164–173.

T108. ter Borg EJ, Horst G, Hummee EJ, Limburg PC, Kallenberg CGM. Measurement of increases in anti-double stranded DNA antibody levels as a predictor of disease exacerbation in systemic lupus erythematosus. Arthritis Rheum 1990;33: 634–643.

T109. ter Borg EJ, Horst G, Limburg PC, Kallenberg CGM. Changes in plasma levels of interleukin 2 receptor in relation to disease exacerbations and levels of anti-dsDNA and complement in systemic lupus erythematosus. Clin Exp Immunol 1990;82:21–26.

T110. ter Borg EJ, Horst G, Limburg PC, van Rijswijk MH, Kallenberg CGM. C-reactive protein levels during disease exacerbations and infections in systemic lupus erythematosus: A prospective longitudinal study. J Rheumatol 1990;17:1642–1648.

T111. ter Borg EJ, Janssen S, van Rijswijk MH, Bijzet J, de Jong PE, Elema JD. AA amyloidosis associated with systemic lupus erythematosus. Rheumatol Int 1988;8:141–143.

T112. Terabayashi H, Okuda K, Nomura F, Ohnishi K, Wong P. Transformation of inferior vena caval thrombosis to membranous obstruction in a patient with the lupus anticoagulant. Gastroenterol 1986;91:219–224.

T113. Terada K, Okuhara E, Kawarada Y, Hirose S. Demonstration of extrinsic DNA from immune complexes in plasma of a patient with systemic lupus erythematosus. Biochem Biophys Res 1991;174(1):323–330.

T114. Terai C, Nojima Y, Takano K, Yamada A, Takaku F. Determination of urinary albumin excretion by radioimmunoassay in patients with subclinical lupus nephritis. Clin Nephrology 1987;27:79–83.

T115. Terasaki PI, McClelland JD. Microdroplet assay of human serum cytotoxins. Nature 1964;204:998–1000.

T116. Terasaki PI, Mottironi VD, Barnett EV. Cytotoxins in disease. Autocytotoxins in lupus. N Engl J Med 1970 Oct 1;283: 724–728.

T117. Terato K, Arai H, Shimozura Y, Fukuda T, Tanaka H, Watamabe H, Nagai Y, Fujimoto K, Okubo F, Cho F, Honjo S, Cremer MA. Sex-linked differences in susceptibility of cynomolgus monkeys to type II collagen-induced arthritis. Arthritis Rheum 1989;32:748–758.

T118. Termaat RM, Brinkman K, van Gompel F, Van den Heuvel LP, Veerkamp JH, Smeenk RJ, Berden JH. Cross-reactivity of monoclonal anti-DNA antibodies with heparan sulfate is mediated via bound DNA/histone complexes. J Autoimmun 1990; 3:531–545.

T119. Terman DS, Buffaloe G, Mattioli C, Cook G, Tillquist R, Sullivan M, Ayus JC. Extracorporeal immunoadsorption: initial experience in human systemic lupus erythematosus. Lancet 1979 Oct 20;2(8147):824–827.

T120. Ternynck T, Avrameas S. Murine natural monoclonal autoantibodies. A study of their polyspecificities and the affinities. Immunol Rev 1986;94:99–112.

T121. Terr AI, Moss RB, Strober S. Effect of total lymphoid irradiation on IgE antibody responses in rheumatoid arthritis and systemic lupus erythematosus. J Allergy Clin Immunol 1987 Dec;80(6):798–802.

T122. Terres G, Morrison SL, Habicht GS. A quantitative differences in the immune response between male and female mice. Proc Exp Biol Med 1968;127:664–667.

T123. Tett SE, Cutler DJ, Day RO, Brown KF. Bioavailability of hydroxychloroquine tablets in healthy volunteers. Br J Clin Pharmacol 1989 Jun;27(6):771–779.

T124. Tetta C, Bussolino F, Modena V, Montrucchio G, Segoloni G, Pescarmona G, Camussi G. Release of platelet-activity factor in systemic lupus erythematosus. Int Arch Allergy Immunol 1990;91:244–256.

T125. Thanavala YM, Roitt IM. Monoclonal anti-idiotypic antibodies as surrogates for hepatitis B surface antigen. Intern Rev Immunol 1986;1:27.

T126. Theissen H, Elzerodt M, Reuter R, Schneider C, Lottspeich F, Argos P, Luhrmann R, Philipson L. Cloning of the human cDNA for the U1 RNA-associated 70K protein. Embo J 1986; 5:3209–3217.

T127. Theofilopoulos AN. Evaluation and clinical significance of circulating immune complexes. Prog Clin Immunol 1980;4: 63–106.

T128. Theofilopoulos AN, Balderas RS, Gozes Y, Fidler JM, Liu FT, Ahmed A, Dixon FJ. Surface and fucntional characteristics of B cells from lupus-prone murine strains. Clin Immunol Immunopath 1982;23:224–244.

T129. Theofilopoulos AN, Balderas R, Shawler DL, Izui S, Kotzin BL, Strober S, Dixon FJ. Inhibition of T cell proliferation and SLE-like syndrome of MRL/l mice by whole body or total lymphoid irradiation. J Immunol 1980;125:2137–2142.

T130. Theofilopoulos AN, Dixon FJ. Murine models of SLE. Adv Immunol 1985;37:269–285.

T131. Theofilopoulos AN, Dixon FJ. Experimental murine systemic lupus erythematosus. In: Lahita RG, editor. Systemic lupus erythematosus. 1987:121–202.

T132. Theofilopoulos AN, Dixon FJ. Immune complexes in human diseases. Am J Pathol 1980;100:529–594.

T133. Theofilopoulos AN, Dixon FJ. Etiopathogenesis of murine systemic lupus erythematosus. Immunol Rev 1981;55:179–216.

T134. Theofilopoulos AN, Kofler R, Singer PA, Dixon FJ. Molecular genetics of murine lupus models [review]. Adv Immunol 1989;46:61–109.

T135. Theofilopoulos AN, Shawler DL, Eisenberg RA, Dixon FJ. Splenic immunoglobulin-secreting cells and their regulation in autoimmune mice. J Exp Med 1980 Feb 1;151(2):446–466.

T136. Theofilopoulos AN, Wilson CB, Dixon FJ. The Raji cell radioimmunoassay for immune complexes in human sera. J Clin Invest 1976;57:169–182.

T137. Thiagarajan D, Wongsurawat N. Systemic lupus erythematosus associated with adrenal insufficiency. J Kans Med Soc 1978 Oct;79(10):565–566.

T138. Thiagarajan P, Pengo V, Shapiro SS. The use of the dilute russell viper venon time for the diagnosis of lupus anticoagulants. Blood 1986;68:869.

T139. Thiagarajan P, Shapiro SS, De Marco L. Monoclonal immunoglobulin M Lambda coagulation inhibitor with phospholipid specificity. Mechanism of lupus anticoagulant. J Clin Invest 1980 Sep;66:397.

T140. Thibodeau A, Ruiz-Carrillo A. The globular region of histone H5 Is equally accessible to antibodies in relaxed and condensed chromatin. J Biol Chem 1988; 263:16236–16241.

T141. Thies W. Recent experiences in treatment of chronic discoid lupus erythematosus with atabrine and chloroquine, particularly with local and combined therapy. Hautarzt 1955 Aug; 6:227–232.

T142. Thivolet J, Nicolas JF, Kanitakis J, Lyonnet S, Chouvet B. Recombinant interferon alpha 2a is effective in the treatment of discoid and subacute cutaneous lupus erythematosus. Br J Dermatol 1990 Mar;122(3):405–409.

T143. Thoma F, Koller T, Klug A. Involvement of histone H1 in the organization of the nucleosome and of the salt-dependent superstructures of chromatin. J Cell Biol 1979; 83:403–427.

T144. Thomas DB. Antibodies specific for human T lymphocytes in cold agglutinin and lymphocytotoxic sera. Eur J Immunol 1973;3:824–828.

T145. Thomas JO, Wilson CM, Hardin JA. The major core histone antigenic determinants in systemic lupus erythematosus are in the trypsin-sensitive regions. FEBS Lett 1984;169:90–96.

T146. Thomas JR 3d, Su WP. Concurrence of lupus erythematosus and dermatitis herpetiformis. Arch Dermatol 1983 Sep; 119(9):740–745.

T147. Thomas JW, Vertkin A, Nell LJ. Antiinsulin antibodies and clinical characteristics of patients with systemic lupus erythematosus and other connective tissue diseases with steroid induced diabetes. J Rheumatol 1987 Aug;14(4):732–735.

T148. Thomas ML. The leukocyte common antigen family. Ann Rev Immunol 1989;7:339–369.

T149. Thomas ML, Reynolds PJ, Chain A, Ben-Neriah Y, Trowbridge IS. B-cell variant of mouse T200 (Ly-5). Evidence for alternative mRNA splicing. Proc Natl Acad Sci USA 1987;84:5360–5363.

T150. Thomas MM, Tischer CC, Robinson RR. Influence of pregnancy on lupus nephritis. Kidney Int 1978;14:665.

T151. Thomas R, Vane DW, Grosfeld JL, Faught PR. The effect of chloroquine and hyperthermia on murine neuroblastoma. J Pediatr Surg 1990 Sep;25(9):929–932.

T152. Thomas T, Gunnia UB, Serbold JR, Thomas TJ. Restoration of the DNA binding activity of estrogen receptor in MRL/lpr mice by a polyamine biosynthesis inhibitor. Arthritis Rheum 1991;36:55–62.

T153. Thomas TJ, Messner RP. Effect of lupus-inducing drugs on the B to Z transition of synthetic DNA. Arthritis Rheum 1986; 29:638–645.

T154. Thompson AW, Horne CHW. Biological and clinical significance of pregnancy-associated a_2-glyco-protein (a_2-PAG)—a review. Invest Cell Pathol 1980;3:295–309.

T154a. Thompson BJ, Watson ML, Liston WA, Lambie AT. Plasmapheresis in a pregnancy complicated by acute systemic lupus erythematosus. Case report. Br J Obstet Gynaecol 1985 May;92(5):532–534.

T155. Thompson CB, Neiman PE. Somatic diversification of the chicken immunoglobulin light chain gene is limited to the rearranged variable segment. Cell 1987;48:369–378.

T156. Thompson PJ, Dhillon DP, Ledingham J, Turner-Warwick M. Shrinking lungs, diaphragmatic dysfunction and systemic lupus erythematosus. Am Rev Respir Dis 1985;132:926–928.

T157. Thompson S, Gutierrez D, Quismorio FP Jr. Bullous lupus: Clinical and immunopathological studies [abstract]. Arthritis Rheum 1989 Apr;32(4) Suppl:S116.

T158. Thompson SW. Ballistic movements of the arm in systemic lupus erythematosus. Dis Nerv Syst 1976 Jun;37(6):331–332.

T159. See T154a.

T160. Thorn GW, Boyles TB, Massell BF, Forsham PH, Hill SR Jr, Smith S, Warren JE. Medical progress: Studies on the relation of pituitary-adrenal function to rheumatic disease [published erratum N Engl J Med 1949 Dec 29;241:1057]. N Engl J Med 1949 Oct 6;2451:529–537.

T161. Thorn GW, Forsham PH, Frawley TF, Hill SR Jr, Roche M, Staehelin D, Wilson DL. Medical progress: The clinical usefulness of ACTH and cortisone. N Engl J Med 1950 May;242: 824–834.

T162. Thorner A, Walldius G, Nillson E, Hadell K, Gullberg R. Beneficial effects of reduced intake of polyunsaturated fatty acids in the diet for one year in patients with systemic lupus erythematosus [letter]. Ann Rheum Dis 1990 Feb;49(2):134.

T163. Tikhonov-Bugrov VD. Case of familial dermatitis with clinical picture of acute lupus erythematosus type. Vestn Derm Vener (Russian) 1951;4:38–41.

T164. Tilden AV, Abo T, Balch CM. Suppressor cell function of human granular lymphocytes identified by the HNK-1 (Leu 7) monoclonal antibody. J Immunol 1983;130:1171.

T165. Tiwari JL, Terasaki PI, editors. HLA and Disease Association. New York: Springer-Verlag, 1985.

T166. Tobin DR, Krohel GB, Rynes RI. Hydroxychloroquine: Seven-year experience. Arch Ophthalmol 1982 Jan;100(1): 81–83.

T167. Todd I, Pujol-Borrell R, Bottazzo GF, Londel M, Feldmann M. Autoantigen presentation by target cells: its possible role in determining autoantibody specificity. A I P Immunol 1986; D137:168–173.

T168. Todd JA, Acha-Orbea H, Bell JI, Chao N, Fronek Z, Jacob CO, McDermott M, Sinha AA, Timmerman L, Steinman L, McDevitt HO. A molecular basis for MHC class II-associated autoimmunity. Science 1988;240:1003–1008.

T169. Todd JA, Bell JI, McDevitt HO. HLA-DQ beta gene contributes to susceptibility and resistance to insulin-dependent diabetes mellitus. Nature 1987;329:599–604.

T170. Toder V, Nebel L, Gleicher N. Studies of natural killer cells in pregnancy. I. Analysis at the single cell level. J Clin Lab Immunol 1984;14:123.

T171. Toivanen P, Malta K, Suolanen R, Tykkylainen R. Effect of estrone and progesterone on adjuvant arthritis in rats. Medicine et Pharmacologia Experimentalis 1967;17:33–42.

T172. Tokano Y, Murashima A, Takasaki Y, Hashimoto H, Okumura K, Hirose S. Relation between soluble interleukin 2 receptor and clinical findings in patients with systemic lupus erythematosus. Ann Rheum Dis 1989;48:803–809.

T173. Tokano Y, Yagita H, Iida N, Hashimoto H, Okumura K,

Hirose S. Relation between the level of IgG subclasses and infections in patients with systemic lupus erythematosus. Int Arch Allergy Appl Immunol 1988;87(1):55–58.

T174. Tokuda Y, Inokuma T, Hidaka A, Matsuda K, Katsushima S, Onishi Y, Taniguchi T, Omoto J, Kawaguchi Y, Honda T. Development of adrenal cortical carcinoma in systemic lupus erythematosus: a case report. Nippon Naida Gakkai Zasshi 1986;75:676–680.

T175. Tokunaga K, Imoto K, Akaza T, Akiyama N, Amemiya H, Naito S, Sasazuki T, Satoh H, Juji T. Haplotype study on C4 polymorphism in Japanese. Associations with MHC alleles, complotypes, and HLA-complement haplotypes. Immunogenetics 1985;22:359–365.

T176. Toll JB, Andersson RG. Effects of mecaprine and p-bromophenacyl bromide on anti-IgE and phospholipase A2-induced histamine release from human basophils. Agents Actions 1986 Aug;18(5–6):518–523.

T177. Tollefson G, Rodysill K, Cusulos M. A circulating lupus-like coagulation inhibitor induced by chlorpromazine. J Clin Psych Pharmacol 1984 Feb;4:49–51.

T178. Tollervey D, Mattaj IW. Fungal small nuclear ribonucleoproteins share properties with plant and vertebrate U-snRNPs. Embo J. 1990;6:469–476.

T179. Tomasi TB. The gamma A globulins: First line of defense. Hosp Practice 1967 Jul;2:26–35.

T180. Tomura T, Van Lancker JL. Procainamide-DNA interaction. J Rheumatol 1988;15:59–64.

T181. Tona L, Ng YC, Akera T, Brody TM. Depressant effects of chloroquine on the isolated guinea-pig heart. Eur J Pharmacol 1990 Mar;178(3):293–301.

T182. Tonegawa S. Somatic generation of antibody diversity. Nature 1983;302:575–581.

T183. Tonks NK, Charbonneau H, Diltz CD, Fischer EH, Walsch KA. Demonstration that the leukocyte common antigen CD45 is a protein tyrosine phosphatase. Biochemistry 1988;27: 8695–8701.

T184. Tonks NK, Diltz CD, Fischer EH. CD45, an integral membrane protein tyrosine phosphatase; characterization of enzyme activity. J Biol Chem 1990;265:10674–10680.

T185. Tooke AF, Stuart RA, Maddison PJ. The prevalence of autonomic neuropathy in systemic lupus erythematosus. Br J Rheumatol 1990;30 Suppl 1:22.

T186. Toomey JM, Snyder GG, Maenza RM. Acute epiglottitis due to systemic lupus erythematosus. Laryngoscope 1974;84: 522–527.

T187. Toone EC Jr, Irby R, Pierce EL. The L.E. cell in rheumatoid arthritis. Am J Med Sci 1960 Nov;240:599–608.

T188. Torda T, Yamaguchi I, Hirata F, Kopin IJ, Axelrod J. Quinacrine-blocked desensitization of adrenoceptors after immobilization stress or repeated injection of isoproterenol in rats. J Pharmacol Exp Ther 1981 Feb;216(2):334–338.

T189. Torda T, Yamaguchi I, Hirata F, Kopin IJ, Axelrod J. Mepacrine treatment prevents immobilization-induced desensitization of beta-adrenergic receptors in rat hypothalamus and brain stem. Brain Res 1981 Feb 2;205(2):441–444.

T190. Torrelo A, Espana A, Medina S, Ledo A. Danazol and discoid lupus erythematosus [letter]. Dermatologica 1990; 181(3):239.

T191. Torry DS, Faulk WP, McIntyre JA. Regulation of immunity to extra embryonic antigens in human pregnancy. Am J Reprod Immunol 1989;21(3–4):76–81.

T192. See T241a.

T193. Totoritis MC, Tan EM, McNally EM, Rubin RL. Association of antihistone (H2A-H2B) complex antibody with symptomatic procainamide induced lupus [abstract]. N Engl J Med 1988;318:1431–1436.

T194. Tovar Z, Dauphinee MJ, Talal N. Defective induction of T-cell help and natural killing following anti-CD3 stimulation of autoimmune lymphocytes. J Autoimmun 1988;1:327–337.

T195. Towbin H, Gordon J. Immunoblotting and dot immunobinding - current status and outlook. J Immunol Methods 1984; 72:313–340.

T196. Towbin H, Staehelin T, Gordon J. Immunoblotting in the clinical laboratory. J Clin Chem Clin Biochem 1989;27: 495–501.

T197. Towner SR, Michet CJ, O'Fallon WM, Nelson AM. The epidemiology of juvenile arthritis in Rochester, Minnesota 1960–1970. Arthritis Rheum 1983;26:1208.

T198. Townes AS, Stewart CR, Osler AG. Immunologic studies of systemic lupus erythematosus. I. Quantitative estimations of nucleoprotein reactive gamma globulin in systemic lupus erythematosus and other diseases. Bull Johns Hopkins Hosp 1963;112:183–201.

T199. Toxic Epidemic Syndrome Study Group. Toxic epidemic syndrome, Spain 1981. Lancet 1982;2:697–702.

T200. Tozman ECS, Urowitz MB, Gladman DD. Systemic lupus erythematosus and pregnancy. J Rheumatol 1980;7:624–632.

T201. Tozman ECS, Urowitz MB, Gladman DD. Prolonged complete remission in previously severe SLE. Ann Rheum Dis 1982 Feb;41:39–40.

T202. Trachtman H, Ginzler E, Tejani A, Rao M, Herrod L, Finberg L. Abnormal antidiuretic hormone secretion in patients with systemic lupus erythematosus. Nephron 1987;46(1): 67–72.

T203. Traeger J, Laville M, El Habib R, Moskortchenko JF, Coulet PR, Gautheron DC. Extracorporeal immunoadsorption of DAN antibodies on DNA-coated collagen films: First results in systemic lupus erythematosus. In: Nose Y, editor. Plasmapheresis. Cleveland:ISAO Press, 1983:155–166.

T204. Train J, Hertz I, Cohen BA, Samach M. Lupus vasculitis: Reversal of radiographic findings after steroid therapy. Am J Gastroent 1981;76:460–463.

T205. Trambert J, Reinitz E, Buchbinder S. Ruptured hepatic artery aneurysms in a patient with systemic lupus erythematosus [case report]. Cardiovasc Intervent Radiol 1989 Jan–Feb; 12(1):32–34.

T206. Trasler D. Aspirin-induced cleft lip and other malformations in mice. Lancet 1965;1:606–607.

T207. Travers R, Hughes GR. Salicylate hepatotoxicity in systemic lupus erythematosus: a common occurrence. BMJ 1978 Dec 2;2(6151):1532–1533.

T208. Travers RL, Hughes GR. Oral contraceptive therapy and systemic lupus erythematosus. J Rheumatol 1978 Winter; 5(4):448–451.

T209. Travers RL, Pinching AJ, Hughes GR, Jones T, Moss S. Detection of cerebral involvement in systemic lupus erythematosus by using 15-oxygen brain scanning. Arthritis Rheum 1978 Jun;21:598.

T210. Treadwell BV, Mankin HJ. The synthetic processes of articular cartilage. Clin Orthop 1980;213:50–61.

T211. Tremaine MJ. Subacute Pick's disease (polyserositis) with polyarthritis and glomerulonephritis: report of two fatal cases. N Engl J Med 1934 Oct 25;211:754–759.

T212. Trenholme GM, Carson PE. Therapy and prophylaxis of malaria. J Am Med Assoc 1978;240:2293–2295.

T213. Trentham DE, Belli JA, Bloomer WD, Anderson RJ, Lane H, Reinherz EL, Austen KF. 2,000-centiGray total lymphoid irradiation for refractory rheumatoid arthritis. Arthritis Rheum 1987 Sep;30(9):980–987.

T214. Trepicchio W Jr, Barrett KJ. Eleven MR1-pr/1pr anti-DNA autoantibodies are encoded by genes from four Vh gene families. A potentially biased usage of Vh genes. J Immunol 1987; 138:2323–2331.

T215. Trepicchio W Jr, Maruya A, Barrett KJ. The heavy chain genes of a lupus anti-DNA autoantibody are encoded in the germ line of a nonautoimmune strain of mouse and conserve in strains of mice polymorphic for this gene locus. J Immunol 1987 Nov;139(9):3139–3145.

T216. Trevor RP, Sondhemier FK, Fessel WJ, Wolpert SM. Angiographic demonstration of major cerebral vessel occlusion in systemic lupus erythematosus. Neuroradiology 1972;4: 202–207.

T217. Trimble M, Bell DA, Brien W, Hachinski V, O'Keefe B, McLay C, Black J. The antiphospholipid syndrome: prevalence among patients with stroke and transient ischemic attacks. Am J Med 1990 Jun;88(6):593–597.

T218. Trinchieri G, Matsumoto-Kobayashi M, Clark SC, Sjeehra J, London L, Perussia B. Response of resting human peripheral blood natural killer cells to interleukin-2. J Exp Med 1984; 160:1147.

T219. Trinchieri G, Santoli D. Antiviral activity induced by culturing lymphocytes with tumor-derived or virus-transferred cells. Enhancement of human natural killer cell activity by interferon and inhibition of susceptibility of target cells to lysis. J Exp Med 1978 May 1;147:1314.

T220. Triplett DA, Brandt JT, Kaczor D, Schaeffer J. Laboratory diagnosis of lupus inhibitors: A comparison of the tissue thromboplastin inhibition procedure with a new platelet neutralization procedure. Am J Clin Pathol 1983 Jun;79:678.

T221. Triplett DA, Brandt JT, Musgrave KA, Orr CA. The relationship between lupus anticoagulants and antibodies to phospholipid. JAMA 1988 Jan 22–29;259(4):550–554.

T222. Trist DG, Weatherall M. Inhibition of lymphocyte transformation by mepacrine and chloroquine. J Pharm Pharmacol 1981 Jul;33(7):434–438.

T223. Tromovitch TA, Hyman AB. Systemic lupus erythematosus with hemorrhagic bullae. A case with L.E. cells recovered from the bullae. Arch Dermatol 1961 Jun;83:910–914.

T224. Tron F, Bach J-F. Immunological tests in the diagnosis and prognosis of disseminated lupus erythematosus before treatment [original in French]. Nouv Presse Med 1977 Sep 10; 6:2573–2578.

T225. Tron F, Ganeval D, Droz D. Immunologically-mediated acute renal failure of non-glomerular origin in the course of systemic lupus erythematosus. Am J Med 1979 Sep;67: 529–532.

T226. Trowsdale J, Hanson I, Mockridge I, Beck S, Townsend A, Kelly A. Sequences encoded in the class II region of the MHC related to the ABC superfamily of transporters. Nature 1990; 348:741–747.

T227. Truccone NJ, Mariona FG. Prenatal diagnosis and outcome of congenial complete heart block: the role of fetal echocardiography. Fetal Ther 1986;1:210–216.

T228. Truhan AP, Ahmed AR. Corticosteroids: a review with emphasis on complications of prolonged systemic therapy. Ann Allergy 1989;62:375–390.

T229. Trujillo MA, Yebra M, Mulero J, Gea JC, Ferrer J. Antimitochondrial antibodies and the antiphospholipid syndrome [letter]. J Rheumatol 1990 May;17(5):718–719.

T230. Truneh A, Albert F, Golstein P, Schmitt-Velhulst AM. Early steps of lymphocyte activation bypassed by synergy between calcium ionophores and phorbol ester. Nature 1985;313: 318–320.

T231. Tsakeris DA, Marbet GA, Makris PE, Settas L, Duckert F. Impaired fibrinolysis as essential contribution to thrombosis in patients with lupus anticoagulant. Thromb Heamost 1989; 61:175–177.

T232. Tsankov NK, Lazarova AZ, Vasileva SG, Obreshkova EV. Lupus erythematosus-like eruption due to D-penicillamine in progressive systemic sclerosis. Int J Dermatol 1990; 29: 571–574.

T233. Tsao BP, Ebling FM, Roman C, Panosian-Sahakian N, Calame K, Hahn BH. Structural characteristics of the variable regions of immunoglobulin genes encoding a pathogenic autoantibody in murine lupus. J Clin Invest 1990 Feb;85(2): 530–540.

T234. Tsao BP, Ohnishi K, Hahn BH. A potential mechanism by which pathogenic autoantibodies escape tolerance [abstract]. Arthritis Rheum 1991;34:S34.

T234a. Tsao BP, Ohnishi K, Cheroutre H, Mitchell B, Teitell M, Mixter P, Kronenberg M, Hahn BH. Failed self tolerance and autoimmunity in IgG anti-DNA transgene mice. J Immunol 1992 In press.

T235. Tsianos EB, Tzioufas AG, Kita MD, Tsolas O, Moutsopoulos HM. Serum isoamylases in patients with autoimmune rheumatoid diseases. Clin Exp Rheumatol 1984 Jul–Sep;2(3): 235–238.

T236. Tsokas GC. Biochemical and molecular abnormalities in the pathogenesis of systemic lupus erythematosus. Clin Exp Rheumatol 1991;9:533–539.

T237. Tsokos GC. Overview of cellular immune function in systemic lupus erythematosus. In: Lahita RJ, editor. Systemic lupus erythematosus. New York: Churchill Livingston, 1991. In Press.

T238. Tsokos GC, Balow JE. Cytotoxic responses to alloantigens in systemic lupus erythematosus. J Clin Immunol 1981;1:208.

T239. Tsokos GC, Balow JE. Phenotypes of T lymphocytes in systemic lupus erythematosus: decreased cytotoxic/suppressor subpopulation is associated with deficient allogenic cytotoxic responses rather than with concanavalin A-induced suppressor cells. Clin Immunol Immunopathol 1983 Feb;26: 267–276.

T240. Tsokos GC, Balow JE. Cellular immune response in systemic lupus erythematosus. Prog Allergy 1984;35:93.

T241. Tsokos GC, Balow JE, Huston DP, Wei N, Decker JL. Effect of plasmapheresis on T and B lymphocyte functions in patients with systemic lupus erythematosus: A double blind study. Clin Exp Immunol 1982 May;48(2):449–457.

T241a. Tsokos GC, Caughman SW, Klippel JH. Successful treatment of generalized discoid skin lesions with azathioprine. Its use in a patient with systemic lupus erythematosus. Arch Dermatol 1985 Oct;121:1323–1325.

T242. Tsokos GC, Gorden P. Antonovych T, Wilson CB, Balow JE. Lupus nephritis and other autoimmune features in patients with diabetes mellitus due to autoantibody in insulin receptors. Ann Intern Med 1985 Feb;102(2):176–181.

T243. Tsokos GC, Moutsopoulos HM, Steinberg AD. Muscle involvement in systemic lupus erythematosus. JAMA 1981 Aug 14;246(7):766–768.

T244. Tsokos GC, Rook AH, Djeu JY, Balow JE. Natural killer cells and interferon responses in patients with systemic lupus erythematosus. Clin Exp Immunol 1982 Nov;5:239–245.

T245. Tsokos, GC, Smith PL, Christian CB, Lipnick RN, Balow JE, Djeu JY. Interleukin-2 restores the depressed allogeneic cell-mediated lympholysis and natural killer cell activity in patients with systemic lupus erythematosus. Clin Immunol Immunopathol 1985 Mar;34:379–386.

T246. Tsokos GC, Tsokos M, le Riche NG, Klippel JH. A clinical and pathologic study of cerebrovascular disease in patients with systemic lupus erythematosus. Semin Arthritis Rheum 1986 Aug;16(1):70–78.

T247. Tsokos GC, Boumpas DT, Smith PL, Djeu JY, Balow JE, Rook AH. Deficient gamma-interferon production in patients with systemic lupus erythematosus. Arthritis Rheum 1986;29: 1210–1215.

T248. Tsoulfa G, Rook GAW, Bahr GM, Sattar MA, Behbehani K, Young DB, Mehlert A, Van Ebden JDA, Hay FC, Isenberg DA, Lydard PM. Elevated IgG antibody levels to the mycobacterial 65-kDa heat shock protein are characteristic of patients with rheumatoid arthritis. Scand J Immunol 1989;30: 519–528.

T249. Tsubata T, Nishikawa S, Katsura Y, Kumagai S, Imura H. B cell repertoire for anti-DNA antibody in normal and lupus mice: Differential expression of precursor cells for high and low affinity anti-DNA antibodies. Clin Exp Immunol 1988;71: 50–55.

T250. Tsuboi R, Taneda A, Ogawa H. Coexistent systemic lupus erythematosus and urate deposition [letter]. J Am Acad Dermatol 1986 Nov;15(5 Pt 1):1050–1051.

T251. Tsuchiya N, Mitamura T, Goto M, Moroi Y, Kinoshita M, Yokohari R, Miyamoto T. 2-dimensional flow cytometric analysis of peripheral blood T lymphocytes from patients with systemic lupus erythematosus: preferential expression of HLA-DR antigen on the surface of Leu 2a + cells. J Rheumatol 1988; 15:946–951.

T252. Tsukahara M, Matsuo K, Kojima H. Protein losing enteropathy in a boy with systemic lupus erythematosus. J Pediatr 1990;97:778–780.

T253. Tsukamoto H, Ueda A, Nagasawa K, Tada Y, Niho Y. Increased production of the third component of complement (C3) by monocytes from patients with systemic lupus erythematosus. Clin Exp Immunol 1990;82:257–261.

T254. Tu BY. Combined treatment using traditional Chinese medicine and Western medicine of lupus crisis: a report of 10 cases [English abstract]. Chung Hsi I Chieh Ho Tsa Chih 1986 Apr;6(4):215–217.

T255. Tu WH, Shearn MA. Systemic lupus erythematosus and latent renal tubular dysfunction. Ann Intern Med 1967 Jul; 67(1):100–109.

T256. Tuaillon N, Muller S, Pasquali JL, Bordigoni P, Youinou P, Van Regenmortel MH. Antibodies from patients with rheumatoid arthritis and juvenile chronic arthritis analyzed with core histone synthetic peptides. Int Arch Allergy Appl Immunol 1990;91:297–305.

T257. Tuchinda M, Newcomb RW, DeVald BT. Effect of prednisone treatment on the human response to keyhole limpet hemocyanin. Int Arch Allergy 1972;42:533–544.

T258. Tuffanelli D. Chronic cutaneous (Discoid) Lupus Erythematosus. In: Wallace DJ, Dubois EL, editors. Dubois' Lupus Erythematosus, 3d ed, Philadelphia: Lea & Febiger, 1987: 283–301.

T259. Tuffanelli DL. Acanthosis nigricans with lupoid hepatitis. JAMA 1964 Aug 17;189:584–585.

T260. Tuffanelli DL. Scleroderma, immunological and genetic disease in three families. Dermatologica 1969;13:893.

T261. Tuffanelli DL. Lupus erythematosus panniculitis (profundus) clinical and immunologic studies. Arch Dermatol 1971 Mar;103:231–242.

T262. Tuffanelli DL. Lupus erythematosus. Arch Dermatol 1972; 106:553–566.

T263. Tuffanelli DL. Lupus panniculitis. Semin Dermatol 1985; 4:79–81.

T264. Tuffanelli DL, Dubois EL. Cutaneous manifestations of systemic lupus erythematosus. Arch Dermatol 1964 Oct;90: 377–386.

T265. Tuffanelli DL, Kay D, Fukuyama K. Dermal-epidermal junction in lupus erythematosus. Arch Dermatol 1969 Jun;99: 652–662.

T266. Tufanelli DL, Kay DM. Morphological and immunological studies of necrotizing vasculitis in systemic lupus erythematosus (SLE) [abstract]. Clin Res 1969;17:278.

T267. Tuffanelli DL, Levan NE, Dubois EL. Unusual cutaneous disorders in familial lupus erythematosus. Arch Dermatol 1964 Mar;89(3):324–327.

T268. Tuffanelli DL, Winkelmann RK. Systemic scleroderma. A

clinical study of 727 cases. Arch Dermatol 1961 Sep;84: 359–371.

T269. Tumiati B, Bellelli A, Portioli I, Prandi S. Kikucki's disease in systemic lupus erythematosus: an independent or dependent event. Clin Rheumatol 1991;10:90–93.

T270. Tumulty PA. The clinical course of systemic lupus erythematosus. JAMA 1954 Nov 6;156:947–953.

T271. Tung K. Immunopathology and male infertility. Hosp Pract (Off) 1988 Jun 15;23(6):191–206.

T272. Tunkel AR, Shuman M, Popkin M, Seth R, Hoffman B. Minoxidil-induced systemic lupus erythematosus. Arch Intern Med 1987;147:599–600.

T273. Turner B, Rapp U, App H, Greene M, Dobashi K, Reed J. Interleukin 2 induces tyrosine phosphorylation and activation of p72–74 Raf-1 kinase in a T-cell line. Proc Natl Acad Sci USA 1991;88:1227–1231.

T274. Turner BM, O'Neill LP, Allan IM. Histone H4 acetylation in human cells. Frequency of acetylation at different sites defined by immunolabelling with site-specific antibodies. FEBS Lett 1989;253:141–145.

T275. Turner DA, Templeton AC, Selzer PM, Rosenberg AG, Petasnick JP. Femoral capital osteonecrosis: MR finding of diffuse marrow abnormalities without focal lesions. Radiology 1989 Apr;171(1):135–140.

T276. Turner G, Collins E. Fetal effects of regular salicylate ingestion in pregnancy. Lancet 1975;2:338–339.

T277. Turner JC. Dermatomyositis. A study of 3 cases. N Engl J Med 1937 Jan 28;216:158–161.

T278. Turner R, Lipshutz W, Miller W, Rittenberg G, Schumacher HR, Cohen S. Esophageal dysfunction in collagen disease. Am J Med Sci 1973 Mar;265(3):191–199.

T279. Turner SJ, Levine L, Redman A. Lupus erythematosus and pregnancy. Obstet Gynecol 1956;8:601–609.

T280. Turner-Stokes L, Cambridge G, Corcoran T, Oxford JS, Snaith ML. In vitro response to influenza immunization by peripheral blood mononuclear cells from patients with systemic lupus erythematosus and other autoimmune diseases. Ann Rheum Dis 1988 Jul;47(7):532–535.

T281. Turner-Stokes L, Cambridge G, Snaith ML. In vitro lymph node and peripheral blood lymphocyte responses to influenza immunization in patients with systemic lupus erythematosus. Clin Exp Rheumatol 1989 Jan–Feb;7(1):71–74.

T282. Turner-Stokes L, Isenberg DA. Immunization of patients with rheumatoid arthritis and systemic lupus erythematosus. Ann Rheum Dis 1988 Jul;47(7):529–531.

T283. Twomey JJ, Laughter AH, Steinberg AD. A serum inhibitor of immune regulation in patients with systemic lupus erythematosus (SLE). J Clin Invest 1978 Sep;62:713–715.

T284. Tye K, Steitz JA. U3, U8, and U13 comprise a new class of mammalian snRNPs localized in the cell nucleolus. Embo J 1989;8:3113–3119.

T285. Tye MJ, White H, Appel B, Ansell HB. Lupus erythematosus treated with a combination of quinacrine, hydroxychloroquine and chloroquine. N Engl J Med 1959 Jan 8;260(2): 63–66.

U

U1. Uberbacher EC, Bunick GJ. Structure of the nucleosome core particle at 8 A resolution. J Biomol Struct Dynamics 1989; 7:1–18.

U2. Uberbacher EC, Harp JM, Wilkinson-Singley E, Bunick GJ. Shape analysis of the histone octamer in solution. Science 1986; 232:1247–1249.

U3. Uchino K, Hasegawa O, Matsumaru K, Ochiai H, Yakuwa H, Miyamoto K, Sekine S, Tomiyama M, Miyakawa T. A case of retroperitoneal fibrosis associated with systemic lupus erythematosus. Nippon Naika Gakkai Zasshi 1986 May;75(5): 666–669.

U4. Uddin MS, Lynfield YL, Grosberg SJ, Steifler R. Cutaneous reaction to spironolactone resembling lupus erythematosus. Cutis 1979;24:198–200.

U5. Ueda T, Chueh SH, Noel MW, Gill DL. Influence of inositol 1,4,5-triphosphate and guanine nucleotides on intracellular calcium release within the N1E-115 neuronal cell line. J Biol Chem 1986;261:3184–3192.

U6. Ueki H, Wolf HH, Braun-Falco O. Cutaneous localization of human globulins in lupus erythematosus. Electron micropsy study using the peroxidase-labeled antibody technique. Arch Dermatol Res 1974;248:297.

U7. Uetrecht JP. Reactivity and possible significance of hydroxylamine and nitroso metabolites of procainamide. J Pharmacol Exp Ther 1985;232:420–425.

U8. Uetrecht JP. Metabolism of drugs by activated lymphocytes: implications for drug-induced lupus and other drug hypersensitivity reactions. In: Witmer CM, editor. Biological Reactive Intermediates IV. New York: Plenum Press, 1990:121–132.

U9. Uetrecht JP, Sweetman BJ, Woosley RL, Oates JA. Metabolism of procainamide to a hydroxylamine by rat and human hepatic microsomes. Drug Metab Dispos 1984;12:77–81.

U10. Ueyama H, Hashimoto Y, Uchino M, Sasaki Y, Uyama E, Okajima K, Akari S. Progressing ischemic stroke in a homozygote with variant antithrombin III. Stroke 1989;20:815–818.

U11. Uhl MD, Werner BE, Romano TJ, Zidar BJ. Normal pressure hydrocephalus in a patient with systemic lupus erythematosus [case report]. J Rheumatol 1990 Dec;17(12):1689–1691.

U12. Uitto J, Santa-Cruz DJ, Eisen AJ, Leone P. Verrucous lesions in patients with discoid lupus erythematosus: Clinical, histopathological and immunofluorescence studies. Br J Dermatol 1978;98:507–520.

U13. Uko G, Dawkins RL, Kay P, Christiansen FT, Hollingsworth PN. CR1 deficiency in SLE: acquired or genetic? Clin Exp Immunol 1985;62:329–336.

U14. Ullberg S, Lindquist NG, Sjostrand SE. Accumulation of chorioretinotoxic drugs in the foetal eye. Nature 1970;227:1257–1258.

U15. Umbert P, Winkelman RK. Concurrent localized scleroderma and discoid lupus erythematosus. Cutaneous 'mixed' or 'overlap' syndrome. Arch Dermatol 1978 Oct;114(10):1473–1478.

U16. Umland S, Lee R, Howard M, Martens C. Expression of lymphokine genes in splenic lymphocytes of autoimmune mice. Mol Immunol 1989;26:649–656.

U17. Umland SP, Go NF, Cupp JE, Howard M. Responses of B cells from autoimmune mice to IL-5. J Immunol 1989;142:1528–1535.

U18. Umland SP, Smith SR, Straussner HR. Production of and responsiveness to interleukin 2 in autoimmune BXSB mice. Cell Immunol 1987;107:158–171.

U19. Unander AM, Norberg R, Hahn L, Arfors L. Anticardiolipin antibodies and complement in ninety-nine women with habitual abortion. Am J Obstet Gynecol 1987;156:114–119.

U20. Underwood JR, Pederson JS, Chalmers PJ, Toh BH. Hybrids from normal, germ free, nude and neonatal mice produce monoclonal autoantibodies to eight different intracellular structures. Clin Exp Immunol 1985;60:417–426.

U21. Unkeless JC, Scigliano E, Freedman VH. Structure and function of human and murine receptors for IgG. Ann Rev Immunol 1988;6:251–281.

U22. Unni KK, Holley KE, McDuffie FC, Titus JL. Comparative study of NZB mice under germ-free and conventional conditions. J Rheumatol 1975;2:36–44.

U23. Unterweger B, Klein G, Fleishchhacker WW. Plasma exchange for cerebral lupus erythematosus [letter]. Biol Psychiatry 1988 Dec;24(8):946–947.

U24. Urbain J, Wuilmart C. Some thoughts on idiotypic networks and immunoregulation. Immunol Today 1982;3:88–93.

U25. Urbain J, Wuilmart C, Cazenave PA. Idiotypic regulation in immune networks. Contemp Top Mol Immunol 1981;8:113.

U26. Urban JL, Kumar V, Kono DH, Gomerz C, Horvath SJ, Clayton J, Ando DG, Sercarz EE, Hood L. Restricted use of T cell receptor V genes in murine autoimmune encephalomyelitis raises possibilities for antibody therapy. Cell 1988;54:577–592.

U27. Urban RC Jr, Cotlier E. Corticosteroid-induced cataracts. Survey Ophthal 1986;31:102–110.

U28. Urbanski A, Schwarz T, Nuener P, Krutmann J, Kirknbauer R, Koch A, Luger TA. Ultraviolet light induces increased circulating interleukin-6 in humans. J Invest Dermatol 1990;94:808–811.

U29. Urizar RE, Tinglof B, McIntosh R, Litman N, Barnett E, Wilkerson J, Smith F, Vernier RL. Immunosuppressive therapy of proliferative glomerulonephritis in children. Am J Dis Child 1969;118:411–425.

U30. Urman JD, Abeles M, Houghton AN, Rothfield N. Aseptic necrosis presenting as wrist pain in SLE. Arthritis Rheum 1977;20:825–828.

U31. Urman JD, Lowenstein MB, Abeles M, Weinstein A. Oral mucosal ulceration in systemic lupus erythematosus. Arthritis Rheum 1978 Jan–Feb;21(1):58–61.

U32. Urman JD, Rothfield NF. Corticosteroid treatment in systemic lupus erythematosus: Survival studies. JAMA 1977 Nov 21;238:2272–2276.

U33. Urowitz MB. Late mortality and morbidity. In: Proceedings of the Second International Conference on Systemic Lupus Erythematosus, Tokyo, 1989:190.

U34. Urowitz MB, Bookman AAM, Koehler BE, Gordon DA, Smythe HA, Ogryzlo MA. The bimodal mortality pattern of systemic lupus erythematosus. Am J Med 1976 Feb;60:221–225.

U35. Urowitz MB, Gladman DD. Late mortality in SLE: the price we pay for control. J Rheumatol 1980;7:412.

U36. Urowitz MB, Gladman D, Rubin L. Mortality in SLE: A review of 51 cases. Clin Res 1985;33:783A.

U37. Urowitz MB, Gladman DD, Chalmers A, Ogryzlo MA. Nail lesions in systemic lupus erythematosus. J Rheumatol 1978 Winter;5(4):441–447.

U37a. Urowitz MB, Gladman DD, Tozman ECS, Goldsmith CH. The lupus activity criteria count (LACC). J Rheumatol 1984 Dec;11:783–787.

U38. Uter W, Proksch E, Schauder S. Chilblain-lupus erythematosus [English abstract]. Hautarzt (Ger) 1988 Sep;39(9):602–605.

U39. Utsinger PD, Yount WJ. Phytohemagglutinin response to systemic lupus erythematosus. Reconstitution experiments using highly purified lymphocyte subpopulations and monocytes. J Clin Invest 1977 Sep;60:626–638.

U40. Utsinger PD, Zvaifler NJ, Bluestein HG. Hypocomplementemia in procainamide associated systemic lupus erythematosus. Ann Intern Med 1976 Mar;84:293–296.

U41. Uwatoko S, Mannik M. Low-molecular weight C1q-binding immunoglobulin G in patients with systemic lupus erythematosus consists of autoantibodies to the collagen-like region of C1q. J Clin Invest 1988;82:816–824.

U42. Uytdehaag F, Claassen I, Bunschoten H, Loggen H, Ottenhoff T, Teeuwsen V, Osterhaus A. Human anti-idiotypic lymphocyte clones are activated by autologous anti-rabies virus antibodies presented in association with HLA-DQ molecules. J Mol Cell Immunol 1987;3:145.

U43. Uytdehaag FGCM, Osterhaus ADME. Induction of neutralizing antibody in mice against Poliovirus type II with monoclonal anti-idiotypic antibody. J Immunol 1984;134:1225.

V

V1. Vachtenheim J, Grossman J. Methyl-thiouracil induced lupus erythematosus. Cas Lek Cesk 1963;102:1413–1416.

V2. Vachtenheim J, Grossman J. Perforation of the nasal septum in systemic lupus erythematosus. BMJ 1969 Apr 12;2:98.

V3. Vakil M, Kearney JF. Regulatory influences of neonatal multispecific antibodies on the developing B cell repertoire. Int Rev Immunol 1988;3:117–131.

V4. Valencia ME, Molano J, Vazquez JJ, Lavilla P, Khamashta MA, Pintado V, Barbado FJ, Aguado AG. Determining beta-2 macroglobulin levels in patients with systemic lupus erythematosus. A clinical and biochemical correlation. Rev Clin Esp 1987; 181:310–313.

V5. Valentijn RM, Daha MR, Van Es LA. Clinical significance of laboratory investigations for immune complexes. Clin Immunol Allergy 1985;5:649–660.

V6. Valentijn RM, Overhagen HV, Hazevoet HM, Hermans J, Cats A, Daha MR, Van Es LA. The value of complement and immune complex determinations in monitoring disease activity in patients with systemic lupus erythematosus. Arthritis Rheum 1985;28:904–913.

V7. Valent P, Ashman LK, Hinterberger W, Eckersberger F, Majdic O, Lechner K, Bettelheim P. Mast cell typing: Demonstration of a distinct hematopoietic cell type and evidence for immunophenotypic relationship to mononuclear phagocytes. Blood 1989;73:1778–1785.

V8. Valesini G, Priori R, Borsetti A, Tiberti A, Moncada A, Pivetti-Pezzi P. Clinical serological correlations in the evaluation of Sjogren's syndrome. Clin Exp Rheumatol 1989 Mar–Apr;7(2): 197–202.

V9. Valesini G, Tincani A, Harris EN, Mantelli PG, Allegri F, Palmieri F, Hughes GR, Balsano F, Ballestrieri G. Use of monoclonal antibodies to identify shared idiotypes on anti-cardiolipin and anti-DNA antibodies in human sera. Clin Exp Immunol 1987; 70:18–25.

V10. Vallois H, Debien J, Merchak M, Commissionat Y. Oral manifestations of lupus [original in French]. Actualites Odonto-Stomatologique 1978;124:513–537.

V11. Van Buren C, Bach F, editors. Update on immunonutrition. Nutrition 1990;6:1.

V12. Van Coppenolle F, Vallat M, Smolick J, Treves R, Duprat F, Detre J, Mathon C. Bilateral blindness caused by disseminated arterial lupus erythematosus. Bull Soc Ophthalmol Fr 1989 Feb;89(2):207–209.

V13. van Dam A, Wekking EM, Ovmen HAPC. Psychiatric symptoms as features of systemic lupus erythematosus. Reprint Psychotherapy and Psychosomatics, Psychother Psychosom (Switzerland) 1991;55:132–140.

V14. van Dam A, Winkel I, Zijlstra-Baalbergen J, Smeenk R, Cuypers HT. Cloned human snRNP proteins B and B′ differ only in their carboxy-terminal part. Embo J 1989;8:3853–3860.

V15. van Dam AP, Winkel I, Smeenk R, Cuypers HT. The snRNP protein B and B′ are alternative splicing variants encoded by the same gene. Thesis (van Dam) in the Department of Autoimmune Diseases of the Central Laboratory of the Netherlands Red Cross Blood Transfusion Service and the Laboratory for Experimental and Clinical Immunology of the University of Amsterdam, The Netherlands, 1990:125–133.

V16. van de Laar MA, Meenhorst PL, van Soesbergen RM, Olsthoorn PG, van der Korst JK. Polyarticular Salmonella bacterial arthritis in a patient with systemic lupus erythematosus. J Rheumatol 1989 Feb;16(2):231–234.

V17. van den Brink H, Vroom TM, van de Laar MAF, van Soesber-

gen RM, van der Korst JK. Superior vena cava syndrome caused by systemic lupus erythematosus in a patient with longstanding rheumatoid arthritis. J Rheumatol 1990 Feb; 17(2):240–243.

V18. Van der Straeten C, Wei N, Rothschild J, Goozh JL, Klippel JH. Rapidly fatal pneumococcal septicemia in systemic lupus erythematosus. J Rheumatol 1987 Dec;14(6):1177–1180.

V19. Van der Tempel H, Tulleke JE, Limburg PC, Muskiet FAJ, van Rijswijk MH. Effects of fish oil supplementation in rheumatoid arthritis. Ann Rheum Dis 1990;49:76–80.

V20. Van de Wiel TWM, Van de Wiel-Dorfmeyer H, Van Loghem JJ. Studies on platelet antibodies in man. Vox Sang 1961 Nov 6:64.

V21. Van de Winkel JGJ, Anderson CL. Biology of human immunoglobulin G Fc receptors. J Leukocyte Biol 1991;49: 511–524.

V22. Van de Winkel JGJ, Ernst LK, Anderson CL, Chiu I-M. Gene organization of the human high affinity receptor for IgG, FcγRI (CD64): Characterization and evidence for a second gene. J Biol Chem 1991;266:13449–13455.

V23. Van de Winkel JGJ, van Duijnhoven JLP, Van Ommen R, Capel PJA, Tax WJM. Selective modulation of two human monocyte Fc receptors for IgG by immobilized immune complexes. J Immunol 1988;140:3515–3521.

V24. Van der Woude FJ, Van der Giessen M, Kallenberg GM, Ouwehand W, Beekhuis H, Beelan JM, van Son WJ, Hoedemaeker P J, van der Hem GK, The TH. Reticuloendothelial Fc receptor function in SLE patients. I. Primary HLA linked defect or acquired dysfunction secondary to disease activity. Clin Exp Immunol 1984;55:473–480.

V25. van der Woude FJ. Anticytoplasmic antibodies in Wegener's granulomatosis [letter]. Lancet 1985; 2:48.

V26. Vandre DD, Davis FM, Rao PN, Borisy GG. Distribution of cytoskeletal proteins sharing a conserved phosphorylated epitope. Eur J Cell Biol 1986;41:72–81.

V27. Vane JR, Auggard EE, Botting RM. Mechanisms of disease: regulating functions of the vascular endothelium. N Engl J Med 1990;323:27–36.

V28. Van Eden W, Holoshitz J, Nevo A, Frankel A, Klajman A. Arthritis induced by a T-lymphocyte clone that responds to Mycobacterium tuberculosis and to cartilage protoglycans. Proc Nat Acad Sci USA 1985;82:5117–5120.

V29. Van Elven EH, Van Der Veen FM, Rolink AG, Issa P, Duin TM, Gleichmann E. Diseases caused by reactions of T lymphocytes against incompatible structures of the major histocompatibility complex. V. High titers of IgG autoantibodies to double-stranded DNA. J Immunol 1983;127:2435–2458.

V30. van Es J, Gmelig Meyling FHJ, van de Akker WRM, Aanstoot H, Derksen RHWM, Logtenberg T. Somatic mutations in the variable regions of a human IgG anti-ds DNA autoantibody suggest a role for antigen in the induction of systemic lupus erythematosus. J Exp Med 1991;173:461–470.

V31. van Es JH, Meyling FH, van de Akker WR, Aanstoot H, Derksen RS, Logtenberg T. Somatic mutations in the variable regions of a human IgG anti-double-stranded DNA autoantibody suggest a role for antigen in the induction of SLE. J Exp Med 1991;173:461–470.

V32. Vanheule BA, Carswell F. Sulphasalazine-induced systemic lupus erythematosus in a child. Eur J Pediatr 1983 Mar;140: 66–68.

V33. Van Joost T, van der Sluis JJ, Vuzevski VD, van der Kwast TH. Oral lupus erythematosus: markers of immunologic injury. J Cutaneous Pathology 1985;12:500–505.

V34. van Loenen HJ, Dijkmans BA, de Vries E. Concentration dependency of cyclosporin and chloroquine as inhibitors of cell proliferation and immunoglobulin production upon mitogen stimulation of mononuclear cells. Clin Exp Rheumatol 1990 Jan–Feb;8(1):59–61.

V35. van Rappard-van Der Veen FM, Rolink AG, Gleichmann E. Disease caused by reactions of T lymphocytes towards incompatible structures of the major histocompatibility complex. J Exp Med 1982;155:1555–1560.

V36. Van Snick J. Interleukin 6; an overview. Ann Rev Immunol 1990;8:253–278.

V37. Van Snick JL, Van Roost E, Markowetz R, Cambiaso CL, Masson PL. Enhancement by IgM rheumatoid factor of in vitro ingestion of macrophages and in vivo clearance of aggregated IgG or antigen antibody complexes. Eur J Immunol 1978;8(4):279–285.

V38. Van Steenbergen W, Beyls J, Vermylen J, Fevery J, Marchal G, Desmet V, De Groote J. Lupus anticoagulant and thrombosis of the hepatic veins (Budd-Chiari syndrome). Report of three patients and review of the literature. J Hepatol 1986;3(9):87–94.

V39. Van Story-Lewis PE, Roberts MW, Klippel JH. Oral effects of steroid therapy in a patient with systemic lupus erythematosus: report of a case. J Am Dent Assoc 1987 Jul;115(1):49–51.

V40. Van-Sweden B. Toxic "ictal" confusion in middle age: treatment with benzodiazepines. J Neurol Neurosurg Psychiatry 1985 May;48(5):472–476.

V41. van Venrooij WJ, Sillekens PTG. Small nuclear RNA associated proteins: autoantigens in connective tissue diseases. Clin Exp Rheumatol 1989;7:635–645.

V42. Van Wauwe JP, DeMey JR, Goossens JG. OKT3: A monoclonal anti-human T lymphocyte antibody with potent mitogenic properties. J Immunol 1980;124:2708–2713.

V43. Vaquer S, Salmeron I, Salmeron BO, Moix P, Marquez JA, Molto L, Alvarez de los Heros JI,Salmeron, O, Alvarez-Mon M. Immunobiology of materno-fetal relations. Revista Espanola de Fisiologia 1989;45 Suppl:359–369.

V44. Varga J, Heiman-Patterson TD, Emery DL, Griffin R, Lally EV, Uitto JJ, Jimenez SA. Clinical spectrum of the systemic manifestations of the eosinophilia-myalgia syndrome. Semin Arthritis Rheum 1990;19:313–328.

V45. Varga J, Lopatin M, Boden G. Hypoglycemia due to antiinsulin receptor antibodies in systemic lupus erythematosus [case report]. J Rheumatol 1990(9);17:1226–1229.

V46. Varga J, Peltonen J, Uitto J, Jimenez S. Development of diffuse fasciitis with eosinophilia during L-tryptophan treatment: Demonstration of elevated type I collagen gene expression in affected tissues. A clinicopathologic study of four patients. Ann Intern Med 1990;112:344–351.

V47. Varner MW, Meehan RT, Syrop CH, Strottmann MP, Goplerud CP. Pregnancy in patients with systemic lupus erythematosus. Am J Obstet Gynecol 1982;145:1025–1040.

V48. Vasey H. Arguments in favor of the intervention of a genetic factor in transmission of systemic lupus erythematosus. I. Generalities. Pathol Biol (Paris) 1964;12:1211.

V49. Vasey H. Arguments in favor of the intervention of a genetic factor in transmission of systemic lupus erythematosus. II. Study of 16 families of patients with systemic lupus erythematosus. Pathol Biol (Paris) 1964;12:1211.

V50. Vaughan JH, Bayles TB, Savour CB. The response of serum gammaglobulin level and complement titer to adrenocorticotrophic hormone therapy in lupus erythematosus disseminatus. J Lab Clin Med 1961;37:698–702.

V51. Vaughn M, Taylor M, Mohanakumar T. Characterization of human IgG Fc receptors. J Immunol 1985;135:4059–4065.

V52. Vaughn RY, Bailey JP Jr, Field RS, Loebl DH, Mealing HG Jr, Jerath RS, Dorlon RE. Diffuse nail dyschromia in black patients with systemic lupus erythematosus. J Rheumatol 1990 May;17(5):640–643.

V53. Vaughton KC, Walker DR, Sturridge MF. Mitral valve replacement for mitral stenosis caused by Libman-Sacks endocarditis. Br Heart J 1979;41:730–735.

V54. Vazquez JJ, Dixon FJ. Immunohistochemical analysis of lesions associated with "fibrinoid change." Arch Pathol 1958 Oct;66:504–517.

V55. Vazquez-Cruz J, Traboulssi H, Rodriguez-De la Serna A, Geli C, Roig C, Diaz C. A prospective study of chronic or recurrent headache in systemic lupus erythematosus. Headache 1990; 30:232–235.

V56. Vazquez Rodriguez JJ, Garcia Seoane J, Gial Aguado A, Sobrino JA, Arnalich Barbado FJ, Arnaiz Villena A. Complete heart block and the HLA system. Ann Intern Med 1982;96:126.

V57. Vecht CJ, Markusse HM. Lupus anticoagulant and late onset seizures [letter%mment on: Acta Neurol Scand 1989 Feb;79(2):114–118]. Acta Neurol Scand 1990 Jan;81(1):88–89.

V58. Veille JC, Sunderland C, Bennett RM. Complete heart block in a fetus associated with maternal Sjogren's syndrome. Am J Obstet Gynecol 1985;151:660.

V59. Velayos EE, Leidholt JD, Smyth CJ, Priest R. Arthropathy associated with steroid therapy. Ann Intern Med 1966 Apr; 64(4):759–771.

V60. Velayos EE, Robinson H, Porciuncula FU, Masi AT. Clinical correlation analysis of 137 patients with Raynaud's phenomenon. Am J Med Sci 1971;262:347–356.

V61. Velthuis PJ, Kater L, van der Tweel I, Meyling FG, Derksen RH, Hene RJ, van Geutselaar JA, Baart de la Faille H. In vivo antinuclear antibody of the skin: diagnostic significance and association with selective antinuclear antibodies. Ann Rheum Dis 1990 Mar;49(3):163–167.

V62. Velthuis PJ, van Weelden H, van Wichen D, Baart de la Faille H. Immunohistopathology of light-induced skin lesions in lupus erythematosus. Acta Dermatovener (Stockh) 1990; 70(2):93–98.

V63. Venables PJ, Baboonian C, Horsfall AC, Halliday D, Maini RN, Teo CG. The response to Epstein-Barr virus infection in Sjogren's syndrome. J Autoimmunity 1989;2:439–448.

V64. Venables PJ, Teo CG, Baboonian C, Griffin BE, Hughes RA. Persistence of Epstein-Barr virus in salivary gland biopsies from healthy individuals and patients with Sjogren's syndrome. Clin Exp Immunol 1989;75:359–364.

V65. Venegoni C, Chevallard M, Mele G, Banfi G, Carrabba M. The coexistence of rheumatoid arthritis and systemic lupus erythematosus. Clin Rheumatol 1987 Sep;6(3):439–445.

V66. Venkatraman JT, Gohill J, Fritzler MJ, Lefebvre YA. A histone 1-like antigen is a component of the nuclear envelope. Biochem Biophys Res Commun 1988;156:675–680.

V67. Verheul HAM, Schot LPC, Schuurs AHWN. Therapeutic effects of nandrolone deconate, tibolone, lynsternol and ethylesternol on Sjorgen's syndrome-like disorders in NZB/W mice. Clin Exp Immunol 1986;64:243–248.

V68. Verheul HAM, Stimson WH, den Hollander FL, Schuurs AHWN. Effects of nandrolone, testosterone and their decanoate esters on murine lupus. Clin Exp Immunol 1981;44:11–17.

V69. Verlin M, Laros RK JR, Penner JA. Refractory thrombocytopenic purpura treated successfully with cyclophosphamide [abstract]. Blood 1972;40:971.

V70. Vermess M, Bernstein RM, Bydder GM, Steiner RE, Yound IR, Hughes GR. Nuclear magnetic resonance (NMR) imaging of the brain in systemic lupus erythematosus. J Comput Assist Tomogr 1983 Jun;7(3):461–467.

V71. Vernon Roberts B. The effects of steroid hormones on macrophage activity. Int Rev Cytol 1969;25:131–159.

V72. Verroust PJ, Wilson CB, Cooper NR, Edginton TS, Dixon FJ. Glomerular complement components in human glomerulonephritis. J Clin Invest 1974;53:77–84.

V73. Verztman L, De Paola D, Gandelman L. "Delayed" cutaneous hypersensitivity to leukocytes in patients with systemic lupus erythematosus (SLE). AIR 1962 Dec;5:498–506.

V74. Via CS, Allen RC, Blelton RC. Direct stimulation of neutrophil oxygen activity by serum from patients with systemic lupus erythematosus: a relationship to disease activity. J Rheumatol 1984 Dec;11:745–753.

V75. Via CS, Sharrow SO, Shearer GM. Role of cytotoxic T lymphocytes in the prevention of lupus-like disease occurring in a murine model of graft-vs-host disease. J Immunol 1987;139: 1840–1849.

V76. Via CS, Shearer GM. T-cell interaction in autoimmunity: insights from a murine model of graft-versus-host disease. Immunol Today 1988;9:207–213.

V77. Vicencio GP, Chung-Park M, Ricanati E, Lee KN, DeBaz BP. SLE with interstitial cystitis, reversible hydronephrosis and intestinal manifestations [letter]. J Rheumatol 1989 Feb;16(2): 250–251.

V78. Victor KD, Randen I, Thompson K, Forre O, Natvig JB, Fu SM, Capra JD. Rheumatoid factors isolated from patients with autoimmune disorders are derived from germline genes distinct from those encoding the Wa, Po and Bla cross-reactive idiotypes. J Clin Invest 1991;87:1603–1613.

V79. Victor-Kobrin C, Barak ZT, Bonilla FA, Kobrin B, Sanz I, French D, Rothe J, Bona C. A molecular and structural analysis of the V_H and V_K regions of monoclonal antibodies bearing the A48 regulatory idiotype. J Immunol 1990;144:614.

V80. Vidailhet M, Piette JC, Wechsler B, Bousser MG, Brunet P. Cerebral venous thrombosis in systemic lupus erythematosus. Stroke 1990 Aug;21(8):1226–1231.

V81. Videbaek A. Auto-immune haemolytic anaemia in systemic lupus erythematosus. Acta Med Scand 1962;171 Fasc (2): 187–194.

V82. Vien CV, Gonzalez-Cabello R, Bado I, Gergely P. Effect of vitamin A treatment on the immune reactivity of patients with systemic lupus erythematosus. J Clin Lab Immunol 1988 May; 26(1):33–35.

V83. Viljaranta S, Ranki A, Kariniemi A-L, Nieminen P, Johansson L. Distribution of natural killer cells and lymphocyte subclasses in Jessner's lymphocyte infiltration of the skin and in cutaneous lesions of discoid and systemic lupus erythematosus. Br J Dermatol 1977;116:831–838.

V84. Vilppula A. Muscular disorders in some collagen diseases. A clinical, electromyographic and biopsy study. Acta Med Scand 1972;540 Suppl:1–47.

V85. Vincente P, Kennelly MA, Golden CJ, Kane R, Sweet J, Moses JA, Cardellino JP, Templeton R, Graber B. The relationship of the Halstead-Reitan neuropsychological battery and the Luria-Nebraska neuropsychological battery [preliminary report]. Clin Neuropsychol 1980;2:140–141.

V86. Vine AK, Barr CC. Proliferative lupus retinopathy. Arch Ophthalmol 1984 Jun;102(6):852–854.

V87. Violi F, Valesini G, Iuliano L, Ghiselli A, Falco M, Balsano F. Anticardiolipin antibodies and prostacyclin synthesis. Thromb Haemost 1987;57:374.

V88. Virchow R. Historical note on lupus [original in German]. Arch Pathol Anat 1865 Jan;32:139–143.

V89. Vischer TL, Jeannet M. Lymphocytotoxic antibodies in rheumatoid arthritis: relation to HLA-DR2 and rheumatoid factors. Clin Exp Rheumatol 1986;4:139–142.

V90. Vismara A, Meroni PL, Tincani A, Harris EN, Barcellini W, Brucato A, Khamashta M, Hughes GR, Zanussi C, Balestrieri G. Relationship between anti-cardiolipin and anti-endothelial cell antibodies in systemic lupus erythematosus. Clin Exp Immunol 1988 Nov;74(2):247–253.

V91. Vital Statistics of the United States. Vol II. Mortality, Part A.

US Department of Health, Education and Welfare, Rockville, MD. 1972:1976.

V92. Vitali C, Giuggioli C, Monti P, Rossi G, Wu DH, d'Ascanio A, Chiellini S, Gabriele M, Bombardieri S. Statistical evaluation of different clinical and serological parameters for the diagnosis of Sjogren's syndrome. Clin Exp Rheumatol 1989 Mar–Apr; 7(2):191–195.

V93. Vitebsky E, Rose NR, Terplan K, Paine JR, Egan RW. Chronic thyroiditis and autoimmunization. JAMA 1957 Jul 27;164: 1439–1447.

V93a. Vitetta ES, Uhr JW. Cell surface immunoglobulin. V. Release from murine splenic lymphocytes. J Exp Med 1972;136: 676–696.

V94. Vivas J, Tiliakos NA. Sacroiliitis in male systemic lupus erythematosus. Scand J Rheumatol 1985;14:441.

V95. Vivas J, Tiliakos NA. Sacroiliitis in male systemic lupus erythematosus. Bol Assoc Med P Rico 1985;77:271–272.

V96. Vivier E, Morin P, O'Brien C, Druker B, Schlossman SF, Anderson P. Tyrosine phosphorylation of the Fc gamma RIII (CD16): zeta complex in human natural killer cells. Induction by antibody-dependent cytotoxicity but not by natural killing. J Immunol 1991;146:206–210.

V97. Vivino FB, Schumacher HR Jr. Synovial fluid characteristics and the lupus erythematosus cell phenomenon in drug-induced lupus. Findings in three patients and review of pertinent literature. Arthritis Rheum 1989 May;32(5):560–568.

V98. Voiculetz N, Smith KC, Kaplan HS. Effect of quinacrine on survival and DNA repair in x-irradiated Chinese hamster cells. Cancer Res 1974 May;34:1038–1044.

V99. Voippio H. Incidence of chloroquine retinopathy. Ophthalmologica 1964;148:442–452.

V100. Volc-Platzer B, Wolff K. Treatment of subacute cutaneous lupus erythematosus with thalidomide. Der Hautarzt 1983;34: 175–178.

V101. Volk HD, Kopp J, Koerner IJ, Jahn S, Grunow R, Barthelmes H, Fiebig H. Correlation between the phenotype and the functional capacity of activated T cells in patients with active systemic lupus erythematosus. Scand J Rheumatol 1986;24:109–114.

V102. Volkow ND, Warner N, McIntyre R, Valentine A, Kulkarni M, Mullani N, Gould L. Cerebral involvement in systemic lupus erythematosus. Am J Physiol Imaging 1988;3(2):91–98.

V103. von Bilsen M, van der Vusse GJ, Willemsen PH, Coumans WA, Roemen TH, Reneman RS. Effects of nicotinic acid and mepacrine on fatty acid accumulation and myocardial damage during ischemia and reperfusion. J Mol Cell Cardiol 1990;22: 155–163.

V104. von Bonsdorff M, Friman C, Honkanen E, Pettersson T, Konttinen YT. Plasma exchange in the treatment of systemic lupus erythematosus. Scand J Rheumatol 1988;67 Suppl: 44–46.

V105. von Brauchitsch H. Antinuclear factor in psychiatric disorders. Am J Psychiatry 1972 Jun;128:1552–1554.

V106. Von dem Brone AEG Kr, Helmerhorst FM, Van Leeuwen EF, Pegels HG, Von Riesz E, Engelfriet CP. Autoimmune thrombocytopenia: detection of platelet autoantibodies with the suspension immunofluorescence test. Br J Haematol 1980 Jun; 45:319–327.

V107. Vonderheid EC, Koblenzer PJ, Ming PML, Burgoon CF Jr. Neonatal lupus erythematosus. Report of four cases with review of the literature. Arch Dermatol 1976;112:698–705.

V108. Vonderheid EC, Tan ET, Kantor AF, Shrager L, Micdily B, Van Scott EJ. Long-term efficacy, curative potential, and carcinogenicity of topical mechlorethamine chemotherapy in cutaneous T cell lymphoma. J Am Acad Dermatol 1989 Mar; 20(3):416–428.

V109. Von Feldt J, Ostrov BE. The use of cyclophosphamide in the treatment of CNS lupus [abstract]. Arthritis Rheum 1990 May;33(5) Suppl:R21.

V110. von Holt C. Histones in perspective. Bio Essays 1985;3: 120–124.

V111. Von Keyserlingk H, Meyer-Sabellek W, Arnzt R, Haller H. Plasma exchanged treatment in autoimmune hemolytic anemia of the warm antibody type with renal failure. Vox Sang 1987;52:598–600.

V112. von Pirquet CL. Allergy. Arch Intern Med 1911;7: 259–288.

V113. Von Wussow P, Jakschies D, Hartung K, Deicher H. Presence of interferon and anti-interferon in patients with systemic lupus erythematosus. Rheum Int 1988;8:225–230.

V114. Vormittag W, Weninger M, Scherak O, Kolarz G. Dermatoglyphics and systemic lupus erythematosus. Scand J Rheumatol 1981;10(4):296–298.

V115. Vos GH, Petz LD, Fudenberg HH. Specificity and immunoglobulin characteristics of autoantibodies in acquired hemolytic anemia. J Immunol 1971 May;106:1172–1176.

V116. Vreugdenhil G, Swaak AJG. Anaemia in rheumatoid arthritis: pathogenesis, diagnosis and treatment. Rheumatol Int 1990;9:243–257.

V117. Vroninks P, Remans J, Kahn MF, de Seze S. Aseptic bony necrosis in systemic lupus erythematosus. Report of 7 new cases [original in French]. Sem Hop Paris 1972 Nov 14;48(46): 3001–3009.

V118. Vyakarnam A, Brenner MK, Reittie JE, Houlker CH, Lachmann PJ. Human clones with natural killer function can activate B cells and secrete B cell differentiation factors. Eur J Immunol 1985;15:606.

V119. Vyas CK, Bhatnagar V, Taiwar KK, Sharma SK. Steroid-induced benign intracranial hypertension. Postgrad Med J 1981 Mar;57:181–182.

W

W1. Wade P, Sack B, Schur PH, Anticentromere antibodies—Clinical correlates 1988;15:1759–1763.

W2. Waer M, Van Damme B, Leenaerts P, Roels L, Van der Schueren E, Van de Putte M, Michielsen P. Treatment of murine lupus nephritis with cyclophosphamide or total lymphoid irradiation. Kidney Int 1988;34:678–682.

W3. Waddell CC, Brown JA. The lupus anticoagulant in 14 males male patients. JAMA 1982 Nov 19;248:2493–2495.

W4. Waga S, Tan EM, Rubin RL. Identification and isolation of soluble histones from bovine mild and serum. Biochem J 1987;144:675–682.

W5. Wagemans MA, Bos PJ. Angle-closure glaucoma in a patient with systemic lupus erythematosus. Doc Ophthalmol 1989 Aug;72(3–4):201–207.

W6. Wagenhals CO, Burgeson PA. Systemic lupus erythematosus in identical twins. N Y J Med 1958 Jan 1;58:98–101.

W7. Wagner-Weiner L, Magilavy DB, Emery HM. Flare of childhood lupus nephritis after discontinuing treatment with intravenous pulse cyclophosphamide (IVCY) [abstract]. Arthritis Rheum 1988 Apr;31(4) Suppl:S117.

W8. Wahl SM, Hunt DA, Wong HL, Dougherty S, McCartney-Francis N, Wahl LM, Ellingsworth L, Schmidt JA, Hall G, Roberts AB, Sporn MB. Transforming growth factor-is potent immunosuppressive agent that inhibits IL-1 dependent lymphocyte proliferation. J Immunol 1988;140:3026.

W9. Wahlin B, Perlman P. Characterization of human K cells by surface antigens and morphology at the single cell level. J Immunol 1983;131:2340–2347.

W10. Walaert B, Aerts C, Bart F, Hartron P, Dracon M, Tonnel AB, Voisin C. Alveolar macrophage dysfunction in systemic lupus erythematosus. Am Rev Respir Dis 1987;136:293–297.

W11. Walker IR, Zapf PW, Mackay IR. Cyclophosphamide, cholinesterase, anaesthesia. Aust NZ J Med 1972 Aug;2:247–251.

W12. Walker RJ, Bailey RR, Swainson CP, Lynn KL. Lupus nephritis: a 13 year experience. N Z Med J 1986;99:894–896.

W13. Walker SA, Benditt EP. Serum proteins in diseases of the connective tissue; an electrophoretic study. J Invest Dermatol 1950 Feb;14:113–120.

W14. Walker SE, Bole GG. Augmented incidence of neoplasia in female New Zealand black-New Zealand white NZB/NZW mice treated with long-term cyclophosphamide. J Lab Clin Med 1971;78:978 and 1973;82:619.

W15. Walker SE, Gray RH, Fulton M, Wigley RD, Schnitzer B. Palmerson North mice, a new animal model of systemic lupus erythematosus. J Lab Clin Med 1978:932–945.

W16. Walker SE, Hewett JE. Responses to T-cell and B-cell mitogens in autoimmune Palmerson North and NZB/NZW mice. Clin Immunol Immunopathol 1984;30:469–478.

W17. Wallace C, Schaller JG, Emery H, Wedgewood R. Prospective study of childhood systemic lupus erythematosus. Arthritis Rheum 1978 Jun;21:599–600.

W18. Wallace D. Discoid lupus. Submitted for publication.

W19. Wallace D. Personal correspondence, 1991 Sep.

W20. Wallace D, Metzger A, Piftiner M, Nessim S. Lupus erythematosus in the 1980; A survey of 570 patients. Semin Arthritis Rheum 1991 Aug;21(1):55–64.

W21. Wallace DJ. Personal communication.

W22. Wallace DJ. The role of stress and trauma in rheumatoid arthritis and systemic lupus erythematosus. Semin Arthritis Rheum 1987 Feb;16(3):153–157.

W23. Wallace DJ. Does hydroxychloroquine sulfate prevent clot formation in systemic lupus erythematosus? [letter] Arthritis Rheum 1987 Dec;30(12):1435–1436.

W24. Wallace DJ. The use of quinacrine (Atabrine) in rheumatic diseases: a reexamination. Semin Arthritis Rheum 1989 May; 18(4):282–296.

W25. Wallace DJ. Lupus, acquired immunodeficiency syndrome, and antimalarial agents [letter]. Arthritis Rheum 1991 Mar; 34(3):372–373.

W26. Wallace DJ, Dubois EL. Drugs that exacerbate and induce systemic lupus erythematosus. In: Wallace DJ, Dubois EL, editors. Dubois' lupus erythematosus. 3rd ed. Philadelphia: Lea & Febiger, 1987:450–469.

W27. Wallace DJ, Dubois EL, editors. Differential diagnosis. In: Dubois' Lupus Erythematosus. 3d ed. Philadelphia: Lea & Febiger, 1987:470–487.

W28. Wallace DJ, Dubois EL, editors. Dubois' Lupus Erythematosus. 3d ed. Philadelphia: Lea & Febiger, 1987.

W29. Wallace DJ, Goldfinger D, Bluestone R, Klinenberg JR. Plasmapheresis in lupus nephritis with nephrotic syndrome. A long-term follow-up. J Clin Apheresis 1982;1(1):42–45.

W30. Wallace DJ, Goldfinger D, Nichols S, Goodman D, Fichman M, Stewart M, Klinenberg JR. A controlled study on the use of plasmapheresis in steroid/immunosuppressive resistant systemic lupus erythematosus with nephrotic syndrome. In: Uda T, Shiokawa Y, Inoue N, editors. Proceedings of the First International Congress of the World Apheresis Association; Cleveland (OH): ISAO Press, 1987;91–102.

W31. Wallace DJ, Goldfinger D, Savage G, Nichols S, Goodman D, Fichman M, Stewart M, Klinenberg JR. Predictive value of clinical, laboratory, pathologic and treatment variables in steroid/immunosuppressive resistant lupus nephritis. J Clin Apheresis 1988;4(1):30–34.

W32. Wallace DJ, Klinenberg JR. Apheresis. DM 1984 Jun;30(9): 1–45.

W33. Wallace DJ, Klinenberg JR, Morham D, Berlanstein B, Biren PC, Callis G. Coexistent gout and rheumatoid arthritis. Case report and literature review. Arthritis Rheum 1979 Feb;22(1): 81–86.

W34. Wallace DJ, Margolin K, Waller P. Fibromyalgia and interleukin-2 therapy malignancy [letter]. Ann Intern Med 1988 Jun;108(6):909.

W35. Wallace DJ, Medici MA, Nichols S, Klinenberg JR, Bick M, Gatti R, Goldfinger D. Plasmapheresis versus lymphoplasmapheresis in rheumatoid arthritis: immunologic comparisons and literature review. J Clin Apheresis 1984;2(2): 184–189.

W36. Wallace DJ, Metzger AL. Positive LE preps and negative ANAs in brothers with systemic lupus erythematosus (SLE): Is there still a role for the LE cell Prep? J Rheumatol In press.

W37. Wallace DJ, Metzger AL, Klinenberg JR. NSAID usage patterns by rheumatologists in the treatment of SLE. J Rheumatol 1989 Apr;16(4):557–560.

W38. Wallace DJ, Metzger AL, Stecher VJ, Turnbull BA, Kern PA. Cholesterol-lowering effect of hydroxychloroquine in patients with rheumatic disease: reversal of deleterious effects of steroids on lipids. Am J Med 1990 Sep;89(3):322–326.

W39. Wallace DJ, Podell T, Weiner J, Klinenberg JR, Forouzesh S, Dubois EL. Systemic lupus erythematosus— survival patterns. Experience with 609 patients. JAMA 1981 Mar 6;245(9): 934–938.

W40. Wallace DJ, Podell TE, Weiner JM, Cox MB, Klinenberg JR, Forouzesh S, Dubois EL. Lupus nephritis. Experience with 230 patients in a private practice from 1950 to 1980. Am J Med 1982 Feb;72(2):209–220

W41. Wallach HW. Lupus-like syndrome associated with carcinoma of the breast. Arch Intern Med 1977 Apr;137(4): 532–535.

W42. Wallaert B, Aerts C, Bart F, Hatron PY, Dracon M, Tonnel AB, Voisin C. Impaired in vitro bacterial activity from alveolar macrophages in systemic lupus erythematosus [abstract]. Ann Rev Resp Dis 1986;133:A138.

W43. Wallenburg HCS, Makovitz JW, Dekker GA, Rotmans P. Low-dose aspirin prevents pregnancy-induced hypertension and preeclampsia in angiotensin-sensitive primigravidae. Lancet 1986;1:1–3.

W44. Wallenburg HCS, Rotmans P. Prophylactic low-dosage aspirin and dipyridamole in pregnancy. Lancet 1988;1:939.

W45. Wallenburg HCS, Rotmans P. Prevention of recurrent idiopathic fetal growth retardation by low-dose aspirin and dipyridamole. Am J Obstet Gynecol 1987;157:1230–1235.

W46. Waller RK, Race RR. Six blood-group antibodies in the serum of transfused patient. Br Med J 1951 Feb 3;1:225–226.

W47. Wallis PJ, Clark CJ. Visceral leishmaniasis complicating systemic lupus erythematosus. Ann Rheum Dis 1983 Apr; 42(2):201–202.

W48. Walport M, Ng YC, Lachmann PJ. Erythrocytes transfused into patients with SLE and haemolytic anaemia lose complement receptor type 1 from their cell surface. Clin Exp Immunol 1987;69:501–507.

W49. Walport MJ. Pregnancy and antibodies to phospholipids. Ann Rheum Dis 1989 Oct;48(10):795–797.

W50. Walport MJ, Hubbard WN, Hughes GR. Reversal of aplastic anaemia secondary to systemic lupus erythematosus by high-dose intravenous cyclophosphamide. BMJ Clin Res 1982 Sep 18;285(6344):769–770.

W51. Walport MJ, Lachmann PJ. Erythrocyte complement receptor type 1, immune complexes, and the rheumatic diseases. Arthritis Rheum 1988;31:153–158.

W52. Walport MJ, Peters AM, Elkon KB, Pusey CD, Lavender JP, Hughes GR. The splenic extraction ratio of antibody-coated erythrocytes and its response to plasma exchange and pulse methylprednisolone. Clin Exp Immunol 1985 Jun;60(3): 465–473.

W53. Walport MJ, Ross GD, Mackworth-Young C, Watson JV, Hogg N, Lachmann PJ. Family studies of erythrocyte complement type 1 levels: Reduced levels in patients with SLE are acquired, not inherited. Clin Exp Immunol 1985;59:547–554.

W54. Walravens P, Chase HP. The prognosis of childhood systemic lupus erythematosus. Am J Dis Child 1976 Sep;130: 929–933.

W55. Walsh CM, Nardi M, Karpatkin S. On the mechanism of thrombocytopenic purpura in sexually active homosexual men. N Engl J Med 1984 Sep 6;311:635–639.

W56. Walsh JR, Zimmerman HJ. Demonstration of the "L.E." phenomenon in patients with penicillin hypersensitivity. Blood 1985 Jan;8:65–71.

W57. Walsh SW. Pre-eclampsia: an imbalance in placental prostacyclin and thromboxane production. Am J Obstet Gynecol 1985;152:335–40.

W58. Walshe JM. Penicillamine-induced SLE [letter]. Lancet 1981;2:1416.

W59. Walter MA, Sorti V, Hofker MH, Cox DW. The physical organization of the human immunoglobulin heavy chain gene complex. EMBO J 1990;9:3303–3313.

W60. Walter TS, Triplett DA, Javed N, Musgrave K. Evaluation of lupus anticoagulants: antiphospholipid antibodies, endothelium associated immunoglobulin, endothelial prostacyclin secretion, and antigenic protein S levels. Thromb Res 1988;51: 267–281.

W61. Walton A, Snaith M, Isenberg D. Successful treatment of SLE by dietary modification. Br J Rheumatol 1988;27 Suppl 2: 8.

W62. Walton AJE, Snaith ML, Locniskar M, Cumberland AG, Morrow WJW, Isenberg DA. Dietary fish oil and the severity of symptoms in patients with systemic lupus erythematosus. Ann Rheum Dis 1991;50:463–466.

W63. Walton J, Watson BS, Ney RL. Alternate-day vs shorter-integral steroid administration. Arch Intern Med 1970 Oct; 126:601–607.

W64. Walts AE, Dubois EL. Acute dissecting aneurysm of the aorta as a fatal event in systemic lupus erythematosus. Am Heart J 1977 Mar;93:378–381.

W65. Walz B, Ho Ping Kong H, Silver R. Adrenal failure and the primary antiphospholipid syndrome [case report]. J Rheumatol 1990;17(6):836–837.

W66. Walz-LeBlanc BA, Urowitz EM, Gladman DD, Goodman PH. Serologically active, clinically quiescent systemic lupus erythematosus. Predictors of clinical flares. Arthritis Rheum 1991;34 Suppl:S100.

W67. Wang BX, Yuan ZZ. A tablet of Tripterygium wilfordii in treating lupus erythematosus. Chung Hsi I Chieh Ho Tsa Chih 1989 Jul;9(7):407–408.

W68. Wang H, Horwitz DA. Profile of Cytokine genes expressed by human circulating blood mononuclear cells: preferential IL-2 specific message in active SLE. Arthritis Rheum 1991;34 Suppl:S161.

W69. Wang ZY. Clinical and laboratory studies of the effect of an antilupus pill on systemic lupus erythematosus [English abstract]. Chung Hsi I Chieh Ho Tsa Chih 1989 Aug;9(8):452, 465–468.

W70. Wanner WR, Irvin WS. Disopyramide and antinuclear antibodies [letter]. Am Heart J 1981 May;101:687–689.

W71. Wanzhane Q, Chenghuane L, Shumei Y, Guangdon Z, Kunyuan FL, Shufang F, Guantian T, Zhiming G, Hongtu W, Chengzhn L, Huiming J, Gusheng Z, Yongde S, Jiahe D, Peng L, Caiyi Z, Kegang Z, Guowei Q. Tripterygium wilfordii hook F in systemic lupus erythematosus. Report of 103 cases. Chinese Med J 1981;94:827–834.

W72. Wapner RJ, Cowchock S, Shapiro SS. Successful treatment in two women with antiphospholipid antibodies and refractory pregnancy losses with intravenous immunoglobulin infusions. Am J Obstet Gynecol 1989;161:1271–1272.

W73. Ward MM, Dawson DV, Pisetsky DS. Serum immunoglobulin levels in systemic lupus erythematosus: The effects of age, sex, race and disease duration. J Rheumatol 1991;18:540–544.

W74. Ward MM, Dooley MA, Christenson VD, Pisetsky DS. The relationship between soluble interleukin 2 receptor levels and antidouble stranded DNA antibody levels in patients with systemic lupus erythematosus. J Rheumatol 1991;18:234–240.

W75. Ward MM, Polisson RP. A meta-analysis of the clinical manifestations of older-onset systemic lupus erythematosus. Arthritis Rheum 1989 Oct;32(10):1226–1232.

W76. Ward MM, Pisetsky DS, Christenson VD. Antidouble stranded DNA antibody assays in systemic lupus erythematosus: correlations of longitudinal antibody measurements. J Rheumatol 1989 May;16(5):609–613.

W77. Ward MM, Studenski S. Systemic lupus erythematosus in men: a multivariate analysis of gender differences in clinical manifestations. J Rheumatol 1990;17(2):220–224.

W78. Ward MM, Studenski S. Age associated clinical manifestations of systemic lupus erythematosus: A multivariate regression analysis. J Rheumatol 1990;17(3):476–481.

W79. Wardle EN. Reticuloendothelial clearance studies in the course of horse serum induced nephritis. Br J Exp Pathol 1974;55:149–152.

W80. Warmerdam PAM, van de Winkel JGJ, Gosselin EJ, Capel PJA. Molecular basis for a polymorphism of human Fcγ receptor II (CD32). J Exp Med 1990;172:19–25.

W81. Warmerdam PAM, van de Winkel JGJ, Vlug A, Westerdaal NAC, Capel PJA. A single amino acid in the second Ig-like domain of the human Fcγ receptor II plays a critical role in human IgG2 binding. J Immunol 1991;144:1338–1343.

W82. Warn-Cramer BJ, Almus FE, Rapaport SI. Studies of the factor (extrinsic pathway inhibitor) from cell supernates of cultured human umbilical vein endothelial cells. Thromb Haemost 1989;61:101–105.

W83. Warren MK, Vogel SN. Opposing effects of glucocorticoids on interferon-γ-induced murine macrophage Fc receptor and Ia antigen expression. J immunol 1985;134:2462–2469.

W84. Warren RW, Caster SA, Roths JB, Murphy ED, Pisetsky DS. The influence of the lpr gene on B cell activation: Differential antibody expression in lpr congenic mouse strains. Clin Immunol Immunopathol 1984;31:65–77.

W85. Warren RW, Kredich DW. Transverse myelitis and acute central nervous system manifestations of systemic lupus erythematosus. Arthritis Rheum 1984 Sep;27(9):1058–1060.

W86. Warrier RP, Sahney S, Walker H. Hemoglobin sickle cell disease and systemic lupus erythematosus. J Natl Med Assoc 1984 Nov;76:1030–1031.

W87. Warrington RJ. Interleukin-2 abnormalities in systemic lupus erythematosus and rheumatoid arthritis. A role for overproduction of interleukin-2 in human autoimmunity? J Rheumatol 1988;15:616–620.

W88. Warrington RJ, Rutherford WJ. Normal mitogen-induced suppression of the interleukin-6 (IL-6) response and its deficiency in systemic lupus erythematosus. J Clin Immunol 1990; 10:52–60.

W89. Warrington RJ, Sauder PJ, Homik J, Ofosu-Appiah W. Reversible interleukin-2 response defects in systemic lupus erythematosus. Clin Exp Immunol 1989;77:163–167.

W90. Wasicek CA, Maddison PJ, Reichlin M. Occurrence of antibodies to single-stranded DNA in ANA negative patients. Clin Exp Immunol 1979 Aug;37(2):190–195.

W91. Wasichek CA, Reichlin M. Clinical and serological differences between systemic lupus erythematosus patients with antibodies in Ro versus patients without antibodies to Ro and La. J Clin Invest 1982 Apr;69:835–843.

W92. Wasner CK. Ibuprofen meningitis and systemic lupus erythematosus. J Rheumatol 1978;5:182.

W93. Wasner CK, Fries JF. Treatment decisions in systemic lupus erythematosus. Arthritis Rheum 1980 Mar;23:283–286.

W94. Waters H, Konrad P, Walford RL. The distribution of HL-A histocompatibility factors and genes in patients with systemic lupus erythematosus. Tissue Antigens 1971;1:68–73.

W95. Waterworth RF. Systemic lupus erythematosus occurring with congenital complete heart block. N Z Med J 1980;92: 311–312.

W96. Watsky MS, Lynfield YL. Lupus erythematosus exacerbated by griseofulvin. Cutis 1976;17:361.

W97. Watson DE. Chloroquine protection against virus induced cell damage without inhibition of virus growth. J Gen Virol 1972;14:100–102.

W98. Watson J, Godfrey D, Stimson WH, Belch JJ, Sturrock RD. The therapeutic effects of dietary fatty acid supplementation in the autoimmune disease of the MRL-mp-lpr/lpr mouse. Int J Immunopharmacol 1988;10:467–471.

W99. Watson JI, Mandl MA, Rose B. Disseminated histoplasmosis occurring in association with systemic lupus erythematosus. Can Med Assoc J 1968 Nov 16;99:958–962.

W100. Watson R. Cutaneous lesions in systemic lupus erythematosus. Med Clin North Am 1989;73:1091–1111.

W101. Watson RM, Braunstein BL, Watson AJ, Hochberg MC, Provost TT. Fetal wastage in women with anti-Ro(SSA) antibody. J Rheumatol 1986;13:90–94.

W102. Watson RM, Kang JE, May M, Hudak M, Kickler T, Provost TT. Thrombocytopenia in the neonatal lupus syndrome. Arch Dermatol 1988;124:560–563.

W103. Watson RM, Lane AT, Barnett NK, Bias WB, Arnett FC, Provost TT. Neonatal lupus erythematosus: a clinical, serological and immunogenetic study with review of the literature. Medicine 1984 Nov;63:362–378.

W104. Watson RM, Talwar P, Alexander E, Bias WB, Provost TT. Subacute cutaneous lupus erythematosus—Immunogenetic associations. J Autoimmunity 1991;4:73–85.

W105. Watson WJ, Katz VL, Bowes WA Jr. Plasmapheresis during pregnancy. Obstet Gynecol 1990 Sep;76(3 Pt 1):451–457.

W106. Watts R, Ravirajan CT, Staines NA, Isenberg DA. A human fetal monoclonal DNA-binding antibody shares idiotypes with fetal and adult murine monoclonal DNA-binding antibodies. Immunology 1990;69:348–354.

W107. Watts RA, Isenberg DA. Pancreatic disease in the autoimmune rheumatic disorders. Semin Arthritis Rheum 1989 Dec; 19(3):158–165.

W108. Watts RA, Isenberg DA. Autoantibodies and antibacterial antibodies: from both sides now. Ann Rheum Dis 1990; 49: 961–965.

W109. Watts RA, Ravirajan CT, Wilkinson LS, Williams W, Griffiths M, Butcher D, Horsfall AT, Staines NA, Isenberg DA. Detection of human and murine common idiotypes of DNA antibodies in tissues and sera of patients with autoimmune diseases. Clin Exp Immunol 1991;83:267–273.

W110. Watzl B, Watson RR. Immunomodulation by cocaine-a neuroendocrine mediated response. Life Sci 1990;46: 1319–1329.

W111. Waxman FJ, Hebert LA, Cornacoff JB, Van Aman M, Smead W, Kraut ER, Birmingham DJ, Taguian JM. Complement depletion accelerates the clearance of immune complexes from the circulation of primates. J Clin Invest 1984;74:1329–1340.

W112. Waxman FJ, Hebert LA, Cosio FG, Smead WL, Van Aman ME, Taguiam JM, Birmingham DJ. Differential binding of immunoglobulin A and immunoglobulin G1 immune complexes to primate erythrocytes in vivo: Immunoglobulin A immune complexes bind less well to erythrocytes and are preferentially deposited in glomeruli. J Clin Invest 1986;77:82–89.

W113. Ways SC, Blair PB, Bern HA, Staskawitz MO. Immune responsiveness of adult mice exposed neonatally to diethylstilbestrol, steroid hormones or vitamin A. J Environ Pathol Toxicol 1980;3:207–220.

W114. Weatherhead L, Adam J. Discoid lupus erythematosus. Coexistence with porphyria cutanea tarda. Int J Derm 1985 Sep;24:454–456.

W115. Webb S, Segura F, Cervantes F, Darnell A, Soriano E, Ribas-Mundo M, Garcia-San Miguel J. Systemic lupus erythematosus and amyloidosis. Arthritis Rheum 1979 May;22(5):554–556.

W116. Webel ML, Ritts RE Jr, Taswell HF, Donadio JV Jr, Woods JE. Cellular immunity after intravenous administration of methylprednisolone. J Lab Clin Med 1973;83:383–392.

W117. Webster J, Williams BD, Smith AP, Hall M, Jessop JD. Systemic lupus erythematosus presenting as pneumococcal septicaemia and septic arthritis [case report]. Ann Rheum Dis 1990 Mar;49(3):181–183.

W118. Wechsler B, Le Thi Huong Du, Vignes B, Piette JC, Chomette G, Godeau P. Toxoplasmosis and disseminated lupus erythematosus: Four case reports and a review of the literature [English abstract]. Ann Med Interne (Paris) 1986;137(4):324–330.

W119. Wechsler HL, Stavrides A. Systemic lupus erythematosus with anti-Ro antibodies: Clinical, histologic and immunologic findings. J Am Acad Dermatol 1982;6:73–83.

W120. Weening JJ, Hoedemaeker PHJ, Bakker WW. Immunoregulation and anti-nuclear antibodies in mercury-induced glomerulopathy in the rat. Clin Exp Immunol 1981;45:64–71.

W121. Weetman AP, So AK, Roe C, Walport MJ, Foroni L. T-cell receptor alpha chain V region polymorphism linked to primary autoimmune hypothyroidism but not Grave's disease. Hum Immunol 1987;20:167–173.

W122. Weetman AP, Walport MJ. The association of autoimmune thyroiditis with systemic lupus erythematosus. Br J Rheumatol 1987 Oct;26(5):359–361.

W123. Wegelius O. Amyloidosis of the kidneys, adrenals and spleen as a complication of acute disseminated lupus erythematosus treated with ACTH and cortisone. Acta Med Scand 1956;156(2):91–95.

W124. Wei N, Klippel JH, Huston DP, Hall RP, Lawley TJ, Balow JE, Steinberg AD, Decker JL. Randomized trial of plasma exchange in mild systemic lupus erythematosus. Lancet 1983 Jan 1;1(8314–5):17–21.

W125. Wei N, Wu T, Klippel JH. False positive pregnancy tests in systemic lupus erythematosus. J Rheumatol 1982;9:303–304.

W125a. Weidmann CE, Wallace DJ, Peter JB, Knight PJ, Bear MB, Klinenberg JR. Studies of IgG, IgM and IgA antiphospholipid antibody isotypes in systemic lupus erythematosus. J Rheumatol 1988;15:74–79.

W126. Weigand DA. Lupus band test: Anatomically regional variations in discoid lupus erythematosus. J Am Acad Dermatol 1986 Aug;14(2 Pt 1):426–428.

W127. Weigand DA. Cutaneous immunofluorescence. Med Clin North Am 1989 Sep;73(5):1263–1274.

W128. Weigle WO. Immunological unresponsiveness. Adv Immunol 1973;16:61–122.

W129. Weiler I, Weiler C, Sprenger R, Cosenza H. Idiotype suppression by maternal influences. Eur J Immunol 1977;7:531.

W130. Weill BJ, Menkes CJ, Cormier C, Louvel A, Dougados M, Houssin D. Hepatocellular carcinoma after danazol therapy. J Rheumatol 1988 Sep;15(9):1447–1449.

W131. Weinberg A, Kaplan JG, Myers AR. Extensive soft tissue calcification (calcinosis universalis) in systemic lupus erythematosus. Ann Rheum Dis 1979 Aug;38:384–386.

W132. See W131.

W133. Weinblatt ME, Coblyn JS, Fox DA, Fraser PA, Holdsworth DE, Glass DN, Trentham DE. Efficacy of low-dose methotrexate in rheumatoid arthritis. N Engl J Med 1985 Mar 28;312:818–822.

W134. Weiner AL. Disseminated lupus erythematosus treated by sulfanilamide: report of 4 cases. Arch Dermat & Syph 1940 Mar;441:534–544.

W135. Weiner DK, Allen NB. Large vessel vasculitis of the central nervous system in systemic lupus erythematosus: Report and review of the literature. J Rheumatol 1991;18(5):748–751.

W136. Weiner ES, Abeles M. Aseptic necrosis and glucocorticosteroids in systemic lupus erythematosus: a reevaluation. J Rheumatol 1989 May;16(5):604–608.

W137. Weinreich J. Thrombocytopenias and platelet antibodies. Vox Sang 1957 Sep;2:294–300.

W138. Weinrib L, Sharma OP, Quismorio FP Jr. A long term study of interstitial lung disease in systemic lupus erythematosus. Semin Arthritis Rheum 1990;16:479–481.

W139. Weinshank RL, Luster AD, Ravetch JV. Function and regulation of a murine macrophage-specific IgG Fc receptor, FcR-alpha. J Exp Med 1988;167:1909–1925.

W140. Weinstein A. Drug-induced systemic lupus erythematosus. Prog Clin Immunol 1980;4:1–21.

W141. Weinstein A, Bordwell B, Stone B, Tibbetts C, Rothfield NF. Antibodies to native DNA and serum complement (C3) levels. Application to diagnosis and classification of systemic lupus erythematosus. Am J Med 1983 Feb;74:206–216.

W142. Weinstein C, Miller MH, Axtens R, Buchanan R, Littlejohn GO. Livedo reticularis associated with increased titers of anticardiolipin antibodies in systemic lupus erythematosus. Arch Dermatol 1987 May;123(5):596–600.

W143. Weinstein C, Miller MH, Axtens R, Littlejohn GO, Dorevitch AP, Buchanan R. Lupus and non-lupus cutaneous manifestations in systemic lupus erythematosus. Aust NZ J Med 1987 Oct;17(5):501–506.

W144. Weinstein CL, Littlejohn GO, Thomson NM, Hall S. Severe visceral disease in subacute cutaneous lupus erythematosus. Arch Dermatol 1987;123:638–640.

W145. Weinstein L. Syndrome of hemolysis, elevated liver enzymes, and low platelet count: A severe consequence of hypertension in pregnancy. Am J Obstet Gynecol 1982;142:159–167.

W146. Weinstein Y, Berkovich Z. Testosterone effect on bone marrow, thymus and suppressor T cells in the NZB × NZW F1 mice: it's relevance to autoimmunity. J Immunol 1981;128:998–1002.

W147. Weinstock I, Lee SL. Hypogammaglobulinemia in systemic lupus erythematosus: Report of a case in a nine-year-old child. J Dis Child 1960 Feb;99:242–247.

W148. Weintraub MI. Chorea in childhood systemic lupus erythematosus [letter]. JAMA 1977;283:855.

W149. Weis LS, Pachman LM, Potter EV, Lewy PR, Jennings RB, Herdson PB. Occult lupus nephropathy: a correlated light, electron and immunofluorescent microscopic study. Histopathology 1977 Nov;1:401–419.

W150. Weisbart RH, Colburn K. Effect of corticosteroids on serum antinuclear antibodies in man. Immunopharmacology 1984 Apr;8:97–101.

W151. Weisbart RH, Noritake DT, Wong AL, Chan G, Kacena A, Colburn KK. A conserved anti-DNA antibody idiotype associated with nephritis in murine and human systemic lupus erythematosus. J Immunol 1990 Apr 1;144(7):2653–2658.

W152. Weisbart RH, Yee WS, Colburn KK. Antiguanosine antibodies: A new marker for procainamide-induced systemic lupus erythematosus. Ann Intern Med 1986;104:310–313.

W153. Weisberg LA. The cranial computed tomographic findings in patients with neurologic manifestations of systemic lupus erythematosus. Comput Radiol 1986 Jan–Feb;10(1): 63–68.

W154. Weisberg LA, Chutorian AM. Pseudotumor cerebri of childhood. Am J Dis Child 1977;131(11):1243–1248.

W155. Weisberger AS, Wessler S, Avioli LV. Mechanisms of action of chloramphenicol. JAMA 1969 Jul 7;209:97–103.

W156. Weisman M, Zvaifler NJ. Cryoimmunoglobulinemia in Felty's syndrome. Arthritis Rheum 1976 Jan–Feb;19(1): 3–110.

W157. Weisman MH, Albert D, Mueller MR, Zvaifler NJ, Hesketh SA, Shragg GP. Gold therapy in patients with systemic lupus erythematosus. Am J Med 1983 Dec 30;75 Suppl 6A:157–164.

W158. Weisman MH, McDanald EC, Wilson CB. Studies of the pathogenesis of interstitial cystitis, obstructive uropathy and intestinal malabsorption in a patient with systemic lupus erythematosus. Am J Med 1981 Apr;70(4):875–881.

W159. Weismann G. Labilization and stabilization of lysosomes. Fed Proc 1964;23:1038–1044.

W160. Weiss HG, Rosove MH, Lages BA, Kaplan KL. Acquired storage pool deficiency with increased platelet-associated IgG. Am J Med 1980;69:711–717.

W161. Weiss MJ, Daley JF, Hodgdon JC, Reinherz EL. Calcium dependency of antigen-specific (T3-Ti) and alternative (T11) pathways of human T-cell activation. Proc Natl Acad Sci USA 1984;81:6836–6840.

W162. Weiss S, Bogen B. B-lymphoma cells process and present their endogenous immunoglobulin to major histocompatibility complex-restricted T cells. Proc Natl Acad Sci USA 1989; 86:282.

W163. Weissel M, Scherak O, Fritzsche H, Kolarz G. Serum beta-2 microglobulin and SLE. Arthritis Rheum 1976;Sep–Oct 19: 968.

W164. Weissman BN, Rappoport AS, Sosman JL, Schur PH. Radiographic findings in the hands of patients with systemic lupus erythematosus. Radiology 1978;126:313–317.

W165. Weissmann G, Rothfield N, Thomas L. Cutaneous hyperreactivity to vitamin A in systemic lupus erythematosus (SLE) [abstract]. Arthritis Rheum 1962–5:665.

W166. Wekking EM, Nossent JC, van Dam AP, Swaak AJG. Cognitive and emotional disturbances in systemic lupus erythematosus. Psychother Psychosom 1991;55:126–131.

W167. Wekking EM, Vingerhoets AJJM, van Dam JC, Swaak AJG. Daily stressors and systemic lupus erythematosus: a longitudinal analysis. Psychother Psychosom 1991;55:108–113.

W168. Welch GR, Wong HL, Wahl SM. Selective induction of FcγRIII on human monocytes by transforming growth factor-β. J Immunol 1990;144:3444–3448.

W169. Welch TR, Beischel L, Berry A, Forristal J, West CD. The effect of null Cr alleles on complement function. Clin Immunol Immunopathol 1985;34:316–325.

W170. Welch TR, Beischel LS, Balakrishnan K, Quinlan M, West CD. Major histocompatibility complex extended haplotypes in systemic lupus erythematosus. Dis Markers 1988;6: 247–255.

W171. Wellborne FR, Claypool RG, Copley JB. Nephrotic range pseudoproteinuria in a tolmetin-treated patient. Clin Nephrol 1983 Apr;19(4):211–212.

W172. Welsh AL. Lupus erythematosus; treatment by combined use of massive amounts of pantothenic acid and vitamin E. Arch Dermat & Syph 1954 Aug;70:181–198.

W173. Wen L, Peakman M, Lobo-Yeo A, McFarlane BM, Mowat AP, Mieli-Vergani G, Vergani D. T-cell-directed hepatocyte damage in autoimmune chronic active hepatitis. Lancet 1990 Dec 22–29;336(8730):1527–1530.

W174. Wendling D, Saint-Hillier Y, Hory B, Saunier F, Perol C, Breton JL, Blanc D. Legionnaires' in the course of severe lupus. Rev Rheum Mal Osteoartic 1986 Feb;53(2):137.

W175. Wener WH, Mannik M, Schwartz MM, Lewis EJ. Relationship between renal pathology and the size of circulating immune complexes in patients with systemic lupus erythematosus. Medicine 1987;66:85–97.

W176. Wenger ME, Bole GG. Nitrobule tetrazolium (NBT) dye reduction by peripheral leukocytes from patients with rheumatoid arthritis (RA) and systemic lupus erythematosus (SLE). J Lab Clin Med 1973 Sep;82:513–521.

W177. Werfer T, Witter W, Gotze O. CD11b and CD11c antigens are rapidly increased in human natural killer cells upon activation. J Immunol 1991;147:2423.

W178. Werner G, von dem Borne AEGKr, Bos MJE, Tromp JF, van der Plas-van Dalen CM, Visser FJ, Engelfriet CP, Tetteroo PA. Localization of the human NA1 alloantigen on neutrophils to Fcγ receptors. In: Reinherz EL, Haynes BF, Nadler LM, Bernstein ID, editors. Leucocyte Typing II, Volume 3, New York: Springer Verlag, 1985:109–121.

W179. Wernet P, Kunkel HG. Demonstration of specific T-lymphocyte membrane antigens associated with antibodies inhibiting the mixed leukocyte culture in man. Transplant Proc 1973;5:1875–1881.

W180. Wernet P, Kunkel HG. Antibodies to a specific surface antigen on T cells in human sera inhibiting mixed leukocyte culture reactions. J Exp Med 1973 Oct 1;138:1021–1026.

W181. Wernick R, Lospalluto JJ, Fink CW, Ziff M. Serum IgG and IgM rheumatoid factors by solid phase radioimmunoassay. Arthritis Rheum 1981 Dec;24:1501–1511.

W182. Werth V, Franks A Jr. Treatment of discoid skin lesions with azathioprine [letter]. Arch Dermatol 1986 Jul;122(7): 746–747.

W183. Werth VP, Sanchez M, White W, Franks AG Jr. Aloecia areata with lupus erythematosus (LE)[abstract]. Arthritis Rheum 1989 Jan;32(1) Suppl:R17.

W184. Werthamer S, Govindara JS, Amaral L. Placenta, transcortin and localized immune responses. J Clin Invest 1976;57: 1000.

W185. Wessel G, Abendroth K, Wisheit M. Malignant transformation during immunosuppressive therapy (azathioprine) of rheumatoid arthritis and systemic lupus erythematosus. A retrospective study. Scand J Rheumatol 1988;67 Suppl:73–75.

W186. West CD, McAdams AJ. The chronic glomerulonephritides of childhood. Part I. J Pediatr 1978;93:1–12.

W187. West S, Andersen P. Usefulness of immunologic tests of the cerebrospinal fluid (CSF) in central nervous system (CNS) lupus [abstract]. Arthritis Rheum 1984 Apr;27(4) Suppl:S4.

W188. West SG, Emlen JW, Werner MH, Kotzin BL. Central nervous system lupus (CNS): A ten year, prospective study, Arthritis Rheum 1990 Sep;33(9) Suppl:S29.

W189. West SG, Johnson SC. Danazol for the treatment of refractory autoimmune thrombocytopenia in systemic lupus erythematosus. Ann Intern Med 1988;108:703–706.

W190. West SG, Johnson SC, Andersen PA, Nordstrom DM. Danazol for the treatment of refractory autoimmune thrombocytopenia in systemic lupus erythematosus (SLE)[abstract]. Arthritis Rheum 1986 Apr;29(4) Suppl:S44.

W191. West SG, McMahon M, Portanova JP. Quinidine-induced lupus erythematosus. Ann Intern Med 1984;100:840–842.

W192. West WH, Cannon GD, Kay HD, Blonnard GD, Herberman RB. Natural cytotoxic reactivity of human lymphocytes against a myeloid cell line: Characterization of the effector cells. J Immunol 1977;118:355.

W193. Westberg G, Tarkowski A. Effect of Ma-EPA in patients with SLE. A double-blind, crossover study [abstract]. Kidney Intern 1989;35:235.

W194. Westberg G, Tarkowsky A, Svalender C. Effect of eicosapentaenoic acid rich menhaden oil and Nax EPA on the autoimmune disease of MRL/l mice. Int Arch Allergy Appl Immunol 1988;88:454–461.

W195. Westerink MAJ, Campagnari AA, Wirth MA, Apicella MA. Development and characterization of an anti-idiotype antibody to the capsular polysaccharide of Neisseria meningitis serogroup C. Infect Immunol 1988;56:1120.

W196. Westerman E, Sundstrom W. Antiphospholipid antibody arterial vasculopathy involving the cerebral vascular system: Brain biopsy [abstract]. Arthritis Rheum 1991 May;34(5) Suppl:R8.

W197. Westermann J, Pabst R. Lymphocyte subsets in the blood: a diagnostic window on the immune system? Immunol Today 1990;11:406–410.

W198. Weston WL. Topical corticosteroids in dermatologic disorders. Hosp Pract (Office) 1984 Jan;19(1):159–172.

W199. Weston WL, Harmon C, Peebles C, Manchester D, Franco HL, Huff JC, Norris DA. A serological marker for neonatal lupus erythematosus. Br J Dermatol 1982;107:377–382.

W200. Wetterholm DH, Winter FC. Histopathology of chloroquine retinal toxicity. Arch Ophthalmol 1964 Jan;71:82–87.

W201. Whalley LJ, Roberts DF, Wentzel J, Watson KC. Antinuclear antibodies and histocompatibility antigens in patients on long-term lithium therapy. J Affective Disord 1981; 3: 123–130.

W202. Whicher JT, Gilbert AM, Westacott C, Hutton C, Dieppe PA. Defective production of leucocytic endogenous mediator (interleukin 1) by peripheral blood leucocytes of patients with systemic sclerosis, systemic lupus erythematosus, rheumatoid arthritis and mixed connective tissue disease. Clin Exp Immunol 1986;65:80–89.

W203. Whisnant JP, Espinosa RE, Kierland RR, Lambert EH. Chloroquine Neuromyopathy. Proc Mayo Clin 1963;38:501–513.

W204. White EM, Shapiro DL, Allis CD, Gorovsky MA. Sequence and properties of the message encoding Tetrahymena hv1, a highly evolutionarily conserved histone H2A variant that is associated with active genes. Nucleic Acids Res 1988; 16: 179–198.

W205. White PC, New MI, Dupont B. Cloning and expression of cDNA encoding a bovine adrenal cytochrome p-450 specific for steroid 21-hydroxylation. Proc Nat Acad Sci USA 1984;81: 1986–1990.

W206. White RG, Bass BH, Williams E. Lymphadenoid goiter and the syndrome of systemic lupus erythematosus. Lancet 1961 Feb 18;1:368–373.

W206a. White W. Lupus erythematosus. Polymyositis. Proc Roy Soc Med 1959;52:1035–1036

W207. White WB, Desbonnet CR, Ballow M. Immunoregulatory effects of IV immune serum globulin therapy in common variable hypogammaglobulinemia. Am J Med 1987;83:431–439.

W208. Whiting-O'Keefe Q, Henke JE, Shearn MA, Hopper J, Brava CG, Epstein WV. The information content from renal biopsy in systemic lupus erythematosus: Stepwise linear regression analysis. Ann Intern Med 1982 Jun;96:718–723.

W209. Whiting-O'Keefe Q, Riccardi PJ, Henke JE, Shearn MA, Hopper J Jr, Epstein WV. Recognition of information in renal biopsies of patients with lupus nephritis. Ann Intern Med 1982 Jun;96:723–727.

W210. Whitsed HM, Penny R. IgA/IgG cryoglobulinemia with vasculitis. Clin Exp Immunol 1971 Aug;9:183–191.

W211. Whittingham A, Propert DN, Mackay IR. A strong association between the antinuclear antibody anti-La (SS-B) and the kappa chain allotype Km(1). Immunogenetics 1984;19: 295–299.

W212. Whittingham S, Balazs NDH, Mackay IR. The effect of corticosteroid drugs on serum iron levels in systemic lupus erythematosus and rheumatoid arthritis. Med J Aust 1967 Sep 30;2:639–641.

W213. Whittingham S, Mackay IR. Systemic lupus erythematosus induced by procaine amide. Australs Ann Med 1970 Nov;19: 358–361.

W213a. Whittingham S, Mackay IR. The "pemphigus" antibody and immunopathies affecting the thymus. Br J Dermatol 1971; 84:1–6.

W214. Whittingham S, Mackay IR, Tait BD. Autoantibodies to small nuclear ribonucleoproteins. A strong association between anti-SS-B(La), HLA-B8 and Sjogren's syndrome. Aust N Z J Med 1983;23:565–570.

W215. Whittingham S, Matthews JD, Schonfield MS, Tait BD, Mackay IR. Interaction of HLA and Gm in autoimmune chronic active hepatitis. Clin Exp Immunol 1981;43:80.

W216. Whittingham S, Matthews JD, Schonfield MS, Tait BD, Mackay IR. HLA and Gm genes in systemic lupus erythematosus. Tissue Antigens 1983;21:50–51.

W217. Whittum J, Goldschneider I, Greiner D, Zurier R. Developmental abnormalities of terminal deoxynucleotidyl transferase positive bone marrow cells and thymocytes in New Zealand mice: effects of prostaglandin El. J Immunol 1985 Jul; 135(1):272–280.

W218. Widener HL, Littman BH. Ibuprofen induced meningitis in systemic lupus erythematosus. JAMA 1978 Mar 13;239: 1062–1064.

W219. Wiegand DA. Cutaneous immunofluorescence. Med Clin North Am 1989;73:1263–1274.

W220. Wiegand DA. The lupus band test: A re-evaluation. J Am Acad Dermatol 1984 Aug;11(2 Pt 1):230–234.

W221. Wiener-Kronish JP, Solinger AM, Warnock ML, Churg A, Ordonez N, Golden JA. Severe pulmonary involvement in mixed connective tissue disease. Am Rev Respon Dis 1981 Oct;124:499–503.

W222. Wiernik PH, Duncan JH. Cyclophosphamide in human milk. Lancet 1971;1:912.

W223. Wigfall DR, Sakai RS, Wallace DJ, Jordan SC. Interleukin-2 receptor expression in peripheral blood lymphocytes from systemic lupus erythematosus patients: relationship to clinical activity. Clin Immunol Immunopathol 1988;47:354–362.

W224. Wiland E, Siemieniako B, Trzeciak WH. Binding of low mobility group protein from rat liver chromatin with histones studied by chemical cross-linking. Biochem Biophys Res Commun 1990;166:11–21.

W225. Wilcox MH, Powell RJ, Pugh SF, Balfour AH. Toxoplasmosis and systemic lupus erythematosus [case report]. Ann Rheum Dis 1990 Apr;49(4):254–257.

W226. Wilcox PG, Stein HB, Clarke SD, Pare PD, Pardy RL. Phrenic nerve function in patients with diaphragmatic weakness and systemic lupus erythematosus. Chest 1988;93:352–358.

W227. Wild G, Watkins J, Ward A, Hughes P, Hume A, Rowell NR. C4a anaphylatoxin levels an indicator of disease activity in systemic lupus erythematosus. Clin Exp Immunol 1990;80: 167–170.

W228. Wiljasalo M, Ikkala E. Lymphography in systemic lupus erythematosus. Ann Clin Res 1971 Aug;3:231–235.

W229. Wilke WS, Krall PL, Mazanec DJ, Scheetz RJ, Segal AM, Clough JD. Methotrexate (MTX) for systemic lupus erythematosus (SLE): Steroid-sparing? [abstract] Arthritis Rheum 1988 Apr;31(4) Suppl:S55.

W230. Wilkens KW, Hoffman GS. Massive ascites in systemic lupus erythematosus. J Rheumatol 1985;12:571–574.

W231. Wilks D, Walter LC, Habeshaw JA, Youle M, Gazzard B, Dalgleish AG. Anti-CD4 autoantibodies and screening for anti-idiotypic antibodies to anti-CD4 monoclonal antibodies in HIV-seropositive people. AIDS 1990;4:113–118.

W232. Omitted.

W233. Willems van Dijk K, Schroeder HW Jr, Perlmutter RM,

Milner ECB. Heterogeneity in the human Ig V$_H$ locus. J Immunol 1989;142:2547–2554.

W234. Williams B, Hull DS. Lupus erythematosus keratoconjunctivitis. South Med J 1986 May;79(5):631–632.

W235. Williams DG. Recombinant autoantigens. Ann Rheum Dis 1990; 49:445–451.

W236. Williams GM, Mazne G, McQueen CA, Shimada T. Genotoxicity of the antihypertensive drugs hydralazine and dihydralazine. Science 1980 Oct;210:329–330.

W237. Williams GW, Bluestein HG, Steinberg AD. Brain-reactive lymphocytotoxic antibody in cerebrospinal fluid of patients with systemic lupus erythematosus: correlation with central nervous system involvement. Clin Immunol Immunopathol 1981 Jan;18(1):126–132.

W238. Williams GW, Steinberg AD, Reinertsen JL. Influenza immunization in SLE: A double-blind trial. Ann Intern Med 1978; 88:729–741.

W239. Williams GW, Steinberg AD, Reinersten JL, Klassen LW, Decker JL, Dolin R. Influenza immunization in systemic lupus erythematosus. A double-blind trial. Ann Intern Med 1978 Jun; 88(6):729–734.

W240. Williams IA, Mitchell AD, Rothman W, Tallett P, Williams K, Pitt P. Survey of the long-term incidence of osteonecrosis of the hip and adverse medical events in rheumatoid arthritis after high dose intravenous methylprednisolone. Ann Rheum Dis 1988 Nov;47(11):930–933.

W241. Williams RC. Rheumatoid factors. Human Pathol 1983 May;14:386–391.

W242. Williams RC Jr, Bankhurst AD, Montano JD. IgG anti-lymphocyte antibodies in SLE detected by ^{125}I protein A. Arthritis Rheum 1976 Nov–Dec;19:1261–1270.

W243. Williams RC Jr, Hughes GRV, Smith ML, Parry HF, Diao E, Greaves MF. Lymphocyte antigens in systemic lupus erythematosus studies with heterologous antisera. J Clin Invest 1980 Feb;65:379–389.

W244. Williams RC Jr, Lies RB, Messner RP. Inhibition of mixed leukocyte culture responses by serum and gamma globulin fractions from certain patients with connective tissue disorders. Arthritis Rheum 1973 Sep–Oct;16:597–605.

W245. Williams RE, Mackie RM, O'Keefe R, Thomson W. The contribution of direct immunofluorescence to the diagnosis of lupus erythematosus. J Cutan Pathol 1989 Jun;16(3):122–125.

W246. Williams W, Zumla A, Behrens R, Lockniskar M, Voller A, McAdam PWG, Isenberg D. Studies of common idiotype PR4 in autoimmune rheumatic disease. Arthritis Rheum 1988;31:1097–1104.

W247. Williams WV, Guy HR, Rubin DH, Robey F, Myers JN, Kieber-Emmons T, Weiner DB, Greene MI. Sequences of the cell-attachment sites of reovirus type 3 and its anti-idiotypic/anti-receptor antibody: modeling of their three-dimensional structures. Proc Natl Acad Sci USA 1988;85:6488.

W248. Williamson GG, Pennebaker J, Boyle JA. Clinical characteristics of patients with rheumatic disorders who posses antibodies against ribonucleoprotein particles. Arthritis Rheum 1985;26:509–515.

W249. Williamson J, Paterson RWW, McGavin DDM, Jasani MK, Boyle JA, Doig WM. Posterior subcapsular cataracts and glaucoma associated with long-term oral corticosteroid therapy in patients with rheumatoid arthritis and related conditions. Br J Ophthalmol 1969 Jun;53:361.

W250. Williamson RA, Karp LE. Azathioprine teratogenicity: Review of the literature and case report. Obstet Gynecol 1981; 58:247–250.

W251. Willis WH. Experience with some unusual diseases occurring in families. Henry Ford Hosp Med Bull 1955;3:44.

W252. Willkens RF, Healey LA Jr. The nonspecificity of synovial leukocyte inclusions. J Lab Clin Med 1966;68:628–635.

W253. Wilmers MJ, Russell PA. Autoimmune haemolytic anaemia in an infant treated by thymectomy. Lancet 1963 Nov 2; 2:915–917.

W254. Wilske KR, Shalit IE, Willkins RF, Decker JL. Findings suggestive of systemic lupus erythematosus in subjects on chronic anticonvulsive therapy. Arthritis Rheum 1965 Apr;8: 260–266.

W255. Wilson AP, Jordan JW. Relationship of chronic discoid and disseminated lupus erythematosus. N Y J Med 1950 Oct 15;50:2449–2452.

W256. Wilson CB, Dixon FJ. Quantitation of acute and chronic serum sickness in the rabbit. J Exp Med 1975;134:7s–18s.

W257. Wilson DN. Systemic lupus Erythematosus in a woman with mental handicap. Br J Psychiatry 1991;158:427–429.

W258. Wilson FE, Bergin JJ. Recurrent sunlight induced intravascular hemolysis. Case report. South Med J 1970 Apr;63: 460–461.

W259. Wilson HA, Hamilton ME, Spyker DA, Brunner CM, O'Brien WM, Davis JS IV, Winfield JB. Age influences the clinical and serologic expression of systemic lupus erythematosus. Arthritis Rheum 1981 Oct;24:1230–1235.

W260. Wilson HA, Winfield JB, Lahita RG, Koffler D. Association of IgG anti-brain antibodies with central nervous system dysfunction in systemic lupus erythematosus. Arthritis Rheum 1979 May;22:458–462.

W261. Wilson JD, Booth RJ, Bullock JY. Antinuclear factor in patients on prazosin [letter]. BMJ 1979 Feb;1:553–554.

W262. Wilson JD, Bullock JY, Sutherland DC, Main C, O'Brien KP. Antinuclear antibodies in patients receiving non-practolol beta blockers. BMJ 1978 Jan 7;1:14–16.

W263. Wilson JG, Andriopoulos NA, Fearon DT. CR1 and the cell membranes that bind C3 and C4. A basic and clinical review. Immunol Res 1987;6:192–209.

W264. Wilson JG, Fearon DT. Altered expression of complement receptors as a pathogenic factor in systemic lupus erythematosus. Arthritis Rheum 1984 Dec;27:1321–1328.

W265. Wilson JG, Murphy EE, Wong WW, Klickstein LB, Weis JH, Fearon DT. Identification of a restriction fragment length polymorphism by a CR1 cDNA that correlates with the number on erythrocytes. J Exp Med 1986;164:50–59.

W266. Wilson JG, Ratnoff WD, Schur PH, Fearon DT. Decreased expression of the C3b/C4b receptor (CR1) and the C3d receptor (CR2) on B lymphocytes and of CR1 on neutrophils of patients with systemic lupus erythematosus. Arthritis Rheum 1986;29:739–747.

W267. Wilson JG, Wong WW, Murphy EE, Schur PH, Fearon DJ. Deficiency of the C3b/C4b receptor (CR1) of erythrocytes in systemic lupus erythematosus: Analysis of the stability of the defect and of a restriction fragment length polymorphism of the CR1 gene. J Immunol 1987;138:2706–2710.

W268. Wilson JG, Wong WW, Schur PH, Fearon DT. Mode of inheritance of decreased C3b receptors on erythrocytes of patients with systemic lupus erythematosus. N Engl J Med 1982 Oct 14;307(16):981–986.

W269. Wilson K, Katz J, Abeles M. The use of methotrexate in systemic lupus erythematosus. Arthritis Rheum 1991 May; 34(5) Suppl:R39.

W270. Wilson RK, Lai E, Concannon P, Barth K, Hood L. Structure, organization and polymorphism of murine and human T-cell receptor alpha and beta chain families. Immunol Rev 1988;101:149–172.

W271. Wilson RM, Abbott RR, Miller DK. The occurrence of L.E. cells and hematoxylin bodies in the naturally occurring cutaneous lesions of systemic lupus erythematosus. Am J Med Sci 1961 Jan;241:31–43.

W272. Wilson RM, Maher JF, Schreiner GE. Lupus nephritis: Clinical and histologic survey. Arch Intern Med 1963 Apr;111: 429–438.

W273. Wilson RW, Provost TT, Bias WB, Alexander EL, Edlow DW, Hochberg MC, Stevens MB, Arnett FC. Sjogren's syndrome. Influence of multiple HLA-D region alloantigens on clinical and serologic expression. Arthritis Rheum 1984;27: 1245–1253.

W274. Wilson WA, Hughes GRV. Rheumatic disease in Jamaica. Ann Rheum Dis 1979;38:20.

W275. Wilson WA, Perez MC, Aramantis PE. Partial C4A deficiency is associated with susceptibility to systemic lupus erythematosus in black Americans. Arthritis Rheum 1988;31: 1171–1175.

W276. Wilson WA, Scopelitis E, Michalski JP. Association of HLA-DR with both antibody to SS-A (Ro) and disease susceptibility in blacks with systemic lupus erythematosus. J Rheumatol 1984;11:653.

W277. Winchester RJ. Genetic aspects. In: Schur PH, editor. The clinical management of systemic lupus erythematosus. Orlando: Grune & Stratton, 1983.

W278. Winchester RJ, Fu SM, Hoffman TJ, Kunkel HG. IgG on lymphocyte surfaces: Technical problems and the significance of a third cell population. J Immunol 1975;114:1210–1212.

W279. Winchester RJ, Nunez-Roldan A. Some genetic aspects of systemic lupus erythematosus. Arthritis Rheum 1982 Jul;25: 833–837.

W280. Winchester RJ, Winfield JB, Siegal F, Wernet P, Bentwich Z, Kunkel HG. Analyses of lymphocytes from patients with rheumatoid arthritis and systemic lupus erythematosus. J Clin Invest 1974;54:1082–1092.

W281. Winer LH, Kling DH, Levin GH. Ecchymosis in arthritis patients on prolonged corticosteroids. A histologic study. Arch Dermatol 1961 Nov;86:654–662.

W282. Winfield JB. Cryoglobulinemia. Hum Pathol 1983 Apr;14: 350.

W283. Winfield JB. Stress proteins, arthritis, and autoimmunity. Arthritis Rheum 1989;32:1497–1504.

W284. Winfield JB, Brunner CM, Koffler D. Serologic studies in patients with systemic lupus erythematosus and central nervous system dysfunction. Arthritis Rheum 1978 Apr;21(3): 289–294.

W285. Winfield JB, Davis JS. Anti-DNA antibody in procainamide-induced lupus erythematosus. Arthritis Rheum 1974;17: 97–110.

W286. Winfield JB, Faiferman I, Koffler D. Avidity of anti-DAN antibodies in serum and IgG glomerular eluates from patients with systemic lupus erythematosus. Association of high avidity antinative DNA antibody with glomerulonephritis. J Clin Invest 1977 Jan;59(1):90–96.

W287. Winfield JB, Koffler D, Kunkel HG. Specific concentration of polynucleotide immune complexes in cryoprecipitates of patients with systemic lupus erythematosus. J Clin Invest 1975 Sep 56:563–570.

W288. Winfield JB, Lobo PI, Singer A. Significance of anti-lymphocyte antibodies in systemic lupus erythematosus. Arthritis Rheum 1978 Jun;21 Suppl;S215-S221.

W289. Winfield JB, Shaw M, Lengowski K, Christianson R, Silverman L. Evidence for intrathecal IgG synthesis and blood brain barrier impairment in CNS lupus [abstract]. Arthritis Rheum 1982 Apr;25(4) Suppl:S30.

W290. Winfield JB, Shaw M, Minota S. Modulation of IgM anti-lymphocyte antibody-reactive T cell surface antigens in systemic lupus erythematosus. J Immunol 1986;136;3246–3253.

W291. Winfield JB, Shaw M, Yamada A, Minota S. Subset specificity of anti-lymphocyte antibodies in systemic lupus erythematosus. II. Preferential reactivity with T4 + cells is associated with relative depletion of autologous T4 + cells. Arthritis Rheum 1987;30:162–168.

W292. Winfield JB, Winchester RJ, Kunkel HG. Association of cold-reactive anti-lymphocyte antibodies with lymphopenia in systemic lupus erythematosus. Arthritis Rheum 1975 Nov–Dec;18:587–594.

W293. Winfield JB, Winchester RJ, Wernet P, Fu SM, Kunkel HG. Nature of cold-reactive antibodies to lymphocyte surface determinants in systemic lupus erythematosus. Arthritis Rheum 1975 Jan–Feb;18:1–8.

W294. Winfield JB, Winchester RJ, Wernet P, Kunkel HG. Specific concentrations of anti-lymphocyte antibodies in the serum cryoprecipitates of patients with systemic lupus erythematosus. Clin Exp Immunol Mar 1975 Mar;19:399–406.

W295. Winfield JB 3d, Shaw M, Silverman LM, Eisenberg RA, Wilson HA, Koffler D. Intrathecal IgG synthesis and blood brain-barrier impairment in patients with systemic lupus erythematosus and central nervous system dysfunction. Am J Med 1983 May;74(5):837–844.

W296. Winkelmann RK. Diagnosis and treatment of lupus erythematosus, dermatomyositis, and scleroderma, with emphasis on cutaneous findings. J Chronic Dis 1961 May;13: 401–410.

W297. Winkelmann RK. Panniculitis and systemic lupus erythematosus. JAMA 1970 Jan 19;211:472–475.

W298. Winkelmann RK. Panniculitis in connective tissue disease. Arch Dermatol 1983 Apr;119(4):336–344.

W299. Winkelmann RK, Jordan RE, de Moragas JM. Immunofluorescent studies of dermatomyositis. Dermatologica 1972;145: 42–47.

W300. Winkelmann RK, Merwin CF, Brunsting LA. Antimalarial therapy of lupus erythematosus. Ann Intern Med 1961 Nov; 55:772–776.

W301. Winkelmann RK, Peters MS. Lupus panniculitis. Dermatol Update 1982:135.

W302. Winkler A, Jackson RW, Kay DS, Mitchell E, Carmignani S, Sharp GC. High-dose intravenous cyclophosphamide treatment of systemic lupus erythematosus-associated aplastic anemia [letter]. Arthritis Rheum 1988 May;31(5):693–694.

W303. Winkler RB, Nora AH, Nora JJ. Familial congenital complete heart block and maternal systemic lupus erythematosus. Circulation 1977;56:1103.

W304. Winkler TH, Henscchel TA, Kalies I, Baenkler HW, Skvaril F, Kalden JR. Constant isotype pattern of anti-dsDNA antibodies in patients with systemic lupus erythematosus. Clin Exp Immunol 1988;72:434–439.

W305. Winn DM, Wolfe JF, Lindberg DA, Fistoe FA, Kingsland L, Sharp GC. Identification of a clinical subset of systemic lupus erythematosus by antibodies to the Sm antigen. J Clin Invest 1979 Sep;22:1334–1337.

W306. Winocour PD, Kinlough-Rathbone RL, Mustard JF. The effect of phospholipase mepacrine inhibitor on platelet aggregation, the platelet release reaction and fibrinogen binding to the platelet surface. Thromb Haemost 1981 Jun 30;45(3): 257–262.

W307. Winslow WA, Ploss LN, Loitman B. Pleuritis in systemic lupus erythematosus: Its importance as an early manifestation in diagnosis. Ann Intern Med 1958 Jul;49:70–88.

W308. Wise RA, Wigley F, Newball HH, Stevens MB. The effect of cold exposure on diffusing capacity in patients with Raynaud's phenomenon. Chest 1982 Jun;81(6):695–698.

W309. Wisnieski JJ, Naff GB. Serum IgG antibodies to C1q in hypocomplementemic urticarial vasculitis syndrome. Arthritis Rheum 1989 Sep;32(9):1119–1127.

W310. Witebsky E, Rose NR, Terplan K, Paine JR, Egan RW. Chronic thyroiditis and autoimmunization. JAMA 1957 Jul 27; 164:1439–1447.

W311. Witman G, Davis R. A Lupus erythematosus syndrome induced by clonidine hydrochloride. R I Med J 1981;64: 147–150.

W312. Witten VH. Newer dermatologic methods for using corticosteroids more efficaciously. Med Clin North Am 1961 Jul; 45:857–868.

W313. Woch B. Altered form of albumin excreted by patients with systemic lupus erythematosus. Acta Med Pol 1977;18(3): 191–197.

W314. Wofsy D. Administration of monoclonal anti-T cell antibodies retards murine lupus in BXSB mice. J Immunol 1986; 136:4554–4560.

W315. Wofsy D. The role of Lyt-2+ T cells in the regulation of autoimmunity in murine lupus. J Autoimmun 1988;1: 207–217.

W316. Wofsy D. Treatment of murine lupus with monoclonal antibody to L3T4. I. Effects on the distribution and function of lymphocyte subsets and on the histopathology of autoimmune disease. J Autoimmun 1988;1:415–431.

W317. Wofsy D, Chiang NY. Proliferation of LY-1 B cells in autoimmune NZB and (NZB × NZW)F1 mice. Eur J Immunol 1987 Jun;17(6):809–814.

W318. Wofsy D, Ledbetter JA, Hendler PL, Seaman WE. Treatment of murine lupus with monoclonal anti-T cell antibody. J Immunol 1985;134:852.

W319. Wofsy D, Seaman WE. Successful treatment of autoimmunity in NZB/NZW F1 mice with monoclonal antibody to L3T4. J Exp Med 1985 Feb 1;161(2):378–391.

W320. Wofsy D, Seaman WE. Reversal of advanced murine lupus in NZB/NZW F1 mice by treatment with monoclonal antibody to L3T4. J Immunol 1987 May 15;138(10):3247–3253.

W321. Wohlgelernter D, Loke J, Matthay RA, Siegel NJ. Systemic and discoid lupus erythematosus: analysis of pulmonary function. Yale J Biol Med 1978 Mar–Apr;51:157–164.

W322. Wohlgethan JR, Smith HR. Nonsteroidal anti-inflammatory drugs and the lupus anticoagulant [letter]. Arthritis Rheum 1990 Jul;33(7):1061–1062.

W323. Wolf RE, Brelsford WG. Soluble interleukin-2 receptors in systemic lupus erythematosus. Arthritis Rheum 1988;31: 729–733.

W324. Wolfe JF, Takasugi S, Kingsland L, Londberg DAB, Winn DM, Sharp GC. Objective derivation of clinical discriminators for mixed connective tissue diseases. Arthritis Rheum 1979 Jun;22:675–676.

W325. Wolfe MJ, Cordero JF. Safety of chloroquine in chemosuppression of malaria during pregnancy. BMJ 1985;290: 1466–1467.

W326. Wolin SL, Steitz JA. The Ro small cytoplasmic ribonucleoproteins: identification of the antigenic protein and its binding site on the Ro RNAs. Proc Natl Acad Sci USA 1984;81: 1996–2000.

W327. Wolina V, Beensen H, Kitler L, Schaarschmidt H, Knopf B. PUVA treatment of human cultured fibroblasts from psoriatic skin enhances the binding of antibodies to SSA(Ro). Arch Dermatol Res 1987;279:206–208.

W328. Wolkove N, Frank H. Lupus pericarditis. Can Med Assoc J 1974;11:1331–1334.

W329. Wolkowitz OM, Reus VI, Weingartner H, Thompson K, Breier A, Doran A, Rubinow D, Pickar D. Cognitive effects of corticosteroids. Am J Psychiatry 1990;147:1297–1303.

W330. Wollheim FA. Acute and long-term complications of corticosteroid pulse therapy. Scand J Rheumatol 1983 Sep 16; 54 Suppl:27–32.

W331. Wolska H, Blaszczyk M, Jablonska S. Phototests in patients with various forms of lupus erythematosus. Int J Dermatol 1989;28:98–103.

W332. Wolstenholme GEW. Epithelioma arising on lupus erythematosus. Br J Dermatol 1949 Apr;61:126–130.

W333. Wong DW, Bentwich Z. Martinez-Tarquino C, Seidman JG, Duby AD, Quertermous T, Schur PH. Nonlinkage of the T Cell Receptor α, β, and γ genes to systemic lupus erythematosus in multiplex families. Arthritis Rheum 1988;31: 1371–1376.

W334. Wong K, Hei P, Chan JC, Chan Y, Ha S. The acute lupus hematophagocytic syndrome. Ann Intern Med 1991;114: 387–390.

W335. Wong KC, Li PKT, Nicholls MG, Lai KN. The adverse effects of recombinant human erythropoietin therapy. Adverse Drug React Acute Poisoning Rev 1990;9:183–206.

W336. Wong KL, Chan FY, Lee CHP. Outcome of pregnancy in patients with systemic lupus erythematosus. Arch Intern Med 1991;151:2690–2273.

W337. Wong KL, Tai YT, Loke SL, Woo EK, Wong WS, Chan MK, Ma JT. Disseminated zygomycosis masquerading as cerebral lupus erythematosus. Am J Clin Pathol 1986 Oct;86(4): 546–549.

W338. See W333.

W339. Wong WW, Wilson JG, Fearon DT. Genetic regulation of a structural polymorphism of human C3b receptor. J Clin Invest 1983;72:685.

W340. Woo KT, Junor BJR, Salem H, D'Apice AJF, Whiteworth JA, Kincaid Smith P. Beta thromboglobulin and platelet aggregation in glomerulonephritis. Clin Nephrol 1980;14:92–95.

W341. Wood G, Rucker M, Davis JR, Entwistle R, Anderson B. Interaction of plasma fibronectin with selected cryoglobulins. Clin Exp Immunol 1980 May;40:358–364.

W342. Woodland DL, Happ MP, Gollob KJ, Palmer E. An endogenous retrovirus mediating deletion of alpha beta T cells ? Nature 1991;349:529–530.

W343. Woodland R, Cantor H. Idiotype-specific T helper cells are required to induce idiotype-positive B memory cells to secrete antibody. Eur J Immunol 1978:600.

W344. Woodley DT, Burgeson RE, Lunstrum G, Bruckner-Tuderman L, Reese MJ, Briggaman RA. Epidermolysis bullosa acquisita antigen is the globular carboxyl terminus of type VII procollagen. J Clin Invest 1988 Mar;81(3):683–687.

W345. Woods VL, Oh EH, Mason D, McMillan R. Autoantibodies against the platelet glycoprotein IIb/IIIa complex in patients with chronic ITP. Blood 1984;63:368–373.

W346. Wooley PH, Griffin J, Panayi GS, Batchelor JR, Welsh KI, Gibson TJ. HLA-DR antigens and toxic reaction to sodium thiomalate and D-penicillamine in patients with rheumatoid arthritis. N Engl J Med 1980;303:300–302.

W347. Woolf A, Croker B, Osofski SG, Kredich DW. Nephritis in children and young adults with systemic lupus erythematosus and normal urinary sediment. Kidney Int 1978 Dec;14:667.

W348. Woosley RL, Drayer DE. Reidenberg MM, Nios AS, Carr K, Oates JA. Effect of acetylator phenotype on the rate at which procainamide induces antinuclear antibodies and the lupus syndrome. N Engl J Med 1978;298:1157–1159.

W349. Woppmann A, Rinke J, Luhrmann R. Direct cross-linking of snRNP proteins F and 70K to snRNAs by ultra-violet radiation in situ. Nucleic Acids Res 1988;16:10985–11004.

W350. Worlledge SM. Annotation: The interpretation of a positive direct antiglobulin test. Br J Haematol 1978 Jun;39: 157–168.

W351. Worlledge S. Auto-immunity and blood diseases. Practitioner 1967 Aug;199:171–179.

W352. Worrall JG, Snaith ML, Batchelor JR, Isenberg DA. SLE: A rheumatological view. Analysis of clinical features, serology, and immunogenetics of 100 SLE patients during long-term follow-up. Q J Med 1990;74:319–330.

W353. Worth H, Grahn S, Lakomek HJ, Bremer G, Goeckenjan

G. Lung function disturbances versus respiratory muscle fatigue in patients with systemic lupus erythematosus. Respiratory 1988;53:81–90.

W354. Wright ET, Winer LH. Histopathology of allergic solar dermatitis. J Invest Dermatol 1960 Feb;34:103–106.

W355. Wright FS, Adams P Jr, Anderson RC. Congenital atrioventricular dissociation due to complete or advanced atrioventricular heart block. Am J Dis Child 1959;98:72.

W356. Wright-Sandor L, Reichlin M, Tobin SL. Alternation by heat shock and immunological characterization of Drosophila small nuclear ribonucleoproteins. J Cell Biol 1990;108: 2007–2016.

W357. Wu GG, Gelbart DR, Hasbargen JA, Inman R, McNamee P, Oreopoulus DG. Reactivation of systemic lupus in three patients undergoing CAPD. Peritoneal Dialysis Bull 1986;6: 6–9.

W358. Wu J, Manley JL. Base pairing between U2 and U6 snRNAs is necessary for splicing of a mammalian pre-mRNA. Nature 1991;352:818–821.

W359. Wu RS, Panusz HT, Hatch CL, Bonner WM. Histones and their modifications. CRC Crit Rev Biochem 1986;20:201–263.

W360. Wu-fei C, Nai-Chung K, Ken-Heng T, Ch'ing-Jung C, Teh-Jung S, Yi-Ching W. The inhibition of immunologic response by chloroquine. Chinese Med J 1964;83:531–535.

W361. Wyle FA, Kent JR. Immunosuppression by sex steroid hormones. Clin Exp Immunol 1977;27:407–415.

W362. Wyllie AH, Kerr JFR, Currie AR. Cell death: the significance of apoptosis. Int Rev Cytol 1980;68:251–306.

W363. Wyllie AH, Morris RG, Smith AL, Dunlop D. Chromatin cleavage in apoptosis: association with condensed chromatin morphology and dependence on macromolecular synthesis. J Pathol 1984;142:67–77.

W364. Wynn V, Rob CG. Water intoxication; differential diagnosis of the hypotonic syndromes. Lancet 1954 Mar 20;1: 587–594.

W365. Wysenbeek AJ, Block DA, Fries JF. Prevalence and expression of photosensitivity in systemic lupus erythematosus. Ann Rheum Dis 1989 Jun;48(6):461–463.

W366. Wysenbeek AJ, Leibovici L, Zoldan J. Acute central nervous system complications after pulse steroid therapy in patients with systemic lupus erythematosus. J Rheumatol 1990 Dec;17(12):1695–1696.

W367. Wysenbeek AJ, Mandel DR, Mayes MD, Clough JD. Autoantibodies in systemic lupus erythematosus of late onset. Cleve Clin Q 1985 Summer;52(2):119–122.

W368. Wysocka K, Daniel B, Marcinkowska M, Andrejewski W. CT diagnosed cortical blindness in systemic lupus erythematosus. Akt Rheumatol 1988;13:31–33.

X

X1. Xu R, Gu Y. Detection of circulating immune complexes with polyethylene glycol precipitation F(ab')$_2$ anti-C$_3$ ELISA. J Immunol Meth 1990;135:225–231.

Y

Y1. Yager TD, McMurray CT, Van Holde KE. Salt-induced release of DNA from nucleosome core particles. Biochemistry 1989; 28:2271–2281.

Y2. Yakub YN, Freeman RB, Pabico RC. Renal transplantation in systemic lupus erythematosus. Nephron 1981;27(4–5): 197–201.

Y3. Yakura H, Ashida T, Kawabata I, Katagiri M. Alleviation of autoimmunity in BXSB mice by monoclonal alloantibody to Ly-5 (CD45). Eur J Immunol 1989;19:1505–1508.

Y4. Yam P, Petz LD, Spath P. Detection of IgG sensitization of red cells with 125 I staphylococcal protein A. Am J Hematol 1982;12(4):337–346.

Y5. Yamada A, Cohen PL, Winfield JB. Subset specificity of anti-lymphocyte antibodies in systemic lupus erythematosus. Preferential reactivity with cells bearing the T4 and autologous erythrocyte receptor phenotypes. Arthritis Rheum 1985 Mar; 28:262–270.

Y6. Yamada A, Shaw M, Winfield JB. Surface antigen specificity of cold-reactive IgM antilymphocyte antibodies in systemic lupus erythematosus. Arthritis Rheum 1985 Jan;28:44–51.

Y7. Yamada A, Winfield JB. Inhibition of soluble antigen-induced T cell proliferation by warm-reactive antibodies to activated T cells in systemic lupus erythematosus. J Clin Invest 1984 Dec;74:1948–1960.

Y8. Yamada M, Watanabe A, Minori A, Nakano K, Takeuchi F, Matsuta K, Tanimoto K, Miyamoto T, Yukiyama Y, Tokunaga K, Yokohari R. Lack of gene deletion for complement C4A deficiency in Japanese patients with systemic lupus erythematosus. J Rheumatol 1990;17:1054–1057.

Y9. Yamada Y, Dekio S, Jidol J, Ozasa S. Lupus erythematosus profundus—report of a case treated with dapsone. J Dermatol 1989 Oct;16(5):379–382.

Y10. Yamagata H, Harley JB, Reichlin M. Molecular properties of the Ro/SS-A antigen and enzyme-linked immunosorbent assay for quantitation of antibody. J Clin Invest 1984;74:625-633.

Y11. Yamaguchi M, Kumada K, Sugiyama H, Okamoto E, Ozawa K. Hemoperitoneum due to a ruptured gastroepiploic artery aneurysm in systemic lupus erythematosus. A case report and literature review. J Clin Gastroenterol 1990 Jun;12(3):344-346.

Y12. Yamakado T, Tanaka F, Hidaka H. Mepacrine-induced inhibition of human platelet cyclic-GMP phosphodiesterase. Biochim Biophys Acta 1984 Sep 7;801(1):111–116.

Y13. Yamamoto K, Miura H, Moroi Y, Yoshinoya M, Goto M, Nishioka K, Miyamoto T. Isolation and characterization of a complementary DNA expressing human U1 small nuclear ribonucleoprotein C polypeptide. J Immunol 1988;140: 311–317.

Y14. Yamamoto K, Mori A, Nakahama T, Ito M, Okudaira H, Miyamoto T. Experimental treatment of autoimmune MRL-lpr/lpr mice with immunosuppressive compound FK506. Immunology 1990;69:222–227.

Y15. Yamamoto KR. Steroid receptors regulated transcription of specific genes and gene networks. Annu Rev Genet 1985;19: 209–152.

Y16. Yamamoto M, Watanabe K, Ando Y, Iri H, Murakami H, Sato K, Ideda Y, Toyama K. Further evidences that lupus anticoagulants are anti-phospholipid antibodies. Thromb Haemost 1985 Jul;54:276.

Y17. Yamamoto T, Wilson CB. Binding of anti-basement membrane antibody to alveolar basement membrane after intratracheal gasoline instillation in rabbits. Am J Pathol 1987;126: 497–505.

Y18. Yamanashi Y, Kakiuchi T, Mizuguchi J, Yamamoto T, Toyoshima K. Association of B cell antigen receptor with protein tyrosine kinase Lyn. Science 1991;251:192–194.

Y19. Yamasaki K, Niho Y, Yanase T. Granulopoiesis in systemic lupus erythematosus. Arthritis Rheum 1983 Apr;26:516–521.

Y20. Yamasaki K, Niho Y, Yanase T. Erythroid colony forming cells in systemic lupus erythematosus. J Rheumatol 1984 Apr; 11:167–171.

Y21. Yamashita N, Clement LT. Phenotypic Characterization of the post-thymic differentiation of human alloantigen- specific CD8+ cytotoxic T lymphocytes. J Immunol 1989;143: 1518–1523.

Y22. Yamashita Y, Imai Y, Osawa T. Poly[N-acetyl- lactosamine]-

type sugar chains in CD45 antigens of abnormal T cells of lpr mice are different from those of normal T cells and B cells. Mol Immunol 1989;26:905–913.

Y23. Yamasu K, Senshu T. Reassembly of nucleosomal histone octamers during replication of chromatin. J Biochem 1987; 101:1041–1049.

Y24. Yamauchi K, Arimori S. Effective methylprednisolone "pulse" therapy in myeloerythyroid aplasia associated with systemic lupus erythematosus: case report and literature review. Tokai J Exp Clin Med 1987;12:337-341.

Y25. Yamauchi K, Suzuki Y, Arimori S. "Renal Raynaud's" phenomenon" in systemic lupus erythematosus: measurement of the glomerular filtration rate with 99 m technetium-DTPA [letter]. Arthritis Rheum 1989 Nov;32(11):1487–1488.

Y26. Yamauchi Y, Litwin A, Adams LE, Zimmer H, Hess EV. Induction of antibodies to nuclear antigens in rabbits by immunization with hydralazine-human serum albumin conjugates. J Clin Invest 1975 Oct;56:958–969.

Y27. Yamura W, Hattori S, Morrow WJ, Mayes DC, Levy JA, Shirai T. Dietary fat and immune function. II. Effects on immune complex nephritis in (NZB × NZW)F1 mice. J Immunol 1985;135:3864–3868.

Y28. Yanagi Y, Hirose S, Nagasawa R, Shirai T, Mak TW, Tada T. Does the deletion within T cell receptor beta-chain gene of NZW mice contribute to autoimmunity in (NZB × NZW)F1 mice? Eur J Immunol 1986 Sep;16(9):1179–1182.

Y29. Yancey CL, Doughty RA, Athreya BH. Central nervous system involvement in childhood systemic lupus erythematosus. Arthritis Rheum 1981 Nov;24(11):1389-1395.

Y30. Yancey CL, Zmijewski C, Athreya BH, Doughty RA. Arthropathy of Down's syndrome. Arthritis Rheum 1984 Aug;27(8): 929–934.

Y31. Yaneva M, Arnett FC. Antibodies against Ku protein in sera from patients with autoimmune diseases. Clin Exp Immunol 1989;76:366–372.

Y32. Yaneva M, Ochs R, McRorie DK, Zweiz S, Busch H. Purification of an 80–70 kD nuclear DNA-associated protein complex. Bochem Biophys Acta 1985;841:22–29.

Y33. Yang HT, Zhang JR. Treatment of systemic lupus erythematosus with saponin of ginseng fruit (SPGF): an immunological study [English abstract]. Chung Hsi I Chieh Ho Tsa Chih 1986 Mar;6(3):157–159.

Y34. Yaoita Y, Takahashi M, Azuma C, Kanai Y, Honjo T. Biased expression of variable region gene families of the immunoglobulin heavy chain in autoimmune-prone mice. J Biochem 1988;104:337–343.

Y35. Yap AS, Powell EE, Yelland CE, Mortimer RH, Perry-Keene DA. Lupus anticoagulant [letter]. Ann Intern Med 1989 Aug 1; 111(3):262–263.

Y36. Yasuda H, Logan KA, Bradbury EM. Antibody against globular domain of H1o histone. FEBS Lett 1984;166:263–266.

Y37. Yasuda M, Takasaki Y, Matsumoto K, Kodama A, Hashimoto H, Hirose S. Clinical significance of IgG anti-IgG antibodies in patients with systemic lupus erythematosus. J Rheumatol 1990;17:469–475.

Y38. Yasue T. Livedoid vasculitis and central nervous system involvement in systemic lupus erythematosus. Arch Dermatol 1986 Jan;122(1):66–70.

Y39. Yee AM, Buyon JP, Yip YK. Interferon alpha associated with systemic lupus erythematosus is not intrinsically acid labile. J Exp Med 1989;169:987–993.

Y40. Yemini M, Shoham Z, Dgani R, Lancet M, Mogilner BM, Nissim F, Bar-Khayim Y. Lupus-like syndrome in a mother and newborn following administration of hydralazine; a case report. Eur J Obstet Gynecol Reprod Biol 1989;30:193–197.

Y41. Yerevanian BI, Olafsdottir H, Milanese E, Russotto J, Mallon P, Baciewicz G, Sagi E. Normalization of the dexamethasone suppression test at discharge from hospital. J Affect Disord 1983;5:191–197.

Y42. Yeung CK, Ng WL, Wong WS, Wong KL, Chan MK. Acute deterioration in renal function in systemic lupus erythematosus. Q J Med 1985;56:393–402.

Y43. Yeung CK, Wong KL, Wong WS, Chan KH. Beta-2 microglobulin and systemic lupus erythematosus. J Rheumatol 1986;13:1053–1058.

Y44. Yocum MW, Rossman J, Waterhouse C, Abraham CN, May AG, Condemi JJ. Monozygotic twins discordant for systemic lupus erythematosus. Arthritis Rheum 1975;18:193.

Y45. Yokohari R, Tsunematsu T. Application to Japanese patients, of the 1982 American Rheumatism Association revised criteria for the classification of systemic lupus erythematosus. Arthritis Rheum 1985 Jun;28:693–698.

Y46. Yoo TJ, Kim S-Y, Stuart JM, Floyd RA, Olson GA, Cramer MA, Kang AH. Induction of arthritis in monkeys by immunization with type II collagen. J Exp Med 1988;168:777–782.

Y47. Yood RA, Smith TW. Inclusion body myositis and systemic lupus erythematosus. J Rheumatol 1985 Jun;12(3):568-570.

Y48. Yoshida H, Fossati L, Yoshida M, Abdelmoula M, Herrera S, Merino J, Lambert PH, Izui S. Igh-C allotype-linked control of anti-DNA production and clonotype expression in mice infected with Plasmodium yoelii. J Immunol 1988 Sep 15; 141(6):2125–2131.

Y49. Yoshida H, Kohno A, Ohta K, Hirose S, Maruyama N, Shirai T. Genetic studies of autoimmunity in New Zealand mice III. Associations among anti-DNA antibodies, NTA and renal disease in (NZB × NZW) F1 × NZW backcross mice. J Immunol 1981 Aug;127(2):433–437.

Y50. Yoshida H, Yoshida M, Izui S, Lambert PH. Distinct clonotypes of anti-DNA antibodies in mice with lupus nephritis. J Clin Invest 1985 Aug;76(2):685–694.

Y51. Yoshida K. Post mammaplasty disorder as an adjuvant disease of man. Shikoku Igaku Zasshi 1973;29:318–332.

Y52. Yoshida K, Yukiyama Y, Miyamoto T. Quantification of the complement receptor function on polymorphonuclear leukocytes: its significance in patients with systemic lupus erythematosus. J Rheumatol 1987:14:490–496.

Y53. Yoshida S, Castles JJ, Gershwin ME. The pathogenesis of autoimmunity in New Zealand mice. Semin Arthritis Rheum 1990;19:224–242.

Y54. Yoshida S, Dorshkind K, Bearer E, Castles JJ, Ahmed A, Gershwin ME. Abnormalities of B lineage cells are demonstrable in long term lymphoid bone marrow cultures of NZB mice. J Immunol 1987;139:1454–1458.

Y55. Yoshikawa T, Suzuki H, Kato H, Yano S. Effects of prostaglandin E1 on collagen diseases with high levels of circulating immune complexes [case report]. J Rheumatol 1990 Nov; 17(11):1513–1514.

Y56. Youinou P, Baron A, Garre M, Jouquan J, Poles JM. Autoantibodies and protein-calorie malnutrition [letter]. J Rheumatol 1981 Jan–Feb;8(1):174–175.

Y57. Youinou P, Dorval JC, Cledes J, Leroy JP, Mossec P, Masse R. A study of familial lupus erythematosus-like disease and hereditary angio-oedema treated with danazol. Br J Dermatol 1983;108:717–722.

Y58. Youinou P, Williams W, LeGoff P, Tuaillon N, Jouquan J, Muller S, Isenberg DA. Serological abnormalities, including common idiotype PR4, in families with rheumatoid arthritis. Ann Rheum Dis 1989;48:898.

Y59. Young SM, Fisher M, Sigsbee A, Errichetti A. Cardiogenic brain embolism and lupus anticoagulant. Ann Neurol 1989 Sep;26(3):390–392.

Y60. Yu CL, Ziff M. Effects of long-term procainamide therapy on immunoglobulin synthesis. Arthritis Rheum 1985 Mar;28: 276–284.

Y61. Yu MIu, Folomeev IuV. The use of androgens in multiple modality therapy of men with systemic lupus erythematosus. Ter Arkh 1986;58:111–114.

Y62. Yu SF. Direct immunofluorescent technic of analyzing fibrinogen in the differential diagnosis of certain diseases of the oral mucous membrane [English abstract]. Chung Hua Kou Chiang Hsueh Tsa Chih 1989 Jan;24(1):22–23, 62.

Y63. Yu VYH, Waller CA, MacLennan ICM, Baum JD. Lymphocyte reactivity in pregnant women and newborn infants. BMJ 1975;1:428–430.

Y64. Yuan ZZ, Feng JC. Observation on the treatment of systemic lupus erythematosus with a Gentiani macrophylla complex tablet and a minimal dose of prednisone [English abstract]. Chung Hsi Chieh Ho Tsa Chih 1989 Mar;9(3):133–134, 156–157.

Y65. Yurchak PM, Levine SA, Gorlin R. Constrictive pericarditis complicating disseminated lupus erythematosus. Circulation 1965 Jan;31:113–118.

Z

Z1. Zacharias W, Koopman WJ. Lupus-inducing drugs alter the structure of supercoiled circular DNA domains. Arthritis Rheum 1990;33:366–374.

Z2. Zamansky GB. Sunlight-induced pathogenesis in systemic lupus erythematosus [editorial]. J Invest Dermatol 1985 Sep;85(3):179–180.

Z3. Zamansky GB. Recovery from UV-induced potentially lethal damage in systemic lupus erythematosus skin fibroblasts. Int J Radiat Biol 1986 Aug;50(2):305–312.

Z4. Zamansky GB, Minka DF, Deal CL, Hendricks K. The in vitro photosensitivity of systemic lupus erythematosus skin fibroblasts. J Immunol 1985 Mar;134:1571–1576.

Z5. Zamora JM, Beck WT. Chloroquine enhancement of anticancer drug cytotoxicity in multiple drug resistant human leukemic cells. Biochem Pharmacol 1986 Dec 1;35(23):4303–4310.

Z6. Zamora-Quezada JC, Dinerman H, Stadecker MJ, Kelly JJ. Muscle and skin infarction after free-basing cocaine (crack). Ann Intern Med 1988;108:564–566.

Z7. See Z14.

Z8. Zanetti M, Glotz D, Rogers J. Perturbation of the autoimmune network. II. Immunization with isologous idiotype induces auto-anti-idiotypic antibodies and suppresses the autoantibody response elicited by antigen: a serologic and cellular analysis. J Immunol 1986;137:3140.

Z9. Zanetti M, Rogers J. Independent expression of a regulatory idiotype on heavy and light chain: further immunochemical analysis with anti-heavy and anti-light chain antibodies. J Immunol 1987;139:720.

Z10. Zanetti M, Rogers J, Katz DH. Induction of autoantibodies to thyroglobulin by anti-idiotypic antibodies. J Immunol 1984;133:240.

Z11. Zarafonetis CJD. Therapeutic possibilities of para- aminobenzoic acid. Ann Intern Med 1949 Jun;30:1188- 1211.

Z12. Zarafonetis CJD, Grekin RH, Curtis AC. Further studies on the treatment of lupus erythematosus with sodium para-aminobenzoate. J Invest Dermatol 1984;11:359–381.

Z13. Zarling JM, Clouse JA, Biddison WE, Kung PC. Phenotypes of human natural killer cells populations detected with monoclonal antibodies. J Immunol 1981;127:2575–2580.

Z14. Zarrabi MH, Zucker S, Miller F, Derman RM, Romano GS, Hartnett JA, Varma AO. Immunologic and coagulation disorders in chlorpromazine-treated patients. Ann Intern Med 1979 Aug;91(2):194–199.

Z15. Zashin SJ, Lipsky PE. Pericardial tamponade complicating systemic lupus erythematosus. J Rheumatol 1989;16:374–377.

Z16. Zeilhofer HU, Mollenhauer J, Brune K. Selective growth inhibition of ductal pancreatic adenocarcinoma cells by the lysosomotropic agent chloroquine. Cancer Lett 1989 Jan;44(1):61–66.

Z17. Zein N, Ganuza C, Kushner I. Significance of serum C- reactive protein elevation in patients with systemic lupus erythematosus. Arthritis Rheum 1979 Jan;22:7–12.

Z18. Zeis BM, Schulz EJ, Anderson R, Kleeberg HH. Mononuclearucocyte function in patients with lichen planus and cutaneous lupus erythematosus during chemotherapy with clofazimine. S Afr Med J 1989 Feb 18;75(4):161–162.

Z19. Zeller J, Weissbarth E, Baruth B, Mielke H, Deicher H. Serotonin content of platelets in inflammatory rheumatic disease. Arthritis Rheum 1983;26:532–540.

Z20. Zeller R, Nyffenegger T, De Robertis EM. Nucleocytoplasmic distribution of snRNPs and stockpiled snRNA-binding proteins during oogenesis and early development in Xenopus laevis. Cell 1983;32:425–434.

Z21. Zetterstrom R, Berglund G. Systemic lupus erythematosus in childhood: A clinical study. Acta Paediat 1956;45:189–203.

Z22. Zhang N-Z, Chen WZ. Antineuronal antibodies in Chinese patients with neuropsychiatric SLE. Proceedings of the Second International Conference on Systemic Lupus Erythematosus. Tokyo, Professional Postgraduate Services, 1989:109.

Z23. Zhang XH, Yan YH, Liang ZQ, Cui XL, Jiang M. Changes in neutrophil elastase and alpha 1-antitrypsin in systemic lupus erythematosus. Proc Chin Acad Med Sci Peking Union Med Coll 1989;4:26–29.

Z24. Zheng RQH, Abney E, Chuc CQ, Field M, Grubeck-Loebenstein B, Maini RN, Feldmann M. Detection of interleukin-6 and interleukin-1 production in human thyroid epithelial cells by non-radioactive in situ hybridization and immunohistochemical methods. Clin Exp Immunol 1991;83:314–319.

Z25. Ziboh VA. Biochemical basis for the anti-inflammatory action of g-linolenic acid. In: Omega-6 essential fatty acids: pathophysiology and roles in clinical medicine. Alan R Liss, Inc. 1990;187–201.

Z26. Ziegler G, Medsger TA. Serial complement levels in SLE pregnancies. Arthritis Rheum 1984;27 Suppl:S130.

Z27. Ziff M, Esserman P, McEwen C. Observations on the course and treatment of SLE. Arthritis Rheum 1956;7:332–350.

Z28. Ziff M, Helderman JH. Dialysis and transplantation in end-stage lupus nephritis [editorial]. N Engl J Med 1983 Jan 27;308(4):218–219.

Z29. Zimmerman B, Lally EV, Sharma SC, Schoen FJ, Kaplan SR. Severe aortic stenosis in systemic lupus erythematosus and mucopolysaccharidosis Type II (Hunter's Syndrome). Clin Cariol 1988;11:723–725.

Z30. Zimmerman SW, Jenkins PG, Shelp WD, Bloodworth JMB Jr, Burholder PM. Progression from minimal or focal to diffuse proliferative lupus nephritis. Lab Invest 1975;32(5):665- 672.

Z31. Zingale SB, Sanchez Avalos JC, Andrada JA, Stringa SG, Manni JA. Appearance of anticoagulant factors and certain "autoimmune' antibodies following antigenic stimulation and blood group substances in patients with systemic lupus erythematosus. Arthritis Rheum 1963 Oct;6:581–598.

Z32. Zinkernagel RM, Doherty PC. MHC-restricted cytotoxic T cells: Studies on the biological role of polymorphic major transplantation antigens determining T cell restriction specificity, function and responsiveness. Adv Immunol 1979;27:52–180.

Z33. Zizic TM. Gastrointestinal manifestations. In: P Schur, editor. The clinical management of systemic lupus erythematosus. New York: Grune & Stratton, 1983:153–166.

Z34. Zizic TM. Systemic lupus erythematosus. X: corticosteroid therapy and its complications. Md State Med J 1984 May; 33(5):370–381.

Z35. Zizic TM. Avascular necrosis of bone. Curr Opin Rheumatol 1990 Feb;2(1):26–37.

Z36. Zizic TM, Classen JN, Stevens MB. Acute abdominal complications of systemic lupus erythematosus and polyarteritis nodosa. Am J Med 1982 Oct;73(4):525–531.

Z37. Zizic TM, Conklin JJ, Hungerford DS, Dansereau J-Y, Alderson PO, Gober A, Wagner NH, Stevens MB. Sensitivity of quantitative scintigraphy in the early detection of ischemic necrosis of bone [abstract]. Arthritis Rheum 1981;24:S62.

Z38. Zizic TM, Hungerford DS, Dansereau J-Y, Stevens MB. Corticosteroid associated ischemic necrosis of bone in SLE [abstract]. Arthritis Rheum 1982 Apr;25(4) Suppl:S82.

Z38a. Zizic TM, Hungerford DS, Stevens MB. Ischemic bone necrosis in systemic lupus erythematosus. II. The early diagnosis of ischemic necrosis of bone. Medicine 1980 Mar;59: 134–142.

Z38b. Zizic TM, Hungerford DS, Stevens MB. Ischemic bone necrosis in systemic lupus erythematosus. II. The treatment of ischemic necrosis of bone in systemic lupus erythematosus. Medicine 1980 Mar;59:143–148.

Z39. Zizic TM, Lewis CG, Marcoux C, Hungerford DS. The predictive value of hemodynamic studies in preclinical ischemic necrosis of bone. J Rheumatol 1989 Dec;16(12):1559–1564.

Z40. Zizic TM, Marcoux C, Hungerford DS, Dansereau JY, Stevens MB. Corticosteroid therapy associated with ischemic necrosis of bone in systemic lupus erythematosus. Am J Med 1985 Nov;79(5):596–604.

Z41. Zizic TM, Marcoux C, Hungerford DS, Stevens MB. The early diagnosis of ischemic necrosis of bone. Arthritis Rheum 1986 Oct;29(10):1177–1186.

Z42. Zizic TM, Thomas SC, Hungerford DS. Advanced ischemic necrosis of the hip treated by core decompression [abstract]. Arthritis Rheum 1984 Apr;27(4) Suppl:S31.

Z43. Zlatanova JS. Immunochemical approaches to the study of histone H1 and high mobility group chromatin proteins. Mol Cell Biochem 1990;92:1–22.

Z44. Zone JJ, Provost T. Circulating immune complexes in urticarial vasculitis with systemic lupus erythematosus [abstract]. Clin Res 1980;28:137a.

Z45. Zouali M, Eyquem A. Idiotypic restriction in human autoantibodies in DNA in systemic lupus erythematosus. Immunol Lett 1984;7:187–193.

Z46. Zouali M, Madaio Py M, Canoso RT, Stollar BD. Restriction fragment length polymorphism analysis of the V kappa locus in human lupus. Eur J Immunol 1989;19(9):1757–1760.

Z47. Zouali M, Migliorini P, Mackworth-Young CG, Stollar BD. Nucleic acid-binding specificity and idiotypic expression of canine anti-DNA antibodies. Eur J Immunol 1988;18: 923–927.

Z48. Zubler RH, Lange G, Lambert PH, Miescher PA. Detection of immune complexes in unheated sera by a modified ^{125}I-C1q binding test. Effect of heating on the binding of C1q by immune complexes and application of the test to systemic lupus erythematosus. J Immunol 1976;116:232–235.

Z49. Zucker S, Zarrabi MH, Romano GS, Miller F. IgM inhibitors of the contact phase of coagulation in chlorpromazine treated patients. Br J Hematol 1978;40:447–457.

Z50. Zuckner J, Baldassare H. The nonspecific rheumatoid subcutaneous nodule: its presence in fibrositis and scleroderma [case report]. Am J Med Sci 1976 Jan–Feb;271(1):69–75.

Z51. Zuehlke RL, Lillis PJ, Tice A. Antimalarial therapy for lupus erythematosus: an apparent advantage of quinacrine. Int J Dermatol 1981 Jan–Feb;20(1):57–61.

Z52. Zulman JI, Talal N, Hoffman GS, Epstein WV. Problems associated with the management of pregnancies in patients with systemic lupus erythematosus. J Rheumatol 1980;7:37-49.

Z53. Zupanski B, Thompson EE, Merry AH. Fc receptors for IgG1 and IgG3 on human mononuclear cells—an evaluation with known levels of erythrocyte-count IgG. Vox Sang 1986;50: 97–103.

Z54. Zuraw BL, O'Hair CH, Vaughan JH, Mathison DA, Curd JG, Katz DH. Immunoglobulin E-rheumatoid factor in the serum of patients with rheumatoid arthritis, asthma, and other diseases. J Clin Invest 1981 Dec;68:1610–1613.

Z55. Zurier RB. Reduction of phagocytosis and lysosomal enzyme release from human leukocytes by serum from patients with systemic lupus erythematosus. Arthritis Rheum 1976 Jan– Feb;19:73–78.

Z56. Zurier RB. Prostaglandin E1: Is it useful? [editorial] J Rheumatol 1990 Nov;17(11):1439–1441.

Z57. Zurier RB, Argyros TG, Urman JD, Warren J, Rothfield NF. Systemic lupus erythematosus. Management during pregnancy. Obstet Gynecol 1978;51:178–180.

Z58. Zurier RB, Baker DG, De Marco D, Fantone JC, Paposata M, Santoli D, Tate G. Anti-inflammatory effects of gamma-linolenic acid: studies in animals and in cultured cells. In: Omega-6 essential fatty acids: pathophysiology and roles in clinical medicine. Alan R Liss, Inc. 1990;203–221.

Z59. Zurier RB, Damjanov I, Sayadoff DM, Rothfield NF. Prostaglandin E1 treatment of NZB/NZW F1 hybrid mice. II. Prevention of glomerulonephritis. Arthritis Rheum 1977;20:1449.

Z60. Zurier RB, Sayadoff DM, Torrey SB, Rothfield NF. Prostaglandin E1 treatment of NZB/NZW mice. I. Prolonged survival of female mice. Arthritis Rheum 1977;20:723.

Z61. Zvaifler NJ. The subcellular localization of chloroquine and its effects on lysosomal disruption [abstract]. Arthritis Rheum 1964;7:760–761.

Z62. Zvaifler NJ. Etiology and Pathogenesis of Systemic Lupus Erythematosus. In: Kelley WN, Harris ED, Ruddy S, Sledge CB, editors. Textbook of Rheumatology. Vol. II. Philadelphia: Saunders 1981:1079–1105.

Z63. Zvaifler NJ, Block DJ. Rheumatoid factor—an inhibitor of the complement fixation reaction [abstract]. Arthritis Rheum 1962;5(1):127.

Z64. Zvaifler NJ, Bluestein HG. Lymphocytotoxic antibody activity in cryoprecipitates from serum of patients with SLE. Arthritis Rheum 1976 Mar;19:844–850.

Z65. Zwaal RFA. Membrane and lipid involvement in blood coagulation. Biochem Biophys Acta 1978;515:163–205.

Z66. Zweiman B. Theoretical mechanisms by which immunoglobulin therapy might benefit myasthenia gravis. Clin Immunol Immunopathol 1989;53:S83.

Z67. Zweiman B, Hildreth K. In vivo and in vitro anti- nuclear reaction in lupus patients. Arthritis Rheum 1968;11:660–662.

Z68. Zweiman B, Kornblum J. Cornog J, Hildreth EA. The prognosis of lupus nephritis. Role of clinical- pathological correlations. Ann Intern Med 1968 Sep;69(3):441–462.

Z69. Zwillich SH, Lipsky PE. Molecular mimicry in the pathogenesis of rheumatic diseases. Rheum Dis Clin North Am 1987; 13:339–352.

Z70. Zysset MK, Montgomery MT, Redding SW, Dell'Italia LJ. Systemic lupus erythematosus: a consideration for antimicrobial prophylaxis. Oral Surg Oral Med Oral Pathol 1987 Jul; 64(1):30–34.

AUTHOR CITATION INDEX

Aanstoot H: S209, V30, V31
Aarcon GS: A87
Aarden LA: A1, B411, S782, S783, S779, S780
Abbal M: A46
Abbey H: M176
Abbott G: K277
Abadi I: R263, S660
Abbott RJ: C218
Abbott RL: B162
Abbott RR: W271
Abdelaal M: C405
Abdelmonla M: Y48
Abd-Elrazak M: B163
Abdou NI: A2–A5, B156, B157, S15
Abdou NL: A4
Abdulla M: H16
Abe H: T35
Abe M: H329
Abe R: A6
Abe S: S88
Abe T: A7, A8, H319, I59, M575, M576, M579, M582, N7, T18, T19
Abeles M: A9, A10, F104, U30, U31, W136, W269
Abels R: L292
Abendroth K: W185
Aber VR: H150
Abildagaard CF: S456
Abitbol C: S727
Abiyou GO: B266
Abney E: Z24
Abo T: T164
Abo W: A12, B39
Abramovits W: A70
Abraham AA: G311
Abraham AS: S554
Abraham CN: Y44
Abraham GN: L372, L374
Abraham JP: R22
Abraham N: A196
Abraham NG: M670
Abraham S: P140
Abrahamson SB: A13, A14
Abramovici B: S556
Abramowsky CR: A16, A16
Abrams DI: B353
Abrams PG: O53
Abrams SB: A17
Abramson S: A18, B192, R198, R217, R218
Abramson SB: A19, H414
Abrass CK: A20
Abruzzo JL: D360, F170
Abruzzo LV: A20
Absalon BI: A22
Abud-Mendoza C: A23
Abuaf N: A22, D295

Abud-Mendoza C: A93, A94, D198
Accardo S: C462, C463
Accinni L: A221
Acevedo M: P330
Acevedo-Vazquez E: M469
Acha-Orbea H: A24, A25, J14, M4, T168
Acheson EJ: C11
Acheson JF: A340
Achiron A: A26
Achten M: D283
Ackad A: S656
Ackerman GL: A27, A28
Acra DJ: P127
Acritidis NC: A216
Acton RT: R169, R176
Acuto O: P138
Adachi M: A29
Adam J: W114
Adams DA: D291
Adams DD: K320, M94
Adams DO: D102
Adams EM: A30
Adams J: S449
Adams JL: A31
Adams JP: R331
Adams L: B555
Adams LE: A32, G260, G258, G338, L333, L334, R244, S542, S587, Y26
Adams P Jr: W355
Adams S: A33
Adams-Black A: A34
Adamson JW: A35
Adara F: D134
Addison IE: A140, S701
Ade M: F100
Adelman DC: A36
Adelman NE: A37
Adelsberg BR: K176, K177
Adelstein E: 0132
Adelstein S: A38, G291, G292
Adelusi SA: A39
Ader R: A40
Adeyemi EO: A41
Ad Hoc Neuropsychiatric Lupus Workshop Group: S463
Adinolfi M: A42, A43
Adler DC: D325a
Adler J: M640
Adler M: H239
Adler MK: A44, D253
Adler S: C416
Adler SG: S482
Adler SJ: A45
Adlercreutz H: P1
Adler-Stortz C: K169
Adoue D: A46
Adrianakos AA: A47

Adu D: A48, A49, M589
Aegerter E: A50
Aerts C: W10, W42
Affolter M: A52, R417
Afifi AK: A51
Agarwal A: S632
Agelli M: T94
Agnello V: A53–A58, A371, G4, K110, K336, K337, K462, L37, M456, S670
Agnew JE: M304
Agodoa LC: S109
Agodoa LYC: A59
Agopian MS: A60
Agostoni G: S273
Agostino N: B400
Agrawal N: G331
Aguado AG: V4
Aguado MT: A61, D347, H97
Agudelo CA: A62, G56
Aguirre C: A63
Agulhow F: F195
Agus B: A64, A65, G305, P25, R311
Ahearn JM: A66, A169, H347
Ahern MJ: B332, C329
Ahles TA: A67
Ahlfors E: S65
Ahmad AR: A69–A70, A182
Ahmad M: A159, S248
Ahmad MAM: E90
Ahmed A: B466, B467, G101, O34, T128, T228, Y54
Ahmed SW: M517
Ahn YS: A71–A75, M683
Aho K: K386
Ahren B: E69, L421
Ahuja GH: A76
Aikat BK: P29
Ainsworth SK: C227, F42
Airo P: G306
Aisen AM: A77, M259, M260
Aisen PS: A78
Aisenberg AC: A79
Aiso S: J14
Aitcheson CT: A80
Ait-Kaci A: A81
Ait-Kaci M: G165
Aito SN: K44
Aiuti F: D23
Akagaki Y: I14
Akama H: H402
Akari S: U10
Akashi K: A82
Akaza T: T175
Akbar AN: A83
Akbar S: A84
Arbaraly JP: L185
Akbarian M: D57, D58

841

SUBJECT CITATION INDEX

Antituberculous drugs (see also listings under specific agents), L109, W26

Anus ulcers, R369

Aplastic anemia (see anemia)

Apheresis, A2, B201, C283, C285, C286, C309, C340, D53, D166, E73, E156, F309, H44, H78, H117, H182, H276, H469, J110–J113, J115, J129, K43, K240, K373, K403, K426, L411, M308, P16, P26, P228, S60, S154, S184, S328, S599, S678, S772, T64, T119, T159, T203, T241, V109, W29–W32, W35, W52, W105, W124

Aromatic amines and hydrazines, F235, H353, P114, P116, P134, R125, R128

Arthritis,
    Clinical features, A289, B614, D340, F256, G385, R294, S680
    Feet in, B171, L13, M492, M591
    Hand in, A93, B342, B615, D290, E139, E159, G168, K16, K407, L3, M115, M166, M169, M658, N121, R294, S438, S792, W164
    History, K65
    Knees in, D132, D133
    Neck in, B5, K280
    Sacroiliac in, D178, G310, N37, V94, V95
    Temporomandibular joint and, G81, J124, L278

Ascites, A281, A364, B38, B316, D340, E147, H179, I46, J117, M395, M420, R193, R294, S157, S168, W230

Aspergillosis, K110, Q2

Aspirin, B20, B386, C406, D310, E70, F263, G64, H110, K85, K214, K220, K224, L402, M280, O92, P165, R35, R52, S134, S239, S240, S460, S554, T207, W37, W198,

Atabrine (also see antimalarials), Intralesional, L53

Ataxia (see CNS lupus, chorea)

Autoantibodies,
    Pathogenic (A, P), A222, D62, D174, D197, G74, H43, M135, M137, O42, S191, S377, S378
    Natural, A230, A279, B7, B182, C7, D63, D209, G423, H339, M110, S77, S259, T120

Autoimmune hemolytic anemia (see anemia)

Autoimmune vestibulitis (see ear in SLE)

Autonomic neuropathy (see neuropathies autonomic)

Avascular necrosis (also see antiphospholipid antibodies) A10, A17, D22, D24, D198, D218, D240, D323, D330, D340, F57, F81, F113, F114, F117, G383, H114, H347, J109, K25, K310, D313, L128, L286, L298, L388, L492, M219, M401, M219, N5, N99, P216, P321, R408, S223, S421, S504, U30, V59, V117, W136, W240, Z34, Z35, Z37–Z42, Z38a, Z38b
    Imaging in, B195, G88, G30, K40, M481, R152, S82, S223, S743, T275, Z33
    Treatment, G30, H114, K25, P321, Z35, Z38b, Z42

Azathioprine (see also pregnancy), H83, M478, P21
    Activity, C300, F6, P79, T67
    In nonrenal lupus, C36, L227, M10, M478, M674, P280, S327, S346, S779, S803, T241a, W182

Nephritis studies, A360, B63, B65, C1, C36, D258, D291, F56, G158, H23, H33, K307, K308, L300, N146, S636

Toxicity in SLE, A360, B65, G160, H412, K308, N38, N148, N152, R22, R157, S619, W185

B Cell,
    Activation, A181, A262, B402, B532, B537, C420, C421, D51, D174, E15, E59, E60, E63, E65, E67, F53, G113, G155, H97, H317, I44, I70, J93, J147, K41, K294, K298–K302, K339, L46, M135, M537, P37, P196, P319, R38, R66, R280, R400, S33, S218, S376, S377, S391, S527, S687, T167, V31, V78, W91
    Antibody production, B66, B127, B159, B330, B372, D51, E15, E60, E63, H5, H30, K296, K298, P37, S18
    Cross reactivity, D174, F232, K100, K291, K295, M190, M228, M540,P11, P31, S376, S377, S500, S708, T214, U113
    Defective clonal deletion, C420, E131, K294, K296, K303, M103, M634, R66, T130, T234a, T249
    General, D209, G423
    In SLE, B372, B557, C90, F25, F53, F106, G155, H30, H220, I44, I91, K33, K292, K296, K299, K298, K303, K452, L203, L226, M103, M634, N95, P37, P318, Q18, S33, S100, S521, S635, S639, S644, T31, T54, T81, T133, W207, W238, Z62
    Intrinsic abnormalities, R66, Y54
    Lineage, H218, H308, J70, K244, K335, L320
    Overview, B330, 557, G113, G155, G184, G291, M404, M601, S384, S647a, T19, T25, T130, W320
    Subsets, C125, C126, H125, H126, H219–H221, H270, K297, S410, S773, V3, W317
    Tolerance, influencing factors, A38, D51, E16, G291–G293, H49, H209, K252, K293, K299, K301, K302, K304, K305, K363, K458, L35, M634, N65, S533, U17, W286

Bacteria, pathogenetic for autoimmunity, C165, K345, P86

Baker's cyst, R132

Ballismus (see CNS lupus, chorea)

Basophils, E41, H197

Benoxaprofen, S524

Beta carotene, D335, H16, N71

Beta-2 microglobulin, serum or synovial, E136, F14, F153, K364, M368, V4, W163, Y43

Biliary abnormalities, L39, N70, R12, S787

Biliary cirrhosis and SLE, C280, I7, K434, M510, S38

Biopterin, H19

Birth control pills (see oral contrapceptives)

Bismuth, B250, P58

Bladder (see cystitis)

Blepharospasm (see eye in SLE)

Blood type and transfusion, A35, B52, C28, C29, D340, G358, H262, K447, L22, L142, L292, M387, M677, P166, P195, W46, W335, Z31

Bone in SLE, G196, L1, L199

Bone marrow, B578, M387, Y2

Brain evoked potentials, B309, F187, M544

Brain scanning,
    CT scans, C83, D54, G77, K7, N124, O80, R146, S253, W153
    Magnetic resonance imaging, A77, C362, G373, J30, M259, M260, S296, S407, S692, S771, V70
    SPECT and PET, C76, G437, H319, M378, P192, S691, S712, S713, T209, V102
    Technetium and xenon fluorescence, A8, A369, B207, D336, F46, G124, G385, K449, K482, K483, S253, T55

Bronchoalveolar lavage, B41, J48, P147, W10

Breast (see silica, silcone, and silcane), K268

Breast feeding, A212, B246, B512, B530, F93, J87, K112, L104, L230, M304, N45, N51, O112, S423a, S531, T77, W222

Bromocriptine, J53, R2

Budd-Chiari (see liver, vascular lesions)

Bullous lupus erythematosus, B110, B296, B382, C42–C44, C249, D13, D340, D278, F27, F147, G25, G27, G145, H58, H255, J128, K129, K181, L34, L40, M170, M423, N83, O52, P108, R47, R300, S277, S702, T157, T223, W114, W119, W213a, W344

BXSB/MPJ mouse, A225, C342, D121, D353, E62, E64, G52, G55, H310, H366, I6, I64, M71, M655, M666, M667, S234, S508, S641, U18, W314, Y53

C-reactive protein in SLE, B154, B265, B464, D177, H302, H311, H405, I25, K242, L92, M218, M607, P80, R356, S358, S483, T110, Z21

Cadmium, J133, O33, P276

Calcification (calcinosis) of tissue, B554, C82, G393, J83, L106, N119, W313

Camoquin (see also antimalarials)

Campylobacteria, D381

Canada-Cronkhite syndrome, K441

Candida, B163, F136, G234, S345

Captopril, C128, P66, P188, R127, S311, S411

Carbamazepine, A121, B120, B276, D118, D171, J65, K361, P5, P13, T177, Z7, Z14, Z49

Carcinoma (see malignancy)

Carcinoma in SLE,
    General surveys, H46, K86, L248, O64, R173, R321, S741, U32, U34, W39
    Cervical atypia, G160, N152
    Lymphoproliferative, B80, C370, G349, M416, R82, S598
    Miscellaneous reports, B93, B597, D104, D300, G355, G412, H333, I53, J126, J131, K15, K274, K286, L326, M408, M627, O69, P34, R356, T35, T174, S39, S106, S276, S539

Cardiac (see heart in SLE)

Carprofen, O6

Cataracts (see also corticosteroids)

Cat lupus, in A356, H67, H356

Cathespin D, P173

Central nervous system lupus, K149
    Ataxia, S470
    Ballismus, T158
    Childhood SLE, A287, A321, B227, B402, B546, B551, C2, C75, C83, C147, D143, D206, F46, G124, G226, G285, G403, H274, K232, L165, L319, L371, M341, N131, P36, S781, W85, W148, Y29, W21

INDEX

Page numbers in *italics* indicate illustrations; numbers followed by "t" indicate tables.